Nutrition and Diagnosis-Related Care

SIXTH EDITION

Nutrition and Diagnosis-Related Care

SIXTH EDITION

Sylvia Escott-Stump, MA, RD, LDN

Dietetic Programs Director
East Carolina University
Greenville, North Carolina
and
Consulting Dietitian
Nutritional Balance
Winterville, North Carolina

Wolters Kluwer Health | Lippincott Williams & Wilkins
Philadelphia • Baltimore • New York • London
Buenos Aires • Hong Kong • Sydney • Tokyo

Editor: David B. Troy
Managing Editor: Matthew J. Hauber
Marketing Manager: Marisa A. O'Brien
Production Editor: Eve Malakoff-Klein
Compositor: Maryland Composition
Printer: R.R. Donnelley & Sons

351 West Camden Street
Baltimore, Maryland 21201-2436 USA

530 Walnut Street
Philadelphia, PA 19106

The publisher is not responsible (as a matter of product liability, negligence, or otherwise) for any injury resulting from any material contained herein. This publication contains information relating to general principles of medical care that should not be construed as specific instructions for individual patients. Manufacturers' product information and package inserts should be reviewed for current information, including contraindications, dosages, and precautions.

Printed in the United States of America

First Edition, 1985
Second Edition, 1988
Third Edition, 1992
Fourth Edition, 1997
Fifth Edition, 2002

Library of Congress Cataloging-in-Publication Data

Escott-Stump, Sylvia.
Nutrition and diagnosis-related care / Sylvia Escott-Stump. — 6th ed.
p. ; cm.
Includes bibliographical references and index.
ISBN-13: 978-0-7817-9845-7
ISBN-10: 0-7817-9845-0
1. Diet therapy—Handbooks, manuals, etc. 2. Nutrition—Handbooks, manuals, etc. I. Title.
[DNLM: 1. Diet Therapy—Handbooks. 2. Nutrition—Handbooks. WB 39 E74n 2008]
RM217.2.E83 2008
615.8′54—dc22

2006024804

The publishers have made every effort to trace the copyright holders for borrowed material. If they have inadvertently overlooked any, they will be pleased to make the necessary arrangements at the first opportunity.

To purchase additional copies of this book, call our customer service department at **(800) 638-3030** or fax orders to **(301) 824-7390.** International customers should call **(301) 714-2324.**

Visit Lippincott Williams & Wilkins on the Internet: http://www.LWW.com. Lippincott Williams & Wilkins customer service representatives are available from 8:30 am to 6:00 pm, EST.

06 07 08 09 10
1 2 3 4 5 6 7 8 9 10

FOREWORD

This book is a valuable resource for registered dietitians, dietetic students, and other health care professionals involved or interested in medical nutrition therapy (MNT). Given the increasing time demands confronting health care professionals, efficient time management is essential for delivering high-quality patient care. The ever-changing health care environment necessitates that registered dietitians efficiently and effectively maintain their high level of practice skills. Maintaining and growing practice skills in a time-effective manner are essential to provide maximum time for patient-care activities. This book "fits the bill" as a key resource for prioritizing patient care and appropriately planning a nutrition treatment course. The guidance provided by *Nutrition and Diagnosis-Related Care* will be of immense value in charting the clinical course for each patient. It will be of great value for both routine and familiar cases and especially valuable in dealing with clinical conditions that the practitioner does not routinely treat.

Notable features of the book include an extensive array of clinical conditions that are dealt with routinely in dietetic practice including normal nutrition situations such as pregnancy and lactation. This book presents an extensive compilation of nutrition care information in a most succinct way. An impressive attribute is that the germane information required by dietitians is presented in a single resource. This greatly simplifies the development of nutrition care plans for patients. Thus, this book provides dietetic practitioners with superb guidance they can use to maintain outstanding practice skills. This book is a resource that can help achieve excellence in dietetic practice.

Penny Kris-Etherton, PhD, RD
Pennsylvania State University

Karen Kubena, PhD, RD
Texas A & M University

PREFACE

Health care professionals must identify all elements of patient care capable of affecting nutritional status and outcomes. With limitations on length of hospital stay, the registered dietitian must provide nutritional care in a practical, efficient, timely, and effective manner in any setting. Various environments provide unique and special considerations for the nutrition counselor. The astute dietitian is sensitive to the patient/client's current status in the continuum of care and adapts the nutritional care plan accordingly. The most important element is communication between staff of different facilities to save time in screenings and assessments. Data and summary reports should be shared from one practitioner to the next, regardless of setting. Confidential, computerized medical records enable the dietetic practitioner to maintain current updates for all patients in a readily accessible format.

Nutrition and Diagnosis-Related Care was developed to supplement other texts and references used by practitioners, instructors, interns, and students to quickly assimilate and implement medical nutrition therapy (MNT) for numerous disorders. This manual can be used to help write protocols, to establish priorities in nutritional care, to demonstrate therapies at lower cost than certain medications and total parenteral nutrition (TPN), and to categorize disorders in which nutritional input can reduce costs by lessening complications, further morbidity, mortality, and lengthy hospital stays. Adequate nutritional intervention often results in financial savings for the patient, the family, and the health care system.

The sixth edition includes the latest guidance in medical nutrition therapy. Each section of the book was thoroughly reviewed by leading practitioners in the field. New diagnostic terminology is used, including standardized language used by the dietetic profession. In addition, the format of the book continues to use an effective style that allows easier navigation of the text and quick retrieval of information.

The new Dietary Reference Intakes have been used throughout the text. To find the new data, access the search at the Institute of Medicine website (http://wwwsearch.nationalacademies.org/). Appendix A summarizes the nutrients and their major food sources and functions.

Appendix B has been extensively revised according to the new Nutrition Care Process approved for the profession of dietetics. Sample forms are included, including language related to A-D-I (assessment, nutrition diagnosis, interventions) charting, with M-E (monitoring and evaluation) as follow-up documentation. A thorough Laboratory Assessment table has been added to meet practitioner needs for a handy reference.

Appendix C provides Case Studies and encourages use of the new Standardized Language and an updated concept map format. The cases are designed to encourage practice within all sections of the text. They are designed to be used in either individual or group learning sessions. The cases are especially useful for classes in which problem-based learning (PBL) is available since they require thinking about the additional information needed for assessment, as well as interventions and follow-up care.

An updated Nutritional Acuity Level Ranking for dietitian services is found in Appendix D. It is the consensus from a survey of over 75 clinical nutrition managers and practitioners. This acuity ranking may be used to identify or to negotiate nutrition staffing patterns, to identify key patients at moderate to high nutritional risk, and to plan adequate follow-up services from one site to another.

Complementary nutrition is now described more fully in Section 2, and herbal and botanical tables are available in Appendix E. This information is critical for dietitians to know because of the use by the public and interest within the medical community. Side effects are often unknown; when evidence from clinical trials is available, information is included.

Nutrition care plans, goals, and interventions must be created individually for each patient. The reader is encouraged to maintain current educational knowledge and skills in order to revise localized nutrition guidance as new evidence suggests. Evidence-based practice and use of this manual as a tool serve as the stimulus for improving medical nutrition therapy in all settings. The profession of dietetics continues to evolve and to serve as the role model and leader for its members.

ASSUMPTIONS ABOUT THE READER

For this text, the following assumptions have been made:

1. The reader has an adequate background in nutritional sciences, physiology and pathophysiology, medical terminology, biochemistry, and interpretation of laboratory data to understand the abbreviations, objectives, and interventions.
2. An individualized drug history review is required for all patients; only a few commonly used medications are listed in this manual.
3. Herbs and botanicals and dietary supplements are included because they are often used without prior consultation with a dietitian or a physician; they may have side effects as well as perceived or real benefits.
4. The Patient Education section assumes that the reader will acquire or provide appropriate diet information sheets and tools. Other tips are available from this guide to prepare the patient for independent functioning. The nutrition counselor will share all relevant information, as deemed appropriate, with the patient and significant other(s).
5. Shortened lengths of stay have forced health care practitioners to prioritize nutritional care during hospital stays. Dietitians have new roles in ambulatory centers, extended care facilities, subacute or rehabilitative centers, private practices, grocery stores, web-based practices, and home care. This "seamless" flow affords the possibility of

lifelong patient connections, a reality that promotes more effective patient tracking and follow-up.

6. The Clinical Indicators section for each condition lists tests, disease markers, and common biochemical evaluations reviewed by physicians or dietitians for that condition. Because few laboratory tests are available in nonhospital settings for monitoring nutritional status, assessment tools (such as weight changes) remain the most essential screening factor. Physical changes and signs of malnutrition are important for assessment purposes and should be identified whenever possible.
7. A current diet manual and medical nutrition therapy text should be used to acquire complete lists of diet modifications since full lists are not included with this book.
8. Use of evidence-based guides from The American Dietetic Association is recommended to provide predictable types of interventions over multiple visits, especially when reimbursement is expected. Use the website to determine current guidelines for practice.
9. Except when specifically noted for children, medical nutrition therapy plans are for adults over the age of 18.
10. Vitamin and mineral supplements are needed in cases of a documented or likely deficiency. However, in large doses, they may cause food–drug interactions. Plan meals and nourishments carefully to avoid the need for individual supplements. Use of a general multivitamin-mineral supplement may be beneficial for many adults; monitor intakes judiciously from all food and supplemental sources. Athletes, women, elderly individuals, and vegetarians tend to take vitamin and mineral supplements more often than other individuals and may be at risk for overdoses if not carefully monitored
11. Much evidence points to the benefits of whole foods to acquire known and yet unknown phytochemicals and substances. Healthy persons should obtain nutrients from a balanced diet as much as possible.
12. In general, use a well-balanced, varied diet with the USDA MyPyramid Food Guidance System as the basis for dietary plans. There are many ethnic, vegetarian, pediatric, geriatric, and diabetes food guides for menu planning and design.
13. Ethics, cultural sensitivity, and a concern for patient rights should be considered and practiced at all times. When available, the wishes and advanced directives of the patient are to be followed. This may preclude aggressive use of artificial nutrition.
14. Interesting and varied websites have been included for the reader to use to acquire additional insights into various diseases, conditions, and nutritional interventions. While this list is not comprehensive, it was current at the time of manuscript development.

ACKNOWLEDGMENT

Thanks to Matthew Dallas, MS, RD, who helped with edits for this edition and to Pam Charney, PhD, RD, and all reviewers who made valuable suggestions for changes.

Sylvia Escott-Stump, MA, RD, LDN

REVIEWERS

SECTION 1

Pam Charney	All
Monica Meadows	All
Brenda Malinauskas	Sports Nutrition only
Kris Clark	Sports Nutrition only
Lisa Dorfman	Sports Nutrition only
Kathleen Niedert	Elderly Nutrition only

SECTION 2

Pam Charney	All
Rachel Trevethan	All
Ruth DeBusk	Complementary Nutrition only
Robert Earl	Cultural and Religious Patterns, Food Allergies, Food Safety only
Jan Patenaude	Food Allergies only
Polly Carroll	Food Allergies only
Debora Indorato	Food Allergies only
Diane Lesnick	Jewish Dietary Practices only
Rabbi Allen Berkowitz	Jewish Dietary Practices only
Kavitha Felix	Hindu Dietary Practices only
Ghadah Al-Habib	Muslim Dietary Practices only
Kathleen Niedert	Pressure Ulcers only

SECTION 3

Pam Charney	All
Josephine Cialone	All
Mary Anne Burkhardt	All
Patricia Edwards-Hare	All
Ancy George	All
Ginger Hester	All
Frances Van Geyte	All
Kathy Kolasa	Overweight in Childhood only
Christine Salaita	Overweight in Childhood only

SECTION 4

Pam Charney	All

SECTION 5

Carrie Donovan	All
Karla Kennedy-Hagan	All

SECTION 6

Laura Crist	All
Karla Kennedy-Hagan	All
Susan Kraus	All
Debra Krummel	All
Chris Biesemeier	Coronary Artery Disease/Atherosclerosis only
Penny Kris-Etherton	Coronary Artery Disease/Atherosclerosis only
Joanne Shearer	Coronary Artery Disease/Atherosclerosis only

SECTION 7

Pete Beyer	All
Angela Sullivan	All

SECTION 8

Donna Smith Becker	All
Mary Russell	All
Jane Uzcategui	All

SECTION 9

Marion Franz	Diabetes only
Cindy Polich	Diabetes only
Dr. Lynn Mack-Shipman	Diabetes only
Dr. James Lane	Diabetes only
Susan Perry	Diabetes only
Zara Shah-Rowlands	Diabetes only
Sherri Shafer	All

SECTION 10

Dorothy Chen-Maynard	All
Hale Deniz-Venturi	All

SECTION 11

Susan Kennedy	All
John Anderson, PhD	Bone Health only
Kristine Duncan, RD	Rheumatic Disorders only

SECTION 12

Tracy Stopler, MS, RD	All

SECTION 13

Valerie Kogut, MS, RD	All
Nicole Fox	All
Stephanie Giraulo	All

SECTION 14

Linda Griffith	All
Lisa Trombley	All

SECTION 15

Christine Salaita	HIV/AIDS only
Marcia Nahikian-Nelms	All
Roni Finkelstein	All

SECTION 16

Elaine Fontenot Molaison	All
Jessie Pavlinac	All
Krista Clark	All

SECTION 17

Sara Post	All
Karyn Voulalas	All

APPENDIX A
Matthew Dallas

APPENDIX B
Esther Myers
Mary Jane Oakland
Pat Splett
Mary Russell

APPENDIX C
Pam Charney
Mandy Foust Mitzae

APPENDIX D
Matthew Dallas

APPENDIX E
Ruth DeBusk

COMMON ABBREVIATIONS

AA	amino acid
abd	abdomen, abdominal
ABW	average body weight
ACE	angiotensin-converting enzyme
ACTH	adrenocorticotropic hormone
ADA	American Dietetic Association
Alb	albumin
Alk phos	alkaline phosphatase
ALT	alanine aminotransferase
amts	amounts
ARF	acute renal failure
ASHD	atherosclerotic heart disease
AST	aspartate aminotransferase
ATP	adenosine triphosphate
BCAAs	branched-chain amino acids
BEE	basal energy expenditure
BF	breastfeeding
BMR	basal metabolic rate
BP	blood pressure
BS	blood sugar
BSA	body surface area
BUN	blood urea nitrogen
BW	body weight
bx	biopsy
C	cup(s)
C	coffee
CA	cancer
Ca++	calcium
CABG	coronary artery bypass grafting
CBC	complete blood count
CF	cystic fibrosis
CHD	cardiac heart disease
CHF	congestive heart failure
CHI	creatinine-height index
CHO	carbohydrate
Chol	cholesterol
Cl−	chloride
CNS	central nervous system
CO_2	carbon dioxide
CPK	creatine phosphokinase
CPR	cardiopulmonary resuscitation
CrCl	creatine clearance
CRP	C-reactive protein
CT	computed tomography
Cu	copper
CVA	cerebrovascular accident
DAT	diet as tolerated
dec	decreased
decaf	decaffeinated
def	deficiency
DJD	degenerative joint disease
dL	deciliter
DM	diabetes mellitus
DNA	deoxyribonucleic acid
DOB	date of birth
DRI	dietary reference intakes
DV	daily value
Dx	diagnosis
D5W	5% dextrose solution in water
EAA	essential amino acid
ECG, EKG	electrocardiogram
EEG	electroencephalogram
EFAs	essential fatty acids
Elec	electrolytes
EN	enteral nutrition
ESRD	end-stage renal disease
ETOH	ethanol/ethyl alcohol
Fe++	iron
F & V	fruits and vegetables
FSH	follicle-stimulating hormone
FTT	failure to thrive
FUO	fever of unknown origin
G, g	gram(s)
GA	gestational age
GBD	gallbladder disease
GE	gastroenteritis
gest	gestational
GFR	glomerular filtration rate
GI	gastrointestinal
Gluc	glucose
GN	glomerular nephritis
GTT	glucose tolerance test
H & H	hemoglobin and hematocrit
HBV	high biological value
HBW	healthy body weight
HCl	hydrochloric acid
Hct	hematocrit
HDL	high-density lipoprotein
HbA1c	hemoglobin A1c test (glucose)
HLP	hyperlipoproteinemia or hyperlipidemia
HPN, HTN	hypertension
ht	height
Hx	history
I	infant
I & O	intake and output
IBD	inflammatory bowel disease
IBS	irritable bowel syndrome
IBW	ideal body weight
IEM	inborn error of metabolism
INR	international normalized ratio
IU	international units
IUD	intrauterine device
IV	intravenous
K+	potassium
kcal	food kilocalories
kg	kilogram(s)
L	liter(s)
lb	pound(s)
LBM	lean body mass
LBV	low biological value

LBW	low birth weight
LCT	long-chain triglycerides
LDH	lactate dehydrogenase
LDL	low-density lipoproteins
LE	lupus erythematosus
LGA	large for gestational age
LH	luteinizing hormone
lytes	electrolytes
M	milk
MAC	midarm circumference
MAMC	midarm muscle circumference
MAO	monoamine oxidase
MBF	meat-base formula
MCH	mean cell hemoglobin
MCT	medium-chain triglycerides
MCV	mean cell volume
MI	myocardial infarction
Mg^{++}	magnesium
mg	milligram(s)
μg	micrograms
mm	millimeter(s)
MODS	multiple organ dysfunction syndrome
MSG	monosodium glutamate
MUFA	monounsaturated fatty acids
N&V	nausea and vomiting
N	nitrogen
Na	sodium
NCEP	National Cholesterol Education Program
NCP	Nutrition Care Process
NEC	necrotizing enterocolitis
NG	nasogastric
NPO	nil per os (nothing by mouth)
NSI	Nutrition Screening Initiative
O_2	oxygen
OP	out-patient
OT	occupational therapist
oz	ounce(s)
P	phosphorus
PCM	protein–calorie malnutrition
pCO_2	partial pressure of carbon dioxide
PG	pregnant, pregnancy
PKU	phenylketonuria
PN	parenteral nutrition
pO_2	partial pressure of oxygen
prn	pro re nata (as needed)
Prot	protein
PT	prothrombin time or physical therapy
PTH	parathormone
PUFA(s)	polyunsaturated fatty acid(s)
PVD	peripheral vascular disease
RAST	radioallergosorbent test
RDA	recommended dietary allowance (specific)
RBC	red blood cell count
RDS	respiratory distress syndrome
REE	resting energy expenditure
RQ	respiratory quotient
Rx	treatment
SFA	saturated fatty acids
SGA	small for gestational age
SI	small intestine
SIADH	syndrome of inappropriate antidiuretic hormone
SIDS	sudden infant death syndrome
SOB	shortness of breath
Sub	substitute
Sx	symptoms
t	teaspoon(s)
T	tablespoon
TB	tuberculosis
TF	tube feeding; tube fed
TIBC	total iron-binding capacity
TLC	total lymphocyte count
TPN	total parenteral nutrition
TG	triglycerides
TSF	triceps skinfold
UA	uric acid
UTI	urinary tract infection
UUN	urinary urea nitrogen
VMA	vanillylmandelic acid
VO_{2max}	maximum oxygen intake
WBC	white blood cell count
WNL	within normal limits
Zn	zinc

LIST OF TABLES

SECTION 9

SECTION 10

SECTION 11

SECTION 12

SECTION 13

SECTION 14

SECTION 15

SECTION 16

SECTION 17

APPENDIX A

APPENDIX B

APPENDIX C

APPENDIX D

APPENDIX E

LIST OF FIGURES

CONTENTS

SECTION 8

HEPATIC, PANCREATIC, AND BILIARY DISORDERS 433

SECTION 9

ENDOCRINE DISORDERS 473

SECTION 10

WEIGHT MANAGEMENT, UNDERNUTRITION, AND MALNUTRITION 549

SECTION 11

MUSCULOSKELETAL AND COLLAGEN DISORDERS 581

SECTION 12

HEMATOLOGY: ANEMIAS AND BLOOD DISORDERS 623

SECTION 13

CANCER 657

SECTION 14

SURGICAL DISORDERS 727

SECTION 15

AIDS AND IMMUNOLOGY, INFECTIONS, BURNS, AND TRAUMA 749

SECTION 16

RENAL DISORDERS 785

SECTION 17

ENTERAL AND PARENTERAL NUTRITION INTERVENTIONS 821

APPENDIX A

APPENDIX B

APPENDIX C

APPENDIX D

APPENDIX E

ALPHABETICAL LIST OF TOPICS

SECTION 1

Normal Life-Cycle Conditions

CHIEF ASSESSMENT FACTORS

- Key Screening Factors: Unintentional Weight Loss and Appetite Changes in Adults, Protein-Energy Deficiency or Growth Retardation in Chidren
- General State of Health: Recent Surgery/Hospitalizations, Weight History, Percentage of Body Mass Index (BMI) or Healthy Body Weight (HBW) for Height, Loss of Lean Body Mass (LBM), Previous Weight Percentile or Curve, Weight Changes, Waist–Hip Ratio and Waist Circumference
- Educational Background, Socioeconomic Status, Level of Food Security
- Fatigue, Weakness, Cachexia
- Chills, Sweating, Tremors, Anorexia, Nausea, Diarrhea, Vomiting, Blood Pressure, Temperature or Fever, Pulse
- Hair or Nail Changes, Skin Rashes, Itching, Lesions, Turgor, Petechiae, Pallor
- Hearing Screen, Chronic Otitis Media, Glasses, Blurring of Vision, Glaucoma, Cataracts or Macular Degeneration, Altered Sense of Smell, Nasal Obstruction, Sinusitis
- Headache, Seizures, Convulsions, Altered Speech, Paralysis, Gait, Anxiety, Memory Loss, Sleep Patterns, Depression, Substance Abuse, Motivation
- Dental Screening, Dentures, Loose or Missing Teeth, Caries, Bleeding Gums, Oral Hygiene, Taste Alterations, Dysphagia
- Chest Pain, Dyspnea, Wheezing, Cough, Hemoptysis, Ventilator Support, Blood Gas Levels
- Electrolyte Balance, Hypertension, Cyanosis, Edema, Ascites, Cardiac Output
- Anemias, Heart Rate, Arrhythmias, Blood Loss
- Appetite, Jaundice, Constipation, Indigestion, Ulcers, Hemorrhoids, Melena, Stool Characteristics, Special Diets
- Skinfold Measurements, Visceral Proteins, Estimated Basal Energy Expenditure, Nitrogen Balance
- Vitamin/Mineral Intake, Nutritional Support, Blood Glucose, Dietary Patterns and Typical Intake, Alcohol Intake
- Use of Herbs/Botanicals/Supplements, Over-the-Counter and Prescribed Medications, Side Effects, Food–Drug Interactions, Therapies Such as Radiation or Chemotherapy and Effects on Nutritional Status
- Hematuria, Fluid Requirements, Specific Gravity, Urinary Tract Infections, Renal Disease or Stones
- Hormone Balance, Goiter, Glucose Intolerance, Cellular Immunity
- Food Allergy, Sensitivity, Intolerances
- Pain, Arthritis, Numbness, Amputations, Range of Motion, Muscular Strength
- Knowledge of Food and Nutrition (see Fig. 1-1)

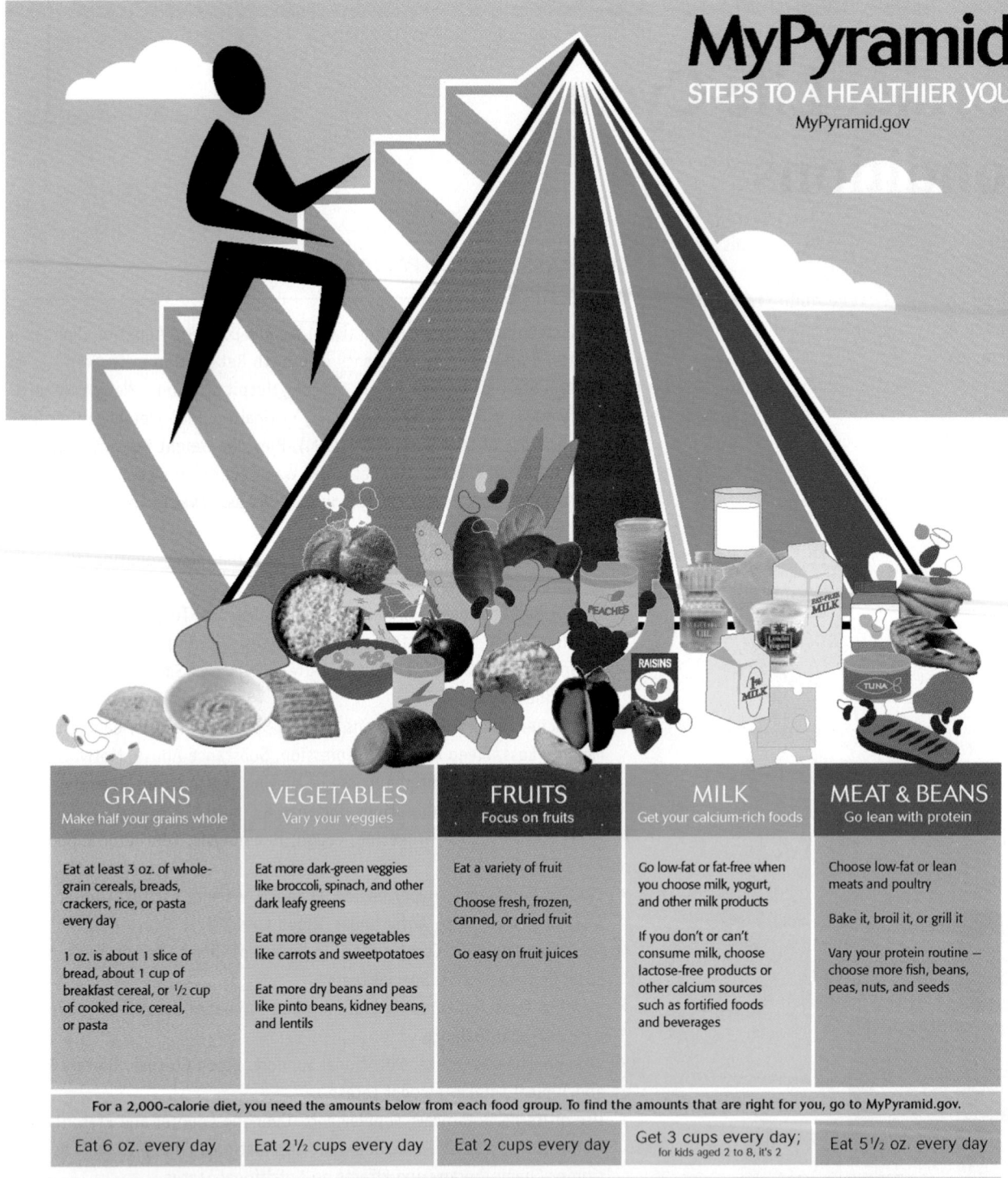

GRAINS Make half your grains whole	VEGETABLES Vary your veggies	FRUITS Focus on fruits	MILK Get your calcium-rich foods	MEAT & BEANS Go lean with protein
Eat at least 3 oz. of whole-grain cereals, breads, crackers, rice, or pasta every day 1 oz. is about 1 slice of bread, about 1 cup of breakfast cereal, or 1/2 cup of cooked rice, cereal, or pasta	Eat more dark-green veggies like broccoli, spinach, and other dark leafy greens Eat more orange vegetables like carrots and sweetpotatoes Eat more dry beans and peas like pinto beans, kidney beans, and lentils	Eat a variety of fruit Choose fresh, frozen, canned, or dried fruit Go easy on fruit juices	Go low-fat or fat-free when you choose milk, yogurt, and other milk products If you don't or can't consume milk, choose lactose-free products or other calcium sources such as fortified foods and beverages	Choose low-fat or lean meats and poultry Bake it, broil it, or grill it Vary your protein routine – choose more fish, beans, peas, nuts, and seeds
For a 2,000-calorie diet, you need the amounts below from each food group. To find the amounts that are right for you, go to MyPyramid.gov.				
Eat 6 oz. every day	Eat 2 1/2 cups every day	Eat 2 cups every day	Get 3 cups every day; for kids aged 2 to 8, it's 2	Eat 5 1/2 oz. every day

Find your balance between food and physical activity

- Be sure to stay within your daily calorie needs.
- Be physically active for at least 30 minutes most days of the week.
- About 60 minutes a day of physical activity may be needed to prevent weight gain.
- For sustaining weight loss, at least 60 to 90 minutes a day of physical activity may be required.
- Children and teenagers should be physically active for 60 minutes every day, or most days.

Know the limits on fats, sugars, and salt (sodium)

- Make most of your fat sources from fish, nuts, and vegetable oils.
- Limit solid fats like butter, stick margarine, shortening, and lard, as well as foods that contain these.
- Check the Nutrition Facts label to keep saturated fats, *trans* fats, and sodium low.
- Choose food and beverages low in added sugars. Added sugars contribute calories with few, if any, nutrients.

Figure 1-1. MyPyramid Food Guidance System. Source: Federal government: http://www.mypyramid.gov/downloads/MiniPoster.pdf.

Life Cycle–Specific Assessments

- Pregnancy: Obesity, Smoking, Drinking Alcohol, Insufficient Intake of Folic Acid, Changes That Take Place Over Time
- Lactating Women: Mother's Intake and Breastfeeding Practices; Extent to Which Infant Is Breastfeeding; Infant Intakes May Be Supplemented with Nutrients or Foods; Composition of Milk Varies with Use of Medications
- Infants: Breast Milk; Formula Intake; Mixed Feedings with Other Foods; Variable Eating Patterns
- Preschool Children: Intakes That Vary Day to Day; Food Jags
- School Children: Limited Ability to Recall Foods Eaten; Limited Attention Span; Use of Any Medications or Special Therapies
- Adolescents: Intakes Change Rapidly with Growth Spurts; Meal Skipping; Dieting; Fasting; Disordered Eating; Abuse of Drugs or Alcohol or Laxatives
- Adults: Literacy May Be a Problem; Reporting May Be Biased Because of Fear of Noncompliance; Failure to Report Use of Herbs, Alcohol, Supplements; Unusual Work Patterns Such as Shift Work
- Elderly: Recall May Be Limited; Limitations in Hearing or Sight; Chronic Illness May Affect Intake

For More Information on MyPyramid Food Guidance System

- Ethnic and regional practices for diabetes
  http://www.eatright.org/catalog/diabetes/html
- MyPyramid Food Guidance System Tools
  http://www.MyPyramidFoodGuidanceSystem.gov/professionals/index.html
  http://www.mypyramid.gov/downloads/MyPyramid_Calorie_Levels.pdf
  http://www.mypyramid.gov/downloads/MyPyramid_Food_Intake_Patterns.pdf
- MyPyramid Food Guidance System Tracker
  http://www.mypyramid.gov/professionals/food_tracking_wksht.html
- New Americans Project
  http://www.monarch.gsu.edu/nutrition/download/htm

TABLE 1-1 Public Health: Ten Services and Ten Achievements

10 Essential Public Health Services

- Monitor health status to identify community health problems.
- Diagnose and investigate health problems and hazards in the community.
- Inform, educate, and empower people about health issues.
- Mobilize community partnerships to identify and solve health problems.
- Develop policies and plans that support individual and community health efforts.
- Enforce laws and regulations that protect health and ensure safety.
- Link people to needed personal health services and assure the provision of health care when otherwise unavailable.
- Assure competent public health and personal health care workforce.
- Evaluate effectiveness, accessibility, and quality of personal and population-based health services.
- Research for new insights and innovative solutions to health problems.

10 Public Health Achievements in the 20th Century

- Development of vaccines
- Increased motor vehicle safety
- Safer workplaces
- Control of infectious diseases
- Decline in deaths from coronary artery disease and stroke
- Safer and healthier foods
- Healthier mothers and babies
- Better family planning
- Fluoridation of drinking water
- Recognition of tobacco as a health hazard

From: http://www.astdhpphe.org/WebStatementMSI.htm and *Morbidity and Mortality Weekly Report,* June 1999.

TABLE 1-2 Dietary Guideline Systems

The International Conference on Nutrition (ICN), which convened years ago by the Food and Agriculture Organization (FAO) and the World Health Organization (WHO) in Rome, suggested strategies and actions to improve nutritional well-being and food consumption throughout the world. This group suggested that all food-based dietary guidelines should be developed by an interdisciplinary group of representatives working in agriculture, health, education and communication, and food and nutritional science, as well as the food industry and consumers. While many countries have identified guidelines specific for their population, basic principles remain steadfast. Several sample sets of guidelines from different countries follow the list of basic principles.

Source: http://www.fao.org/WAICENT/FAOINFO/ECONOMIC/ESN/fbdg/fbdg.htm

Energy

- Nutritional guidelines should aim to prevent the consequences of either energy deficit or excess.
- Food-based dietary guidelines should promote appropriate energy intakes by encouraging adequate food choices, including a good balance of foods containing carbohydrates, fats, proteins, vitamins, and minerals.
- The role of physical activity in the energy balance equation should also be addressed.

Protein

- For high-quality proteins, requirements for most people can be met by providing 8–10% of total energy as protein.
- For predominantly vegetable-based, mixed diets, which are common in developing country settings, 10–12% is suggested to account for lower digestibility and increased incidence of diarrhea disease.
- In the case of the elderly, where energy intake is low, protein should represent 12–14% of total energy.

Fat

- In general, adults should obtain at least 15% of their energy intake from dietary fats and oils.
- Women of childbearing age should obtain at least 20% to better ensure an adequate intake of essential fatty acids needed for fetal and infant brain development.
- Active individuals who are not obese may consume up to 35% fat energy as long as saturated fatty acids do not exceed 10% of energy intake.
- Sedentary individuals should limit fat to not more than 30% of energy intake.
- Saturated fatty acids should be limited to less than 10% of intake.

Carbohydrate

- Carbohydrates are the main source of energy in the diet (>50%) for most people.
- Grain products, tubers, roots, and some fruits are rich in complex carbohydrates. Generally, they need to be cooked before they are fully digestible.
- Sugars usually increase the acceptability and energy density of the diet, and total sugar intake is often inversely related to total fat intake. Moderate intakes of sugar are compatible with a varied and nutritious diet, and no specific limit for sugar consumption is proposed in the report.

Micronutrients

- Vitamins and minerals include compounds with widely divergent metabolic activities and are essential for normal growth and development and optimal health.
- Micronutrients may also be important in preventing infectious and chronic diseases. Epidemiological, clinical, and experimental studies can help to define the role of specific foods and nutrients in disease development and prevention.

Dietary Guidelines

Americans:

An evidence-based approach was used to determine updates to the 2005 Dietary Guidelines for Americans (Nicklas et al, 2005). This included a scientific, systematic approach. The guidelines are:

<u>Balance Nutrients With Calories</u>

Eat a variety of nutrient-dense foods and beverages within and among the basic food groups.

Choose foods that limit the intake of saturated and trans fats, cholesterol, added sugars, salt, and alcohol.

Meet recommended intakes within energy needs by adopting a balanced eating pattern, such as the U.S. Department of Agriculture (USDA) Food Guide or the Dietary Approaches to Stop Hypertension (DASH) Eating Plan.

(continued)

TABLE 1-2 Dietary Guideline Systems *(continued)*

Manage Weight

To maintain body weight in a healthy range, balance calories from foods and beverages with calories expended.

To prevent gradual weight gain over time, make small decreases in food and beverage calories and increase physical activity.

Maintain Physical Activity

Engage in regular physical activity and reduce sedentary activities to promote health, psychological well-being, and a healthy body weight.

To reduce the risk of chronic disease in adulthood, engage in at least 30 minutes of moderate-intensity physical activity, above usual activity, at work or home on most days of the week. For most people, greater health benefits can be obtained by engaging in physical activity of more vigorous intensity or longer duration.

To help manage body weight and prevent gradual, unhealthy body weight gain in adulthood, engage in approximately 60 minutes of moderate- to vigorous-intensity activity on most days of the week, while not exceeding caloric intake requirements.

To sustain weight loss in adulthood, participate in at least 60–90 minutes of daily physical activity.

Achieve physical fitness by including cardiovascular conditioning, stretching exercises for flexibility, and resistance exercises or calisthenics for muscle strength and endurance.

Food Groups to Emphasize

Consume 9 ½-cup servings of fruits and vegetables daily (2 cups of fruit and 2 ½ cups of vegetables for reference 2000-calorie intake).

Choose a variety of fruits and vegetables each day. In particular, select from all five vegetable subgroups (dark green, orange, legumes, starchy vegetables, and other vegetables) several times a week.

Consume ≥3-oz equivalents of whole-grain products per day, with the rest of the recommended grains coming from enriched or whole-grain products. In general, at least half the grains should come from whole grains.

Consume 3 cups per day of fat-free or low-fat milk or equivalent milk products.

Eat the Right Fats

Aim for 20–35% of total calories from fats, mostly from polyunsaturated and monounsaturated sources, such as fish, nuts, and vegetable oils.

Consume less than 10% of calories from saturated fatty acids and less than 300 mg/d of cholesterol, and keep trans fatty acid consumption as low as possible.

When selecting and preparing meat, poultry, dry beans, and milk or milk products, make choices that are lean, low fat, or fat free.

Carbohydrates Do Matter

Choose fiber-rich fruits, vegetables, and whole grains.

Choose and prepare foods and beverages with little added sugars or caloric sweeteners, such as amounts suggested by the USDA Food Guide and the DASH Eating Plan.

Practicing good oral hygiene by consuming sugar- and starch-containing foods and beverages less frequently.

Less Sodium and More Potassium

Consume less than 2300 mg (approximately 1 teaspoon of salt) of sodium per day. Choose and prepare foods with little salt. Eat more potassium-rich foods, such as fruits and vegetables.

Take It Easy on Alcoholic Beverages

Those who choose to drink alcoholic beverages should do so in moderation—up to one drink per day for women and up to two drinks per day for men.

Alcoholic beverages should not be consumed by some individuals, including those who cannot restrict their alcohol intake, women of childbearing age who may become pregnant, pregnant and lactating women, children and adolescents, individuals taking medications that can interact with alcohol, and those with specific medical conditions.

Alcoholic beverages should be avoided by individuals engaging in activities that require attention, skill, or coordination, such as driving or operating machinery.

Keep Food Safe

Wash hands, food contact surfaces, and fruits and vegetables. Meat and poultry should not be washed or rinsed.

Separate raw, cooked, and ready-to-eat foods while shopping, preparing, or storing foods.

Cook foods to a safe temperature to kill micro-organisms.

Chill (refrigerate) perishable food promptly and defrost foods properly.

Avoid raw (unpasteurized) milk or any products made from unpasteurized milk, raw or partially cooked eggs or foods containing raw eggs, raw or undercooked meat and poultry, unpasteurized juices, and raw sprouts.

Sources: Federal government (http://www.health.gov/dietaryguidelines/dga2005/document); Kris-Etherton and Weber, 2005; and Nicklas et al, 2005.

(continued)

TABLE 1-2 Dietary Guideline Systems *(continued)*

Canada's Food Guide to Healthy Eating

- Provide energy consistent with the maintenance of body weight within the recommended range.
- Include essential nutrients in amounts specified in the Recommended Nutrient Intakes.
- Include no more than 30% of energy as fat (33 g/1000 kcal or 39 g/5000 kJ) and no more than 10% as saturated fat (11 g/1000 kcal or 13 g/5000 kJ).
- Provide 55% of energy as carbohydrate (138 g/1000 kcal or 165 g/5000 kJ) from a variety of sources.
- Be reduced in sodium content.
- Include no more than 5% of total energy as alcohol, or 2 drinks daily, whichever is less.
- Contain no more caffeine than the equivalent of 4 cups of regular coffee per day.
- Use community water supplies that are fluoridated.

Source: http://www.hc-sc.gc.ca/hpfb-dgpsa/onpp-bppn/food_guide_rainbow_e.html.

Chinese Nutrition Society Food-Based Dietary Guidelines (1997)

- Eat a variety of foods, with grains as the staple food.
- Eat more vegetables, fruits, and tubers.
- Eat milk and legumes, and their products, every day.
- Increase appropriately the consumption of fish, poultry, egg, and/or lean, meat, and decrease the consumption of fat meat and/or animal fat.
- Keep balance between the amount of food consumed and physical activity in order to maintain a healthy body weight.
- Eat a diet with less fat/oil and salt.
- For those who consume alcohol, be moderate.
- Do not eat putrid and deteriorated foods.

Source: http://www.afic.org/National%20Dietary%20Guidelines%20for%20China.htm.

European Food-Based Guidelines

- A varied diet, consisting mainly of plant foods
- Daily intake of bread, grains, rice, potatoes, and/or pasta every day
- Daily intake of fresh and local vegetables and fruits
- Healthy body mass index (BMI) range and physical activity
- Low fat intake (total and saturated)
- Intake of lean meat, poultry, fish, and legumes
- Intake of low-fat milk and low-fat dairy products
- Low sugar intake
- Low salt intake
- Limited alcohol intake
- Hygienic preparation of food
- Exclusive breastfeeding

Source: http://www.gla.ac.uk/departments/humannutrition/students/resources/jscott/guidelines.html.

Greek Food-Based Guidelines

- Do not exceed the optimal body weight for your height.
- Eat slowly, preferably at regular times during the day and in a pleasant environment.
- Prefer fruits and nuts as snacks, instead of sweets or candy bars.
- Prefer whole-grain bread or pasta.
- Always prefer water over soft drinks.
- Healthy adults, with the exception of pregnant women, do not need dietary supplements (vitamins, minerals, etc.) when they follow a balanced diet.
- Light foods are not a substitute for physical activity when it comes to controlling excess body weight; furthermore, their consumption in high quantities has been shown to promote obesity.
- Although the indicated model diet is the ultimate goal, gradual adoption may be more realistic for some people.

Source: http://www.nut.uoa.gr/english/GreekGuid.htm#diatr8.

(continued)

TABLE 1-2 Dietary Guideline Systems *(continued)*

South African Dietary Guidelines

- Enjoy a variety of foods; this is difficult but necessary in developing countries.
- Be active.
- Make starchy foods the basis of most meals.
- Eat plenty of vegetables and fruits every day.
- Eat more legumes for better overall health.
- Foods from animals can be eaten every day.
- Eat fats sparingly—implications for health and disease.
- Eat salt sparingly—sprinkle, don't shake!
- Drink water—the neglected nutrient.
- If you drink alcohol, drink sensibly.

Source: http://www.sahealthinfo.org/nutrition/safoodbased.htm.

References for cited sources in this table are as follows: Kris-Etherton PM, Weber JA. Dietary Guidelines 2005: contributions of registered dietitians to the evolution and dissemination of the guidelines. *J Am Diet Assoc.* 105:1362, 2005; and Nicklas TA, et al. The 2005 Dietary Guidelines Advisory Committee: developing a key message. *J Am Diet Assoc.* 105:1418, 2005.

Pregnancy and Lactation

PREGNANCY

NUTRITIONAL ACUITY RANKING: LEVEL 1 (UNCOMPLICATED); LEVEL 3 (HIGH RISK PREGNANCY)

DEFINITIONS AND BACKGROUND

Pregnancy is an anabolic state that affects maternal tissues using hormones synthesized to support successful pregnancy. Progesterone induces fat deposition to insulate the baby, supports energy reserves, and relaxes smooth muscle, which will cause a decrease in intestinal motility for greater nutrient absorption. Estrogen increases tremendously during pregnancy for growth promotion, uterine function, and water retention. Progesterone and estrogen secreted during pregnancy in combination also help prepare for successful lactation. Figure 1-2 shows the signs of pregnancy.

Adequate weight gain is needed to ensure optimal fetal outcome. Energy costs of pregnancy vary by BMI of the mother (Butte et al, 2004). Tissue growth in pregnancy: breast, 0.5 kg; placenta, 0.6 kg; fetus, 3–3.5 kg; amniotic fluid, 1 kg; uterus, 1 kg; increase in blood volume, 1.5 kg; and extracellular fluid, 1.5 kg.

Higher maternal weight before pregnancy increases the risk of late fetal death, although it protects against the delivery of a small for gestational age (SGA) infant. Obesity is associated with increased risk of first trimester or recurrent miscarriages (Lashen et al, 2004) and the need for caesarean delivery (Weiss et al, 2004). Underweight is associated with SGA or preterm deliveries. In addition, maternal obesity may actually promote obesity in children aged 2–4 (Whitaker, 2004). Women who have had previous bariatric surgery are not at risk for adverse perinatal outcome (Sheiner et al, 2004); which is important since many obese women seek that surgery to improve their health or to enhance the likelihood of sustaining a pregnancy.

A short span between pregnancies or an early pregnancy within 2 years of menarche increases the risk for preterm birth and growth-retarded infants; maternal nutrient depletion of energy and protein leads to poor maternal nutritional status at conception and altered pregnancy outcomes (King, 2003). Poor maternal iron and folate status has been associated with preterm births and intrauterine growth retardation, two outcomes for which women with early or closely spaced pregnancies are at high risk (King, 2003).

Several of the major diseases of later life, including CHD, HPN, and type 2 diabetes, may originate from impaired intrauterine growth and development (Dempsey et al, 2004; Godfrey and Barker, 2000). Such diseases may be consequences of a programmed stimulus or insult at a critical, sensitive time. People who are small or disproportionate (thin or short) at birth may have high rates of CHD, high BP, high cholesterol concentrations, and abnormal glucose-insulin metabolism, independent of length of gestation (Godfrey and Barker, 2000). Interestingly as well, HDL cholesterol levels in women tend to decline after multiple pregnancies (Gunderson et al, 2004).

Bulimia nervosa during pregnancy can lead to miscarriage, inappropriate weight gain (excessive or inadequate), complicated delivery, low birth weight, prematurity, infant malformation, low Apgar scores, and other problems; it must be identified and carefully addressed (Morrill and

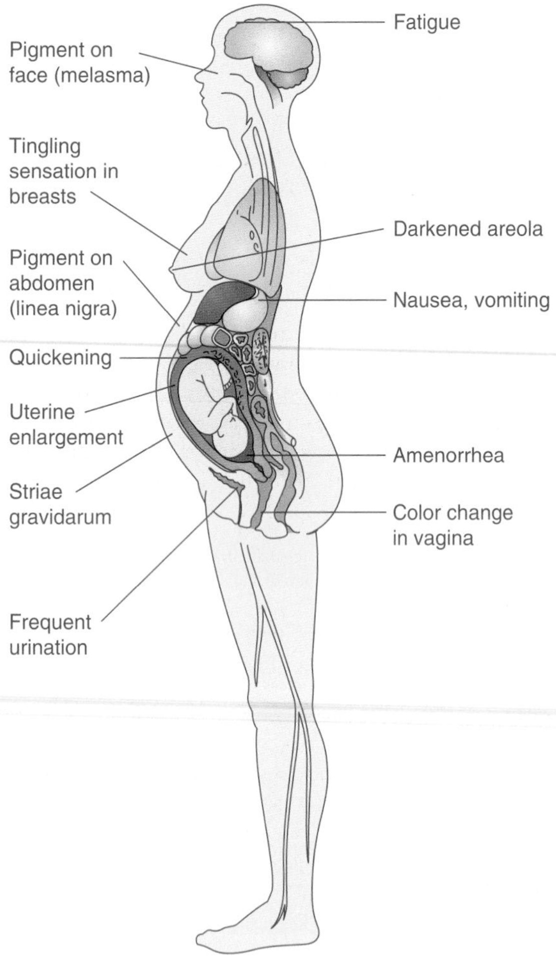

Figure 1-2 Signs of pregnancy. (From Pillitteri A. *Maternal and child nursing.* 4th ed. Philadelphia: Lippincott, Williams & Wilkins, 2003.)

Nickols-Richardson, 2001). Another concern during pregnancy is PKU; women with untreated PKU often have poor reproductive outcomes. Early maintenance of maternal plasma Phe concentrations and mean protein intake greater than RDA with adequate energy intake are important (Acosta et al, 2001). Women with PKU seem to have a higher number of babies who are born with congenital heart disease; prevention requires initiation of the low Phe diet before conception or early in pregnancy, with metabolic control no later than the eighth gestational week (Levy et al, 2001).

Nutritional deficits are also serious in pregnancy. Planned pregnancies usually have the most favorable outcomes. Continuous dietary monitoring of pregnant women and pregnant teens is essential, especially for calcium, folate, magnesium, iron, and vitamin E (Pobocik et al, 2003); fiber, zinc, and vitamin D should also be monitored (Giddens et al, 2000). Biotin deficiency should also be avoided during pregnancy (Zempleni and Mock, 1999).

Table 1-3 lists risk assessments and indicators of potentially poor maternal or fetal outcomes. To prevent small for gestational age (SGA) births, a mother is encouraged not to smoke, to manage any cardiac disease or conditions such as elevated blood pressure, and to gain sufficient weight (Cheng et al, 2004). Women who are HIV positive may experience undesirable weight loss (Villamore, 2004). Approximately 35% of major cardiac defects may be prevented by maternal use of multivitamins during the periconceptual period (Botto et al, 2000).

For twin and multiple pregnancies, twice-monthly visits, sufficient energy intake, multimineral supplementation, and patient education may reduce complications such as low birth weight and neonatal morbidity (Luke et al, 2003). The American Dietetic Association has suggested three visits for medical nutrition therapy in high-risk pregnancies.

INTERVENTION: OBJECTIVES

- Prevent prematurity and low birth weight deliveries.
- Provide adequate weight gain during course of pregnancy. American Dietetic Association standards (2002) state that underweight women (BMI < 18.5) should gain 28–40 lb. Normal weight women (BMI $= 19–24.9$) should gain 25–35 lb total. Overweight women (BMI $= 25–29.9$) should gain 15–25 lb. Obese women (BMI > 30) should gain less than 15 lb; obesity is a major risk for neural tube defects (Scialli, 2006).
- Encourage proper rate of weight gain: 2–4 lb first trimester, 10–11 lb second trimester, and 12–13 lb third trimester. More weight should be gained if patient is be-

TABLE 1-3 Prenatal Risk Assessments and Indicators of Potentially Poor Outcomes

Prepregnancy

- Adolescence (poor eating habits, greater needs).
- History of three or more pregnancies in past 2 years, especially miscarriages.
- History of poor obstetrical/fetal performance.
- Overweight and obesity, which can cause a higher risk for gestational diabetes, preeclampsia, eclampsia, C-section, and/or delivery of infant with macrosomia (Baeten et al, 2001).

Prepregnancy or During Pregnancy

- Economic deprivation.
- Food faddist; smoker; user of drugs/alcohol; practice of pica with related iron or zinc deficiencies; anorexia nervosa or bulimia.
- Modified diet for chronic systemic diseases.
- Prepartum weight of less than 85% or more than 120% of IBW (may reflect inability to attain proper weight or poor dietary habits).
- Deficient Hgb (less than 11 g) or hematocrit (Hct) (less than 33%).
- Any weight loss during PG or gain of less than 2 lb/month in the last two trimesters; dehydration; hyperemesis.
- Risk of toxemia (2-lb weight gain per week or more).
- Poorly managed vegetarian diet.
- Poor nutrient or energy intakes over the course of the pregnancy–assess intakes over the duration.
- Poor intake of magnesium, zinc, calcium, and other key nutrients.

low ideal weight range before pregnancy; this is especially true for young women. Adolescents are at high risk of gaining an excessive amount of weight during pregnancy and should be closely monitored (Howie et al, 2003).

- Provide additional nutrients and energy (net cost of pregnancy varies from 20,000–80,000 kcal total). Women carrying more than one fetus must add extra kilocalories to support multiple births. Energy deficit may contribute to low infant birth weight. Women will need to meet increased needs for fetus and tissues.
- Prevent or correct hypoglycemia and ketosis.
- Provide adequate amino acids to meet fetal and placental growth. Approximately 950 g of protein are synthesized for fetus and placenta. Low protein intake may lead to a reduced infant head circumference (Ivanovic et al, 2004; Thame et al, 1997).
- Promote development of an adequate fetal immune system, especially during first trimester (Stene et al, 2004).
- Prevent or correct deficiencies of iron or folic acid, which are common in 50–75% of pregnancies. Folate deficiency may cause miscarriage and neural tube defects. Iron deficiency may cause low infant birth weight and premature birth (Luke, 2005). A woman with a history of spontaneous abortion in her immediate prior pregnancy may be at increased risk for a pregnancy affected by a neural tube defect; short interpregnancy interval increases this risk (Todoroff and Shaw, 2000). In addition, neural tube defects, stillbirth, and clubfoot may be related to elevated homocysteine levels (Vollset et al, 2000).
- Vitamin A deficiency is strongly associated with depressed immune system and higher morbidity and mortality due to infectious diseases such as measles, diarrhea, and respiratory infections. Vitamin A deficiency is often related to mother to infant HIV transmission (Fawzi et al, 2004). On the other hand, avoid excesses of vitamin A; doses of 10,000–30,000 IU/d can cause birth defects (Miller et al, 1998).
- Calcium is important. Supplementation with calcium during pregnancy does not necessarily prevent preeclampsia. In the Calcium for Preeclampsia Prevention Study, 4314 women were followed during pregnancy; 7.6% had preeclampsia, and 17% had pregnancy-associated hypertension. High BMI and race were more commonly related to these conditions than any of the 23 nutrients that were also studied (Morris et al., 2001).
- Avoid vitamin D deficiency, which may lead to a low infant birth weight (Fuller, 2000).
- Supply sufficient iodine to prevent cretinism with mental and physical retardation (Angermayr and Clar, 2004).
- Provide requirements of zinc to prevent congenital malformations, such as neural tube defects (Groenen et al, 2003).
- Only extremely high serum levels of paraxanthine (a caffeine metabolite) are associated with spontaneous abortion (Signorello and McLaughlin, 2004). Therefore, moderate caffeine intake is unlikely to cause an increased risk of miscarriage. Limit caffeinated beverage intake to two cups daily.
- Avoid alcohol. Mothers who drink relatively high levels of alcohol around the time of conception increase the risk of orofacial clefts in their offspring (Shaw and Lammer, 1999).
- Maintain adequate gestational duration and avoid preterm delivery.
- Develop or improve good eating habits to prevent or delay onset of chronic health problems postnatally. Support the individual patient; pregnant women who are fatigued, stressed, and anxious tend to consume more macronutrients and may be consuming decreased intakes of important micronutrients (Hurley et al, 2005).
- Monitor blood pressure and blood glucose regularly to prevent or to identify complications such as preeclampsia or gestational diabetes. Avoid or treat other complications, such as nausea and vomiting of pregnancy (NVP) and hyperemesis gravidarum. See Table 1-3 for a list of risk factors. See also the appropriate entries.
- Women should drink plenty of fluids to remain adequately hydrated (Klein, 2005).
- Multiple gestation creates new challenges and magnified nutritional requirements (Luke, 2005). There are more risks for adverse outcomes, including diabetes, hypertension, eclampsia, delivery of a premature or low birth weight (LBW) infant (Klein, 2005; Luke, 2005). For twins, weight gain should reflect the period of gestation and prepartum BMI (Luke, Hediger et al, 2003); 35–45 lb is often recommended with twins, and 50 lb overall is recommended for triplets (Brown and Carlson, 2000).

INTERVENTION: FOOD AND NUTRITION

- Include in diet: 1 g protein/kg body weight daily (or 10–15 g above recommended dietary allowances for age). Young teens: 11–14 years (1.7 g/kg); 15–18 years (1.5 g/kg); over 19 years of age (1.7 g/kg); high risk (2 g/kg).
- Energy: In women of normal weight, energy requirements increase minimally in the first trimester, by 350 kcal/d in the second trimester, and by 500 kcal/d in the

SAMPLE NUTRITION DIAGNOSTIC STATEMENT

Pica in Pregnancy

PES: Harmful beliefs/attitudes about food or nutrition-related topics related to intake of unsafe substances as evidenced by reports of consuming laundry starch 2 times daily as recommended by grandmother.

Assessment Data: Food records; adverse side effects; weight and prenatal growth charts; lab reports for H & H, serum ferritin.

Intervention: Education and counseling about appropriate dietary and substance intake for pregnancy; dangers of consuming nonfood substances.

Monitoring and Evaluation: Weight and prenatal growth charts; successful pregnancy outcome for infant and mother; lab reports for H & H, serum ferritin.

third trimester (Butte et al, 2004). Add more or less, depending on level of physical activity. Evaluate teens individually according to age and prepregnancy weight. With twins, dietary prescription of 3000 to 4000 kcal/d may be needed (Luke et al, 2003).

- The diet should include 27 mg of ferrous iron (diet plus supplements) and 5-mg increase in intake of zinc (easily obtained from meats). Women who have previously given birth to an infant with a neural tube defect should consume up to 4–5 mg/d of dietary folate (American Dietetic Association, 2002). Otherwise, the 600 μg folate daily throughout pregnancy should be sufficient (Klein, 2005).
- The recommended intake of calcium in pregnancy is 1000 mg for women over age 19 and 1300 mg for women under age 19.
- Encourage use of vitamin C foods with iron-rich foods or an iron sulfate supplement. While supplemental vitamins C and E do not always prevent preeclampsia (Duley, 2003), daily intake of 1000 mg vitamin C and 400 IU vitamin E can be recommended for women with a history of preeclampsia in a prior pregnancy (Klein, 2005).
- Use adequate vitamins A and D. Avoid hypervitaminosis, which may lead to fetal damage. Monitor use of dietary supplements carefully.
- Be sure to use iodized salt, but avoid excessive salt intake.
- Desired pattern of food intake: 2–3 servings of milk-yogurt-cheese group (for calcium, protein); 6 oz of meat or protein substitute (protein, iron, zinc); 3 fruits and 4 vegetables, including citrus (vitamin C) and rich sources of vitamin A and folacin; 9 servings of grains and breads, 3 of which are whole-grain or enriched breads/substitutes (iron, energy); 3 servings of fat.
- Omit alcohol. Reduce caffeine intake to the equivalent of two cups of coffee; this includes intake from colas, chocolate, and tea.
- Use cereal grains, nuts, black beans, green vegetables, and seafood for extra magnesium. Magnesium seems to play a role in preventing or correcting high blood pressure in susceptible women (Dawson et al, 2000).

SAMPLE NUTRITION DIAGNOSTIC STATEMENT

Normal Pregnancy

PES: Excessive energy intake related to misinformation of nutrition needs during pregnancy as evidenced by dietary recall showing eating of high-calorie foods and by 3-pound body weight gain per week during the second trimester and a total 20-pound weight gain by the middle of the second trimester.

Assessment Data: Summary of dietary history that reflected high-caloric foods referenced in the PES statement, patient statements reflecting misinformation, dates of weights and statement about rate of weight gain compared to recommended rate of weight gain.

Intervention: Education on food and nutrient needs during pregnancy. Referral to WIC if eligible financially and medically.

Monitoring and Evaluation: Plan at monthly appointment would include diet history and weight gain.

SAMPLE NUTRITION DIAGNOSTIC STATEMENT

Multiple Gestation

PES: Inadequate protein intake related to estimated needs for pregnancy with twins as evidenced by dietary intake records meeting 60% of goal and slow growth on prenatal growth grid.

Assessment Data: Dietary recall; labs such as albumin, BUN, and H & H; prenatal growth grid.

Intervention: Education and counseling tips on protein and protein-sparing kcals during pregnancy for twins, snacks

Monitoring and Evaluation: Changes in dietary intake, improved lab values, improved weight gain on prenatal growth grid, successful pregnancy outcome for infants and mother.

- Essential fatty acids from fats, such as corn oil or safflower oil and walnuts, should equal 1–2% of daily calories. Fish and seafood (e.g., tuna, mackerel, salmon) should be encouraged for their omega-3 fatty acids several times weekly, if there are no related allergies.
- Extra vitamin B_6 and copper will be needed. These are readily obtained from a planned diet.
- **Vegan vegetarians** will need a vitamin B_{12} supplement and probably zinc, calcium, and vitamin D as well.
- In cases of **severe gastrointestinal problems,** as in women with inflammatory bowel disease, pancreatitis, or anorexia nervosa, total parenteral nutrition (TPN) may be needed. Adequate lipids (10–20% of energy) are needed for the fetus, as well as protein and carbohydrate. Check blood sugar regularly. Be sure to use adequate fluid (2–3 L for some). Complications of TPN in pregnancy may include bacteremia, decreased renal function with preexisting disease, neonatal hypoglycemia, and possible subclavian vein thrombosis.
- Avoidance of common food allergens during pregnancy does not seem to play a significant role in the incidence of atopic eczema during the first 12–18 months of the infant's life (Kramer and Kakuma, 2003). Women may use their own discretion if they have food allergies themselves.
- For **multiple gestation**, diet therapy with a diabetic regimen of 20% of calories from protein, 40% of calories from carbohydrate, and 40% of calories from fat may be particularly useful (Luke, 2005). Supplement with calcium, magnesium, and zinc, as well as multivitamins and essential fatty acids (Luke, 2005).
- For **hyperemesis gravidarum** (intractable vomiting), hospitalization with tube feeding may be needed (Quinla and Hill, 2003). When eating orally, liquids taken between meals, extra B-complex vitamins and vitamin C, and limited fat may be beneficial. Hyperemesis affects 20% of pregnancies. Low birth weight and greater length of hospital stay are common with these pregnancies (Paauw et al, 2005). Electrolyte imbalances must be avoided. Metoclopramide (Reglan) may help some women. Aggressive treatment, including nutrition support, should be offered early (Paauw et al, 2005). Tips may include:
  - Don't force eating; suck on ice chips or other frozen items. Make up lost calories later.

SAMPLE NUTRITION DIAGNOSTIC STATEMENT

Hyperemesis Gravidarum (morning sickness)

PES: Involuntary weight loss related to prolonged inadequate intake of oral food and beverages as evidenced by weight loss of 3 pounds since last medical visit and dietary intake of 50% of goal for stage of pregnancy.

Assessment Data: Dietary recall, weight records, frequency reports of nausea and emesis.

Intervention: Enteral feedings, counseling tips on managing hyperemesis (odors, cooking, cold vs. hot foods).

Monitoring and Evaluation: Weight and dietary intake records, decrease in frequency or termination of nausea or emesis, successful pregnancy outcome for infant and mother.

- Eat dry food items, such as crackers or dry bread, before getting out of bed.
- Suggest eating meals and snacks in a well-ventilated area, free of odors; avoid strong spices and aromas.
- Eating and drinking should be done slowly, and resting after meals is helpful.
- Frequent, small meals should be eaten separately from fluids; high-protein snacks, such as cheese or lean meat, are helpful.
- Use dry foods; avoid very sweet or fried or fatty foods.
- Avoid lying down after eating.
- Avoid skipping meals; nausea may be more intense on an empty stomach.

CLINICAL INDICATORS

Clinical/History

- Gravida (number of pregnancies)
- Para (number of births)
- Abortus (number of abortions)
- Multiple gestation?
- Height
- Prepregnancy weight (% standard)
- Weight grid or prenatal BMI (19.8–20.0)
- Present weight for gestational age
- Desired weight at term
- Diet history
- Hx of births with neural tube defects, preterm delivery, multiple births
- Uterine or cervical abnormalities?
- Current use of alcohol
- Smoking habits and drug use
- Exposure to the medication diethylstilbestrol (DES)?
- Nausea (frequency, duration, impact on intake)
- Vomiting (frequency, duration, impact on intake)
- Pica?
- Blood pressure (BP)
- Hx of domestic violence, stress, lack of social support

Lab Work

- Hemoglobin and hematocrit (H & H)
- Serum Fe
- Urea N
- Glucose (by 24–28 weeks)
- Ca^{++}, Mg^{++}
- Albumin (Alb)
- Transferrin
- Ceruloplasmin
- T3, T4
- Blood urea nitrogen (BUN)
- Creatine
- Cholesterol (may be increased)
- Alkaline phosphatase (alk phos) (may be increased)
- Total iron-binding capacity (TIBC) (often increased in late pregnancy)

Common Drugs Used and Potential Side Effects

- After the fourth month, encourage use of a basic vitamin-mineral supplement between meals (with liquids other than milk, coffee, or tea) for better utilization. Supplements vary greatly; read labels carefully. Iron is the only nutrient that cannot be met from diet alone (30 mg needed after the first trimester). Discuss the relevance of tolerable upper intake levels (ULs) from the latest dietary reference intakes of the National Academy of Sciences. These levels were set to protect individuals from receiving too much of any nutrient from diet and dietary supplements.
- Avoid taking iron supplements with antacids. Bedtime is a good time to take an iron supplement.
- Avoid taking isotretinoin (Accutane) or 13-*cis*-retinoic acid (CRA) for acne; they have been linked to birth defects. There is some review of the overall safety of isotretinoin at this time as well.
- Avoid excesses of vitamin A, especially in the first trimester. Be wary of 10,000 IU of vitamin A or more; birth defects may result.
- Insulin may be needed with consistently high blood glucose levels over 120 mg/dL; monitor overfeeding.
- Antiemetic agents may be used to control NVP and include ondansetron (Zofran), cyclizine (Marezine), buclizine (Bucladin-S), metoclopramide (Reglan), meclizine (Antivert), prochlorperazine (Compazine), promethazine (Phenergan), or antihistamines such as Benadryl. Side effects vary but may include sedation, dizziness, changes in blood pressure, and/or tachycardia. Diclectin and Bendectin (doxylamine with vitamin B_6) are only available in Canada at this time; they are safe for the fetus (Baggley et al, 2004).
- Women who develop preterm labor are often treated with one of several drugs (tocolytics) to stop premature labor. Drugs include calcium channel blockers, terbutaline, ritodrine, magnesium sulfate, indomethacin, ketorolac, and sulindac. Use is short term, and side effects are not significant.

Herbs, Botanicals, and Supplements

- Pregnant women should not use herbs, botanical supplements, and herbals teas (American Dietetic Association, 2002). Women who are using such supplements should stop immediately when they discover they are pregnant. There are no rigorous scientific studies of the safety of dietary supplements during pregnancy, and the Teratology Society has stated that it should not be assumed that they are safe for the embryo or fetus (Marcus and Snodgrass, 2005).

- Pregnant women should not take herbal and botanical supplements containing aloe, apricot kernel, black cohosh, borage, calendula, chaparral, chasteberry, comfrey, dong quai, ephedra, euphorbia, feverfew, foxglove, gentian, ginseng, golden seal, hawthorne, horehound, horseradish, juniper, licorice root, nettle, plantain, pokeroot, prickly ash, red clover, rhubarb, sassafras, saw palmetto, senna, skullcap, St. John's wort, tansy, wild carrot, willow, wormwood, yarrow, or yohimbe (American Dietetic Association, 2002). Willow bark, which contains salicilin, may cause stillbirth, prolonged gestation, and low birth weight.
- Initial treatment of nausea and vomiting should be conservative and should involve dietary changes, emotional support, and perhaps alternative therapy such as ginger (Quinla and Hill, 2003). Sips of ginger ale or use of small amounts of ginger in cooking may be useful. Ginger may be an effective treatment for nausea and vomiting in pregnancy (Borrelli et al, 2005). However, when taking blood thinners or preparing for surgery, discontinue use.

	Recommendation		
Nutrient	**Age 18 Years or Under**	**Ages 19–30 Years**	**Ages 31–50 Years**
Energy	1st tri = +0 kcal/d; 2nd tri = +340 kcal/d; 3rd tri = +452 kcal/d	1st tri = +0 kcal/d; 2nd tri= +340 kcal/d; 3rd tri= +452 kcal/d	1st tri = +0 kcal/d; 2nd tri = +340 kcal/d; 3rd tri = +452 kcal/d
Protein	71 g/d	71 g/d	71 g/d
Calcium	1300 mg/d	1000 mg/d	1000 mg/d
Iron	27 mg/d	27 mg/d	27 mg/d
Folate	600 μg/d	600 μg/d	600 μg/d
Phosphorus	1250 mg/d	700 mg/d	700 mg/d
Vitamin A	750 μg	770 μg	770 μg
Vitamin C	80 mg/d	85 mg/d	85 mg/d
Thiamin	1.4 mg/d	1.4 mg/d	1.4 mg/d
Riboflavin	1.4 mg/d	1.4 mg/d	1.4 mg/d
Niacin	18 mg/d	18 mg/d	18 mg/d

Data from: Food and Nutrition Board, Institute of Medicine. *Dietary reference intakes for energy, carbohydrate, fiber, fat, fatty acids, cholesterol, protein, and amino acids (macronutrients)*. Washington, DC: National Academy Press, 2002.

INTERVENTION: NUTRITION EDUCATION, COUNSELING, CARE MANAGEMENT

- The March of Dimes has launched a 5-year campaign to raise public awareness and reduce rates of preterm birth and increase research to find the cause. The March of Dimes recommends the following to reduce the risk and/or effects of a premature birth (http://www.modimes.org/prematurity/13454_5810.asp). Women should:
  - Consume a multivitamin containing 400 μg of the B vitamin folic acid before and in the early months of pregnancy.
  - Stop smoking.
  - Stop drinking and/or using illicit drugs or prescription or over-the-counter drugs (including herbal preparations) not prescribed by a doctor aware of the pregnancy.
  - Once pregnant, get early regular prenatal care, eat a balanced diet with enough calories (usually about 300 more than a woman normally eats), and gain enough weight (25–35 pounds is usually recommended).
  - Talk to their doctor about signs of premature labor and what to do if any of the warning signs are evident.
- Describe an adequate pattern and rate of weight gain in pregnancy; explain the rationale. Individualize according to goals (e.g., short women at lower range of gain). Excess equals more than 6.5 lb gained monthly after 20 weeks. Inadequate intake equals less than 2 lb gained monthly after the first trimester.
- Nausea and vomiting of pregnancy (NVP; or morning sickness) affects 80% of pregnancies (Koren and Maltepe, 2004); share tips and handouts. Try lemonade and potato chips rather than just ginger ale and saltines; minimize offensive odors (Erick and Bunnell, 2000). Avoid large meals and spicy and high-fat foods if not tolerated. Eat dry crackers before rising in the morning. If necessary, drink fluids between meals rather than with meals. Multivitamin-mineral supplements may also trigger NVP; it may be helpful to try a different brand. Rehydration may be essential. NVP often abates by 17 weeks of pregnancy, which can be reassuring.

- Encourage adequate calcium intake. Discuss what to do for milk allergy/intolerance and lactose intolerance, suggesting alternative foods and ways to include calcium.
- Discourage use of trendy diets and fads, low–nutrient density foods, and the habit of skipping breakfast. Discuss ketosis from low glucose levels and its effect on the fetus (e.g., brain development).
- Encourage stress reduction, which has an effect on nitrogen and calcium. Encourage pleasant mealtimes and a healthy appetite.
- Encourage breastfeeding (except for women who are HIV positive). Explain reasons for doing so (e.g., immunological benefits, bonding, and weight stabilization).
- For excessive weight gain, the goal should be to restore eating patterns to match a normal growth curve. Severe calorie restriction should be avoided, and at least 175 g of CHO will be needed.
- Discuss fluoride and iodine intake from water, table salt, and related sources (such as seafood). A balance of both nutrients is needed, but excesses are to be avoided.
- Discuss effects of drug use (cocaine, alcohol, and marijuana), such as decreased birth weight and congenital malformations (Reynolds and Bada, 2003). Discourage tobacco smoking because of the effect on the fetus.
- Aspartame and other sweeteners may be used in moderation throughout the day (Hueston et al, 1995).
- Eligible women should be referred to participate in the WIC Program (Black et al, 2004), especially to decrease low birth weight (Lazariu-Bauer et al, 2004). Many barriers hinder low-income women's participation in nutrition education programs, including lack of transportation or child care. Facilitated discussions, support groups, cooking classes, and a website are preferred methods of nutrition education for WIC participants (Birkett et al, 2004).
- For constipation, extra fiber, activity, and fluid are recommended (2–3 quarts, or 35–40 cc/Kg). Avoid use of laxatives.
- For swelling of ankles, hands, and legs, become more physically active; avoid excessive salt at the table but do not restrict salt severely.
- For heartburn, eat smaller meals more frequently, eat slowly, and cut down on spicy or high-fat foods. Avoid antacids unless approved by the physician.
- Pica prevalence is sometimes identified among women enrolled in WIC and is associated with ice, freezer frost, baking soda, baking powder, cornstarch, laundry starch, baby powder, clay, or dirt (Rainville, 1998). Pica practices are associated with significantly lower hemoglobin levels at delivery; counselors must be aware. Discussion of pica practices should be nonjudgmental because pica may have strong cultural implications (Corbett et al, 2003). Food cravings and aversions usually subside after pregnancy.
- All infections are cause for concern among pregnant women because they pose a risk to the health of the baby. Women should have a periodontal evaluation to rule out gum disease and to eliminate infection; prostaglandins may stimulate early labor and cause delivery of an LBW infant.
- Postpartum concerns should be discussed, including physical activity, breastfeeding, anemia, and control of hyperglycemia. Adherence to dietary guidelines may be limited in low-income, postpartum women because of neglect of self-care, weight-related distress, negative body image, stress, and depressive symptoms (George et al, 2005). Attention to psychosocial needs may help to improve dietary intakes.

Patient Education—Food Safety

- Nausea and vomiting of pregnancy affects approximately 80% of pregnant women, and *Helicobacter pylori* should be suspected as one possible cause (Quinla and Hill, 2003). Careful hand washing is recommended.
- Hepatitis A, *Salmonella, Shigella, Escherichia coli,* and *Cryptosporidium* are common causes of diarrhea during pregnancy (American Dietetic Association, 2002).
- Avoid soft cheeses such as feta, brie, camembert, Roquefort, and Mexican soft cheese; they may have been contaminated with *Listeria,* which can cause fetal death or premature labor. If they are used, cook until boiling first.
- Avoid raw or partially cooked eggs, raw or undercooked fish or shellfish, and raw or undercooked meats because of potential foodborne illnesses.
- Do not eat or drink raw (unpasteurized) milk or products made from it.
- Avoid eating unpasteurized juices and raw sprouts.
- Pregnant women should not eat shark, swordfish, king mackerel, and tilefish. These long-lived larger fish contain the highest levels of methyl mercury, which may harm an unborn baby's developing nervous system. Pregnant women should select a variety of other kinds of fish, such as shellfish, canned fish, smaller ocean fish, and farm-raised fish. They can safely eat 12 oz of cooked fish per week, with a typical serving size being 3–6 oz. Keep fish and shellfish refrigerated or frozen until ready to use.

For More Information

- American College of Nurse-Midwives (ACNM)
  http://www.midwife.org
- American Academy of Periodontology
  http://www.perio.org/consumer/mbc.baby.htm
- Department of Defense—Program for WIC Overseas
  www.tricare.osd.mil/wic/default.htm
- Farmers' Markets, Agricultural Marketing Service of USDA
  www.ams.usda.gov/farmersmarkets/
- National Healthy Mothers, Healthy Babies Coalition
  http://www.hmhb.org/
- Healthy Start, Grow Smart
  http://www.ed.gov/parents/earlychild/ready/healthystart/index.html
- American Association of Birth Centers
  http://www.birthcenters.org/
- National Center for Education in Maternal-Child Health
  http://www.ncemch.org/
- National Council on Folic Acid
  http://www.hmhb.org/ncfa.html
- National Foundation—March of Dimes
  http://www.modimes.org/
- National Women's Health Information Center
  www.4woman.gov

- WIC Program—Supplemental Food Programs Division
http://www.fns.usda.gov/wic/
- WIC Electronic Health Model
http://www.wmich.edu/wic/startframe.html

PREGNANCY—CITED REFERENCES

Acosta P, et al. Intake of major nutrients by women in the Maternal Phenylketonuria (MPKU) Study and effects on plasma phenylalanine concentrations. *Am J Clin Nutr.* 73:792, 2001.

American Dietetic Association. Position of the American Dietetic Association: nutrition and lifestyle for a healthy pregnancy outcome. *J Am Diet Assoc.* 102:1479, 2002.

Angermayr L, Clar C. Iodine supplementation for preventing iodine deficiency disorders in children. *Cochrane Database Syst Rev.* 2:CD003819, 2004.

Baeten JM, et al. Pregnancy complications and outcomes among overweight and obese nulliparous women. *Am J Public Health.* 91:436, 2001.

Baggley A, et al. Determinants of women's decision making on whether to treat nausea and vomiting of pregnancy pharmacologically. *J Midwifery Womens Health.* 49:350, 2004.

Birkett D, et al. Reaching low-income families: focus group results provide direction for a behavioral approach to WIC services. *J Am Diet Assoc.* 104: 1277, 2004.

Black MM, et al. Special Supplemental Nutrition Program for Women, Infants, and Children participation and infants' growth and health: a multisite surveillance study. *Pediatrics* 114:169, 2004.

Borrelli F, et al. Effectiveness and safety of ginger in the treatment of pregnancy-induced nausea and vomiting. *Obstet Gynecol.* 105:849, 2005.

Botto LD, et al. Occurrence of congenital heart defects in relation to maternal multivitamin use. *Am J Epidemiol.* 151:878, 2000.

Brown JE, Carlson M. Nutrition and multifetal pregnancy. *J Am Diet Assoc.* 100:343, 2000.

Butte NF, et al. Energy requirements during pregnancy based on total energy expenditure and energy deposition. *Am J Clin Nutr.* 79:1078, 2004.

Cheng CJ, et al. Body mass index change between pregnancies and small for gestational age births. *Obstet Gynecol.* 104:286, 2004.

Corbett RW, et al. Pica in pregnancy: does it affect pregnancy outcomes? *Am J Matern Child Nurs.* 28:183, 2003.

Dawson EB, et al. Blood cell lead, calcium, and magnesium levels associated with pregnancy-induced hypertension and preeclampsia. *Biol Trace Elem Res.* 74:107, 2000.

Dempsey JC, et al. Maternal birth weight in relation to plasma lipid concentrations in early pregnancy. *Am J Obstet Gynecol.* 190:1359, 2004.

Duley L. Pre-eclampsia and the hypertensive disorders of pregnancy. *Br Med Bull.* 67:161, 2003.

Erick M, Bunnell MK. Nausea and vomiting of pregnancy: manifestations and current interventions. *Female Patient* 25:59, 2000.

Fawzi WW, et al. A randomized trial of multivitamin supplements and HIV disease progression and mortality. *N Engl J Med.* 351:23, 2004.

Fuller KE. Low birth-weight infants: the continuing ethnic disparity and the interaction of biology and environment. *Ethn Dis.* 10:432, 2000.

George GC, et al. Compliance with dietary guidelines and relationship to psychosocial factors in low-income women in late postpartum. *J Am Diet Assoc.* 105:916, 2005.

Giddens JB, et al. Pregnant adolescent and adult women have similarly low intakes of selected nutrients. *J Am Diet Assoc.* 100:1334, 2000.

Godfrey KM, Barker DJ. Fetal nutrition and adult disease. *Am J Clin Nutr.* 71S: 1344, 2000.

Groenen PM, et al. Maternal myo-inositol, glucose, and zinc status is associated with the risk of offspring with spina bifida. *Am J Obstet Gynecol.* 189: 1713, 2003.

Gunderson EP, et al. Long-term plasma lipid changes associated with a first birth: the Coronary Artery Risk Development in Young Adults study. *Am J Epidemiol.* 159:1028, 2004.

Howie LD, Parker JD, Schoendorf KC. Excessive maternal weight gain patterns in adolescents. *J Am Diet Assoc.* 103:1653, 2003.

Hueston WJ, et al. Common questions patients ask during pregnancy. *Am Fam Physician.* 51:1465, 1995.

Hurley KM, et al. Psychosocial influences in dietary patterns during pregnancy. *J Am Diet Assoc.* 105:963, 2005.

Ivanovic DM, et al. Head size and intelligence, learning, nutritional status and brain development. Head, IQ, learning, nutrition and brain. *Neuropsychologia* 42:1118, 2004.

King JC. The risk of maternal nutritional depletion and poor outcomes in early or closely spaced pregnancies. *J Nutr.* 133:1732S, 2003.

Klein L. Nutritional recommendations for multiple pregnancy. *J Am Diet Assoc.* 105:1050, 2005.

Koren G, Maltepe C. Pre-emptive therapy for severe nausea and vomiting of pregnancy and hyperemesis gravidarum. *J Obstet Gynaecol.* 24:530, 2004.

Kramer M, Kakuma R. Maternal dietary antigen avoidance during pregnancy and/or lactation for preventing or treating atopic disease in the child. *Cochrane Database Syst Rev.* 4:CD000133, 2003.

Lashen H, et al. Obesity is associated with increased risk of first trimester and recurrent miscarriage: matched case-control study. *Hum Reprod.* 19:1644, 2004.

Lazariu-Bauer V, et al. A comparative analysis of effects of early versus late prenatal WIC participation on birth weight. *Matern Child Health J.* 8:77, 2004.

Levy H, et al. Congenital heart disease in maternal phenylketonuria: report from the Maternal PKU Collaborative Study. *Pediatr Res.* 49:636, 2001.

Luke B. Nutrition and multiple gestation. *Semin Perinatol.* 29:349, 2005.

Luke B, et al. Specialized prenatal care and maternal and infant outcomes in twin pregnancy. *Am J Obstet Gynecol.* 189:934, 2003.

Luke B, Hediger ML, et al. Body mass index–specific weight gains associated with optimal birth weights in twin pregnancies. *Reprod Med.* 48:217, 2003.

Marcus DM, Snodgrass WR. Do no harm: avoidance of herbal medicines during pregnancy. *Obstet Gynecol.* 105:1119, 2005.

Miller RK, et al. Periconceptional vitamin A use: how much is teratogenic? *Reprod Toxicol.* 12:75, 1998.

Morrill ES, Nickols-Richardson HM. Bulimia nervosa during pregnancy: a review. *J Am Diet Assoc.* 101:448, 2001.

Morris CD, et al. Nutrient intake and hypertensive disorders of pregnancy: evidence from a large prospective cohort. *Am J Obstet Gynecol.* 184:643, 2001.

Quinla JD, Hill DA. Nausea and vomiting of pregnancy. *Am Fam Physician.* 68: 121, 2003.

Paauw JD, et al. Hyperemesis gravidarum and fetal outcome. *J Parenter Enteral Nutr.* 29:93, 2005.

Pobocik RS, et al. Pregnant adolescents in Guam consume diets low in calcium and other micronutrients. *J Am Diet Assoc.* 3:611, 2003.

Rainville A. Pica practices of pregnant women are associated with lower maternal hemoglobin level at delivery. *J Am Diet Assoc.* 98:293, 1998.

Reynolds EW, Bada HS. Pharmacology of drugs of abuse. *Obstet Gynecol Clin North Am.* 30:501, 2003.

Scialli AR. 2005 Josef Warkany lecture: clinicians. *Birth Defects Res A Clin Mol Teratol.* 76:1, 2006.

Shaw GM, Lammer EJ. Maternal periconceptional alcohol consumption and risk for orofacial clefts. *J Pediatr.* 134:298, 1999.

Sheiner E, et al. Pregnancy after bariatric surgery is not associated with adverse perinatal outcome. *Am J Obstet Gynecol.* 190:1335, 2004.

Signorello LB, McLaughlin JK. Maternal caffeine consumption and spontaneous abortion: a review of the epidemiologic evidence. *Epidemiology* 15: 229, 2004.

Stene LC, et al. Perinatal factors and development of islet autoimmunity in early childhood: the diabetes autoimmunity study in the young. *Am J Epidemiol.* 160:3, 2004.

Thame M, et al. Relationship between maternal nutritional status and infant's weight and body proportions at birth. *Eur J Clin Nutr.* 51:134, 1997.

Todoroff K, Shaw GM. Prior spontaneous abortion, prior elective termination, interpregnancy interval, and risk of neural tube defects. *Am J Epidemiol.* 151:505, 2000.

Villamore E, et al. Weight loss during pregnancy is associated with adverse pregnancy outcomes among HIV-1 infected women. *J Nutr.* 134:1424, 2004.

Vollset SE, et al. Plasma total homocysteine level and complications and outcomes of pregnancy. *Am J Clin Nutr.* 71:962, 2000.

Weiss JL, et al. Obesity, obstetric complications and cesarean delivery rate—a population-based screening study. *Am J Obstet Gynecol.* 190:1091, 2004.

Whitaker RC. Predicting preschooler obesity at birth: the role of maternal obesity in early pregnancy. *Pediatrics* 114:29, 2004.

Zempleni J, Mock DM. Biotin biochemistry and human requirements. *J Nutr Biochem.* 10:128, 1999

LACTATION

NUTRITIONAL ACUITY RANKING: LEVEL 1

DEFINITIONS AND BACKGROUND

Breastfeeding should be supported and encouraged because of its immunological, physiological, economic, social, and hygienic effects on mother and infant. Exclusive breastfeeding for the first 6 months of life provides the best form of nutrition (James et al, 2005). Because maternal intake and breastfeeding practices vary over the duration of lactation, assess regularly and determine whether or not the infant needs supplemental foods or nutrients. Only rarely is supplementation needed. In fact, adding formula or solids to the diet of the exclusively breastfed infant almost guarantees lactation failure. Unless mom is severely malnourished, she can keep making good milk.

Breastfeeding is an anabolic state, requiring extra energy. The composition of breast milk varies over time. Colostrum contains mainly immunological factors (days 1–4); a short transition occurs (days 5–9); breast milk secreted between days 9 and 28 is primarily nutritional; and breast milk content is equally valuable for immunity and nutrition between days 28 and 84 (Montagne et al, 2000).

Human milk is better digested and absorbed by infants than other forms of milk; it has more DHA and arachidonic acid for normal cognitive and visual development (Innis, 2003) and carnitine for mitochondrial oxidation of these long-chain fatty acids. It also has less sodium and a proper protein ratio. In women who have diabetes, DHA and arachidonic acid levels are lower; insulin resistance is higher among their infants (Min et al, 2005).

Breast milk has 1.5 times as much lactose as cow's milk; consequently, protein is absorbed better. The whey to casein ratio of 80:20 is more desirable than that of many formulas. In comparison, cow's milk has twice as much protein and mineral content. The composition of breast milk also changes to meet the baby's changing needs (i.e., the fat content decreases over time). See Table 1-4 about the content of human milk and Figure 1-3 for the physiology of the breast.

Food allergies are less frequent in infants who are exclusively breastfed (Muraro et al, 2004). Protection is even greater when maternal diets are higher in omega-3 fatty acids (Hanson et al, 2003). Compared with cow's milk formulas, breast milk has more antibodies and over 45 bioactive factors such as digestive enzymes, hormones, immune factors, and growth factors. The promotion of nearly universal breastfeeding has played an important role in improving child health by providing optimum nutrition and protection against common childhood infections and by promoting child spacing (Weinberg, 2000).

Breast milk is a living fluid. Infants receive beneficial nucleotides, macrophages, leukocytes, lymphocytes, and neutrophils from human milk, which protect against diarrhea, allergies (Muraro et al, 2004; Wright et al, 2001), ear infections, necrotizing enterocolitis, urinary tract infection, and pneumonia (Department of Health and Human Services, 2000). Bacterial flora of breastfed infants are generally *Lactobacillus*, not *Escherichia coli* like those of formula-fed infants. Formula-fed infants may be more prone to wheezing, GE reflux, urinary tract infection, influenza, sepsis, and *Giardia*, and exclusive breastfeeding for 6 months is highly recommended (Hanson et al, 2003; Yu, 2002; Sikorski et al, 2002).

Reasons not to breastfeed include if the mother uses alcohol or illicit drugs, if the mother is receiving chemotherapy, if the infant has galactosemia, or if the mother is human immunodeficiency virus (HIV) positive. Unfortunately, breastfeeding by HIV-infected mothers increases pediatric HIV infection; even early use of medication may not help (Taha et al, 2004). In developing nations, where adequate sanitary replacement feeding is not available, the decision to withhold breastfeeding so as to decrease HIV transmission may lead to increased rates of child morbidity and mortality from diarrheal and respiratory diseases and malnutrition (Weinberg, 2000); waiting 6 months to use breast milk from the infected mother may balance out the risks (Ross and Labbok, 2004). Women must be fully informed about the risks of breastfeeding transmission of HIV and the expense and availability of obtaining formula.

Women should be encouraged to breastfeed as long as mutually desirable (American Academy of Pediatrics, 2004) until the child is 1 year of age. In developing countries, mothers may be encouraged to increase the breastfeeding time to 2 years (Lauer et al, 2004), but mothers should not deprive themselves. The volume of milk decreases in a poorly nourished mother. New mothers who are breastfeeding should try not to lose weight rapidly during lactation. In addition, women who are obese before pregnancy may need extra encouragement to breastfeed (Li et al, 2003). Prolonged breastfeeding tends to lower postpartum weight, which is desirable for many women (Kac et al, 2004); this benefit may slow as the mother's age increases.

The long-term effects of breastfeeding an infant include possibly lower incidences of type 2 diabetes, Crohn's disease, some types of cancer, allergies, and neurological disabilities. The intake of several minerals and peptides found in milk has a blood pressure–lowering effect, which may play a protective role later in life for the infant (Groziak and Miller, 2000; Singhal et al, 2001). There is indication that adult ischemic disease may also be reduced by breastfeeding, but more studies are needed (Rich-Edwards et al, 2004).

Better cognitive development in the infant is also a benefit of breastfeeding. Breastfeeding is associated with higher cognitive development than formula feeding; the enhancement remains until about age 15 years of age (Anderson et al, 1999). Long-chain fatty acids (DHA and EPA) are important in this role (Helland et al, 2003). Breastfed infants are often more mature, secure, and assertive and tend to score

TABLE 1-4 Content of Mature Human Milk

Nutrient	Units	1 Cup/246.000 g
Proximates		
Water	g	215.250
Energy	kcal	171.125
Protein	g	2.534
Total lipid (fat)	g	10.775
Carbohydrate	g	16.949
Fiber, total dietary	g	0.000
Minerals		
Calcium, Ca	mg	79.212
Iron, Fe	mg	0.074
Magnesium, Mg	mg	8.364
Phosphorus, P	mg	33.702
Potassium, K	mg	125.952
Sodium, Na	mg	41.574
Zinc, Zn	mg	0.418
Copper, Cu	mg	0.128
Manganese, Mn	mg	0.064
Selenium, Se	μg	4.428
Vitamins		
Vitamin C	mg	12.300
Thiamin	mg	0.034
Riboflavin	mg	0.089
Niacin	mg	0.435
Pantothenic acid	mg	0.549
Vitamin B_6	mg	0.027
Folate	μg	12.792
Vitamin B_{12}	μg	0.111
Vitamin A, IU	IU	592.860
Vitamin A, RE	μg	157.440
Vitamin D	IU	9.840
Vitamin E	mg	2.214
Lipids		
Fatty acids, saturated	g	4.942
Fatty acids, monounsaturated	g	4.079
Fatty acids, polyunsaturated	g	1.223
Cholesterol	mg	34.194
Amino acids		
Tryptophan	g	0.042
Threonine	g	0.113
Isoleucine	g	0.138
Leucine	g	0.234
Lysine	g	0.167
Methionine	g	0.052
Cystine	g	0.047
Phenylalanine	g	0.113
Tyrosine	g	0.130
Valine	g	0.155
Arginine	g	0.106
Histidine	g	0.057
Alanine	g	0.089
Aspartic acid	g	0.202
Glutamic acid	g	0.413
Glycine	g	0.064
Proline	g	0.202
Serine	g	0.106

From: U.S. Department of Agriculture, November 1999.

higher on developmental tests. Healthy People 2010 includes a goal of increasing to 75% the proportion of mothers who breastfeed upon discharge from the hospital and increasing to 50% the proportion of infants still breastfeeding at 6 months of age.

Billions of dollars would be saved if breastfeeding were increased to those levels recommended by the U.S. Surgeon General; this figure represents cost savings from the treatment of three childhood illnesses alone: otitis media, gastroenteritis, and necrotizing enterocolitis (Weimer, 2001). Breastfeeding also reduces the risk of breast and ovarian cancers, protects bone density in the mother, improves glucose profiles in gestational diabetes, and saves money not spent on formula (James et al, 2005). While it has been proposed that breastfeeding helps adults maintain a desirable BMI, this needs further evaluation (Owen et al, 2005).

There is an essential role for dietetics professionals in promoting and supporting breastfeeding by providing up-to-date, practical information to pregnant and postpartum women, involving family and friends in breastfeeding education and counseling, removing institutional barriers to breastfeeding, collaborating with community organizations that promote and support breastfeeding, and advocating for policies that position breastfeeding as the norm (James et al, 2005). In a survey of physicians about their

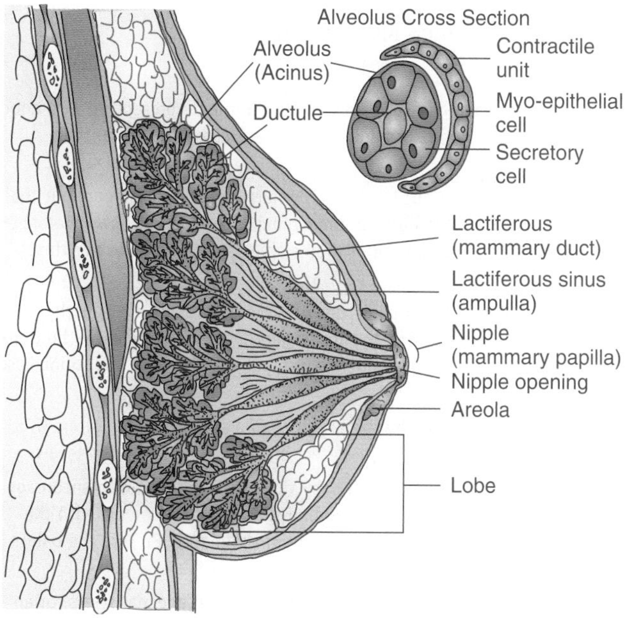

Figure 1-3 Physiology of the Breast. (From Pillitteri A. *Maternal and child nursing.* 4th ed. Philadelphia: Lippincott, Williams & Wilkins, 2003.)

breastfeeding promotion practices, over half indicated that they had had little or no education about breastfeeding, and problem solving was the main area in which they suggested more education be available (Krogstrand and Parr, 2005).

The nutrition counselor should encourage the mother as much as possible to continue breastfeeding for 6–12 months, and somewhat longer in developing countries. The Ten Steps to Successful Breastfeeding (WHO/UNICEF) provide an evidence-based standard used to assess individual hospitals and their support for mothers to breastfeed (Grizzard et al, 2006). See Table 1-5 for common problems that occur during breastfeeding.

INTERVENTION: OBJECTIVES

- Provide for adequate lactation (usual secretion, 750–800 mL/d). Human milk provides 67 kcal/dL. Good energy intake improves milk production, especially in undernourished women.
- Breast milk can meet nutrient needs during the first 6 months, with possible exception of vitamin D and iron in certain populations (Dewey, 2001).
- Exclusive breastfeeding for 6 months has many nutritional benefits (Butte et al, 2002). Have the mother continue breastfeeding for up to 1 year when possible. Exclusive breastfeeding should be encouraged for at least 4–6 months in infants at both high and low risk of atopy and irrespective of a history of maternal asthma (Friedman and Zeigler, 2005).
- Decrease nutritional risks from use of alcohol, stimulants, and medications while mother is breastfeeding. Alcohol intake inhibits the letdown reflex from oxytocin (Silva et al, 2002). Discourage excessive use of stimulants, including caffeine from coffee (limit to 2 cups daily) and from tea, colas, and chocolate.
- Omit known food allergens while breastfeeding if infant shows signs of colic (Hill et al, 2005). Eliminate cow's milk, eggs, peanuts, tree nuts, wheat, soy, and fish, especially if members of the immediate family have allergies.
- Promote adequate infant growth and development, including bone mineralization. Lactation doubles normal daily loss of calcium for the mother. Lactation is generally considered to be beneficial for protecting bone health (Chantry et al, 2004).
- Normalize body composition gradually so that the mother returns to ideal weight. Promote gradual weight loss even in obese women. In overweight women who are exclusively breastfeeding, weight loss of 0.5 kg per week between 4–14 weeks after delivery does not affect the growth of their infants (Lovelady et al, 2000).
- Support brain health and visual acuity by including fatty acids in the diet (Anderson et al, 2005; Lauritezen et al, 2005).

	Recommendation		
Nutrient	**Age 18 Years or Under**	**Ages 19–30 Years**	**Ages 31–50 Years**
Energy	1st 6 mos = +330 kcal/d; 2nd 6 mos = 400 kcal/d	1st 6 mos = +330 kcal/d; 2nd 6 mos = 400 kcal/d	1st 6 mos = +330 kcal/d; 2nd 6 mos = 400 kcal/d
Protein	61 g/d or 1.1 g/kg/d	61 g/d or 1.1 g/kg/d	61 g/d or 1.1 g/kg/d
Calcium	1200 mg/d	1300 mg/d	1300 mg/d
Iron	10 mg/d	9 mg/d	9 mg/d
Folate	500 μg/d	500 μg/d	500 μg/d
Phosphorus	1250 mg/d	700 mg/d	700 mg/d
Vitamin A	1200 μg	1300 μg	1300 μg
Vitamin C	115 mg/d	120 mg/d	120 mg/d
Thiamin	1.4 mg/d	1.4 mg/d	1.4 mg/d
Riboflavin	1.6 mg/d	1.6 mg/d	1.6 mg/d
Niacin	17 mg/d	17 mg/d	17 mg/d

Data from: Food and Nutrition Board, Institute of Medicine. *Dietary reference intakes for energy, carbohydrate, fiber, fat, fatty acids, cholesterol, protein, and amino acids (macronutrients)*. Washington, DC: National Academy Press, 2002.

TABLE 1-5 Common Problems in Breastfeeding and Reasons Why Women Discontinue Breastfeeding

Colic and Fussiness: A randomized, controlled trial of a low-allergen maternal diet was conducted among exclusively breastfed infants presenting with colic; when mothers excluded cow's milk, eggs, peanuts, tree nuts, wheat, soy, and fish from their diet, crying/fuss duration was reduced by a substantially greater amount in the low-allergen group (Hill et al, 2005).

Engorgement: The best way to prevent engorgement is to begin breastfeeding as soon as possible after birth followed by nursing regularly throughout the day. Rapid filling of the breasts and blocked mammary ducts may cause a painful engorgement. Frequent nursing, breast massage or warm shower before feedings, use of cold packs shortly after nursing, wearing a firm bra that is not too tight, and avoiding the use of nipple shields can help alleviate this condition.

Inadequate Milk Supply: Poor milk supply can be a cause of failure to thrive in breastfeeding infants. Maternal causes of poor milk supply are hypothyroidism, excessive antihistamine use, smoking, oral contraceptive use, illness, inadequate intake after gastric bypass surgery, poor diet, decreased fluid intake, infrequent nursing, or fatigue. Correction of any of these causes may improve milk supply. Increasing frequency of nursing is the best way to increase milk supply.

Jaundice: Breast milk jaundice occurs in about 1% of the population of breastfeeding newborns, is caused by the presence of a substance that alters liver function, and may cause red cell hemolysis. Mothers should be encouraged to breastfeed 10–12 times per day to correct elevated serum bilirubin levels.

Latching On: For problems with baby latching on, the trick is to have the baby open his or her mouth wide. Brush baby's lips with the nipple to encourage him or her to open wide, as if yawning. Once baby's mouth is open wide, *quickly* pull the baby onto the breast by pulling the baby toward mom with the arm that is holding him or her (not moving mom towards the baby). Baby's gums should cover an inch of the aerola behind the nipple. Be sure the baby's lips are everted and not inverted (turned in). Almost the entire areola should be in the baby's mouth.

Mastitis: Breast infection causes fever, chills, redness, flu-like symptoms, and breast sensitivity. A clogged mammary duct, maternal anemia, stress, or an infection carried from the baby may cause mastitis. The primary goal is emptying the infected breast; frequent nursing (every 1–3 hours during the day and 2–3 hours at night) is encouraged. The physician should be notified so that antibiotics or pain relievers can be prescribed. Application of heat to the breast, drinking plenty of fluids, and adequate rest are useful measures for treatment.

Nipple Confusion: Infants who are breastfeed may refuse to take a bottle as the weaning of breastfeeding occurs. Mothers should be encouraged to continue attempts at breastfeeding.

Sore Nipples: Frequent, short nursing, repositioning the infant at the breast, applying cold packs or heat to breasts, avoiding irritating soaps or lotions on nipples, air-drying nipples after nursing, exposing nipples to direct sunlight or 60-watt bulb for 15 minutes several times per day, applying vitamin E squeezed from capsules or ointment such as vitamin A and D or pure lanolin cream to nipples, and avoiding the use of nipple shields may help ease the pain. Occasionally, sore nipples are caused by *Candida albicans*; the breasts may not appear to have a fungal infection, but cultures of nipple surfaces will be positive for *Candida albicans*.

Reasons Why Women Discontinue Lactation

Hospital practices that do not support breastfeeding (Grizzard et al, 2006); physician and nurse apathy or misinformation

Acute infections in the mother (Rempel, 2004)

Mother's chronic illness (e.g., tuberculosis, severe anemia, chronic fevers, cardiovascular or renal disease) and/or use of medications (Della-Giustina and Chow, 2003)

Maternal depression (Taveras et al, 2003)

Mother's inability to provide 50% of the infant's needs

Mother's return to work by 12 weeks postpartum (Taveras et al, 2003)

Infant's inability to nurse due to weakness or oral anomalies

Lack of information and support and/or inadequate preparation

Lack of part-time jobs, flexible scheduling, and convenient day care for mothers who must work

Obesity: poor infant feeding behavior and reduced hormonal responses in the early postpartum period result in delayed lactogenesis and early cessation of breastfeeding (Lovelady, 2005; Hilson et al, 2004; Li et al, 2003).

INTERVENTION: FOOD AND NUTRITION

- In the first 6 months, increase the mother's energy by 330 kcal over RDA for age. In the next 6 months, increase energy by 400 kcal over RDA for age. Recommendations may vary because individuals vary in prepregnancy weights, activity levels, and rates of weight gain (Shabert, 2004).
- Consider the special needs of adolescents or women older than 35 years of age. Energy and nutrient requirements will change accordingly.
- Increase the mother's intake of protein (approximately 65 grams daily). Encourage intake of sources of high-quality protein.
- Encourage intake of usual sources of vitamins and minerals. Intake of calcium should be 1200–1300 mg/d. Increases of B-complex vitamins (thiamine and vitamin B_6) and of vitamins A and C should be included in the diet. Supplementation may be needed for women with poor dietary intakes or chronic illnesses.
- Adequate vitamin D will be needed if maternal intake is poor or if infant receives little sunshine exposure. Dark-skinned, breastfed infants should be given vitamin D sup-

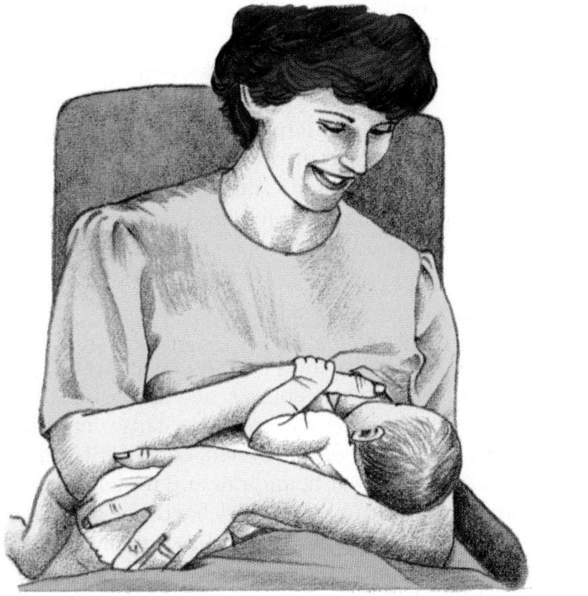

Figure 1-4 Breastfeeding mother. (Barnes ME, et al. *Nursing procedures.* 4th ed. Philadelphia: Lippincott Williams & Wilkins, 2004.)

plements to prevent nutritional rickets (Kreiter et al, 2000).
- Levels of both iron and copper decrease with progression of lactation; there is no evident need for supplementation in the first 6 months of lactation (Dorea, 2000).
- Increase intake of fluids. Omit alcohol unless permitted by physician.
- Beyond 3 months of lactation, the mother should increase her energy intake if her weight loss has been excessive.
- Women who follow vegan diets may need zinc, calcium, vitamin D, or vitamin B_{12} supplementation. These diets also may be low in carnitine.
- If tube feeding is needed using breast milk, some fat losses can occur. Formula enhancers may be added if long-term use is required.
- Breastfeeding by adolescent mothers is associated with greater bone mineral density (BMD) during young adulthood; lactation may be protective to the bone health of adolescent mothers (Chantrey et al, 2004). See Figure 1-4 for a breastfeeding mother.

CLINICAL INDICATORS

Clinical/History

- BP
- Smoking
- Height
- Current weight
- Weight history
- Prepregnancy weight
- Healthy body weight range for height
- Date of birth (DOB) for infant
- Goal for return to usual body weight
- Diet History

Lab Work

- Glucose
- Albumin (Alb) or transthyretin (if needed)
- H & H, serum Fe
- Alk phos
- Protime or INR
- Chol
- Triglycerides (Trig)
- Ca++
- Serum phosphorus

Common Drugs Used and Potential Side Effects

- Discuss the relevance of tolerable upper intake levels (ULs) from the latest dietary reference intakes of the National Academy of Sciences. These levels were set to protect individuals from receiving too much of any nutrient from diet and dietary supplements. Lactating mothers should be especially aware of what they are consuming between diet and supplements. Be careful to avoid hypervitaminosis A and D. Read supplement labels carefully.
- Alcohol, smoking, and most drugs are transmitted through breast milk to infants. Their use should be discouraged unless permitted by a physician. Cigarette smoking also reduces the amount of milk produced. Moderate amounts of caffeine are acceptable (equivalent of 2 cups of coffee is the usual recommendation).
- Cimetidine, Prozac, lithium, cyclosporine, cold medicines, and some other drugs may be contraindicated. Otherwise, the majority of prescribed medications may be used under supervision of the doctor. Drugs that may be used during breastfeeding include acetaminophen, some antibiotics and antihistamines, codeine, decongestants, insulin, quinine, ibuprofen, and thyroid medications.
- Parlodel (bromocriptine mesylate) inhibits secretion of prolactin (decreases lactation) and is used for this purpose for women who do not wish to breastfeed. Constipation or anorexia may result.

Herbs, Botanicals, and Supplements

- Herbs and botanical supplements should not be used without first discussing with the physician. In general, these supplements have not been proven to be safe for breastfeeding mothers and their infants. Fenugreek, anise, fennel, garlic, and echinacea have been suggested for breastfeeding but have not been studied in this population for side effects. Lactating women should not take kava, chasteberry, dong quai, Asian ginseng, licorice root, or saw palmetto.
- IgM-, IgA-, and IgG-secreting cells are higher in infants who are breastfed exclusively for at least for 3 months and supplemented with probiotics compared with breastfed infants receiving placebo; use of probiotics during breastfeeding may positively influence gut immunity (Rinne et al, 2005).

INTERVENTION: NUTRITION EDUCATION, COUNSELING, CARE MANAGEMENT

- Self-esteem is key. Help mom believe that she can do it! Use positive feedback, and help mom handle negative comments from others. Support can prevent early discontinuation. Self-efficacy questions may be useful during counseling (Dennis, 2003).
- Help mom address barriers, such as work-related barriers (e.g., short maternity leave, lack of private places to pump, coworker comments), health care barriers (e.g., lack of support from doctor or nurses), and old wives' tales (e.g., breastfeeding spoils the baby, restrictive diet).

- "Best practice" counseling includes one prenatal and one postpartum home contact and telephone consultation by a lactation consultant (Bonuck et al, 2005). Explain the composition of breast milk, the benefits of breastfeeding, nipple care, and what to do during illness or infection.
- Women who are at risk for delayed onset of lactation need additional support during the first week postpartum (Taveras et al, 2003). Frequent nursing should be recommended to establish the pattern.
- To be sure baby receives enough milk, mom should be nursing at least eight times in each 24-hour period. Baby should be able to rest for about 2 hours between feedings. Nursing should not take longer than 1 hour each time.
- Breastfed infants should have five wet diapers (minimally) in each 24 hours. Discuss how stools of breastfed babies differ from formula-fed infants (such as being more loose). By day 4, there should be three stools a day, yellowish in hue.
- Explain the meaning of a balanced diet. Encourage the mother to normalize weight after delivery, but while the mother is nursing, she should not be placed on a weight loss program. Other than postpartum diuresis, average loss is 0.67 kg/month.
- Guidance for lactating women should stress food sources of nutrients likely to be limited in their diets: calcium, zinc, folate, and vitamins E, D, and B_6 (Mackey et al, 1998). Lactation has been associated with some decreased bone mineral density and bone loss; careful attention is needed for adequacy of calcium and vitamin D (Grimes and Wimalawansa, 2003). Vegetarian women should be counseled about vitamin B_{12} to prevent neurological damage resulting from deficiency (Weiss et al, 2004).
- Explain the requirements of infant nutrition after weaning. Refer eligible infants to the WIC program, if available (Chatterji and Brooks-Gunn, 2004).
- Amounts of food antigens in breast milk may be controlled by modifying the maternal diet (Hill et al, 2005). Infants fed formulas of intact cow's milk or soy protein compared with breast milk have a higher incidence of atopic dermatitis and wheezing illnesses in early childhood; exclusive breastfeeding should be encouraged for at least 4–6 months (Friedman and Zeigler, 2005). Breastfeeding 4 months or longer reduces risk for eczema and onset of allergy (Kull et al, 2005).
- Infant feeding methods do not alter the rate of postpartum weight loss (but total weight gained during pregnancy does). Mothers should not attempt rapid losses during the breastfeeding period; they should try to maintain their postpartum weight during lactation. Weight loss should not be initiated until breastfeeding is discontinued, with no more than 1 lb/wk.
- With permission of the physician at a postpartum visit, moderate exercise seems to have no adverse effects on breastfeeding among healthy mothers (McCrory, 2001). Extra energy intake may be needed if vigorous exercise is pursued (Lovelady, 2004).
- Exercise alone is not always sufficient to promote the desired level of weight reduction; once lactation is established, overweight women may be able to restrict energy intake by 500 kcal to allow gradual weight loss of 0.5 kg/wk (Lovelady, 2004).
- Lactating women are at high risk of energy and nutrient inadequacies, especially in low-income communities. Strategies to ensure adequate intakes must be planned.
- Depressive symptoms in postpartum mothers should be identified and addressed (Hatton et al, 2005).
- Discuss issues related to safe handling of breast milk (see the following Food Safety recommendations).

Patient Education—Food Safety

- Avoid soft cheeses such as feta, brie, camembert, Roquefort, and Mexican soft cheese; they may have been contaminated with *Listeria,* which can cause fetal death or premature labor. If they are used, cook until boiling first.
- Avoid raw eggs, raw fish, and raw and undercooked meats because of potential viral and bacterial foodborne illnesses. *Helicobacter pylori* should be suspected as one possible cause of nausea or vomiting (Quinla and Hill, 2003). Careful hand washing is recommended.
- Nursing mothers should not eat shark, swordfish, king mackerel, and tilefish. These long-lived larger fish contain the highest levels of methyl mercury, which may harm a baby's developing nervous system. Nursing women should select a variety of other kinds of fish, such as shellfish, canned fish, smaller ocean fish, or farm-raised fish. They can safely eat 12 oz of cooked fish per week, with a typical serving size being 3–6 oz.
- After expressing milk, it should be stored in a clean, tightly enclosed container. An opaque container may help to protect riboflavin more than a clear container if there is any exposure to light.
- Human milk can be stored safely if refrigerated but not at room temperature because bacterial growth and lipolysis are rapid. Milk to be used within 48 hours can be refrigerated; if milk is to be used after 48 hours, try freezing (up to 6 months) immediately.

For More Information

- ABCs of Breastfeeding
  http://www.mymidwife.org/caring/breastfeeding.cfm
- American Academy of Pediatrics
  http://www.aap.org/
- Breastfeeding a Cleft-Lip/Palate Baby
  http://www.cleft.org/breastfeeding.htm
- Breastfeeding Basics Course
  University Hospitals of Cleveland
  http://www.breastfeedingbasics.org/
- Breastfeeding Promotion Committee
  Healthy Mothers, Healthy Babies National Coalition
  http://www.hmhb.org/
- CDC Breastfeeding topics
  http://www.cdc.gov/breastfeeding/
- Center for Breastfeeding Information
  La Leche International
  847-519-7730
  http://www.lalecheleague.org/
- Got Mom: Breastfeeding Resources
  http://www.gotmom.org/

- Human Milk Banking Association of North America
  http://www.hmbana.org/
- International Lactation Consultant Association Directory
  http://www.breastfeeding.com/directory/lcdirectory.html
- Keep Kids Healthy
  http://www.keepkidshealthy.com/breastfeeding/
- Lactation Institute and Breastfeeding Clinic
  http://www.lactationinstitute.org/
- Medline Plus
  http://www.nlm.nih.gov/medlineplus/ency/article/002452.htm
- Mother's Best
  http://www.breastfeeding.com/
- National Women's Health Information Center
  Breastfeeding
  http://www.4woman.gov/Breastfeeding/

LACTATION—CITED REFERENCES

American Academy of Pediatrics Committee on Nutrition. *Pediatric nutrition handbook.* 5th ed. Elk Grove, IL: American Academy of Pediatrics, 2004.

Anderson JG, et al. Can prenatal N-3 fatty acid deficiency be completely reversed after birth? Effects on retinal and brain biochemistry and visual function in rhesus monkeys. *Pediatr Res.* 58:865, 2005.

Anderson JW, Johnstone BM, Remley DT. Breast-feeding and cognitive development: a meta-analysis. *Am J Clin Nutr.* 70:525, 1999.

Bonuck KA, et al. Randomized, controlled trial of a prenatal and postnatal lactation consultant intervention on duration and intensity of breastfeeding up to 12 months. *Pediatrics* 116:1413, 2005.

Butte NF, et al. Nutrient adequacy of exclusive breastfeeding for the term infant during the first six months of life. Geneva, Switzerland: World Health Organization, NLM Classification WS 125, 2002.

Chantry CJ, Auinger P, Byrd RS. Lactation among adolescent mothers and subsequent bone mineral density. *Arch Pediatr Adolesc Med.* 158:650, 2004.

Chatterji P, Brooks-Gunn J. WIC participation, breastfeeding practices, and well-child care among unmarried, low-income mothers. *Am J Public Health.* 94:1324, 2004.

Della-Giustina K, Chow G. Medications in pregnancy and lactation. *Emerg Med Clin North Am.* 21:585, 2003.

Dennis CL. The breastfeeding self-efficacy scale: psychometric assessment of the short form. *J Obstet Gynecol Neonatal Nurs.* 32:734, 2003.

Department of Health and Human Services. Blueprint for action on breastfeeding. Washington, DC: U.S. Department of Health and Human Services, 2000; available at http://www.cdc.gov/breastfeeding/pdf/bluprntbk2.pdf#search='Department%20of%20Health%20and%20Human%20Services.%20Blueprint%20for%20action%20on%20breastfeeding'.

Dewey KG. Nutrition, growth and complementary feeding of the breastfed infant. *Pediatr Clin North Am.* 48:87, 2001.

Dorea JG. Iron and copper in human milk. *Nutrition* 16:209, 2000.

Friedman NJ, Zeigler RS. The role of breast-feeding in the development of allergies and asthma. *J Allergy Clin Immunol.* 115:1238, 2005.

Grimes JP, Wimalawansa SJ. Breastfeeding and postmenopausal osteoporosis. *Curr Womens Health Rep.* 3:193, 2003.

Grizzard TA, et al. Policies and practices related to breastfeeding in Massachusetts: hospital implementation of the ten steps to successful breastfeeding. *Matern Child Health J.* 10:247, 2006.

Groziak SM, Miller GD. Natural bioactive substances in milk and colostrum: effects on the arterial blood pressure system. *Br J Nutr.* 84: 119S, 2000.

Hanson LA, et al. Breast-feeding, infant formulas, and the immune system. *Ann Allergy Asthma Immunol.* 90:59S3, 2003.

Hatton DC, et al. Symptoms of postpartum depression and breastfeeding. *J Hum Lact.* 21:444, 2005.

Helland IB, et al. Maternal supplementation with very-long-chain n-3 fatty acids during pregnancy and lactation augments children's IQ at 4 years of age. *Pediatrics* 111:e39, 2003.

Hill DJ, et al. Effect of a low-allergen maternal diet on colic among breastfed infants: a randomized, controlled trial. *Pediatrics* 116:709, 2005.

Hilson JA, et al. High prepregnant body mass index is associated with poor lactation outcomes among white, rural women independent of psychosocial and demographic correlates. *J Hum Lact.* 20:18, 2004.

Innis SM. Perinatal biochemistry and physiology of long-chain polyunsaturated fatty acids. *J Pediatr.* 143:1S, 2003.

James DC, Dobson B, American Dietetic Association. Position of The American Dietetic Association: Promoting and supporting breast feeding. *J Am Diet Assoc.* 105:810, 2005.

Kac G, et al. Breastfeeding and postpartum weight retention in a cohort of Brazilian women. *Am J Clin Nutr.* 79:487, 2004.

Kreiter SR, et al. Nutritional rickets in African American breast-fed infants. *J Pediatr.* 137:153, 2000.

Krogstrand KS, Parr K. Physicians ask for more problem-solving information to promote and support breastfeeding. *J Am Diet Assoc.* 105:1943, 2005.

Kull I, et al. Breast-feeding reduces the risk for childhood eczema. *J Allergy Clin Immunol.* 116:657, 2005.

Lauer JA, et al. Breastfeeding patterns and exposure to suboptimal breastfeeding among children in developing countries: review and analysis of nationally representative surveys. *BMC Med.* 2:26, 2004.

Lauritezen L, et al. Maternal fish oil supplementation in lactation: effect on developmental outcome in breast-fed infants. *Reprod Nutr Dev.* 45:535, 2005.

Li R, et al. Maternal obesity and breastfeeding practices. *Am J Clin Nutr.* 77: 931, 2003.

Lovelady CA. Is maternal obesity a cause of poor lactation performance? *Nutr Rev.* 63:352, 2005.

Lovelady CA. The impact of energy restriction and exercise in lactating women. *Adv Exp Med Biol.* 554:115, 2004.

Lovelady CA, et al. The effect of weight loss in overweight, lactating women on the growth of their infants. *N Engl J Med.* 342:449, 2000.

Mackey A, et al. Self-selected diets of lactating women often fail to meet dietary recommendations. *J Am Diet Assoc.* 98:297, 1998.

McCrory MA. Does dieting during lactation put infant growth at risk? *Nutr Rev.* 59:18, 2001.

Min Y, et al. Unfavorable effect of type 1 and type 2 diabetes on maternal and fetal essential fatty acid status: a potential marker of fetal insulin resistance. *Am J Clin Nutr.* 82:1162, 2005.

Montagne PM, et al. Dynamics of the main immunologically and nutritionally available proteins of human milk during lactation. *J Food Comp Anal.* 13:127, 2000.

Muraro A, et al. Dietary prevention of allergic diseases in infants and small children. *Pediatr Allergy Immunol.* 15:291, 2004.

Owen CG, et al. The effect of breastfeeding on mean body mass index throughout life: a quantitative review of published and unpublished observational evidence. *Am J Clin Nutr.* 82:1298, 2005.

Quinla JD, Hill DA. Nausea and vomiting of pregnancy. *Am Fam Physician.* 68: 121, 2003.

Rempel LA. Factors influencing the breastfeeding decisions of long-term breastfeeders. *J Hum Lact.* 20:306, 2004.

Rich-Edwards JW, et al. Breastfeeding during infancy and the risk of cardiovascular disease in adulthood. *Epidemiology* 15:550, 2004.

Rinne M, et al. Effect of probiotics and breastfeeding on the bifidobacterium and *Lactobacillus/Enterococcus* microbiota and humoral immune responses. *J Pediatr.* 147:186, 2005.

Ross JS, Labbok MH. Modeling the effects of different infant feeding strategies on infant survival and mother-to-child transmission of HIV. *Am J Public Health.* 94:1174, 2004

Shabert J. Nutrition during pregnancy and lactation. In: Mahan K, Escott-Stump S, eds. *Krause's food, nutrition and diet therapy.* 11th ed. Philadelphia: WB Saunders, 2004.

Sikorski J, et al. Support for breastfeeding mothers. *Cochrane Database Syst Rev.* 1:CD001141, 2002.

Silva SM, et al. Prolonged alcohol intake leads to irreversible loss of vasopressin and oxytocin neurons in the paraventricular nucleus of the hypothalamus. *Brain Res.* 925:76, 2002.

Singhal A, et al. Early nutrition in preterm infants and later blood pressure: two cohorts after randomised trials. *Lancet* 357:413, 2001.

Taha TE, et al. Nevirapine and zidovudine at birth to reduce perinatal transmission of HIV in an African setting: a randomized controlled trial. *JAMA.* 292:202, 2004.

Taveras EM, et al. Clinician support and psychosocial risk factors associated with breastfeeding discontinuation. *Pediatrics* 112:108, 2003.

United States Department of Agriculture. USDA Nutrient Database for Standard Reference, Release 13 (November 1999). Available at http://www.nal.usda.gov/fnic/foodcomp/Data/SR13/sr13.html.

Weimer J. The economic benefits of breastfeeding: A review and analysis. ERS Food Assistance and Nutrition Research Report No. 13, March 2001.

Weinberg GA. The dilemma of postnatal mother-to-child transmission of HIV: to breastfeed or not? *Birth* 27:199, 2000.
Weiss R, Fogelman Y, Bennett M. Severe vitamin B12 deficiency in an infant associated with a maternal deficiency and a strict vegetarian diet. *J Pediatr Hematol Oncol.* 26:270, 2004.
Wright AL, et al. Factors influencing the relation of infant feeding to asthma and recurrent wheeze in childhood. *Thorax* 56:192, 2001.
Yu VY. Scientific rationale and benefits of nucleotide supplementation of infant formula. *J Paediatr Child Health.* 38:543, 2002.

INFANCY, CHILDHOOD, AND ADOLESCENCE

INFANT, NORMAL (0–6 MONTHS)

NUTRITIONAL ACUITY RANKING: LEVEL 1

DEFINITIONS AND BACKGROUND

Normal gestation is 40 weeks. The average birth weight of an infant ranges between 5.5 and 10 lb; the average is approximately 7–7.5 lb. Healthy, full-term infants lose some weight in the first days after birth but tend to regain it within approximately 1 week (Shabert, 2004). Infants often double their birth weight by 4–6 months and triple it within 1 year (Shabert, 2004). Head circumference increases about 40% during the first year, and brain weight should almost double. Infants are composed of approximately 75–80% water, whereas adults are composed of 60–65% water. Infants may become dehydrated easily, especially in hot weather or after bouts of diarrhea.

For assessment of an infant, monitoring growth is the best way to evaluate intake. See Figure 1-5 for evaluating a healthy infant.

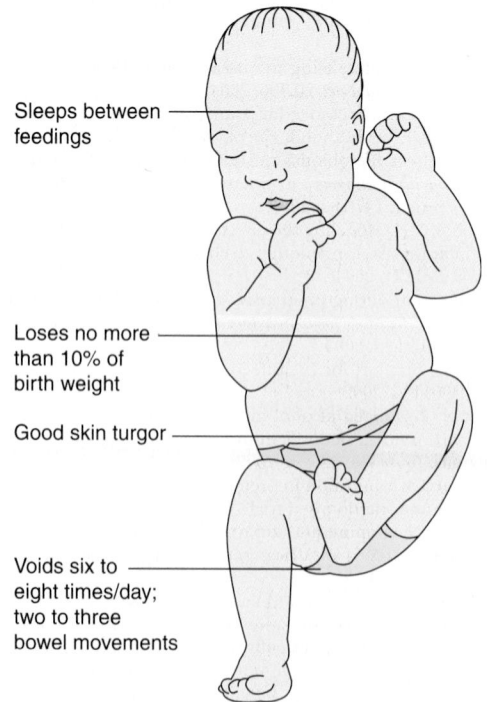

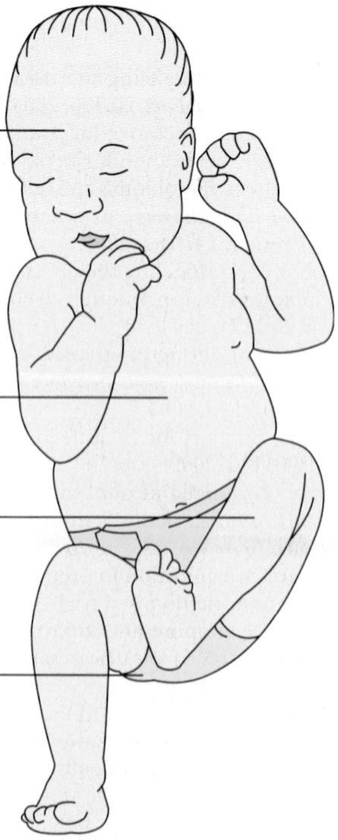
Sleeps between feedings
Loses no more than 10% of birth weight
Good skin turgor
Voids six to eight times/day; two to three bowel movements

Figure 1-5 Assessing healthy infant status. (From Pillitteri A. *Maternal and child nursing.* 4th ed. Philadelphia: Lippincott, Williams & Wilkins, 2003.)

When infants are ill, special techniques (doubly labeled water studies or test weighing) may be used for determining intakes of breast milk. Mixed feedings of formula, breast milk, and foods complicate the process in older infants, and eating patterns vary from one month to the next because appetite regulates growth.

Mineral status should be carefully assessed. Infants are born with a 4- to 6-month supply of iron if maternal stores were adequate during gestation and if the mother was not anemic during pregnancy. Correcting iron deficiency anemia may prevent developmental and behavioral delays (Algarin et al, 2003; Lozoff et al, 2003). Calcium is another important mineral during infancy. Optimizing calcium and bone status during the first year of life sets the stage for healthy bones later (Koo and Warren, 2003). Infants of vegan mothers may require zinc, calcium, and vitamin B_{12} supplementation (Weiss et al, 2004; American Dietetic Association and Dietitians of Canada, 2003). Hypoxia, nicotine exposure, and, possibly, low levels of magnesium may contribute to sudden infant death syndrome; magnesium deficiency may cause inability to lift the neck muscles from a prone position in infants who are at risk (Caddell, 2001).

A common problem in infancy is low vitamin D intake during pregnancy and lactation and the increasing risk of rickets among infants (Hollis and Wagner, 2004; Molgaard and Michelsen, 2003). Growth failure, lethargy, and irritability are early signs of deficiency (Molgaard and Michaelsen, 2003). Oversupplementation should also be avoided.

Breastfeeding takes longer than cup or bottle feeding but has the most benefits and is the preferred method. When breastfeeding is not possible or not desired, formula feeding is used. For formula feedings in infants with oral or developmental problems, administration times, amounts ingested, and physiological stability of infants are similar when newborn infants are fed using a bottle or a cup. If using a cup, use a small plastic medicine cup and stroke the lower lip to stimulate rooting (Howard et al, 1999). Section 3 describes conditions where alternative feeding methods may be needed.

The Committee on Nutrition of the American Academy of Pediatrics supports the following practices during infancy (American Academy of Pediatrics, 1998):

- Exclusively breastfeed for the first 6 months. Supplement with vitamin D from birth and use iron supplementation as ferrous sulfate drops or iron-fortified cereal after 4 months of age. Fluoride supplementation may be required after 6 months of age depending on the fluoride content of the city water. Feeding of iron-fortified commercial infant formula may be done for the first year as an alternative to breastfeeding.

- Delay the use of whole cow milk until after 1 year of age. Early introduction of whole cow milk protein during infancy may contribute to iron deficiency anemia by increasing gastrointestinal blood loss. Whole cow milk has an increased renal solute load compared to infant formulas.
- Reduced-fat milks should be delayed until after the second year of life. Adequate fat intake is important for the developing brain, and milk is usually the primary source of fat for infants and toddlers.
- Delay the introduction of semisolid foods until 4–6 months of age or until the infant demonstrates signs of developmental readiness, such as head control and ability to sit with support.

INTERVENTION: OBJECTIVES

- Promote normal growth and development: assess sleeping, eating, and attentiveness habits. Compare infant's growth to the chart of normal growth patterns. Weight for length (height) is the most meaningful measurement. Use updated Centers for Disease Control (CDC) growth charts and monitor growth trends, not a singular value. Malnutrition results in decreased weight, then height, and then head circumference (if chronic).
- Overcome any nutritional risk factors or complications, such as otitis media or dehydration.
- Evaluate use and discourage early introduction of solids and cow's milk.
- Encourage the mother to use breast milk as the infant's main source of nutrition for the first 6 months, introducing solids and juices slowly beginning at approximately 4 months of age.
- If the infant is breastfed, assess the mother's prepregnancy nutritional status and risk factors, weight gain pattern, food allergies, and medical history (such as preeclampsia, chronic illnesses, or anemia). Discuss any current conditions that may affect lactation (e.g., smoking, use of alcohol, family history of allergies).
- If the infant is formula fed, the mother should learn about early childhood caries (ECC) prevention and about potential overfeeding problems. Overnutrition is associated with subsequent fatness (Martorelli et al., 2001).
- Promote growth and development through adequate fatty acid intake, especially for visual acuity—linoleic acid n-6 and linolenic n-3 (Hoffman et al, 2004).
- Effects of soy formulas on the thyroid must be monitored in infants with hypothyroidism. Iodine has been added to most infant formulas; check labels.

INTERVENTION: FOOD AND NUTRITION

- Fluid requirements may include the following: 60–80 mL/kg water in newborns; 80–100 mL/kg by 3 days of age; 125–150 mL/kg up to 6 months of age. Assess individual needs according to status.
- Energy needs are estimated to decrease between birth and 6 months; this can be met in about 28–32 oz of human milk or infant formula.
- Protein requirement is generally 1.52 g/kg, or about 9.1 g/d. Sick infants may need a higher ratio. Usen the nutrient recommendation chart (see below).

Nutrient	**Recommendation for Infants Ages 0–6 Months**
Energy	570 kcal/d males; 520 kcal/d females
Protein	9.1 g/d or 1.52 g/kg/d
Calcium	210 mg/d
Iron	0.27 mg/d
Folate	65 mg/d
Phosphorus	100 mg/d
Vitamin A	400 μg
Vitamin C	40 mg
Thiamin	0.2 mg/d
Riboflavin	0.3 mg/d
Niacin	2 mg/d

Data from: Food and Nutrition Board, Institute of Medicine. *Dietary reference intakes for energy, carbohydrate, fiber, fat, fatty acids, cholesterol, protein, and amino acids (macronutrients)*. Washington, DC: National Academy Press, 2002.

- If infant is breastfed, discourage the mother from using drugs and alcohol; keep caffeine intake limited to the equivalent of 2 cups of coffee per day. Teach parents about use of diluted fruit juice (perhaps apple) at 4 months of age. Breastfed infants may require vitamin D, fluoride, and sometimes iron supplements (at about 3 months of age). Mothers of infants predisposed to allergies should avoid fish, cow's milk, and nuts. Do not introduce cow's milk before 12 months of age.
- Formula-fed infants: type of formula—milk-based, soy, etc. Check list of significant ingredients and amount used for 24 hours. No calorie-containing formula should be given in the crib, only water. Sweetened beverages should not be used between meals or at bedtime. Be careful in warming bottles because folic acid and vitamin C may be destroyed. Iron-fortified formula is often used after 2–3 months (American Academy of Pediatrics, 1999).
- The inhibitory effect of calcium and phosphorus on iron absorption is not clinically important in infants fed iron-fortified formulas (Dalton et al., 1997). No fluoride supplement is needed unless the water supply provides less than 0.3 ppm. Discourage use of evaporated milk formula, which is low in vitamin C and high in protein, sodium, and potassium; it is not for use with infants.
- Standard formulas have a 60:40 whey to casein ratio, which is desirable in a formula; they provide 20 kcal/oz. Breast milk yields an 80:20 whey to casein ratio and approximately the same calories. Standard formulas include Enfamil, Similac, Gerber Formula, Good Start, and others.
- Special formulas are available for special needs, such as ProSobee, Carnation Alsoy, or Isomil for cow's milk allergies; soy formulas are fortified with zinc and iron. Alimentum, Portagen, or Pregestimil are available for malabsorption and inclusion of medium-chain triglycerides

(MCT); Nutramigen, Alimentum, or Pregestimil are available for other complex gastrointestinal (GI) problems. Nutramigen may also be used for allergies to both soy and cow's milk protein. Contact nutritional formula companies for updated information.
- Soy formulas now include carnitine, which generally is available in breast milk.
- At 4–6 months, introduce plain (not mixed, sweetened, or spiced) strained or pureed baby cereals, then nonallergenic vegetables (such as carrots or green beans), and then fruits. Start with 1–2 teaspoons, and progress as appetite indicates. Try a single new item for 7–10 days to detect any signs of food allergy. The intake of solids should not decrease breast milk or formula intake to less than 32 oz daily. Avoid giving too much juice; 4–6 oz daily is sufficient (Marshall et al, 2003; Dewey, 2001).
- Ensure that the daily requirements are being met for all other nutrients for each stage of growth. Vitamin D fortification in milk may be unpredictable, for example, and signs of any problem should be noted. When in doubt, a multivitamin-mineral supplement is advisable (Dewey, 2001).
- For tube-fed infants, PediaSure, Kindercal, Nutren Junior, and Resource Just for Kids are specifically for pediatrics. If an elemental diet is needed for severe protein intolerance or cow's milk allergy, Pediatric Vivonex, Neocate One Plus, and Elecare may be useful. Monitor carefully for hydration; don't modify nutrients because of changing osmolality. Breast milk has an osmolality of 285 mOsm/kg; formulas vary from 150–380 mOsm/kg. Formulas with over 400 mOsm/kg can cause diarrhea or vomiting. Formula should contain 10–20% protein, 30–40% fat, and 40–60% carbohydrates. Fat should not be excessive so that the infant does not experience ketosis.
- Minimal enteral feeding (MEF) favors secretion of gastrointestinal hormones in sick premature infants. Early MEF seems to be preferable to late feeding since it protects against necrotizing entercolitis and other infections (Berseth et al, 2003; Clark et al, 2003). See Low Birth Weight entry in Section 3.
- For special conditions, TPN may be used. Inclusion of 1–2% essential fatty acids (EFAs) may be necessary to prevent signs of deficiency, such as inadequate wound healing, growth, immunocompetence, and platelet formation. Linoleic and linolenic acids are required.

CLINICAL INDICATORS

Clinical/History		Lab Work
Birth weight Birth length Present weight for gestational age	BP Head circumference Diet/intake history	H & H Other lab work as needed

Herbs, Botanicals, and Supplements

- Infants and children may be even more susceptible to some of the adverse effects and toxicity of these products because of differences in physiology, immature metabolic enzyme systems, and dose per body weight (Tomassoni and Simone, 2001). Herbs and botanical supplements should not be used without discussing with the physician. In general, these types of supplements have not been proven to be safe for infants (Gardiner and Kemper, 2000).
- Most topical preparations are benign; however, garlic poultices can cause burns. Internal use of herbs containing saturated pyrrolizidine alkaloids (comfrey) should be avoided.
- Discuss the relevance of tolerable upper intake levels (ULs) from the latest dietary reference intakes of the National Academy of Sciences. These levels were set to protect adults from receiving too much of any nutrient from diet and dietary supplements; infants are especially at risk for toxicities.

INTERVENTION: NUTRITION EDUCATION, COUNSELING, CARE MANAGEMENT

- Explain the proper timing and sequence of feeding. Discuss successful feeding as trusting and responding to cues from the infant about timing, pace, and eating capacity.
- Explain growth patterns (e.g., an infant who is 4–6 months of age should double his or her birth weight). Discuss problems related to inadequate growth (e.g., for children with atopic dermatitis, the method of feeding does not seem to affect growth rate; other factors may be involved by ages 6–12 months) (Agostoni et al, 2000).
- Emphasize the importance of adequate bonding with mother and child.
- Explain the proper care of infant's teeth, including risks of early childhood caries (ECC). Ad lib nocturnal feeding should be discontinued after the first teeth erupt. Bottle-fed infants should not be put to sleep with the bottle.
- Explain the proper timing and sequence of solid food introduction. Avoid use of stringy foods or foods like peanut butter that are hard to swallow. Hard candies, grapes, and similar foods may increase the risk of aspiration.
- Discuss the rationale for delaying introduction of cow's milk (risks for allergy, gastrointestinal bleeding).
- Discuss why fluid intake is essential, and explain that infant needs are much greater than adult needs, as compared with total body weight.
- If the infant is breastfed, discuss the normalcy of 4–6 soft stools each day. Compare the normal stool with symptoms of diarrhea.
- Infants who use pacifiers and sleep on their backs may be more protected against sudden infant death syndrome.
- For special feeding problems, see Table 1-6.

Patient Education—Food Safety

- Hand washing with soap and hot water is recommended before breastfeeding or before formula preparation. Use clean utensils and containers for mixing formula. Wash the top of the can before opening.
- Before using tap water for formula preparation or to give as a beverage, let cold tap water run for 2 minutes to remove any lead that may be in the pipes.

TABLE 1-6 Special Problems in Infant Feeding[a]

Spitting Up or Reflux. If there is no weight loss concern, just offer encouragement that the problem will resolve in a few months. Positioning is an important consideration during feeding. Feed more slowly and burp often. Use feeding volumes and a schedule that is set. Avoid exposure to second-hand smoke. Offer parental reassurance.

Regurgitation. Position the infant in an upright, 40–60° position after feeding for approximately 30 minutes; have the doctor rule out other problems. Use smaller, more frequent feedings to avoid overfeeding. Thickening of formula with a small amount of cereal has been recommended; now there are prethickened formulas available if the doctor thinks it is necessary.

Diarrhea. Replace fluids and electrolytes (for example, Pedialyte) as directed by the doctor. After an extended period of time, have the doctor rule out allergy. Monitor weight loss and fluid intake carefully. The FDA has approved a vaccine (RotaTeq) aimed at preventing rotavirus, which causes severe diarrhea and fever and dehydration in infants and results in many hospitalizations each year (Glass and Parashar, 2006).

Pale, oily stools. Check for fat malabsorption. Use an MCT-containing formula if necessary.

Constipation. The doctor will make a careful assessment and may suggest adding 1 t of a carbohydrate source to 4 oz of water or formula, one to two times daily. Avoid use of honey and corn syrup to prevent infant botulism.

Colic. Check for hunger, food allergy, incorrect formula temperature, stress, or other underlying problems. Give small, frequent feedings and parental encouragement. Colic is equally common in breastfed or formula-fed infants. If breastfed, continue to breastfeed. Rarely, removal of cow's milk products from the mother's diet is useful. If formula fed, expensive elemental formulas should be discontinued if symptoms do not improve. Curved bottles allow infants to be fed while they are held upright. Collapsable bags decrease swallowing of air. Infants should be burped regularly during feedings.

Allergy. Primary prevention through a hypoallergenic diet may reduce the prevalence of food allergy, eczema, and urticaria (Halken, 2004). Breastfeeding should be recommended for all children. Introduce new foods at the appropriate age and singly; try for at least 7 days before introducing any new foods. Discuss any symptoms with the doctor immediately. Avoid cow's milk strictly, and delay introduction of egg, nuts, wheat, and fish (Arshad, 2001).

[a]See also: American Dietetic Association references including *Pediatric Manual of Clinical Dietetics* and *Children with Special Health Care Needs: NutritionCare Handbook*.

- Well water should not be used since it may contain bacteria.
- Follow the 2-hour rule: discard any formula that has been left at room temperature for 2 hours or longer. Do not reuse.
- Do not use honey in the diets of infants to decrease potential exposure to botulism.
- Avoid using raw or partially cooked eggs, raw or undercooked fish or shellfish, and raw or undercooked meats because of potential foodborne illnesses.
- Avoid using raw (unpasteurized) milk or products made from it.
- Avoid using unpasteurized juices and raw sprouts.

For More Information

- American Academy of Pediatrics
  http://www.aap.org/
- American Academy of Pediatrics Breastfeeding Advocacy
  http://www.aap.org/advocacy/bf/aapbrres.htm
- Bright Futures–Babies
  http://www.nal.usda.gov/wicworks/Learning_Center/BF_babies.pdf
- Clinical Practice Guidelines (constipation, gastroenteritis, etc.)
  http://www.aap.org/policy/paramtoc.html
- Feeding Kids Newsletter
  http://www.nutritionforkids.com/Feeding_Kids.htm
- Growth Charts
  http://www.cdc.gov/growthcharts
- Infant Nutrition
  http://www.nal.usda.gov/fnic/etext/000106.html
- Kids Health
  http://www.kidshealth.org/
- Mead Johnson (products for infants)
  http://meadjohnson.com/products_store.html
- Nestle
  http://www.verybestbaby.com/
- National Perinatal Association
  http://www.nationalperinatal.org/
- Pediatric Nutrition Practice Group
  http://www.pediatricnutrition.org/
- Ross Laboratories (products for infants)
  http://rosslabs.com
- Sudden Infant Death Syndrome
  SIDS Hotline: 800-221-SIDS
  http://www.sidscenter.org/
  http://www.nichd.nih.gov/publications/pubs/sidsfact.htm
  http://www.nichd.nih.gov/womenshealth/sids_research.cfm
- USDA/ARS Children's Nutrition Research Center
  1100 Bates Street, Houston, TX 77030; Phone: 713-798-7971
  http://www.bcm.tmc.edu/cnrc/
- WIC Topics A-Z
  http://www.nal.usda.gov/wicworks/Topics/Infant_Nutrition.html
- World Health Organization
  http://www.who.int/child-adolescent-health/NUTRITION/infant.htm

Manufacturers

- Beech Nut
  800-523-6633
  http://www.babycenter.com/solidfoods/product.jhtml
- Gerber
  800-4-gerber
  http://www.gerber.com/
- Heinz
  800-USA-BABY
  http://www.heinzbaby.com/

INFANT, NORMAL (0–6 MONTHS)—CITED REFERENCES

Agostoni C, et al. Growth pattern of breastfed and nonbreastfed infants with atopic dermatitis in the first year of life. *Pediatrics* 106:73E, 2000.

Algarin C, et al. Iron deficiency anemia in infancy: long-lasting effects on auditory and visual system functioning. *Pediatr Res.* 53:217, 2003.
American Academy of Pediatrics Committee on Nutrition. Iron fortification of infant formulas. *Pediatrics* 104:119, 1999.
American Academy of Pediatrics Committee on Nutrition. Soy protein-based formulas: recommendations for use in infant feeding. *Pediatrics* 101:148, 1998.
American Dietetic Association and Dietitians of Canada. Position of the American Dietetic Association and Dietitians of Canada: vegetarian diets. *J Am Diet Assoc.* 103:748, 2003.
Arshad SH. Food allergen avoidance in primary prevention of food allergy. *Allergy* 67:113S, 2001.
Berseth CL, et al. Prolonging small feeding volumes early in life decreases the incidence of necrotizing enterocolitis in very low birth weight infants. *Pediatrics* 111:529, 2003.
Caddell JL. Magnesium deficiency promotes muscle weakness, contributing to the risk of sudden infant death (SIDS) in infants sleeping prone. *Magnes Res* 14:39, 2001.
Clark RH, et al. Nutrition in the neonatal intensive care unit: how do we reduce the incidence of extrauterine growth restriction? *J Perinatol.* 23:337, 2003.
Dalton M, et al. Calcium and phosphorus supplementation of iron-fortified infant formula. *J Am Diet Assoc.* 97:921, 1997.
Dewey KG. Nutrition, growth and complementary feeding of the breastfed infant. *Pediatr Clin North Am.* 48:87, 2001.
Gardiner P, Kemper KJ. Herbs in pediatric and adolescent medicine. *Pediatr Rev.* 21:44, 2000.
Glass RI, Parashar UD. The promise of new rotavirus vaccines. *N Engl J Med.* 354:75, 2006.
Halken S. Prevention of allergic disease in childhood: clinical and epidemiological aspects of primary and secondary allergy prevention. *Pediatr Allergy Immunol.* 16:4S, 2004.
Hoffman DR, et al. Maturation of visual acuity is accelerated in breast-fed term infants fed baby food containing DHA-enriched egg yolk. *J Nutr.* 134:2307, 2004.
Hollis BW, Wagner CL. Assessment of dietary vitamin D requirements during pregnancy and lactation. *Am J Clin Nutr.* 79:717, 2004.
Howard CR, et al. Physiologic stability of newborns during cup and bottle-feeding. *Pediatrics* 104:1204, 1999.
Koo WW, Warren L. Calcium and bone health in infants. *Neonatal Netw.* 22:23, 2003.
Lozoff B, et al. Behavioral and developmental effects of preventing iron-deficiency anemia in healthy full-term infants. *Pediatrics* 112:846, 2003.
Marshall TA, et al. Dental caries and beverage consumption in young children. *Pediatrics* 112:e184, 2003.
Martorelli R, et al. Early nutrition and later adiposity. *J Nutr.* 131:874S, 2001.
Molgaard C, Michaelsen KF. Vitamin D and bone health in early life. *Proc Nutr Soc.* 62:823, 2003.
Shabert J. Nutrition during pregnancy and lactation. In: Mahan K, Escott-Stump S, eds. *Krause's food, nutrition and diet therapy.* 11th ed. Philadelphia: WB Saunders, 2004.
Tomassoni AJ, Simone K. Herbal medicines for children: an illusion of safety? *Curr Opin Pediatr.* 13:162, 2001.
Weiss R, et al. Severe vitamin B12 deficiency in an infant associated with a maternal deficiency and a strict vegetarian diet. *J Pediatr Hematol Oncol.* 26:270, 2004.

INFANT, NORMAL (6–12 MONTHS)

NUTRITIONAL ACUITY RANKING: LEVEL 1–2

DEFINITIONS AND BACKGROUND

Infants older than 6 months of age are beginning the developmental stages that will lead to walking and talking. Many of the same principles associated with infant feeding during the first 6 months will continue with the greater use of solids. The growth pattern of breastfed and formula-fed infants differs in the first 12 months of life. The new CDC growth charts were developed with a larger proportion of breastfed infants. Growth indices in breastfed groups, which are high at birth and closer than expected to the reference at 12 months, may reflect differences in genetic factors, intrauterine conditions, or both (Agostoni et al, 2000). Overall, infant feeding mode (i.e., breastfeeding or formula) is associated with differences in body composition in early infancy that do not persist into the second year of life (Butte et al, 2000).

Timing of the introduction of complementary foods (solids) is an important consideration. The Feeding Infants and Toddlers Study (FITS) evaluated the introduction of complementary foods into the diets of young children, and the findings show that health care professionals play an important role in improving feeding practices (Stang, 2006).

Early introduction is considered to be at 3–4 months of age, and late introduction is considered to be at 6 months of age. A study that monitored the effect of introduction of complementary foods on iron and zinc status among formula-fed infants at 12, 24, and 36 months of age found that overall iron and zinc status were not influenced by timing of the introduction of complementary foods (Kattelmann et al, 2001). Many foods that are introduced are of low nutritional value, including sweetened beverages, cookies, processed meats, cakes, and pies (Stang, 2006).

Introduction of cow's milk at 12 months of age brings new problems and risks related to essential fatty acid deficiency if low-fat or skim milks are used. It seems that long-chain fatty acids are useful in normal growth and development of infants and young children. It is not necessary to alter the diets of young children to prevent heart disease, lower cholesterol, etc.

Studies support inclusion of fatty acids in the diets of infants (Helland et al, 2003; Koo, 2003). Breastfed and formula-fed infants maintain a characteristic serum cholesterol ester fatty acid pattern after age 7 months even after they begin to receive solid food; the breastfed infants have higher levels of arachidonic acid and docosahexaenoic acid and tend to have better cognitive development (Daniels et al, 2004).

Growth and development at this stage are affected by underlying or acute illnesses, nutritional intake, and related factors. In children with severe atopic dermatitis, for example, a progressive impairment in growth occurs regardless of the early type of feeding (Agostoni et al, 2000). Breast-fed infants have a strong prevalence of bifidobacteria and lactobacilli, which stimulate formation of oligosaccharides that have a prebiotic effect that can be protective for the immune system (Coppa et al, 2004).

Lead poisoning should be monitored in growing children, especially children who live in older homes or spend time in older buildings where there are day care centers. Tod-

TABLE 1-7 Staging of Infant Feeding

Age and Stage	Skills	Serve
Birth through 4 months	Babies can only suck and swallow. Tongue thrust reflex. Poor control of head, neck, and trunk.	**Liquids only:** Breast milk or iron-fortified formula
4 months through 6 months	May enjoy new tastes. Babies draw in lower lip as spoon is removed from mouth. Sitting with support. Swallowing spoonful of pureed or strained foods without choking. Position control for food in mouth. Mouth opens when food is seen.	**Add strained foods:** Infant (rice) cereal with iron; cooked, pureed, or strained potato, squash, green beans, sweet potato; cooked, pureed, or strained peaches, applesauce, or pears; pureed bananas
5 months through 9 months	Babies mimic up and down munching movement. Sitting alone begins (6–7 months). Pincer grasp at 8–9 months.	**Add semisolid foods:** Mashed or diced fruit, such as bananas; mashed or soft-cooked vegetables such as broccoli, peas, cauliflower, and potatoes; cooked and strained meat, poultry, and boneless fish; dried beans and lentils; egg yolk; tofu
8 months through 11 months	Babies move tongue side to side. Begin spoon feeding self with help. Begin chewing and some teeth. Begin holding food and using fingers to feed self. Drink from a cup with help.	**Add modified table foods:** Mashed cooked egg yolk; finger foods such as soft cheese cubes, sliced bread, pears, peaches, kiwi, plums, melons, soft-cooked vegetables, toast, crackers, cooked pasta, cereal; juice in a cup; mashed beans and lentils
10 months through 12 months	Babies use rotary chewing (grinding). Begin to put spoon in mouth. Begin to hold cup. Reaches for food. Encourage self-feeding.	**Add table food:** Chopped food and small pieces of soft, cooked table foods

Adapted from: University of Maine, Extension Program, http://www.umext.maine.edu/onlinepubs/PDFpubs/4061.pdf.

dlers may eat lead-based paint that is chipping away from walls. Lead depletes iron and replaces calcium in the bone; deposition may be seen in x-rays of the knee, ankle, or wrist.

Sodium and chloride intakes may be higher than desirable in infants and toddlers; delaying the introduction of cows' milk, limiting the amount of salt used in food processing and preparation, and increasing intake of fruits and vegetables are reasonable measures that can be applied (Heird et al, 2006). Overall, the design of interventions for improving the diets of young children should focus on breastfeeding and the whole continuum of childhood diets in order to promote healthy guidelines (Couch and Falciglia, 2006).

INTERVENTION: OBJECTIVES

- Continue to promote normal growth and development during this second stage of very rapid growth. Use updated CDC growth charts. Monitor trends in growth, not a singular value.
- Prevent significant weight losses from illness or inadequate feeding. Malnutrition results in decreased weight, then height, and then head circumference.
- Avoid dehydration.
- Prevent or correct such complications as diarrhea, constipation, and otitis media. Otitis media is more common in bottle-fed infants (Brown and Magnuson, 2000).
- Introduce new solids, at appropriate periods of time, singly. Support feeding skills development; see Table 1-7 for tips.
- Begin to encourage greater physical activity; prepare for walking by ensuring adequate energy intake.
- Continue to emphasize the role of good nutrition in the development of healthy teeth.
- Delay allergenic foods until 12 months of age (e.g., citrus, egg white, cow's milk, corn). Be wary of peanut and nut butters because they can be highly allergenic.
- Use of follow-up formulas with higher percentage of kilocalories from protein and carbohydrates (CHO) and less from fat have questionable benefits at this time.
- Prevent nutrient deficiencies upon weaning (e.g., zinc, iron). Iron supplementation, even during breastfeeding, may be beneficial for healthy development (Friel et al, 2003).

INTERVENTION: FOOD AND NUTRITION

The following guidelines are from Start Healthy Feeding Guidelines for Infants and Toddlers (Butte et al, 2004; http://www.bcm.edu/cnrc/consumer/nyc/vol_2004_3/guidelines_ADA.pdf).

- Repeated exposure to a particular food is usually necessary before it is accepted by the infant or toddler. Studies show that up to 10–15 exposures may be necessary before a specific food is accepted. Introduction of a variety of flavors in the first 2 years of life may lead to acceptance of a wider variety of flavors in later childhood and may increase the likelihood of children trying new foods.
- After 6 months, most breastfed infants need complementary foods to meet current recommendations (DRI) for energy, manganese, iron, fluoride, vitamin D, vitamin B_6, niacin, zinc, vitamin E, magnesium, phosphorus, biotin, and thiamin. Amounts of energy and nutrients needed from complementary foods will vary depending upon the intake of human milk or formula. Although iron-fortified infant formula provides the recommended intakes of energy and nutrients until about 1 year of age depending on intake, all infants need complementary foods for exposure to flavors and textures as well as to master eating skills.
- Provision of complementary foods such as meats and fortified cereals contribute significant amounts of iron; this is helpful in preventing deficiency, which is common in toddlers under the age of 2 years.
- Because rickets due to vitamin D deficiency has been observed recently in dark-skinned, breastfed infants and other infants without adequate sun exposure, 200 IU of vitamin D is recommended as a supplement for breastfed infants and infants receiving less than 500 mL of formula per day. Intakes of the essential fatty acids may require emphasis once breast milk or formula is replaced with cow's milk.
- The introduction of the major food allergens, such as eggs, milk, wheat, soy, peanuts, tree nuts, fish, and shellfish, should be delayed until well after the first year of life. Those foods that are associated with lifelong sensitization (e.g., peanuts, tree nuts, and shellfish) should not be introduced until even later years.
- While there is no evidence that physical activity in infants or toddlers is related to activity or health in later years, age-appropriate, daily physical activity in a safe, nurturing environment may help promote physical development and movement skills and teach the healthy habit of activity. Encourage parents and caregivers to promote enjoyment of movement and motor skill confidence at an early age. Motor skills, like cognitive skills, flourish when the infant is exposed to a stimulating environment. Early childhood is a key period for promoting physical activity because during this time, fundamental motor skills (e.g., walking, running, jumping, etc.) begin to develop. When activity is encouraged, these skills can further develop into advanced patterns of motor coordination. Television viewing should be discouraged for children under 2 years of age.
- Hungry toddlers may point at foods or beverages, ask for foods or beverages, or reach for foods. Full toddlers may slow the pace of eating, become distracted or notice surroundings more, play with food, throw food, want to leave the table or chair, and/or not eat everything on the plate. To help avoid underfeeding or overfeeding, parents and caregivers must be sensitive to the hunger and satiety cues of the healthy infant and young child.
- There is no evidence for a benefit to introducing complementary foods in any specific sequence or at any specific rate. However, it is generally recommended that the first solid foods be single-ingredient foods and that they be started one at a time at 2- to 7-day intervals. The order of introduction of complementary foods is not critical, except for providing nutrients required from complementary foods. Meat and fortified infant cereals provide many of these nutrients. Combination foods (instead of single-ingredient foods) may be given to older infants after tolerance for the individual components has been established.
- Children often eat small frequent meals and snacks throughout the day, customarily three regular meals and two to three appropriate, healthy snacks. Portions should provide essential nutrients but not exceed energy requirements for the child.
- Studies show that occasional picky eating is not associated with changes in nutrient intake or height and weight. Consuming a single food or foods for extended periods of time is called a food jag. The health consequences of persistent picky eating or food jags on nutritional status or growth are not known. Occasional picky eating can be a normal stage of development. Provide multiple and varied options of new and familiar foods, and allow the toddler to choose. Offer foods again and again to enhance acceptance. If a particular food is rejected, move on and try it again later; avoid forcing toddlers to eat or finish foods. Monitor growth more frequently if a food jag persists for a long time.

Other Guidelines

For energy needs, the current DRI recommends about 743 kcal/d for males and 676 kcal/d for females. Monitor according to the CDC growth charts, and identify problems early.

Nutrient	Recommendation for Infants Ages 6 Months to 1 Year
Energy	743 kcal/d males; 676 kcal/d females
Protein	13.5 g/d
Calcium	270 mg/d
Iron	11 mg/d
Folate	80 mg/d
Phosphorus	275 mg/d
Vitamin A	500 μg
Vitamin C	50 mg/d
Thiamin	0.3 mg/d
Riboflavin	0.4 mg/d
Niacin	4 mg/d

Data from: Food and Nutrition Board, Institute of Medicine. *Dietary reference intakes for energy, carbohydrate, fiber, fat, fatty acids, cholesterol, protein, and amino acids (macronutrients)*. Washington, DC: National Academy Press, 2002.

- Fluid requirements may include approximately 125–150 mL/kg up to 1 year old. Fluid needs may decline slightly during this stage.
- Continue to provide breast milk or iron-fortified formula during this stage. The presence of docosahexaenoic acid (DHA) and arachidonic acid (ARA) in human milk but not in infant formula, along with lower plasma and brain

lipid contents of DHA in formula-fed compared with breastfed infants and reports of higher IQ in individuals who were breastfed versus formula fed as infants, suggest that exogenous DHA and ARA may be essential for optimal development (Heird and Lapillone, 2005).

- Avoid use of excessively sweetened beverages. The use of special milk substitutes is not necessary unless there is an allergy to soy protein or cow's milk.
- Protein requirement for an infant 6 months old is generally 1.5 g/kg and changes as the infant grows. This equals about 13.5 g/d. By 12 months, the need is only 1.1 g/kg. See nutrient recommendations chart.
- Introduce more solids (Table 1-7 provides a guideline). Toddler or junior foods may be used, but selection of those items that are single foods rather than mixed dishes may be more appropriate (for example, some mixed dishes are primarily starch and not meat). Read labels carefully. Figure 1-6 shows a toddler who is able to hold her own sippy cup that contains fruit juice.
- Avoid raw vegetables and fruits (other than ripe banana or soft peeled apple). Beware of foods that may cause choking (e.g., hot dogs, popcorn, nuts, grapes, seeds) because toddlers do not have molars for proper chewing (Morley et al, 2004).
- As tolerated, introduce coarsely ground table foods by 10–12 months of age.
- Introduce cow's milk at 12 months of age, ensuring that intake does not go above 1 quart daily to prevent anemia. Use whole milk to include sufficient access to fatty acids.
- Whole egg may be offered at 12 months of age, using caution because of potential allergy to the egg whites.
- Begin to offer fluids by cup at approximately 9–12 months of age; weaning often occurs by about 1 year of age. Avoid sweetened beverages at this age whenever possible.
- Spicy foods often are not liked or not tolerated. Taste buds are very acute at this stage. This is also affected by culture and the seasoning of foods that are introduced.
- Continue use of iron-fortified baby cereal after 12 months of age to ensure adequate intake (Briefel et al, 2004).
- Adult cereals often are inappropriate for infants and children younger than 4 years of age. Approximately 10 mg of iron is required. WIC-approved cereals are iron fortified.

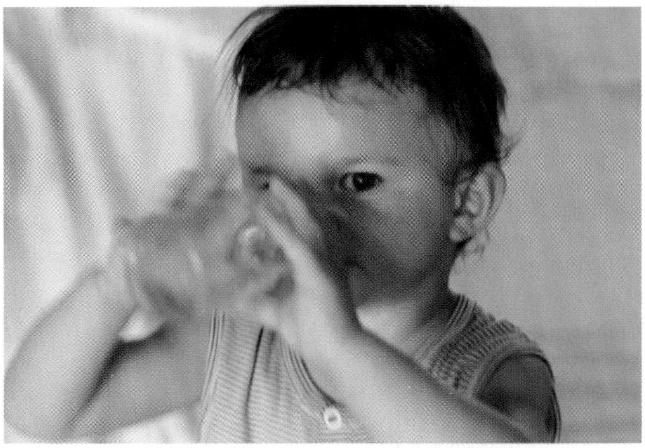

Figure 1-6 Toddler drinking from a sippy cup.

- Discourage use of low-density foods that are relatively high in energy, such as carbonated beverages, French fries, candy, and other sweets (Briefel et al, 2004).
- Generally, healthy infants and toddlers can achieve recommended levels of intake from food alone; encourage caregivers to use foods rather than supplements as the primary source of nutrients in children's diets (Briefel et al, 2006).
- Vitamin and mineral supplements can help infants and toddlers with special nutrient needs or marginal intakes achieve adequate intakes; avoid excessive intakes of vitamin A, zinc, and folate, which are commonly fortified in the food supply (Briefel et al, 2006).
- Children who require tube feeding require specialty care. If the infant needs a tube feeding (e.g., for poor weight gain, low volitional intake, 5th percentile or lower for weight for height and age, slow and prolonged feeding times over 4–6 hours because of oral/motor problems), a standard isotonic tube feeding formula that provides 30 kcal/oz of intact proteins may be used. If necessary, lactose-free and gluten-free formulas are available. Added fiber and a mix of long-chain and medium-chain fatty acids may be useful. Osmolality of 260–650 mOsm/kg is common; monitor tolerances regularly. Be sure to use sufficient water. The infant may tolerate bolus feedings in the day and continuous feedings at night.

CLINICAL INDICATORS

Clinical/History

Length
Current weight
Birth length/weight
Percentile weight/length
Diet/intake history
Age in months
Head circumference
Developmental stage
Hydration status
Tooth development
Physical handicaps
Appetite
Intake and output (I & O)
Persistent vomiting
Diarrhea

Lab Work

Glucose
Serum Fe or H & H (if needed)
Alb (if needed)

Herbs, Botanicals, and Supplements

- Infants and children may be even more susceptible to some of the adverse effects and toxicity of these products because of differences in physiology, immature metabolic enzyme systems, and dose per body weight (Tomassoni and Simone, 2001). Herbs and botanical supplements should not be used without discussing with the physician. In general, these types of supplements have not been proven to be safe for infants (Gardiner and Kemper, 2000).
- Discuss the relevance of tolerable upper intake levels (ULs) from the latest dietary reference intakes of the National Academy of Sciences. These levels were set to protect adults from receiving too much of any nutrient from diet and dietary supplements; infants are even more at risk for toxicities.

INTERVENTION: NUTRITION EDUCATION, COUNSELING, CARE MANAGEMENT

- Early childhood is a critical time for development of appropriate food choices and eating habits, which are complex processes for parents to understand (Stang, 2006).
- Discuss adequate weight pattern: infants generally double or triple birth weight by 12 months of age; body length increases by about 55%; head circumference increases by about 40%; and brain weight doubles.
- Discuss the healthy guidelines that are available (Butte et al, 2004; Pac et al, 2004).
- For lunches at home, parents will need suggestions about appropriate and easy to serve foods, homemade or commercial, for toddler lunches and snacks (Ziegler et al, 2006).
- Special attention and counseling tips should be given to assist mothers who have less than a college education, who are unmarried, whose child is in day care, or who are enrolled in the Special Supplemental Nutrition Program for Women, Infants, and Children (Hendricks et al, 2006).
- Assure parents and caregivers that, while infants and toddlers have an innate ability to regulate energy intake, there is potential for environmental cues to diminish natural hunger-driven eating behaviors, even among young toddlers (Fox et al, 2006). Overfeeding may result if children are not taught to recognize their natural cues about hunger and satiety (Briefel et al, 2004).
- Encourage consumption of milk at home and other locations, such as restaurants and friends' homes, in place of fruit-flavored drinks or other sweetened beverages (Ziegler et al, 2006).
- All day care providers should be encouraged to use menu planning aids, such as those available from the U.S. Department of Agriculture (Ziegler et al, 2006).
- Discuss iron intake, fluid intake, and other nutritional factors related to normal growth and development, including calcium for bone health (Specker, 2004).
- Plan toddler snacks to complement meals by including additional fruits, vegetables, and whole grains that are culturally appropriate rather than fruit drinks, cookies, and crackers; this will increase fiber intake and limit fat and sugar intakes (Ziegler, Hanson et al, 2006).
- To develop healthful eating patterns, introduce toddlers to foods 8 to 10 times to increase food acceptance and the likelihood of establishing healthful eating patterns (Ziegler, Hanson et al, 2006).
- Discuss role of fat-soluble vitamins and their presence in whole milk. Discuss also the role of essential fatty acids in normal growth and development of the nervous system (Fewtrell et al, 2004).
- Bottled waters are not a substitute for formula. Hyponatremia may result.
- Fluoridated water is recommended; check the community status. Be wary of use of fluoride supplements when the water is fluoridated and the infant receives adequate water from this source. Note that well water is not fluoridated and that supplementation may be needed in this case, if prescribed by the physician.
- When brushing teeth, be carefully not to use a large amount of fluoridated toothpaste. A very small amount suffices.
- For planning vegan diets in infancy, breast milk should be the sole food, with soy-based formula as an alternative; breastfed vegan infants may need supplements of vitamin B_{12}, zinc, and vitamin D (Reed Mangels and Messina, 2001). Protein sources for older infants may include tofu and dried beans.

Patient Education—Food Safety

- Hand washing with soap and hot water is recommended before breastfeeding or before formula preparation. Use clean utensils and containers for mixing formula. Wash the top of the can before opening.
- Before using tap water for formula preparation or to give as a beverage, let cold tap water run for 2 minutes to remove any lead that may be in the pipes.
- Well water should not be used since it may contain bacteria.
- Follow the 2-hour rule: discard any formula, beverage, or food that has been left at room temperature for 2 hours or longer. Do not reuse.
- Do not use honey in the diets of infants to decrease potential exposure to botulism.
- Avoid using raw or partially cooked eggs, raw or undercooked fish or shellfish, and raw or undercooked meats because of potential foodborne illnesses.
- Do not use raw (unpasteurized) milk or products made from it.
- Avoid using unpasteurized juices and raw sprouts.
- For hospital preparation of infant formula, use available guidelines (Robbins and Beker, 2004).

For More Information

- American Academy of Pediatrics
  http://www.aap.org/
- Bright Futures–Babies
  http://www.nal.usda.gov/wicworks/Learning_Center/BF_babies.pdf
- Clinical Practice Guidelines (constipation, gastroenteritis, etc).
  http://www.aap.org/policy/paramtoc.html
- Feeding Kids Newsletter
  http://www.nutritionforkids.com/Feeding_Kids.htm
- Growth Charts
  http://www.cdc.gov/growthcharts
- Infant Nutrition
  http://www.nal.usda.gov/fnic/etext/000106.html
- Kids Health
  http://www.kidshealth.org/
- Mead Johnson (products for infants)
  http://www.meadjohnson.com/products_store.html
- Nestle
  http://www.verybestbaby.com/
- National Perinatal Association
  http://www.nationalperinatal.org/
- Pediatric Nutrition Practice Group
  http://www.pediatricnutrition.org/
- Ross Laboratories (products for infants)
  http://rosslabs.com
- Sudden Infant Death Syndrome
  SIDS Hotline: 800-221-SIDS
  http://www.sidscenter.org/

- USDA/ARS Children's Nutrition Research Center
  1100 Bates Street, Houston, TX 77030; Phone: 713-798-7971
  http://www.bcm.tmc.edu/cnrc/
- WIC Topics A-Z
  http://www.nal.usda.gov/wicworks/Topics/Infant_Nutrition.html
- World Health Organization
  http://www.who.int/child-adolescent-health/NUTRITION/infant.htm
- Vegetarian Baby Food (Homemade)
  http://www.vrg.org/recipes/babyfood.htm

Manufacturers

- Beech Nut
  http://www.babycenter.com/solidfoods/product.html
- Gerber
  http://www.gerber.com/
- Heinz
  http://www.heinzbaby.com/

INFANT, NORMAL (6–12 MONTHS)—CITED REFERENCES

Agostoni C, et al. Growth pattern of breastfed and nonbreastfed infants with atopic dermatitis in the first year of life. *Pediatrics* 106:73E, 2000

Briefel R, et al. Feeding infants and toddlers study: do vitamin and mineral supplements contribute to nutrient adequacy or excess among US infants and toddlers? *J Am Diet Assoc.* 106:52S, 2006.

Briefel R, et al. Toddlers' transition to table foods: impact on nutrient intakes and food patterns. *J Am Diet Assoc.* 104:s38, 2004.

Brown CE, Magnuson B. On the physics of the infant feeding bottle and middle ear sequela: ear disease in infants can be associated with bottle feeding. *Int J Pediatr Otorhinolaryngol.* 54:13, 2000.

Butte NF, et al. Infant feeding mode affects early growth and body composition. *Pediatrics* 106:1355, 2000.

Butte NF, et al. The Start Healthy Feeding Guidelines for infants and toddlers. *J Am Diet Assoc.* 104:442, 2004.

Coppa GV, et al. The first prebiotics in humans: human milk oligosaccharides. *J Clin Gastroenterol.* 38:S80, 2004.

Couch SC, Falciglia GA. Improving the diets of the young: considerations for intervention design. *J Am Diet Assoc.* 106:10S, 2006.

Daniels JL, et al. Fish intake during pregnancy and early cognitive development of offspring. *Epidemiology* 15:394, 2004.

Fewtrell MS, et al. Randomized, double-blind trial of long-chain polyunsaturated fatty acid supplementation with fish oil and borage oil in preterm infants. *J Pediatr.* 144:471, 2004.

Fox MK, et al. Relationship between portion size and energy intake among infants and toddlers: evidence of self-regulation. *J Am Diet Assoc.* 106:77S, 2006.

Friel JK, et al. A double-masked, randomized control trial of iron supplementation in early infancy in healthy term breast-fed infants. *J Pediatr.* 143:582, 2003.

Gardiner P, Kemper KJ. Herbs in pediatric and adolescent medicine. *Pediatr Rev.* 21:44, 2000.

Heird WC, et al. Current electrolyte intakes of infants and toddlers. *J Am Diet Assoc.* 106:43S, 2006.

Heird WC, Lapillone A. The role of essential fatty acids in development. *Annu Rev Nutr.* 25:549, 2005.

Helland IB, et al. Maternal supplementation with very-long-chain n-3 fatty acids during pregnancy and lactation augments children's IQ at 4 years of age. *Pediatrics* 111:e39, 2003.

Hendricks K, et al. Maternal and child characteristics associated with infant and toddler feeding practices. *J Am Diet Assoc.* 106:135S, 2006.

Kattelmann KK, et al. Effect of timing of introduction of complementary foods on iron and zinc status of formula fed infants at 12, 24 and 36 months of age. *J Am Diet Assoc.* 101:443, 2001.

Koo WW. Efficacy and safety of docosahexaenoic acid and arachidonic acid addition to infant formulas: can one buy better vision and intelligence? *J Am Coll Nutr.* 22:101, 2003.

Morley RE, et al. Foreign body aspiration in infants and toddlers: recent trends in British Columbia. *J Otolaryngol.* 33:37, 2004.

Pac S, et al. Development of the Start Healthy Feeding Guidelines for infants and toddlers. *J Am Diet Assoc.* 104:455, 2004.

Reed Mangels A, Messina V. Considerations in planning vegan diets: infants. *J Am Diet Assoc.* 101:670, 2001.

Robbins ST, Beker L. *Infant feedings: guidelines for preparation of formula and breastmilk in health care facilities.* Chicago: American Dietetic Association, 2004.

Specker B. Nutrition influences bone development from infancy through toddler years. *J Nutr.* 134:691S, 2004.

Stang J. Improving the eating patterns of infants and toddlers. *J Am Diet Assoc.* 106:7S, 2006.

Tomassoni AJ, Simone K. Herbal medicines for children: an illusion of safety? *Curr Opin Pediatr.* 13:162, 2001.

Ziegler P, et al. Nutrient intakes and food patterns of toddlers' lunches and snacks: influence of location. *J Am Diet Assoc.* 106:124S, 2006.

Ziegler P, Hanson C, et al. Feeding infants and toddlers study: meal and snack intakes of Hispanic and non-Hispanic infants and toddlers. *J Am Diet Assoc.* 106:107S, 2006.

CHILDHOOD

NUTRITIONAL ACUITY RANKING: LEVEL 1–2

DEFINITIONS AND BACKGROUND

The American Dietetic Association (2004) has taken the position that children between the ages of 2 and 11 years should have appropriate eating habits so they can achieve optimal physical and cognitive development, a healthy weight, and enjoyment of their meals. Children are not "little adults" and should be treated individually.

Conversation with an adult is usually required to discuss actual food intake by a child; the ability to recall by children is often limited because of vocabulary and attention span. Even if reporting within 90 minutes after eating school lunch, children have difficulty reporting what they have eaten; accuracy decreases markedly the longer the time span after eating (Baxter and Domel, 1997). Macronutrient intake reports may be more accurate if the children are trained in advance (Weber et al, 2004).

Growth during this stage involves changes in appetite, physical activity, and frequency of illnesses. The CDC growth charts provide a guideline for monitoring successful growth related to weight, height, and age. Body mass index (BMI) calculations are now available for use with children, and calculations may be used to identify underweight, potential stunting, or obesity. Prevalence for low height for age (stunting) and low weight for age (wasting) can be high among children from persistently poor families (Miller and Korenman, 1994); more studies are needed to determine the physiological and psychological effects of food insecurity on children's overall health status (Matheson et al, 2002).

During the early years of life, eating occurs primarily as a result of hunger and satiety cues. Evidence suggests that, by the time children are 3 or 4 years old, eating is no longer driven by real hunger but is influenced by a variety of environmental factors, including presentation of larger portions (Rolls et al, 2000) and parenting behaviors (Golan and Crow, 2004). Girls with mothers who are dieting have more ideas about dieting than girls with moms who do not diet (Abramovitz and Birch, 2000). Restricting young girls' access to palatable foods may promote greater intake, thereby generating negative feelings about their consumption (Orlet Fisher and Birch, 2000).

Children from underserved, ethnically diverse population groups may have increased risk for obesity (Hoelscher et al, 2004), increased serum lipids, and dietary consumption patterns that do not meet suggested dietary guidelines (Bronner, 1996). Intake of dairy products, fruits, and vegetables tends to be significantly lower (Lindquist et al, 2000).

In the past few decades, children's dietary intakes have changed dramatically, and children are eating more meals away from home (Nicklas et al, 2004). Children are becoming more overweight and less active; type 2 diabetes usually affects those over age 45 years, but more children are given a diagnosis of diabetes. Prevalence and incidence of type 2 diabetes estimates vary depending on age and ethnicity; adolescence is an especially prevalent time for onset (O'Brien et al, 2004). For more information, see Obesity, Childhood in Section 3.

Almost 23% of children under the age of 18 in the United States live in poverty; some may be exposed to lead poisoning, and iron deficiency anemia is the biggest risk. Because even mild undernutrition affects brain growth and function (Peters et al, 2004), food assistance programs should be used whenever possible. It is also essential that school-aged children have adequate snacks to eliminate transient hunger, which tends to interfere with classroom performance. Attention is easily diverted at this age; total intake may vary. Scheduling of lunch after recess results in greater intake of all foods and energy (Getlinger et al, 1996).

Misconceptions must be corrected, such as "good foods/bad foods" or "foods that are good for you taste bad." Dietary fat restriction may compromise growth and should not be implemented. There is no proof of long-term safety and efficacy for restricting fat in children's diets; lowered calcium, zinc, magnesium, phosphorus, vitamins E and B_{12}, thiamin, niacin, and riboflavin intakes can be a problem when fat intake is limited (Olson, 2000).

The National Academy of Sciences has recommended that adequate dietary intake of calcium is necessary in children and adolescents for the development of peak bone mass and prevention of fractures and osteoporosis later in life (Food and Nutrition Board, 2002). The current recommended adequate intake for children 9–18 years of age is 1300 mg/d, based largely on the results of calcium-balance studies that show that, in healthy children of this age, maximal net calcium balance is achieved with this intake (Food and Nutrition Board, 2002).

Adequate calcium and vitamin D are essential during growth and into puberty, especially during rapid bone growth and mineralization (Weisberg et al, 2004). Current mean dietary intakes are below desired levels; children may need encouragement to increase their intakes of skim and low-fat dairy products (Rajeshwari et al, 2004). According to the American Academy of Pediatrics, families may need information about appropriate inclusion of calcium supplements (American Academy of Pediatrics, 1999; Greer and Krebs, 2006). Dietary calcium needs of children who take medications that alter bone metabolism are uncertain; provide at least RDA levels for calcium and for vitamin D. Rickets is becoming more common in childhood, even in the developed nations (Wharton and Bishop, 2003).

Iron deficiency is a major concern in young children (Skalicky et al, 2006). Participation in WIC programs may be helpful because of increased access to and use of iron-rich foods (Altucher et al, 2005). Dietary intake of foods that are less healthful than desired (such as sugar-sweetened beverages, high-fat foods, and refined carbohydrates) plays a role in displacing nutrient-dense foods and can contribute to the risk of childhood obesity, type 2 diabetes, and adult chronic diseases (Stroehla et al, 2005).

Estimates suggest that malnutrition (measured as poor weight status) is associated with about 50% of all deaths among children, with diarrhea and pneumonia being primary concerns (Lopez, 2004; Caulfield et al, 2004). Infectious diseases of childhood may be related to poor nutrition, especially lack of vitamin C (Seaton and Devereux, 2000), zinc, and vitamin A (Lopez, 2004). Children who are prone to repetitive illness may benefit from a basic multivitamin-mineral supplement in addition to a carefully planned diet.

INTERVENTION: OBJECTIVES

- Assess growth patterns, feeding skills, dietary intake, activity patterns, inherited factors, and cognitive development. Promote adequate growth and development patterns such as increased independence at 12–18 months (stop bottle, begin eating with a spoon) and growth slowdown from 18 months–2 years (less interest in food, begin eating with utensils); energy intake varies from 2–3 years (control exerted), and brain growth triples by age 6.
- Avoid food deprivation, which may decrease ability to concentrate, cause growth failure or anemia, aggravate stunting, and lead to easy fatigue (Connell et al, 2004).
- Monitor long-term drug therapies and related side effects (e.g., use of anticonvulsants and the effects on folate, growth, etc.).
- Assess nutritional deficiencies, especially iron. If possible, detect and correct pica (eating nonfood items or any one food to the exclusion of others—even ice chips). Prevent "milk anemia," which may originate from drinking too much milk with meals and not consuming enough iron-rich meats (Murphy and Allen, 2003), grains, and vegetables.
- Evaluate status of the child's dental health. Prevent dental decay.
- Support adequate nutritional immunity through a balanced diet, and encourage vaccinations to prevent infectious diseases such as measles, mumps, and tetanus.
- Promote adequate intake of calcium, vitamin D (Greer and Krebs, 2006; Abrams and O'Brien, 2004; Weisberg et

al, 2004), fiber, and zinc, which are nutrients that are often poorly consumed by young children.

- Help reduce onset of chronic diseases later in life by prudent menu planning and meal intakes. Early lesions of atherosclerosis begin in childhood; diet, obesity, exercise, and certain inherited dyslipidemias influence the progression of such lesions (American Heart Association, 2006; Holmes and Kwiterovich, 2005). Good nutrition, a physically active lifestyle, and absence of tobacco use contribute to lower risk and can delay or prevent the onset of cardiovascular disease (American Heart Association, 2006; American Dietetic Association, 2004).
- Avoid mislabeling overweight children as "fat," which may trigger an eating disorder later. To advise an overweight or obese child, see appropriate entries in this text.
- The school, parents, and the community have equal responsibility for achieving integrity of school food service (American Dietetic Association, 2003). For example, access to sweetened soft drinks should be limited (Grimm et al, 2004).
- To promote proper growth, especially for stature, parents and caretakers should limit sweetened beverage intake to 12 fl oz/d (Dennison et al, 1999). Fruit juice should be limited to 4–6 oz daily for proper dental health (Marshall et al, 2003) and to encourage sufficient calcium intake from dairy beverages (Fisher et al, 2004). Excesses of juice containing malabsorbed carbohydrate may also cause diarrhea (Moukarzel et al, 2002).
- Emphasize food variety to reduce fear of new foods (neophobia), which may reduce nutritional status (Falciglia et al, 2000). Introduction of many new foods and flavors before age 4 may be an important way to enhance children's acceptance of new food items (Nicklas et al, 2005).

INTERVENTION: FOOD AND NUTRITION

- Energy and nutrient requirements vary by age and sex; see charts below.

	Recommendation		
Nutrient	**Ages 1–3 Years**	**Ages 4–8 Years**	**Ages 9–13 Years**
Energy	1046 kcal/d	1742 kcal/d	2279 kcal/d males; 2071 kcal/d females
Protein	13 g/d or 1.1 g/kg	19 g/d or 0.95 g/kg	34 g/d or 0.95 g/kg
Calcium	500 mg/d	800 mg/d	1300 mg/d
Iron	7 mg/d	10 mg/d	8 mg/d
Folate	150 μg/d	200 μg/d	300 μg/d
Phosphorus	460 mg/d	500 mg/d	1250 mg/d
Vitamin A	300 μg	400 μg	600 μg
Vitamin C	15 mg/d	25 mg/d	45 mg/d
Thiamin	0.5 mg/d	0.6 mg/d	0.9 mg/d
Riboflavin	0.5 mg/d	0.6 mg/d	0.9 mg/d
Niacin	6 mg/d	8 mg/d	12 mg/d
Fiber	19 g	25 g	26 g females; 31 g males
Sodium	$<$1500 mg	$<$1900 mg	$<$2200 mg
Potassium	3000 mg	3800 mg	4500 mg

Data from: Food and Nutrition Board, Institute of Medicine. *Dietary reference intakes for energy, carbohydrate, fiber, fat, fatty acids, cholesterol, protein, and amino acids (macronutrients)*. Washington, DC: National Academy Press, 2002; and American Heart Association, 2006.

- Carbohydrates should be 45–65% of total energy (American Dietetic Association, 2004). Added sugars should not exceed 25% of energy intake; less is actually better.
- Protein needs are 1.1 g/kg for ages 1–3, decreasing to 0.95 g/kg for ages 4–8 and 9–13. The meal plan should include 5–20% of energy from protein for young children and 10–30% for older children (American Dietetic Association, 2004). Include protein with 50% high biological value when possible.
- Provide fat as 30–40% total energy for ages 1–3 years and as 25–35% total energy in ages 4–18 years (American Dietetic Association, 2004). Use of saturated fats and trans fatty acids should be low while maintaining nutritional adequacy (American Dietetic Association, 2002). Where there is evidence or high risk for cardiovascular disease, start with a diet low in total and saturated fat and cholesterol, use water-soluble fiber and plant sterols, and promote weight control and exercise (Holmes and Kwiterovich, 2005). Select some lower fat foods, use low-fat cooking techniques, or spread jelly on bread instead of butter.
- Follow the guidelines of the American Heart Association (2006) for a successful meal plan:

  Balance dietary calories with physical activity to maintain normal growth.

  60 minutes of moderate to vigorous play or physical activity daily.

Daily Estimated Calories and Recommended Servings for Grains, Fruits, Vegetables, and Milk/Dairy by Age and Gender

	1 Year	2–3 Years	4–8 Years	9–13 Years	14–18 Years
Kilocalories[a]	900	1000			
Female			1200	1600	1800
Male			1400	1800	2200
Fat, % of total kcal	30–40	30–35	25–35	25–35	25–35
Milk/dairy, cups[b]	2[c]	2	2	3	3
Lean meat/beans, oz	1.5	2		5	
Female			3		5
Male			4		6
Fruits, cups[d]	1	1	1.5	1.5	
Female					1.5
Male					2
Vegetables, cups[d]	3/4	1			
Female			1	2	2.5
Male			1.5	2.5	3
Grains, oz	2	3			
Female			4	5	6
Male			5	6	7

Calorie estimates are based on a sedentary lifestyle. Increased physical activity will require additional calories: increase of 0–200 kcal/d if moderately physically active and increase of 200–400 kcal/d if very physically active.

[a]For youth 2 years and older; adapted from Tables 2 and 3 and Appendix A-2 in U.S. Department of Health and Human Services, U.S. Department of Agriculture. *Dietary guidelines for Americans*. 6th ed. Washington, DC: U.S. Government Printing Office, 2005; www.healthierus.gov/dietaryguidelines. Nutrient and energy contributions from each group are calculated according to the nutrient-dense forms of food in each group (e.g., lean meats and fat-free milk).

[b]Milk listed is fat free (except for children under the age of 2 years). If 1%, 2%, or whole-fat milk is substituted, this will use, for each cup, 19, 39, or 63 kcal of discretionary calories and add 2.6, 5.1, or 9.0 g of total fat, of which 1.3, 2.6, or 4.6 g are saturated fat, respectively.

[c]For 1-year-old children, calculations are based on 2% fat milk. If 2 cups of whole milk are substituted, 48 kcal of discretionary calories will be utilized. The American Academy of Pediatrics recommends that low-fat/reduced-fat milk not be started before 2 years of age.

[d]Serving sizes are 1/4 cup for 1 year of age, 1/3 cup for 2–3 years of age, and 1/2 cup for ≥4 years of age. A variety of vegetables should be selected from each subgroup over the week.

Reference: American Heart Association, 2006. Website accessed February 7, 2006, http://pediatrics.aappublications.org/cgi/content/full/117/2/544/T3.

Eat vegetables and fruits daily; limit juice intake.

Use vegetable oils and soft margarines low in saturated fat and trans fatty acids instead of butter or most other animal fats in the diet.

Eat whole-grain breads and cereals rather than refined-grain products.

Reduce the intake of sugar-sweetened beverages and foods.

Use nonfat (skim) or low-fat milk and dairy products daily.

Eat more fish, especially oily fish, broiled or baked.

Reduce salt intake, including salt from processed foods.

- Offer calcium as indicated in nutrient charts to increase mineral density. Yogurt, plain or flavored milks, calcium-fortified juices or soy milk, soft-serve ice cream, and cheeses are generally well accepted by children. If dairy foods are not used, children can include foods such as 1 oz of cooked dried beans (161 mg), 10 figs (169 mg), spinach (120 mg), 1 packet of oatmeal (100 mg), 1 medium orange (50 mg), ½ cup of mashed sweet potato (44 mg), or ½ cup of cooked broccoli (35 mg).
- Phosphorus intake should be relatively similar to calcium intake.
- Encourage exposure to sunlight and monitor dietary intake of vitamin D. Adequate folate, magnesium, selenium, and vitamin E are important to obtain from dietary sources.
- Day care meals given for a 4- to 8-hour stay should provide for one third to one half of daily needs. School lunch programs generally provide one third of daily needs. Meals at home should be planned carefully to make up the differences.
- Give 50–60 mL/kg of fluids daily. Milk, fruit juice, vegetable juices, and water should be the basic fluids offered. Cut out carbonated beverages as much as possible.
- To increase fiber in the diet, provide 19 g/d for 1- to 3-year olds and 25 g/d for 4- to 8-year olds. Boys aged 9–13 need 31 g/d; girls aged 9–13 need 26 g/d (American Dietetic Association, 2004). Fiber from fruits, vegetables, grains, and legumes may help to prevent or alleviate constipation. Ensure that adequate fluid is consumed each day as well.

CLINICAL INDICATORS

Clinical/History		Lab Work
Age	Appetite	Glucose
Weight	Hydration (I & O)	H & H, serum Fe
Height	Triceps skinfold (TSF)	Chol, Trig (check family history of heart disease)
Growth percentile for age	Midarm muscle circumference (MAMC),	Alk phos
Diet/intake history	midarm circumference (MAC)	Ca++
Dental status		Alb (if needed)
Physical handicaps		

Common Drugs Used and Potential Side Effects

- Anticonvulsants may cause problems with the child's growth and normal body functions. Diet should be adjusted carefully.
- Corticosteroids may cause growth stunting if given over an extended time in large doses.
- Drug therapy with inhibitors of hydroxymethylglutaryl CoA reductase, bile acid sequestrants, and cholesterol absorption inhibitors may be considered in those with a positive family history of premature coronary artery disease and a low-density lipoprotein cholesterol level above 160 mg/dL after dietary and lifestyle changes (Holmes and Kwiterovich, 2005).
- Nutritional supplements should be taken only when prescribed by a physician, although over-the-counter use is common. Avoid serving cereals to children that fulfill the adult RDAs for vitamins and minerals. Poly-Vi-Fluor contains fluoride; use caution in areas where water is fluoridated. Too much can cause fluorosis.
- Stimulants like methylphenidate (Ritalin) or dextroamphetamine (Dexedrine) may cause anorexia, growth stunting, nausea, stomach pain, and weight loss; frequent snacks may be useful (Harding, 2003). Strattera (atomoxetine) works on the norepinephrine, whereas stimulants primarily work on dopamine; these neurotransmitters are believed to play a role in attention-deficit hyperactivity disorder (ADHD). Strattera may decrease appetite.
- Tofranil (imipramine) may be used for bedwetting. Dry mouth may result.

Herbs, Botanicals, and Supplements

- Herbs and botanical supplements have not been proven to be safe for children. While not needed or desirable, use of nutrient supplements is still common in the first 2 years of life (Eichenberger Gilmore et al, 2005).
- Discuss the relevance of tolerable upper intake levels (ULs) from the dietary reference intakes of the National Academy of Sciences. These levels were set to protect individuals from receiving too much of any nutrient from diet and dietary supplements.
- Children are more prone to toxicity than adults. For example, jinbuhuan causes bradycardia and CNS and respiratory depression and is to be avoided in children; fenugreek may trigger asthma in susceptible individuals.

INTERVENTION: NUTRITION EDUCATION, COUNSELING, CARE MANAGEMENT

- Education, with the support of the health care community, combined with health policy and environmental change to support optimal nutrition and physical activity are central to the health strategy of "primordial prevention" in children (American Heart Association [AHA], 2006). The general dietary recommendations of the AHA for those aged 2 years and older stress a diet that primarily relies on fruits and vegetables, whole grains, low-fat and nonfat dairy products, beans, fish, and lean meat, and specific AHA tips for parents include the following (AHA, 2006):
  Reduce added sugars, including sugar-sweetened drinks and juices.
  Use canola, soybean, corn, safflower, or other unsaturated oils in place of solid fats during food preparation.
  Use recommended portion sizes on food labels when preparing and serving food.
  Use fresh, frozen, and canned vegetables and fruits and serve at every meal; be careful with added sauces and sugar.
  Introduce and regularly serve fish as an entree.
  Remove the skin from poultry before eating.
  Use only lean cuts of meat and reduced-fat meat products.
  Limit high-calorie sauces such as Alfredo sauce, cream sauces, cheese sauces, and hollandaise.
  Eat whole-grain breads and cereals rather than refined products; read labels and ensure that "whole grain" is the first ingredient on the food label of these products.
  Eat more legumes (beans) and tofu in place of meat for some entrees.
  Breads, breakfast cereals, and prepared foods, including soups, may be high in salt and/or sugar; read food labels for content and choose high-fiber, low-salt/low-sugar alternatives.
- The most recent Dietary Guidelines for Americans (for those 2 years of age and older) and the American Academy of Pediatrics Nutrition Handbook provide important supporting reference information with regard to overall diet composition, appropriate caloric intakes at different ages, macronutrients, micronutrients, portion size, and food choices.
- Children should be treated respectfully. Initiate conversation with the child rather than only talking with parents or caregivers. As with any counseling relationship, a personalized conversation elicits the most effective response.

- Be aware of developmental phase of the child. For example, toddler (1–3 years of age): autonomy; preschooler (4–6 years of age): initiative; and school-age child (6–12 years of age): industry (Erikson, 1963). It is helpful to include games, projects, or tasks that are age appropriate for learning nutrition concepts.
- Explain the age-appropriate diet for children. Encourage parents to use finger foods for toddlers. Young children have food jags, and they often prefer single foods. Older children need nutritious snacks; cheese cubes are good snacks for the teeth, and iron-rich desserts can be served on occasion. Avoid use of empty-calorie foods (Schulze et al, 2004).
- Encourage a relaxed atmosphere at mealtime. There should be no pressure to eat, hurry, or finish meals.
- Explain to parents that bribery or rewards for eating should never be used. Rewards can actually decrease acceptance. Parents must be careful about "control" issues around meals or foods to avoid promoting disordered eating.
- With toddlers, continued use of iron-fortified cereal can be beneficial. Include juices that are naturally high in vitamin C.
- Children should be allowed to vary in their food acceptance, choices, and intakes, just as adults do. An authoritative feeding style is generally more effective than an authoritarian style (Patrick et al, 2005).
- Proper atmosphere is important to children since their eating patterns are strongly influenced by both the physical and social environment. Children are more likely to eat foods that are available and easily accessible; they tend to eat greater quantities when larger portions are provided; and structured family mealtimes are important factors related to children's eating patterns (Patrick and Nicklas, 2005).
- Many children skip breakfast each day. Discuss the importance of eating breakfast for enhancing the abilities to concentrate, learn, and retain new information. Consumption of a healthy breakfast each day is recommended, especially breakfasts containing a variety of foods with emphasis on high-fiber and nutrient-rich whole grains, fruits, and dairy products (Rampersaud et al, 2005).
- Promote healthy meals at school (Briggs et al, 2003). It is essential that school-aged children have adequate meals to eliminate transient hunger, which interferes with classroom performance (Ivanovic et al, 2004). Attention is easily diverted at a young age; total intake may vary. Scheduling of lunch after recess results in greater intake of all foods and energy (Getlinger et al, 1996).
- Establish at least one "champion" for nutrition issues at school (e.g., a parent, the principal, the foodservice manager), and promote teamwork (Making It Happen, 2004). Discuss the role of competitive foods, and work toward standards for children to have access to nutritious choices. Both school and the community have a shared responsibility to provide students with high-quality foods and school-based nutrition services (American Dietetic Association, 2006).
- Knowledge and training are needed to improve food consumption patterns as children consume foods away from home and as they take on greater responsibility for meal preparation and food selection.
- Promote healthy forms of activity, using the USDA Kids' Activity MyPyramid Food Guidance System as a guide. Refer to website at http://www.usda.gov/cnpp/KidsPyra/.
- Encourage intake of whole grains from breakfast cereals and breads (Thane et al, 2005).
- Vegan children should be encouraged to consume adequate sources of vitamin B_{12}, riboflavin, zinc, and calcium, and vitamin D if sun exposure is not adequate (Messina and Reed Mangels, 2001).
- Children who have chronic illnesses fare better if parents give them responsibilities, such as meal planning and taking their own medications. Tasks should be age appropriate. Section 3 addresses pediatric illnesses in greater detail. Special considerations for children are found in Table 1-8.
- A dramatic increase in childhood obesity is related to many things, including decreased physical activity and fitness levels and minimal physical education in schools (Lucas, 2001). See Table 1-9 for more suggestions for childhood activities. All providers should be aware of the problems of childhood obesity and refer accordingly (O'Brien et al, 2004).

TABLE 1-8 Special Considerations for Children

Lead Poisoning: Lead poisoning remains the most common environmental health problem affecting American children. Lead is a confirmed neurotoxicant (Canfield et al, 2004). Data show an inverse relationship between blood lead concentration and scores on four measures of cognitive functioning: arithmetic scores, reading scores, nonverbal reasoning, and short-term memory; deficits occur at blood lead concentrations lower than 5 mg/dL (Lanphear et al, 2000). Lead exposure occurs through ingestion of lead-contaminated household dust and soil in older housing containing lead-based paint. Lead replaces calcium in the bone; deposition may be seen in x-rays of the knee, ankle, or wrist. Anemia may also occur. Nutritional interventions involve provision of regular meals with adequate amounts of calcium and iron supplementation for iron deficiency. Educational efforts address parental awareness of lead exposure pathways, hygiene, and housekeeping measures to prevent ingestion of dust and soil. Use drinking water from the cold tap, not hot water tap; bottled water is not guaranteed as a safe alternative. Blood lead screening is often recommended universally at ages 1 and 2 years. For more information, visit the following website: http://www.cdc.gov/nceh/lead/lead.htm.

Measles and Blindness in Children: Measles blindness is the single leading cause of blindness in low-income countries (Semba and Bloem, 2004). In high-income countries, lesions of the optic nerve and higher visual pathways predominate as causes of blindness; retinopathy from prematurity occurs in middle-income countries (Gilbert and Foster, 2001). In the United States, as many as 15 million individuals may lack humoral immunity against measles (Hutchins et al, 2001). Control of blindness in children is a priority within the World Health Organization's VISION 2020 program; strategies are region specific and based on activities to prevent blindness in the community. Measles immunization, health education, control of vitamin A deficiency, and provision of eye care facilities for conditions that require specialists are part of this plan.

TABLE 1-9 Tips for Encouraging Children to Enjoy Nutrition and Physical Activity

1. Children should be empowered to make food choices that reflect the Dietary Guidelines for Americans.
2. Good nutrition and physical activity are essential to children's health and educational success.
3. School meals that meet the Dietary Guidelines for Americans should appeal to children and taste good.
4. Programs must build upon the best science, education, communication, and technical resources available.
5. School, parent, and community teamwork is essential to encouraging children to make food and physical activity choices for a healthy lifestyle.
6. Messages to children should be age appropriate and delivered in a language they speak, through media they use, and in ways that are entertaining and actively involve them in learning.
7. Focusing on positive messages regarding food choices children can make.
8. It is critical to stimulate and support action and education at the national, state, and local levels to successfully change children's eating behaviors.

Source: USDA Team Nutrition, http://www.fns.usda.gov/tn; accessed January 15, 2005.

- Too much time in front of the television or computer results in low energy expenditure, which is a problem for overweight children (Marshall et al, 2004). See Figure 1-7 for a photo of children at play.

Patient Education—Food Safety

- Children should be taught to wash their hands before eating and after use of the toilet, sneezing, etc., to prevent foodborne illness and the spread of various infections.
- Children can be taught to avoid food and beverages that have an unusual flavor or odor.
- Avoid raw or partially cooked eggs, raw or undercooked fish or shellfish, and raw or undercooked meats because of potential foodborne illnesses.
- Five of the most commonly eaten varieties of fish are low in mercury (shrimp, canned light tuna, salmon, pollack, and catfish); AHA continues to recommend two servings of fish weekly (American Heart Association, 2006).
- Do not use raw (unpasteurized) milk or products made from it.
- Avoid serving unpasteurized juices and raw sprouts.
- Only serve certain deli meats and frankfurters that have been reheated to steaming hot temperature.
- Child Care Centers should follow guidelines for safe food handling and for inclusion of nutritious meals and snacks (American Dietetic Association, 2005). A safe and sanitary setting is needed.

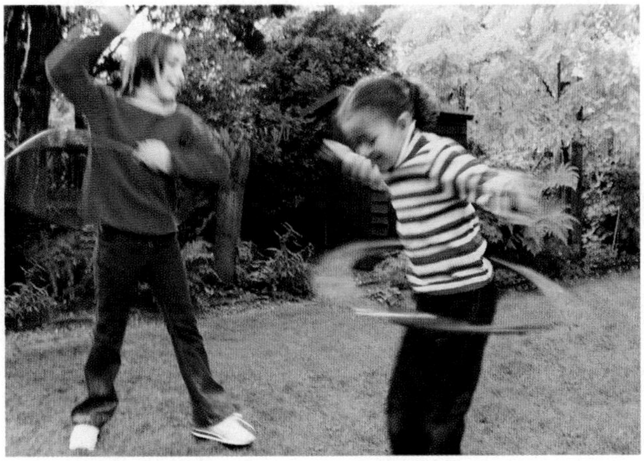

Figure 1-7 Children at play.

For More Information

- American Academy of Pediatrics
  http://www.aap.org/
- American School Foodservice Association
  http://www.asfsa.org/
- Bright Futures
  http://www.brightfutures.org
- Children's Nutrition Research Center – Baylor University
  http://www.bcm.tmc.edu/cnrc/
- Gerber
  http://www.gerber.com/
- Growth Charts
  http://www.cdc.gov/growthcharts
- Healthy School Meals
  http://schoolmeals.nal.usda.gov/
- Heinz
  http://www.heinzbaby.com/
- Mead Johnson (products for infants)
  http://www.meadjohnson.com/products_store.html
- Pediatric Nutrition Practice Group
  http://www.pediatricnutrition.org/whatsnew/conference.htm

SAMPLE NUTRITION DIAGNOSTIC STATEMENT

Lead Poisoning in Childhood

PES: Excessive bioactive substance intake related to lead consumption from lead-based paint exposure in environment as evidenced by high serum lead levels, documented iron deficiency anemia, and deposition seen on x-rays.

Assessment Data: Dietary recall; labs such as H & H, serum ferritin, and serum lead levels; growth charts.

Intervention: Education and counseling tips on avoiding accidental lead intake; increasing sources of iron and calcium in the diet; tips on reducing environmental lead sources; running water awhile before drinking.

Monitoring and Evaluation: Reduced intake of sources of lead; improved lab values, improved weight gain on growth grid; successful growth and development.

- Ross Laboratories (products for infants)
  http://rosslabs.com

- USDA Kids Food MyPyramid Food Guidance System
  http://www.usda.gov/cnpp/KidsPyra/

CHILDHOOD—CITED REFERENCES

Abramovitz BA, Birch LL. Five-year-old girls' ideas about dieting are predicted by their mothers' dieting. *JAMA.* 100:1157, 2000.

Abrams SA, O'Brien KO. Calcium and bone mineral metabolism in children with chronic illnesses. *Annu Rev Nutr.* 24:13, 2004.

Altucher K, et al. Predictors of improvement in hemoglobin conventration among toddlers enrolled in the Massachusetts WIC program. *J Am Diet Assoc.* 105:709, 2005.

American Academy of Pediatrics Committee on Nutrition. Calcium requirements of infants, children, and adolescents. *Pediatrics* 104:1152, 1999.

American Dietetic Association. Position of The American Dietetic Association: child and adolescent food and nutrition programs. *J Am Diet Assoc.* 103:887, 2003.

American Dietetic Association. Position of The American Dietetic Association: dietary guidance for healthy children ages 2 to 11 years. *J Am Diet Assoc.* 104:660, 2004.

American Dietetic Association. Position of The American Dietetic Association: local support for nutrition integrity in schools. *J Am Diet Assoc.* 106: 122, 2006.

American Heart Association. Dietary recommendations for children and adolescents: a guide for practitioners. *Pediatrics* 117:544, 2006.

Baxter SD, et al. Impact of gender, ethnicity, meal component, and time interval between eating and reporting on accuracy of fourth-graders' self-reports of school lunch. *J Am Diet Assoc.* 97:1293, 1997.

Briggs M, et al. Position of the American Dietetic Association, Society for Nutrition Education, and American School Food Service Association. Nutrition services: an essential component of comprehensive school health programs. *J Am Diet Assoc.* 103:505, 2003.

Bronner Y. Nutritional status outcomes for children: ethnic, cultural, and environmental contexts. *J Am Diet Assoc.* 96:891, 1996.

Canfield RL, et al. Impaired neuropsychological functioning in lead-exposed children. *Dev Neuropsychol.* 26:513, 2004.

Caulfield LE, et al. Undernutrition as an underlying cause of child deaths associated with diarrhea, pneumonia, malaria, and measles. *Am J Clin Nutr.* 80:193, 2004.

Connell CL, et al. Food security of older children can be assessed using a standardized survey instrument. *J Nutr.* 134:2566, 2004.

Dennison BA, et al. Children's growth parameters vary by type of fruit juice consumed. *J Am Coll Nutr.* 18:346, 1999.

Eichenberger Gilmore JM, et al. Longitudinal patterns of vitamin and mineral supplement use in young white children. *J Am Diet Assoc.* 105:763, 2005.

Erikson E. *Childhood and society.* 2nd ed. New York: WW Norton & Company, 1963.

Falciglia GA, et al. Food neophobia in childhood affects dietary variety. *J Am Diet Assoc.* 100:1474, 2000.

Fisher JO, et al. Meeting calcium recommendations during middle childhood reflects mother-daughter beverage choices and predicts bone mineral status. *Am J Clin Nutr.* 79:698, 2004.

Food and Nutrition Board. Institute of Medicine. *Dietary reference intakes for energy, carbohydrate, fiber, fat, fatty acids, cholesterol, protein, and amino acids (macronutrients).* Washington, DC: National Academy Press, 2002.

Getlinger MJ, et al. Food waste is reduced when elementary school lunch children have recess before lunch. *J Am Diet Assoc.* 96:906, 1996.

Gilbert C, Foster A. Childhood blindness in the context of VISION 2020—the right to sight. *Bull World Health Organ.* 79:227, 2001.

Golan M, Crow S. Parents are key players in the prevention and treatment of weight-related problems. *Nutr Rev.* 62:39, 2004.

Greer FR, Krebs N. Optimizing bone health and calcium intakes of infants, children, and adolescents. *Pediatrics* 117:578, 2006.

Grimm GC, et al. Factors associated with soft drink consumption in school-aged children. *J Am Diet Assoc.* 104:1244, 2004.

Harding KL, et al. Outcome-based comparison of Ritalin versus food-supplement treated children with AD/HD. *Altern Med Rev.* 8:319, 2003.

Hoelscher DM, et al. Measuring the prevalence of overweight in Texas schoolchildren. *Am J Public Health.* 94:1002, 2004.

Holmes KW, Kwiterovich PO Jr. Treatment of dyslipidemia in children and adolescents. *Curr Cardiol Rep.* 7:445, 2005.

Hutchins SS, et al. National serologic survey of measles immunity among persons 6 years of age or older, 1988-1994. *Med Gen Med.* 24:E5, 2001.

Ivanovic DM, et al. Head size and intelligence, learning, nutritional status and brain development. Head, IQ, learning, nutrition and brain. *Neuropsychologia* 42:1118, 2004.

Lanphear BP, et al. Cognitive deficits associated with blood lead concentrations <10 microg/dL in US children and adolescents. *Pub Health Rep.* 115:521, 2000.

Lindquist CH, et al. Role of dietary factors in ethnic differences in early risk of cardiovascular disease and type 2 diabetes. *Am J Clin Nutr.* 71:725, 2000.

Lopez A. Malnutrition and the burden of disease. *Asia Pac J Clin Nutr.* 13:S7, 2004.

Lucas B. Ensuring healthy and well-nourished children. *J Am Diet Assoc.* 101: 628, 2001.

Making It Happen. School nutrition success stories. Accessed in 2004 at http://www.fns.usda.gov/tn/Healthy/execsummary_makingithappen.html.

Marshall SJ, et al. Relationships between media use, body fatness and physical activity in children and youth: a meta-analysis. *Int J Obes Relat Metab Disord.* 28:1238, 2004.

Marshall TA, et al. Dental caries and beverage consumption in young children. *Pediatrics* 112:e184, 2003.

Matheson DM, et al. Household food security and nutritional status of Hispanic children in the fifth grade. *Am J Clin Nutr.* 76:210, 2002.

Messina V, Reed Mangels A. Considerations in planning vegan diets: children. *J Am Diet Assoc.* 101:661, 2001.

Miller J, Korenman S. Poverty and children's nutritional status. *Am J Epidemiol.* 140:233, 1994.

Moukarzel AA, et al. Irritable bowel syndrome and nonspecific diarrhea in infancy and childhood—relationship with juice carbohydrate malabsorption. *Clin Pediatr (Phila).* 41:145, 2002

Murphy SP, Allen LH. Nutritional importance of animal source foods. *J Nutr.* 133:3932S, 2003.

Nicklas TA, et al. A prospective study of food variety seeking in childhood, adolescence and early adult life. *Appetite* 44:289, 2005.

Nicklas TA, et al. Children's meal patterns have changed over a 21-year period: the Bogalusa Heart Study. *J Am Diet Assoc.* 104:753, 2004.

O'Brien SH et al. Identification, evaluation, and management of obesity in an academic primary care center. *Pediatrics* 114:154, 2004.

Olson R. Is it wise to restrict fat in the diets of children? *J Am Diet Assoc.* 100: 28, 2000.

Orlet Fisher J, Birch LL. Parents' restrictive feeding practices are associated with young girls' negative self-evaluation of eating. *J Am Diet Assoc.* 100: 1341, 2000.

Patrick H, et al. The benefits of authoritative feeding style: caregiver feeding styles and children's food consumption patterns. *Appetite* 44:243, 2005.

Patrick H, Nicklas TA. A review of family and social determinants of children's eating patterns and diet quality. *J Am Coll Nutr.* 24:83, 2005.

Peters A, et al. The selfish brain: competition for energy resources. *Neurosci Biobehav Rev.* 28:143, 2004.

Rajeshwari R, et al. Longitudinal changes in intake and food sources of calcium from childhood to young adulthood: the Bogalusa heart study. *J Am Coll Nutr.* 23:341, 2004.

Rampersaud GC, et al. Breakfast habits, nutritional status, body weight and academic performance in children and adolescents. *J Am Diet Assoc.* 105: 743, 2005.

Rolls B, Engell D, Birch LL. Serving portion size influences 5-year-old but not 3-year old children's food intakes. *J Am Diet Assoc.* 100:232, 2000.

Schulze MB, et al. Sugar-sweetened beverages, weight gain, and incidence of type 2 diabetes in young and middle-aged women. *JAMA.* 292:927, 2004.

Seaton A, Devereux G. Diet, infection and wheezy illness: lessons from adults. *Pediatr Allergy Immunol.* 13:37, 2000.

Semba RD, Bloem MW. Measles blindness. *Surv Ophthalmol.* 49:243, 2004.

Skalicky A, et al. Child food insecurity and iron deficiency anemia in low-income infants and toddlers in the United States. *Matern Child Health J.* 10:177, 2006.

Stroehla BC, et al. dietary sources of nutrients among rural Native American and white children. *J Am Diet Assoc.* 105:1908, 2005.

Thane CW, et al. Whole-grain intake of British young people aged 4-18 years. *Br J Nutr.* 94:825, 2005.

Weber JL, et al. Validity of self-reported dietary intake at school meals by American Indian children: the Pathways Study. *J Am Diet Assoc.* 104:746, 2004.

Weisberg P, et al. Nutritional rickets among children in the United States: review of cases reported between 1986 and 2003. *Am J Clin Nutr.* 80:1697S, 2004.

Wharton B, Bishop N. Rickets. *Lancet* 362:1389, 2003.

ADOLESCENCE

NUTRITIONAL ACUITY RANKING: LEVEL 2

DEFINITIONS AND BACKGROUND

According to Erickson's psychological stages of development (1968), teens (12–18 years of age) are working on "identity." For cognitive development, the concrete, "here and now" stage lasts from ages 11–14 years in girls and from ages 13–15 years in males. Early abstract thinking and daydreams are common among 15- to 17-year-old females and 16- to 19-year-old males. True abstract thinking and idealism (faith, trust, and spirituality) occur for young women at ages 18–25 years and for males at 20–26 years of age.

Adolescents need to consume food and beverages that provide adequate energy and nutrients to reduce risk for poor outcomes including growth retardation, iron deficiency anemia, poor academic performance, development of psychosocial difficulties, and an increased likelihood of developing chronic diseases such as heart disease and osteoporosis during adulthood (American Dietetic Association, 2003b). Breakfast consumption is important to enhance cognitive function related to memory, test grades, and school attendance (Rampersaud et al, 2005).

Physiological growth is more accurately assessed by using Tanner Stages than by chronological age alone. Girls often start their growth spurt by age 10–11 and generally stop by age 15, whereas boys begin at 12–13 and generally stop by age 19.

Teens require increased nutrients to provide for the accelerated growth that takes place; nutritional deficiencies in adolescence can lead to loss of height, osteoporosis, and delayed sexual maturation (Herbold and Frates, 2000). The brain also continues developing through late adolescence, especially with the nerve fiber system that transmits messages from one hemisphere to the other. There is an increase in gray matter at the onset of adolescence, followed by a substantial loss in the frontal lobes from the mid-teens through the mid-twenties, where inhibiting impulses and regulating emotions may be altered. Teens are encouraged to make the most of their brains during this time, when they can "hard wire" their ability to process skills in academics, sports, and music.

Skeletal growth is unpredictable, and girls may gain 3.5 inches in 1 year, and boys may gain 4 inches in 1 year. When the teen years begin, the adolescent has achieved 80–85% of final height, 53% of final weight, and 52% of final skeletal mass. Teens may almost double their weight and can add 15–20% in height. Maintaining adequate calcium intake during childhood and adolescence is necessary for the development of peak bone mass, which may be important in reducing the risk of fractures and osteoporosis later in life (Greer and Krebs, 2006).

Some teens develop more rapidly than others (early maturers), while others may develop more slowly (late maturers). Girls who mature early may be prone to depression, eating disorders, and anxiety. Obesity is an increasing trend, as noted in the National Longitudinal Study of Adolescent Health (Gordon-Larsen et al, 2004). Parental pressure and weight status concerns are evident among girls who are "picky eaters" (Galloway et al, 2005).

With longer life expectancy due to antibiotics, better medical care, and sanitation than in past decades, more teens today can expect to live into their late 70s (http://original-ghr15.com/secrets.html; accessed September, 22, 2004).

Intakes change often during teen years, especially during growth spurts and varying stages of physical maturation. Sociocultural influences are known to affect adolescent eating patterns and behaviors (i.e., some teens reject a meat-based diet to become vegetarians; others take up dieting to lose weight or develop an eating disorder) (Herbold and Frates, 2000). Meal skipping, snacks at odd hours, laxative or diuretic use, fasting, bulimia, self-induced vomiting, and sports requirements are issues that should be addressed in a nutritional assessment. Dietary recalls are challenging. More than 60% of the incidence of obesity in children and teens may be related to excessive time spent watching television (i.e., 5 or more hours compared with 2 or fewer hours in those not overweight) (Gortmaker et al, 1996).

Daily requirement tables establish preteen years as ages 9–13 years and teen years as ages 15–18 years. The growth spurt of girls occurs at 9 1/2 to 13 1/2 years of age; menarche generally is at 12 1/2 years. For boys, the growth spurt occurs during the ages of 11 3/4 to 14 1/2 years. Sexual maturation occurs at ages 10–12 years for girls and at ages 12–14 years for boys. The increase in percentage of total body fat in girls is 1.5–2 times that of boys at this time. Boys have greater increases in lean body mass (muscle) and greater increases in height before epiphyseal closure of long bones occurs. Most skeletal growth is completed by 19 years of age. Girls have more total body fat and less total body water than boys.

Dietary intake and body size influence age at menarche and growth patterns in teen girls. Puberty comes early for some girls because of a gene (*CYP1B1*) that speeds up the body's breakdown of androgens. Age at menarche is also inversely related to percentage of energy intake from dietary protein at ages 3–5 years; fat intake at ages 1–2 years and percentage of energy from animal protein at ages 6–8 years influence age at peak growth (Berkey et al, 2000). These factors may have implications for later development of diseases whose risks are associated with adolescent growth, including breast cancer and heart disease.

INTERVENTION: OBJECTIVES

- Provide adequate energy for growth and development. Modify diet to meet the needs of an ongoing or potential growth spurt.
- Evaluate the patient's weight status. Offer appropriate guidance.
- Prevent or correct nutritional anemias. Determine a girl's sexual maturity, onset of menstruation, and growth spurts, which are often associated with depletion of iron (Ilich-Ernst et al, 1998). Alter diet accordingly to provide sufficient vitamins and minerals.

- Evaluate use of fad diets, skipping meals, unusual eating patterns, or tendency toward eating disorders. If problems are noted, seek immediate assistance. Family therapy may be beneficial.
- To prevent obesity in a teen whose parents are obese, a family approach focused on regular breakfast consumption is most beneficial (Fiore et al, 2006).
- Prevent future tendency toward osteoporosis. Because of the influence of the family's diet on the diet of children and adolescents, adequate calcium intake by all members of the family is important; low-fat dairy products, fruits, and vegetables and appropriate physical activity are important for achieving good bone health (Greer and Krebs, 2006).
- Introduce food changes one at a time; reassure patient regarding nutrition and fast foods.
- Encourage healthy food choices according to the factors of greatest interest to teens (taste and appearance). Health, energy, and price are often not viewed as essential at this stage.
- Vegetarians should be encouraged to consume adequate sources of vitamin B_{12}, riboflavin, zinc, iron, calcium, protein, and energy for growth. Cobalamin deficiency, in the absence of hematologic signs, may lead to impaired cognitive performance in adolescents (Louwman et al, 2000). Vegan children tend to have higher intakes of fiber and lower intakes of saturated fatty acids and cholesterol than omnivore children; they may need to increase intake of omega-3 fatty acids (Messina and Reed Mangels, 2001).
- Girls may have higher total cholesterol concentration than boys, which is somewhat related to differences in male and female hormones.

INTERVENTION: FOOD AND NUTRITION

- The MyPyramid Food Guidance System: 4 cups of milk or equivalent source of calcium; 2–3 servings of meat or equivalent; 6–12 servings from the bread group; 2–4 servings of fruit or juices; 3–5 servings from vegetable group.
- For energy needs, see nutrient recommendation charts. Snacks should be planned as healthy inclusions in the diet.

	Recommendation	
Nutrient	**Males 14–18 Years**	**Females 14–18 Years**
Energy	3152 kcal/d	2368 kcal/d
Protein	52 g/d or 0.85 g/kg/d	46 g/d or 0.85 g/kg/d
Calcium	1300 mg/d	1300 mg/d
Iron	12 mg/d	15 mg/d
Folate	400 μg/d	400 μg/d
Phosphorus	1250 mg/d	1250 mg/d
Vitamin A	900 mg	700 mg
Vitamin C	75 mg/d	75 mg/d
Thiamin	1.2 mg/d	1.0 mg/d
Riboflavin	1.3 mg/d	1.0 mg/d
Niacin	16 mg/d	14 mg/d

Data from: Food and Nutrition Board, Institute of Medicine. *Dietary reference intakes for energy, carbohydrate, fiber, fat, fatty acids, cholesterol, protein, and amino acids (macronutrients)*. Washington, DC: National Academy Press, 2002.

- Protein intake should be sufficient to support growth.
- Adequate zinc and iodine are needed for growth and sexual maturation; use iodized salt and foods such as meat and dairy.
- Calcium is needed for bone growth; vitamins D and A are also essential in this age group. Iron is needed for menstrual losses in girls; obese teens may be an at-risk group that is often not considered (Nead et al, 2004).
- Debut age of drinking (alcohol) is important. If drinking begins before age 15, there is twice the risk of substance abuse and four times the risk of dependence.
- Diet for athletes: an acceptable diet for the athlete would be a normal diet for age, sex, and level of activity plus adequate intake of carbohydrates and fluids. Avoid excesses of protein and inadequate replacement of electrolytes (see Sports Nutrition entry).
- For pregnant teens, follow guidelines listed in Table 1-10.

CLINICAL INDICATORS

Clinical/History		Lab Work
Age Height Weight Weight/height percentile BMI or healthy body weight Waist to hip ratio Recent changes (height, weight) Diet history	Tanner stage of sexual maturation Hydration status (I & O) Physical activity level or athletics Physical handicaps Disordered eating patterns Gastrointestinal (GI) complaints	H & H, serum Fe Glucose Chol Trig Albumin (if needed) Retinol-binding protein (RBP) Na+, K+ Ca++, Mg++, phosphorus

Common Drugs Used and Potential Side Effects

- Vitamin-mineral supplements are not needed, except for pregnant teens or teens whose diets are generally inadequate (such as those following an unplanned vegetarian pattern or restricted energy plans). The majority of American teens do not use supplements; those who do use them tend to eat a more nutrient-dense diet than those who do not. Vitamins A and E, calcium, and zinc tend to be low regardless of use of supplements among all teens (Stang, 2000). In addition, excesses of these nutrients are not recommended and may lead to toxic levels of vitamins A and D if taken indiscriminately.
- Discuss the relevance of tolerable upper intake levels (ULs) from the dietary reference intakes of the National Academy of Sciences. These levels were set to protect individuals from receiving too much of any nutrient from diet and dietary supplements.
- Monitor use of nonprescription medications (such as aspirin, cold remedies, etc.) and use of illegal drugs, including marijuana and alcohol. Side effects may in-

TABLE 1-10 Special Considerations for Adolescent Pregnancy

Issue	Comments
Mother is still growing	Check gynecological age (chronological age less age of menarche) to determine future potential growth of the mother.
Low birth weight (LBW) and prematurity are common.	Fetuses grow more slowly in 10- to 16-year olds. Increased weight in the last trimester is helpful in lessening the incidence of LBW.
Goal: optimal fetal growth and maintain an optimal nutritional status during and after gestation for the growing mother	By the end of the pregnancy, the mother's desired weight gain should be between 25 and 35 lb. Add the desired increments for energy for requirements of same-age nonpregnant teens, or monitor the weight gain pattern to assess the adequacy of the present diet. Adolescents are at high risk of gaining an excessive amount of weight during pregnancy and should be monitored during pregnancy by dietetics professionals (Howie et al, 2003).
Protein requirements	Protein requirement is 1.1 g/kg body weight for most adolescents.
Problem nutrients include calcium, zinc, iron, and vitamins A and C	The physician will prescribe prenatal vitamins.
Meal patterns	Diet may include 5 cups of milk, 3 servings of meat, 4 servings of fruits/vegetables, and 4 servings of breads/cereals. Three snacks daily will be needed.
Nutrients needed	Consume a wide variety of foods, including nutrient-dense choices: Vitamin A: chicken liver, cantaloupe, mango, spinach, apricots. Vitamin C: citrus fruits and juices, broccoli, spinach, melon, strawberries. Calcium: low-fat milk, yogurt, broccoli, cheddar cheese, low-fat shakes, skim-milk cheeses. Iron: liver, rice, whole milk, raisins, baked potatoes, enriched cereal. Vitamin B_6: white meats, bananas, potatoes, egg yolks. Folacin: wheat germ, spinach, asparagus, strawberries. Zinc: apples, chicken, peanut butter, tuna, rice, whole milk.
Bad habits, cravings, and aversions	Discourage skipping of meals. Cravings are common, especially for chocolate, fruit, fast foods, pickles, and ice cream. Watch for aversions to meat, eggs, and pizza during this time.
Iron deficiency anemia (IDA) during pregnancy	Women who conceive during or shortly after adolescence are likely to enter pregnancy with low or absent iron stores. IDA during pregnancy is associated with significant morbidity for mothers and infants; supplementation during adolescence is a strategy to improve iron balance in pregnant teens (Lynch, 2000).
Smoking	Pregnant teens are more likely to smoke, to deliver preterm infants, and to have their infants die in the first year than other mothers (Markovitz et al, 2005). Counseling methods must consider that they are still teens.
Dietitian as another authoritarian adult	Encourage the teen to see herself as having a key role in providing good nutritional support for her new family. Allow her to express her feelings and concerns openly.
WIC Program	Encourage enrollment in organized programs such as WIC where an individualized nutrition risk profile is developed for each pregnant teen, and a specific nutrition rehabilitation program is effective. Positive outcomes are noted in birth weight, rates of low or very low birth weight, preterm delivery, maternal morbidity, and perinatal morbidity/mortality (Dubois et al, 1997).

clude poor oral dietary intakes of several nutrients. Smoking cigarettes tends to decrease serum levels of vitamin C.

Herbs, Botanicals, and Supplements

- Herbs and botanical supplements should not be used without discussing with the physician. In general, these supplements have not been proven to be safe for adolescents. There may be subgroups who are at risk for inappropriate use of these products (e.g., individuals with eating disorders and athletes).
- In a study (Bell et al, 2004) of the use of supplements by teens, the most popular were multivitamin-mineral preparations. More males than females used both creatine and diuretics. Females consume herbal weight control products significantly more than males. Athletes reported supplementing with creatine and protein. There may be misguided beliefs in performance enhancement by these products.

INTERVENTION: NUTRITION EDUCATION, COUNSELING, CARE MANAGEMENT

- Explain the MyPyramid Food Guidance System and the rationale behind the concepts. Use of the Healthy Eating Index may be a good way of assessing usual intake of healthful and less healthful foods (Feskanich et al, 2004).
- Explain the relation of diet to the needs of the adolescent athlete, as well as its influence on skin, weight control, and general appearance. Educate about desirable snacks, especially fruits and vegetables. School-based interventions to promote healthy choices are often beneficial (French et al, 2004).

- Help the family recognize the adolescent's need for independence. This may include choosing meals and snack items.
- Emphasize dental health and oral hygiene in relation to diet.
- Diets of teens are often low in vitamins A and C, folate, and iron. Discuss the concept of nutrient density; food comparison charts are useful. Encourage a minimum of five servings of fruits and vegetables daily.
- Discuss body image, heroes, and peer pressure. Boys generally want larger biceps, shoulders, chests, and forearms. Girls often want smaller hips, waistlines, and thighs, and larger bustlines.
- Emphasize the importance of not skipping meals, especially breakfast. Discourage obsessions with dieting and weight (Neumark-Sztainer et al, 2004). Promote safe dieting practices when needed (Calderon et al, 2004). The 5-year period between adolescence and adulthood is a time of potential weight gain (Gordon-Larsen et al, 2004).
- Discuss calcium and vitamin D; many adolescent girls consume inadequate amounts. Assess current intake by asking questions such as: How many times a day do you drink milk or eat cheese and yogurt? Have you had any bone fractures? Low-fat dairy products may be helpful for maintaining or achieving a healthy body weight; use 3–4 servings daily (Lappe et al, 2005; Novotny et al, 2004). Teens who live in northern climates may need to be extra careful about increasing vitamin D intake (Sullivan et al, 2005).
- Teens respond well to discussions that respect their independence, sense of justice, and idealism. One of their roles is to establish a clear identity of how they fit into the world. Teens spend increased amounts of time with their friends but still tend to conform to parental ideals when it comes to values, education, and long-term life plans.
- Teens often feel that "it can't happen to me," prompting them to take unnecessary risks like drinking and driving ("I won't crash this car"), having unprotected sex ("I can't possibly get pregnant"), or smoking ("I can't possibly get cancer"). Effects of various nutrients on appearance or energy levels may be helpful since approaches that highlight future diseases are less meaningful to this age group.
- Parents need to be aware of the availability of soft drinks in school vending machines and to express their opinions to the local school authorities (Hendel-Paterson et al, 2004). Encourage family meals but also discuss options for nourishing meals eaten away from home ("portable foods").
- Consumption of fast food is common and may contribute to weight gain if not carefully monitored (Ebbeling et al, 2004). Figure 1-8 shows meal planning using food models.

Patient Education—Food Safety Tips

- Since teens may not think about the consequences of their actions, gentle reminders about hand washing and safe food handling may be important. Use of hand sanitizers may be popular among teen girls.
- Avoid raw or partially cooked eggs, raw or undercooked fish or shellfish, and raw or undercooked meats because of potential foodborne illnesses.
- Do not use raw (unpasteurized) milk or products made from it.
- Avoid serving unpasteurized juices and raw sprouts.

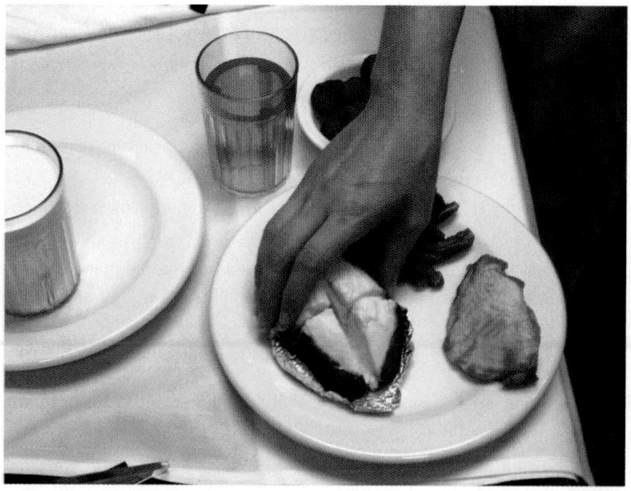

Figure 1-8 Planning a healthy meal using food models. (Permission provided by R. High.)

- Only serve processed deli meats and frankfurters that have been reheated to steaming hot temperature.
- Safe food handling is an important part of school food service (American Dietetic Association, 2003a).

For More Information

- American Academy of Child and Adolescent Psychology
  http://www.aacap.org/
- Attention Deficit Hyperactivity Disorder
  http://www.nimh.nih.gov/publicat/adhd.cfm#adhd14
- Body Image
  http://www.focusas.com/BodyImage.html
- Bright Futures—Adolescence
  http://brightfutures.aap.org/web/
- Center for Adolescent and Family Studies
  http://www.indiana.edu/~cafs/
- Food Safety for Teens
  http://www.fsis.usda.gov/food_safety_education/for_kids_&_teens/index.asp
- Good Parents.com
  http://www2.goodparentsinc.com/res_articles.htm
- Vegetarian Nutrition for Teens
  http://www.vrg.org/nutrition/teennutrition.htm

ADOLESCENCE—CITED REFERENCES

American Dietetic Association. Position of the American Dietetic Association: nutrition services: an essential component of comprehensive health programs. *J Am Diet Assoc.* 103:505, 2003a.

American Dietetic Association. Position of The American Dietetic Association: child and adolescent food and nutrition programs. *J Am Diet Assoc.* 103:887, 2003b.

Bell A, et al. A look at nutritional supplement use in adolescents. *J Adolesc Health.* 34:508, 2004.

Berkey CS, et al. Relation of childhood diet and body size to menarche and adolescent growth in girls. *Am J Epidemiol.* 152:446, 2000.

Calderon LL, et al. Dieting practices in high school students. *J Am Diet Assoc.* 104:1369, 2004.

Dubois S, et al. Ability of the Higgins Nutrition Intervention Program to improve adolescent pregnancy outcome. *J Am Diet Assoc.* 97:871, 1997.

Ebbeling CB, et al. Compensation for energy intake from fast food among overweight and lean adolescents. *JAMA.* 291:2828, 2004.

Erikson EH. *Identity youth and crisis.* New York: W. W. Norton, 1968.

Feskanich D, et al. Modifying the Healthy Eating Index to assess diet quality in children and adolescents. *J Am Diet Assoc.* 104:1375, 2004.
Fiore H, et al. Potentially protective factors associated with healthful body mass index in adolescents with obese and nonobese parents: a secondary data analysis of the third national health and nutrition examination survey, 1988-1994. *J Am Diet Assoc.* 106:55, 2006.
French SA, et al. An environmental intervention to promote lower-fat food choices in secondary schools: outcomes of the TACOS Study. *Am J Public Health.* 94:1507, 2004.
Galloway AT, et al. Parental pressure, dietary patterns and weight status among girls who are "picky eaters." *J Am Diet Assoc.* 105:541, 2005.
Gordon-Larsen P, et al. Five-year obesity incidence in the transition period between adolescence and adulthood: the National Longitudinal Study of Adolescent Health. *Am J Clin Nutr.* 80:569, 2004.
Gortmaker S, et al. Television viewing as a cause of increasing obesity among children in the United States, 1986–1990. *Arch Pediatr Adolesc Med.* 1996; 150:356.
Greer FR, Krebs N. Optimizing bone health and calcium intakes of infants, children, and adolescents. *Pediatrics* 117:578, 2006.
Hendel-Paterson M, et al. Parental attitudes towards soft drink vending machines in high school. *J Am Diet Assoc.* 104:1597, 2004.
Herbold NH, Frates SE. Update of nutrition guidelines for the teen: trends and concerns. *Curr Opin Pediatr.* 12:303, 2000.
Howie LD, et al. Excessive maternal weight gain patterns in adolescents. *J Am Diet Assoc.* 103:1653, 2003.
Ilich-Ernst JZ, et al. Iron status, menarche, and calcium supplementation in adolescent girls. *Am J Clin Nutr.* 68:880, 1998.
Lappe JM, et al. Girls on a high-calcium diet gain weight at the same rate as girls on a normal diet: a pilot study. *J Am Diet Assoc.* 104:1361, 2004.
Louwman MW, et al. Signs of impaired cognitive function in adolescents with marginal cobalamin status. *Am J Clin Nutri.* 72:762, 2000.
Lynch SR. The potential impact of iron supplementation during adolescence on iron status in pregnancy. *J Nutri.* 130:448, 2000.
Markovitz BP, et al. Socioeconomic factors and adolescent pregnancy outcomes: distinctions between neonatal and post-neonatal deaths? *BMC Public Health.* 5:79, 2005.
Messina V, Reed-Mangels A. Considerations in planning vegan diets: children. *J Am Diet Assoc.* 101:661, 2001.
Nead KG, et al. Overweight children and adolescents: a risk group for iron deficiency. *Pediatrics* 114:104, 2004.
Neumark-Sztainer D, et al. Weight-control behaviors among adolescent girls and boys: implications for dietary intake. *J Am Diet Assoc.* 104:913, 2004.
Novotny R, et al. Dairy intake is associated with lower body fat and soda intake with greater weight in adolescent girls. *J Nutr.* 134:1905, 2004.
Rampersaud GC, et al. Breakfast habits, nutritional status, body weight and academic performance in children and adolescents. *J Am Diet Assoc.* 105: 743, 2005.
Stang J, et al. Relationships between vitamin and mineral supplement use, dietary intake, and dietary adequacy among adolescents. *J Am Diet Assoc.* 100:905, 2000.
Sullivan SS, et al. Adolescent girls in Maine are at risk for vitamin D insufficiency. *J Am Diet Assoc.* 105:971, 2005.

PHYSICAL FITNESS AND STAGES OF ADULTHOOD

SPORTS NUTRITION

NUTRITIONAL ACUITY RANKING: LEVEL 2

DEFINITIONS AND BACKGROUND

Many athletes are involved in running, jogging, weight lifting, or wrestling (active sports) when they seek nutritional guidance. Weight control guidance, disordered eating patterns, and wellness guidance are common; only a few athletes have a true clinical concern such as diabetes or gastrointestinal problems. During high physical activity, energy and protein intakes must be met to maintain body weight, replenish glycogen stores, and provide adequate protein for building and repairing tissues (American Dietetic Association, 2000).

The needs of child athletes have not been well studied. Sports training does not appear to affect growth, maturation, or nutritional status during puberty in most cases (Fogelholm et al, 2000). Use of carbohydrate drinks may be essential to maintain energy intake and to prevent dehydration (Unnithan and Goulopoulu, 2004).

Female children and adolescent athletes may develop nonanemic iron deficiency (Unnithan and Goulopoulu, 2004), disordered eating, menstrual dysfunction, or decreased bone mineral density; and pediatricians need to carefully monitor their health closely (American Academy of Pediatrics, Committee on Sports Medicine and Fitness, 2000). Recreational athletes should be screened for iron deficiency using serum ferritin, serum transferrin receptor, and hemoglobin (Sinclair and Hinton, 2005).

Female athletes are under intense pressure to have a low percentage of body fat for performance, which may result in a vulnerable athlete resorting to disordered eating and subsequently developing amenorrhea and osteoporosis, the "female athlete triad" (Sanborn et al, 2000). The consequences of lost bone mineral density can be devastating; premature osteoporotic fractures can occur, and lost bone mineral density may never be regained (Hobart and Smucker, 2000). Winter sports may be more protective of bone density than some other types of sports because of the vigor required (Meyer et al, 2004).

The female athlete triad is a serious syndrome that requires a multidisciplinary approach. Perfectionism is the trait most likely to suggest risk for disordered eating, especially in varsity athletes (Hopkinson and Lock, 2004). Prevention efforts require de-emphasis of a low percentage of body fat and an adequate emphasis on good nutrition.

The primary fuel for athletic events using less than 50% VO_{2max} (or aerobic capacity) is fat. Muscle glycogen and blood glucose supply half of the energy for aerobic exercise during a moderate workout (at or below 60% of VO_{2max} or aerobic capacity) and nearly all the energy during a hard workout (above 80% of aerobic capacity). In short-duration events of more than 70% VO_{2max} (as in events like swimming or sprint running), glycogen is the key fuel. In long-duration events or activities of more than 70% VO_{2max} (such as long-distance running, cycling, or swimming), muscle glycogen can be depleted in 100–120 minutes; maintaining a high-carbohydrate daily diet while training for adequate glycogen replenishment is necessary in these cases.

Carbohydrate (CHO) ingestion during prolonged exercise and CHO loading before exercise can have different effects on fuel substrate kinetics. The glycemic index of the carbohydrates consumed during the immediate postexercise period might not be important as long as sufficient carbohydrate is consumed; high insulin concentrations following a high–glycemic index meal later in the recovery period could facilitate further muscle glycogen resynthesis (Stevenson et al, 2005). Elite athletes may metabolize CHO more effectively than nonathletes, but nutritional factors still affect glycemic control. It appears that elite power athletes appear to be more insulin resistant than elite endurance athletes (Chou et al, 2005).

Performance in endurance events is dependent upon maximal aerobic power as sustained by the availability of substrates (carbohydrates and fats). Protein has the role of maintaining and repairing muscle mass and tissues; a sufficient but not excessive intake is important. Excessive protein intakes may cause dehydration. In a study of gymnasts, it was found that they had a lower weekly calorie intake but a higher intake from dietary protein than nonathletes. Gymnasts are often at risk of malnutrition, which when compounded with intense physical exercise, could lead to immunosuppression in these athletes (Lopez-Varela et al, 2000).

Fatigue is associated with reduced muscle glycogen; increasing muscle glycogen or blood glucose prolongs performance, while increasing fat and decreasing CHO decreases performance. This has led to an emphasis on CHO intake in athletes in endurance sports, which quite often leads to low energy intake (Pendergast et al, 2000). Trained individuals have higher levels of fat oxidative capacity, which spares glycogen during endurance sports. Use of isocaloric high-fat diets (42–55%) maintains adequate CHO levels compared to diets composed of low fat intake (10–15%). Endurance runners who eat a low-fat diet may not consume enough energy, essential fatty acids (EFAs), and some minerals, especially zinc; these inadequate intakes may compromise their performance (Horvath et al, 2000). Pendergast et al (2000) suggest consideration of a diet comprising 20% protein, 30% CHO, and 30% fat, with the remaining 20% of the energy distributed between CHO and fat based on the intensity and duration of the sport.

Athletes should be well hydrated before the start of exercise and should drink enough fluid during and after exercise to balance fluid losses. Consumption of sports drinks containing carbohydrates and electrolytes during exercise will provide fuel for the muscles, help maintain blood glucose and the thirst mechanism, and decrease the risk of dehydration or hyponatremia (American Dietetic Association, 2000).

INTERVENTION: OBJECTIVES

- Promote healthy, safe eating habits and activities that can be continued throughout life. Aerobic activity is especially beneficial, as is resistance (weight) training. Participation in sports activity can be an important component of obesity prevention programs (Alfano et al, 2002).
- Promote improved performance.
- Correct faddist beliefs, participation in dangerous dieting trends, meal skipping, and other unhealthy eating behaviors.
- Prevent or correct amenorrhea, which may result from poor energy and fat intake. Monitor or correct eating disorders, such as bulimia and anorexia nervosa.
- Help prevent injuries, dehydration, overhydration, and hyponatremia.
- Meet extra energy requirements created by a higher BMR for metabolically active muscle mass.
- Enhance overall health and fitness. Maintain healthy body weight; evaluate body fatness and counsel accordingly (Table 1-11).
- Protect bone density and immune function. Prolonged exercise can depress the immune system, and it is recommended that a balanced diet be consumed (Gleeson et al, 2004). Intake of 30–60 g of carbohydrate during sustained and intensive exercise seems to limit the rise in stress hormone levels (Gleeson et al, 2004).

TABLE 1-11 Body Fat Standards

A certain amount of fat is essential to bodily functions. Fat regulates body temperature, cushions and insulates organs and tissues, and is the main form of energy storage. Ranges of body fat standards have been established by the American Council on Exercise and are listed below.

Stages	Men	Women
Essential for life	4–5%	10–12%
Athletes	6–13%	14–20%
Acceptable	18–25%	25–31%
Clinical obesity	25%	32%
Childlren's reference levels[a]	14% newborn	14% newborn
	13% 10-year-old boy	19% 10-year-old girl

Source: American Council on Exercise, http://www.acefitness.org/fitfacts/fitfacts_list.aspx; accessed December 20, 2005.

[a] From: Shils M, et al. *Modern nutrition in health and disease*. 9th ed. Philadelphia: Lippincott Williams & Wilkins, 1999, p. 799.

INTERVENTION: FOOD AND NUTRITION

- For active individuals, use a normal diet for age and sex with special attention to energy needs for the specific activity and frequency; 50–60% CHO is generally a good target. Athletes do not always consume sufficient levels of carbohydrate and protein, although males are more likely to do so than females, especially because females often want to lose weight (Hinton et al, 2004).
- Protein requirements should be calculated by age and sex, with a slightly higher requirement in endurance sports activity (Gleeson, 2005). Avoid excesses of protein, but be aware of the role that an adequate protein to calorie ratio plays in preventing amenorrhea and in maintaining an adequate iron status. It is important to avoid running out of glycogen, when protein would be used for energy. Table 1-12 provides estimates of protein needs for athletes.
- Extra riboflavin may be needed to meet muscle demands (Manore, 2000). Inclusion of dairy foods should be sufficient for all except the most strenuous activities.
- Fluid replacement may be essential with a calculation of 1 mL/kcal used for an average. Do not dilute sports

TABLE 1-12 Protein Needs by Type of Athletics

Protein Needed by Type of Athletics	Grams Protein Per Kilogram Body Mass Per Day
Athlete undertaking general training program	1.0
Endurance athlete undertaking moderate to heavy training	1.2–1.6
Endurance athlete undertaking extreme training program or competition	2.0
Strength athlete undertaking heavy training program	1.2–1.7
Adolescent athletes	2.0

Source: Australian Institute of Sport, www.ais.org.au/nutrition.

drinks because they have been formulated to have between 6 and 8% CHO along with an appropriate amount of electrolytes.

- Electrolytes must be carefully monitored and replaced. Newer sports drinks on the market contain glucose polymers with lower osmolality than sugared drinks or fruit juice. Gatorade and other recently formulated sports drink products are acceptable.
- Avoid fads such as omission of meat from the diet. Heme iron is important, and meat is also a good source of zinc. Dried beans and enriched cereals are also good suggestions for iron.
- Ensure adequate calcium intake for women (1–1.5 g/d) to prevent osteoporosis and to reduce muscle cramping and stress fractures. Weight-bearing exercises, such as walking and running in moderation, tend to be especially beneficial for bone mineral density accumulation.
- Maintain total fat intake at a level determined by age, medical status, and type of performance and endurance required.
- Prevent meal skipping. Breakfast is especially important in maintaining homeostasis. Small meals or frequent small snacks are useful for some individuals.
- There is some evidence that antioxidant foods may be useful for correcting "oxidative stress." Supplemental sources are not recommended in lieu of foods rich in these substances.
- Because athletes train almost daily, glucose loading is not recommended for endurance activities. Based on time spent training, most athletes should consume 6–10 g of CHO per kg of body weight on a daily basis (Berning, 2004). In addition, complex CHO in the form of starch can help with glycogen storage; see Table 1-13 for tips on planning meals before and after events. Figure 1-9 shows a runner.

CLINICAL INDICATORS

Clinical/History

Height
Weight
Goal weight
BMI
Healthy body weight range for height
Diet/intake history
Hydration (I & O)

Lab Work

H & H, serum Fe
Transferrin
Na+, K+, chloride
Serum glucose
BP
Alb, transthyretin (if needed)
Chol—high-density lipoprotein (HDL), low-density lipoprotein (LDL), total
Trig
Serum insulin
Ca++, Mg++
Alk phos

Common Drugs Used and Potential Side Effects

- If an athlete is in a sport that requires drug testing, check first with the U.S. Olympic Committee or the National Collegiate Athletic Association (NCAA) before using any drug. Androstenedione and anabolic steroids do promote muscle mass enhancement but are not allowed. Steroids affect numerous nutritional parameters. Take a careful drug history and discuss all side effects as appropriate.
- Salt tablets should be discouraged. A balanced sports drink is more desirable.
- Discuss the relevance of tolerable upper intake levels (ULs) from the latest dietary reference intakes of the National Academy of Sciences. These levels were set to protect individuals from receiving too much of any nutrient from diet and dietary supplements. Discuss the fact that excessive use of vitamin-mineral supplements can lead to toxicity, especially for vitamins A and D.

Herbs, Botanicals, and Supplements

- Herbs and botanical supplements should not be used without discussing with the physician, especially for underlying medical conditions. Use of supplements is common in athletes, and there may be undesirable side effects (Burns et al, 2004). The Food and Drug Administration (FDA) has proposed new guidelines for stricter monitoring of dietary supplements.
- Some supplements may be contaminated with banned substances, and if the athlete is found to have a banned substance in their system, actions will be taken by the regulatory agency (International Olympic Committee, NCAA, and other sports sanctioned agencies). Athletes must be aware that the supplements they are taking may be contaminated. The FDA has announced major regulatory initiatives to implement the Dietary Supplementation Health and Education Act (DSHEA) more effectively.
- Ergogenic aids are expensive and not necessary; use with caution only. A well-balanced diet will suffice for most athletic events (American Dietetic Association, 2000).
- Creatine supplementation increases the capacity of skeletal muscle to perform work during periods of alternating intensity exercises, possibly because of increased aerobic phosphorylation and flux through the creatine kinase system (Rico-Sanz and Mendez Marco, 2000). Creatine supplements have a slight beneficial effect with strength training (Becque et al, 2000).
- Ginseng may be used for performance enhancement. It should not be taken with warfarin, insulin, oral

TABLE 1-13 Guidelines for Planning Pre- and Postevent Meals

Pregame

- Eat lightly before an athletic competition.
- Eat complex carbohydrates, keep protein and fat intakes low because these slow digestion.
- Avoid bulky foods (raw fruits and vegetables, dry beans and peas, and popcorn), which may stimulate bowel movements.
- Avoid gas-forming foods such as vegetables from the cabbage family and cooked dry beans.
- Eat slowly and chew well.
- Drink water to be adequately hydrated: drink 2 cups of cool water 1–2 hours before the event and 1–2 cups of fluid 15 minutes before the event.
- Avoid drastic changes in normal diet routine immediately prior to competition. Some athletes prefer to focus on favorite foods.

Athlete Nutrition Guidelines Postgame Rules

- Consume carbohydrate-rich foods and beverages as soon as possible after competition to replenish glycogen stores quickly and get the athlete back into performance shape. Fruits, juices, and high-carbohydrate drinks are examples.
- Athletes training hard for several hours per day should consume 1.5 g of CHO per kg within 30 minutes postexercise followed by an additional 1.5 g of CHO per kg 2 hours later for glycogen synthesis.
- Replace fluids that have been lost. For every pound that is lost, drink 2 cups of fluids.
- Replace any potassium or sodium that has been lost during competition or training by using foods. Fruits and vegetables are excellent sources of potassium. Replace sodium by eating salty foods, and if activity was vigorous and exceeded 2 hours, a sports beverage may be useful.
- Return to normal high-carbohydrate diet at the next meal. The following chart provides some useful estimates for carbohydrate and protein intake.

	Protein (grams)	Carbohydrate (grams)
200 CALORIES		
2 Starch Servings	6	30
1 Fruit Serving	0–4	6–15
Total	6–10	36–45
600 CALORIES		
4 Starch Servings	8	60
2 Fruits or 6 Vegetables	0–12	30
1 cup Fruit Juice or 4 oz Tofu	0–9	3–15
1 tsp Preserves or Syrup	0	13
Total	8–29	106–118

	Protein (grams)	Carbohydrate (grams)
400 CALORIES		
3 Starch Servings	6	45
1 Fruit or Vegetable	0–2	5–15
1 cup Fruit Juice or 4 oz Tofu	0–9	3–15
Total	6–17	53–75
800 CALORIES		
5 Starch Servings	10	75
3 Fruits or 6 Vegetables	0–12	30–45
1 cup Fruit Juice or 4 oz Tofu	0–9	3–15
1 tsp Preserves or Syrup	0	13
Total	10–31	121–148

One Starch Serving:

1/3 cup cooked rice, legumes, sweet potato

1/2 cup corn, potato, cooked cereal, pasta (cooked)

3/4 cup ready-to-eat cereal

3/4 cup winter squash

1 slice bread, 6-inch tortilla, 4-inch pancake

1/2 bagel, bun, English muffin; 6-inch pita bread

One Vegetable Exchange:

1/2 cup non-starchy vegetable

One Fruit Serving:

1 average piece fruit

1/2 banana or mango

1/2 cup fruit, canned fruit, or fruit juice

2 tbsp raisins, 3 prunes, 7 apricot halves

Sources: Adapted from Linda Boeckner, Extension Nutrition Specialist, University of Nebraska Panhandle Research and Extension Center; and the Vegetarian Resource Guidelines at http://www.vrg.org/nutshell/athletes.htm.

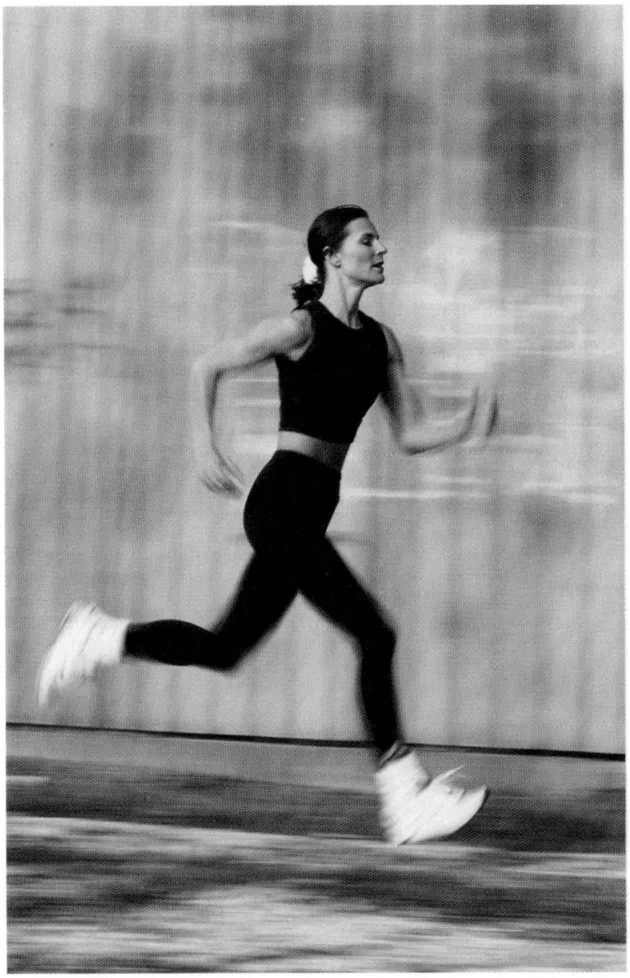

Figure 1-9 The running athlete. (Copyright 1999. Artville, LLC. All rights reserved.)

hypoglycemics, CNS stimulants, caffeine, steroids, hormones, antipsychotics, aspirin, or antiplatelet drugs.
- L-tryptophan, the precursor to serotonin, has sometimes been used to enhance performance. It should not be used with monoamine oxidase (MAO) inhibitors, antidepressants, or serotonin receptor antagonists. It can lead to symptoms of psychosis.
- Zinc supplements are sometimes taken to enhance performance. Zinc should not be taken with immunosuppressants, fluoroquinolones, and tetracycline.

INTERVENTION: NUTRITION EDUCATION, COUNSELING, CARE MANAGEMENT

- Dispel such myths as "milk is for children only," "meat is bad for you," "carbohydrates are fattening," and "dieting is the key to fluid control." Discuss appropriate alternatives.
- If the client is an adult child of alcoholic parents, he or she may need help in reducing such traits as perfectionism, compulsive or controlling behaviors, and the need for attention. Many athletes are driven by such traits and can cope more effectively with personalized counseling; refer to the appropriate health provider as needed.
- For weight control problems, address not only body weight but also family genetics and body type. Body fatness is another key issue; see Table 1-11. Parenting styles, socioeconomic issues, and environmental cues also play important roles in managing weight.
- Pre-event diets should be eaten up to an hour before the activity (Berning, 2004). Complex carbohydrates should be consumed, using less fat and protein because of their effect on digestive processes. See Table 1-13. After an event, recovery carbohydrate intake is suggested.
- Discuss how to obtain a high-calorie, high–complex carbohydrate diet with attention to the individual's preferences. In vigorous training programs, 3000–6000 kcal may be needed, especially for ultramarathons.
- Water is necessary to avoid dehydration. Drink fluids before, during, and after exercising. Weigh before and after events. Drink 1–2 cups of cool fluids 2 hours before the event, 4–8 oz immediately after the event, 8–16 oz after exercise, 8 oz of fluid between meals, and 8 oz of fluid with meals; replacement drinks should contain 80–120 mg of sodium per 8 oz (Berning, 2004).
- Alcoholic beverages do nothing to promote performance and may negatively affect neurologic and cardiac systems. Caffeine promotes mild physical endurance and alertness but is limited in competitive sports.
- There is no such thing as "quick energy." The habit of eating candy before a game can cause an insulin overshoot, leading to hypoglycemia. A balanced diet is more practical.
- Although female athletes with subclinical eating disorders tend to have dietary intakes of energy, protein, CHO, and certain micronutrients below desired levels, micronutrient status appears relatively unaffected (Hinton et al, 2004), probably due to use of supplements (Beals and Manore, 1998). Instituting an appropriate diet and moderating the frequency of exercise may result in return of menses (Hobart and Smucker, 2000).
- Some populations may have lower resting metabolic rates (RMRs), total daily expenditures, and physical activity energy expenditures than others. If these findings are confirmed, targeted interventions designed to decrease energy intake and to increase physical activity may become especially important to reduce the high obesity rates and associated metabolic disorders (Gannon et al, 2000).
- Women who are breastfeeding can exercise reasonably without adverse effects and may find that return to normal weight is easier than while being sedentary (Lovelady et al, 2004).

Patient Education—Food Safety Tips

- Reminders about hand washing and safe food handling may be important, especially for athletes with busy lifestyles.
- Use of scented hand sanitizers is often popular among teens and can be encouraged.

For More Information

- American Academy of Family Physicians
  Nutrition Prescription
  http://familydoctor.org/298.xml
- American College of Sports Medicine
  http://www.acsm.org/
- American Council on Exercise
  http://www.acefitness.org
  Recipes: http://www.acefitness.org/getfit/recipes.aspx

- American Alliance for Health, Physical Education, Recreation and Dance
  http://www.aahperd.org
- American Dietetic Association
  Sports and Cardiovascular Nutritionists
  http://www.scandpg.org/
- Centers for Disease Control Nutrition and Physical Activity
  http://www.cdc.gov/nccdphp/dnpa/
- Food and Nutrition Information Center
  http://www.nal.usda.gov/fnic/etext/000054.html
- Gatorade Sports Science Institute
  http://www.gssi.com
- National Institutes of Health
  http://www.nlm.nih.gov/medlineplus/exerciseandphysicalfitness.html
- Penn State University Fitness and Sports Nutrition
  http://nirc.cas.psu.edu/fitness.cfm
- President's Council on Physical Fitness and Sports
  http://www.fitness.gov/
- Sports Science Peer Reviewed Information
  http://www.sportsci.org/index.html?jour/03/03.htm&1
- U.S. Olympic Committee
  http://www.olympic-usa.org/
- Vanderbilt Medical center
  http://www.mc.vanderbilt.edu/health/wellness/child_nutrition.html
- Women's Sports Foundation
  http://www.womenssportsfoundation.org/

SPORTS NUTRITION—CITED REFERENCES

Alfano CM, et al. History of sport participation in relation to obesity and related health behaviors in women. *Prev Med.* 34:82, 2002.

American Academy of Pediatrics, Committee on Sports Medicine and Fitness. Medical concerns in the female athlete. *Pediatrics* 106:610, 2000.

American Dietetic Association. Position of the American Dietetic Association and the Canadian Dietetic Association: nutrition for physical fitness and performance for adults. *J Am Diet Assoc.* 100:1543, 2000.

Beals KA, Manore MM. Behavioral, psychological, and physical characteristics of female athletes with subclinical eating disorders. *Int J Sport Nutr Exerc Metab.* 10:128, 2000.

Becque MD, et al. Effects of oral creatine supplementation on muscular strength and body composition. *Med Sci Sport Exerc.* 32:654, 2000.

Berning J. Nutrition in athletic performance. In: Mahan K, Escott-Stump S, eds. *Krause's food, nutrition, and diet therapy.* 11th ed. Philadelphia: WB Saunders, 2004.

Burns RD, et al. Intercolleagiate student athlete use of nutritional supplements and the role of athletic trainers and dietitians in nutrition counseling. *J Am Diet Assoc.* 104:246, 2004.

Chou SW, et al. Characteristics of glycemic control in elite power and endurance athletes. *Prev Med.* 40:564, 2005.

Fogelholm M, et al. Growth, dietary intake, and trace element status in pubescent athletes and school children. *Med Sci Sport Exerc.* 32:738, 2000.

Gannon B, et al. Do African Americans have lower energy expenditure than Caucasians? *Int J Obes Relat Metab Disord.* 24:4, 2000.

Gleeson M. Interrelationship between physical activity and branched-chain amino acids. *J Nutr.* 135:1591S, 2005.

Gleeson M, et al. Exercise, nutrition and immune function. *J Sports Sci.* 22: 115, 2004.

Hinton PS, et al. Nutrient intakes and dietary behaviors of male and female collegiate athletes. *Int J Sport Nutr Exerc Metab.* 14:389, 2004.

Hobart JA, Smucker DR. The female athlete triad. *Am Fam Physician.* 61:3357, 2000.

Hopkinson RA, Lock J. Athletics, perfectionism, and disordered eating. *Eat Weight Disord.* 9:99, 2004.

Horvath PJ, et al. The effects of varying dietary fat on performance and metabolism in trained male and female runners. *J Am Coll Nutr.* 19:52, 2000.

Lopez-Varela S, et al. Nutritional status of young female elite gymnasts. *Int J Vitam Nutri Res.* 70:185, 2000.

Lovelady C, et al. Immune status of physically active women during lactation. *Med Sci Sports Exerc.* 36:1001, 2004.

Manore MM. Effect of physical activity on thiamine, riboflavin, and vitamin B-6 requirements. *Am J Clin Nutr.* 72:598S, 2000.

Meyer NL, et al. Bone mineral density of olympic-level female winter sport athletes. *Med Sci Sports Exerc.* 36:1594, 2004.

Pendergast DR, et al. A perspective on fat intake in athletes. *J Am Col Nutri.* 19:345, 2000.

Rico-Sanz J, Mendez Marco MT. Creatine enhances oxygen uptake and performance during alternating intensity exercise. *Med Sci Sports Exerc.* 32:379, 2000.

Sanborn CF, et al. Disordered eating and the female athlete triad. *Clin Sports Med.* 19:199, 2000.

Sinclair LM, Hinton PS. Prevalence of iron deficiency with and without anemia in recreationally active men and women. *J Am Diet Assoc.* 105:975, 2005.

Stevenson E, et al. The metabolic responses to high carbohydrate meals with different glycemic indices consumed during recovery from prolonged strenuous exercise. *Int J Sport Nutr Exerc Metab.* 15:291, 2005.

Unnithan VB, Goulopoulou S. Nutrition for the pediatric athlete. *Curr Sports Med Rep.* 3:206, 2004.

ADULTHOOD

NUTRITIONAL ACUITY RANKING: LEVEL 2

DEFINITIONS AND BACKGROUND

The period of young adulthood is generally 18–40 years old (careers are a priority); and middle adulthood is 40–65 years old (family is the primary focus). A healthy life expectancy measures the distribution of health status within a population. The World Health Organization has found that people living in poor countries face lower life expectancies than those in richer countries and also live a higher proportion of their lives in poor health (Mathers et al, 2004).

As important as it is to improve poor dietary habits, a review of family history and genetics related to the potential for chronic disease is also essential. Polymorphisms in genes can lead to differences in the level of susceptibility of individuals to adverse environmental issues, such as exposure to chemicals, or to reproductive success (Cummings and Kavlock, 2004). Effects on male reproduction attributable to gene–environment interaction involve infertility as a result of either organophosphorous (OP) pesticide interaction with the polymorphic paraoxonase (*PON1*) gene or antiandrogenic agent interaction with the androgen receptor (Cummings and Kavlock, 2004).

Female fertility has nutritional relationships in many cases. Methylenetetrahydrofolate reductase (MTHFR), folate metabolism, and dietary folic acid are considered in conjunction with preeclampsia and early pregnancy loss (Cummings and Kavlock, 2004). Male subfertility may also have nutritional relationships; zinc and folate both play an important role in healthy DNA and RNA synthesis (Wong et al, 2000), as may vitamin C and lycopene.

Healthy People 2010 supports changes in health and nutritional behaviors to improve quality of life and to increase longevity; peer pressure and persuasion may help promote long-term changes in adult behavior (Satia et al, 2001). For example, men can prevent a decline in sexual function by exercising vigorously, keeping weight in check, not smoking (or quitting smoking), and maintaining healthy vascular health (Esposito et al, 2004). Peer support may be helpful to start and maintain lifestyle changes.

Weight control is a major concern among adults. Over the past 40 years, BMI and weight have increased for both sexes, all ethnic groups, and all ages; mean height has also increased for most ages and for both sexes (Ogden et al, 2004). There are health implications with this average increase of 24 pounds (Ogden et al, 2004). Low physical activity level, high carbohydrate intake, and current smoking habits are associated with an increased risk of having metabolic syndrome that predisposes to cardiovascular events (Zhu et al, 2004). Both men and women should attempt to maintain a healthy body weight. If overweight, loss of 10 pounds can be an effective starting point to lower risks.

Prehypertension is now identified at lower levels of blood pressure, and up to 60% of adults may be affected, especially among African Americans, older people, low–socioeconomic status groups, and overweight individuals (Wang and Wang, 2004). Lifestyle modifications and use of appropriate medications may be needed.

Both genetics and conditioning influence taste preferences and intake. Taste seems to be innate, and responses to odors are more conditioned. The influence of genetic variation in taste on food intake depends on how perceptible sweet, fat, or bitter components are in foods and beverages as well as the value of convenience on personal dietary choices (Duffy and Bartoshuk, 2000). Female "supertasters" of bitterness may avoid high-fat or sweet foods because these oral sensations are too intense and thus less pleasant. Supertasters may taste more bitterness in vegetables but still enjoy eating them because of healthfulness and because condiments can be added (Duffy and Bartoshuk, 2000). It is important to work with individuals to employ sensory perceptions to identify foods that will help to achieve healthy eating patterns.

TABLE 1-14 Special Nutrition-Related Concerns of Adult Women[a]

Fibrocystic Breast Conditions: Fibrocystic breast conditions, formerly considered benign breast or fibrocystic breast disease, actually affect about half of all women and present with breast nodularity, swelling, and pain (Horner and Lampe, 2000). Excessive estrogen or sensitivity is the dominant theory. Randomized controlled studies have failed to support these nutrition interventions: decreased sodium or fluid and caffeine; increased use of primrose oil, herbal teas, vitamins A, C, E, and B_6, iodine, omega-3 fatty acids, and selenium. Overall, use of a low-fat (15–20% kcal), adequate fiber diet (30 g/d) and soy isoflavones seems to be useful (Horner and Lampe, 2000). Fruit and vegetable intake should be high (Wu et al, 2004). Figure 1-10 shows fibrocystic tissue.

[a] See specific entries for Anemia, Cancers, Cardiovascular Diseases, Diabetes, Eating Disorders, Osteoporosis, Overweight and Obesity, and Table 1-15 also.

Nutrition is involved in the 10 leading causes of death in women. Heart disease is the number one disabler and killer of women in the United States, whereas cancer is the leading cause of premature death. Table 1-14 lists special considerations for women, and Table 1-15 lists some concerns for men.

When adults are hospitalized, nutritional declines occur and lead to higher hospital charges (about $15,000 more) with more complications (Braunschweig et al, 2000). Refusal to follow dietary prescriptions can be frustrating to the nutrition professional. Longstanding dietary habits from childhood, confusion about orally communicated instructions or facts, coexisting depression, inadequate referral or information, literacy deficits, social influences and barriers, and even the right to refuse treatments all play a role (Stein, 2005). Understanding the reasons why patients refuse to follow a diet prescription is the first step in overcoming these obstacles and helping them achieve a healthier lifestyle.

INTERVENTION: OBJECTIVES

- Maintain quality of nutrition while compensating for energy needs lower than during periods of growth.
- Prevent obesity resulting from a sedentary lifestyle where relevant. Highly sedentary people lose 20–24% of overall muscle mass and strength. Every adult should accumulate

TABLE 1-15 Leading Causes of Death for Men in the United States in 2000 and Their Nutritional Implications

1. **Heart Disease:** hyperlipidemia and hypertension are commonly related (see appropriate entries).
2. **Cancer:** prostate, testicular, esophageal, and stomach cancers have special nutritional implications (see appropriate entries). Increasing intake of soy products, fruits, and vegetables and reducing red meat intake may be beneficial.
3. **Stroke:** high intake of sodium and alcohol are problematic, as is chronic hypertension that is untreated (see appropriate entry).
4. **Accidents:** excessive alcohol intake may be related (see appropriate entry).
5. **Chronic lower respiratory diseases:** weight loss or gain may aggravate breathing problems.
6. **Diabetes:** carbohydrate intake should be consistent and consumed at regular intervals.
7. **Influenza and pneumonia:** infectious diseases burn more energy, and weight loss can occur if intake is poor.
8. **Suicide:** depression and excessive alcohol intake may play a role (see appropriate entries).
9. **Kidney disease:** many renal diseases have implications for control of protein, sodium, electrolytes, and fluid. Kidney stones are more common in men than in women and drinking plenty of fluids and consuming adequate calcium may prevent onset or recurrence (see appropriate entries).
10. **Chronic liver disease and cirrhosis:** excessive alcohol intake is often related (see appropriate entry).

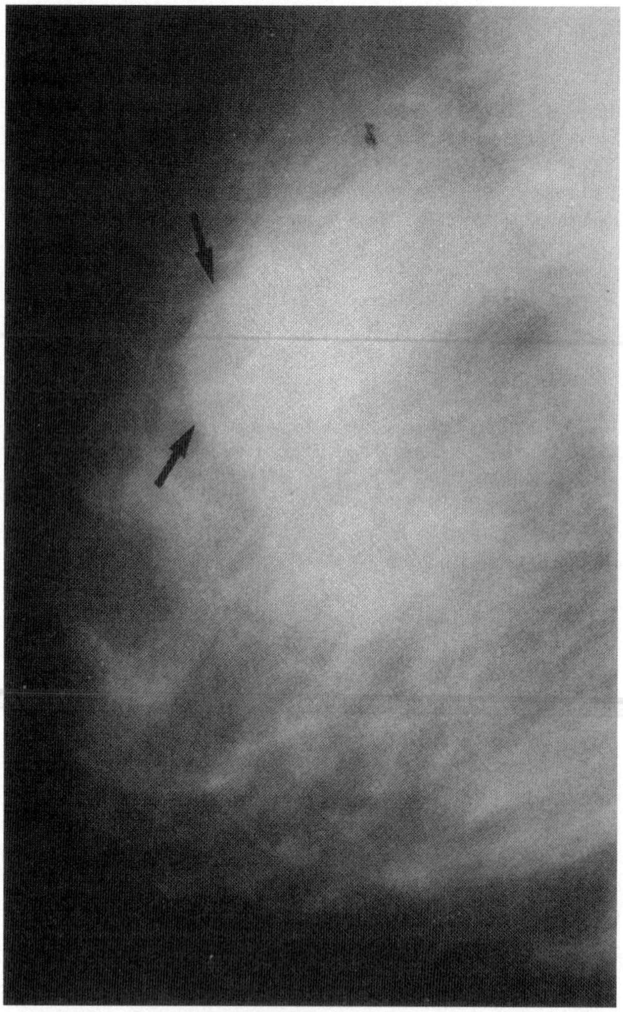

Figure 1-10 Fibrocystic breast tissue.

30 minutes or more of moderate-intensity physical activity on most days of the week. Also useful are strength training (resistance or weight training with 8–12 repetitions), isotonics, and aerobics (20 minutes of walking, jogging, swimming, or bicycling).

- Maintain a healthy lifestyle, which offers greater longevity than genetics alone. Losing excess weight, exercising, and eating a nearly meat-free diet are tips shared by many centenarians.
- Prevent or delay the onset of medical conditions (e.g., hypertension, osteoporosis, cardiovascular disease, diabetes, renal disorders, Alzheimer's disease, and cancers). Focus on a plant-based diet, rich in colorful fruits and vegetables plus nuts, seeds, and whole grains. Include fish and sources of omega-3 fatty acids, including walnuts, flaxseed, and dark-green leafy vegetables. A Mediterranean style of diet may be a good pattern to follow (Knoops et al, 2004).
- Improve nutrient density of meals, especially those eaten away from home. The average American eats 3–4 meals away from home each week. Making "each calorie count more" is a new concept message that encourages selecting foods that offer more per "bite." The Naturally Nutrient Rich (NNR) approach is helpful; encourage use of foods such as salmon, blueberries, bananas, whole-wheat grains, fat-free yogurt, broccoli, and top round steak (Drewnoski, 2004). These are "super foods."
- Use of a multivitamin-mineral supplement can assure that the basics are met, but a balanced diet provides other beneficial nutrients. For example, lutein and zeaxanthin from food are preferable over supplements for protection against age-related eye diseases such as macular degeneration.
- Promote adequate bone mass density, which peaks at 25–30 years of age. Osteopenia is common, and testing of bone density is recommended, especially in women over age 40.
- Iron deficiency affects approximately one half of all women. Correct through diet as far as possible. Avoid excesses, especially in men.
- Identify problems with food insecurity and their relationship to available foods and consumption patterns. For example, food insecurity is common among migrant workers and farmworker households (Quandt et al, 2004) and among those families with incomes below $15,000 (Stuff et al, 2004). Hunger is related to a variety of factors, including participation in food banks, dependence on family members and friends outside of the household for food, inadequate transportation, and not having a garden (Holben et al, 2004).
- **Infertility and Spontaneous Abortions:** High caffeine intake has been reported to delay conception in fertile women (Tolstrup et al, 2003), but evidence is inconclusive (Signorello et al, 2004). Body mass index that is high (over 35) or low (below 20) reduces the possibility of achieving pregnancy (American Dietetic Association, 2004). A normal female needs to have body fat levels that are suitable for reproduction; avoid having either too much or too little body fat (Fedorcsak et al, 2004). Infertility may be related to a number of factors, including male factor (25–40%), ovulation defect (20–30%), fallopian tube defect (20–30%), unexplained or other causes (10–24%), and endometriosis (5–10%) (Gharib, 2003). Among the polymorphic genes and environmental interactions related to prenatal development are P-glycoprotein (multidrug resistance protein); methylenetetrahydrofolate reductase (MTHFR), an enzyme in folate metabolism; transforming growth factor alpha (TGFα) and cigarette smoke; and alcohol dehydrogenase (ADH) and cytochrome P-450 (CYP)

SAMPLE NUTRITION DIAGNOSTIC STATEMENT

Fibrocystic Disease

PES: Inadequate fiber intake related to low intake of fruits, vegetables, and whole grains as evidenced by diet history indicating use of sandwiches from fast food restaurants 6 days per week.

Assessment Data (sources of info): Dietary recall, nutrient analysis of fiber intake, food and symptom diary, use of soy.

Intervention: Education and counseling about sources of fiber and how to obtain 30 grams daily; use of adequate fluid.

Monitoring and Evaluation: Food and symptom diary indicating fewer symptoms, and less density.

SAMPLE NUTRITION DIAGNOSTIC STATEMENT

Infertility

PES: Imbalance of nutrients related to low micronutrient intake (vitamins A and C, magnesium, and potassium) as evidenced by consistent omission of fruits and vegetables in dietary intake records and poor nutritional lab values.

Assessment Data: Dietary recall, nutrient analysis for vitamins and minerals, laboratory analyses.

Intervention: Counseling and education about a healthy diet for promoting optimal reproductive health.

Monitoring and Evaluation: Dietary intake records, increased intake of fruits and vegetables, improved nutritional lab reports.

SAMPLE NUTRITION DIAGNOSTIC STATEMENT

Menopause

PES: Harmful beliefs about food/nutrition related to regular intake of dietary supplements as evidenced by dietary recall indicating use of large doses of Chinese herbal remedies that are unsubstantiated by medical efficacy.

Assessment Data: Dietary recall, assessment of identified side effects from taking multiple herbs.

Intervention: Education and counseling about safe use of herbs and supplements for menopausal symptoms (soy, black cohosh, multivitamin-mineral supplements).

Monitoring and Evaluation: Dietary recall and dietary supplement usage pattern, side effect reports, improvement of symptoms of menopause.

2E1 in association with alcohol consumption (Cummings and Kavlock, 2004). Not only is it important to stop smoking and drinking alcohol, but adequate intakes of folate and vitamin B_{12} are essential for maintaining a successful pregnancy (American Dietetic Association, 2004).

- **Premenstrual Syndrome (PMS) and Premenstrual Dysphoric Disorder (PMDD):** Up to 40% of women experience symptoms including edema, migraines, depression, and mastalgia, and thus far, calcium supplementation has been found to be of greatest benefit (American Dietetic Association, 2004). Herbal supplements have no supporting evidence (Johnson, 2004). The doctor may recommend a general multivitamin-mineral supplement to assure adequacy of all nutrients.
- **Perimenopause:** Women who are undergoing the 2- to 10-year stage before menopause can experience many symptoms, including hot flashes, night sweats, fatigue, insomnia, weight gain, loss of libido, irregular periods, fibroids or heavy bleeding, breast pain, mood swings and irritability, cravings for sweets or alcohol, digestive problems, hair loss, stiffness or joint pain, anxiety, and depression. Women can maintain or add exercise, as well as assuring a healthy diet (see following item on menopause). Herbal remedies are available but not always effective.
- **Menopause:** Needs during menopause change because of declining levels of estrogens and other hormones and because of cessation of menstrual periods. This change decreases the need for extra iron. Hormone replacement therapy may promote development of cancer, so it is no longer the mainstay for preventing postmenopausal osteoporosis and fractures. Exercise, calcium, and vitamin D are important for this role. Encourage regular physical examinations as well. Because a healthy diet provides so many benefits, it is useful to consume a diet that is moderate in carbohydrate to avoid insulin shifts and that is adequate in lean proteins and moderate in fat to avoid weight gain. Vitamins C and E are important for their antioxidant properties. Whole grains, flax seed, and other omega-3 fatty acids may reduce inflammatory processes, which may aggravate hot flashes. While phytoestrogens such as soy and red clover do not seem to clearly make any difference in symptoms of menopause (Krebs, 2004), there have been positive results in some women. Isoflavones, lignans, and coumestans in soy foods and flaxseed can be included in most diets. Avoid large amounts of soy if breast cancer is a known risk. Botanical products such as black cohosh may have undesirable side effects (see herbal guidelines).
- **Postmenopause:** Older women may be at risk for poor nutritional intake because their diets tend to be more limited; they may have difficulty chewing; and they may no longer enjoy cooking (American Dietetic Association, 2004). Nutrient supplementation may be beneficial, especially for calcium, zinc, and vitamins found in fruits and vegetables.

INTERVENTION: FOOD AND NUTRITION

- Ensure intake from the MyPyramid Food Guidance System: 2–3 servings of milk, 2–3 servings of meat or substitute, 3–5 servings of vegetables, 2–4 servings of fruits, and 6–12 bread group servings. Fats, oils, sugars, and sweets are to be controlled as needed to increase or decrease energy intake. Be aware that foods from the fats/sweets/alcohol group often replace nutrient-dense foods in the American diet. Limit or eliminate foods that contain trans fatty acids whenever possible.
- Follow the dietary guidelines (see Table 1-2). Modify diet as needed for special medical conditions, such as hypertension, heart disease, and osteoporosis.
- Energy needs will vary by sedentary or active status; 30 kcal/kg/d is average and may range as low as 25 kcal/kg/d when weight loss is desired to 40 kcal/kg/d when weight gain is needed. Most adults are encouraged to maintain weight rather than gaining weight decade by decade after reaching adulthood. See nutritional recommendation charts.
- For most healthy adults, 0.8 g of protein/kg will suffice. Use fish, poultry, and nonmeat entrees (e.g., dry beans, peas, nuts as tolerated) regularly instead of just meat-centered meals. Soy products such as tofu, textured soy protein, soynut butter, or tempeh can be useful. The Continuing Survey of Food Intakes by Individuals (CSFII) has found that households with higher income tend to use more chicken and less beef and pork (Guenther et al, 2005).
- For carbohydrate, the Institute of Medicine has set the minimum intake at 130 g daily. In general, use of whole

grains, fresh fruits or vegetables, and low-fat dairy products will provide high-quality carbohydrate. Refined carbohydrates in sweetened beverages, desserts, and candy should be used less often.

- Mineral and phytochemical balance is important, including sodium, potassium, calcium, and magnesium. The DASH diet may be useful for designing meal patterns to lower blood pressure and lipids, when needed (Most, 2004).
- Eat a balanced diet. The most recent national study of What We Eat in America (United States Department of Agriculture, 2006) identified that vitamins A, C, and E and magnesium tend to be low in most diets; teen girls and older men and women tend to be low in zinc intakes; and potassium, calcium, vitamin D, vitamin K, and fiber are low as well.
- Hyperhomocysteinemia, the rise of plasma homocysteine levels above 15 μmol/L, is accepted as an independent risk factor for cardiovascular disease in men and women, and the B-complex vitamins are especially important to correct this (Aguilar et al, 2004).
- Adequate vitamins A, C, and E and selenium foods should be consumed for their antioxidant properties. Foods rather than supplements are recommended because of the phytochemical and biological properties that may be beneficial. For example, quercetin (found in apples, broccoli, oranges, tomatoes, kale, and onions) may help protect against cataracts.
- Phytochemicals are now recognized for their potential effect on prevention of chronic disorders. Soybeans, fruits, and vegetables seem to yield the greatest risk reductions. Soy protein, as in tofu and meat extenders, may reduce serum cholesterol and possibly reduce risks of some forms of cancer. Consume polyphenols (flavonoids from tea, cocoa, red wine, Concord grape juice, blueberries, and chocolate) that are protective of heart health. Arginine, sometimes recommended for enhancement of libido, is available from foods such as nuts, seeds, whole grains, and chocolate. Phytosterols are helpful; sunflower seeds, pistachio nuts, sesame seeds, and wheat germ are good sources.
- Women of childbearing age should include foods rich in folic acid, now available through fortification of grains, to prevent neural tube defects. Men may need to eat more folic acid–rich foods to lower risk for colorectal cancer. Cold cereals, cooked pinto or navy beans, asparagus, spinach, orange juice, lentils, and avocado should be planned into the diet regularly. Low folic acid, vitamin B_{12}, and vitamin B_6 can lead to high serum homocysteine levels; high levels are not only a cardiac risk factor, but also may contribute to Alzheimer's disease.
- Fiber-rich foods may help protect against heart disease, stroke, diabetes, high blood pressure, some types of cancer, constipation, and diverticulosis. They are also helpful with management of weight by increasing satiety with meals. Soluble fiber is found in pectins, gums, plums, apples, berries, figs, broccoli, potatoes, and okra. Insoluble fibers are found in bran cereal, whole-wheat bread, brown rice, legumes, vegetables, and many fruits. Nuts and seeds are also good sources of fiber.
- Favorable dietary habits promote health, whereas unfavorable habits are linked to various chronic diseases; an individual's "sense of coherence" (SOC) is reported to correlate with prevalence of some diseases to which dietary habits are linked (Lindmark et al, 2005).
- Functional food ingredients, including fortified, enriched, or enhanced foods, have a potentially beneficial effect on health when consumed as part of a varied diet on a regular basis (Hasler et al, 2004). Plant sterols and stanols are products that help to lower serum cholesterol levels; while these dietary products are more costly than the equivalent products, they are less expensive than statin drugs.
- A Mediterranean-style diet can enhance the effect of cholesterol-lowering statins in men (Gotto, 2003). It may be useful to plan menus accordingly. See Table 1-16 for a list of other functional foods to include regularly in the diet. Each food or ingredient should be assessed individually for its relative merit.
- Use spices and herbs liberally in cooking. Oregano, cinnamon, dill, savory, coriander, cumin, and other herbs have potent antioxidant properties.
- Family meals are often associated with positive dietary intakes and healthy behaviors. Family interaction can lower risks for loneliness-based eating for comfort. A positive atmosphere is encouraged. Information is available at http://www.cfs.purdue.edu/CFF/promotingfamilymeals/index.html.

	Recommendations	
Nutrient	**Males 19–50 Years**	**Males 51–70 Years**
Energy	3067 kcal/d	3067 kcal/d
Protein	56 g/d or 0.8 g/kg/d	56 g/d or 0.8 g/kg/d
Calcium	1000 mg/d	1200 mg/d
Iron	8 mg/d	8 mg/d
Folate	400 mg/d	400 mg/d
Phosphorus	700 mg/d	700 mg/d
Vitamin A	900 μg/d	900 μg/d
Vitamin C	90 mg/d	90 mg/d
Thiamin	1.2 mg/d	1.2 mg/d
Riboflavin	1.3 mg/d	1.3 mg/d
Niacin	16 mg/d	16 mg/d

	Recommendations	
Nutrient	**Females 19–50 Years**	**Females 51–70 Years**
Energy	2043 kcal/d	2043 kcal/d
Protein	46 g/d	46 g/d
Calcium	1000 mg/d	1200 mg/d
Iron	18 mg/d	8 mg/d
Folate	400 mg/d	400 mg/d
Phosphorus	700 mg/d	700 mg/d
Vitamin A	700 μg/d	700 μg/d
Vitamin C	75 mg/d	75 mg/d
Thiamin	1.1 mg/d	1.1 mg/d
Riboflavin	1.1 mg/d	1.1 mg/d
Niacin	14 mg/d	14 mg/d

Data from: Food and Nutrition Board, Institute of Medicine. *Dietary reference intakes for energy, carbohydrate, fiber, fat, fatty acids, cholesterol, protein, and amino acids (macronutrients)*. Washington, DC: National Academy Press, 2002.

TABLE 1-16 Functional Foods List

Food	Function
Almonds	Lower LDL and total cholesterol to reduce heart disease. Source of potassium, vitamin E, riboflavin, magnesium, and zinc.
Apples	Good source of fiber, quercetin in the skin.
Apricots	Good source of vitamins A and C, as well as lycopene. Cancer prevention.
Avocado	Reduces risk of heart disease, high blood pressure, and osteoporosis. Contains vitamins B_6 and E, folate, potassium, and fiber.
Bananas	Good source of potassium and magnesium, which are helpful to prevent heart disease, bone loss, and hypertension.
Barley	Good whole grain source.
Blueberries, and other berries	Reduce risk of cancer; may improve cognitive function. Contain vitamin C as well as anthocyanins, fiber, and ellagic acid.
Brazil nuts	Supply of selenium, which is a cancer preventive. Use no more than 2 per day.
Broccoli	Reduces risk of cancer and maintains healthy immune system. Sulforaphane detoxifies carcinogens.
Brown rice	Rich whole grain with phosphorus and potassium in greater amounts than white rice.
Brussels sprouts	Source of sulforaphane to prevent cancer; also good source of vitamin K.
Cabbage	Contains sulforaphane; consume often as a cancer prevention measure.
Canola oil	Good source of fatty acids, which reduce heart disease and cancer.
Cantaloupe	Great source of beta-carotene and vitamin C.
Carrots	Rich source of beta-carotene.
Cauliflower	Rich in sulforaphane and vitamin C; may protect against cancer.
Cheese	May decrease risk of colon cancer because of calcium content.
Chicken or turkey breast	Skinless poultry is a great source of protein and zinc; turkey is also high in B vitamins and selenium.
Chocolate	May decrease risk for cardiovascular disease; flavonoid content is a powerful antioxidant.
Citrus fruits	Limonoids reduce risk of certain cancers.
Cocoa	Rich source of flavonols; reduces risk of cancer and heart disease.
Collard greens and kale	Great source of carotenoids, vitamin C, lutein, sulforaphane, and calcium.
Cranberries	Improves urinary tract health and prevents infection; reduces risk of heart disease; may reduce periodontitis/gingivitis.
Cruciferous vegetables	Sulforaphane content helps to prevent cancer. Brussels sprouts, cauliflower, broccoli, and bok choy are in this family.
Edamame	Green soybeans, a staple in Asia. They can lower LDL cholesterol and may protect against colon cancer.
Fatty fish	Source of omega-3 fatty acids; helpful for brain, eye, and neurological health.
Flaxseed	Reduces risk of heart disease, high blood pressure, and osteoporosis. Provides lignans and alpha linolenic acid, an omega-3 fatty acid.
Garlic	Reduces risk of cancer; lowers cholesterol levels and blood pressure.
Kale	High in antioxidants lutein and zeaxanthin; protects eye health.
Kiwifruit	High in potassium, vitamin C, fiber, folate, magnesium, vitamin E, copper, and lutein. Great antioxidant fruit.
Legumes and beans	Lentils, dried beans, and peas provide folate, which reduces DNA damage and helps with cancer prevention. Rich in fiber, magnesium, potassium, protein, and iron.
Milk, non-fat	Reduces risk of osteoporosis, high blood pressure, and colon cancer. Good source of vitamin D, calcium, and potassium.
Oatmeal	Reduces total and LDL cholesterol levels.
Olive oil	Good source of monounsaturated fatty acids (MUFA), which reduce heart disease risk by improving cholesterol levels.
Onions	Sulfur-rich and full of quercetin (red or yellow are richer). Blood thinning to help lower blood pressure and LDL cholesterol levels.
Oranges	Great source of potassium and vitamin C.
Peaches	Good source of vitamin C, carotenoids, niacin, and potassium.
Peanut butter	Good source of protein, MUFA, and niacin.
Pork loin	Leanest cut of "red meat" sources. Protein, zinc, and iron source.
Prunes	Great source of antioxidants, fiber, potassium, and vitamins A and B_6.
Quinoa	Seed containing high amounts of protein, fiber, magnesium, potassium, vitamin E, riboflavin, zinc, copper, and iron.
Salmon, sardines, mackerel	Improve mental and visual function; reduce risk of heart disease and may prevent cancers. Rich omega-3 fatty acid source.
Shredded wheat	Great source of whole-grain fiber, as well as magnesium; helpful in maintaining normal blood glucose levels.
Soy	Reduces risk of heart disease by lowering LDL cholesterol; eases menopausal symptoms. Isoflavones have weak estrogenic effects.

TABLE 1-16 Functional Foods List *(continued)*

Food	Function
Spinach and romaine lettuce	Great source of lutein, carotenoids, and vitamin C; maintain healthy vision.
Squash, acorn	Rich in carotenoids, folate, vitamin C, and potassium; all helpful in reducing heart disease and cancer risk.
Strawberries	May lower blood pressure, reduce the risk of heart disease and some cancers, and improve memory.
Tea, black, green, or white	Reduces risk for stomach, esophageal, and skin cancers, and heart disease. Flavonoids neutralize free radicals.
Tofu	Great meat substitute; rich in protein and isoflavones and may be high in calcium.
Tomatoes	Reduce risk of prostate cancer and heart attack; rich in lutein, lycopene, and vitamin C. Lycopene protects cell membranes.
Tuna	Reduces risk of heart disease; high in vitamins B_6 and B_{12}, omega-3 fatty acids, and protein.
Walnuts	Lower total and LDL cholesterol and reduces risk of heart disease. Good source of vitamin E, alpha linolenic acid, minerals, and folate.
Whey protein	Immune-enhancing properties including lactoferrin, beta-lactoglobulin, alpha-lactalbumin, and immunoglobulins. Useful for intracellular conversion of cysteine to glutatione, a powerful antioxidant. Whey protein is found naturally in milk.
Whole grains	Reduce risk of certain cancers and heart disease. Contain saponins, flavonoids, and lignans.
Wine, red and grapes/grape juice	Reduce risk of cardiovascular disease and cancer because of resveratrol, a flavonoid (polyphenol).
Winter squash	Butternut squash is one example. Good source of beta-carotene, calcium, potassium, and folate.
Yogurt	Improves intestinal health because of bacterial (probiotic) content; reduces risk of cancer; lowers cholesterol. Rich source of calcium, vitamin B_{12}, magnesium, and protein. May also use cultured dairy products.

From: Marshall K. Therapeutic applications of whey protein. *Altern Med Rev.* 9:136, 2004; Functional Foods List, http://www.mealsmatter.org/EatingForHealth/FunctionalFoods/func_list.aspx; accessed January 31, 2006; Tufts University Health and Nutrition Letter, 23:1S, August 2005; Environmental Health newsletters, 2002–2006; and Produce for Better Health Foundation, http://www.5aday.com/; accessed January 31, 2006.

CLINICAL INDICATORS

Clinical/History

BP
Height
Weight, current
Weight, usual
BMI and waist to hip ratio
Recent weight changes
Healthy body weight (HBW) range
Diet history
Body fat analysis
Smoking
Alcohol use

Lab Work

Glucose
Chol—HDL, LDL, total
Trig
Na+, K+
Mg++, Ca++
H & H, serum Fe
Serum homocysteine
Serum folic acid and vitamin B_{12}
C-reactive protein (CRP)
Alb, transthyretin (if needed)
BUN, Creat

Common Drugs Used and Potential Side Effects

- In general, discuss the relevance of tolerable upper intake levels (ULs) from the latest dietary reference intakes of the National Academy of Sciences. These levels were set to protect individuals from receiving too much of any nutrient from diet and dietary supplements.

For Women of Childbearing Years

- Contraceptive steroids may decrease serum levels of vitamin B_6, vitamin B_{12}, folic acid, and vitamin C and increase serum levels of vitamin A, copper, and lipids; adjust diet accordingly. There is a reduction in the risk of endometrial and ovarian cancer, a possible small increase in the risk for breast and cervical cancer, and an increased risk of liver cancer from use of contraceptive steroids (Burke et al, 2004).
- Users of intrauterine devices should increase their intake of iron and vitamin C to counteract increased menstrual losses.
- For chronic interstitial cystitis (IC), acidic foods and beverages such as coffee, alcoholic beverages, fruit juices, carbonated beverages, tomato products, and other foods and beverages may cause irritation. Use of buffering products such as Prelief may reduce symptoms. Pain relievers may also be useful. More information is available at the Interstitial Cystitis Association website (www.ichelp.org).

For Menopausal Women

- Low doses of Megace (megestrol acetate) may be used to decrease hot flashes in postmenopausal women who cannot take estrogen. Megace can cause increased appetite, edema, and sodium retention.
- Alendronate (Fosamax) may be used to maintain bone density without breast cancer risk.

For Men—Erectile Dysfunction

- Sildenafil citrate (Viagra) and tadalafil (Cialis) have been widely used to treat erectile dysfunction (ED), but they are not without potential health risks (Mulhall, 2000). Studies and clinical trials of similar drugs are under way.

For Men—Baldness

- Note: Androgenic alopecia (baldness) may suggest higher risk for prostate cancer (Giles et al, 2002) or for early, severe coronary heart disease (Matilainen et al, 2001)
- Use of Rogaine (minoxidil) to treat baldness may cause diarrhea, low blood pressure, nausea, vomiting, and weight gain; it is a vasodilator. A low-sodium, low-calorie diet may be beneficial.
- 5-Alpha reductase catalyzes the conversion of testosterone to dihydrotestosterone; disturbances in 5-alpha reductase activity in skin cells might contribute to male pattern baldness, acne, or hirsutism. The discovery of a plant homolog of human 5-alpha reductase may lead to new drugs.

For Men—Prostate Problems

- Proscar (finasteride) and other medications are used with some relief. Monitor blood pressure and other side effects. No nutritional side effects are noted. There is evidence that saw palmetto may be useful (see following herb section).
- Antioxidants including selenium may help protect against prostate cancer (Kranse et al, 2005). Brazil nuts, seafood, and whole grains are natural sources and may provide greater benefits than supplements. Lycopene is another useful protective factor; dietary sources (tomato-based items) are preferable at this time over supplements. Finally, intake of broccoli and cauliflower can reduce prostate cancer risk significantly (Joseph et al, 2004).

Herbs, Botanicals, and Supplements

- Herbs, botanical products, and supplements should not be used without discussing with a physician, especially with underlying medical conditions (Boullata, 2005; American Dietetic Association, 2001). The Food and Drug Administration will be implementing new guidelines for DSHEA; information can be found at http://www.fda.gov/bbs/topics/news/2004/NEW01130.html. Knowing that supplement use is common among middle-aged men and women in the United States, it should be recognized that micronutrient intakes of vitamins A, C, and E, niacin, folate, and iron are often higher than from foods alone (Archer et al, 2005). Section 2 provides an extensive list of herbs and botanicals for consideration; see Table 2-1.
- For alternatives to hormone replacement therapy, a useful website that reviews studies is http://www.cognis.com/veris/ScientificReports/Hormone_Replacement_Therapy.pdf.
- No studies have confirmed efficacy for the following herbs and botanicals:
  - For endometriosis: soybean, peanut, flax, and alfalfa.
  - For impotence: fava bean, anise, gingko, yohimbe, and cardamom.
  - For infertility: cauliflower, ginseng, spinach, ginger, guava, and sunflower.
  - For insomnia: lemon balm, lavender, chamomile, and hops.
  - For menopause: alfalfa and licorice.

INTERVENTION: NUTRITION EDUCATION, COUNSELING, CARE MANAGEMENT

- Help plan a diet in accordance with individual lifestyle. Nutrient density, food cost, and portion sizes should be explained. Meal and snack patterns may be markers for nutrient intakes and diet quality (Kerver et al, 2006).
- Explain the benefits of weight management for adults to prevent or delay the onset of chronic diseases (Kerver et al, 2003; Savoca et al, 2004; Winters et al, 2004). Start with body mass index and select a healthy body weight goal if needed. Successful weight losers tend to follow a low-fat, high-carbohydrate food plan with high levels of physical activity; they eat breakfast regularly.
- Popular low-carbohydrate, high-protein diet plans may contribute to problems such as kidney stones and are not advised for most adults. The South Beach diet recommends olive oil and use of fatty fish, which are more similar to recommendations of the Mediterranean diet plan than the Atkins plan.
- Encourage planned meals. Skipping breakfast may lead to overeating later at night.
- Describe the effects of the "business lunch" with alcohol on nutritional status; alcohol intake may equal 300 calories or more. Discourage intake of more than two alcoholic drinks per day for men and one drink for women.
- Being physically fit can improve the odds against cancer (Vainio et al, 2002). Goal setting may be an effective strategy for planning physical activity (Shilts et al, 2004). The Surgeon General recommends 1 hour daily of physical activity. Many people have found that using a pedometer to count steps is very motivating; "10,000 steps a day" is the popular goal. Each mile is approximately 2000 steps. Other forms of exercise should be encouraged as well (for example, pilates). Tai chi has been found to help increase flexibility.
- Water intake is often lower than desirable. Dehydration can contribute to kidney stones, strain on the heart and cardiovascular system, drug toxicity, and other conditions. Encourage intake of 8–10 glasses of water or other liquids each day. Both coffee and tea seem to be preventive against cancers, diabetes, heart disease, and Parkinson's disease, and their inclusion in moderate amounts each day is recommended.
- Asking for the right medical tests during annual doctor visits is a good idea. For example, cholesterol and blood pressure screening should start at age 20 for a baseline; dental check-ups and Pap smears should be planned as well. Women aged 35 years and older should be tested for thyroid status (as with the TSH test). Women should schedule mammograms at least every 3 years or more frequently with family risk. Periodic EKGs and fasting blood glucose are useful after age 40. After age 50, a fecal occult blood test, bone density scan, and prostate-specific antigen test might be needed. Vaccines for tetanus, flu, and pneumonia are useful after age 60.
- Functional foods may reduce the risk of coronary heart disease, cancers, hypertension, and osteoporosis (Klotzbach-Shimomura, 2001). A list of functional foods is found in Table 1-16.

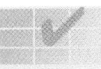

- Help clarify conflicting information about diet. Some of this confusion is related to the difference between a "serving" and a "portion" as noted on food labels.
- The American Council on Science and Health (ACSH) ranks consumer magazines as sources of reliable nutrition information. *Parents*, *Cooking Light*, and *Good Housekeeping* tend to rank highly for accuracy.
- Discuss food choices when eating away from home. For travelers who experience jet lag, adjust meal times to match new time zone, which may help the liver adjust more readily.
- Discuss calcium alternatives for people who exclude milk products. There are calcium-fortified foods and beverages, such as fortified orange juice, cereals, mineral waters, and margarine.
- For persons who live in northern climates, taking vitamin D may be especially important after age 50.
- Discuss the role of managing blood pressure and how diet can help. Ignoring high blood pressure can set the stage for stroke, dementia, and heart disease later in life. Intensive diet and physical activity modifications can greatly reduce disease risk (Aldana et al, 2005).
- For infertility, advise that smoking can reduce the ability of sperm to bind to an egg and can also reduce fertility in women (Bordel et al, 2006). Oxidative stress is detrimental to sperm function and a significant factor in the etiology of male infertility; there are benefits from dietary and supplementary intake of the antioxidants vitamin C, vitamin E, and beta-carotene on sperm chromatin integrity (Silver et al, 2005).
- Discuss fiber, nonmeat vegetarian meals, cooking methods for nutrient preservation, and phytochemicals. Nutrition messages that lead to increased consumption of dietary fiber need to be strengthened; good taste and convenience are critical components (Auld et al, 2000). Peer education seems to be effective in increasing fruit and vegetable intakes in adults (Butler et al, 2000). See Table 1-17 for ways in which to include more fruits and vegetables in the diet.
- Determine psychological readiness for dietary and lifestyle change and the individual's current stage. The Transtheoretical Model for Stages of Change (precontemplation, contemplation, preparation, action, maintenance, or termination) is a useful tool that defines motivation as a dynamic process (Prochaska and DiClemente, 1982). Persons in the action stages tend to display healthier eating; demographic and psychosocial factors help to mediate readiness to change dietary factors; and precontemplators need individually tailored interventions (Vallis et al, 2003). Many primary care patients are ready to lose weight, improve diet, and increase exercise (Wee et al, 2005). Concentrate on small changes with the client.

TABLE 1-17 Five to Nine a Day for Better Health

Tips for Eating More Fruits and Vegetables

- Eat at least one vitamin A–rich fruit or vegetable, such as apricots, cantaloupe, carrots, sweet potatoes, spinach, collards, or broccoli each day.
- Eat at least one vitamin C–rich fruit or vegetable such as oranges, strawberries, green peppers, or tomatoes each day.
- Eat several high-fiber fruits or vegetables, such as apples, grapefruit, broccoli, or cauliflower, each day.
- Eat berries often; blueberries have been highly rated for their antioxidant properties (anthocyanins). Other berries are equally nutritious and contain fiber, quercetin, and other flavonoids.
- Eat cabbage family vegetables, such as cauliflower, broccoli, Brussels sprouts, and cabbage, several times every week.
- Add fruit to cereal or plain yogurt.
- Use fruit juice instead of water when preparing cakes and muffins.
- Drink 100% fruit juice instead of soda.
- Eat a piece of fruit for a morning snack; choose a grapefruit or an orange for an afternoon snack.
- Choose the darkest green or red leaf lettuce greens for salads; add carrots, red cabbage, and spinach.
- Add more vegetables to soups and stews; add tomato juice to soups and stews for more vitamins A and C.
- Choose pizza with extra green pepper, onion, broccoli, and tomatoes.
- Munch on raw vegetables with a low-fat dip for an afternoon snack.
- When eating out, choose a side dish of vegetables.
- Fill up most of the plate with vegetables at lunch or dinner.
- Choose fortified foods and beverages such as juice with added calcium.
- Snack on dried fruits, such as dried apricots, peaches, raisins, or "craisins."
- Use dried plums (prunes) for a natural laxative.
- Use dried plum puree as a butter or margarine substitute in recipes to reduce fat; use half the measure required.

Refer clients to:

- *The Color Code: A Revolutionary Eating Plan for Optimum Health* by James A. Joseph, PhD; Daniel A. Nadeau, MD; and Anne Underwood.
- Produce for Better Health Foundation, http://www.5aday.com/.

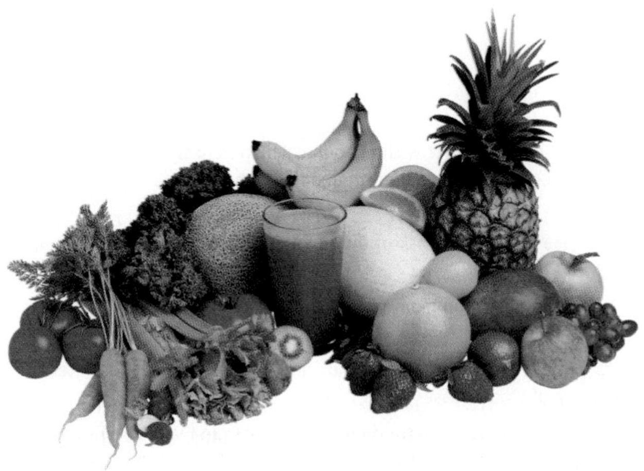

Figure 1-11 Figure shows a healthy grouping of fruits and vegetables.

- The "Slow Food" movement is trying to counter the fast-food culture by returning to traditional foods, having pleasurable mealtimes, and enjoying the aroma and flavors of foods more fully.
- If needed, provide advice on resources to alleviate food insecurity (American Dietetic Association, 2002).
- Nutrition information on packaged food labels is useful to teach point-of-purchase tips, and adults can be encouraged to use them (Satia et al, 2005). Most adults do not know how to use the food label as well as they might (Levy et al, 2000). Label reading may be a marker for other dietary behaviors that predict healthful food choices and should be discussed. See Tables 1-18 and 1-18A through 1-18C.

Patient Education—Food Safety Tips

- Reminders about hand washing and safe food handling may be important, especially for those adults who prepare and serve meals for others.
- Avoid food preparation when sick with viral or bacterial infections. Use latex gloves if there are any cuts on the hands. Thoroughly cook meat, poultry, and fish entrees. Keep cold foods cold and hot foods hot.
- Bacteria are commonly found on foods such as green onions (scallions), cantaloupe, cilantro, and many types of imported produce. Wash all fresh fruits and vegetables. Scrub the outside of produce such as melons and cucumbers before cutting.
- Avoid tap water and ice made from tap water, uncooked produce such as lettuce, and raw or undercooked seafood when traveling (American Dietetic Association, 2003). Use of alcoholic beverages in moderation may prevent foodborne illness; studies are under way to determine why.
- Airline water may not be free from contamination. Use of bottled water is recommended. Coffee and tea may not be hot enough to kill all bacteria.
- Throw out cooked foods that have been at room temperature for longer than 2 hours.
- Consumption of sulforaphane in foods such as broccoli, cauliflower, cabbage and Brussels sprouts may reduce the presence of *Helicobacter pylori.*
- Avoid raw or partially cooked eggs, raw or undercooked fish or shellfish, and raw or undercooked meats because of potential foodborne illnesses.
- Do not use raw (unpasteurized) milk or products made from it.
- Avoid serving unpasteurized juices and raw sprouts.
- Only serve processed deli meats and frankfurters that have been reheated to steaming hot temperature.

For More Information

- American Association of Family and Consumer Sciences
  http://www.aafcs.org/
- American Pregnancy Association: Preconceptual Nutrition
  http://www.americanpregnancy.org/gettingpregnant/preconceptionnutrition.html
- American Public Health Association
  http://www.apha.org/
- Centers for Disease Control and Prevention
  http://www.cdc.gov/
- Dietary Supplements
  http://www.cfsan.fda.gov/~dms/supplmnt.html#about
- Eating Well
  http://www.eatingwell.com

TABLE 1-18 Food Labeling Terms and Health Claims

Because consumers are confronted with a vast array of food and dietary supplement products claiming to improve health, manage conditions, and reduce disease risks, health professionals should know and share the legal requirements, regulatory processes, and scientific evaluation of these label statements (Turner et al, 2005). The U.S. Food and Drug Administration (FDA) regulates labeling. Current regulations cover three categories of health-related statements: health claims, structure/function claims, and nutrient content claims (Turner et al, 2005).

Labeling Terms

% Fat Free	Food must be a low-fat or fat-free food to include this value
Free	Food contains 0% of the indicated nutrient
Good Source	Contains 10–19% of the daily value (DV) for a nutrient
High	Contains 20% or more DV for a nutrient
Lean	Food (meat) is no more than 10% fat by weight, not calories; contains 10 g fat or less and 95 mg cholesterol or less (extra lean 5% fat by weight)
Less	Food contains 25% less than original food
Light/Lite	Food contains fewer calories or 50% less fat than original food OR description of color (if indicated on the label)
Low	Low fat as 3 g or less; low sodium as 140 mg or less; very low sodium as 35 mg or less; low cholesterol as 20 mg or less; low calorie as 40 calories or less
More	Food contains 110% or more DV than original food
Reduced	Product has been altered to contain 25% less of a nutrient or the usual calories of that food
Reduced cholesterol	The food contains 75% or less of the cholesterol found in the original product

Source: U.S. Food and Drug Administration.

TABLE 1-18A Authorized Health Claims

Diet	Disease	Model Claim
Calcium	Osteoporosis	Regular exercise and a healthful diet with enough calcium help teens and young adult white and Asian American women maintain good bone health and may reduce their risk of osteoporosis.
Sodium	Hypertension	Diets low in sodium may reduce the risk of high blood pressure, a disease associated with many factors.
Dietary fat	Cancer	Development of cancer depends on many factors. A diet low in total fat may reduce the risk of some cancers.
Dietary saturated fat and cholesterol	Coronary heart disease	While many factors affect heart disease, diets low in saturated fat and cholesterol may reduce the risk of this disease.
Fiber-containing grain products, fruits, and vegetables	Cancers	Low-fat diets rich in fiber-containing grain products, fruits, and vegetables may reduce the risk of some types of cancer, a disease associated with many factors.
Fruits, vegetables, and grain products that contain fiber, particularly soluble fiber	Coronary heart disease	Diets low in saturated fat and cholesterol and rich in fruits, vegetables, and grain products that contain some types of dietary fiber, particularly soluble fiber, may reduce the risk of heart disease, a disease associated with many factors.
Fruits and vegetables	Cancer	Low-fat diets rich in fruits and vegetables may reduce the risk of some types of cancer, a disease associated with many factors.
Folate	Neural tube birth defects	Healthful diets with adequate daily folate may reduce a woman's risk of having a child with a brain or spinal cord birth defect.

Health claims must be supported by significant scientific agreement among experts that the proclaimed benefit of a food or food component on a disease or health-related condition is true (Turner et al, 2005). Table 1-18A shows diet–disease relationships mandated for review by the U.S. Food and Drug Administration under the Nutrition Labeling and Education Act and currently approved as health claims.

Reprinted with permission from: Hasler CM. Functional foods: benefits, concerns and challenges—a position paper from the American Council on Science and Health. *J Nutr.* 132:3772–3781, 2002.

TABLE 1-18B Authorized Health Claims after Petition

Diet	Disease	Approved Health Claim
Sugar alcohols	Dental caries	"Frequent eating of foods high in sugars and starches as between-meal snacks can promote tooth decay. The sugar alcohol [name of product] used to sweeten this food may reduce the skin of dental caries."
Foods that contain fiber from whole-oat products	Coronary heart disease	"Diets low in saturated fat and cholesterol that include soluble fiber from whole oats may reduce the risk of heart disease."
Foods that contain fiber from psyllium	Coronary heart disease	"Diets low in saturated fat and cholesterol that include soluble fiber from psyllium seed husk may reduce the risk of heart disease."
Soy protein	Coronary heart disease	"Diets low in saturated fat and cholesterol that include 25 grams of soy protein a day may reduce the risk of heart disease. One serving of [name of food] provides 6.25 grams of soy protein."
Plant sterol/stanol esters	Coronary heart disease	Plant sterols: "Foods containing at least 0.65 grams per serving of plant sterols, eaten twice a day with meals for a daily total intake of at least 1.3 grams, as part of a diet low in saturated fat and cholesterol, may reduce the risk of heart disease. A serving of [name of the food] supplies ___ grams of vegetable oil sterol esters." Plant stanol esters: "Foods containing at least 1.7 grams per serving of plant stanol esters, eaten twice a day with meals for a total daily intake of at least 3.4 grams, as part of a diet low in saturated fat and cholesterol, may reduce the risk of heart disease. A serving of [name of the food] supplies ___ grams of plant stanol esters."

When significant scientific agreement is lacking, qualifying statements may be required on the label to describe the strength of the evidence that supports the claim (Turner et al, 2005). Table 1-18B lists health claims approved by the U.S. Food and Drug Administration following petitions submitted by the food industry.

Reprinted with permission from: Hasler CM. Functional foods: benefits, concerns and challenges—a position paper from the American Council on Science and Health. *J Nutr.* 132:3772–3781, 2002.

TABLE 1-18C **Qualified Health Claims That Are Not Approved by FDA**

Diet-Disease Relationship	Disease	Qualified Health Claim
Omega-3 fatty acids	Coronary heart disease	Consumption of omega-3 fatty acids may reduce the risk of coronary heart disease. FDA evaluated the data and determined that, although there is scientific evidence supporting the claim, the evidence is not conclusive.
Folic acid, B_6, B_{12}	Vascular disease	As part of a well-balanced diet that is low in saturated fat and cholesterol, Folic Acid, Vitamin B_6 and Vitamin B_{12} may reduce the risk of vascular disease. FDA evaluated the above claim and found that, while it is known that diets low in saturated fat and cholesterol reduce the risk of heart disease and other vascular diseases, the evidence in support of the above claim is inconclusive.
Selenium	Cancer	Selenium may reduce the risk of certain cancers. Some scientific evidence suggests that consumption of selenium may reduce the risk of certain forms of cancer. However, FDA has determined that this evidence is limited and not conclusive.
Phosphatidylserine	Dementia	Very limited and preliminary scientific research suggests that phosphatidylserine may reduce the risk of dementia [cognitive dysfunction] in the elderly. FDA concludes that there is little scientific evidence supporting this claim.

Qualified health claims, where FDA has found some support but not enough clear evidence to allow an approved health claim.

Reprinted with permission from: Hasler CM. Functional foods: benefits, concerns and challenges—a position paper from the American Council on Science and Health. *J Nutr.* 132:3772–3781, 2002.

- Family Mealtimes
  http://www.eatsmart.org
  http://www.cfs.purdue.edu/CFF/promotingfamilymeals
- Food and Drug Administration
  http://www.fda.gov/
- Foundation for Better Health Care–Menopause
  http://fbhc.org/modules/menopause.cfm
- Health Statistics
  http://www.cdc.gov/nchs/fastats/Default.htm
- International Food Information Council
  http://ific.org/
- Men's Health
  http://www.nlm.nih.gov/medlineplus/menshealth.html
- MyPyramid Food Guidance System
  http://www.mypyramid.gov/
- National Center for Complementary and Alternative Medicine
  http://nccam.nih.gov/
- National Institutes of Health
  http://www.nih.gov/
- National Women's Health Resource Center
  http://www.4woman.org/
- Novartis Men's Health Page
  http://www.healthandage.com/Home/gc=28
- Recipes:
  http://www.deliciousdecisions.org
  http://www.cookinglight.com
  http://www.mealsforyou.com
  http://www.allrecipes.com
- Shape Up America
  http://www.shapeup.org/
- Slow Food Movement
  http://slowfood.com
- Sustainable Food Systems
  http://www.localharvest.org
- Women's Health Initiative
  http://www.nhlbi.nih.gov/whi/index.html

ADULTHOOD—CITED REFERENCES

Aguilar B, et al. Metabolism of homocysteine and its relationship with cardiovascular disease. *J Thromb Thrombolysis.* 18:75, 2004.

Aldana SG, et al. Effects of an intensive diet and physical activity modification program on the health risks of adults. *J Am Diet Assoc.* 105:371, 2005.

American Dietetic Association. Position of the American Dietetic Association: domestic food and nutrition security. *J Am Diet Assoc.* 102:1840, 2002.

American Dietetic Association. Position of the American Dietetic Association: food and water safety. *J Am Diet Assoc.* 103:1203, 2003.

American Dietetic Association. Position of the American Dietetic Association: food fortification and dietary supplements. *J Am Diet Assoc.* 101:115, 2001.

American Dietetic Association. Position of the American Dietetic Association and Dietitians of Canada: women's health and nutrition. *J Am Diet Assoc.* 104:984, 2004.

Archer SL, et al. Association of dietary supplement use with specific micronutrient intakes among middle-aged American men and women: the INTERMAP study. *J Am Diet Assoc.* 105:1106, 2005.

Auld GW, et al. Reported adoption of dietary fat and fiber recommendations among consumers. *J Am Diet Assoc.* 100:52, 2000.

Bordel R, et al. Nicotine does not affect vascularization but inhibits growth of freely transplanted ovarian follicles by inducing granulose cell apoptosis. *Hum Reprod.* 21:610, 2006.

Boullata J. Natural health product interactions with medication. *Nutr Clin Pract.* 20:33, 2005.

Braunschweig C, et al. Impact of declines in nutritional status on outcomes in adult patients hospitalized for more than 7 days. *J Am Diet Assoc.* 100:1316, 2000.

Burke R, et al. Safety concerns and health benefits associated with oral contraception. *Am J Obstet Gynecol.* 190:S5, 2004.

Butler DB, et al. Randomized trial testing the effect of peer education at increasing fruit and vegetable intake. *J Natl Cancer Inst.* 91:1491, 2000.

Cummings AM, Kavlock RJ. Gene-environment interactions: a review of effects on reproduction and development. *Crit Rev Toxicol.* 34:461, 2004.

Drewnoski A. Indices of nutrient density: making each calorie count. Lecture, American Dietetic Association Symposium, Anaheim, CA, October 5, 2004.

Duffy VB, Bartoshuk LM. Food acceptance and genetic variation in taste. *J Am Diet Assoc.* 100:647, 2000.

Esposito K, et al. Effect of lifestyle changes on erectile dysfunction in obese men: a randomized controlled trial. *JAMA.* 291:2978, 2004.

Fedorcsak P, et al. Impact of overweight and underweight on assisted reproduction treatment. *Hum Reprod.* 19:2523, 2004.

Gharib SD, ed. *Infertility: a guide to evaluation, treatment and counseling.* Boston: Brigham and Women's Hospital, 2003.

Giles GG, et al. Androgenetic alopecia and prostate cancer: findings from an Australian case-control study. *Cancer Epidemiol Biomarkers Prev.* 11:549, 2002.

Gotto AM. Antioxidants, statins, and atherosclerosis. *J Am Coll Cardiol.* 41:1205, 2003.

Guenther PM, et al. Sociodemographic, knowledge, and attitudinal factors related to meat consumption in the United States. *J Am Diet Assoc.* 105:1266, 2005.

Hasler CM, et al. American Dietetic Association. Position of the American Dietetic Association: functional foods. *J Am Diet Assoc.* 104:814, 2004.

Holben DH, et al. Food security status of households in Appalachian Ohio with children in Head Start. *J Am Diet Assoc.* 104:238, 2004.

Horner NK, Lampe JW. Potential mechanisms of diet therapy for fibrocystic breast conditions show inadequate evidence of effectiveness. *J Am Diet Assoc.* 100:1368, 2000.

Johnson SR. Premenstrual syndrome, premenstrual dysphoric disorder, and beyond: a clinical primer for practitioners. *Obstet Gynecol.* 104:845, 2004.

Joseph MA, et al. Cruciferous vegetables, genetic polymorphisms in glutathione s-transferases m1 and t1, and prostate cancer risk. *Nutr Cancer.* 50:206, 2004.

Kerver JM, et al. Dietary patterns associated with risk factors for cardiovascular disease in healthy US adults. *Am J Clin Nutr.* 78:1103, 2003.

Kerver JM, et al. Meal and snack patterns are associated with dietary intake of energy and nutrients in US adults. *J Am Diet Assoc.* 106:46, 2006.

Klotzbach-Shimomura. Functional foods: the role of physiologically active compounds in relation to disease. *Top Clin Nutri.* 16:68, 2001.

Knoops KTB, et al. Mediterranean diet, lifestyle factors, and 10-year mortality in elderly European men and women: The HALE Project. *JAMA.* 292:1433, 2004.

Kranse R, et al. Dietary intervention in prostate cancer patients: PSA response in a randomized double-blind placebo-controlled study. *Int J Cancer.* 113:835-840, 2005.

Krebs EE. Phytoestrogens for treatment of menopausal symptoms: a systematic review. *Obstet Gynecol.* 104:824, 2004.

Levy L, et al. How well do consumers understand percentage daily value on food labels? *Am J Health Promotion.* 14:157, 2000.

Lindmark U, et al. Food selection associated with sense of coherence in adults. *Nutr J.* 4:9, 2005.

Mathers CD, et al. Global patterns of healthy life expectancy in the year 2002. *BMC Public Health.* 4:66, 2004.

Matilainen VA, et al. Early onset of androgenetic alopecia associated with early severe coronary heart disease: a population-based, case-control study. *J Cardiovasc Risk.* 8:147, 2001.

Most MM. Estimated phytochemical content of the Dietary Approaches to Stop Hypertension (DASH) Diet is higher than in the control study diet. *J Am Diet Assoc.* 104:1725, 2004.

Mulhall JP. Current concepts in erectile dysfunction. *Am J Manag Care.* 6:S625, 2000.

Ogden CL, et al. Mean body weight, height, and body mass index, United States 1960-2002. *Adv Data.* 347:1, 2004.

Prochaska JO, DiClemente CC. Transtheoretical therapy: toward a more integrative model of change. *Psychotherapy: Theory, Research and Practice* 19:276, 1982.

Quandt SA, et al. Household food security among migrant and seasonal Latino farmworkers in North Carolina. *Public Health Rep.* 119:568, 2004.

Satia JA, et al. Food nutrition label use is associated with demographic, behavioral, and psychosocial factors and dietary intake among African Americans in North Carolina. *J Am Diet Assoc.* 105:392, 2005.

Satia JA, et al. Motivations for healthful dietary change. *Public Health Nutr.* 4:953, 2001.

Savoca MR, et al. Food habits are related to glycemic control among people with type 2 diabetes mellitus. *J Am Diet Assoc.* 104:560, 2004.

Shilts MK, et al. Goal setting as a strategy for dietary and physical activity behavior change: a review of the literature. *Am J Health Promot.* 19:81, 2004.

Signorello LB, et al. Maternal caffeine consumption and spontaneous abortion: a review of the epidemiologic evidence. *Epidemiology* 15:229, 2004.

Silver EW, et al. Effect of antioxidant intake on sperm chromatin stability in healthy nonsmoking men. *J Androl.* 26:550, 2005.

Stein K. Refusal to follow dietary prescriptions. *J Am Diet Assoc.* 105:1188, 2005.

Stuff JE, et al. High prevalence of food insecurity and hunger in households in the rural lower Mississippi Delta. *J Rural Health.* 20:173, 2004.

Tolstrup JS, et al. Does caffeine and alcohol intake before pregnancy predict the occurrence of spontaneous abortion? *Hum Reprod.* 18:2704, 2003.

Turner RE, et al. Label claims for foods and supplements: a review of the regulations. Label claims for foods and supplements: a review of the regulations. *Nutr Clin Pract.* 20:21, 2005.

United States Department of Agriculture. What We Eat in America, 2001-2002. Accessed January 2, 2006 at http://www.ars.usda.gov/Services/docs.htm?docid=7674.

Vainio H, et al. Weight control and physical activity in cancer prevention: international evaluation of the evidence. *Eur J Cancer Prev.* 11:94S, 2002.

Vallis M, et al. Stages of change for healthy eating in diabetes: relation to demographic, eating-related, health care utilization, and psychosocial factors. *Diabetes Care.* 26:1468, 2003.

Wang Y, Wang QJ. The prevalence of prehypertension and hypertension among US adults according to the new joint national committee guidelines: new challenges of the old problem. *Arch Intern Med.* 164:2126, 2004.

Wee CC, et al. Stage of readiness to control weight and adopt weight control behaviors in primary care. *J Gen Intern Med.* 20:410, 2005.

Winters BL, et al. Dietary patterns in women treated for breast cancer who successfully reduce fat intake: the Women's Intervention Nutrition Study (WINS). *J Am Diet Assoc.* 104:551, 2004.

Wong WY, et al. Male factor subfertility: possible causes and the impact of nutritional factors. *Fertil Steril.* 73:435, 2000.

Wu C, et al. A case-control study of risk factors for fibrocystic breast conditions: Shanghai Nutrition and Breast Disease Study, China, 1995-2000. *Am J Epidemiol.* 160:945, 2004.

Zhu C, et al. Lifestyle behaviors associated with lower risk of having the metabolic syndrome. *Metabolism* 53:1503, 2004.

GERIATRIC NUTRITION

NUTRITIONAL ACUITY RANKING: LEVEL 2

DEFINITIONS AND BACKGROUND

Aging involves a progression of physiological changes with cell loss and organ decline; decreased glomerular filtration rate (GFR) and creatinine-height index (CHI), constipation, decreased glucose tolerance, and lowered cell-mediated immunity can occur. The need for energy as related to basal metabolism can decrease as much as 10% for ages 50–70 years and by 20–25% thereafter. After 70 years of age, body weight generally declines; physical activity can prevent unnecessary losses in lean body mass.

It is estimated that most of the older population have one or more chronic conditions that would benefit from nutrition interventions. Challenges of nutritional assessment in older adults include limited recall, hearing and vision losses, changes in attention span, and variations in dietary intake from day to day. The inability to perform activities of daily living can be of major concern in the geriatric population. Older adults may need assistance with shopping, meal preparation, and in ensuring adequate intake. Figure 1-12 shows a healthy senior citizen in her eighth decade.

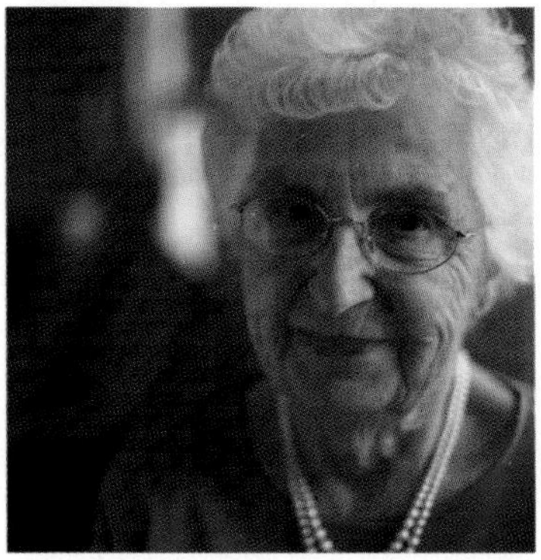

Figure 1-12 Healthy senior citizen.
(Miller CA. *Nursing for wellness in older adults: theory and practice*. 4th ed. Philadelphia: Lippincott Williams & Wilkins, 2004.)

Although the term "life span" describes the maximal potential for humans (estimated to be between 120–140 years), life expectancy is the mean length of life projected for a population at a given age (Harris, 2004). The oldest age attained by humans seems to be 114 years. Nutritional well-being is an integral part of successful aging; a broad set of culturally appropriate food and nutrition services are available and should be customized to the individual's needs (American Dietetic Association, 2005).

Essentially, older persons consume less food than younger persons, about one third few calories than younger people. Protein intake is estimated at below the desired levels for 10% of older men and 20% of older women. Over 30% of older persons consume less energy than recommended levels, and 50% have low mineral and vitamin intakes. Lower food intake by the geriatric populations appears to be a result of smaller meals eaten at a slower rate.

Energy restriction with a high-quality diet may increase longevity when initiated in a healthy younger adult (Smith et al, 2004). However, many gerontologists prefer to have patients start out a little overweight than too underweight to support the immune system.

According to the U.S. Census Bureau, persons older than 65 years of age comprise 13% of the United States population. Only about 5% of elderly individuals are in nursing homes, the others live in the community, often alone. Approximately 20–50% of hospital admissions are malnourished, especially among the elderly (Robinson et al, 2003; Correia and Campos, 2003; Guigoz et al, 2002). Although the stress response to surgery (decrease in albumin and transferrin) is not affected by age, serum protein levels return to normal more slowly in older individuals; this factor must be considered for older surgical patients.

The term "frail elderly" refers to individuals with low lean body mass, often far below the desired range for height. Up to 25% of persons older than age 65 are frail and exhibit loss of muscle strength, easy fatigue, physical inactivity, slow or unsteady gait, poor appetite, unintentional loss of weight, impaired cognition, and depression; they die sooner (Vanitallie, 2003). Research suggests that resistance training improves strength, and there are studies under way about the use of hormones such as growth hormone (GH) for improvements in appetite and intake (Morgan et al, 2004; Vanitallie, 2003). Nutrition alone is not sufficient to rebuild lost muscle mass; some sort of physical activity seems to be needed.

Loss of teeth is common among older individuals. According to CDC, in 1997, edentulism was more common among persons aged ≥ 75 years (26.7%) than among persons aged 65–74 years (22.9%) (http://www.cdc.gov/epo/mmwr/preview/mmwrhtml/00056723.htm). Decreased salivation and absorption, as well as declining taste and smell, are also common.

BMR declines 2% with each decade of life; LBM declines 6% with each decade and generally is replaced by fat. Being too thin is risky to the immune system of elderly individuals. In general, weight loss in elderly individuals is not desirable because it usually is difficult for them to recover lost LBM (Pichard et al, 2004).

In long-term care facilities, residents may be undernourished. In testimony before the U.S. Senate Special Committee on Aging, evidence from various studies was cited that between one-quarter and one-third of all nursing home residents have a low Body Mass Index, and many experience significant weight loss (http://www.cms.hhs.gov/medicaid/). Protein-energy undernutrition may contribute to pressure ulcers, immune dysfunction, infections, hip fractures, anemia, muscle weakness, fatigue, edema, cognitive changes, and mortality. While weight loss, depression, dehydration, and feeding problems are the easiest to detect, elevated CRP levels should also be corrected. Where possible, include activity and exercise to help stimulate an improved appetite. Use of appetite enhancers may help improve poor nutritional intake; a variety of medications are now available.

Increased intakes of vitamins E, B_{12}, and B_6 and folate, calcium, and zinc may be needed to counteract gastric atrophy, decreased levels of hydrochloric acid, and poor nutrient intakes. Evidence for the role of folate in depression and dementia in the aged is increasing, although mechanisms are not well understood (D'Anci and Rosenberg, 2004). Because of limited exposure to sunshine, some older persons may benefit from supplemental vitamin D (Dawson-Hughes, 2004). Multivitamin-mineral supplementation in healthy older persons may be beneficial (D'Anci and Rosenberg, 2004; Hercberg et al, 2004; Wolters et al, 2004).

Precipitously declining cholesterol (<150 mg/dL) appears to be a marker for mortality, often from cancer, congestive heart failure (Kalantar-Zadeh K et al, 2004), chronic pulmonary disease, or critical illness. Higher cholesterol may indicate protection from fat-soluble antioxidants, may result in enhanced delivery of lipids to cells during the immune response or tissue repair, or may enhance defense against endotoxins and viruses (Jacobs and Iribarren, 2000). Low cholesterol may suggest poor nutrition, as from depression; more research is needed, especially among the elderly.

At the opposite end of the cholesterol issue, the Cardiovascular Health Study found that modifiable behavioral factors (physical activity, smoking, and obesity) and cardiovascular risk factors (diabetes, HDL cholesterol, and blood pressure) are generally associated with maintenance of good health in older adults (Burke et al, 2001). High homocysteine levels should be lowered for heart disease prevention, and for mental agility. High levels of homocysteine can damage the blood vessels in the brain (Marengoni et al, 2004).

TABLE 1-19 Nutrition Assessment Tools for the Elderly

1. Nutrition Screening Initiative (NSI) DETERMINE Checklist

The NSI is targeted for identification of elderly individuals who are at nutritional risk. The following are warning signs for malnutrition that should be addressed (Nutrition Screening Initiative, 1994).[a]

D Disease (illness affects nutritional intake)

E Eating poorly, especially fewer than two meals daily

T Tooth loss, mouth pain, chewing difficulty

E Economic hardship (too few dollars to buy food)

R Reduced social contact; eating meals alone

M Multiple medicines (three or more prescribed or over-the-counter medications)

I Involuntary weight loss or gain (10 lb in 6 months)

N Needs assistance with self-care (shopping, cooking, eating)

E Elderly years (older than 80 years of age), with increasing frailty

2. Mini Nutrition Assessment (MNA) (Nestle)

The MNA is a reliable and easy-to-use nutritional assessment tool. It allows physicians, dieticians, medical students, or nurses to quickly evaluate the nutritional status of a subject. This tool is composed of 18 questions grouped in four categories: anthropometric assessment (weight, height, and weight loss); general assessment (6 questions related to lifestyle, medication, and mobility); dietary assessment (8 questions related to number of meals, food and fluid intake, and autonomy of feeding); and subjective assessment (self-perception of health and nutrition). The interactive tool may be found at the following website: http://www.mna-elderly.com/clinical-practice.htm.

- Asks questions relating to the last 3 months
- Food intake, digestive problems, chewing or swallowing difficulties
- Weight loss
- Mobility problems
- Psychological stress or acute disease
- Dementia or depression
- BMI

3. Subjective Global Assessment (SGA)

The SGA classification technique can aid in the recognition of undernutrition by assessing a patient's nutritional status based on features of the medical history and physical examination (see Section 13 for examples).

4. Malnutrition in Older People—Screening Issues[b]

Impaired protein synthesis

Decline of the protein reserve of the body

Diminished capacity to meet the extra demand of protein synthesis associated with disease or injury

Increased frailty

Falls

Illness

Hospitalization

Immobilization

Sarcopenia

Decreased nutrition intake ("anorexia of aging")

Nonphysiological causes of undernutrition in older people

Social factors

Poverty

Inability to shop

Inability to prepare and cook meals

Inability to feed oneself

Living alone, social isolation, or lack of social support network

Failure to cater to ethnic food preferences

Psychological factors

Alcoholism

Bereavement

Depression

Dementia or Alzheimer's disease

Dietary cholesterol phobia

Medical factors (mediated through anorexia, early satiation, malabsorption, increased metabolism, cytokine-mediated and impaired functional status)

Cancer

Alcoholism

Cardiac failure

Chronic obstructive pulmonary disease

Infection

Dysphagia

Rheumatoid arthritis

Parkinson disease

Hypermetabolism (e.g., hyperthyroidism)

Malabsorption syndromes

Gastrointestinal symptoms: dyspepsia, atrophic gastritis, vomiting, diarrhea

Constipation

Poor dentition

5. Council on Nutrition Appetite Questionnaire[c]

A. My appetite is

1. Very poor
2. Poor
3. Average
4. Good
5. Very good

B. When I eat, I feel full after

1. Eating only a few mouthfuls
2. Eating about a third of a plate/meal
3. Eating over half of a plate/meal
4. Eating most of the food
5. Hardly ever

C. I feel hungry

1. Never
2. Occasionally
3. Some of the time
4. Most of the time
5. All of the time

(continued)

TABLE 1-19 Nutrition Assessment Tools for the Elderly *(continued)*

D. Food tastes
1. Very bad
2. Bad
3. Average
4. Good
5. Very good

E. Compared to when I was 50, food tastes
1. Much worse
2. Worse
3. Just as good
4. Better
5. Much better

F. Normally, I eat
1. Less than one regular meal a day
2. One meal a day
3. Two meals a day
4. Three meals a day
5. More than three meals a day (including snacks)

G. I feel sick or nauseated when I eat
1. Most times
2. Often
3. Sometimes
4. Rarely
5. Never

H. Most of the time my mood is
1. Very sad
2. Sad
3. Neither sad nor happy
4. Happy
5. Very happy

Scoring

Total the score by adding the numbers associated with the patient's response. A score of less than 28 is cause for concern. If the total is 8–16, then the patient is at risk for anorexia and needs nutrition counseling. If the total score is 17–28, then the patient needs frequent reassessment. If the total score is >28, then the patient is not at risk at this time.

[a] Reprinted with permission by the Nutrition Screening Initiative, a project of the American Academy of Family Physicians, The American Dietetic Association and the National Council on the Aging, Inc., and funded in part by a grant from Ross Products Division, Abbott Laboratories Inc.

[b] Adapted from: Australian College of Royal General Practitioners. SNAP: a population guide to be behavioural risk factors in general practice. *Australian Family Physician.* 33:1, 2004.

[c] Source: http://medschool.slu.edu/agingsuccessfully/pdfsurveys/appetitequestionnaire.pdf.

A major cause of weight changes, particularly weight loss in the geriatric population, is the effects of drugs. Many of the medications that cause anorexia are commonly used in this age group. These include drugs such as digoxin, furosemide, fentanyl patch, warfarin, paroxetine, nifedipine, ranitidine, theophylline, amlodipine, ciprofloxacin, and sertraline.

Before ordering lab work, decide if labs are truly warranted and cost effective and determine what they will suggest; for example, albumin would be expected to be low in a person with a draining wound. According to findings documented by the Nutrition Screening Initiative (http://www. aafp.org/), medical nutritional therapies save $11,000–$16,000 *per patient, per hospital stay* if cost-effective nutritional therapy were provided. Studies completed by the American Dietetic Association for the Nutrition Screening Institute also demonstrate that for every dollar spent on nutrition screening and intervention, at least $3.25 is saved in health care costs (http://www.aafp.org/x16093.xml). Nutritional risk assessments used for older citizens are in Table 1-19.

INTERVENTION: OBJECTIVES

- Monitor carefully for signs of malnutrition since prevalence increases with age, is more common in institutionalized individuals, and is associated with greater susceptibility to infection, longer hospital stay, and increased mortality (Hudgens and Langkamp-Henken, 2005). An eight-item Council on Nutrition Appetite Questionnaire (CNAQ) and its four-item derivative, the Simplified Nutritional Appetite Questionnaire (SNAQ), are short, simple appetite assessment tools that predict anorexia-related weight loss in community-dwelling adults and long-term care residents (Wilson et al, 2005).
- Provide proper nutrition for weight control, healthy appetite, and prevention of acute illness or complications of chronic diseases (e.g., osteoporosis, fractures, anemias, obesity, diabetes, heart disease, and cancers).
- Correct existing nutritional deficiencies. Malnutrition may be caused by poverty, ignorance, depression, chronic disease, poor dietary intake, polypharmacy, and mental or physical disability. Avoid restrictive diets as much as possible (Niedert, 2005). Malnourished elderly patients receiving oral supplemental beverages gain more fat-free mass and make more new proteins when compared to those not receiving any supplements (Bos et al, 2000).
- Recognize cachexia syndromes that are not reversible by hypercaloric feeding. Determine if failure of nonpharmacologic therapy warrants consideration of orexigenic drug therapy.
- Determine baseline functional level and evaluate changes over time.
- Provide foods of proper consistency by status of dentition. Dentures alter the taste of foods (Duffy et al, 1999). Dentures increase bitter and sour taste sensations. In addition, elderly individuals have fewer taste buds, especially for sweets and salt. More sweet flavorings and salty foods (or equivalent seasoning) may be required to satisfy the appetite.

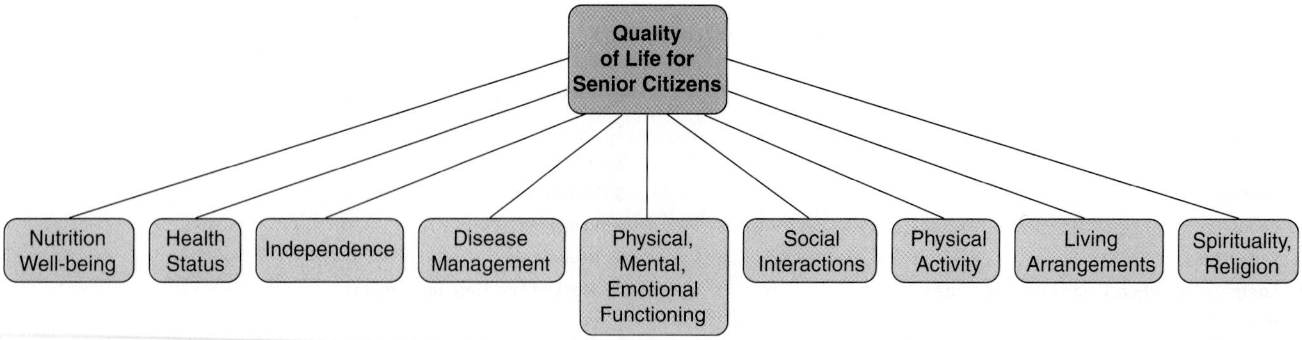

Figure 1-13. Quality of life factors in aging.
(Figure created from American Dietetic Association. Position of The American Dietetic Association: Nutrition across the spectrum of aging. *J Am Diet Assoc.* 105:616, 2005.)

- Evaluate for laxative or enema overuse or abuse. Recommend suitable alternatives and interventions.
- Evaluate for alcohol abuse; suggest appropriate referrals if needed.
- Provide a diet of correct texture. For example, it may need to exclude hard, sticky foods that are difficult to chew and swallow.
- Choose an appropriate regimen: "if the gut works, use it." Maintain weight through oral diet. However, for individuals who are unable to regain significant lost weight, artificial nutrition may be needed. Review advance directives accordingly.
- Investigate all major shifts in body weight. Ensure adequate hydration. Diminishing thirst mechanisms and incontinence play a part in dehydration, a common reason for hospital admissions (Feinsod et al, 2004). A general recommendation suggests that this population should ingest 1500–2000 mL of fluids per day.
- Assess the environment and social situation (i.e., Who shops? Who cooks? How are finances handled? How often are meals eaten away from home? Is this person dependent or independent?). Evaluate the need for various types of assistance.
- Correct frailty, which is similar to "failure to thrive" in infants and children (Vanitallie, 2003). Evaluate family and social support. Depression, use of multiple medications, underlying medical illnesses, and other factors should be addressed. For example, persons with low total cholesterol levels (<189 mg/dL) are at higher risk of dying even when many related factors have been taken into account; physicians may want to regard very low levels of cholesterol as potential warning signs of occult disease or as signals of rapidly declining health (Brescianini et al, 2003).
- Encourage physical activity, especially resistance training, to maintain metabolically active tissue, to stimulate appetite, to improve sleep, to correct mild constipation, to improve cognitive function, to enhance nitrogen balance, and to promote positive outcomes in psychological factors such as depression, memory, self-esteem, and independence. Figure 1-13 shows many factors that influence the quality of life among older individuals.

Nutrient	Recommendation for Males over 70 Years	Recommendation for Females over 70 Years	Comments
Energy	2100 kcal/d	1900 kcal/d	Declining compared with younger adults
Protein	56 g/d	46 g/d	Remains the same as for younger adults
Calcium	1200 mg/d	1200 mg/d	Ability to absorb declines; bones lose calcium
Iron	8 mg/d	8 mg/d	Smaller amount needed, especially for women
Folate	400 mg/d	400 mg/d	Keeps homocysteine levels down
Phosphorus	700 mg/d	700 mg/d	Same level as for younger adults
Vitamin A	900 μg/d	700 μg/d	Use caution not to consume excesses
Vitamin C	90 mg/d	75 mg/d	Maintains healthy gums and collagen
Thiamin	1.2 mg/d	1.1 mg/d	Requirements drop if kcals or carbohydrates are down
Riboflavin	1.3 mg/d	1.1 mg/d	Helps keep skin and oral tissues healthier
Niacin	16 mg/d	14 mg/d	Maintains cardiovascular health
Vitamin D	600 IU/d	600 IU/d	Needed to metabolize calcium properly
Vitamin B_6	1.7 mg/d	1.5 mg/d	May help maintain brain function and antibodies

Data from: Food and Nutrition Board, Institute of Medicine. *Dietary reference intakes for energy, carbohydrate, fiber, fat, fatty acids, cholesterol, protein, and amino acids (macronutrients)*. Washington, DC: National Academy Press, 2002.

INTERVENTION: FOOD AND NUTRITION

- Ensure intake of the MyPyramid Food Guidance System: 3–4 servings of milk, dairy products, or calcium substitutes; 2–3 servings of protein foods (meat or substitute); 3–5 servings of vegetables; 2–4 servings of fruits; and 6–12 bread group servings. Fats, oils, sugars, and sweets are to be controlled to increase or decrease energy intake, as appropriate for the individual.
- Diet should provide adequate intake of protein: 0.8–1 g/kg body weight (Morse et al, 2001). This may mean 63 g for men and 50 g for women. Consider liver and renal impairments and decrease as needed. Increase for pressure ulcers, cancers, and other conditions requiring a higher protein intake.
- Energy: 25–35 kcal/kg. The Institute of Medicine suggests that the average 75-year-old female and male need 2403 and 3067 kcal, respectively, if ambulatory. Fewer kcals are needed if nonambulatory (e.g., living in an institution). Nutritional supplements may provide needed energy and protein for elderly nursing home residents (Avenell and Handoll, 2005).
- Consume 1200 mg of calcium (from milk, yogurt, and related dairy products when possible). Include sources of the B vitamins and zinc. Iron needs are lower in women after menopause, but the minimum should still be included. Ensure sufficiency of other nutrients according to the patient's age and sex, using the DRI tables.
- If patient has cardiovascular disease, encourage lower intake of saturated fat and use the DASH diet. Liberalize where possible to keep intake at a sufficient level. Extra natural vitamin E may be useful from nuts, some vegetable oils, and more fruits and vegetables.
- The consistency of the food should be altered (i.e., ground, pureed, or chopped) only as required. Try to maintain whole textures as often as possible to enhance the food's appeal and to increase chewing with saliva. Significant data exist demonstrating that, often, mechanically altered diets are not necessary, may have been started inappropriately, and are ineffective. These diets often compromise taste and acceptability of food and also have the potential to compromise micronutrient intake.
- Adequate fiber and fluid intakes are necessary. Prudent increases in fiber (e.g., from prunes and bran) can reduce laxative abuse. Dehydration is a common cause of confusion and should be identified or avoided.
- Adoption of a low-fat, vegan diet is associated with significant weight loss in overweight postmenopausal women, even with the absence of prescribed limits on portion size or energy intake (Barnard et al, 2005). If obesity is present, this change may be helpful in improving health status.
- Adequate amounts of vitamins C and D, folic acid, and iron are needed; these nutrients frequently are deficient in the diets of elderly individuals. Vitamin C levels must be increased for those individuals who smoke.
- When taste and olfactory sensations are weak, the diet should provide adequate intake of zinc, folate, and vitamins A and B_{12}. Season with herbs and spices; add butter-flavored seasonings, garlic, maple or vanilla extract, and cheese or bacon-flavored seasonings. Consider all possible taste enhancers.
- About 10–30% of people over the age of 50 may have protein-bound vitamin B_{12} malabsorption; these people need to consume a majority of their needs from synthetic forms rather than from food form (Ho et al, 1999).
- Increased thiamin may be needed because of decreased metabolic efficiency. Men are especially susceptible.
- Reduce intake of excessive carbohydrates such as sweets; poor glucose tolerance and insulin resistance are common after 65 years of age.
- If early satiety is a problem, having the main meal at noon may help.
- Encourage socialization at mealtimes. Healthy individuals have recorded food intakes much greater when eating with other people. Higher food intakes are reported to occur when women eat with men and when both sexes dine with family or friends.
- Offer substitutes for major foods not consumed. If the individual resides in an institution, it is recommended to try other menu alternatives before offering a nutritional supplement as a meal replacement. Be sure to consult a dietitian if intake is chronically poor. If absolutely necessary, liquid supplements can provide needed energy, protein, and micronutrients (Milne et al, 2002).
- Tips for eating alone: plan menus and shop accordingly. Cook in batches and freeze extras.
- For hospice patients, provide comfort foods and liquids as requested.

SAMPLE NUTRITION DIAGNOSTIC STATEMENT

Elderly Resident in Long-Term Care

PES: Involuntary weight loss related to inadequate food and beverage intake as evidenced by 24-pound weight loss and dining room food records indicating intake at less than 50% of meals.

Assessment: Intake reports and food preferences, I & O records, weight changes, lab values, psychological issues.

Intervention: Offer more favorite foods; promote consumption of between-meal nourishments, collaboration with social worker.

Monitoring and Evaluation: Changes in weight, verbalized improvement in appetite, dining room food intake records.

SAMPLE NUTRITION DIAGNOSTIC STATEMENT

End of Life Nutrition

PES: Inadequate food and beverage intake related to patient's choice to withdraw nutritional support as evidenced by minimal oral intake and palliative care status.

Assessment Data (sources of info): MD order for palliative care.

Intervention: Make food and fluids available upon patient or family request

Monitoring and Evaluation: Check on measures taken for meeting patient or family requests.

CLINICAL INDICATORS

Clinical/History		Lab Work
Age	Urinary incontinence	Glucose
Height (actual)	Hx of surgery, radiation, chemotherapy	C-reactive protein (CRP)
Weight, current	Mini-Mental State Examination	Ca++, Mg++
Weight, usual	Incontinence, indwelling catheter	Urinary N
Recent weight changes	Hydration status, I & O	Na+, K+
BMI and waist to hip ratio	Clinical signs of malnutrition	H & H, serum Fe
Diet history	DXA to evaluate for sarcopenia or osteopenia	Serum vitamin B_{12}, methylmalonic acid
Temperature (hypothermia is more common)	Changes in appetite	Serum folate
BP	Nausea, vomiting, indigestion	Serum homocysteine
Dentition	Pain	Chol, Trig
Eyesight	Infection	Alb or transthyretin (may be deceptively high in dehydration)
Hearing	Abnormal motor coordination	TSF, MAC, MAMC
Difficulty in chewing		BUN, Creat
Dysphagia		Transferrin
Constipation, diarrhea, fecal impaction, changes in bowel habits		TLC
Skin condition and pressure ulcers		Protime (PT) or international normalized ratio (INR)

Common Drugs Used and Potential Side Effects

- Many drugs affect the nutritional status of the patient. A thorough drug history is needed. Polypharmacy is common in elderly individuals, especially those living in institutionalized settings. Evidence exists that a long-term, high-carbohydrate, low-protein diet may be undesirable with drug therapies of many types due to the amount of protein-bound drugs prescribed. Drug metabolism is slowed down, which is a potentially dangerous occurrence. Many drugs cause undesirable side effects:
  - Nausea/vomiting: antibiotics, opiates, digoxin, theophylline, nonsteroidal anti-inflammatory agents (NSAIDs).
  - Anorexia: antibiotics, digoxin.
  - Decreased sense of taste: metronidazole, calcium channel blockers, angiotensin-converting enzyme (ACE) inhibitors, metformin.
  - Early satiety: anticholinergic drugs, sympathomimetic agents.
  - Reduced feeding ability: sedatives, opiates, psychotropic agents.
  - Dysphagia: potassium supplements, NSAIDs, bisphosphonates, prednisolone.
  - Constipation: opiates, iron supplements, diuretics.
  - Diarrhea: laxatives, antibiotics.
  - Hypermetabolism: thyroxine, ephedrine.
- Drug metabolism and detoxification require an adequate diet containing methionine; vitamins A, C, and E; choline; folacin; selenium; other sulfur amino acids; and vitamin B_{12}.
- Amphetamines, anorexic agents, and barbituates of all kinds may be highly addictive in older adults and are not recommended for use in this population (except phenobarbital).
- Aspirin in large doses can decrease serum folate, vitamin C, and iron.
- Cardiac drugs (such as amiodarone, guanethidine, guanadrel, doxazosin, nifedipine, and clonidine) can cause hypotension upon standing from a seated position.
- Cimetidine (Tagamet) can decrease vitamin B_{12} levels and may cause confusion.
- Digoxin: decreased clearance from the kidneys can increase risks for toxicity.
- Diuretic therapy is one central pharmacologic therapy of heart insufficiency and hypertension. Diuretics not only lead to an increased urinary excretion of electrolytes but also of water-soluble vitamins. Thiamin deficiency is a real risk; a low-dose thiamin supplement may be useful to prevent subclinical beri-beri in older subjects on diuretics (McCabe-Sellers et al, 2005). Diuretics can also decrease serum levels of potassium, magnesium, calcium, and zinc.
- Indomethacin has many adverse CNS side effects.
- Mineral oil should be discouraged as a laxative because it decreases absorption of fat-soluble vitamins and calcium.
- Sulfonamides decrease levels of vitamin K and the B-complex vitamins.
- Discuss the relevance of tolerable upper intake levels (ULs) from the latest dietary reference intakes of the National Academy of Sciences. These levels were set to protect individuals from receiving too much of any nutrient from diet and dietary supplements.

Herbs, Botanicals, and Supplements

- Herbs and botanical supplements should not be used without discussing with the physician, especially for underlying medical conditions. Older people should be encouraged to report the use of herbs and nutritional supplements to their doctors, and doctors should provide comprehensive and current information about potential herb–drug interactions (Canter and Ernst, 2004). Among the elderly, herbal supplement users are more likely to perceive their supplements as safe and to consider conventional medicine to be less effective than nonusers (Shahrokh et al, 2005).
- Age-associated increase in prostaglandin E2 production contributes to the decline in T-cell–mediated function with age. Black currant seed oil rich in both gamma and alpha linoleic acids has a moderate immune-enhancing effect related to its ability to reduce production of prostaglandin E2 (Wu et al, 1999).

- Creatine supplements have been used to increase strength in some older individuals. More studies are needed because results are mixed.
- Echinacea may be used as an immune system stimulant. It should not be taken with steroids, cyclosporine, or immunosuppressants. It may aggravate allergies in susceptible individuals.
- Gingko biloba has been studied for its beneficial effects on memory. While some studies have demonstrated some effectiveness for treatment of age-related memory loss or dementia, others have not (Van Dongen et al, 2000).
- Ginseng may be used for stress adaptation, performance enhancement, impotence, or as a digestive aid. It should not be taken with warfarin, insulin, oral hypoglycemics, CNS stimulants, caffeine, steroids, hormones, antipsychotics, aspirin, or antiplatelet drugs.
- Kava is sometimes used as a sleep aid; avoid use with sedatives, alcohol, antipsychotics, or other CNS depressants. Discourage use.
- Vitamin E supplements may ward off colds or flu in older people (Meydani et al, 2004).

INTERVENTION: NUTRITION EDUCATION, COUNSELING, CARE MANAGEMENT

- Efforts to correct malnutrition in the elderly are beneficial and cost-effective measures (Rypkema et al, 2004). Numerous tools are available and can be used in a variety of settings (Delacorte et al, 2004). Dietitians can and should serve as case managers for handling the discharge planning nutrition needs of the elderly (Baker and Wellman, 2005).
- When needed, senior citizens may increase their protein intake after appropriate counseling is offered (Rousset et al, 2006).
- Emphasize the need to consume adequate amounts of calcium, folic acid, vitamins A and E, and often vitamin D (DiDaniele et al, 2004). Review the desired nutrient intake with the client; supplemental iron is not often needed unless there is documented anemia. Vitamin B_{12} and thiamin may be needed, depending on medications used and concurrent chronic disease.
- Be aware of income limitations when planning a menu—less expensive protein sources may be necessary. Discuss shopping and meal preparation tips.
- Prevent excessive use of caffeine (e.g., coffee, colas, and tea), which may prevent intake of other desirable juices and beverages. Three 6- to 9-oz cups of coffee per day pose no specific health risk; monitor effects of anxiety, medications, etc. Caffeine may also promote improved cognition.
- Ensure that the diet uses sources of fluid and fiber to alleviate constipation. Discuss exercises such as walking and resistance training.
- Make every effort to determine whether the patient is using alcohol because multiple deficiencies may result, especially thiamin, vitamin B_{12}, folacin, and zinc deficiencies. Make appropriate referrals. Remember, older adults may not admit to the true amount of alcohol being consumed.
- Encourage participation in Meals on Wheels, food stamps, congregate feeding programs, and Senior Farmers' Market programs.
- Ensure adequate fluid intake where permitted.
- Encourage exercise as prescribed (e.g., strength conditioning). Walking may be especially beneficial to reduce the likelihood of falls. Yoga may help to prevent weight gain with aging.
- Discuss adding herbs, spices, and other flavor enhancers to foods. Olfactory decline is more common than once believed (Landis et al, 2004). Flavorful foods may release endorphins, which help boost the immune system (Duffy et al, 1999).
- Hypothermia is common in the elderly (i.e., body temperature of 95°F or lower). Fatigue, weakness, poor coordination, lethargy, slurred speech, and drowsiness can occur. Give hot beverages and place in a warm bed. When body temperature reaches 90°F, death is likely.
- Restorative dining may require specialized attention from a dietitian. The American Dietetic Association has suggested three visits for medical nutrition therapy for restorative dining procedures.
- For patients with a history of, current status of, or risk for dehydration, the American Dietetic Association has recommended two medical nutrition therapy visits.
- Because depression affects 20–40% of older Americans but is not a normal part of aging and because it causes a lot of weight loss in nursing homes and in the community, it must be identified and treated (Tolmunen et al, 2004). Tables 1-20, 1-21, and 1-22 can be used to determine weight and stature among the elderly.
- Support intake of antioxidants to protect the aging brain (Petot and Friedland, 2004). A key list of important nutrients in fruits and vegetables is provided in Table 1-23. Top choices include: grape juice, blueberries, papaya, kiwifruit, cantaloupe, mango, apricot, broccoli, spinach, tomato, sweet potato, and collards.

Patient Education—Food Safety Tips

- Reminders about hand washing and safe food handling may be important, especially for adults who prepare and serve meals for the elderly.
- Avoid food preparation when sick with viral or bacterial infections; use gloves if needed.
- Thoroughly cook meat, poultry, and fish entrees. Keep cold foods cold and hot foods hot.
- Because bacteria are commonly found on foods such as green onions (scallions), cantaloupe, cilantro, and imported produce, wash all fresh fruits and vegetables. Scrub the outside of produce such as melons and cucumbers before cutting.
- When traveling, avoid tap water and ice made from tap water, uncooked produce such as lettuce, and raw or undercooked seafood.
- Airline water may not be free from contamination. Use of bottled water is recommended. Coffee and tea may not be hot enough to kill all bacteria.
- Throw out cooked foods that have been at room temperature for longer than 2 hours.
- Consumption of sulforaphane in foods such as broccoli, cauliflower, cabbage, and Brussels sprouts may reduce the presence of *Helicobacter pylori*, which is beneficial.

TABLE 1-20 Weight Table for Men Aged 70 and Over

Height (inches)	Ages 70–74	Ages 75–79	Ages 80–84	Ages 85–89	Ages 90–94	Ages Over 94
61	128–156	125–153	123–151	120–145	118–142	113–139
62	130–158	127–155	125–153	122–148	119–143	114–140
63	131–161	129–157	127–155	122–150	120–146	115–141
64	134–164	131–161	129–157	124–152	122–148	116–142
65	136–166	134–164	130–160	127–155	125–153	117–143
66	139–169	137–167	133–163	130–158	128–156	120–146
67	140–172	140–170	136–166	132–162	130–160	122–150
68	143–175	142–174	139–169	135–165	133–163	126–154
69	147–179	146–178	142–174	139–169	137–167	130–158
70	150–184	148–182	146–178	143–175	140–172	134–164
71	155–189	152–186	149–183	148–180	144–176	139–169
72	159–195	156–190	154–188	153–187	148–182	143–173
73	164–200	160–196	158–192	157–189	156–187	155–177
74	169–205	165–201	163–197	162–190	160–188	158–181

Adapted from *Journal of the American Medical Association*, Vol. 177, p. 658, with permission of American Medical Association, Copyright 1960. American Medical Association.

- Avoid raw or partially cooked eggs, raw or undercooked fish or shellfish, and raw or undercooked meats because of potential foodborne illnesses.
- Do not use raw (unpasteurized) milk or products made from it.
- Avoid serving unpasteurized cider, juices, and raw sprouts because they may contain *Escherichia coli.*
- Only serve processed deli meats and frankfurters that have been reheated to steaming hot temperature. If the patient is immunocompromised, it may be best to avoid deli meats and ready-to-eat meat and poultry products; smoked fish; and soft cheese such as brie and blue-veined varieties because of the risk for *Listeria.* Homemade egg nog, cookie and cake batter, and other foods prepared

TABLE 1-21 Weight Table for Women Aged 70 and Over

Height (inches)	Ages 70–74	Ages 75–79	Ages 80–84	Ages 85–89	Ages 90–94	Ages Over 94
55	117–143	106–132	107–132	94–113	86–108	85–107
56	118–144	108–134	108–133	95–114	88–110	87–109
57	119–145	110–136	109–134	96–115	90–112	89–110
58	120–146	112–138	111–135	97–118	94–115	93–114
59	121–147	114–140	112–136	100–122	99–121	98–120
60	122–148	116–142	113–139	106–130	102–124	101–123
61	123–151	118–144	115–141	109–133	104–128	103–129
62	125–153	121–147	118–144	112–136	108–132	107–131
63	127–155	123–151	121–147	115–141	112–136	107–131
64	130–158	126–154	123–151	119–145	115–141	108–132
65	132–162	130–158	126–154	122–150	120–146	112–136
66	136–166	132–162	128–157	126–154	124–152	116–142
67	140–170	136–166	131–161	130–158	128–156	120–146
68	143–175	140–170	137–164	134–162	131–160	124–150
69	148–180	144–176	NA*	NA	NA	NA

Adapted from *Journal of the American Medical Association*, Vol. 177, p. 658, with permission of American Medical Association, Copyright 1960. American Medical Association.

*NA, not available.

TABLE 1-22 Formula for Calculating Stature Using Knee Height

Knee height can be used to estimate standing height in a bedridden or handicapped person. Knee height is not affected by aging. Different populations may require the use of different equations; equations derived from taller statured populations (e.g., Caucasians) may be less accurate when applied to shorter statured populations. Sample formulas are as follows:

Stature for Caucasian men $= 64.19 - (0.04 \times \text{age in years}) + (2.02 \times \text{knee height in cm})$

Stature for Japanese men $= 71.16 - (0.56 \times \text{age in years}) + (2.61 \times \text{knee height in cm})$

Stature for Caucasian women $= 84.88 - (0.24 \times \text{age in years}) + (1.83 \times \text{knee height in cm})$

Stature for Japanese women $= 63.06 - (0.34 \times \text{age in years}) + (2.38 \times \text{knee height in cm})$

Sources: Chumlea, 1984; Chumlea et al, 1994; Knous and Arisawa, 2002; and Mendoza-Nunez et al, 2002.

TABLE 1-23 Key Nutrients in Fruits and Vegetables[a]

Food	Vitamin A, >500 IU	Vitamin C, >6 mg	Folate, >0.04 mg	Potassium, >350 mg	Dietary Fiber, >2 g
Fruits					
Apple, with skin (1 medium)		X			X
Apricot, dried (3)	X	X		X	X
Banana (1 medium)		X		X	X
Blackberries (1/2 cup)					X
Blueberries (1 cup)		X			X
Cantaloupe (1 cup)	X	X		X	
Grapefruit (1/2 medium)		X			
Grapefruit juice (3/4 cup)		X		X	
Grapes (1/2 cup)		X			
Honeydew melon (1 cup)		X		X	X
Kiwifruit (2 medium)		X	X	X	X
Mango (1 medium)	X	X			X
Nectarine (1 medium)	X	X			X
Orange (1 medium)		X	X		X
Orange juice (3/4 cup)		X	X	X	
Papaya (1 medium)	X	X	X	X	X
Peach, with skin (1 medium)	X	X			X
Pear, with skin (1 medium)		X			X
Pineapple (two 3/4″ slices)		X			X
Plum, with skin (2 medium)		X			X
Prunes (4) (dried plums)	X				X
Raspberries (1 cup)		X			X
Strawberries (1/2 cup)		X			X
Watermelon (1 cup)	X	X			

(continued)

TABLE 1-23 Key Nutrients in Fruits and Vegetables[a] *(continued)*

Food	Vitamin A, >500 IU	Vitamin C, >6 mg	Folate, >0.04 mg	Potassium, >350 mg	Dietary Fiber, >2 g
Vegetables					
Artichokes (1 medium)					X
Asparagus (5 spears)		X	X		X
Beans, kidney (1/2 cup)			X	X	X
Beans, lima (1/2 cup)			X	X	X
Black-eyed peas (1/2 cup)			X		X
Bok choy (1 cup cooked)		X			
Broccoli (1/2 cup)	X	X	X		X
Brussels sprouts (1/2 cup)		X			
Carrots (1 medium)	X	X			X
Cauliflower (1 cup)		X	X		X
Collards (1/2 cup)	X	X	X		X
Corn (1 cup)		X	X	X	X
Green beans (1/2 cup)		X			X
Green pepper (1 medium)	X	X			X
Kale (1/2 cup)	X	X			X
Lentils (1/2 cup)			X	X	X
Peas, green (1/2 cup)		X	X		X
Peas, split (1/2 cup)			X	X	X
Potato (1 medium)		X		X	
Potato, with skin (1 medium)		X		X	X
Romaine lettuce (6 leaves)	X	X	X		
Spinach, cooked (1/2 cup)	X	X	X	X	X
Squash, winter (1/2 cup)	X	X		X	X
Sweet potato (1 medium)	X	X		X	X
Tomato (1 medium)	X	X		X	
Turnip greens (1/2 cup)	X	X	X		

Adapted from *Supermarket Savvy* newsletter, Linda McDonald Associates Inc., www.supermarketsavvy.com. Used with permission.

[a] X indicates that the item provides 10% or more of the daily value in the serving size specified or at least 2 grams of dietary fiber.

with raw eggs should be avoided because of the risks of *Salmonella*.

- Raw seafood such as oysters, clams, and mussels may contain *Vibrio* bacteria. Caution or avoidance is recommended.

For More Information

- American Association of Retired Persons (AARP)
  http://www.aarp.org/
- Administration on Aging
  http://www.aoa.dhhs.gov/
- Aging with Dignity
  http://www.agingwithdignity.org/
- American Federation for Aging Research
  http://www.afar.org/
- American Geriatrics Society
  http://www.americangeriatrics.org/
- American Society on Aging
  http://www.asaging.org/
- Centers for Medicare and Medicaid (Nursing Homes)
  http://www.cms.hhs.gov/medicaid/
- Elder Care
  http://www.eldercare.com/
- The Gerontological Society of America
  http://www.geron.org/
- Government Page for Seniors
  http://www.firstgov.gov/Topics/Seniors.shtml
- Health and Age
  http://www.eldercare.com/
- Homecare Online
  http://www.nahc.org/
- Meals on Wheels
  http://www.mowaa.org/
- Medicare Information
  http://www.medicare.gov/
- National Association Directors of Nursing Administration in Long Term Care
  http://www.nadona.org/

- National Association of Nutrition and Aging Services Programs
http://www.nanasp.org/

- National Council on Aging (NCOA)
http://www.ncoa.org/

- National Institute on Aging (NIA)
31 Center Drive, MSC 2292, Building 31, Room 5C27
Bethesda, MD 20892
http://www.nih.gov/nia/

- National Policy and Resource Center on Nutrition and Aging
http://nutritionandaging.fiu.edu/

- New York State Aging
http://agingwell.state.ny.us/eatwell/index.htm

- Novartis Health and Age Page
http://www.healthandage.com/

- Nursing Statement: Foregoing Food and Nutrition
http://nursingworld.org/readroom/position/ethics/etnutr.htm

- Nutrition Screening Initiative (NSI)
1010 Wisconsin Avenue, NW, Suite 800
Washington, DC 20007
http://www.aafp.org/x16081.xml

- Okinawa Centenarians Study
http://www.okicent.org/

- U.S. Senate Committee on Aging
http://aging.senate.gov/

GERIATRIC NUTRITION—CITED REFERENCES

American Dietetic Association. Position of the American Dietetic Association: nutrition across the spectrum of aging. *J Am Diet Assoc.* 105:616, 2005.

Avenell A, Handoll HH. Nutritional supplementation for hip fracture aftercare in older people. *Cochrane Database Syst Rev.* 2:CD001880, 2005.

Baker EB, Wellman NS. Nutrition concerns in discharge planning for older adults: a need for multidisciplinary collaboration. *J Am Diet Assoc.* 105:603, 2005.

Barnard ND, et al. The effects of a low-fat, plant-based dietary intervention on body weight, metabolism, and insulin sensitivity. *Am J Med.* 118:991, 2005.

Bos C, et al. Short-term protein and energy supplementation activates nitrogen kinetics and accretion in poorly nourished elderly subjects. *Am J Clin Nutr.* 71:1129, 2000.

Brescianini S, et al. Low total cholesterol and increased risk of dying: are low levels clinical warning signs in the elderly? Results from the Italian Longitudinal Study on Aging. *J Am Geriatr Soc.* 51:991, 2003.

Burke GL, et al. Factors associated with healthy aging: the cardiovascular health study. *J Am Geriatr Soc.* 49:254, 2001.

Canter PH, Ernst E. Herbal supplement use by persons aged over 50 years in Britain: frequently used herbs, concomitant use of herbs, nutritional supplements and prescription drugs, rate of informing doctors and potential for negative interactions. *Drugs Aging.* 21:597, 2004.

Chumlea WC. Methods of assessing body composition in nonambulatory persons. In: *Body composition assessment in youths and adults.* Report of the Sixth Ross Conference on Medical Research. Columbus, OH: Ross Laboratories, 1984, pp. 86–90.

Chumlea WC, et al. Prediction of stature from knee height for black and white adults and children with application to mobility-impaired or handicapped persons. J *Am Diet Assoc.* 94:1385, 1994.

Correia MI, Campos AC; ELAN Cooperative Study. Prevalence of hospital malnutrition in Latin America: the multicenter ELAN study. *Nutrition* 19:823, 2003.

D'Anci KE, Rosenberg IH. Folate and brain function in the elderly. *Curr Opin Clin Nutr Metab Care.* 7:659, 2004.

Dawson-Hughes B. Racial/ethnic considerations in making recommendations for vitamin D for adult and elderly men and women. *Am J Clin Nutr.* 80:1763S, 2004.

Delacorte RR, et al. Mini-nutritional assessment score and the risk for undernutrition in free-living older persons. *J Nutr Health Aging.* 8:531, 2004.

DiDaniele N, et al. Effect of supplementation of calcium and vitamin D on bone mineral density and bone mineral content in peri- and post-menopause women: a double-blind, randomized, controlled trial. *Pharmacol Res.* 50:637, 2004.

Duffy V, et al. Measurement of sensitivity to olfactory flavor: application in a study of aging and dentures. *Chem Senses.* 24:671, 1999.

Feinsod FM, et al. Dehydration in frail, older residents in long-term care facilities. *J Am Med Dir Assoc.* 5:35S, 2004.

Guigoz Y, et al. Identifying the elderly at risk for malnutrition. The Mini Nutritional Assessment. *Clin Geriatr Med.* 18:737, 2002.

Harris N. Nutrition in aging. In: Mahan LK, Escott-Stump S, eds. *Krause's food, nutrition, and diet therapy.* 11th ed. Philadelphia: WB Saunders, 2004.

Hercberg S, et al. The SU.VI.MAX Study: a randomized, placebo-controlled trial of the health effects of antioxidant vitamins and minerals. *Arch Intern Med.* 164:2335, 2004.

Ho C, et al. Practitioners' guide to meeting the vitamin B12 Recommended Dietary Allowance for people aged 51 and older. *J Am Diet Assoc.* 99:725, 1999.

Hudgens J, Langkamp-Henken B. The mini nutritional assessment as an assessment tool in elders in long-term care. *Nutr Clin Pract.* 19:463, 2005.

Jacobs DR, Iribarren C. Invited commentary: low cholesterol and nonatherosclerotic disease risk: a persistently perplexing question. *Am J Epidemiol.* 151:748, 2000.

Kalantar-Zadeh K, et al. Reverse epidemiology of conventional cardiovascular risk factors in patients with chronic heart failure. *J Am Coll Cardiol.* 43:1439, 2004.

Knous BL, Arisawa M. Estimation of height in elderly Japanese using region-specific knee height equations. *Am J Hum Biol.* 14:300, 2002.

Landis BN, et al. A study on the frequency of olfactory dysfunction. *Laryngoscope* 114:1764, 2004.

Marengoni A, et al. Homocysteine and disability in hospitalized geriatric patients. *Metabolism* 53:1016, 2004.

McCabe-Sellers B, et al. Diuretic medication therapy use and low thiamin intake in homebound older adults. *J Nutr Elder.* 24:57, 2005.

Mendoza-Nunez VM, et al. Equations for predicting height for elderly Mexican Americans are not applicable for elderly Mexicans. *Am J Hum Biol.* 14:351, 2002.

Meydani SN, et al. Vitamin E and respiratory tract infections in elderly nursing home residents: a randomized controlled trial. *JAMA.* 292:828, 2004.

Milne AC, et al. Protein and energy supplementation in elderly people at risk from malnutrition. *Cochrane Database Syst Rev.* 3:CD003288, 2002.

Morgan RO, et al. Low-intensity exercise and reduction of the risk for falls among at-risk elders. *J Gerontol A Biol Sci Med Sci.* 59:1062, 2004.

Morse MH, et al. Protein requirement of elderly women: nitrogen balance responses to three levels of protein intake. *J Gerontol A Biol Sci Med Sci.* 56:724, 2001.

Niedert K. Position of the American Dietetic Association: liberalized diets for older adults in long-term care. *J Am Diet Assoc.* 105:1955, 2005.

Petot GJ, Friedland RP. Lipids, diet and Alzheimer disease: an extended summary. *J Neurol Sci.* 226:31, 2004.

Pichard C, et al. Nutritional assessment: lean body mass depletion at hospital admission is associated with an increased length of stay. *Am J Clin Nutr.* 79:613, 2004.

Robinson MK, et al. Improving nutritional screening of hospitalized patients: the role of transthyretin. *J Parenter Enteral Nutr.* 27:389, 2003.

Rousset S, et al. Change in protein intake in elderly French people living at home after a nutritional information program targeting protein consumption. *J Am Diet Assoc.* 106:253, 2006.

Rypkema G, et al. Cost-effectiveness of an interdisciplinary intervention in geriatric inpatients to prevent malnutrition. *J Nutr Health Aging.* 8:122, 2004.

Shahrokh LE, et al. Elderly herbal supplement users less satisfied with medical care than nonusers. *J Am Diet Assoc.* 105:1138, 2005.

Smith J, et al. Energy restriction and aging. *Curr Opin Clin Nutr Metab Care.* 7:615, 2004.

Tolmunen T, et al. Association between depressive symptoms and serum concentrations of homocysteine in men: a population study. *Am J Clin Nutr.* 80:1574, 2004.

Van Dongen MC, et al. The efficacy of gingko for elderly people with dementia and age-associated memory impairment: new results of a randomized clinical trial. *J Am Geriatr Soc.* 48:1183, 2000.

Vanitallie TB. Frailty in the elderly: contributions of sarcopenia and visceral protein depletion. *Metabolism* 52:22S, 2003.

Wilson MM, et al. Appetite assessment: simple appetite questionnaire predicts weight loss in community-dwelling adults and nursing home residents. *Am J Clin Nutr.* 82:1074, 2005.

Wolters M, et al. Cobalamin: a critical vitamin in the elderly. *Prev Med.* 39:1256, 2004.

Wu D, et al. Effect of dietary supplementation with black currant seed oil on the immune response of healthy elderly subjects. *Am J Clin Nutr.* 70:536, 1999.

S E C T I O N

Dietary Practices and Miscellaneous Conditions

2

CHIEF ASSESSMENT FACTORS

- Cultural Patterns
- Vegetarian Diets
- Religious Preferences and Special Diets or Practices
- Mouth: Dental Problems, Periodontal Diseases, Dentures (Ill-Fitting), Missing or Loose Teeth, Caries, Dental Care, Increased Salivation, Dryness, Lesions
- Problems with Self-Feeding
- Vision: Cataracts, Visual Field Changes, Diplopia, Glaucoma, Macular Degeneration, Blindness
- Skin: Texture or Color Changes, Dryness, Ecchymoses, Lesions, Masses, Petechiae, Pressure Ulcers
- Signs of Vitamin Deficiencies
- Food Allergies or Intolerances
- Complementary and Alternative Medicine, Including Use of Herbs, Spices, and Botanical Products
- Head/Face: Pain, Past Trauma, Syncope, Unusual or Frequent Headaches
- Ears: Problems, Discharge, Infections, Tinnitus or Vertigo
- Food-Borne Illnesses

For More Information

- American Dietetic Association–Nutrition Education for the Public
  http://www.nepdpg.org/
- Centers for Disease Control–Index for Consumer Questions
  http://www.cdc.gov/health/diseases.htm
- Evidence-Based Practice Centers
  http://www.ahrq.gov/clinic/epcquick.htm
- Federal Consumer Information Center
  http://www.pueblo.gsa.gov/food.htm
- Federal Trade Commission
  http://www.ftc.gov/
- Health Finder
  http://www.healthfinder.gov/
- Health Fraud and Quackery
  http://www.quackwatch.com/
- Health Statistics
  http://www.cdc.gov/nchswww/
- Healthy People 2010
  http://web.health.gov/healthypeople/
- Human Anatomy Online
  http://www.innerbody.com/
- International Food Information Council–Functional Foods
  http://www.ific.org/nutrition/functional/index.cfm
- PubMed
  http://www.ncbi.nlm.nih.gov/PubMed/
- Tufts University Nutrition Navigator
  http://navigator.tufts.edu/
- USDA
  Food Composition Tables
  http://www.nal.usda.gov/fnic/foodcomp/Data/HG72/hg72.html
  Nutrient Data Tables
  http://www.ars.usda.gov/main/site_main.htm?modecode=12354500

COMPLEMENTARY NUTRITION

COMPLEMENTARY NUTRITION

NUTRITIONAL ACUITY RANKING: LEVEL 2 (DIETARY ADAPTATIONS, ADVISEMENT)

DEFINITIONS AND BACKGROUND

The philosophy that food can be health promoting beyond its nutritional value has gained acceptance within the public arena. Botanical supplement use is going up, whereas supporting evidence for these herbs is not as clear (Shah and Grant, 2000). About 34% of Americans take a vitamin-mineral supplement daily (Thomson et al, 2005).

In the arena of dietary supplements, dietitians are uniquely qualified to translate sound scientific evidence into practical applications. Dietitians consider themselves knowledgeable about use of functional foods and nutrient supplements, but only 10% have felt confident about the roles of herbs in prevention and treatment of illnesses (Lee et al, 2000).

Education and training are useful tools for the dietetic practitioner in preparing to answer questions about complementary nutrition. Dietitians should be able to describe implications of FDA structure/function claims, explain how to read labels, identify sound resources, associate common dietary supplements and their appropriate uses, and assess the science behind the supplement claims (Thomson et al, 2005).

Because this text focuses on the herbs, spices, and botanical products and does not cover the extensive additional concepts and practices that are available (e.g., homeopathy, acupuncture, traditional Chinese or Indian medicine), the reader may wish to seek an update from other resources.

Functional foods are foods that provide health benefits beyond basic nutrition and are adjunctive to a balanced diet (Hasler et al, 2004). Fish provides fish oils; fermented dairy products have probiotics; and beef has conjugated linoleic acid. Many plants contain biologically active chemicals known as phytochemicals. Phenolic phytochemicals are the largest group of phytochemicals, with the most important subgroups being flavonoids, phenolic acids, and polyphenols. Phenolics are biologically active compounds that may possess some disease-prevention properties (King and Young, 1999). Oats provide beta-glucan, soy provides isoflavones, flaxseed provides lignins and alpha-linolenic acid, garlic provides organosulfur compounds, broccoli and cruciferous vegetables provide isothiocyanates and indoles, citrus fruits provide liminoids, cranberry provides polymeric compounds, tea provides cachectin, and wine provides phenolics (Hasler et al, 2004).

Increasing numbers of patients use herbal medicines but do not tell their health care providers. Consumers are testing many new products, and some are more effective than others. There are 29,000 different dietary supplements available to consumers, and an average of 1000 new products are added yearly according to the Food and Drug Administration (FDA) (Stein, 2000). Natural health products often interfere with medications, and the knowledge about the specific effects is still incomplete (Boullata, 2005). Caution should be the approach. About 15 million Americans are at risk for drug–supplement interactions (Boullata, 2005).

Nutrition is an integral part of many complementary therapies for cancer, arthritis, chronic back pain, human immunodeficiency virus (HIV), gastrointestinal (GI) problems, and eating disorders (Hamilton, 1998). Chinese herbal formulations may reduce some symptoms of patients with irritable bowel syndrome (Bensoussan et al, 1998). Dried culinary herbs (e.g., oregano, sage, peppermint, garden thyme, lemon balm, clove, allspice, and cinnamon) contain very high concentrations of antioxidants (i.e., >75 mmol/100 g), and dietary intake of herbs may contribute significantly to the total intake of plant antioxidants (Dragland et al, 2003).

USP-verified logo on products means that the products have the approval of the Dietary Supplement Verification Program (website: www.uspverified.org). Adverse reactions are discovered after marketing through case studies versus clinical trials for pharmaceuticals. There are excellent references available for use, including a *Physican's Desk Reference* specifically for herbal products (*Physician's Desk Reference for Herbal Medicines*, 2004), Tyler's *Honest Herbal* text (1999), and a reference from the American Dietetic Association (Sarubin-Fragakis, 2003). In Appendix E, Table E-1 provides a more complete list of potential interactions between botanicals and drugs. Table 2-1 provides more detail.

INTERVENTION: OBJECTIVES

The White House Commission on Complementary and Alternative Medicine Policy Executive Summary (2002) supports the following 10 guiding principles in counseling individuals about the use of complementary and alternative medicine (CAM) therapies and herbs or botanical products:

- Apply a "wholeness orientation" in health care delivery. Health involves all aspects of life—mind, body, spirit, and environment.
- Evaluate for evidence of safety and efficacy. Promote the use of science and appropriate scientific methods to help identify safe and effective CAM services and products.
- Identify the healing capacity of the individual person. People have a remarkable capacity for recovery and self-healing; support and promote this capacity.
- Respect individuality, recognizing that each person is unique and has the right to health care that is appropriately responsive to him or her, respecting preferences and preserving dignity.
- Recognize patient rights. Each has the right to choose treatment; to choose freely among safe and effective care or approaches; and to choose among qualified practitioners who are accountable for their claims and actions and responsive to the person's needs.
- Support health promotion, self-care, and early intervention for maintaining and promoting health.
- Develop partnerships. Good health care requires teamwork among patients, health care practitioners (conventional and CAM), and researchers committed to creating optimal healing environments and to respecting the diversity of all health care traditions.
- Educate about prevention, healthy lifestyles, and the power of self-healing.
- Disseminate comprehensive and timely information. The quality of health care can be enhanced by promoting efforts that thoroughly and thoughtfully examine the evidence on which CAM systems, practices, and products are based and make this evidence widely, rapidly, and easily available.
- Integrate public involvement. The input of informed consumers and other members of the public must be incorporated in setting priorities for health care and health care research and in reaching policy decisions, including those related to CAM, within the public and private sectors.

INTERVENTION: FOOD AND NUTRITION

- Promote the appropriate use of herbal and botanical products that have shown efficacy and safety. The best strategy for promoting optimal health and for reducing chronic disease is to choose a wide variety of foods (American Dietetic Association, 2005).
- Dietetics professionals are trained to assess dietary adequacy and the need for dietary modifications (American Dietetic Association, 2005). Sometimes there are individuals who need dietary supplements because of disease states, certain life stages, or chronic conditions. It is important to respect those cultural patterns and habits in which herbs and botanicals have been used without negative side effects and to teach the potential side effects of herbals and botanical products when used with medications.
- Functional foods are available that have health benefits beyond basic nutrition (e.g., omega-3–enriched eggs, stanol- and sterol-fortified soft chews and related margarines, or high-flavanol chocolate snacks). Use often.
- Special attention may be needed for intake of iron and folic acid for females in teen and childbearing years; vitamin B_{12} for adults over age 50; and vitamin D for older adults, those with dark skin, and those exposed to ultraviolet radiation (American Dietetic Association, 2005).

Herbs, Botanicals, and Supplements

Many cultures use herbs and botanicals as part of their meal patterns, rituals, and celebrations. Herbs commonly used by WIC children include aloe vera, chamomile, garlic, peppermint, lavender, cranberry, ginger, echinacea, and lemon; they are recommended by family or friends (Lohse et al, 2006). Identify those that are used and monitor for potential side effects. Because herbs with safety issues, such as St. John's wort, dong quai, and kava, may also be used, herbal education is highly recommended for WIC clinics, especially for Latinos (Lohse et al, 2006).

The National Center for Complementary and Alternative Medicine is one of many reliable resources. HerbMed, an interactive, electronic herbal database, provides hyperlinked access to the scientific data including clinical trials and efficacy. More specific information is listed in Sections 1 and 13, and more general information is available in Appendix E.

Table 2-1 was developed from multiple resources, including the American Botanical Council; the hazardous herbs list was derived from the U.S. Consumer Product Safety Commission (CSPC).

INTERVENTION: NUTRITION EDUCATION, COUNSELING, CARE MANAGEMENT

- Demonstrate respect for the beliefs, values, and practices of the patient and family members.
- Discuss evidence that is known about different types of herbs and botanical products.

TABLE 2-1 Herbs, Botanicals, Spices, and Commentary

Herb, Botanical, Spice	Commentary
Alfalfa (*Medicago sativa*)	Used for diuretic properties in asthma, diabetes, thyroid gland malfunction, arthritis, high cholesterol, peptic ulcers. Said to promote menstruation and lactation. Rats fed with this are prone to colon cancer. Fatalities reported due to ingestion of contaminated alfalfa.
Alpha Lipoic Acid	Used to prevent cancer, HIV, AIDS, and liver disease. Used to lower triglycerides by reducing endothelial dysfunction. Most studies have been done with rats, and more human studies are needed. Contained in broccoli, spinach, tomato. Its antioxidant activity may antagonize the effects of chemotherapy.
Aloe Vera	Topical administration of aloe vera gel for burns is generally safe. It may help reduce radiation-induced skin changes, but clinical trials are inconsistent. Aloe vera is derived from the leaves of the plant *Aloe barbadensis*. FDA rules that it is not safe as a stimulant laxative. Causes strong GI cramping. Chronic use can lead to loss of potassium. Do not use with diuretics, corticosteroids, or antihyperglycemic or cardiovascular agents.
Arnica (*Arnica montana*)	Used as a topical ointment for bruises, osteoarthritis. If taken orally, causes hypotension and shortness of breath and can be fatal. In homeopathy preparations, these features are not seen.
Artemesia (Wormwood)	Used as an antimalarial; also used in cancer, fever, infections. GI upset is a common side effect. It's to be avoided by people with hyperacidity.
Avlimil	Used to alleviate symptoms of female sexual dysfunction. Contains cloves, capsicum, black cohosh, ginger, and licorice. It is contraindicated in women having hormone-sensitive cancers. Stomach upset is an adverse reaction.
Ayurveda	Used in diabetes, rheumatoid arthritis (RA), Parkinson's disease, obesity, and cancer. World bank is funding research in India to evaluate ayurvedic treatment for anemia, edema, and postpartum complications of pregnancy. Effects of meditation in reducing anxiety, lowering blood pressure, and enhancing general well-being have been confirmed. The components of the herbs show antioxidant, antitumor, antimicrobial, hypoglycemic, and anti-inflammatory properties. Lead poisoning is a potential complication.
Bilberry (*Vaccinium myrtillus*)	Used in Europe as an antioxidant to prevent diabetic retinopathy; improves visual acuity and retinal function. Used for cataracts, cancer, circulatory disorders, diabetic retinopathy, glaucoma, macular degeneration, hemorrhoids, varicose veins. Relative of blueberry. Do not use with anticoagulants or antiplatelet medications. No adverse reactions reported.
Bitter Melon (*Momordica charantia*)	Used in cancer prevention, diabetes, fever, HIV, infections, menstrual disorders. Contraindicated in children and pregnant women because it causes bleeding, contraction of the uterus, and abortion. Adverse reactions include hypoglycemia and hepatotoxicity, headache, fever, abdominal pain, and coma.
Black Cohosh (*Cimicifuga racemosa*)	Often suggested for use with hot flashes, headaches, vaginal dryness, mood swings, cough, dysmenorrhea, RA, sedation. It functions as an antispasmodic, sedative, or relaxant. Black cohosh may cause hypotension, vomiting, headache, dizziness, GI distress, and limb pain. Still controversial whether black cohosh possesses estrogenic activity. GI upset can occur. May increase the toxicity of doxorubicin and docetaxel. May interact with drugs that are metabolized by CYP3A4 enzyme. **Warning: should not be confused with blue cohosh (*Caulophyllum thalictroides*), which can be toxic** and may be used in an attempt to induce abortion.
Borage Oil (*Borago officinalis*)	Used for RA, infantile seborrheic dermatitis, cough, chest congestion, menopausal symptoms. Borage oil contains pyrrolizidine alkaloid and amabiline, which are hepatotoxic. Unsafe during pregnancy due to teratogenic effects and premature labor. Adverse effects include constipation and hepatotoxicity after chronic administration.
Boswellia (*Boswellia serrata*)	Used for arthritis, asthma, colitis, inflammation, menstrual cramps. Long-term affects on humans are unknown, but it has cytotoxic activities.
Brewer's Yeast	Used as a natural source of chromium. Brewer's yeast should not be taken with MAO inhibitors such as Nardil, Parnate.
Bromelain (sulfhydryl proteolytic enzyme)	Used for arthritis, bruises, burns, cancer prevention and treatment, edema, indigestion, and circulatory disorders. Bromelain is obtained from pineapple. Adverse reactions include diarrhea, GI disturbances, allergic reactions.
Bupleurum (*Bupleurum chinense, B. scoizone—raefolium*)	Used for colds, fever, infections, cirrhosis, hepatitis, liver disease, malaria, cancer treatment. Warning: may be associated with interstitial pneumonitis as an ingredient of shosaiko. Adverse reactions include nausea, vomiting, edema, GI disturbance.
Burdock (*Arctium majus*)	Used for arthritis, HIV, AIDS, psoriasis, diabetes, eczema, and anorexia; no human studies on these proposed claims. Promotes urination. Contraindications include pregnant or lactating women and those allergic to chrysanthemum. Warning: burdock tea sometimes is contaminated with belladonna alkaloids.
Butcher's Broom (*Ruscus aculeatus*)	Used for hemorrhoids, varicose veins, circulatory diseases, lymphedema, leg cramps, constipation, inflammation. Diarrhea is an adverse effect.
Calendula (*Calendula officinalis*)	Used for conjunctivitis, eczema, GI disturbance, inflammation, menstrual cramps, radiation therapy. Contraindications include pregnancy and lactation. Adverse reactions include possible allergic reactions.
Capsicum, Capsaicin (*Capsicum frutescens* and *C. annuum*)	Used as a circulatory stimulant to aid in digestion. Used externally to relieve pain, as from arthritis, circulatory disorders, diabetic and herpes zoster neuropathy, high cholesterol, motion sickness, muscle pain, toothache. Avoid contact with eyes and irritated or broken skin. Adverse reactions include burning skin, urticaria, and contact dermatitis. Drug interactions: increases the incidence of cough associated with ACE inhibitors.

(continued)

TABLE 2-1 Herbs, Botanicals, Spices, and Commentary *(continued)*

Herb, Botanical, Spice	Commentary
Cascara (*Rhamnus purshiana*)	Used for cancer treatment and constipation. Often found in over-the-counter laxatives. Avoid use with cardiovascular agents. Cascara is used to relieve constipation; FDA rules that cascara is not safe as a stimulant laxative. Contraindications: should not be used in intestinal obstruction or undiagnosed abdominal symptoms; patients with inflammatory bowel disease should use caution while using this supplement. Adverse reactions include vomiting, intestinal cramps; excessive use can cause diarrhea, weakness, and rarely cholestatic hepatitis. Drug interactions: excess loss of $K+$ with digoxin as it may potentiate the cardiac effects.
Cayenne	Used for muscle spasms and relief of pain in arthritis. Large doses may lead to chronic gastritis and kidney or liver damage. Do not use with anticoagulants or antiplatelet medications.
Chamomile (*Matricaria recutita*)	Used for colic, GI disturbance, hemorrhoids, infections, skin ulcers, mucositis. Chamomile soothes indigestion, flatulence. Topical and oral administration are safe except in patients with allergies to ragweed or chrysanthemum. Adverse reactions include contact dermatitis to anaphylaxis in those allergic to it. Drug interactions: increases anticoagulant effects due to its coumarin content.
Chasteberry (*Vitex agnus castus*)	Used for premenopausal symptoms, dysmenorrhea, or menopause. Should not be taken with hormone replacement therapy or oral contraceptives; an itchy rash can occur. It may interact with dopamine antagonists. Adverse reactions include GI upset, nausea, rash, urticaria, and headache.
Chinese Asparagus (*Asparagus cochinchinensis*)	Used for cancer treatment, constipation, cough, hepatitis. No adverse reactions and drug interactions reported.
Chitosan	Used as an ingredient in many weight loss supplements, with claims to bind and trap dietary fat. It is clinically insignificant (Gades and Stern, 2005).
Cholesterol Spinach (*Gynura crepioides*)	Used for control of high cholesterol; no scientific evidence. Contraindications: immunocompromised patients due to the possibility of contamination.
Chondroitin	Used to support healthy connective tissue and synovial fluid that lubricates joints. Improves functional status of people with hip or knee osteoarthritis, relieves pain, and reduces joint swelling and stiffness. Used with glucosamine in many products. Third most widely used supplement by elderly (Wold et al, 2005).
Chromium Picolinate	May have some merit in diabetes management, but more studies are needed. Naturally found in mushrooms, nuts, bread, yeast. Use may lead to impaired iron and zinc metabolism, GI intolerance, nephritis, or chromosomal damage. Often used by athletes.
Cinnamon	Used daily to increase sensitivity of insulin and to help manage diabetes (Anderson et al, 2004).
Chrysanthemum (*Chrysanthemum morifolium*)	Used for angina, hypertension, fever, common cold. No human studies. Contraindications: those with allergy to ragweed. Adverse reactions include contact dermatitis, photosensitivity.
Coenzyme Q10	Used for patients with heart failure or early signs of Parkinson's disease. Coenzyme Q10, superoxide dismutase (SOD), S-adenosyl-L-methionine methionine (SAM-e), and other products have not been proven to reduce the effects of aging.
Cone Flower (*Echinacea purpurea, E. pallida, E. augustifolia*)	Used for common cold, immunostimulation, infections, viral infections, wound healing. Contraindications: patients with autoimmune disorders (systemic lupus erythematosus, RA, multiple sclerosis, tuberculosis, HIV). Adverse reactions include headache, dizziness, nausea, rash, dermatitis, anaphylaxis.
Cranberry	Used to prevent urinary tract infection caused by *Escherichia coli* bacteria, especially after menopause.
Creatine	Used to increase strength in some older individuals and in athletes. More studies are needed. Heavy use may lead to cardiomyopathy, hypertension, renal impairment.
Curcumin and Curry	Used for antioxidant effects in cystic fibrosis, cognitive function in Alzheimer's disease, cancer prevention, and other conditions.
Dandelion (*Taraxacum mongolicum*)	Used for diabetes, lactation stimulation, promote urination, rheumatoid arthritis, liver disease. Used as salad greens and in teas. Only a few clinical studies. Contraindication in patients with obstruction of the bile duct or gallbladder. Adverse reactions include allergic reactions, contact dermatitis, dyspepsia. Drug interactions: additive effect on hypoglycemic activity
Da Qing Ye (*Isatis tinctoria*)	Used for cancer treatment, diarrhea, GI disorders, hepatitis, HIV and AIDS, respiratory infections. Adverse reactions include nausea, vomiting, hematuria following injection.
Devil's Claw (*Harpagophytum procumbens*)	Used for analgesic, anti-inflammatory, osteoarthritis, muscle pain, GI disturbances. Contraindication in pregnancy. Adverse reactions include dyspepsia, diarrhea, bradycardia.
Dong Quai (*Angelica sinensis*)	Used as Chinese tonic for menstrual cramps, peripheral vasodilator, and pain reliever. It has not shown effectiveness for reducing hot flashes. It should not be used in pregnancy. Do not use with anticoagulants or antiplatelet medications because it has Coumadin-like substances. Increased doses are carcinogenic. Adverse effects are bloating, loss of appetite, diarrhea, photosensitivity, gynecomastia.

(continued)

TABLE 2-1 Herbs, Botanicals, Spices, and Commentary *(continued)*

Herb, Botanical, Spice	Commentary
Echinacea (see Cone Flower)	Used as an immune system stimulant. Echinacea is no more effective for upper respiratory tract infections than placebo. It should not be taken with corticosteroids, cyclosporine, or immunosuppressants. It may trigger allergies since it is related to the ragweed family (as are butterbur, chamomile, goldenrod, and yarrow). Avoid taking for longer than 2 months at a time.
Eucalyptus	Used for asthma, coughs, arthritis in small doses. Overdoses can be fatal.
Evening Primrose Oil (*Oenothera biennis*)	Used for RA, mastalgia, eczema, fatigue, diabetic neuropathy, premenstrual syndrome, menopausal symptoms, cancer treatment. Contraindication: pregnant women. Adverse reactions are headache, nausea, GI upset. Drug interactions: may lower the seizure threshold in patients taking phenothiazines. Contains essential fatty acid known as gamma linolenic acid (GLA), which may be useful in cardiac or arthritic conditions. Avoid use also with chlorpromazine, fluphenazine, and mesoridazine. Do not use with anticoagulants or antiplatelet medications.
Fenugreek (*Trigonella foenum-graecum*)	Used for laxatives, lactation stimulation, diabetes, high cholesterol, wounds, alopecia, arthritis, GI disturbance, induce child birth. Contraindication: infants and pregnant women. Adverse reactions: flatulence, diarrhea, bleeding, bruising, hypoglycemia.
Feverfew (*Tanacetum parthenium*)	Used for migraine, psoriasis, arthritis, dysmenorrhea. Avoid use with nonsteroidal anti-inflammatory drugs (NSAIDs) because they negate its usefulness (Miller, 1998). Avoid use with warfarin, antiplatelet, or with other migraine headache medicines. Contraindication in those who are allergic to ragweed or marigold. Adverse reactions are mouth ulcers; withdrawal causes anxiety, muscle stiffness, and pain.
Flaxseed (*Linum usitatissimum*)	Used for cancer prevention, constipation, high cholesterol, menopausal symptoms, periodontal diseases, radiation therapy. Adverse reactions: affects radiation therapy.
Folk remedy oils	Used for childhood ailments in Mexican culture. May cause pneumonia in infants and children.
Forskolin (*Coleus forskohlii*)	Used for cancer treatment, glaucoma, asthma, heart failure, weight loss, allergy. Adverse reactions are hypotension, tachycardia. Drug interactions: additive hypotensive effect with beta blockers and calcium channel blockers and additive platelet inhibiton with anticoagulants.
Gamma Linolenic Acid (GLA)	Used for reducing signs of PMS or menopause. Black currant oil contains GLA. Do not use with anticonvulsants or anabolic steroids. Liver toxicity may occur.
Garcinia cambogia (hydroxycitric acid)	Used as ingredient of many weight loss products.
Garlic	Used to help lower cholesterol. Antibacterial, antifungal, antiviral, and hypotensive benefits have also been noted. Avoid using capsules with warfarin and with diabetes medications (may cause drop in blood glucose). Fourth most widely used supplement by elderly (Wold et al, 2005). Garlic appears to induce cytochrome P450 3A4 and may enhance metabolism of many medications such as cyclosporine and saquinavir.
Ginger (*Zingiber officinale*)	Used as a treatment for nausea, motion sickness, vomiting, anorexia, drug withdrawal, RA. Do not use with anticoagulants or antiplatelet medications. Adverse reactions include heartburn, dermatitis, CNS affects, depression, arrhythmias. Drug interactions: increases risk of bleeding if used with anticoagulant; additive effects on hypoglycemic drugs and histamine antagonists.
Gingko Biloba	Used to improve blood flow to the brain; to help with memory, hearing loss, dementias, circulatory disturbance, Raynaud's disease, sexual dysfunction, stress, tinnitus, asthma. Avoid use with warfarin, antihyperglycemic agents, vitamin E, or aspirin. Second most widely used supplement by elderly (Wold et al, 2005). Warning: to be discontinued before surgery. Adverse reactions include headache, dizziness, GI upset, diarrhea, and seizures in patients predisposed to seizures or on medications that lower seizure threshold. Gingko biloba may cause allergic skin reactions or bleeding.
Ginseng	Used for stress adaptation, cognitive or performance enhancement, impotence, or as a digestive aid. It should not be taken with warfarin, insulin, oral hypoglycemics, CNS stimulants, caffeine, steroids, hormones, antipsychotics, aspirin, cardiovascular agents, warfarin, or other antiplatelet drugs. May interfere with digoxin action (Miller, 1998). It does not enhance psychological well-being. Ginseng may add to the effects of estrogens or corticosteroids and can elevate BP. Do not take if pregnant or lactating. Siberian ginseng (*Acanthopanax senticosus*) uses: chemotherapy side effects, health maintenance, strength and stamina, and immunostimulation. Contraindicated in patients with hypertension (HTN) and premenopausal women.
Glehnia (*Glehnia littoralis*)	Used for bronchitis, chest congestion, whooping cough. Contraindicated in radiation therapy. No adverse reactions have been reported, but photosensitivity may occur due to psoralens component.
Glucosamine Sulfate	Used to build new cartilage, rebuild old cartilage, lubricate joints, mount a healthy inflammatory response, and ease symptoms of osteoarthritis. It is often taken with chondroitin. Side effects are mild. Most widely used supplement by elderly (Wold et al, 2005).
Gotu Kola (*Centella asiatica, Hydrocotyle asiatica*)	Used for burns, cancer treatment, circulatory disorders, GI disorders, hypertension, memory loss, psoriasis, scars, sedation, varicose veins. Gotu kola should not be confused with kolanut; gotu kola does not contain any caffeine and has not been shown to have stimulant properties. There are wide variations in terpenoid concentrations depending on the location in which gotu kola is grown. Products should be standardized as to asiaticoside, asiatic acid, madecassic acid, and madecassoside content. Adverse effects: contact dermatitis, pruritus, photosensitization, and headache; reduced fertility may occur in women wishing to become pregnant. With toxic levels, hyperglycemia, hyperlipidemia, and sedation have occurred.

(continued)

TABLE 2-1 Herbs, Botanicals, Spices, and Commentary *(continued)*

Herb, Botanical, Spice	Commentary
Green Tea	Used for activation of thermogenesis, fat oxidation, or both (Dulloo et al, 1999). Green tea is popular in several cultures. Both black and green tea may be preventive for cancers and strokes; they are also a good source of fluoride. Green tea contains a class of polyphenols called catechins, which consist mainly of epigallocatechin gallate (EGCG), epicatechin gallate, and gallocatechin gallate. Catechins have been reported to have various physiological and pharmacological properties over the years. Green tea extract (GTE) may be a useful tool for improving endurance capacity and possibly for weight loss (Nagao et al, 2005). GTE boosts exercise endurance, utilizing fat as energy source, accompanied by lower respiratory quotients and higher rates of fat oxidation; results come from the equivalent of about 4 cups of tea a day. Avoid use with MAO inhibitors and warfarin since green tea contains vitamin K. Avoid use in pregnancy and infants.
Guggul	Used to treat osteoarthritis and bone fractures; suppresses the nuclear factor-κB activation induced by various carcinogens (Ichikawa and Aggarwal, 2006). Guggul may induce CYP3A4 activity. Not enough scientific evidence to support the use of guggul for any medical condition. Guggul may cause stomach discomfort or allergic rash. It should be avoided in pregnancy and lactation and in children.
Hawthorn (*Crataegus monogyna*)	Used for angina, atherosclerosis, congestive heart failure (CHF), HTN, indigestion. Contraindications: pregnancy, lactation. Adverse reactions: nausea, sweating, fatigue, hypotension, arrhythmia. Because hawthorn lowers blood pressure and cholesterol levels, never take with digoxin. It seems to be safe for long-term use. In high doses, it can cause hypotension and sedation and should be monitored carefully. Avoid use with cardiovascular agents.
Horseradish	Used as a natural decongestant.
Huang Lian (*Coptis chinensis*)	Used for diarrhea, hypertension, bacterial and viral infections, ear infections, and cancer treatment. Contraindications: not to be administered to jaundiced neonates. Adverse reactions: nausea, vomiting, dyspnea. Toxicity: seizures, hepatotoxicity, cardiac toxicity.
Indirubin (*Indigofera tinctoria*)	Used for cancer treatment, inflammation. There are limited clinical data. Adverse reactions: nausea, vomiting, abdominal pain. Long-term treatment caused pulmonary arterial hypertension and cardiac insufficiency in a few patients.
Juniper	Used as a diuretic or for indigestion in some cultures. Avoid in pregnancy and kidney disease.
Karela	Used to lower blood glucose. Because it affect blood glucose levels, it should not be used by patients with diabetes mellitus (DM).
Kudzu (*Pueraria mirifica*, *P. thunbergiana*, *P. montana* var. *lobata*, *P. montana* var. *thomsonii*)	Used for estrogenic effects. Promoted for alcoholism, common cold, diabetes, eye pain, fever, menopausal symptoms, neck pain. Individuals with hormone-sensitive cancers and those taking tamoxifen should avoid it. Those with hypersensitivity to kudzu and patients with estrogen receptor–positive (ER+) breast cancer should also avoid kudzu.
Kyushin	Used as a cardiotonic medicine in China. Kyushin may interfere with digoxin action (Miller, 1998).
Licorice (*Glycyrrhiza glabra*, *G. uralensis*)	Used for bronchitis, chest congestion, constipation, GI disorders, hepatitis, inflammation, menopausal symptoms, microbial infection, peptic ulcers, primary adrenocortical insufficiency, prostate cancer. Licorice should not be consumed by those with renal or liver dysfunction or women who are pregnant or breastfeeding. Active ingredient (glycyrrhizin) has an anti-inflammatory role. May interfere with digoxin action (Miller, 1998). Licorice can offset the pharmacological effect of spironolactone. Large doses can produce headache or lethargy, as well as high blood pressure. May increase potassium losses when used with thiazide diuretics. Avoid use with liver cirrhosis, hypertension, cholestatic liver disease, hypokalemia, kidney failure.
Lycium (*Lycium barbarum*; *L. chinense*; *L. europeaum*)	Used for anemia, burns, cancer treatment, cough, inflammation, pain, sedation, skin infections, visual acuity. May prolong bleeding time in some individuals.
Mayapple	Used for venereal warts (condyloma acuminata); it contains podophyllotoxins. Common in Native American medicine.
Melatonin	Used as a sleep aid or a jet lag adjuster. Avoid use with CNS depressants such as alcohol, barbiturates, corticosteroids, or immunosuppressants.
Milk Thistle (silymarin)	Used for acoholic liver disease, cirrhosis, infectious hepatitis, drug-induced hepatitis. It may have a mild laxative effect or can cause uterine or menstrual stimulation. Best administered by injection. Serves as a natural antidote for death-cap mushroom poisoning.
Mint	Used in oil form for colds, bronchitis, fever, indigestion. Mild GI distress may result. Worsens gastroesophageal reflux disease (GERD) or hiatal hernia symptoms.
Mushrooms, Edible	Used to prevent cancer but results are vague. AHCC obtained from mycelia of several species of basidiomycetes mushrooms. May enhance resistance to *Klebsiella pneumoniae* due to its antioxidant effects. *Agaricus blazei*, an edible mushroom native to Brazil and Japan, used to treat arteriosclerosis, hepatitis, hyperlipidemia, diabetes, dermatitis, and cancer. One randomized study showed oral administration of *Agaricus* extract improved the natural killer cell activity and quality of life in gynecological cancer patients undergoing chemotherapy.
Oregano	Used for antioxidant effect and for destroying *Helicobacter pylori* bacteria or *Giardia*.
N-Acetyl-L-Cysteine (NAC)	Used to fight aging, alleviate allergies, and fight viruses. It may work as an an antiodixant to protect against sun damage and skin lesions.

(continued)

TABLE 2-1 Herbs, Botanicals, Spices, and Commentary *(continued)*

Herb, Botanical, Spice	Commentary
Parsley	Used for flatulence, indigestion, topical antibiotic. Avoid use in pregnancy as it may stimulate uterine contractions. May work as a diuretic in large doses. Breath freshener after a meal.
Peppermint	Used to relieve excess gas as a digestive aid (Koretz and Rotblatt, 2004). It has antispasmodic action. There may be some usefulness for irritable bowel syndrome and cramping.
Policosanols	Used to protect against cancers, cardiovascular disease, and obesity (Awika and Rooney, 2004) by reducing platelet aggregation and hepatic synthesis of cholesterol (Varady et al, 2003). Policosanols are phytochemicals extracted from sugar cane.
Probiotics	Used in inflammatory bowel disease and other GI disorders and to replenish gut flora after antibiotic use. "Good bacteria" such as *Lactobacillus* and *Lactobacillus acidophilus* can reduce presence of harmful bacteria in the gut and decrease vaginal infections. Select yogurt and products made with live cultures.
Psyllium	Use as a laxative to alleviate chronic constipation. Avoid use with cardiovascular agents.
Red Clover	Used for hot flashes because it contains isoflavones. However, current evidence suggests that it has no effectiveness (Krebs et al, 2004). It may also be used for coughs, eczema, and psoriasis.
Rhodiola (*Rhodiola rosea*), arctic root	Used for depression, fatigue. Side effects are insomnia and irritability.
Rhubarb or Da-Huang (*Rheum palmatum, R. officinale*)	Used for cancer treatment, constipation, fever, hypertension, immunosuppression, inflammation, microbial infection, peptic ulcers. Stimulant laxative products such as rhubarb should not be used for prolonged periods (over 7 days) without medical supervision. Patients with arthritis, kidney or hepatic dysfunction, history of kidney stones, inflammatory bowel disease, or intestinal obstruction should not take this herb. Rhubarb may cause uterine stimulation and therefore should not be consumed by women who are pregnant. Reported effects include abdominal cramps, nausea, vomiting, diarrhea with possible hypokalemia, anaphylaxis, and renal and hepatic damage.
Rice Bran Oil	Used for powerful antioxidant properties. Rice bran oil contains tocotrienols, powerful antioxidants that belong to the vitamin E family and protect against coronary heart disease (CHD) and some forms of cancer (McCaskill and Zhang, 1999).
Rosemary	Used for antioxidant and anticarcinogenic potential (Oluwatuyi et al, 2004). Often used for lowering blood pressure. Do not use in pregnancy in large doses.
Royal Jelly	Used as cancer prevention. Apalbumin 1 (Apa1) is the major royal jelly and honey glycoprotein and has various biological properties. It seems to stimulate macrophages to release TNF-α. It is a milky substance secreted by young worker honey bees. Avoid use with asthma; may cause allergic reactions.
Saw Palmetto	Used with benign prostatic hyperplasia. The extract can increase urine flow. Tannic acids are present. Saw palmetto should not be taken with oral contraceptives, estrogens, or anabolic steroids. Can cause GI upset in rare cases.
Schisandra (*Schisandra chinensis*)	Used for asthma, cough, influenza, diarrhea, indigestion, liver disease, premenstrual syndrome, strength, and stamina. Adverse reactions include depression and heartburn.
Senna	Used as a laxative herb; it contains anthraquinone, which stimulates bowel contractions. Safe for constipation, but dependence or obstruction can occur with long use. Fluid and electrolyte losses may be too severe. Avoid during pregnancy and lactation. Psyllium and other naturally high-fiber foods (such as prunes), extra fluids, and exercise are better choices.
Sheep Sorrel (*Rumex acetosella*)	Used for cancer treatment, diarrhea, scurvy, fever, inflammation. Contraindications: patients with kidney stones should not use this herb. Adverse reactions: abdominal cramps, gastroenteritis, diarrhea leading to hypokalemia, adrenal and liver damage.
Slippery Elm (*Ulmus rubra*)	Used for bronchitis, cancer treatment, cough, diarrhea, fever, inflammation, peptic ulcer, skin abscess, skin ulcers, sore throat. Adverse reactions: none known, but no human studies have been done to evaluate its actions.
Spirulina (Blue-green algae)	Used to treat cancers, viral infections, weight loss, oral leucoplakia, increased cholesterol, attention-deficit hyperactivity disorder (ADHD). Sold as an immune enhancer or to lower cholesterol levels. Adulterated form can cause allergies or gastroenteritis. Expensive as a protein source. Adverse effects are uncommon unless contaminated; if contaminated, it is hepato-, nephro-, and neurotoxic.
Stillingia (*Stillingia sylvatica*)	No clinical data to support its uses in bronchitis, chest congestion, cancer treatment, hemorrhoids, constipation, skin abscess, laryngitis, spasm, syphilis. Warning: the diaterpene esters in this herb are irritants to the skin and mucous membranes. Adverse reactions: vertigo, burning sensation over the mucous membrane, diarrhea, nausea, vomiting, pruritus, skin eruptions, cough, fatigue, and sweating.
St. John's Wort (*Hypericum perforatum*)	Used to alleviate anxiety and nervousness. It may function like an MAO inhibitor but has not been found to alleviate depression. Avoid use with statins, blood pressure medications, donepezil, antidepressants, other CNS medications, and chemotherapy. It can reduce the effectiveness of other prescription drugs and may inhibit iron absorption.
Tannins and Saponins (*Acacia pennata, Hibiscus* spp., *Lasianthica africana, Gouania lupiloides*)	Used for dental hygiene and to treat gingivitis.
Tea Tree Oil	Used for acne treatment, wound healing, or as an antiseptic for thrush (as in HIV infection). Topical use only; toxic if consumed. Allergy is possible in sensitive individuals. Natural fungicide.

(continued)

TABLE 2-1 Herbs, Botanicals, Spices, and Commentary *(continued)*

Herb, Botanical, Spice	Commentary
Tribulus terrestris	Used by athletes. Contains steroidal glycosides and saponins that cause secretion of luteinizing hormone, testosterone. It is phototoxic, cytotoxic, and neurotoxic.
Tryptophan	Used to promote sleep or to correct depression. L-tryptophan is the precursor to serotonin. It should not be used with MAO inhibitors, antidepressants, or serotonin receptor antagonists. It can exaggerate conditions of psychosis.
Turmeric (*Curcuma longa*)	Used for immune system enhancement, correcting anorexia, carcinoma prevention, reducing infections (such as reducing *H. pylori*) and inflammation, kidney stones. Warning: breast cancer patients on cyclophosphamide should restrict intake because it inhibits the antitumor action of chemotherapeutic agents. Contraindications: patients with bile duct obstruction, gallstones, GI disorders.
Ukrain (*Chelidonium majus* alkaloid-theophosphoric acid derivative)	Used for cancer prevention and treatment, hepatitis, HIV and AIDS, immunostimulation. Warning: it is not regulated by FDA. Adverse reactions: soreness at the injection site, nausea, diarrhea, dizziness, fatigue, drowsiness, polyuria, hematological side effects, and tumor bleeding were reported in a recent trial.
Valerian (*Valeriana officinalis*, *Valerianae radix*, garden heliotrope)	Used for insomnia, anxiety, colic, menstrual cramps, migraine treatment, sedation, spasms, stomach and intestinal gas. Effective as a sleep aid and is not habit forming. Benzodiazepines, sedatives, alcohol, antipsychotics, and antidepressants should not be used at the same time because of the risk of additional sedation. Long-term use can cause headaches, sleeplessness, cardiac dysfunction, hepatotoxicity. Patients should be warned not to drive or operate dangerous machinery when taking valerian. Valerian should be stopped about 1 week before surgery because it may interact with anesthesia. Headache, uneasiness, cardiac disturbances, morning drowsiness, and impaired alertness can occur.
Vanadium (*vanadyl sulfate*)	Used to mimic insulin; it may restore plasma DHEA and seems to improve insulin action. There may be a role for its use in the metabolic syndrome. Found in mushrooms and shellfish. May cause GI bleeding.
Vitex (chaste tree)	Used for relief of menstrual disorders. Fruits are used; approved for use in Germany.
White Willow	Used for fever, headache, pain, and rheumatic complaints. GI irritation or stomach ulcers can occur with long-term use; similar reactions as aspirin (aspirin is derived from white willow). Avoid use with alcohol, methotrexate, phenytoin, and valproate. Do not use in pregnancy or lactation.
Wild Yam (*Dioscorea villosa*)	Used for amenorrhea, dysmenorrhea, colic, cough, GI symptoms, rheumatoid arthritis, menopausal symptoms, urinary tract disorders, sexual dysfunction, spasms. Warning: efficacy of its hormonal actions is not proved, and some topical creams that say that they contain yam extracts as a source of natural progesterone should not be believed.
Willow Bark (*Salix alba*)	Used for fever, headache, inflammation, influenza, muscle pain. Adverse reactions: nausea, vomiting, GI bleed, tinnitus, renal damage. Drug interactions: increases risk of bleeding with anticoagulants and GI bleed with NSAIDs.
Witch Hazel	Used as astringent with bruises or varicose veins. Approved for use with hemorrhoid products.
Yew (*Taxus baccata*, *T. wallachiana*, *T. media*)	Used in treatment of some breast tumors. Cultivated varieties are being used to prepare triterpenoid precursors which are used to create paclitaxel and docetaxel, which in turn, have an antiestrogenic effect.
Zinc	Used to prevent viral illness, enhance performance, and correct male infertility. It should not be taken with immunosuppressants, fluoroquinolones, or tetracycline. Large doses may also conflict with copper metabolism.
Herbs to Discontinue before Surgery	Ephedra, feverfew, garlic, ginger, gingko biloba, ginseng, goldenseal, St. John's wort, and valerian should be discontinued about 2 weeks before planned surgery.
Hazardous Products	**Definitely Hazardous** • **Aristolochic acid** (*Aristolochia*, birthwort, snakeroot, snakeweed, snagree root, sangrel, serpentary, wild ginger). They list this as having caused documented human cancers, and it is linked to kidney failure. • **Belladonna** causes GI pain and spasms; contains toxic alkaloids, which can cause coma and death. **Very Likely Hazardous:** These are banned in other countries, have an FDA warning, or show adverse effects in studies: • **Androstenedione** (4-androstene-3, 17-dione, andro, androstene). Increased cancer risk and decrease in "good" HDL cholesterol have been reported. • **Chaparral** (*Larrea divaricata*, creosote bush, greasewood, hediondilla, jarilla, larreastat). Abnormal liver function and hepatitis or even cirrhosis have been linked to use. Often used for anti-inflammatory and anticancer effects, arthritis, carcinoma treatment, inflammation, spasm. • **Comfrey** (*Symphytum officinale*, ass ear, black root, blackwort, bruisewort, *Consolidae radix*, consound, gum plant, healing herb, knitback, knitbone, salsify, slippery root, *Symphytum radix*, wallwort). Used for bronchitis, cancer treatment, rheumatoid arthritis, wound healing. Abnormal liver function or damage, often irreversible. It contains pyrrolizidine alkaloids and causes hepatic veno-occlusive disease or death. To be avoided in infants. If pregnant women use it, it is transmitted during lactation to the newborn. FDA asked all manufacturers to remove products containing comfrey because it is hepatotoxic. • **DHEA** is used as an immune enhancer or to prevent heart disease. No evidence that it works. Can actually aggravate heart disease and have effects like steroids; may promote cancers in breast, prostate, or ovaries.

(continued)

TABLE 2-1 Herbs, Botanicals, Spices, and Commentary *(continued)*

Herb, Botanical, Spice	Commentary
Hazardous Products *(continued)*	• **Ephedra** (ma huang) contains cardiac toxins linked to dozens of deaths from myocardial infarction. Banned by FDA. Ephedra can cause stroke, insomnia, hypertension, or heart attack. Avoid taking with caffeine, sedatives, antipsychotics, antidepressants, antihyperglycemic agents, decongestants, and cardiovascular agents. • **Germander** (*Teucrium chamaedrys*, wall germander, wild germander). Abnormal heart and liver function have been linked to use. Germander contains flavinoids. • **Goldenseal** (*Hydrastis canadensis*) is used for anorexia, heart disease, coughs, upset stomach, menstrual problems, and arthritis. It has long been used by Native Americans for antiseptic and wound-healing properties. It can raise blood pressure, complicating treatment for those taking beta-blockers. For patients taking medication to control diabetes or kidney disease, this herb can cause dangerous electrolyte imbalance. Patients with hypertension or cardiovascular disease and women who are pregnant should not take this herb. GI complaints are common side effects. With toxicity: stomach ulcerations, constipation, convulsions, hallucinations, nausea, vomiting, depression, nervousness, bradycardia, respiratory depression, seizures. • **Kava** (*Piper methysticum*, ava, awa, gea, gi, intoxicating pepper, kao, kavain, kawa-pfeffer, kew, long pepper, malohu, maluk, meruk, milik, rauschpfeffer, sakau, tonga, wurzelstock, yagona, yangona). Abnormal liver function has been linked to use. • **Kelp:** if ingested as a source of iodine, it may interfere with thyroid replacement therapies. May worsen hyperthyroidism. • **Red yeast rice** is the fermented product of rice on which red yeast has been grown. A dietary staple in Asian countries to lower total cholesterol levels (Heber et al, 1999), it has been removed from the market in the United States. Avoid use with grapefruit juice or niacin. **Likely Hazardous:** These have adverse event reports or theoretical risks: • **Astragalus** is used in Chinese and Indian medicine for its immune enhancement. Do not take with antihyperglycemic agents. Not recommended for use, especially in immunosuppressed patients. • **Bitter orange** (*Citrus aurantium*, green orange, kijitsu, neroli oil, Seville orange, shangzhou zhiqiao, sour orange, zhi oiao, zhi xhi). High blood pressure and increased risk of heart arrhythmias, heart attack, and stroke are risks associated with use. • **Borage** may cause liver toxicity or even cancers. • **Horse chestnut** (*Aesculus hippocastanum*; aescin 50 mg). Studies have shown clinical efficacy in chronic venous insufficiency, but no data support the reversal of varicose veins. Patients with compromised renal or hepatic functions should not consume horse chestnut. It may also interact with anticoagulants and increase the risk of bleeding. • **Kombucha tea** can cause liver damage or intestinal problems or death. It is sometimes suggested for acne or insomnia or in AIDS. • **Lobelia** (*Lobelia inflata*, asthma weed, bladderpod, emetic herb, gagroot, lobelie, Indian tobacco, pukeweed, vomit wort, wild tobacco). Difficulty breathing and rapid heart rates are thought to be associated with lobelia. Large doses can lead to rapid heartbeat, paralysis, coma, or death. To be avoided by children, infants, pregnant women, smokers, and people with cardiac diseases. • **Mistletoe/Eurixor** (*Viscum album*) may be used for arthritis, cancer treatment, hepatitis, HTN, spasm, immunostimulation. Warning: berries and leaves are highly poisonous. Contraindication in pregnancy. Adverse reactions include fever, headache, chest pain, bradycardia, hypotension, coma. • **Organ/glandular extracts** (brain/adrenal/pituitary/placenta/other gland "substance" or "concentrate"). Theoretical risk of mad cow disease, particularly from brain extracts. • **Passion flower** is sometimes recommended for sedative use. It can cause seizures, hypotension, hallucinations. • **Pennyroyal oil** (*Hedeoma pulegioides*, lurk-in-the-ditch, mosquito plant, piliolerial, pudding grass, pulegium, run-by-the-ground, squaw balm, squawmint, stinking balm, tickweed). Liver and kidney failure, nerve damage, convulsions, abdominal tenderness, and burning of the throat are risks; deaths have been reported. • **Poke root** may cause low blood pressure and respiratory depression. Extremely toxic. • **Sassafras** (*Sassafras albidum*) is a stimulant; produces sweat, and contains safrole, which is banned as a carcinogen. Used for detoxification, inflammation, health maintenance, rheumatoid arthritis, mucositis, sprain, syphilis, urinary tract disorders. Warning: risk of liver cancer with prolonged use, so it is not safe to use. Adverse reactions: hot flashes, diaphoresis, hallucinations, hypertension, tachycardia, liver cancer, and death. • **Skullcap** (*Scutellaria lateriflora*, *S. baicalensis*, baikal, blue pimpernel, helmet flower, hoodwort, mad weed, mad-dog herb, mad-dog weed, quaker bonnet, scutelluria, scullcap). Uses: epilepsy, hepatitis, infections, cancer. Toxicity causes stupor, confusion, seizures. Adverse reactions include hepatotoxicity and pneumonitis. • **Wheat grass** (*Triticum aestivum*) is used for carcinoma treatment, chronic fatigue syndrome, immunostimulation, ulcerative colitis. Adverse reactions: nausea because of contamination. An antioxidant. No safety guidelines available. • **Yohimbe** (*Pausinystalia yohimbe*, johimbi, yohimbehe, yohimbine, yohimbe bark). Blood pressure changes, heartbeat irregularities, heart attacks, and paralysis have been reported. It causes CNS stimulation and vasodilation. In high doses, it is an MAO inhibitior. It is to be avoided in individuals with hypotension, CHF, diabetes, and kidney and liver diseases. Yohimbe is not effective for male impotence and can cause side effects such as hypertension and kidney failure; it can also aggravate bipolar disorder or decrease antidepressant effectiveness.

- Practitioners who refer their patients to a medical herbalist should assess for specific skills, educational background, national qualifications, experience, hours of supervised clinical practice, professionalism, association memberships, and willingness to communicate openly with the referring practitioner (Libster, 1999). It is also important to find out whether he/she sells particular brands of herbal products and bases clinical decisions on information provided by the manufacturer.
- Alcohol interacts with many medications and possibly with herbs. Mix with caution.

Patient Education—Food Safety

- Discuss food handling, preparation, and storage of herbs and botanical products.
- Because bacteria are commonly found on foods such as green onions (scallions), cilantro, and imported produce, wash all fresh fruits and vegetables.
- Store spices as directed and discard after shelf-life expiration. Spices such as paprika are easily contaminated.

For More Information

- American Botanical Council
  http://www.herbalgram.org/
- American Council on Science and Health
  http://www.acsh.org/
- American Dietetic Association
  http://www.eatright.org/
- American Heart Association, Position on Vitamin and Mineral Supplements
  http://www.americanheart.org/presenter.jhtml?identifier=4788
- American Herbal Products Association
  http://www.ahpa.org/
- Alternative Medicine Foundation
  http://www.amfoundation.org/
- Alternative Medicines
  http://www.ftc.gov/bcp/conline/pubs/health/whocares/altmeds.htm
- Botanical Dietary Supplements
  http://ods.od.nih.gov/factsheets/BotanicalBackground.asp
- CAM on PubMed—Searchable database
  http://www.nlm.nih.gov/nccam/camonpubmed.html
- Cochrane Collaboration–Complementary Medicine
  http://www.compmed.umm.edu/cochrane/index.html
- Consumer Lab.com
  http://www.consumerlab.com/
- Dietary Supplements
  http://vm.cfsan.fda.gov/~dms/supplmnt.html
- Facts about Dietary Supplements
  http://www.cc.nih.gov/ccc/supplements/intro.html
- Federal Trade Commission (FTC)
  Consumer Response Center: Toll Free: (877) 382-4357
  http://www.ftc.gov/ftc/who.htm
- FDA/CFSAN Regulations for DSHEA
  http://www.cfsan.fda.gov/~dms/ds3strat.html
- Food and Nutrition Information Center (FNIC)
  http://www.nal.usda.gov/fnic/etext/000015.html
- Herbal Monographs and Frequently Asked Questions on Herbs from RxList.com
  http://www.rxlist.com/alternative.htm#herbal_mon
- HerbMed–Interactive, electronic herbal database
  http://www.herbmed.org/
- Herb Research Foundation
  http://www.herbs.org/
- Herbs and Cultural Uses
  http://asiarecipe.com/herb.html
- Intelihealth, Vitamin and Nutrition Resource Center
  http://www.intelihealth.com/IH/ihtIH/WSIHW000/325/325.html
- Institute of Food Technologists
  http://www.ift.org/
- International Food Information Council – Functional Foods
  http://www.ific.org/nutrition/functional/index.cfm
- Mayo Clinic
  http://www.mayohealth.org/
- MEDLINE, Vitamin and Mineral Supplements
  http://www.nlm.nih.gov/medlineplus/vitaminandmineralsupplements.html
- National Center for Complementary and Alternative Medicine (NCCAM)
  http://altmed.od.nih.gov/
- National Institutes of Health, Office of Dietary Supplements
  http://ods.od.nih.gov/
- PubMed
  http://www.ncbi.nlm.nih.gov/entrez/query.fcgi
- Special Nutritionals Adverse Event Monitoring System–Searchable database from the FDA
  http://www.fda.gov/medwatch/how.htm
- Supplement Use
  http://www.cfsan.fda.gov/~dms/ds-take.html
- U.S. Pharmacopeia
  http://www.usp.org/
- USP Verified Program
  http://www.uspverified.org/

COMPLEMENTARY NUTRITION—CITED REFERENCES

American Dietetic Association. Position of the American Dietetic Association: fortification and nutritional supplements. *J Am Diet Assoc.* 105:1300, 2005.

Anderson RA, et al. Isolation and characterization of polyphenol type-A polymers from cinnamon with insulin-like biological activity. *J Agric Food Chem.* 52:65, 2004.

Awika JM, Rooney LW. Sorghum phytochemicals and their potential impact on human health. *Phytochemistry* 65:1199, 2004.

Bensoussan A, et al. Treatment of irritable bowel syndrome with Chinese herbal medicine: a randomized controlled trial. *JAMA.* 280:1585, 1998.

Boullata J. Natural health product interactions with medication. *Nutr Clin Pract.* 20:33, 2005.

Dragland S, et al. Several culinary and medicinal herbs are important sources of dietary antioxidants. *J Nutr.* 133:1286, 2003.

Dulloo A, et al. Efficacy of a green tea extract rich in catechin polyphenols and caffeine in increasing 24-hr energy expenditure and fat oxidation in humans. *Am J Clin Nutri.* 70:1040, 1999.

Gades MD, Stern JS. Chitosan supplementation and fat absorption in men and women. *J Am Diet Assoc.* 105:72, 2005.

Hamilton K. An overview of herbal and nutritional integrative medicine: a registered dietitian's perspective. *Support Line.* 20:5, 1998.

Hasler CM, et al. Position of The American Dietetic Association: functional foods. *J Am Diet Assoc.* 104:814, 2004.

Heber D, et al. Cholesterol-lowering effects of a proprietary Chinese red-yeast-rice dietary supplement. *Am J Clin Nutri.* 69:231, 1999.
Ichikawa H, Aggarwal BB. Guggulsterone inhibits osteoclastogenesis induced by receptor activator of nuclear factor-kappaB ligand and by tumor cells by suppressing nuclear factor-kappaB activation. *Clin Cancer Res.* 12:662, 2006.
King A, Young G. Characteristics and occurrence of phenolic phytochemicals. *J Am Diet Assoc.* 99:21, 1999.
Koretz RL, Rotblatt M. Complementary and alternative medicine in gastroenterology: the good, the bad, and the ugly. *Clin Gastroenterol Hepatol.* 2:957, 2004.
Lee Y, et al. The knowledge, attitudes, and practices of dietitians licensed in Oregon regarding functional foods, nutrient supplements, and herbs as complementary medicine. *J Am Diet Assoc.* 100:543, 2000.
Libster M. Guidelines for selecting a medical herbalist for consultation and referral: consulting a medical herbalist. *J Altern Complement Med.* 5:457, 1999.
Lohse B, et al. Survey of herbal use by Kansas and Wisconsin WIC participants reveals moderate, appropriate use and identifies herbal education needs. *J Am Diet Assoc.* 106:227, 2006.
McCaskill D, Zhang F. Use of rice bran oil in foods. *Food Technol.* 53:50, 1999.
Miller L. Herbal medicinals: selected clinical considerations focusing on known or potential drug–herb interactions. *Arch Intern Med.* 158:2200, 1998.
Nagao T, et al. Ingestion of a tea rich in catechins leads to a reduction in body fat and malondialdehyde-modified LDL in men. *Am J Clin Nutr.* 81:122, 2005.
Oluwatuyi M, et al. Antibacterial and resistance modifying activity of *Rosmarinus officinalis. Phytochemistry* 65:3249, 2004.
Physician's Desk Reference for Herbal Medicines. 3rd ed. Montvale, NJ: Medical Economics Company, 2004.
Sarubin-Fragakis A. *A health professional's guide to popular dietary supplement.* 2nd ed. Chicago: The American Dietetic Association, 2003.
Shah P, Grant K. An overview of common herbal supplements. *Support Line.* 22:3, 2000.
Stein K. Herbal supplements or prescription drugs: a risky combination? *J Am Diet Assoc.* 100:412, 2000.
Thomson CA, et al. Practice paper of the American Dietetic Association: dietary supplements. *J Am Diet Assoc.* 105:460, 2005.
Tyler V. *The honest herbal: a sensible guide to the use of herbs and related remedies.* 4th ed. New York: Pharmaceutical Products Press, 1999.
Varady KA, et al. Role of policosanols in the prevention and treatment of cardiovascular disease. *Nutr Rev.* 61:376, 2003.
White House Commission on Complementary and Alternative Medicine Policy. Final report. Available at http://www.whccamp.hhs.gov, 2002.
Wold RS, et al. Increasing trends in elderly persons' use of nonvitamin, nonmineral dietary supplements and concurrent use of medications. *J Am Diet Assoc.* 105:54, 2005.

CULTURAL FOOD PATTERNS, VEGETARIANISM, RELIGIOUS PRACTICES

CULTURAL FOOD PATTERNS

NUTRITIONAL ACUITY RANKING: LEVEL 2 (DIETARY ADAPTATIONS, ADVISEMENT)

DEFINITIONS AND BACKGROUND

Varied dietary intakes by age, culture, gender, and years in the United States are known and accepted (Kim et al, 2000). Assessment of a patient's cultural food preferences is essential to determine adequacy of nutritional intake (Stein, 2004). Nutrition planning for immigrant and minority patients will be more effective if tailored to the level of dietary acculturation; the ability to accurately assess dietary acculturation is an important component of nutrition education, interventions, and counseling in these populations (Satia et al, 2001).

Adoption of U.S. dietary patterns that tend to be high in fat and low in fruits and vegetables is not positive. The process by which immigrants adopt the dietary practices is multidimensional, dynamic, and complex; in addition, it varies considerably, depending on a variety of personal, cultural, and environmental attributes (Unger et al, 2004).

In addition to planning for individual patients, effective prevention initiatives require use of available findings about individual cultures. Reinforcement of positive traditional dietary habits, adaptation of healthy Western food items, and development of strategies that will effectively correct likely deficiencies in diet are important intervention goals (Kim et al, 2000). Dietetics practitioners can use the information presented here to study nutrition-related chronic diseases in public health planning and in nutrition education efforts directed toward ethnic-specific groups (Bermudez et al, 2000).

It is important to become aware of indigenous/tribal/ethnic minorities from different parts of the world, including the extent of their diversity, importance of their traditions, and knowledge of local food resources (Kuhnlein et al, 2003). Finally, knowledge of integrative medicine in corporates herbal and botanical products that are used for preventive or medicinal purposes. Different cultures ap ply different herbs and practices, traditionally known as folk medicine. See Appendix E for more detailed infor mation.

INTERVENTION: OBJECTIVES

- Become aware of one's own cultural values; avoid imposing them on others. For example, the desire to be thin is more common among Caucasians than people from other ethnic backgrounds.
- Assess values, attitudes, beliefs, practices, and rituals of the patient/client before attempting to discuss any lifestyle changes. Observe and interact appropriately.
- Provide individualization for cultural patterns that differ from the standard in the region. Do not assume that each person fits a typical pattern but be prepared to understand the differences from the "typical American" diet.
- Determine which habits, if any, are detrimental for healthy lifestyles. In addition, review any patterns or food intakes that aggravate existing or predisposing chronic or acute conditions for each person. Build on healthy practices.
- Correct the diet for deficits, such as calcium and riboflavin, in dietary patterns in which dairy products or milk are excluded or not tolerated. Identify other nutrients that are at risk for insufficiency.

- Offer suggestions for changes in food preparation (e.g., ways for reducing fat or salt) rather than changing the foods themselves, whenever possible.
- Understand and interpret customs, festive occasions, fasting, and ceremonial activities, and offer reasonable suggestions (Satia-Abouti et al, 2002).
- Functional foods, including whole foods and fortified, enriched, or enhanced foods have a potentially beneficial effect on health when consumed as part of a varied diet on a regular basis at effective levels (Hasler et al, 2004). Each culture may have foods that have special attributes.

DIETARY PATTERNS

It is important to review and identify specific ethnic and religious food patterns. Table 2-2 describes religious dietary patterns and common practices. A brief overview of common food patterns is listed here. More extensive information can be found on the internet.

- Asian patterns. Asian diets vary from one country to another. Diets may be low in calcium and riboflavin because milk often is not tolerated or consumed. Encourage use of tofu, green vegetables, and fish containing small bones. Diet may be high in sodium if monosodium glutamate (MSG) and soy sauces are used. The traditional Chinese diet is 80% grains, legumes, and vegetables (Earl, 2004). Stir-frying, deep fat frying, and steaming are common cooking methods. Pork is the preferred meat. Hot peppers may be used daily. "Hot" and "cold" foods may be used during pregnancy or illness; these terms do not refer to food temperatures. Korean Americans tend to have a greater intake of carbohydrates and vitamins A and C and a lower intake of total fat, cholesterol, and saturated fat (Kim et al, 2000).
- Hmong (Southeast Asian) patterns. Milk is seldom used and is often related to lactose intolerance, and calcium may be a problem. Fish, chicken, and pork are common entrees. Rice may be eaten at nearly every meal. A highly salted fish sauce is used. Snacking is rare in the family diet. Anemia may result from parasite infestation because many individuals have been refugees (Earl, 2004). Like Chinese patterns, hot–cold patterns are sometimes observed (American Dietetic Association, 1999a). A website for Vietnamese food is available at http://www.ivietbusiness.com/vietnamese-food-recipe.htm.
- Hispanic (Mexican and Latin American) patterns. Whole milk may be used rarely, but cheese is a common additive to meals. Fruits and vegetables may be viewed as luxuries, but chili peppers, mangos, and avocados are common. The main starch is corn or flour tortilla. The diet may be high in sugar and saturated fat (lard). A common main dish is beans with rice. Hot and cold foods are concepts commonly found. Salsa or sofrito seasonings are used frequently. Rice is the major contributor of energy among the elderly; more acculturated Hispanic elders consume fewer ethnic foods and more foods related to the non-Hispanic white eating patterns than those less acculturated (Bermudez et al, 2000). Obesity, type 2 diabetes, cardiovascular disease, dental caries, and undernutrition may be problems in this population (Stein, 2004; Lin et al, 2003). Snacking becomes more common with higher levels of acculturation.
- Indian/Pakistani patterns. India has some of the most diverse populations and diets in the world. Cancer rates in India are lower than those seen in Western countries, but

TABLE 2-2 Common Religious Food Practices

	Seventh-Day Adventist	Buddhist	Eastern Orthodox	Hindu	Jewish	Mormon	Moslem	Roman Catholic
Beef	A	A		X				
Pork	X	A		A	X		X	
All Meat	A	A	R	A	R		R	R
Eggs/Dairy	O	O	R	O	R			
Fish	A	A	R	R	R			
Shellfish	X	A	O	R	X			
Alcohol	X			A		X	X	
Coffee/Tea	X					X	A	
Meat and Dairy at Same Meal					X			
Leavened Foods					R			
Ritual Slaughter of Meats					+		+	
Moderation	+	+					+	
Fasting*		+	+	+	+	+	+	+

X, prohibited or strongly discouraged; A, avoided by the most devout; R, some restrictions regarding types of foods or when a food may be eaten; O, permitted, but may be avoided at some observances; +, practiced.
* Fasting varies from partial (abstention from certain foods or meals) to complete (no food or drink).
Used with permission from http://asiarecipe.com/religion.html.

they are rising with increasing migration of rural population to the cities, increasing life expectancy, and changes in lifestyles (American Dietetic Association, 1996). In India, rates for oral and esophageal cancers are high; the rates for colorectal, prostate, and lung cancers are low (Sinha et al, 2003). Indian immigrants in the United States are largely Hindi. Pakistani immigrants are mostly Muslims. Vegetarianism is the primary practice among Indians, deriving from religious beliefs in which the cow is sacred. Lentils and legumes are a primary source of protein; in some families, eggs, fish, shrimp, and milk are consumed. Sattvic foods are believed to create a healthy life; these include milk products (except cheese made from rennet), rice, wheat, and legumes. Rajasic foods are believed to contribute to aggression; these include meats, eggs, and rich or very salty foods. Tamasic foods are believed to contribute to slothfulness or dullness; these include garlic, pickled foods, stale or rotten foods, and alcohol used for pleasure or to excess. Lack of portion control may be a factor in diabetes, which is common in this population. Combination foods include biryani (grain, meat), samosas (grain, vegetable, meat, fat), kheer "rice pudding" (grain, milk), and curry (meat, vegetable). For cancer prevention, turmeric (curcumin), an ingredient in common Indian curry spice, is under study (Sinha et al, 2003).

- Mediterranean diet patterns. The Mediterranean patterns reflect the habits of populations of Italy, Crete, and Greece. Research suggests that this dietary pattern has advantages for reducing cardiac disease and cancers (Simopoulos, 2004; Trichopoulou et al, 2004). Olive oil; fish, poultry, and eggs rather than beef; breads, fruits, and vegetables in abundance; and lots of beans/legumes, yogurt, and cheeses make up this pattern. Exercise and wine are also mainstays. The Mediterranean diet pattern (MDP) is more often found among older people and people in rural areas, among males more than females, and among people who are more physically active (Tur et al, 2004; Scali et al, 2001). Urban young people should be encouraged to return to this pattern. Recent studies suggest that the Mediterranean diet counters onset of the metabolic syndrome. A Mediterranean-style diet rich in whole grains, fruits, vegetables, legumes, walnuts, and olive oil is effective in reducing both the prevalence of the metabolic syndrome and its associated cardiovascular risks (Knoops et al, 2004).
- Middle Eastern patterns. Countries usually include Egypt, Iran, Jordan, Lebanon, Saudi Arabia, and Turkey. Pork is eaten only by Christians. Lamb and beef are consumed. Yogurt and cheese provide calcium sources. Lactose intolerance is common. Because olive oil is commonly used, lower blood pressure may be present (Stein, 2004). For Muslim food habits, see appropriate entry.
- Native American patterns (American Indian and Alaskan Native). Food has great religious and social significance and is commonly part of many celebrations (Earl, 2004). Fried foods, fried bread, corn, mutton, and goat are foods frequently used by American Indians, whereas seafood and game are more common among Alaskan natives. Obesity and type 2 diabetes are very common in these populations (American Dietetic Association, 1999b).

Herbs, Botanicals, and Supplements

- Many cultures use herbs and botanicals as part of their meal patterns, rituals, and celebrations. Identify those that are used and monitor for potential side effects. HerbMed, an interactive, electronic herbal database, provides hyperlinked access to the scientific data including clinical trials and efficacy. The National Center for Complementary and Alternative Medicine is also one of many reliable resources.

INTERVENTION: NUTRITION EDUCATION, COUNSELING, CARE MANAGEMENT

- Culturally appropriate counseling and awareness of religious practices are important for improving health issues, such as obesity (Wang and Tussing, 2004) and increasing intake of fruits and vegetables (Hart et al, 2004). Different methods may be needed for dietary modification for obesity, diabetes, and hypertension, taking into account differences in cultural understanding and food practices (Sharma and Cruickshank, 2001). First, demonstrate respect for the beliefs, values, and practices of the patient and family members.
- Interpreters may be needed. Bilingual staff or community volunteers are helpful. Speak directly to the individual and not to the interpreter during sessions to show respect.
- Alternative solutions to dietary patterns must be gently offered. There is no "one right way" for dietary patterns.
- Understanding background, health problems, statistics, social issues, and disease patterns is useful when providing multicultural education.
- Build relationships through sensitivity and communication. Remove assumptions and stereotypes; cultures are changing, growing, and dynamic.
- Family beliefs and behaviors may sabotage a client's efforts; be aware and be helpful. Development of an intuitive counseling style may be beneficial (Curry, 2000).
- Offer tips on food selection, preparation, and storage; identify available resources, ethnic stores, and agencies.
- Interpreting food labels and preparing unfamiliar foods can be part of the educational session.

Patient Education—Food Safety

- Discuss food handling, preparation, and storage within a cultural context.
- When traveling, avoid tap water and ice made from tap water, uncooked produce such as lettuce, and raw or undercooked seafood.
- Avoid raw or partially cooked eggs, raw or undercooked fish or shellfish, and raw or undercooked meats because of potential foodborne illnesses.
- Do not use raw (unpasteurized) milk or products made from it.
- Avoid serving unpasteurized juices and raw sprouts.

For More Information

- Center for Cross-Cultural Health
  http://www.crosshealth.com/links.htm
- Cultural Food Pyramids
  http://www.semda.org/info/

- Food History Timeline
  http://www.foodtimeline.org/
- Food Habits and Anthropology
  http://www.foodhabits.info/
- Food and Nutrition Information Center
  Agricultural Research Service, USDA
  National Agricultural Library
  http://www.nal.usda.gov/fnic/
- Georgia State Nutrition Handouts
  http://monarch.gsu.edu/multiculturalhealth
- National Center for Cultural Competence
  http://gucchd.georgetown.edu/nccc/index.html
- Ohio State University Extension Fact Sheets
  http://ohioline.osu.edu/hyg-fact/5000/index.html
- Oldways Cultural Food Pyramids
  http://www.oldwayspt.org/
- Religious Food Practices
  http://asiarecipe.com/religion.html#help
- Seventh Day Adventist Foodways
  http://www.andrews.edu/NUFS/veggiediet.html
- Transcultural Health Care
  http://www.lww.com/promos1/rosdahl/images/s_sample_chapter.pdf
- University of Michigan, Multicultural Content
  http://www.med.umich.edu/multicultural/ccp/topic.htm
- USDA Food Pyramid–Ethnic and Cultural Versions
  http://www.nal.usda.gov/fnic/Fpyr/pyramid.html

CULTURAL FOOD PATTERNS—CITED REFERENCES

American Dietetic Association. *Ethnic and regional food practices: Indian and Pakistani food practices, customs, and holidays.* Chicago: American Dietetic Association, 1996.

American Dietetic Association. *Ethnic and regional food practices: Hmong American food practices, customs, and holidays.* Chicago: American Dietetic Association, 1999a.

American Dietetic Association. *Ethnic and regional food practices: northern plains Indian food practices, customs, and holidays.* Chicago: American Dietetic Association, 1999b.

Bermudez O, et al. Intake and food sources of macronutrients among older Hispanic adults: association with ethnicity, acculturation, and length of residence in the United States. *J Am Diet Assoc.* 100:665, 2000.

Curry KR. Multicultural competence in dietetics and nutrition. *J Am Diet Assoc.* 100:1142, 2000.

Earl R. Guidelines for dietary planning. In: Mahan K, Escott-Stump S, eds. *Krause's food, nutrition, and diet therapy.* 11th ed. Philadelphia: WB Saunders, 2004.

Hart A, et al. Is religious orientation associated with fat and fruit/vegetable intake? *J Am Diet Assoc.* 104:1292, 2004.

Hasler CM, et al. Position of The American Dietetic Association: functional foods. *J Am Diet Assoc.* 104:814, 2004.

Kim K, et al. Nutritional status of Korean Americans: implications for cancer risk. *Oncol Nurs Forum.* 27:1573, 2000.

Knoops KTB, et al. Mediterranean diet, lifestyle factors, and 10-year mortality in elderly European men and women: the HALE Project. *JAMA.* 292:1433, 2004.

Krebs EE, et al. Phytoestrogens for treatment of menopausal symptoms: a systematic review. *Obstet Gynecol.* 104:824, 2004.

Kuhnlein HV, Johns T; IUNS Task Force on Indigenous Peoples' Food Systems and Nutrition. Northwest African and Middle Eastern food and dietary change of indigenous peoples. *Asia Pac J Clin Nutr.* 12:344, 2003.

Lin H, et al. Dietary patterns of Hispanic elders are associated with acculturation and obesity. *J Nutr.* 133:3651, 2003.

Satia J, et al. Development of scales to measure dietary acculturation among Chinese-Americans and Chinese-Canadians. *J Am Diet Assoc.* 101:548, 2001.

Satia-Abouta J, et al. Dietary acculturation: applications to nutrition research and dietetics. *J Am Diet Assoc.* 102:1105, 2002.

Scali J, et al. Diet profiles in a population sample from Mediterranean southern France. *Public Health Nutri.* 4:173, 2001.

Sharma S, Cruickshank JK. Cultural differences in assessing dietary intake and providing relevant dietary information to British African-Caribbean populations. *J Hum Nutr Diet.* 14:449, 2001.

Simopoulos AP. The traditional diet of Greece and cancer. *Eur J Cancer Prev.* 13:219, 2004.

Sinha R, et al. Cancer risk and diet in India. *J Postgrad Med.* 49:222, 2003.

Stein K. Cultural literacy in health care. *J Am Diet Assoc.* 104:1657, 2004.

Trichopoulou A, et al. Adherence to a Mediterranean diet and survival in a Greek population. *N Engl J Med.* 348:2599, 2003.

Tur JA, et al. Adherence to the Mediterranean dietary pattern among the population of the Balearic Islands. *Br J Nutr.* 92:341, 2004.

Unger JB, et al. Acculturation, physical activity, and fast-food consumption among Asian-American and Hispanic adolescents. *J Community Health.* 29:467, 2004.

Wang Y, Tussing L. Culturally apppropriate approaches are needed to reduce ethnic disparity in childhood obesity. *J Am Diet Assoc.* 104:1664, 2004.

VEGETARIANISM

NUTRITIONAL ACUITY RANKING: LEVEL 2 (FOR MEAL PLANNING)

DEFINITIONS AND BACKGROUND

Vegetarian diets are basically plant-based diets, with fruits, vegetables, legumes, seeds, and nuts (American Dietetic Association, 2003). There are three major categories of vegetarianism: vegan, a very strict vegetarian food pattern ("pure" vegetarianism); lacto, a vegetarian food pattern using milk; and lacto-ovo, a vegetarian food pattern using milk and eggs. Conscious combining of complementary protein sources does not appear to be necessary (American Dietetic Association, 2003). Approximately 2.5% of adults in the United States and 4% of adults in Canada follow vegetarian diets (American Dietetic Association, 2003).

Dietary quality from intakes studied in the Continuing Survey of Food Intake by Individuals (CSFII) 1994–1996 have been reviewed. Diets that were high in carbohydrates and low to moderate in fat tended to be lower in energy; the lowest energy intakes and BMIs were found among those on a vegetarian diet (Kennedy et al, 2001).

Vegetarian diets can be healthful when carefully planned and monitored. These diets can improve obesity, constipation, diabetes, hypertension, and diverticular disease. Long-term vegetarians have a better antioxidant status and coronary heart disease risk profile than do apparently healthy omnivores; plasma ascorbic acid is a useful marker of overall health status (Szeto et al, 2004). Vegetarian diets also may reduce the incidence of breast cancer, colon cancer, and gallstones.

There may be fewer kidney stones among vegetarians. A balanced diet with a moderate animal protein and purine content, an adequate fluid intake, and a high-alkali load with fruits and vegetables results in the lowest risk of uric acid crystallization compared to the omnivorous diets (Siener and Hesse, 2003).

Vegetarians tend to have less appendicitis, hiatal hernia, irritable bowel syndrome, hemorrhoids, and varicose veins. The National Cancer Institute recommends intake of 25–35 g of fiber per day; vegetarian diets can easily provide this level.

Vegetarians usually consume less saturated fats and cholesterol and generally have more favorable lipid levels (Bederova et al, 2000). Vegetarian diets usually provide higher levels of polyunsaturated fatty acids and vitamins E and C. Vegetarians tend to have significantly higher levels of all antioxidant vitamins as a result of a higher consumption of vegetables, fruits, plants, fat, and sprouts (Bederova et al, 2000).

Hindus and other religious groups suggest following a vegetarian lifestyle. A relevant website for more details may be found at: http://www-unix.oit.umass.edu/~efhayes/ hindu.htm or at http://monarch.gsu.edu/WebRoot$/multiculturalhealth/handouts/Hindi/Hindi_food_pyramid.pdf.

INTERVENTION: OBJECTIVES

- Encourage use of a wide variety of foods in adequate quantity and balance of amino acids to achieve a balance of amino acids throughout the day (Table 2-3).
- Provide nutritionally adequate menus with sufficient energy for weight maintenance/idealization. Discourage excessive use of sweets.
- Monitor fiber intake because excesses may interfere with absorption of calcium, zinc, and iron.
- Monitor the diet carefully if the patient is a pregnant woman or lactating mother. In addition, monitor elderly persons following a vegetarian diet.
- Infants, children, and teens on vegan diets should be monitored closely to ensure adequate energy intake and mineral and vitamin intakes (Perry, 2002). High-fiber diets may replace calories and cause some stunting or other growth deficits.
- Prevent or correct anemia.
- Be aware of the limiting amino acids in typical protein foods: wheat (lysine), rice (lysine and threonine), corn (lysine and tryptophan), beans (methionine), and chickpeas (methionine). Vary the choices, e.g., bread and milk, rice and cheese, or pasta and cheese; rice and beans, bread and beans, or corn and beans; garbanzo beans and sesame seeds (as in dips) and beans (as in roasted snacks). Serve vegetables with nuts, dairy products, rice, sunflower seeds, or wheat germ. Different food combinations provide essential amino acids that produce higher quality proteins (American Dietetic Association, 2003).
- Plant sources of protein can provide adequate amounts of essential amino acids. Using a variety of plant foods is key, and energy needs should readily be met. Although vegetarian diets are lower in total protein and a vegetarian's protein needs may be somewhat elevated because of the lower quality of some plant proteins, protein intake in both lacto-ovo-vegetarians and vegans appears to be adequate (Messina and Messina, 1996).
- Where desired, use of soy foods can be useful to reduce elevated cholesterol levels as part of a healthy vegetarian diet (Rosell et al, 2004).

INTERVENTION: FOOD AND NUTRITION

The American Dietetic Association recommends consultation with a registered dietitian or other qualified nutrition professional, especially during periods of growth, breastfeeding, pregnancy, or recovery from illness.

- For a balanced diet, minimize intake of less nutritious foods such as sweets and fatty foods. Choose whole or unrefined grain products instead of refined products. Choose a variety of nuts, seeds, legumes, fruits, and vegetables, including good sources of vitamin C to improve

TABLE 2-3 Potential Complications of a Vegetarian Diet

Iron Deficiency Anemia. Females should be sure to obtain an adequate amount of absorbable iron (Sharma et al, 2003). The iron in dairy, eggs, and plant foods is largely nonheme, of which only about 2–20% is absorbed.

Vitamin B_{12} Deficiency. An individual following a vegan diet should use supplements to obtain this vitamin (Stabler and Allen, 2004).

Vitamin D Deficiency or Rickets. The human body can synthesize vitamin D from sunlight, but this is only possible when the sun reaches a certain intensity level. For many people who live in North America, this means that for a few months of the year, they will have to seek other sources of vitamin D because the sun is not intense enough. Milk is generally fortified with vitamin D, but for vegans who do not consume dairy products, supplements are necessary (Outila et al, 2000). A very low-fat vegan diet can be nutritionally adequate with the exception of vitamin D; supplementation is needed (Dunn-Emke et al, 2005).

Excess Bulk. In some circumstances, this regimen can restrict energy intake in the first few years of life (Murphy and Allen, 2003). This is also true for adults who consume large amounts of fiber to the extent that many other nutrients are not able to be absorbed in the small intestine.

Omega-3 Fatty Acids and essential amino acids **methionine** and **lysine** are found in significantly lower amounts in vegetarian diets (Mezzano et al, 2000).

Calcium absorption may be inhibited in vegetarians as a consequence of the presence of phytates in plant foods; vegetarian nutrition represents a risk for pregnant women, children, and adolescents if the values of iron and calcium are not carefully planned.

Zinc intake may be lower in vegetarian diets (Hunt, 2003).

iron absorption. Choose low-fat or nonfat varieties of dairy products, if they are included in the diet.
- Follow the new food guide for North American vegetarians. Include:

6–12 servings from the bread group
2–3 servings of legumes, nuts, or seeds, or eggs (if used)
2–3 servings from the dairy group (if used); tofu, yogurt, or fortified soy milk may be substituted
4 or more servings of vegetables
3 or more servings of fruits
2–3 servings of fats and oils, including olives and avocado

CLINICAL INDICATORS

Clinical/History	hematocrit (H & H)	Glucose (gluc)
Height	Mean cell volume (MCV)	Serum folate
Weight	Serum Fe	Serum B_{12}
BMI	Transferrin	Ca++, Mg++
Diet history	Albumin (alb), transthyretin	Na+, K+
Lab Work	Cholesterol (chol), Trig	Serum zinc
Hemoglobin and		Alkaline phosphatase (alk phos)
		Serum vitamin D

Herbs, Botanicals, and Supplements

- Many cultures use herbs and botanicals as part of their meal patterns, rituals, and celebrations. Identify those that are used and monitor side effects.
- Counsel about use of herbal teas, especially regarding toxic substances.

INTERVENTION: NUTRITION EDUCATION, COUNSELING, CARE MANAGEMENT

- Beneficial changes to diet may occur on changing to a self-selected vegetarian diet; for example, it is one way of achieving a better blood lipid profile (Robinson et al, 2002).
- Explain patterns of food intake that provide complementary amino acids. Whole grains, legumes, seeds, nuts, and vegetables contain sufficient essential and nonessential amino acids if taken in the right combinations.
- Emphasize the importance of a balanced diet.
- Describe the role vegetarian diets play in lowering serum cholesterol, triglycerides, and glucose. These are beneficial changes that can result after starting a vegetarian diet pattern (Phillips et al, 2004).
- Counsel about appropriate products for infants and children (e.g., fortified soy formula). Protein may be the

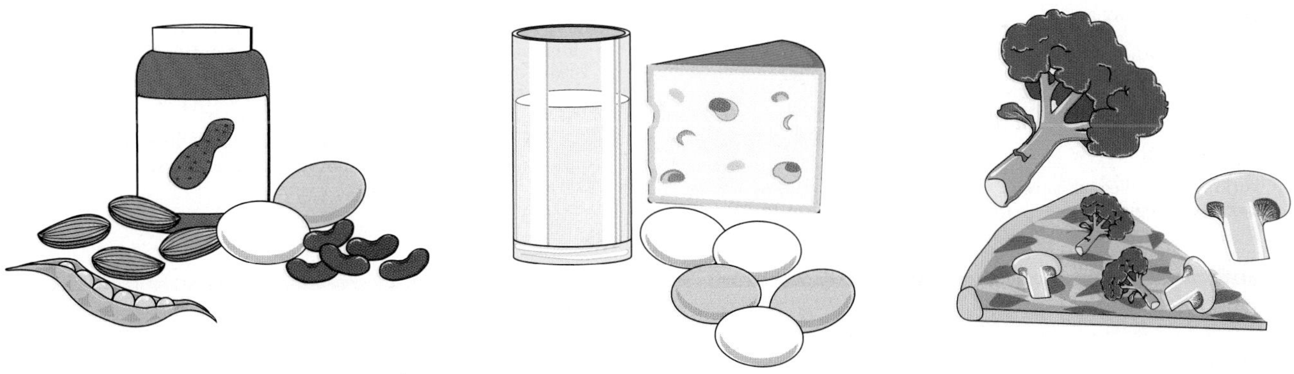

Nutrients to focus on for vegetarians

- **Protein** has many important function in the body and is essential for growth and maintenance. Protein needs can easily be met by eating a variety of plant-based foods. Combining different protein sources in the same meal is not necessary. Sources of protein for vegetarians include beans, nuts, nut butters, peas, and soy products (tofu, tempeh, veggie burgers). Milk products and eggs are also good protein sources for lacto-ovo vegetarians.
- **Iron functions** primarily as a carrier of oxygen in the blood. Iron sources for vegetarians include iron-fortified breakfast cereals, spinach, kidney beans, black-eyed peas, lentils, turnip greens, molasses, whole wheat breads, peas, and some dried fruits (dried apricots, prunes, raisins).
- **Calcium** is used for building bones and teeth and in maintaining bone strength. Sources of calcium for vegetarians include fortified breakfast cereals, soy products (tofu, soy-based beverages), calcium-fortified orange juice, and some dark green leafy vegetables (collard greens, turnip greens, bok choy, mustard greens). Milk products are excellent calcium sources for lacto vegetarians.
- **Zinc** is necessary for many biochemical reactions and also helps the immune system function properly. Sources of zinc for vegetarians include many types of beans (white beans, kidney beans, and chickpeas), zinc-fortified breakfast cereals, wheat germ, and pumpkin seeds. Milk products are a zinc source for lacto vegetarians.
- **Vitamin B_{12}** is found in animal products and some fortified foods. Sources of vitamin B_{12} for vegetarians include milk products, eggs, and foods that have been fortified with vitamin B_{12}. These include breakfast cereals, soy-based beverages, veggie burgers, and nutritional yeast.

Figure 2-1 Vegetarian guidance.

biggest problem. Soy milk also should be fortified with calcium and vitamin B_{12}.
- Unless otherwise advised by a doctor, those taking dietary supplements should limit the dose to 100% of the Daily Reference Intakes (Recommended Daily Allowances).

Patient Education—Food Safety

- Discuss food handling, preparation, and storage, especially careful washing of fruits and vegetables.
- Starches such as hot cereals and rice should not be prepared and held in large batches because of the risks of *Bacillus cereus.*

For More Information

- North American Vegetarian Society
http://www.navs-online.org/
- Oldways Preservation and Trust
http://www.oldwayspt.org/
- Seventh-Day Adventist Dietetic Association
http://www.adventist.org/
- Seventh-Day Adventist Foodways
http://www.andrews.edu/NUFS/veggiediet.html
- UCLA Vegetarian Nutrition
http://apps.medsch.ucla.edu/nutrition/vegetarianism.htm
- Vegetarian Cuisine
http://vegweb.com/
- Vegetarian Network (Victoria, Australia)
http://www.vnv.org.au/
- Vegetarian Resource Group
http://www.vrg.org/
- Vegetarian Society of the United Kingdom
http://www.vegsoc.org/
- World Guide to Vegetarianism
http://www.veg.org/veg/

VEGETARIANISM—CITED REFERENCES

American Dietetic Association. Position of The American Dietetic Association: vegetarian diets. *J Am Diet Assoc.* 103:748, 2003.

Bederova A, et al. Comparison of nutrient intake and corresponding biochemical parameters in adolescent vegetarians and nonvegetarians. *Cas Lek Cesk.* 139:396, 2000.

Dunn-Emke SR, et al. Nutrient adequacy of a very-low-fat vegan diet. *J Am Diet Assoc.* 105:1442, 2005.

Hunt JR. Bioavailability of iron, zinc, and other trace minerals from vegetarian diets. *Am J Clin Nutr.* 78:633S, 2003.

Kennedy E, et al. Popular diets: correlation to health, nutrition, and obesity. *J Am Diet Assoc.* 101:411, 2001.

Messina M, Messina V. *The dietitian's guide to vegetarian diets: issues and applications.* Gaithersburg, MD: Aspen Publishers, 1996.

Mezzano D, et al. Cardiovascular risk factors in vegetarians. Normalization of hyperhomocysteinemia with vitamin B(12) and reduction of platelet aggregation with omega-3 fatty acids. *Thromb Res.* 100:153, 2000.

Murphy SP, Allen LH. Nutritional importance of animal source foods. *J Nutr.* 133:3932S, 2003.

Outila TA, et al. Dietary intake of vitamin D in premenopausal, healthy vegans was insufficient to maintain concentrations of serum 25-hydroxyvitamin D and intact parathyroid hormone within normal ranges during the winter in Finland. *J Am Diet Assoc.* 100:434, 2000.

Perry CL, et al. Adolescent vegetarians: how well do their dietary patterns meet the Healthy People 2010 objectives? *Arch Pediatr Adolesc Med.* 156: 431, 2002.

Phillips F, et al. Effect of changing to a self-selected vegetarian diet on anthropometric measurements in UK adults. *J Hum Nutr Diet.* 17:249, 2004.

Robinson F, et al. Changing from a mixed to self-selected vegetarian diet—influence on blood lipids. *J Hum Nutr Diet.* 15:323, 2002.

Rosell MS, et al. Soy intake and blood cholesterol concentrations: a cross-sectional study of 1033 pre- and postmenopausal women in the Oxford arm of the European Prospective Investigation into Cancer and Nutrition. *Am J Clin Nutr.* 80:1391, 2004.

Sharma JB, et al. Effect of dietary habits on prevalence of anemia in pregnant women of Delhi. *J Obstet Gynaecol Res.* 29:73, 2003.

Siener R, Hesse A. The effect of a vegetarian and different omnivorous diets on urinary risk factors for uric acid stone formation. *Eur J Nutr.* 42:332, 2003.

Stabler SP, Allen RH. Vitamin B12 deficiency as a worldwide problem. *Annu Rev Nutr.* 24:299, 2004.

Szeto YT, et al. Effects of a long-term vegetarian diet on biomarkers of antioxidant status and cardiovascular disease risk. *Nutrition* 20:863, 2004.

EASTERN RELIGIOUS DIETARY PRACTICES

NUTRITIONAL ACUITY RANKING: LEVEL 2 (ADVISEMENT/PLANNING)

DEFINITIONS AND BACKGROUND

Hinduism, Jainism, and Sikhism

Hindus may be vegetarian while adhering to *ahimsa,* related to nonviolence as applied to the infliction of pain on animals. Beef is never eaten (the cow is considered sacred), and pork is usually avoided. Foods prohibited may include snails, crab, poultry, cranes, ducks, camels, boars, and some types of fish.

The Brahmins, "high caste" folk, have stricter rules and practices, and there are differences between the North Indian Brahmins and the South Indian Brahmins. Some foods promote purity of the body, mind, and spirit. Devout Hindus avoid alcoholic beverages and foods that stimulate the senses, such as garlic and onions.

Feast days include Holi, Dusshera, Pongal, and Divali (varying each year according to the lunar calendar). In addition, personal feast days include the anniversaries of birthdays, marriages, and deaths. Fasting depends on a person's social standing (caste), family, age, gender, and degree of orthodoxy. Fasting can be complete, adopting a completely vegetarian diet, or it can be abstaining from favorite foods.

Jainism is a branch of Hinduism that also promotes the nonviolence of ahimsa. Devout Jains are complete vegans. They avoid blood-colored foods (tomatoes) and avoid root vegetables, which may result in the death of insects clinging to the vegetable when it is harvested.

Sikhs participate in Hindu practices. They differ by their belief in a single God. Sikhs abstain from beef and alcohol, but pork is permitted.

Buddhism

Buddhist dietary customs vary considerably depending on sect (Theravada or Hinayana, Mahayana, Zen) and on country of origin. Most Buddhists also subscribe to the concept of ahimsa, and many are lacto-ovo-vegetarians. Some eat fish, whereas some only abstain from beef. Some believe that unless they personally slaughter an animal, they may eat its meat.

Buddhist monks fast completely on the days of the new moon and full moon each lunar month; they also avoid eating any solid food after the noon hour. Buddhist feasts vary from one region to another. Celebrations include the birth, enlightenment, and death of Buddha in Mahayana Buddhism; the 3 days are unified into the single holiday of Vesak for Theravada Buddhism.

Buddhist vegetarian diets tend to allow more natural insulin sensitivity, so diabetes is less common (Kuo et al, 2004). However, serum homocysteine should be monitored because of possibly lower intakes of vitamin B_{12} (Hung et al, 2002).

INTERVENTION: OBJECTIVES

- Serve appropriate menu choices, and omit foods or beverages that are not permitted.
- Respect traditions and preferences of patient and family members.

INTERVENTION: FOOD AND NUTRITION

- Support dietary practices as followed by the individual and family members.
- Counsel about specific nutritional changes according to the medical diagnosis and current condition.

CLINICAL INDICATORS

Clinical/History		
Height	Diet history	Chol, Trig
Weight	Blood pressure (BP)	Serum Na+, K+
BMI		Ca++, Mg++
Recent weight changes	**Lab Work**	Alk phos
	Gluc	H & H, serum Fe

Herbs, Botanicals, and Supplements

- Many cultures use herbs and botanicals as part of their meal patterns, rituals, and celebrations. Identify those that are used and monitor side effects.
- Counsel about use of herbal teas, especially regarding toxic substances.

INTERVENTION: NUTRITION EDUCATION, COUNSELING, CARE MANAGEMENT

- Show the patient how to prepare foods to reduce cholesterol, fat, or sodium if heart disease or hypertension is present.
- Various types of cancer may prevail in different parts of the world and in different cultures. Discuss diet in relationship to what is common.

Patient Education—Food Safety

- Discuss safe preparation and storage of foods to reduce likelihood of bacterial contamination.

For More Information

- Asian Foods
  http://www.asiafood.org/
- Asian Society
  http://www.asiasociety.org/
- Asia Source
  http://www.asiasource.org/links/
- Buddhism
  http://www.buddhanet.net/
- Ethnic Recipes
  http://asiarecipe.com/religion.html
- Hinduism
  http://www.hindunet.org/healthlifestyle/
- International Studies
  http://www.internationaled.org/

EASTERN RELIGIOUS DIETARY PRACTICES—CITED REFERENCES

Hung CJ, et al. Plasma homocysteine levels in Taiwanese vegetarians are higher than those of omnivores. *J Nutr.* 132:152, 2002.

Kuo CS, et al. Insulin sensitivity in Chinese ovo-lactovegetarians compared with omnivores. *Eur J Clin Nutr.* 58:312, 2004.

WESTERN RELIGIOUS DIETARY PRACTICES

NUTRITIONAL ACUITY RANKING: LEVEL 2 (ADVISEMENT/PLANNING)

DEFINITIONS AND BACKGROUND

Judaism (Edited by Rabbi Allan Bernstein)

Jewish congregations in the United States are either identified as Orthodox, Conservative, or Reform. Orthodox Jews believe the laws are the direct commandments of God, to be explicitly followed by the faithful. Reform Jews follow the moral law but believe that the laws are still being interpreted (some are considered dated or currently irrelevant) and may be observed selectively. Conservative Jews fall in between the other congregations in their beliefs and adherence to the laws. About 25–30% of Jews in America keep kosher to one extent or another (http://www.jewfaq.org/kashrut.htm).

Jewish dietary laws are known as *Kashrut* and are among the most complex of all religious food practices. The term *kosher*, or *kasher*, means "fit" and describes all foods that are permitted for consumption. Kosher is loosely used to identify Jewish dietary laws, and to "keep kosher" means that the laws are followed. The dietary laws are complex. Briefly, they include what foods are fit to eat, what foods are prohibited (a lengthy list that includes pork, shellfish, and other foods), how animals must be slaughtered, how they must be prepared, and when they may be consumed (specifically, rules regarding when milk products can be consumed with meat products).

Jewish feast days include Rosh Hashanah, Sukkot, Hanukkah, Purim, Passover, and Shavout (dates vary because Judaism uses a lunar calendar). Specific foods are associated with the feasts but may differ nationally. Complete fast days (no food or water from sunset to sunset) include Yom Kippur and Tisha b'Av. Partial fast days (no food or water from sunrise to sunset) include Tzom Gedaliah, Tenth of Tevet and Seventeenth of Tamuz, Ta'anit Ester, and Ta'anit Bechorim. Special kosher laws are observed during Passover, including the elimination of any products that can be leavened.

INTERVENTION: OBJECTIVES

- Observe dietary practices as followed by the laws of Judaism: meats are limited to cud-chewing animals with cloven hooves (cows and sheep) that are properly slaughtered. Pork (including ham and all pork products), shellfish, and scavenger fish are forbidden.
- Separate utensils are used for preparation and eating and especially for separating meat and milk foods.
- Monitor the kosher diet, which tends to be high in cholesterol, saturated fats, and sodium. Encourage application of the DASH diet principles where possible, but reduce lactose and sodium if necessary.

INTERVENTION: FOOD AND NUTRITION

The Jewish dinner table follows these guidelines (http://www.jewfaq.org/kashrut.htm):

- Certain animals may not be eaten at all. This restriction includes the flesh, organs, eggs, and milk of the forbidden animals. No pork, ham, bacon, pork products, rabbit, shellfish, or eel may be eaten.
- Of the animals that may be eaten, the birds and mammals must be killed in accordance with Jewish law. All blood must be drained from the meat or broiled out of it before it is eaten. Certain parts of permitted animals may not be eaten. Sheep, cattle, goats, and deer are kosher.
- Meat (the flesh of birds and mammals) cannot be eaten with dairy. Fish, eggs, fruits, vegetables, and grains can be eaten with either meat or dairy. According to some views, fish may not be eaten with meat.
- Dairy: Milk may be consumed before a meal, but once meat is eaten, 3–6 hours (depending on individual traditions) must pass before dairy products can be consumed. Omit lactose if not tolerated; provide other sources of calcium and riboflavin.
- Utensils that have come into contact with meat may not be used with dairy and vice versa. Utensils that have come into contact with non-kosher food may not be used with kosher food.
- Fruits, vegetables, and grains can be used, except that breads made with milk products are forbidden with meat meals. Grape products made by non-Jews may not be eaten.
- Leavened (raised) bread is forbidden during Passover. Matzoh bread or crackers may be used. Haroset and fried matzoh are traditional Passover foods. Seder plates and other items appropriate for the Seder dinner are important additions to the menu at this time.
- Common food choices include matzoh ball soup, chicken soup with kreplach, gefilte fish with beet horseradish, cheese blintz with sour cream, flanken tzimmes, chopped liver, noodle Kugel, and kishka. Frozen kosher meals may be available in some areas.
- Fasting is common during Yom Kippur.
- Traditional Hanukkah foods include latkes and sour cream or applesauce.

CLINICAL INDICATORS

Clinical/History		
Height	Diet history	Serum Na+, K+
Weight	BP	Ca++, Mg++
BMI	**Lab Work**	Alk phos
Recent weight changes	Gluc	H & H, serum Fe
	Chol, Trig	

INTERVENTION: NUTRITION EDUCATION, COUNSELING, CARE MANAGEMENT

- Show the patient how to limit foods high in cholesterol/fat if weight and elevated lipid levels are a problem.
- Discuss sodium and obesity in relationship to hypertension, as appropriate. Recommend other herbs, spices, and cooking methods.
- Low-fat cheeses should be substituted for high-fat cheeses such as cream cheese.
- Note that food labels with a "U" with an "O" encircling it are considered kosher. Many other foods are considered kosher, but an inquiry should be made.
- Discuss holiday preferences and alternatives when needed.

Patient Education—Food Safety

- Discuss safe preparation and storage of foods to reduce likelihood of bacterial contamination.

For More Information

- Determining Kosher
  http://www.ou.org/kosher/primer.html
- Hebrew Food Pyramid
  http://monarch.gsu.edu/WebRoot$/multiculturalhealth/handouts/hebrew//Hebrew_food_pyramid.pdf
- Judaism 101
  http://www.jewfaq.org/kashrut.htm
- Kashrut–Dietary Laws
  http://www.myjewishlearning.com/daily_life/Kashrut.htm
- Kosher certification
  http://www.okkosher.com/
- Kosherfest
  http://www.kosherfest.com/
- Union for Traditional Judaism
  http://www.utj.org/

DEFINITIONS AND BACKGROUND

Christianity

There are three major branches of the Christian faith: Roman Catholicism, Eastern Orthodox Christianity, and Protestantism. Dietary practices vary; some are minimal.

(1) **Roman Catholicism:** Devout Catholics observe several feast and fast days during the year. Feast days include Christmas, Easter, the Annunciation (March 25th), Palm Sunday (the Sunday before Easter), the Ascension (40 days after Easter), and Pentecost Sunday (50 days after Easter). Catholics in each country observe many food traditions. Fasting (one full meal per day permitted; snacking according to local custom) and/or abstinence (meat is prohibited, but eggs, dairy products, and condiments with animal fat are permitted) may be practiced during Lent, on the Fridays of Advent, and Ember Days (at the beginning of the seasons) by some Catholics; some fast or abstain only on Ash Wednesday and Good Friday. Today, Catholics avoid meat only on the Fridays of Lent (40 days before Easter). Food and beverages (except water) should be avoided for 1 hour before communion is taken.

(2) **Eastern Orthodox Christianity:** The 14 self-governing churches that form the Orthodox Church differ from Catholicism in their interpretation of the Biblical theology, including the use of leavened bread instead of unleavened wafers in communion. Numerous feast and fast days are observed (dates vary according to whether the Julian or Gregorian calendar is used). Feast days include Christmas, Theophany, Presentation of the Lord into the Temple, Annunciation, Easter, Ascension, Pentecost Sunday, the Transfiguration, Dormition of the Holy Theotokos, Nativity of the Holy Theotokos, and Presentation of the Holy Theotokos. In addition, Meat Fare Sunday is observed the third Sunday before Easter (all meat in the house is consumed, and none is eaten again until Easter); Cheese Fare Sunday is observed on the Sunday before Easter (all cheese, eggs, and butter are consumed); and on the next day, Clean Monday, the Lenten fast begins. Food and drink are avoided before communion.

Meat and all animal products (milk, eggs, butter, and cheese) are prohibited on fast days; fish is avoided, but shellfish is permitted. Some devout followers may avoid olive oil on fast days, too. Fast days include every Wednesday and Friday (except for three fast-free weeks each year), the Eve of Theophany, the Beheading of John the Baptist, and Elevation of the Holy Cross. Fast periods include Advent, Lent, the Fast of the Apostles, and Fast of the Dormition of the Holy Theotokos.

(3) **Protestantism:** The only feast days common in most Protestant religions are Christmas and Easter. Few practice fasting. The only denominations with dietary laws fundamental to their faith are Mormons (Church of Jesus Christ of Latter Day Saints) and Seventh-Day Adventists. **Mormons** avoid alcoholic beverages, hot drinks (coffee and tea), and caffeine-containing drinks. Followers are encouraged to eat mostly grains and to limit meats. Some Mormons fast 1 day a month and donate their food money to the poor. **Seventh-Day Adventists** avoid overeating; most are lacto-ovo-vegetarians, but when meat is consumed, most avoid pork. Tea, coffee, and alcoholic beverages are prohibited. Water is consumed before and after meals, and eating between meals is discouraged. Strong seasonings and condiments, such as pepper and mustard, are avoided.

INTERVENTION: OBJECTIVES

- Observe dietary practices as followed by the individual.
- Assist immigrants in maintaining their own healthy dietary practices and religious traditions, as appropriate (Kaplan et al, 2004).
- Discuss the role of special meals, fasting, or events and plan menus accordingly.

INTERVENTION: FOOD AND NUTRITION

- Promote a healthy diet. For example, application of the principles of a Mediterranean diet may be suitable for many individuals (Bilenko et al, 2005).
- Fasting may be common during special holidays. Discuss concerns related to pregnancy or malnourished status.

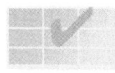

- Some individuals avoid caffeine and alcohol as part of their religious preferences; honor those wishes.
- Determine if any foods are avoided on special days of the week and plan alternatives accordingly.

CLINICAL INDICATORS

Clinical/History	Diet history	Serum Na+, K+
Height	BP	Ca++, Mg++
Weight		Alk phos
BMI	**Lab Work**	H & H, serum Fe
Recent weight changes	Gluc	C-reactive protein (CRP)
	Chol, Trig	

INTERVENTION: NUTRITION EDUCATION, COUNSELING, CARE MANAGEMENT

- Show the patient how to limit foods high in cholesterol/fat if weight and elevated lipid levels are a problem.
- Discuss sodium and obesity in relationship to hypertension, as appropriate. Recommend other herbs, spices, and cooking methods.
- Discuss holiday preferences and alternatives where needed.
- There tend to be few specific relationships between religion, fat intake, and physical activity in contemporary U.S. society; religion may play only a small role in the context of how diet and exercise are developed and maintained (Kim and Sobal, 2004).

Patient Education—Food Safety

- Discuss safe preparation and storage of foods to reduce likelihood of bacterial contamination.

For More Information

- Andrews University–Seventh-Day Adventist Practices http://www.andrews.edu/NUFS/resource.html

WESTERN RELIGIOUS DIETARY PRACTICES—CITED REFERENCES

Bilenko N, et al. Mediterranean diet and cardiovascular diseases in an Israeli population. *Prev Med.* 40:299, 2005.

Kaplan MS, et al. The association between length of residence and obesity among Hispanic immigrants. *Am J Prev Med.* 27:323, 2004.

Kim KH, Sobal J. Religion, social support, fat intake and physical activity. *Pub Health Nutr.* 7:773, 2004.

MIDDLE EASTERN RELIGIOUS DIETARY PRACTICES

NUTRITIONAL ACUITY RANKING: LEVEL 2 (ADVISEMENT/PLANNING)

DEFINITIONS AND BACKGROUND

Islam is an Arabic word that means submission, surrender, and obedience; it also means peace, as it is derived from the word "Salam," which means peace. As a religion, Islam stands for complete submission and obedience to God. Followers of the Islamic faith are known as Muslims. Muslims promote the concept of eating to live, not living to eat. They advise sharing food.

Prohibited foods as described in the Koran are called *haram*; those in question are *mashbooh.* Pork and birds of prey are haram; meats must be slaughtered properly. Alcohol is prohibited, and stimulants, such as coffee and tea, are allowed. *Halal* is the term for all permitted foods. The flesh of animals must be slaughtered according to Islamic law or *halal*; kosher items may be used for this reason. Feast days (dates vary according to the lunar calendar) include Eid al-Fitr, Eid al-Azha, Nau-Roz (a Persian holiday), Al-Ghadeer, and Maulud n'Nabi.

Fasting is considered an opportunity to earn the approval of Allah, to wipe out sins, and to understand the suffering of the poor. Fasting includes abstention from all food and drink from dawn to sunset. Voluntary fasting is common on Mondays and Thursdays; it is undesirable to fast on certain days of the month and on Fridays. Muslims are required to fast during the entire month of Ramadan and are encouraged to fast 6 days during the month of Shawwal, on the Al-Ghadeer day, and on the 9th day of Zul Hijjah.

INTERVENTION: OBJECTIVES

- During fasting, eating occurs only before dawn and after sunset. Plan accordingly.
- Monitor dietary patterns, which include fasting 3 days a month. Pregnant and breastfeeding mothers need not fast.
- Monitor need for vitamin D in women if sun exposure is minimal.

INTERVENTION: FOOD AND NUTRITION

- Pork and pork products are forbidden, including gelatin.
- Alcohol is not used, even in vanilla extract and other preparations.

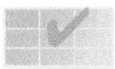

- Foods such as dates, seafood, honey, sweets, yogurt, milk (goat's milk also), meat, and olive or vegetable oils are encouraged. Beef, chicken, and lamb are commonly used. Couscous, pita bread, rice, millet, and bulgur are frequently included. Eggplant, cucumbers, green peppers, pomegranates, and tomatoes are readily available.
- Typical combination foods include: falafel (grain, fat), hummus (grain, fat), kibbeh (meat, grain, fat), tabouli (vegetable, grain, fat), baba ghanouj (vegetable, fat), pilaf (grain, fat), stuffed grape leaves (meat, grain, fat), and shawarma (meat, grain, fat). Khoresh is a stew with meats (lamb, beef, or veal), poultry, or fish with vegetables; fresh or dried fruits; beans, grains, and even nuts.

CLINICAL INDICATORS

Clinical/History	Diet history	Serum Na+, K+
Height	BP	Ca++, Mg++
Weight		Alk phos
BMI	**Lab Work**	H & H, serum Fe
Recent weight changes	Gluc	
	Chol, Trig	

INTERVENTION: NUTRITION EDUCATION, COUNSELING, CARE MANAGEMENT

- If diet is low in heme iron, anemia may occur. Discuss options if necessary.
- Fasting is not recommended for persons who have diabetes, cancer, or HIV/AIDS. Discuss menu planning for religious occasions.
- Discuss useful dietary changes for managing obesity and diabetes.

For More Information

- Catering for Muslim Patients
  http://www.healthandnutrition.co.uk/hffhk/pages/ARTICLES/muslim.htm
- Iranian Cooking
  http://www.asiafood.org/persiancooking/index.cfm
- Islamic Food and Nutrition Council of America
  http://www.ifanca.org/
- Muslim Consumer group
  http://www.muslimconsumergroup.com/hfs.htm

OROFACIAL CONDITIONS

DENTAL DIFFICULTIES AND ORAL DISORDERS

NUTRITIONAL ACUITY RANKING: LEVEL 2–3

DEFINITIONS AND BACKGROUND

Diet and nutrition impact on many oral diseases, in particular dental caries (Moynihan, 2005a). Cell turnover is rapid in the tongue and oral mucosa; therefore, the oral cavity is one of the first areas where signs of systemic disease appear. Health professionals should monitor changes in the oral/dental health of a patient. Assessment of the teeth should include missing, loose teeth; presence of dentures and whether they fit well; and presence of rampant tooth decay.

Tooth loss can prevent proper bite and may lessen the ability to chew foods properly. Dietary advice given at the time of denture provision results in increased consumption of fruits and vegetables and positive movement through the stages of change (Moynihan, 2005a).

Many Americans lack fluoridated water, an effective safeguard against dental cavities. Those who are poor or have no dental insurance are also at risk for caries. Studies show that water fluoridation can reduce caries in baby teeth by as much as 60% and can reduce tooth decay in permanent adult teeth by nearly 35% (http://www.ada.org/public/topics/fluoride/facts/index.asp).

Two oral infectious diseases are diet related; dental caries (tooth decay) is influenced by numerous factors, including diet composition and frequency, and periodontal disease is associated with malnutrition (Touger-Decker et al, 2003). In dental caries, chronic infectious disease leads to progressive destruction of tooth substances from interactions between bacteria and organic tooth compounds. *Streptococcus mutans* and *Lactobacillus* are common culprits; acid forms between 20 seconds and 30 minutes after contact. Erosion of tooth enamel may occur in patients who chronically consume acidic beverages and/or keep such beverages or foods in the mouth for a period of time (e.g., sucking lemons, chewing vitamin C tablets, chewing lemon hard candies).

Some dental problems are age specific. Infants should be monitored for early childhood caries (ECC); dental decay often occurs during the growth spurts of adolescents; and older patients should be monitored for changes in eating habits and use of an inadequate diet, as well as caries. Elderly persons who wear dentures are more prone to malnutrition (de Oliveria and Frigerio, 2004). In addition, problems with oral health (chewing, swallowing, and mouth pain) often precede hospitalizations in older persons (Bailey et al, 2004).

Poor oral hygiene can increase the likelihood of gingival abnormalities when vitamin C and vitamin D intakes have been poor. Some conditions, such as diabetes, can also make individuals prone to dry mouth and dental decay. An increase in water intake, extra care with oral hygiene, chewing sugarless gum, and prevention of periodontal disease are important steps.

With tongue disorders, mastication of food may be affected. The ability to push mashed food with the tongue and anterior hard palate will be affected. Other oral problems may cause pain, problems with chewing, dysphagia, mouth dryness, or infection including aphthous stomatitis, cheilosis, oral cancer, lichen planus, oral herpes, candidiasis, thrush, or xerostomia. Many of these conditions occur because of altered immunity and debility, as in cancer or HIV/AIDS.

Fracture of the lower jaw (mandible) is a common injury, and treatment involves intermaxillary fixation (wiring). Patients with wired jaws face a whole new lifestyle for up to 6 weeks following maxillofacial surgery. Patients have to eat liquefied meals, and proper presurgical patient education is essential.

Proper nutrition is essential. Table 2-4 provides a list of the key nutrients needed for healthy oral mucosa and teeth. Plasma ascorbate and plasma retinol are significant (Sheiham et al, 2001); prevention and treatments of leukoplakias are implicated (Scully, 2000). Treatment with beta-carotene or retinoids is recommended for leukoplakia (Lodi et al, 2004).

Table 2-5 lists dental problems, treatment, and prevention. Figure 2-2 shows the anatomy of a normal tooth.

INTERVENTION: OBJECTIVES

Broken or Wired Jaw

- Provide adequate nourishment to allow healing while reducing jaw movement.
- Decrease complications such as fever, nausea, and vomiting.
- Prevent excessive weight loss; up to 10% is common.
- Maintain a patent airway.

Dental Caries

- Alter dietary habits; deprive bacteria of substrate; reduce acid; keep pH at 7.0.
- Maintain frequent fluoride contact with tooth surfaces as directed by a dental professional.

Early Childhood Caries (ECC)

- ECC is a preventable dental disease.
- Enamel erodes, and tooth surface is permanently damaged from long exposure to liquid carbohydrate sources.
- Education is the biggest factor. Children with significant risk factors for caries (e.g., inadequate home dental care and poor oral hygiene, a mother with a high number of cavities, a high sugar intake, enamel defects, premature birth, special health care needs, low socioeconomic status) should be referred to a dentist (Douglass et al, 2004).

Edentulism

- Provide proper consistency to allow the patient to eat.
- Monitor for deficiencies in fiber and vitamins A and C if whole grains, fruits, and vegetables are not consumed (Touger-Decker, 2004).

Mouth Ulcers or Pain

- Lessen mouth soreness to increase dietary intake; some mouth sprays may be available to lessen pain while eating.

TABLE 2-4 Nutrients Needed for Proper Oral Tissue Synthesis and Dental Care

Protein	Needed for healthy tissue growth and maintenance.
Vitamin A	Necessary for epithelial tissue and enamel. Beta-carotene may play a role in oral cancer prevention (Lodi et al, 2004).
Vitamin B-Complex	Deficiencies show a bright scarlet tongue and stomatitis in niacin deficiency; magenta tongue, glossitis, and angular cheilitis in riboflavin deficiency; smooth tongue in vitamin B_{12} deficiency.
Folate	Needed for a healthy blood supply.
Vitamin C	Enables connective tissue cells to elaborate intercellular substances. Deficiency can lead to easy bleeding or swelling of gums and gingivitis. Forms collagen; helps to heal wounds and bleeding gums.
Vitamin K	Aids with calcium absorption in bone; adequate blood clotting; helps in healing.
Vitamin D	Protects against chronic inflammation of the gums, which can lead to gingivitis or periodontal disease (Dietrich et al, 2004). Necessary for dentin, bony tissue synthesis; mineralization; and jawbone sufficiency.
Calcium and Phosphorus	Necessary for dentin and bony tissue synthesis. Poor mineralization occurs with deficiency. Maintains jawbone sufficiency.
Chromium	Needed for proper glucose metabolism. Controlled intake of carbohydrates helps to maintain healthier gums and overall health status (Moynihan, 2005b).
Copper	Needed for production of blood and nerve fibers.
Fluoride	Consumption of fluoridated water coupled with a reduction in nonmilk sugar intake is an effective means of caries prevention (Moynihan, 2005a; American Dietetic Association, 2000). Keeps bones healthy. Drinking water should contain 1 ppm; toothpaste, mouth rinses, and topical treatments also help.
Iron	Helps produce red blood cells; promotes resistance to disease; improves health of the teeth, skin, and bones. Maintains energy.
Magnesium	Helps in bone development. Enhances use of vitamin C. Deficiency may lead to calcium resorption.
Potassium	Needed for muscle contraction and proper nerve function.
Zinc	Regulates the inflammatory process; aids in wound healing. Deficiencies can lead to poor healing, susceptibility to infection, loss of taste, and altered metabolism.

TABLE 2-5 Dental Problems, Treatment, and Prevention

Symptoms	Likely Cause	Treatment	Prevention
Bad Breath			
Odor from mouth; bad, metallic taste; coated tongue	Food caught around and between teeth; infection in gums; improper brushing; sinusitis; digestive problems, such as preulcerative conditions; diabetes	Practice good oral hygiene, including rinsing with mouthwash; brush tongue often; see dentist to evaluate throat, sinuses, tongue, and possible gum infection, and professionally clean teeth and gums; review diet	Regular dental visits; flossing, brushing, and rinsing; good nutrition
Broken Tooth or Filling			
Tooth feels sharp; tooth sensitivity to temperature and pressure	Accidental trauma; decay; weak tooth from grinding or improper bite	Do not irritate; place piece of soft dental wax from drugstore over cracked or fractured tooth; see a dentist immediately	Regular dental checkups to discover possible weak teeth, decay, or large, unstable fillings
Canker Sores			
Painful red circular area that develops on the tongue, gums, lips, or cheeks; in certain phases, sores have a yellow or white center area; sore to touch; sensitivity to spicy, salty foods	Bacterial or viral infection; trauma from denture in mouth; stress	Use over-the-counter remedies recommended by the dentist; coat lesions after meals; see dentist to make sure there is no infection or for additional medication if pain persists; the dentist will evaluate dentures for weight-bearing points to be certain the problem does not exist there	Avoid irritating the area; avoid spicy, acidic foods while mouth is sore
Dental Abscess (swelling around tooth or cheek)			
Pain, throbbing in gum or tooth; swelling; sensitive bite; loose teeth; sensitivity to heat	Tooth decay; initial eruption of tooth through the gums or fractured tooth; tooth nerve damage	Rinse with salt water solution; use mouthwash; avoid eating on or near tooth; see dentist immediately; may require antibiotics or root canal treatment to prevent spread of infection	Regular dental checkups; good oral hygiene; brushing, flossing, and rinsing
Discolored Teeth			
Teeth have unsightly and discolored appearance; single tooth begins to turn yellow or gray	Surface stain from certain foods, such as tea and coffee; internal staining from tooth nerve damage or from rheumatic fever; stains from tetracycline	Improve oral hygiene; brush frequently; diminish coffee or tea intake; rinse with peroxide; consult dentist to check nerve in darkened tooth; consider supervised tooth bleaching/whitening	Good oral hygiene; avoid foods and liquids that can stain teeth, such as tea and coffee
Gum Disease			
Gum pain; nonthrobbing ache; swelling; gum bleeding; blood in saliva when brushing; metallic taste	Food debris between teeth; tartar beneath gums; infection; poor bite may worsen this condition	Improve oral hygiene by brushing often and flossing; rinse with mouthwash; consult dentist to evaluate extent of condition; treatment by removing plaque and tartar may require surgery and/or bite adjustment	Good oral hygiene; regular dental checkups and cleanings
Red Inflamed Gums			
Color of gums around teeth progresses from pink to red with swelling or puffiness; dry mouth; snoring	Mouth breathing; some medications, such as antihistamines, blood pressure medications, and antidepressants, decrease salivary flow	Use oral salivary rinses and toothpastes for dry mouth; improve oral hygiene; consult dentist because this condition can lead to tooth decay, advanced gum disease, or other mouth infections	Ask physician if medications can be changed; consult dentist about obtaining oral rinses and a snoreguard

(continued)

TABLE 2-5 Dental Problems, Treatment, and Prevention *(continued)*

Symptoms	Likely Cause	Treatment	Prevention
Loose Teeth			
Teeth move; spongy feel to bite; teeth sensitive or even painful when chewing	Gum disease; tooth grinding; orthodontic appliances too tight; cyst, tumor, abscess, or trauma to teeth	See dentist as soon as possible to determine cause; practice good oral hygiene; be aware of tooth grinding or clenching and use appliance to prevent grinding	Regular dental visits; good oral hygiene; have your dentist evaluate your bite; use a bite appliance if your dentist advises
Lumps Under Jaw or Neck Muscle			
Neck sore to touch or movement; swelling in neck; sore throat; difficulty swallowing	Cold/flu; tooth abscess or infection; tumor	Treat cold/flu symptoms; limit neck movement; check temperature; take pain relievers such as aspirin; see a dentist if symptoms persist to evaluate the extent of swelling and infection	Regular dental checkups; patients should pay special attention to any growth or changes in the head or neck
Toothache (tooth pain on biting or chewing)			
Tooth pain related to temperature change or touch or from chewing or biting; dark brown spots on teeth may indicate new decay	Bacterial acids; large filling broken out of tooth; tooth grinding	Rinse mouth often with vanilla extract to soothe discomfort; avoid chewing on tooth; see a dentist as soon as possible to determine cause and further treatment	Regular dental visits for prevention; the sooner examined, the better the chance of success
Tooth Sensitivity to Temperature Change			
Breathing outside in cold air causes pain; waking up with toothache; pain when eating/drinking cold things	Inflamed gums; gum recession that exposes root surfaces; tooth decay; teeth clenching or grinding that has worn away tooth enamel	Use desensitizing toothpaste on a daily basis; use a soft bristle brush; avoid temperature differences; consult dentist for appropriate treatment	Good oral hygiene; apply fluoride gel; use desensitizing toothpaste; avoid food temperature differences; avoid hard bristle toothbrushes; become aware of and avoid tooth grinding or squeezing teeth together; have fillings bonded to seal areas of sensitivity; dentist may recommend a biteguard for grinding

Adapted with permission from Rhode Island Dental Association, 200 Centerville Road, Warwick, RI 02886; Phone: (401) 732-6833; http://www.ridental.com/dentalproblems.cfm, accessed January 10, 2005.

- Promote healing for a return to normal eating patterns.
- Prevent weight loss or other consequences.

Tongue Disorders

- Provide adequate nourishment despite acute or chronic disability.

Tube Feeding

- Children on tube feedings often have dental problems; therefore, these children should receive more attention to oral hygiene than those fed orally.
- Adults will require special attention to oral hygiene and mouth care while on tube feedings.

Xerostomia

- Dry mouth may be more severe after radiation therapy than with other causes such as diabetes.
- Artificial saliva agents may be useful for some, but not all patients find relief. Reduced saliva affects patient perception of swallowing ability and changes dietary choices (Logemann et al, 2003).
- Good oral hygiene may prevent dental decay.

INTERVENTION: FOOD AND NUTRITION

Broken or Wired Jaw

- A diet of pureed and strained foods and liquids of high protein/calorie content are necessary.
- Adequate amounts of vitamin C should be taken to aid healing.
- Monitor food temperatures carefully.
- Six to eight meals are needed.
- Follow meals with salt water rinse.
- Use supplemental beverages that are high in calories (perhaps 2 kcal/mL). Double-strength milk may also be used to keep protein intake at a high level.

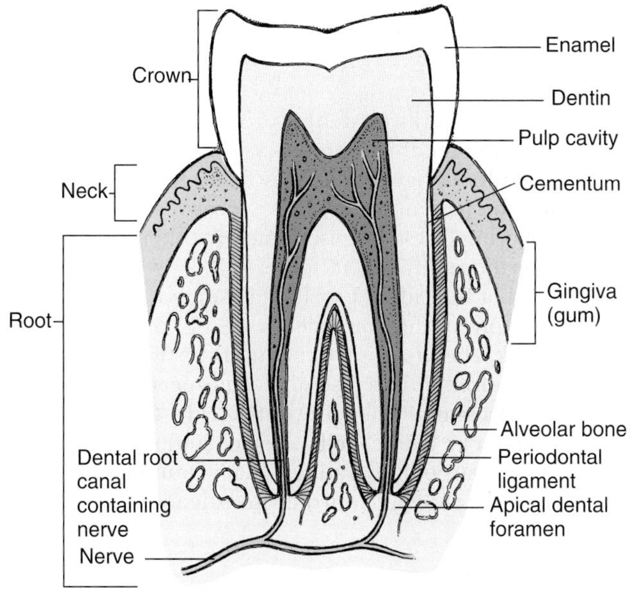

Figure 2-2 Anatomy of a tooth. (From *Stedman's medical dictionary*, 27th ed. Baltimore: Lippincott Williams & Wilkins, 2000.)

Dental Caries

- Decrease sucrose and cooked or sticky starches, as well as the frequency of snacking and duration of exposure time. *Streptococcus mutans* is a common bacterial culprit; others include *Lactobacillus casein* and *Streptococcus sanguis* (Touger-Decker, 2004).
- Use a balanced diet, eating sweets or starches with meals.
- Fluoride exposure should be adequate, including from water supplies.
- The sequence of eating foods, the combination of foods, the form of foods and beverages consumed, and nutrient composition of foods/beverages must be evaluated and altered accordingly (Touger-Decker, 2004).

Early Childhood Caries (ECC)

The following are guidelines for prevention (The American Academy of Pediatric Dentistry, 2005-2006; Clarke et al, 2006; Wagner, 2006):

- Don't allow a child to fall asleep with a bottle containing milk, formula, fruit juices, or other sweet liquids. Never let a child walk with a bottle in his/her mouth.
- Comfort a child who wants a bottle between regular feedings or during naps with a bottle filled with cool water.
- Always make sure a child's pacifier is clean, and never dip a pacifier in a sweet liquid.
- Introduce children to a cup as they approach 1 year of age. Children should stop drinking from a bottle soon after their first birthday.
- Notify the parent of any unusual red or swollen areas in a child's mouth or any dark spot on a child's tooth so that the parent can consult the child's dentist.
- Never put an infant or child to bed with a bottle that is filled with sugar-containing beverages, including fruit juice or Kool-Aid. Good oral hygiene is needed. Wean children by age 2 years.
- Monitor for iron deficiency anemia, which is common (Clarke et al, 2006).

Edentulism

- A chopped, ground, strained, or pureed diet should be followed as required. Use the least restricted diet and progress as tolerated.
- Identify potential solutions such as obtaining new dentures, repairing current dentures, etc.

Mouth Ulcers or Pain

- Foods low in acid and spices should be consumed (e.g., citrus juices are not allowed).
- Supplement the diet with vitamin C, protein, and calories to speed the rate of healing.
- Small, frequent meals and oral supplements may be beneficial to prevent weight loss.
- Moist foods and blenderized foods with additional liquid are helpful.
- Soft, cold foods such as canned fruits, ice cream, popsicles, yogurt, cottage cheese, or cold pasta dishes may be used.
- Use of a straw may be helpful.
- Cut or grind meats or vegetables.
- Extra butter, mild sauces, and gravies may be needed.
- Follow meals by brushing teeth to reduce possibility of dental caries.

Tongue Disorders

- If the patient is unable to chew, tube feeding should be considered (Fig. 2-3).
- Liquids may be added to the diet as tolerated. Many foods are tolerated if liquefied and blenderized.

Tube Feeding

- Good oral hygiene and mouth care will be needed, even if a patient is not fed by mouth. Tube feeding should include all key nutrients to meet patient needs. See Section 17.

Xerostomia

- Moisten foods, adding water or milk when possible. Use sauces or gravies if needed.
- Avoid too many added spices.

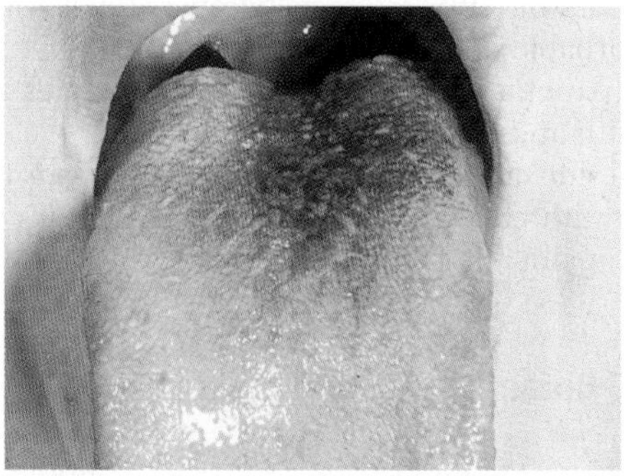

Figure 2-3 Hairy tongue. (From Bickley LS, Szilagyi P. *Bates' guide to physical examination and history taking*. 8th ed. Philadelphia: Lippincott Williams & Wilkins, 2003.)

SAMPLE NUTRITION DIAGNOSTIC STATEMENT

Dental Problems

PES: Inadequate energy intake related to inability to chew foods from poor dentition as evidenced by weight loss of 6 pounds in 14 days.

Assessment Data (sources of info): Food records and intake calculations; dental evaluations, if available.

Intervention: Recommend dental referral if needed for dentures or correcting poor dentition, alter diet to reduce need for chewing (chopped or ground meats, cooked vs. fresh fruits and vegetables, etc.).

Monitoring and Evaluation: Intake records, reduction in chewing problems, improved weight records.

- Avoid excessively chewy foods like steak, crumbly foods like crackers or cake, dry foods like chips, or sticky foods such as peanut butter (Touger-Decker, 2004).

CLINICAL INDICATORS

Clinical/History		Lab Work
Height	Caries	Alb, transthyretin
Weight	Missing or loose teeth	Serum Na+, K+
BMI	Taste alterations	Ca++, Mg++
Recent weight changes	Sore or bleeding gums	Alk phos
Diet history	Dentures, especially poorly fitting	H & H, serum Fe
Mouth or tongue lacerations		X-rays (such as mandible)
		Serum folate

Common Drugs Used and Potential Side Effects

- Luride is a fluoride supplement for children to strengthen teeth against tooth decay. Avoid use with calcium or dairy products because it may form a nonabsorbable product.
- For patients with cancer, various therapies affect the mouth and gums. Monitor closely.
- Oral side effects of drugs are adverse effects that interfere with client function and increase risks for infection, pain, and possible tooth loss (Spolarich, 2000).

Herbs, Botanicals, and Supplements

- Herbs and botanicals may be used; identify and monitor side effects.
- Counsel about use of herbal teas, especially regarding unsuitable products such as comfrey tea.

INTERVENTION: NUTRITION EDUCATION, COUNSELING, CARE MANAGEMENT

- If needed for oral or dental problems, blended foods and/or tube feedings should be prepared. Sometimes, using a bulb syringe to feed may be useful.
- Provide the patient with creative ideas for the seasoning and flavoring of foods. Discuss acceptable restaurant options for those who are at home.
- Ensure that fluoride is provided in some way by the diet, water supply, or dental office.
- Read milk labels to ensure vitamin D fortification.
- Consideration of dental status is an especially important part of assessment and preventive care for the elderly (Sahyoun et al, 2003; Sheiham et al, 2001).
- Feasible means of integrating dietary counseling into the dental setting warrants further investigation (Moynihan, 2005a).

To prevent caries:

- Encourage good habits in oral hygiene and diet: detergent foods (e.g., raw fruits and vegetables) should be recommended rather than sticky or impactant foods (e.g., soft cookies, bread, sticky sweets, dried fruits, etc.).
- Avoid cariogenic foods such as dried fruits, candy, cookies, pies, cakes, ice cream, canned fruit, soft drinks, fruit drinks, lemonade, gelatin desserts, snack crackers, pretzels or chips, and muffins.
- Cariostatic foods should be encouraged, such as cheese, raw fruits and vegetables, peanuts, and cocoa.
- Use cheese after meals or sugary snacks to normalize pH.

Patient Education—Food Safety

- When traveling, avoid ice made from tap water. Airline water may not be free from contamination. Use of bottled water is recommended for brushing teeth in countries where water is not safe.

For More Information

- American Academy of Pediatric Dentistry
  http://www.aapd.org/
- American Academy of General Dentistry
  http://www.agd.org/
- American Academy of Periodontology
  http://www.perio.org/
- American Dental Association
  http://www.ada.org/
- Colgate
  http://www.colgate.com/app/Colgate/US/OralCare/HomePage.cvsp
- Dentistry Online
  http://www.floss.com/dental_nutrition.htm
- International Association for Disability and Oral Health
  http://www.iadh.org/
- National Institute of Dental and Craniofacial Research (NIDCR)
  http://www.nidcr.nih.gov/
- National Oral Health Information Clearinghouse
  http://www.healthfinder.gov/orgs/HR2457.htm

- Oral Health America
  http://www.oralhealthamerica.org/
- USDA Fluoride Content
  http://www.nal.usda.gov/fnic/foodcomp/Data/Fluoride/fluoride.pdf

DENTAL DIFFICULTIES AND ORAL DISORDERS—CITED REFERENCES

American Academy of Pediatric Dentistry. Policy on early childhood caries (ECC): classifications, consequences, and preventive strategies. *Pediatr Dent.* 27:31, 2005-2006.

American Dietetic Association. Position of The American Dietetic Association: the impact of fluoride on health. *J Am Diet Assoc.* 100:1208, 2000.

Bailey RL, et al. Persistent oral health problems associated with comorbidity and impaired diet quality in older adults. *J Am Diet Assoc.* 104:1273, 2004.

Clarke M, et al. Malnourishment in a population of young children with severe early childhood caries. *Pediatr Dent.* 28:254, 2006.

de Oliveria TR, Frigerio ML. Association between nutrition and the prosthetic condition in edentulous elderly. *Gerodontology* 21:205, 2004.

Dietrich T, et al. Association between serum concentrations of 25-hydroxyvitamin D3 and periodontal disease in the US population. *Am J Clin Nutr.* 80:108, 2004.

Douglass JM, et al. A practical guide to infant oral health. *Am Fam Physician.* 70:2113, 2004.

Lodi G, et al. Interventions for treating oral leukoplakia. *Cochrane Database Syst Rev.* 3:CD001829, 2004.

Logemann JA, et al. Xerostomia: 12-month changes in saliva production and its relationship to perception and performance of swallow function, oral intake, and diet after chemoradiation. *Head Neck.* 25:432, 2003.

Moynihan P. The interrelationship between diet and oral health. *Proc Nutr Soc.* 64:571, 2005a.

Moynihan P. The role of diet and nutrition in the etiology and prevention of oral diseases. *Bull World Health Org.* 83:694, 2005b.

Sahyoun NR, et al. Nutritional status of the older adult is associated with dentition status. *J Am Diet Assoc.* 103:61, 2003.

Scully C. Advances in oral medicine. *Prim Dent Care.* 7:55, 2000.

Sheiham A, et al. The relationship among dental status, nutrient intake, and nutritional status in older people. *J Dent Res.* 80:408, 2001.

Spolarich A. Managing the side effects of medications. *J Dent Hyg.* 74:57, 2000.

Touger-Decker R. Oral and dental health. In: Mahan K, Escott-Stump S, eds. *Krause's food, nutrition, and diet therapy.* 11th ed. Philadelphia: WB Saunders, 2004.

Touger-Decker R, Mobley C, American Dietetic Association. Position of the American Dietetic Association: oral health and nutrition. *J Am Diet Assoc.* 103:615, 2003.

Wagner R. Early childhood caries. *J Am Dent Assoc.* 137:150, 2006.

PERIODONTAL DISEASE AND GINGIVITIS

NUTRITIONAL ACUITY RANKING: LEVEL 1–2

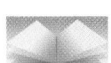

DEFINITIONS AND BACKGROUND

Tissues that support teeth in the jaws are collectively known as the periodontium (gums, alveolar bone, periodontal membrane). Any abnormality that leads to a visible change or loss of integrity of any component of the supporting tissue is listed as a periodontal disease. Periodontal disease is a painless, chronic inflammatory disease generally caused by dental plaque and microbial flora. Usually, dental caries and periodontal disease are not present in the same patients because the microbial flora differs.

A poor diet and inadequate dental hygiene can cause destruction of the jawbone. Osteoporosis and inflammation-associated bone degradation, such as in periodontitis, have a pathogenesis that involves communication between osteoclasts and osteoblasts during osteogenesis (Serhan, 2004). Periodontal disease is evident approximately 10 years before osteoporosis.

Periodontal disease most commonly manifests as pyorrhea alveolaris. In the United States, periodontal disease affects a large portion of the population, especially after age 55. Genetic predisposition affects 30% of those afflicted with periodontal disease (http://www.perio.org/consumer/2a.html#causes).

At risk in particular are pregnant women, women after menopause, obese individuals, diabetics, alcoholics, smokers, persons with immune system conditions (including AIDS or rheumatoid arthritis), persons with respiratory ailments, and persons on certain medications including heart medicines, antidepressants, and antihistamines. Periodontal disease can start in the second decade, and wisdom teeth are a breeding ground for bacteria that cause problems. Children and teens are at risk if their oral and dental health needs are not met (Cummins, 2006).

Nutrient deficiencies may be related. Immune-enhancing nutrients include protein, zinc, vitamin C, vitamin E, calcium, and the B-complex vitamins. Smokers are especially vulnerable to vitamin C deficiency and risk of periodontal disease (Nishida et al, 2000).

Periodontitis involves a gross breakdown of supporting tissues with progressive loosening and loss of teeth; it is a major cause of tooth loss in adults. See Figure 2-4. *Periodontoclasia* involves destruction of tissues around the teeth.

Gingivitis involves minor inflammatory change; it may be acute or chronic, local or generalized. Vitamin C deficiency is implicated. *Acute necrotizing ulcerative gingivitis* (Vincent's disease or trench mouth) is an acute ulceration affecting marginal gingiva with inflamed or necrotic interdental papillae. The onset is abrupt and painful with slight fever, malaise, excess salivation, and bad breath. It can be caused by systemic disease. Vitamin D has been found to be important in reducing gingivitis because of its anti-inflammatory action (Dietrich et al, 2005).

There have been advances in evidence-based periodontology over the past decade, such as adjunctive antimicrobial therapy, regenerative periodontal surgery, periodontal plastic surgery, bone regeneration surgery and implant treatment, and advanced soft tissue management at implant sites (Tonetti, 2000). Periodontal disease and bacterial pneumonia may be related, so treatment is important.

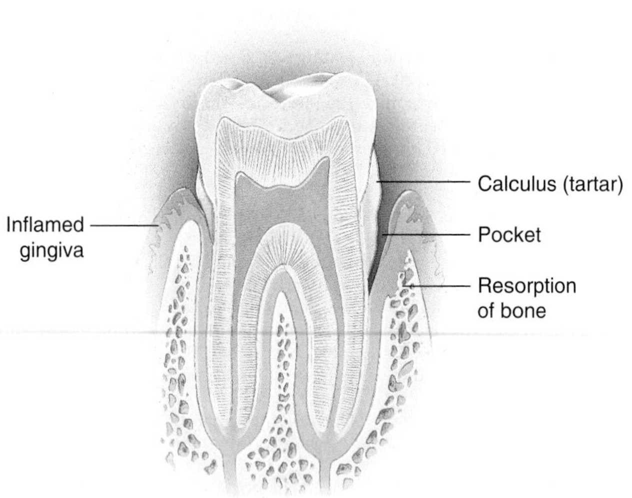

Figure 2-4 Periodontal disease. Asset provided by Anatomical Chart Co.

INTERVENTION: OBJECTIVES

- Reduce inflammation and promote healing.
- Reduce obesity, which may be causative (Mohammed et al, 2003).
- Correct poor nutritional habits that can lead to chronic subclinical nutritional deficiencies in levels of vitamin C, amino acids, vitamin D, riboflavin, folacin, vitamin A, zinc, and calcium.
- Prevent further decline in status of bones and gums.
- Protect the jawbone with adequate calcium and vitamin D (Hildebolt et al, 2004), especially after menopause in women.
- Review medications and consider alternatives to those causing dry mouth or other problems.
- Pregnant women with this condition are at risk for preterm birth and other adverse obstetric outcomes, such as preeclampsia and low birth weight; they should be closely monitored with prenatal medical and dental care.

INTERVENTION: FOOD AND NUTRITION

- Ensure adequate intake of calcium, protein, zinc, and phosphorus. Ensure adequate intake of vitamin C, fluoride, and vitamin A. A multivitamin-mineral supplement is usually needed.
- Vitamin D–fortified milk should be used.
- Use high-detergent foods (firm, fresh fruits and raw vegetables or those that are lightly cooked). Include cranberries, blueberries, and other foods rich in antioxidants
- If needed, a plan should be designed to control timing and frequency of meals and snacks to reduce exposure of susceptible gum tissue and teeth to the acids that form plaque.
- Control blood glucose in persons who have diabetes.

CLINICAL INDICATORS

Clinical/History	Lab Work
Height Weight BMI Diet history Gums—color, friability Oral examination for tooth mobility, calculus Presence of dental caries Missing teeth Mouth sores Overall nutritional status	Serum Na+, K+ Ca++, Mg++ Serum ascorbic acid H & H, serum Fe Alb, transthyretin CRP

Common Drugs Used and Potential Side Effects

- Sodium bicarbonate may be used as a mouthwash. Patients with high blood pressure should not swallow this wash.
- Peridex is an oral rinse to control bleeding gums. Taste changes may occur with its use.
- Triclosan-containing dentifrices may slow periodontal disease progression (Niederman, 2004).
- Antibiotic treatment of periodontitis includes amoxicillin/clavulanic acid, metronidazole, and clindamycin.

Herbs, Botanicals, and Supplements

- Herbs and botanicals may be used; identify and monitor side effects. For gingivitis, bloodroot, Echinacea, purslane, chamomile, licorice, and sage have been recommended but not confirmed for efficacy.
- Counsel about use of herbal teas, especially those containing toxic substances.
- A "Connective Tissue Nutrient Formula" that contains vitamins A, C, and D, glucosamine sulfate, magnesium, oligoproanthocyanidins, copper, zinc, manganese, boron, silicon, and calcium may be prescribed to enhance the integrity of key connective tissue elements.
- Naturopathic physicians prescribe *Panax ginseng, Withania somnifera,* and *Eleutherococcus senticosus* to reverse the impact of bacterial and psychosocial stressors. A clinical trial is being designed to study the effects of these therapies (http://www.clinicaltrials.gov/).

INTERVENTION: NUTRITION EDUCATION, COUNSELING, CARE MANAGEMENT

- Encourage a proper diet, especially calcium and vitamins C and D. Control weight if obesity is an issue; encourage exercise where possible.
- Recommend meticulous oral hygiene and regular dental examinations to maintain dental hygiene. Brush often and floss after eating sticky foods such as candy, sticky buns, and fruit rolls. Drink lots of water.
- Encourage pregnant women and persons with dentures, diabetes, cancer, HIV/AIDS, rheumatoid arthritis, or leukemia to pay special attention to oral hygiene.

For More Information

- American Academy of Periodontology
  http://www.perio.org/index.html
- Dental Societies
  http://www.perio.org/links/links.html#dental
- Periodontal Societies
  http://www.perio.org/links/links.html#perio

PERIODONTAL DISEASE AND GINGIVITIS—CITED REFERENCES

Cummins D. The impact of research and development on the prevention of oral diseases in children and adolescents: an industry perspective. *Pediatr Dent.* 28:118, 2006.

Dietrich T, et al. Association between serum concentrations of 25-hydroxyvitamin D and gingival inflammation. *Am J Clin Nutr.* 82:575, 2005.

Hildebolt CF, et al. Estrogen and/or calcium plus vitamin D increase mandibular bone mass. *J Periodontol.* 5:811, 2004.

Mohammed S, et al. Obesity and periodontal disease in young, middle-aged, and older adults. *J Periodontol.* 74:610, 2003.

Niederman R. Triclosan-containing dentifrice may slow periodontal disease progression. *Evid Based Dent.* 5:107, 2004.

Nishida M, et al. Dietary vitamin C and the risk for periodontal disease. *J Periodontol.* 71:1215, 2000.

Serhan CN. Clues for new therapeutics in osteoporosis and periodontal disease: new roles for lipoxygenases? *Expert Opin Ther Targets.* 8:643, 2004.

Tonetti M. Advances in periodontology. *Prim Dent Care.* 7:149, 2000.

TEMPOROMANDIBULAR JOINT DYSFUNCTION

NUTRITIONAL ACUITY RANKING: LEVEL 1

DEFINITIONS AND BACKGROUND

Temporomandibular joint (TMJ) disorders result from local or systemic causes, such as rheumatoid or osteoarthritis and connective tissue disorders. The TMJ is a diarthrodial joint with moving elements (mandible) and fixed elements (temporal bone). With this dysfunction, overuse or abuse of any part of normal action affects the mastication process. Patients with temporomandibular disorder pain dysfunction syndrome have toothaches or facial pains, which often lead to food intake problems (Irving et al, 1999).

The National Institute of Dental and Craniofacial Research (2004) indicates that 10.8 million people in the United States suffer from TMJ problems at any given time. Osteoarthrosis and internal derangement may coexist in the same joint in about 33% of cases; pathological tissue changes should be examined in patients with TMJ (Dimitroulos, 2005).

Women between the ages of 30 and 60 years account for 75% of all cases. Signs and symptoms include pain; clicking noise; stiffness of neck, face, or shoulders; locking of affected joint; trismus; and mandibular deviation—often from repetitive overloading (stress or habit such as gum chewing, grinding), from functional masseter muscle coordination problems, or from incorrect occlusion (as with missing teeth). Structural problems are treated by surgery (e.g., fusion can be treated by removing the area of fused bone and replacing it with silicon rubber). Sometimes an artificial joint is the answer; but surgery is recommended for only a few patients. Undue muscle tension causes most TMJ, with some other problems stemming from inadequate bite (as from a high filling or a malocclusion). People with TMJ will benefit from a visit to their dentist or other specialists (e.g., ear, nose, and throat specialists). See Figure 2-5.

INTERVENTION: OBJECTIVES

- Reduce repetitive overloading by use of a splint or by breaking bad habits such as grinding (bruxism).
- Reduce stress with relaxation techniques. Relieve pain and muscle spasms.
- Prevent or correct malnutrition or weight loss.
- Ensure adequate intake of soft, nonchewy sources of fiber.
- Reduce any existing inflammation and prevent complications such as mitral valve prolapse.

INTERVENTION: FOOD AND NUTRITION

- Use a normal diet with soft foods to prevent pain while chewing.
- Cut food into small, bite-sized pieces. Avoid chewy foods such as caramel, nuts, toffee, chewy candies, and gummy bread and rolls.
- Avoid opening mouth widely, as for large and thick sandwiches. Grate vegetables (e.g., carrots) to reduce chewing.
- Use adequate sources of vitamin C for adequate gingival health.

Herbs, Botanicals, and Supplements

- Herbs and botanicals may be used; identify and monitor side effects.
- Counsel about use of herbal teas, especially avoiding toxic ingredients.

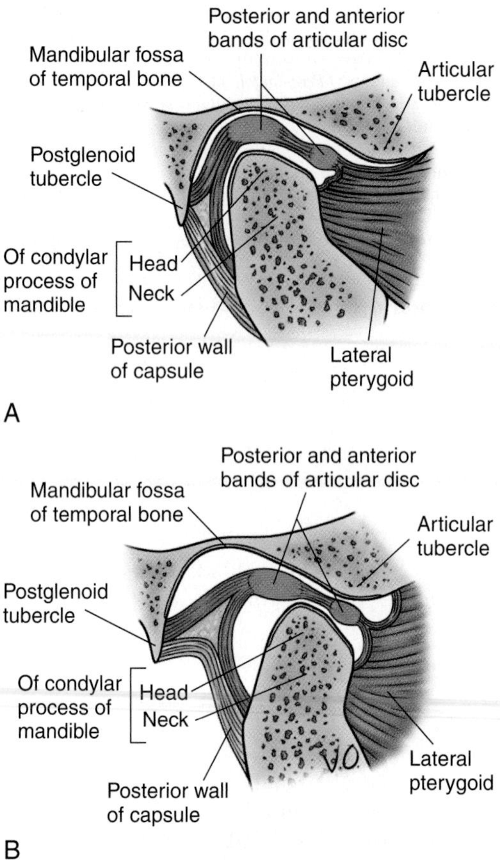

Figure 2-5 Views of the temporomandibular joint (TMJ). (From Moore KL, Agur A. *Essential clinical anatomy*. 2nd ed. Philadelphia: Lippincott Williams & Wilkins, 2002.)

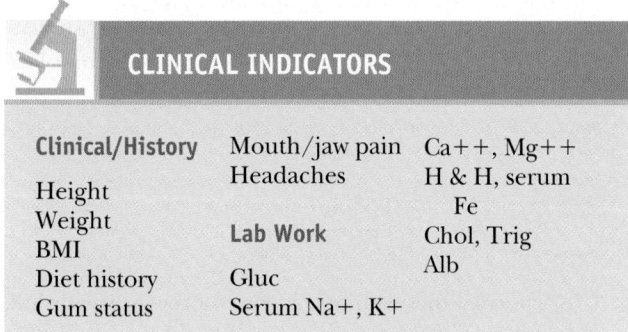

CLINICAL INDICATORS

Clinical/History		
Height	Mouth/jaw pain	Ca++, Mg++
Weight	Headaches	H & H, serum Fe
BMI	**Lab Work**	Chol, Trig
Diet history	Gluc	Alb
Gum status	Serum Na+, K+	

INTERVENTION: NUTRITION EDUCATION, COUNSELING, CARE MANAGEMENT

- Discuss the role of dental care in maintaining adequate health.
- Monitor for any tooth or gum soreness; advise the dentist as necessary. Regular oral hygiene must be continued despite mouth pain.
- Physical therapy may be needed to correct functioning of muscles and joints.
- Nail biting, gum chewing, use of teeth to cut thread, or similar habits should be stopped.
- Smoking is often a cause of bruxism, and programs to stop smoking should be considered if needed.

For More Information

- Jaw Joints and Allied Musculoskeletal Disorders Foundation
  http://www.tmjoints.org/
- Temporomandibular Joint Disorder
  http://www.tmj.org/

TEMPOROMANDIBULAR JOINT DYSFUNCTION—CITED REFERENCES

Dimitroulos G. The prevalence of osteoarthrosis in cases of advanced internal derangement of the temporomandibular joint: a clinical, surgical and histological study. *Int J Oral Maxillofac Surg.* 34:345, 2005.

Irving J, et al. Does temporomandibular disorder pain dysfunction syndrome affect dietary intake? *Dent Update.* 26:405, 1999.

National Institute of Dental and Craniofacial Research. TMJ diseases and disorders. Accessed December 22, 2004 at http://www.tmj.org/basics.asp.

VISION AND SELF-FEEDING PROBLEMS

VISION AND SELF-FEEDING PROBLEMS

NUTRITIONAL ACUITY RANKING: LEVEL 1–2 (VARIES BY SEVERITY)

DEFINITIONS AND BACKGROUND

The medical assessment, which includes a self-feeding, vision changes, hearing, continence, gait and balance, and cognition evaluation, can provide additional information to performance status and potential complications (Rao et al, 2004). Three areas of concern that can limit self-feeding (part of the activities of daily living) are low vision or blindness, coordination problems, and chewing problems. Where appropriate, these factors are also mentioned in relation to specific disorders in other sections. Dysphagia is a fourth problem that is described in detail in Section 7.

Low vision or blindness can affect any age, and children with developmental disabilities may have low vision just as older persons may have cataracts or macular degeneration. The World Health Organization defines "low vision" as visual acuity between 20/70 and 20/400, with the best possible correction, or a visual field of 20 degrees or less. "Blindness" is defined as a visual acuity worse than 20/400, with the best possible correction. Someone with a visual acuity of 20/70 can see at 20 feet what someone with normal sight can see at 70 feet. Someone with a visual acuity of 20/400 can see at 20 feet what someone with normal sight can see at 400 feet. Normal visual field is about 160–170 degrees horizontally.

Age-related macular degeneration (AMD) and cataract are the leading causes of visual impairment and blindness in the United States. Both diseases increase dramatically after age 60. Although excellent treatments for cataract are available, there are no equivalent treatments for AMD, a vascular condition that damages the retina.

The Age-Related Eye Disease Study (AREDS), sponsored by the Federal government's National Eye Institute (http://www.nei.nih.gov/amd), has found that taking high levels of antioxidants and zinc can reduce the risk of developing advanced age-related macular degeneration (AMD) by about 25%. The specific daily amounts used by the study researchers were 500 mg of vitamin C; 400 IU of vitamin E; 15 mg of beta-carotene (equivalent to 25,000 IU of vitamin A); 80 mg of zinc as zinc oxide; and 2 mg of copper as cupric oxide. Copper was added to the formulations containing zinc to prevent copper deficiency anemia.

Persons who consume more fish in their diet are less likely to have **dry eye syndrome** (Miljanovic et al, 2005) or macular degeneration than those who consume less fish. EPA and DHA from fish, four or more times per week, are suggested for good visual health (Cho et al, 2001). However, studies suggest that ALA may actually increase the risk of macular degeneration. Diets high in saturated fat, animal fat, linoleic acid, and trans fatty acids may promote higher risk of AMD (Seddon et al, 2003; Cho et al, 2001). Abdominal obesity has also been implicated. Protective foods include nuts, fish (Seddon et al, 2003), and lycopene (pink grapefruit, tomato sauce, tomato juice, and watermelon). Smokers should not take beta-carotene supplements (Age-Related Eye Disease Research Group, 2001).

Glaucoma is another eye disorder with nutritional implications. In chronic glaucoma, risk factors include age over 40, a family history of glaucoma, diabetes, and myopia. African Americans have a higher incidence, and 1–2% of people over 40 have chronic glaucoma. Acute glaucoma may occur in persons with a family history of acute glaucoma, older age, presbyopia, and the use of systemic anticholinergic medications. Prostagladins regulate inner eye pressure, so type of fat in the diet makes a difference; glaucoma may be related to a higher intake ratio of omega-3 fatty acids to omega-6 fatty acids (Kang et al, 2004). Soybean, safflower, and sunflower oils may also be protective.

Coordination problems may also occur in any age group. Hand–eye coordination is needed for self-feeding, and when this is not working properly, assistance will be needed. Other types of coordination problems include: falling forward, feet not touching the floor, leaning to one side, poor balance while sitting, and poor neck control. Sometimes, it is possible to adjust table height, offer pillows or other positioning equipment, offer a footstool, or adjust pedals on a wheelchair. It is recommended to work with an occupational therapist for the proper types of adjustments to allow for better mealtime food intake. Conditions that can cause coordination problems are many. They include Alzheimer's disease, alcohol abuse, attention deficit disorder, brain cancer, chorea, Down syndrome, encephalitis, fetal alcohol syndrome, progressed HIV infection, hydrocephaly, multiple sclerosis, Parkinson's disease, Rett syndrome, stroke, and Wilson's disease.

Chewing problems may cause inability to consume enough food or foods of varying texture. Total edentulism without dentures may contribute to deterioration in the systemic health of the elderly. Without chewing, there is less production of saliva and food is not properly mixed before swallowing.

Dry mouth, from a variety of causes, can interfere with chewing and swallowing; it should be corrected where possible to allow for proper chewing and swallowing of foods.

INTERVENTION: OBJECTIVES

- Promote independence in self-feeding, when possible.
- Address all nutritional deficiencies and complications individually. Select nutrient-dense foods.
- Promote overall wellness and health.
- Increase interest in eating.
- Prevent malnutrition and weight loss.
- Decrease instances in which constipation, anorexia, or other problems affect nutritional status.
- Increase pleasure associated with mealtimes.
- Educate the caregiver about adaptive equipment, utensils, and special food modifications.

INTERVENTION: FOOD AND NUTRITION

Blindness or Low Vision

- Provide special plate guards, utensils, double handles, and compartmentalized plates with foods placed in similar locations at each meal. Explain placement of foods. Open packets if needed.
- Work with occupational therapist (OT) or family to practice kitchen safety and to determine ability to have independence at mealtimes.
- Create a feeling of usefulness by delegating appropriate tasks related to mealtime, such as drying dishes and assisting with simple meal tasks that are safe for the individual.
- The individual may benefit from companionship during meals, especially if any problems occur or if anything else is needed.
- Use straws for beverages if there are no problems with dysphagia.

Coordination Problems

- Self-feeding requires the ability to suck, to sit with head and neck balanced, to bring hand to mouth, to grasp cup and utensil, to drink from a cup, to take food from a spoon, to bite, to chew, and to swallow.

- Each person should be assessed individually to determine which, if any, aspects of coordination have been affected by his or her condition. Adjust self-feeding accordingly.
- Use of clothing protectors at mealtime may be useful for maintaining dignity.
- Assist with feeding if needed. Adjust table or chair height; use adaptive feeding equipment as needed (such as weighted utensils, large-handled cups, larger or smaller silverware than standard).

Chewing Problems

- Dentures should fit well and be adjusted or replaced as needed, such as after weight loss.
- Decrease texture in foods as necessary (e.g., use a mechanical soft, pureed, or liquid diet as needed). Season as desired for individual taste. Try to progress in textures if possible because chewing is important for saliva production and for proper digestion of foods.
- Liquid or blenderized foods may be beneficial. If needed, use a tube feeding.
- For some persons, a straw may be helpful; for others, it is not. Speech therapists may help in assessment of this ability.
- Protein foods such as tofu, cottage cheese, peanut butter, eggs, cheese, and milk products can be used when meats or nuts cannot be chewed.
- If fruits and vegetables cannot be consumed in raw form, use canned sources or juices. Decrease texture if needed to pureed form.
- If whole grain breads and cereals are not tolerated, cooked cereals are generally well accepted. Use caution with rice and foods with particles if dysphagia is also present (see Section 7).

CLINICAL INDICATORS

Clinical/History		
Height	Diet history	Dentures, especially poorly fitting
Weight	Mouth or tongue lacerations	Blindness or vision problems
BMI	Missing or loose teeth	
Recent weight changes	Sore or bleeding gums	

TABLE 2-6 Nutrients for Healthy Vision[a]

Protein and Amino Acids	Protein undernutrition is associated with increased risk of cataract. Low protein intake may induce deficiencies of specific amino acids that are needed to maintain the health of the lens, or other nutritional deficiencies, particularly niacin, thiamin, and riboflavin (Delcourt et al, 2005).
Vitamin A and Lutein	Vitamin A is needed for healthy cornea and conjunctiva. Cataract patients tend to be deficient in vitamin A and the carotenes, lutein, and zeaxanthin (Head, 2001).
	Antioxidants, especially carotenoids are most associated with reduced risk of macular degeneration (Krinsky et al, 2003; Seddon et al, 2003). Good sources include kale, collards, spinach, turnip greens, broccoli, yellow corn, peas, egg yolk, tangerine, and orange bell peppers. Lutein is facilitated with ascorbic acid supplementation (Tanumihardjo et al, 2005). Eggland's Best eggs contain 185 mg of lutein.
Thiamin	For normal retinal and optic nerve functioning. Protective against cataracts (Jacques et al, 2005).
Riboflavin	For corneal vascularization. Protective against cataracts (Jacques et al, 2005). Riboflavin appears to play an essential role as a precursor to flavin adenine dinucleotide (FAD), a cofactor for glutathione reductase activity (Head, 2001).
Niacin	For healthy vision. Avoid excesses, which can cause nicotinic acid maculopathy (Spirn et al, 2003).
Folate	A strong protective influence on cortical cataract from use of folate or vitamin B_{12} supplements is a recent finding (Kuzniarz et al, 2001).
Vitamin B_6	For healthy conjuntiva. Untreated homocystinuria is known to cause ocular changes; vitamin B_6 can help to lower homocysteine levels.
Vitamin B_{12}	For retinal and nerve fibers. Protective against cataract (Kuzniarz et al, 2001). Found only in animal foods such as meat and milk.
Vitamin C	For healthy conjuntiva and vitreous humor. Long-term use of adequate vitamin C may delay or prevent early age-related lens opacity (Ferrigno et al, 2005; Valero et al, 2002). Orange and grapefruit juices, cantaloupe, oranges, green peppers, tomato juice, broccoli, kiwifruit, and strawberries are good sources.
Vitamin E	Important for antioxidant properties. May slow the onset of cataracts. Long-term use of supplements may be beneficial (Jacques et al, 2005). Vitamin E is found in almonds, peanuts, peanut butter, sunflower seeds, safflower oil, margarines, and creamy salad dressings.
Omega-3 Fatty Acids	Omega-3 fatty acids and fish are protective against age-related macular degeneration (Cho et al, 2001). Eating fish (sardines, salmon, herring, tuna, fortified eggs) weekly and cutting back on saturated fatty acids may be helpful in reducing age-related macular degeneration (Smith et al, 2000). Infants need a supply of DHA for up to a year for healthy visual development (Hoffman et al, 2004). Avoid use of large doses of alpha linolenic acid.
Omega-6 Fatty Acids	Omega-6 fatty acids in soybean, safflower, and sunflower oils may be protective against glaucoma (Kang et al, 2004) but not against cataracts. High doses of canola, flaxseed, and soybean oils may actually increase the risk of cataracts (Jacques et al, 2005).
Selenium	Pathophysiological mechanisms of cataract formation include deficient glutathione levels contributing to a faulty antioxidant defense system within the lens of the eye; nutrients that increase glutathione levels and activity include selenium (Flohe, 2005; Head, 2001).
Sodium	Sodium-restricted diets may be protective against development of cataracts (Cumming et al, 2000).
Zinc	For healthy retina and optic nerve. Found in beef, chicken, oysters, mixed nuts, and milk.

[a] Long-term use of multivitamin, B group, and vitamin A supplements is associated with reduced prevalence of either nuclear or cortical cataract (Kuzniarz et al, 2001).

Chewing problems	Coordination problems	Serum Na+, K+
Dysphagia (see Section 7)		Ca++, Mg++
Signs of dehydration or edema	**Lab Work**	I & O
	Alb, transthyretin	H & H, serum Fe
		X-rays (such as mandible)

Herbs, Botanicals, and Supplements

- Nutrients and botanicals that may prevent cataracts include folic acid, melatonin, and bilberry (Head, 2001). Flavonoids, particularly quercetin, and ginkgo biloba may increase circulation to the optic nerve (Head, 2001). Curcumin is also under study.
- Herbs and botanicals may be used; identify and monitor side effects. For glaucoma, oregano, jaborandi, kaffir potato, and pansy have been recommended but not confirmed as effective. For cataract, rosemary, catnip, and capers have not been found to be effective.
- Counsel about use of herbal teas, especially avoiding intake of toxic substances.

INTERVENTION: NUTRITION EDUCATION, COUNSELING, CARE MANAGEMENT

- Discuss the importance of various therapies and medications for recovery.
- Discuss the role of nutrition in health, weight control, and recovery or repair processes.
- Provide instruction regarding simplified meal planning and preparation.
- Refer to agencies such as Meals-on-Wheels, as needed.
- For healthy eyes, nutrition plays an essential role. See Table 2-6 for a description of this role.

For More Information

- Age-Related Macular Degeneration Alliance
  http://www.amdalliance.org/
- American Association of Ophthalmology
  http://www.eyenet.org/
- American Council for the Blind
  Phone: (800) 424-8666
  http://www.acb.org/
- American Occupational Therapy Association
  http://www.aota.org/
- American Optometric Association
  http://www.aoanet.org/conditions/eye_coordination.asp
- Low Vision
  http://www.lowvision.org/
- National Center for Education in Maternal and Child Health
  http://www.brightfutures.org/physicalactivity/issues_concerns/10.html
- National Library Service for the Blind and Physically Handicapped (NLS)
  The Library of Congress
  http://www.loc.gov/nls
- National Eye Institute, NIH
  http://www.nei.nih.gov/
- Prevent Blindness America
  http://www.preventblindness.org/

VISION AND SELF-FEEDING PROBLEMS—CITED REFERENCES

Age-Related Eye Disease Research Group. A randomized, placebo-controlled, clinical trial of high-dose supplementation with vitamins C and E, beta-carotene, and zinc for age-related cataract and vision loss. AREDS Report No. 9. *Arch Ophthalmol.* 119:1439, 2001.

Cho E, et al. Prospective study of dietary fat and the risk of age-related macular degeneration. *Am J Clin Nutri.* 73:209, 2001.

Cumming R, et al. Dietary sodium intake and cataract: the Blue Mountains Eye Study. *Am J Epidemiol.* 151:624, 2000.

Delcourt C, et al. Albumin and transthyretin as risk factors for cataract: the POLA study. *Arch Ophthalmol.* 123:225, 2005.

Ferrigno L, et al. Associations between plasma levels of vitamins and cataract in the Italian-American Clinical Trial of Nutritional Supplements and Age-Related Cataract (CTNS): CTNS Report #2. *Ophthalmic Epidemiol.* 12:71, 2005.

Flohe L. Selenium, selenoproteins and vision. *Dev Ophthalmol.* 38:89, 2005.

Head KA. Natural therapies for ocular disorders, part two: cataracts and glaucoma. *Altern Med Rev.* 6:141, 2001.

Hoffman DR, et al. Maturation of visual acuity is accelerated in breast-fed term infants fed baby food containing DHA-enriched egg yolk. *J Nutr.* 134:2307, 2004.

Jacques PF, et al. Long-term nutrient intake and 5-year change in nuclear lens opacities. *Arch Ophthalmol.* 123:517, 2005.

Kang JH, et al. Dietary fat consumption and primary open-angle glaucoma. *Am J Clin Nutr.* 79:755, 2004.

Krinsky NI, et al. Biologic mechanisms of the protective role of lutein and zeaxanthin in the eye. *Annu Rev Nutr.* 23:171, 2003.

Kuzniarz M, et al. Use of vitamin supplements and cataract: the Blue Mountains Eye Study. *Am J Ophthalmol.* 132:19, 2001.

Miljanovic B, et al. Relation between dietary n-3 and n-6 fatty acids and clinically diagnosed dry eye syndrome in women. *Am J Clin Nutr.* 82:887, 2005.

Rao AV, et al. Geriatric assessment and comorbidity. *Semin Oncol.* 31:149, 2004.

Seddon JM, et al. Progression of age-related macular degeneration: association with dietary fat, transunsaturated fat, nuts, and fish intake. *Arch Ophthalmol.* 121:1728, 2003.

Smith W, et al. Dietary fat and fish intake and age-related maculopathy. *Arch Ophthalmol.* 118:401, 2000.

Spirn MJ, et al. Optical coherence tomography findings in nicotinic acid maculopathy. *Am J Ophthalmol.* 135:913, 2003.

Tanumihardjo SA, et al. Lutein absorption is facilitated with cosupplementation of ascorbic acid in young adults. *J Am Diet Assoc.* 105:114, 2005.

Valero MP, et al. Vitamin C is associated with reduced risk of cataract in a Mediterranean population. *J Nutr.* 132:1299, 2002.

Skin Conditions, Pressure Ulcers, and Vitamin Deficiencies

SKIN DISORDERS

NUTRITIONAL ACUITY RANKING: LEVEL 1

DEFINITIONS AND BACKGROUND

The skin is affected by both internal and external influences, which may lead to photo aging, inflammation, immune dysfunction, imbalanced epidermal homeostasis, and other skin disorders (Boelsma et al, 2001). The skin often reflects problems such as GI disturbances, alcoholism, or general malnutrition. In many respects, human skin fulfills the requirements for being the largest, independent peripheral endocrine organ of the body (Zouboulis, 2000).

Nutritional factors continue to be studied for their impact on skin properties such as hydration, sebum production, and elasticity and on prevention of skin cancer (Greenwald, 2001). For example, a low-fat diet and use of foods rich in vitamin D and carotenoids may be protective against some forms of skin cancer and actinic keratoses (Millen et al, 2004).

Enzymes of the cytochrome P450 (P450 or CYP) family are important as a class of drug-metabolizing enzymes that are induced in skin in response to xenobiotic exposure; they also play important roles in metabolism of fatty acids, eicosanoids, sterols, steroids, vitamin A, and vitamin D (Ahmad and Mukhtar, 2004). In psoriasis, for example, many of these CYP enzymes are elevated, and further investigation is needed.

Retinoids are a group of naturally occurring and synthetic compounds with vitamin A biological activity; they have benefits for skin diseases and reversal of photo aging. Supplementation with vitamins, carotenoids, and polyunsaturated fatty acids has been shown to provide protection against ultraviolet light; however, sunscreens are more important overall (Boelsma et al, 2001). Erythema after tanning may be lessened by taking supplements with carotenoids plus vitamin E (Stahl et al, 2000).

Acne affects many young people and may cause psychological distress. Iodine can aggravate acne; one study suggests that milk and dairy products contain a high level of iodine, and more studies are needed (Arbesman, 2005). However, changes in diet are not the primary solution. Benzoyl peroxide is efficacious in mild to moderate acne. Adapalene and tretinoin are better for acne of greater severity. Green tea polyphenols have been found to be beneficial for their anti-inflammatory effects. Green tea and tea tree extracts in topical creams may also have benefit. See Figure 2-6.

Atopic dermatitis (AD), or eczema, causes itchy, inflamed skin. It usually affects the insides of the elbows, backs of the knees, and the face, but can cover much of the body. AD falls into a category of diseases called atopic, a term originally used to describe the allergic conditions of asthma and hay fever. AD often affects people who either suffer from asthma and/or hay fever or have family members who do (the "atopic triad"). AD tends to flare when the person is exposed to trigger factors, such as dry skin, irritants, allergens, emotional stress, heat and sweating, and infections; avoiding triggers is the key. Because essential fatty acids (EFAs) form an important component of cell membranes, are eicosanoid precursors, and are required for both the structure and function of every cell, EFAs may benefit persons who have AD or psoriasis (Das, 1999). Figure 2-7 shows AD.

Dermatitis herpetiformis (DH or Durhing's disease) is related to celiac disease (Karpati, 2004). There is the presence of villous atrophy and endomysial antibodies (EMAs). EMAs are found to be a marker both in celiac disease (CD) and in DH (Kumar et al, 2001). A gluten-restricted diet is used in these conditions.

Epidermolysis bullosa is a hereditary condition in which blistering of the skin occurs with even slight trauma. It affects 2 out of every 100,000 live births, occurring in both sexes and all ethnic groups. Nail dystrophy can occur, with rough, thickened, or absent fingernails or toenails. There may be problems with the soft tissue inside the mouth, and blisters may occur there as well. In this condition, protein–calorie malnutrition, stunting, anemia, and vitamin and mineral deficiencies are common. Treatment involves careful skin and wound care, as well as prevention of infections.

Nickel dermatitis affects 8–15% of women and 1% of men. Less exposure to nickel is needed in these cases. Sensitization to nickel, the most frequently identified allergen on patch testing, is associated with ear piercing (Garner, 2004). In severe cases, reduced exposure to foods exposed to nickel may be helpful (Antico and Soana, 1999).

Nummular eczematous dermatitis occurs as a rash in individuals, and the etiology is unknown. The rash is coin shaped and worsens in very hot or cold weather. It is not known if food or medication allergies are the cause, but it is hard to resolve. Wool, soaps, frequent bathing (more

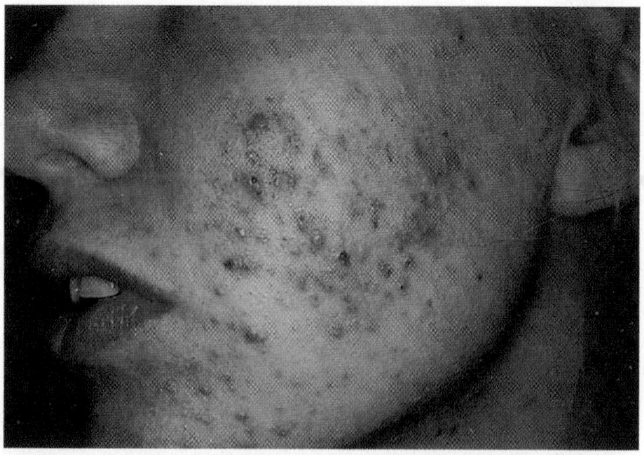

Figure 2-6 Severe acne. (From Sauer GC, Hall JC. *Manual of skin diseases*. 7th ed. Philadelphia: Lippincott-Raven Publishers, 1996.)

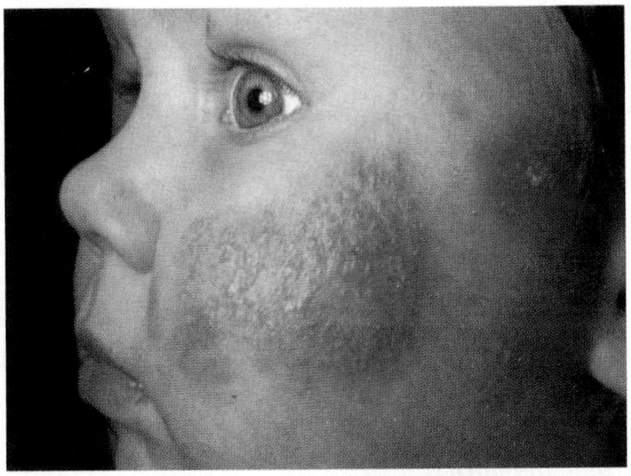

Figure 2-7 Atopic dermatitis. (From Sauer GC, Hall JC. *Manual of skin diseases*. 7th ed. Philadelphia: Lippincott-Raven Publishers, 1996.)

than once a day), detergents, and rough clothing may be irritating. No special diet is needed unless food allergies are identified.

Psoriasis is a skin disorder with patches of scaly red skin that may burn, itch, or bleed. See Figure 2-8. Calcitriol and vitamin D analogs are useful, along with controlled exposure to sunlight (Lehmann et al, 2004; May et al, 2004). The addition of omega-3 fatty acids (specifically EPA) to a drug regimen of etretinate and topical corticosteroids may improve symptoms of psoriasis. Enbrel (etanercept), a tumor necrosis factor alpha (TNFα) inhibitor, relieves the clinical symptoms of psoriasis and may also clear up the depression and fatigue common among those with this disease.

Rosacea is a disorder of the central portion of the facial skin with onset in the third decade and peak onset in the fourth or fifth decade. A chronic and progressive condition of flare-ups and remissions, rosacea can be disfiguring if left untreated. Rosacea resembles other dermatological conditions, especially acne vulgaris. It affects one in 20 people, or 13 million people in the United States. Members of the same family tend to be affected; fair-skinned individuals of Northern and Eastern European descent (English, Scottish, Welsh, or Scandinavian) are most commonly affected (Litt, 1997). Green tea extract in creams may have benefit; research is under way. See Figure 2-9.

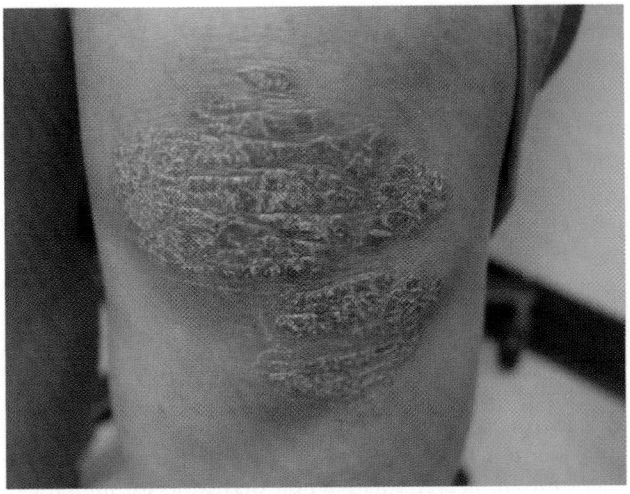

Figure 2-8 Psoriasis. (Image provided by *Stedman's*.)

INTERVENTION: OBJECTIVES

- Reduce inflammation, redness, and edema where present.
- Apply nutritional principles according to the particular condition.
- Prevent further exacerbations of the condition.
- Identify any offending foods and omit from the diet where relevant (such as with allergies).

INTERVENTION: FOOD AND NUTRITION

- **Acne.** Encourage intake of adequate zinc and vitamin A. This condition is hormone dependent. It is less common in non-Western societies, so a high-fat diet that is low in fruit and vegetable intake should be avoided (Cordain et al, 2002). Drinking green tea can be highly recommended.
- **Acrodermatitis enteropathica.** Supplement with zinc because absorption of zinc is impaired in this condition. Use protein of high biological value. Decrease excess fiber, if necessary, to normalize bowel function.
- **Atopic dermatitis.** According to the National Eczema Association, dietary therapies do not work well. Reduce use of salicylates (berries and dried fruits), aspirin, penicillin, food molds, some herbs and spices, and FD&C yellow 5. In infants, problems may result from hypersensitivity to milk, egg albumin, or wheat, or there may be a linoleic acid metabolic defect. Control energy excess in obese infants. Avoid herbal products, such as chamomile tea, for which allergy is possible, but use of green tea is safe and recommended.
- **Dermatitis herpetiformis.** A gluten-free diet is quite successful in treating this condition. See entry in Section 7.
- **Epidermolysis bullosa.** Gastrostomy feeding may be needed in severe cases. Otherwise, a balanced diet that includes a multivitamin-mineral supplement would be most useful. Highlight the skin nutrients that are beneficial, including omega-3 fatty acids, vitamin A, and zinc.

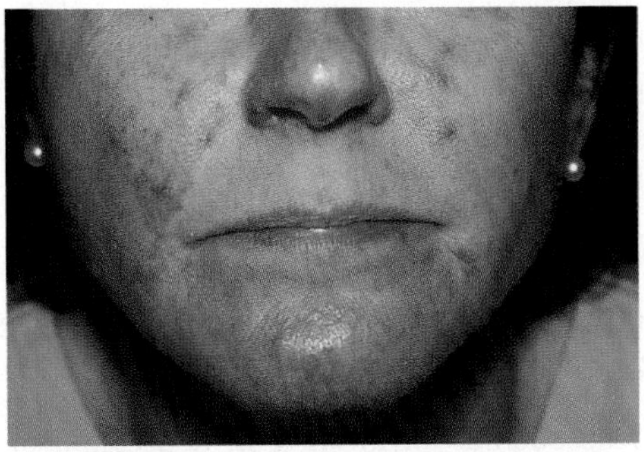

Figure 2-9 Rosacea. (From Goodheart HP. *Goodheart's photoguide of common skin disorders*. 2nd ed. Philadelphia: Lippincott Williams & Wilkins, 2003.)

- **Nickel dermatitis.** Avoid canned foods, such as tuna fish, tomatoes, corn, spinach, and other canned vegetables. Do not cook with stainless steel utensils. Chocolate, nuts, and beans may have slightly higher naturally occurring nickel than other foods; avoid large quantities (Christensen et al, 1999).
- **Psoriasis.** Psoriasis may precede arthritis by months or years because both are inflammatory processes. Because of their antiproliferative effects, calcitriol and other vitamin D analogs are highly efficient in the treatment of psoriasis vulgaris (Lehmann et al, 2004; May et al, 2004). In addition, the known therapeutic effect of UVB light therapy in the treatment of psoriasis may be related to its skin synthesis of calcitriol.
- **Rosacea.** Consumption of alcoholic beverages (especially red wine), spicy foods, hot beverages, some fruits and vegetables, marinated meats, and dairy products may trigger flare-ups. Avoid as needed. Change spices and herbs as necessary. For example, reduce use of all forms of pepper, paprika, chili powder, and curry. Substitute with cumin, oregano, sage, thyme, marjoram, turmeric, cinnamon, basil, and milder spices. Drinking green tea can be highly recommended.

CLINICAL INDICATORS

Clinical/History

Height
Weight
BMI
Growth pattern in children
Diet history

Lab Work

Alb (decreased in exfoliative dermatitis)
Transthyretin
Serum zinc
Serum histamine
Skin tests for allergies
Rashes, blisters, pustules
Thyroid-stimulating hormone (TSH), T4 level
H & H, serum Fe
Gluc
Chol, Trig
Serum Na+, K+
Ca++, Mg++
Serum carotene
Retinol-binding protein (RBP)
CRP

Common Drugs Used and Potential Side Effects

When using cortisone ointments, use just a little and massage in well. Application once daily does as much good as using it more often. The potential for long-term use to suppress the adrenal gland exists (Woo and McKenna, 2003; Matsuda et al, 2000).

Acne

- Isotretinoin (Accutane) may be used for acne. Watch for a decrease in high-density lipoprotein (HDL) and an increase in triglycerides. Controversy exists; side effects such as an increase in depression or suicide attempts seem to be correlated. Avoid vitamin A supplements. Dry mouth can occur. Do not use during pregnancy.
- Retin A (retinoic acid) is useful for moderate cases of acne. Side effects are not as pronounced as with Accutane.
- Antibiotics are used in acne for their anti-inflammatory effect, not for their antibacterial impact. Tetracycline should not be taken within 2 hours of use of milk products or calcium supplements. Excesses of vitamin A can cause headaches or hypertension. Use more riboflavin, vitamin C, and calcium in the diet. Protein and iron malabsorption may result from prolonged use. Diarrhea is the major gastrointestinal (GI) effect. Minocycline causes less GI distress and does not affect calcium metabolism as dramatically.

Atopic Dermatitis

- Topical cortisone (steroid) creams, such as Aclovate, usually have a mild effect on the nutritional status of the patient. Stronger brands or dosages may act like oral steroids and can suppress the adrenal system if taken for prolonged periods.

Psoriasis

- Calcitriol and other vitamin D analogs are often highly effective. Topical products such as tazarotene (Tazorac) and calcipotriene, a form of vitamin D, have been available for years.
- Enbrel (enteracept), Humira (adalimumab), or Remicade (infliximab) are used for severe chronic plaque psoriasis. Other tumor necrosis factor inhibitors such as efalizumab (Raptiva) yield less frequent itching and better quality of life (Ricardo et al, 2004).

Rosacea

- Antibiotic creams such as metronidazole (MetroCream) and azelaic acid (Finacea) are commonly prescribed.
- Tetracycline may also be prescribed. Avoid taking within an hour of dairy or calcium-related supplements.
- Taking an antihistamine about 2 hours before a meal may counter the effects of histamine.
- Aspirin may reduce the effects of niacin-containing foods in sufferers affected by the flushing effect of these foods. Monitor multivitamin supplements and intakes carefully.

Herbs, Botanicals, and Supplements

- Counsel about use of herbal teas, especially related to potentially toxic ingredients. Herbs and botanicals may be used; identify and monitor side effects.
- Tea tree oil topical solutions may be beneficial for **acne** because of their anti-inflammatory effects (Koh et al, 2002; Liao, 2001). Bacterial infections of skin have positive results for an ointment containing tea leaf extract in impetigo contagiosa infections, acne, and methicillin-resistant *Staphylococcus aureus*; results are equivalent to conventional treatments (Martin and Ernst, 2003).
- There is insufficient evidence to make recommendations for prevention of **atopic dermatitis** through use of Chinese herbs, dietary restrictions, homeopathy, house

dust mite reduction, massage therapy, hypnotherapy, evening primrose oil, emollients, topical coal tar, and topical doxepin (Hoare et al, 2000). Calendula may be recommended but is not proven effective; it might also be best to avoid extracts of arnica (*Arnica montana*), chamomile (*Chamomilla recutita*), tansy (*Tanacetum vulgare*), and feverfew (*Tanacetum parthenium*) because of potential allergic reactions.

- **Psoriasis:** bishop's weed, avocado, licorice, red pepper, Brazil nut, and purslane have been proposed but not confirmed. Red clover is sometimes used for dermatitis or psoriasis; avoid use with warfarin or hormone replacement therapy.
- For **scabies:** evening primrose, onion, neem, and mountain mint have been proposed. No confirming studies are available.
- For **sunburn:** eggplant, plantain, and calendula have been proposed. Aloe is used for sunburn and mild burns; it causes GI cramping and hypokalemia if ingested.

INTERVENTION: NUTRITION EDUCATION, COUNSELING, CARE MANAGEMENT

- Encourage the patient to read food, medication, and supplement labels. A symptom and food diary may be quite useful to identify any relationship between diet, allergies, or skin flare-ups.
- Help the patient modify his or her diet as specifically indicated by the condition.
- Encourage adequate fluid intake. Hydration of the skin is important. Drinking green tea can be highly recommended.
- Discuss avoidance of topical or specialty products, except as prescribed by the doctor.
- Discuss the roles of nutrients in skin care. Sunscreens may prevent vitamin D from penetrating the skin, especially formulas with higher protective factors. Therefore, if dietary intakes are low in vitamin D, a supplement may be needed. Protein, vitamin A, and zinc are also important nutrients for healthy skin; describe good sources.
- Discuss the effect of essential fatty acids on membrane function and how to include them in the diet. Omega-3 fatty acids may play a role in reducing inflammation for some skin conditions.

For More Information

- Acne Hotline
  http://www.niams.nih.gov/hi/topics/acne/acne.htm
- Acne Resources
  http://www.acne-resource.org/
- American Academy of Dermatology
  http://www.aad.org/
- Dystrophic Epidermolysis Bullosa Research Association of America
  http://www.debra.org/
- National Eczema Association
  http://www.nationaleczema.org/home.html
- National Psoriasis Foundation
  http://www.psoriasis.org/
- National Quality Measures Clearinghouse
  http://www.qualitymeasures.ahrq.gov/
- National Rosacea Society
  http://www.rosacea.org/
- NIH–Dermatitis
  http://www.niams.nih.gov/hi/topics/dermatitis/
- NIH–Eczema
  http://www.nlm.nih.gov/medlineplus/eczema.html

SKIN DISORDERS—CITED REFERENCES

Ahmad N, Mukhtar H. Cytochrome p450: a target for drug development for skin diseases. *J Invest Dermatol.* 123:417, 2004.

Antico A, Soana R. Chronic allergic-like dermatopathies in nickel-sensitive patients. Results of dietary restrictions and challenge with nickel salts. *Allergy Asthma Proc.* 20:235, 1999.

Arbesman H. Dairy and acne—the iodine connection. *J Am Acad Dermatol.* 53:1102, 2005.

Boelsma E, et al. Nutritional skin care: health effects of micronutrients and fatty acids (review). *Am J Clin Nutr.* 73:853, 2001.

Christensen JM, et al. Nickel concentrations in serum and urine of patients with nickel eczema. *Toxicol Lett.* 108:185, 1999.

Cordain L, et al. Acne vulgaris: a disease of Western civilization. *Arch Dermatol.* 138:1584, 2002.

Das U. Essential fatty acids in health and disease. *J Assoc Physicians India.* 47:906, 1999.

Garner LA. Contact dermatitis to metals. *Dermatol Ther.* 17:321, 2004.

Greenwald P. From carcinogenesis to clinical interventions for cancer prevention. *Toxicology.* 166:37, 2001.

Hoare C, et al. Systematic review of treatments for atopic eczema. *Health Technol Assess.* 4:1, 2000.

Karpati S. Dermatitis herpetiformis: close to unravelling a disease. *J Dermatol Sci.* 34:83, 2004.

Koh KJ, et al. Tea tree oil reduces histamine-induced skin inflammation. *Br J Dermatol.* 147:1212, 2002.

Kumar V, et al. Tissue transglutaminase and endomysial antibodies-diagnostic markers of gluten-sensitive enteropathy in dermatitis herpetiformis. *Clin Immunol.* 98:378, 2001.

Lehmann B, et al. Vitamin D and skin: new aspects for dermatology. *Exp Dermatol.* 13:11S, 2004.

Liao S. The medicinal action of androgens and green tea epigallocatechin gallate. *Hong Kong Med J.* 7:369, 2001.

Litt J. Rosacea: how to recognize and treat an age-related skin disease. *Geriatrics* 52:39, 1997.

Martin KW, Ernst E. Herbal medicines for treatment of bacterial infections: a review of controlled clinical trials. *J Antimicrob Chemother.* 51:241, 2003.

Matsuda K, et al. Adrenocortical function in patients with severe atopic dermatitis. *Ann Allergy Asthma Immunol.* 85:35, 2000.

May E, et al. Immunoregulation through 1,25-dihydroxyvitamin D3 and its analogs. *Curr Drug Targets Inflamm Allergy.* 3:377, 2004.

Millen AE, et al. Diet and melanoma in a case-control study. *Cancer Epidemiol Biomarkers Prev.* 13:1042, 2004.

Ricardo RR, et al. Clinical benefits in patients with psoriasis after efalizumab therapy: clinical trials versus practice. *Cutis* 74:193, 2004.

Stahl W, et al. Carotenoids and carotenoids plus vitamin E protect against ultraviolet light-induced erythema in humans. *Am J Clin Nutr.* 71:795, 2000.

Woo WK, McKenna KE. Iatrogenic adrenal gland suppression from use of a potent topical steroid. *Clin Exp Dermatol.* 28:672, 2003.

Zouboulis C. Human skin: an independent peripheral endocrine organ. *Horm Res.* 54:230, 2000.

PRESSURE ULCER

NUTRITIONAL ACUITY RANKING: LEVEL 2–3 (STAGES 1–2), LEVEL 4 (STAGES 3 OR 4)

DEFINITIONS AND BACKGROUND

Patients with severe malnutrition are at risk for many types of complications, including the incidence, progression, and severity of pressure ulcers (Thomas et al, 2000). Pressure, friction, or shear and a lack of oxygen and nutrition to an affected area have often been associated with the development of pressure ulcers. They can occur over bony or cartilaginous prominences (e.g., hip, sacrum, elbow, heels, back of the head).

Pressure ulcers are common among patients with protein-energy malnutrition (as in HIV infection, pulmonary and cardiac cachexia, rheumatological cachexia, cancers, and renal diseases) and among bedridden or paralyzed patients. With immobility and loss of lean body mass (muscle and skin), which lead to lowered immunity, the risk of pressure ulcers increases by 74% (Harris and Fraser, 2004).

Many patients with pressure ulcers are below their usual body weight, have a low transthyretin level, and are not taking in enough nutrition to meet their needs (Guenter et al, 2000). Poor nutritional status and decreased oxygen perfusion are predictors of pressure ulcers; nutritional status and length of stay are predictors of ulcer severity in institutions (Williams et al, 2000).

Risk factors for pressure ulcer development should be assessed frequently. Risks include unintentional weight loss, incontinence, immobility, poor circulation (as in diabetes, peripheral vascular disease, or anemia), infection, poor nutritional status, prolonged pressure, drugs, and serum albumin below 3.4 g/dL. Reduced functional ability, poor oral intake of less than 50% of meals over 3 days compared with usual intakes, chewing or swallowing problems, low serum albumin with normal hydration, and cholesterol levels below 160 mg/dL (as from use of low-fat tube feedings or diets) may be found. Use of the mini-nutritional assessment (MNA) with older adults is a useful tool, with better results than using visceral proteins alone (Langkamp-Henken et al, 2005).

Common causes of malnutrition in the elderly that should be carefully monitored include (Harris and Fraser, 2004): decreased appetite, requirement of any amount of assistance with meal intake, impaired cognition and/or communication, poor positioning, frequent acute illnesses with gastrointestinal losses, medications that decrease appetite or increase nutrient losses, polypharmacy, decreased thirst response, decreased ability to concentrate urine, intentional fluid restriction because of fear of incontinence, fear of choking if dysphagic, psychosocial factors such as isolation and depression, monotony of diet, and higher nutrient density requirements.

Reversible protein-energy malnutrition should be treated. Use of the following "MEALS ON WHEELS" mnemonic is helpful in determining individuals who are at risk (Morley and Thomas, 2004:)

Medications
Emotional problems
Anorexia/alcoholism
Late-life paranoia
Swallowing disorders
Oral problems
Nosocomial infections
Wandering and other dementia behaviors
Hyperthyroidism/hypercalcemia/hypoadrenalism
Enteric problems
Eating problems
Low-salt, low-cholesterol diets
Stones (cholelithiasis)

Overall, the MNA and MNA Screening Form provide advantages over using visceral proteins in screening and assessing nutritional status of elderly people with pressure ulcers (Langkamp-Henken et al, 2005).

Wound healing is complex and has three distinct phases. In each phase of wound healing, energy and macronutrients are required, and animal studies have established a specific role for certain nutrients: the amino acid arginine; vitamins A, B, and C; and the minerals selenium, manganese, zinc, and copper (Mathus-Vliegen, 2004). Careful administration of nutrition is an important part of wound healing.

Medicare costs attributable to pressure ulcer treatment are over $2 billion annually. The cost of caring for these preventable pressure ulcers may now be as high as $60,000 per patient (Edlich et al, 2004). The development of pressure ulcers in the hospital affects 10% of admissions, especially among the elderly (Harris and Fraser, 2004).

Mortality, usually secondary to sepsis, may be quite high in patients with pressure ulcers (Brem et al, 2003). Pain, amputations, and osteomyelitis may result. In most cases, it is difficult to determine whether a pressure ulcer led to a terminal event such as sepsis or whether the process of dying (i.e., decreased cardiac output, severe catabolic state) led to an unpreventable pressure ulcer (Braden, 1996).

INTERVENTION: OBJECTIVES

- Restore to a healthy nutritional status. Correct protein and energy malnutrition; this is of paramount importance.
- Monitor scores on the risk assessment scales. Nutrition risks evaluate the person's usual food intake pattern; intake of 3–5 days can be useful.
- Improve low-grade infections, fever, diarrhea, and vomiting. Support the patient's immune system to prevent new infections.
- Heal the pressure ulcer and prevent further tissue breakdown; Table 2-7 indicates staging. Assess healing by scales such as the Sessing scale (see Table 2-8). Figure 2-10 shows a stage 4 pressure ulcer.

TABLE 2-7 Skin Changes with Aging and Pressure Ulcer Stages

Skin Change	Consequences
Thinning of epidermis	Increased vulnerability to trauma and skin tears
Decreased epidermal proliferation	Slower production of new skin cells
Atrophy of dermis	Underlying tissue more vulnerable to injury; decreased wound contraction
Decreased vascularity of dermis	Easy bruising and injury; decreased wound capillary growth
Compromised vascular response	Impaired immune and inflammatory responses
Fragility	Easy bruising and tearing
Staging of Pressure Ulcers	
Stage I	Redness and warmth; nonblanchable erythema of intact skin
Stage II	Shallow ulcer with distinct edges; partial-thickness skin loss
Stage III	Full-thickness loss of skin involving damage or necrosis of subcutaneous tissue
Stage IV	Full-thickness skin loss with extensive destruction, tissue necrosis, or damage to muscle, bone, and supporting structures

Data from: AHCPR, 2006, and Mulder et al, 1999.

INTERVENTION: FOOD AND NUTRITION

- Provide a high-quality protein diet (Mathus-Vliegen, 2004). The AHCPR Guidelines for the Treatment of Pressure Ulcers (2006) recommend 1.0–1.5 g protein/kg body weight. A deep ulcer or multiple sites may require 1.5–2 g/kg. It may be necessary to add protein powders to beverages, casseroles, tube feedings, and liquid supplements to get the adequate amount. Intake of protein greater than 2 g/kg of body weight may not be metabolized to increase protein synthesis.

TABLE 2-8 Sessing Scale of Healing (Ferrell, 1997)

0	Normal skin, but at risk
1	Skin completely closed, but may lack pigmentation or may be reddened
2	Wound edges and center are filled in
3	Wound bed filling with pink granulating tissue; slough present; free of necrotic tissue; minimal drainage and odor
4	Moderate-to-minimal granulating tissue; slough and minimal necrotic tissue; moderate drainage and odor
5	Presence of heavy drainage and odor, eschar, and slough; surrounding skin reddened or discolored
6	Breaks in skin around primary ulcer; purulent discharge; foul odor; necrotic tissue and/or eschar; may have sepsis

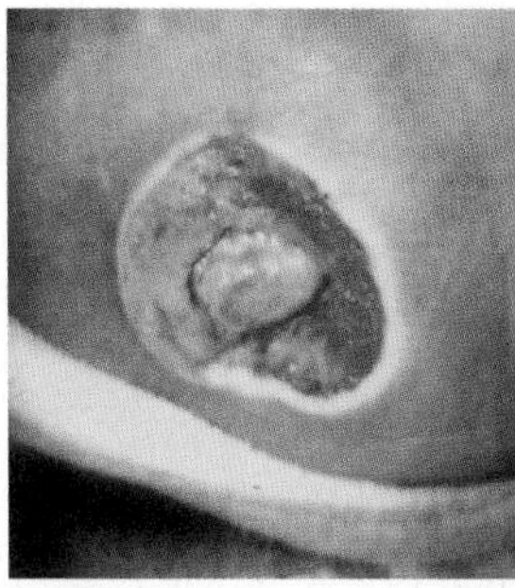

Figure 2-10 Stage 4 pressure ulcer. (From Nettina SM. *The Lippincott manual of nursing practice*. 7th ed. Philadelphia: Lippincott Williams & Wilkins, 2001.)

- Recommended calorie levels for wound healing vary from 25–35 kcal/kg body weight; use lower levels for obese patients and higher levels for underweight patients. Whether or not pressure ulcers are preventable remains controversial, but removing nutritional deficits is one key element (Thomas, 2006).
- Feed by tube if necessary. With a large sacral pressure ulcer, total parenteral nutrition (TPN) may be the only way to feed if bowel incontinence is present. Essential fatty acid deficiencies must be prevented with TPN.
- Provide small, frequent feedings if oral intake is poor, 4–6 times daily.
- Supplement diet with a general multivitamin-mineral supplement to supply adequate B vitamins, vitamin A, vitamin C, zinc, and copper; excesses are wasteful and do not necessarily speed the healing process and may harm the immune system (AHCPR, 2006).

Common Drugs Used and Potential Side Effects

- Monitor the drug profile for potential side effects, depletion of serum proteins, and blood-forming nutrients. Categories of drugs that can affect skin are antibacterials, antihypertensives, analgesics, tricyclic antidepressants, antihistamines, antineoplastic agents, antipsychotic agents, corticosteroids, diuretics, and hypoglycemic agents.

SAMPLE NUTRITION DIAGNOSTIC STATEMENT

Pressure Ulcer

PES: Inadequate protein intake related to poor appetite and low intake of milk, meat, eggs, and cheese as evidenced by a stage 2 and stage 4 pressure ulcer this past month.

Assessment Data (sources of info): Food intake records, weight records, pressure ulcer team reports.

Intervention: Counseling about good food sources of protein, enhancing menu items with protein powders or liquid supplements, supplements with Med Pass, adequate fluid intake.

Monitoring and Evaluation: Increased healing of pressure ulcers within 14 days, improved intake of protein foods to meet needs that are higher than normal.

CLINICAL INDICATORS

Clinical/History

Height
Weight
Weight changes
BMI
Diet history
Stage of ulcer(s)
Size of ulcer(s)
Exudate
Infection
Pain
Abnormal motor coordination
Diagnoses
Changes in appetite
Prognostic Inflammatory and Nutritional Index (PINI)
Braden scale—intense or prolonged pressure (activity, mobility, sensory perception) and tissue tolerance for pressure (nutrition, moisture, friction, and shear); scores range from 6–23, with lower scores suggesting higher risk
Norton scale (physical condition, mental status, activity, mobility, and incontinence); rating of 16 or higher suggests onset of risk
Anorexia
Nausea/vomiting
Indigestion
Diarrhea
Bowel function
Recent or frequent surgeries

Lab Work

C-reactive protein
Serum Chol
Blood urea nitrogen (BUN), Creat
Serum Na+, K+ Ca++, Mg++
H & H, serum Fe
Total protein (TP)
Alb, transthyretin
RBP (usually decreased)
N balance
Gluc
Transferrin
Total lymphocyte count (TLC)
Protime or INR
Serum zinc
Serum B_{12}

- Antibiotics may be needed in sepsis; monitor specific effects.
- Recommend, if needed, an appetite stimulant. Unintentional weight loss may be corrected by using dronabinol or Marinol (cannabinoids); megestrol acetate (Megace); oxymetholone; and other drugs still undergoing research evaluation.

Herbs, Botanicals, and Supplements

- Herbs and botanicals may be used; identify and monitor side effects and potential drug interactions.
- Counsel about use of herbal teas, especially regarding ingredients that may be toxic or ineffective.

INTERVENTION: NUTRITION EDUCATION, COUNSELING, CARE MANAGEMENT

- Instruct nursing personnel and patient's family about the importance of adequate nutrition for healing of tissues.
- Discuss importance of maintaining healthy, intact skin. Skin should be kept clean and dry; avoid massage over bony prominences.
- Provide teaching tools in regard to high-protein diets and the appropriate calorie level.
- Where possible, improve ambulation and circulation to all tissues. Exercise may also help improve appetite.
- Discuss the role of nutrition in wound healing (i.e., collagen and fibroblasts require protein, zinc, and vitamin C for proper formation).
- Discuss degree of assistance needed at mealtimes and provide ideas for self-help devices to increase overall intake (wet cloth under plate, curved flatware, two-handled cup, etc.).

Patient Education—Food Safety

- Hand washing will be important for caretakers or nurses before and after serving meals to patients who have pressure ulcers of stage 2 or greater.

For More Information

- Agency for Healthcare Research and Quality
  Clinical Practice Guidelines–Pressure Ulcer Treatment
  http://www.ahcpr.gov/
  http://www.ncbi.nlm.nih.gov/books/bv.fcgi?rid=hstat2.chapter.4409
- Centers for Medicare and Medicaid Services
  http://www.cms.hhs.gov/
- European Pressure Ulcer Advisory Panel
  http://www.epuap.org/
  Nutrition Guidelines: http://www.epuap.org/guidelines/english1.html
- National Decubitus Foundation
  http://www.decubitus.org/links/links.html
- National Pressure Ulcer Advisory Panel
  http://www.npuap.org/
- Wound Care Network
  http://www.woundcarenet.com/index.html

PRESSURE ULCERS—CITED REFERENCES

AHCPR. Executive summary. Accessed July 26, 2006 at http://www.ncbi.nlm.nih.gov/books/bv.fcgi?rid=hstat2.section.4502.

Braden B. Using the Braden scale for predicting pressure sore risk. *Support Line.* XVIII:14, 1996.

Edlich RF, et al. Pressure ulcer prevention. *J Long Term Eff Med Implants.* 14:285, 2004.

Ferrell BA. The Sessing Scale for measurement of pressure ulcer healing. *Adv Wound Care.* 10:78, 1997.

Guenter P, et al. Survey of nutritional status in newly hospitalized patients with stage III or stage IV pressure ulcers. *Adv Skin Wound Care.* 13:164, 2000.

Harris CL, Fraser C. Malnutrition in the institutionalized elderly: the effects on wound healing. *Ostomy Wound Manage.* 50:54, 2004.

Langkamp-Henken B, et al. Mini nutritional assessment and screening scores are associated with nutritional indicators in elderly people with pressure ulcers. *J Am Diet Assoc.* 105:1590, 2005.

Mathus-Vliegen EM. Old age, malnutrition, and pressure sores: an ill-fated alliance. *J Gerontol A Biol Sci Med Sci.* 59:355, 2004.

Morley JE, Thomas DR. Update: guidelines for the use of oregigenic drugs in long-term care. *Supplement to the Annals of Long-Term Care.* St. Louis: St. Louis University, 2004.

Mulder GD, Haberer PA, Jeter KF, eds. *Clinicians' pocket guide to chronic wound repair.* 4th ed. Springhouse, PA: Springhouse Corporation, 1999, pp. 21–22.

Thomas DR. Prevention and treatment of pressure ulcers. *J Am Med Dir Assoc.* 7:46, 2006.

Thomas DR, et al. Nutritional management in long-term care: development of a clinical guideline. *J Gerontol Med Sci.* 55:725, 2000.

Williams D, et al. Patients with existing pressure ulcers admitted to acute care. *J Wound Ostomy Continence Nurs.* 27:216, 2000.

VITAMIN DEFICIENCIES

NUTRITIONAL ACUITY RANKING: LEVEL 3

DEFINITIONS AND BACKGROUND

Vitamins are a part of a healthy diet. If a person eats a variety of foods, deficiency is less likely. However, people who follow restricted diets may not get enough of one or more particular nutrients. Deficiencies may be primary (self-induced by inadequate diet) or secondary to disease process. They are especially common in alcoholics, people who live alone and eat poorly, and among those who follow restrictive food fads. Vegetarians are also susceptible, especially for vitamin B_{12} deficiency. Appendix A provides greater detail about the vitamins and their sources, toxicities, and deficiencies.

Vitamin A deficiency is common among children. Night blindness and eye changes are often early signs. There is evidence now that many infections (such as measles) may cause vitamin A deficiency. Vitamin A helps form and maintain healthy teeth, mucous membranes, skeletal and soft tissues, and skin. The form known as retinol generates the pigments in the retina. Vitamin A promotes good vision (especially in dim light) and is required for healthy reproduction and lactation. Because beta-carotene is a precursor for vitamin A and because so many carotenoids play a role in maintaining good health, deficiencies of these phytochemicals may play an even larger role in maintaining vitamin A adequacy in the body.

Thiamin deficiency commonly occurs in alcoholics, patients with heart failure, and persons with poor-quality diets. Thiamin helps convert carbohydrate (CHO) into energy, so a high-CHO diet will deplete thiamin unless replaced. It is also important for proper functioning of the heart, nervous system, and muscles; it may be useful to replace thiamin when conditions affect those systems.

Niacin and riboflavin deficiencies often occur in conjunction with other B-complex vitamin deficiencies. Riboflavin (B_2) is important for growth, red cell production, and releasing energy from carbohydrates. Niacin assists in the functioning of the digestive system, skin, and nerves; it is important in the conversion of food to energy. A deficient diet or failure of the body to absorb niacin or tryptophan can cause signs of deficiency or pellagra. It is common in certain parts of the world where people consume large quantities of corn and is characterized by dermatitis, diarrhea, and schizophrenia-like dementia. It sometimes develops after gastrointestinal diseases or among alcoholics.

Vitamin B_6 deficiency decreases conversion of tryptophan to niacin. It can occur after surgery or as a result of poor diet. Vitamin B_6 deficiency is being studied for its role in cardiac disorders (atrial fibrillation, hyperhomocysteinemia, etc.) and inflammation (Friso et al, 2004) and in dopamine release in the brain. Because vitamin B_6 plays a role in the synthesis of antibodies and red blood cells, a healthy immune system and circulatory system depend on it. The higher the protein intake, the more need there is for vitamin B_6; a high protein–low CHO diet may deplete vitamin B_6.

Folic acid deficiency may result in a megaloblastic anemia; adequate supplementation is needed (see Section 12 on anemias). Folic acid acts as a coenzyme with vitamins C and B_{12} in the metabolism and synthesis of proteins. It is needed to make red blood cells, to synthesize DNA, and to support tissue growth and cell function. Research continues to identify roles for folic acid in disease prevention (e.g., neural tube defects, cancers, heart disease).

Vitamin B_{12} deficiency may also result in megaloblastic anemia (see Section 12 on anemias). Peripheral neuropathy and a positive Schilling test are needed to indicate B_{12} deficiency. Folic acid supplementation may mask a B_{12} deficiency, so if one is given, the other should also be given.

Pantothenic acid and biotin deficiencies are not common. Pantothenic acid is essential for metabolism and in the synthesis of hormones and cholesterol. Biotin is also essential for metabolism of proteins and carbohydrate and the synthesis of hormones and cholesterol.

Choline deficiency may occur in long-term TPN use without lipid replacement. Otherwise, it is thought to be rare.

Vitamin C deficiency occurs overtly with scurvy after 3 months without intake of ascorbic acid due to lack of consumption of fresh fruits and vegetables. Hypovitaminosis C can occur in the elderly and the homeless, among those who live alone or have psychiatric diseases, and in those who follow food fads. It is more common than realized in the general population. Long-term deficiency can be a concern for people who acquire some forms of cancer or cataracts.

Vitamin D deficiency and insufficiency may be a concern. Insufficiency is defined as a low threshold value for plasma 25-OHD (50 nmol/L). Secondary hyperparathyroidism, increased bone turnover, bone mineral loss, and seasonal variations in plasma PTH can occur with insufficiency. Vitamin D deficiency is defined as 25-OHD values below 25 nmol/L. Vitamin D deficiency is common among community-dwelling elderly who live in higher latitudes and among institutionalized elderly, geriatric patients, and patients with hip fractures. Vitamin D is produced in the skin by exposure to the sun and is found in fortified milk and other foods. For individuals who are not getting enough vitamin D in the diet, supplements may be helpful. The average adult under 50 needs 200 IU of vitamin D a day; 1 cup of vitamin D–fortified milk provides 50 IU of vitamin D (Surgeon General's Report, 2004). Recent studies suggest a role for vitamin D in autoimmune disorders, including multiple sclerosis (Mark and Carson, 2006).

Vitamin E deficiency is considered to be rare. It is an antioxidant, protects body tissue from the damage of oxidation, helps form red blood cells, and supports the use of vitamin K. Abetalipoproteinemia is the most severe deficiency and occurs mainly in premature and sick children. Problems occur with fat malabsorption in a deficiency state, especially in children.

Vitamin K deficiency is rare except in intestinal problems and short gut syndromes because intestinal bacteria in the healthy gut can make vitamin K. Healthy bones require it, so it is now believed that prevention of osteoporosis requires sufficient vitamin K.

INTERVENTION: OBJECTIVES

- Replenish the deficient nutrient and restore normal serum levels.
- Prevent or correct signs, symptoms, and effects of nutrient deficiency:
- **Vitamin A.** Reduced growth, night blindness leading progressively to xerophthalmia, changes in epithelial tissue, failure of tooth enamel and/or degeneration, and loss of taste and smell. Reduced immunity and high maternal and child mortality occur in populations at risk for deficiency (Cox et al, 2006).
- **B-Complex Vitamins:**
  Thiamin. Impairment of cardiovascular, nervous, and gastrointestinal systems.
  Riboflavin. Magenta tongue, angular stomatitis, and cheilosis.
  Niacin. Dermatitis, diarrhea, depression, and (sometimes) death.
  Folic Acid. Decrease in number of all types of blood cells; large red blood cells. Pregnancy-induced anemias; neural tube defects (Tamura and Picciano, 2006). Cardiovascular disease with elevated homocysteine levels.
  Vitamin B_6. Convulsions or intractable seizures in infants and young children (Gospe, 2006); anemias; nerve and skin disorders.
  Vitamin B_{12}. Pernicious anemia and other anemias; poor vision; some psychiatric symptoms.
  Biotin. Inflammation of the lips and skin.
  Choline. Liver damage and altered DNA function.
- **Vitamin C.** Delay in wound healing can occur. Clinical signs include weakness, myalgia, arthralgia, vascular purpura, gingivorragia, and loss of teeth. Biological signs include anemia, hypocholesterolemia, and hypoalbuminemia.
- **Vitamin D.** Abnormal bone growth and repair; rickets in children; osteomalacia in adults; muscle spasms. Decreased immunity with possible relationships with HIV infection (Villamor, 2006), type 1 diabetes or hypertension (Holick, 2006), and ovarian cancer (Zhang et al, 2006).
- **Vitamin E.** Rupture of red blood cells; nerve damage.
- **Vitamin K.** Poor wound healing may occur because of the role in blood clotting. Bone health is also related; osteopenia can result (Duggan et al, 2004).

INTERVENTION: FOOD AND NUTRITION

- **Vitamin A deficiency.** Use a diet including foods high in vitamin A and carotene: carrots, sweet potatoes, squash, apricots, collards, broccoli, cabbage, dark leafy greens, liver, kidney, cream, butter, and egg yolk.
- **B-Complex Vitamins:**
  - Thiamin deficiency or beri-beri. Use a diet including foods high in thiamin: pork, whole grains, enriched cereal grains, nuts, potatoes, legumes, green vegetables, fish, meat, fruit, and milk in quantity. A high-protein/high-carbohydrate intake should be included.
  - Riboflavin deficiency. Use a diet including foods high in riboflavin: milk, eggs, liver, kidney, and heart. Caution against losses resulting from cooking and exposure to sunlight.
  - Niacin deficiency or pellagra. Use a diet including foods high in niacin and other B vitamins: yeast, milk, meat, peanuts, cereal bran, and wheat germ.
  - Folic acid deficiency. Use fresh, leafy green vegetables, fruits such as oranges and orange juice, liver and other organ meats, and dried yeast.
  - Vitamin B_6 deficiency. Use dried yeast, liver, organ meats, whole-grain cereals, fish, and legumes.
  - Vitamin B_{12} deficiency. Use liver, beef, pork, organ meats, eggs, milk, and dairy products.
  - Biotin deficiency. Use liver, kidney, egg yolks, yeast, cauliflower, nuts, and legumes.
  - Pantothenic acid deficiency. Use live yeast and vegetables.
  - Choline. Include eggs, liver, beef, milk, oatmeal, soybeans, peanuts, and iceberg lettuce.
- **Vitamin C deficiency or scurvy**. Use a diet high in citrus fruits, tomatoes, strawberries, green peppers, cantaloupe, and baked potatoes.
- **Vitamin D deficiency**. Use fortified milk, fish liver oils, and egg yolks. Expose skin to sunlight if possible.
- **Vitamin E deficiency**. Use vegetable oil, wheat germ, leafy vegetables, egg yolks, margarine, and legumes.
- **Vitamin K deficiency**. Use a diet high in leafy vegetables, pork, liver, and vegetable oils.

CLINICAL INDICATORS

Clinical/History

Height
Weight
BMI
Diet history
Neurological changes
Hepatic or renal changes
Signs of malnutrition in hair, eyes, skin, mouth, gums, tongue, teeth (see Appendix A also):

- Vitamin A – night blindness, Bitot's spots, xerophthalmia, follicular hyperkeratosis
- Vitamin C – follicular hyperkeratosis, petechiae, ecchymosis, coiled hairs, inflamed and bleeding gums, perifollicular hemorrhages, joint effusions, arthralgia, and impaired wound healing
- Vitamin D – widening at ends of long bones, rachitic rosary in children, rickets, osteomalacia
- Riboflavin – sore throat, hyperemia, edema of pharyngeal and oral mucous membranes, cheilosis, angular stomatitis, glossitis, seborrheic dermatitis, and normochromic, normocytic anemia with pure erythrocyte cytoplasia of the bone marrow

- Niacin – symmetrical, pigmented rash on areas exposed to sunlight, bright red tongue, pellagra
- Vitamin B_6 – seborrheic dermatitis, stomatitis, cheilosis, glossitis, confusion, depression
- Vitamin B_{12} – tingling and numbness in extremities, diminished vibratory and position sense, motor disturbances including gait disturbances
- Folic acid – signs such as depapillation of the tongue are uncommon
- Choline – there are no visible physical signs of note

Lab Work

- Vitamin A–serum retinol < 0.35 mmol/L
- Vitamin C – plasma concentrations <0.2 mg/dL
- Vitamin D – 25-OHD values <25 nmol/L
- Vitamin E – plasma alpha-tocopherol <18 μmol/g
- Vitamin K – elevated prothrombin time, altered INR
- Thiamin – erythrocyte transketolase activity >1.20 μg/mL/h; AST is often decreased
- Riboflavin – erythrocyte glutathione reductase >1.2 IU/mg hemoglobin
- Niacin – *N*-methyl-nicotinamide excretion <5.8 μmol/d
- Vitamin B_6 – plasma pyridoxal 5′phosphate <20 nmol/L
- Vitamin B_{12} – serum concentration <180 pmol/L; elevated homocysteine
- Folic acid – serum concentration <7 nmol/L; red cell folate <315 nmol/L
- Choline – plasma choline and phosphatidylcholine concentrations fall when humans are fed a choline-deficient diet, but otherwise there are no clear lab techniques at this time; abnormal liver function tests may occur with deficiency

Common Drugs Used and Potential Side Effects or Toxicity

Note: The new DRI "tolerable upper intake levels" (UL) address the toxic side.

- **Vitamin A.** Absorption of vitamin A depends on bile salts in the intestinal tract. Controlled high doses may be prescribed for a short period of time. Beware of doses greater than the recommended upper limit per day for a long time, especially for children.
- **Thiamin.** A common dose is 5–10 mg/d of thiamin; anorexia and nausea may be common at the beginning of treatment. Intravenous therapy may be better tolerated.
- **Riboflavin.** Achlorhydria may precipitate a deficiency and may preclude successful correction. Alkaline substances destroy riboflavin.
- **Niacin.** Treatment with niacin may cause flushing. Niacinamide is a better choice; 200–400 mg of niacin or niacin equivalents may be used for a short time. Nicotinic acid can cause nausea, vomiting, and diarrhea.
- **Vitamin B_6.** Pyridoxine hydrochloride is the common content.
- **Pantothenic acid.** Pantholin is a drug that is prescribed as needed.
- **Choline.** Choline hydrochloride salt may be degraded by intestinal bacteria and cause a fishy body odor. This does not occur when lecithin is eaten in the diet.
- **Vitamin C.** Excesses can cause false-positive glucosuria tests. Cevalin or Cevita are drug sources; 50–300 mg/d may be given to correct scurvy. Excesses may have an antihistamine effect or cause diarrhea.
- **Vitamin D.** Calderol, Rocaltrol, Hytakerol, and Calciferol are common drug sources. Be sure to use vitamin D_3 [25-hydroxyvitamin D (25-OHD)] for greater effectiveness.
- **Vitamin E.** Aquasol E has no adverse side effects if used within measured dosage for age and daily requirements.
- **Vitamin K.** Vitamin K is usually injected to correct deficiency rather than using diet alone. Synkayvite, Mephyton, and Konakion are trade names.

Herbs, Botanicals, and Supplements

- Herbs and botanicals may be used by many individuals; identify and monitor side effects.
- Counsel about use of herbal teas, especially regarding ingredients that may be toxic.

INTERVENTION: NUTRITION EDUCATION, COUNSELING, CARE MANAGEMENT

- Explain where sources of the specific nutrient may be found.
- Demonstrate methods of cooking, storage, etc., that prevent losses.
- Help the patient plan a menu incorporating his or her preferences.
- Discuss the use of vitamin and mineral supplements. Although they may be appropriate to correct a deficiency state, they may not be warranted for continuous or long-term use.

For More Information

- Food and Nutrition Information Center
  http://www.nal.usda.gov/fnic/etext/000068.html
- NIH Office of Dietary Supplements
  http://www.cc.nih.gov/ccc/supplements/intro.html
- Nutrient Data Laboratory
  http://www.nal.usda.gov/fnic/foodcomp/
- Nutrition Information
  http://www.nutrition.org/
- U.S. Department of Health and Human Services
  http://www.dhhs.gov/
- Vitamin Information, VERIS Online Service
  http://www.cognis.com/veris/verisdefault.htm

VITAMIN DEFICIENCIES—CITED REFERENCES

Cox SE, et al. Vitamin A supplementation increases ratios of proinflammatory to anti-inflammatory cytokine responses in pregnancy and lactation. *Clin Exp Immunol.* 144:392 2006.

Duggan P, et al. Vitamin K status in patients with Crohn's disease and relationship to bone turnover. *Am J Gastroenterol.* 99:2178, 2004.

Friso S, et al. Low plasma vitamin B-6 concentrations and modulation of coronary artery disease risk. *Am J Clin Nutr.* 79:992, 2004.

Gospe SM. Pyridoxine-dependent seizures: new genetic and biochemical clues to help with diagnosis and treatment. *Curr Opin Neurol.* 19:148, 2006.

Holick MF. High prevalence of vitamin D inadequacy and implications for health. *Mayo Clin Proc.* 81:353, 2006.

Mark BL, Carson JA. Vitamin D and autoimmune disease—implications for practice from the multiple sclerosis literature. *J Am Diet Assoc.* 106:418, 2006.

Surgeon General's Report on Bone Health. By 2020, one in two Americans over age 50 will be at risk for fractures from osteoporosis or low bone mass. Available at http://www.hhs.gov/news/press/2004pres/20041014.html; 2004.

Tamura T, Picciano MF. Folate and human reproduction. *Am J Clin Nutr.* 83:993, 2006.

Villamor E. A potential role for vitamin D on HIV infection? *Nutr Rev.* 64:226, 2006.

Zhang X, et al. Vitamin D receptor is a novel drug target for ovarian cancer treatment. *Curr Cancer Drug Targets.* 6:229, 2006.

FOOD ALLERGY AND MÉNIÈRE'S SYNDROME

FOOD ALLERGY AND INTOLERANCES

NUTRITIONAL ACUITY RANKING: LEVEL 2–3 (SIMPLE); LEVEL 3–4 (COMPLEX)

DEFINITIONS AND BACKGROUND

True food allergy is an immune response, generally from immunoglobulin E (IgE); a reaction usually occurs within 2 hours. Immediate (1 minute–2 hours) or delayed reactions (2–48 hours) may also occur. A food allergy results from hypersensitivity to an antigen of food source (usually protein); however, any food product is capable of producing an intolerance. The manifestations of the allergy are caused by the release of histamine and serotonin. It is important to distinguish food allergies from intolerances caused by toxins or drugs and metabolic disorders such as lactase deficiency or celiac disease.

Ingestion is the principal route for food allergens, yet some highly sensitive individuals may also react through skin contact or inhalation (Tan et al, 2001). According to the Food and Drug Administration and the American Academy of Allergy, Asthma, and Immunology, over 90% of food allergies are caused by eight foods: eggs, milk, wheat, soy, fish, shellfish, peanuts, and tree nuts. Allergy to peanuts and tree nuts (TNs) is the leading cause of fatal and near-fatal food allergic reactions (Sicherer, 2003).

Allergic tendencies are inherited but not necessarily to a specific antigen (i.e., a parent with a genetic predisposition to severe bee sting reactions could have a child with a bee sting allergy, food allergy, or other allergy). People who have a tendency toward allergy may develop sensitivity to new foods. Approximately 6% of children younger than age 3 and 1.5% of the general population have true food allergies (Food and Drug Administration, 2001). Prevalence in the United States is now about 6–7 million people.

There is a pattern of immune deviation and disturbed gut motility in children with multiple food allergies, along with a maternal history of autoimmunity (Latcham et al, 2003). Interestingly, the American Academy of Allergy, Asthma, and Immunology has reported that children who have a fever before age 1 are less likely to develop allergies by age 6–7 years; exposure to dogs at an early age is also preventive; and consumption of omega-3 fatty acids can reduce the severity of asthma symptoms (http://www.aaaai.org/media/news_releases/).

Activation of nuclear transcription factor-κB has been linked with a variety of inflammatory diseases, including allergy and asthma; research has shown that the pathway that activates this transcription factor can be interrupted by phytochemicals derived from spices such as turmeric (curcumin); red pepper (capsaicin); cloves (eugenol); ginger (gingerol); cumin, anise, and fennel (anethol); basil and rosemary (ursolic acid); garlic (diallyl sulfide, S-allylmercaptocysteine, ajoene); and pomegranate (ellagic acid) (Aggarwal and Shishodia, 2004).

Food allergy can manifest as urticaria/angioedema, anaphylaxis, atopic dermatitis, respiratory symptoms, or gastrointestinal disorder (Garcia-Careaga and Kerner, 2005). The most common symptoms of food allergies are gastrointestinal (GI): diarrhea, nausea, vomiting, cramping, and abdominal distention and pain. GI allergic manifestations can be classified as IgE mediated (immediate GI hypersensitivity and oral allergy syndrome); "mixed" GI allergy syndromes (involving some IgE components and some non-IgE or T-cell–mediated components); or eosinophilic gastroenteritis (Garcia-Careaga and Kerner, 2005).

The greatest danger in food allergy comes from anaphylaxis, a violent allergic reaction that involves many parts of the body. Signs include itchy lips, tongue, or palate; metallic taste; flushing and itching or urticaria of skin; angioedema and edema of lips and tongue; nausea, vomiting, or diarrhea; tightness in chest or throat; dysphagia; hoarseness; dry cough; shortness of breath or wheezing; rhinorrhea or congestion; bronchospasm; syncope; chest pain; and hypotension. Anaphylaxis occurs when a person is exposed to an allergen after being sensitized by a previous exposure.

Anaphylaxis is life threatening and potentially fatal; severe asthma may cause respiratory arrest, shock, and death (Frankland and Pumphrey, 2002). Peanuts, tree nuts, shellfish, milk, eggs, and fish are the most common causes. Even miniscule amounts of the offending food have caused deaths. Peanut allergy is the most serious due to its persistence and high risk of severe anaphylaxis (Scurlock and Burks, 2004; Shimamoto and Bock, 2002).

Histamine is a primary mediator of anaphylaxis by triggering a cascade of inflammatory mediators (Winbery and Lieberman, 2002). Histamine occurs in foods such as cheese, red wines, spinach, eggplant, and yeast extract; it can elicit a response, including urticaria, gastrointestinal irritability, nausea, and flushing (Maher, 2002). A nonallergic reaction may occur from eating spoiled (scombroid) fish, which tends to be high in histamine; it may cause a reaction similar to anaphylaxis. Histamine also appears to play a role in chronic idiopathic urticaria (CIU), or hives. Persons with CIU may have a subclinical impairment of small bowel enterocyte function that could induce higher sensitivity to histamine-producing foods (Guida et al, 2000).

Food-dependent exercise-induced anaphylaxis (FDEIA) is an allergic reaction characteristically induced by intense exercise combined with the ingestion of causative food (Matsuo et al, 2005). FDEIA is often associated with celery, chicken, shrimp, oyster, peaches, and wheat. Exercise and aspirin may facilitate allergen absorption from the gastrointestinal tract (Matsuo et al, 2005). Nutrient deficiencies will depend on the foods involved and omitted.

Alcoholic beverages may also contribute to hypersensitivity reactions: flushing syndrome, anaphylactoid reactions of urticaria/angioedema, asthma, food allergy, or exercise-induced anaphylaxis in susceptible subjects (Gonzalez-Quintela et al, 2004). Alcohol intake may play a role as a promoter of the development of IgE-mediated hypersensitivity to different allergens; alcohol abuse and even moderate alcohol consumption are associated with increased total serum IgE levels (Gonzalez-Quintela et al, 2004).

Oral allergy syndrome (OAS) involves direct contact of the oral mucosa with an offending food, causing oral itching, lip swelling, and labial angioedema as a result of hypersensitivity to pollens (Pastorello and Ortolani, 1997). There is a rapid onset of symptoms, and it is rarely progressive. Patients with OAS may react to allergens (lipid transfer proteins) that are shared by botanically unrelated fruits such as nuts, peanuts, legumes, tomato, and plum (Asero, 1999).

The Food Allergen Labeling and Consumer Protection Act (FALCPA) became effective January 1, 2006. Food ingredient labeling is the first line of defense for those with food allergies and their caregivers. Food ingredient labeling should be read every time a food is purchased and used. Under FALCPA, food labels are to provide clear, consistent, and reliable ingredient labeling information by including "common English" names of the top eight major food allergens in food labeling.

The FALCPA legislation requires one of two options for food labeling with these common terms. The first is to list the food allergen in parentheses following the required ingredient term; for example, "whey (milk)" or "semolina (wheat)." The second option is to follow the ingredient declaration with a statement such as "contains flounder, pecan, wheat, and soy." Additionally, all spices, flavors, and incidental additives that contain or are derived from a major food allergen will be labeled with the name of an allergen under either ingredient labeling option. For example, a flavor that contains an ingredient derived from milk might say "natural butter flavor (milk)."

Genetically modified (GM) foods are the product of biotechnology. Genetic bioengineering may, eventually, be able to reduce the level of allergens in the food supply (Lehrer, 2004), a common concern among members of the public (Celec et al, 2005). For GM foods, possible allergenicity of proteins is evaluated by comparison of their amino acid sequence with that of known allergens and determination of their stability during processing (Martens, 2000). GM crops that have been grown commercially are regularly evaluated for allergenic properties (Goodman et al, 2005). Overall, biotechnology can enhance the safety, nutritional value, and variety of foods without promoting allergies (American Dietetic Association, 2006).

INTERVENTION: OBJECTIVES

- Careful clinical history, diagnostic studies, endoscopy, or double-blind food challenge may be needed. Assist as needed in obtaining information; teach how to keep a food diary to track reactions to food.
- The main therapy remains avoidance of incriminating foods and education to deal with inadvertent exposures. Exclude or avoid the offending allergen. If it is not known, use an elimination diet to discover the cause. Note that "rotation diets" are not effective and are potentially dangerous.
- Monitor the onset of reactions, which may be delayed or immediate. If delayed, the onset of the reaction may take from several hours to as long as 5 days. An immediate response is more common with raw foods; patient history may include diarrhea, urticaria, dermatitis, rhinitis, and asthma. (See the Asthma entry in Section 5.)
- Treatment of GI allergic disorders includes strict dietary elimination of offending food, use of protein hydrolysates, and use of L-amino acid–based formula when protein hydrolysates fail (Garcia-Careaga and Kerner, 2005).
- Children with atopic dermatitis could have a food allergy that can be diagnosed using a skin prick test and double-blind food challenge.
- Ensure extensive nutrition counseling and health education for those who have food allergies to avoid nutrient deficiencies, to limit unnecessary restrictions, and to prevent reactions.
- Breastfeeding should be promoted for primary prevention of allergic infants (Isolauri et al, 1999). If breastfeeding is not possible, use from birth of hydrolysate formulas may prevent atopic disease in the infants of families who have allergies (Garcia-Careaga and Kerner, 2005).
- Education on reading ingredient labeling is essential.
- Treat nutritional deficiencies or ensure adequate supplementation. Children who have multiple food allergies, for example, tend to have growth problems (Christie et al, 2002). The nutritional consequences of food allergy by various allergens are listed in Table 2-9.

INTERVENTION: FOOD AND NUTRITION

- The most common allergens in infants are eggs, wheat, milk, and fish. For children, cow's milk, eggs, soy,

TABLE 2-9 Major Food Allergens and Nutritional Consequences

Most Common	Nutrients of concern
Milk	Check for deficiencies in protein, riboflavin, calcium, and vitamins A and D.
Eggs	Check for iron from other sources.
Fish and Shellfish	Other protein sources will be needed. Niacin, vitamin B_6, vitamin B_{12}, omega-3 fatty acids, phosphorus, and selenium should be available from other foods.
Nuts, Tree	Protein, fatty acids, and other nutrients will be needed from other sources in the diet. Often, children outgrow a tree nut allergy.
Peanuts	Protein, fatty acids, and other nutrients will be needed from other sources in the diet.
Soy	Protein and other nutrients may be needed from other sources.
Wheat	Check for sufficiency of B vitamins and iron from other sources.
Less Common	Most frequently tied to adverse reactions that can be confused with food allergy are yellow dye number 5, monosodium glutamate (MSG), and sulfites.
Food Additives: Tartrazine (not a true food allergen)	Yellow dye number 5 can cause hives, although rarely. FD&C Yellow No. 5, or tartrazine, is used to color beverages, dessert powders, candy, ice cream, custards, and other foods. The color additive may cause hives in fewer than one out of every 10,000 people. By law, whenever the color is added to foods or taken internally, it must be listed on the label so those who may be sensitive to FD&C Yellow No. 5 can avoid it (http://www.cfsan.fda.gov/~dms/qa-top.html).
Monosodium Glutamate (MSG) (not a true food allergen)	Dietary glutamate is a major energy source for the intestines and placenta. The brain is well protected against a flux of glutamate, and it is not toxic. Glutamate is found naturally in foods such as tomatoes and cheeses and is released in protein hydrolysis during stock or soup preparation. It is added to foods in crystalline form as monosodium glutamate (MSG). MSG, which is 14% sodium, is used as a flavor enhancer, known as "umami." Glutamate helps to stimulate the vagus nerve and helps to facilitate digestion and nutrient absorption (Fernstrom and Garattini, 2000). MSG enhances flavor, but when consumed in large amounts, it can cause flushing, sensations of warmth, lightheadedness, headache, facial pressure, and chest tightness; these effects are temporary. These adverse reactions, "Chinese restaurant syndrome," have not been confirmed in double-blind studies (Geha et al, 2000).
Mustard	Mustard allergy is not as uncommon as previously believed (Figueroa et al, 2005). There is a relationship with mugwort pollinosis and plant-derived food allergies. A relationship between this syndrome and food-dependent exercise-induced anaphylaxis has also been reported (Figueroa et al, 2005).
Rice	Certain ethnic groups may have sensitivities to foods that may not be as allergenic for other populations. An example is an Asian person who develops an allergy to rice. Some of this may be dose-related exposure.
Spices	Spices may cause delayed-typed contact allergic or immediate allergic reaction. Sesame seed is a fairly common allergen. Carmine/cochineal is another minor allergen.
Sulfites (not a true food allergen)	Although not an IgE-mediated allergic response, sulfites can produce life-threatening reactions similar to the major food allergens. To help sulfite-sensitive people avoid problems, FDA requires the presence of sulfites in processed foods to be declared on the label and prohibits the use of sulfites on fresh produce intended to be sold or served raw to consumers (FDA Consumer: http://vm.cfsan.fda.gov/~dms/wh-alrg1.html). Foods such as wine, beer, dried fruits and vegetables, maraschino cherries, and dried or frozen potatoes may contain sulfites. No specific nutrient deficits are likely if omitted from the diet.

TABLE 2-10 Food Processing Concerns

Manufacturing processes	The food industry has taken steps to address the needs of consumers with food allergies, including changes to manufacturing processes to reduce the potential for cross contact with major food allergens. Under existing good manufacturing practice (GMP) regulations, reasonable precautions must be taken to prevent cross contact with major allergenic proteins. In instances when cross contact cannot be avoided, even when complying, food and ingredient manufacturers use labeling that informs the food allergic consumer of the possible presence of allergens in the food. Food manufacturers label the ingredients in their products in accordance with existing regulatory requirements. The rule is, "no protein, no problem."
Oils in processing	Most oils used in food processing and for sale to the public contain no protein and are extracted from the oilseed or nut using solvents and then are degummed, refined, bleached, and deodorized. Some oils are mechanically extracted (cold pressed) and left unrefined to purposely maintain the flavor; these oils may contain protein and be allergenic.
Product recalls	Undeclared food allergens have been responsible for many food product recalls during the past decade, and the food industry has made significant investment, effort, and improvements in allergen control during this time (Hefle and Taylor, 2004). More research will be important.

TABLE 2-11 Specifics of Food Allergies

Egg	Reactions are usually mild. Flu shots may contain egg albumin. Yolks are often tolerated. ALWAYS CONTAINS IT: Eggs, egg whites, dried eggs, egg solids, egg nog, albumin, cake, some candies or creamed foods, cookies, custard, doughnuts, egg rolls, some frostings, hollandaise sauce, some ice creams, lecithin, mayonnaise, meringue, some puddings, pretzels, Simplesse sweetener, souffle, waffles. MAY CONTAIN IT: Egg may appear as "albumin" in marshmallows, frozen dinners, and dry food mixes. Egg washes are often used on bakery goods to make them look shiny. Eggs are often used in glazes and icings.
Fish and shellfish	Avoid seafood restaurants. Abalone, clams, crab, crawfish, lobster, oysters, scallops, shrimp, cockle (sea urchin), and mussels are the shellfish that should be avoided. ALWAYS CONTAINS IT: Fish, shellfish, agar, alginic acid, ammonium alginate, anchovies, calcium alginate, caviar, disodium ionsinate, potassium alginate, propylene glycol alginate sodium alginate, imitation crab or "surimi," roe. MAY CONTAIN IT: Asian sauces, Caesar salad dressing, omega-3 fatty acid capsules or oils; Chinese, Vietnamese, Japanese, Indian, Indonesian, and Thai foods; fried foods, i.e., french fries, chicken nuggets (often cooked in the same oil as fish/shellfish); steak or Worcestershire sauces.
Latex	Natural rubber latex contains more than 35 proteins that may be related to type IgE–mediated allergy (Perkin, 2000). Latex-specific IgF may be responsible. Cross-reactivity has been documented with banana, avocado, kiwi, and European chestnuts; less commonly with potatoes; tomatoes; and peaches, plums, cherries, and other pitted fruits. Individuals with latex allergy also tend to report food allergies, including fish and shellfish (Kim and Hussain, 1999). Children with spina bifida and atopic dermatitis are a high-risk group for latex sensitization. Increasing age, additional sensitization to ubiquitous inhaled allergens, and enhanced total serum IgE values seem to be important variables for latex sensitization and further sensitization to the latex-associated foods (Tucke et al, 1999).
Milk	ALWAYS CONTAINS IT: Casein, caseinates, lactalbumins, lactoglobulins, lactose, nougat, rennet, milk, milk solids, nonfat or powdered milks, buttermilk, evaporated milk, condensed milk, yogurt, cream, cream cheese, sour cream, cheese, cheese sauces, cottage cheese, butter, butter fat, curds, whey, white sauces. MAY CONTAIN IT: Artificial butter flavor. Caramel color or flavoring, flavorings or seasonings, puddings, custards, sauces, sherbet. It may be necessary to acquire sufficient calcium from greens and broccoli or clams, oysters, shrimp, and salmon if not allergic to fish. Calcium supplementation may also be warranted. Persons with a milk allergy can add vanilla or other flavorings to soy milk. Goat's milk has less lactalbumin, vitamin D, and folacin than cow's milk and supplements may be required. Some people may also be allergic to goat's milk, so caution must be used. Avoid early introduction of cow's milk in infancy.
Nuts, tree	Tree nuts include almonds, Brazil nuts, cashews, chestnuts, filberts, hazelnuts, hickory nuts, macadamia nuts, pecans, pine nuts, pistachios, and walnuts. Monitor food labels for nut paste, nut oil, and nut extracts. Avoid nut butters also. Read labels for ground or mixed nuts.
Peanut	Peanuts are a type of legume, but a person is more likely to be allergic to tree nuts than to beans, peas, and lentils. Avoid nut butters also; aflatoxins can cause an allergic-like reaction. For the food industry, new inexpensive kits are available to test for presence of peanut proteins in cookies, cereal, ice cream, and milk chocolate. Despite severity and reaction frequency to peanut and tree nut allergy, only 74% of children and 44% of adults in a large study sought evaluation for the allergy, and fewer than half who did were prescribed self-injectable epinephrine (Sicherer et al, 2003). It may be recommended that those children who outgrow their peanut allergy be encouraged to eat peanut frequently and carry epinephrine until they demonstrate true peanut tolerance (Fleischer et al, 2004). ALWAYS CONTAINS IT: Peanuts, mixed nuts, peanut butter, peanut oil, peanut flour, ground or mixed nuts, artificial nuts, nougat, many types of candy or cookies, ethnic dishes made with peanut oil, some egg rolls, marzipan. MAY CONTAIN IT: Peanut butter may be used to keep egg rolls from falling apart or in chili as a thickener.
Soybean	Some people are also allergic to legumes such as chickpeas, navy beans, kidney beans, black beans, pinto beans, lentils, and peanuts. ALWAYS CONTAINS IT: Soybeans, soybean oil, margarines made from soybean oil, soy sauce, soy nuts, soy milk. Reading food labels will be very important. COMMON SOURCES: Soy protein, textured vegetable protein, hydrolyzed plant protein, lecithin, miso, soy sauce, Worcestershire sauce, tofu, tempeh, some vegetable broths.
Wheat	Wheat-dependent, exercise-induced anaphylaxis (WDEIA) and baker's asthma are different clinical forms of wheat allergy (Mittag et al, 2004). ALWAYS CONTAINS IT: Whole-wheat or enriched flour, high-gluten flour, high-protein flour, bran, farina, bulgur, durum, wheat malt, wheat starch, modified starch, wheat germ, graham flour, wheat gluten, matzoh/matzoh meal, semolina, bread crumbs, cereal extract, dextrin, malt flavoring, modified starch. COMMON SOURCES: Baby food, baked goods, baking mixes, breaded foods, processed meats, pastas, snack foods, soups, breads, cookies, cakes and other baked goods made with wheat flour; crackers, many cereals, some couscous, cracker meal, pasta, gelatinized starch, hydrolyzed vegetable protein, wheat gluten, vegetable gum, vegetable starch.

peanuts, wheat, tree nuts, and fish are often a problem. For adults, common allergens include shellfish, peanuts, and tree nuts. Peanuts are implicated in approximately one third of all cases of anaphylaxis.

- After medical testing (RAST or skin testing), a double-blind, placebo-controlled food challenge (DBPCFC) can be useful (Perry et al, 2004). This should only be used under the guidance of a physician in case there are immediate or severe reactions.
- For an elimination diet, use an unflavored elemental diet as a hypoallergenic base to which other foods are added as test challenges. Foods that seldom cause an allergic reaction include apples, apricots, artichokes, carrots, gelatin, lamb, lettuce, peaches, pears, rice, squash, and turkey; they may be used in this protocol.
- Read labels of foods prepared for the patient. Check all menu items served to patients. See Table 2-10.
- Monitor food preparation methods to exclude possible cross contact with the allergen.
- Monitor nutrient needs specific for the patient's age; evaluate for possible "hidden" ingredients.
- For infants, exclusive breastfeeding is best (American Academy of Pediatrics, 2000). Breast milk generally is nonallergenic.
- Lactating mothers may need to omit cow's milk from their own diets, as well as eggs, fish, and nuts. Infants with cow's milk allergy may exhibit eczema, rhinorrhea, abdominal pain, diarrhea, and otitis media appearing from 2–80 hours after their mothers have consumed cow's milk (Jarvinen et al, 1999). Infants who are allergic to cow's milk and soy may need Nutramigen or another hydrolyzed formula. See Table 2-11.
- Persons with rhinitis may be sensitive to monosodium benzoate in fruit juice, pie filling, pickles, olives, salad dressings, and fruit drinks.

CLINICAL INDICATORS

Clinical/History	BMI	Diet history
Height	Recent weight changes	BP
Weight		Temperature
Chronic GI distress, diarrhea	Serum tryptase (elevated)	false-positive rate but very reliable for negative tests)
Asthma or rhinitis	Serum histamine	Patch tests for delayed hypersensitivity reactions
Angioedema, urticaria	Radioallergosorbent test (RAST) or CAP RAST test	CRP
Double-blind food challenge test	Allergen-specific IgE levels: prick skin tests (50%	Alb, transthyretin
Lab Work		BUN, creatinine
H & H, serum Fe		

SAMPLE NUTRITION DIAGNOSTIC STATEMENT

Food Allergies

PES: Intake of unsafe food related to knowledge deficit as evidenced by anaphylaxis reaction after consumption of peanuts.

Assessment: Food diaries, food history, history of previous anaphylaxis and known food allergens.

Intervention: Education and counseling about identified food allergies, food labeling, recipes, and ingredients; evaluation of nutritional adequacy.

Monitoring and Evaluation: Review of food diaries and reports of no further admissions or problems with anaphylactic reactions to foods.

Common Drugs Used and Potential Side Effects

- Aspirin may trigger skin reactions, which are associated with the inhibition of cyclooxygenase-1 (COX-1) and characterized by overproduction of cysteinyl leukotrienes; these reactions are due to the interference of aspirin-like drugs with arachidonic acid metabolism (Mastalerz, 2005).
- Cyclosporine, when used, can be steroid sparing; monitor BUN, creatinine, and blood pressure (Kaplan, 2004).
- Epinephrine is a synthetic version of a naturally occurring adrenaline. It is the first line of defense for anaphylaxis and often requires an emergency room visit. Injectable epinephrine should be carried by those who are prone to allergic reactions to food and other allergens. An Epi-Pen provides a single dose; the Ana-Kit provides two doses.
- Treatment with topical or systemic steroids is used if all dietary measures are unsuccessful (Garcia-Careaga and Kerner, 2005).
- Oral antihistamines, such as Benadryl or Atarax or Vistaril, should be taken with food. Dry mouth, constipation, and GI distress are potential side effects.
- Anti-IgE antibodies are being studied for their possible use in treatment of food allergy.
- H_1-antihistamines are adjunctive treatment therapy for acute anaphylactoid reactions, but they have a slow onset of action when compared with epinephrine, the medication of choice (Winbery and Lieberman, 2002). Oral H_1-antihistamines are a mainstay of therapy for urticaria; those that are nonsedating at recommended doses (fexofenadine, loratadine, and desloratadine) may be selected (Monroe, 2005).

Herbs, Botanicals, and Supplements

- Bee pollen does not prevent allergies and may, in fact, cause asthma, urticaria, rhinitis, or anaphylaxis after eating plants that cross-react with ragweed, such as sunflowers or dandelion greens.
- Food/plant sensitivities are common (e.g., melon/ragweed, apple/birch, wheat/grasses). Be wary of herbal teas; some may contain toxic substances.

- Garlic, jewelweed, parsley, ginger, stinging nettle, amaranth, gingko, chamomile, and feverfew have been proposed for use in allergies or with hives, but no long-term studies prove efficacy.
- Sweeteners are not usually allergenic. After reviewing scientific studies, the FDA determined in 1981 that aspartame is safe for use in foods. Persons who have phenylketonuria (PKU) should not use it because it is made from phenylalanine (http://vm.cfsan.fda.gov).

INTERVENTION: NUTRITION EDUCATION, COUNSELING, CARE MANAGEMENT

Tips to share with individuals who have allergies are as follows (adapted from: http://www.enjoylifefoods.com/cart/PDF_files/allergen_free_bro.pdf).

(1) Hints for shopping in food stores:

DELI: Ask to have the deli slicer cleaned before preparing the order. Avoid prepared foods because they often share bins and serving utensils. Request that clean gloves be worn.

ICE CREAM SHOPS: Make sure they don't share scoops for different flavors.

PACKAGED FOODS: Read labels to detect hidden allergens. Choose foods made in facilities that don't make other problematic products. Re-read labels often as ingredients may change; if unsure, call the manufacturer.

SALAD BARS: Be careful with severe allergies because food can drop from one container into another.

(2) Hints for dining out:

AVOID FRIED FOODS, which often share oil with other problem foods.

INQUIRE AHEAD if possible and consult the chef on best menu picks for safe dining.

USE A PLEASANT BUT ASSERTIVE MANNER in explaining the situation to wait staff. Let them know that eating even a small amount of a certain food(s) will make you severely ill.

BE CAREFUL of sauces and soups. Make sure you know exactly what's in them before eating.

REGULAR PATRONAGE. Choose a favorite eatery that accommodates well and visit often.

(3) Hints for children and schools:

EDUCATE. Schools need to educate their entire staff, improve prevention and avoidance measures, make sure epinephrine is readily available and that the staff knows how to administer it, and use consumer agency resources (Munoz-Furlong, 2004). The Food Allergy Network has educational kits targeted at schools to assist in the training of the staff on food allergies.

MEDIC ALERT. Students should be encouraged to wear a Medic-Alert bracelet.

CAFETERIA MEALS. Food allergy continues to rise in childhood, and careful meal planning is needed.

(4) At home:

KEEP A FOOD DIARY. Identify all symptoms, timing, and foods eaten.

READ FOOD LABELS every time a food is purchased and used.

FIND RECIPE BOOKS THAT PROVIDE ALTERNATIVES. Recipe books are available from formula companies, food manufacturers, the Food Allergy and Anaphylaxis Network, and registered dietitians.

PATIENT OR PARENT EDUCATION. Patients and parents must stay informed about how to handle allergic reactions (Stone, 2004).

(5) At the doctor's office:

TESTING. Cytotoxic testing, sublingual provocative tests, pulse tests, kinesiologic testing, yeast hypersensitivity, and brain allergy theories should be dismissed entirely.

(6) After anaphylaxis:

To work with anaphylaxis, remember the "3 Rs": RECOGNIZE symptoms; REACT quickly; REVIEW what happened to prevent it from happening again.

For More Information

- American Academy of Allergy, Asthma, and Immunology
  http://www.aaaai.org/
- American College of Allergy, Asthma, and Immunology
  http://www.acaai.org/
- Asthma and Allergy Foundation of America
  http://www.aafa.org/
- Cherrybrook Kitchens: Allergy free
  https://www.cherrybrookkitchen.com/index.html
- Enjoy Life Foods
  http://www.enjoylifefoods.com/cart/PDF_files/allergen_free_bro.pdf
- Food Allergy and Anaphylaxis Network
  http://www.foodallergy.org/
- Food Allergies Database
  http://allergyadvisor.com/
- Food Allergy Initiative
  http://www.foodallergyinitiative.org/
- Food and Nutrition Information Center
  http://www.nal.usda.gov/fnic/pubs/bibs/gen/allergy.htm
- FDA Consumer–Food Allergy Page
  http://vm.cfsan.fda.gov/~dms/wh-alrg1.html
- Food Labeling
  http://www.fda.gov/fdac/special/foodlabel/food_toc.html
- Food Products Association
  http://www.fpa-food.org/
- International Food Information Council Foundation
  http://ific.org
- Kids with Allergies
  http://www.kidswithfoodallergies.org
- Mayo Clinic
  http://mayohealth.org
- Medem Allergy Clinic
  http://www.medem.com/medlb/sub_detaillb.cfm?parent_id=78&act=disp
- Medline: Food Allergy
  http://www.nlm.nih.gov/medlineplus/foodallergy.html
- National Institute on Allergy and Infectious Diseases
  http://www.niaid.nih.gov/

- RAST Testing
  http://www.labtestsonline.org/understanding/analytes/allergy/test.html
- Teen Allergies
  http://kidshealth.org/teen/food_fitness/nutrition/food_allergies.html

FOOD ALLERGY AND INTOLERANCES—CITED REFERENCES

Aggarwal BB, Shishodia S. Suppression of the nuclear factor-kappaB activation pathway by spice-derived phytochemicals: reasoning for seasoning. *Ann N Y Acad Sci.* 1030:434, 2004.

American Academy of Pediatrics, Committee on Nutrition. Hypoallergenic infants' formulas. *Pediatr.* 106:346, 2000.

American Dietetic Association. Position of the American Dietetic Association: agricultural and food biotechnology. *J Am Diet Assoc.* 106:285, 2006.

Asero R. Detection and clinical characterization of patients with oral allergy syndrome caused by stable allergens in *Rosaceae* and nuts. *Ann Allergy Asthma Immunol.* 83:377, 1999.

Celec P, et al. Biological and biomedical aspects of genetically modified food. *Biomed Pharmacother.* 59:531, 2005.

Christie L, et al. Food allergies in children affect nutrient intake and growth. *J Am Diet Assoc.* 102:1648, 2002.

Food and Drug Administration. Food allergies: when food becomes the enemy. *FDA Consumer Magazine.* Washington, DC: USDA Food and Drug Administration, July–August, 2001.

Fernstrom J, Garattini S. International symposium on glutamate: proceedings of a symposium held October 12–14, 1998 in Bergamo, Italy. *J Nutri.* 130:891S, 2000.

Figueroa J, et al. Mustard allergy confirmed by double-blind placebo-controlled food challenges: clinical features and cross-reactivity with mugwort pollen and plant-derived foods. *Allergy* 60:48, 2005.

Fleischer DM, et al. Peanut allergy: recurrence and its management. *J Allergy Clin Immunol.* 114:1195, 2004.

Frankland AW, Pumphrey RS. Acute allergic reactions to foods and cross reactivity between foods. In: Brostoff J, Challacombe S, eds. *Food allergy and intolerance.* 2nd ed. London: Saunders, 2002.

Garcia-Careaga M Jr, Kerner JA Jr. Gastrointestinal manifestations of food allergies in pediatric patients. *Nutr Clin Pract.* 20:526, 2005.

Geha R, et al. Review of alleged reaction to monosodium glutamate and outcome of a multicenter double-blind placebo-controlled study. *J Nutri.* 130:1058S, 2000.

Gonzalez-Quintela A, et al. Alcohol, IgE and allergy. *Addict Biol.* 9:195, 2004.

Goodman RE, et al. Assessing genetically modified crops to minimize the risk of increased food allergy: a review. *Int Arch Allergy Immunol.* 137:153, 2005.

Guida B, et al. Histamine plasma levels and elimination diet in chronic idiopathic urticaria. *Euro J Clin Nutri.* 54:155, 2000.

Hefle SL, Taylor SL. Food allergy and the food industry. *Curr Allergy Asthma Rep.* 4:55, 2004

Isolauri E, et al. Breastfeeding of allergic infants. *J Pediatr.* 134:27, 1999.

Jarvinen K, et al. Cow's milk challenge through human milk evokes immune responses in infants with cow's milk allergy. *J Pediatr.* 135:506, 1999.

Kaplan AP. Chronic urticaria: pathogenesis and treatment. *J Allergy Clin Immunol.* 114:465, 2004.

Kim K, Hussain H. Prevalence of food allergy in 137 latex-allergic patients. *Allergy Asthma Proc.* 20:95, 1999.

Latcham F, et al. A consistent pattern of minor immunodeficiency and subtle enteropathy in children with multiple food allergy. *J Pediatr.* 143:39, 2003.

Lehrer SB. Genetic modification of food allergens. *Ann Allergy Asthma Immunol.* 93:S19, 2004.

Maher TJ. Pharmacological actions of food and drink. In Brostoff J, Challacombe S. *Food allergy and intolerance.* 2nd ed. London: Saunders, 2002.

Martens M. Safety evaluation of genetically modified foods. *Int Arch Occup Environ Health.* 73:S14, 2000.

Mastalerz L, et al. Mechanism of chronic urticaria exacerbation by aspirin. Mechanism of chronic urticaria exacerbation by aspirin. *Curr Allergy Asthma Rep.* 5:277, 2005.

Matsuo H, et al. Exercise and aspirin increase levels of circulating gliadin peptides in patients with wheat-dependent exercise-induced anaphylaxis. *Clin Exp Allergy.* 35:461, 2005.

Mittag D, et al. Immunoglobulin E-reactivity of wheat-allergic subjects (baker's asthma, food allergy, wheat-dependent, exercise-induced anaphylaxis) to wheat protein fractions with different solubility and digestibility. *Mol Nutr Food Res.* 48:380, 2004.

Monroe E. Review of H1 antihistamines in the treatment of chronic idiopathic urticaria. *Cutis* 76:118, 2005.

Munoz-Furlong A. Food allergy in schools: concerns for allergists, pediatricians, parents, and school staff. *Ann Allergy Asthma Immunol.* 93:S47, 2004.

Pastorello EA, Ortolani C. Oral allergy syndrome. In: Metcalf D, et al, eds. *Food allergy: adverse reactions to foods and food additives.* 2nd ed. Cambridge: Blackwell Science, 1997.

Perkin J. The latex and food allergy connection. *J Am Diet Assoc.* 100:1381, 2000.

Perry TT, et al. Risk of oral food challenges. *J Allergy Clin Immunol.* 114:1164, 2004.

Scurlock AM, Burks AW. Peanut allergenicity. *Ann Allergy Asthma Immunol.* 93:S12, 2004.

Shimamoto SR, Bock SA. Update on the clinical features of food-induced anaphylaxis. *Curr Opin Allergy Clin Immunol.* 2:211, 2002.

Sicherer SH, et al. Prevalence of peanut and tree nut allergy in the United States determined by means of a random digit dial telephone survey: a 5-year follow-up study. *J Allergy Clin Immunol.* 112:1203, 2003.

Stone KD. Advances in pediatric allergy. *Curr Opin Pediatr.* 16:571, 2004.

Tan B, et al. Severe food allergies by skin contact. *Ann Allergy Asthma Immunol.* 86:583, 2001.

Tucke J, et al. Latex type I sensitization and allergy in children with atopic dermatitis. Evaluation of cross-reactivity to some foods. *Pediatr Allergy Immunol.* 10:160, 1999.

Winbery SL, Lieberman PL. Histamine and antihistamines in anaphylaxis. Histamine and antihistamines in anaphylaxis. *Clin Allergy Immunol.* 17:287, 2002.

MÉNIÈRE'S SYNDROME

NUTRITIONAL ACUITY RANKING: LEVEL 1

DEFINITIONS AND BACKGROUND

A rare disease of unknown origin, Ménière's syndrome affects the inner ear and causes disturbed balance. Signs and symptoms include rapid onset, fluctuating hearing loss, tinnitus with roaring sensation, vertigo, nausea and vomiting, and blurred vision. Patient may have a history of otitis media, smoking, allergies, leukemia, or atherosclerosis. Attacks may last from a few hours to several days. Vertigo causes disability in many patients with Ménière's disease.

Sodium restriction and diuretic treatment are early management measures for Ménière's disease (Minor et al, 2004; Devaiah and Ator, 2000). Patients with possible Ménière's disease should be treated with aggressive medical therapy to prevent disease progression.

INTERVENTION: OBJECTIVES

- Correct nausea and vomiting; replace any electrolyte losses.
- Avoid or decrease edema.
- Decrease fluid retention, which can aggravate an attack.
- Omit any known food allergens from the diet.

INTERVENTION: FOOD AND NUTRITION

- Low-sodium diet may be useful.
- Restrict fluid to reduce pressure on the labyrinth, unless contraindicated for other reasons (such as history of dehydration).
- Use a multivitamin-mineral supplement and foods that are nutrient dense. Intakes of vitamins A, B-complex (especially B_{12}), C, and D, riboflavin, niacin, folate, magnesium, and calcium may be important as well. Calcium and vitamin D strengthen the bones of the inner ear. Folate and vitamins B_6 and B_{12} reduce high levels of homocysteine, which can reduce blood flow to the cochlea. Vitamin B_{12} also protects the nerves of the ear.
- Provide a diet that is free of known allergens and is specific for the individual. Some people report feeling better after eliminating caffeine, for example.

CLINICAL INDICATORS

Clinical/History		
Height	Temp	H & H, serum Fe
Weight	BP	Alb
BMI	**Lab Work**	Electrocochleography
Diet history	Chol, Trig	Serum Na++, K+
Known allergies	IgE	I & O

Common Drugs Used and Potential Side Effects

- Diuretics are used to reduce edema in the ear.
- Gentamicin has been shown to be useful (Minor et al, 2004).
- Anticholinergics, such as atropine or epinephrine, may be used. Cardiac output is increased through an increased heart rate.
- Diazepam (Valium) may cause nausea, fatigue, and other effects. Limit caffeine.
- Antihistamines may be used. Antivert (Meclizine HCl) is an antihistamine that helps with dizziness. Dry mouth may result.
- Vasodilators may be used to dilate the blood vessels.
- Chronic use of nonsteroidal anti-inflammaotry drugs (ibuprofen, etc.) and antibiotics may damage the inner ear, which should be avoided.

Herbs, Botanicals, and Supplements

- Herbs and botanicals may be used; identify and monitor side effects. For earache: ephedra, goldenseal, forsythia, gentian, garlic, honeysuckle, and Echinacea are sometimes recommended but have not been proven as effective. For tinnitus: black cohosh, sesame, goldenseal, and spinach have been suggested; no long-term studies are on record that prove effectiveness.
- Gingko biloba is approved for use to treat tinnitus in Europe. More research is needed.
- Counsel about use of herbal teas, especially regarding toxic substances.

INTERVENTION: NUTRITION EDUCATION, COUNSELING, CARE MANAGEMENT

- Discuss how a balanced diet can affect general health status.
- Discuss sources of sodium and hidden ingredients that could aggravate the condition.
- Relaxation and biofeedback techniques may be useful for enhancing pain tolerance.

For More Information

- Ear Surgery Center
  http://www.earsurgery.org/meniere.html

MÉNIÈRE'S SYNDROME—CITED REFERENCES

Devaiah A, Ator G. Clinical indicators useful in predicting response to the medical management of Ménière's disease. *Laryngoscope* 110:1861, 2000.

Minor LB, et al. Ménière's disease. *Curr Opin Neurol.* 17:9, 2004.

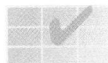

FOODBORNE ILLNESS

FOODBORNE ILLNESS

NUTRITIONAL ACUITY RANKING: LEVEL 1 (PREVENTIVE COUNSELING); LEVEL 2 (CORRECTIVE THERAPY)

DEFINITIONS AND BACKGROUND

True cases of foodborne illness are gastrointestinal insults or infections/intoxications resulting from contaminated beverages or food. Millions of cases occur annually, but only a few hundred are reported. The Centers for Disease Control report that there are millions of cases each year in the United States (http://www.cdc.gov/). Most vulnerable to foodborne diseases are elderly people, pregnant women, immune-compromised people, and children. Bacterial pathogens cause the largest percentage of outbreaks; chemical agents, viruses, and parasites are often implicated. In addition, multistate outbreaks caused by contaminated produce and outbreaks caused by *Escherichia coli* O157:H7 remain a concern (Olsen, 2000). See Table 2-12.

TABLE 2-12 **Bacteria That Cause Foodborne Illness**

Source of illness: Raw and undercooked meat and poultry

Symptoms: Abdominal pain, diarrhea, nausea, and vomiting

Bacteria: *Campylobacter jejuni, Escherichia coli* 0157:H7, *Listeria monocytogenes, Salmonella*

Source of illness: Raw (unpasteurized) milk and dairy products, such as soft cheeses

Symptoms: Nausea and vomiting, fever, abdominal cramps, and diarrhea

Bacteria: *L. monocytogenes, Salmonella, Shigella, Staphylococcus aureus, C. jejuni*

Source of illness: Raw or undercooked eggs. Raw eggs may not be recognized in some foods such as homemade hollandaise sauce, caesar and other salad dressings, tiramisu, homemade ice cream, homemade mayonnaise, cookie dough, and frostings.

Symptoms: Nausea and vomiting, fever, abdominal cramps, and diarrhea

Bacteria: *Salmonella enteriditis*

Source of illness: Raw or undercooked shellfish

Symptoms: Chills, fever, and collapse

Bacteria: *Vibrio vulnificus, V. parahaemolyticus*

Source of illness: Improperly canned goods and smoked or salted fish

Symptoms: Double vision, inability to swallow, difficulty speaking, and inability to breathe (seek medical help right away!)

Bacteria: *Clostridium botulinum*

Source of illness: Fresh or minimally processed produce

Symptoms: Diarrhea, nausea, and vomiting

Bacteria: *E. coli* 0157:H7, *L. monocytogenes, Salmonella, Shigella, Yersinia enterocolitica*, viruses, and parasites

Source: http://digestive.niddk.nih.gov/ddiseases/pubs/bacteria/#10, accessed February, 1, 2006.

Pathogens often transmitted via food contaminated by infected food handlers are *Salmonella typhi* and other species, *Shigella, Staphylococcus aureus, Streptococcus pyogenes*, hepatitis A virus, norovirus, *Listeria*, and *E. coli* O157:H7. Personal hygiene is one of the most important steps in food safety. The Centers for Disease Control and most health departments require that food handlers and preparers with gastroenteritis ***not*** work until 2 or 3 days after they feel better. Strict hand washing after using the bathroom and before handling food items is important in preventing contamination. Food handlers who were recently sick can be given different duties in the foodservice operation so that they do not have to handle food.

An outbreak occurs when when two or more individuals develop the same symptoms over the same time period. Infants and children younger than age 6, people with chronic illnesses (such as HIV infection or cancer), pregnant women, and elderly individuals are most at risk. Nausea, vomiting, diarrhea, abdominal cramping, vision problems, fever, chills, dizziness, and headaches may occur. Some people attribute their symptoms mistakenly to "stomach flu." Table 2-13 lists the most common foodborne illnesses and their onset and duration.

INTERVENTION: OBJECTIVES

- Allow the GI tract to rest after rehydration; progress diet as tolerated.
- Prepare and store all foods using safe food-handling practices and good personal hygiene. Temperatures should be maintained below 40°F or above 140°F for safe handling, storage, and holding.
- Teach the importance of handwashing, care of food contact surfaces, and insect or rodent extermination. This is especially important in foodservice operations where members of the public are fed.
- Any person operating a foodservice operation should know and use Hazard Analysis and Critical Control Point (HACCP) procedures to evaluate critical control points where foodborne illness risk is high and use precautions and safeguards (McCluskey, 2004). Careful monitoring is recommended. For the aging population in particular, barriers against the use of HACCP should be minimized (Strohbehn et al, 2004).
- Sanitize all surfaces before food preparation; sanitize after each food item is prepared when using the same surface (e.g., cutting boards and slicers). See Table 2-14 for more safe food practices. A consumer website is available as well at http://www.cfsan.fda.gov/~dms/qa-topfd.html.

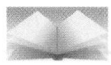

TABLE 2-13 Types of Foodborne Illness

Illness	Signs and Symptoms	Onset and Duration	Causes and Prevention	Comments
Bacillus cereus	Watery diarrhea, abdominal cramping, vomiting.	6–15 hours after consumption of contaminated food. Duration = 24 hours in most instances.	Meats, milk, vegetables, and fish have been associated with the diarrheal type. Vomiting-type outbreaks have generally been associated with rice products; potato, pasta, and cheese products. Food mixtures such as sauces, puddings, soups, casseroles, pastries, and salads may also be a source.	*Bacillus cereus* is a gram-positive, aerobic spore former.
Campylobacter jejuni	Diarrhea (often bloody), fever, and abdominal cramping are the key symptoms.	2–5 days after exposure. Duration = 2–10 days.	Drinking raw milk or eating raw or undercooked meat, shellfish, or poultry. To prevent exposure, avoid raw milk and cook all meats and poultry thoroughly. It is safest to drink only pasteurized milk. The bacteria may also be found in tofu or raw vegetables. Hand washing is important for prevention. Wash hands with soap before handling raw foods of animal origin, after handling raw foods of animal origin, and before touching anything else. Prevent cross-contamination in the kitchen. Proper refrigeration and sanitation are also essential.	Top source of foodborne illness. Some people develop antibodies to it, but others do not. In persons with compromised immune systems, it may spread to the blood stream and cause sepsis. It may lead to arthritis or to Guillain-Barré syndrome (GBS); 40% of GBS cases in the United States are caused by campylobacteriosis, which affects the nerves of the body beginning several weeks after the diarrheal illness, can lead to paralysis that lasts several weeks, and usually requires intensive care.
Clostridium botulinum	Muscle paralysis caused by the bacterial toxin: double or blurred vision, drooping eyelids, slurred speech, difficulty swallowing, dry mouth, and muscle weakness. Infants with botulism appear lethargic, feed poorly, are constipated, and have a weak cry and poor muscle tone.	In foodborne botulism, symptoms generally begin 18–36 hours after eating contaminated food; can occur as early as 6 hours or as late as 10 days. Duration = days or months.	Home-canned foods with low acid content, such as asparagus, green beans, beets, and corn. Outbreaks have occurred from more unusual sources such as chopped garlic in oil, chile peppers, tomatoes, improperly handled baked potatoes wrapped in aluminum foil, and home-canned or fermented fish. Persons who do home canning should follow strict hygienic procedures to reduce contamination of foods. Oils infused with garlic or herbs should be refrigerated. Potatoes that have been baked while wrapped in aluminum foil should be kept hot until served or refrigerated. Because high temperatures destroy the botulism toxin, persons who eat home-canned foods should boil the food for 10 minutes before eating.	If untreated, these symptoms may progress to cause paralysis of the arms, legs, trunk, and respiratory muscles; long-term ventilator support may be needed. Throw out bulging, leaking, or dented cans and jars that are leaking. Safe home canning can be obtained from county extension services or from the U.S. Department of Agriculture. Honey can contain spores of *Clostridium botulinum* and has been a source of infection for infants; children younger than 12 months old should not be fed honey.

(continued)

TABLE 2-13 Types of Foodborne Illness *(continued)*

Illness	Signs and Symptoms	Onset and Duration	Causes and Prevention	Comments
Clostridium perfringens	Nausea with vomiting, diarrhea, and signs of acute gastroenteritis lasting 1 day.	Within 6–24 hours from the ingestion.	Ingestion of canned meats, contaminated dried mixes, gravy, stews, refried beans, meat products, and unwashed vegetables. Cook foods thoroughly. Leftovers must be reheated properly or discarded.	
Cryptosporidium parvum	Watery stools, diarrhea, nausea, vomiting, slight fever, and stomach cramps.	2–10 days after being infected.	Contaminated food from poor handling. Hand washing is important.	Protozoa cause diarrhea among immunocompromised patients.
Enterotoxigenic *Escherichia coli* (ETEC)	Watery diarrhea, abdominal cramps, low-grade fever, nausea, and malaise.	With high infective dose, diarrhea can be induced within 24 hours.	Contamination of water with human sewage may lead to contamination of foods. Infected food handlers may also contaminate foods. Dairy products such as semi-soft cheeses may cause problems, but this is rare.	More common with travel to other countries. In infants or debilitated elderly persons, electrolyte replacement therapy may be necessary.
E. coli 0157:H7; enterohemorrhagic *E. coli* (EHEC)	Hemorrhagic colitis (painful, bloody diarrhea).	Onset is slow, usually approximately 3–8 days after ingestion. Duration = 5–10 days.	Undercooked ground beef and meats, from unprocessed apple cider, or from unwashed fruits and vegetables. Sometimes water sources. Alfalfa sprouts, unpasteurized fruit juices, dry-cured salami, lettuce, game meat, and cheese curds. Cook meats thoroughly, use only pasteurized milk, and wash all produce well.	Antibiotics are not used because they spread the toxin further. The condition may progress to hemolytic anemia, thrombocytopenia, and acute renal failure requiring dialysis and transfusions. Hemolytic uremic syndrome can be fatal, especially in young children. There are several outbreaks each year, particularly from catering operations, church events, and family picnics. *E. coli* 0157:H7 can survive in refrigerated acid foods for weeks (Mayerhauser, 2001).
Listeria monocytogenes (LM)	Mild fever, headache, vomiting, and severe illness in pregnancy; sepsis in the immunocompromised patient; meningoencephalitis in infants; and febrile gastroenteritis in adults.	Onset is 2–30 days. Duraction is variable.	Processed, ready-to-eat products such as undercooked hot dogs, deli or lunchmeats, and unpasteurized dairy products. Postpasteurization contamination of soft cheeses such as feta or Brie, milk, and commercial coleslaw. Cross-contamination between food surfaces has also been a problem. Use pasteurized milk and cheeses; wash produce before use. Reheat foods to proper temperatures. Wash hands with hot, soapy water after handling these ready-to-eat foods. Discard foods by their expiration dates.	May be fatal. Caution must be used by pregnant women, who may pass the infection on to their unborn child (Woteki, 2001).

(continued)

TABLE 2-13 Types of Foodborne Illness *(continued)*

Illness	Signs and Symptoms	Onset and Duration	Causes and Prevention	Comments
Norovirus	Gastroenteritis with nausea, vomiting, and/or diarrhea accompanied by abdominal cramps. Headache, fever/chills, and muscle aches may also be present.	24–48 hours after ingestion of the virus, but can appear as early as 12 hours after exposure.	Foods can be contaminated either by direct contact with contaminated hands or work surfaces that are contaminated with stool or vomit, or by tiny droplets from nearby vomit that can travel through air to land on food. Although the virus cannot multiply outside of human bodies, once on food or in water, it can cause illness. Most cases occur on cruise ships.	Symptoms are usually brief and last only 1 or 2 days. However, during that brief period, people can feel very ill and vomit, often violently and without warning, many times a day. Drink liquids to prevent dehydration.
Salmonella	Diarrhea, fever, and abdominal cramps.	12–72 hours after infection. Duration = usually 4–7 days.	Ingestion of raw or undercooked meat, poultry, fish, eggs, unpasteurized dairy products; unwashed fruits and raw vegetables (melons and sprouts). Prevent by thorough cooking, proper sanitation, and hygiene.	There are many different kinds of *Salmonella* bacteria. *Salmonella typhimurium* and *Salmonella enteritidis* are the most common in the United States. Most people recover without treatment, but some have diarrhea that is so severe that the patient needs to be hospitalized. This patient must be treated promptly with antibiotics. The elderly, infants, and those with impaired immune systems are more likely to have a severe illness.
Shigellosis	Bloody diarrhea, fever, and stomach cramps.	24–48 hours after exposure. Duration = 4–7 days.	Milk and dairy products; cold mixed salads such as egg, tuna, chicken, potato, and meat salads. Proper cooking, reheating, and maintenance of holding temperatures should aid in prevention; careful hand washing is essential.	This is caused by a group of bacteria called *Shigella*. May be severe in young children and the elderly. Severe infection with high fever may be associated with seizures in children younger than 2 years old.
Staphylococcus aureus	Nausea, vomiting, retching, abdominal cramping, and prostration.	Within 1–6 hours; rarely fatal. Duration = 1–2 days.	Meat, pork, eggs, poultry, tuna salad, prepared salads, gravy, stuffing, cream-filled pastries. Cooking does not destroy the toxin. Proper handling and hygiene are crucial for prevention.	Refrigerate foods promptly during preparation and after meal service.
Streptococcus pyogenes	Sore and red throat, pain on swallowing, tonsillitis, high fever, headache, nausea, vomiting, malaise, rhinorrhea; occasionally a rash occurs.	Onset = 1–3 days.	Milk, ice cream, eggs, steamed lobster, ground ham, potato salad, egg salad, custard, rice pudding, and shrimp salad. In almost all cases, the foodstuffs were allowed to stand at room temperature for several hours between preparation and consumption.	Entrance into the food is the result of poor hygiene, ill food handlers, or the use of unpasteurized milk. Complications are rare. Treated with antibiotics.

(continued)

TABLE 2-13 Types of Foodborne Illness *(continued)*

Illness	Signs and Symptoms	Onset and Duration	Causes and Prevention	Comments
Vibrio vulnificus	Vomiting, diarrhea, or both. Illness is mild.	Gastroenteritis occurs about 16 hours after eating contaminated food. Duration = about 48 hours.	Seafood, especially raw clams and oysters, that has been contaminated with human pathogens. Although oysters can only be harvested legally from waters free from fecal contamination, even these can be contaminated with *V. vulnificus* because the bacterium is naturally present.	This is a bacterium in the same family as those that cause cholera. It yields a norovirus. It may be fatal in immunocompromised individuals.
Yersinia enterocolitica	Common symptoms in children are fever, abdominal pain, and diarrhea, which is often bloody. In older children and adults, right-sided abdominal pain and fever may be predominant symptom and may be confused with appendicitis.	1–2 days after exposure. Duration = 1–3 weeks or longer.	Contaminated food, especially raw or undercooked pork products. Postpasteurization contamination of chocolate milk, reconstituted dry milk, pasteurized milk, and tofu are also high-risk foods. Cold storage does not kill the bacteria. Cook meats thoroughly; use only pasteurized milk. Proper hand washing is also important.	Infectious disease caused by the bacterium *Yersinia*. In the United States, most human illness is caused by *Y. enterocolitica*. It occurs most often in young children. In a small proportion of cases, complications such as skin rash, joint pains, and spread of bacteria to the bloodstream can occur.

From: http://www.cdc.gov/az.do and http://www.cfsan.fda.gov/~mow/intro.html.

- Figure 2-11 provides a Food Safety Pyramid of how issues are handled by health departments and the Centers for Disease Control and Prevention (CDC).

INTERVENTION: FOOD AND NUTRITION

- For patients with extreme diarrhea or vomiting, feed with intravenous glucose (NPO) until progress has been made. Oral rehydration therapy may be a useful adjunct treatment in the recovery process.
- Start with bland or soft foods and then progress to a normal diet. Prolonged inability to eat orally may require tube feeding.

CLINICAL INDICATORS

Clinical/History

Height
Weight
BMI
Usual weight
Weight loss/changes during illness
Diet history
Vomiting
Diarrhea
Nausea
Abdominal cramps
Blood in stools?
Presence of parasites in stool?
Fever?
Timing of symptoms after suspected meal
Signs of dehydration; I & O

Lab Work

Na+, K+
Chloride (Cl−)
H & H, serum Fe

Common Drugs Used and Potential Side Effects

- Hydrochloric acid protects the body against pathogens ingested with food or water. A gastric fluid pH of 1 to 2 is deleterious to many microbial pathogens; however, the neutralization of gastric acid by antacids or the inhibition of acid secretion by various drugs can alter stomach pH and may increase the risk of acquiring food- or waterborne illnesses (Smith, 2003).
- Octreotide (Sandostatin) may be used parenterally only. It may alter fat absorption and fat-soluble vitamin absorption.
- Puromycin, erythromycin, or a fluoroquinolone may be prescribed.
- For *Salmonella*, ampicillin, gentamicin, trimethoprim/sulfamethoxazole, or ciprofloxacin may be used.
- *V. vulnificus* infection is treated with doxycycline or ceftazidime.

TABLE 2-14 Safe Food Handling and Food Safety Guidelines

Food Preparation

- Clean hands, food contact surfaces, and fruits and vegetables. Meat and poultry should not be washed.
- Because bacteria are commonly found on foods such as cantaloupe, cilantro, and imported produce, wash all fresh fruits and vegetables. Scrub the outside of produce such as melons and cucumbers before cutting. Scallions have been linked to hepatitis A outbreak; cook them thoroughly.
- Discard cracked eggs; avoid using products from dented cans.
- Avoid food preparation when sick with viral or bacterial infections; use gloves if needed.
- Sanitize work surfaces and sponges daily with a mild bleach solution (2 teaspoons per quart of water is sufficient). However, if a work surface comes into contact with raw food, it should be sanitized after contact with each food, just like cutting boards.
- Separate raw, cooked, and ready-to-eat foods while shopping, preparing, and storing foods.
- Sanitize work surfaces after each food. Ideally, keep one board for poultry, another for meats, and another for produce to prevent cross-contamination. Discard cutting boards that are badly damaged.
- Chill (refrigerate) perishable food promptly and defrost foods properly. Thaw meats and poultry in the refrigerator, not at room temperature. If necessary, thaw in a sink with cold running water that allows continuous drainage or thaw quickly in the microwave and use immediately.
- Do not partially cook meat or poultry in advance of final preparation. Bacteria may still grow rampantly.
- Cook foods to a safe temperature to kill micro-organisms. Cook beef to proper internal temperature of 160°F, pork to 165°F, and poultry to 175°F. Cook hamburger to the proper temperature of 165°F; "pink in the middle, cooked too little." Monitor internal temperatures with an accurate food thermometer placed correctly into the meat or poultry.
- Boil water used for drinking when necessary; hold at boiling temperature for 1 minute.
- Avoid raw or partially cooked eggs, raw or undercooked fish or shellfish, and raw or undercooked meats because of potential foodborne illnesses.
- Avoid raw (unpasteurized) milk or products made from it.
- Avoid serving unpasteurized juices and raw sprouts.

Holding and Serving Foods

- Hold and serve foods at 140–165°F during meal service.
- Reheat foods to at least 165°F. Discard leftovers after the first reheating process.
- Keep hot foods above 140°F and cold foods below 40°F.
- Discard cooked foods that are left at room temperature for more than 2 hours.
- Reheat home-canned foods appropriately. In institutional settings, do not allow home-cooked foods at all.
- Only serve certain deli meats and frankfurters that have been reheated to steaming hot temperature.
- Keep pet foods and utensils separate from those for human use.
- Use clean plates and separate utensils between raw and cooked foods.
- Cool foods quickly in shallow pans (2–4 inches deep). Temperature should reach 70°F within 2 hours. If food has not cooled to that level, place in the freezer for a short time. Then, wrap lightly and return to refrigerator.

Other Tips

- When traveling, avoid tap water and ice made from tap water, uncooked produce such as lettuce, and raw or undercooked seafood.
- Airline water may not be free from contamination. Use of bottled water is recommended. Coffee and tea may not be hot enough to kill all bacteria.
- See also the Fight BAC guidelines at http://www.fightbac.org/.

Herbs, Botanicals, and Supplements

- Note that herbs and botanicals themselves could be a source of foodborne bacteria and thus exacerbate an existing foodborne infection. If herbs and botanicals are used, identify and monitor for potential contamination and side effects.
- Counsel about use of herbal teas, especially regarding toxic substances.

INTERVENTION: NUTRITION EDUCATION, COUNSELING, CARE MANAGEMENT

- Encourage safe methods of food handling (see Table 2-15). More males, African Americans, and adults between 30 and 54 years consumed raw/undercooked ground beef than any other demographic segments; males, Caucasians, Hispanics, and young adults between 18 and 29 years old were more likely to engage in poor hygienic

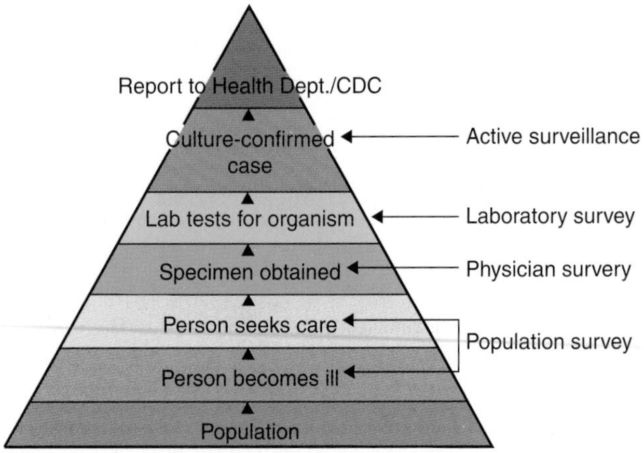

Figure 2-11 Food safety pyramid for Health Departments and the Centers for Disease Control and Prevention (CDC).

practices in a meta-analysis of practices (Patil et al, 2004). Errors in methods of washing hands, utensils, and preparation surfaces between food preparation tasks are common, and many do not use thermometers to evaluate doneness (Kendall et al, 2004).

- Monitor water supply for odors or color changes that are unexpected; report to authorities.
- Discuss ways to prevent further episodes of foodborne illness. See Table 2-14 for food safety guidelines.
- Teach awareness that commercial mayonnaise, salad dressings, and sauces appear to be safe due to their content of acetic acid and lesser amounts of citric or lactic acids (Smittle, 2000).
- For prevention of parasite infestation (such as *Giardia*), sewage treatment, proper hand washing, and consumption of bottled water can be preventive (Kucik et al, 2004). See Section 7 for more details.
- Some consumers are concerned about the safety of food irradiation, genetically modified foods (GMOs), and allergens. Biotechnology has developed food crops that are more resistant to pests and have better nutritional value as well as having longer shelf-life for food safety. Detailed information is available at the government website http://vm.cfsan.fda.gov/~lrd/bioeme.html. Nutrition professionals should feel comfortable addressing these issues to reassure the public.

TABLE 2-15 Recommended Refrigerator Food Storage

Food	Time Period
Butter	1–3 months
Cheese, hard	6 months unopened; 3–4 weeks opened
Cheese, soft	1 week
Chicken, turkey	1–2 days
Eggs in shell	3–5 weeks
Eggs, raw	2–4 days
Fish, cooked	3–4 days
Fish, raw	1–2 days
Gravy	1–2 days
Hamburger, raw	1–2 days
Juices, chilled	3 weeks unopened, 7–10 days opened
Luncheon meat	3–5 days opened, 2 weeks in sealed package
Margarine	4–5 months
Milk	1 week
Pizza	3–4 days
Roast or steak	3–5 days (uncooked)
Sausage, raw	1–2 days
Sausage, smoked	1 week
Shellfish, fresh	1–2 days
Soups, stews	3–4 days
Yogurt	1–2 weeks

For More Information

- American Dietetic Association Home Food Safety Program
  http://www.homefoodsafety.org/index.jsp
- Biotechnology and Genetic Engineering of Foods
  http://vm.cfsan.fda.gov/~lrd/bioeme.html
- Bioterrorism and Food Safety Legislation
  http://www.cfsan.fda.gov/~dms/fsterr.html
- Botulism
  http://www.cdc.gov/ncidod/dbmd/diseaseinfo/botulism_g.htm
- Federal USDA—Food Safety Research
  http://www.nal.usda.gov/fsrio/new/release.htm
- Foodborne Diseases Active Surveillance Network
  CDC's Emerging Infections Program
  http://www.cdc.gov/foodnet/
- Food and Drug Administration
  Center for Food Safety and Applied Nutrition (CFSAN)
  http://www.cfsan.fda.gov/list.html
- Food and Drug Administration Seafood Hotline
  http://vm.cfsan.fda.gov/seafood1.html
- Fight BAC
  http://www.fightbac.org/
  http://www.pueblo.gsa.gov/cic_text/food/fight-back/fightbac.htm
- Government–Nutrition and Food Safety Information
  http://www.nutrition.gov/
- Government Food Safety Website
  http://www.foodsafety.gov/
- International Food Safety Sites
  http://www.foodsafety.gov/?7Efsg/fsgintl.html
- National Food Safety Programs
  http://www.foodsafety.gov/~dms/fs-toc.html
- North Carolina State University
  http://www.ces.ncsu.edu/depts/foodsci/agentinfo/
- USDA Food borne Illness Education Information Center
  http://www.nal.usda.gov/fnic/foodborne/about.html
- USDA Meat and Poultry Hotline
  http://www.fsis.usda.gov/Food_Safety_Education/USDA_Meat_&_Poultry_Hotline/index.asp
- US Food Safety and Inspection Service (FSIS)
  http://www.fsis.usda.gov/
- Water Quality Association
  http://www.wqa.org/

FOODBORNE ILLNESS—CITED REFERENCES

Kendall PA, et al. Observation versus self-report: validation of a consumer food behavior questionnaire. *J Food Prot.* 67:2578, 2004.

Kucik CJ, et al. Common intestinal parasites. *Am Fam Physician.* 69:1161, 2004.

Mayerhauser C. Survival of enterohemorrhagic *Escherichia coli* O157:H7 in retail mustard. *J Food Prot.* 64:783, 2001.

McCluskey KM. Implementing hazard analysis critical control points. *J Am Diet Assoc.* 104:1699, 2004.

Olsen S, et al. Surveillance for food borne disease outbreaks–United States, 1993–1997. *Morbid Mortal Wkly Rep CDC Surveil Sum.* 49:1, 2000.

Patil SR, et al. An application of meta-analysis in food safety consumer research to evaluate consumer behaviors and practices. *J Food Prot.* 67:2587, 2004.

Smith JL. The role of gastric acid in preventing foodborne disease and how bacteria overcome acid conditions. *J Food Prot.* 66:1292, 2003.

Smittle R. Microbiological safety of mayonnaise, salad dressings, and sauces produced in the United States. *J Food Protection.* 63:1144, 2000.

Strohbehn CH, et al. Food safety practice and HACCP implementation: perceptions of registered dietitians and dietary managers. *J Am Diet Assoc.* 101:1692, 2004.

Woteki C. Dietitians can prevent listeriosis. *J Am Diet Assoc.* 101:285, 2001.

SECTION 3

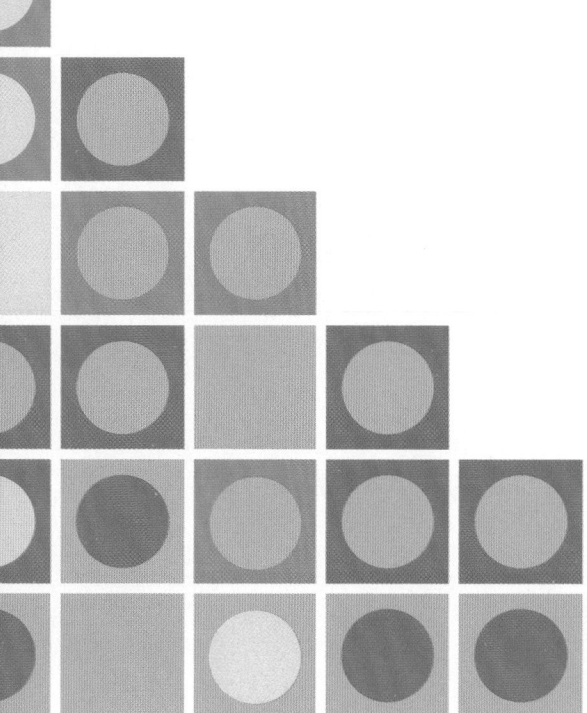

Pediatrics: Birth Defects and Genetic and Acquired Disorders

CHIEF ASSESSMENT FACTORS (SEE ALSO TABLES 3-1 AND 3-2)

Anthropometric:

- Birth Data (Weight, Length, Head Circumference, Size, Gestational Age)
- Growth Parameters: Current Height and Weight
  - Wt/age less than 10th percentile or more than 95th percentile
  - Ht/age less than 5th percentile
  - Wt/ht less than 5th percentile or more than 90th percentile
  - Head circumference less than 5th percentile (under 3 years of age)
- Birth Defects, Physical
- Unintentional Weight Loss
- Pubertal Staging (Tanner Stages), Skeletal Maturity Staging (Fig. 3-1 shows how to measure length of an infant properly)

Clinical:

- Congenital or Chromosomal Abnormalities, Inborn Errors of Metabolism
- Chronic Illnesses (Diabetes, Failure to Thrive, Developmental Delay, Kidney Disease, Malabsorption, HIV/AIDS, Trauma)
- Oral Lesions
- Recent Trauma, Surgery, Hospitalizations, and Acute Illnesses
- Symptoms of Depression, Pain or Dyspnea
- Recent Chemotherapy, Radiation, Surgery
- Protein–Energy Malnutrition
- Gastrointestinal Functioning, Nausea, Vomiting, Diarrhea, or Constipation, Other Digestive Problems or Poor Appetite Longer Than 3 Days
- Medications, Especially Anticonvulsants (affect vitamins C, K, D, and B-complex, and calcium); Stimulants Such as Ritalin (affect energy and protein intake, growth, appetite); Diuretics (affect potassium, magnesium, calcium, energy, and can cause GI problems); Antibiotics (affect energy, protein, minerals and can cause GI problems); Corticosteroids (affect calcium, phosphorus, glucose levels, and can cause weight gain or stifle growth); Sulfonamides (affect vitamin C, protein, folate, and iron); Tranquilizers (affect energy intake and can cause weight gain)

Dietary Issues and Feeding Skill:

- Feeding: Persons Involved, Length of Time, Feeding Method, Skill Level (*Continued on page 139*)

TABLE 3-1 Overview of Pediatric Disorder Assessments

Newborn Screening:

Mandated state newborn screening programs for the approximately 4 million infants born each year in the United States involve components of: (1) initial screening, (2) immediate follow-up testing of the screen-positive newborn, (3) diagnosis confirmation (true positive vs. false positive), (4) care, immediate and long term, and (5) evaluation of process and outcomes measures (Desposito et al, 2001).

Nutritional Screening and Assessment of Hospitalized Children:

Nutritional status affects a child's response to illness. Good nutrition is important for achieving normal growth and development. About 10–15% of children in the United States have special health care needs that require medical attention. Nutritional screening and assessment, where indicated, should be an integral part of the care for every pediatric patient (Mascarenhas et al, 1998). Simple nutritional risk screening tools can help identify children at risk for malnutrition during hospital stays. Malnutrition may exist in 25–33% of children admitted to a hospital. Nutritionally at risk patients may benefit from determination of resting energy expenditure by indirect calorimetry (Mascarenhas et al, 1998). Use of the age-, gender-, and disease-specific growth charts from the Centers for Disease Control and Prevention (CDC) is essential in assessing nutritional status and monitoring nutrition interventions. Accuracy is better when using trained personnel and appropriate equipment. Proper interventions and referrals are important for growth and optimal development. Efforts should be made to enhance appetite and intake in children who cannot eat at home with their families. Familiarity is important; hospitalized children enjoy home-like meals. Finally, it is important to screen for use of medications and dietary supplements, since their use is common (Harris, 2005; Nardella, 2002; Trahms and Pipes, 1997).

Serum cholesterol for children and adolescents should be monitored. If it is above 200 mg/dL, a fasting lipid profile is needed. If serum cholesterol is 170–199 mg/dL, take another total serum cholesterol, and average the two together. The goal is to achieve a total serum cholesterol less than 170 mg/dL (Carson et al, 2005).

Birth Defects (from March of Dimes, 2004):

Both genetic and environmental factors can cause birth defects. However, the causes of about 60–70% of birth defects currently are unknown. Some birth defects can be diagnosed before birth, using one or more prenatal tests including ultrasound, amniocentesis, and chorionic villus sampling (CVS). Ultrasound can help diagnose structural birth defects, such as spina bifida and heart and urinary tract defects. Amniocentesis and CVS are used to diagnose chromosomal abnormalities, such as Down syndrome. They also can detect, or rule out, numerous genetic birth defects that may be suspected because of family history or ethnic background. Estimated incidence of structural, metabolic, and other defects is as follows.

Structural:

Heart defects: 8–12 in 1000 births
Muscles and skeleton: 1 in 130 births
Genital and urinary tract: 1 in 135 births
Nervous system and eye: 1 in 235 births
Chromosomal syndromes: 1 in 600 births
Club foot: 1 in 735 births
Down syndrome (trisomy 21): 1 in 900 births
Respiratory tract: 1 in 900 births
Cleft lip/palate: 1 in 700 births
Anencephaly: 1 in 8000 births
Spina bifida: 1 in 2000 births

Metabolic:

Metabolic disorders: 1 in 3500 births
PKU: 1 in 15,000 births

Other:

Fetal alcohol syndrome: 1 in 1000 births
Untreated syphilis: 1 in 2000 births

(continued)

TABLE 3-1 Overview of Pediatric Disorder Assessments *(continued)*

Chronic Diarrhea:

Chronic diarrhea in infants under age 3 months may indicate inappropriate formulas, infection, use of too much juice, disaccharide deficiency, cow's milk or soymilk protein intolerance, cystic fibrosis, or immunodeficiency state. In infants aged 3–18 months, it might mean celiac disease, lactose deficiency, or inflammatory bowel disease. But gastrointestinal (GI) infection is the most common cause in children of all ages. Watery, explosive stools indicate sugar intolerance; foul-smelling, bulky stools indicate fat malabsorption. Marked weight loss indicates malabsorption, inflammatory bowel disease (IBD), hyperthyroidism, or malignancy.

Developmental Disabilities:

Proper assessment of nutritional status, feeding skills, and feeding behaviors, including positioning, is important. Various disability screening tools have been developed, which should screen for all major disabilities (i.e., physical, motor, sensory, and developmental delays). Gradually rewarding behaviors as they begin to match desired behaviors is known as "shaping" and is used commonly for these children. For those in whom measurement of height is difficult, arm span may be a reasonable substitute. Three developmental disabilities do not have mental retardation as a component—cerebral palsy, autism, and epilepsy. Plan care around the individual person: design the desired outcomes, determine necessary resources, and seek regular feedback on progress or obstacles. The roles of personal control, independence, and choice must be considered in all care plans.

For estimating energy needs of children with very low energy requirements (such as Down syndrome or Prader-Willi syndrome), use: low 7–9 kcal/cm; moderate 9–11 kcal/cm; or high 12–15 kcal/cm (Lucas, 2004, p. 41). In children whose weight is hard to maintain, catch-up growth is important with an emphasis on energy and protein.

Estimating Daily Energy Requirements (EER) and Total Energy Expenditure (TEE) (Institute of Medicine, 2002; Lucas, 2004)

Age (months)	Equation
0–3	$(89 \times Wt - 100) + 175$
4–6	$(89 \times Wt - 100) + 56$
7–12	$(89 \times Wt - 100) + 22$
13–35	$(89 \times Wt - 100) + 20$
Boys: Age (years)	**Equation**
3–8	$EER = 88.5 - 61.9 \times age\ (y) + PA \times (26.7 \times Wt + 903 \times Ht) + 20$
9–19	$EER = 88.5 - 61.9 \times age\ (y) + PA \times (26.7 \times Wt + 903 \times Ht) + 25$
3–19, overweight	$TEE = -114 - 50.9 \times age\ (y) + PA\ (19.5 \times Wt + 116.4 \times Ht)$
Girls: Age (years)	**Equation**
3–8	$EER = 135.3 - 30.8 \times age\ (y) + PA \times (10.0 \times Wt + 934 \times Ht) + 20$
9–19	$EER = 135.3 - 30.8 \times age\ (y) + PA \times (10.0 \times Wt + 934 \times Ht) + 25$
3–19, overweight	$TEE = 389 - 41.2 \times age\ (y) + PA \times (15.0 \times Wt + 701 \times Ht)$

Physical Activity (PA) Coefficients for Boys Aged 3–19 Years

Activity Level	Coefficient	
	Normal Wt	Overweight
Sedentary	1.0	1.0
Low active	1.13	1.12
Active	1.26	1.24
Very Active	1.42	1.45

Physical Activity (PA) Coefficients for Girls Aged 3–19 Years

Activity Level	Coefficient	
	Normal Wt	Overweight
Sedentary	1.0	1.00
Low active	1.16	1.18
Active	1.31	1.35
Very Active	1.56	1.60

(continued)

TABLE 3-1 Overview of Pediatric Disorder Assessments *(continued)*

Acceptable Macronutrient Ranges

	Range (% of energy)		
Age	CHO	Fat	Protein
Full-term infant	35–65	30–55	7–16
1–3 years	45–65	30–40	5–20
4–18 years	45–65	25–35	10–30

Pediatric Tube Feedings and TPN (see Section 17 also):

Tube feedings may be needed for children with prematurity, developmental delays, orofacial defects, cerebral palsy, anorexia nervosa, cystic fibrosis, inborn errors of metabolism, renal failure, HIV infection, and inflammatory bowel disorders. Home tube feeding promotes catch-up growth in most children (Kang et al, 1998). Many specific pediatric tube feedings are available. A percutaneous endoscopic gastrostomy may be a good alternative to a nasogastric tube in children with cholestasis and mild portal hypertension (Duche et al, 1999). Mothers of children with tube feedings expressed greater stress than mothers who did not have tube feedings to provide; they also received less support from family and friends. Include fathers, friends, etc., in training so this can be changed (Adams et al, 1999).

For TPN, special pediatric solutions are available. It may be possible to wean from TPN to tube or oral feeding in some conditions; for others, parenteral nutrition may be permanent. Consider that children cannot tolerate fasting as long as adults. Parenteral nutrition may be needed for children with biliary atresia, Hirschsprung's disease with enterocolitis, Crohn's disease or ulcerative colitis, short-bowel syndrome, GI ischemia, GI fistulas, severe burns or trauma, and bowel transplantation.

Neonatal Intensive Care Units:

Although there are almost 800 neonatal intensive care units (NICUs) in the United States, only about three quarters involve a registered dietitian (RD) in patient care, and one quarter have no RD involvement. In one survey, it was found that NICUs without RD involvement were more likely to provide full-term feedings to very low birth weight infants, a practice that can be detrimental for these patients (Olsen et al, 2005). In addition, the survey found that NICUs with full-time or part-time RD involvement provided fewer kcals and more protein in parenteral nutrition and more kcals and protein enterally (Olsen et al, 2005).

TABLE 3-2 Nutritional Risk Factors Associated with Selected Pediatric Disorders

	Underweight	Overweight	Short Stature	Low Energy Needs	High Energy Needs	Feeding Problems	Constipation	Chronic Meds
Autism spectrum disorders	X				X	X		X
Bronchopulmonary dysplasia	X	X			X	X		X
Cerebral palsy	X	X	X	X	X	X	X	X
Cystic fibrosis	X		X		X	X		
Down syndrome		X		X		X		
Fetal alcohol syndrome	X		X					
Heart disease, congenital	X				X	X		X
HIV infection, AIDS	X				X			X
Phenylketonuria	X					X		
Prader-Willi syndrome		X	X	X				
Prematurity, low birth weight	X		X		X	X		
Seizure disorder								X
Spina bifida; neural tube defects	X	X	X	X			X	X

Adapted from Baer M, Harris A. Pediatric nutrition assessment: identifying children at risk. *J Am Diet Assoc.* 97:107A, 1997.

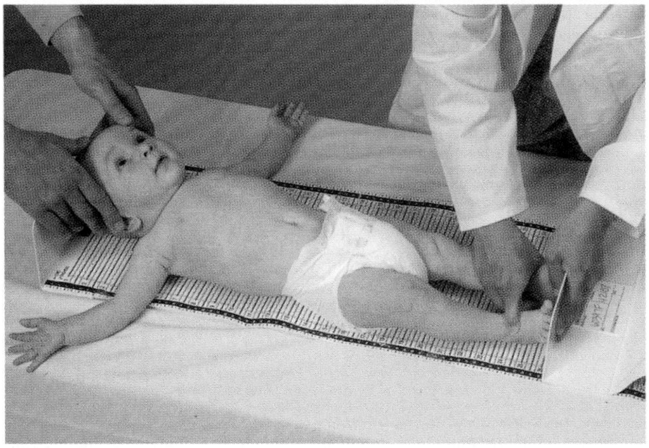

Figure 3-1 Measuring an infant. (From Bickley LS, Szilagyi, P. *Bates' guide to physical examination and history taking*. 8th ed. Philadelphia: Lippincott Williams & Wilkins, 2003.)

- Avoidance of Foods That Are Readily Aspirated
- Difficulty Chewing or Swallowing, Requiring Texture Modifications
- Coordination for Safe and Proper Chewing, Sucking, Swallowing
- Food Intake, Ability to Eat and Retain Food
- Preferences, Intolerances
- Multiple or Severe Food Allergies
- Special Formula or Supplements, Tube Feeding or Parenteral Nutrition

Behavioral and Psychosocial:

- Growth and Development Milestones
- Hunger and Satiety—Use of Food for Reward or as Pacifier
- Home Environment and Family Economics That Affect Access to Food
- Developmental Disorders: Chronic Disorders of Mental Development with Onset in Childhood; Such Disorders Are Now Classified as Mental Retardation, Learning Disorders, Motor Skills Disorder, Communication Disorders, or Pervasive Developmental Disorders

CITED REFERENCES

Adams R, et al. Maternal stress in caring for children with feeding disabilities: implications for health care providers. *J Am Diet Assoc.* 99:962, 1999.

Carson JAS, et al. *Cardiovascular nutrition: disease management and prevention.* Chicago: The American Dietetic Association, 2005.

Desposito F, et al. Survey of pediatrician practices in retrieving statewide authorized newborn screening results. *Pediatrics* 108:22, 2001.

Duche M, et al. Percutaneous endoscopic gastrostomy for continuous feeding in children with chronic cholestasis. *J Pediatr Gastroenterol Nutr.* 29:42, 1999.

Harris AB. Evidence of increasing dietary supplement use in children with special health care needs: Strategies for improving parent and professional communication. *J Am Diet Assoc.* 105:34, 2005.

Institute of Medicine. *Dietary reference intakes for energy, carbohydrate, fiber, fat, fatty acids, cholesterol, protein, and amino acids.* Washington, DC: National Academy of Sciences, 2002

Kang A, et al. Catch-up growth in children treated with home enteral nutrition. *Pediatrics* 102:951, 1998.

Lucas B, ed. *Children with special care needs: nutrition care handbook.* Chicago: The American Dietetic Association, 2004.

March of Dimes. March of Dimes homepage. Accessed December 27, 2004 at http://www.modimes.org/.

Mascarenhas M, Zemel B, Stallings V. Nutritional assessment in pediatrics. *Nutrition* 14:105, 1998.

Nardella M, et al. *Nutrition interventions for children with special health care needs.* Olympia, WA: Washington State Department of Health, 2002.

Olsen IE, et al. Dietitian involvement in the neonatal intensive care unit: more is better. *J Am Diet Assoc.* 105:1224, 2005.

Trahms CM, Pipes PL. *Nutrition in infancy and childhood.* 6th ed. New York, WCB-McGraw Hill, 1997

For More Information About Birth Defects and Genetic Disorders

- CDC Birth Defects Research
  http://www.cdc.gov/ncbddd/bd/research.htm
- March of Dimes
  http://www.modimes.org/
- National Center for Education in Maternal and Child Health
  http://www.ncemch.org/
- National Dissemination Center for Children with Disabilities
  http://www.nichcy.org/
- National Folic Acid Campaign
  http://www.cdc.gov/ncbddd/folicacid/council.htm

For More Information About Feeding Problems and Assistance

- American Occupational Therapy Association, Inc.
  http://www.aota.org/
- The Oley Foundation for Home Enteral/Parenteral Therapy
  http://www.oley.org/

For More Information About Foods and Formula

- Low-Protein Foods:
  Cambrooke Foods: http://www.cambrookefoods.com/
  Dietary Specialties: http://www.dietspec.com/
  Ener-G Foods: http://www.ener-g.com/
  Glutino: http://www.glutino.com/
  Kingsmill Foods: http://www.kingsmillfoods.com/
  Loprofin (SHS): http://www.shsna.com/pages/loprofin.htm
  MedDiet: http://www.med-diet.com/
- Mead Johnson
  http://www.meadjohnson.com
  Phone: 812-429-6399
- Novartis
  http://www.novartis.com
  Phone: 800-333-3785
- Ross Laboratories Pediatric Products
  http://www.rosslabs.com/productHandbook/pedNut.asp
  Phone: 800-986-8510
- Scientific Hospital Supply, SHS North America
  http://www.shsna.com
  Phone: 800-636-2283

For More Information About Health Laws Affecting Families/Children with Special Health Care Needs

- National Health Law Program
  http://www.healthlaw.org

For More Information About Pediatric Journals

- http://www.angelfire.com/in/pedscapes/index.html

For More Information About Rare Disorders

- Alliance of Genetic Support Groups
  http://geneticalliance.org/
- FDA—National Information Center for Orphan Drugs and Rare Diseases
  http://www.fda.gov/orphan/rdid/index.htm
- Genes and Disease
  http://www.ncbi.nlm.nih.gov/books/bv.fcgi?rid=gnd
- Genetics Home Reference
  http://ghr.nlm.nih.gov/
- National Organization for Rare Disorders
  http://www.rarediseases.org/
- Office of Rare Diseases
  National Institutes of Health
  http://rarediseases.info.nih.gov/

ABETALIPOPROTEINEMIA

NUTRITIONAL ACUITY RANKING: LEVEL 2–3

DEFINITIONS AND BACKGROUND

Abetalipoproteinemia (Bassen-Kornzweig syndrome) is a rare, inherited disease characterized by the inability to make lipoproteins (low-density lipoproteins [LDL], very low–density lipoproteins [VLDL], and chylomicrons) or to fully absorb dietary fats through the gut. Other names for this condition are acanthocytosis or apolipoprotein B deficiency. Acanthocytosis refers to the altered shape of the normal erythrocyte into one with a few irregularly shaped external projections that are thorny in appearance (Rampoldi et al, 2003; Wong, 2004).

Infants present with failure to thrive and fatty and pale stools that are frothy and foul smelling. They may also have a protruding abdomen, developmental delays, poor muscle coordination and weakness after age 10, slurred speech, and problems with balance and coordination. Prognosis is related to progression of neurological and visual problems; severe forms of the disease lead to irreversible neurological disease before age 30 and often to blindness. Mental deterioration and scoliosis can also occur.

The progressive ataxic neuropathy and retinopathy are thought to be due to oxidative damage resulting from deficiencies of vitamins E and A (Granot and Kohen, 2004). Nutritional supplementation is an essential part of treatment.

Treatments such as stem-cell therapy and gene product replacement are being evaluated.

INTERVENTION: OBJECTIVES

- Decrease rapid progression of disorder by giving large doses of fat-soluble vitamin supplements. This may help prevent deterioration of vision and degeneration of the retina.
- Avoid use of long-chain triglycerides; use medium-chain triglycerides (MCT) instead.
- Prevent nutrient deficiency symptoms and conditions.

INTERVENTION: FOOD AND NUTRITION

- The diet should contain no more than 5 ounces of lean meat, fish, or poultry per day.
- Use skim milk instead of whole milk. Reduce other types of fat from dairy products.
- Use MCT oil in food preparation and with gravies, sauces, and other cooked foods.
- The diet should be supplemented with fat-soluble vitamins A, D, E, and K to prevent deficiency. Water-miscible forms will be needed.

CLINICAL INDICATORS

Clinical/History

- Height
- Weight
- Growth chart
- Diet/intake history
- Scoliosis
- Retinal degeneration, retinitis pigmentosa
- Low vision or blindness
- Developmental delay?

Lab Work

- CBC with abnormal, thorny-shaped cells
- Serum apolipoprotein B levels (low or absent)
- Albumin (Alb)
- Cholesterol (Chol)
- VLDL (may be low)
- Fatty acid profile
- Triglycerides (Trig)
- Fecal fat study (high levels); steatorrhea
- Serum vitamins A, E, K
- Alkaline phosphorus (for vitamin D status)
- Ca++, Mg++
- EMG or nerve conduction velocity testing (demyelination of peripheral nerves)
- Hemoglobin and hematocrit (H & H)

Common Drugs Used and Potential Side Effects

- Large doses of supplemental vitamins A and E may be needed and will be prescribed by the physician (Chowers et al, 2001).

Herbs, Botanicals, and Supplements

- Herbs and botanicals are not recommended for this condition because there are no clinical trials proving efficacy.

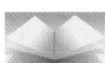

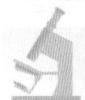

INTERVENTION: NUTRITION EDUCATION, COUNSELING, CARE MANAGEMENT

- Advise that MCT products should be eaten slowly to avoid side effects such as diarrhea.
- Discuss the need for intake of sources of essential fatty acids; a multivitamin-mineral supplement may also be recommended. Identify food sources of the fat-soluble vitamins and discuss how the disorder prevents use of these vitamins accordingly.
- For persons with low vision, teaching with food models or large pictures may be more beneficial than use of text. Audiotapes may also be developed.

Patient Education—Food Safety

- Hand washing with soap and hot water is recommended before preparing formula or meals. Use clean utensils and containers for mixing formula.
- Before using tap water for formula preparation or to give as a beverage, let cold tap water run for 2 minutes to remove any lead that may be in the pipes.
- Follow the 2-hour rule: discard any beverage or food that has been left at room temperature for 2 hours or longer.
- Do not use honey in the diets of infants to decrease potential risk of botulism.

For More Information

- Prevent Blindness
  http://www.preventblindness.org/
- Prevent Blindness Foundation
  http://www.pbf.org.au/

ABETALIPOPROTEINEMIA—CITED REFERENCES

Chowers I, et al. Long-term assessment of combined vitamin A and E treatment for the prevention of retinal degeneration in abetalipoproteinaemia and hypobetalipoproteinaemia patients. *Eye* 15:525, 2001.
Granot E, Kohen R. Oxidative stress in abetalipoproteinemia patients receiving long-term vitamin E and vitamin A supplementation. *Am J Clin Nutr.* 79:226, 2004.
Rampoldi D, et al. Clinical features and molecular bases of neuroacanthocytosis. *J Mol Med.* 80:475, 2002.
Wong P. A basis of the acanthocytosis in inherited and acquired disorders. *Med Hypotheses.* 62:966, 2004.

ATTENTION-DEFICIT DISORDERS

NUTRITIONAL ACUITY RANKING: LEVEL 1

DEFINITIONS AND BACKGROUND

Attention-deficit disorder (ADD) and attention-deficit hyperactivity disorder (ADHD) were formerly called childhood hyperkinesis. Today, it is known that adults may have symptoms as well and may find relief from certain medications and therapies. ADD is a neurobiological condition characterized by developmentally inappropriate level of attention, concentration, activity, distractibility, and impulsivity (Wender, 2002). There are no concrete explanations for ADHD, but there are numerous theories.

ADHD is the most commonly diagnosed behavioral disorder of childhood, affecting an estimated 7.5% of school-aged children (Schonwald, 2005). Three types have been noted in children and are designated by level of inattentiveness, impulsivity, or hyperactivity. There may be a small familial link, but there is not a specific gene noted at this time. ADD is more common in males than in females.

Glucose is the brain's energy source. In ADD, brain regions that inhibit impulses and control attention actually use less glucose; this decreased activity in the brain leads to inattention. PET scan comparisons between the brain of a normal child and the brain of an ADHD child show a significant difference. Children should be assessed for seizure disorders, which may cause inattention and sleep disturbances (Schubert, 2005).

Iron deficiency causes abnormal dopaminergic neurotransmission and may contribute to the physiopathology of ADD (Konofal et al, 2004). Children with ADHD may have low levels of certain essential fatty acids (including EPA and DHA) in their bodies. In a study of nearly 100 boys, those with lower levels of omega-3 fatty acids demonstrated more learning and behavioral problems (such as temper tantrums and sleep disturbances) than boys with normal omega-3 fatty acid levels. In animal studies, low levels of omega-3 fatty acids have been shown to lower the concentration of certain brain chemicals (such as dopamine and serotonin) related to attention and motivation. Studies that examine the ability of omega-3 supplements to improve symptoms of ADHD are still needed. At this point in time, eating foods high in omega-3 fatty acids is a reasonable approach for someone with ADHD.

Most ADHD is identified by age 6 in children. The Preschool ADHD Treatment Study (PATS), funded by the National Institute of Mental Health, will provide important clinical guidance for diagnostic considerations and intervention strategies for children with ADHD who are between the ages of 3 and 5.

INTERVENTION: OBJECTIVES

- Prevent nutrient deficiency symptoms and conditions if diet is inadequate or if there are extensive documented food allergies.
- Address poor intake and appetite, where present. Offer foods that are liked along with one to two new tastes to encourage expanding preferences.

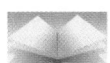

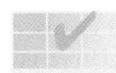

- Correct iron deficiency anemia, where indicated. Rule out lead poisoning in susceptible children. Provide sufficient intake of omega-3 fatty acids.

INTERVENTION: FOOD AND NUTRITION

- The diet should be balanced and sufficient in energy and protein for age and sex. The MyPyramid food guide should be the basis for planning (see Section 2).
- Omit any food allergens that have been medically diagnosed and verified. Elimination of sugar is not required, but moderation in use for all children is a reasonable guideline to ensure adequate intake of other nutrients.
- Essential fatty acid (EFA) deficiency is being researched; supplemental use of EFA may be useful in some cases (Murphy et al, 2005; Schnoll et al, 2003). Include good sources of omega-3 fatty acids, such as tuna, mackerel, herring, sardines, and salmon.
- While there is no benefit to reduction of specific carbohydrates, ensuring a wholesome diet with plenty of whole grains, low-fat dairy, fruits, and vegetables in greater proportion than sugary foods will provide more micronutrients and phytochemicals.
- Discuss good food sources of iron, especially for children who are following a limited diet or food jags. They may not eat meats, poultry, fish, eggs, and iron-fortified cereals in sufficient amounts.

CLINICAL INDICATORS

Clinical/History

- Height
- Weight
- Growth chart
- Diet/intake history
- Mental retardation, other developmental delay?
- Seizures or hx of epilepsy?
- EEG

Lab Work

- Glucose (Gluc)
- Alb
- Chol
- Liver function tests
- H & H
- Serum Fe
- Serum lead

Common Drugs Used and Potential Side Effects

- Drugs such as Ritalin (methylphenidate) have been used for many years. Newer, long-acting medications are coming to the market, and they will alleviate the burden on individuals with ADD (Connor and Steingard, 2004).
- Antiepileptic drugs may be used when there are seizures. They do not adversely affect attention and behavior, with the exception of phenobarbital, gabapentin, and topiramate (see Table 4-8). Some antiepileptic drugs, such as lamotrigine and carbamazepine, may even have beneficial effects on attention span.
- Medications such as Strattera (atomoxetine) are used to increase attention and the ability to focus. However, long-term use may cause liver damage; monitor carefully.
- Other drugs such as mood stabilizers, beta-blockers, or serotonin reuptake inhibitors may be helpful in managing symptoms related to aggression or self-injury. There are many side effects that are specific to the medication (such as weight gain or loss, elevation of glucose with possible diabetes, gastrointestinal [GI] distress, etc.). Monitor closely.

Herbs, Botanicals, and Supplements

- Herbs and botanicals are not recommended for this condition because there are no clinical trials proving efficacy.

INTERVENTION: NUTRITION EDUCATION, COUNSELING, CARE MANAGEMENT

- Many parents believe that food dyes or other food additives cause hyperactivity; correct this misinformation. There are many different causes of the symptoms of ADD, including allergies or food intolerances, anxiety, depression, family problems, poor discipline, and even some forms of illness. A healthy, balanced diet is important (Marcason, 2005).
- Since glucose is the brain's source of energy, a sufficient intake of carbohydrate is needed; assure that healthy choices are made from dairy, fruit and vegetable, and bread and cereal items. Reduced intake of sugary sweets, beverages, and snacks is a commonsense approach that most parents or caregivers will understand.
- Essential fatty acids are important. Include adequate amounts of fats in the daily diet. Zinc intake may also play a role (Arnold and DiSilvestro, 2005).
- Individual psychotherapy may be quite beneficial. Encourage full participation. ADD is a challenge, not an "excuse."

Patient Education—Food Safety

- Hand washing with soap and hot water is recommended before preparing formula or meals. Use clean utensils and containers for mixing formula.
- Before using tap water for formula preparation or to give as a beverage, let cold tap water run for 2 minutes to remove any lead that may be in the pipes.
- Follow the 2-hour rule: discard any beverage or food that has been left at room temperature for 2 hours or longer.
- Do not use honey in the diets of infants to decrease potential risk of botulism.

For More Information

- Attention Deficit Disorder Association
  http://www.add.org/
- National Institute for Mental Health
  http://www.nimh.nih.gov/publicat/adhd.cfm

ATTENTION-DEFICIT DISORDERS—CITED REFERENCES

Arnold LE, DiSilvestro RA. Zinc in attention-deficit/hyperactivity disorder. *J Child Adolesc Psychopharmacol.* 15:619, 2005.

Connor DF, Steingard RJ. New formulations of stimulants for attention-deficit hyperactivity disorder: therapeutic potential. *CNS Drugs.* 8:1011, 2004.

Konofal E, et al. Iron deficiency in children with attention-deficit/hyperactivity disorder. *Ach Pediatr Adolesc Med.* 158:1113, 2004.

Marcason W. Can dietary intervention play a part in the treatment of attention deficit and hyperactivity disorder? *J Am Diet Assoc.* 105:1161, 2005.

Murphy P, et al. Effect of the ketogenic diet on the activity level of Wistar rats. *Pediatr Res.* 57:353, 2005.

Schnoll R, et al. Nutrition in the treatment of attention-deficit hyperactivity disorder: a neglected but important aspect. *Appl Psychophysiol Biofeedback.* 28:63, 2003.

Schonwald A. Update: attention deficit/hyperactivity disorder in the primary care office. *Curr Opin Pediatr.* 17:265, 2005.

Schubert R. Attention deficit disorder and epilepsy. *Pediatr Neurol.* 32:1, 2005.

Wender P. *ADHD: attention-deficit hyperactivity disorder in children and adults.* Oxford, United Kingdom: Oxford University Press, 2002.

AUTISM SPECTRUM DISORDERS

NUTRITIONAL ACUITY RANKING: LEVEL 1–2

DEFINITIONS AND BACKGROUND

Autism spectrum disorders (ASDs) begin in childhood and are developmental disabilities caused by abnormalities in the brain. Generalized enlargement of gray and white matter cerebral volumes, but not cerebellar volumes, are present at 2 years of age in autism; increased rate of brain growth may have its onset postnatally in the latter part of the first year of life (Hazlett et al, 2005).

People with ASDs have problems with social and communication skills, even though they may speak. They like to repeat certain behaviors and do not want change in their daily activities. Many people with ASDs also have unusual ways of learning, paying attention, or reacting to different sensations. Rather than being insensitive or indifferent, the person with an ASD may be hypersensitive to sensory stimuli (e.g., tastes, smells, sounds, sights) and withdraw to reduce what is perceived as distressing or painful. They may repeat back what has been said, rather than conversing in a dialogue fashion; this is called echolalia. Up to 40% of persons with an ASD do not speak.

The ASDs are part of a broader category of pervasive developmental disorders (PDD). Over 500,000 individuals in the United States are affected with some type of PDD. New technology and studies are under way to identify and treat ASDs. Many solutions are being tested.

Autism is considered to be the most genetic of the neuropsychiatric disorders, affecting one in every 500 children (White, 2003). In addition, there may be environmental factors, such as exposure to toxins, infections (such as measles, mumps, or rubella), or diet (White, 2003), that play a role. High levels of serotonin may be found in the brain of persons with autism. Persons with autism may have trouble maintaining a conversation.

Mental retardation and seizures of mild to moderate intensity can be present in autism, especially in the condition identified as **fragile X syndrome** (found mostly in males). **Rett syndrome** disorder occurs primarily in girls and is evident by repetitive hand movements. If a diagnosis is not clear, it may be identified primarily as atypical autism or a type of PDD. In **Asperger's disorder**, speech occurs at the usual time, and intelligence is normal or above average. Social skills are stunted, and interests may be limited or obsessive.

At this time, there is no clear evidence that megadoses of nutrients are helpful (Nye and Brice, 2002). Feeding problems may prevail. Pica is often a concern, such as eating paper, string, or dirt; anemia is one possible consequence. Ritualistic eating behaviors and food limitations are common, and variety in texture or colors may not be accepted. Food jags are also common; actual food intake may be low. The individual may swallow food without chewing, so foods that could cause choking should be avoided. A quiet environment for eating is best tolerated. Messy eating habits are common.

INTERVENTION: OBJECTIVES

- Prevent or lessen complications of the disorder, such as feeding problems. Offer consistency in food textures and tastes to prevent sensory overload.
- Evaluate carefully and analyze which nutrients should be replaced in the diet. If the diet has been severely limited, nutritional status may be at risk.
- Correct constipation if fiber intake is low and if symptoms are present.
- Work with other therapies, such as speech therapy or occupational therapy, to determine how to best offer foods of greater texture and variety that can be consumed by the child or offered by the caregiver.
- Monitor food jags, pica, history of choking on foods, and intolerances for varied textures, and adapt meals and menu items accordingly.

INTERVENTION: FOOD AND NUTRITION

- Offer foods of texture and variety that are desired by the child. Follow usual pattern and enhance with nutrient-dense additives in food preparation that will not alter flavor and texture. For example, if a multivitamin-mineral supplement is needed, use one that is acceptable in taste to the individual.

- There are theories that gluten elimination or the addition of vitamin B_6 may make a difference in behavior; their potential benefits cannot be ruled out. However, there are no trials that show real efficacy from these treatments (Nye and Brice, 2002), and deficiencies of tyrosine and tryptophan can be an undesirable result (Arnold et al, 2003).
- Offer extra energy if weight is low, a common finding. Assess needs according to activity levels, weight and nutritional status, and medications that are prescribed.
- Since the brain requires omega-3 fatty acids for membrane integrity and to reduce inflammation, it might be beneficial to include them in the diet regularly or to use them in supplemental form. Autism seems to be related to altered immunity (Ashwood et al, 2004).

CLINICAL INDICATORS

Clinical/History

Height
Weight
Growth chart
Diet/intake history
Childhood Asperger Syndrome Test (CAST), a parental questionnaire
MRI or CT scan of the brain
Pica?

Lab Work

Gluc
H & H
Serum Fe
Fatty acid profile
Alb
Chol, Trig
Serum lead (with pica)
C-reactive protein (CRP)

Common Drugs Used and Potential Side Effects

- Medications to control seizures may be needed (Tuchman, 2004).
- If fenfluramine is used to lower serotonin levels, anorexia or GI distress may result.
- If clonidine, clomipramine, haloperidol, naltrexone, or desipramine is prescribed for behavioral or learning problems, monitor for GI side effects, nausea, and diarrhea.
- D-cycloserine treatment may improve social withdrawal (Posey et al, 2004). No significant side effects have been noted.
- There are National Institutes of Health (NIH) clinical trials studying donepezil (Aricept) and citalopram (Celexa) (may cause anorexia, dehydration, dry mouth, and weight changes). Olanzapine (Zyprexa) may cause weight gain, dry mouth, and constipation. Fluoxetine (Prozac) may cause anorexia or weight loss, GI distress, and diarrhea. Human secretin is also being evaluated.

Herbs, Botanicals, and Supplements

- Herbs and botanicals are not recommended for these conditions because there are no clinical trials proving efficacy.
- Vitamin megadoses may have been used for these individuals; discuss the implications and potential risks.

INTERVENTION: NUTRITION EDUCATION, COUNSELING, CARE MANAGEMENT

- Vaccines have been implicated in the onset of autism (e.g., measles-mumps-varicella), but most evidence suggests that there is no correlation. Reassure parents and offer reasonable advice about managing the condition.
- Evaluate for behaviors such as pica; discuss how this may lead to anemia.
- Assist with tips on how to handle picky eaters and rigid food behaviors. Nutrient deficiency may result.
- Discuss various ways to include nutrient-dense foods in the diet.
- Discuss the importance of maintaining a quiet environment with few interruptions or distractions to allow for better food intake.
- Keep language simple and concrete; do not offer abstract text. Pictures and simple words are more effective when working with the older child or teen personally.

Patient Education—Food Safety

- Hand washing with soap and hot water is recommended before preparing formula or meals. Use clean utensils and containers for mixing formula.
- Before using tap water for formula preparation or to give as a beverage, let cold tap water run for 2 minutes to remove any lead that may be in the pipes.
- Follow the 2-hour rule: discard any beverage or food that has been left at room temperature for 2 hours or longer.

For More Information

- Asperger's Syndrome
  http://www.aspergers.com/
- Asperger Syndrome Coalition of the United States
  http://www.irsc.org/
- Autism Society of America
  http://www.autism-society.org/
- CDC–About Autism
  http://www.cdc.gov/ncbddd/autism/
- Center for Collaborative Genetic Studies on Mental Disorders
  http://www.nimhgenetics.org
- National Fragile X Foundation
  http://www.nfxf.org/
- Report to Congress on Autism
  http://www.nimh.nih.gov/autismiacc/autismreport2004.pdf
- Rett Syndrome
  http://www.rettsyndrome.org/

AUTISM SPECTRUM DISORDERS—CITED REFERENCES

Arnold GL, et al. Plasma amino acids profiles in children with autism: potential risk of nutritional deficiencies. *J Autism Dev Disord.* 33:449, 2003.
Ashwood P, et al. Spontaneous mucosal lymphocyte cytokine profiles in children with autism and gastrointestinal symptoms: mucosal immune activation and reduced counter regulatory interleukin-10. *J Clin Immunol.* 24:664, 2004.

Chez MG, et al. Immunizations, immunology, and autism. *Semin Pediatr Neurol.* 11:214, 2004.
Hazlett HC, et al. Magnetic resonance imaging and head circumference study of brain size in autism: birth through age 2 years. *Arch Gen Psychiatry.* 62:1366, 2005.
Nye C, Brice A. Combined vitamin B6-magnesium treatment in autism spectrum disorder. *Cochrane Database Syst Rev.* 4:CD003497, 2002.
Posey DJ, et al. A pilot study of D-cycloserine in subjects with autistic disorder. *Am J Psychiatry.* 161:2115, 2004.
Tuchman R. AEDs and psychotropic drugs in children with autism and epilepsy. *Ment Retard Dev Disabil Res Rev.* 10:135, 2004.
White JF. Intestinal pathophysiology in autism. *Exp Biol Med (Maywood).* 228:639, 2003.

BILIARY ATRESIA

NUTRITIONAL ACUITY RANKING: LEVEL 2–3

DEFINITIONS AND BACKGROUND

Unconjugated hyperbilirubinemia occurs in approximately 60% of normal-term infants and in 80% of preterm infants; persistence beyond 2 weeks of age demands evaluation (Gubernick et al, 2000). Biliary atresia (neonatal hepatitis) is a serious condition, affecting one in 15,000 births. Incidence is highest in the Asian population.

Complete degeneration or incomplete development of one or more of the bile duct components occurs due to arrested fetal development. CD4(1) lymphocytes and CD56(1) (natural killer [NK] cells) predominate in the liver of infants with extrahepatic biliary atresia (Davenport et al, 2001). Lymphocyte-mediated inflammatory damage of the bile ducts plays a role (Shinkai et al, 2006), as does altered *HLA-DR* gene expression in bile ductules (Feng et al, 2004).

Biliary atresia results in persistent jaundice, enlarged spleen, liver damage, portal hypertension, clay-colored stools, dark urine, irritability, and swollen abdomen. The condition becomes evident between 2 and 6 weeks after birth. Treatment involves having a surgical procedure done, the Kasai procedure, which bypasses the ducts to connect the liver to the small intestine. It is more successful if performed early. Complications of the surgery can include liver failure, infections, and sepsis.

If a donor is available, the patient may be a candidate for a liver transplantation. This is the most common disease in childhood that requires liver transplantation. Malnutrition is a critical predictor of mortality and morbidity in children with biliary atresia who undergo transplantation (Bucuvalas et al, 1996). Immunosuppressive drugs are then necessary to overcome organ rejection.

INTERVENTION: OBJECTIVES

Preoperatively:

- Correct malabsorption and alleviate steatorrhea from decreased bile.
- Correct malnutrition of fat-soluble vitamins and zinc.
- Prevent hemorrhage from high blood pressure if there is portal hypertension.
- Prevent rickets, visual disturbances, peripheral neuropathy, and coagulopathies by having surgery.
- Prepare for surgery or transplantation.

Postoperatively:

- Support proper wound healing by providing all necessary nutrients (e.g., vitamin C, zinc) using appropriate and tolerated feeding method.
- Promote normal growth and development.
- Provide regular nutritional assessments to evaluate progress and improvement or decline.

INTERVENTION: FOOD AND NUTRITION

Preoperative:

- Infants need 1.5–3.0 g protein/kg dry weight to avoid protein catabolism, dependent on enteral versus parenteral source. This translates to 2–2.5 g/kg for parenteral nutrition (PN) and 2.5–3 g/kg for enteral nutrition, 1–1.5 g/kg if encephalopathic.
- Check for products enriched with branched-chain amino acids. Small, frequent feedings may be useful.
- Use low total fat from the diet. Supplement with oil high in medium-chain triglycerides (MCTs). Add essential fatty acids (EFAs) for age and body size. Portagen is available for infants but provides only minimal EFAs. Pregestimil or Alimentum or other elemental formulas may be needed.
- Decrease fiber intake to prevent hemorrhage from anywhere along the GI tract.
- With edema, limit intake of sodium to 1–2 g/d.
- Supplement with vitamins A, D, E, and K. Intravenous supplementation may be necessary, or water-miscible forms can be used.
- Serum levels of minerals, such as selenium, zinc, and iron, tend to be low. Avoid use of copper in total parenteral nutrition (TPN) or supplements.
- Failing nutrition should prompt aggressive support (Utterson et al, 2005). Tube feed especially if recurrent or prolonged bleeding from the GI tract occurs. If nasogastric (NG) feeding is not tolerated, a percutaneous gastrostomy (PEG) tube may be used (Duche et al, 1999).

Postoperative:

- Control sodium, protein, and other nutrients only if necessary based on symptoms such as edema and renal failure.
- Carefully monitor vitamin and mineral requirements.

- For needed catch-up growth, tube feeding may be beneficial (Holt et al, 2000). Assure that all key nutrients are included over a long-term basis.

CLINICAL INDICATORS

Clinical/History

- Birth weight
- Height
- Growth (%)
- Diet/intake history
- Dark urine
- Steatorrhea
- Edema
- Jaundice
- Clay-colored stools
- Nuclear HIDA test
- Liver biopsy

Lab Work

- Alb
- Transthyretin
- H & H
- Alk phos
- Chol
- Trig
- Transferrin
- Blood urea nitrogen (BUN)
- Aspartate aminotransferase (AST)
- Alanine aminotransferase (ALT)
- Alpha-1 antitrypsin deficiency
- Protime (PT) or international normalized ratio (INR)
- Serum zinc
- Serum copper

Common Drugs Used and Potential Side Effects

- Ursodiol (Actigall, Urso) promotes bile flow and may be used after surgery. Side effects are minimal.
- Phenobarbital and cholestyramine are often used to control the hyperlipidemia of this disorder, as well as pruritus. Increase vitamin D and calcium intakes; also increase vitamin B_{12} and folate. Constipation can result.
- Corticosteroids may be needed to stimulate independent bile flow. Long-term use can deplete stores of calcium and phosphorus; may elevate glucose, cause stunting, or cause weight gain.
- Diuretics may be used; monitor carefully. Potassium, magnesium, calcium, and folate may be depleted. Appetite may decline.
- Antibiotics such as Bactrim or Septra may be needed to manage cholangitis, a common complication following the Kasai procedure. Anorexia, nausea, or vomiting may result. Use of acidophilus and probiotic products may alleviate loss of intestinal bacteria.
- Growth hormone may be useful to promote catch-up growth.

Herbs, Botanicals, and Supplements

- Herbs and botanicals are not recommended with this condition because the liver is not able to perform its usual role of detoxification.
- Probiotics may be helpful; more studies are needed.

INTERVENTION: NUTRITION EDUCATION, COUNSELING, CARE MANAGEMENT

- Teach parents about proper feedings and supplements.
- If bile flow improves after surgery or transplantation, a regular diet may be used, although continuing use of MCT oil may be better tolerated for awhile.
- Teach that the fat-soluble vitamins A, D, E, and K can be used only when they are bound to fat. It may be important to take supplements by mouth.

Patient Education—Food Safety

- Hand washing with soap and hot water is recommended before preparing formula or meals. Use clean utensils and containers for mixing formula.
- Before using tap water for formula preparation or to give as a beverage, let cold tap water run for 2 minutes to remove any lead that may be in the pipes.
- Follow the 2-hour rule: discard any beverage or food that has been left at room temperature for 2 hours or longer.
- Do not use honey in the diets of infants to decrease potential risk of botulism.

For More Information

- American Liver Foundation
  http://www.liverfoundation.org/
- Canadian Liver Foundation
  http://www.liver.ca/Home.aspx
- Children's Liver Association for Support Services
  Phone: 877-679-8256
  http://www.classkids.org/library/biliaryatresia.htm

BILIARY ATRESIA—CITED REFERENCES

Bucuvalas J, et al. Growth hormone insensitivity in children with biliary atresia. *J Pediatr Gastroenterol Nutr.* 23:135, 1996.

Davenport M, et al. Immunohistochemistry of the liver and biliary tree in extrahepatic biliary atresia. *J Pediatr Surg.* 36:1017, 2001.

Duche M, et al. Percutaneous endoscopic gastrostomy for continuous feeding in children with chronic cholestasis. *J Pediatr Gastroenterol Nutr.* 29:42, 1999.

Feng J, et al. The aberrant expression of HLA-DR in intrahepatic bile ducts in patients with biliary atresia: an immunohistochemistry and immune electron microscopy study. *J Pediatr Surg.* 39:1658, 2004.

Gubernick J, et al. U.S. approach to jaundice in infants and children. *Radiographics* 20:173, 2000.

Holt R, et al. Nasogastric feeding enhances nutritional status in pediatric liver disease but does not alter circulating levels of IGF-I and IGF binding proteins. *Clin Endocrinol.* 52:217, 2000.

Shinkai M, et al. Increased CXCR3 expression associated with CD3-positive lymphocytes in the liver and biliary remnant in biliary atresia. *J Pediatr Surg.* 41:950, 2006.

Utterson EC, et al. Biliary atresia: clinical profiles, risk factors, and outcomes of 755 patients listed for liver transplantation. *J Pediatr.* 147:180, 2005.

BRONCHOPULMONARY DYSPLASIA

NUTRITIONAL ACUITY RANKING: LEVEL 3–4

DEFINITIONS AND BACKGROUND

Bronchopulmonary dysplasia (BPD) is a chronic lung disease with abnormal growth of the lungs, usually following respiratory distress syndrome of prematurity. Nutrition plays a critical role in the prevention and management of BPD and growth failure (Biniwale and Ehrenkranz, 2006). Dexamethasone, which is used to facilitate extubation and treat severe BPD, is known to have adverse effects on growth. Very low birth weight (VLBW) infants should be given adequate nutritional attention (e.g., parenteral or enteral nutrition, fluid restriction) from the first day of life to enhance growth and minimize respiratory morbidity (Biniwale and Ehrenkranz, 2006).

Respiratory failure, supplemental oxygen use, mechanical ventilation, endotracheal intubation, and congenital heart disease are part of the etiology (D'Angio and Maniscalco, 2004). Slow growth occurs as a result, and feeding problems are common. Long-term chronic care is required. Infants with BPD may benefit from comprehensive nutrition and feeding therapy, which provides adequate energy, parental support and education, and feeding evaluation (Biniwale and Ehrenkranz, 2006). Between 10% and 25% of preterm infants with BPD have malnutrition after 2 years of age, and 30–60% of them will continue to suffer from persistent airway obstruction or asthma (Bott et al, 2004).

VLBW infants, who develop severe respiratory disease, may have special nutrient requirements to enhance utilization of nutrients for epithelial cell repair and to support catch-up growth (Atkinson, 2001). Poor vitamin A status during the first month of life significantly increases the risk of developing BPD (Spears et al, 2004). Vitamin A provides benefit in these patients (Biniwale and Ehrenkranz, 2006; Darlow and Graham, 2000).

Glutamine is the main source for lung energy; inositol is necessary for surfactant synthesis; vitamin E and selenium have antioxidant effects (Bott et al, 2004). Long-chain polyunsaturated fatty acids, surfactant replacement therapy, and retinol (vitamin A) therapy are being used to prevent BPD in susceptible infants (D'Angio and Maniscalco, 2004). More controlled nutritional trials are needed to verify efficacy of these therapies (Biniwale and Ehrenkranz, 2006).

INTERVENTION: OBJECTIVES

- Achieve desirable growth. Infants with BPD tend to have delayed development (Bott et al, 2004). High energy needs persist (approximately 25–50% above normal needs). Correct malnutrition and anorexia from respiratory distress and ventilator support.
- Provide optimal amounts of protein for linear growth, development, and resistance to infection. Increase lean body mass if depleted.
- Spare protein by providing extra energy from fat and carbohydrate. Excesses of carbohydrate can increase CO_2 and prevent extubation; calculate needs carefully.
- Replace lost electrolytes, especially chloride, which may lead to death if not corrected.
- Provide essential fatty acids and inositol.
- Correct gastroesophageal reflux, which is common. Be sure to position an infant carefully if formula fed.
- Avoid overfeeding, which can lead to too rapid a weight gain for length and result in obesity.
- Prevent progressive pulmonary disease and complications, such as aspiration pneumonia or choking during feeding, through proper positioning.
- Improve tolerance for therapies and medications through adequate nutrition.
- Fluid restriction may be needed if fluid retention is noted; monitor closely.
- Prevent metabolic bone disease by including sufficient calcium intake.

INTERVENTION: FOOD AND NUTRITION

- Energy requirements will be 25% above normal; intake should be 120–160 kcal/kg to achieve optimal weight. Within the first few days of life, TPN or tube feeding may be required, if possible. Initially: 70 (PN) or 95 (enteral) kcal/kg, increasing to 120–130 kcal/kg; ongoing (after acute sickness): 130–180 kcal/kg.
- Protein requirements may be slightly higher than usual for infants with BPD. Infants with BPD may have improved protein status with careful formula management (Puangco and Schanler, 2000). Initially, use 2.0 g protein/kg, increasing to 2.5–3.5 g/kg.
- Decrease total carbohydrate (CHO) intake if glucose intolerance develops; monitor blood glucose levels. Increasing energy intake may improve growth and respiratory functioning by correcting some nutritional deficits (Lai et al, 2006).
- Provide at least the normal recommended allowances for antioxidant and other important nutrients. Include vitamins A, D, and E (use water-miscible sources if necessary); provide adequate calcium, phosphorus, and iron if needed. Nutrient or energy-enriched infant formulas may be needed for catch-up growth.
- Fluid intake (may be restricted to <150 cc/kg/d) and sodium levels may need to be restricted if there is pulmonary edema or hypertension.
- Infants can tolerate most formulas. Nocturnal tube feeding may be useful, especially with growth failures. With gastroesophageal (GE) reflux, a gastrostomy feeding tube may be more comfortable than a nasogastric (NG) tube.
- With decreased suck and swallowing ability, tube feeding may be better tolerated.

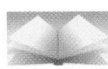

- Increase fat:CHO ratio with respiratory distress. To meet essential fatty acid needs, start with 0.5–1 g/kg and progress to 3 g/kg.
- Omega-3 fatty acids, selenium, inositol, and vitamin E have been suggested for use with infants who have chronic pulmonary insufficiency; only vitamin A has been confirmed (Biniwale and Ehrenkranz, 2006; Bott et al, 2004; Atkinson, 2001).
- When ready to progress to oral diet, use of solids may be better tolerated than liquids. If necessary, thicken liquids or formula (e.g., with baby cereal or other thickeners). Use a supine position to avoid aspiration.

CLINICAL INDICATORS

Clinical/History

- Gestational age
- Length
- Body mass index (BMI)
- Growth chart for height and weight (LBW and VLBW charts are available)
- Diet/intake history
- Size for gestational age (use intrauterine growth chart if available)
- Head circumference
- Emesis
- Stool pattern
- Urinary output
- Pulmonary hypertension

Lab Work

- H & H
- pH
- Chol, Trig
- K+ (tends to be low)
- Na+
- Cl− (tends to be low)
- Alb
- Alkaline phosphatase (alk phos)
- White blood cell count (WBC)
- PT or INR
- Gluc
- Oxygen saturation levels
- Partial pressure of carbon dioxide (pCO_2)
- Partial pressure of oxygen (pO_2)
- Ca++, Mg++
- Urine-specific gravity

Common Drugs Used and Potential Side Effects

- Exogenous steroid therapy (dexamethasone or methylprednisone) is limited to improving pulmonary compliance in ventilated premature infants (Grier and Halliday, 2005). This may compromise vitamin A status and restrict somatic and bone mineral growth (Atkinson et al, 2001). Sodium retention, anorexia, edema, hypertension, and potassium losses are common side effects. Take with food to decrease GI effects. Use more protein and less sodium; enhance potassium if needed.
- Antibiotics are needed during infections. Use of acidophilus and probiotic products may alleviate losses of intestinal bacteria.
- Bronchodilators or caffeine may be used for apnea of prematurity. Anorexia can occur.
- Diuretics may be needed to lessen pulmonary edema. Monitor those that deplete serum potassium, such as furosemide (Lasix). Magnesium, calcium, and folate may be also depleted; appetite may decline.
- Antiarrhythmics may be used.

Herbs, Botanicals, and Supplements

- Herbs and botanicals should not be used for BPD because the lungs are not able to perform their role in oxygenation of cells.
- Use of acidophilus and probiotic products may be useful with chronic antibiotic therapy.

INTERVENTION: NUTRITION EDUCATION, COUNSELING, CARE MANAGEMENT

- Diet must be reevaluated periodically to reflect growth and disease process. Assure adequacy of vitamins and related nutrients for lung health (for example, vitamin A).
- Ensure that all foods and beverages are nutrient dense.
- New foods may be introduced gradually; thicken as needed to avoid aspiration.
- Fluid intake should be adequate to meet needs but not excessive.
- Discuss signs of overhydration and dehydration with the parent/caregiver.
- Oral–motor skills may be delayed from long-term ventilator use; discuss how to make adjustments with caregiver.

Patient Education—Food Safety

- Hand washing with soap and hot water is recommended before preparing formula or meals. Use clean utensils and containers for mixing formula.
- Before using tap water for formula preparation or to give as a beverage, let cold tap water run for 2 minutes to remove any lead that may be in the pipes.
- Follow the 2-hour rule: discard any beverage or food that has been left at room temperature for 2 hours or longer.
- Do not use honey in the diets of infants to decrease potential risk of botulism.

For More Information

- American Lung Association
  http://www.lungusa.org/site/pp.asp?c=dvLUK9O0E&b=35017
- National Blood, Heart, and Lung Institute
  http://www.nhlbi.nih.gov/health/dci/Diseases/Bpd/Bpd_WhatIs.html

BRONCHOPULMONARY DYSPLASIA—CITED REFERENCES

Atkinson S. Special nutritional needs of infants for prevention of and recovery from bronchopulmonary dysplasia. *J Nutr.* 131:942S, 2001.

Biniwale MA, Ehrenkranz RA. The role of nutrition in the prevention and management of bronchopulmonary dysplasia. *Semin Perinatol.* 30:200, 2006.

Bott L, et al. Nutrition and bronchopulmonary dysplasia. *Arch Pediatr.* 11:234, 2004.

D'Angio CT, Maniscalco WM. Bronchopulmonary dysplasia in preterm infants: pathophysiology and management strategies. *Paediatr Drugs.* 6:303, 2004.

Darlow B, Graham P. Vitamin A supplementation for preventing morbidity and mortality in very-low-birth-weight infants. *Cochrane Database Syst Rev.* 2:CD000501, 2000.

Grier DG, Halliday HL. Management of bronchopulmonary dysplasia in infants: guidelines for corticosteroid use. *Drugs* 65:15, 2005.

Johnson D, et al. Nutrition and feeding in infants with bronchopulmonary dysplasia after initial hospital discharge: risk factors for growth failure. *J Am Diet Assoc.* 98:649, 1998.

Lai N, et al. The role of nutrition in the prevention and management of bronchopulmonary dysplasia. *Semin Perinatol.* 30:200, 2006.
Puangco M, Schanler R. Clinical experience in enteral nutrition support for premature infants with bronchopulmonary dysplasia. *J Perinatol.* 20:87, 2000.
Spears K, et al. Low plasma retinol concentrations increase the risk of developing bronchopulmonary dysplasia and long-term respiratory disability in very-low-birth-weight infants. *Am J Clin Nutr.* 80:1589, 2004.

CEREBRAL PALSY

NUTRITIONAL ACUITY RANKING: LEVEL 3

DEFINITIONS AND BACKGROUND

Cerebral palsy (CP) is a neurological dysfunction resulting from brain damage to motor centers before, during, or after birth. Human epidemiological data suggest a relationship between CP and cytokines or inflammation (Gaudet and Smith, 2001). One out of 500 live births may be affected; 1200–1500 preschool-age children in the United States are identified each year with CP.

CP causes physical and mental disabilities and is considered to be nonprogressive. Seizures, mental retardation, hyperactive gag reflex, tongue thrust, poor lip closure, and inability to chew properly are common problems. Behavioral problems and visual or auditory problems may occur. Infants may present with early abnormal rolling, stiffness, irritability, and developmental delays (see Table 3-3).

Symptoms may be mild or more severe and vary from one person to the next. Skeletal maturation is frequently delayed in children with CP (Ihkkan and Yalcin, 2001). Types of palsy include **spastic** (difficult, stiff movement), **athetoid** (involuntary worm-like movement), **ataxic** (impaired coordination and balance), and **mixed**. Approximately, 70–80% of those with CP have the spastic form, with uncontrolled shaking and stiffness; 10–20% have athetosis, with continuous worm-like movement; 5–10% have ataxia; and many have mixed forms (Ekvall, 1993).

Wasting of voluntary muscles, which is common in CP, contributes to reduced resting energy needs (Hogan, 2004). The potential for malnutrition is real. Indirect calorimetry is a useful tool for measuring actual energy requirements (Hogan, 2004).

INTERVENTION: OBJECTIVES

- Alleviate malnutrition resulting from the patient's inability to close lips, suck, bite, chew, or swallow.
- Promote independence through use of adaptive feeding devices. Eye–hand coordination is often lacking, and grasp may not be strong.
- Assess appropriate energy and nutrient needs.
- Promote mealtimes in a quiet, unhurried environment. When adequately nourished, children and adolescents with CP appear more tranquil and require decreased feeding time (Hogan, 2004).
- Correct nutritional deficits, altered growth rate, developmental delays, or retardation. For example, sufficient magnesium sulfate may reduce the risk of death in very preterm infants (Crowther et al, 2003).
- Correct constipation, which may be common.
- Prevent aspiration pneumonia and gastroesophageal reflux.
- Prevent or correct pressure ulcers.

INTERVENTION: FOOD AND NUTRITION

- Energy requirements of children and adolescents with CP appear to be disease specific, varying depending on functional capacity, degree of mobility, severity of disease, and level of altered metabolism (Hogan, 2004). Breast milk is recommended (Vohr et al, 2006).
  (a) Reduce energy intake for spastic patients or those with severely limited activity, 11 kcal/cm for ages 5–11. For moderately active patients, use 14 kcal/cm for ages 5–11.
  (b) Increase energy intake (up to 45 kcal/kg) to accommodate for the added movements of the athetoid patient over age 18. In adults with CP, athetosis may increase energy needs by as much as 524 kcal/d (Johnson et al, 1995).
- Feeding gastrostomy tubes are a reasonable alternative for severe feeding and swallowing problems and poor weight gain (Rogers, 2004; Sullivan et al, 2004). Night feedings may allow more normal daytime routines. Daytime bolus feedings of high-calorie, high-protein formulas at scheduled times may also be needed to provide adequate nutrition in some cases.
- For chewing problems, eliminate coarse, stringy foods. Puree foods as needed.
- For frequent vomiting, assess actual intake. Medications may be needed.
- For constant dribbling, add cereal or yogurt to fluids. Replace fluids; thickened liquids may be needed.
- For constipation, use laxative foods, high-fiber foods, or bran in the diet. Provide extra fluids. In younger children, too much fiber can displace intake of adequate nutrition.
- For swallowing problems, tube feed if necessary.
- Supplement with a general multivitamin-mineral supplement, especially for B-complex vitamins and for calcium and vitamin D (Henderson et al, 2005).
- For pressure ulcers or skin breakdown from the same positioning of the body, ensure adequate protein, vitamins C and A, and zinc.

TABLE 3-3 Warning Signs of Cerebral Palsy

At Birth:	*At 6 Months:*
Difficult breathing	Cannot sit without help
Trouble eating	Does not laugh or make sounds
Trouble eliminating	Does not actively reach for toys
Lack of certain reflexes	
At 3 Months:	*At 7–8 Months:*
Doesn't respond to your voice	Doesn't follow toys with both eyes at both near and far ranges
Doesn't follow toys with his or her eyes	Doesn't actively reach for toys
Doesn't use facial expressions	Doesn't bear some weight on his or her legs
Has unusually stiff or floppy muscles	Doesn't try to attract attention through actions
Consistently uses one side of his body more often than the other	Doesn't babble
Doesn't enjoy being around people	Won't play games
At 4–5 Months:	
Has difficulty getting objects to his or her mouth	
Doesn't turn head to locate sounds	
Doesn't smile spontaneously	

Source: http://www.cerebralpalsy.org/.

CLINICAL INDICATORS

Clinical/History		Lab Work
Low birth weight (LBW)	Dentition problems	Skull x-ray
Height, weight	Seizures	Gluc
Growth (%)	Gastro-esophageal reflux disease (GERD)	Alb
Diet/intake history	Constipation	Serum Ca++, Mg++
Low 5-minute Apgar score (below 7)		Transferrin
		Alk phos
		H & H

Common Drugs Used and Potential Side Effects

- Dantrolene (Dantrium) is used to control muscle spasms and cramps. It inhibits the release of calcium in muscle and skeletal tissue, preventing muscle cramping and spasms. Diarrhea, changes in blood pressure, weight loss, and constipation may all occur.
- Klonopin (clonazepam) is a benzodiazepine used to slow down the central nervous system (CNS) in the treatment of spasticity. Side effects may include constipation or diarrhea, dizziness, drowsiness, clumsiness or unsteadiness, a "hangover" effect, headache, nausea, and vomiting.
- Antibiotics such as baclofen may cause or aggravate diarrhea. Use of acidophilus and probiotic products may alleviate loss of intestinal bacteria.
- Laxatives may often be needed; monitor for fiber and fluid needs. Milk of Magnesia can be used safely in a pediatric dosage. Avoid using laxatives containing mineral oil.
- Anticonvulsants may increase risk of osteomalacia if calcium and vitamin D are insufficiently supplemented. Nutrient deficiencies are common: vitamins D, B_6, B_{12}, and K, folate, calcium, and biotin are often insufficient.

Herbs, Botanicals, and Supplements

- Herbs and botanicals should not be used for CP because there are no controlled trials to prove efficacy.
- Probiotics may be used to alleviate loss of intestinal bacteria. Encourage natural sources such as yogurt or acidophilus milk if tolerated.

INTERVENTION: NUTRITION EDUCATION, COUNSELING, CARE MANAGEMENT

- Remind patients to keep lips closed to avoid losing food from their mouths as they try to chew.
- Fortify the diet with dry or evaporated milk, wheat germ, and other foods when intake is inadequate.
- If special training is needed for a specific feeding procedure (e.g., a preemie nipple for poor sucking), it should be provided.

- Help parent or caretaker with problems relating to dental caries, drugs, constipation, pica, or weight.
- Allow extra time for feedings. Use of adaptive feeding equipment may be beneficial.
- Tube feeding may be needed. Ensure proper positioning.

Patient Education—Food Safety

- Hand washing with soap and hot water is recommended before preparing formula or meals. Use clean utensils and containers.
- Before using tap water for formula preparation or to give as a beverage, let cold tap water run for 2 minutes to remove any lead that may be in the pipes.
- Follow the 2-hour rule: discard any beverage or food that has been left at room temperature for 2 hours or longer.
- Do not use honey in the diets of infants to decrease potential risk of botulism.

For More Information

- American Academy of Developmental Medicine and Dentistry
  http://www.aadmd.org
- American Association on Health and Disabilities
  http://www.aahd.us/
- American Cerebral Palsy Information Center
  http://www.cerebralpalsy.org
- CP Connection
  http://www.cpconnection.com/
- CP Resource Center
  http://twinenterprises.com/cp/
- Developmental Disabilities Nurses Association
  http://www.ddna.org/
- Disability Resource Network
  http://www.d-r-d.com/
- Easter Seals
  http://www.easter-seals.org
- Exceptional Parent Magazine
  http://www.exceptionalparent.com/
- Hemiplegic Cerebral Palsy
  http://www.hemikids.org/
- Telability
  http://www.telability.org
- United Cerebral Palsy Association, Inc.
  http://www.ucpa.org/

CEREBRAL PALSY—CITED REFERENCES

Crowther CA, et al. Australasian Collaborative Trial of Magnesium Sulphate (ACTOMg SO4) Collaborative Group. Effect of magnesium sulfate given for neuroprotection before preterm birth: a randomized controlled trial. *JAMA*. 290:2669, 2003.

Ekvall S. *Pediatric nutrition in chronic diseases and developmental disorders.* New York: Oxford University Press, 1993.

Gaudet L, Smith G. Cerebral palsy and chorioamnionitis: the inflammatory cytokine link. *Obstet Gynecol Surv.* 56:433, 2001.

Henderson RC. Longitudinal changes in bone density in children and adolescents with moderate to severe cerebral palsy. *J Pediatr.* 146:769, 2005.

Hogan SE. Energy requirements of children with cerebral palsy. *Can J Diet Pract Res.* 65:124, 2004.

Ihkkan D, Yalcin E. Changes in skeletal maturation and mineralization in children with cerebral palsy and evaluation of related factors. *J Child Neurol.* 16:425, 2001.

Johnson R, et al. Athetosis increases resting metabolic rate in adults with cerebral palsy. *J Am Diet Assoc.* 95:145, 1995.

Rogers B. Feeding method and health outcomes of children with cerebral palsy. *J Pediatr.* 145:S28, 2004.

Sullivan PB, et al. Impact of gastrostomy tube feeding on the quality of life of carers of children with cerebral palsy. *Dev Med Child Neurol.* 46:796, 2004,

Vohr BR, et al. Beneficial effects of breast milk in the neonatal intensive care unit on the developmental outcome of extremely low birth weight infants at 18 months of age. *Pediatrics* 118:115, 2006.

CLEFT LIP AND PALATE (OROFACIAL CLEFTS)

NUTRITIONAL ACUITY RANKING: LEVEL 3

DEFINITIONS AND BACKGROUND

Cleft lip and palate are congenital malformations occurring during the embryonic period of development. They result in a fissure in the lip and roof of the mouth, which may be unilateral or bilateral. Incidence is approximately 1 in 700 births in Caucasians, or about 5000 births annually in the United States. Infants with cleft palate are often smaller in size and weight than other infants (Spyropoulos and Burdi, 2001).

Periconceptional folate and folic acid intake prevents orofacial clefts (OFC) (Krapels et al, 2004; Bienengraber et al, 2001). Other nutrients also play a role, and many mothers who eat poorly risk having a baby with OFC. Improved preconceptual intake of macronutrients and key micronutrients (e.g., ascorbic acid, iron, magnesium, vegetable protein, and fiber) may decrease OFC risk (Krapels et al, 2006). Vitamin A may also play an important role in proper formation of the palate during pregnancy (Mitchell et al, 2003).

INTERVENTION: OBJECTIVES

- Cleft palate is more of a problem than cleft lip. Compensate for the patient's inability to suck because of the air space between the mouth and nose.
- Prevent choking, air swallowing, coughing, and fatigue as much as possible.
- Encourage breastfeeding where possible to protect against otitis media (Aniansson et al, 2002).

- Supply the child with energy to heal and to grow; offer tips for meal planning and resources because feeding will be a challenge (Redford-Badwal et al, 2003).
- For surgery, allow extra energy and protein for healing; use a multivitamin supplement. Before surgery, a custom retainer device may be placed in the mouth and is intended to gradually pull the edges of the cleft closer to achieve better lip repair. The device also aids in the feeding process.

INTERVENTION: FOOD AND NUTRITION

- Provide a normal diet in accordance with the patient's age and dietary recommendations. Monitor diet carefully because mother may have had a poor diet during preconceptual period and pregnancy.
- For infant feeding, use a medicine dropper or plastic bottle with a soft nipple and enlarged hole. The use of a squeezable, collapsible bottle (Shaw et al, 1999) with a longer nipple and a large crosscut opening, which allows parents to control the flow of milk, can help. Release formula or milk a little at a time, in coordination with the infant's chewing movements. Burp infant frequently to release swallowed air. Feed the infant in an upright position to prevent aspiration.
- When the infant is 4–6 months of age, begin to add solids in the diet. Pureed baby foods can be used, or the infant can be spoon fed with milk used to dilute the baby foods. Feed solids from a spoon and avoid use of a bottle or commercial syringe feeder, unless prescribed for unique circumstances.
- Avoid fruit peelings, nuts, peanut butter, leafy vegetables, heavy cream dishes, popcorn, grapes, biscuits, cookies, and chewing gum as they may get lodged in the palate. Avoid spicy, acidic foods if they cause irritation.

CLINICAL INDICATORS

Clinical/History		Lab Work
Length (height) Growth (%) Weight Weight changes Diet/intake history Head circumference	Cleft type (unilateral or bilateral; complete or incomplete) Otitis media or other infections Chewing difficulty	Gluc Alb H & H Serum Ca++, Mg++

Herbs, Botanicals, and Supplements

- Herbs and botanicals should not be used for cleft palate because there are no controlled trials to prove efficacy.

INTERVENTION: NUTRITION EDUCATION, COUNSELING, CARE MANAGEMENT

- Explain how to feed the infant with a special nipple as needed.
- Indicate that solids may be fed starting at 4–6 months. Follow usual pattern, using baby food and pureed foods as tolerated.
- Supplement the diet with vitamin C if citrus juices are not taken well.
- Have the parents use small amounts of liquid when they are feeding an infant. To prevent choking, slow swallowing should be encouraged and proper positioning should be taught.
- Discuss the impact of surgery and how to promote effective healing by using a nutrient-dense diet with adequate amounts of vitamins A and C and zinc.
- Because of the types of problems that may occur (teeth in the area of the cleft may be missing or improperly positioned, which affects chewing ability; speech difficulties; frequent colds, sore throats, otitis media, tonsillitis), assistance from a variety of therapists and professionals is needed. The dietitian can assist with nutrition and feeding-related issues. Nutrient density and texture assessments should be ongoing.

Patient Education—Food Safety

- Hand washing with soap and hot water is recommended before preparing formula or meals. Use clean utensils and containers for mixing formula.
- Before using tap water for formula preparation or to give as a beverage, let cold tap water run for 2 minutes to remove any lead that may be in the pipes.
- Follow the 2-hour rule: discard any beverage or food that has been left at room temperature for 2 hours or longer.
- Do not use honey in the diets of infants; this will decrease the risk of botulism.

For More Information

- AboutFace USA
http://www.aboutfaceusa.org/
- About Smiles
http://www.aboutsmiles.org/
- American Cleft Palate-Craniofacial Association
http://www.cleftline.org/
- Center for Craniofacial Development and Disorders
http://www.hopkinsmedicine.org/craniofacial/Home/Index.cfm
- Cleft Lip and Palate Resources
http://www.widesmiles.org/
- Cleft Palate Foundation
http://www.cleftline.org/aboutclp/
- FACES: The National Craniofacial Organization
http://www.faces-cranio.org/
- Federation for Children with Special Needs
http://www.faces-cranio.org/
- Forward Face: The Charity for Children with Craniofacial Conditions
http://www.nffr.org/ForwardFace.htm
- Smile Train
http://www.smiletrain.org/library/PublicLibrary.html

CLEFT LIP AND PALATE—CITED REFERENCES

Aniansson G, et al. Otitis media and feeding with breast milk of children with cleft palate. *Scand J Plast Reconstr Surg Hand Surg.* 36:9, 2002.
Bienengraber V, et al. Is it possible to prevent cleft palate by prenatal administration of folic acid? An experimental study. *Cleft Palate Craniofac J.* 38:393, 2001.
Krapels IP, et al. Nutrition and genes in the development of orofacial clefting. *Nutr Rev.* 64:280, 2006.
Mitchell LE, et al. Retinoic acid receptor alpha gene variants, multivitamin use, and liver intake as risk factors for oral clefts: a population-based case-control study in Denmark, 1991-1994. *Am J Epidemiol.* 158:69, 2003.
Redford-Badwal DA, et al. Impact of cleft lip and/or palate on nutritional health and oral-motor development. *Dent Clin North Am.* 47:305, 2003.
Shaw W, et al. Assisted feeding is more reliable for infants with clefts—a randomized trial. *Cleft Palate Craniofac J.* 36:262, 1999.
Spyropoulos M, Burdi A. Patterns of body and visceral growth in human prenates with clefts of the lip and palate. *Cleft Palate Craniofac J.* 38:341, 2001.

CONGENITAL HEART DISEASE

NUTRITIONAL ACUITY RANKING: LEVEL 2

DEFINITIONS AND BACKGROUND

Persons born with congenital heart disease (CHD) may have associated noncardiac anomalies (25%); a small percentage (6%) are small for gestational age at birth. Usually, some developmental defect occurred between weeks 5 and 8 of pregnancy (e.g., from rubella). Incidence is approximately 700 in 100,000 births. Patients with CHD are at increased risk for malnutrition and growth failure. Pulmonary hypertension seems to be a concern (Varan et al, 1999).

Growth disturbance is generally related to an anatomical lesion and is most severe in infants and children with congestive heart failure (Leitch, 2001). Cyanotic CHD causes more growth retardation than acyanotic CHD from chronic hypoxemia, which reduces serum insulin-like growth factor-I (IGF-I) concentrations (Dundar et al, 2000).

Energy expenditure appears to be significantly elevated in this population (Leitch, 2001). Feeding difficulties are related to the organic condition; professional support may be required for mothers of infants with CHD to maintain feeding routines and to deal with the difficulties that arise (Clemente et al, 2001). Supplementary oxygen is often needed, and the child will not grow if oxygen is inadequate. During feeding, many desaturate and need oxygen.

Presently, surgical repair in this population is often delayed in order to permit increased weight gain. Surgery is performed when a patient reaches an ideal weight and age or when failure to thrive precludes further waiting.

INTERVENTION: OBJECTIVES

- Support normal growth and weight gains. These infants or children tend to have growth failure, especially with associated congestive heart failure.
- Improve oral intake. Poor sucking may occur in infants, but it is possible to breastfeed with education and support of the mother (Barbas and Kelleher, 2004).
- Lessen fatigue associated with mealtimes.
- Meet caloric needs from increased metabolic rate and from need for catch-up growth, without creating excessive cardiac burden.
- Avoid excessive renal solute overload.
- Assure adequate oxygen replacement, especially during feeding.
- Improve appetite, which can be decreased from the medications.

INTERVENTION: FOOD AND NUTRITION

- Determine and provide calories as needed for age (e.g., 100 kcal/kg in second year of life, etc.). See RDA tables. Most formulas contain 67 kcal/dL or 20 kcal/oz. Severe cases may need an extra 30–60 kcal/kg/d over RDA; follow standard mixing recommendations for formula concentration and add modular products to reach desired level. For infants, a formula up to 90–100 kcal/dL can be used while carefully monitoring adequacy of fluid ingestion.
- PEG tube feeding can be a useful adjunctive therapy, especially formulas with a lower mineral to protein ratio (e.g., partially demineralized whey).
- Energy should contain approximately 10% protein (avoid overloading), 35–50% fat as vegetable oils (known to be readily absorbed), and 40–55% CHO.
- Sodium intake should be approximately 6–8 mEq daily, dependent on diuretic use and cardiopulmonary status.
- Continuous 24-hour NG tube feeding may be useful. If extended tube feeding is needed, a PEG tube is more comfortable.

CLINICAL INDICATORS

Clinical/History		Lab Work
Height Weight Head circumference Growth pattern Diet/intake history	Blood pressure (BP) Weight changes Intake and output (I & O) Ultrasound Echocardiography	Urinary Osm Na+, K+ BUN, creatinine (Creat) Chol Trig

Common Drugs Used and Potential Side Effects

- Drugs are specific to the individual patient's requirements. See Table 3-4. For some patients, angiotensin-converting enzyme inhibitors (ACEIs) and beta-blockers may be needed; GI distress or nausea may result. Long-term use of corticosteroids can deplete stores of calcium and phosphorus and may elevate glucose, cause stunting, or cause weight gain. With diuretics, potassium, magnesium, calcium, and folate may be depleted, and appetite may decline.
- Nesiritide is now used for congestive heart failure to cause diuresis; hypotension may result (Feingold and Law, 2004).
- Infective endocarditis (IE) among children with *Staphylococcus aureus* bacteremia may require treatment with antibiotics. Use of acidophilus and probiotic products may alleviate loss of intestinal bacteria.

Herbs, Botanicals, and Supplements

- Herbs and botanicals should not be used for CHD because there are no controlled trials to prove efficacy.
- With prolonged use of antibiotic therapy, probiotic products may be useful. Encourage intake of yogurt, acidophilus milk, and related products.

TABLE 3-4 Medications for Congenital Heart Disease

Generic Name	Brand Name
Acebutol	Sectral
Atenolol	Tenormin
Azathioprine	Imuran
Baby aspirin	Bayer
Captopril	Capoten
Cisapride	Propulsid
Digoxin	Lanoxin
Enalapril	Vasotec
Furosemide	Lasix
Hydrochlorothiazide	Hydrodiuril
Lisinopril	Zestril
Metoprolol	Lopressor
Prednisone	Deltasone
Propranolol	Inderal
Spironolactone	Aldactone
Warfarin	Coumadin

INTERVENTION: NUTRITION EDUCATION, COUNSELING, CARE MANAGEMENT

- Discuss the role of nutrition in achieving adequate growth and controlling heart disease.
- Discuss growth patterns and goals.
- Provide support for breastfeeding mothers who wish to continue as long as possible.

Patient Education—Food Safety

- Hand washing with soap and hot water is recommended before preparing formula or meals. Use clean utensils and containers for mixing formula.
- Before using tap water for formula preparation or to give as a beverage, let cold tap water run for 2 minutes to remove any lead that may be in the pipes.
- Follow the 2-hour rule: discard any beverage or food that has been left at room temperature for 2 hours or longer.
- Do not use honey in the diets of infants to decrease potential risk of botulism.

For More Information

- Cardiac Information–C.S. Mott Children's Hospital
  http://www.med.umich.edu/1libr/chheart/chhear00.htm
- Children's Cardiomyopathy Foundation
  http://www.childrenscardiomyopathy.org/site/overview.php
- Children's Heart Institute
  http://www.childrenheartinstitute.org/educate/heartwrk/elechhse.htm
- Children's Organ Transplant Network
  http://www.cota.org/customsites/cota/index.asp
- Congenital Heart Defects
  http://www.congenitalheartdefects.com/
- Congenital Heart Disease Online Handbook
  http://my.execpc.com/~markc/congenit.html
- Congenital Heart Information Network
  http://www.tchin.org/
- Heart Center Encyclopedia
  http://www.cincinnatichildrens.org/health/heart-encyclopedia/default.htm
- Heart Institute for Children
  http://www.thic.com/Default.htm
- Kids with Heart, National Association for Children's Heart Disorders, Inc
  http://kidswithheart.org/
- United Hearts
  http://kidswithheart.org/

CONGENITAL HEART DISEASE—CITED REFERENCES

Barbas KH, Kelleher DK. Breastfeeding success among infants with congenital heart disease. *Pediatr Nurs.* 30:285, 2004.
Clemente C, et al. Are infant behavioral feeding difficulties associated with congenital heart disease? *Child Care Health Dev.* 27:47, 2001.
Dundar B, et al. Chronic hypoxemia leads to reduced serum IGF-I levels in cyanotic congenital heart disease. *J Pediatr Endocrinol Metab.* 13:431, 2000.
Feingold B, Law YM. Nesiritide use in pediatric patients with congestive heart failure. *J Heart Lung Transplant.* 23:1455, 2004.
Leitch C. Growth, nutrition and energy expenditure in pediatric heart failure. *Prog Pediatr Cardiol.* 11:195, 2001.
Varan B, et al. Malnutrition and growth failure in cyanotic and acyanotic congenital heart disease with and without pulmonary hypertension. *Arch Dis Child.* 81:49, 1999.

CYSTINOSIS AND FANCONI'S SYNDROME

NUTRITIONAL ACUITY RANKING: LEVEL 3

DEFINITIONS AND BACKGROUND

Accumulation of cystine (cystinosis) results in multiple organ damage, with renal damage being the most severe. Transplantation of the kidney may be needed.

There are three distinct forms of cystinosis. **Infantile nephropathic cystinosis** is the most severe form and is a lysosomal membrane transport defect. Failure to thrive, rickets, metabolic acidosis, and unexplained glucosuria of renal tubular origin may occur by age 1. Abnormal sensitivity to light and loss of color in the retina of the eyes can appear as early as 6–12 months of age. Crystals of cystine are deposited throughout the body. The affected gene is *CTNS*. If left untreated, this form of the disease may lead to kidney failure by age 9–10. Toxic accumulations of copper in the brain and kidney account for neurological symptoms. Manifestations are also seen in hereditary fructose intolerance.

In people with **intermediate cystinosis** (juvenile/adolescent), kidney and eye symptoms typically become apparent during the teenage years or early adulthood. Polyuria, growth retardation, rickets, acidosis, and vomiting are present. In **benign or adult cystinosis**, crystalline cystine accumulates primarily in the cornea of the eyes. Adults also present with acidosis, hypokalemia, polyuria, and osteomalacia. Cystinosis may also be caused by lead poisoning at any age.

Fanconi's syndrome is generalized tubular dysfunction and can be acquired or inherited. Valproate, often used for managing epilepsy, may cause Fanconi's syndrome in rare cases (Knorr et al, 2004). Renal Fanconi's syndrome demonstrates impaired kidney function with excessive urination (polyuria), excessive thirst (polydipsia), and abnormally low levels of potassium in the blood (hypokalemia). Myopathy in nephropathic cystinosis results in restrictive lung disease in adults who have not received long-term cystine depletion; whether or not oral cystamine therapy can prevent this complication remains to be determined (Anikster et al, 2001).

INTERVENTION: OBJECTIVES

- Prevent bone demineralization and kidney failure.
- Correct hypokalemia.
- Adapt to swallowing dysfunction.
- Support growth, which tends to be stunted in infants and children.
- Prevent or delay corneal damage.
- Provide large volumes of water and supplemental nutrients.
- Prepare for renal transplantation if needed.
- Postoperatively, promote wound healing and prevent graft rejection.

INTERVENTION: FOOD AND NUTRITION

- Use a diet low in cystine, with PFD1 or PFD2 (Mead Johnson).
- Provide sufficient fluid intake. Input and output should be checked by standards for age.
- Supplement with vitamin D (cannot convert 25-dihydroxycholecalciferol to the 1,25 form); give phosphate and calcium as appropriate. Bicarbonate is also needed.
- Provide sufficient sodium and potassium replacements.
- Alter consistency (liquids, solids) as needed.

CLINICAL INDICATORS

Clinical/History

Birth weight
Present weight
Length
Growth (%)
Diet/intake history
Head circumference
Abnormal sensitivity to light
Loss of color in the retina
Rickets
Dehydration
Dysphagia
Patchy brown skin

Lab Work

Ca++, Mg++
Phosphorous (P) (decreased)
Na+
K+ (decreased)
CO_2
Alb
H & H
Serum Fe
Serum vitamin D
I & O
Uric acid (decreased)
BUN
Creat
Ceruloplasmin
White blood cells

Common Drugs Used and Potential Side Effects

- Sodium bicarbonate or citrate should be used to correct acidosis. Take separately from iron supplements. Edema is one side effect for some patients.
- Cysteamine (Cystagon), administered orally, can halt glomerular destruction and halts the cystine content in cells.
- Long-term growth hormone treatment can be safe and effective in young children with nephropathic cystinosis; it should be started early in the course of the disease (Wuhl et al, 2001).

Herbs, Botanicals, and Supplements

- Herbs and botanicals should not be used for this condition because there are no controlled trials to prove efficacy.
- Use of Chinese herbs may be problematic in susceptible individuals, causing some forms of cystinosis. Discourage use.

INTERVENTION: NUTRITION EDUCATION, COUNSELING, CARE MANAGEMENT

- Emphasize the importance of correcting fluid and electrolyte imbalances.
- Discuss any necessary changes in consistency.
- Discuss diet for managing renal failure if necessary.
- If transplantation is needed, discuss guidelines for managing side effects such as graft–host resistance.

Patient Education—Food Safety

- Hand washing with soap and hot water is recommended before preparing formula or meals. Use clean utensils and containers for mixing formula.
- Before using tap water for formula preparation or to give as a beverage, let cold tap water run for 2 minutes to remove any lead that may be in the pipes.
- Follow the 2-hour rule: discard any beverage or food that has been left at room temperature for 2 hours or longer.
- Do not use honey in the diets of infants to decrease potential risk of botulism.

For More Information

- American Foundation for Urologic Disease
  http://www.afud.org
- Cystinosis Central
  http://medicine.ucsd.edu/cystinosis/Index.htm
- Cystinosis Foundation
  http://www.cystinosisfoundation.org/
- Cystinosis Research Foundation
  http://www.cystinosis.org/

CYSTINOSIS AND FANCONI'S SYNDROME—CITED REFERENCES

Anikster Y, et al. Pulmonary dysfunction in adults with nephropathic cystinosis. *Chest.* 119:394, 2001.

Knorr M, et al. Fanconi syndrome caused by antiepileptic therapy with valproic acid. *Epilepsia* 45:868, 2004.

Wuhl E, et al. Long-term treatment with growth hormone in short children with nephropathic cystinosis. *J Pediatr.* 138:880, 2001.

DOWN SYNDROME

NUTRITIONAL ACUITY RANKING: LEVEL 2

DEFINITIONS AND BACKGROUND

Down syndrome (DS) is a congenital defect in which patients carry altered chromosomes. Trisomy 21 patients are those with an extra chromosome 21. See Figure 3-2.

There is a direct correlation between the incidence of the syndrome and maternal age. Children with this condition have short stature, decreased muscle tone, constipation, intestinal defects, weight changes, and mental retardation. There is a higher risk for congenital heart disease, gum disease, celiac disease, Hirschsprung's disease, hypothyroidism, a rare form of leukemia, respiratory problems, gastroesophageal reflux, and Alzheimer's disease.

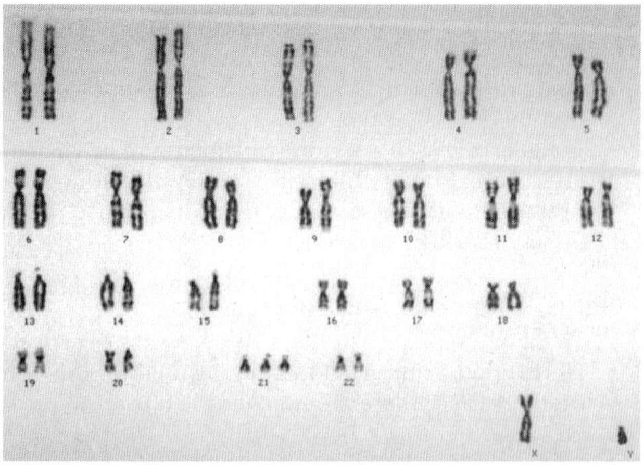

Figure 3-2 Trisomy 21. (From Rubin E, Farber JL. *Pathology*. 3rd ed. Philadelphia: Lippincott Williams & Wilkins, 1999.)

There is convincing epidemiological evidence of chronic oxidative stress in individuals with DS; these individuals develop Alzheimer-like changes in the brain in their 30s and 40s, autoimmune diseases, and cataracts (Jovanovic et al, 1998). Antioxidants, such as vitamins C and E, are under study. Research suggests that folate may also have a relationship to DS but does not cure it (James et al, 1999). Any woman of childbearing age should consume a food source or supplement of 400 mg of folic acid daily (Trissler, 2000).

Supplementation may help prevent DS (Rosenblatt, 1999), especially iron and folic acid when used in the first month of pregnancy (Czeizel and Puho, 2005). Compared to other individuals, individuals with DS may have lower levels of vitamin A, thiamin, folate, vitamin B_{12}, vitamin C, magnesium, manganese, selenium, zinc, carnitine, carnosine, and choline; excesses of copper, cysteine, phenylalanine, and superoxide dismutase are sometimes encountered (Thiel and Fowkes, 2004). In addition, disorders of metabolism involving vitamin B_6, vitamin D, calcium, and tryptophan may play a role, and further examination is needed (Thiel and Fowkes, 2004).

INTERVENTION: OBJECTIVES

- Provide adequate energy and nutrients for growth. Use DS growth charts; short stature is not caused by nutritional deficiencies.

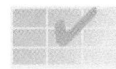

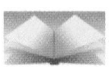

- To avoid lowering already inadequate intakes of several vitamins and minerals, treatment of obesity in children with DS should combine a balanced diet without energy restriction, vitamin and mineral supplementation, and increased physical activity.
- Assist with feeding problems. Tongue thrust and poor suck are common problems in infants. Use proper positioning for feeding.
- Prevent emotional problems that may lead to overeating. Overfeeding should be avoided.
- Counteract constipation, diarrhea, gluten enteropathy, or urinary tract infections.
- Correct gum and periodontal diseases, which are common.
- Monitor introduction of solid food, which is often delayed. Fruits and vegetables may not be consumed in adequate amounts (Hopman et al, 1998).
- Prevent osteoporosis and bone disease, which are common in individuals with DS.

INTERVENTION: FOOD AND NUTRITION

- Tube feed if the patient is unable to eat orally. Gradually wean to solids when possible.
- Supply adequate amounts of energy for age; for children ages 5–11 years, use 14.3 kcal/cm for girls and 16.1 kcal/cm for boys (Lucas, 2004, p. 41).
- Use protein according to RDA (age dependent).
- Use a gluten-free diet if celiac disease is present (Hill et al, 2005).
- Monitor for pica, overeating, and idiosyncrasies.
- Provide supplemental sources of folate, vitamin A, vitamin E, zinc, iron, and calcium (Hopman, 1998) if intake of fruits, vegetables, meats, dairy products, or whole grains is limited.
- Provide feeding assistance if needed.
- Provide extra fluid for losses in drooling, diarrhea, or spillage.
- Encourage complex carbohydrates, prune juice, etc., if constipation is a problem.

CLINICAL INDICATORS

Clinical/History		Lab Work
Length or height	Eye slant	Gluc
Birth weight	Hyperextensibility of joints	Uric acid (increased)
Present weight	History of prematurity?	Plasma zinc
BMI	Large tongue	Chol, Trig
Diet/intake history	Endocardial defects?	Na+, K+
Head circumference	Developmental delay	Ca++, Mg++
DS growth chart	Small nose with flat bridge	I & O
Growth (%)		

Common Drugs Used and Potential Side Effects

- Aricept, a drug used in Alzheimer's disease, may have some benefit in individuals with DS. Nausea or diarrhea are sometimes side effects. Improvements in learning and language may result. Larger trials are needed.

Herbs, Botanicals, and Supplements

- Herbs and botanicals should not be used for DS because there are no controlled trials to prove efficacy.

INTERVENTION: NUTRITION EDUCATION, COUNSELING, CARE MANAGEMENT

- Explain feeding techniques that may be beneficial.
- Help control or increase energy intake and physical activity.
- Discuss use of self-feeding utensils if needed.
- Never rush mealtime.
- Encourage socialization.
- Discuss how growth patterns differ from usual and how problems such as failure to thrive (Krugman and Dubowitz, 2003) or excessive weight gain can result as the child grows older.

Patient Education—Food Safety

- Hand washing with soap and hot water is recommended before preparing formula or meals. Use clean utensils and containers for mixing formula.
- Before using tap water for formula preparation or to give as a beverage, let cold tap water run for 2 minutes to remove any lead that may be in the pipes.
- Follow the 2-hour rule: discard any beverage or food that has been left at room temperature for 2 hours or longer.
- Do not use honey in the diets of infants to decrease potential risk of botulism.

For More Information

- Down Syndrome
  http://www.nas.com/downsyn/
- Down Syndrome Health Issues
  http://www.ds-health.com
- Down Syndrome Quarterly
  http://www.denison.edu/dsq
- Drexel University
  Down Syndrome Growth Charts
  http://www.growthcharts.com/
  http://www.growthcharts.com/charts/DS/charts.htm
- National Association for Down Syndrome
  http://www.nads.org/
- National Down Syndrome Society
  http://www.ndss.org/content.cfm
- Special Olympics
  http://www.specialolympics.org/Special+Olympics+Public+Website/default.htm

DOWN SYNDROME—CITED REFERENCES

Czeizel AE, Puho E. Maternal use of nutritional supplements during the first month of pregnancy and decreased risk of Down's syndrome: case-control study. *Nutrition* 21:698, 2005.
Hill ID, et al. Guideline for the diagnosis and treatment of celiac disease in children: recommendations of the North American Society for Pediatric Gastroenterology, Hepatology and Nutrition. *J Pediatr Gastroenterol Nutr.* 40:1, 2005.
Hopman E, et al. Eating habits of young children with Down syndrome in The Netherlands: adequate nutrient intakes but delayed introduction of solid food. *J Am Diet Assoc.* 98:79, 1998.
James S, et al. Abnormal folate metabolism and mutation in the methylenetetrahydrofolate reductase gene may be maternal risk factors for Down syndrome. *Am J Clin Nutr.* 70:495, 1999.
Jovanovic S, et al. Biomarkers of oxidative stress are significantly elevated in Down syndrome. *Free Radic Biol Med.* 25:1044, 1998.
Krugman SD, Dubowitz H. Failure to thrive. *Am Fam Physician.* 68:879, 2003.
Lucas B, ed. *Children with special care needs: nutrition care handbook.* Chicago: The American Dietetic Association, 2004.
Thiel RJ, Fowkes SW. Down syndrome and epilepsy: a nutritional connection? *Med Hypotheses.* 62:35, 2004.
Trissler R. Folic acid and Down syndrome. *J Am Diet Assoc.* 100:159, 2000.

FAILURE TO THRIVE

NUTRITIONAL ACUITY RANKING: LEVEL 4

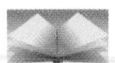

DEFINITIONS AND BACKGROUND

Failure to thrive (FTT) is a diagnostic term used to describe infants and children who fail to grow and develop at a normal rate; it is also another term for protein–energy malnutrition. In many pediatric centers, one third of the referred children are malnourished. Vitamin-mineral depletion is also found with protein–energy malnutrition. Adequate hydration is needed. Prompt diagnosis and intervention are important for preventing malnutrition and developmental delays (Krugman and Dubowitz, 2003). Careful attention must be paid to plotting growth parameters and completing thorough medical histories (Krugman and Dubowitz, 2003).

About 25% of normal infants will shift to a lower growth percentile in the first 2 years of life and then follow that percentile; this is not FTT (Krugman and Dubowitz, 2003). Note that infants with Down syndrome, intrauterine growth retardation, or premature birth follow different growth patterns than normal infants, and monitor carefully (Krugman and Dubowitz, 2003).

Feeding disorders can lead to FTT, susceptibility to chronic illness, and death. FTT is a complex problem that can be caused by many medical or social factors. Prevention is suggested by giving children a wide range of foods before reaching 15–18 months, keeping healthy foods available, teaching children to communicate hunger by relating food intake to appetite, and reinforcing good mealtime behaviors (Stein, 2000).

The growth percentiles of an infant or child who fails to thrive are at the fifth percentile or below for weight and length of infants the same age. Other indices include a small head circumference, muscular wasting, apathy, weight loss, or poor weight gain. Learning failure (e.g., slow to talk, behavior problems) can occur in children with FTT. Weight is the most reliable marker for FTT and its associated problems (Raynor and Rudolf, 2000). According to the American Academy of Pediatrics (2004), FTT is established when weight (or weight/height) is less than 2 standard deviations below the mean for sex and age and/or the weight curve has dropped more than 2 percentile lines on the National Center for Health Statistics growth charts after having achieved a previously stable pattern.

Primary FTT originates from social/environmental deficits, inadequate feeding procedures, or caretaker behaviors. Adolescent mothers may need a lot of support and teaching. If FTT results from a problematic infant–mother interaction, there may also be a physiological basis to the behaviors that are exhibited by these infants (Steward et al, 2001). Children with feeding disorders exhibit more withdrawal during feeding. Proximity and touch are especially disturbed in feeding disorders (i.e., mothers provide less touch that supports growth), and children demonstrate signs of touch aversion (Feldman et al, 2004). Early interventions by trained home visitors can promote a more nurturing environment and reduce developmental delays in primary FTT (Black et al, 1995).

Secondary FTT originates from some disease states (e.g., cancer, allergies, chronic infections, cystic fibrosis, cleft lip or palate, Down syndrome, or other physical or mental disability). Growth failure plus fever of unknown origin and anemia in older children or teens may suggest the onset of Crohn's disease; evaluation is recommended.

About half of the causes of FTT are organic; the other 50% are from inorganic causes. The American Dietetic Association promotes at least five medical nutrition therapy visits for infants and children with pediatric FTT.

INTERVENTION: OBJECTIVES

- All children with FTT need additional calories for catch-up growth at about 150% of the energy requirement for their expected, not actual, weight (Krugman and Dubowitz, 2003). There are calculation formulas for determining needs in the *Pediatric Manual of Clinical Dietetics* (Nevin-Folino, 2003).
- Provide optimal nutrition compatible with normal growth pattern. Achieve daily gains (30 g for young infants is about average weight gain; extra may be desirable for catch-up).
- Identify and correct causes, which may include decreased intake, increased nutrient losses, increased metabolic

demands, and decreased growth efficiency. Determine if malnutrition is primary (from faulty feeding patterns or dietary inadequacy) or secondary (from disease process interfering with intake).

- Teach the parent or caretaker how to properly feed and how to determine needs. Parenting advice about nurturing during feeding is often useful.
- Provide adequate schedule of feeding for infant's age.
- Support catch-up growth. See Table 3-5 for comparison with growth rates of normal children for height and weight.

INTERVENTION: FOOD AND NUTRITION

- Conduct a thorough nutrition assessment and acquire actual intake records when possible. Evaluate the child's nutritional history and growth in comparison to the percentiles of normal children. Discuss with parent or caretaker. If special growth charts are needed, use those instead (as for Down syndrome, etc.).
- Calculate diet according to infant's age for energy and protein. While not always possible or practical, resting energy expenditure (REE) may be measured in young infants and children with moderate to severe FTT when knowledge of caloric needs is required (Sentongo et al, 2000). Protein intake should be assessed carefully as well (Sullivan et al, 2002; Queen and Lang, 1993).
- Check recommended dietary needs for all nutrients and provide adequate zinc and vitamin B_6, as determined by the infant's age. Using slightly higher levels (such as 130%) is a common practice.
- Monitor growth (weight) and feeding behaviors. Weekly weights may be needed, especially in young infants.
- If the infant is in a state of dehydration, provide adequate amounts of water.
- FTT can be aggravated by excessive consumption of fruit juice and sweetened beverages (often 12–30 oz daily). This amount may replace other nutrient-dense foods. Limit to 4–6 oz daily until overall dietary quality and growth rate have improved.
- Parents should provide meals and snacks at scheduled times to avoid the habit of grazing. Provide a comfortable social and emotional environment at mealtimes. Family meals and allowing children to be a part of meal preparation are also important.
- In FTT children who are strictly vegan, monitor carefully for vitamins B_{12}, D, B_6, and B_2, iron, zinc, and calcium deficiencies.
- Tube feeding may be useful or necessary as a supplemental or alternative feeding method to oral intake. Night feeding is an effective recommendation for many.

CLINICAL INDICATORS

Clinical/History

- Height
- Birth weight
- Weight, goal weight
- Growth grid
- Percent height for age (actual height/expected height)
- Diet/intake history
- Head circumference
- Skinfold thickness
- Apgar scores
- Food allergies
- Medical history
- Premature or small for gestational age?
- Breastfed or bottle fed?
- Solid food introduction pattern
- Diarrhea or vomiting?
- Constipation
- Signs of dehydration?
- Sources of income for food
- Feeding schedule and timing

Lab Work

- H & H
- Serum Fe
- Iron deficiency anemia
- Alb
- Gluc
- Chol, Trig
- BUN
- Thyroid function tests
- I & O
- Sweat test?

TABLE 3-5 Normal Growth Rates for Height and Weight in Children

Age	Growth in Length or Height (mm/d)[a]	Growth in Length or Height (inches/yr)
0–6 months	1.06 declining to 0.77	7–10
6–12 months	0.47	6–7
1–2 years	0.35 declining to 0.30	4–5
2–3 years	—	3–4
3–4 years	—	2–3
4–10 years	—	2
Age	**Daily Growth in Weight (oz/d)[a]**	**Growth in Weight**
0–4 months	1.0 declining to 0.61	1 1/2 lb/mo
4–10 months	0.61 declining to 0.47	1 lb/mo
10–24 months	0.47 declining to 0.25	1/2 lb/mo
2–8 years	—	3-4 lbs/yr

Adapted from: [a]Nevin-Folino, 2003; and http://www.magicfoundation.org/.

Common Drugs Used and Potential Side Effects

- Evaluate all medications given for any reason to determine if some or all affect nutritional intake. Adjust diet as needed.
- Endogenous cannabinoids or other appetite enhancers are being studied for their safety and effectiveness in FTT.

Herbs, Botanicals, and Supplements

- Herbs and botanicals should not be used for FTT because there are no controlled trials to prove efficacy.
- Probiotics may be useful; these are live micro-organisms that confer a health benefit. Medical conditions that have been reportedly treated or have the potential to be treated with probiotics include many GI disorders, cancer, infant allergies, FTT, and infections (Brown and Valiere, 2004).
- Zinc supplementation is being studied for catch-up growth in malnourished children; studies are not yet conclusive (Castillo-Duran and Weisstaub, 2003).

INTERVENTION: NUTRITION EDUCATION, COUNSELING, CARE MANAGEMENT

- Describe the appropriate nutritional intake according to age of the child. Describe the predisposing medical conditions when appropriate.
- Encourage the use of appropriate growth charts at home to monitor success.
- Develop a progress chart for developmental milestones. Growth spurts follow sustained weight gains. Monitor growth frequently.
- Offer simple, specific instructions such as mechanics of breastfeeding and typical intakes for children of same age. If formula is given, improper mixing of formula is common; help correct any misunderstandings.
- Discuss nutrient density (e.g., milk vs. sweetened carbonated beverages).
- Explain proper use of over-the-counter vitamin-mineral supplements.
- Address unusual dietary beliefs (Feld and Hyams, 2004).
- Practical suggestions should be offered regarding nurturing and emotional support for the child. Parenting classes may be beneficial. Referral to child welfare services may be needed in some cases where neglect is suspected (Block et al, 2005).
- Follow-up should be provided at outpatient clinics or by home visits. Refer to WIC programs and other resources, such as La Leche League or food stamps, if possible.

Patient Education—Food Safety

- Hand washing with soap and hot water is recommended before preparing formula or meals. Use clean utensils and containers for mixing formula.
- Before using tap water for formula preparation or to give as a beverage, let cold tap water run for 2 minutes to remove any lead that may be in the pipes.
- Follow the 2-hour rule: discard any beverage or food that has been left at room temperature for 2 hours or longer.
- Do not use honey in the diets of infants; this will decrease the potential risk of botulism.

For More Information

- Kids Health
  http://kidshealth.org/parent/nutrition_fit/nutrition/failure_thrive.html

FAILURE TO THRIVE—CITED REFERENCES

American Academy of Pediatrics. *Pediatric nutrition handbook.* 5th ed. Elk Grove Village, IL: American Academy of Pediatrics, 2004.

Black M, et al. A randomized clinical trial of home intervention for children with failure to thrive. *Pediatrics* 95:807, 1995.

Block RW, et al. Failure to thrive as a manifestation of child neglect. *Pediatrics* 116:1234, 2005.

Brown AC, Valiere A. Probiotics and medical nutrition therapy. *Nutr Clin Care.* 7:56, 2004.

Castillo-Duran C, Weisstaub G. Zinc supplementation and growth of the fetus and low birth weight infant. *J Nutr.* 133:1494S, 2003.

Feld LG, Hyams JS, eds. *Growth assessment and growth failure. Consensus in pediatrics.* Evansville, IN: Mead Johnson & Company, 2004.

Feldman R, et al. Mother-child touch patterns in infant feeding disorders: relation to maternal, child, and environmental factors. *J Am Acad Child Adolesc Psychiatry.* 43:1089, 2004.

Krugman SD, Dubowitz H. Failure to thrive. *Am Fam Physician.* 68:879, 2003.

Nevin-Folino N, ed. *Pediatric manual of clinical dietetics.* 2nd ed. Chicago: The American Dietetic Association, 2003, pp. 775-776.

Queen PM, Lang CE. *Handbook of pediatric nutrition.* Gaithersburg, MD: Aspen Publishers, Inc, 1993.

Raynor P, Rudolf M. Anthropometric indices of failure to thrive. *Arch Dis Child.* 82:364, 2000.

Sentongo TA, et al. Resting energy expenditure and prediction equations in young children with failure to thrive. *J Pediatr.* 136:345, 2000.

Stein K. Children with feeding disorders: an emerging issue. *J Am Diet Assoc.* 100:1000, 2000.

Steward D, et al. Biobehavioral characteristics of infants with failure to thrive. *J Pediatr Nurs.* 16:162, 2001.

Sullivan PB, et al. Impact of feeding problems on nutritional intake and growth: Oxford Feeding Study II. *Dev Med Child Neurol.* 44:461, 2002.

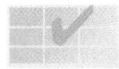

FETAL ALCOHOL SYNDROME

NUTRITIONAL ACUITY RANKING: LEVEL 1–2

DEFINITIONS AND BACKGROUND

Generally noted shortly after birth, fetal alcohol syndrome (FAS) is a syndrome in infants with developmental delay, ocular anomalies, LBW, tremors, short stature, retardation of intellect, seizures, and microcephaly. FAS is the third leading cause of mental retardation in the United States and is considered to be the most preventable (Centers for Disease Control, 2004). There is now a continuum of these disorders, recognized as fetal alcohol spectrum disorders (FASD). CDC analyzed data for women aged 18–44 years from the 2002 Behavioral Risk Factor Surveillance System (BRFSS) survey; approximately 10% of pregnant women used alcohol, and 2% engaged in binge drinking or frequent use of alcohol (Centers for Disease Control, 2004).

No level of alcohol consumption during pregnancy is safe (Centers for Disease Control, 2004). Exposure to alcohol during brain development can permanently alter the physiology of the hippocampal formation, thus promoting epileptic activity and facilitating spreading of depression (Bonthius et al, 2001). In addition, disrupted cholesterol homeostasis may contribute to neurotoxicity; the developing brain requires cholesterol for proper cell proliferation (Guizzetti and Costa, 2005). Children with milder fetal alcohol effects (FAE) perform better on motor ability tests than those with FAS and have a slightly better weight status (Alvear et al., 1998).

Heavy prenatal alcohol exposure with or without physical features of FAS leads to IQ defects (Mattson et al, 1997). Women who are pregnant or who might become pregnant should abstain totally from use of alcohol (Centers for Disease Control, 2004). Sometimes blood tests are better to detect at-risk pregnant women rather than self-reported alcohol intakes (Stoler et al, 1998). Acetaldehyde may play a role in the damage from alcohol (Eriksson, 2001). The steady concurrent use of tobacco and alcohol by young women emphasizes the need for enhanced efforts to reduce initial tobacco and alcohol use by young people. Women who report abuse of tobacco or alcohol should be evaluated for abuse of both substances, and interventions should address abuse of both substances, especially to prevent FAS (Ebrahim et al, 2000).

Early assessment of children at risk is important to offer needed services. In many communities, it may be difficult to find and treat children who have the indicators of FASD. Using the combination of weight and head circumference below the 10th percentile at birth is a useful methodology for identifying children at substantial risk for growth and developmental delays from FAS (Weiss et al, 2004). Children with FAS may have more social and medical needs; they often have more facial dysmorphology, growth deficiency, central nervous system dysfunction, muscular problems, hospitalizations for otitis media, pneumonia, dehydration, and anemia (Kvigne et al, 2004).

INTERVENTION: OBJECTIVES

- Promote effective family coping skills and effective parental bonding.
- Prevent additional retardation and developmental delays, blindness, etc.
- Improve intake and nutritional status.
- Prevent or correct vomiting and other problems.
- Improve cardiac symptoms.
- Encourage normal growth patterns; prevent problems such as failure to thrive. Distorted eating perception can occur, with underweight a possible outcome.

INTERVENTION: FOOD AND NUTRITION

- Provide a diet appropriate for age and status (see Low Birth Weight entry).
- Ensure adequate protein and energy for catch-up growth.
- If necessary, provide tube feeding or TPN while hospitalized. Some infants may require additional nutrition support in the home setting to promote better growth and development.

CLINICAL INDICATORS

Clinical/History	Head circumference (often under 10th percentile)	Lab Work
Birth weight	Seizures	Alb
Current weight (often below 10th percentile)	Physical growth delay?	Na+, K+
Length	Functional deficits (motor, social, memory, etc.)	Gluc
Growth (%)		H & H
Diet/intake history		Serum Fe
		Ca++, Mg++
		Serum folate

Common Drugs Used and Potential Side Effects

- Anticonvulsants may be needed to correct seizures. Monitor for depletion of vitamins C, D, B_6, B_{12}, and K, folic acid, and calcium.

Herbs, Botanicals, and Supplements

- Herbs and botanicals should not be used for FAS because there are no controlled trials to prove efficacy.

INTERVENTION: NUTRITION EDUCATION, COUNSELING, CARE MANAGEMENT

- Discuss appropriate feeding techniques for age of infant.
- Discuss importance of diet in aiding normal growth and development.
- Encourage mother's participation in alcohol rehabilitation if needed. Discuss her future plans for additional pregnancies and encourage counseling to avoid continued alcohol intake during that time.

Patient Education—Food Safety

- Hand washing with soap and hot water is recommended before preparing formula or meals. Use clean utensils and containers for mixing formula.
- Before using tap water for formula preparation or to give as a beverage, let cold tap water run for 2 minutes to remove any lead that may be in the pipes.
- Follow the 2-hour rule: discard any beverage or food that has been left at room temperature for 2 hours or longer.
- Do not use honey in the diets of infants; this will decrease potential risk of botulism.

For More Information

- CDC–Division of Birth Defects and Developmental Disabilities, FAS Site
http://www.cdc.gov/ncbddd/fas/
- CDC Diagnosis and Referral Guide
http://www.cdc.gov/ncbddd/fas/documents/FAS_guidelines_accessible.pdf
- Fetal Alcohol and Drug Unit
http://depts.washington.edu/fadu
- Fetal Alcohol Syndrome Handbook
http://www.usd.edu/cd/publications/fashandbook.cfm
- Fetal Alcohol Syndrome websites
http://www.come-over.to/FAS/faslinks.htm
- FAS Community Resource Center
http://www.come-over.to/FASCRC/
- National Center for Family Support
http://www.familysupport-hsri.org/
- National Clearinghouse for Alcohol and Drug Information (NCADI)
http://www.health.org/
- National Council on Alcoholism and Drug Dependence (NCADD)
http://www.ncadd.org/
- National Organization of Fetal Alcohol Syndrome
http://www.nofas.org/

FETAL ALCOHOL SYNDROME—CITED REFERENCES

Alvear J, et al. Fetal alcohol syndrome and fetal alcohol effects: importance of early diagnosis and nutritional treatment. *Rev Med Chil.* 126:407, 1998.

Bonthius D, et al. Alcohol exposure during the brain growth spurt promotes hippocampal seizures, rapid kindling, and spreading depression. *Alcohol Clin Exp Res.* 25:734, 2001.

Centers for Disease Control. Alcohol consumption among women who are pregnant or who might become pregnant–United States, 2002. *MMWR Morb Mortal Wkly Rep.* 53:1178, 2004.

Ebrahim S, et al. Combined tobacco and alcohol use by pregnant and reproductive-aged women in the United States. *Obstet Gynecol.* 96:767, 2000.

Eriksson C. The role of acetaldehyde in the actions of alcohol (update 2000). *Alcohol Clin Exp Res.* 25:15S, 2001.

Guizzetti M, Costa LG. Disruption of cholesterol homeostasis in the developing brain as a potential mechanism contributing to the developmental neurotoxicity of ethanol: an hypothesis. *Med Hypotheses.* 64:563, 2005.

Kvigne VL, et al. Characteristics of children who have full or incomplete fetal alcohol syndrome. *J Pediatr.* 145:635, 2004.

Mattson S, et al. Heavy prenatal alcohol exposure with or without physical features of fetal alcohol syndrome leads to IQ defects. *J Pediatr.* 131:718, 1997.

Stoler J, et al. The prenatal detection of significant alcohol exposure with maternal blood markers. *J Pediatr.* 133:346, 1998.

Weiss M, et al. The Wisconsin Fetal Alcohol Syndrome Screening Project. *WMJ.* 103:53, 2004.

HIRSCHSPRUNG'S DISEASE (CONGENITAL MEGACOLON)

NUTRITIONAL ACUITY RANKING: LEVEL 4

DEFINITIONS AND BACKGROUND

Hirschsprung's disease (HD) is characterized by the absence of ganglion cells and the presence of hypertrophic nerve trunks in the distal bowel (Yoneda et al, 2001). HD is also known as jejunal gangliosus or congenital megacolon. Incidence is one in 5000 live births. HD may reoccur in other babies born to the same family with a child with HD (Stewart and von Allmen, 2003).

As a congenital malformation, HD interferes with normal mass peristalsis and functional obstruction. Normally, ganglia stimulate the gut and allow peristalsis to occur. In HD, the ganglia are missing, and segments of bowel become obstructed. This creates abdominal distention, which can cause failure to pass meconium stool, vomiting, and constipation. If not diagnosed until the child is older, growth failure may be a presenting sign.

TABLE 3-6 Clinical Grading System for Hirschsprung's-Associated Enterocolitis

Grade	Clinical Symptoms
I	Mild explosive diarrhea, mild or moderate abdominal distention, and no systemic manifestations
II	Moderate explosive diarrhea, moderate to severe abdominal distention, and mild systemic symptoms
III	Severe explosive diarrhea, marked abdominal distention, and shock or impending shock

From: Elhalaby et al, 1995.

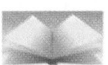

Surgical removal may be required to prevent bowel obstruction and may be followed by a temporary colostomy. The usual complications after a definitive pull-through procedure for HD include stricture formation, enterocolitis, and occasionally, wound infection (Finck et al, 2001). Often, removal of the affected area and reconnection of the colon occurs at age 6 months or older. Over the long term, one in five patients will have continuation of constipation, occasional soiling, and incontinence, and one in 10 patients may have severe problems. A special type of enterocolitis, HD-associated enterocolitis (HAE), may also be a concern (Nofech-Mozes et al, 2004). The condition can be life threatening, and signs include hypoalbuminemia, diarrhea and vomiting, and anorexia and weight loss. See Table 3-6.

INTERVENTION: OBJECTIVES

- Provide adequate nutrition for the patient's age and development. Growth may be inhibited.
- Replace electrolytes and fluids, especially with diarrhea and enterocolitis.
- Compensate for poor absorption of nutrients; water-miscible forms of fat-soluble vitamins may be needed.
- Prevent complications after surgery, especially constipation, incontinence, or enterocolitis.

INTERVENTION: FOOD AND NUTRITION

- Use a high-energy/high-protein diet. Enteral products, oral supplements, or TPN can be used if required.
- Monitor serum electrolytes, especially potassium, if laxatives are used. Encourage a diet high in fiber and fluid to wean off medication if possible.
- Provide fluids adequate for the patient's age and hydration status.
- Provide TPN if large sections of the bowel are removed. Advance infant feedings as tolerated using human milk or preterm or standard infant formulas, and then gradually progress to soft/bland foods.
- Monitor calcium, magnesium, and other nutrients if long-term TPN is needed.

CLINICAL INDICATORS

Clinical/History		Lab Work
Birth weight	Watery diarrhea (newborn)	H & H
Length	Constipation	Serum Fe
Present weight	Temperature	Alb
FTT	Vomiting	Na+, K+
Growth (slow)	Abdominal distention	Ca++, Mg++
Diet/intake history	Dehydration; I & O	Gluc
Failure to pass meconium after birth	Abdominal x-ray	
	Barium enema	
	Malabsorption	

Common Drugs Used and Potential Side Effects

- Antibiotics may be needed if perforation has occurred or when there is enterocolitis. Monitor for side effects.
- In constipation, laxatives can deplete numerous nutrient reserves; monitor carefully. Encourage a diet high in fiber and fluid to wean off medication if possible.

Herbs, Botanicals, and Supplements

- Herbs and botanicals should not be used for megacolon because there are no controlled trials to prove efficacy.

INTERVENTION: NUTRITION EDUCATION, COUNSELING, CARE MANAGEMENT

- Teach patient about sources of protein, energy, potassium, and other key nutrients from diet.
- Discuss wound healing or colostomy procedures after surgery.
- For constipation and bowel incontinence, a high-fiber diet may be useful, but discuss signs and symptoms of obstruction to report immediately to a doctor. Extra fluids will be needed with high-fiber intake.

Patient Education—Food Safety

- Hand washing with soap and hot water is recommended before preparing formula or meals. Use clean utensils and containers for mixing formula.
- Before using tap water for formula preparation or to give as a beverage, let cold tap water run for 2 minutes to remove any lead that may be in the pipes.
- Follow the 2-hour rule: discard any beverage or food that has been left at room temperature for 2 hours or longer.
- Do not use honey in the diets of infants to decrease potential risk of botulism.

For More Information

- Digestive Health Matters
  http://www.aboutkidsgi.org/publications.html
- The Hirschsprung's & Motility Disorders Support Network
  http://www.hirschsprungs.info/index.html
- International Foundation for Functional Gastrointestinal Disorders
  http://www.iffgd.org/
- National Digestive Diseases Clearinghouse
  http://digestive.niddk.nih.gov/
- Pull-Through Network
  http://www.pullthrough.org/Hirschsprungs.html
- United Ostomy Association
  http://uoa.org/

HIRSCHSPRUNG'S DISEASE—CITED REFERENCES

Elhalaby EA, et al. Enterocolitis associated with Hirschsprung's disease: a clinical-radiological characterization based on 168 patients. *J Pediatr Surg*. 30:76, 1995.

Finck C, et al. Presentation of carcinoma in a patient with a previous operation for Hirschsprung's disease. *J Pediatr Surg.* 36:E5, 2001.
Nofech-Mozes Y, et al. Difficulties in making the diagnosis of Hirschsprung disease in early infancy. *J Paediatr Child Health.* 40:716, 2004.
Stewart DR, von Allmen D. The genetics of Hirschsprung disease. *Gastroenterol Clin North Am.* 32:819, 2003.
Yoneda A, et al. Cell-adhesion molecules and fibroblast growth factor signaling in Hirschsprung's disease. *Pediatr Surg Int.* 17:299, 2001.

HIV INFECTION, PEDIATRIC

NUTRITIONAL ACUITY RANKING: LEVEL 4

DEFINITIONS AND BACKGROUND

There are unique considerations related to HIV infection in infants, children, and adolescents. With the use of highly active antiretroviral therapy (HAART), there is minimal mother-to-child transmission of HIV infection in developed countries (i.e., 1–2% only) (King et al, 2004; Newell and Thorne, 2004). In developed nations, HIV infection is more of a chronic disease, with extensive medications, costs, and side effects to consider. A high proportion of HIV-infected individuals are African or African American.

Worldwide, more than 1900 children are infected with HIV each day (2004 Report on the Global AIDS Epidemic/UNAIDS Fourth Global Report, July 2004). Developing nations still have a battle to address. Infants who are breastfed by HIV-infected mothers still have the risk of acquiring the infection. In addition, HIV-infected mothers may transmit opportunistic pathogens to their infants.

In children with AIDS, failure to thrive (FTT) and protein–calorie malnutrition (PCM) are common; regular monitoring and interventions are needed (Gorbea-Robles et al, 1998). Every child with HIV infection should be assessed at baseline and every 4–6 months thereafter to determine risk of nutritional compromise. Severity or degree of nutritional risk is measured in anthropometric, biochemical, dietary intake, and medical data. Height for age, weight for age, clinical class, somatic protein stores, mid-arm circumference, weight for height, serum albumin, immunological status, body mass index (BMI), energy intake, and evidence of opportunistic infections are reliable indicators of status (Heller, 2000).

Salivary gland disease is a common finding related to HIV infection; gland enlargement or xerostomia may present, and the reduction in saliva must be addressed (Pinto and DeRossi, 2004).

INTERVENTION: OBJECTIVES

- Achieve a normal growth pattern; allow for catch-up growth if needed. Monitor patterns closely.
- Support efforts for prevention of opportunistic infections by improving or maintaining immune status with good nutrition.
- Alleviate effects of wasting syndrome, diarrhea, and other symptoms. Prevent malabsorption, enteric infections, malnutrition, and immune deficiency.
- Preserve lean body mass.

INTERVENTION: FOOD AND NUTRITION

- Use a high-protein diet. Enteral products, oral supplements, and frequent snacks should be used if required. Protein needs are 1.5–2 times the usual for age and gender (Heller, 1997; Heller, 2000).
- Energy needs may vary from 50–200% of the usual requirements. Children with severe encephalopathy may be bed bound and require fewer total calories.
- Assure adequacy of fluid intake, especially because there are so many medications to be taken each day.
- A multivitamin supplement is needed to provide at least 100% of the daily needs. Poor absorption may be a problem for vitamins A, C, B_6, and B_{12}, folate, iron, selenium, and zinc. Calcium is needed to prevent loss of bone mass, which may persist (O'Brien et al, 2001).
- Naturally occurring antioxidants are safe when consumed in normal amounts. For example, include nuts for vitamin E and selenium and citrus fruits for vitamin C. Be aware of excesses from pills and other supplemental forms because excesses are not proven to be of benefit. Megadoses are considered to be 10 times the RDA (American Academy of Pediatrics, 2004, p. 684) and have not proven to be of benefit.
- Early identification of children with HIV/AIDS is essential, and aggressive nutritional support is critical. Nocturnal, continuous feedings may be useful.

CLINICAL INDICATORS

Clinical/History	Diet/intake history	Lab Work
Height Weight Growth percentile and pattern	Head circumference (infants) Stunting FTT	H & H Serum Fe Alb Na+, K+ Ca++, Mg++ Gluc

Common Drugs Used and Potential Side Effects

- For a list of FDA-approved medications used in pediatric HIV infection, see Section 15.

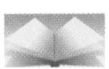

- HIV-infected mothers may transmit opportunistic pathogens to their infants. There may be antibiotics or antiviral agents prescribed accordingly that should be closely monitored for nutritional and GI side effects. Children's adherence to complex antiretroviral (HAART) therapy requires addressing developmental, psychosocial, and family factors (Mellins et al, 2004).
- Few HIV medicines are produced in pediatric formulations. Those drugs available as syrups have limitations, such as short shelf-life, objectionable taste, difficult measuring of correct doses, and expense.

Herbs, Botanicals, and Supplements

- Herbs and botanicals should not be used for HIV because there are no clinical trials proving efficacy.
- HIV-infected individuals may be attracted to the many possible supplements on the market. Carefully review all items and discuss their viability or potential for harm.
- Use of acidophilus and probiotic products may alleviate loss of intestinal bacteria.

INTERVENTION: NUTRITION EDUCATION, COUNSELING, CARE MANAGEMENT

- There will be a need to manage medications, a nutrient-dense diet, doctor visits, and other interventions or therapies. Provide support to the child and family or caregivers.
- Encourage formula feeding if mother has HIV infection.
- Discuss HIV infection prevention strategies, especially with noninfected teens.
- Children should receive all of the usual vaccinations to prevent other illnesses or complications.

Patient Education—Food Safety

- Hand washing with soap and hot water is recommended before preparing formula or meals. Use clean utensils and containers for mixing formula.
- Before using tap water for formula preparation or to give as a beverage, let cold tap water run for 2 minutes to remove any lead that may be in the pipes.
- Follow the 2-hour rule: discard any beverage or food that has been left at room temperature for 2 hours or longer.
- Do not use honey in the diets of infants to decrease potential risk of botulism.

For More Information

- AIDSinfo
  www.aidsinfo.nih.gov
- AIDS Vaccine Advocacy Coalition (AVAC)
  www.avac.org
- American Foundation for AIDS Research (amFAR)
  www.amfar.org
- Baylor International Pediatric AIDS Initiative
  http://bayloraids.org/
- CDC National Prevention Information Network (NPIN)
  http://www.cdcnpin.org/scripts/index.asp
- International AIDS Society (IAS)
  www.ias.se
- Johns Hopkins University School of Medicine AIDS Site
  www.hopkins-aids.edu/
- National Institute of Allergy and Infectious Diseases (NIAID)
  www.niaid.nih.gov/daids/
- National Pediatric AIDS Network
  http://www.npan.org/
- Pediatric AIDS Foundation
  http://www.pedaids.org/
- U.S. Coalition for Child Survival
  www.child-survival.org

HIV INFECTION, PEDIATRIC—CITED REFERENCES

American Academy of Pediatrics. *Pediatric nutrition handbook.* 5th ed. Elk Grove Village, IL: American Academy of Pediatrics, 2004.
Gorbea-Robles M, et al. Nutrition assessment in pediatric patients infected with the human immunodeficiency virus. *Nutr Clin Pract.* 13:172, 1998.
Heller L. Nutrition support for children with HIV/AIDS. *J Am Diet Assoc.* 97:473, 1997.
Heller L, et al. Development of an instrument to assess nutritional risk factors for children infected with human immunodeficiency virus. *J Am Diet Assoc.* 100:323, 2000.
King SM, et al. Evaluation and treatment of the human immunodeficiency virus-1–exposed infant. *Pediatrics* 114:497, 2004.
Mellins CA, et al. The role of psychosocial and family factors in adherence to antiretroviral treatment in human immunodeficiency virus-infected children. *Pediatr Infect Dis J.* 23:1035, 2004.
Newell ML, Thorne C. Antiretroviral therapy and mother-to-child transmission of HIV-1. *Expert Rev Anti Infect Ther.* 2:717, 2004.
O'Brien K, et al. Bone mineral content in girls perinatally infected with HIV. *Am J Clin Nutr.* 73:821, 2001.
Pinto A, De Rossi SS. Salivary gland disease in pediatric HIV patients: an update. *J Dent Child.* 71:33, 2004.

HOMOCYSTINURIA

NUTRITIONAL ACUITY RANKING: LEVEL 3–4

DEFINITIONS AND BACKGROUND

Homocystinuria (HCU) is an autosomal recessive metabolic disorder, a disorder of amino acid metabolism caused by a missing cystathionine enzyme. There are three forms of HCU: cystathionine beta-synthase (CBS) deficiency, defective cobalamin coenzyme synthesis, and 5,10-methylenetetrahydrofolate reductase deficiency. HCU is more common than previously thought, and newborn screening has been recommended (Refsum, Fredriksen et al, 2004).

Homocystinuria due to **deficiency of CBS** is inherited as an autosomal recessive trait. The disorder results from changes (mutations) of a gene on the long arm (q) of chromosome 21 (21q22.3) that regulates the production of the CBS enzyme. Human CBS is an *S*-adenosylmethionine–regulated enzyme that plays a key role in the metabolism of homocysteine (Shan et al, 2001). It occurs in one in 20,000 to one in 200,000 births in the United States. If untreated, it may lead to mental retardation, seizures, altered growth, hepatic disease, osteoporosis, thromboses, glaucoma, cataracts, and strokes. Individuals with HCU may be unusually tall in stature, with long arms and legs. This tall stature suggests that overgrowth is directly mediated by homocysteine and that it may be prevented by optimal metabolic control (Topaloglu et al, 2001). Dietary restriction of methionine is only helpful in the CBS deficiency; in the others, it is harmful to restrict.

Deranged vitamin B_6 metabolism or low levels of reductase enzyme may also cause HCU (methionine to cysteine conversion). A single biochemical test is not available; abnormal urinary tHcy response after methionine loading is the most sensitive test (Guttormsen et al, 2001). Urinary excretion of homocysteine occurs but is unusual, which is a marker for one of these disorders.

Inborn errors of cobalamin transport and metabolism present with HCU and methylmalonic aciduria, either alone or in combination; they share many of the clinical features of nutritional cobalamin deficiency (Rosenblatt and Whitehead, 1999). Patients may have dramatic reduction of plasma-free homocysteine and urine methylmalonic acid excretion after initiation of therapy with carnitine and intramuscular hydroxocobalamin; growth and microcephaly may also be improved (Andersson et al, 1999).

5,10-Methylene-tetrahydrofolate reductase deficiency (MTHFR) affects many enzyme systems. It can present with mental retardation, microcephaly, gait disturbance, psychiatric disturbances, seizures, abnormal EEG, and limb weakness. Therapy usually involves administration of folinic acid to enhance enzyme activity; 5-methyl-tetrahydrofolate to replace the missing end product; and betaine, hydroxycobalamin, carnitine, and riboflavin to assist with related enzymatic actions.

For some patients, medications can help reduce the excretion of homocysteine in the urine, increase body weight, and improve mental function and symptoms. Methionine may be given to correct lowered serum levels, and pyridoxine may lower serum homocysteine levels if needed. If some individuals are not responsive to combinations of these drugs, supportive care is offered to reduce symptoms.

INTERVENTION: OBJECTIVES

- Prevent further mental retardation, growth delays, fractures, etc. Fractures are common because of defective collagen formation. The eye is affected since the lens may become dislocated (in CBS deficiency).
- Prevent cardiovascular complications (arterial and venous thrombosis).
- Supplement with essential nutrients. Low folic acid intakes aggravate the symptoms.
- **In CBS deficiency:** Reduce methionine in the diet to prevent accumulation of homocysteine.
- **Inborn errors of cobalamin** will require intramuscular vitamin B_{12}.

INTERVENTION: FOOD AND NUTRITION

- **For CBS (B_6 nonresponsive):** Dietary control of methionine intake is the mainstay of therapy. Use a low-protein diet with a supplement of cystine to supply sulfur. Reduce intake of methionine; no meat, poultry, fish, or eggs. Soy products (e.g., Isomil, ProSobee, Soyalac) can be used. XMET Maxamaid (SHS North America, Gaithersburg, MD), Hominex 1 for infants or Hominex 2 for children (Ross Laboratories), or Product HOM 1 or HOM 2 (Mead Johnson) are also useful.
- **In MTHFR:** Vitamins B_6 and B_{12}, riboflavin, choline, and betaine are useful supplements. Monitor intake from all sources.
- **For inborn errors of cobalamin transport and metabolism:** Intramuscular vitamin B_{12} is needed; dietary vitamin B_{12} will not be used, and supplementation will not be effective.
- Increase fluid intake.

CLINICAL INDICATORS

Clinical/History		
Birth weight	Blood clots in veins?	Plasma methionine (often increases more than 1 mg/dL)
Present weight	Mental retardation or psychiatric problems?	Serum homocysteine
Length	**Lab Work**	Urinary tHcy after methionine load
FTT?	ALT, AST	Serum folate
Growth (%)	Gluc	Serum B_6
Diet/intake history	Serum B_{12}	Serum Ca++, Mg++
Scoliosis	Urinary methylmalonic acid	
Long limbs, tall stature?		
Nearsightedness?		
Lens dislocation?		

Common Drugs Used and Potential Side Effects

- Dipyridamole may be used to decrease thrombosis.
- Pyridoxine therapy (vitamin B_6) for longer than 1 month is useful for some forms of the condition. The doctor may prescribe 100–500 mg or higher.
- Folic acid and vitamin B_{12} should be supplied if low serum levels are detected.
- Choline and betaine may be useful for some patients (Busby et al, 2005; Alfthan et al, 2004).

Herbs, Botanicals, and Supplements

- Herbs and botanicals should not be used for homocystinuria because there are no controlled trials to prove efficacy.

INTERVENTION: NUTRITION EDUCATION, COUNSELING, CARE MANAGEMENT

- Emphasize the importance of controlling diet, snacks, etc.
- Discuss good food sources of folic acid and other B-complex vitamins.
- Newborn screening for tHcy might be useful to detect vitamin B_{12} deficiency or HCU (Refsum et al, 2004).
- Because of increased incidence of osteoporosis in persons with HCU, it has become evident that high serum homocysteine levels interfere with collagen cross-linking (McLean et al, 2004). Controlling the levels of homocysteine in serum is an important factor in this disorder for bone health.

Patient Education—Food Safety

- Hand washing with soap and hot water is recommended before preparing formula or meals. Use clean utensils and containers for mixing formula.
- Before using tap water for formula preparation or to give as a beverage, let cold tap water run for 2 minutes to remove any lead that may be in the pipes.
- Follow the 2-hour rule: discard any beverage or food that has been left at room temperature for 2 hours or longer.
- Do not use honey in the diets of infants to decrease potential risk of botulism.

For More Information

- Cerebral Folate Deficiency
  http://www.folates.com/mthfr_def.html
- Children Living with Inherited Metabolic Diseases
  http://www.climb.org.uk/
- Save Babies
  http://www.savebabies.org/diseasedescriptions/homocystinuria.php

HOMOCYSTINURIA—CITED REFERENCES

Alfthan G, et al. The effect of low doses of betaine on plasma homocysteine in healthy volunteers. *Br J Nutr.* 92:665, 2004.

Andersson H, et al. Long-term outcome in treated combined methylmalonic acidemia and homocystinemia. *Genet Med.* 1:146, 1999.

Busby MG, et al. Choline- and betaine-defined diets for use in clinical research and for management of trimethylaminuria. *J Am Diet Assoc.* 105:1836, 2005.

Guttormsen A, et al. Disposition of homocysteine in subjects heterozygous for homocystinuria due to cystathionine beta-synthase deficiency: relationship between genotype and phenotype. *Am J Med Genet.* 100:204, 2001.

McLean RR, et al. Homocysteine as a predictive factor for hip fracture in older persons. *N Engl J Med.* 350:2042, 2004.

Refsum H, et al. Screening for serum total homocysteine in newborn children. *Clin Chem.* 50:1769, 2004

Refsum H, Fredriksen A, et al. Birth prevalence of homocystinuria. *J Pediatr.* 144:830, 2004.

Rosenblatt D, Whitehead V. Cobalamin and folate deficiency: acquired and hereditary disorders in children. *Semin Hematol.* 36:19, 1999.

Shan X, et al. Mutations in the regulatory domain of cystathionine beta synthase can functionally suppress patient-derived mutations in cis. *Hum Mol Genet.* 10:635, 2001.

Topaloglu A, et al. Influence of metabolic control on growth in homocystinuria due to cystathionine b-synthase deficiency. *Pediatr Res.* 49:796, 2001.

INBORN ERRORS OF CARBOHYDRATE METABOLISM

NUTRITIONAL ACUITY RANKING: LEVEL 4

DEFINITIONS AND BACKGROUND

An inherited, defective gene that prevents a normal step in carbohydrate metabolism causes these rare inborn error disorders. Several congenital defects of sugar metabolism are caused by aberrant transporter genes (e.g., the glucose–galactose malabsorption syndrome, *SGLT1*; the glucose transporter 1 deficiency syndrome; and the Fanconi-Bickel syndrome, *GLUT2*) (Scheepers et al, 2004).

Incidence is estimated to be one in 5000 live births. Diagnosis of these conditions is usually during infancy or childhood, with hypoglycemia, hepatomegaly, poor physical growth, and deranged biochemical profiles. Persons with delayed development, seizures, stroke-like episodes, cerebellar hypoplasia, and demyelinating neuropathy should be assessed for CHO-deficient syndromes (Patterson, 1999).

Fructosemia results from a defect in the enzyme converting fructose to glucose (1-phosphofructaldolase). It is inherited as an autosomal recessive disease and is as common as one in 20,000 persons in some European countries. Ingesting fructose causes profound hypoglycemia, and if left untreated, progressive liver disease results.

Sucrose/maltose intolerance requires omission of sucrose and maltose from the diet.

Congenital glucose–galactose malabsorption (CGGM) is a rare disorder thought to be an autosomal recessive trait. Watery, profuse diarrhea occurs because of the defective sodium-coupled cotransport of glucose and galactose in the intestinal mucosa. Removal of lactose, sucrose, and glucose is needed. A fructose-based solid diet will be needed for older children. There is no cure.

Galactosemia, also known as galactose-1-phosphate uridylyltransferase deficiency or GALT deficiency, causes cataracts, hepatomegaly, and mental retardation. The enzyme galactokinase is being studied for its role in causing this condition (Holden et al, 2004). There may be high levels of the sugar alcohol form, galactitol (Ning et al, 2001). Failure to thrive is the initial clinical symptom; vomiting or diarrhea begins within a few days of milk ingestion. Long-term treatment does not always prevent retardation, and bone density may decline over time (Panis et al, 2004). It occurs in one out of 60,000 births. People with galactosemia are unable to fully metabolize the simple sugar galactose.

Hepatic glycogen storage diseases (GSDs) are rare genetic disorders in which glycogen cannot be metabolized to glucose in the liver because of enzyme deficits. If severe, liver transplantation may be needed. Table 3-7 lists the various types of glycogen storage diseases and related details.

INTERVENTION: OBJECTIVES

- Prevent hypoglycemia, where indicated.
- Prevent essential fatty acid (EFA) deficiency since children with chronic liver diseases have a high risk of EFA deficiency (Abdel-Ghaffar et al, 2003).
- Eliminate the offending nutrient that cannot be digested. Alter other nutrient intakes to promote growth and maintenance.
- Read labels carefully. Note that galactose is not always reported on labels.
- Fructose intolerance is rare and can cause GI discomfort, nausea, malaise, and growth failure.
- For galactosemia, correct diet to prevent physical and mental retardation, cataracts, portal hypertension, and cirrhosis. Vitamin E seems to have positive, protective effects.
- For glycogen storage disease, maintain glucose homeostasis, prevent hypoglycemia, promote positive nitrogen balance and growth, and correct or prevent fatty liver.
- Sucrose intolerance occurs rarely as a genetic defect or temporarily after GI flu or irritable bowel distress. Sucrase deficiency may be combined with maltase deficiency. Eliminate the carbohydrate(s) to decrease osmotic diarrhea.

INTERVENTION: FOOD AND NUTRITION

Fructosemia

- Diet must exclude fructose, sucrose, sorbitol, invert sugar, maple syrup, honey, and molasses.
- Read labels carefully.
- Be careful when using tube feedings or intravenous solutions that may contain sources of fructose.

Galactosemia

- Use a lactose and galactose-free diet—no milk, milk products, soybeans, peaches, lentils, liver, brains, or breads or cereals containing milk or cream cheese. Fresh blueberries and honeydew melon should be excluded from the diets of these persons; however, fresh cherries, citrus, mango, red plums, and strawberries are allowed (Stepnick-Gropper et al, 2000).
- For infants with the condition, try formulas such as Isomil or ProSobee, Elecare, or Nutramigen, or formulas containing casein hydrolysate.
- Supplement with calcium, vitamin D, vitamin E, and riboflavin. In some forms of galactosemia, galactose can often be reintroduced later in life.

TABLE 3-7 Glycogen Storage Diseases (GSDs)

Disease	Description
GSD type I: glucose-6 phosphatase deficiency (G6PD), Von Gierke's disease	Caused by a deficiency of the enzyme that normally converts glycogen to glucose. Hemolytic anemia due to G6PD deficiency is another name for the condition. Problems include slow or stunted growth, enlarged liver, delayed or absent pubertal development, gout, kidney failure, and a poor ability to withstand fasting due to low blood sugar. Patients with this condition may be prone to frequent infections or inflammatory bowel disease. Brain damage may result from low glucose availability to the brain (Melis et al, 2004). In the past, early death was common. Treatment of GSD type I by portacaval shunt may need to be considered in patients with height for age below the 3rd percentile (Corbeel et al, 2000).
GSD type II: alpha-glucosidase deficiency, Pompe's disease	Onset in infancy is the most severe; most patients present with hypotonia and cardiomyopathy. The recombinant human GAA (rhGAA) is currently in clinical trials for enzyme replacement therapy of Pompe's disease (Raben et al, 2005).
GSD type III: debrancher enzyme deficiency, Cori's disease	There may be low bone density and a high risk for osteoporosis (Cabrera-Abreu et al, 2004).
GSD type IV: brancher enzyme deficiency, Anderson's disease	This is a disorder due to glycogen branching enzyme (GBE) deficiency and resulting in the accumulation of an amylopectin-like polysaccharide. It presents with liver disease, progressing to lethal cirrhosis (Bruno et al, 2004).
GSD type V: muscle glucagon phosphorylase deficiency, McArdle's disease	This is an X-linked liver glycogenosis (XLG) and is one of the most common forms of glycogen storage disease (Burwinkel et al, 1998). It is characterized by low levels of phosphorylase with resulting abnormal storage of glycogen in muscle tissue, with muscle pain, cramping and stiffness, and poor exercise tolerance. Avoidance of strenuous exercise is recommended. Onset is often in adulthood.
GSD type VI: liver phosphorylase deficiency, Hers' disease	Gross hepatomegaly may result along with hypoglycemia with reduced liver phosphorylase activity.
GSD type VII: muscle phosphofructokinase deficiency, Tarui's disease	This syndrome presents often with exertional myopathy and hemolytic syndrome.
GSD type VIII	This type is rare and is related to ineffective glycogenosis. Cirrhosis or hepatic tumors may result.
GSD type IX: liver glycogen phosphorylase kinase deficiency	Growth retardation, abdominal distention, and hepatomegaly may be presenting signs (Schippers et al, 2003). Liver transplantation results in normal fasting glucose production and normal glucose and insulin concentrations.

- Be careful when using tube feedings or intravenous solutions that may contain sources of lactose.
- Read labels carefully; galactose is not reported on labels. Formulas labeled "low lactose" are *not* good substitutes; they contain lactose in amounts that can seriously harm patients with galactosemia.

CGGM

- Use a diet free from sucrose, lactose, and glucose.
- A CHO-free formula, to which fructose is incrementally added, may be tolerated (Abad-Sinden et al, 1997). Fructose may be used in a solid diet for older children; the other CHO sources should be avoided.

GSDs

- Increase protein intake to increase muscle strength (Bembi et al, 2003).
- Use small, frequent feedings and, if steroids are used in treatment, a low-sodium diet. Long-term use of steroids can deplete stores of calcium and phosphorus and may elevate glucose, cause stunting, or cause weight gain.
- Avoid lactose and sucrose. Glucose may be used; check labels. Cornstarch is used to prevent hypoglycemia.
- Concentrated sweets may be restricted unless made with pure glucose syrup.
- Sometimes, night feedings with additional daytime meals work effectively. Giving Vivonex or cornstarch/uncooked starch at night may help the liver to maintain a normal blood glucose level (sometimes allowing omission of parenteral nutrition).
- A multivitamin-mineral supplement with vitamin C, iron, and calcium may be needed because fruits and milk are limited. If necessary, use parenteral nutrition to replete lost nutrient stores, such as vitamin B_{12}, folate, calcium, and iron (Kishnani et al, 1999).

Sucrose/Maltose Intolerance

- Omit sucrose and maltose from the diet.
- For nongenetic form, gradually add these sugars back into the diet.
- Be careful when using tube feedings or intravenous solutions because they may contain sources of sucrose or maltose.

CLINICAL INDICATORS

Clinical/History	Lab Work	
Height or length	Trig, Chol (elevated in Von Gierke's disease)	Gluc (may decrease in fructosemia)
Weight	Liver function tests: ALT, AST, CK	Acetone
BMI	Urinary and serum galactose or fructose	Serum phosphate
Growth (%)		Serum lactate
Diet/intake history		Serum ammonia
Infections		Serum bilirubin
Nausea and vomiting		Uric acid
Jaundice		Alb
Head circumference		
Edema		

Common Drugs Used and Potential Side Effects

- For persons with galactosemia, eliminate drugs containing lactose and supplement with calcium and riboflavin.
- Sucrose and maltose are added to many drugs; check carefully.
- All vitamin-mineral supplements must be free of the nontolerated carbohydrates.
- If liver transplantation is needed, support the immunosuppressants with appropriate nutrition interventions. Changes in fluid or sodium or other nutrients may be required.

Herbs, Botanicals, and Supplements

- Herbs and botanicals should not be used for these conditions because there are no controlled trials to prove efficacy.

INTERVENTION: NUTRITION EDUCATION, COUNSELING, CARE MANAGEMENT

- Explain which sources of carbohydrate are allowed specific to the disorder.
- Read labels carefully. Many foods contain milk solids, galactose (e.g., luncheon meats, hot dogs), and other sugars. Omit according to the disorder.
- Contact formula companies regarding special product updates. More research is being conducted regarding these conditions.

Patient Education—Food Safety

- Hand washing with soap and hot water is recommended before preparing formula or meals. Use clean utensils and containers for mixing formula.
- Before using tap water for formula preparation or to give as a beverage, let cold tap water run for 2 minutes to remove any lead that may be in the pipes.
- Follow the 2-hour rule: discard any beverage or food that has been left at room temperature for 2 hours or longer.
- Do not use honey in the diets of infants to decrease potential risk of botulism.

For More Information

- Association for Glycogen Storage Disease–United Kingdom
  http://www.agsd.org.UK/
- Association for Glycogen Storage Disease–United States
  http://www.agsdus.org/
- Diseases of the Liver
  http://cpmcnet.columbia.edu/dept/gi/disliv.html
- Genetics Education Center
  http://www.kumc.edu/gec/
- International Pompe Association
  http://www.worldpompe.org/
- March of Dimes
  http://www.marchofdimes.com
- McArdle's Disease
  http://members.aol.com/itsgumby/
- Rare Genetic Disorders
  http://www.med.nyu.edu/rgdc/homenew.htm

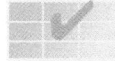

INBORN ERRORS OF CARBOHYDRATE METABOLISM—CITED REFERENCES

Abad-Sinden A, et al. Nutrition management of congenital glucose-galactose malabsorption: a case study. *J Am Diet Assoc.* 97:1417, 1997.
Abdel-Ghaffar YT, et al. Essential fatty acid status in infants and children with chronic liver disease. *East Mediterr Health J.* 9:61, 2003.
Bembi EB, et al. Efficacy of multidisciplinary approach in the treatment of two cases of nonclassical infantile glycogenosis type II. *Inherit Metab Dis.* 26:675, 2003.
Bruno C, et al. Clinical and genetic heterogeneity of branching enzyme deficiency (glycogenosis type IV). *Neurology* 63:1053, 2004.
Burwinkel B, et al. Variability of biochemical and clinical phenotype in X-linked liver glycogenosis with mutations in the phosphorylase kinase PHKA2 gene. *Hum Genet.* 102:423, 1998.
Cabrera-Abreu J, et al. Bone mineral density and markers of bone turnover in patients with glycogen storage disease types I, III and IX. *J Inherit Metab Dis.* 27:1, 2004.
Corbeel L, et al. Long-term follow-up of portacaval shunt in glycogen storage disease type 1B. *Eur J Pediatr.* 159:268, 2000.
Holden HM, et al. Galactokinase: structure, function and role in type II galactosemia. *Cell Mol Life Sci.* 61:2471, 2004.
Kishnani PS, et al. Nutritional deficiencies in a patient with glycogen storage disease type Ib. *J Inherit Metab Dis.* 22:795, 1999.
Melis D, et al. Brain damage in glycogen storage disease type I. *J Pediatr.* 144:637, 2004.
Ning C, et al. Galactose metabolism in mice with galactose-1-phosphate uridyltransferase deficiency: sucklings and 7-week-old animals fed a high-galactose diet. *Mol Genet Metab.* 72: 306, 2001.
Panis B, et al. Bone metabolism in galactosemia. *Bone* 35:982, 2004.
Patterson M. Screening for "prelysosomal disorders": carbohydrate-deficient glycoprotein syndromes. *J Child Neurol.* 14:S16, 1999.
Raben N, et al. Replacing acid alpha-glucosidase in Pompe disease: recombinant and transgenic enzymes are equipotent, but neither completely clears glycogen from type II muscle fibers. *Mol Ther.* 11:48, 2005.
Scheepers A, et al. The glucose transporter families SGLT and GLUT: molecular basis of normal and aberrant function. *JPEN J Parenter Enteral Nutr.* 28:364, 2004.
Schippers HM, et al. Characteristic growth pattern in male X-linked phosphorylase-b kinase deficiency (GSD IX). *J Inherit Metab Dis.* 26:43, 2003.
Stepnick-Gropper S, et al. Free galactose content of fresh fruits and strained fruit and vegetable baby foods: more foods to consider for the galactose-restricted diet. *J Am Diet Assoc.* 100:573, 2000.

LARGE FOR GESTATIONAL AGE INFANT (INFANT MACROSOMIA)

NUTRITIONAL ACUITY RANKING: LEVEL 1–3

DEFINITIONS AND BACKGROUND

High birth weight (3300–4000 g) at 40 weeks is termed large for gestational age (LGA). These infants are considered to be over the 90th percentile of appropriate weight for gestational age. Macrosomia in newborns raises the risk for birth-related problems (Samaras et al, 2004). Problems may include hypoglycemia, respiratory distress, aspiration pneumonia, bronchial paralysis, macrosomia, and facial paralysis.

LGA infants are most often born to mothers who are obese or have diabetes, multiparous women, or mothers with genetic predispositions for excessive birth weight. Obesity and pregestational diabetes are independently associated with increased risk of LGA delivery (Ehrenberg et al, 2004). Because fewer women are smoking as often during pregnancy, birth weights are increasing in many cases (Surkan et al, 2004). LGA neonates have higher body fat and lower lean body mass than appropriate for gestational age (AGA) infants; impaired maternal glucose tolerance enhances these body composition changes (Hammami et al, 2001).

Cord plasma adiponectin and leptin levels, but not insulin level, tend to be significantly higher in LGA infants compared with AGA infants (Tsai et al, 2004). It would seem that adiponectin may be involved in regulating fetal growth. Fetal growth standards are more appropriate in predicting the impact of birth weight or prematurity than are neonatal growth standards; the risks of preterm birth in LGA infants are 2–3 times greater than the risks among AGA infants (Lackman et al, 2001).

Controlling maternal weight gain remains an important goal for successful pregnancy outcome. High birth weight may lead to greater adult obesity, cancer, and chronic disease (Samaras et al, 2004). Much research is taking place in this area of study. Table 3-8 lists potential risks for fetal macrosomia.

TABLE 3-8 Risk Factors for Fetal Macrosomia and LGA Births

Maternal diabetes	Excessive maternal weight gain
Maternal impaired glucose intolerance	Male fetus
Multiparity	Parental stature
Previous macrosomic infant	Need for labor augmentation
Prolonged gestation	Prolonged second stage
Beckwith's syndrome	Genetic predisposition
Transposition of the great vessels	
Miscalculation of expected day of confinement	
Rh isoimmunization	
Maternal obesity	

From: Zamorski and Briggs, 2001; American Pediatric Association, 1999, p. 45.

INTERVENTION: OBJECTIVES

- Allow adequate growth rate and development.
- Prevent hypoglycemia.
- Maintain energy intake at desired level while allowing adequate growth in the infant. Prevent obesity and its consequences for the infant as much as possible.
- Monitor serum lipid levels as deemed necessary.

INTERVENTION: FOOD AND NUTRITION

- Feed the infant often, as indicated by infant's appetite and goal weight pattern.
- Control source of energy, avoiding excessive glucose intake if infant shows signs of hyperglycemia.
- Alter intake of fat as determined by a lipid profile.
- Maintain sufficient level of protein if energy needs to be restricted from CHO or fat.

CLINICAL INDICATORS

Clinical/History		Lab Work
Head circumference	Neonatal Growth Assessment Scores	Serum Gluc (maternal and infant)
Length	Brazelton Neonatal Behavior Assessment Scale (motor maturity, autonomic stability, and withdrawal)	Serum insulin (maternal and infant)
Birth weight		Chol, Trig
Growth pattern		Alb
Diet/intake history		H & H
Respirations		
Urinary acetone		
BP		
I & O		

Common Drugs Used and Potential Side Effects

- Insulin may be necessary to control hyperglycemia. Beware of any excesses of insulin, which could aggravate hypoglycemia.

Herbs, Botanicals, and Supplements

- Herbs and botanicals should not be used for LGA infants because there are no controlled trials to prove efficacy for any related problems.

INTERVENTION: NUTRITION EDUCATION, COUNSELING, CARE MANAGEMENT

- Signs of hyperglycemia and hypoglycemia should be discussed.
- Discuss normal growth patterns as appropriate for the infant, reviewed in concert with the pediatrician.
- Review risks inherent in another pregnancy, especially if the mother has diabetes.

Patient Education—Food Safety

- Hand washing with soap and hot water is recommended before preparing formula or meals. Use clean utensils and containers for mixing formula.
- Before using tap water for formula preparation or to give as a beverage, let cold tap water run for 2 minutes to remove any lead that may be in the pipes.
- Follow the 2-hour rule: discard any beverage or food that has been left at room temperature for 2 hours or longer.
- Do not use honey in the diets of infants to decrease potential risk of botulism.

For More Information

- American College of Obstetricians and Gynecologists http://www.acog.org

LARGE FOR GESTATIONAL AGE INFANT—CITED REFERENCES

American Pediatric Association. *Handbook of pediatric nutrition.* 2nd ed. Gaithersburg, MD: Aspen, 1999, p. 45.

Ehrenberg HM, et al. The influence of obesity and diabetes on the prevalence of macrosomia. *Am J Obstet Gynecol.* 191:964, 2004.

Hammami M, et al. Disproportionate alterations in body composition of large for gestational age neonates. *J Pediatr.* 138:817, 2001.

Lackman F, et al. The risks of spontaneous preterm delivery and perinatal mortality in relation to size at birth according to fetal versus neonatal growth standards. *Am J Obstet Gynecol.* 184:946, 2001.

Samaras TT, et al. Is short height really a risk factor for coronary heart disease and stroke mortality? A review. *Med Sci Monit.* 10:63, 2004.

Surkan PJ, et al. Reasons for increasing trends in large for gestational age births. *Obstet Gynecol.* 104:720, 2004.

Tsai PJ, et al. Cord plasma concentrations of adiponectin and leptin in healthy term neonates: positive correlation with birthweight and neonatal adiposity. *Clin Endocrinol (Oxf).* 61:88, 2004.

Zamorski MA, Briggs WS. Management of suspected fetal macrosomia. *Am Fam Physician.* 63:302, 2001.

LEUKODYSTROPHIES

NUTRITIONAL ACUITY RANKING: LEVEL 1

DEFINITIONS AND BACKGROUND

Leukodystrophies (peroxisome biogenesis disorders) are genetic disorders that affect the myelin sheath. A list of multiple related conditions is available at http://www.ulf.org/types/types.html. The genetic defect and biochemical abnormalities have been defined; there is a wide range of phenotypic expression (Moser et al, 2005). Neonatal adrenoleukodystrophy and infantile Refsum's disease are mild phenotypes (Suzuki et al, 2001). The most severe form is Zellweger's syndrome, which may be fatal and is characterized by an enlarged liver, high serum levels of iron and copper, and visual changes. Noninvasive and presymptomatic diagnosis and prenatal diagnosis are available; family screening and genetic counseling are key to disease prevention (Moser et al, 2005).

X-linked adrenoleukodystrophy (X-ALD) is an autosomal recessive disorder with an enzymatic defect in very long–chain fatty acid (VLFA) oxidation, which is usually abundant in sphingomyelin. Ultimately, the myelin sheath surrounding the nerves is destroyed, causing demyelination and neurological problems; adrenal gland malfunction causes Addison's disease (adrenal insufficiency). Accumulation of saturated VLFA, especially hexacosanoate (C26:0), occurs because there is a missing or defective protein (ALD protein) to process that fatty acid. The incidence of X-ALD, estimated to be one in 17,000 in all ethnic groups, approximates that of phenylketonuria (Moser et al, 2005).

Onset of X-ALD is usually in childhood, with a rapid, progressive demyelination of the central nervous system, hypotonia, and psychomotor retardation. However, at least half of patients with X-ALD are adults with somewhat milder manifestations, and women who are carriers may become symptomatic (Moser et al, 2005). X-ALD is often misdiagnosed as attention-deficit hyperactivity disorder in boys and as multiple sclerosis in men and women and may cause Addison's disease (Moser et al, 2005). Prognosis is poor and death may occur up to a decade after onset.

The observation that dietary fatty acids affect membrane composition has led to the use of modified diets in these conditions. Lorenzo's oil is a mixture of oleic and erucic (rapeseed, or canola) oils. This oil often prevents the onset of the disease by reducing the production of VLFA, whose buildup leads to demyelination. Lymphocytopenia and depression of natural killer cells have been observed in patients with ALD treated with Lorenzo's oil, an indication of increased cellular immunity (Pour et al, 2000). During treatment, C22:6 content increases in red blood cells and in the brain membranes, as considerable neurological and electrophysiological improvement suggests. Early oral administration helps infants and children with the neonatal form (Suzuki, 2001).

An omega-3 fatty acid, DHA, is present in large amounts in infant brains. DHA is present in fatty fish (e.g., salmon, tuna, mackerel) and mother's milk but is not usually present in infant formulas. Because DHA deficiencies have been noted in ALD (Horrocks and Yeo, 1999), intake of omega-3 fatty acids is now recommended.

Genetic and biochemical analysis, neuroimaging, and the ability to create animal models have led to advances in the field of leukodystrophy research (Berger et al, 2001). Studies are showing some success with bone marrow transplantations in boys with early symptoms of X-ALD (Moser et al, 2004).

INTERVENTION: OBJECTIVES

- Decrease rapid progression of demyelination of CNS by offering sufficient fatty acids.
- Prevent or lessen complications of the disorder, including adrenal dysfunction.
- Alter type of dietary fat to limit progression of the disease. Use more omega-3 fatty acids also. Overall, maintain total VLFA levels while altering sources.
- Support the physical therapy by maintaining strength with an adequate diet.

INTERVENTION: FOOD AND NUTRITION

- Increase endogenous VLFA synthesis of monounsaturated fatty acids by restricting exogenous (dietary) VLFA (C26:0) to less than 3 mg and by increasing oleic acid (C18:1). The typical American diet yields 35–40% total energy from fat with 12–40 mg C26:0 daily.
- Offer a low- to very low–fat diet, with supplementation of specific unsaturated fatty acids such as oleic and erucic acids (Lorenzo's oil) and DHA. For this diet, use the VLFA C26:0-restricted diet, with the addition of 60 mL of oleic acid. Lorenzo's oil is similar to olive oil (87% C18:1, 4.8% linoleic acid) but lacks measurable fatty acids with a chain length greater than C20. It can be used in cooking, as a supplement in juice, as an oil for salad dressings, or in food preparation instead of margarine, butter, mayonnaise, or shortening.
- To reduce the need to digest VLFA present in fatty foods and in cutin (outer layer of plants, fruits, vegetables, and nuts), use these items less often in the diet. For example, peel fruits and vegetables before serving. Use alternative cooking methods besides frying.
- If the patient requires tube feeding, a formula can be developed that contains nonfat milk, specialty oil, corn syrup or sugar, and a vitamin-mineral supplement.
- Studies are not conclusive regarding special vitamin E, selenium, or carnitine requirements.
- Include sources of omega-3 fatty acids, such as salmon, tuna, or mackerel, for older children and adults.

CLINICAL INDICATORS

Clinical/History	Lab Work	
Height	Plasma phosphatidylcholine	Plasma sphingomyelin
Weight	Fatty acid profile	H & H
Growth chart	Alb	Pipecolic acid testing
Diet/intake history	Chol	
Bronzing of skin (Addison's disease)	Trig	

Common Drugs Used and Potential Side Effects

- It may be necessary to treat Addison's disease with prednisone and spironolactone or related medications. Side effects may include hyperglycemia, osteoporosis, and other conditions that have to be closely monitored.
- NIH is studying the effects of cholic acid, chenodeoxycholic acid, and ursodeoxycholic acid in patients with ALD. Lovastatin is also being tested.

Herbs, Botanicals, and Supplements

- Herbs and botanicals should not be used for this condition because there are no clinical trials proving efficacy.

INTERVENTION: NUTRITION EDUCATION, COUNSELING, CARE MANAGEMENT

- The whole family can be instrumental in accepting the diet; it can be adapted for everyone.
- Restaurant dining can be a problem. Some special meals may have to be developed for travel.
- If nausea occurs, the oil can be taken in an emulsion.

Patient Education—Food Safety

- Hand washing with soap and hot water is recommended before preparing formula or meals. Use clean utensils and containers for mixing formula.
- Before using tap water for formula preparation or to give as a beverage, let cold tap water run for 2 minutes to remove any lead that may be in the pipes.
- Follow the 2-hour rule: discard any beverage or food that has been left at room temperature for 2 hours or longer.
- Do not use honey in the diets of infants to decrease potential risk of botulism.

For More Information

- Dr. Hugo Moser, Kennedy Krieger Institute
  Phone: 800-873-3377
- National Institute of Neurological Disorders and Stroke
  http://www.ninds.nih.gov/disorders/adrenoleukodystrophy/adrenoleukodystrophy.htm
- The Myelin Project
  http://www.myelin.org/
- United Leukodystrophy Foundation
  http://www.ulf.org/

LEUKODYSTROPHIES—CITED REFERENCES

Berger J, et al. Leukodystrophies: recent developments in genetics, molecular biology, pathogenesis and treatment. *Curr Opin Neurol.* 14:305, 2001.

Horrocks L, Yeo Y. Health benefits of docosahexaenoic acid (DHA). *Pharmacol Res.* 40:211, 1999.

Moser HW, et al. Adrenoleukodystrophy: new approaches to a neurodegenerative disease. *JAMA.* 294:3131, 2005.

Moser HW, et al. Progress in X-linked adrenoleukodystrophy. *Curr Opin Neurol.* 17:263, 2004.

Pour R, et al. Enhanced lymphocyte proliferation in patients with adrenoleukodystrophy treated with erucic acid (22:1)-rich triglycerides. *J Inherit Metab Dis.* 2000;23:113.

Suzuki Y. The clinical course of childhood and adolescent adrenoleukodystrophy before and after Lorenzo's oil. *Brain Dev.* 23:30, 2001.

Suzuki Y, et al. Clinical, biochemical, and genetic aspects and neuronal migration in peroxisome biogenesis disorders. *J Inherit Metab Dis.* 24:151, 2001.

LOW BIRTH WEIGHT OR PREMATURITY

NUTRITIONAL ACUITY RANKING: LEVEL 3–4

DEFINITIONS AND BACKGROUND

Every newborn is classified as one of the following: premature (<37 weeks of gestation), full-term (37–42 weeks of gestation), or postterm (>42 weeks of gestation). **Prematurity** is generally correlated with low birth weight. **Low birth weight (LBW)** infants may be small for date, have intrauterine growth retardation, or have dysmaturity. LBW infants weigh less than 2500 g or 5.5 lb (<10th percentile for gestational age) at birth. Very low birth weight (VLBW) infants (<1300–1500 g) are especially prone to nutritional deficits. Infants who weigh 1000 g are sometimes called "micropreemies."

According to the March of Dimes (2005), LBW infants comprise 7–8% of all live births; preterm birth rate was highest for black infants (17.6%), followed by Native Americans (12.9%), Hispanics (11.4%), whites (10.7%), and Asians (10.2%). In the United States, infants born to mothers less than 20 or over 35 years old are more likely to be preterm than infants born to mothers 20 to 35 years old (March of Dimes, 2005). Finally, 15% of those infants born prematurely are from multiple births (twins, etc.).

Because early motherhood is associated with LBW infants and is avoidable, public health strategies need to be developed to educate women about delaying pregnancy (Okosun et al, 2000). Infants of women with hypertension or preeclampsia, who smoke, or who use of an antihypertensive agent or prednisone during pregnancy are at increased risk of LBW, preterm birth, diseases of prematurity, and death (Ray et al, 2001). Low weight and BMI at conception or delivery, as well as poor weight gain during pregnancy, are associated with LBW, prematurity, and maternal delivery complications (Ehrenberg et al, 2003). In addition, women who have periodontal disease are 7 times more likely to have a baby born too early and too small; very high levels of prostaglandin are found in severe cases, and this may be the culprit (March of Dimes, 2004).

Typical problems of the LBW or premature infant include hypoglycemia, hypothermia, jaundice, dry skin, decreased subcutaneous fat, and anemia. Admission to neonatal intensive care units (NICUs) is common, especially for respiratory distress. Loss of body water occurs in healthy preterm babies and those with respiratory distress syndrome; adequate nutrition support almost immediately after birth is important (Tang et al, 1997).

Preterm infants have lower energy expenditure when they are fed breast milk than when they are fed preterm infant formula (Lubeztsky et al, 2003). For these infants, the immunological and GI benefits of human milk compared with those of preterm infant formula outweigh the risks associated with slower growth (Schanler et al, 1999). Interventions to support breastfeeding in the hospital and at home are indicated to improve brainstem maturation (Amin et al, 2000).

Breastfeeding is very beneficial for these infants, even if the process is difficult. Several studies suggest that "on demand" feeding is best for premature infants (Crosson and Pickler, 2004). However, careful and frequent monitoring of growth patterns among LBW infants will be needed to prevent developmental delays. If weight gain by 4 months is not adequate, aggressive nutritional therapy should be offered (Kennedy et al, 1999). During the first months after discharge, VLBW babies need to have nutrition support to help promote early catch-up growth and mineralization. These babies are at risk of postnatal growth deficiency and osteopenia (Rigo et al, 2000).

Early feeding increases intestinal lactase activity in preterm infants; lactase activity is a marker of intestinal maturity and may influence clinical outcomes. Infants who begin enteral feedings early have 100% greater lactase activity at age 10 days and 60% greater levels at age 28 days than infants who start after delays (Shulman et al., 1998). Parenteral glutamine supplementation, while probably not harmful, does not show evidence of decreasing sepsis or onset of other problems such as necrotizing enterocolitis (Poindexter et al, 2004). Selenium supplementation may be beneficial for reducing sepsis (Darlow and Austin, 2003).

There has been much research about the role of omega-3 fatty acids for a healthy pregnancy and for healthy infants (Fewtrell et al, 2004). The need for increased maternal dietary intake of DHA has been suggested for pregnancy. Brain, retina, and other neural tissues are rich in DHA and arachidonic acid (ARA). By providing gamma linolenic acid as a source of ARA, preterm boys showed efficacy for growth and for neurodevelopment with no adverse effects (Fewtrell et al, 2004). The role of supplementation in premature infants remains controversial.

In LBW infants, although the full-term sucking pattern is not necessary for successful oral feeding, an infant's feeding proficiency and efficiency at the first oral feeding are reliable predictors of early independent oral feeding (Lau et al, 1997). Nonnutritive sucking before bottle feedings may improve oxygen saturation, behavior state, and feeding behavior of preterm infants (Pickler et al, 1996). Premature breast milk has higher electrolyte, protein, and MCT levels than mature breast milk.

In 2001, charges for hospital stays for infants with any diagnosis of prematurity were estimated at $13.6 billion (March of Dimes, 2005). The American Dietetic Association recommends at least five medical nutrition therapy visits for taking care of high-risk, premature infants. Table 3-9 lists the nutritional deficits found in premature or LBW infants.

INTERVENTION: OBJECTIVES

- Begin feedings of distilled water or colostrum as soon as possible for infants without respiratory distress. Early feeding (3–5 days after birth) tends to allow babies to mature faster than those fed later. Early-fed babies have fewer days of intolerance, a shorter hospital length of stay, and earlier tolerance of full feedings.
- Encourage the mother to breastfeed, especially to provide milk with the higher preterm protein level. If tube feeding is needed, mother can express milk to be given to the infant. Consider adding that breast milk can also be supplemented for increased needs.
- Supplement the infant's diet as needed with EFAs. EFA deficiency increases antioxidative susceptibility of red blood cells (RBCs) in VLBW infants (Tomsits et al, 2000). DHA supplementation, while not absolutely supported by evidence, may become a requirement.
- Gradually increase energy and protein to meet the needs of rapid growth. For proteins, ensure a proper whey to casein ratio.
- Promote normal growth and development. Prevent illness, rickets, respiratory distress, hypoglycemia or hyperglycemia, necrotizing enterocolitis, infections, obstructive jaundice, and tyrosinemia.
- Assure adequate intake of folate and vitamin B_{12} to reduce anemias, when indicated.

TABLE 3-9 Nutritional Deficits in the Premature or LBW Infant

- Marginal nutrient stores at birth, including fat, glycogen, and minerals such as calcium and phosphorus.
- Limited ability to consume adequate amounts of nutrient caused by delayed oral neuromuscular development and small gastric capacity.
- Immaturity at the cellular level with consequent alteration of biochemical needs.
- Higher metabolic demands and rate of growth.
- Malabsorption from underdeveloped digestive/absorptive abilities.
- Risk from poor nutritional intake of the mother where relevant (e.g., pregnant women who are folate deficient are more likely to give birth to LBW infants).
- Risk of essential fatty acid deficiency with less growth, more renal and lung changes, fatty liver, impaired water balance, RBC fragility, and dermatitis.

- With parenteral feeding, include amino acids in proper amounts, especially cysteine, taurine (Wharton et al, 2004), tyrosine, glycine, and arginine (Wu et al, 2004). American McGaw makes intravenous TrophAmine for parenteral nutrition (PN).
- Be sure an adequate amount of selenium is provided (Darlow and Austin, 2003).
- Omit aluminum from products where possible. Prolonged intravenous (IV) feeding with solutions containing aluminum is associated with impaired neurological development (Bishop, 1997).
- When possible, advance from PN or tube feedings to oral intake to reduce cholestasis and osteopenia.

INTERVENTION: FOOD AND NUTRITION

- While in the radiant warmer, feed the infant 60–80 mL/kg body weight (BW)/d of water. Gradually increase to 150 mL/kg BW. Add electrolytes (sodium, potassium, and chloride on at least the second day).
- Day 1: Breastfeed or give glucose at 6–8 mg/kg/min. Advance by no more than 20 mL/kg daily.
- Progress to special formulas such as Similac Special Care 24 or Enfamil Premature Formula (24 kcal/oz) to yield 120–150 mL/kg up to 180–200 mL/kg/d. NeoSure or Enfacare are helpful for transition to home (22 kcal/oz with added Ca++ and phosphorus).
- Within 7 days, the diet should provide 120–150 kcal/kg BW daily; carbohydrate should be 40–45% total kcal (10–30 g/kg). Protein should be age specific.
- Tube feeding initiation: Start at 10–15 mL/hr at one-quarter strength. Progress as tolerated to desired rate. Specialty products have been developed for VLBW infants, such as Mead Johnson's Enfamil Human Milk Fortifier (Berseth et al, 2004). See Table 3-10 for estimated energy calculations.

TABLE 3-10 Enteral Energy Needs (Preterm Infant)

Basal needs	40–50 kcal/kg
+ activity	5–15 kcal/kg
+ cold stress	0–10 kcal/kg
+ fecal losses	10–15 kcal/kg
+ SDA (specific dynamic action)	10 kcal/kg
+ growth	20–30 kcal/kg
Total Energy Needs	85–130 kcal/kg
Evaluate for special needs and increase energy accordingly.	
Add extra energy for:	
Fever	7% per 1° elevation
Cardiac failure	15–25%
Major surgery	20–30%
Severe sepsis	40–50%
Protein:	
Calorie malnutrition (PCM)	50–100%
Growth failure	60%
Burns	100%

- Use TPN if not fed by day 3; the glucose infusion rate in the neonatal intensive care unit (NICU) is often 15 mg/kg/min. TPN needs are similar to enteral nutrition (EN) needs. Modern crystalline amino acid infusions promote positive nitrogen balance by use of 1 g/kg/d as soon as possible. Use up to 3 g/kg/d of lipid infused continuously or early enteral feeding to prevent cholestatic liver disease. Carnitine deficiency may also occur with PN therapy (Bonner et al, 1995). See Table 3-11 for recommended parenteral vitamin and mineral intakes.
- There may be subtle and delayed hunger cues from the infant. If poor sucking or swallowing instincts exist, the infant may need gavage feeding. Feed every 2 hours or use continuous drip feeding and change to bolus feedings when full strength is tolerated.
- Feeding style: If infant weighs 1000–1750 g, feed more vigorously; if infant weighs 1750 g or more, feed as a normal-term infant.
- The micronutrient needs of a stable, preterm LBW infant may be as follows: high levels of calcium (140–160 mg/100 kcal), 120–230 mg/kg; 25 IU of vitamin E (water soluble) daily, 6.0–12.0 mg/kg; 2.5 mg iron/100 kcal in formula (necessary only if stores are depleted); 300–500 IU of vi-

TABLE 3-11 Parenteral Vitamin and Mineral Needs (preterm infant)

Nutrient	Recommended Intake for Infants <2.5 kg	Recommended Intake for Infants >2.5 kg
Vitamin A	280 μg	700 μg
Vitamin D	160 IU	400 IU
Vitamin E	2.8 mg	7 mg
Vitamin K	80 μg	200 μg
Vitamin C	32 mg	80 mg
Thiamin	0.48 mg	1.2 mg
Riboflavin	0.56 mg	1.4 mg
Niacin	6.8 mg	17 mg
Pyridoxine (B_6)	0.40 mg	1.0 mg
Folic acid	56 μg	140 μg
Vitamin B_{12}	0.40 μg	1 μg
Biotin	8 μg	20 μg
Pantothenate	2 mg	5 mg
Calcium	80–100 mg/kg	80–100 mg/kg
Phosphorus	43-62 mg/kg	43-62 mg/kg
Magnesium	6–10 mg/kg	6–10 mg/kg
Chromium	0.2 μg/kg	0.2 μg/kg
Copper	20 μg/kg	20 μg/kg
Iodide	1 μg/kg	1 μg/kg
Manganese	1 μg/kg	1 μg/kg
Molybdenum	0.25 μg/kg	0.25 μg/kg
Selenium	2 μg/kg	2 μg/kg
Zinc	400 μg/kg	400 μg/kg

Note: Needs are estimated for use with a solution of 2.5 g/dL of amino acids infused at 120–150 mL/kg/dL.
Derived from Cross, 2005.

tamin D, 400 IU/d; adequate folic acid, 25–50 μg/kg; adequate sodium (3 mEq/d) to avoid hyponatremia, 2–3 mEq/kg; 30–50 mg/d vitamin C, 18–24 mg/kg; and 95–108 mg phosphorus/100 kcal given (60–140 mg/kg).
- Monitor need for vitamin B_{12}. Other nutrients should be provided according to the DRI tables for the newborn. Note that magnesium, zinc, selenium, and copper may be low. Evidence suggests that vitamin A should be supplemented (Wardle et al, 2001; Shenai et al, 2000).
- Total fat should be 5–7 g/kg to meet half of energy needs without excess carbohydrate. Soybean oil can provide EFAs (1–2% EFAs needed) in the form of linoleic acid. Exogenous carnitine may be needed to take EFAs into the mitochondria. Inositol (in membrane phospholipids) may also be needed to decrease respiratory distress, but this is under study.

CLINICAL INDICATORS

Clinical/History		
Birth weight	Sucking reflex	Transferrin (8-day half-life)
Gestational age	Apgar scores	ALT, AST
Birth length	I & O	Serum folic acid and vitamin B_{12}
Percentage of weight/length	**Lab Work**	Serum phosphorus
Diet/intake history	Gluc	Lecithin to sphingomyelin ratio (L:S ratio)
Swallowing reflex	H & H	Bilirubin
Temperature (often decreased)	Alb	
	Ca++, Mg++	
	Na+, K+	
	Respiratory distress syndrome (RDS)	
	Transthyretin	

Common Drugs Used and Potential Side Effects

- VLBW babies often experience hyperkalemia and hyperglycemia and are given insulin to manage these problems (Ditzenberger et al, 1999). Insulin may also be needed if hyperglycemia results from TPN. Continuous intravenous infusion is best tolerated.
- Other medications may be used for specific underlying disease states. Monitor for side effects.
- Use caution with introduction of vitamin supplements. Early vitamin supplementation seems to promote increased risk for asthma in black children and food allergies in exclusively formula-fed children (Milner et al, 2004).

Herbs, Botanicals, and Supplements

- Herbs and botanicals should not be used for LBW or premature infants because there are no controlled trials to prove efficacy for any related problems. There may be allergic or asthmatic reactions that are undesirable.

INTERVENTION: NUTRITION EDUCATION, COUNSELING, CARE MANAGEMENT

- Teach the caretaker or parent about increased nutrient needs of infant. Special formulas have 80 kcal/dL compared with the usual 67 kcal/dL and have MCT, extra protein, calcium, phosphorus, and sodium.
- Emphasize the normal progression of infant feeding after the infant achieves adequate growth pattern and weight. Catch-up is common by 2–3 years for LBW or premature infants. Note that chronic lung disease, prolonged parenteral nutrition, delayed initiation of enteral feeding, severe intraventricular hemorrhage, necrotizing enterocolitis, or late-onset sepsis may delay weight gain in VLBW infants (Ehrenkrantz, 1999).
- VLBW infants experience catch-up growth and attain predicted genetic height during adolescence, if they were not small for gestational age (Anderson, 2004). VLBW infants who survive without major neurodevelopmental disability attain lower growth during adolescence than normal birth weight infants; sexual maturation and relative body composition will be similar (Peralta-Carcelen et al, 2000).
- Emphasize the importance of nutrient density for growth (e.g., zinc, vitamin B_6, and vitamin E).
- Do not overfeed. Excess nonprotein energy is stored as fat regardless of its source (fat or carbohydrate); therefore, high-energy or MCT intake in otherwise healthy, growing preterm infants does not promote nitrogen retention and should be avoided (Romero et al, 2004). Monitor for the tendency to aspirate, for lactose intolerance, and for other problems.
- The child may benefit from the WIC program if available.
- Follow-up clinic or home visits are recommended. Offer tips such as using small, frequent feedings; using a quiet, calm environment for feeding; supporting the jaw; and trying special feeding equipment if needed (angle-neck bottle).

Patient Education—Food Safety

- Hand washing with soap and hot water is recommended before preparing formula or meals. Use clean utensils and containers for mixing formula.
- Before using tap water for formula preparation or to give as a beverage, let cold tap water run for 2 minutes to remove any lead that may be in the pipes.
- Follow the 2-hour rule: discard any beverage or food that has been left at room temperature for 2 hours or longer.
- Do not use honey in the diets of infants to decrease potential risk of botulism.

For More Information

- March of Dimes–Prematurity
http://www.modimes.org/prematurity/
- Prematurity
http://www.prematurity.org/
- UNICEF
http://www.unicef.org

LOW BIRTH WEIGHT OR PREMATURITY—CITED REFERENCES

Amin S, et al. Brainstem maturation in premature infants as a function of enteral feeding type. *Pediatrics* 106:318, 2000.

Anderson D. Nutrition in the care of the low-birth-weight infant. In: Mahan K, Escott-Stump S, eds. *Krause's food, nutrition, and diet therapy.* 11th ed. Philadelphia: WB Saunders, 2004.

Berseth CL, et al. Growth, efficacy, and safety of feeding an iron-fortified human milk fortifier. *Pediatrics.* 114:e699, 2004.

Bishop N, et al. Aluminum neurotoxicity in preterm infants receiving intravenous-feeding solutions. *N Engl J Med.* 336:1557, 1997.

Bonner C, et al. Effects of parenteral L-carnitine supplementation on fat metabolism and nutrition in premature neonates. *J Pediatr.* 126:287, 1995.

Cross S. Meeting the vitamin and mineral needs of the preterm infant. *Support Line.* 27:3, 2005.

Crosson DD, Pickler RH. An integrated review of the literature on demand feedings for preterm infants. *Adv Neonatal Care.* 4:216, 2004.

Darlow BA, Austin NC. Selenium supplementation to prevent short-term morbidity in preterm neonates. *Cochrane Database Syst Rev.* 4:CD003312, 2003.

Ditzenberger G, et al. Continuous insulin intravenous infusion therapy for VLBW infants. *J Perinat Neonatal Nurs.* 13:70, 1999.

Ehrenberg HM, et al. Low maternal weight, failure to thrive in pregnancy, and adverse pregnancy outcomes. *Am J Obstet Gynecol.* 189:1726, 2003.

Ehrenkrantz R, et al. Longitudinal growth of hospitalized very low birth weight infants. *Pediatrics.* 104:280, 1999.

Fewtrell MS, et al. Randomized, double-blind trial of long-chain polyunsaturated fatty acid supplementation with fish oil and borage oil in preterm infants. *J Pediatr.* 144:471, 2004.

Kennedy T, et al. Growth patterns and nutritional factors associated with increased head circumference at 18 months in normally developing, low-birth-weight infants. *J Am Diet Assoc.* 99:1522, 1999.

Lau C, et al. Oral feeding in low birth weight infants. *J Pediatr.* 130:561, 1997.

Lubeztsky R, et al. Energy expenditure in human milk- versus formula-fed preterm infants. *J Pediatr.* 143:750, 2003.

March of Dimes. Born too soon and too small in the United States. Accessed January 1, 2005 at http://www.marchofdimes.com/peristats/prematurity.aspx?reg=99.

March of Dimes. Periodontal disease and preterm birth. Accessed December 30, 2004 at http://www.marchofdimes.com/files/MP_PeriodontalDiseaseAndPretermBirth031004.pdf.

Milner JD, et al. Early infant multivitamin supplementation is associated with increased risk for food allergy and asthma. *Pediatrics* 114:27, 2004.

Okosun I, et al. Ethnic differences in the rates of low birth weight attributable to differences in early motherhood: a study from the Third National Health and Nutrition Examination Survey. *J Perinatol.* 20:105, 2000.

Peralta-Carcelen M, et al. Growth of adolescents who were born at extremely low birthweight without major disability. *J Pediatr.* 136:633, 2000.

Pickler R, et al. Effects of nonnutritive sucking on behavioral organization and feeding performance in preterm infants. *Nurs Res.* 45:132, 1996.

Poindexter BB, et al. Parenteral glutamine supplementation does not reduce the risk of mortality or late-onset sepsis in extremely low birth weight infants. *Pediatrics* 113:1209, 2004.

Ray J, et al. MOS HIP: McMaster Outcome Study of Hypertension in Pregnancy. *Early Hum Dev.* 64:129, 2001.

Rigo J, et al. Bone mineral metabolism in the micropreemie. *Clin Perinatol.* 27:147, 2000.

Romero G, et al. Energy intake, metabolic balance and growth in preterm infants fed formulas with different nonprotein energy supplements. *J Pediatr Gastroenterol Nutr.* 38:407, 2004.

Schanler R, et al. Feeding strategies for premature infants: beneficial outcomes of feeding fortified human milk versus preterm formula. *Pediatrics.* 103:1150, 1999.

Shenai J, et al. Vitamin A status and postnatal dexamethasone treatment in bronchopulmonary dysplasia. *Pediatrics.* 106:547, 2000.

Shulman R, et al. Early feeding, feeding tolerance, and lactase activity in preterm infants. *J Pediatr.* 133:645, 1998.

Tang W, et al. Influence of respiratory distress syndrome on body composition after preterm birth. *Arch Dis Child Fetal Neonatal Ed.* 77:28, 1997.

Tomsits E, et al. Effects of early nutrition on free radical formation in VLBW infants with respiratory distress. *J Am Col Nutr.* 19:237, 2000.

Wardle S, et al. Randomized controlled trial of oral vitamin A supplementation in preterm infants to prevent chronic lung disease. *Arch Dis Child Fetal Neonatal Ed.* 84:F9, 2001.

Wharton BA, et al. Low plasma taurine and later neurodevelopment. *Arch Dis Child Fetal Neonatal Ed.* 89:497, 2004.

Wu G, et al. Arginine deficiency in preterm infants: biochemical mechanisms and nutritional implications. *J Nutr Biochem.* 15:442, 2004.

MAPLE SYRUP URINE DISEASE

NUTRITIONAL ACUITY RANKING: LEVEL 3–4

DEFINITIONS AND BACKGROUND

Maple syrup urine disease (MSUD) results from an autosomal recessive trait, causing an inborn error of metabolism in which branched-chain alpha-keto acid dehydrogenase (BCKD) is missing (Riazi et al, 2004). Because of the missing enzyme, the branched-chain amino acids (BCAAs; leucine, isoleucine, valine) and their byproducts, called ketoacids, become elevated. It is these elevations that cause an infant or child with MSUD to become symptomatic.

In the United States, MSUD occurs in one in 225,000 births. The Mennonite population from eastern Pennsylvania has a high percentage of births with this disorder. MSUD also occurs in other populations throughout the world. Another name for the condition is leucinosis.

Onset of disease occurs in children between the ages of 1 and 8 years. Symptoms in an infant include poor sucking reflex, anorexia, failure to thrive, listlessness, irritability, and a characteristic odor (sweet, burnt maple syrup odor of the urine and sweat). They have a high-pitched cry and may alternate between limp and rigid.

Without treatment, symptoms progress rapidly to seizures, coma, and death (Schonberger et al, 2004). With earlier diagnosis and treatment, there is a lower risk of permanent damage, such as peripheral neuropathy. Nutrition therapy is lifelong; omission of the BCAAs from the diet is essential. Note that thiamin is the coenzyme for BCAAs and should be made available. Alpha-keto acids have a role in MSUD along with transport of glutamate (Reis et al, 2000).

There are four classifications used to identify the types of MSUD: classic, intermediate, intermittent, and thiamin-responsive; these refer to the amount and type of enzyme activity present. See Table 3-12.

TABLE 3-12 Types and Nutrition Interventions for Maple Syrup Urine Disease (MSUD)

Type	Nutrition Intervention
Classic MSUD	Most common. Little or no enzyme activity (usually <2% of normal). Protein from branched-chain amino acids (BCAAs) must be severely restricted.
Intermediate MSUD	Higher level of enzyme activity (approximately 3–8% of normal). Tolerance for leucine is slightly better. Management is the same as for the classic form.
Intermittent MSUD	Milder form; greater enzyme activity (8–15% of normal). Few symptoms until 12–24 months of age, often in response to an illness or larger protein intake. During episodes of illness or fasting, the BCAA levels elevate, the characteristic odor becomes evident, and the child can go into a metabolic crisis.
Thiamin-responsive MSUD	Rare form. Giving large doses of thiamin to the thiamin-responsive child will increase the enzyme activity. Moderate protein restriction is needed.

Derived from data available at http://www.msud-support.org/overv.htm; accessed January 2, 2005.

INTERVENTION: OBJECTIVES

- Prevent endogenous protein catabolism (Morton et al, 2002).
- Prevent toxic concentrations of BCAAs (Riazi et al, 2004) by using an appropriate medical formula, special intravenous feeding, or low-BCAA diet. Monitor serum levels of BCAAs frequently to determine current status.
- Support normal growth and development with adequate protein synthesis and prevention of essential amino acid deficiencies.
- Control intake of BCAAs for life. As the child grows, add BCAAs individually in a controlled manner.
- Maintain normal serum osmolality (Morton et al, 2002).
- In emergencies, hemodialysis is sometimes necessary (Hmiel et al, 2004).
- Overcome any difficulty with feeding related to poor sucking reflex.

INTERVENTION: FOOD AND NUTRITION

- Restrict intake of BCAAs in the diet to 45–62 mg/d (Riazi et al, 2004). Use Mead Johnson's MSUD powder or Ross Laboratories' Maxamaid MSUD. Use the latter with PFD1 or PFD2 (Mead Johnson) because it contains no cholesterol or fat.
- When BCAA levels are high (during illness or fasting), it may be necessary to use a specific IV solution that allows the excess leucine, valine, and isoleucine to be used for protein synthesis in the body, thereby rapidly decreasing the elevated levels.
- Provide adequate energy intake from CHO and fat to spare amino acids for building tissue, etc.
- Use small amounts of milk in the diet to support growth. Cow's milk contains 350 mg of leucine, 228 mg of isoleucine, and 245 mg of valine per 100 mL.
- Avoid eggs, meat, nuts, and other dairy products. Gelatin, a form of protein low in BCAAs, may be used in the diet.
- If hemodialysis is needed, monitor fluid, protein, and electrolytes carefully.

CLINICAL INDICATORS

Clinical/History	Lab Work	
Length (height)	Plasma leucine, isoleucine, valine (therapeutic range of 100–300 µmol/L)	Urinary excretion of ketoacids
Birth weight	Plasma L-alloisoleucine 0.5 µmol/L (most specific and most sensitive for MSUD)	Urinary odor of burnt maple syrup
Present weight		Alb
Growth (%)		Globulin
Diet/intake history		Uric acid (increased?)
Perspiration that has maple odor		H & H
Grand mal seizures?		Serum Fe
Hypertonicity		Serum osmolality
Cerebral edema?		

Common Drugs Used and Potential Side Effects

- Sometimes insulin or a similar agent is given to speed up the utilization of excess BCAAs where needed.
- The doctor may prescribe large doses of thiamin for children who are thiamin responsive.
- Avoid use of aspirin with MSUD; individuals with this condition may be more prone to Reye's syndrome.

Herbs, Botanicals, and Supplements

- Herbs and botanicals should not be used for MSUD because there are no controlled trials to prove efficacy for any related problems.

INTERVENTION: NUTRITION EDUCATION, COUNSELING, CARE MANAGEMENT

- Educate caregiver and patient that the diet must be maintained for life.
- Discuss the diet's total energy and protein intake that are appropriate for the patient's age and stage of development.
- Illness or infection can cause elevations in the BCAAs. This can lead to vomiting, diarrhea, irritability, sleepiness, unusual breathing, staggering, hallucinations, and slurred speech. This is an emergency and must be treated immediately.
- With knowledge of the pathophysiology of MSUD and understanding of what to do for cerebral edema, fluid and electrolyte management, nutrition, and psychosocial issues, a full life is possible (Robinson and Drumm, 2001).

Patient Education—Food Safety

- Hand washing with soap and hot water is recommended before preparing formula or meals. Use clean utensils and containers for mixing formula.
- Before using tap water for formula preparation or to give as a beverage, let cold tap water run for 2 minutes to remove any lead that may be in the pipes.
- Follow the 2-hour rule: discard any beverage or food that has been left at room temperature for 2 hours or longer.
- Do not use honey in the diets of infants to decrease potential risk of botulism.

For More Information

- Clinic for Special Children
  http://www.clinicforspecialchildren.org/
- MSUD Dietary Resource List
  http://www.msud-support.org/resource_dietary.htm
- MSUD Family Support Group
  http://www.msud-support.org/
- National Newborn Screening
  http://genes-r-us.uthscsa.edu/
- Screening
  http://www.msud-support.org/testing.htm

MAPLE SYRUP URINE DISEASE—CITED REFERENCES

Hmiel SP, et al. Amino acid clearance during acute metabolic decompensation in maple syrup urine disease treated with continuous venovenous hemodialysis with filtration. *Pediatr Crit Care Med.* 5:278, 2004.

Morton DH, et al. Diagnosis and treatment of maple syrup disease: a study of 36 patients. *Pediatrics* 109:999, 2002.

Reis M, et al. Chloride-dependent inhibition of vesicular glutamate uptake by alpha-keto acids accumulated in maple syrup urine disease. *Biochem Biophys Acta.* 1475:114, 2000.

Riazi R, et al. Total branched-chain amino acids requirement in patients with maple syrup urine disease by use of indicator amino acid oxidation with L-[1-13C]phenylalanine. *Am J Physiol Endocrinol Metab.* 287:142, 2004.

Robinson D, Drumm LA. Maple syrup disease: a standard of nursing care. *Pediatr Nurs.* 27:255, 2001.

Schonberger S, et al. Dysmyelination in the brain of adolescents and young adults with maple syrup urine disease. *Mol Genet Metab.* 82:69, 2004.

MEDIUM-CHAIN ACYL-COA DEHYDROGENASE DEFICIENCY

NUTRITIONAL ACUITY RANKING: LEVEL 4

DEFINITIONS AND BACKGROUND

Medium-chain acyl-coenzyme A (CoA) dehydrogenase deficiency (MCADD) is a rare, hereditary (autosomal recessive) disease that is caused by the lack of an enzyme required to convert fat to energy. Children with MCADD cannot use medium-chain triglycerides (MCTs) to make energy, so the body begins to malfunction when they fast (i.e., they have no more long-chain dietary fats available from the diet).

MCADD occurs in approximately one in every 10,000 live births. MCADD occurs mostly among Caucasians of Northern European background. It is estimated that about one in 100 sudden infant death syndrome (SIDS) deaths are probably a result of undiagnosed MCADD.

Symptoms typically begin in infancy or early childhood, often with simple lethargy. While some affected individuals have no symptoms at birth, disorders such as hypoglycemia, seizures, coma, brain damage, or cardiac arrest can occur very quickly with illness.

If not detected and treated appropriately, MCADD can result in death. Over half of MCADD individuals die from their first crisis if it occurs after the age of 2 years. Untreated MCADD can lead to mental retardation and death. Early detection of this disorder allows treatment and a normal life expectancy.

INTERVENTION: OBJECTIVES

- Avoid periods of fasting.
- Use of IV glucose is required when food cannot be tolerated (such as with colds, flu, etc.).

INTERVENTION: FOOD AND NUTRITION

- Restrict periods of fasting by offering small, frequent feedings.
- A balanced diet with avoidance of MCTs will be needed. For example, do not use enteral formulas that contain MCTs.
- Supplemental carnitine has been recommended for some children.

CLINICAL INDICATORS

Clinical/History	Diet/intake history	Alb
Length (height)	Seizures?	Chol
Birth weight	**Lab Work**	Trig
Present weight	Gluc	H & H
Growth (%)		Serum Fe

Herbs, Botanicals, and Supplements

- Herbs and botanicals should not be used for MCADD because there are no controlled trials to prove efficacy for any related problems.

INTERVENTION: NUTRITION EDUCATION, COUNSELING, CARE MANAGEMENT

- Educate about the dangers of fasting, including periods during illness.
- Share information about frequent feedings and how to avoid MCTs from supplemental products.

Patient Education—Food Safety

- Hand washing with soap and hot water is recommended before preparing formula or meals. Use clean utensils and containers for mixing formula.
- Before using tap water for formula preparation or to give as a beverage, let cold tap water run for 2 minutes to remove any lead that may be in the pipes.
- Follow the 2-hour rule: discard any beverage or food that has been left at room temperature for 2 hours or longer.
- Do not use honey in the diets of infants to decrease potential risk of botulism.

For More Information

- Fatty Oxidation Disorder
  http://www.fodsupport.org/
- MCADD
  http://www.mcadangel.com/mcad-links.html
- National Newborn Screening
  http://genes-r-us.uthscsa.edu/

MYELOMENINGOCELE

NUTRITIONAL ACUITY RANKING: LEVEL 2–3

DEFINITIONS AND BACKGROUND

Myelomeningocele (MMC) is one of the most severe forms of birth defects of the brain and spinal cord. The bones of the spine do not completely form, and the spinal canal is incomplete. This allows the spinal cord and meninges (the membranes covering the spinal cord) to protrude from the child's back. Myelomeningocele accounts for about 75% of all cases of spina bifida; it affects one out of every 800 infants. Pregnant women who are tested will usually show a positive alpha-fetoprotein level during prenatal testing in a triple screen.

MMC is a severe neural tube defect that includes external protrusion of meninges, spinal fluid and cord, and the nerve roots. Neural tube defects (NTDs) may be caused by a variety of genetically caused defects in developmental mechanisms that are responsible for elevation of the neural folds (Harris and Juriloff, 1999). The cause of MMC is unknown; folic acid deficiency is thought to play a part in all NTDs. Daily consumption of 400 μg of folic acid before conception and during early pregnancy dramatically reduces the occurrence of NTDs (Honein et al, 2001) (see also Spina Bifida and Neural Tube Defects entry).

Protrusion of the spinal cord and meninges damages the spinal cord and nerve roots, causing a decrease or lack of function of body areas controlled at or below the defect. Symptoms are related to the anatomic level of the defect. Most defects occur in the lower lumbar or sacral areas of the back (the lowest areas of the back) because this area is normally the last part of the spine to close. Symptoms include partial or complete paralysis of the legs with corresponding partial or complete lack of sensation and loss of bowel or bladder control. The exposed spinal cord is susceptible to infections such as meningitis. Congenital disorders, such as hydrocephalus and hip dislocation, may also be present. Sometimes, surgery to repair the hydrocephaly improves the condition.

MMC patients are usually wheelchair bound or will wear braces or be on crutches. Patients with MMC are often overweight because of complex interactive factors that are not strictly related to energy intake (Fiore et al, 1998), such as decreased active muscle tissue. Obesity can increase likelihood of pressure ulcers or make ambulation and surgery more difficult.

INTERVENTION: OBJECTIVES

- Manage feeding problems, which are common. Assure proper positioning for all feedings.
- Control weight; metabolic rate may only be 50% of usual rate for age (Grogan and Ekvall, 1999).
- Prevent or heal pressure ulcers.
- Reduce impact of the defect. Promote any and all possible ambulation or activity.
- Correct infections; prevent or correct sepsis.
- Correct nutrient deficiencies.
- Alter diet to prevent or correct constipation, obesity, and urinary tract infections.

INTERVENTION: FOOD AND NUTRITION

- Decrease energy to control weight; as low as 7 kcal/cm may be needed, especially if weight loss is needed. To

maintain weight, 9–11 kcal/cm may be used. Use of standard CDC growth charts is not beneficial in this population; refer to special growth charts.
- Low-calorie snacks should be the only between-meal snacks allowed.
- For infants, ensure at least RDA for kcals and protein to prevent nutrient deficiencies and follow growth curve
- For healing of any pressure ulcers, adequate zinc, vitamins A and C, and protein are required. A multivitamin with minerals should be recommended for those who lack variety in their diets. For females who are of childbearing age, pay attention to folic acid and iron needs.
- Ensure adequate fiber intake and fluid to prevent or correct problems with diarrhea or constipation.
- Use of cranberry juice may help reduce urinary tract infections; use a low-calorie brand to reduce energy intake if needed.

CLINICAL INDICATORS

Clinical/History

- Height, weight
- Birth weight/length
- Weight changes
- Diet/intake history
- Temperature
- Spinal x-rays or computed tomography (CT) scan
- Diarrhea
- Constipation
- Skin integrity
- Triceps skinfold (TSF)
- Hydrocephaly

Lab Work

- Gluc
- Alb, transthyretin
- H & H
- Serum Fe
- Chol
- Na+, K+
- Ca++, Mg++

Common Drugs Used and Potential Side Effects

- Be cautious when using zinc and iron (especially with parenteral administration) with infections or sepsis; these are bacterial nutrients.
- Botulinum-A toxin injections have been used in cases of neurogenic detrusor overactivity to manage some bladder incontinence (Leippold et al, 2003). Otherwise, medications for managing urinary incontinence may be used; monitor for side effects.
- Certain medications prescribed commonly to this patient population may affect the utilization of certain vitamins and minerals. These medications include antibiotics, anticonvulsants, antihypertensives, cathartics, corticosteroids, stimulants, sulfonamides, and tranquilizers. Vitamin and mineral supplements are recommended in some cases to compensate for the specific nutrient alteration (Samour and King, 2005).

Herbs, Botanicals, and Supplements

- Herbs and botanicals should not be used for MMC because there are no controlled trials to prove efficacy for any related problems.

INTERVENTION: NUTRITION EDUCATION, COUNSELING, CARE MANAGEMENT

- Behavior modification, low-calorie food and snack preparation, rewards, and activity/exercise factors should be reviewed with the parent/caretaker.
- Food lists with green "go" foods, red "stop" foods, and yellow "caution" foods have been used with some success for weight management.
- Discuss some potential medical conditions, such as fractures, seizures, lazy eye, early puberty, and allergy to latex. Bone health and allergies can be managed with some nutritional interventions.

Patient Education—Food Safety

- Hand washing with soap and hot water is recommended before preparing formula or meals. Use clean utensils and containers for mixing formula.
- Before using tap water for formula preparation or to give as a beverage, let cold tap water run for 2 minutes to remove any lead that may be in the pipes.
- Follow the 2-hour rule: discard any beverage or food that has been left at room temperature for 2 hours or longer.
- Do not use honey in the diets of infants to decrease potential risk of botulism.

For More Information

- Association for Spina Bifida and Hydrocephalus
  www.asbah.org
- Management of Myelomenigocele Study
  http://www.spinabifidamoms.com/english/index.html
- Spina Bifida Association
  www.sbaa.org

MYELOMENINGOCELE—CITED REFERENCES

Fiore P, et al. Nutritional survey of children and adolescents with myelomeningocele (MMC): overweight associated with reduced energy intake. *Eur J Pediatr Surg.* 1:34S, 1998.

Grogan CB, Ekvall SM. Body composition of children with myelomeningocele, determined by 40K, urinary creatinine and anthropometric measures. *J Am Coll Nutr.* 18:316, 1999.

Harris M, Juriloff D. Mini-review: toward understanding mechanisms of genetic neural tube defects in mice. *Teratology* 60:292, 1999.

Honein M, et al. Impact of folic acid fortification of the U.S. food supply on the occurrence of neural tube defects. *JAMA.* 285:2981, 2001.

Leippold T, et al. Botulinum toxin as a new therapy option for voiding disorders: current state of the art. *Eur Urol.* 44:165, 2003.

McDonnell G, McCann J. Issues of medical management in adults with spina bifida. *Childs Nerv Syst.* 16:222, 2000.

Samour PQ, King K. *Handbook of pediatric nutrition.* 3rd ed. Sudbury, MA: Jones and Bartlett Publishers, 2005.

NECROTIZING ENTEROCOLITIS

NUTRITIONAL ACUITY RANKING: LEVEL 4

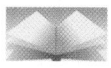

DEFINITIONS AND BACKGROUND

Necrotizing enterocolitis (NEC) involves ischemia of the intestinal tract and invasion of the mucosa with enteric pathogens. This is a common GI problem in preterm infants with tissue injury and inflammation. These kinds of infections are very common in VLBW infants (Stoll et al, 2004). Decreased interleukin levels may contribute to the pathogenesis of NEC by allowing bacteria to escape host defenses (Goepfert et al, 2004; Nadler et al, 2001). NEC has been seen in infants with congenital heart disease (Fatica et al, 2000), in small, asphyxiated preterm infants after exchange transfusions, and in infants with Hirschsprung's disease.

Symptoms and signs include a distended abdomen, lethargy, respiratory distress, pallor, hyperbilirubinemia, vomiting, diarrhea, grossly bloody stools, and sepsis. NEC is the leading cause of short bowel syndrome in infancy; it is a medical emergency. NEC affects about 1–5% of all admissions to neonatal intensive care units (NICUs). Signs of thrombocytopenia within the first 3 days after a diagnosis of NEC suggests a higher likelihood of bowel gangrene, morbidity, and mortality (Kenton et al, 2005).

Feeding intolerance can be rather significant. It seems to be beneficial to use breast milk rather than formula in the prevention of NEC. Infants with colitis induced by protein in their infant formula may not respond to casein hydrolysate formula; symptoms may resolve when given amino acid hydrolysate infant formula (Vanderhoof et al, 1997). There is no conclusive evidence about the use of special formulas that include glutamine or arginine (Wilmore, 2004; Shah and Shah, 2004).

Preventive strategies include amino acid or polyunsaturated fatty acid administration (Reber and Nankervis, 2004).

INTERVENTION: OBJECTIVES

- Allow bowel to rest; avoid stimulants. These measures are usually temporary.
- Prevent or correct starvation, diarrhea, and further malnutrition.
- Prepare patient for bowel surgery, for wound healing, and for the possibility of ostomy feeding if surgery becomes necessary, as for perforation or after peritonitis.
- Prevent or correct hypoglycemia.
- Because breastfeeding is more protective than formula feeding, promote and encourage breastfeeding or use of donor milk when possible (Updegrove, 2004).

INTERVENTION: FOOD AND NUTRITION

- Acute: No oral feedings. Use IVs and TPN as appropriate.
- Recovery: Use 2 times RDA of protein; 25% more kcal than normal for age; frequent feedings.
- Where possible, offer donor milk if mother cannot breastfeed (Updegrove, 2004).
- Some partially elemental formulas are available, such as Pregestimil or Nutramigen, or more elemental nutrients may be required if the digestive tract has not recovered fully. Among infants between 1000 and 2000 g at birth, giving feedings at 30 mL/kg/d seems to be a safe practice and is faster than using 20 mL/kg/d (Caple et al, 2004).
- Ensure adequate iron and zinc. Iron-fortified products may reduce the need for blood transfusions in VLBW infants (Berseth et al, 2004).
- Copper seems to protect against TPN-related liver damage from intrauterine growth deficits (Zambrano et al, 2004).
- Occasionally, a colostomy or ileostomy must be performed, and tube feeding may be needed.

CLINICAL INDICATORS

Clinical/History	Lab Work	
Height/length	H & H (decreased)	K+ (increased)
Weight/birth weight	Abdominal x-ray	Platelets (decreased)
Diet/intake history	PT (prolonged), INR	Gluc
Head circumference	Guaiac test for blood in stools	Elevated WBCs
Vomiting	Na+ (decreased)	Lactic acidosis
Diarrhea?		Thrombocytopenia (low platelet count)
		Neutropenia

Common Drugs Used and Potential Side Effects

- Aggressive treatment of hyperglycemia may be needed, as with insulin (Hall et al, 2004). Monitor for side effects.
- There are some studies about the possible use of probiotics for this condition (Henry and Moss, 2004).

Herbs, Botanicals, and Supplements

- Herbs and botanicals should not be used for NEC because there are no controlled trials to prove efficacy for any related problems.

INTERVENTION: NUTRITION EDUCATION, COUNSELING, CARE MANAGEMENT

- Promote continuation of breastfeeding when possible (Updegrove, 2004).
- Ensure that the parent/caretaker understands the differences between ready-to-feed and concentrated formula (i.e., hypertonicity of the solution).
- If surgery was needed and short-gut syndrome is evident, long-term TPN may be needed.
- Careful monitoring of growth is important. Besides bowel sequelae, VLBW infants who survive NEC are at risk for impairment of growth and neurodevelopment (Yeh et al, 2004).
- Monitor weight and stool changes; advise physician when necessary.

Patient Education—Food Safety

- Hand washing with soap and hot water is recommended before preparing formula or meals. Use clean utensils and containers for mixing formula.
- Before using tap water for formula preparation or to give as a beverage, let cold tap water run for 2 minutes to remove any lead that may be in the pipes.
- Follow the 2-hour rule: discard any beverage or food that has been left at room temperature for 2 hours or longer. Powdered infant formulas are not sterile and may contain pathogenic bacteria; milk products are also media for bacterial proliferation (Agostoni et al, 2004).
- Do not use honey in the diets of infants to decrease potential risk of botulism.

For More Information

- Merck Manual
  http://www.merck.com/mrkshared/mmanual/section19/chapter260/260n.jsp
- Necrotizing Enterocolitis
  http://www.pediatrie.be/NECROT_%20ENTEROCOL.htm

NECROTIZING ENTEROCOLITIS—CITED REFERENCES

Agostoni C, et al. Preparation and handling of powdered infant formula: a commentary by the ESPGHAN Committee on Nutrition. *J Pediatr Gastroenterol Nutr.* 39:320, 2004.

Berseth CL, et al. Growth, efficacy, and safety of feeding an iron-fortified human milk fortifier. *Pediatrics* 114:e699, 2004.

Caple J, et al. Randomized, controlled trial of slow versus rapid feeding volume advancement in preterm infants. *Pediatrics* 114:1597, 2004.

Fatica C, et al. A cluster of necrotizing enterocolitis in term infants undergoing open heart surgery. *Am J Infect Control.* 28:130, 2000.

Goepfert AR, et al. Umbilical cord plasma interleukin-6 concentrations in preterm infants and risk of neonatal morbidity. *Am J Obstet Gynecol.* 191:1375, 2004.

Hall NJ, et al. Hyperglycemia is associated with increased morbidity and mortality rates in neonates with necrotizing enterocolitis. *J Pediatr Surg.* 39:898, 2004.

Henry MC, Moss RL. Current issues in the management of necrotizing enterocolitis. *Semin Perinatol.* 28:221, 2004.

Kenton AB, et al. Severe thrombocytopenia predicts outcome in neonates with necrotizing enterocolitis. *J Perinatol.* 25:14, 2005.

Nadler E, et al. Intestinal cytokine gene expression in infants with acute necrotizing enterocolitis: interleukin-11 mRNA expression inversely correlates with extent of disease. *J Pediatr Surg.* 36:1122, 2001.

Reber KM, Nankervis CA. Necrotizing enterocolitis: preventative strategies. *Clin Perinatol.* 31:157, 2004.

Shah P, Shah V. Arginine supplementation for prevention of necrotising enterocolitis in preterm infants. *Cochrane Database Syst Rev.* 4:CD004339, 2004.

Stoll BJ, et al. Neurodevelopmental and growth impairment among extremely low-birth-weight infants with neonatal infection. *JAMA.* 292:2357, 2004.

Updegrove K. Necrotizing enterocolitis: the evidence for use of human milk in prevention and treatment. *J Hum Lact.* 20:335, 2004.

Vanderhoof J, et al. Intolerances to protein hydrolysate infant formulas: an unrecognized cause of gastrointestinal symptoms in infants. *J Pediatrics.* 131:741, 1997.

Wilmore D. Enteral and parenteral arginine supplementation to improve medical outcomes in hospitalized patients. *J Nutr.* 134:2863S, 2004.

Yeh TC, et al. Necrotizing enterocolitis in infants: clinical outcome and influence on growth and neurodevelopment. *J Formos Med Assoc.* 103:761, 2004.

Zambrano E. Total parenteral nutrition induced liver pathology: an autopsy series of 24 newborn cases. *Pediatr Dev Pathol.* 7:425, 2004.

OBESITY, CHILDHOOD

NUTRITIONAL ACUITY RANKING: LEVEL 3–4 (COUNSELING)

DEFINITIONS AND BACKGROUND

Obesity does not have one set definition, and different ages use different indicators. The prevalence of overweight is increasing for children and adolescents in the United States. "At risk for overweight" is defined by the sex- and age-specific ≥85th percentile cutoff points of the National Center for Health Statistics (NCHS)/Centers for Disease Control and Prevention (CDC) growth charts or of BMI for age; overweight or obese is defined as ≥95th percentile of growth charts or BMI for age. Obesity has been identified as an epidemic by the CDC; rates of unhealthy body weight among children and adolescents have tripled since the 1980s to 15% (Evans et al, 2005). According to the National Health and Nutrition Examination Surveys (NHANES) data, the prevalence of overweight among 12–19 year olds is 15.5% compared with 10.5% from 1988 to 1994 (Pender and Pories, 2005).

BMI increases during the first year of life and then decreases; it begins to rise again at 6–6.5 years of age. BMI tables are not useful before age 2; they are a screening tool and do not reflect body composition well. While BMI tables have limitations, they are considered a reasonable place to begin for further evaluations (Wang, 2004). An increase in BMI of 3–4 units is a reason to investigate.

The preferred weight gain pattern in childhood is as follows. The usual weight gain pattern in an infant is that the infant doubles birth weight by 6 months and triples birth weight at 12 months. Tripling birth weight before 1 year is associated with increased risk of obesity. In year 2, gain is

8–10 lb (3.5–4.5 kg); in year 3, gain is 4.5–6.5 lb (2–3 kg); annually thereafter, the gain is about 4.5–6.5 lb (2–3 kg).

Until 6 years of age, the number of fat cells increases (hyperplasia). After 6 years of age, the size of fat cells increases (hypertrophy). In addition, hormones play a role in establishing obesity in childhood. Leptin, insulin, and adiponectin regulate lipid metabolism in childhood; adiponectin seems to affect lipid alterations as seen in obesity (Gil-Campos et al, 2004). More research in this area is needed.

The European Avon Longitudinal Study of Pregnancy and Childhood (ALSPAC) has found that fetal growth is influenced by both genes and maternal factors (Ong and Dunger, 2004). Interaction between genes in the fetus and maternal environmental factors related to either overnutrition or undernutrition may be relevant. Women who are obese should attempt healthy weight loss before they become pregnant because maternal obesity appears to influence not only the outcome of pregnancy but also fetal, neonatal, childhood, and adult health and mortality (Martorell et al, 2001; Kral, 2004).

Women should be encouraged to breastfeed for many reasons, including protecting the child against obesity later in life (Arenz et al, 2004; Gillman et al, 2001). After birth, overfeeding for catch-up growth in a premature or underweight child can contribute to obesity; weight gain proceeds at a rate that is too fast for linear growth. Overnutrition, resulting from high birth weight or gestational diabetes, is also associated with subsequent fatness in the child. Three critical periods for prevention of adult obesity are: ages 5–7 years, adolescence, and pregnancy.

Many formerly "adult-onset" disorders are showing up in obese children, including heart disease (Li et al, 2004), insulin resistance (Viner et al, 2005; Eisenmann et al, 2004), type 2 diabetes, hypertension, dyslipidemia (Kral, 2004), and gallbladder disease. Other problems include asthma, sleep apnea, maturity-onset diabetes of youth (MODY), Cushing's syndrome, hypothyroidism, polycystic ovary syndrome, and Prader-Willi syndrome. In addition, obesity is the single most significant risk factor for the development of nonalcoholic fatty liver disease (NAFLD) in children and adults; NAFLD occurs in approximately 53% of obese children (Blackburn and Mun, 2004). Despite evidence that both genetics and environment play a role, social factors in childhood strongly influence adult obesity. Most prevention programs include at least one of the following (Caballero, 2004): dietary changes, physical activity, behavior modification, family participation, and school-based prevention programs.

Dietary recommendations for families include providing children with access to nutrient-dense foods and beverages and high-fiber foods; reducing children's access to high-calorie, nutrient-poor beverages and foods both when eating at home and at restaurants; avoiding excessive food restriction or use of food as a reward; and encouraging children to eat breakfast on a daily basis (Ritchie et al, 2005).

While it is not clear what the ideal treatment is, successful management of preadolescent obesity seems to be successful when it is started during preschool years. Counseling will need to consider the differences between "simple obesity" and severe or "morbid" obesity in the child, as well as comorbidities. Major attitudinal changes are often needed in parents or caretakers when a child has reached the severe/morbid phase. Recent guidelines, listed in Table 3-13, suggest a pattern for when to initiate dietary weight loss plans.

TABLE 3-13 When to Initiate Weight Loss Diets

Children aged 2–7 years	BMI: 85th to 94th percentiles; BMI greater than the 95th percentile with no complications	Maintain weight
	BMI is above the 95th percentile with mild complications (mild hypertension, dyslipidemia, insulin resistance)	Gradual weight loss is recommended
	Patients with acute complications such as pseudotumor cerebri, sleep apnea, obesity hypoventilation syndrome, or orthopedic problems	Refer to a pediatric obesity center
Children 7 years of age and older	BMIs between the 85th and 94th percentiles with no complications	Maintain weight
	If the BMI is between the 85th and 94th percentiles with mild complications or the BMI is equal to or above the 95th percentile	Gradual weight loss is recommended

Source: Marcason W. At what age should an overweight child follow a calorie-restricted diet? *J Am Diet Assoc.* 104:834, 2004.

INTERVENTION: OBJECTIVES

Health Supervision Recommendations (from Krebs et al, 2003; American Academy of Pediatrics, 2005)

- Identify and track patients at risk by virtue of family history, birth weight, or socioeconomic, ethnic, cultural, or environmental factors. Calculate and plot BMI once a year in all children and adolescents; use change in BMI to identify rate of excessive weight gain relative to linear growth. Develop a weight maintenance or weight loss plan that is individualized for the child.
- Encourage parents and caregivers to promote healthy eating patterns by offering nutritious snacks, such as vegetables and fruits, low-fat dairy foods, and whole grains; encouraging children's autonomy in self-regulation of food intake and setting appropriate limits on choices; and modeling healthy food choices.
- Routinely promote physical activity, including unstructured play at home, in school, in child care settings, and throughout the community. Recommend limitation of television and video time to a maximum of 2 hours per day (Caballero, 2004).
- Recognize and monitor changes in obesity-associated risk factors for adult chronic disease, such as hypertension, dyslipidemia, hyperinsulinemia, impaired glucose tolerance, and symptoms of obstructive sleep apnea syndrome.

Other Objectives

- Create an environmental–behavioral synergy through directed changes to promote a healthy weight trajectory according to the CDC BMI charts that are age appropriate (Koplan et al, 2005).

- Discuss behavioral tips that are easily handled by the dietetics professional; refer complex cases to a behavioral specialist. Discourage the use of sweets and foods to reward behavior. Avoid the "clean plate" theory, but be wary about withholding food, which can have the opposite effect.
- Help the child "find" the right body for him or her. Encourage self-recognition of hunger cues (e.g., stop eating when feeling "full").

Advocacy Objectives (From Krebs et al, 2003; American Academy of Pediatrics, 2005)

- Help parents, teachers, coaches, and others who influence youth to discuss health habits, not body build, as part of their efforts to control overweight and obesity.
- Enlist policy makers from local, state, and national organizations and schools to support a healthful lifestyle for all children, including proper diet and adequate opportunity for regular physical activity.
- Encourage organizations that are responsible for health care and health care financing to provide coverage for effective obesity prevention and treatment strategies.
- Encourage public and private sources to direct funding toward research on effective strategies to prevent overweight and obesity and to maximize limited family and community resources to achieve healthful outcomes for youth.
- Support and advocate for social marketing intended to promote healthful food choices and increased physical activity.

INTERVENTION: FOOD AND NUTRITION

- Determine approximate needs for the child according to age and sex: kcals, protein, and other nutrients. A balanced diet for children includes protein at 10–35%, fat at 25–40%, and CHO at 45–65% according to the Institute of Medicine (2002).
- Plan a diet with basal calories, calculated according to age, activity, and likelihood of growth spurts. For family teaching, it is better to discuss behavioral changes that are easy and to place less emphasis on a specific calorie level. Portion sizes should be a primary teaching focus.
- Emphasize low-fat, low-cholesterol foods when hypercholesterolemia is present. According to some studies, the use of plant stanols and sterols may be beneficial for the dietary management of elevated total cholesterol and low-density lipoprotein (LDL) cholesterol in the pediatric population.
- Reduce the energy intake by reducing the energy density of foods, increasing fresh fruits and nonstarchy vegetables, using low-calorie versions of products, and reducing offering of energy-dense food items (Caballero, 2004).
- Decrease the use of sweets as snack foods or dessert. Decrease the use of fatty or fried foods.
- Check for anemia; correct diet accordingly to include more sources of iron, B-complex vitamins, vitamin C, and protein.
- Limit milk to a reasonable amount daily for age. Be sure others foods are consumed in addition to milk. Use low-fat or skim milk after 2 years of age.
- Limit juice to 6 oz for young children. Limit sugar-sweetened beverages in general. Added sugars should comprise no more than 25% of total calories consumed.
- Control between-meal snacks. Good snacks include fresh fruit or vegetables, plain crackers, pretzels, plain popcorn, cooked egg slices, unsweetened fruit or vegetable juices, and low-fat cheese cubes. Age appropriateness of snacks is important; younger children can choke on popcorn and fresh carrots, etc.
- Avoid grazing; give small helpings at meals and allow more small helpings until "full." Discuss "hunger cues" and "satiety cues."
- Ensure that the family has adequate fluoride protection, as dental caries are common.

CLINICAL INDICATORS

Clinical/History

Height
Birth length
Birth weight
Present weight
Weight hx
Diet/intake history
BMI 85–94% = at risk of continuing overweight into adulthood
BMI ≥95% = overweight with need for in-depth assessment
Family hx of CHD, diabetes mellitus, hypertension, overweight/obesity
Breastfed vs. formula or other milk (young child)
Maternal gestational diabetes
Gestational age at birth
BP
Acanthosis nigricans
Amount of TV watching
Inactive lifestyle?
Skipping meals?

Lab Work

H&H, Serum Fe
Chol, Trig (elevated)?
Serum homocysteine
Gluc
Alk phos
Alb
Ca++, Mg++
Na+, K+
Liver function tests
Serum insulin

Common Drugs Used and Potential Side Effects

- Discourage the use of drugs for weight loss; no diet medicines are safe for children under age 16 years. The addition of sibutramine to a comprehensive behavioral program for teens can induce significant weight loss; however, medications for weight loss should be used only on an experimental basis in adolescents and children until further clinical trials have been completed (Berkowitz et al, 2003).
- Antidepressants are sometimes prescribed for childhood depression, which is more common than once realized. Monitor for side effects such as changes in metabolism and appetite, which can contribute to obesity in some cases.

Herbs, Botanicals, and Supplements

- Herbs and botanicals should not be used for obesity in children because there are no controlled trials to prove efficacy or safety. Physicians may ask dietitians to discuss herbs, botanicals, life cycle, and disease-specific and obesity guidance with their patients.

INTERVENTION: NUTRITION EDUCATION, COUNSELING, CARE MANAGEMENT

- Intervention should start early and focus on the family, not the child. Educate parents about the dangers of medical complications.
- Many parents innocently overfeed their children. Discuss age-appropriate portions and snacks. Showing child-sized plates and utensils with sample portion sizes may be quite helpful. Try to eliminate one "problem food" per visit (e.g., regular soda pop or sugar-sweetened fruit punch). Diluting juice, substituting lower calorie beverages, and giving tips on how many calories are saved can be quite effective. Reading labels may also be a useful skill to evaluate products for overall energy and nutrient quality.
- Tailor treatment and prevention efforts to each particular ethnicity; integrate culturally appropriate approaches and strategies (Wang and Tussing, 2004). For example, bilingual professionals might develop culturally sensitive wellness programs targeted at immigrant Hispanic families to encourage moderate-intensity physical activity and more frequent consumption of lower calorie foods (McArthur et al, 2004).
- A good example should be set in the home. Encourage regular family meals whenever possible; limit unplanned or habitual snacking. Between meals, ice water can be offered as a special treat instead of sweetened beverages.
- Since many children who enter adolescence overweight will become overweight or obese adults (Magarey et al, 2003; Ferraro et al, 2003), encourage healthy eating habits and increased physical activity. Simple things like using dance videos can be an easy activity to do at home, especially for children who are self-conscious about exercising in public.
- Discuss the relationship of food, weight, and energy balance. Metabolic rates may be low while watching television. In elementary school–aged children, limit television and nonproductive computer time to <2 hours daily (American Academy of Pediatrics, 2005; Hancox et al, 2004). Encourage activity, such as jogging, ball games, swimming, bike riding, and school-based physical activities (Datar and Sturm, 2004).
- Discourage potentially dangerous weight-control schemes or practices.
- Responsibilities should be shared; parents are responsible for a proper emotional setting and for what is offered; the child is responsible for what and how much is eaten (Satter, 2005). Emphasis becomes *supporting each child's normal growth* (Satter, 2005).
- A system for "traffic light" foods can be used for younger children: green for "go" foods, yellow for "caution" foods, and red for "stop" foods. While weight loss is occurring, maintain the child's self-image through positive reinforcement.
- Parents who practice restrained eating with their children tend to be overly indulgent later (fast/feast); the result is chronic anxiety. Eating can become very controlled, inconsistent, and emotional. Highlight non–food-related achievements; avoid nagging about diet or food.
- See Table 3-14 for more tips.

Patient Education—Food Safety

- Hand washing with soap and hot water is recommended before preparing meals.
- Before using tap water as a beverage, let cold tap water run for 2 minutes to remove any lead that may be in the pipes.
- Follow the 2-hour rule: discard any beverage or food that has been left at room temperature for 2 hours or longer.

For More Information

- American Academy of Family Physicians
  http://familydoctor.org/344.xml
- American Dietetic Association
  Position Paper: Dietary guidance for healthy children aged 2 to 11 years (2004)
  http://www.eatright.org/Public/Other/index_adap0199.cfm
- Centers for Disease Control and Prevention
  http://www.cdc.gov/nchs/products/pubs/pubd/hestats/overwght99.htm
- CDC Charts for BMI in Children and Teens
  http://www.cdc.gov/nccdphp/dnpa/bmi/bmi-for-age.htm
- Ellyn Satter Institute
  http://www.ellynsatter.com/

TABLE 3-14 Components of Successful Weight Loss For Children

Component	Comment
Reasonable weight loss goal	Initially, a rate of 1 lb per month if >95th or >85th percentile with comorbidity, based on age.
Dietary management	Guide family choices rather than dictating; encourage child to eat when hungry and to eat slowly. Encourage family meals. Avoid using food as reward or withholding as punishment. Drink plenty of water and limit sugar-sweetened beverages. Plan healthy snacks. Aim for 5 servings of fruits and vegetables each day. Promote healthy breakfast each day. Consume milk with dinner instead of soft drinks.
Physical activity	Begin according to child's fitness level, with ultimate goal of 60 minutes of moderate activity daily.
Behavior modification	Teach self-monitoring, nutritional education, control of cues, modification of eating habits, physical activity, attitude change, reinforcements, and rewards.
Family involvement	Review family activity and television viewing patterns; involve parents in nutrition counseling.

Adapted from: Mullen and Shield, 2004.

- Institute of Medicine–Childhood Obesity and Role of Parents
  http://www.iom.edu/news.asp?id=22902
- International Food Information Council
  http://ific.org/
  http://ific.org/nutrition/obesity/index.cfm
- NIDDK Weight Control Network
  http://win.niddk.nih.gov/publications/over_child.htm

OBESITY, CHILDHOOD—CITED REFERENCES

American Academy of Pediatrics. Overweight and obesity. Accessed March 2, 2005 at http://www.aap.org/healthtopics/overweight.cfm.

Arenz S, et al. Breast-feeding and childhood obesity—a systematic review. *Int J Obes Relat Metab Disord.* 28:1247, 2004.

Berkowitz RI, et al. Behavior therapy and sibutramine for the treatment of adolescent obesity: a randomized controlled trial. *JAMA.* 289:1805, 2003.

Blackburn GL, Mun EC. Effects of weight loss surgeries on liver disease. *Semin Liver Dis.* 24:371, 2004.

Caballero B. Obesity prevention in children: opportunities and challenges. *Int J Obes Relat Metab Disord.* 28:S90, 2004.

Datar A, Sturm R. Physical education in elementary school and body mass index: evidence from the early childhood longitudinal study. *Am J Public Health.* 94:1501, 2004.

Eisenmann JC, et al. Stability of variables associated with the metabolic syndrome from adolescence to adulthood: the Aerobics Center Longitudinal Study. *Am J Hum Biol.* 16:690, 2004.

Evans WD, et al. Public perceptions of childhood obesity. *Am J Prev Med.* 28:26, 2005.

Ferraro KF, et al. The life course of severe obesity: does childhood overweight matter? *J Gerontol B Psychol Sci Soc Sci.* 58:S110, 2003.

Gil-Campos M, et al. Hormones regulating lipid metabolism and plasma lipids in childhood obesity. *Int J Obes Relat Metab Disord.* 28:S75, 2004.

Gillman M, et al. Risk of overweight among adolescents who were breastfed as infants. *JAMA.* 285:2461, 2001.

Hancox RJ, et al. Association between child and adolescent television viewing and adult health: a longitudinal birth cohort study *Lancet.* 364:257, 2004.

Institute of Medicine. Dietary references intakes: macronutrients. Available at http://www.iom.edu/report.asp?id=4340, 2002.

Koplan JP, et al. Preventing childhood obesity: health in the balance, executive summary. *J Am Diet Assoc.* 105:131, 2005.

Kral JG. Preventing and treating obesity in girls and young women to curb the epidemic. *Obes Res.* 12:1539, 2004.

Krebs NF, et al. Prevention of pediatric overweight and obesity. *Pediatrics* 112:424, 2003.

Li X, et al. Childhood adiposity as a predictor of cardiac mass in adulthood: the Bogalusa Heart Study. *Circulation* 110:3488, 2004.

Magarey AM, et al. Predicting obesity in early adulthood from childhood and parental obesity. *Int J Obes Relat Metab Disord.* 27:505, 2003.

Marcason W. At what age should an overweight child follow a calorie-restricted diet? *J Am Diet Assoc.* 104:834, 2004.

Martorell R, et al. Early nutrition and later adiposity. *J Nutr.* 131:874S, 2001.

McArthur LH, et al. Are household factors putting immigrant Hispanic children at risk of becoming overweight: a community-based study in eastern North Carolina. *J Comm Health.* 29:387, 2004.

Mullen MC, Shield J. *Childhood and adolescent overweight: the health professional's guide to identification, treatment and prevention.* Chicago, IL: American Dietetic Association, 2004.

Ong KK, Dunger DB. Birth weight, infant growth and insulin resistance. *Eur J Endocrinol.* 151:131S3, 2004.

Pender JR, Pories WJ. Epidemiology of obesity in the United States. *Gastroenterol Clin N Am.* 34:1, 2005.

Ritchie LD, et al. Family environment and pediatric overweight: what is a parent to do? *J Am Diet Assoc.* 105:70S, 2005.

Satter E. Accessed January 2, 2005 at http://www.ellynsatter.com.

Viner RM, et al. Prevalence of the insulin resistance syndrome in obesity. *Arch Dis Child.* 90:10, 2005.

Wang Y, Epidemiology of childhood obesity—methodological aspects and guidelines: wht is new? *Int J Obes Relat Metab Disord.* 28:S21, 2004.

Wang Y, Tussing L. Culturally appropriate approaches are needed to reduce ethnic disparity in childhood obesity. *J Am Diet Assoc.* 104:1664, 2004.

OTITIS MEDIA

NUTRITIONAL ACUITY RANKING: LEVEL 1

DEFINITIONS AND BACKGROUND

Acute otitis media (OM; acute middle ear infection) is common in children. There is a bacterial or viral infection of the fluid of the middle ear that leads to production of pus, excess fluid, or even bleeding in the middle ear. The drainage system (the eustachian tube) becomes clogged. The eustachian tube of the ear of a child is shorter and less slanted than in adults. This allows bacteria and viruses to find their way into the middle ear more easily, resulting in pus building up in the middle ear. See Figure 3-3, which shows OM.

Pressure from fluids associated with OM may cause the eardrum to rupture. This can also result in ear infection by allowing bacteria or viruses direct entry to the middle ear. Ear infections often occur along with respiratory infections or with blocked sinuses and eustachian tubes caused by allergies. OM with effusions (OME) can lead to significant hearing loss in children if not properly treated.

Recent illness of any type and lowered immunity; crowded or unsanitary living conditions; genetic factors (susceptibility to infection may run in families); cold climate and high altitude; and bottle feeding of infants (can allow fluid to pool in the throat near the eustachian tube) may be causative factors.

Breast milk is more protective than formula feeding. Breast milk contains protective factors such as lactoferrin; oligosaccharides function to support microbial receptors preventing mucosal attachment, the initial step of most infections (Hanson et al, 2002). Premature cessation of feeding with breast milk may contribute to an increased incidence of acute and secretory OM, especially in children at risk, such as those with cleft palate (Aniansson et al, 2002).

The prevalence of early-onset and repeated OM continues to increase among preschool children; an increase in prevalence of allergic conditions among poor children is one concern (Auinger et al, 2003). Breastfeeding should be encouraged to reduce onset of celiac disease or allergies (Hanson et al, 2002).

In older children, chewing xylitol gum or lozenges helps to prevent OM by preventing growth of pneumococci (Uhari et al, 1998). Studies are under way to determine if the use of antioxidants or other nutrients makes any difference in healing.

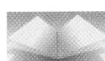

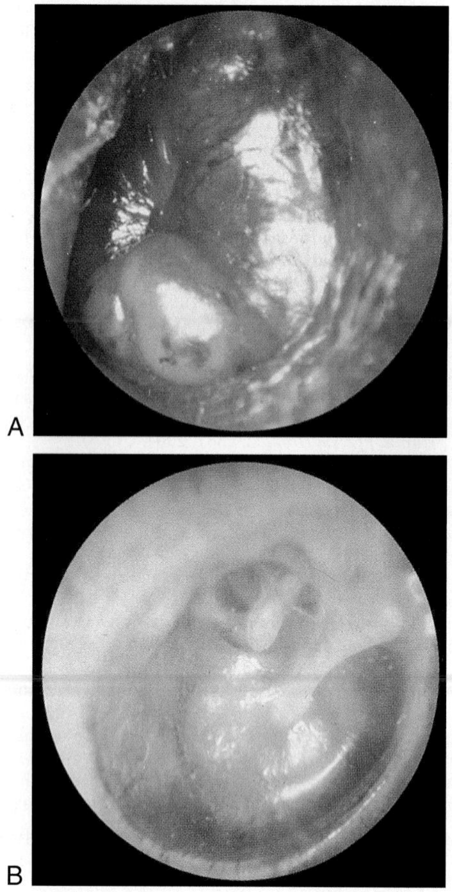

Figure 3-3 Otitis media. (From Moore KL, Dalley AF II. *Clinical oriented anatomy*. 4th ed. Baltimore: Lippincott Williams & Wilkins, 1999.)

INTERVENTION: OBJECTIVES

- Promote breastfeeding of newborns, especially for 6 months or longer.
- If formula fed, babies should be positioned in a semi-upright position so that the milk will flow downward into the baby's stomach and not wash up and into the baby's nasal passages and up through the eustachian tubes. Always position the infant's head higher than the stomach.
- In older children, monitor nutrient density of the diet to maintain a healthy immune system. Inclusion of a children's multivitamin-mineral supplement may be needed for poor eaters or during food jags.

INTERVENTION: FOOD AND NUTRITION

- Determine the recommended allowances for the child's age group: kcal, protein, and other nutrients. Plan a reasonable menu pattern accordingly.
- Highlight foods that include sufficient levels of iron, vitamins A and C, and zinc to support a healthy immune system to fight further infections.
- If child has food allergies, discuss options for maintaining a healthy diet, especially if large food group categories must be eliminated.

CLINICAL INDICATORS

Clinical/History	I & O	Lab Work
Height Birth length Birth weight Present weight Diet/intake history Family history of asthma, allergies	Fever? Irritability, fussiness? Exposure to cigarette smoking? Audiometry	H & H Serum Fe Chol, Trig Gluc Alb Na+, K+

Common Drugs Used and Potential Side Effects

- Antibiotics such as penicillin are often prescribed for bacterial infections; side effects may include rash, vomiting, and diarrhea. Viral infections have to run their course. Use of probiotics in foods such as yogurt can help to replenish the gut and support healthy immunity.

Herbs, Botanicals, and Supplements

- Herbs and botanicals should not be used for OM because there are no controlled trials to prove efficacy.

INTERVENTION: NUTRITION EDUCATION, COUNSELING, CARE MANAGEMENT

- Explain to parents that overfeeding can aggravate asthma, which is often triggered by bouts of OM.
- Discuss the role of nutrition and immunity.
- If needed, teach principles for managing food allergies and asthma.
- Chronic recurrence should be addressed with an ear-nose-throat specialist to prevent hearing loss and speech delay.
- Smoking around the child should be discontinued, especially to avoid recurrent infections (Lieu and Feinstein, 2002).
- Older children may benefit from chewing xylitol gum (Uhari et al, 1998).

For More Information

- Family Doctor
  http://familydoctor.org/055.xml
- I-tonsil
  http://www.itonsil.com/index.html

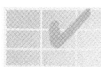

OTITIS MEDIA—CITED REFERENCES

Aniansson G, et al. Otitis media and feeding with breast milk of children with cleft palate. *Scand J Plast Reconstr Surg Hand Surg.* 36:9, 2002.

Auinger P, et al. Trends in otitis media among children in the United States. *Pediatrics* 112:514, 2003.

Hanson LA, et al. Breast-feeding, a complex support system for the offspring. *Pediatr Int.* 44:347, 2002.

Lieu JE, Feinstein AR. Effect of gestational and passive smoke exposure on ear infections in children. *Arch Pediatr Adolesc Med.* 156:147, 2002.

Uhari M, et al. A novel use of xylitol sugar in preventing acute otitis media. *Pediatrics* 102:879, 1998.

PHENYLKETONURIA

NUTRITIONAL ACUITY RANKING: LEVEL 4

DEFINITIONS AND BACKGROUND

Phenylketonuria (PKU) is a rare, inherited condition that occurs in one in 10,000 births. PKU is caused by an inborn error that results from a mutation in the phenylalanine hydroxylase gene. As a result, phenylalanine (Phe) is not metabolized to tyrosine. Infants are tested for this disorder after birth and after the first feeding and again if levels of Phe are above given cutoff levels (≥6 mg/dL).

If very strict diets are followed early and continually, normal development and life span are possible. Children with PKU who follow their special diet for life have fewer intellectual and neurological deficits (Weglage et al, 2001). The diet should not be totally discontinued at any age. Referral to a metabolic dietitian and special programs at the state level may be required.

Desirable serum Phe levels are below 10 mg/dL. Higher levels are associated with declining IQ. There is international consensus that patients with Phe levels <360 μM on a free diet do not need Phe-lowering dietary treatment, whereas patients with levels >600 μM do; different recommendations exist for patients with mild hyperphenylalaninemia (Weglage et al, 2001). In general, however, "diet for life" is the rule, especially for women with PKU who are considering pregnancy (de la Cruz and Koch, 2001).

Tyrosine is an essential amino acid in patients with PKU because of the limited Phe converted to tyrosine (Bross et al, 2000). In depressed individuals with PKU, treatment with large neutral amino acid supplements may help to correct low or deficient blood concentrations of both tyrosine and tryptophan, which are precursors for dopamine and serotonin (Koch et al, 2003).

Serum lipids are usually under good control because of the vegetarian-type diet needed for PKU (Schulpis et al, 2003). However, micronutrient status of folic acid and vitamins B_6 and B_{12} can be low, and there may be a risk for coronary artery disease (Schulpis et al, 2002; Robinson et al, 2000). Individuals who follow diets low in natural proteins (as in PKU) should be advised to take selenium (VanBakel et al, 2000) and iron supplements (Acosta et al, 2004).

INTERVENTION: OBJECTIVES

- Prevent toxic buildup of abnormal metabolites.
- Prevent mental retardation. Promote normal intellectual and social development.
- Establish the child's daily requirement for Phe, protein, and energy according to age. The appropriate Phe intake for age is as follows: infants 0–3 months, 60–90 mg/kg; infants 4–6 months, 40 mg/kg; infants 7–9 months, 35 mg/kg; infants 10–12 months, 30 mg/kg; children 1–2 years, 25 mg/kg; and children 2+ years, 20 mg/kg body weight. Maximal Phe intake for children with PKU should be no higher than 20 mg/kg (Courtney-Martin et al, 2002).
- Provide a diet aiding growth and development. A high energy to protein ratio is needed to spare protein.
- Introduce solids and textures at usual ages. Encourage self-feeding when it is possible for the infant to do so.
- Establish a positive attitude toward the diet in the parent or caretaker and in the child.
- Monitor for deficiency in nutrients, such as vitamin B_{12}, folic acid, selenium, and iron.

INTERVENTION: FOOD AND NUTRITION

- Use a diet low in Phe. Use special milk substitutes made from casein hydrolysate, corn oil, corn syrup, tapioca starch, minerals, and vitamins. Special formulas, Phenyl-free, or Maxamaid XP can be used. Phenyl-free does not provide total nutritional needs. A new product, Phlexy-10, may appeal to some individuals; it is available from SHS North America.
- Some milk and Lofenalac formula should be used to provide for the infant's needs (use Lofenalac for 85–100% of an infant's needs). Subtract Phe requirement in formula from total needs (the difference is that which is provided by solid foods).
- Initially, the infant's tolerance must be assessed individually, and progress in treatment must develop accordingly.
- Determine if serum iron, vitamin B_{12}, folic acid, selenium, or other nutrient levels are low and enhance diet or use a multivitamin-mineral supplement as needed.
- Introduce solids and textures at the appropriate ages. Omit meat, fish, poultry, bread, milk, cheese, legumes, and peanut butter from the diet of older children. Flavors can be added to the formula to continue its use as a beverage.
- To add calories, try jam, jelly, sugar, honey, molasses, syrups, cornstarch, and oils that are Phe-free.
- Try using low-protein bread, pasta, crackers, cookies, and muffin mixes.

SAMPLE NUTRITION DIAGNOSTIC STATEMENT

Phenylketonuria (PKU)

PES: Inappropriate intake of amino acids related to low comprehension of nutrition care plan as evidenced by serum phenylalanine level of 28 mg/dL, whereas >8 mg/dL indicates loss of dietary control in PKU.

Assessment Data (sources of info): Diet intake records, serum lab values of phenylalanine, previous education on appropriate diet for PKU management.

Intervention: Counseling on phenylalanine in diet, use of special formulas and products, referral to State Health Department for resources and financial support, referral to child health clinics.

Monitoring and Evaluation: Serum phenylalanine reports, changes in mental health status and alertness.

CLINICAL INDICATORS

Clinical/History

- Birth weight
- Present weight
- Growth (%)
- Diet/intake history
- Mental retardation
- Mousy odor in urine and sweat
- Length/height
- Dermatitis

Lab Work

- Electroencephalograms (EEGs)
- Plasma Phe
- Urinary Phe
- Plasma tyrosine
- H & H
- Serum Fe
- Serum pyridoxine
- Serum vitamin B_{12}
- Serum folic acid

Common Drugs Used and Potential Side Effects

- Antianxiety or psychotropic medications are used to help patients manage their behaviors. Behavioral redirection may be useful to help them socialize better.

Herbs, Botanicals, and Supplements

- Herbs and botanicals should not be used for PKU because there are no controlled trials to prove efficacy.

INTERVENTION: NUTRITION EDUCATION, COUNSELING, CARE MANAGEMENT

- Because initial acceptance of formula may be poor due to its strong taste, the mother should be careful not to express her own distaste. Recommend appropriate recipes and cookbooks.
- Monitor the calculation of Phe in the diet.
- Avoid items sweetened with aspartame (NutraSweet), including diet sodas.
- Self-management should begin by 7–8 years of age, at least for formula preparation. By 12 years of age, the child should begin calculating his or her own intake of Phe from foods.
- For women of childbearing age, it is important to note that women who have PKU tend to give birth to children with microcephaly, mental retardation, congenital heart defects, and intrauterine growth retardation with LBW (Rouse et al, 2000). Metabolic control by the end of the first trimester is, therefore, important as a goal. Treatment at any time during pregnancy may reduce the severity of delayed development (Waisbren et al, 2000). Referral to a dietetics professional is highly recommended (Kaiser et al, 2002).

Patient Education—Food Safety

- Hand washing with soap and hot water is recommended before preparing formula or meals. Use clean utensils and containers for mixing formula.
- Before using tap water for formula preparation or to give as a beverage, let cold tap water run for 2 minutes to remove any lead that may be in the pipes.
- Follow the 2-hour rule: discard any beverage or food that has been left at room temperature for 2 hours or longer.
- Do not use honey in the diets of infants to decrease potential risk of botulism.

For More Information

- Children's PKU Network
  http://www.kumc.edu/gec/support/pku.html
- Diet Tips for PKU
  http://www.pkunews.org/
- National Coalition for PKU and Allied Disorders
  http://www.pku-allieddisorders.org/
- PKU News
  www.pkunews.org

PHENYLKETONURIA—CITED REFERENCES

Acosta P, et al. Iron status of children with phenylketonuria undergoing nutrition therapy assessed by transferrin receptors. *Genet Med.* 6:96, 2004.

Bross R, et al. Tyrosine requirements in children with classical PKU determined by indicator amino acid oxidation. *Am J Physiol Endocrinol Metab.* 278:195, 2000.

Courtney-Martin G, et al. Phenylalanine requirement in children with classical PKU determined by indicator amino acid oxidation. *Am J Physiol Endocrinol Metab.* 283:1249, 2002

de la Cruz F, Koch R. Genetic implications for newborn screening for phenylketonuria. *Clin Perinatol.* 28:419, 2001.

Kaiser LL, et al. Position of the American Dietetic Association: nutrition and lifestyle for a healthy pregnancy outcome. *J Am Diet Assoc.* 102:1479, 2002.

Koch R, et al. Large neutral amino acid therapy and phenylketonuria: a promising approach to treatment. *Mol Genet Metab.* 79:110, 2003.

Robinson M, et al. Increased risk of vitamin B12 deficiency in patients with phenylketonuria on an unrestricted or relaxed diet. *J Pediatr.* 136:545, 2000.

Rouse B, et al. Maternal phenylketonuria syndrome: congenital heart defects, microcephaly, and developmental outcomes. *J Pediatr.* 136:57, 2000.

Schulpis KH, et al. Effect of diet on plasma total antioxidant status in phenylketonuric patients. *Eur J Clin Nutr.* 57:383, 2003.

Schulpis KH, et al. Homocysteine and other vascular risk factors in patients with phenylketonuria on a diet. *Acta Paediatr.* 91:905, 2002.
VanBakel M, et al. Antioxidant and thyroid hormone status in selenium-deficient phenylketonuric and hyperphenylalaninemic patients. *Am J Clin Nutri.* 72:976, 2000.
Waisbren S, et al. Outcome at age 4 years in offspring of women with maternal phenylketonuria: the Maternal PKU Collaborative Study. *JAMA.* 283:756, 2000.
Weglage J, et al. Normal clinical outcome in untreated subjects with mild hyperphenylalaninemia. *Pediatr Res.* 49:532, 2001.

PRADER-WILLI SYNDROME

NUTRITIONAL ACUITY RANKING: LEVEL 3–4

DEFINITIONS AND BACKGROUND

Prader-Willi syndrome (PWS) is a disorder caused by DNA abnormalities of chromosome 15. Major characteristics are infant hypotonia, hypogonadism, mental retardation (average IQ is around 70), small hands and feet, atypical facial features, and obesity because of insatiable appetite in early childhood. Short stature is part of the syndrome and is not nutritional in origin. PWS patients have increased fasting ghrelin levels.

The incidence of PWS is one in 8000 births in the United States. Onset occurs at birth, but symptoms begin by 1–4 years of age. These children often present with absence of crying, poor suck, lethargy, and floppy muscle tone (hypotonia) as infants. Motor development is delayed; learning disability or retardation may occur. Individuals with PWS are not able to control their food sneaking, stealing, and gorging behaviors. They have little or no gag reflex, do not vomit, and may eat contaminated or inedible food combinations (Dykens, 2000).

Because they are difficult to manage, approximately 75% of these patients live in group homes. Lifelong morbidities of PWS include osteoporosis, type 2 diabetes mellitus, respiratory disorders, and cardiorespiratory failure related to obesity and hypotonia (Allen and Carrel, 2004). Sexual development is incomplete; most PWS individuals are infertile.

Treatment with growth hormone (GH) has been shown to increase height velocity in children with PWS, decrease weight-for-height index values and body fat mass, and have a positive effect on lean body mass during at least the first year of therapy (Eiholzer and Whitman, 2004). Biliopancreatic diversion is not an adequate treatment alone for weight loss for those with this syndrome (Grugni et al, 2000). Behavioral manifestations, including deficit in appetite control and cognitive limitations, require long-term multidisciplinary management (Eiholzer and Whitman, 2004).

INTERVENTION: OBJECTIVES

- Reduce excess weight. Monitor weight weekly.
- In preschool children, prevent obesity.
- Maintain recommended dietary intakes for all nutrients and protein to promote growth and development.
- Provide feeding assistance if needed.
- Prevent complications like CHD, hypertension (HPN), diabetes mellitus (DM), sleep apnea, dental problems, and pneumonia.
- Correct serum lipid levels if elevated.
- Minimize unusual food-seeking behaviors such as eating food from the trash or eating inappropriate or unpalatable food combinations. Correct pica and related nutritional deficits (iron, etc.).
- Promote an exercise program.

INTERVENTION: FOOD AND NUTRITION

- Often, these children start with failure to thrive (FTT) and then become obese; identify where the child is in this continuum.
- Use a low-calorie diet to reduce weight: 10–11 kcal/cm height to maintain; 8.5 kcal/cm for slow weight loss (Lucas, 2004, p. 41). For older teens, reduce the total calorie level to 800–1200 kcal/d (about 7–8 kcal/cm for weight loss or 10–14 kcal/cm to maintain). Patients' needs are about 60% of those without PWS.
- Ensure that the diet provides adequate protein and nutrients. Follow RDAs for age but reduce overall fat and energy intake. Follow the Prader-Willi pyramid pattern; see Figure 3-4.

SAMPLE NUTRITION DIAGNOSTIC STATEMENT

Prader-Willi Syndrome

PES: Overweight related to excessive nutrient intake as evidenced by BMI of 35 and nutrition history indicating consumption of 2900 kcal/d and sneaking of foods between meals.

Assessment Data: Diet, weight, and physical activity histories.

Intervention: Interventions would address appropriate nutrient intake, enhancing physical activity, and keeping logs. Using stoplight teaching for "Go-Caution-No" foods in color-coded system.

Monitoring and Evaluation: Having patient return in 1 month to assess weight and review diet and activity logs.

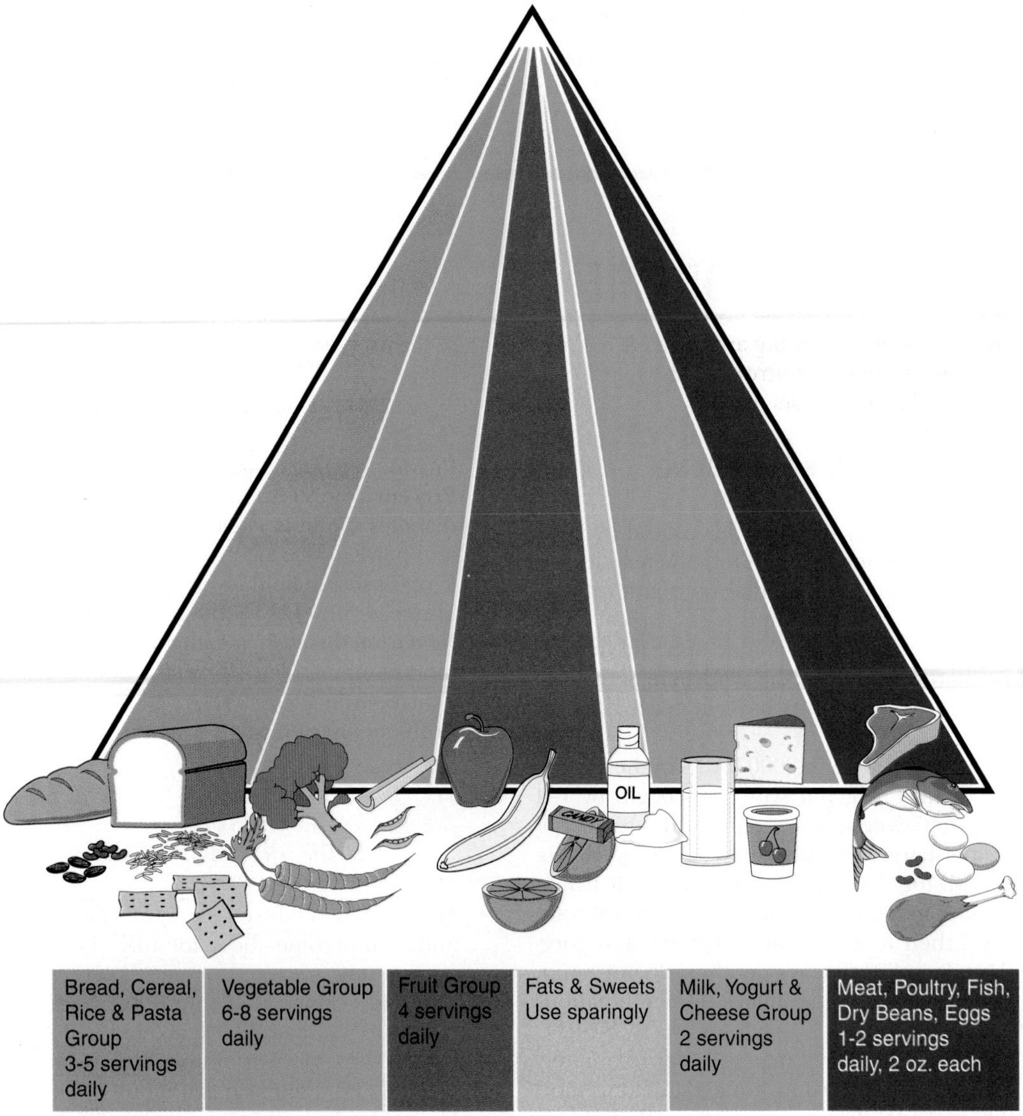

Figure 3-4 Adaptation of the Prader-Willi Food Pyramid following the format of USDA's MyPyramid. (Based on information from http://www.pwsausa.org/syndrome/foodpyramid.htm.)

CLINICAL INDICATORS

Clinical/History

- Height
- Birth weight
- Present weight
- Goal weight
- Diet/intake history
- Mental retardation
- Small head, hands, feet
- Sleep apnea?
- Asthma or other respiratory problems?
- Hypotonia

Lab Work

- Gluc, Glucose tolerance test (GTT)
- Alb
- BP
- Chol, Trig
- Liver function tests
- pCO_2, pO_2
- H & H
- Serum Fe

Common Drugs Used and Potential Side Effects

- Weight loss products have not proven to be useful in this population. Drugs may react differently and are, therefore, not recommended.
- Growth hormone may be used to correct short stature, and hormone replacement therapy may be used to improve signs of osteopenia or osteoporosis (Allen and Carrel, 2004).
- With outbursts of temper or repetitive behaviors, medications may be needed.

Herbs, Botanicals, and Supplements

- Persons with PWS may be more sensitive, and small doses of herbs and drugs may cause a greater reaction than in other people (see http://www.pwsausa.org/syndrome/herbal.htm).
- Herbs and botanicals should not be used for PWS because there are no controlled trials to prove efficacy.

INTERVENTION: NUTRITION EDUCATION, COUNSELING, CARE MANAGEMENT

- Encourage the patient to be active and to exercise daily. Discuss feeding practices plus activity factors.
- Behavior modification is an important part of treatment. Help the patient lose weight with specific behavior modification techniques. Effective systems promote a green/yellow/red (go/caution/stop) method of food choices.
- Main elements of concern in the diet are sugars and fats.
- Record keeping and calorie counting are generally better than use of exchange systems. Control of excess intake is the main goal; locked refrigerators or cupboards may be needed in the household.
- An interdisciplinary approach is useful (Eiholzer and Whitman, 2004).
- There is a need to reduce guilt and depression. Self-monitoring is the eventual goal.

For More Information

- Heimlich Maneuver–for choking
  http://www.heimlichinstitute.org/howtodo.html#chokingAnchor
- Prader-Willi Syndrome Association
  http://www.pwsausa.org/

PRADER-WILLI SYNDROME—CITED REFERENCES

Allen DB, Carrel AL. Growth hormone therapy for Prader-Willi syndrome: a critical appraisal. *J Pediatr Endocrinol Metab.* S17:1297S, 2004.

Dykens E. Contaminated and unusual food combinations: what do people with Prader-Willi syndrome choose? *Ment Retard.* 38:163, 2000.

Eiholzer U, Whitman BY. A comprehensive team approach to the management of patients with Prader-Willi syndrome. *J Pediatr Endocrinol Metab.* 17:1153, 2004.

Grugni G, et al. Failure of biliopancreatic diversion in Prader-Willi syndrome. *Obes Surg.* 10:179, 2000.

Lucas B, ed. *Children with special care needs: nutrition care handbook.* Chicago, IL: The American Dietetic Association, 2004.

RICKETS, NUTRITIONAL

NUTRITIONAL ACUITY RANKING: LEVEL 3

DEFINITIONS AND BACKGROUND

Vitamin D insufficiency and deficiency during pregnancy lead to lower maternal weight gain and disturbed skeletal homeostasis in the infant, with reduced bone mineralization, radiologically evident rickets, and fractures (Pawley and Bishop, 2004). Specifically, nutritional rickets is caused by calcium, phosphorus, and vitamin D deficiency.

Nutritional rickets can be seen in children or premature infants, including up to 30–70% of LBW and VLBW infants. It is also seen in breastfed children from multiple births and those living in higher latitudes with darker skin pigmentation (Kreiter et al, 2000; Pugliese et al, 1998). Factors that may have contributed to the increase in numbers of children with nutritional rickets include: more African American women breastfeeding, fewer infants receiving vitamin D supplements, and mothers and children exposed to less sunlight (Kreiter et al, 2000). It may also occur in malabsorption syndromes (vitamin D is fat soluble) with steatorrhea; anticonvulsant use; renal failure; and biliary cirrhosis.

Features of nutritional rickets include leg bowing, inability to walk or stand, poor linear growth, seizures, irritability, abnormal serum calcium and phosphorus, and abnormal alkaline phosphatase levels. Sunlight is important to skin production of vitamin D, and environmental conditions where sunlight exposure is limited may reduce access. Vitamin D supplementation and sunlight are effective treatments (Kaper et al, 2000).

The American Academy of Pediatrics (AAP) recently recommended the following: (1) a minimal intake of 200 IU/d of vitamin D for all infants, beginning in the first 2 months of life; (2) a vitamin D supplement for breastfed infants who do not consume at least 500 mL of a vitamin D–fortified beverage; (3) education about the higher risk of rickets among children who are dark skinned or have little sun exposure; and (4) education about the importance of weaning children to a diet adequate in both vitamin D and calcium (Weisberg et al, 2004). In addition, newborns should receive a vitamin K injection to support bone health (Collier et al, 2004).

INTERVENTION: OBJECTIVES

- Correct body mineral status; prevent further problems and deformity. Vitamin D participates in mineral homeostasis, regulation of gene expression, and cell differentiation. Complement drug therapy with adequate diet.
- Prevent or correct tetany, hypocalcemia, and other complications.
- Identify and treat other problems such as dental caries or bone fractures, which may also be common.
- Promote growth, since short stature can result if not treated early enough.

INTERVENTION: FOOD AND NUTRITION

- Use a balanced diet appropriate for age and sex. If diet is inadequate in the specific nutrients, ensure intake of a sufficient level of vitamin D, calcium, and phosphorus for age and sex. Ensure that phytate intake is not excessive.

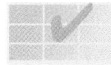

- Use milk if no milk or lactose intolerances exist; increase appropriately while monitoring serum values.
- There may be additional use of such calcium-containing foods as cheeses, yogurt, and fortified juice, if milk is not tolerated.
- If necessary, early tube feeding (TF) with extra calcium and phosphorus may be useful.
- With PN, there may be inadequate use of calcium and phosphorus; monitor carefully.
- With steatorrhea, check serum levels of vitamin D and calcium, and supplement appropriately.

CLINICAL INDICATORS

Clinical/History

Height
Weight
Growth (%)
Diet/intake history
Decreased linear growth
Steatorrhea
Muscle spasm
Chvostek's sign (facial spasm)
Metabolic acidosis
DEXA scan for bone density
Wrist radiographs
Radiographs for fractures

Lab Work

Urinary Ca^{++} (elevated)
Urinary phosphorus (P)
Alk phos (increased)
Serum P (decreased)
Serum Ca^{++} (often low)
Mg^{++}, Na^{+}, K^{+}

Common Drugs Used and Potential Side Effects

- Calciferol 1500–3000 IU daily by mouth helps in 2–4 weeks; some maintenance doses may also be required over time. Monitor use with dietary calcium. Calcitriol may be needed in renal disorders that cause deficiency.
- Vitamin D: A large dose may be given upon diagnosis; with long-term use (3 months or longer), administer according to causative factors. Be wary of toxic effects of vitamin D (hypercalcemia, nausea, vomiting, anorexia, malaise, renal problems, or hypertensive problems). For anticonvulsant use, vitamin D will be supplemented at 1000–2000 IU/d.
- Furosemide (Lasix): May cause rickets in some cases; hypercalciuria may occur.
- Antacid excess may cause a phosphorus deficiency; monitor carefully and correct. Use alternative measures.
- Rickets may also occur secondary to anticonvulsant use. A vitamin D supplement will be needed.

Herbs, Botanicals, and Supplements

- Herbs and botanicals should not be used for rickets because there are no controlled trials to prove efficacy.

INTERVENTION: NUTRITION EDUCATION, COUNSELING, CARE MANAGEMENT

- Discuss needed alterations of the diet in conjunction with drug therapy.
- Discuss the role of sunlight in vitamin D metabolism.
- Good posture and positioning are important aspects of treatment.
- The recommended intake of 200 IU/d may not be enough; more data are needed to support the adequacy of the present daily recommended intake and possibly even higher recommended vitamin D daily intakes (Greer, 2004).

Patient Education—Food Safety

- Hand washing with soap and hot water is recommended before preparing formula or meals. Use clean utensils and containers for mixing formula.
- Before using tap water for formula preparation or to give as a beverage, let cold tap water run for 2 minutes to remove any lead that may be in the pipes.
- Follow the 2-hour rule: discard any beverage or food that has been left at room temperature for 2 hours or longer.
- Do not use honey in the diets of infants to decrease potential risk of botulism.

For More Information

- Vanderbilt - History of Rickets
  http://www.mc.vanderbilt.edu/biolib/hc/nh8.html

RICKETS, NUTRITIONAL—CITED REFERENCES

Collier S, et al. Nutrition for the pediatric office: update on vitamins, infant feeding and food allergies. *Curr Opin Pediatr.* 16:314, 2004.

Greer FR. Issues in establishing vitamin D recommendations for infants and children. *Am J Clin Nutr.* 80:1759S, 2004.

Kaper B, et al. Nutritional rickets: report of four cases diagnosed at orthopedic evaluation. *Am J Orthop.* 29:214, 2000.

Kreiter S, et al. Nutritional rickets in African American breastfed infants. *J Pediatr.* 137:153, 2000.

Pawley N, Bishop NJ. Prenatal and infant predictors of bone health: the influence of vitamin D. *Am J Clin Nutr.* 80:1748S, 2004.

Pugliese M, et al. Nutritional rickets in suburbia. *J Am Col Nutri.* 17:637, 1998.

Weisberg P, et al. Nutritional rickets among children in the United States: review of cases reported between 1986 and 2003. *Am J Clin Nutr.* 80:1697S, 2004.

SMALL FOR GESTATIONAL AGE INFANT

NUTRITIONAL ACUITY RANKING: LEVEL 3

DEFINITIONS AND BACKGROUND

Each year, about 40,000 infants born at term in the United States are small for gestational age (SGA), and they are at risk for preterm delivery (Zaw et al, 2003). Infants may be SGA at birth because of genetic or nongenetic factors. Nongenetic causes may retard intrauterine growth but are not often apparent before 32–34 weeks of gestation. Growth retardation due to nongenetic factors may cause malnutrition while sparing growth of the brain and long bones. Some other genetic disorders and congenital infections result in total growth retardation, in which height, weight, and head circumference are equally affected. There may be wide ranges in weight gains after birth in SGA infants.

SGA usually occurs because of intrauterine growth retardation (IUGR) from placental insufficiency. This insufficiency may result from maternal diseases (hyperemesis, preeclampsia, primary hypertension, renal disease, or diabetes); from infections such as cytomegalovirus, rubella virus, or *Toxoplasma gondii*; or if the mother is a narcotic or cocaine addict or heavy user of alcohol or tobacco (Dodds et al, 2006). The term SGA should be used for an infant who has failed to achieve a weight threshold (usually defined as the 10th percentile), whereas an IUGR infant has not reached his or her genetic growth potential due to an insult that has occurred during pregnancy (Bamberg and Kalache, 2004).

If IUGR was caused by chronic placental malnutrition, SGA infants may demonstrate remarkable catch-up growth within the first 2–3 years after delivery if they are provided with adequate nutrition. The rates of catch-up growth vary according to many factors including birth weight, gestational age, parental size, adequacy of intrauterine growth, neurological impairment, clinical course, and nutrition (Carver, 2005).

Fetal growth restriction is associated with greater morbidity than among infants born within a normal size range. Insulin-like growth factor has a critical role in mediating fetal and postnatal growth (Randhawa and Cohen, 2005).

Common complications in SGA infants include hypoglycemia, perinatal asphyxia, meconium aspiration, polycythemia, respiratory distress syndrome, and necrotizing enterocolitis (Dodds et al, 2006; Zaw et al, 2003). Prognosis is quite serious for infants who have perinatal asphyxia or congenital conditions.

INTERVENTION: OBJECTIVES

- Correct body mineral status; prevent further problems and deformity.
- Complement any necessary drug therapy with adequate diet. Monitor carefully for side effects.
- Identify and treat underlying congenital problems.
- Promote catch-up growth, since short stature can result if not treated early enough. compensatory catch-up growth may continue into adolescence and adulthood (Carver, 2005).
- Prevent or correct hypoglycemia and other complications.
- Prevent long-term consequences, such as hypertension, insulin resistance and metabolic syndrome, type 2 diabetes mellitus, cardiovascular disease, short stature, and polycystic ovary syndrome (van Weissenbruch et al, 2005; Regev and Reichman, 2004).

INTERVENTION: FOOD AND NUTRITION

- Promote exclusive breastfeeding whenever possible to promote cognitive development. At least 6 months is needed.
- While nutrient-enriched formulas that provide 22 kcal/oz are often prescribed for VLBW preterm infants after hospital discharge, promoting greater rates of catch-up growth and increases in head circumference, studies are not as clear in SGA infants (Carver, 2005).
- Use a balanced diet appropriate for older children. Include reasonable snacks with high-quality nutritional value.
- If diet is inadequate in the specific nutrients, ensure intake of a sufficient level of vitamin D, calcium, and phosphorus for age and sex.

CLINICAL INDICATORS

Clinical/History		Lab Work
Height	Decreased linear growth	Glucose
Weight	I & O	BUN, creatinine
Growth (%)	BP	Serum phosphorus
Diet/intake history	Temperature	Serum Ca++

Common Drugs Used and Potential Side Effects

- Growth hormone (GH) therapy for improving height in these children has been approved by the FDA; it promotes growth acceleration and normalization of height during childhood. High doses can affect carbohydrate metabolism and cause hyperglycemia.

Herbs, Botanicals, and Supplements

- Herbs and botanicals should not be used in children.

INTERVENTION: NUTRITION EDUCATION, COUNSELING, CARE MANAGEMENT

- Help families adjust to special requirements for their child. The child may have diabetes and other chronic consequences from being born SGA. Children born SGA without postnatal catch-up are shorter and have higher weight than children of similar age, height, and sex (Carrascosa et al, 2004).

Patient Education—Food Safety

- Hand washing with soap and hot water is recommended before preparing formula or meals. Use clean utensils and containers for mixing formula.
- Before using tap water for formula preparation or to give as a beverage, let cold tap water run for 2 minutes to remove any lead that may be in the pipes.
- Follow the 2-hour rule: discard any beverage or food that has been left at room temperature for 2 hours or longer.
- Do not use honey in the diets of infants to decrease potential risk of botulism.

SMALL FOR GESTATIONAL AGE—CITED REFERENCES

Bamberg C, Kalache KD. Prenatal diagnosis of fetal growth restriction. *Semin Fetal Neonatal Med.* 9:387, 2004.
Carrascosa A, et al. Fetal growth regulation and intrauterine growth retardation. *J Pediatr Endocrinol Metab.* 17:435S, 2004.
Carver JD. Nutrition for preterm infants after hospital discharge. *Adv Pediatr.* 52:23, 2005.
Dodds L, et al. Outcomes of pregnancies complicated by hyperemesis gravidarum. *Obstet Gynecol.* 107:285, 2006.
Randhawa R, Cohen P. The role of the insulin-like growth factor system in prenatal growth. *Mol Genet Metab.* 86:84, 2005.
Regev RH, Reichman B. Prematurity and intrauterine growth retardation—double jeopardy? *Clin Perinatol.* 31:453, 2004.
van Weissenbruch MM, et al. Fetal nutrition and timing of puberty. *Endocr Dev.* 8:15, 2005.
Zaw W, et al. The risks of adverse neonatal outcome among preterm small for gestational age infants according to neonatal versus fetal growth standards. *Pediatrics* 111:1273, 2003.

SPINA BIFIDA AND NEURAL TUBE DEFECTS

NUTRITIONAL ACUITY RANKING: LEVEL 3

DEFINITIONS AND BACKGROUND

Neural tube defects (NTDs) are serious birth defects of the spine (spina bifida) and brain (anencephaly), affecting approximately 3000 pregnancies each year in the United States; periconceptional consumption of folic acid (400 mg daily) reduces the occurrence of NTDs by 50–70% (Centers for Disease Control, 2004).

Spina bifida includes any congenital defect involving insufficient closure of the spine (usually laminae of the vertebrae). Approximately 2500–3000 children are born each year with either spina bifida or anencephaly. Myelomeningocele may affect as many as one out of every 800 infants (see Myelomeningocele entry). The rest of the cases are most commonly spina bifida occulta (where the bones of the spine do not close, the spinal cord and meninges remain in place, and skin usually covers the defect) and meningoceles (where the meninges protrude through the vertebral defect but the spinal cord remains in place).

Spina bifida occurs in 150 of 100,000 births; the lumbar section generally is affected. Clubfoot, dislocated hip, scoliosis, and other musculoskeletal deformities may also be present. Spina bifida cystica is more severe. Spina bifida occulta is seen in approximately 10% of children and adults; the defect is usually discovered accidentally on x-ray. There are diverse disabilities among adults with spina bifida (McDonnell and McCann, 2000).

A majority of serious birth defects of the spine and brain could be prevented if women consumed adequate daily amounts of folate in their diets, especially in the months preceding pregnancy. Women who plan to become pregnant should be certain that their diets contain sufficient amounts of folate. Clinical trials indicate that periconceptual use of folic acid supplements (400–800 μg/d) can reduce up to 70% of the NTDs (Gross et al, 2001). Use of folic acid supplements and fortified foods are even more effective than eating high-folate foods (Cuskelly et al, 1996).

Women at risk for having a baby with NTDs are of English/Irish ancestry or Hispanic ancestry, are of lower socioeconomic status, have diabetes mellitus, are obese, have poor dietary habits, or take medications that are folate antagonists such as anticonvulsant medications (e.g., phenytoin), metformin, sulfasalazine, triamterene, and methotrexate (http://www.getfolic.com/). It also seems important to take in sufficient amounts of magnesium, niacin, plant proteins, and iron during the periconceptual period (Groenen et al, 2004).

INTERVENTION: OBJECTIVES

- Control side effects (i.e., hydrocephalus and possibly sepsis).
- Increase independence and self-care potentials.
- Improve nutritional status.
- Achieve and maintain ideal body mass index for age. There are decreased energy needs because of short stature and limited mobility. Obesity is common.
- Preserve brain function, as far as possible, with hydrocephalus.
- Initiate treatment or surgical intervention as appropriate.
- Correct constipation, pressure ulcers, swallowing prob-

lems (from Arnold-Chiari malformation of the brain), and other concerns.

INTERVENTION: FOOD AND NUTRITION

- Individualize diet for proper nutrition to achieve a desirable weight and monitor carefully.
- For children under age 8 who are minimally active, use 9–11 kcal/cm or 50% fewer calories than recommended for child of similar age; to promote weight loss, use 7 kcal/cm (Lucas, 2004, p. 41). For older teens or adults, 7 kcal/cm may be needed for weight loss; generally, needs are about 50% of normal.
- Provide adequate protein, B-complex vitamins, zinc, and other nutrients for age. Folic acid has been implicated in etiology.
- Provide adequate nutrients for wound healing if surgery has been performed.

CLINICAL INDICATORS

Clinical/History	Temperature	Alb
Height	I & O	H & H
Weight	Vertebral defect	Serum Fe
Growth percentile	**Lab Work**	Na+, K+
Diet/intake history	Serum folic acid	
	Gluc	

Common Drugs Used and Potential Side Effects

- Antibiotics may be required if the patient develops sepsis. Use of acidophilus and probiotic products may alleviate loss of intestinal bacteria.
- Use of oral contraceptives depletes folic acid; change diet and supplement as needed.
- Sulfonamides may crystallize vitamin C in the bladder; extra vitamin C, protein, iron, and folate may be needed.

Herbs, Botanicals, and Supplements

- Herbs and botanicals should not be used for spina bifida because there are no controlled trials to prove efficacy.

INTERVENTION: NUTRITION EDUCATION, COUNSELING, CARE MANAGEMENT

- Family counseling may be needed in preparation for future pregnancies.
- Referral to a local chapter of the March of Dimes may be beneficial.

Patient Education—Food Safety

- Hand washing with soap and hot water is recommended before preparing formula or meals. Use clean utensils and containers for mixing formula.
- Before using tap water for formula preparation or to give as a beverage, let cold tap water run for 2 minutes to remove any lead that may be in the pipes.
- Follow the 2-hour rule: discard any beverage or food that has been left at room temperature for 2 hours or longer.
- Do not use honey in the diets of infants to decrease potential risk of botulism.

For More Information

- Centers for Disease Control
  Folic Acid National Campaign
  http://www.cdc.gov/ncbddd/Folicacid
- Food and Drug Administration
  "How Folate Can Help Prevent Birth Defects"
  http://www.cfsan.fda.gov/~dms/fdafolic.html
- Spina Bifida Association of America
  http://www.sbaa.org/

SPINA BIFIDA AND NEURAL TUBE DEFECTS—CITED REFERENCES

Centers for Disease Control. Use of vitamins containing folic acid among women of childbearing age–United States, 2004. *MMWR Morb Mortal Wkly Rep.* 53:847, 2004.

Cuskelly G, et al. Effect of increasing dietary folate on red-cell folate: implications for prevention of neural tube defects. *Lancet.* 347:657, 1996.

Groenen PM, et al. Low maternal dietary intakes of iron, magnesium, and niacin are associated with spina bifida in the offspring. *J Nutr.* 134:1516, 2004.

Gross S, et al. Inadequate folic acid intakes are prevalent among young women with neural tube defects. *J Am Diet Assoc.* 101:342, 2001.

Lucas B, ed. *Children with special care needs: nutrition care handbook.* Chicago: The American Dietetic Association, 2004.

McDonnell G, McCann J. Issues of medical management in adults with spina bifida. *Childs Nerv Syst.* 16:222, 2000.

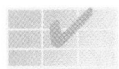

TYROSINEMIA

NUTRITIONAL ACUITY RANKING: LEVEL 4

DEFINITIONS AND BACKGROUND

Hereditary tyrosinemia type I (HTI), a severe disease affecting primarily the liver, is caused by a deficiency of fumarylacetoacetate hydrolase (FAH). Tyrosine, phenylalanine, and methionine build up. The condition is acute, often causing death within the first year of life. Type I needs to be treated with diet for life and is a much more severe disease than other types. This condition results in liver failure or severe nodular cirrhosis with renal tubular involvement. Tyrosine accumulation can be aggravated by vitamin C deficiency, a high-protein diet, or liver immaturity.

In type II, recalcitrant keratitis may be the presenting sign; a tyrosine-restricted and phenylalanine-restricted diet in infancy is most effective in preventing cognitive impairment (McSai et al, 2001).

Prenatal diagnosis is possible and can be performed by measuring succinyl acetone in the amniotic fluid or FAH in amniotic fluid cells, allowing for genetic counseling (Liver Foundation, 2005). Liver transplantation is the best treatment at this time.

INTERVENTION: OBJECTIVES

- Restrict phenylalanine and tyrosine from the diet.
- Promote normal growth and development for age.
- Provide adequate vitamin C for conversion processes.

INTERVENTION: FOOD AND NUTRITION

- Initially, feed a phenylalanine/tyrosine hydrolysate to infants, with small amounts of milk added to provide the minimum requirements of tyrosine and phenylalanine. Mead Johnson product TYROS and 3200-AB; Ross product Maxamaid XPHEN, TYR; or TYROMEX-1 or TYREX from SHS can be used.
- If blood methionine levels are elevated, try PFD1 or PFD2 (Mead Johnson). Use carbohydrate supplements, vitamins, and minerals.
- Supplement with vitamin C appropriate to the patient's age.

CLINICAL INDICATORS

Clinical/History

Birth weight, present weight
Growth (%)
Diet/intake history
Abdominal distention
Hyperpigmentation
Dermatitis
"Cabbage-like" odor
Rancid butter–like odor (type I)
FTT

Lab Work

Phosphate
Gluc (low?)
Alb (often low)
FAH (very low?)
Plasma phenylalanine
Methionine
H & H
Serum Fe
Plasma tyrosine
Liver function tests (elevated)
Bilirubin (elevated)
PT and INR

Common Drugs Used and Potential Side Effects

- Antibiotics may be needed to correct infections. Use of acidophilus and probiotic products may alleviate loss of intestinal bacteria.

Herbs, Botanicals, and Supplements

- Herbs and botanicals should not be used for tyrosinemia because there are no controlled trials to prove efficacy.

INTERVENTION: NUTRITION EDUCATION, COUNSELING, CARE MANAGEMENT

- Provide sources of tyrosine and phenylalanine in the diet determined appropriately for age and body size.
- Adjust intake of energy and nutrients according to the patient's age.
- Discuss desirable intake of protein (avoid excesses) and encourage adequate intake of vitamin C to meet recommended levels.

Patient Education—Food Safety

- Hand washing with soap and hot water is recommended before preparing formula or meals. Use clean utensils and containers for mixing formula.
- Before using tap water for formula preparation or to give as a beverage, let cold tap water run for 2 minutes to remove any lead that may be in the pipes.
- Follow the 2-hour rule: discard any beverage or food that has been left at room temperature for 2 hours or longer.

- Do not use honey in the diets of infants to decrease potential risk of botulism.

For More Information

- American Liver Foundation
  http://www.liverfoundation.org/

TYROSINEMIA—CITED REFERENCES

Liver Foundation. Accessed January 3, 2005 at http://www.liverfoundation.org/

Macsai MS, et al. Tyrosinemia type II: nine cases of ocular signs and symptoms. *Am J Ophthalmol.* 132:522, 2001.

UREA CYCLE DISORDERS

NUTRITIONAL ACUITY RANKING: LEVEL 2–4

DEFINITIONS AND BACKGROUND

As a group, urea cycle disorders occur in one in 25,000 newborns. Statewide newborn screening does not always screen for these conditions. However, screening is important for all newborns, especially if there is a family history of any of these disorders. It is believed that some cases of sudden infant death syndrome may be related to urea cycle disorders.

The urea cycle disorders are manifested most often in the newborn between ages 1 and 5 days, when they are often initially thought to be septic. With later onset, patients have partial enzyme deficiencies and are recognized after a clinical episode months or years later. Ornithine transcarbamylase (OTC) deficiency is the most common disorder. Except for OTC, which is X-linked, all of the other disorders are autosomal recessive. All are genetic diseases associated with lack of a protein or enzyme activity in the urea cycle: Table 3-15 describes the urea cycle disorders.

Hyperammonemia is a deadly neurotoxin. Chronic hyperammonemia also results in increased L-tryptophan metabolites including serotonin. Concentrations of ammonia above 60 μmol/L lead to anorexia, irritability, lethargy, vomiting, somnolence, disorientation, asterixis, cerebral edema, coma, and death (Cohn and Roth, 2004).

When they present in childhood, adolescence, and adulthood, there is often FTT, persistent vomiting, developmental delay, behavioral changes, hyperammonemia, irritability, somnolence, seizures, and coma; if not treated rapidly, they

TABLE 3-15 Urea Cycle Disorders (UCD)

UCD	Enzyme Deficiency	Symptoms/Comments
Type I hyperammonemia	Carbamoylphosphate synthetase I (CPS I)	Within 24–72 hours after birth, infant becomes lethargic, needs stimulation to feed, vomiting, increasing lethargy, hypothermia and hyperventilation; without measurement of serum ammonia levels and appropriate intervention, infant will die; treatment with arginine, which activates N-acetylglutamate synthetase
N-acetylglutamate synthetase deficiency	N-acetylglutamate synthetase (NAGS)	Severe hyperammonemia, mild hyperammonemia associated with deep coma, acidosis, recurrent diarrhea, ataxia, hypoglycemia, hyperornithinemia: treatment includes administration of carbamoyl glutamate to activate CPS I
Type 2 hyperammonemia	Ornithine transcarbamylase (OTC)	Most commonly occurring UCD, only X-linked UCD, ammonia and amino acids elevated in serum, increased serum orotic acid due to mitochondrial carbamoylphosphate entering cytosol and being incorporated into pyrimidine nucleotides, which leads to excess production and consequently excess catabolic products; treat with high-carbohydrate, low-protein diet, ammonia detoxification with sodium phenylacetate or sodium benzoate
Classic citrullinemia	Argininosuccinate synthetase (ASS)	Episodic hyperammonemia, vomiting, lethargy, ataxia, seizures, eventual coma; treat with arginine administration to enhance citrulline excretion, also with sodium benzoate for ammonia detoxification
Argininosuccinic aciduria	Argininosuccinate lyase (argininosuccinase) (ASL)	Episodic symptoms similar to classic citrullinemia, elevated plasma and cerebral spinal fluid argininosuccinate; treat with arginine and sodium benzoate
Hyperargininemia	Arginase	Rare UCD, progressive spastic quadriplegia and mental retardation, ammonia and arginine high in cerebral spinal fluid and serum; arginine, lysine, and ornithine high in urine; treatment includes diet of essential amino acids excluding arginine, low-protein diet

Adapted from: http://web.indstate.edu/thcme/mwking/nitrogen-metabolism.html.

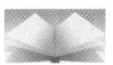

may cause irreversible neuronal damage (Mathias et al, 2001). Diagnosis of urea cycle disorder should be considered in any patient with unexplained neurological and psychiatric disorders with selective anorexia, unexplained coma with cerebral edema, and respiratory alkalosis, even in adulthood (Legras et al, 2002).

Appetite and nutrition problems are common; one concern is the early identification and management of chronic catabolism, which is difficult to treat (Wilcken, 2004). Any patient on a low-protein diet should be monitored clinically, with appropriate laboratory tests and an emergency plan (Leonard, 2001). The outcome of untreated or poorly treated patients with urea cycle disorders is universally bad (Summar, 2001). Hemodialysis may be needed to bring down ammonia levels rapidly (Mathias et al, 2001).

Diet is one of the main treatments of these disorders; protein intake should be adjusted according to the inborn error, severity, patient's age, growth rate, and preferences (Wilcken, 2004). Most patients, except those with arginase deficiency, will need supplements of arginine, but the value of other supplements, including citrate and carnitine, is unclear (Wilcken, 2004).

The prospect of gene therapy "cures" for these diseases, striving for the best possible outcome in the critical newborn period, is a worthy goal (Summar, 2001). Liver transplantation is another treatment that shows promise.

INTERVENTION: OBJECTIVES

- Restrict total protein from the diet to minimize endogenous ammonia production and protein catabolism. Limit one or more essential amino acids while providing adequate energy and nutrients (Trahms, 2004).
- Promote anabolism with normal growth and development for age; use energy from nonprotein sources in amounts to spare protein for other purposes.
- Normalize blood ammonia levels and reduce the effects of hyperammonemia, which may cause neuronal damage. Elevated levels of ammonia can come from muscle breakdown or diet; evaluate to determine which process is the problem.
- Administer desired substrates of the urea cycles. If necessary, support dialysis if blood ammonia levels are 3–4 times above normal.

INTERVENTION: FOOD AND NUTRITION

- Initially, feed a protein-controlled diet (often 1.0–1.5 g/kg daily) with use of special formulas. For example, Cyclinex (Ross Labs) with specific supplements of arginine or PFD1 or PFD2 (Mead Johnson) is used for arginosuccinic aciduria. For OTC deficiency, a low-protein diet is needed, with additives such as Moducal (Mead Johnson) to give extra energy.
- Add extra energy sources if needed to support growth and development. Weight gain is the best measure of success in infants and children.
- If dehydration occurs, intravenous fluids and glucose may be needed.

CLINICAL INDICATORS

Clinical/History		
Birth weight, present weight	Hyperactivity, irritability	Alb
Growth (%)	Seizures or coma	Plasma amino acid levels (specific to disorder)
Diet/intake history	Developmental delay	Plasma ammonia
FTT	**Lab Work**	H & H
Vomiting	Phos	Blood gases
	Gluc	Na+, K+, Cl−
		Ketonuria

Common Drugs Used and Potential Side Effects

- Protein restriction is used in conjunction with medications to remove ammonia from the blood. Medications are given by way of tube feedings, either via gastrostomy tube or NG tube. To provide alternative route for ammonia, what is given depends on where the defect in the urea cycle has occurred. Arginine is often supplemented (400–700 mg/d), except for arginine deficiency (Trahms, 2004). For argininosuccinate synthetase and argininosuccinate lyase deficiencies, 0.4–0.7 g arginine/kg/d is given; 0.17 g/kg/d of citrulline is given for carbamyl phosphate synthetase deficiency.
- Sodium phenylbutyrate may also be used to normalize serum ammonia by diverting nitrogen to alternative paths for excretion (Scaglia et al, 2004).

Herbs, Botanicals, and Supplements

- Herbs and botanicals should not be used for urea cycle disorders because there are no controlled trials to prove efficacy.

INTERVENTION: NUTRITION EDUCATION, COUNSELING, CARE MANAGEMENT

- Provide sources of all essential amino acids in the diet, determined appropriately for age and body size. There are tables available for these purposes (Trahms, 2004).
- Adjust intake of energy and nutrients according to the patient's age.
- Comprehensive newborn screening is recommended for families who have had the birth of one or more children with these disorders.

Patient Education—Food Safety

- Hand washing with soap and hot water is recommended before preparing formula or meals. Use clean utensils and containers for mixing formula.
- Before using tap water for formula preparation or to give as a beverage, let cold tap water run for 2 minutes to remove any lead that may be in the pipes.

- Follow the 2-hour rule: discard any beverage or food that has been left at room temperature for 2 hours or longer.
- Do not use honey in the diets of infants to decrease potential risk of botulism.

For More Information

- My Special Diet
  http://www.myspecialdiet.com/
- National Urea Cycle Disorders Foundation
  http://www.nucdf.org
- Organic Acidemia Association
  http://www.oaanews.org/
- UCD Kids Network
  http://www.geocities.com/ucdkidsnet/index.html

UREA CYCLE DISORDERS—CITED REFERENCES

Cohn RM, Roth KS. Hyperammonemia, bane of the brain. *Clin Pediatr (Phila).* 43:683, 2004.
Legras A, et al. Late diagnosis of ornithine transcarbamylase defect in three related female patients: polymorphic presentations. *Crit Care Med.* 30:241, 2002.
Leonard JV. The nutritional management of urea cycle disorders. *J Pediatr.* 138:S40, 2001.
Mathias R, et al. Hyperammonemia in urea cycle disorders: role of the nephrologist. *Am J Kidney Dis.* 37:1069, 2001.
Scaglia F, et al. Effect of alternative pathway therapy on branched chain amino acid metabolism in urea cycle disorder patients. *Mol Genet Metab.* 81:S79, 2004.
Summar M. Current strategies for the management of neonatal urea cycle disorders. *J Pediatr.* 138:S30, 2001.
Trahms C. Metabolic disorders. In: Mahan K, Escott-Stump S, eds. *Krause's food, nutrition, and diet therapy.* 11th ed. Philadelphia: WB Saunders, 2004.
Wilcken B. Problems in the management of urea cycle disorders. *Mol Genet Metab.* 81:S86, 2004.

WILSON'S DISEASE (HEPATOLENTICULAR DEGENERATION)

NUTRITIONAL ACUITY RANKING: LEVEL 3

DEFINITIONS AND BACKGROUND

An autosomal recessive disorder, Wilson's disease causes abnormal transport and storage of copper, resulting in hepatolenticular degeneration, neurologic damage, and damage to the kidney, brain, and cornea. Onset occurs at birth, but symptoms may appear from 5–40 years old.

The major physiological role of copper is to serve as a cofactor to a number of key metabolic enzymes. Copper is a trace element essential for normal cell homeostasis, promoting iron absorption for hemoglobin synthesis and for formation of bone and myelin sheath. In hepatic tissues, 90% of the copper in the copper-albumin complex is converted to ceruloplasmin. Tissue deposition occurs instead of formation of ceruloplasmin in Wilson's disease.

Wilson's disease may lead to severe pathologies, including neurodegeneration, liver lesions, and behavior abnormalities. Three types of neurological symptoms can occur: dystonic syndrome (dystonic postures and choreoathetosis); ataxic syndrome (postural and intentional tremor and ataxia of the limbs); and parkinsonian syndrome (hypokinesia, rigidity, and resting tremor). Shortened attention span, slurring of speech, and depression may be early symptoms.

A low-copper diet is seldom essential but implemented when other therapies are unsuccessful (e.g., copper-chelating agents). Other dietary treatments under study include the use of increased histidine, specific polyunsaturated fatty acids, low soy, and other plans.

If not diagnosed until onset of fulminant failure, the patient will die. Without treatment, patients may die by age 30. Liver transplantation is the best, most permanent treatment.

INTERVENTION: OBJECTIVES

- Keep optimal balance of copper in patient.
- Decrease serum copper levels, generally with drug chelation. Enhance urinary excretion of excesses.
- Prevent or reverse damage to body tissues and liver.
- Watch caloric intake to prevent obesity.
- Monitor changes in gag reflex or dysphagia.
- Provide sufficient zinc to chelate excess copper under doctor's supervision.
- Prepare for transplantation if necessary.

INTERVENTION: FOOD AND NUTRITION

- A normal diet provides 2–5 mg/d of copper. To lower copper in the diet (to 1–2 mg), use limited amounts of liver, kidney, shellfish, nuts, raisins and other dried fruits, dried legumes, brain, oysters, mushrooms, chocolate, poultry, and whole-grain cereals.
- A lacto-ovo-vegetarian diet may be useful to increase content of fiber and phytates. Copper is less available in vegetarian diets (Brewer et al, 1993).
- Control energy intake, food textures, and other nutrients if necessary.
- Increase fluid intake but avoid alcoholic beverages.
- Increase zinc from meat, poultry, fish, eggs, and milk if deemed appropriate for the patient.

CLINICAL INDICATORS

Clinical/History		
Height Weight BMI Diet/intake history Enlarged liver Swallowing difficulty Drooling? Easy bruising Jaundice? Kayser-Fleischer ring (gold or gray-brown opacity of peripheral cornea) Fixed pseudo-smile Postural tremor of arms Rigidity Abrupt personality change	**Lab Work** Ceruloplasmin (often low) Alb H & H BUN, Creat Serum P PT or INR Serum Cu (abnormal) Liver copper levels Urinary Cu	ALT, AST [low transaminases (100–500 IU/L)] Bilirubin (>300 μmol/L) Alk phos, low (<600 IU/L) Serum zinc

Common Drugs Used and Potential Side Effects

- D-penicillamine (Cuprimine or Depen), a copper-chelating agent, should be taken orally before meals. A vitamin B_6 supplement is needed with this drug; usually a dose of 25 mg.
- Zinc acetate may be used to chelate copper with fewer side effects than D-penicillamine. Doses of 75–150 mg are often prescribed. Oral zinc is a suitable alternative to penicillamine as long-term maintenance therapy.
- Laxatives or stool softeners may be needed. Encourage a diet high in fiber and fluid to wean off medication if possible.
- Tetrathiomolybdate is being evaluated for effectiveness (Murray et al, 2003).
- Corticosteroids and immunosuppressive therapy are used for autoimmune hepatitis. Side effects can be significant, including hyperglycemia, osteopenia, and nutrient depletion.

Herbs, Botanicals, and Supplements

- A neurological disorder has been noted after taking Chinese herbs; it is best to avoid them in Wilson's disease (Wang and Yang, 2003). Herbs and botanicals should not be used because there are no controlled trials to prove efficacy.

INTERVENTION: NUTRITION EDUCATION, COUNSELING, CARE MANAGEMENT

- Teach the patient about the copper and zinc content of foods. Explain that breast milk has higher copper levels than cow's milk to those individuals who need to know.
- Help the patient with feeding at mealtimes, if poor muscular control is demonstrated.
- Discuss effective coping mechanisms, community resources, and genetic counseling.
- Discuss the importance of maintaining prescribed drug therapy, which is essential for life.

Patient Education—Food Safety

- Hand washing with soap and hot water is recommended before preparing formula or meals. Use clean utensils and containers for mixing formula.
- Before using tap water for formula preparation or to give as a beverage, let cold tap water run for 2 minutes to remove any lead that may be in the pipes.
- Follow the 2-hour rule: discard any beverage or food that has been left at room temperature for 2 hours or longer.
- Do not use honey in the diets of infants to decrease potential risk of botulism.

For More Information

- Euro Wilson
  http://www.eurowilson.org/
- National Institute of Neurological Disorders and Stroke
  http://www.ninds.nih.gov/disorders/wilsons/wilsons.htm
- Wilson's Disease Association
  http://www.wilsonsdisease.org/
- Wilson's Disease Center
  http://www.wilsonsdiseasecenter.org/

WILSON'S DISEASE—CITED REFERENCES

Brewer G, et al. Does a vegetarian diet control Wilson's disease? *J Am Col Nutri.* 12:527, 1993.

Murray KF, et al. Current and future therapy in haemochromatosis and Wilson's disease. *Expert Opin Pharmacother.* 4:2239, 2003.

Wang XP, Yang RM. Movement disorders possibly induced by traditional Chinese herbs. *Eur Neurol.* 50:153, 2003.

SECTION 4

Neurological and Mental Conditions

CHIEF ASSESSMENT FACTORS

- Loss of Consciousness, Seizures
- Dizziness, Vertigo, Weakness, Drowsiness
- Headaches, Pain
- Numbness, Paralysis, Sensory Pain
- Bowel or Bladder Dysfunction
- Disturbed Taste, Smell, Changes in Vision
- Dysphagia; Coughing or Choking While Eating/Swallowing
- Status of Food in Oral Cavity
- Easy Aspiration of Food into Lungs
- Hallucinations, Tremors; Tics, Spasms, Ataxia
- Nervousness, Irritability
- Depression, Anxiety
- Stress (may speed up aging process because of protein kinase C)
- Confusion, Memory Loss; Disorientation Regarding Place and Time
- Problems with Abstract Thinking, Personality Changes
- Poor or Weaker Judgment; Difficulty Performing Familiar Tasks
- Mood Swings, Behavioral Changes, Psychotic Delusions
- Extremities: Coldness, Stiffness, Limited Movement, Discoloration, Pain
- Marked Disturbance in Eating Behaviors, Pica
- Impulse Control Disorders
- Blunting of Emotions, Apathy, Egocentricity

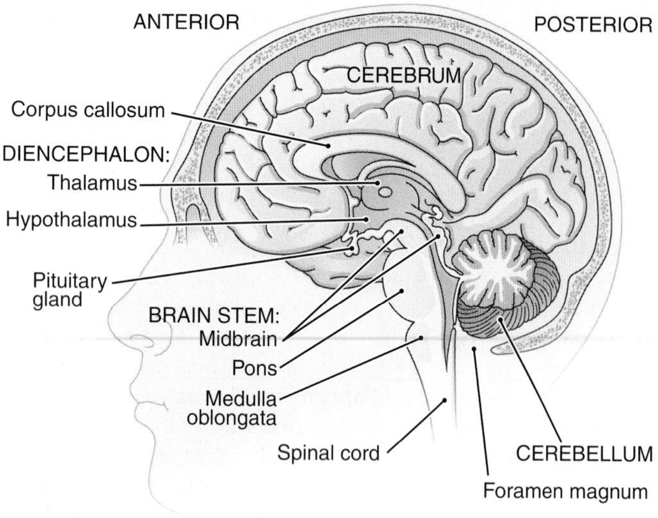

Figure 4-1 Brain. (Reprinted with permission from Cohen BJ. *Memmler's the human body in health and disease*. 10th ed. Baltimore: Lippincott Williams & Wilkins, 2005.)

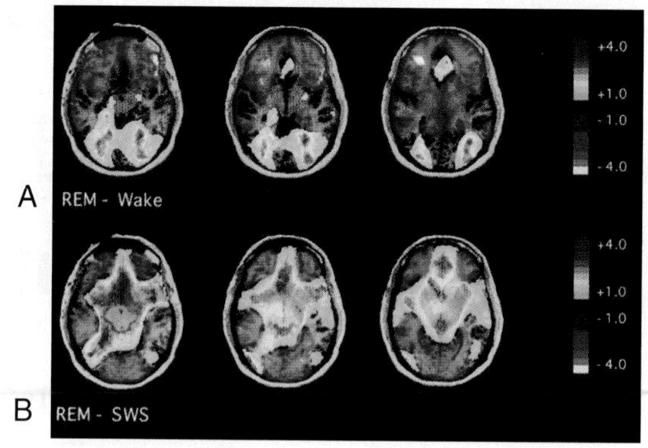

Figure 4-2 PET scan (http://www.mayoclinic.com/health/petscan/CA00052).

OVERVIEW OF NEUROLOGICAL AND MENTAL DISORDERS

The central nervous system (CNS) consists of the brain and the spinal cord. The brain has three main sections: the cerebrum, the cerebellum, and the brainstem. Figure 4-1 shows the brain and its parts. The normal adult brain weighs 3 pounds; it grows steadily until 20 years of age and then loses weight for the rest of life. Grey matter consists of CNS tissue rich in neuronal cell bodies, their dendrites, axons, and glial cells; it includes the cerebral cortex, the central spinal cord, the cerebellar cortex, and the hippocampal cortex. White matter refers to large axon tracts in the brain and spinal cord involved with the cerebral hemispheres, the cerebellum, and the hippocampus. Figure 4-2 shows a positron emission tomography (PET) scan of the brain. Figure 4-3 shows how an electroencephalogram (EEG) is completed.

A steady stream of neurotransmitters is needed for good mental and neurological health. The neurotransmitters serotonin, dopamine, norepinephrine, and acetylcholine are subject to dietary manipulation (Remig, 2004). Increases or decreases in dietary precursors affect nerve functioning. "Brain foods" aim at preventing as well as treating a growing number of stress-related mental disorders since stress increases activity of serotonergic neurons in the brain (Takeda, 2004).

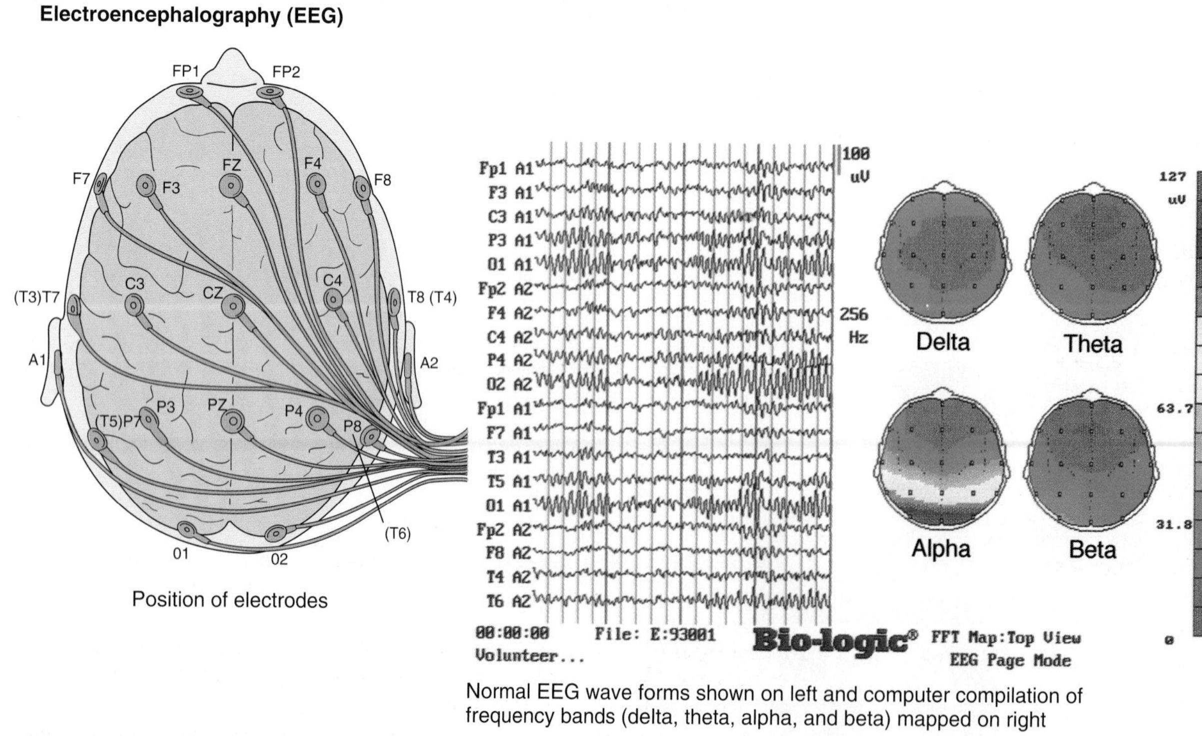

Figure 4-3 Electroencephalogram (EEG). (From Willis MC. *Medical terminology: a programmed learning approach to the language of health care*. Baltimore: Lippincott Williams & Wilkins, 2002.)

Lipids are an essential part of brain and neuron functioning. Lipid peroxidation is a major outcome of free radical–mediated injury to brain, where it directly damages membranes and generates a number of oxidized products; brain lipid peroxidation is a potential therapeutic target early in the course of Alzheimer's disease and Huntington's disease (Montine et al, 2004). In addition, understanding of the molecular mechanisms involved in fatty acid metabolism and COX-2 upregulation will help to clarify age-related changes that lead to various neurological disorders (Wu and Meydani, 2004).

Liu et al (2004) have identified the emerging role for cytochrome P-450 enzymes and their metabolic end products in the pathogenesis and treatment of central nervous system disorders (stroke), chronic neurodegenerative disease (Alzheimer's disease, Parkinson's disease, epilepsy, multiple sclerosis), and psychiatric disorders (anxiety and depression). Brain P-450 enzymes catalyze the formation of neurosteroids and eicosanoids and metabolize substrates such as vitamins A and D, cholesterol, and bile acids (Liu et al, 2004). Clearly, research into the mechanisms and substrates in the brain will continue to be important.

There is an emerging association between psychiatric and metabolic disorders that suggests a fundamental biological link between these two systems (Bazar et al, 2006). Nearly 20% of Americans will experience a mental disorder during their lifetime. Insulin resistance, diabetes, hypertension, metabolic syndrome, obesity, attention-deficit hyperactivity disorder (ADHD), depression, psychosis, sleep apnea, inflammation, autism, and schizophrenia may operate through common pathways, and treatments used exclusively for one of these conditions may prove beneficial for the others (Bazar et al, 2006).

Affective spectrum disorders (ASD) represents a group of psychiatric and medical conditions known to respond to antidepressant medications and hence possibly linked by common heritable abnormalities, including major depressive disorder (MDD), ADHD, bulimia nervosa, dysthymic disorder, fibromyalgia, generalized anxiety disorder, irritable bowel syndrome, migraine, obsessive-compulsive disorder, panic disorder, posttraumatic stress disorder, premenstrual dysphoric disorder, and social phobia (Hudson et al, 2003). With this in mind, dietetic professionals should be prepared to understand the complexities of neuropsychiatric conditions within the context of their scope of practice.

A multidisciplinary approach is most effective. Psychotherapy addresses the will to change, responsibility for self, and search for meaning and identity. Psychiatrists focus on the medical and chemical management of prescribed drugs. Social workers assist with family and relationship issues. Dietitians focus on overall health status, medical issues, prescribed medicines and alternative therapies, and appropriate dietary treatments. Nutritional assessment must include careful review of histories, including medications and treatments, a positive approach, prevention of malnutrition, use of the team concept for treatment, and restoration of feeding abilities and satisfaction.

This chapter provides an overview of neurological and psychiatric disorders that have nutritional implications. A few disorders are found in other relevant sections (e.g., ADHD, mental retardation, and developmental disorders are found in Section 3; cerebrovascular disease [stroke] is found in Section 6; dysphagia is found in Section 7; and effects of anesthesia from surgery are found in Section 14). The primary neurological disorders are separated from those indicated as psychiatric disorders because there is need for referral to a qualified psychologist, psychiatrist, and team for the latter.

Table 4-1 shows the brain and its functions more completely. Table 4-2 lists the cranial nerves and highlights those that affect chewing and swallowing. Table 4-3 lists mental health disorders and their relevance to nutrition. Table 4-4 lists neurotransmitters and their nutritional relevance. Table 4-5 describes nutrients important for brain health.

TABLE 4-1 Brain Parts and Their Functions

Parts	Relevant Nerves	Functions
FOREBRAIN		
Cerebrum–Temporal Lobe	8th cranial nerve	Controls hearing, expressive language, music and rhythm. Contains the hippocampus. Diseases that affect this area include Alzheimer's disease, depression, and mania.
Cerebrum–Frontal Lobe		Controls personality, mood, behavior, reasoning, emotional control, and cognition. Diseases affecting this area include Alzheimer's disease, depression, mania, and Huntington's disease.
Cerebrum–Parietal Lobe		Comprehension of written language and oral speech; sensory stimulation such as pain, touch, smell, hearing, and heat; body position. Alzheimer's disease affects this area; epilepsy and stroke may also impact this area.
Cerebrum–Occipital Lobe	2nd cranial nerve	Vision
Thalamus		Relays sensory information to the cerebral cortex.
Hypothalamus		Lies beneath the thalamus. Secretes corticotropin-releasing hormone, affecting metabolism by its influence on pituitary gland. Secretes vasopressin, which regulates sleep and wake cycles.
Limbic system	System of nerve pathways	**Amygdala** affects depression. **Hippocampus** may affect mania, depression, and Alzheimer's. Located inside the temporal lobe (humans have two hippocampi, one in each side of the brain). Part of the limbic system. Plays a part in memory, learning, and navigation.
MIDBRAIN	3rd cranial nerve	Site between hindbrain and forebrain. Controls oculomotor nerve; eye movement. Affected in Parkinson's disease and some strokes.

(continued)

TABLE 4-1 Brain Parts and Their Functions *(continued)*

Parts	Relevant Nerves	Functions
HINDBRAIN		
Cerebellum	3rd–5th cranial nerves	Found at bottom rear of the head. Posture and balance; voluntary movements such as sitting, standing, and walking. Directing attention and measuring time; other motor and cognitive functions. Stroke often affects this area.
Pons	4th–7th cranial nerves	Connects brainstem with cerebellum. Receives information from visual areas to control eye and body movements. Controlling patterns of sleep and arousal; coordination of muscular movements; helps maintain equilibrium. Affects sleep disorders.
Medulla Oblongata	8th–12th cranial nerves	Hearing, balance, some taste, some swallowing. Movement of the tongue. Involuntary functions such as heartbeat, circulation, muscle tone, and breathing. Stroke often affects this area.
SPINAL CORD		Sends and receives messages to and from brain and body parts.

Developed from Brainexplorer: http://www.brainexplorer.org; accessed January 26, 2005.

TABLE 4-2 Cranial Nerves and Those Specifically Affecting Mastication and Swallowing

	Nerve	Function	Affected Part of Body
I	Olfactory	Smell	Olfactory bulbs
II	Optic	Vision	Retina
III	Oculomotor	Eyeball movement	4 eyeball muscles and 1 eyelid muscle
		Lens accommodation	
	Oculomotor	Pupil constriction	
IV	Trochlear	Eyeball movement	Superior oblique muscles
V	Trigeminal[a]	Sensations	Face, scalp, teeth, lips, eyeballs, nose and throat lining
		General sensory from tongue	Anterior two thirds of tongue
		Proprioception	Jaw muscles for mastication
	Trigeminal	Chewing	Muscles of mastication
VI	Abducens	Eyeball movement	Lateral rectus muscle
VII	Facial[a]	Taste	Anterior two thirds of tongue
		Proprioception	Face and scalp
	Facial	Facial expressions	Muscles of the face
	Facial	Salivation and lacrimation	Salivary and lacrimal glands via submandibular and pterygopalatine ganglia
VIII	Vestibulocochlear	Balance	Vestibular apparatus of internal ear
		Hearing	Cochlear of internal ear
IX	Glossopharyngeal[a]	Taste	Posterior two thirds of tongue
		Proprioception for swallowing	Throat muscles
		Blood pressure receptors	Carotid sinuses
	Glossopharyngeal	Swallowing and gag reflex	Throat muscles
		Tear production	Lacrimal glands
	Glossopharyngeal	Saliva production	Parotid glands
X	Vagus	Chemoreceptors	Blood oxygen concentration, aortic bodies
		Pain receptors	Respiratory and digestive tracts
		Sensations	External ear, larynx, and pharynx
		Taste	Tongue

(continued)

TABLE 4-2 Cranial Nerves and Those Specifically Affecting Mastication and Swallowing *(continued)*

	Nerve	Function	Affected Part of Body
	Vagus	Heart rate and stroke volume	Pacemaker and ventricular muscles
		Peristalsis	Smooth muscles of digestive tract
		Air flow	Smooth muscles in bronchial tubes
		Speech and swallowing	Muscles of larynx and pharynx
XI	Spinal Accessory	Head rotation	Trapezius and sternocleidomastoid muscles
XII	Hypoglossal[a]	Speech and swallowing	Tongue and throat muscles

Adapted from http://www.teaching-biomed.man.ac.uk/resources/wwwcal/cranial_nerves/page2.asp; accessed January 16, 2005.
[a] Cranial nerves affecting chewing and swallowing.

TABLE 4-3 Disorders of Mental Health (DSM-IV)

Mental Health Disorders	Explanation or Relevance to Nutrition
Acute stress disorder	Development of anxiety and dissociative and other symptoms within 1 month following exposure to an extremely traumatic event; other symptoms include reexperiencing the event and avoidance of trauma-related stimuli.
Adjustment disorder	Maladaptive reaction to identifiable stressful life events.
Amnestic disorder	Mental disorder characterized by acquired impairment in the ability to learn and recall new information, sometimes accompanied by inability to recall previously learned information, and not coupled to dementia or delirium.
Anxiety disorders	A group of mental disorders in which anxiety and avoidance behavior predominate, including panic disorders, agoraphobia, specific phobia, social phobia, obsessive-compulsive disorder, posttraumatic stress disorder, acute stress disorder, generalized anxiety disorder, and substance abuse anxiety disorder.
Attention-deficit disorder	Mental disorder characterized by inattention (such as distractibility, forgetfulness, not finishing tasks, and not appearing to listen), by hyperactivity and impulsivity (such as fidgeting and squirming, difficulty in remaining seated, excessive running or climbing, feelings of restlessness, difficulty awaiting one's turn, interrupting others, and excessive talking), or by both types of behavior. See Section 3 for details.
Autistic disorder	Severe pervasive developmental disorder with onset usually before 3 years of age and a biological basis related to neurological or neurophysiological factors. Characterized by qualitative impairment in reciprocal social interaction (e.g., lack of awareness of the existence of feelings of others, failure to seek comfort at times of distress, lack of imitation), in verbal and nonverbal communication, and in capacity for symbolic play and by restricted and unusual repertoire of activities and interests.
Binge eating disorder	An eating disorder characterized by repeated episodes of binge eating, as in bulimia nervosa, but not followed by inappropriate compensatory behavior such as purging, fasting, or excessive exercise.
Bipolar disorders	Mood disorders characterized by a history of manic, mixed, or hypomanic episodes, usually with concurrent or previous history of one or more major depressive episodes.
Body dysmorphic disorder	A mental disorder in which a normal-appearing person is either preoccupied with some imagined defect in appearance or is overly concerned about some very slight physical anomaly.
Catatonic disorder	Catatonia due to the physiological effects of a general medical condition and neither better accounted for by another mental disorder nor occurring exclusively during delirium.
Childhood disintegrative disorder	Pervasive developmental disorder characterized by marked regression in a variety of skills, including language skills, social skills or adaptive behavior, play, bowel or bladder control, and motor skills, after at least 2, but less than 10, years of apparently normal development.
Circadian rhythm sleep disorder	A sleep disorder consisting of a lack of synchrony between the schedule of sleeping and waking required by the external environment and that of a person's own circadian rhythm.
Conduct disorder	A type of disruptive behavior disorder of childhood and adolescence characterized by a persistent pattern of conduct in which rights of others or age-appropriate societal norms or rules are violated, with misconduct including aggression to people or animals, destruction of property, deceitfulness or theft, and serious violations of rules.
Conversion disorder	Mental disorder characterized by conversion symptoms (loss or alteration of voluntary motor or sensory functioning suggesting physical illness, such as seizures, paralysis, dyskinesia, anesthesia, blindness, or aphonia) having no demonstrable physiological basis.

(continued)

TABLE 4-3 Disorders of Mental Health (DSM-IV) *(continued)*

Mental Health Disorders	Explanation or Relevance to Nutrition
Delusional disorder	Mental disorder marked by well-organized, logically consistent delusions but lacking other psychotic symptoms. Most functioning is not markedly impaired, the criteria for schizophrenia have never been satisfied, and symptoms of a major mood disorder have been present only briefly if at all.
Depersonalization disorder	Dissociative disorder characterized by one or more severe episodes of depersonalization (feelings of unreality and strangeness in one's perception of the self or one's body image) not due to another mental disorder, such as schizophrenia. The perception of reality remains intact; patients are aware of their incapacitation. Episodes are usually accompanied by dizziness, anxiety, fears of going insane, and derealization.
Depressive disorders	Mood disorders in which depression is unaccompanied by manic or hypomanic episodes.
Disruptive behavior disorders	Group of mental disorders of children and adolescents consisting of behavior that violates social norms, is disruptive, and may be illegal, often distressing others more than it does the person with the disorder.
Dissociative disorders	Mental disorders characterized by sudden, temporary alterations in identity, memory, or consciousness, segregating normally integrated memories or parts of the personality from the dominant identity of the individual.
Dissociative identity disorder	A dissociative disorder characterized by the existence in an individual of two or more distinct personalities, each having unique memories, characteristic behavior, and social relationships. Multiple personality disorder.
Dysthymic disorder	Mood disorder characterized by depressed feeling (sad, blue, low), by loss of interest or pleasure in one's usual activities, and by at least some of the following: altered appetite, disturbed sleep patterns, lack of energy, low self-esteem, poor concentration or decision-making skills, and feelings of hopelessness. Symptoms have persisted for more than 2 years but are not severe enough to meet the criteria for major depressive disorder.
Eating disorder	Any of several disorders in which abnormal feeding habits are associated with psychological factors; in DSM-IV, these include anorexia nervosa, bulimia nervosa, pica, and rumination disorder.
Factitious disorder	Mental disorder characterized by repeated, intentional simulation of physical or psychological signs and symptoms of illness for no apparent purpose other than obtaining treatment.
Generalized anxiety disorder	Anxiety disorder characterized by the presence of excessive, uncontrollable anxiety and worry about two or more life circumstances, for 6 months or longer, accompanied by some combination of restlessness, fatigue, muscle tension, irritability, disturbed concentration or sleep, and somatic symptoms.
Impulse control disorders	Group of mental disorders characterized by repeated failure to resist an impulse to perform some act harmful to oneself or to others.
Learning disorders	Group of disorders characterized by academic functioning that is substantially below the level expected on the basis of the patient's age, intelligence, and education, interfering with academic achievement or other functioning. Included are reading disorder, mathematics disorder, and disorder of written expression.
Mental disorder	Any clinically significant behavioral or psychological syndrome characterized by the presence of distressing symptoms, impairment of functioning, or significantly increased risk of suffering death, pain, disability, or loss of freedom. Mental disorders are assumed to be the manifestation of a behavioral, psychological, or biological dysfunction in the individual.
Motor skills disorder	Any disorder characterized by inadequate development of motor coordination severe enough to limit locomotion or restrict the ability to perform tasks, schoolwork, or other activities.
Obsessive-compulsive disorder	Anxiety disorder characterized by recurrent obsessions or compulsions, which are severe enough to interfere significantly with personal or social functioning. Performing compulsive rituals may release tension temporarily, and resisting them causes increased tension.
Oppositional defiant disorder	A type of disruptive behavior disorder characterized by a recurrent pattern of defiant, hostile, disobedient, and negativistic behavior directed toward those in authority, including such actions as defying the requests or rules of adults, deliberately annoying others, arguing, spitefulness, and vindictiveness that occur much more frequently than would be expected on the basis of age and developmental stage.
Pain disorder	A somatoform disorder characterized by a chief complaint of severe chronic pain that causes substantial distress or impairment in functioning; the pain is neither feigned nor intentionally produced, and psychological factors appear to play a major role in its onset, severity, exacerbation, and maintenance.
Panic disorder	Anxiety disorder characterized by recurrent panic (anxiety) attacks, episodes of intense apprehension, fear, or terror associated with somatic symptoms such as dyspnea, palpitations, dizziness, vertigo, faintness, or shakiness and with psychological symptoms such as feelings of unreality (depersonalization or derealization) or fears of dying, going crazy, or losing control; there is usually chronic nervousness and tension between attacks. It is almost always associated with agoraphobia.
Personality disorders	Mental disorders characterized by enduring, inflexible, and maladaptive personality traits that deviate markedly from cultural expectations, are self-perpetuating, pervade a broad range of situations, and either generate subjective distress or result in significant impairments in social, occupational, or other functioning. Onset is by adolescence or early adulthood.
Pervasive developmental disorders	Group of disorders characterized by impairment of development in multiple areas, including the acquisition of reciprocal social interaction, verbal and nonverbal communication skills, and imaginative activity and by stereotyped interests and behaviors; included are autism, Rett's syndrome, childhood disintegrative disorder, and Asperger's syndrome.
Premenstrual dysphoric disorder	Premenstrual syndrome viewed as a psychiatric disorder.

(continued)

TABLE 4-3 Disorders of Mental Health (DSM-IV) *(continued)*

Mental Health Disorders	Explanation or Relevance to Nutrition
Reading disorder	Learning disorder in which the skill affected is reading ability, including accuracy, speed, and comprehension.
Rumination disorder	Eating disorder seen in infants under 1 year of age; after a period of normal eating habits, the child begins excessive regurgitation and rechewing of food, which is then ejected from the mouth or reswallowed; if untreated, death from malnutrition may occur.
Schizoaffective disorder	A mental disorder in which a major depressive episode, manic episode, or mixed episode occurs along with prominent psychotic symptoms characteristic of schizophrenia, the symptoms of the mood disorder being present for a substantial portion of the illness, but not for its entirety, and the disturbance not being due to the effects of a psychoactive substance.
Seasonal affective disorder	A cyclically recurring mood disorder characterized by depression, extreme lethargy, increased need for sleep, hyperphagia, and carbohydrate craving; it intensifies in one or more specific seasons, most commonly the winter months, and is hypothesized to be related to melatonin levels. In DSM-IV terminology, it is called "mood disorder with seasonal pattern."
Separation anxiety disorder	Excessive, prolonged, developmentally inappropriate anxiety and apprehension in a child concerning removal from parents, home, or familiar surroundings.
Shared psychotic disorder	A delusional system that develops in one or more persons as a result of a close relationship with someone who already has a psychotic disorder with prominent delusions.
Sleep disorders	Chronic disorders involving sleep. Primary sleep disorders comprise dyssomnias and parasomnias; causes of secondary sleep disorders may include a general medical condition, mental disorder, or psychoactive substance.
Speech disorder	Defective ability to speak; it may be either psychogenic or neurogenic.
Substance-related disorders	A variety of behavioral or psychological anomalies resulting from ingestion of or exposure to a drug of abuse, medication, or toxin.

Adapted from Merck Manual; http://www.mercksource.com/pp/us/cns/cns_home.jsp; accessed February 17, 2005.

TABLE 4-4 Neurotransmitters and Nutritional Relevance

Type	Neurotransmitter	Postsynaptic Effect	Functions and Nutritional Relevance
Biogenic amine	Acetylcholine	Excitatory	Affected by choline from the diet (eggs, soybeans), especially related to cognitive function. Main neurotransmitter in the parasympathetic nervous system that controls heart rate, digestion, secretion of saliva, and bladder function. Drugs that affect cholinergic activity produce changes in these body functions. Some antidepressants act by blocking cholinergic receptors; this anticholinergic activity is an important cause of dry mouth. Alzheimer's disease seems to be related to a malfunction in this neurotransmitter. Botulism suppresses release of acetylcholine, and nicotine increases receptors for acetylcholine.
Amino acids	Gamma aminobutyric acid (GABA)	Inhibitory	Glutamate is a precursor. Pyridoxal phosphate is a cofactor for both synthesis and break-down.
	Glycine	Inhibitory	Glycine has the ability to inhibit neurotransmitter signals in the CNS. Very available from proteins in the diet, but most contain only small amounts (exception is collagen). May have a unique role as a type of antioxidant.
	Glutamate	Excitatory	No specific dietary precursors. Primarily synthesized in the brain from alpha-keto glutarate and glucose. Glutamate is generally considered to be the most important neurotransmitter for normal brain function; it is estimated that over half of the neurons in the brain release glutamate. Glutamate is also important in the brain because it can be used to synthesize glutamine (by taking up ammonia), which readily diffuses into the blood thus reducing excessive ammonia levels in the brain, which can alter amino acid metabolism in the brain. Glutamate is a precursor of gamma-aminobutyric acid in the brain. The process of ammonia removal via glutamine is important in diseases such as hepatic encephalopathy, which elevates blood ammonia levels. The sodium salt of glutamic acid, monosodium glutamate (MSG), is responsible for one of the five basic tastes of the human sense of taste, umami, and MSG is extensively used as a food additive.
	Aspartate	Excitatory	No specific dietary precursors. Synthesized primarily from glutamate. Acidic analog of asparagine.

(continued)

TABLE 4-4 Neurotransmitters and Nutritional Relevance *(continued)*

Type	Neurotransmitter	Postsynaptic Effect	Functions and Nutritional Relevance
Biogenic amines (monoamines)	Dopamine	Excitatory	Synthesized from phenylalanine and tyrosine. Dopamine is a monoamine neurotransmitter, concentrated in the basal ganglia. It is widely distributed throughout the brain in the nigrostriatal, the mesocorticolimbic, and the tuberohypophyseal pathways. A decreased brain dopamine concentration is a contributing factor in Parkinson's disease, while an increase in dopamine concentration has a role in the development of schizophrenia.
Epinephrine	Excitatory		Secreted by the adrenal medulla. Affects fight or flight reactions; secreted in greater quantity during anger and fear, with resulting increase in heart rate and hydrolysis of glycogen to glucose. Used as a stimulant in cardiac arrest, as a vasoconstrictor in shock, as a bronchodilator in asthma, and to lower intraocular pressure in glaucoma.
	Noradrenaline	Excitatory	Synthesized from phenylalanine and tyrosine. A monoamine neurotransmitter that affects "fight or flight," attention and arousal, and blood pressure.
	Serotonin	Excitatory	Synthesized from tryptophan in the diet. Affects mood control, regulation of sleep, pain perception, body temperature, blood pressure, and hormonal activity. Also affects gastrointestinal and cardiovascular systems.
	Histamine	Excitatory	A potent agent believed to be involved in sleep–wake cycles.

Developed from the following websites: http://www.brainexplorer.org/neurological_control/Neurological_index.shtml and http://en.wikipedia.org/wiki/Neurotransmitter.

TABLE 4-5 Nutrients for Brain Health

Nutrient	Role in the Brain	Comments
Aromatic amino acids (tryptophan, tyrosine, and phenylalanine)	Precursors of serotonin, dopamine, and norepinephrine	Increase in brain tryptophan from eating a carbohydrate-rich/protein-poor meal causes parallel increases in the amounts of serotonin released into synapses. Tryptophan can induce sleep from high-carbohydrate (CHO) meals, whereas high-protein meals tend to increase alertness.
Corticotropin-releasing hormone	Disturbances occur in periods of stress in the hypothalamic pituitary-adrenal axis	Eating is often suppressed during stress due to anorectic effects of corticotropin-releasing hormone and increased during recovery from stress due to appetite-stimulating effects of residual cortisol. Night eating syndrome is related to cortisol levels.
Cytokines	Influence sleep and eating behaviors; involved in a number of infectious, inflammatory, neoplastic, metabolic, and degenerative illnesses (Malek-Ahmadi, 2004)	Implicated in depressive and anxiety disorders; schizophrenic disorders (chronic and acute); autistic disorder; eating disorders; and obsessive-compulsive disorder.
Dietary antioxidants	Improve cognitive functioning	Fruits, vegetables, coffee, and tea. Strong inverse relationship between coffee intake and risk of suicide (Takeda et al, 2004). Quercetin (in red apples with skins, onions, blueberries, cranberries, strawberries) seems to protect against brain-cell damage (Silva et al, 2004).
Endocannabinoids	Endocannabinoids are a class of lipids including amides, esters, and ethers of long-chain polyunsaturated fatty acids (Battista et al, 2004). The presence and function of CB2 central nervous system neurons receptors in are ontroversial; they are activated by a CB2 receptor agonist, arachidonoylglycerol, and by elevated endogenous levels of endocannabinoids (Van Sickle et al, 2005).	Anandamide (N-arachidonoylethanolamine; AEA) and 2-arachidonoylglycerol are the main endogenous agonists of cannabinoid receptors, able to mimic several pharmacological effects of delta(9)-tetrahydrocannabinol, the active principal component of *Cannabis sativa* preparations like hashish and marijuana (Battista et al, 2004). There is a possibility of nonpsychotropic therapeutic interventions using enhanced endocannabinoid levels in localized brain areas (Van Sickle et al, 2005).
Essential fatty acids (EFA)	Fluidity of neuronal membrane, synthesis and functions of brain neurotransmitters, immune system integrity (Yehuda et al, 2005)	The blood–brain barrier determines the bioavailability, and the myelination process determines the efficiency of brain and retinal functions of EFA. Since they must be supplied from the diet, a decreased bioavailability is bound to induce major disturbances (Yehuda et al, 2005).

(continued)

TABLE 4-5 Nutrients for Brain Health *(continued)*

Nutrient	Role in the Brain	Comments
Omega-3 fatty acids (DHA, EPA)	Control inflammatory and autoimmune processes; part of the brain lipid membranes. DHA depletion leads to losses in neuronal function (Lim et al, 2005).	Helpful in depression, bipolar disorder, multiple sclerosis, and other neurological conditions. DHA and arachidonic acid (AA) may not distribute evenly in the brain. There are age-induced regional changes in fatty acid composition of brain phospholipids; alpha linolenic acid deficiency induces regional depletion and recovery of DHA in the brain. Many studies are ongoing.
Omega-6 polyunsaturated fatty acids (ALA, GLA)	Part of the brain lipid membranes	Useful in anorexia nervosa and several neurological conditions. May reduce risk for Parkinson's disease (de Lau et al, 2005).
Uridine	A pyrimidine nucleoside that is formed when uracil is attached to a ribose ring	Component of RNA. Its nucleotides participate in the biosynthesis of polysaccharides and some polysaccharide-containing compounds. Foods containing uridine are thought to play a role in alleviating depression (Carlezon et al, 2005).
Vitamins and minerals	Vitamins B_6, B_{12}, and folic acid lower elevated amounts of homocysteine. Vitamin D has nuclear hormone receptors that regulate gene expression and nervous system development (MacKay-Sim et al, 2004). Vitamin D has been found to delay onset of multiple sclerosis and effects of depression (especially seasonal affective disorder). It is being studied in schizophrenia. Vitamins C and E function as antioxidants. Iron and zinc are important for the brain as well.	These play a role in many neurological conditions.

A balanced mood can be protected by ensuring that diets provide adequate amounts of complex carbohydrates, essential fats, amino acids, vitamins and minerals, and water; many anecdotal, clinical, and controlled studies point to the importance of diet as one part of the jigsaw in the prevention of poor mental health and the promotion of good mental health (Mental Health Foundation, 2006).

CITED REFERENCES

Bazar KA, et al. Obesity and ADHD may represent different manifestations of a common environmental oversampling syndrome: a model for revealing mechanistic overlap among cognitive, metabolic, and inflammatory disorders. *Med Hypotheses.* 66:263, 2006.

Battista N, et al. Endocannabinoids and their involvement in the neurovascular system. *Curr Neurovasc Res.* 1:129, 2004.

Carlezon WA Jr, et al. Antidepressant-like effects of uridine and omega-3 fatty acids are potentiated by combined treatment in rats. *Biol Psychiatry.* 57:343, 2005.

de Lau LM, et al. Dietary fatty acids and the risk of Parkinson disease: the Rotterdam study. *Neurology* 64:2040, 2005.

Hudson JI, et al. Family study of affective spectrum disorder. *Arch Gen Psychiatry.* 60:170, 2003.

Lim SY, et al. N-3 fatty acid deficiency induced by a modified artificial rearing method leads to poorer performance in spatial learning tasks. *Pediatr Res.* 58:741, 2005.

Liu M, et al. Cytochrome P450 in neurological disease. *Curr Drug Metab.* 5:225, 2004.

MacKay-Sim A, et al. Schizophrenia, vitamin D, and brain development. *Int Rev Neurobiol.* 59:351, 2004.

Malek-Ahmadi P. Role of cytokines in psychopathology: therapeutic implications. *Drug News Perspect.* 11:271, 1998.

Mental Health Foundation. Accessed February 7, 2006 at http://www.mentalhealth.org.uk/html/content/feedingminds_exec_summary.pdf.

Montine KS, et al. Isoprostanes and related products of lipid peroxidation in neurodegenerative diseases. *Chem Phys Lipids.* 128:117, 2004.

Remig T. Nutrition in neurologic disease. In: Mahan K, Escott-Stump S, eds. *Krause's food, nutrition, and diet therapy.* 11th ed. Philadelphia: WB Saunders, 2004.

Silva BA, et al. Neuroprotective effect of *H. perforatum* extracts on beta-amyloid-induced neurotoxicity. *Neurotox Res.* 6:119, 2004.

Takeda E. Stress control and human nutrition. *J Med Invest.* 51:139, 2004.

Van Sickle MD, et al. Identification and functional characterization of brainstem cannabinoid CB2 receptors. *Science* 310:329, 2005.

Wu D, Meydani SN. Mechanism of age-associated up-regulation in macrophage PGE2 synthesis. *Brain Behav Immun.* 18:487, 2004.

Yehuda S, et al. Essential fatty acids and the brain: from infancy to aging. *Neurobiol Aging.* 26:98S, 2005.

For More General Information

- American Academy of Neurology
  http://www.aan.com
- American Association of Neuroscience Nurses
  http://www.aann.org
- American Neurological Association
  http://www.aneuroa.org
- American Society of Neurorehabilitation
  http://www.asnr.com
- Brain Research Foundation
  http://brainresearchfdn.org/
- Mental Health Foundation–United Kingdom
  http://www.mentalhealth.org.uk/
- Recipes for Good Mental Health
  http://www.mentalhealth.org.uk/page.cfm?pagecode=PRFMRE
- Society for Neuroscience
  http://www.sfn.org
- The Brain Matters
  http://www.thebrainmatters.org/index.cfm?key=1.1.1

NEUROLOGICAL DISORDERS

ALZHEIMER'S DISEASE AND DEMENTIAS

NUTRITIONAL ACUITY RANKING: LEVEL 3

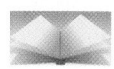

DEFINITIONS AND BACKGROUND

Dementias include multiple cognitive defects with memory loss; they often involve aphasia, apraxia, agnosia, and disturbed daily functioning. Risk factors for dementia include diabetes, cardiovascular diseases such as stroke and hypertension, head injury, aging, depression, and family history. Of over 50 common dementias, **Alzheimer's disease (AD)** is the most common neurodegenerative dementia (Schliebs, 2005). AD involves a progressive deterioration of intellect, memory, personality, and self-care, leading to severe degeneration of nerve cells. Other conditions should be ruled out before choosing AD as a diagnosis; medical evaluation is important. Early stages of AD manifest with short-term memory loss; problems finding the appropriate word; asking the same questions over and over; difficulty making decisions and planning ahead; suspiciousness; changes in senses of smell and taste; denial; depression; loss of initiative; personality changes; and problems with abstract thinking.

The hallmark pathological changes in AD are abundant plaque and tangle formation, especially in the temporal lobes and hippocampus; a lifetime history of major depression may precede the neuropathological changes in AD (Rapp et al, 2006). AD is characterized by deposition of extracellular neuritic, beta-amyloid peptide-containing plaques (senile plaques) in cerebral cortical regions and presence of intracellular neurofibrillary tangles in cerebral pyramidal neurons (Schliebs, 2005). Acetylcholine-containing neurons are especially affected by AD. Acetylcholine normally triggers breakdown of a beta-amyloid precursor protein (APP) in brain cells; this factor is missing in AD. Basal forebrain cholinergic dysfunction may cause the cognitive deficits seen with this dementia (Schliebs, 2005).

Impaired cerebral energy metabolism and pyruvate dehydrogenase activity are associated with neurodegenerative disorders including AD, suggesting that this enzyme is an important link in the pathophysiology of chronic neurodegeneration (Martin et al, 2005). Insulin and associated signaling molecules begin to disappear from the brain during early AD, suggesting the possibility of a form of "type 3 diabetes." The suspicion that AD is a neuroendocrine disease continues to be studied (Lester-Coll et al, 2006).

A lifetime of depression may contribute to AD (Ownby et al, 2006). Depression should be considered a risk factor for the disease. Alzheimer's disease is similar to mood disorders, with onset from the sixth to seventh decades. Mood instability and increased distractibility, irritability, agitation, and irregular sleep can be present. Behavioral changes, such as aggressive behavior, psychosis, and overactivity, occur frequently and often determine the need for institutionalization. Mood stabilizers may be indicated when behavior is hard to manage.

Severe depression can be treated with medication, and electroconvulsive therapy (ECT) is also used when patients are refractory to medications. When depression is adequately treated either with medications or ECT, appetite frequently improves. In addition, fear and paranoia can exist and be quite emotionally painful. Paranoia can include fear that food is being poisoned, and until treatment becomes effective, receiving food in closed containers (such as individual yogurt containers) can be helpful.

Patients with AD may have dysfunctional mechanisms of body weight regulation or changes in their brain that lead to weight loss. Declining body mass over time is strongly linked to the risk of developing AD with aging, and greater losses of weight have the strongest correlation (Buchman et al, 2005). People losing approximately one unit of BMI per year may have a 35% greater risk of developing AD than people with no change in BMI over time (Buchman et al, 2005). Weight loss tends to increase with severity and progression of AD and is a predictor of mortality among AD patients (Power et al, 2001).

Circadian patterns of food intake are associated with measures of functional and cognitive deterioration in seniors with AD; disturbed eating patterns may occur, with altered macronutrient selection (Greenwood et al, 2005). Psychomotor disturbances (including irritability, agitation, and disinhibition) are strongly associated with shifts in eating patterns toward carbohydrate and away from protein, placing individuals with these conditions at risk for protein deficiency (Greenwood et al, 2005). Since amino acids are the building blocks of all brain neurotransmitters, enhancing protein intake is important in this population.

Studies of the nutrients and antioxidants suggest that free radical–induced oxidative stress occurs in AD; zinc and iron may play a role. In addition, changes in the distribution of the serum copper components seem to be characteristic of AD (Squitti et al, 2005). Glycogen synthase kinase-3 (GSK-3) is an enzyme in various cellular pathways for proteins; it has been implicated in the pathophysiology and treatment of AD, diabetes, and bipolar disorder (Gould et al, 2003).

Nutrients that increase the levels of brain catecholamines and protect against oxidative damage are important. Moderately high dietary intake of vitamins C and E and selenium is helpful (Engelhart et al, 2002; Reichman, 2000). Antioxidants in foods such as blueberries, cranberries, strawberries, kale, and spinach may improve cognitive function. In addition, vitamins B_6 and B_{12} and folate lower elevated levels of homocysteine, which affects circulation in the brain. Folic acid in doses of 800 μg daily seems to help older adults maintain cognitive functioning. Curry, cumin, and turmeric may block beta-amyloid plaque formation in the brain; studies are under way.

The way the brain uses energy is an area of additional research. The disease affects primarily the frontal lobe of the cerebral cortex, the temporal lobe, and the parietal lobe. Dietary interventions to maintain adequate energy intake, restore energy balance, and maintain skeletal muscle mass are important because these patients have high daily energy expenditures and low energy intakes (Poehlman & Dvorak, 2000).

Apolipoprotein E (apoE) is an important determinant of plasma lipoprotein metabolism and the risk of diseases characterized by oxidative damage, such as coronary heart disease and AD (Dietrich et al, 2005). ApoE genotypes also influence cognitive function and decline. Prevention of cardiovascular disease may limit the onset of AD (Kang et al, 2005). In addition, decreased serum insulin-like growth factor I (IGF-I) levels and the progression of carotid atherosclerosis could also play a role as independent risk factors for dementia (Wantanabe et al, 2005).

Comprehensive treatment of AD requires thorough caregiver support and thoughtful and informed use of medications for cognition enhancement, neuroprotection, and the treatment of disturbed behavior (Reichman, 2000). The current prognosis for AD is improving, but death most often occurs from renal, pulmonary, or cardiac complications between 2 and 20 years after onset of symptoms. Pneumonia is a common cause of morbidity and death in patients with AD; risk for pneumonia is related to dysphagia, aspiration, altered mobility, decreased nutritional status, and lowered host immune response (Chouinard, 2000).

INTERVENTION: OBJECTIVES

- To effectively enhance intake, interventions must work with individuals' changing needs and intake patterns (Young et al, 2005). Prevent weight loss from altered activity levels, poor eating habits, depression, impaired memory, and insufficient self-feeding ability.
- Walking 90 minutes per week helps to maintain lean body mass and can possibly help with appetite problems.
- Avoid constipation or impaction; support continence through proper schedules.
- Encourage self-feeding at mealtimes as long as possible.
- Prevent or correct dehydration.
- Monitor dysphagia and aspiration. Nourish by appropriate methods such as tube feeding, especially in early stages. While the terminal stage of AD is generally indicated by the inability to swallow, the potential role of enteral feeding in patients with advanced AD is limited (Chouinard, 2000).
- Protect patient from injuries; provide emotional support.
- Use creative feeding strategies. Offer frequent snacks, even at night if desired.
- Prevent pressure ulcers and other signs of nutritional decline.

INTERVENTION: FOOD AND NUTRITION

- Ensure a healthy diet, including protein and increased calories for age, sex, and activity, especially for "wanderers" and those who pace. Persons with AD may need 35 kcal/kg of body weight or more.
- Include nutrient-dense foods that are high in antioxidants and omega-3 fatty acids and mixed nuts. One alcohol-containing beverage per day may be used, such as red wine for flavonols. Use more color-rich fruits and vegetables (blueberries, cranberries, strawberries, spinach, kale, broccoli, and oranges and other citrus fruits). Eat more oily fish such as salmon, halibut, trout, and tuna for omega-3 fatty acids; a daily fish oil capsule may also be useful. Cocoa and red wine contain flavonols that increase blood flow to the brain. Adequate vitamin E, selenium, and other antioxidants are essential in management of this disorder (Reichman, 2000).
- Vitamins B_6 and B_{12} and folate lower elevated levels of homocysteine; include dietary sources. Extra folic acid may also lessen decline of cognitive function. Leafy greens, orange juice, and other nutrient-dense food choices should be made available.
- Foods high in copper may be warranted. Liver, kidney, shellfish such as oysters, nuts, dried beans and legumes, cocoa, eggs, prunes, and potatoes are recommended sources.
- Offer meals at regular and consistent times each day. Allow sufficient time for eating.
- Offer one course at a time (first salad, then entree, then fruit dessert) to prevent confusion. Avoid distractions and include soft background music that is calming. Cueing is also useful.
- Use dishes without a pattern. White is a good choice. Use a simple place setting and a single eating utensil. Use a bowl for easier scooping and special spoons or adaptive equipment as needed. Serve soup in mugs.
- Finger foods, such as sandwiches cut into four, cheese cubes, halved hard cooked eggs, chicken strips, julienne vegetables, and brownies (vs. apple pie), may be easier to eat, helping the patient to maintain weight.
- Providing a high-carbohydrate meal for dinner increases food intake in seniors at later stages of the disease who are experiencing cognitive and behavioral difficulties; this reflects a shift in preference for high-carbohydrate foods (Young et al, 2005). Knowing this allows nutrition staff to plan menus accordingly. For example, because sweets are well liked, offer nutrient-dense desserts (such as fruit tarts, puddings topped with fruit, and custards).
- Tube feed or use texture-altered foods with thickened liquids as needed to compensate for dysphagia.
- Choline may be beneficial (Michel et al, 2006). Use of foods such as soybeans or eggs will provide choline in the form useful to the body; lecithin tablets do not increase acetylcholine levels adequately.
- Adequate fluid intake is essential. Offer regular drinks of water, juice, milk, and other fluids to avoid dehydration.
- Cut back on saturated fats, which may increase brain beta-amyloid levels and the effects of AD. High-fat dairy products, fast food, fried foods, and processed foods should be eaten less often.

CLINICAL INDICATORS

Clinical/History

- Height, weight
- Current BMI
- Changes in BMI over time
- Subtle weight loss
- Dietary/intake history
- Anorexia and poor intake
- Nausea, vomiting
- Diarrhea
- Bowel incontinence
- Intake and output (I & O)
- Electroencephalogram (EEG)
- Loss of sense of smell
- ApoE genotype
- Computed tomography (CT) scan or brain

magnetic resonance imaging (MRI)
Medial temporal lobe thickness (often thinned)
Mini-Mental State Examination
Severe Impairment Battery and Global Deterioration Scale
Mattis Dementia Rating Scale
Behavioral disturbances: Neuropsychiatric Inventory
Behavioral function: London Psychogeriatric Rating Scale

Lab Work

Cerebrospinal fluid biomarkers (T-τ and Aβ42)
Choline acetyltransferase activity (ChAT)
Serum homocysteine levels (tHcy), often elevated
C-reactive protein (CRP)
Cholesterol (chol) (may be high)
Glucose (gluc)
Serum folate
Serum vitamin B_{12}
Serum zinc
Serum copper
Alanine aminotransferase (ALT)
Aspartate aminotransferase (AST)
Dopamine (DA)
Cerebral spinal fluid (CSF) pyruvate and lactate levels
Na+, K+
Blood urea nitrogen (BUN)
Creatinine (creat)
H & H
Serum Fe
Albumin or transthyretin

Common Drugs Used and Potential Side Effects

- See Table 4-6.

Herbs, Botanicals, and Supplements

- Gingko biloba has some evidence of efficacy in reducing memory decline, possibly by inhibiting cellular oxidation and enhancing circulation. It interacts with anticoagulants and antiplatelets such as aspirin, warfarin, and dipyridamole. There is a clinical trial under way for testing its efficacy in AD.
- Coenzyme Q10, choline, and lecithin may be useful. More studies are planned.
- Huperzine A (Chinese club moss) may prevent breakdown of acetylcholine. Research is under way.
- Phosphatidylserine, acetyl-L-carnitine, horse balm, Brazil nut, rosemary, dandelion, and sage have been promoted but have not been proven for efficacy; side effects have not been clearly identified.

INTERVENTION: NUTRITION EDUCATION, COUNSELING, CARE MANAGEMENT

- A nutrition education program intended for caregivers of AD patients can yield positive effects on patient weights and cognitive function (Riviere et al, 2001).

TABLE 4-6 Medications for Alzheimer's Disease and Possible Side Effects

Medication	Side Effects
Antidepressants	Minimal improvements have been noted. Mirtazapine may be useful in the treatment of the comorbid symptoms of weight loss, insomnia, and anxiety, a reflection of its enhancement of brain serotonergic and noradrenergic neurotransmission (Raji and Brady, 2001). Large, randomized controlled trials (RCTs) are needed.
Atypical antipsychotics	The efficacy of risperidone and olanzapine for the treatment of psychotic symptoms has been demonstrated by large RCTs in Alzheimer's disease (Hoeh et al, 2003).
Cholinesterase inhibitors donepezil (Aricept), rivastigmine (Exelon), memantine (Namenda)	Can slow agitation and the progression of cognitive and functional deficits in Alzheimer's disease in early stages. Rivastigmine tartrate (Exelon) improves cognitive function, behavior, and daily functioning. Memantine (Namenda) limits actions of glutamate. Nausea or diarrhea may occur.
Coenzyme Q10	Studies are inconclusive at this time.
Cognex (tacrine hydrochloride)	May cause abdominal pain, increased liver function tests, constipation, diarrhea, indigestion, anorexia, vomiting, or weight loss. Does not yield significant improvements.
Galanthamine (Reminyl)	Blocks acetylcholine breakdown; looks promising.
Hydergine	Relieves symptoms of declining mental capacity. Nausea and gastrointestinal (GI) distress are common.
Ibuprofen and other nonsteroidal, anti-inflammatory drugs	May reduce the risk of development of Alzheimer's disease, according to studies at Johns Hopkins; reduction of the inflammatory process occurs.
Insulin	If Alzheimer's disease is related to diabetes, it may be important to assure that adequate levels of insulin are maintained in the brain. Research continues in this area.
Laxatives	To control constipation. Offer high-fiber foods and sufficient fluid.
Mood stabilizers (lithium)	Low doses may be useful when combined with antipsychotics. Lithium regulates amyloid-beta precursor protein processing (Su et al, 2004).
Selegiline (Eldepryl)	Selegiline should not be used with ginseng, ma huang (ephedra), yohimbe, or St. John's wort.
Statins	People taking statin drugs may have lower blood cholesterol and less incidence of Alzheimer's disease. They may have the ability to break down plaque-building amyloid protein.
Vitamin E	In one study, 2000 IU alpha-tocopherol (vitamin E) was shown to delay the progression of nursing home admission in patients with mild-to-moderate Alzheimer's disease (Reichman, 2000). In another study, vitamin E had no benefit in patients with mild cognitive impairment (Petersen et al, 2005).

- A DASH diet may be useful, especially if serum lipids are high. Encourage use of fruits such as blueberries and other berries. Exercise and an antioxidant-rich diet may be protective against further cognitive decline.
- Encourage routines such as regular mealtimes, good mouth care, etc. Reduce distractions at mealtime.
- Refer family or caretakers to support groups. Long-term care or home care may be needed at some point in time.
- Special feeding methods may be needed. If the patient must be spoon fed, gently holding his or her nose will force the mouth open.
- Liquid supplements can add extra calories and protein without excessive expense. Baking nutritious cookie bars or snacks enhances calorie intake and addresses the need for sensory stimulation.
- Use unbreakable dishes and utensils to avoid injury. Cutting and preparing foods for the patient are useful.

Patient Education—Foodborne Illness

- Careful food handling will be important. The same is true for hand washing.

For More Information

- Alzheimer's Association
  http://www.alz.org/
- Alzheimer's Disease Education and Referral (ADEAR) Center
  http://www.alzheimers.org
- Alzheimer's Disease International
  http://www.alz.co.uk/
- American Academy of Neurology–Alzheimer's Disease
  http://www.aan.com/professionals/practice/pdfs/dem_pat.pdf

ALZHEIMER'S DISEASE AND DEMENTIAS—CITED REFERENCES

Buchman AS, et al. Change in body mass index and risk of incident Alzheimer disease. *Neurology* 65:892, 2005.

Chouinard J. Dysphagia in Alzheimer disease: a review. *J Nutr Health Aging.* 4:214, 2000.

Dietrich M, et al. Associations between apolipoprotein E genotype and circulating F2-isoprostane levels in humans. *Lipids* 40:329, 2005.

Engelhart MJ, et al. Dietary intake of antioxidants and risk of Alzheimer disease. *JAMA.* 287:3223, 2002.

Gould TD, et al. Effects of a glycogen synthase kinase-3 inhibitor, lithium, in adenomatous polyposis coli mutant mice. *Pharmacol Res.* 48:49, 2003.

Greenwood CE, et al. Behavioral disturbances, not cognitive deterioration, are associated with altered food selection in seniors with Alzheimer's disease. *J Gerontol A Biol Sci Med Sci.* 60:499, 2005.

Hoeh N, et al. Pharmacologic management of psychosis in the elderly: a critical review. *J Geriatr Psychiatry Neurol.* 16:213, 2003.

Kang JH, et al. Apolipoprotein E, cardiovascular disease and cognitive function in aging women. *Neurobiol Aging.* 26:475, 2005.

Lester-Coll N, et al. Intracerebral streptozotocin model of type 3 diabetes: relevance to sporadic Alzheimer's disease. *J Alzheimers Dis.* 9:13, 2006.

Martin E, et al. Pyruvate dehydrogenase complex: metabolic link to ischemic brain injury and target of oxidative stress. *J Neurosci Res.* 79:240, 2005.

Michel V, et al. Choline transport for phospholipid synthesis. *Exp Biol Med (Maywood).* 231:490, 2006.

Ownby RL, et al. Depression and risk for Alzheimer disease: systematic review, meta-analysis, and metaregression analysis. *Arch Gen Psychiatry.* 63:530, 2006.

Petersen RC, et al. Vitamin E and donepezil for the treatment of mild cognitive impairment. *N Engl J Med.* 352:2379, 2005.

Poehlman E, Dvorak R. Energy expenditure, energy intake, and weight loss in Alzheimer disease. *Am J Clin Nutri.* 71:650S, 2000.

Power DA, et al. Circulating leptin levels and weight loss in Alzheimer's disease patients. *Dement Geriatr Cogn Disord.* 12:167, 2001.

Raji MA, Brady SR. Mirtazapine for treatment of depression and comorbidities in Alzheimer disease. *Ann Pharmacother.* 35:1024, 2001.

Rapp MA, et al. Increased hippocampal plaques and tangles in patients with Alzheimer disease with a lifetime history of major depression. *Arch Gen Psychiatry.* 63:161, 2006.

Reichman W. Alzheimer's disease: clinical treatment options. *Am J Manag Care.* 6:1125S, 2000.

Riviere S, et al. A nutritional education program could prevent weight loss and slow cognitive decline in Alzheimer's disease. *J Nutr Health Aging.* 5:295, 2001.

Schliebs R. Basal forebrain cholinergic dysfunction in Alzheimer's disease: interrelationship with beta-amyloid, inflammation and neurotrophin signaling. *Neurochem Res.* 30:895, 2005.

Squitti R, et al. Excess of serum copper not related to ceruloplasmin in Alzheimer disease. *Neurology* 64:1040, 2005.

Su Y, et al. Lithium, a common drug for bipolar disorder treatment, regulates amyloid-beta precursor protein processing. *Biochemistry* 43:6899, 2004.

Wantanabe T, et al. Relationship between serum insulin-like growth factor-1 levels and Alzheimer's disease and vascular dementia. *J Am Geriatr Soc.* 53:1748, 2005.

Young KW, et al. A randomized, crossover trial of high-carbohydrate foods in nursing home residents with Alzheimer's disease: associations among intervention response, body mass index, and behavioral and cognitive function. *J Gerontol A Biol Sci Med Sci.* 60:1039, 2005.

AMYOTROPHIC LATERAL SCLEROSIS

NUTRITIONAL ACUITY RANKING: LEVEL 3

DEFINITIONS AND BACKGROUND

Amyotrophic lateral sclerosis (ALS) is a progressive motor neuron disease of adult life that destroys nerve cells from the spinal cord to muscle cells. Men are more often affected than women; the disease affects 20,000 people in the United States, and ALS usually occurs after age 40. It is also known as progressive spinal muscular atrophy or Lou Gehrig's disease.

Symptoms and signs of ALS include muscular wasting and atrophy, drooling, loss of reflexes, respiratory infections or failure, spastic gait, and weakness. Respiratory failure occurs as a result of bulbar, cervical, and thoracic loss of motor neurons; inspiratory muscles are affected. Management of respiratory failure includes the use of strategies that limit aspiration pneumonia, the reduction in secretions, positioning of the patient to a maximal mechanical advantage, and use of noninvasive positive pressure ventilation. The decision to undertake invasive mechanical ventilation should be made prior to the development of symptoms that might warrant this intervention (Hardiman, 2000).

Nutrition is an independent, prognostic factor for survival and disease complications in ALS; individualized nutritional management of symptoms is critical (Cameron and Rosenfeld, 2002). Malnutrition is present in 16–50% of ALS patients (Desport et al, 2000). It is thought to be caused by elevated metabolic needs and swallowing dysfunction from involvement of the lower sets of cranial nerves. Standard equations for calculating needs in ALS patients are not useful because they overestimate energy expenditure but underestimate requirements; indirect calorimetry is suggested (Sherman et al, 2004).

Malnutrition produces neuromuscular weakness and adversely affects patients' quality of life. In later stages of the disease, percutaneous endoscopic gastrostomy (PEG) confers a significant survival benefit in some patients but not all (Hardiman, 2000; Desport et al, 2000). Consider patient preferences and advance directives (American Dietetic Association, 2002).

While dietary factors have been suspected of being risk factors for ALS, few human studies have been reported. Lycopene and magnesium are important nutrients (Oyanagi et al, 2006; Longnecker et al, 2000). Energy metabolism by the brain is affected in ALS; one theory implicates glutamate excitotoxicity in the pathogenesis of ALS (Nelson et al, 2000).

Familial amyotrophic lateral sclerosis (FALS) shows mutations in the gene for superoxide dismutase-1 (Shibata, 2001). Proposed mechanisms of motor neuron degeneration have been suggested such as oxidative injury, superoxide dismutase-1 aggregation, and apoptosis. Creatine significantly increases longevity and motor performance of mice and improves function of the glutamate transport system, which has a high demand for energy and is susceptible to oxidative stress (Andreassen et al, 2001).

There is no known cure at this time. Research has shown some evidence that a form of ALS can improve or disappear with some of the antiviral drug therapies used in AIDS (MacGowan et al, 2001). ALS has a 50% fatality rate at 2 to 5 years from pneumonia or renal failure; 10% of patients with ALS live 10 years or longer. At the end of life, ALS patients often have respiratory distress, anxiety, pain, and choking (Bradley et al, 2001).

INTERVENTION: OBJECTIVES

- Maintain good nutrition to prevent further complications.
- Reduce difficulties in chewing and swallowing. Monitor gag reflex.
- Reduce the patient's fear of aspiration; test swallowing reflexes with water and feed slowly.
- Minimize the possibility of urinary tract infection and constipation.
- Correct negative nitrogen balance and nutritional deficiencies that exist.
- Ease symptoms to try to maintain independence.
- Reduce fatigue from the mealtime process; provide a slower pace to avoid choking.

INTERVENTION: FOOD AND NUTRITION

- In initial stages, use a soft diet. Flaky fish, ground meats, and casseroles should be encouraged, along with foods moistened with gravies and sauces. Provide adequate fiber in the diet, perhaps using Benefiber or psyllium when fibrous foods are no longer tolerated.
- The diet should include 2–3 L of water daily. Thicken liquids as needed with commercial thickeners, gelatin powder, or mashed potato flakes. Sips of liquid are best tolerated between bites of food.
- Place food at side of mouth and tilt head forward to facilitate swallowing, when possible.
- Energy intake should be normal to high. Five to six small meals should be scheduled daily. Increase protein intake to counteract wasting.
- Diet and supplemental feedings should provide an adequate intake of zinc, magnesium, potassium, omega-3 fatty acids, amino acids, lycopene, and phosphorus.
- Foods should be moistened and not dry or crumbly. Cake and crackers should not be served plain, whereas yogurt, applesauce, and pudding generally are acceptable.
- PEG or percutaneous endoscopic jejunostomy (PEJ) tube placement is well tolerated and provides more efficient enteral nutrition than nasogastric tube feeding when dysphagia becomes severe (Cameron and Rosenfeld, 2002; Desport et al, 2000).

CLINICAL INDICATORS

Clinical/History

- Height
- Weight
- Weight changes
- BMI (below 18–20 indicates malnutrition)
- Dietary/intake history
- Difficulty in swallowing
- Temperature
- I & O
- Gag reflex
- ALS Functional Rating Scale (ALSFRS-R)

Lab Work

- H & H
- Serum Fe
- Na+, K+
- Ca++, Mg++
- Albumin (alb), transthyretin
- Transferrin
- BUN, Creat
- Nitrogen (N) balance
- Electromyogram (EMG)
- Gluc
- CRP

Common Drugs Used and Potential Side Effects

- Ceftriaxone alters glutamate and has been found to prolong survival in animal models of ALS.
- Riluzole (a glutamate release inhibitor and membrane stabilizer) has been used to block nerve cell destruction. It seems to slow the disease but not curb its progress. Reports from patient databases describe experience with increased survival with riluzole over time. Adding vitamin E to this therapy does not seem to cause any improvement (Graf et al, 2005).
- Antiviral drugs such as nelfinavir, zidovudine, and lamivudine have shown evidence of being effective in

one patient with HIV infection (MacGowan et al, 2001).

- Studies suggest that magnesium, lycopene, and anti-inflammatory drugs may be beneficial.
- A large, multicenter clinical trial has shown that a family of antibiotics that includes penicillin may help prevent nerve damage and death in ALS by increasing the transporters of glutamate from the nerves. Minocycline may also slow progression of ALS by blocking caspases.
- Baclofen reduces muscle spasm and may lessen muscle cramping. It may elevate glucose levels.

Herbs, Botanicals, and Supplements

- No specific herbs and botanical products have demonstrated efficacy in ALS. However, taking supplements of various kinds may be common in this population (Cameron and Rosenfeld, 2002).
- Creatine significantly increases longevity and motor performance of mice and improves function of the glutamate transport system (Andreassen et al, 2001). It is not clear whether supplemental creatine is indicated for ALS.

INTERVENTION: NUTRITION EDUCATION, COUNSELING, CARE MANAGEMENT

- Dietary counseling is important, but oral intake rapidly becomes insufficient, particularly in bulbar-onset ALS, where enteral nutritional support is then necessary (Desport et al, 2000). Discuss care plan in front of patient; include the patient as much as possible.
- In early stages, discuss adding fiber to the diet to prevent constipation. Explain which foods have fiber.
- Encourage the planning of small, adequately balanced meals.
- Carefully monitor the patient's weight loss; 10% loss is common.
- Lightweight utensils are beneficial. A referral to an occupational therapist is recommended.
- Minimize chewing, but avoid use of baby food, which can be insulting. Puree adult foods, especially preferred foods that are seasoned as usual for the individual.
- In later stages, decide if enteral nutrition will be used. If care will be given at home, teach family members what they can do to provide the feedings.

Patient Education—Foodborne Illness

- Careful food handling will be important. The same is true for sanitizing work area before and after preparing tube feedings to prevent contamination. Formula companies have good information on safe handling of formula in the home and institution.

For More Information

- ALS Association
  http://www.alsa.org/
- ALS Therapy Development Foundation
  http://www.als.net/
- Practice Guidelines
  http://www.neurology.org/cgi/reprint/52/7/1311.pdf

AMYOTROPHIC LATERAL SCLEROSIS—CITED REFERENCES

American Dietetic Association. Position of The American Dietetic Association: ethical and legal issues in nutrition, hydration and feeding. *J Am Diet Assoc.* 102:716, 2002.

Andreassen O, et al. Increases in cortical glutamate concentrations in transgenic amyotrophic lateral sclerosis mice are attenuated by creatine supplementation. *J Neurochem.* 77:383, 2001.

Bradley WG, et al. Current management of ALS: comparison of the ALS CARE Database and the AAN Practice Parameter. The American Academy of Neurology. *Neurology.* 57:500, 2001.

Cameron A, Rosenfeld J. Nutritional issues and supplements in amyotrophic lateral sclerosis and other neurodegenerative disorders. *Curr Opin Clin Nutr Metab Care.* 5:631, 2002.

Desport J, et al. Nutritional assessment and survival in ALS patients. *Amyotroph Lateral Scler Other Motor Neuron Disord.* 1:91, 2000.

Graf M, et al. High dose vitamin E therapy in amyotrophic lateral sclerosis as add-on therapy to riluzole: results of a placebo-controlled double-blind study. *J Neural Transm.* 112:649–660, 2005.

Hardiman O. Symptomatic treatment of respiratory and nutritional failure in amyotrophic lateral sclerosis. *J Neurol.* 247:245, 2000.

Longnecker M, et al. Dietary intake of calcium, magnesium, and antioxidants in relation to risk of amyotrophic lateral sclerosis. *Neuroepidemiology.* 19:210, 2000.

MacGowan D, et al. An ALS-like syndrome with new HIV infection and complete response to antiretroviral therapy. *Neurology.* 57:1094, 2001.

Nelson L, et al. Population-based case-control study of amyotrophic lateral sclerosis in western Washington state. *Am J Epidemiol.* 151:164, 2000.

Oyanagi K, et al. Magnesium deficiency over generations in rats with special references to the pathogenesis of the Parkinsonism-dementia complex and amyotrophic lateral sclerosis of Guam. *Neuropathology* 26:115, 2006.

Sherman MS, et al. Standard equations are not accurate in assessing resting energy expenditure in patients with amyotrophic lateral sclerosis. *J Parenter Enteral Nutr.* 28:442, 2004.

Shibata N. Transgenic mouse model for familial amyotrophic lateral sclerosis with superoxide dismutase-1 mutation. *Neuropathology.* 21:82, 2001.

BRAIN TRAUMA

NUTRITIONAL ACUITY RANKING: LEVEL 4

DEFINITIONS AND BACKGROUND

Traumatic brain injury (TBI) results from head injury after motor vehicle or industrial accidents, falls, fights, explosions, and gunshot wounds (with 40% involving alcohol use). Any sudden impact or blow to the head (with or without unconsciousness) may cause a TBI. Two thirds of patients with TBI die before reaching a hospital.

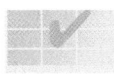

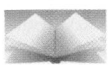

A TBI is classified by location, effect, and severity. **Hypothalamic lesions** can aggravate hyperphagia. Lateral lesions can aggravate aphasia and cachexia. **Frontal lobe damage** may result in loss of voluntary motor control and expressive aphasia. **Occipital lobe damage** may impair vision. **Temporal lobe damage** could result in receptive aphasia and hearing impairments. The term TBI is not used for persons who are born with a brain injury or for injuries that happen during the birth process.

Immediate signs of concussion (seen within seconds or minutes) include any loss of consciousness, impaired attention, vacant stare, delayed responses, inability to focus, slurred or incoherent speech, lack of coordination, disorientation, unusual emotional reactions, and memory problems. Later signs of concussion (hours, days, or even weeks after head injury) include persistent headache, dizziness with vertigo, poor attention or concentration, memory problems, nausea or vomiting, easy fatigue, irritability, intolerance for bright lights or loud noises, anxiety, depression, and disturbed sleep. Long term, TBI patients may exhibit dyspnea, vertigo, altered consciousness, seizures, vomiting, altered blood pressure, weakness or paralysis, aphasia, and problems with physical control of hands, head, or neck with resulting difficulty in self-feeding.

A TBI can change how a student learns in school, how a person acts, and how thinking and reasoning occur. There are often problems understanding words, learning and remembering things, paying attention, solving problems, thinking abstractly, talking, behaving, walking, seeing, and hearing. Headache, some irritability, and altered thought processes are a general outcome. Longitudinal psychological test results are used to explore the complex relationship between length of coma, time of testing on the recovery curve, and corresponding cognitive status after a TBI (Wong et al, 2001).

Pyruvate dehydrogenase complex (PDHC) is a mitochondrial matrix enzyme complex that catalyzes the oxidative decarboxylation of pyruvate to form acetyl-coenzyme A (CoA), nicotinamide adenine dinucleotide, and CO_2 as the bridge between anaerobic and aerobic cerebral energy metabolism; PDHC enzyme activity and immunoreactivity are lost in selectively vulnerable neurons after cerebral ischemia, and this explains the reduced cerebral glucose and oxygen consumption that occurs after cerebral ischemia (Martin et al, 2005). Brain trauma is accompanied by regional alterations of brain metabolism, overall reduction in metabolic rates, and persistent metabolic crisis (Vespa et al, 2005). Interestingly, mild hypothermia of 12–24 hours in duration after insults will decrease the cerebral metabolic rate for glucose and oxygen; brain ATP breakdown is reduced more than its synthesis (Erecinska et al, 2003).

Severe head injuries also tend to be associated with negative nitrogen balances. Data show that starved head-injured patients lose sufficient nitrogen to reduce weight by 15% per week (Brain Trauma Foundation, 2000).

With severe head injuries (Glasgow Coma Scale of 8), there is an increased tendency for gastric feeding to regurgitate into the upper airway; keeping the patient upright and checking residuals is important in such patients. Jejunal feedings are less apt to be aspirated. If the gastrointestinal tract cannot be used to reach nutritional goals within 3 days, total parenteral nutrition (TPN) is begun within 24–48 hours so as to reach these nutritional goals by either one or both routes by the third or fourth day (Wilson et al, 2001).

Severity of head injury may be closely associated with infections (Minard et al, 2000). Free fatty acids (FFA) and lactic acid are markers of secondary cellular injury following TBI; a creatine (Cr)-enriched diet may provide neuroprotection (Scheff and Dhillon, 2004). The trauma population is also at increased risk of venous thromboembolic disease, a potentially preventable cause of mortality and morbidity (Knudsen and Ikossi, 2004).

INTERVENTION: OBJECTIVES

- Prevent life-threatening complications, such as aspiration pneumonia, meningitis, sepsis, urinary tract infections (UTIs), syndrome of inappropriate antidiuretic hormone (SIADH), hypertension, pressure ulcers, Curling's ulcer, and gastrointestinal (GI) bleeding.
- Assess regularly the substrate needs to prevent malnutrition, cachexia, or overfeeding. Indirect calorimetry to determine the respiratory quotient and resting energy expenditure should be determined twice weekly. It has not been established that any method of feeding is better than another or that early feeding prior to 7 days improves outcome, but based on the level of nitrogen wasting and the nitrogen-sparing effect of feeding, it is a guideline that full nutritional replacement be instituted by day 7 (Brain Trauma Foundation, 2000).
- Prevent or correct hyperglycemia by carefully regulating glucose and insulin intake.
- Provide adequate protein for improving nitrogen balance (serum albumin tends to be low, especially if comatose, and urinary losses may be as high as twice normal). About 100–140% replacement of resting metabolism expenditure with 15–20% nitrogen calories reduces nitrogen loss (Brain Trauma Foundation, 2000).
- Monitor hydration; prevent both dehydration and overhydration.
- Correct any self-feeding problems, breathing and swallowing problems, and other conditions affecting self-care.
- Prevent or reduce seizure activity, convulsions, and intracranial edema.
- Prevent cerebral edema and fluid overload when using TPN, if necessary.
- After patient is stabilized, adapt to residual impairments.

INTERVENTION: FOOD AND NUTRITION

- Enteral feeding (EN) should begin as soon as the patient is hemodynamically stable, attempting to reach 35–45 kcal/kg and a protein intake of 2.0–2.5 g/kg on day 1 or as soon as possible (Wilson et al, 2001). Tube feeding is preferable over parenteral nutrition (PN) in general. In certain patients on EN, malabsorption may promote a persistently low serum albumin and total protein and peripheral edema, and a short course of supplemental PN may help, followed by a normal regimen of EN (Datta et al, 2003).

- While postpyloric feedings or TPN may be required for a long period of time, it is not always essential to use a jejunostomy feeding if aspiration risk is carefully managed (Klodell et al, 2000). The need for surgery or ventilation will have an effect on the ability to progress to any oral intake.
- Patients who are immobile for a long period of time may have a 10% decrease in weight, perhaps from lowered metabolic rate. Energy intake may need to be varied accordingly.
- Increased urinary zinc losses can occur. Otherwise, use normal recommended levels for most vitamins and minerals. Monitor potassium, phosphorus, and magnesium requirements; losses are often high.
- Progress, when possible, to oral intake (perhaps using a thick pureed diet with dysphagia). Use of probiotics (such as yogurt or buttermilk) may be helpful in maintaining GI integrity.
- Over time, a patient may actually gain excessive weight if the brain injury affects the hypothalamus. Some patients forget that they have eaten and indicate constant hunger. Monitor energy needs carefully.

CLINICAL INDICATORS

Clinical/History

Height
Weight
BMI
Dietary/intake history
Blood pressure (BP)
Temperature
Visual field examination
Glasgow Coma Scale
Dysphagia?
Weight changes
Intracranial pressure
CT scan
Skull x-rays
Brain scan
Cerebral angiography
EEG
I & O

Lab Work

Partial pressure of carbon dioxide (pCO_2)
Partial pressure of oxygen (pO_2)
Alb, transthyretin
Urinary urea nitrogen (UUN) excretion (24-hour specimens)
Gluc (increased with ischemia of the brain)
CRP
Folic acid
Serum ethanol/ethyl alcohol (ETOH) levels
Complete blood count (CBC)
Total lymphocyte count (TLC)
Transferrin
H & H
Serum Fe
Na^+, K^+
Ca^{++}, Mg^{++}
AST (increased with brain necrosis)
BUN, Creat
Alkaline phosphatase (alk phos)

Common Drugs Used and Potential Side Effects

- Anticonvulsants may be needed to reduce seizure activity. Watch folic acid levels and other affected nutrients. Presence of food reduces effectiveness of the liquid form of phenytoin (Dilantin). Adjust phenytoin dosage rather than hold feedings, since phenytoin efficacy is amenable to adjustment.
- Reglan may be used as a promotility agent in tube-fed patients to assist in transit time and to decrease the risk of aspiration.
- Soluble fibers or mixed fibers (Benefiber or other soluble fiber supplements used effectively as probiotics for gut regularity and integrity) or laxatives (Metamucil) are often helpful in alleviating constipation. Bloating, nausea, diarrhea, or vomiting may result.
- Analgesics are used for pain. Antacids and Pepcid may then be needed to reduce the onset of stress ulcers.
- Insulin may be needed if hyperglycemia occurs or persists.

Herbs, Botanicals, and Supplements

- Avoid using phenytoin (Dilantin) with evening primrose oil, gingko biloba, and kava.

INTERVENTION: NUTRITION EDUCATION, COUNSELING, CARE MANAGEMENT

- Encourage the patient to chew and swallow slowly, if and when the patient is able to eat solids.
- Gradually relearn self-feeding techniques.
- Be wary of food temperatures, especially if patient has become less sensitized to hot and cold.
- Preparation of colorful and attractive meals is crucial to acceptance.
- The team approach is beneficial, with occupational therapists, speech therapists, psychologists, and physical therapists helping the dietitian with treatment plans.
- Plate guards, long-handled utensils, and other adaptive feeding devices may be useful. Discuss with the occupational therapist.
- Discuss a healthy eating pattern and use of foods such as yogurt for their role as probiotics.
- Emotional changes are common after a head injury. Family should be prepared to address changes that relate to mealtimes, eating patterns, and weight management (Hurley and Taber, 2002). Maintain a consistent, structured routine when possible.
- The National Institutes of Health (NIH) has noted that most brain injury patients do not receive any counseling about the long-term effects of their injury (http://www.headinjury.com/welcome.htm#introduction). Provide written instructions for review later as needed.

Patient Education—Foodborne Illness

- Careful food handling will be important. The same is true for sanitizing work area before and after preparing tube feedings to prevent contamination. Formula companies have good information on safe handling of formula in the home and institution.

For More Information

- Brain Death
  http://aan.com/professionals/practice/pdfs/pdf_1995_thru_1998/1995.45.1012.pdf
- Brain Injury Association
  http://www.biausa.org

- Head Injury Awareness Foundation
  http://www.hiaf.org/
- Head Injury Hotline
  http://www.headinjury.com
- NIH Consensus Statement about Head Injury
  http://consensus.nih.gov/cons/109/109_statement.htm
- Persistent Vegetative State
  http://www.aan.com/professionals/practice/pdfs/pdf_1995_thru_1998/1995.45.1015.pdf

BRAIN TRAUMA—CITED REFERENCES

Brain Trauma Foundation. The American Association of Neurological Surgeons. The Joint Section on Neurotrauma and Critical Care: nutrition. *J Neurotrauma.* 17:539, 2000.

Datta G, et al. The role of parenteral nutrition as a supplement to enteral nutrition in patients with severe brain injury. *Br J Neurosurg.* 17:432, 2003.

Erecinska M, et al. Effects of hypothermia on energy metabolism in Mammalian central nervous system. *J Cereb Blood Flow Metab.* 23:513, 2003.

Hurley R, Taber K. Emotional disturbances following traumatic brain injury. *Curr Treat Options Neurol.* 4:59, 2002.

Klodell C, et al. Routine intragastric feeding following traumatic brain injury is safe and well tolerated. *Am J Surg.* 179:168, 2000.

Knudsen MM, Ikossi DG. Venous thromboembolism after trauma. *Curr Opin Crit Care.* 10:539, 2004.

Martin E, et al. Pyruvate dehydrogenase complex: metabolic link to ischemic brain injury and target of oxidative stress. *J Neurosci Res.* 79:240, 2005.

Minard G, et al. Early versus delayed feeding with an immune-enhancing diet in patients with severe head injuries. *J Parenter Enteral Nutr.* 24:1450, 2000.

Scheff SW, Dhillon HS. Creatine-enhanced diet alters levels of lactate and free fatty acids after experimental brain injury. *Neurochem Res.* 29:469, 2004.

Vespa P, et al. Metabolic crisis without brain ischemia is common after traumatic brain injury: a combined microdialysis and positron emission tomography study. *J Cereb Blood Flow Metab.* 25:763, 2005.

Wilson R, et al. The nutritional management of patients with head injuries. *Neurol Res.* 23:121, 2001.

Wong P, et al. Mathematical models of cognitive recovery. *Brain Inj.* 15:519, 2001.

CEREBRAL ANEURYSM

NUTRITIONAL ACUITY RANKING: LEVEL 2–3

DEFINITIONS AND BACKGROUND

A cerebral aneurysm may involve the dilation of a cerebral artery resulting from a weakness of the blood vessel wall. Epidemiological evidence from multiple sources suggests that most intracranial aneurysms do not rupture; it is important to identify which unruptured intracranial aneurysms (UIAs) are at greatest risk of rupture when considering which to repair (Wiebers et al, 2004).

Symptoms and signs include altered consciousness, drowsiness, confusion, stupor, sometimes coma, headache, facial pain, eye pain, blurred vision, vertigo, tinnitus, hemiparesis, elevated blood pressure, and dilated pupils. Aneurysms may burst and cause hemorrhage. An intracranial hemorrhage is bleeding inside the skull. Head injury is the most common cause. Bleeding within the brain is intracerebral. Hemorrhages between the brain and the subarachnoid space are called subarachnoid hemorrhages; those between the meninges are subdural hemorrhages; and those between the skull and covering of the brain are called epidural hemorrhages. Hemorrhagic stroke may occur (see Section 6 for more information about stroke).

After an aneurysmal subarachnoid hemorrhage, nearly half of patients die, and the half who survive suffer from irreversible cerebral damage (Chen et al, 2004).

INTERVENTION: OBJECTIVES

- Omit fluids if necessary to reduce cerebral edema.
- Rest is essential. Avoid constipation and straining at stool.
- Lower hypertension if possible.
- Prevent further complications or problems such as lingering neurological problems.
- Prepare for surgery if safe and possible.
- Gradually encourage self-feeding.

INTERVENTION: FOOD AND NUTRITION

- Nothing by mouth unless ordered; appropriate IVs should be used. Upon verification of progress, the physician should order a diet appropriate for condition.
- Restrict sodium and dietary cholesterol if deemed necessary.
- Alter dietary fiber intake, as appropriate.
- Control fluid if required.

CLINICAL INDICATORS

Clinical/History		
Height	I & O	Alb, transthyretin
Weight	BP (increased)	Gluc
BMI	**Lab Work**	Na+, K+
Weight changes	Chol	H & H
Dietary/intake history	Triglycerides (trig)	Serum Fe
		MRI
		CT scan results

Common Drugs Used and Potential Side Effects

- Cardiovascular drugs are usually ordered according to significant parameters. Adjust dietary intake accordingly.
- Diuretics may be used. Monitor need for potassium replacement if furosemide is prescribed.

Herbs, Botanicals, and Supplements

- No specific herbs and botanical products have been used for cerebral aneurysm in any clinical trials.

INTERVENTION: NUTRITION EDUCATION, COUNSELING, CARE MANAGEMENT

- Discuss fiber sources from the diet. Foods such as prune juice or bran added to cereal can be helpful in alleviating constipation.
- Counsel regarding self-feeding techniques.
- Discuss role of nutrition in preventing further cardiovascular or neurological problems.

Patient Education—Foodborne Illness

- Careful food handling will be important. The same is true for sanitizing work area before and after preparing tube feedings to prevent contamination. Formula companies have good information on safe handling of formula in the home and institution.

CEREBRAL ANEURYSM—CITED REFERENCES

Chen PR, et al. Natural history and general management of unruptured intracranial aneurysms. *Neurosurg Focus.* 17:e1, 2004.
Wiebers DO, et al. Pathogenesis, natural history, and treatment of unruptured intracranial aneurysms. *Mayo Clin Proc.* 79:1572, 2004.

COMA

NUTRITIONAL ACUITY RANKING: LEVEL 4

DEFINITIONS AND BACKGROUND

Coma is the unconscious state in which the patient is unresponsive to verbal or painful stimuli. Impaired consciousness or coma can occur from a stroke, head injury, meningitis, encephalitis, sepsis, lack of oxygen, epileptic seizure, toxic effects of alcohol or drugs, liver or kidney failure, high or low blood glucose levels, or altered body temperature. Medical staff can use the Glasgow Coma Scale to determine levels of unconsciousness and prognosis. Often, the 1-month performance on measures such as Disability Rating Scale (DRS) and Glasgow Outcome Scale (GOS) scores can help predict status 6 months post injury (Pastorek et al, 2004).

Nutritional support is associated with improved survival in coma (Borum et al, 2000). Most patients are tube fed because it is safer and more practical than hand feeding. Dietitians have an integral role with other members of the team in developing and implementing ethical guidelines for feeding patients (Maillet et al, 2002). Table 4-7 lists the consequences of withholding food and fluid from patients who are terminally ill and whose advance directives indicate no further "heroic measures."

In the United States, there are 14,000–35,000 people in a permanently unconscious state. A patient in a **permanently vegetative state (PVS)** does not have the ability to request or refuse treatment. The doctor determines the diagnosis of PVS. According to the American Dietetic Association position on legal and ethical issues in feeding permanently unconscious patients (Maillet et al, 2002), nutrition, hydration, and the definition of death are central to the dilemma of feeding permanently unconscious patients.

INTERVENTION: OBJECTIVES

- Maintain standards for primary condition.
- When possible, elevate head to prevent aspiration during feeding process.
- Assess daily calorie and fluid requirements.

TABLE 4-7 Consequences of Withholding Food and Fluid in Terminally Ill Patients

Neither nutrition nor hydration in terminal patients increases comfort or quality of life. Physiological adaptation allows patients not to suffer from the absence of food, as follows:

1. Two thirds of the patients who are not fed or hydrated at the end of life feel no hunger. They usually have loss of appetite and reduced enjoyment of food.
2. Thirst and dry mouth are common initially. Use ice chips, lubricating the lips, and small amounts of food and water to reduce the thirst sensations from dehydration.
3. Dehydration eventually results in hemoconcentration and hyperosmolality with subsequent azotemia, hypernatremia, and hypercalcemia. These changes may produce a sedative effect on the brain just before death.
4. Withholding or minimizing hydration can reduce disturbing oral and bronchial secretions, the need for frequent urination, and coughing from diminished pulmonary congestion.

Adapted from Maillet et al, 2002.

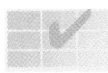

- Prevent or treat pressure ulcers, constipation, and other complications of immobility.
- For terminally ill patients, follow their wishes as directed by their advance directives.

INTERVENTION: FOOD AND NUTRITION

- Immediately give intravenous glucose until the cause is better identified.
- Tube feed (increased energy and protein as appropriate) every 2–3 hours or as ordered by the physician. Parenteral fluids may also be appropriate at this time. Total parenteral nutrition (TPN) may be appropriate for some persons, following evaluation of the original disorder, sepsis, and other complicating factors.
- If tube fed, a formula with fiber can be helpful in preventing or easing constipation; be sure sufficient fluid is included as well.
- Progress, when or if possible, to oral feedings.
- For patients who are terminally ill, gradual withdrawal of food and fluid would be appropriate if directed by the advance directives of the patient.

CLINICAL INDICATORS

Clinical/History

Height
Weight
BMI
Weight changes (bed scale)
Dietary/intake history
Glasgow Coma Scale (13 or higher is mild; 8 or less is severe brain injury); measures eye, motor, and verbal responses
BP

Lab Work

H & H
Serum Fe
pCO_2
pO_2
Chol, full lipid profile (HDL, LDL)
Trig
Alb
Gluc
BUN, Creat
CT scan or MRI
I & O
Urine tests for chemicals, glucose
Serum alcohol level
Serum vitamin B_{12}

Common Drugs Used and Potential Side Effects

- Anticonvulsants, such as phenytoin (Dilantin), may aggravate folic acid metabolism and cause decreased serum levels over time. Avoid use with evening primrose oil, gingko biloba, and kava.
- Steroids may be used with side effects such as increased sodium retention, increased potassium, calcium and magnesium losses, and increased nitrogen depletion.
- Antacids may be needed to prevent stress ulcers.
- Cathartics are often used. Monitor for electrolyte imbalances.

Herbs, Botanicals, and Supplements

- No specific herbs and botanical products have been used in comatose patients in any clinical trials.
- With phenytoin (Dilantin), avoid use with evening primrose oil, gingko biloba, and kava.

INTERVENTION: NUTRITION EDUCATION, COUNSELING, CARE MANAGEMENT

- Discuss with caretaker or family any necessary measures that are completed to provide adequate nourishment. Explain importance of prevention of complications such as aspiration.
- Evaluate self-feeding potentials over time.
- A Medic Alert bracelet or other ID may be useful for persons with disorders that may lead to unconsciousness.

Patient Education—Foodborne Illness

- Careful food handling will be important. The same is true for sanitizing work area before and after preparing tube feedings to prevent contamination. Formula companies have good information on safe handling of formula in the home and institution.

For More Information

- Coma
  http://www.neuroskills.com/coma.shtml
- Glasgow Coma Scale
  http://www.neuroskills.com/glasgow.shtml

COMA—CITED REFERENCES

Borum M, et al. The effect of nutritional supplementation on survival in seriously ill hospitalized adults: an evaluation of the SUPPORT data. Study to Understand Prognoses and Preferences for Outcomes and Risks of Treatments. *J Am Geriatr Soc.* 48:S33, 2000.

Maillet JO, et al. Position of the American Dietetic Association: ethical and legal issues in nutrition, hydration, and feeding. *J Am Diet Assoc.* 102:716, 2002.

Pastorek NJ, et al. Prediction of global outcome with acute neuropsychological testing following closed-head injury. *J Int Neuropsychol Soc.* 10:807, 2004.

EPILEPSY AND SEIZURE DISORDERS

NUTRITIONAL ACUITY RANKING: LEVEL 2

DEFINITIONS AND BACKGROUND

Epilepsy, a paroxysmal disturbance of the nervous system, results in recurrent attacks (seizures) with loss of consciousness, convulsions, motor activity, or behavioral abnormalities. The seizures result from excessive neuronal discharges in the brain. A grand mal seizure involves an aura, a tonic phase, and a clonic phase. A petit mal seizure involves momentary loss of consciousness.

There are many forms of epilepsy, each with its own symptoms. In two thirds of cases, no structural abnormality is found. A single seizure does not imply epilepsy. Incidence is 2–6 in 1000 people; 45,000 children under the age of 15 develop epilepsy each year. It is common with cerebral palsy and spina bifida.

A ketogenic diet should be considered for refractory epilepsy where seizures are difficult to control (Vaisleib et al, 2004; Freeman, 1998). The exact mechanism remains unclear (Papandreou et al, 2006). Several modifications of the original diet have been used (e.g., the medium-chain triglycerides [MCT] diet) in an attempt to overcome the obstacles of compliance and acceptance. A ketogenic diet is 70–90% fat with the remainder as protein and carbohydrates (CHO); in most patients, this produces a ketosis, and seizure activity is reduced or eliminated (Couch et al, 1999).

Modern ketogenic diets have been used with better success as compared with previous attempts (Carroll and Koenigsberger, 1998). Medical nutrition therapy (MNT) with the ketogenic diet for seizure control requires an average of 16 hours per patient (MacCracken and Scalisi, 1999). Seizure reduction and improved behavior control occurs; substantial financial savings are likely (Mandel et al, 2002).

Research suggests that overall caloric restriction improves the efficacy of the ketogenic diet in treating epilepsy as characterized by impaired glutamic acid decarboxylase (GAD) or gamma-aminobutyric acid (GABA) activity (Cheng et al, 2004). One concern, however, is that use of the ketogenic diet slows growth (Peterson et al, 2005). Bone health is another concern after taking antiepileptic drugs (AEDs), and concerns are related to altered hepatic cytochrome P-450 enzyme system, altered metabolism of vitamin D, resistance to parathyroid hormone, inhibition of calcitonin secretion, and impaired calcium absorption (Fitzpatrick, 2004).

Use of an alternative diet that is not as strict promotes use of a low–glycemic index treatment, with more liberal total carbohydrate intake, but use of low–glycemic index foods may allow greater than 90% reduction in seizure frequency in 50% of cases (Pfeifer and Thiele, 2005).

INTERVENTION: OBJECTIVES

- Minimize seizures via medications or lesionectomy surgery.
- Provide a well-balanced diet that avoids excess of food or fluid intake.
- If drug therapy does not work (as in the case of intractable myoclonic or akinetic seizures of infancy), a ketogenic diet may be used to produce ketosis. Ketosis stabilizes convulsions by decreasing restlessness and irritability. Reverse the usual ratio of cholesterol and fat. Beware of changing the diet abruptly; a gradual approach is preferred. This approach works best for children aged 2–5 years. If hyperuricemia or hypercalciuria occurs, increase fluid intake and consider use of diuretics.
- Monitor for deficits of key nutrients.
- Correct nutritional deficits from long-term anticonvulsant medication use (disorders of vitamin D, calcium, and bone metabolism). Phenytoin therapy (PHT) decreases serum folate by half, thereby increasing risk of deficiency.
- Monitor for possible long-term cardiac implications while following the ketogenic diet (Best et al, 2000). Growth retardation in children should also be prevented.

INTERVENTION: FOOD AND NUTRITION

- Provide a diet reflecting the patient's age and activity.
- The high-fat, high-protein, low-carbohydrate Atkins diet, because it is somewhat ketogenic, may be useful in managing medically resistant epilepsy (Kossoff et al, 2003).
- A ketogenic diet is useful but may be unpalatable. The diet follows a ratio of 3:1 or 4:1 of fat to carbohydrate and protein. MCTs are more ketogenic, having more rapid metabolism and absorption. If used in this way, MCTs would provide 60% of kcal (the rest of the diet would consist of 10% other fats, 10% protein, and 20% carbohydrates). Protein should meet basic needs (such as 0.8–1 g/kg body weight).
- If the pure ketogenic diet is not tolerated, try modifying it with low–glycemic index foods (Pfeifer and Thiele, 2005).
- Stimulants such as tea, coffee, colas, and alcohol are not usually recommended with the ketogenic diet.
- Supplements may be needed, especially for calcium, vitamin D, folacin, and vitamins B_6 and B_{12}.
- Add sufficient fiber and fluid for relief of constipation.

CLINICAL INDICATORS

Clinical/History	I & O	Serum Ca++, Mg++
Height	CT scan	Na+, K+
Weight	Skull x-ray	Alb, transthyretin
BMI	EEG	H & H
Dietary/intake history	**Lab Work**	Alk phos
BP	Urinary acetone (AM levels)	Chol, Trig
		Serum folate

Common Drugs Used and Potential Side Effects

- Cough syrups, laxatives, and other medications contain a high CHO content; monitor drug–drug interactions (McGhee and Katyal, 2001).
- Anticonvulsant therapy can cause interference with vitamin D metabolism, leading to a calcium imbalance and possibly rickets or osteomalacia. Therapy with 25-hydroxyvitamin D is recommended. Common anticonvulsants and potential side effects are listed in Table 4-8.

Herbs, Botanicals, and Supplements

- Vitamin B_6 is the vitamin associated with neuronal function. High doses of pyridoxine should not be taken with phenobarbital or phenytoin because seizure control might be compromised. If vitamin B_6 is added to either drug regimen, keep it at the lowest effective dose and monitor serum drug levels.
- St. John's wort is used as a natural antidepressant. Do not use with monoamine oxidase inhibitors (MAOI), selective serotonin reuptake inhibitors (SSRI), cyclosporine, digoxin, oral contraceptives, HIV protease inhibitors, theophylline, warfarin, or calcium channel blockers such as amlodipine, diltiazem, or verapamil. Avoid use with benzodiazepines such as alprazolam, clonazepam, diazepam, and midazolam.
- Psyllium and ginseng should not be used with divalproex sodium (Depakote) and lithium.
- With phenytoin (Dilantin), avoid use with evening primrose oil, gingko biloba, and kava.

INTERVENTION: NUTRITION EDUCATION, COUNSELING, CARE MANAGEMENT

- Ketogenic diets cause nausea and vomiting; a small drink of fruit juice can help relieve the symptoms. Regular monitoring of the diet is crucial.
- An ID tag, such as Medic Alert, is recommended.
- Alcohol should be avoided. A balanced diet is needed.
- To alter fats, the following tips may be helpful: to increase long-chain triglycerides (LCT), add sour cream, whipped cream, butter, margarine, or oils to casseroles, desserts, or other foods; to use MCT, add to salad dressings, fruit juice, casseroles, and sandwich spreads.

TABLE 4-8 Medications Used in Epilepsy

Generic Name	Trade Name	Possible Side Effects
Carbamazepine	Carbatrol, Tegretol XR, Tegretol	Dry mouth, vomiting, nausea, anorexia, low red blood cell and white cell counts.
Clonazepam	Klonopin	Anorexia, weight loss or gain, increased thirst.
Diazepam	Diazepam Intesol, Diastat, Valium	Anorexia, weight loss or gain, increased thirst.
Ethosuximide	Zarontin	Gastrointestinal upset, anemia, and weight loss. Take with food or milk.
Felbamate	Felbatol	Constipation, nausea, vomiting, and anorexia.
Fosphenytoin	Cerebyx	Water-soluble phenytoin. May need vitamin D, calcium, thiamin, magnesium.
Gabapentin	Neurontin	Weight gain and increased appetite occur. Take magnesium supplement separately by 2 hours.
Lamotrigine	Lamictal	Anorexia, weight loss, nausea and vomiting, abdominal pain.
Levetiracetam	Keppra	Anorexia, headache.
Oxcarbazepine	Trileptal	Restrict fluid with hyponatremia.
Phenobarbital	Luminal	Depletes vitamins D, K, B_{12}, B_6, folate, and calcium. Nausea, vomiting, constipation, sedation, and anorexia can occur. Limit caffeine and alcohol. May elevate serum cholesterol levels.
Phenytoin	Dilantin	Gum hyperplasia and carbohydrate intolerance. It binds serum proteins and decreases folate, vitamins B_{12} and C, and magnesium absorption. Be careful with vitamin B_6; excesses can reduce drug effectiveness. Stop tube feedings 30 minutes before and after administration of the medication; nutritional intake may need to be calculated over 21 versus 24 hours.
Primidone	Mysoline	Gastrointestinal upset, anemia, and weight loss. Take with food or milk. Primidone is similar to a barbiturate; vomiting may occur.
Tiagabine	Gabitril	Mouth ulcers, nausea and vomiting may occur.
Topiramate	Topamax	Weight loss, anorexia are common.
Valproate, valproic acid, divalproex sodium	Depacon, Depakote, Depakene, Depakote ER	Nausea, vomiting, anorexia, weight gain, or hair loss.
Vigabatrin	Sabril	Visual field loss can occur.
Zonisamide	Zonegran	Anorexia and weight loss are common.

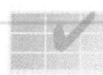

- Pseudo ice cream may be made with frozen, flavored whipped cream.
- Women who have epilepsy and wish to have children will need advice about medications and their possible side effects. Pregnancy itself can increase seizure frequency, and infants can be born with low birth weight, developmental delay, and childhood epilepsy (Yerby et al, 2004).
- Because of the potential for loss of bone mineral density, discuss inclusion of more calcium and vitamin D–rich foods. A multivitamin-mineral supplement may be recommended.

Patient Education—Foodborne Illness

- Careful food handling will be important. Hand washing is key as well.

For More Information

- American Epilepsy Society
  http://aesnet.org
- Citizens United for Research in Epilepsy (CURE)
  http://www.CUREepilepsy.org
- Continuing Medical Education Program
  http://www.cmediscovery.com/epilepsy/
- Epilepsy Foundation
  http://www.EpilepsyFoundation.org

EPILEPSY AND SEIZURE DISORDERS—CITED REFERENCES

Best T, et al. Cardiac complications in pediatric patients on the ketogenic diet. *Neurology* 54:2328, 2000.

Carroll J, Koenigsberger D. The ketogenic diet: a practical guide for caregivers. *J Am Diet Assoc.* 98:316, 1998.

Cheng CM, et al. Caloric restriction augments brain glutamic acid decarboxylase-65 and -67 expression. *J Neurosci Res.* 77:270, 2004.

Couch S, et al. Growth and nutritional outcomes of children treated with the ketogenic diet. *J Am Diet Assoc.* 99:1573, 1999.

Fitzpatrick LA. Pathophysiology of bone loss in patients receiving anticonvulsant therapy. *Epilepsy Behav.* 5:S3, 2004.

Freeman J, et al. The efficacy of the ketogenic diet—1998: a prospective evaluation of intervention in 150 children. *Pediatrics* 102:1358, 1998.

Kossoff EH, et al. Efficacy of the Atkins diet as therapy for intractable epilepsy. *Neurology* 61:1789, 2003.

MacCracken K, Scalisi J. Development and evaluation of a ketogenic diet program. *J Am Diet Assoc.* 99:1554, 1999.

Mandel A, et al. Medical costs are reduced when children with intractable epilepsy are successfully treated with the ketogenic diet. *J Am Diet Assoc.* 102:396, 2002.

McGhee B, Katyal N. Avoid unnecessary drug-related carbohydrates for patients consuming the ketogenic diet. *J Am Diet Assoc.* 101:87, 2001.

Papandreou D, et al. The ketogenic diet in children with epilepsy. *Br J Nutr.* 95:5, 2006.

Peterson SJ. Changes in growth and seizure reduction in children on the ketogenic diet as a treatment for intractable epilepsy. *J Am Diet Assoc.* 105:718, 2005.

Pfeifer HH, Thiele EA. Low-glycemic-index treatment: a liberalized ketogenic diet for treatment of intractable epilepsy. *Neurology* 65:1810, 2005.

Vaisleib II, et al. Ketogenic diet: out patient initiation, without fluid, or caloric restrictions. *Pediatr Neurol.* 31:198, 2004.

Yerby MS, et al. Risks and management of pregnancy in women with epilepsy. *Cleve Clin J Med.* 71:S25, 2004.

GUILLAIN-BARRÉ SYNDROME

NUTRITIONAL ACUITY RANKING: LEVEL 3

DEFINITIONS AND BACKGROUND

Guillain-Barré syndrome (GBS), also known as acute inflammatory demyelinating polyneuropathy, is a neurological syndrome of rapid and increasing weakness, numbness, pain, and paralysis of the legs, arms, and respiratory muscles. It often occurs after recent surgery, a viral infection (*Campylobacter jejuni* from undercooked meat, poultry, or contaminated milk), or immunization. Bloody diarrhea, fever, cramping, and headache occur with *C. jejuni.*

C. jejuni is the most frequently diagnosed bacterial cause of human gastroenteritis in the United States, and there is an association between *Campylobacter* infection and GBS (Rautelin and Hanninen, 2000; Fields and Swerdlow, 1999). Undercooked poultry and cross-contamination of other foods with uncooked meat products are sources of this infection. In general, the role of *C. jejuni* has been greatly underestimated (Schmidt-Ott et al, 2006).

Symptoms and signs of GBS include muscular weakness of lower extremities progressing to arms, trunk, face, and head; respiratory failure; paralysis of lower extremities or quadriplegia; unstable blood pressure; aspiration; dysphagia or difficulty in chewing; impaired speech; muscular pain; low-grade fever; tachycardia; weight loss, anorexia; urinary tract infections (UTIs); and personality changes. Sometimes ventilatory assistance is needed. Most people recover fully, but some may need intensive care support early, followed by wheelchair assistance. There is no treatment that has been totally effective. Prevention of contamination with *C. jejuni* is important.

INTERVENTION: OBJECTIVES

- Meet added energy requirements from any fever.
- Adjust diet or method of feeding for chewing and swallowing problems.
- Wean, as possible, from ventilator dependency.
- Prevent or correct weight loss and resulting malnutrition.
- Improve neurological functioning and overall prognosis.

INTERVENTION: FOOD AND NUTRITION

- Acute: Intravenous fluids will be required. Tube feeding or TPN may be necessary while patient is acutely ill over a period of time. Increased energy intake and protein may be necessary. Alter fat intake if necessary to reduce production of carbon dioxide, especially on ventilator.
- Progression: For some, a thick, pureed diet may be beneficial with dysphagia. When tolerated, the individual can use a soft or general diet.
- Supplement oral intake with frequent snacks, such as shakes or eggnog, if unintentional weight loss has occurred.
- A vitamin–mineral supplement may be beneficial if intake has been poor.

CLINICAL INDICATORS

Clinical/History
Height
Weight
Weight changes
Dietary/intake history
BMI
BP
Temperature
Dysphagia
Vomiting
Bloody diarrhea?
Rapidly ascending weakness
Loss of reflexes (knee, etc.)

Lab Work
CBC
H & H
Serum Fe
Alb
pO_2, pCO_2
Lumbar puncture for CSF protein levels
Gluc

Common Drugs Used and Potential Side Effects

- Antibiotics may be needed if UTIs or other problems are identified.
- Autoimmune globulin may be given.
- Analgesics are used to reduce pain and inflammation.
- Steroids are seldom used except for chronic relapsing polyneuropathy; their effects can be deleterious over time.
- Vasopressors may be used.

Herbs, Botanicals, and Supplements

- Vitamin B_6 is the vitamin associated with neuronal function. High doses of pyridoxine should not be taken with phenobarbital or phenytoin because seizure control might be compromised. If vitamin B_6 is added to either drug regimen, keep it at the lowest effective dose and monitor serum drug levels.
- St. John's wort is used as a natural antidepressant. Do not use with MAOI antidepressants, SSRI antidepressants, cyclosporine, digoxin, oral contraceptives, HIV protease inhibitors, theophylline, warfarin, or calcium channel blockers such as amlodipine, diltiazem, or verapamil. No studies have been conducted for efficacy in GBS.

INTERVENTION: NUTRITION EDUCATION, COUNSELING, CARE MANAGEMENT

- Encourage self-feeding, if possible.
- Discuss adequacy of energy and protein intake to improve weight status and nutritional health.
- Avoid foodborne illnesses, upper respiratory infections, and exposure to other illnesses.
- Arrange for special feeding utensils, if needed by the individual.
- Avoid constipation through use of fruits, vegetables, crushed bran, prune juice, and adequate fluid intake.

Patient Education—Foodborne Illness

- *C. jejuni* may be one cause of GBS, so its prevention is essential. Avoid drinking raw milk or eating raw or undercooked meat, shellfish, or poultry. The bacteria may also be found in tofu and raw vegetables.
- Hand washing is important for prevention. Wash hands with soap before handling raw foods of animal origin.
- Prevent cross-contamination in the kitchen. Proper refrigeration and sanitation are also essential.

For More Information

- Guillain-Barré Foundation International
  http://www.guillain-barre.com/about.html
- National Chronic Care Organization
  http://www.ncccon line.org

GUILLAIN-BARRÉ SYNDROME—CITED REFERENCES

Fields PI, Swerdlow DL. *Campylobacter jejuni. Clin Lab Med.* 19:489, 1999.
Rautelin H, Hanninen ML. *Campylobacters*: the most common bacterial enteropathogens in the Nordic countries. *Ann Med.* 32:440, 2000.
Schmidt-Ott R, et al. Improved serological diagnosis stresses the major role of *Campylobacter jejuni* in triggering Guillain-Barré syndrome. *Clin Vaccine Immunol.* 13:779, 2006.

HUNTINGTON'S DISEASE

NUTRITIONAL ACUITY RANKING: LEVEL 3

DEFINITIONS AND BACKGROUND

Huntington's disease (HD) is a genetic, autosomal dominant, neurodegenerative disorder for which there is no known cure (Sullivan et al, 2001). There is a defective gene on chromosome 4. HD is caused by an abnormal polyglutamine expansion within the protein huntingtin and is characterized by microscopic death of selected neurons (Arrasate et al, 2004). Transglutaminase (TGase) activity is increased in affected regions of brains from patients with HD, and some medications have been designed to alter those levels (Karpuj et al, 2002).

HD develops in middle to late life, with involuntary, spasmodic, irregular movements (chorea) and cerebral degeneration. Cognitive decline and speech difficulties occur. HD differs from AD in that there is loss of control of voluntary movements. Behavioral changes begin 10 years before the movement disorder, which may begin by ages 35 to 40 years.

Nutritional intake may play an important role in prevention or therapy. For example, it is speculated that folic acid plays a role in HD by affecting DNA methylation (Mattson, 2003). In addition, research suggests that restricted-calorie diets may increase the resistance of neurons in the brain to dysfunction and death in experimental models of Huntington's disease through expression of "stress proteins" and neurotrophic factors (Mattson, 2000). Coenzyme Q10, minocycline, and unsaturated fatty acids are among the substances considered investigational for neuroprotection (Bonelli and Wenning, 2006). Clearly, more research is imperative before specific recommendations can be made.

Remotivation therapy may be beneficial; it leads to increased self-awareness, increased self-esteem, and an improved quality of life, even in late-stage HD (Sullivan et al, 2001). Duration of HD is generally 13–15 years before death, which often results from pneumonia or a fatal fall.

INTERVENTION: OBJECTIVES

- Promote normal nutritional status, despite tissue degeneration. Extra energy intake is important (Trejo et al, 2004).
- Encourage the patient to self-feed until this is no longer possible. Swallowing problems are significant in this disorder (see Dysphagia entry in Section 7).
- Avoid aspiration of solids and liquids.
- Avoid gluten if not tolerated.

INTERVENTION: FOOD AND NUTRITION

- Provide a diet that gives sufficient energy and protein to prevent pressure ulcers and other sequelae. Usually 1–1.5 g/kg protein is needed. In late stages, weight gain may be a problem; monitor closely and change diet as needed.
- Use a thick, pureed, or chopped diet as appropriate. Feed slowly to prevent choking. Small, frequent meals are suggested.
- Tube feed when necessary; bolus feedings are usually tolerated.
- Provide adequate fiber (e.g., prune juice or tube feedings that contain fiber) for normal elimination.
- Supplement with a multivitamin-mineral supplement if needed. Folic acid and other B-complex vitamins may be especially important.
- If gluten intolerance occurs, omit gluten from the diet (e.g., wheat, barley, and rye products).

CLINICAL INDICATORS

Clinical/History		
Height	I & O	H & H
Weight	CT scan for changes in the brain	CRP
BMI	Unified Huntington's Disease Rating Scale	Homocysteine levels
Weight changes		Acetylcholine levels
Dietary/intake history	**Lab Work**	Dopamine levels
Ability to self-feed	BUN/Creat	Alb, transthyretin
Chewing or swallowing difficulties	Serum glucose	Serum folate
		Vitamin B_{12}

Common Drugs Used and Potential Side Effects

- Anti-inflammatory drugs such as ibuprofen may be useful.
- Supplemental vitamin E, antioxidants, and omega-3 fatty acids to lower inflammation and use of folic acid with vitamins B_{12} and B_6 to lower serum homocysteine levels may be a future protocol.
- Minocycline may slow the disease process. It blocks caspases from entering the brain.
- Riluzole has been used with some success and few side effects. It is a membrane stabilizer and a glutamate-release inhibitor.

Herbs, Botanicals, and Supplements

- Vitamin B_6 is the vitamin most often linked with neuronal function. High doses of pyridoxine should not be taken with phenobarbital or phenytoin because seizure control might be compromised. If vitamin B_6 is added to either drug regimen, keep it at the lowest effective dose and monitor serum drug levels.

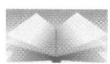

- Creatine is under study for its effectiveness in HD.
- St. John's wort is used as a natural antidepressant. Do not use with MAOI antidepressants, SSRI antidepressants, cyclosporine, digoxin, oral contraceptives, HIV protease inhibitors, theophylline, warfarin, or calcium channel blockers such as amlodipine, diltiazem, or verapamil. No studies have been conducted for efficacy in HD patients.

INTERVENTION: NUTRITION EDUCATION, COUNSELING, CARE MANAGEMENT

- Semisolid foods may be easier to swallow than thin liquids.
- Encourage genetic counseling; each child of an affected parent has a 50% chance of inheriting the disease.
- Teach family or caretakers about the Heimlich maneuver to correct episodes of choking.
- Adding protein and calories through supplements or nutritionally dense foods may be essential.
- If the patient or family wishes to forego tube feeding and hydration, the dietitian should discuss the possible consequences of malnutrition that may occur (Maillet et al, 2002).

Patient Education—Foodborne Illness

- Careful food handling will be important. The same is true for sanitizing work area before and after preparing tube feedings to prevent contamination.
- Formula companies have good information on safe handling of tube feeding formula in the home and institution.

For More Information

- Huntington's Disease Society of America
  http://www.hdsa.org/

HUNTINGTON'S DISEASE—CITED REFERENCES

Arrasate M, et al. Inclusion body formation reduces levels of mutant huntingtin and the risk of neuronal death. *Nature* 431:805, 2004.

Bonelli RM, Wenning GK. Pharmacological management of Huntington's disease: an evidence-based review. *Curr Pharm Des.* 12:2701, 2006.

Karpuj MV, et al. Evidence for a role for transglutaminase in Huntington's disease and the potential therapeutic implications. *Neurochem Int.* 40:31, 2002.

Maillet JO, et al. Position of the American Dietetic Association: ethical and legal issues in nutrition, hydration, and feeding. *J Am Diet Assoc.* 102:716, 2002.

Mattson MP. Methylation and acetylation in nervous system development and neurodegenerative disorders. *Ageing Res Rev.* 2:329, 2003.

Mattson MP. Neuroprotective signaling and the aging brain: take away my food and let me run. *Brain Res.* 886:47, 2000.

Sullivan F, et al. Remotivation therapy and Huntington's disease. *J Neurosci Nurs.* 33:136, 2001.

Trejo A, et al. Assessment of the nutrition status of patients with Huntington's disease. *Nutrition* 20:192, 2004.

MIGRAINE HEADACHE

NUTRITIONAL ACUITY RANKING: LEVEL 1

DEFINITIONS AND BACKGROUND

Migraine is a neurological process of the trigeminovascular system; vascular effects are secondary (Wenzel et al, 2004). Migraine involves paroxysmal attacks of headache, vasospasm, and increased coagulation, often preceded by visual disturbances.

Migraine may be caused by inherited abnormalities in the brain. Migraine headaches affect 12% of the adult population in the United States and cause a significant economic loss due to decreased workplace productivity (Wenzel et al, 2004). Up to 28 million Americans may suffer. Women may be affected as a result of hormones and premenstrual syndrome (PMS) symptoms (Martin et al, 2006).

Low blood levels of serotonin may bring on migraines. A drop in serotonin or estrogen or use of vasodilators (found in some foods) may cause blood vessels to swell and may contribute to migraines in sensitive individuals. In addition, studies are ongoing about the close connection between migraine and epilepsy, as well as sleep disorders.

Diet can also play an important role in children and adolescents with migraine, which may include underage drinking of alcoholic beverages (Millichap and Yee, 2003).

Dietary triggers affect phases of the migraine process by influencing release of serotonin and norepinephrine, causing vasoconstriction or vasodilatation, or by direct stimulation of trigeminal ganglia, brainstem, and cortical neuronal pathways (Millichap and Yee, 2003).

Reactions are often within 24 hours after an implicated food has been consumed. Nausea, vomiting, and acute sensitivity to light or sound may occur. Vascular-amine toxicity causes a rapid increase in blood pressure when high-tyramine foods such as cheese, wine, beer, fava beans, and sauerkraut are eaten in combination with medications such as MAOIs. Use 25 mg/d as the limit on tyramine for menus and for diet instructions, especially for patients on MAOIs.

Lack of food or sleep, exposure to light, anxiety, stress, fatigue, or hormonal irregularities in women can set off a migraine attack. Exercise, relaxation, biofeedback, and other therapies designed to help limit discomfort have a role in migraine treatment. Migraines may be reduced with intake of omega-3 fatty acids from fish oil and from intake of olive oil (Harel et al, 2002).

Treatment begins with a headache and diet diary and the selective avoidance of foods presumed to trigger attacks; omission of all potential triggers is not recommended

(Millichap and Yee, 2003). True immunoglobulin E–mediated food allergy is infrequent.

Stroke is a risk factor in young people who are prone to migraines; they should be monitored carefully. Surgical deactivation of headache trigger sites may be an effective treatment for migraines. Long-term prophylactic drug therapy is appropriate after exclusion of headache-precipitating trigger factors, including dietary factors. Regulation of sleep (improved sleep hygiene), moderation of caffeine, regular exercise, and identification of provocative influences such as stress, foods, and social pressures are essential (Lewis et al, 2005).

INTERVENTION: OBJECTIVES

- Eliminate stressors and other triggers, such as crowds, bright lights, and noises, at vulnerable times.
- Reduce or eliminate use of foods that cause migraines in sensitive individuals.
- Encourage a well-balanced diet, with adequate meal spacing to prevent fasting or skipping of meals.
- Obesity is a risk factor for chronic daily headaches; weight loss may be indicated.

INTERVENTION: FOOD AND NUTRITION

- Promote regular mealtimes and adequate relaxation.
- The list of foods, beverages, and additives that may trigger migraines includes cheese, chocolate, citrus fruits, hot dogs, monosodium glutamate, aspartame, fatty foods, ice cream, caffeine withdrawal, alcoholic drinks, histamine, nitrites, and sulfites (Millichap and Yee, 2003).
- Magnesium and fish oil capsules have been recommended for some cases, especially to curb onset quickly. While magnesium does not alleviate headache in all cases, it has been shown to reduce the number of days of suffering in children (Wang et al, 2003).
- Monitor for cross-reactivity in foods, even if never eaten before.
- Increase intake of fish oils and olive oil from the diet (Harel et al, 2002).
- Limit sensitive foods if identified (see Table 4-9). There is no scientific basis for recommending omission of red wine, tyramine, and phenylethylamine in chocolate for individuals with headache (Jansen et al, 2003).
- Promote exercise and weight loss if needed.

CLINICAL INDICATORS

Clinical/History		
Height	Headache symptoms and duration	Recent illnesses
Weight	Foods eaten in past 24 hours	Signs of dehydration or edema
BMI	History of similar reactions	Migraine Disability Assessment Score
Dietary/intake history		

TABLE 4-9 Foods Implicated in Various Types of Headaches

Food	Description
Alcohol	Champagne and red wine contain both phenols and tyramine; sulfites may also be involved as a trigger. There is not a clear relationship for red wine for migraines (Jansen et al, 2003). Beer is another possible problem.
	Alcoholic beverages: limit yourself to two normal size drinks of choices such as Cutty Sark scotch, Seagram's VO whisky, Riesling wine (National Headache Foundation, 2006).
Caffeine-containing products	Coffee, tea, and cola can trigger caffeine-withdrawal headache from methyl xanthines (18 hours after withdrawal); taper withdrawal gradually. Coffee is the major source of caffeine in adults; soft drinks are the major source for children and teens (Frary et al, 2005).
Cheese and tyramine	Aged cheese that contains tyramine has been implicated. Ripened cheeses: cheddar, emmentaler, stilton, brie, and camembert.
Chocolate	Chocolate contains phenylethylamine (no clear relationship to migraine; Jansen et al, 2003).
Fermented foods	Chicken livers, aged cheese such as cheddar, red wine, pickled herring, chocolate, broad beans, and beer contain tyramine (no clear relationship to migraine; Jansen et al, 2003).
Fruits	Bananas, figs, raisins; some citrus fruits.
Gluten	Celiac disease has been associated with migraine (Bushara, 2005).
Histamine-containing foods	Scombroid fish (slightly spoiled).
Ice cream	
Nuts, peanuts	Some contain vasodilators. Avoid nuts and peanut butter if necessary.
Processed meats	Hot dogs, bacon, ham, and salami contain nitrites.
Sulfites	Some people respond to the sulfites in shrimp, packaged potato products.
Vegetables	Onions, pea pods, lima beans.

Additional Reference: Millichap and Yee, 2003.

Lab Work	time (PT) or international normalized ratio (INR)	Serum Na+, K+ Ca++, Mg++ Gluc
Histamine Prothrombin		

Common Drugs Used and Potential Side Effects

- The particular drug selected for the individual patient requires an appreciation of comorbidities such as affective or anxiety disorders, knowledge of coexistent medical conditions such as asthma or diabetes, and acceptability of potential toxicities such as weight gain, sedation, and tremor (Lewis et al, 2005).
- Antiemetics may be prescribed if there is nausea or frequent vomiting with the headaches.
- Currently there are several large-scale randomized, placebo-controlled clinical trials in progress evaluating the efficacy, optimal dosing, and side effect profile of botulinum toxin A (BoNT/A), a neurotoxin, for treating migraine and other headache types (Dodick et al, 2004).
- Medicines can be used to relieve pain and restore function during attacks. The most promising of these are drugs called triptans (Wenzel et al, 2004). Drugs such as almotriptan, eletriptan, naratriptan, rizatriptan, sumatriptan, and zolmitriptan may be used to enhance the effects of serotonin. Almotriptan has few side effects and is well tolerated.
- Drugs designed to lower blood pressure also may prevent headaches, such as thiazides, beta-blockers, angiotensin-converting enzyme (ACE) inhibitors, and angiotensin II receptor agonists.
- If effective medicines are not found to treat headache with its onset, daily preventive medicines are sometimes used, such as anticonvulsants, nonsteroidal anti-inflammatory drugs (NSAIDs), tricyclic antidepressants, and serotonergic agents.
- If sedatives, tranquilizers, antidepressants, anticonvulsants, or diuretics are used, alter diet accordingly because there may be a number of side effects.
- Valproic acid has benefit for migraine, chronic daily headache, and cluster headache (Frietag, 2003).
- Melatonin is being studied for its possible impact on migraine headaches.
- For some women, hormone therapy may help.
- Capsaicin from hot chili peppers may be used as a source of relief for cluster headache pain. It does not seem to relieve migraines.
- Avoid using aspirin in children under age 15 because of the potential for Reye's syndrome.

Herbs, Botanicals, and Supplements

- Homeopathy may be attempted when medical management fails (Jonas et al, 2003). Feverfew may have some usefulness. Side effects include decreased platelet aggregation if used with warfarin, aspirin, and ticlopidine. NSAIDs (e.g., ibuprofen, indomethacin, etc.) decrease the herb's anti-inflammatory action; do not use together.
- Other herbs and botanicals may be used; identify and monitor side effects. Evening primrose, red pepper, willow, and ginger have been recommended, but no studies prove efficacy. Counsel about avoiding herbal teas, especially if they contain toxic ingredients.
- Omega-3 fatty acids and coenzyme Q10 are being studied for their potential relief of migraines.
- Food/plant sensitivities may exist (e.g., melon/ragweed, carrot/potato, apple/birch, wheat/grasses). Products such as echinacea may cause an allergic reaction.
- Bee pollen does not prevent headache or allergies and may cause asthma, dermatitis, rhinitis, or anaphylaxis after eating plants that cross-react with ragweed, such as sunflowers or dandelion greens.

INTERVENTION: NUTRITION EDUCATION, COUNSELING, CARE MANAGEMENT

- Teach the importance of not skipping meals because fasting can increase likelihood of a headache. Regular mealtimes are important.
- Encourage the patient to identify triggers.
- Teach the patient how to keep an accurate food diary if food sensitivities are implicated. Read food labels. Avoid packaged items containing foods that are problematic.
- Monitor drugs taken in correlation with headache sensitivity.
- Investigate underlying conditions such as asthma and reactive airway disease, hypertension, glaucoma, and ear problems.
- Psychotherapy may be useful for mental and emotional distress. Regular sleeping patterns are needed to alleviate migraines that result from lack of sleep. It may be helpful to evaluate for problems such as insomnia and sleep apnea.
- Discuss the possibility of medication overuse headache or rebound headaches from use of caffeine in the diet or in medicines.
- Biofeedback is used as a treatment modality for migraines. Acupuncture has also been proposed.

Patient Education—Food Safety

- Food storage is a major issue; warmer temperatures and extended holding times, especially in high-protein foods, is a concern. Teach safe food handling.

For More Information

- American Council for Headache Education
  http://www.achenet.org
- American Headache Society
  http://www.ahsnet.org
- Evidence-Based Guideline for Headache in Pediatrics
  http://www.aan.com/professionals/practice/pdfs/Headache_Peds_Physicians.pdf
- Low Tyramine Headache Diet
  http://www.headaches.org/consumer/topicsheets/LowTyramineDiet.pdf
- Medline: Headache
  http://www.nlm.nih.gov/medlineplus/headache.html
- National Headache Foundation
  http://www.headaches.org/
- National Institute of Neurological Disorders and Stroke—Brain Resources and Information Network
  http://www.ninds.nih.gov
- National Migraine Association
  http://www.migraines.org

- Practice Guidelines
  http://www.neurology.org/cgi/reprint/63/12/2215.pdf
- World Headache Alliance
  http://www.w-h-a.org

MIGRAINE HEADACHE—CITED REFERENCES

Bushara KO. Neurologic presentation of celiac disease. Neurologic presentation of celiac disease. *Gastroenterology* 128:92S, 2005.

Dodick D, et al. Botulinum neurotoxin for the treatment of migraine and other primary headache disorders. *Clin Dermatol.* 22:76, 2004.

Frary C, et al. Food sources and intakes of caffeine in the diets of persons in the United States. *J Am Diet Assoc.* 105:110, 2005.

Frietag FG. Divalproex in the treatment of migraine. *Psychopharmacol Bull.* 37:98S, 2003.

Harel Z, et al. Supplementation with omega-3 polyunsaturated fatty acids in the management of recurrent migraines in adolescents. *J Adolesc Health.* 31:154, 2002.

Jansen SC, et al. Intolerance to dietary biogenic amines: a review. *Ann Allergy Asthma Immunol.* 91:233, 2003.

Jonas WB, et al. A critical overview of homeopathy. *Ann Intern Med.* 138:393, 2003.

Lewis DW, et al. The treatment of pediatric migraine. *Pediatr Ann.* 34:448, 2005.

Martin VT, et al. Symptoms of premenstrual syndrome and their association with migraine headache. *Headache* 46:125, 2006.

Millichap JG, Yee MM. The diet factor in pediatric and adolescent migraine. *Pediatr Neurol.* 28:9, 2003.

National Headache Foundation. Website. Summer food may trigger migraines. Accessed February 1, 2006 at http://www.headaches.org/consumer/pressreleases/SummerFoodMayTriggerMigraines0605.doc.

Wang F, et al. Oral magnesium oxide prophylaxis of frequent migrainous headache in children: a randomized, double-blind, placebo-controlled trial. *Headache* 43:601, 2003.

Wenzel R, et al. Migraine treatment. *Headache* 44:1059, 2004.

MULTIPLE SCLEROSIS

NUTRITIONAL ACUITY RANKING: LEVEL 2

DEFINITIONS AND BACKGROUND

Multiple sclerosis (MS) involves scarring and the loss of myelin sheath, the insulating material around nerve fibers. The disease causes progressive or episodic nerve degeneration and disability. The cause is not known. Insufficient vitamin D has been found to play a role, and those persons living in colder climates with less sun exposure are more prone (Esparza et al, 1995). Heredity has also been implicated.

There is evidence implicating proinflammatory cytokines such as tumor necrosis factor-alpha (TNF-α) in the pathogenesis of MS (Mikova et al, 2001). MS has a much higher incidence among Caucasians than in any other race; white females living in colder, wetter areas are more susceptible than those living in warmer areas (Johnson, 2000).

Symptoms and signs of MS include tingling; numbness in arms, legs, trunk, or face; double vision; fatigue; weakness; clumsiness; tremor; stiffness; sensory impairment; loss of position sense; and respiratory problems. Dysphagia is common in MS patients but is not a major complaint and does not usually cause nutritional failure of these patients (Thomas and Wiles, 1999). Spasticity and bladder dysfunction are also common (Klewer et al, 2001).

Onset is usually between 20 and 40 years of age (average age, 27 years old). After diagnosis, 70% of persons with MS are as active as previously. Women seem to have MS more often than men.

Proinflammatory cytokines, pathological iron deposition, and oxidative stress have been implicated in the pathogenesis (Mehindate et al, 2001). Toll-like receptors (TLRs) are part of an innate immune system that instructs the adaptive immune system (T and B cells and other cells and proteins) to launch an attack to suppress the invader (National MS Society, 2005).

Antioxidants may play a protective role. Supplementation with magnesium, vitamin B_6, vitamin B_{12}, zinc, vitamin D, vitamin E, selenium, and omega-3 fatty acids has been suggested (Johnson, 2000). Low vitamin D status has been specifically implicated in the etiology of multiple sclerosis (Kantarci and Wingerchuk, 2006; Munger et al, 2004; Holick, 2003). The optimal level of vitamin D intake required to support optimal immune function is not known but is likely to be at least that required for healthy bones and T-cell function (Cantorna and Mahan, 2004).

Vitamin B_{12} is important for proper myelination of the spinal cord; malnutrition during pregnancy and infancy may play a role in pathophysiology of this disorder (Montanha-Rojas et al, 2005).

The courses of MS are shown in Table 4-10.

INTERVENTION: OBJECTIVES

- During the chronic phase of the disease, treatment centers on reducing the incidence of respiratory infections and UTIs, managing bowel problems, controlling muscle spasms, preventing contractures and pressure ulcers, and correcting constipation and fecal impactions.
- Adjust caloric intake to avoid excessive weight gain, if this becomes a problem.
- Maintain good nutritional status. Since vitamin D seems to play a role in autoimmunity, be sure the diet is supple-

TABLE 4-10 Courses of Multiple Sclerosis

Course	Description
Benign	Few, mild early exacerbations with normal life expectancy and minimal disability (20% of cases).
Exacerbating/ remitting	More frequent early attacks with less complete clearing; long periods of stability, some disability (25% of cases).
Chronic/ relapsing	Fewer and less complete remissions after attacks; greater disability that may plateau after many years (20% will be ambulatory, 20% will be nonambulatory).
Chronic/ progressive	Onset is more insidious and more slowly progressive than chronic/relapsing (15% of cases).

mented with at least the recommended daily dose. Increased vitamin D intakes might decrease the incidence and severity of autoimmune diseases and the rate of bone fracture (Cantorna and Mahan, 2004).
- Reduce fatigue associated with mealtimes.
- During the active phase of the disease, corticosteroids may be used to decrease symptoms. Alter diet accordingly.
- Prevent chronic diseases such as coronary heart disease, which may be a problem with immobilization.

INTERVENTION: FOOD AND NUTRITION

- Normal protein and adequate carbohydrate intakes are recommended. Use olive oil and omega-3 fatty acids more frequently in the diet (Simopoulos, 2002).
- Provide adequate intake of multivitamins, especially vitamins D and B_{12}.
- Laxative foods and liquids may ease constipation.
- Reduce sodium intake during use of steroid therapy. Otherwise, sodium plays a role in lipid/protein transport in myelin tissues.
- Small, frequent meals may be better tolerated than large meals. If swallowing difficulties increase and coordination decreases, foods may need to be liquefied or fed by tube.
- To prevent UTIs, cranberry juice is quite effective (Raz et al, 2004; Howell, 2002).

CLINICAL INDICATORS

Clinical/History	Lab Work	
Height	Alb	Serum Fe
Weight	Chol	Gluc
BMI	Trig (may be low in autoimmune disorders)	MRI scan
Dietary/intake history	Na+, K+	Evoked potentials test
BP	Alk phos	CSF (WBC, γ-globulin are increased)
I & O	H & H	EEG
Edema		L:S ratio
Temperature		

Common Drugs Used and Potential Side Effects

- Interferon injections are useful treatments. Interferon-β1a (Avonex) may cause nausea, diarrhea, liver damage, flu-like symptoms, headache, infections, or anemia. Interferon-β1b (Betaseron) may cause weight changes, abdominal pain, diarrhea, constipation, fever, headache, hypertension, or tachycardia.
- Corticosteroids require controlled sodium intake while these drugs are being used. Glucose intolerance, negative nitrogen balance, and decreased serum zinc, calcium, and potassium may occur.
- Antispasticity drugs such as baclofen (Lioresal) may cause nausea, diarrhea, and constipation. Muscle relaxants may also be used.
- The immunosuppressant azathioprine (Imuran) reduces new brain lesions in relapsing-remitting MS (Massacesi et al, 2005).
- Women who use oral contraceptives for 3 years or longer may have a lower risk of MS.

Herbs, Botanicals, and Supplements

- Many patients with MS seek alternative therapies. The most frequently recommended therapies in one study included diet (52.4%), essential fatty acid supplements (44.6%), vitamin-mineral supplements (33.7%), homeopathy (30.7%), botanicals (22.3%), and antioxidants (18.1%); treatments were "very effective" for the early stages of MS (Shinto et al, 2004). The National MS Society has a useful website (http://www.nationalmssociety.org/Brochures-Vitamins.asp) that describes complementary and alternative medicine (CAM) therapy in this population.
- High doses of pyridoxine should not be taken with phenobarbital or phenytoin because seizure control might be compromised. If vitamin B_6 is added to either drug regimen, keep it at the lowest effective dose and monitor serum drug levels.
- St. John's wort should not be used with MAOI antidepressants, SSRI antidepressants, cyclosporine, digoxin, oral contraceptives, HIV protease inhibitors, theophylline, warfarin, or calcium channel blockers such as amlodipine, diltiazem, or verapamil. No studies have been conducted for efficacy in MS patients.
- Stinging nettle, pineapple, black currant, evening primrose, and purslane have been recommended for MS, but no clinical trials have proven efficacy.

INTERVENTION: NUTRITION EDUCATION, COUNSELING, CARE MANAGEMENT

- Teach the patient how to control caloric intake, especially if inactive.
- Teach the patient about sources of linoleic acid and omega-3 fatty acids in the diet. Discuss the role of fat and vitamin E in myelin sheath formation and maintenance.
- Teach the patient about foods high in fiber.
- Avoid total inactivity. Physical therapy may be beneficial.
- Encourage moderate exposure to sunlight for the vitamin D.
- Utensils with large handles may be useful in food preparation and self-feeding.
- At a restaurant, foods may need to be cut before serving.
- Use tabletop cooking methods and equipment to avoid lifting.
- Allergen-free, gluten-free, pectin-free, fructose-restricted, raw foods diets and liquid diets have been ineffective.
- Avoid smoking.

Patient Education—Foodborne Illness

- Careful food handling will be important. The same is true for sanitizing work area before and after preparing tube feedings to prevent contamination. Formula companies have good information on safe handling of formula in the home and institution.

For More Information

- Consortium of Multiple Sclerosis Centers
http://www.mscare.org
- Multiple Sclerosis Association of America
http://www.msaa.com
- National MS Society
http://www.nmss.org/

MULTIPLE SCLEROSIS—CITED REFERENCES

Cantorna MT, Mahan BD. Mounting evidence for vitamin D as an environmental factor affecting autoimmune disease prevalence. *Exp Biol Med.* 229:1136, 2004.

Esparza M, et al. Nutrition, latitude, and multiple sclerosis mortality: an ecologic study. *Am J Epidemiol.* 142:733, 1995.

Holick MF. Vitamin D: a millenium perspective. *J Cell Biochem.* 88:296, 2003.

Howell AB. Cranberry proanthocyanidins and the maintenance of urinary tract health. *Crit Rev Food Sci Nutr.* 42(suppl):273, 2002.

Johnson S. The possible role of gradual accumulation of copper, cadmium, lead and iron and gradual depletion of zinc, magnesium, selenium, vitamins B2, B6, D, and E and essential fatty acids in multiple sclerosis. *Med Hypotheses.* 55:239, 2000.

Kantarci O, Wingerchuk D. Epidemiology and natural history of multiple sclerosis: new insights. *Curr Opin Neurol.* 19:248, 2006.

Klewer J, et al. Problems reported by elderly patients with multiple sclerosis. *J Neurosci Nurs.* 33:167, 2001.

Massacesi L, et al. Efficacy of azathioprine on multiple sclerosis new brain lesions evaluated using magnetic resonance imaging. *Arch Neurol.* 62:1843, 2005.

Mehindate K, et al. Proinflammatory cytokines promote glial heme oxygenase-1 expression and mitochondrial iron deposition: implications for multiple sclerosis. *J Neurochem.* 77:1386, 2001.

Mikova O, et al. Increased serum tumor necrosis factor alpha concentrations in major depression and multiple sclerosis. *Eur Neuropsychopharmacol.* 11:203, 2001.

Montanha-Rojas EA, et al. Myelin basic protein accumulation is impaired in a model of protein deficiency during development. *Nutr Neurosci.* 8:49, 2005.

Munger KL, et al. Vitamin D intake and incidence of multiple sclerosis. *Neurology* 62:60, 2004.

National MS Society. Toll-like receptors: newly discovered molecules play possible role in MS. Accessed November 28, 2005 at http://www.nationalmssociety.org/Highlights-Toll.asp.

Raz R, et al. Cranberry juice and urinary tract infection. *Clin Infect Dis.* 38:1413, 2004.

Shinto L, et al. Complementary and alternative medicine in multiple sclerosis: survey of licensed naturopaths. *J Altern Complement Med.* 10:891, 2004.

Simopoulos AP. Omega-3 fatty acids in inflammation and autoimmune diseases. *J Am Coll Nutr.* 21:495, 2002.

Thomas F, Wiles C. Dysphagia and nutritional status in multiple sclerosis. *J Neurol.* 246:677, 1999.

MYASTHENIA GRAVIS AND NEUROMUSCULAR JUNCTION DISORDERS

NUTRITIONAL ACUITY RANKING: LEVEL 2

DEFINITIONS AND BACKGROUND

Myasthenia gravis (MG) is an autoimmune disorder caused by autoantibodies against the nicotinic acetylcholine receptor on the postsynaptic membrane at the neuromuscular junction (Thanvi and Lo, 2004; Baraka, 2001). Some types are congenital, but others can be acquired.

The thymus gland is involved in the autosensitization process, and the disease frequently is associated with thymic morphologic abnormalities. There is consensus that removal of the thymus gland is imperative in MG (Juel and Massey, 2005). An early, safe, and complete thymectomy offers benefits to a patient with MG with minimal risk for morbidity and postoperative pain (Meyers and Cooper, 2001).

Symptoms and signs include drooping eyelids, double vision, fatigue, general weakness, dysphagia, weak voice, inability to walk on heels, and pneumonia. MG occurs in 50–125 in 1,000,000 individuals (approximately 25,000 affected people in the United States). Incidence begins with the first peak in the third decade and a second peak in the sixth decade (Thanvi and Lo, 2004). Plasmapheresis can be used during a crisis to remove the abnormal antibodies.

A myasthenic crisis is defined as the need for mechanical ventilatory support; approximately 16% of all patients experience a crisis with progressive weakness, oropharyngeal symptoms, refractoriness to anticholinesterase medication, intercurrent infection, and invasive procedures including needle biopsies of thymic gland masses (Younger and Raksadawan, 2001).

Acquired neuromuscular junction disorders include botulism, autoimmune MG, and drug-induced MG. When MG is suspected, tests will be needed. A tensilon test involves insertion of a small intravenous catheter through which tensilon is given; this very short-acting drug blocks the degradation of acetylcholine. The short-term availability of acetylcholine results in improved muscle function, often in the eye area.

Diabetes, sleep apnea, and thyroid problems are common in persons who have MG. Management of these secondary conditions should be closely monitored.

INTERVENTION: OBJECTIVES

- Increase the likelihood of obtaining adequate nutrition by altering the consistency of foods. This is necessary when muscles used in chewing and swallowing are weakened.
- Feedings should be small to reduce fatigue.
- Prevent permanent structural damage to the neuromuscular system.
- Allow adequate time to complete meals.

INTERVENTION: FOOD AND NUTRITION

- Diet should include frequent, small feedings of easily masticated foods.

- Provide tube feeding when needed.
- Provide adequate potassium supplements.
- If corticosteroids are part of treatment, use a low-sodium diet.
- Use a high-energy diet if weight loss occurs, which is common.
- The use of lecithin and choline has been successful in some cases but has not been documented consistently.
- Avoid giving medications with coffee or fruit juice; give with milk and crackers or bread.

CLINICAL INDICATORS

Clinical/History		
Height	Tensilon test	Acetylcholine antibodies test
Weight	Chest CT scan for thymoma	Electromyogram
BMI	**Lab Work**	Gluc
Dietary/intake history	Na+, K+	Mg++, Ca++
I & O	BP	Alb
Weight changes	CRP	H & H
		Serum Fe

Common Drugs Used and Potential Side Effects

- Control of MG is provided by the use of immunosuppressants, usually prednisone. It is usually started at a high dose every day, and then reduced to every other day. In the event of intolerable side effects or failure of treatment, other immunosuppressants may be used, most commonly azathioprine (Imuran). GI distress, nausea, vomiting, and anorexia may occur.
- Transient symptomatic control can be achieved by the initiation of a medication (pyridostigmine [Mestinon]) that blocks the degradation of acetylcholine at the neuromuscular junction, increasing the level of acetylcholine with better muscle response to stimulation by the nerve. Mestinon is a temporary symptomatic treatment and does not reverse the course of the illness. Limit sodium intake. Anorexia, abdominal cramps, diarrhea, and weakness may result. Long-acting capsules may be needed if morning weakness is persistent.
- Long-term use of antacids negatively affects calcium and magnesium metabolism.

Herbs, Botanicals, and Supplements

- No studies have been conducted for efficacy of herbs or botanicals in MG patients.

INTERVENTION: NUTRITION EDUCATION, COUNSELING, CARE MANAGEMENT

- Show the patient how to prepare foods and nutrient-dense beverages with the use of a blender, if necessary.
- Indicate how to take medication with food or milk. Discuss potential side effects.
- Avoidance of alcohol is important.
- Food and utensils should be arranged within reach of the patient.

Patient Education—Foodborne Illness

- Careful food handling will be important. The same is true for sanitizing work area before and after preparing tube feedings to prevent contamination. Formula companies have good information on safe handling of formula in the home and institution.

For More Information

- Myasthenia Gravis Foundation of America
  http://www.myasthenia.org/
- Neuromuscular Junction Disorders
  http://www.neuro.wustl.edu/neuromuscular/synmg.html

MYASTHENIA GRAVIS AND NEUROMUSCULAR JUNCTION DISORDERS—CITED REFERENCES

Baraka A. Anesthesia and critical care of thymectomy for myasthenia gravis. *Chest Surg Clin N Am.* 11:337, 2001.

Juel VC, Massey SM. Autoimmune myasthenia gravis: recommendations for treatment and immunologic modulation. *Curr Treat Options Neurol.* 7:3, 2005.

Meyers B, Cooper J. Transcervical thymectomy for myasthenia gravis. *Chest Surg Clin N Am.* 11:363, 2001.

Thanvi BR, Lo TC. Update on myasthenia gravis. *Postgrad Med J.* 80:690, 2004.

Younger D, Raksadawan N. Medical therapies in myasthenia gravis. *Chest Surg Clin N Am.* 11:329, 2001.

PARKINSON'S DISEASE

NUTRITIONAL ACUITY RANKING: LEVEL 2

DEFINITIONS AND BACKGROUND

Parkinson's disease (PD) is a neuromuscular disorder resulting from diminished levels of dopamine at the basal ganglia of the brain that causes tremor of hands, arms, legs, jaw, and face; rigidity of limbs and trunk; slowness of gait; and coordination difficulty. Problems with chewing, speaking, or swallowing can occur. Approximately 24 conditions are categorized as PDs. Approximately 1–1.5 million people are affected.

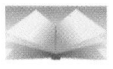

A test for PD progression includes decline in ability to smell, depression, and speed of wrist movements. About 30% of those with PD get depression and dementia-related symptoms (Rodriguez and Arenas, 2001). Figure 4-4 shows effects of PD.

Levodopa must be provided. Men are affected slightly more often than women. The disease is also more common after 60 years of age, and life expectancy is 12.5 years after diagnosis. Studies suggest that there is significant variation in the prevalence of PD between different populations; rates are highest in populations of European origin, suggesting that there may be a genetic link (Muthane et al, 2001).

Causes and pathophysiology are poorly understood. Altered brain energy metabolism occurs. Men with low total and LDL cholesterol levels may have an increased risk of PD. A high intake of unsaturated fatty acids may protect against PD (de Lau et al, 2005).

Long-term exposure to manganese, herbicides, or pesticides and high intake of iron, especially in combination with high manganese intake, may promote onset of PD symptoms (Ascherio et al, 2006; Fitsanakis et al, 2006; Powers et al, 2003). Sometimes, use of medications such as major tranquilizers or metoclopramide can cause PD-like symptoms; cessation of those medications may be needed.

Neuroprotection is being studied as a means of combating PD. If oxidative stress initiates or promotes degeneration of neurons, then antioxidant therapy, such as with vitamin E, may reduce the rate of progression (Prasad, 1999). Drinking 4–5 cups of coffee daily may be preventive (Benedetti, 2000; Honig, 2000; Ross et al, 2000). Because unsaturated fatty acids are important constituents of neuronal cell membranes with neuroprotective, antioxidant, and anti-inflammatory properties, high intake of unsaturated fatty acids might protect against PD (de Lau et al, 2005).

Data suggest that high-calorie diets and elevated homocysteine levels may render the brain vulnerable to neurodegenerative disorders (Mattson, 2003). Folate therapy does not seem to be singularly protective (Chen et al, 2004).

Esophageal motor abnormalities are frequent in PD and may appear at an early stage of the disease (Bassotti et al, 1998). About 60–80% of PD patients also suffer from constipation; constipation appears about 10–20 years prior to motor symptoms (Ueki and Otsuka, 2004).

Unintentional weight loss is common, resulting in increased morbidity and mortality. Weight loss occurs from increased energy expenditure due to tremor, dyskinesias, and rigidity; reduced energy intake due to olfactory dysfunction, cognitive impairment, depression, dysphagia, and disability; and medication-related side effects, including dry mouth, nausea/vomiting, appetite loss, anorexia, insomnia, fatigue, and anxiety (Chen et al, 2003; Holden, 2000).

There are various treatments and algorithms for management of PD (Olanow et al, 2001). PD is progressive. Dietary vitamin E may have a neuroprotective effect attenuating the risk of PD (Etminan et al, 2005). Other nutrients are being studied.

INTERVENTION: OBJECTIVES

- Supply dopamine to the brain with drugs. Monitor diet therapy accordingly.
- Maintain optimal physical and emotional health.
- Exercise may be protective, especially for men (Carne et al, 2005).
- Improve the patient's ability to eat. Use semisolid foods rather than fluids if sucking/swallowing reflexes are reduced. Drooling may also be a problem. (See Dysphagia entry in Section 7.)

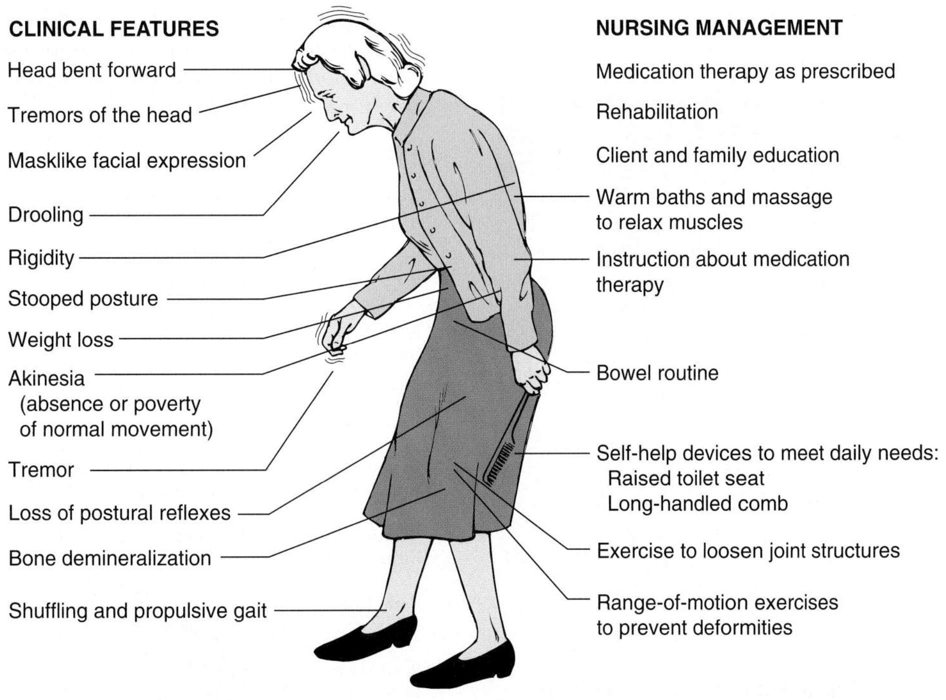

Figure 4-4 Effects of Parkinson's disease. (LifeART image, copyright 2006, Lippincott Williams & Wilkins. All rights reserved.)

- Provide adequate energy to prevent weight loss (Chen et al, 2003). Avoid obesity as well.
- Provide adequate hydration.
- Correct alterations in GI function (i.e., increased transit time, heartburn, and constipation).
- Preserve functioning; delay chronic disability as long as possible.

INTERVENTION: FOOD AND NUTRITION

- A high intake of protein diminishes the effectiveness of levodopa; use 0.5 g/kg body weight. If unplanned weight loss is a problem, 1–1.5 g/kg may be needed. For some, a protein redistribution diet is used (i.e., low-protein breakfast and lunch with high-protein dinner and snack) but this is not always effective.
- In the rare use of levodopa alone, vitamin B_6 foods should be consumed, such as dry skim milk, peas and beans, sweet potatoes, yams, avocado, fortified cereal, bran, oatmeal, wheat germ, yeast, pork, beef organs, tuna, and fresh salmon.
- Query patient about choking. Request a swallow evaluation from a speech therapist to determine proper consistency of foods, and plan diet accordingly. Cut, mince, or soften foods as required. Use small meals if needed.
- Add crushed bran to hot cereal for fiber; prune juice may be needed.
- A multivitamin-mineral supplement may be beneficial, especially for vitamin C (Martin et al, 2002) and B-complex vitamins. Elevated homocysteine levels may play a role in PD; use of folate and vitamins B_6 and B_{12} will be important (Grimble, 2006).
- Highlight foods that are high in vitamin E, such as vegetable oils, salad dressings, and nuts.

CLINICAL INDICATORS

Clinical/History	Lab Work	
Height	Na+, K+	Ca++, Mg++
Weight	N balance	Serum manganese
BMI	H & H	Serum homocysteine
Dietary/intake history	Serum Fe	Serum folate
BP	Alb, transthyretin	Serum B_{12}
I & O	Dopamine	
Dysphagia	Norepinephrine	
Tremors	BUN, Creat	
Depression, anorexia	ALT, AST	
	Gluc	
Constipation	Uric acid	

Common Drugs Used and Potential Side Effects

- See Table 4-11.

Herbs, Botanicals, and Supplements

- No studies have been conducted for efficacy of herbs or botanicals in PD patients; fava bean, evening primrose, St. John's wort, passionflower, velvet bean, and gingko have been suggested but not proven.
- Kava should not be taken in patients with PD because it decreases effectiveness of medications.
- Ginseng, ma huang (ephedra), yohimbe, and St. John's wort should not be used with MAOIs, including selegiline (Eldepryl).

INTERVENTION: NUTRITION EDUCATION, COUNSELING, CARE MANAGEMENT

- Education for the patient and family, access to support groups, regular exercise, and good nutrition are essential (Koller, 2002).
- Explain how to blenderize food and how to make food and beverages more nutrient dense, as needed.
- Help patient to control weight, which may fluctuate from reduced mobility or inability to ingest sufficient quantities.
- Place all foods within easy reach of the patient.
- Braces may help the patient control severe tremors at mealtime.
- Music therapy helps to relieve depression and improves balance.
- Discuss how to resolve issues such as weight loss, constipation, osteopenia, gastroesophageal reflux disease (GERD), side effects of medications, xerostomia, and dehydration.
- There may be a correlation between negativism, pessimism, anxiety, and PD; further studies are needed.

Patient Education—Foodborne Illness

- Careful food handling will be important. The same is true for sanitizing work area before and after preparing tube feedings to prevent contamination. Formula companies have good information on safe handling of formula in the home and institution.

For More Information

- American Parkinson's Disease Association
  http://www.apdaparkinson.org/user/index.asp
- Michael J. Fox Foundation for Parkinson's Research
  http://www.MichaelJFox.org/
- National Parkinson's Foundation
  http://www.parkinson.org/
- Parkinson's Disease Foundation, Inc.
  http://www.pdf.org/
- Parkinson's Disease: Guidelines for MNT
  http://www.nutritionucanlivewith.com/
- Parkinson's Genetic Research Group
  http://depts.washington.edu/pgrgroup/
- Parkinson's Web
  http://pdweb.mgh.harvard.edu
- Society for Neuroscience
  http://web.sfn.org/
- Young Parkinson's
  http://www.youngparkinsons.org/pages/index/siteindex.htm

TABLE 4-11 Medications for Parkinson's Disease and Possible Side Effects

Medication	Side Effects
Antidepressants	Weight gain, dry mouth, or nausea can result.
Anticholinergics: Cogentin (benztropine), Artane (trihexyphenidyl), Kemadrin (procyclidine)	Confusion, agitation, dizziness, sedation, euphoria, tachycardia, hypotension, dry mouth, constipation, nausea, urinary retention, and blurred vision.
Antiviral agent: Symmetrel (amantadine)	Possible adverse effects include anorexia, dry mouth, nausea, constipation, dizziness, insomnia, blurred vision, depression, ataxia, confusion, fatigue, leg/ankle edema, hallucinations, anxiety, and livedo reticularis (skin discoloration).
Catechol-O-methyltransferase inhibitors: Tasmar (tolcapone), Comtan (entacapone)	Diarrhea, orthostatic hypotension, hallucinations, sleep disturbances, dyskinesias, muscle cramping, and vivid dreams.
Dopamine agonists: Permax (pergolide), Parlodel (bromocriptine), Mirapex (pramipexole), Requip (ropinirole)	Possible adverse effects include nausea, headache, fatigue, confusion, hallucinations, somnolence, and "sleep attacks." With ropinirole, fewer side effects, such as dyskinesia, have been identified. Some studies suggest that dopamine agonists, rather than levodopa, should be the initial symptomatic therapy in Parkinson's disease; levodopa is often started first in some patients because of patient age, cognitive status, or cost of drugs (Koller, 2002).
Apokyn (apomorphine hydrochloride)	Approved in 2004 for the treatment of acute, intermittent hypomobility episodes associated with advanced Parkinson's disease.
Ibuprofen	Users of ibuprofen are less likely to develop Parkinson's disease than nonusers.
Levodopa/carbidopa: Sinemet, Sinemet CR, Atamet, Madopar	Possible adverse effects include nausea, dyskinesia, weakness, hallucinations, mental confusion, orthostatic hypotension, fatigue, daytime sleepiness, insomnia, elevated serum glucose and homocysteine, and anemia. Large neutral amino acids block levodopa absorption, both from the gut and at the blood–brain barrier. Levodopa preparations should be taken 30–60 minutes prior to meals, and intake of vitamin B_6 should be limited to RDA levels. Up to 15 mg of vitamin B_6 can be taken daily in either food or supplement form. Today's preparations combine levodopa with carbidopa or benserazide, which prevents peripheral decarboxylation of levodopa. Increase intake of foods rich in vitamin B_{12}, folate (Yasui et al, 2000), and vitamin C.
MAO type B inhibitor: Eldepryl (selegiline)	Insomnia, dry mouth, confusion, hypertension, abdominal pain, and weight loss. Selegiline should not be used with ginseng, ma huang (ephedra), yohimbe, or St. John's wort.

PARKINSON'S DISEASE—CITED REFERENCES

Ascherio A, et al. Pesticide exposure and risk for Parkinson's disease. *Ann Neurol.* 2006. In press.

Bassotti G, et al. Esophageal manometric abnormalities in Parkinson's disease. *Dysphagia* 13:28, 1998.

Benedetti M, et al. Smoking, alcohol, and coffee consumption preceding Parkinson's disease: a case-control study. *Neurology* 55:1350, 2000.

Carne W, et al. Efficacy of a multidisciplinary treatment program on one-year outcomes of individuals with Parkinson's disease. *Neurorehabilitation* 20:161, 2005.

Chen H, et al. Folate intake and risk of Parkinson's disease. *Am J Epidemiol.* 160:368, 2004.

Chen H, et al. Weight loss in Parkinson's disease. *Ann Neurol.* 53:676, 2003.

de Lau LM, et al. Dietary fatty acids and the risk of Parkinson disease: the Rotterdam study. *Neurology* 64:2040, 2005.

Etminan M, et al. Intake of vitamin E, vitamin C, and carotenoids and the risk of Parkinson's disease: a meta-analysis. *Lancet Neurol.* 4:362, 2005.

Fitsanakis VA, et al. The use of magnetic resonance imaging (MRI) in the study of manganese neurotoxicity. *Neurotoxicology* 27:798, 2006.

Grimble RF. The effects of sulfur amino acid intake on immune function in humans. *J Nutr.* 136:1660S, 2006.

Holden K. Unintentional weight loss. In: *Parkinson's disease: guidelines for medical nutrition therapy.* 1st ed. Ft. Collins, CO: Five Star Living, Inc., 2000.

Honig L. Relationship between caffeine intake and Parkinson's disease. *JAMA.* 284:1378, 2000.

Koller WC. Treatment of early Parkinson's disease. *Neurology* 58:S79, 2002.

Martin A, et al. Roles of vitamins E and C on neurodegenerative diseases and cognitive performance. *Nutr Rev.* 60:308, 2002.

Mattson MP. Will caloric restriction and folate protect against AD and PD? *Neurology* 60:690, 2003.

Muthane U, et al. Hunting genes in Parkinson's disease from the roots. *Med Hypotheses.* 57:51, 2001.

Olanow C, et al. An algorithm (decision tree) for the management of Parkinson's disease (2001): treatment guidelines. *Neurology* 56:S1, 2001.

Powers KM, et al. Parkinson's disease risks associated with dietary iron, manganese, and other nutrient intakes. *Neurology* 60:1761, 2003.

Prasad K, et al. Multiple antioxidants in prevention and treatment of Parkinson's disease. *J Am Col Nutr.* 8:413, 1999.

Ross G, et al. Association of coffee and caffeine intake with the risk of Parkinson's disease. *JAMA.* 283:2674, 2000.

Rodriguez J, Arenas A. Variables affecting cognitive deterioration in Parkinson's disease. *Rev Neurol.* 32:107, 2001.

Ueki A, Otsuka M. Life style risks of Parkinson's disease: association between decreased water intake and constipation. *J Neurol.* 251:II18, 2004.

Yasui K, et al. Plasma homocysteine and MTHFR C677T genotype in levodopa-treated patients with PD. *Neurology* 55:437, 2000.

SPINAL CORD INJURY

NUTRITIONAL ACUITY RANKING: LEVEL 3

DEFINITIONS AND BACKGROUND

Spinal cord injury (SCI) is often caused by traffic accidents, falls, diving accidents, sports injury, or gunshot wounds. Partial versus total self-care deficits depend on resulting hemiplegia, diplegia, paraplegia (thoracic or lumbar cord), or quadriplegia (cervical cord).

Classification of SCI usually includes cause, direction of injury, level of injury, stability of vertebral column, and degree of cord involvement. The nervous system of a patient with neurological trauma is vulnerable to glucose and oxygen variations and variations in other nutrients.

Vitamin levels may be related to function, general health, and pressure ulcer incidence in persons with SCI (Moussavi et al, 2003). Vitamin B_{12} deficiency is common and should be managed (Petchkrua et al, 2003). Pressure ulcers are very common in this population. See Section 2 for management of pressure ulcers.

After long-term immobility, SCI patients may require weight loss. There has been success with a 12-week program incorporating psychosocial, behavioral, and dietary interventions (Chen et al, 2006).

INTERVENTION: OBJECTIVES

Immediate

- Monitor for acid–base and electrolyte imbalances. Assess needs on admission and then daily thereafter.
- Reduce the danger of aspiration by avoiding oral feedings if patient has been vomiting.
- Ensure adequate fluid and calcium intake to prevent renal stones.
- Increase opportunities for rehabilitation by monitoring weight changes; loss of 10–30% in the first month is common.
- Prevent UTIs, paralytic ileus, pneumonia, malnutrition, pressure ulcer, constipation, stress ulcer, and fecal impaction. Neurologic deficits can be compounded by complications such as acute respiratory distress syndrome (ARDS) and aspiration pneumonia (Munro, 2000).

Long Term

- Mobilize, prevent complications, and regain independence as far as possible. Monitor for weight gain since excessive weight gain can lead to pressure ulcers and make transfers more difficult. Maintain an ideal body weight.
- Promote neuronal growth and survival, encourage the formation of synapses, enhance the production of myelin, and restore conduction capabilities and thus restore the compromised circuitry in the injured spinal cord.
- Prevent long-term problems. Osteoporosis and risk of fracture increase in this population (Ott, 2001).

INTERVENTION: FOOD AND NUTRITION

- Provide patient with intravenous solutions as soon as possible after injury. Check blood gas measurements and chemistries. Once peristalsis returns, patient may be tube fed. Elevate head of bed 30–45°, if possible, to prevent aspiration.
- Paraplegics initially need 1.5–1.7 g protein/kg. Progress to more normal intake, such as 1.2–1.5 g/kg, when nitrogen balance returns.

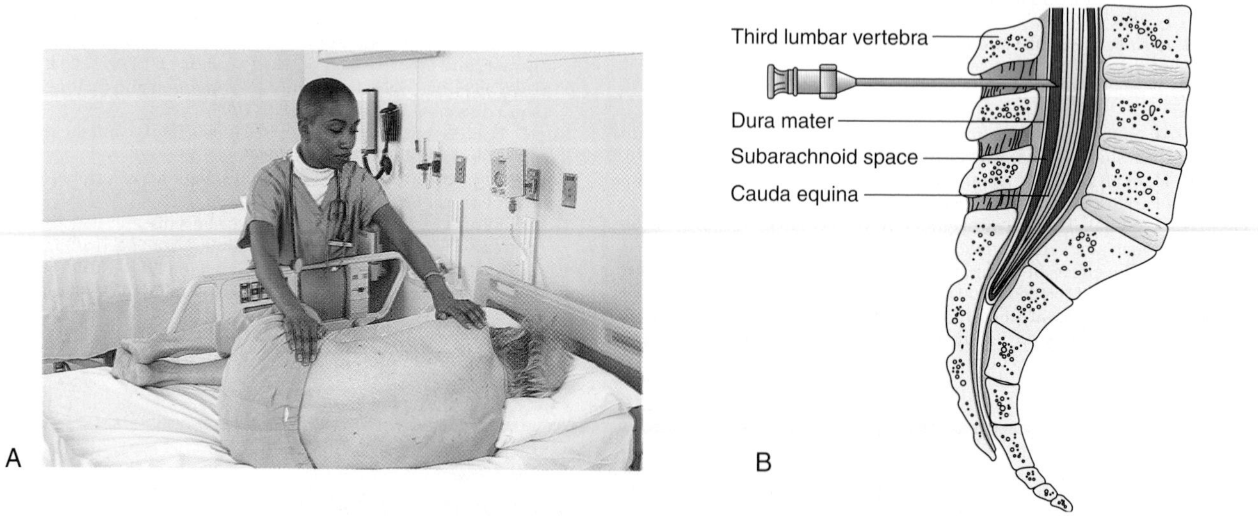

Figure 4-5 Spinal tap. (From Smeltzer SC, Bare BG. *Textbook of medical-surgical nursing.* 9th ed. Philadelphia: Lippincott Williams & Wilkins, 2000.)

- Monitor weight: paraplegics should be at lower end of normal BMI range. Quadriplegics should be about 15–20 lb below ideal body weight.
- Determine energy needs by indirect calorimetry. If unavailable, use these guidelines (O'Brien, 1990):
  - Paraplegic: subtract 5–10% from ideal body weight.
  - Quadriplegic: subtract 10–15% from ideal body weight.
- Ensure adequate CHO and fat intake, including at least 1–2% essential fatty acids (EFA).
- Encourage adequate fluid and fiber. Be careful about gas-forming foods; monitor tolerance.
- Ensure adequate intake of thiamine, niacin, vitamins B_6, B_{12}, and C, and amino acids. Monitor iron stores and adjust diet as needed.
- Provide adequate vitamin D and calcium intake to prevent fractures and osteoporosis, which are common (Ott, 2001).
- With hypertension, the DASH diet may be useful (increases in calcium, potassium, and magnesium are beneficial).
- Monitor intake of antioxidants, which tend to be lower in this population (Burri and Neidlinger, 2002).
- Tube feeding should be used if needed. There are no significant differences between early feeding and delayed feeding (Dvorak et al, 2004). PEG tube is the preferred method (Dwyer et al, 2002).

CLINICAL INDICATORS

Clinical/History	Alb, transthyretin	MRI or CT scan
Height	Na+, K+	pCO_2, pO_2
Weight	Creat (eventually decreased)	PT or INR
BMI	BUN	Ca++, Mg++
Dietary/intake history	Gluc	Hypercalciuria
I & O	Cervical x-rays	Parathormone (may be low)
BP (tends to be elevated)	Somatosensory-evoked potentials	25-hydroxyvitamin D
Lab Work	Myelogram (see Fig. 4-5 for a spinal tap)	N balance
H & H (decreased)		Erythrocyte sedimentation rate (ESR)
Serum Fe		CRP
		Serum B_{12}

Common Drugs Used and Potential Side Effects

- Corticosteroids such as prednisone are used to prevent swelling. Long-term use can cause hyperglycemia and nitrogen, calcium, and potassium losses. Sodium retention occurs.
- Analgesics for pain relief (e.g., aspirin/salicylates) can prolong bleeding time. GI bleeding may eventually result. An increased intake of vitamin C and folacin is needed.
- Laxatives may be used; encourage fiber and fluid instead.
- Anabolic steroids (oxandrolone) are being tested for their ability to help with healing of pressure ulcers. These medications help increase appetite in anorexic persons.
- To protect against fractures, bisphosphonates may help prevent acute bone loss; oral routes must not be used in recumbent patients (Ott, 2001).

Herbs, Botanicals, and Supplements

- Studies have found usefulness in pretreatment of patients with creatine for neuroprotection before spinal surgery; further studies are needed to evaluate the benefit of immediate creatine administration in case of acute spinal cord injury (Hausmann et al, 2002).

INTERVENTION: NUTRITION EDUCATION, COUNSELING, CARE MANAGEMENT

- Provide weight control measures for successful rehabilitation (Chen et al, 2006).
- Teach patient about good sources of iron and other minerals, vitamins, and protein.
- Help promote a structured feeding routine. Feed slowly (over 30–45 minutes). Bites of food should be small.
- Discuss long-term risks of heart disease.
- Encourage participation in weight-bearing exercise to reduce calcium loss and risk of fracture or osteoporosis.

Patient Education—Foodborne Illness

- Careful food handling will be important. The same is true for sanitizing work area before and after preparing tube feedings to prevent contamination. Formula companies have good information on safe handling of formula in the home and institution.

For More Information

- American Association of Spinal Cord Injury Nurses (AASCIN)
  http://www.aascin.org/
- Christopher Reeve Paralysis Foundation
  http://www.christopherreeve.org/
- Cure Paralysis Now
  http://www.cureparalysisnow.org/
- Foundation for Spinal Cord Injury Prevention, Care, & Cure
  http://www.fscip.org/
- Model Spinal Cord Injury System Dissemination Center
  http://www.mscisdisseminationcenter.org/
- National Spinal Cord Injury Association
  http://www.spinalcord.org/
- Paralyzed Veterans of America
  http://www.pva.org
- Spinal Cord Injury Information Network
  http://www.spinalcord.uab.edu/

SPINAL CORD INJURY—CITED REFERENCES

Burri BJ, Neidlinger TR. Dietary intakes and serum concentrations of vitamin E and total carotenoids of healthy adults with severe physical disabilities are lower than matched controls. *J Am Diet Assoc.* 102: 1804, 2002.

Chen Y, et al. Obesity intervention in persons with spinal cord injury. *Spinal Cord.* 44:82, 2006.
Dvorak MF, et al. Early versus late enteral feeding in patients with acute cervical spinal cord injury: a pilot study. *Spine* 29:E175, 2004.
Dwyer KM, et al. Percutaneous endoscopic gastrostomy: the preferred method of elective feeding tube placement in trauma patients. *J Trauma.* 52:26, 2002.
Hausmann ON, et al. Protective effects of oral creatine supplementation on spinal cord injury in rats. *Spinal Cord.* 40:449, 2002.
Moussavi RM, et al. Serum levels of vitamins A, C, and E in persons with chronic spinal cord injury living in the community. *Arch Phys Med Rehabil.* 84:1061, 2003.
Munro N. Pulmonary challenges in neurotrauma. *Crit Care Nurs Clin North Am.* 12:457, 2000.
O'Brien RY. Spinal cord injury. In: Gines DJ, ed. *Nutrition management in rehabilitation.* Rockville, MD: Aspen Publishers, Inc, 1990, p. 165.
Ott SM. Osteoporosis in women with spinal cord injuries. *Phys Med Rehabil Clin N Am.* 12:111, 2001.
Petchkrua W, et al. Vitamin B12 deficiency in spinal cord injury: a retrospective study. *J Spinal Cord Med.* 26:116, 2003.

STROKE (CEREBROVASCULAR ACCIDENT)

NUTRITIONAL ACUITY RANKING: LEVEL 3

DEFINITIONS AND BACKGROUND

A cerebrovascular accident (CVA) (stroke) is caused by damage to a portion of the brain resulting from loss of blood supply due to a blood vessel spasm, clot, or rupture. Transient ischemic attacks (TIAs) are brief episodes of blood loss to the brain from a clot or an embolism; 10% of victims have a major CVA within a year. Stroke patients need to be seen medically within 60 minutes to begin appropriate treatment. Some people recover completely; others may be seriously disabled or die. Strokes cause 10% of all fatalities in the United States. The most common symptoms are listed in Table 4-12.

Hypertension, smoking, diabetes mellitus, atrial fibrillation, and oral contraceptive use are key risk factors for strokes. High HDL cholesterol levels are protective against ischemic stroke in the elderly (Sacco et al, 2001). Obesity and weight gain are important risk factors for ischemic and total stroke but not for hemorrhagic stroke in women, according to the Nurse's Health Study (Rexrode et al, 1997). Figure 4-6 shows an ischemic stroke.

Unconsciousness, paralysis, and other problems may occur depending on the site and extent of the brain damage. Left CVA affects sight and hearing most commonly, including the ability to see where foods are placed on a plate or tray. Patients with a right-hemisphere, bilateral, or brainstem CVA have significant problems with feeding and swallowing of food; speech problems also occur.

Neurogenic deficits may include motor deficits with muscle weakness of the tongue and lips; nerve damage with resulting lack of coordination; apraxia; sensory deficits with inability to feel food in the mouth; and cognitive deficits with difficulty sustaining attention, poor short-term memory, visual field problems, impulsiveness, aphasia, and judgment problems such as not knowing how much food to take or what to do with the food once it reaches the mouth.

A dietary pattern with higher intakes of red and processed meats, refined grains, and sweets and desserts may increase stroke risk, whereas a diet higher in fruits and vegetables, fish, and whole grains may protect against stroke (Fung et al, 2004). Intake of cruciferous and green leafy vegetables and citrus fruits and juice may be especially protective against risk of ischemic stroke (Joshipura et al, 1999). Carotenoids seem to be protective as well (Hak et al, 2004).

Among elderly individuals, consumption of tuna or other broiled or baked fish is associated with lower risk of ischemic stroke, while intake of fried fish or fish sandwiches is associated with higher risk; potential mechanisms and alternate explanations warrant further study (Mozaffarian et al, 2005). Both fish and omega-3 fatty acids seem to prevent thrombotic strokes without increasing hemorrhagic strokes among middle-aged women (Iso et al, 2001).

Risk reductions from controlled trials with vitamin E have not been consistent (Pearce et al, 2000; Eidelman et al, 2004). However, at the cellular level, vitamin E acts by inhibiting smooth muscle cell proliferation, platelet aggregation, monocyte adhesion, and cytokine production, reactions that are implied in the progression of atherosclerosis (Muntaneau et al, 2004). Vitamin E also influences the activity of several enzymes (e.g., PKC, PP2A, COX-2, 5-lipooxygenase,

TABLE 4-12 Most Common Stroke Symptoms

- Sudden numbness or weakness of face, arm, or leg, especially on one side of the body
- Sudden confusion, trouble speaking or understanding
- Sudden trouble seeing in one or both eyes
- Sudden trouble walking, dizziness, loss of balance or coordination
- Sudden severe headache with no known cause

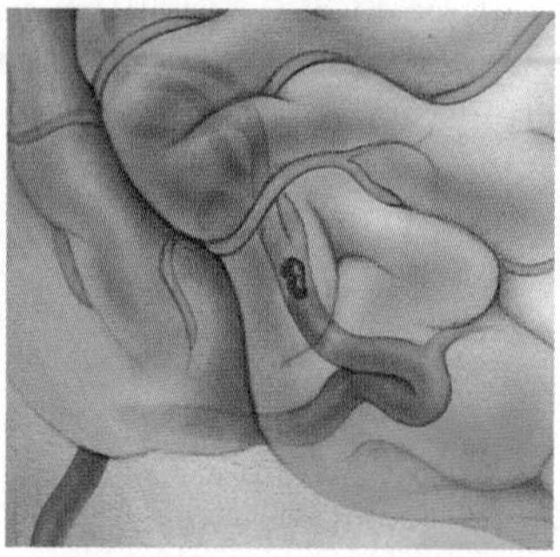

Figure 4-6 Ischemic stroke. (Image provided by Anatomical Chart Co.)

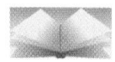

nitric oxide synthase, NADPH-oxidase, superoxide dismutase, and phospholipase A2) and modulates gene expression (Muntaneau et al, 2004). Because of these factors, it is wise to include adequate amounts but not excesses; dietary mayonnaise, margarine, and nuts are useful (Yochum et al, 2000).

Vitamin C levels tend to be lower among stroke patients, probably due to the relationship to inflammation and oxidative stress (Sanchez-Moreno et al, 2004). A high vitamin C intake from supplements is associated with an increased risk of cardiovascular disease mortality in postmenopausal women with diabetes (Lee et al, 2004). Clearly, sufficient intakes but not excesses are to be suggested.

Lowering elevated serum homocysteine is another important factor. For example, homocystinuria is a congenital metabolic disorder that is a known life-threatening risk factor for ischemic stroke. Folate deficiency and resultant hyperhomocysteinemia increase oxidative DNA damage and ischemic lesion size in stroke patients (Endres et al, 2005). Folate intake was not associated with incident of stroke among women participating in the Nurse's Health Study (Al-Delaimy et al, 2004). Intakes of folate and vitamins B_6 and B_{12} should be maintained at DRI levels in populations at risk.

There is good review evidence that dietary advice to those with coronary heart disease can reduce stroke mortality and morbidity, and this is often overlooked by physicians (Spence, 2006). Dietary advice should be individualized and prioritized (Hooper et al, 2004).

INTERVENTION: OBJECTIVES

- Immediate treatment consists of maintaining fluid-electrolyte balance for lifesaving measures.
- Ongoing treatment consists of improving residual effects such as dysphagia, hemiplegia, and aphasia and correcting side effects (i.e., constipation, UTIs, pneumonia, renal calculi, and pressure ulcers).
- If the patient is excessively overweight, weight reduction is necessary to lower elevated blood pressure and lipids and lessen workload of the cardiovascular system.
- Chewing should be minimized for dysphagia, and choking should be prevented. Avoid use of straws.
- Lower elevated serum lipids, especially try to improve low levels of HDL cholesterol.
- Promote self-help, self-esteem, and independence.
- Prevent additional strokes, which may be common. See Table 4-13. Since inflammation may be caused by a response to oxidized low-density lipoproteins, chronic infection, or other factors, monitor markers of this process, such as C-reactive protein (Paoletti et al, 2004).

INTERVENTION: FOOD AND NUTRITION

- Initial treatment: NPO with intravenous fluids for 24–48 hours. Avoid overhydration. Tube feeding may be needed, especially gastrostomy or jejunostomy. If the patient is comatose, tube feeding definitely is required, and the head of the bed should be elevated at least 30° during feeding to prevent aspiration.
- Treatment should progress from NPO to liquids. Enteral sip feeding may improve nutrient intake and nutritional status of stroke patients who do not have swallowing difficulties.
- Thick pureed liquids or a mechanical soft diet may be needed. At first, use easy-to-chew foods and spoon rather than fork foods. Progress slowly.
- Provide adequate energy intake (patient's weight should be checked frequently). Monitor the patient's activity levels. From 25–45 kcal/kg and 1.2–1.5 g protein/kg may be needed, depending on weight status and loss of lean body mass.
- Texture modification to compensate for dysphagia should be made to reduce risk of choking and/or aspiration. Liquids can be thickened with gels. Always start with small amounts of food.
- With dysphagia, avoid foods that cause choking or that are hard to manage (e.g., tart juices and foods, dry or crisp foods, fibrous meats, unboned fish, chewy or stringy meats, sticky peanut butter and bananas, thinly pureed foods that are easily aspirated, foods of varying consistency, excessively sweet drinks or fruits that aggravate drooling, raw vegetables, and mashed potatoes or soft breads for some patients).
- With decreased salivation, moisten foods with small amounts of liquid. Use thickener products to make semisolids out of soup, beverages, juices, and shakes. Test swallowing periodically. When ready, use of a syringe or training cup is beneficial.
- The amount of saturated and trans fatty acids in the diet should be <10% of total calories, and the dietary cholesterol intake should be <300 mg/d. A useful recommendation is to reduce the quantity of fat by 20–25%, reduce animal fats, and decrease the amount of salt added to foods in cooking and at the table (Smith et al, 2004). Replacement of saturated fat with monounsaturated sources is more desirable than replacement with carbohydrates (Tanasescu et al, 2004). Use more olive, soybean, and canola oils and nuts such as walnuts, almonds, macadamias, pecans, and pistachios. Walnuts contain alpha linolenic acid; almonds are a good source of vitamin E. Nuts also contain flavonoids, phenols, sterols, saponins, elegiac acid, folic acid, magnesium, copper, potassium, and fiber. Use of plant sterols and stanols, as from margarines and related products, is useful.
- Increase omega-3 fatty acids from fish (except in hemorrhagic stroke). Compared with other nationalities, Americans tend to eat much less fish; this practice should be changed to protect against further ischemic strokes (Iso et al, 2001). Fish consumption as seldom as 1–3 times per month may be protective (He et al, 2004).
- The Mediterranean diet is a useful diet to follow; in this diet, unsaturated fats replace most of the saturated fat, and fruits and vegetables are highlighted (Spence, 2006).
- Use skim milk products whenever possible. Milk fat is negatively correlated with certain cardiovascular disease risk factors.
- Increase potassium unless using potassium-sparing diuretics or with end-stage renal disease.
- Increasing potassium intake has beneficial effects for reducing the risk of stroke (He and MacGregor, 2003). Fruits and vegetables are the best sources (oranges, bananas, prunes, baked potatoes); milk is another good source.

TABLE 4-13 Strategies Used to Prevent Strokes

- Keep blood pressure at 120/80 or below.
- Exercise moderately each day for at least 30–60 minutes. Brisk walking (about 3 mph) is most protective, but any walking is good as a preventive measure.
- Quit smoking (Voko et al, 2003).
- Primary prevention of stroke, based on recent clinical trial results and clinical guidelines, includes use of a high-dose statin, low to standard doses of antihypertensive therapy, aspirin, omega-3 fish oil, cardiac rehabilitation, and diet (Robinson and Maheshwari, 2005). Dietary measures include recommendations to:
  - Eat a balanced diet.
  - Eat more fruits and vegetables, whole grains, and low-fat dairy products. This will provide more potassium, vitamin C, calcium, and magnesium.
  - Limit sodium from salt shaker, processed meats, pickles, and olives.
  - Include omega-3 fatty acids in foods regularly (fish, flaxseed, and walnuts).
  - Include natural sources of fatty acids and vitamin E, such as mayonnaise, margarine, and nuts.
  - Vitamin K may help to slow hardening of the arteries by curtailing vascular calcification; 500 μg may be what people need for this effect.
  - Take a multivitamin-mineral supplement daily, especially for folic acid and vitamins B_6 and B_{12}, to reduce homocysteine levels and to help lower blood pressure.
  - Achieve and maintain body weight within BMI range for height. Avoid obesity.
  - Maintain serum cholesterol levels of 200 or lower; LDL of 100 or lower; triglycerides of 150 or less; HDL of >60.
  - Drink alcoholic beverages in moderation only (one drink for women, two for men per day). Alcohol boosts HDL and may reduce clot formation.

- Fluid should be given in sufficient quantity if tolerated; estimate needs at 30 mL/kg and increase to 35 mL/kg if dehydration occurs. Give oral beverages at the end of the meal to increase solid food intake.
- The diet should provide adequate fiber from prune juice, bran, whole grains, etc. Metamucil may be useful for persons who are unable to chew fibrous foods; mix with juice to improve acceptance.
- Magnesium, vitamin E, folic acid (He, Merchant et al, 2004), and vitamins B_{12} and B_6 should be included in sufficient quantities to meet at least minimum daily requirements. Following the DASH diet is beneficial (see Section 6).
- Use caution with supplemental vitamin C; excesses may act as a pro-oxidant. Be sure to include levels that meet DRI recommendations.
- Flavonoids such as grapefruit, grape juice, tea, and red wine may be useful when the patient can tolerate a soft diet.
- Increase intake of whole grains (breads, cereals, oatmeal, bran, wheat germ, popcorn, brown rice).

SAMPLE NUTRITION DIAGNOSTIC STATEMENT

Cerebrovascular Accident (CVA)

PES: Swallowing difficulty related to CVA as evidenced by coughing with intake of thin liquids.

Assessment Data (sources of info): Results of swallow study and x-rays, food diary, and problems noted with specific types of liquids/foods; swallow studies and conferences with speech therapist.

Intervention: Alter diet to thicken liquids with all meals, snacks, medication passes, special events, dining out; recipes for use of thickened liquids.

Monitoring and Evaluation: Reduced incidence of aspiration; no hospital admissions for aspiration pneumonia; review of repeat swallow studies.

CLINICAL INDICATORS

Clinical/History

Height
Weight
BMI
Waist to hip ratio
Dietary/intake history
Positron emission tomography (PET) scan
Sleep apnea
Chewing ability
Hand to mouth coordination
Gag reflex—Present or absent?
BP
Temperature
Visual field scan
EEG
Carotid ultrasound
CT scan or MRI
I & O

Lab Work

CRP
PT
INR: 2.0–4.0 desirable
Na+, K+
Ca++, Mg++
Chol (total, HDL, LDL)
Trig
Homocysteine (tHcy)
Serum folate
Ferritin
H & H
Gluc (often increased)
Creatine phosphokinase (CPK)
Serum uric acid

Common Drugs Used and Potential Side Effects

- Angiotensin-converting enzyme inhibitors/angiotensin receptor blockers are commonly used. These may include Atacand, Teveten, Avapro, Cozaar, Benicar, Micardis, or Diovan. They may cause anemia or hyperkalemia. Be careful with salt substitutes. Use with a low-sodium, low-calorie diet. Diarrhea or GI distress can occur.
- Anticoagulants used to prevent thromboembolism, such as warfarin (Coumadin), require a controlled amount of vitamin K. Monitor tube feeding (TF) products and supplements. Limit high–vitamin K foods to 1 per day (e.g., green leafy vegetables, fish, broccoli, kale, Brussels sprouts). Many patients who

are taking warfarin can safely monitor their INR levels at home and adjust their medications accordingly. Monitor supplements containing vitamins A, C, and E with these drugs because of potential side effects. Avoid taking with dong quai, fenugreek, feverfew, excessive garlic, ginger, gingko, and ginseng.

- Aspirin is safer than warfarin and just as effective for treating blocked arteries in the brain (Koroshetz, 2005). Aspirin is often used to prevent future strokes as a blood thinner (generally 1 tablet per day). Monitor for GI bleeding or other chronic side effects; it may decrease serum ferritin by increasing occult blood loss (Fleming et al, 2001).
- Grapefruit juice decreases drug metabolism in the gut (via P450-CYP3A4 inhibition) and can affect medications up to 24 hours later. Consistency of use may be more important than total quantity. Avoid taking with alprazolam, buspirone, cisapride, cyclosporine, statins, tacrolimus, and many others.
- Products containing phenylpropanolamine (PPA) are a risk for stroke. PPA has been pulled from the shelves but may still be available to some people in cough medicines.
- Statins may be quite beneficial. Lipitor, Lescol, Mevacor, Pravachol, Crestor, and Zocor are commonly prescribed. Nausea, abdominal pain, and other GI effects are common. Do not take with grapefruit juice or St. John's wort. Monitor liver enzymes.
- Stool softeners may be used. Tube feeding containing a mix of soluble and insoluble fiber can be used. If a low-residue formula is used, a fiber supplement such as Benefiber can be mixed with water and administered via Y-port.
- Thiazide diuretics, such as Lasix, may be needed. Monitor for potassium depletion.

Herbs, Botanicals, and Supplements

- The patient should not take herbals and botanicals without discussing with the physician.
- Coenzyme Q10 should not be used with statins, gemfibrozil, tricyclic antidepressants, or warfarin. Coenzyme Q10 may act similarly to vitamin K.
- Niacin (nicotinic acid) should not be taken with statins, antidiabetic medications, and carbamazepine because of potentially serious risks of myopathy and altered glucose control.
- Vitamin E should not be taken with warfarin because of the possibility of increased bleeding. Avoid doses greater than 400 IU/d.
- Herbs and botanicals such as garlic, willow, pigweed, gingko, evening primrose, and carrot have been recommended, but no clinical trials have proven efficacy.

INTERVENTION: NUTRITION EDUCATION, COUNSELING, CARE MANAGEMENT

- Help the patient simplify meal preparation. Arrange food and utensils within reach. Discuss the use of appropriate assistive devices.
- Explain which sources of adequate nutrition do not aggravate the patient's condition. Discuss fat, cholesterol, sodium, potassium, calcium, magnesium, specific vitamins, and other nutrients. Correlate with drug therapy.
- Help the patient make mealtime safe and pleasant. Encourage small bites of food and slow, adequate chewing.
- Discuss ways to prevent future strokes; linolenic acid from walnut, canola, and soybean oils may be protective. Increased fruit and vegetable intake is also protective.
- Physical therapy is very important in early stages after a stroke, especially to regain use of limbs such as hands and arms. EXCITE is a multicenter study that is studying the impact of exercise in nonaffected limbs of stroke patients.
- Help to manage depression, which is common after a stroke. Treatments may include patient and family counseling and education, reestablishment of sleep pattern, improving diet, and regular physical activity.
- Future prevention strategies should be taught to stroke patients and their families (Ovbiagele et al, 2004). Modifiable risk factors include hypertension, exposure to cigarette smoke, diabetes, atrial fibrillation and certain other cardiac conditions, dyslipidemia, carotid artery stenosis, sickle cell disease, postmenopausal hormone therapy, poor diet, physical inactivity, and obesity and body fat distribution (Goldstein et al, 2006). Less well-documented or potentially modifiable risk factors include the metabolic syndrome, alcohol abuse, drug abuse, oral contraceptive use, sleep-disordered breathing, migraine headache, hyperhomocysteinemia, elevated lipoprotein A, elevated lipoprotein-associated phospholipase, hypercoagulability, inflammation, and infection (Goldstein et al, 2006).
- The American Heart Association, American Cancer Society, and American Diabetes Association agree that lifestyle changes are essential and that early detection is very essential (Eyre et al, 2004).

Patient Education—Foodborne Illness

- Careful food handling will be important. If tube feeding is needed, discuss proper sanitation of work counters during preparation.
- Hand washing is important, especially for caregivers if the patient is unable to feed himself or herself.

For More Information

- American Academy of Physical Medicine and Rehabilitation
  http://www.aapmr.org/
- American Stroke Association
  http://www.strokeassociation.org/presenter.jhtml?identifier=1200037
- National Aphasia Association
  http://www.aphasia.org
- National Institute of Neurological Disorders and Stroke
  Phone: 800-352-9424
  http://www.ninds.nih.gov/
- National Rehabilitation Awareness Foundation
  http://www.nraf-rehabnet.org/
- National Rehabilitation Hospital
  http://www.nrhrehab.org/

- National Stroke Association
  http://www.stroke.org/
- North Carolina Stroke Association
  http://www.ncstroke.org/
- UCLA Stroke Center
  http://www.stroke.ucla.edu/

STROKE—CITED REFERENCES

Al-Delaimy WK, et al. Folate intake and risk of stroke among women. *Stroke* 35:1259, 2004.

Eidelman RS, et al. Randomized trials of vitamin E in the treatment and prevention of cardiovascular disease. *Arch Intern Med.* 164:1552, 2004.

Endres M, et al. Folate deficiency increases postischemic brain injury. *Stroke* 36:321, 2005.

Eyre H, et al. Preventing cancer, cardiovascular disease, and diabetes: a common agenda for the American Cancer Society, the American Diabetes Association, and the American Heart Association. *Stroke* 35:1999, 2004.

Fleming D, et al. Aspirin intake and the use of serum ferritin as a measure of iron status. *Am J Clin Nutr.* 74:219, 2001.

Fung TT, et al. Prospective study of major dietary patterns and stroke risk in women. *Stroke* 35:2014, 2004.

Goldstein LB, et al. Primary prevention of ischemic stroke: a guideline from the American Heart Association/American Stroke Association Stroke Council: cosponsored by the Atherosclerotic Peripheral Vascular Disease Interdisciplinary Working Group; Cardiovascular Nursing Council; Clinical Cardiology Council; Nutrition, Physical Activity, and Metabolism Council; and the Quality of Care and Outcomes Research Interdisciplinary Working Group. *Circulation* 113:e873, 2006.

Hak AE, et al. Prospective study of plasma carotenoids and tocopherols in relation to risk of ischemic stroke. *Stroke* 35:1584, 2004.

He FJ, MacGregor GA. Potassium: more beneficial effects. *Climacteric* 6:36S, 2003.

He K, et al. Fish consumption and incidence of stroke: a meta-analysis of cohort studies. *Stroke* 35:1538, 2004.

He K, Merchant A, et al. Folate, vitamin B6, and B12 intakes in relation to risk of stroke among men. *Stroke* 35:169, 2004.

Hooper L, et al. Dietetic guidelines: diet in secondary prevention of cardiovascular disease (first update, June 2003). *J Hum Nutr Diet.* 17:337, 2004.

Iso H, et al. Intake of fish and omega-3 fatty acids and risk of stroke in women. *JAMA.* 285:304, 2001.

Joshipura K, et al. Fruit and vegetable intake in relation to risk of ischemic stroke. *JAMA.* 282:1233, 1999.

Koroshetz W. Warfarin, aspirin, and intracranial vascular disease. *N Engl J Med.* 352:1368, 2005.

Lee DH, et al. Does supplemental vitamin C increase cardiovascular disease risk in women with diabetes? *Am J Clin Nutr.* 80:1194, 2004.

Mozaffarian D, et al. Fish consumption and stroke risk in elderly individuals: the cardiovascular health study. *Arch Intern Med.* 165:200, 2005.

Muntaneau A, et al. Anti-atherosclerotic effects of vitamin E—myth or reality? *J Cell Mol Med.* 8:59, 2004.

Ovbiagele B, et al. In-hospital initiation of secondary stroke prevention therapies yields high rates of adherence at follow-up. *Stroke* 35:2879, 2004.

Paoletti R, et al. Inflammation in atherosclerosis and implications for therapy. *Circulation* 109(suppl 1):III20, 2004.

Pearce KA, et al. Update on vitamin supplements for the prevention of coronary disease and stroke. *Am Fam Physician.* 62:1359, 2000.

Rexrode K, et al. A prospective study of body mass index, weight change, and risk of stroke in women. *JAMA.* 277:1539, 1997.

Robinson JG, Maheshwari N. A "poly-portfolio" for secondary prevention: a strategy to reduce subsequent events by up to 97% over five years. *Am J Cardiol.* 95:373, 2005.

Sacco R, et al. High-density lipoprotein cholesterol and ischemic stroke in the elderly. *JAMA.* 285:2729, 2001.

Sanchez-Moreno C, et al. Decreased levels of plasma vitamin C and increased concentrations of inflammatory and oxidative stress markers after stroke. *Stroke* 35:163, 2004.

Smith S, et al. Principles for national and regional guidelines on cardiovascular disease prevention: a scientific statement from the World Heart and Stroke Forum. *Circulation* 109:3112, 2004.

Spence JD. Nutrition and stroke prevention. *Stroke* 2006. In press.

Tanasescu M, et al. Dietary fat and cholesterol and the risk of cardiovascular disease among women with type 2 diabetes. *Am J Clin Nutr.* 79:999, 2004.

Voko Z, et al. Dietary antioxidants and the risk of ischemic stroke: the Rotterdam Study. *Neurology* 61:1273, 2003.

Yochum L, et al. Intake of antioxidant vitamins and risk of death from stroke in postmenopausal women. *Am J Clin Nutr.* 72:476, 2000.

TARDIVE DYSKINESIA

NUTRITIONAL ACUITY RANKING: LEVEL 2

DEFINITIONS AND BACKGROUND

Tardive dyskinesia (TD) refers to involuntary, repetitive, persistent movements caused by the use of drugs that block dopamine receptors (dopamine receptor antagonists [DRAs]). When used in the classic sense, TD refers to a disorder produced by the long-term use of drugs to treat schizophrenia that act by blocking dopamine receptors. TD occurs in 20–40% of all patients receiving long-term antipsychotic drugs.

Psychiatric conditions are often treated with antipsychotic agents, which can be typical or atypical. The typical agents include phenothiazines, butyrophenones, dibenzodiazepines, indolones, diphenylbutylpiperidines, and thioxanthenes. These are more likely to cause TD than the newer antipsychotic agents.

Signs and symptoms of TD include abnormal, involuntary movements (e.g., chorea, athetosis, dystonia, tics, and facial grimacing). Tongue, face, neck, lung muscles, and extremities are usually involved. Patients are often elderly and chronically institutionalized.

Very limited evidence supports the use of vitamin E in the treatment of TD (Zhang et al, 2004). Phenylalanine sensitivity has been speculated as the cause of TD. Amine-depleting agents such as reserpine (Serpalan, Serpasil) and tetrabenazine (Nitoman) deplete dopamine, norepinephrine, and serotonin. Tarvil, a medical food with high branched-chain amino acids, targets excess phenylalanine and has few side effects.

INTERVENTION: OBJECTIVES

- Prevent or correct malnutrition, weight loss, and other problems.
- Identify and assist with feeding problems. Some patients have problems with sucking and puckering of the lips and difficulty in eating.
- Restore eating capacity as far as possible.
- Alter textures as necessary (eating problems are rare or occur late in the condition).

- Prevent stress, which aggravates supersensitivity psychoses.
- Free radicals may be involved in the pathogenesis of TD (Elkashef and Wyatt, 1999).

INTERVENTION: FOOD AND NUTRITION

- Offer the usual diet with soft textures to reduce chewing as needed.
- Decrease energy intake if obese; increase intake if underweight.
- Carbohydrate craving is common from drugs that block histamine receptors; watch overall intake of sweets or offer nutrient-dense varieties.
- Increase dietary choline from foods such as eggs, soybeans, peanuts, and liver.
- Moisten foods with gravy, sauces, and liquids if dry mouth is a problem.
- Alter fiber intake if needed to prevent or correct constipation.
- Ensure adequate intake of antioxidants and omega-3 fatty acids (colorful fruits and vegetables, nuts, fish and seafood).

CLINICAL INDICATORS

Clinical/History	Lab Work	
Height	CRP	Acetylcholine levels
Weight	BUN, Creat	Gluc
BMI	H & H	Alb, transthyretin
Dietary/intake history	Serum Fe	Ceruloplasmin
BP	Serum homocysteine	Serum Cu
Tremors and involuntary movements	Serum folate	Serum phenylalanine
	Serum prolactin (often increased)	

Common Drugs Used and Potential Side Effects

- Incidence of TD with the use of newer atypical antipsychotic agents such as clozapine (Clozaril), olanzapine (Zyprexa), risperidone (Risperdal), and quetiapine (Seroquel) is minimal (Casey, 2006). Risperidone (Risperdal) appears to bring out the symptoms of TD more frequently, as compared to the other newer atypical antipsychotic agents.
- Drugs other than those used to treat psychiatric illnesses can also block the dopamine receptors, and their use has also been found to be linked to TD. These include anticholinergics and SSRIs, which are used to treat depression. Whether other antidepressant medication, such as MAOIs and tricyclics, causes TD is not known.
- Reduction in the use of the drug that caused TD would be desirable. Changing to a different medication, such as an atypical antipsychotic, is recommended. Patients on antipsychotics should be checked regularly for signs of TD (Ananth et al, 2004). Tetrabenazine (Nitoman) appears to be a more effective drug for the treatment of TD, but it is not currently available in the United States.

Herbs, Botanicals, and Supplements

- No studies have been conducted for efficacy of herbs or botanicals in TD.

INTERVENTION: NUTRITION EDUCATION, COUNSELING, CARE MANAGEMENT

- Diet instructions should be offered directly to the patient unless this is not possible.
- Discuss major issues related to nutrition, self-feeding practices, moistening of foods, etc.
- Discuss sources of foods that contain branched-chain amino acids and how to obtain medical foods that may be used.

Patient Education—Foodborne Illness

- Careful food handling will be important. The same is true for hand washing.

For More Information

- We Move–Tardive Dyskinesia
  http://www.wemove.org/td/

TARDIVE DYSKINESIA—CITED REFERENCES

Ananth J, et al. Tardive dyskinesia in 2 patients treated with ziprasidone. *J Psychiatry Neurosci.* 29:467, 2004.

Casey DE. Implications of the CATIE trial on treatment: extrapyramidal symptoms. *CNS Spectr.* 11(suppl 7):25, 2006.

Elkashef A, Wyatt R. Tardive dyskinesia: possible involvement of free radicals and treatment with vitamin E. *Schizophr Bull.* 25:731, 1999.

Zhang XY, et al. The effect of vitamin E treatment on tardive dyskinesia and blood superoxide dismutase: a double-blind placebo-controlled trial. *J Clin Psychopharmacol.* 24:83, 2004.

TRIGEMINAL NEURALGIA

NUTRITIONAL ACUITY RANKING: LEVEL 1–2

DEFINITIONS AND BACKGROUND

Trigeminal neuralgia (tic douloureux) manifests as a disorder of the fifth cranial nerve and is characterized by paroxysms of excruciating pain of a burning nature. The painful periods alternate with pain-free periods. The disorder is rare before 40 years of age and is more common in elderly women. The right side of the face is affected more often; the pain can be incapacitating. Dentists often play a role in identifying this condition (Bagheri et al, 2004).

Loss of taste in patients after surgery for trigeminal neuralgia supports the existence of an accessory gustatory pathway through the trigeminal sensory root and the gasserian ganglion; Bell's palsy is the most common pathology of the peripheral gustatory pathway (Sanchez-Juan and Combarros, 2001).

INTERVENTION: OBJECTIVES

- Control pain with medications, especially before meals.
- Provide appropriate counseling and assistance with consistency of meals (foods and beverages).
- Individualize for preferences and tolerances.
- Maintain body weight within a desirable range.

INTERVENTION: FOOD AND NUTRITION

- Use a normal diet as tolerated, perhaps altering to soft or pureed foods as needed.
- Small, frequent feedings may be better tolerated than large meals.
- Liquids may be preferred if given by straw. Individualize.
- Avoid extremes in temperature.
- Use nutrient-dense foods if weight loss occurs.

CLINICAL INDICATORS

Clinical/History		
Height	PET scan	CT scan or MRI
Weight	Chewing ability	I & O
BMI	BP	
Dietary/intake history	Temperature	**Lab Work**
	EEG	CRP
	Carotid ultrasound	Na+, K+
		Folate

Ca++, Mg++	Trig	H & H
Chol (total, HDL, LDL)	Ferritin	Gluc

Common Drugs Used and Potential Side Effects

- Phenytoin (Dilantin) or carbamazepine (Tegretol), which are anticonvulsants, may be used. Diarrhea, nausea, and vomiting are common. Ensure adequate intake of folate.
- Nonsteroidal anti-inflammatory medications or narcotics may be used to reduce pain.
- There is insufficient evidence from trials to suggest use of nonantiepileptic drugs at this time (He et al, 2006).

Herbs, Botanicals, and Supplements

- No studies have been conducted for efficacy of herbs or botanicals in trigeminal neuralgia.
- With anticonvulsants such as phenytoin (Dilantin), avoid use with evening primrose oil, gingko biloba, and kava.

INTERVENTION: NUTRITION EDUCATION, COUNSELING, CARE MANAGEMENT

- The importance of oral and dental hygiene should be stressed, even with pain. Use pain medications as directed.
- The patient should be encouraged to avoid eating when tense or nervous.
- Relaxation therapy may be beneficial.

Patient Education—Foodborne Illness

- Careful food handling will be important. The same is true for hand washing.

TRIGEMINAL NEURALGIA—CITED REFERENCES

Bagheri SC, et al. Diagnosis and treatment of patients with trigeminal neuralgia. *J Am Dent Assoc.* 135:1713, 2004.

He L, et al. Non-antiepileptic drugs for trigeminal neuralgia. *Cochrane Database Syst Rev.* 3:CD004029, 2006.

Sanchez-Juan P, Combarros O. Gustatory nervous pathway syndromes. *Neurologia* 16:262, 2001.

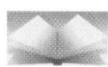

MENTAL DISORDERS–EATING DISORDERS

ANOREXIA NERVOSA

NUTRITIONAL ACUITY RANKING: LEVEL 3

DEFINITIONS AND BACKGROUND

Anorexia nervosa (AN) is an eating disorder (ED) in which the patient severely rejects food, causing extreme weight loss, low basal metabolic rate, and exhaustion. The gene AGRP (agouti-related protein) has been linked with AN susceptibility (Vink et al, 2001). About 6–15% of the population is affected. Five percent of females and 1% of males suffer from EDs (American Dietetic Association, 2001). AN is more common in girls, especially just after the onset of puberty, peaking at 12–13 and 19–20 years old; it also can occur at any age.

Signs include relentless pursuit of thinness, misperception of body image, and restrained eating, binge eating, or purging (see Bulimia and Binge Eating Disorder entries). Generally, cases are separated into "restricting" or "binge-purging" types: anorectic restrictor (AN-R) and anorectic bulimics (AN-B). Fear of fatness and a codependent focus outside of one's self are common in AN. The intense fear of becoming fat (not diminishing as weight loss progresses) has no known physical cause. Patients with EDs may have dermatologic manifestations secondary to starvation; recognition of these signs can lead to early diagnosis and treatment (Glorio et al, 2000).

Weight is 85% or less of former weight; there is usually amenorrhea. Length of amenorrhea, estrogen exposure (age minus age at menarche minus years of amenorrhea), and body weight have independent effects on bone densities; therefore, osteopenia is common (Brooks et al, 1998). Long-term sequelae may include Cushing's disease and osteoporosis. Without treatment, death may occur, usually from cardiac arrhythmias.

Problems commonly found include perfectionism (Castro et al, 2004); denial, impulse control, manipulative behavior, trust issues, power issues within the family, and misinformation are also issues. These individuals may demonstrate low tolerance for change and new situations and fear of growing up and assuming adult responsibilities and lifestyle. Traits include being overly dependent on parents or family, obsessive-compulsive, meticulous, introverted, emotionally reserved, socially insecure, overly rigid in thinking, self-denying, and overly compliant. Group parenting education may be quite helpful (Zucker et al, 2006).

Because patients deny the severity of their illness, they delay seeking psychiatric treatment (Mehler, 2001). Teens with ED often use subterfuge to give the impression that they are cooperating with treatment plans, when they in fact are not. These behaviors prolong treatment and can lead to malnutrition.

Some careers promote a thin body for success (e.g., fashion, air travel, entertainment, and athletics). Many female athletes struggle with an ED. The main concern is inadequate energy intake (Gabel, 2006). Although female athletes with subclinical EDs have dietary intakes of energy, protein, CHO, and certain micronutrients below recommended levels, micronutrient status may be fine due to use of supplements (Beals and Manore, 1998).

Studies suggest that individuals with AN have lower than optimal levels of polyunsaturated fatty acids (including ALA and GLA). To prevent the complications associated with essential fatty acid deficiencies, some experts recommend that treatment programs for AN include polyunsaturated fatty acid (PUFA)–rich foods (Ayton, 2004).

High postprandial levels of cholecystokinin (CCK) observed in AN may aggravate the course of this disease by intensifying nausea and vomiting (Tomasik et al, 2004). High serum levels of cortisol seem to be related to severe undernutrition (Misra et al, 2004). Other altered hormones (such as growth hormone) have been studied, and there are no clear answers at this time regarding cause or effect.

Despite all of this, the majority of patients with EDs make a full recovery (Rock, 1999). Two or more consecutive spontaneous menses implies resumption of menses; this is dependent on body weight but not on body fat levels (Golden, 1997). Insulin-like growth factor I (IGF-I) represents a biochemical marker of malnutrition and a sensitive index of nutritional repletion in patients with EDs (Cargaro et al, 2001).

Dietitians must be able to identify and refer patients with EDs. But medical nutrition therapy for EDs is a specialization that requires training beyond entry level. The American Dietetic Association has recommended eight medical nutrition therapy visits by a trained professional for persons who have EDs.

INTERVENTION: OBJECTIVES

- Restore normal physiological function by correcting starvation and its associated changes, including electrolyte imbalance, bradycardia, and hypotension (Misra et al, 2004).
- Check weight or growth charts to determine difference and to set goals. Promote weight gain of 1–3 lb weekly (in-patient) and 0.5–1 lb weekly (out-patient) to reach a weight closer to a healthy BMI.
- Promote adequate psychotherapy and use of medications to protect the heart, fluid, and electrolytes, which are the most important.
- Obtain diet history to assess bulimia, vomiting, and use of diuretics or laxatives.
- Do not force feedings; rejection of food is part of the illness. Promote normal eating behavior instead.
- Gradually increase intake to a normal or high-energy intake to lessen likelihood of edema and other consequences of malnutrition.
- For young women, promote normal menstrual cycles.
- Reduce preoccupation with weight and food. Erroneous

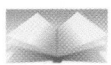

TABLE 4-14 Average Woman Versus "Fashion Woman"

	Average Woman	Barbie Doll	Store Mannequin
Height	5′ 4″	6′ 0″	6′ 0″
Weight	145 lbs	101 lbs	Not available
Dress size	11–14	4	6
Bust	36–37″	39″	34″
Waist	29–31″	19″	23″
Hips	40–42″	33″	34″

From the website: http://www.anred.com/stats.html.

perceptions of "normal" should be alleviated. Promote adequate self-esteem.

- Refer to appropriate care for psychiatric maladies and comorbid conditions, especially insulin-dependent diabetes mellitus (Cartwright, 2004).
- Coordinate nutrition education and counseling with the overall team plan. Table 4-14 shows how average women compare with "fashion women"; counseling will need to be adjusted according to the individual's self-perception.

INTERVENTION: FOOD AND NUTRITION

- Serve attractive, palatable meals in small amounts, observing food preferences. Small, frequent meals are useful. Encourage variety.
- Limit bulky foods during the early stages of treatment; gastrointestinal intolerance may persist for a long time. Assure the patient that constipation will be alleviated.
- Diet should be called a "low-calorie diet for AN" to convince the patient of the counselors' good intentions.
- According to the standards set by the American Psychiatric Association (2005): start at 30–40 kcal/kg (about 1000–1600 kcals/d) and increase as possible. Promote weekly weight gain by gradually attaining intake of up to 70–100 kcal/kg for some patients. Weight maintenance may need to be 40–60 kcal/kg.
- Protein refeeding takes a long time. Repletion may not be complete until weight has returned to normal. Monitor for improved biochemical results (BUN, albumin). In addition, monitor serum cholesterol levels; low levels have been correlated with suicidality (Favaro et al, 2004).
- While not a preferred method, use tube feeding if necessary (i.e., only if the patient weighs 40% of lower end of BMI range for normal). Nocturnal tube feeding may be especially helpful in adolescent males with AN (Silber et al, 2004).
- Help the patient resume normal eating habits. Have the patient measure and record food intake at first; then, gradually lessen the emphasis on food.
- A "no added salt" diet may reduce fluid retention.
- It may be useful to avoid caffeine because of stimulant/diuretic effect.
- A vitamin–mineral supplement may be needed for zinc and other nutrients (Schebendach, 2004).

SAMPLE NUTRITION DIAGNOSTIC STATEMENT

Anorexia Nervosa

PES: Disordered eating pattern related to complaints of being "too fat" as evidenced by current weight of 82 lb and self-limited dietary intake of 450 kcals daily on nutrient analysis.

Assessment Data: BMI charts and current versus desirable weight for height; body fat measurements.

Intervention: Provide meals appropriate for refeeding protocol; education and counseling about appropriate body size, weight, BMI; goal setting for self-management.

Monitoring and Evaluation: Body weight changes; intake records; discussion about perceptions of mealtimes and eating, body image.

- Refeeding may take longer in some patients. A rise in resting energy expenditure (REE) observed during refeeding may be linked to anxiety level, abdominal pain, physical activity, and cigarette smoking; this contributes to resistance to weight gain (Van Wymelbeke et al, 2004).

CLINICAL INDICATORS

Clinical/History

Height
Present weight
Former weight
Recent weight
Percentage of weight changes
BMI
Weight goal/timing
Dietary/intake history
History (Hx) of bulimia or vomiting?
Laxative or diuretic abuse?
BP (low?)
Amenorrhea
Lanugo hair
Edema
Blood in stool?
MRI or CT scan for ventricular enlargement from malnutrition
Dual-energy x-ray absorptiometry (DEXA; after 6 months underweight)
EKG

Lab Work

Luteinizing hormone (LH) (decreased)
Follicle-stimulating hormone (FSH)
IGF-I
Serum estradiol (low)
Serum cortisol (high)
Urinary cortisol (high)
Sex hormone–binding globulin (SHBG)
Alb, transthyretin, N balance
Chol (low?)
Trig
Gluc
BUN (low?)
H & H
Serum Fe
Thyroid-stimulating hormone (TSH)
Leukopenia?
Na+, K+, Cl−
Serum amylase (with vomiting)
Serum Ca++, Mg++
Serum phosphorus
Liver function tests
Leptin decreased, ghrelin increased?

Common Drugs Used and Potential Side Effects

- Pharmacotherapy is not always successful in AN (Williamson et al, 2004). Olanzapine has been tried

with some benefit (Barbarich et al, 2004); significant reductions in depression, anxiety, and ED symptoms, and weight increases have been noted. Dry mouth and constipation are the most common side effects.
- Antidepressants may be prescribed; they sometimes have nutritional side effects that should be monitored carefully. SSRIs are considered to be more effective. However, fluoxetine has failed to demonstrate protection against relapse in AN (Walsh et al, 2006).

Herbs, Botanicals, and Supplements

- No specific herbs and botanical products have been used for AN in clinical trials.

INTERVENTION: NUTRITION EDUCATION, COUNSELING, CARE MANAGEMENT

- See Table 4-15.

Patient Education—Foodborne Illness

- Careful food handling will be important. The same is true for sanitizing work area before and after preparing tube feedings to prevent contamination. Formula companies have good information on safe handling of formula in the home and institution.

For More Information

- Academy for Eating Disorders
  http://www.aedweb.org
- American Anorexia/Bulimia Association
  http://www.aabaphila.org/
- Anorexia Nervosa and Related Eating Disorders (ANRED)
  http://www.anred.com/
- Eating Disorders Anonymous
  http://www.eatingdisordersanonymous.org/
- Eating Disorder Recovery
  http://www.addictions.net/

TABLE 4-15 Tips for Helping Patients with Eating Disorders (EDs)

Goal	Suggested Action
Encourage full participation, especially with in-patient treatment	Treatment is especially important to manage anxiety disorders, which may precede onset of the ED (Kaye et al, 2004). Patients with the binge eating/purging type of anorexia nervosa are significantly less likely to complete in-patienttreatment (Woodside et al, 2004).
	Attachment theory suggests that persons with anorexia nervosa and avoidant personality style may discontinue therapy early (Tasca et al, 2004).
Help the patient become an effective, independently functioning person	Convey principles rather than rigid "rules" to avoid reinforcing the patient's compulsive rituals and preoccupation with food. Perfectionism is a common trait (Castro et al, 2004).
Positive regular habits should be encouraged	Behavioral contracting is useful.
Follow a balanced diet	Discuss how a balanced diet affects weight goals. Encourage healthy snacks. Medical nutrition therapy and education is a cornerstone of therapy; nutrition "expertise" is not an early feature of the disorder and does not likely contribute to its development (Breen and Espelage, 2004).
Identify hunger cues	Discuss signs of hunger and satiety.
Support positive family relationships	Family dynamics play a role. Include family members in nutrition education. Conflict management, support for individuality and personal opinions, and discussion of emotions will be part of the counseling offered by therapists.
Support healthy assertiveness and self-efficacy	Codependent behavior generally is a problem. Helping the individual to develop healthy reconnections and assertiveness is important (Maine, 2004). Computer-based psychosocial counseling may be helpful (Low et al, 2006).
Address social pressure for thinness	Preventive actions during middle school years may be helpful. For older individuals, open discussion of these issues may be useful as well.
Prevent relapse, which is common	Psychiatric abnormalities may continue (Foppiani, 1998). Starvation and self-imposed dieting may lead to binges once food is available. Preoccupation with food and eating, increased emotional lability, dysphoria, and distractibility are common.
Monitor patients who have type 1 diabetes	Monitor for poor control, bulimia, and skipping meals. These individuals are at high risk for hypoglycemia, hyperglycemia, and early onset of complications. Eating disorders are often correlated (Cartwright, 2004).
Support healthy pregnancy if this occurs in a young woman	Successful treatment includes appropriate pattern of weight gain, decreases in bingeing and purging behaviors, and normal infant birth weight. Special guidance is needed to achieve positive fetal outcomes. Team approach is suggested for helping a pregnant woman with an eating disorder (Franko and Spurrell, 2000).
Promote healthy levels of physical activity	Discuss goals for the individual; sometimes exercise is a goal in itself. Therapy may be needed to address this issue along with eating patterns. Excessive exercise and hyperactivity are common in 40–60% of individuals with anorexia nervosa (Holtkamp et al, 2004).

- International Association of Eating Disorders Professionals (IAEDP)
  http://www.iaedp.com/
- National Association of Anorexia Nervosa and Associated Disorders (ANAD)
  http://www.anad.org/
- National Institute for Clinical Excellence: Eating Disorders Guidelines
  http://www.nice.org.uk/page.aspx?o=101239
- Practice Guideline for Eating Disorders
  http://www.psych.org/psych_pract/treatg/pg/prac_guide.cfm
- Relapse Support
  http://www.mirror-mirror.org/relwarn.htm
- Renfrew Centers
  http://www.remudaranch.com/index.asp?flash=yes

ANOREXIA NERVOSA—CITED REFERENCES

American Dietetic Association. Position of The American Dietetic Association: nutrition intervention in the treatment of anorexia nervosa, bulimia nervosa, and eating disorders not otherwise specified (EDNOS). *J Am Diet Assoc.* 101:805, 2001.

American Psychiatric Association. Standards of practice for eating disorders. Accessed January 17, 2005 at http://www.psych.org/psych_pract/treatg/pg/eating_revisebook_3.cfm?pf=y#CIHJAJDG.

Anorexia Nervosa and Related Eating Disorders. Less-well-known eating disorders and related problems. Accessed January 18, 2005 at http://www.anred.com/defslesser.html.

Ayton AK. Dietary polyunsaturated fatty acids and anorexia nervosa: is there a link? *Nutr Neurosci.* 7:1, 2004.

Barbarich NC, et al. An open trial of olanzapine in anorexia nervosa. *J Clin Psychiatry.* 65:1480, 2004.

Beals K, Manore M. Nutritional status of female athletes with subclinical eating disorders. *J Am Diet Assoc.* 98:419, 1998.

Breen HB, Espelage DL. Nutrition expertise in eating disorders. *Eat Weight Disord.* 9:120, 2004.

Brooks E, et al. Compromised bone density 11.4 years after diagnosis of anorexia nervosa. *J Women's Health.* 7:567, 1998.

Cargaro L, et al. Insulin-like growth factor 1 (IGF-1), a nutritional marker in patients with eating disorders. *Clin Nutr.* 20:251, 2001.

Cartwright MM. Eating disorder emergencies: understanding the medical complexities of the hospitalized eating disordered patient. *Crit Care Nurs Clin N Am.* 16:515, 2004.

Castro J, et al. Perfectionism dimensions in children and adolescents with anorexia nervosa. *J Adolesc Health.* 35:392, 2004.

Favaro A, et al. Total serum cholesterol and suicidality in anorexia nervosa. *Psychosom Med.* 66:548, 2004.

Foppiani L, et al. Frequency of recovery from anorexia nervosa of a cohort of patients re-evaluated on a long-term basis following intensive care. *Eat Weight Disord.* 3:90, 1998.

Franko D, Spurrell E. Detection and management of eating disorders during pregnancy. *Obstet Gynecol.* 95:942, 2000.

Gabel KA. Special nutritional concerns for the female athlete. *Curr Sports Med Rep.* 5:187, 2006.

Glorio R, et al. Prevalence of cutaneous manifestations in 200 patients with eating disorders. *Int J Dermatol.* 39:348, 2000.

Golden N, et al. Resumption of menses in anorexia nervosa. *Arch Pediatr Adolesc Med.* 151:16, 1997.

Holtkamp K, et al. The contribution of anxiety and food restriction on physical activity levels in acute anorexia nervosa. *Int J Eat Disord.* 36:163, 2004.

Kaye WH, et al. Comorbidity of anxiety disorders with anorexia and bulimia nervosa. *Am J Psychiatry.* 161:2215, 2004.

Low KG, et al. Effectiveness of a computer-based interactive eating disorders prevention program at long-term follow-up. *Eat Disord.* 14:17, 2006.

Maine M. Altering women's relationships with food: a relational, developmental approach. *J Clin Psychol.* 57:1301, 2004.

Mehler P. Diagnosis and care of patients with anorexia nervosa in primary care settings. *Ann Intern Med.* 134:1048, 2001.

Misra M, et al. Effects of anorexia nervosa on clinical, hematologic, biochemical, and bone density parameters in community-dwelling adolescent girls. *Pediatrics* 114:1574, 2004.

Rock C. Nutritional and medical assessment and management of eating disorders. *Nutr Clin Care.* 2:332, 1999.

Schebendach J. Eating disorders. In: Mahan K, Escott-Stump S, eds. *Krause's food, nutrition, and diet therapy.* 11th ed. Philadelphia: WB Saunders, 2004.

Silber TJ, et al. Nocturnal nasogastric refeeding for hospitalized adolescent boys with anorexia nervosa. *J Dev Behav Pediatr.* 25:415, 2004.

Tasca GA, et al. Attachment predicts treatment completion in an eating disorders partial hospital program among women with anorexia nervosa. *J Pers Assess.* 83:201, 2004.

Tomasik PJ, et al. Cholecystokinin, glucose dependent insulinotropic peptide and glucagon-like peptide 1 secretion in children with anorexia nervosa and simple obesity. *J Pediatr Endocrinol Metab.* 17:1623, 2004.

Van Wymelbeke V, et al. Factors associated with the increase in resting energy expenditure during refeeding in malnourished anorexia nervosa patients. *Am J Clin Nutr.* 80:1469, 2004.

Vink T, et al. Association between agouti-related protein gene polymorphism and anorexia nervosa. *Mol Psychiatry.* 6:325, 2001.

Walsh BT, et al. Fluoxetine after weight restoration in anorexia nervosa: a randomized controlled trial. *JAMA.* 295:2605, 2006.

Williamson DA, et al. Psychological aspects of eating disorders. *Best Pract Res Clin Gastroenterol.* 18:1073, 2004.

Woodside DB, et al. Predictors of premature termination of inpatient treatment for anorexia nervosa. *Am J Psychiatry.* 161:2277, 2004.

Zucker NL, et al. A group parent-training program: a novel approach for eating disorder management. *Eat Weight Disord.* 11:78, 2006.

BINGE EATING DISORDER

NUTRITIONAL ACUITY RANKING: LEVEL 3–4

DEFINITIONS AND BACKGROUND

Binge eating disorder (BED) and subclinical syndromes of disturbed eating and distress are far more prevalent than anorexia nervosa and bulimia nervosa. BED involves recurrent episodes of binge eating (eating in a discrete period of time an amount of food larger than most people would eat in the same time), a sense of lack of control over the eating episodes, rapid or secretive eating, guilt, and shame.

Episodes may involve three or more of the following behaviors: eating more rapidly than normal, eating until uncomfortable, eating when not physically hungry, eating these foods alone, and feeling disgusted, guilty, or depressed. Binge eating occurs an average of 2 days weekly for 6 months or longer without vomiting, purging, fasting, or engaging in excessive exercise after binges.

In BED, the binges do not occur as part of anorexia nervosa or bulimia nervosa. Weight cycling involves weight loss followed by weight regain. Binge eaters report cycling along with psychological distress. Patients in weight control programs may binge at least twice per month.

People who have this disorder may be genetically predisposed to weigh more than the cultural ideal, so they may eat little, get hungry, and then binge in response to that hunger. Binge eating is a serious problem among a subset of the obese. Chronic dieting may predispose vulnerable individuals to binge eating, alcoholism, or drug abuse. Many individuals with this problem have a personal or parental history of substance abuse.

"Clinical" perfectionism involves both the determined pursuit of self-imposed standards and extremely vulnerable self-evaluation (Dunkley et al, 2006). Persons with BED tend to be depressed and overweight. A single traumatic event, several years of unusual stress or pain, an extended period of emotional pain, or mood disorders may be involved. Regardless of actual weight, there are high degrees of psychological distress in this group of individuals (Didie and Fitzgibbon, 2005). In addition, these individuals may have high levels of serum cortisol, which indicates chronic stress (Gluck et al, 2004).

INTERVENTION: OBJECTIVES

- Support the individual's counseling and therapy to identify the causes of binges. Help them follow a step-wise plan:
    - Establish self-monitoring records; establish regular pattern of eating to displace binge eating. Use alternative behaviors to help resist urges.
    - Educate about food, eating, body shape, and weight patterns. Eliminate all aspects of restrained eating.
    - Develop skills for dealing with difficulties that triggered past binges. Identify and challenge problematic ways of thinking. Consider the origins of the binge eating problem and then evaluate family/social factors that can be changed.
    - Plan for the future. Have realistic expectations and strategies ready for when problems occur.
    - Encourage a return to eating that is under the control of the individual.
- Correct any imbalances that have occurred as a result of the binges (e.g., weight, electrolyte imbalances).
- Support therapy, especially if there is a dual diagnosis, such as substance abuse.

INTERVENTION: FOOD AND NUTRITION

- A balanced diet, using principles of the dietary guidelines and the Food Guide Pyramid, should be planned according to age, sex, and goals for BMI.
- A slightly higher protein intake than usual may help reduce binge eating behavior. Less hunger, greater fullness, and lower overall food intake may occur after eating protein more than after eating CHO (Latner and Wilson, 2004).
- Alter diet according to medication therapies, medical recommendations or history, and interdisciplinary care plan. This may include restriction of CHO, protein, fat, sodium, or other nutrients accordingly.

CLINICAL INDICATORS

Clinical/History		Lab Work
Height	Binge pattern and frequency	Serum cortisol (high?)
Weight	Socially Prescribed Perfectionism Scale	Na+, K+, Cl−
BMI	Eating disorder examination	BUN, Creat
% Weight changes		Gluc
Dietary/intake history		Urinary acetone
		Chol, Trig

Common Drugs Used and Potential Side Effects

- Pharmacotherapy is often beneficial in addition to psychotherapy. Antidepressants may be useful; monitor their specific effects.
- Topiramate (Topamax) may be an effective BED treatment; it has mild side effects, such as weight loss, that may be desirable (McElroy et al, 2004; Shapira et al, 2000).
- The antiobesity agent sibutramine significantly reduces binge eating behavior and body weight in BED (Appolinario and McElroy, 2004).

Herbs, Botanicals, and Supplements

- No specific herbs and botanical products have been used for binge eating in any clinical trials.

INTERVENTION: NUTRITION EDUCATION, COUNSELING, CARE MANAGEMENT

- Discuss use of a food diary to record time, place, foods eaten, cues, binge feelings, and other comments.
- Discuss exercise and its effect on sense of well-being.
- Discuss shopping, holidays, and stressors.
- Discuss not skipping breakfast and lunch. This may lead to bingeing late into the evening or night.
- Focus on self-efficacy and proper assertiveness for coping with stressors.

Patient Education—Foodborne Illness

- Careful food handling will be important. The same is true for hand washing.
- Note any unusual behaviors, such as pica, and discuss food safety issues if relevant.

For More Information

- Academy for Eating Disorders
  http://www.aedweb.org
- Eating Disorders Anonymous
  http://www.eatingdisordersanonymous.org/
- National Association of AN and Associated Disorders (ANAD)
  http://www.anad.org/
- National Eating Disorders Association
  http://www.edap.org/

BINGE EATING DISORDER—CITED REFERENCES

Appolinario JC, McElroy SL. Pharmacological approaches in the treatment of binge eating disorder. *Curr Drug Targets.* 5:301, 2004.

Didie ER, Fitzgibbon M. Binge eating and psychological distress: is the degree of obesity a factor? *Eat Behav.* 6:35, 2005.

Dunkley DM, et al. Personal standards and evaluative concerns: dimensions of "clinical" perfectionism: a reply to Shafran et al. (2002, 2003) and Hewitt et al. (2003). *Behav Res Ther.* 44:63, 2006.

Gluck ME, et al. Cortisol, hunger, and desire to binge eat following a cold stress test in obese women with binge eating disorder. *Psychosom Med.* 66:876, 2004.

Latner JD, Wilson GT. Binge eating and satiety in bulimia nervosa and binge eating disorder: effects of macronutrient intake. *Int J Eat Disord.* 36:402, 2004.

McElroy SL, et al. Topiramate in the long-term treatment of binge-eating disorder associated with obesity. *J Clin Psychiatry.* 65:1463, 2004.

Shapira N, et al. Treatment of binge-eating disorder with topiramate: a clinical case series. *J Clin Psychiatry.* 61:368, 2000.

BULIMIA NERVOSA

NUTRITIONAL ACUITY RANKING: LEVEL 3–4

DEFINITIONS AND BACKGROUND

Bulimia nervosa is an eating disorder with food addiction as the primary coping mechanism. Criteria for diagnosis of bulimia include recurrent episodes of binge eating, sense of lack of control, self-evaluation unduly influenced by weight or body shape, and recurrent and inappropriate compensating behavior two times weekly for 3 months or longer (vomiting, use of laxatives or diuretics, fasting, excessive exercise).

In bulimia nervosa, repeated binge episodes increase gastric capacity, which delays emptying, blunts cholecystokinin (CCK) release, and impairs satiety response (Devlin et al, 1997). Purging versus nongorging types have been identified in this condition. When not bingeing, individuals with bulimia nervosa tend to be dieting; when hungry, they might binge again.

Of the 5–30% of the population with bulimia, 85% are college-educated women. Self-worth tends to be associated with thinness in these individuals. They are also more likely to experience loneliness, irritability, passivity, and sadness and to be prone to suicidal behavior. Bulimia nervosa can be fatal if left untreated.

Usually, 60–70% of bulimics have had overweight mothers, and eating may have been taught as a coping mechanism for stress. Codependency, a dysfunctional pattern of relating to one's own feelings, may be present. Individuals with bulimia nervosa focus on others or on things outside of themselves and deny their feelings. Fear, shame, despair, anger, rigidity, denial, and confusion may be integral.

Weight may be normal or near normal. Addictive behavior patterns and impulse control are common; they may shoplift, be promiscuous, and abuse alcohol, drugs, or credit cards. Substance disorders are common in bulimia, with disordered eating occurring for some time before drug or alcohol problems.

Disturbances in neuronal systems have been found to play a role in the modulation of feeding, mood, and impulse control (Barbarich et al, 2003), including neuropeptides (CRH, opioids, neuropeptide-Y [NPY] and peptide YY [PYY], vasopressin and oxytocin, CCK, and leptin) and monoamines (serotonin, dopamine, and norepinephrine). After recovery, there continues to be altered serotonin levels, which may contribute to continued problems with disordered eating.

Cognitive dysfunction, use of food or substance to relieve anxiety or depression, secretiveness, social isolation, and denial are common. Low self-esteem needs to be corrected. Therefore, psychotherapy is of primary importance. The multidisciplinary team approach to the patient with disordered eating is best practice; members include a physician, a nutritionist, and a mental health professional (Joy et al, 2003).

INTERVENTION: OBJECTIVES

- Stabilize fluid and electrolyte imbalances.
- Assess patient thoroughly and create an individualized care plan. Include such factors as weight history, dieting behaviors, binge eating episodes, purging behaviors, eating patterns, and exercise patterns.
- Promote effective weight control while altering lifestress management. Establish a target weight in accordance with desirable BMI, present weight, time frame for recovery, and related factors. Fear of suggesting a diet for obese persons (i.e., that it will lead to an eating disorder) should not prevent care providers from recommending modest energy restrictions (Wadden et al, 2004).
- Correct or prevent edema.

- Counteract lowered metabolic rate with balanced diet and exercise.
- Prevent oral health problems, including tooth enamel decay or erosion (perimolysis), from vomiting and poor eating habits. About one third of persons with this condition will have erosion. Table 4-16 lists oral manifestations and issues of concern in bulimia nervosa.

INTERVENTION: FOOD AND NUTRITION

- Use controlled portions of a regular diet, usually with three meals and two snacks.
- Provide basal energy needs plus 300–400 calories as a beginning stage.
- Decrease sugar and alcohol intake, stressing importance of other key nutrients. Highlight nutrient density and impact on health, appearance, and stamina.
- Encourage exercise along with diet and psychotherapy. Exercise decreases negative mood, improves eating disorders, and leads to more overall weight loss (Fossati et al, 2004).

CLINICAL INDICATORS

Clinical/History

Hx of laxative and diuretic abuse
BP
Height
Weight, current
Usual weight
BMI
Percentage of weight changes
Dietary/intake history
Oral/dental concerns
PET scan

Lab Work

Chol, Trig
Gastrin
LH, FSH (may be low)
Gluc
Alb
Na+, K+, Cl−
Serum cortisol
Serum folate
BP

TABLE 4-16 Assessment of Oral Manifestations in Bulimia Nervosa

Condition	Issues of Concern
Enamel erosion (perimolysis)	Thermal sensitivity and pain
Salivary gland swelling (sialadenosis)	Hypertrophy from regurgitation of acidic contents; malnutrition
Dry mouth (xerostomia)	From vomiting, laxative, or diuretic abuse
Increased serum amylase	2–4 times increased levels occur after binging and vomiting; a marker for bulimia
Mucosal trauma	Abrasions and bleeding from rapid, forceful regurgitation
Gingival recession	From frequent and rigorous tooth brushing
Dental caries	From increased intake of junk foods, candy, sweets

Common Drugs Used and Potential Side Effects

- Opiate antagonists, lithium, and older anticonvulsants are not very effective in bulimia nervosa. One promising medication that requires further study is ondansetron (Kaplan, 2003).
- The new anticonvulsant topiramate has shown good results in both binge and purge symptoms and represents a potential treatment for bulimia nervosa (Hoopes et al, 2003). Topiramate tends to cause anorexic symptoms and weight loss.
- Antidepressants may be used. Monitor side effects such as glucose changes, dry mouth, constipation, increased blood pressure, abdominal cramps, and weight changes. Avoid use with ma huang (ephedra), St. John's wort, and gingko biloba because they may enhance the effects and cause restlessness.
- Laxative and diuretic abuse can cause cardiac arrest and other problems. Discourage this practice.

Herbs, Botanicals, and Supplements

- Alternative medicines are frequently used in this population; many products are available with potentially significant toxicities, especially diet pills and diuretics (Roerig et al, 2003).
- No specific herbs and botanical products have been used for bulimia nervosa in any clinical trials.
- Ma huang (ephedra), St. John's wort, and gingko biloba may enhance the effects of antidepressants and cause restlessness.
- With anticonvulsants such as phenytoin (Dilantin), avoid use with evening primrose oil, gingko biloba, and kava.

INTERVENTION: NUTRITION EDUCATION, COUNSELING, CARE MANAGEMENT

- Use of a biopsychosocial approach offers a means of working toward healing the whole person (Kreipe, 2006). The four elements of successful treatment in adolescents are (Kreipe and Yussman, 2003):
  - Recognizing the disorder and restoring physiological stability early in its course.
  - Establishing a trusting, therapeutic partnership with the adolescent.
  - Involving the family in treatment.
  - Using an interdisciplinary team approach.

SAMPLE NUTRITION DIAGNOSTIC STATEMENT

Bulimia Nervosa

PES: Disordered eating pattern related to harmful belief about food and nutrition (that kcals are not available after using laxatives) as evidenced by use of laxatives after meals.

Assessment Data: Food records.

Intervention: Educate and counsel about food and absorption after meals, dangers of laxative use for weight control.

Monitoring and Evaluation: Food records, self-report of decreased use of laxatives as a weight-control measure.

- The combination of cognitive-behavioral therapy with a nutritional education and a physical activity program helps to decrease depression and anxiety (Fossati et al, 2004).
- Help the patient rediscover the ability to be alone without giving in to the urge to binge. Assertiveness training may be of great benefit.
- Information, as from basic nutrition texts, can also encourage improved habits.
- Discuss the outcomes of electrolyte imbalance, such as muscle spasms, kidney problems, or cardiac arrest.
- Assert that there is "no such thing as a forbidden food." Discuss how to handle the cycle of bulimia: hopelessness or anxiety leading to gorging, leading to fear of fatness, leading to vomiting or drug abuse, leading to release from fear, leading to guilt, etc.
- Stringent oral hygiene after vomiting may reduce dental erosion.
- Self-help groups are often beneficial.
- Table 4-17 describes other disordered eating patterns.

TABLE 4-17 Other Disordered Eating Patterns

Disorder	Description
Anorexia athletica (compulsive exercising)	The person repeatedly exercises beyond the requirements for good health and is a fanatic about weight and diet. Not a formal diagnosis; behaviors are usually a part of anorexia nervosa, bulimia, or obsessive-compulsive disorder. Focuses on challenge and does not savor victory; proud of being an "elite athlete." Rarely satisfied with athletic achievements or performance. Needs a team approach for therapeutic intervention.
Body dysmorphic disorder (BDD)	BDD is thought to be a subtype of obsessive-compulsive disorder. It is not a variant of anorexia nervosa or bulimia nervosa. The person feels "ugly" and suffers from shyness and acts withdrawn in new situations or with unfamiliar people. Often strikes before age 18; affecting 2% of people in the United States. Sufferers are excessively concerned about appearance, in particular perceived flaws of face, hair, and skin. They are convinced these flaws exist despite reassurances from friends and family members who usually can see nothing to justify such intense worry and anxiety. High risk for despair and suicide; may undergo unnecessary, expensive plastic surgery. BDD is treatable and begins with an evaluation by a physician and mental health care provider. Treatments include medication that adjusts serotonin levels in the brain and cognitive-behavioral therapy. A clinician makes the diagnosis and recommends treatment based on the needs and circumstances of each person.
Cyclic vomiting syndrome	Cycles of frequent vomiting, usually (but not always) found in children, often related to migraine headaches. Careful medical assessment is needed. Not a true eating disorder.
Eating disorders not otherwise specified (ED-NOS)	Official diagnosis describing atypical eating disorders where a person meets some but not all criteria for one specific eating disorder. Food behaviors are not normal and healthy; for example, behavior that resembles bulimia nervosa because of purging but without binge eating.
Gourmand syndrome	Person is preoccupied with fine food, including its purchase, preparation, presentation, and consumption. Exceedingly rare; thought to be caused by injury to the right side of the brain (as from tumor, concussion, or stroke). Relationship to addictions or obsessive-compulsive disorder possible. Had normal relationship with food prior to injury. Start with a neurologist evaluation.
Muscle dysmorphic disorder (bigorexia)	Sometimes called bigorexia, muscle dysmorphia is the opposite of anorexia nervosa. People with this disorder obsess about being small and undeveloped. They worry that they are too little and too frail. Even if they have good muscle mass, they believe their muscles are not big enough or are inadequate. Depression is the underlying concern. May understand the risks of steroid use but continue anyway. This condition results in disordered eating with very high protein and very low fat and often very low carbohydrate, often combined with excessive supplements.
Night eating syndrome	Affects 1–2% of general population. Likely that over one quarter of all morbidly obese persons may have this condition. This disorder is being considered for next psychiatric diagnostic classification manual. The person has little or no appetite for breakfast, delays first meal for several hours after waking up, and is often upset about how much was eaten the night before. Most calories are eaten late in the day or during the night. Sertraline, a selective serotonin reuptake inhibitor, may be beneficial in the treatment of night eating syndrome (O'Reardon et al, 2004). Psychotherapy is recommended. Self-help groups such as Overeaters Anonymous or group therapy can help.
Nocturnal sleep-related eating disorder	More of a sleep disorder than a true eating disorder. Individual eats while asleep and may sleep walk. No conscious memory of eating when they awaken again. Much guilt and confusion ensues.
Orthorexia nervosa	Eating the "right" food becomes an important, or even the primary, focus of life. One's worth or goodness is seen in terms of what one does or does not eat. Personal values, relationships, career goals, and friendships become less important than the quality and timing of what is consumed. May be a type of obsessive-compulsive disorder.
Pica	A craving for nonfood items such as dirt, clay, plaster, chalk, or paint chips. Pica may occur in pregnancy, in people whose diets are deficient in minerals found in the substances, in people with psychiatric conditions or developmental disabilities, or in people with family history of similar customs. Sometimes people who diet become hungry and ease their hunger with nonfood substances. May cause a medical emergency if obstruction or severe constipation occurs or if electrolyte imbalances occur.
Rumination syndrome	Person eats, swallows, and then regurgitates food back into the mouth where it is chewed and swallowed again. Process may be repeated several times or for several hours per episode. Process may be voluntary or involuntary. Ruminators report that regurgitated material does not taste bitter and that it is returned to the mouth with a gentle burp, not violent gagging or retching, not even nausea. Consequences range from minor inconveniences to life-threatening crises and include bad breath, indigestion, chapped lips and chin, damage to dental enamel and tissues in the mouth, aspiration pneumonia, failure to grow (children), weight loss, electrolyte imbalance, and dehydration.

From: O'Reardon and Stunkard, 2004; Anorexia Nervosa and Related Eating Disorders, Inc website: http://www.anred.com/defslesser.html; accessed January 18, 2005.

Patient Education—Foodborne Illness

- Careful food handling and hand washing are important. If constant hand washing is a concern, referral to a mental health provider may be useful.

For More Information

- Academy for Eating Disorders
  http://www.aedweb.org
- Anorexia Nervosa and Related Eating Disorders
  http://www.anred.com/
- Eating Disorders Anonymous
  http://www.eatingdisordersanonymous.org/
- National Association of Anorexia Nervosa and Associated Disorders (ANAD)
  http://www.anad.org/
- National Eating Disorders Association
  http://www.edap.org/
- Orthorexia
  http://www.orthorexia.com

BULIMIA NERVOSA—CITED REFERENCES

Barbarich NC, et al. Neurotransmitter and imaging studies in anorexia nervosa: new targets for treatment. *Curr Drug Targets CNS Neurol Disord.* 2:61, 2003.

Devlin M, et al. Postprandial cholecystokinin release and gastric emptying in patients with bulimia nervosa. *Am J Clin Nutr.* 65:114, 1997.

Fossati M, et al. Cognitive-behavioral therapy with simultaneous nutritional and physical activity education in obese patients with binge eating disorder. *Eat Weight Disord.* 9:134, 2004.

Hoopes SP, et al. Treatment of bulimia nervosa with topiramate in a randomized, double-blind, placebo-controlled trial, part 1: improvement in binge and purge measures. *J Clin Psychiatry.* 64:1335, 2003.

Joy EA, et al. The multidisciplinary team approach to the outpatient treatment of disordered eating. *Curr Sports Med Rep.* 2:331, 2003.

Kaplan AS. Academy for Eating Disorders International Conference on Eating Disorders. Denver, CO, USA, May 29-31, 2003. *Expert Opin Invest Drugs.* 12:1441, 2003.

Kreipe RE. The biopsychosocial approach to adolescents with somatoform disorders. *Adolesc Med Clin.* 17:1, 2006.

Kreipe RE, Yussman SM. The role of the primary care practitioner in the treatment of eating disorders. *Adolesc Med.* 14:133, 2003.

O'Reardon JP, Stunkard AJ, Allison KC. Clinical trial of sertraline in the treatment of night eating syndrome. *Int J Eat Disord.* 35:16, 2004.

Roerig JL, et al. The eating disorders medicine cabinet revisited: a clinician's guide to appetite suppressants and diuretics. *Int J Eat Disord.* 33:443, 2003.

Wadden TA, et al. Dieting and the development of eating disorders in obese women: results of a randomized controlled trial. *Am J Clin Nutr.* 80(3):560, 2004.

MENTAL DISORDERS–OTHER

BIPOLAR DISORDER

NUTRITIONAL ACUITY RANKING: LEVEL 1–2

DEFINITIONS AND BACKGROUND

Abnormalities in brain biochemistry and circuits are responsible for the extreme shifts in mood, energy, and functioning that characterize bipolar disorder. Bipolar affective disorders are characterized by mood swings from mania (exaggerated feeling of well-being, stimulation, and grandiosity in which a person can lose touch with reality) to depression (overwhelming feelings of sadness, anxiety, and low self-worth, which can include suicidal thoughts and suicide attempts). The disorders affect men and women equally. Children are rarely affected. See Table 4-18.

The old name for bipolar disorder is manic-depressive illness. The spectrum involves depression with varying degrees of excitatory signs and symptoms. Genetics seem to be involved. Relatives of people with bipolar affective disorder and depression are more likely to be affected. In general, the less severe the case, the later the onset of clinically observable mood disorder.

According to the DSM-IV, bipolar disorder is a severe, recurrent, lifelong illness that affects up to about 7% of Americans. Lifetime prevalence rates for bipolar I and II disorder range up to 2%; for cyclothymia, a milder form of bipolar disorder, prevalence ranges from 3–5%. More recent prevalence estimates are even higher. The World Health Organization reports that bipolar disorder is the sixth leading cause of years lived with disability, worldwide.

For doctors working in a primary care setting, it is important to recognize the signs and symptoms of bipolar disorder; it is commonly misdiagnosed as unipolar depression. Patients with bipolar depression are significantly more likely to report hallucinations, current suicidal ideation, and low self-esteem than patients with unipolar depression but less likely to report disturbed appetite (Das et al, 2005; Olfson et al, 2005).

The cyclical nature of the disorder poses challenges and barriers. Mood swings significantly impair the ability to func-

TABLE 4-18 The Bipolar Spectrum and Symptoms

Bipolar type I	Depression and varying degrees of excitatory signs and symptoms up to full mania	Onset during teens and early adulthood; 60% will have problems with substance abuse.
Bipolar type II	Discrete hypomanic episodes; may appear to have just depression, but mood stabilizers seem to help more than antidepressants	50% will have problems with substance abuse.
Bipolar type III	Hypomania associated with antidepressants and/or psychostimulants	
Bipolar type IV	Hyperthymic temperament	Onset during 4th or 5th decade of life
Bipolar type V	Recurrent depressions without discrete irritability, hypomania, but mixed hypomanic episodes with agitation, and racing thoughts during depression	
Bipolar type VI	Alzheimer's type	Onset in the 6th or 7th decade
Manic symptoms	Severe changes in mood, either extremely irritable or overly silly and elated	
	Overly inflated self-esteem, grandiosity	
	Increased energy	
	Decreased need for sleep, ability to go with very little or no sleep for days without tiring	
	Increased talking, talks too much, too fast; changes topics too quickly; cannot be interrupted	
	Distractibility, attention moves constantly from one thing to the next	
	Hypersexuality, increased sexual thoughts, feelings, or behaviors; use of explicit sexual language	
	Increased goal-directed activity or physical agitation	
	Disregard of risk, excessive involvement in risky behaviors or activities	
Depressive symptoms	Persistent sad or irritable mood	
	Loss of interest in activities once enjoyed	
	Significant change in appetite or body weight	
	Difficulty sleeping or oversleeping	
	Physical agitation or slowing	
	Loss of energy	
	Feelings of worthlessness or inappropriate guilt	
	Difficulty concentrating	
	Recurrent thoughts of death or suicide	

tion in social situations and to hold down a job. Patients often need to take days off from work either due to worsening clinical symptoms or hospitalization. When at work, problems may result from mood episodes such as poor concentration or low motivation during depression and inappropriate behavior during mania.

In mania, a person's behavior is often reckless and self-damaging. During mania, patients may spend excessive amounts of money or may have excessive urges to drive fast. During the depressive phase of the illness, patients may try to self-medicate themselves with alcohol or other substances, leading to problems with abuse or dependence. A series of four or more manic or depressive episodes in 12 months is known as "rapid cycling," a condition that can be more difficult to treat. Patients with bipolar I disorder are ill nearly half the time and have a high probability of relapse; bipolar II is more chronic, more depressive, and associated with more neuroticism and emotional instability between episodes than bipolar I (Keller, 2004).

Magnetic resonance spectroscopy imaging (MRSI) of the brains of patients (before starting medication) shows different patterns in the chemical fingerprint in more severe cases than patients with mild to moderate disease. Severe bipolar disorder requires more aggressive treatment.

Cholesterol levels are lower in manic and depressive phases than in mixed episodes; low cholesterol may be a result rather than a trait (Ghaemi et al, 2000). Individuals treated with omega-3 fatty acids (in combination with their usual mood stabilizing medications) for 4 months experience fewer mood swings and recurrence of either depression or mania (Keck et al, 2006)

For treatment of resistant bipolar disorder, high-dose thyroid hormones, calcium channel blockers, electroconvulsant therapy, omega-3 fatty acids, and various psychosocial strategies have been under active investigation (Gitlkin, 2001). Vitamin D may play a role. While often helpful, electroconvulsive therapy (ECT) may also lead to amnesia.

Comorbid conditions are almost always involved. Anxiety, substance use, and conduct disorders are the most common mental problems; overeating, sexual behavior, attention-deficit hyperactivity, impulse control, autism spectrum disorders, and Tourette's disorder are less common (McElroy, 2004). For these "dual diagnoses," both psychotherapy and appropriate medications are extremely important (Levin and Hennessey, 2004).

The most common general medical comorbidities are migraine, thyroid illness, obesity, type 2 diabetes, and cardiovascular disease (McElroy, 2004). Rates of chronic fatigue syndrome, migraine, asthma, chronic bronchitis, multiple chemical sensitivities, hypertension, and gastric ulcer tend to be significantly higher in the bipolar patient population (McIntyre et al, 2006). Painful physical symptoms are common, and treatment of both physical and emotional symptoms associated with mood disorders may increase a patient's chance of achieving remission; abnormalities of serotonin and noradrenaline are strongly associated (Wise et al, 2005).

INTERVENTION: OBJECTIVES

- Support efforts at maintaining a balance between nutritional intake, physical activity, medications, and well-being.
- Centrally located body fat and obesity are found to be more prevalent in bipolar patients compared to matched population controls (Elmslie et al, 2000). Monitor energy intake; counsel appropriately and offer tips for reducing kcals from meals, snacks, and beverages.
- Monitor for medical problems related to weight gain, such as low HDL and high LDL cholesterol levels, elevated triglyceride levels, hyperglycemia or diabetes, and cardiovascular problems.
- Seek stable periods that are relatively normal ("euthymia"). Reduce stress, which elevates protein kinase C levels in the brain.
- Manage comorbid conditions that occur, such as diabetes, obesity, cardiovascular disease, and thyroid disorders (McElroy, 2004).
- Maintain bone density since losses are common with various medications.

INTERVENTION: FOOD AND NUTRITION

- Persons with bipolar disorder may need an energy-controlled diet if their medication causes weight gain or obesity.
- Snacks that are low in energy or fat may be useful between meals. Offer suggestions on what to keep on hand.
- During episodes of depression, keeping prepared meals on hand, such as frozen dinners or packaged meals that are easy to fix, may be helpful.
- Discuss the inclusion of adequate fluid and fiber if constipation is a problem.
- Include sufficient to higher levels of calcium and vitamin D intake from diet; a multivitamin-mineral supplement may be beneficial.
- Include omega-3 fatty acids. Fish oil–enriched diets increase omega-3 fatty acids in tissue phospholipids; flax oil increases circulating $18{:}3\omega$-3, thereby presenting tissue with this EFA for further elongation and desaturation (Barcelo-Coblijn et al, 2005).

CLINICAL INDICATORS

Clinical/History		
Height	Disordered eating?	Clinical Global Impression Severity and Improvement Scores for Bipolar Disorder (CGI-BP)
Weight	Bipolar symptoms	DEXA scan
BMI	Mood Disorder Questionnaire	
Dietary/intake history	Sheehan Disability Scale	
BP		
I & O		
Constipation		
Food pica?		
Lab Work		
H & H	Trig	Serotonin
Serum Fe	Serum homocysteine	Thyroid tests (T4, TSH)
Alb	CRP	Na+, K+
Chol with full profile	Serum Ca++, Mg++	
	Gluc	

Common Drugs Used and Potential Side Effects

- Because of the risks of treating bipolar disorder with antidepressant monotherapy, physicians should assess their depressed patients for mania before prescribing antidepressants (Olfson et al, 2005). The American Psychiatric Association guideline for the treatment of bipolar disorder recommends optimizing individual medications before switching to combination therapy, especially preventing discontinuation of therapy because of side effects (Bowden, 2004). Depressive symptoms of bipolar disorder have a more negative impact on a patient's life than manic symptoms (Gao and Calabrese, 2005).
- **New antipsychotics** generally appear effective for acute mania, and some may ultimately prove effective in acute depression (e.g., olanzapine combined with fluoxetine, quetiapine) and maintenance (Gao and Calabrese, 2005). Some antipsychotics, particularly olanzapine, clozapine, chlorpromazine, and thioridazine, result in serious weight gain. Energy expenditure is lower in people taking atypical antipsychotics; weight management programs may need to offer 280 kcals less per day (Sharpe et al, 2005). Aripiprazole has been found to be effective and has fewer side effects than some of the other atypical antipsychotics (Perlis et al, 2006).
- **Mood stabilizers**, such as lithium carbonate (Lithane, Lithobid, Lithotabs) and valproate, stabilize mood by significantly decreasing the manic and hypomanic symptoms of bipolar disorder. They may also have effects on depressive symptoms. Lithium causes weight gain in many patients, with up to 25% becoming clinically obese. Lithium requires constancy in sodium intake and limits on caffeine. Metallic taste, nausea, vomiting, and diarrhea may also occur. Valproate increases

testosterone levels in teenage girls and may produce polycystic ovary syndrome; careful monitoring is needed. These medications are contraindicated in pregnancy and lactation; lithium is associated with cardiac malformations, and valproate is associated with neural tube defects.

- **New anticonvulsants** may be useful for aspects of bipolar disorders. Lamotrigine is used for maintenance or for acute bipolar depression. Compared with lithium and divalproex, lamotrigine is more effective in preventing bipolar depression (Gao and Calabrese, 2005). Topiramate may be used for problems related to obesity, bulimia, alcohol dependence, or migraine.
- **Multinutrient combinations** of vitamins, minerals, herbals, and the omega-3 fatty acids EPA and DHA have been found to be somewhat effective (Kidd, 2004). Pramipexole, a dopamine D2/D3 receptor agonist, and omega-3 fatty acids, a polyunsaturated fatty acid, are used to augment mood stabilizers and are excellent in reducing depressive symptoms (Gao and Calabrese, 2005).
- Treatment of comorbid conditions may include use of gabapentin for anxiety or pain and zonisamide for obesity.
- **Medicines that can cause mania** include: amphetamines, Antabuse, anticholinergics, baclofen, benztropine, bromocriptine, bupropion, captopril, cimetidine, corticosteroids, cyclosporine, hydralazine, isoniazid, levodopa, MAOIs such as Nardil or Parnate, Ritalin, Synthroid, opioids, procarbazine, and yohimbe.
- **Medicines that can cause depression** include: acyclovir, alcohol, anticonvulsants, asparaginase, baclofen, barbiturates, benzodiazepines, beta-blockers, bromocriptine, calcium channel blockers, corticosteroids, cycloserine, dapsone, estrogens, fluoroquinolone, histamine H_2–receptor antagonists, interferon, isotretinoin, mefloquine, methyldopa, metoclopramide, narcotics, progestins, statins, sulfonamides.

Herbs, Botanicals, and Supplements

- Licorice, ginger, purslane, rosemary, and ginseng have been suggested, but there are no clinical trials that prove efficacy in bipolar disorders.
- Ginseng and yohimbe should not be used with MAOI antidepressants.
- Gingko biloba interacts with anticoagulants and antiplatelets such as aspirin, warfarin, and dipyridamole.
- L-tryptophan may be tried for insomnia or depression. Do not use with MAOI antidepressants, SSRI antidepressants, or serotonin receptor antagonists.
- Ma huang (ephedra) and kava should not be taken by patients with depression.
- Psyllium and ginseng should not be used with divalproex or lithium.
- St. John's wort is used as a natural antidepressant. Do not use with MAOI antidepressants, SSRI antidepressants, cyclosporine, digoxin, oral contraceptives, HIV protease inhibitors, theophylline, warfarin, or calcium channel blockers such as amlodipine, diltiazem, or verapamil.

INTERVENTION: NUTRITION EDUCATION, COUNSELING, CARE MANAGEMENT

- Teach creative menu planning and food preparation methods that address the side effects and symptoms the patient is experiencing.
- Teach the patient how to moisten foods for dry mouth syndrome resulting from certain medications. Sugar-free candy may help.
- Limit caffeine-containing foods and beverages in the late evening to improve sleep.
- Individuals who are prone to bouts of depression or mania may find it difficult to eat properly. Simple meals and snacks should be readily available.
- Since there is a higher risk for suicide, individuals with bipolar disorder should be carefully monitored for signs of severe depression and should seek help from a mental health professional immediately.
- Functional outcomes are reliable measure of response to treatment. Changes in circadian rhythm and sleep patterns may predict onset of relapse (Keck 2004). Patients and families may benefit from education and therapy.

Patient Education—Foodborne Illness

- Careful food handling will be important. The same is true for hand washing.

For More Information

- Bipolar Help Center
  http://www.bipolarhelpcenter.com/index.jsp
- National Institute for Mental Health
  http://www.nimh.nih.gov/healthinformation/bipolarmenu.cfm
- National Mental Health Information Center
  http://www.mentalhealth.samhsa.gov/
- Suicide Prevention Information
  http://www.nimh.nih.gov/suicideprevention/index.cfm

BIPOLAR DISORDER—CITED REFERENCES

Barcelo-Coblijn G, et al. Dietary alpha-linolenic acid increases brain but not heart and liver docosahexaenoic acid levels. *Lipids* 40:787, 2005.

Bowden CL. Making optimal use of combination pharmacotherapy in bipolar disorder. *J Clin Psychiatry*. 15:21, 2004 (suppl).

Das AK, et al. Screening for bipolar disorder in a primary care practice. *JAMA*. 293:956, 2005.

Elmslie J, et al. Prevalence of overweight and obesity in bipolar patients. *J Clin Psychiatry*. 61:179, 2000.

Gao K, Calabrese JR. Newer treatment studies for bipolar depression. *Bipolar Disord*. 7:13S, 2005.

Ghaemi S, et al. Cholesterol levels in mood disorders: high or low? *Bipolar Disord*. 2:60, 2000.

Gitlin M, et al. Treatment-resistant bipolar disorder. *Bull Menninger Clin*. 65:26, 2001.

Keck PE Jr. Defining and improving response to treatment in patients with bipolar disorder. *J Clin Psychiatry*. 15:25, 2004 (suppl).

Keck PE Jr, et al. Double-blind, randomized, placebo-controlled trials of ethyl-eicosapentanoate in the treatment of bipolar depression and rapid cycling bipolar disorder. *Biol Psychiatry*. 2006. In press.

Keller MB. Improving the course of illness and promoting continuation of treatment of bipolar disorder. *J Clin Psychiatry*. 15:10, 2004 (suppl).

Kidd PM. Bipolar disorder and cell membrane dysfunction. Progress toward integrative management. *Altern Med Rev*. 9:107, 2004.

Levin FR, Hennessey G. Bipolar disorder and substance abuse. *Biol Psychiatry*. 56:738, 2004.

McElroy SL. Diagnosing and treating comorbid (complicated) bipolar disorder. *J Clin Psychiatry*. 15:35, 2004 (suppl).
McIntyre RS, et al. Medical comorbidity in bipolar disorder: implications for functional outcomes and health service utilization. *Psychiatr Serv*. 57: 1140, 2006.
Olfson M, et al. Bipolar depression in a low-income primary care clinic. *Am J Psychiatry*. 162:2146, 2005.
Perlis RH, et al. Atypical antipsychotics in the treatment of mania: a meta-analysis of randomized, placebo-controlled trials. *J Clin Psychiatry*. 67:509, 2006.
Sharpe JK, et al. Resting energy expenditure is lower than predicted in people taking atypical antipsychotic medication. *J Am Diet Assoc*. 105:612, 2005.
Wise TN, et al. Management of painful physical symptoms associated with depression and mood disorders. *CNS Spectr*. 10:1S, 2005.

DEPRESSION

NUTRITIONAL ACUITY RANKING: LEVEL 1 (MILD); LEVEL 2 (NUMEROUS MEDICATIONS)

DEFINITIONS AND BACKGROUND

Depression involves changes in body chemistry (neurotransmitters) after a traumatic event, hormonal changes, altered health habits, the presence of another illness, or substance abuse. Those persons with major depressive disorder have had at least one major depressive episode over a 14-day period or longer. It may be recurrent throughout their lives.

Depression is the leading cause of disability in the United States. About 39% of risk for major depression is inherited; 61% is from environmental factors such as substance abuse. In nursing homes, it is expected that about 50% of individuals will have some form of depression for which medication should be prescribed.

Dysthymia is a chronic, moderate type of depression and is expressed as poor appetite or overeating, insomnia or oversleeping, and low energy or fatigue. Awareness of a problem is low; functioning is usually not greatly impaired, but irritability and high stress are frequent. Seasonal affective disorder (SAD) increases with latitude; vitamin D and sunlight or light therapy may be beneficial.

Postpartum depression and antepartum depression are conditions that negatively affect mother and child and need to be detected as early as possible to limit the use of pharmacological treatments with possible side effects (Campagne, 2004). Careful assessment is needed to determine the specific type of depression and its most effective treatments.

Depression frequently develops between the ages of 25 and 44. Approximately 20 million adult Americans experience depression every day. Diagnosis of depression is indicated by four of eight of the following symptoms: SIGECAPS—Sleep changes, loss of Interest, inappropriate Guilt (hopelessness), Energy decline, Concentration changes, Appetite changes, Psychomotor changes, and Suicidal tendencies. In addition, prolonged sadness and unexplained crying spells, chronic irritability and agitation or anxiety, chronic pessimism or indifference, indecisiveness, social withdrawal, and unexplained aches and pains may also be present.

Men often mask signs of depression by working long hours or drinking too much. Women may have first signs of depression during times of hormonal change (menstruation, pregnancy, miscarriage, the postpartum period, and menopause). Children and teens who experience depression may experience frequent headaches and absences from school. Older individuals may experience depression along with a chronic disease such as heart disease, diabetes, or hypertension. Levels of C-reactive protein tend to be elevated in depression, which may contribute to heart disease (Ford and Erlinger, 2004).

Monitoring physical health, including nutrition, is an important adjunct to medication or psychotherapy. There is some evidence to support psychotherapy as effective as medication for many individuals, even changing brain chemistry after cognitive restructuring. For some persons for whom medications and therapy are not useful, electroconvulsive therapy (ECT) may be helpful. Finally, an experimental pacemaker-like device is under trial that sends electrical stimulations into the vagus nerve of the neck, alleviating depressive symptoms.

Many persons with depression (40%) have a deficiency of brain serotonin. A mixed diet of protein/CHO should provide tryptophan, a precursor of serotonin. Intake of dietary protein high in tryptophan increases the ratio of tryptophan to large neutral amino acids (LNAA) and improves coping ability in stress-vulnerable persons (Markus et al, 2000). Antidepressants that are serotonin reuptake modulators actually promote growth of serotonin innervation in the forebrain (Zhou et al, 2006). Painful physical symptoms commonly exist comorbid with depressive disorders; better recognition and treatment of both physical and emotional symptoms associated with mood disorders may increase a patient's chance of achieving remission; abnormalities of serotonin and noradrenaline are strongly associated with depression and play a role in pain perception (Wise et al, 2005).

Adequate intake of long-chain polyunsaturated fatty acids, especially the omega-3 fatty acids, may reduce depression (Casper, 2004). The omega-3 fatty acids are important components of nerve cell membranes because they help nerve cells communicate with each other. In medicated patients, added treatment with omega-3 fatty acids, particularly EPA, may ameliorate symptoms of major depressive disorder (Casper, 2004).

INTERVENTION: OBJECTIVES

- Provide adequate nutritional intake (e.g., excessive weight loss or shock therapy requires increased energy intake).

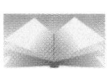

- Monitor weight at least twice monthly to evaluate status and changes.
- Assess usual eating habits and related problems, which may include loneliness, difficulty in activities of daily living, boredom, lack of hobbies and interests, and poor sleep habits. Adequate drug therapy usually helps appetite improve.
- Monitor for consequences such as weight gain from certain antidepressants.
- Assure adequate intake of amino acids, omega-3 fatty acids, folic acid, vitamin D, and related nutrients.
- Reduce stress, which elevates protein kinase C levels in the brain.

INTERVENTION: FOOD AND NUTRITION

- Use a diet providing high-quality protein. Inadequate protein intake may decrease intake of iron, thiamine, riboflavin, niacin, and vitamins B_6 and B_{12} as well.
- Increase intake of omega-3 fatty acids and uridine from foods such as fish, walnuts, molasses, and sugar beets (Carlezon et al, 2005). Supplements may also be used, but diet may be more beneficial.
- Low serum folate is common in many depressed adults, especially women (Tolmunen et al, 2004; Ramos et al, 2004). Intake of 400 μg is needed daily.
- Vitamin D should be supplemented, and calcium intake needs to be sufficient to protect bone density (Mussolino et al, 2004).
- If serum homocysteine levels are high, include more vitamins B_6 and B_{12} in addition to folate.
- Use a tyramine-restricted diet for patients given MAOI drugs. Such a diet excludes aged cheese, beer, red wine, ale, chicken livers, broad bean pods, sausage, salami, pepperoni, commercial gravies, ripe avocado, fermented soy sauce, and pickled or smoked herring.
- If overeating, limit access to food and provide low-calorie diet information. Encourage increased physical activity, which often helps to lift depressive moods.
- Sometimes a craving for carbohydrates occurs; monitor if weight gain is a problem or if overall nutrient density decreases.
- Intake of liquid supplements may be useful because they require less effort.
- TPN is not advised for patients who are suicidal.

CLINICAL INDICATORS

Clinical/History		
	Constipation	Thyroid tests (T4, TSH)
	DEXA scan	Na+, K+
Height		N balance
Weight	**Lab Work**	Serum homocysteine
BMI		Serum folate and B_{12}
Weight changes	H & H	CRP
Dietary/intake history	Serum Fe	
	Alb	
BP	Ca++, Mg++	
Food pica	Gluc	
I & O	Serotonin	

Common Drugs Used and Potential Side Effects

- See Table 4-19.
- Some serotonergic antidepressants (e.g., fluoxetine) reduce hyperglycemia, normalize glucose homeostasis, and increase insulin sensitivity, whereas some noradrenergic antidepressants (e.g., desipramine) exert opposite effects (McIntyre et al, 2006).

Herbs, Botanicals, and Supplements

- Licorice, ginger, purslane, rosemary, and ginseng have been suggested for depression, but there are no clinical trials that prove efficacy.
- Ginseng and yohimbe should not be used with MAOI antidepressants.
- L-tryptophan may be tried for insomnia or depression. Do not use with MAOI antidepressants, SSRI antidepressants, or serotonin receptor antagonists.
- Ma huang (ephedra) and kava should not be used with antidepressants.
- St. John's wort is used as a natural antidepressant. Do not use with MAOI antidepressants, SSRI antidepressants, cyclosporine, digoxin, oral contraceptives, HIV protease inhibitors, theophylline, warfarin, or calcium channel blockers such as amlodipine, diltiazem, or verapamil.

INTERVENTION: NUTRITION EDUCATION, COUNSELING, CARE MANAGEMENT

- Encourage full involvement with psychotherapy, cognitive-behavioral therapy (CBT), or interpersonal therapy (IPT). These are helpful with (or instead of) medication.
- Teach creative menu planning and food preparation methods that address the side effects and symptoms the patient is experiencing.
- Teach the patient how to moisten foods for dry mouth syndrome resulting from certain medications. Sugar-free candy may help.
- Promote exercise, which seems to help reduce symptoms of depression. Teens may be especially vulnerable to depression, and exercise may help improve other health- related behaviors, including eating better (Fulkerson et al, 2004).
- Limit caffeine-containing foods and beverages in the late evening.
- After giving birth, three postpartum mood disorders—postpartum "blues," postpartum depression, and postpartum psychosis—may occur, and education is an important instrument in the treatment of these disorders (Spinelli, 1998). Maternal depression in the prenatal and postnatal periods predicts poorer growth and higher risk of diarrhea in some infants (Rahman et al, 2004).
- In the elderly, "failure to thrive" usually includes: impaired physical function, malnutrition, depression, and cognitive impairment (Robertson and Montagnini, 2004). Treatment of depression may help to improve appetite. Adding breakfast to homebound meals for the elderly may be a good start (Gollub and Weddle, 2004).

TABLE 4-19 **Medications for Depression and Mood Disorders and Possible Side Effects**

Medication	Side Effects
Dual-mechanism antidepressants: Cymbalta (duloxetine), Effexor (venlafaxine)	Approved for the treatment of major depressive disorder in 2004, these are serotonin and norepinephrine reuptake inhibitors. Dual-mechanism antidepressants do not appear to disrupt glucose homeostatic dynamics. Brain-derived neurotrophic factor, which is increased with antidepressant treatment, appears to influence regulation of mood and perception of pain; evidence indicates that dual-acting agents may have an advantage in modulating pain over those agents that increase either serotonin or noradrenaline alone (Wise et al, 2005).
Other antidepressants	Clomipramine (Anafranil) is used in obsessive-compulsive disorders. Dry mouth is common; hard sugarless candy or chewing gum may be useful. Anorexia and abdominal pain are also common. Norpramin (desipramine) may cause abdominal cramps, altered blood glucose levels, and vomiting. Avoid use with ma huang (ephedra), St. John's wort, and ginkgo biloba. Nortriptyline (Aventyl, Pamelor) may cause increased appetite for sweets, GI distress, vomiting, and diarrhea. Wellbutrin (bupropion) tends to have a stimulating effect but may also cause weight loss, dry mouth, nausea, and vomiting. It may be used to help with smoking cessation.
Monoamine oxidase inhibitors: Parnate (tranylcypromine), Nardil (phenelzine), Marplan (isocarboxazid)	Nonselective hydrazine monoamine oxidase inhibitors (e.g., phenelzine) are associated with hypoglycemia and an increased glucose disposal rate (McIntyre et al, 2006). Tyramine is a pressor amine. Tyramine-restricted diet to prevent hypertensive crisis: spoiled, overripe, and aged products are the most problematic. Beware of Chianti wines, beer, fava beans, and sauerkraut. Constipation, weight gain, and GI distress are common side effects. Avoid ginseng, L-tryptophan, yohimbe, St. John's wort, kava, and ma huang (ephedra).
SAMe (S-5-adenosyl-methionine)	Useful for mild depression but may trigger coronary problems. A positive side effect is that it may actually help with degenerative joint disease symptoms.
Selective serotonin reuptake inhibitors (SSRIs): Paxil (paroxetine), Prozac (fluoxetine), Zoloft (sertraline)	May cause abdominal pain, anorexia, diarrhea, and weight changes; SSRIs are used to treat despair and helplessness. Prozac may also cause nausea, vomiting, glucose changes, and decreased sodium. Do not use in pregnancy; neurobehavioral effects have been noted in otherwise healthy infants (Zeskind and Stephens, 2004). Fetal exposure to a mother's antidepressants during pregnancy may leave her newborn in withdrawal, known as neonatal abstinence syndrome (Levinson-Castiel et al, 2006). Zoloft can cause dry mouth and diarrhea; avoid use with St. John's wort and ma huang (ephedra).
Tranquilizers, benzodiazepines: Halcion (triazolam), Versed (midazolam), Serax (oxazepam), Librium (chlordiazepoxide), Xanax (alprazolam), Restoril (temazepam), Ativan (lorazepam), Klonopin (clonazepam), Tranxene (clorazepate) Valium (diazepam), Dalmane (flurazepam)	The main use of the short-acting benzodiazepines is in insomnia, while anxiety responds better to medium- to long-acting substances that will be required all day. Benzodiazepines may cause either weight loss or gain and GI distress. Avoid use with sedatives or chamomile. Increased thirst is common.
Tricyclic antidepressants: Tofranil (imipramine), Elavil (amitriptyline), Asendin (amoxapine), Doxepin (sinequan)	May cause dry mouth, increase in appetite, weight gain, nausea, vomiting, syndrome of inappropriate antidiuretic hormone (SIADH), constipation, anorexia, or stomatitis.

Patient Education—Foodborne Illness

- Careful food handling will be important. The same is true for hand washing.

For More Information

- Academy of Cognitive Therapy
  http://www.academyofct.org
- American Mental Health Counselors Association
  http://www.amhca.org/
- American Psychiatric Association
  http://www.psych.org/
- American Society of Geriatric Psychiatry
  http://www.aagpgpa.org/
- Anxiety Disorders of America
  http://www.adaa.org/
- Depression and Bipolar Support Alliance
  http://www.dbsalliance.org/
- Depression and Related Affective Disorders Association
  http://www.drada.org/
- National Depression Screening
  http://www.mentalhealthscreening.org/events/ndsd/results.htm

DEPRESSION—CITED REFERENCES

Campagne DM. The obstetrician and depression during pregnancy. *Eur J Obstet Gynecol Reprod Biol.* 116:125, 2004.

Carlezon WA Jr, et al. Antidepressant-like effects of uridine and omega-3 fatty acids are potentiated by combined treatment in rats. *Biol Psychiatry.* 57:343, 2005.

Casper RC. Nutrients, neurodevelopment, and mood. *Curr Psychiatry Rep.* 6:425, 2004.

Ford DE, Erlinger TP. Depression and C-reactive protein in US adults: data from the Third National Health and Nutrition Examination Survey. *Arch Intern Med.* 164:1010, 2004.

Fulkerson JA, et al. Depressive symptoms and adolescent eating and health behaviors: a multifaceted view in a population-based sample. *Prev Med.* 38:865, 2004.
Gollub EA, Weddle DO. Improvements in nutritional intake and quality of life among frail homebound older adults receiving home-delivered breakfast and lunch. *J Am Diet Assoc.* 104:1227, 2004.
Levinson-Castiel R, et al. Neonatal abstinence syndrome after in utero exposure to selective serotonin reuptake inhibitors in term infants. *Arch Pediatr Adolesc Med.* 160:173, 2006.
Markus C, et al. The bovine protein alpha-lactalbumin increases the ratio of tryptophan to the other large neutral amino acids, and in vulnerable subjects raises brain serotonin activity, reduces cortisol concentration, and improves mood under stress. *Am J Clin Nutr.* 71:1536, 2000.
McIntyre RS, et al. The effect of antidepressants on glucose homeostasis and insulin sensitivity: synthesis and mechanisms. *Expert Opin Drug Saf.* 5:157, 2006.
Mussolino ME, et al. Depression and bone mineral density in young adults: results from NHANES III. *Psychosom Med.* 66:533, 2004.
Rahman A, et al. Impact of maternal depression on infant nutritional status and illness: a cohort study. *Arch Gen Psychiatry.* 61:946, 2004.
Ramos MI, et al. Plasma folate concentrations are associated with depressive symptoms in elderly Latina women despite folic acid fortification. *Am J Clin Nutr.* 80:1024, 2004.
Robertson RG, Montagnini M. Geriatric failure to thrive. *Am Fam Physician.* 70:343, 2004.
Spinelli M. Antepartum and postpartum depression. *J Gend Specif Med.* 1:33, 1998.
Tolmunen T, et al. Dietary folate and the risk of depression in Finnish middle-aged men. A prospective follow-up study. *Psychother Psychosom.* 73:334, 2004.
Wise TN, et al. Management of painful physical symptoms associated with depression and mood disorders. *CNS Spectr.* 10:1S, 2005.
Zeskind PS, Stephens LE. Maternal selective serotonin reuptake inhibitor use during pregnancy and newborn neurobehavior. *Pediatrics* 113:368, 2004.
Zhou L, et al. Evidence that serotonin reuptake modulators increase the density of serotonin innervation in the forebrain. *J Neurochem.* 96:396, 2006.

SCHIZOPHRENIA

NUTRITIONAL ACUITY RANKING: LEVEL 1–2

DEFINITIONS AND BACKGROUND

Schizophrenia (SCZ) is a group of disorders manifested by disordered thinking, hallucinations, delusions, social withdrawal, and mood and behavioral disturbances (delusional, catatonic, or paranoid). Nearly 1% of the population develops SCZ, with onset generally between ages 15–25 years. Onset is earlier in males.

SCZ has a genetic component. Genetic predisposition likely accounts for a large proportion of the cognitive deficits; five genes are being studied for their role (*COMT, GRM3, G72, DISC1*, and *BDNF*) in SCZ (Roffman et al, 2006). Magnetic resonance imaging studies have identified hippocampal volume reductions in SCZ (Velakoulis et al, 2006). Studies are limited by having small samples, especially early in the disease process.

In the resulting psychosis in SCZ, the individual loses contact with reality. It can be either episodic or chronic and will result in irrational behaviors. When patients are at risk of self-harm or harm to others, hospital treatment is appropriate. Delusions may involve control, persecution, grandiosity, or abnormal fears. Hallucinations are perceptions of an external stimulus without a source in the external world.

Psychotic behavior may also occur in patients with dementia that is caused by cerebral arteriosclerosis or chemical or toxic trauma; this is diagnosed using an Organic Brain Syndrome Scale. Organic forms of psychosis can cause dazed expressions, confused speech, visual hallucinations, bizarre or withdrawn behavior, low self-esteem, appetite changes, and sleep disturbances.

Folate levels may be lower in patients who have SCZ. Glutamate carboxypeptidase II (GCPII) regulates both folate absorption and activation of N-methyl-D-aspartic acid receptors, so it is hypothesized that folate and SCZ may be related (Goff et al, 2004). Some hypotheses suggest that low maternal folate, maternal stress, and childhood infections may lead to SCZ later (Smits et al, 2004). Selenium may also play role (Benton, 2002).

Oxidative stress, oxidative injury, and abnormal membrane phospholipid (essential polyunsaturated fatty acid [PUFA]) metabolism cause reduced levels of antioxidant enzymes in SCZ (Evans et al, 2003). In addition, the normal skin flush response to niacin is attenuated in SCZ and is mediated by prostaglandins that are derived from arachidonic acid (AA) (Messamore, 2003). These data support the hypothesis that relative depletion of AA and other essential fatty acids plays a role. People with SCZ experience an improvement in symptoms when given PUFA (Reddy and Yao, 2003).

Similar to diabetes, conversion of ALA to EPA or DHA is inefficient in SCZ. A tight relationship exists between essential fatty acid status and normal neurotransmission (duBois et al, 2005). These data support the augmentation of antipsychotic treatment by supplementation with a combination of antioxidants and omega-3 fatty acids (Evans et al, 2003; Richardson et al, 2003).

Low vitamin D availability during brain development interacts with susceptibility genes to alter the trajectory of brain development, probably by epigenetic regulation that alters gene expression throughout adult life (MacKay-Sim et al, 2004; McGrath et al, 2004). Vitamin D supplementation during the first year of life is associated with a reduced risk of SCZ in males; preventing hypovitaminosis D during early life may reduce the incidence of SCZ (McGrath et al, 2004).

Effective lipid control may be more difficult to attain for some patients with SCZ; additional research to clarify the barriers to effective lipid management is essential (Weiss et al, 2006).

INTERVENTION: OBJECTIVES

- Provide adequate nourishment to prevent significant weight changes. Weight gain is common with the use of many antipsychotic medications or with the presence of metabolic syndrome.

- Correct any nutritional deficits. Include sufficient levels of folate, vitamins B_6 and B_{12}, and vitamin D.
- Promote a normal pattern of dietary intake and routines.
- Develop a trusting relationship; make expectations clear to the patient.
- Prevent or correct constipation or impaction.
- Manage diabetes and coronary heart disease and their complications, which tend to be common and often underdiagnosed (Henderson, 2005; Peet, 2004). Metabolic syndrome is common in this population (McEvoy et al, 2005).
- Reduce stress, which increases protein kinase C in the brain. This also increases forgetfulness and speeds up aging.

INTERVENTION: FOOD AND NUTRITION

- A balanced diet for age and sex should be used, unless other medical conditions are present, such as diabetes or metabolic syndrome (Peet, 2004). Reduction in sugars and saturated fats may be beneficial if signs of metabolic syndrome are present.
- Adjust calories according to goal weight for patient and medications.
- Reduce potential accidents by avoiding glass containers and serving dishes.
- Vitamins C, D, B_6, and B_{12}, folate, and selenium levels may be low in persons with SCZ; encourage improved intake accordingly.
- Highlight use of antioxidant foods and omega-3 fatty acids (Evans et al, 2003; Richardson et al, 2003).
- Breastfeeding mothers should avoid use of medications as much as possible. Should psychiatric medication be necessary, available information regarding the effects of these medications on the infant should be provided. It is strongly recommended that the infant's pediatrician be involved in monitoring the infant (Burt et al, 2001).

CLINICAL INDICATORS

Clinical/History

- Height
- Weight
- Weight changes
- BMI
- Dietary/intake history
- I & O
- BP
- Dyskinesia
- Global Assessment of Functioning Scale (GAF)
- Positive and Negative Syndrome Scale (PANSS)
- Delusions, auditory hallucinations
- EEG and brain-wave patterns
- MRI or PET scans

Lab Work

- Alb, transthyretin
- Na+, K+
- H & H
- Serum Fe
- Gluc
- Creatine phosphokinase (CPK) (elevated in acute episodes)
- Chol (total profile)
- Trig
- Serum homocysteine
- Serum folate
- Serum B_{12}
- CRP
- Serum insulin
- Serum D_3
- Ca^{++}, Mg^{++}

Common Drugs Used and Potential Side Effects

- Some drugs can cause psychiatric symptoms. Anxiety, mania, hallucinations, suicidal thoughts, and bizarre behavior may result from various medications, and a doctor should be contacted if these occur. A psychiatric response is rare but may include:
  Confusion: acyclovir, propoxyphene (Darvon), and cimetidine (Tagamet)
  Depression: oral contraceptives, ibuprofen, metronidazole (Flagyl), barbiturates, cimetidine, and diazepam (Valium)
  Insomnia: acyclovir and alprazolam
  Paranoia: amphetamines, ibuprofen, cimetidine, and tricyclic antidepressants
  Excitement or agitation: alprazolam, amphetamines, barbiturates, metronidazole, and diazepam
- Antidepressants and medications may be used for some patients; evaluate specific drugs accordingly for possible side effects. See Depression entry.
- To reduce anxiety, Ativan, Xanax, Klonopin, and Paxil have been used. Sometimes, it is useful to offer a beverage or snack to reduce anxiety rather than adding more medications.
- Table 4-20 provides more guidance on medications.

Herbs, Botanicals, and Supplements

- Ginseng should not be used with CNS stimulants, caffeine, hormones, steroids, or antipsychotics. Ginseng and yohimbe should not be used with MAOI antidepressants.
- Gingko biloba interacts with anticoagulants and antiplatelets such as aspirin, warfarin, and dipyridamole.
- Indian snakeroot has been used for mental illness in some cultures. Do not use with digoxin, phenobarbital, levodopa, albuterol, furosemide, thiazide diuretics, MAOI antidepressants, beta-blockers such as atenolol or propranolol, or tranquilizers. Problems include potential sedation, increased blood pressure, arrhythmias, and CNS excitation.
- Kava and valerian should not be taken by patients with SCZ who are using anxiety-reducing drugs (e.g., alprazolam, diazepam, lorazepam).
- L-tryptophan may be tried for insomnia or depression. Do not use with MAOI antidepressants, SSRI antidepressants, or serotonin receptor antagonists.
- Ma huang (ephedra) and kava should not be taken in patients with depression.
- Psyllium and ginseng should not be used with divalproex or lithium.
- St. John's wort should not be used with MAOI antidepressants, SSRI antidepressants, cyclosporine, digoxin, oral contraceptives, HIV protease inhibitors, theophylline, warfarin, or calcium channel blockers such as amlodipine, diltiazem, or verapamil.

INTERVENTION: NUTRITION EDUCATION, COUNSELING, CARE MANAGEMENT

- Teach nutrition principles to the patient or the caregiver.

TABLE 4-20 Antipsychotic Medications and Possible Side Effects

Medication	Side Effects
Tranquilizers	Triavil combines an antidepressant with a tranquilizer. Nausea, diarrhea, and vomiting may result.
Typical antipsychotics: clozapine (Clozaril), butyrophenone (Haldol), thiothixene (Navane)	May cause dizziness, drowsiness, dry mouth, weight gain, edema, nausea, constipation, or vomiting. They help to quiet symptoms and help when the patient is resistant to other drugs and alternatives.
Phenothiazines: perphenazine (Trilafon), fluphenazine (Prolixin), prochlorperazine (Compazine), chlorpromazine (Thorazine)	Chlorpromazine (Thorazine) contains sulfites. It may cause dry mouth, constipation, and weight gain.
Atypical antipsychotics (aAPs): aripiprazole (Abilify), quetiapine (Seroquel), risperidone (Risperdal), olanzapine (Zyprexa), ziprasidone (Geodon)	The phospholipids in the neuronal membranes of the brain are rich in highly unsaturated essential fatty acids (EFAs). With a beneficial effect on dyskinesia as well, EPA is an effective adjunct to antipsychotics (Emsley et al, 2003). Biochemical measures showing depletion of essential fatty acids are generally normalized after 6 months of antipsychotic treatment (Evans et al, 2003). Aripiprazole exhibits high affinity for dopamine, serotonin, and histamine receptors. Ziprasidone is not as likely to cause weight gain as some other antipsychotics. Olanzapine performs modestly better than most other medications, but weight gain can be significant. The availability of long-acting risperidone injection may increase adherence and lead to improved clinical and economic outcomes for individuals with schizophrenia (Edwards et al, 2005). Typical doses may be: olanzapine (schizophrenia: 15 mg; mania: 20 mg); quetiapine (schizophrenia: 750 mg; mania: 800 mg); ziprasidone (schizophrenia and mania: 160 mg); aripiprazole (schizophrenia and mania: 30 mg).
SSRIs and obsessive-compulsive disorder medications	Prozac, Anafranil, Luvox, and Zoloft have been used with some success. Avoid use with ma huang (ephedra) and St. John's wort. Fluvoxamine (Luvox) is an SSRI that may cause anorexia, dry mouth, nausea, diarrhea, and constipation.

- Encourage self-care.
- Successfully terminate client relationship when independence is possible.
- Provide follow-up, especially with any stages of regression. If daily medications are a problem, monthly injectable medications may be useful.
- A quiet environment is often helpful when the patient is agitated. Identify if there are other causes of agitation besides SCZ. For example, trauma, pain, endocrine disorders, infection, and metabolic disorders may be present (Marco and Vaughan, 2005).
- Weight loss programs may be beneficial for patients with SCZ who have experienced weight gain from medications (Menza et al, 2004). In addition, following the National Cholesterol Education guidelines may be needed if lipids are elevated.
- Assist with attempts to quit smoking, which is common in SCZ patients. Because cigarette smoke contains many pro-oxidants that contribute directly to oxidative stress and because PUFAs are very susceptible to oxidative effects of free radicals, smoking should be discontinued (Reddy and Yao, 2003).
- Osteoporosis may be a problem with long-term medication use; monitor carefully (Hummer et al, 2005).

Patient Education—Foodborne Illness

- Careful food handling will be important. The same is true for hand washing.

SCHIZOPHRENIA—CITED REFERENCES

Benton D. Selenium intake, mood and other aspects of psychological functioning. *Nutr Neurosci.* 5:363, 2002.

Burt V, et al. The use of psychotropic medications during breastfeeding. *Am J Psychiatry.* 158:1001, 2001.

duBois TM, et al. Membrane phospholipid composition, alterations in neurotransmitter systems and schizophrenia. *Prog Neuropsychopharmacol Biol Psychiatry.* 29:878, 2005.

Edwards NC, et al. Cost effectiveness of long-acting risperidone injection versus alternative antipsychotic agents in patients with schizophrenia in the USA. *Pharmacoeconomics* 23:75S, 2005.

Emsley R, et al. Clinical potential of omega-3 fatty acids in the treatment of schizophrenia. *CNS Drugs.* 17:1081, 2003.

Evans DR, et al. Red blood cell membrane essential fatty acid metabolism in early psychotic patients following antipsychotic drug treatment. *Prostaglandins Leukot Essent Fatty Acids.* 69:393, 2003.

Goff DC, et al. Folate, homocysteine, and negative symptoms in schizophrenia. *Am J Psychiatry.* 161:1705, 2004.

Henderson DC. Schizophrenia and comorbid metabolic disorders. *J Clin Psychiatry.* 66:11S, 2005.

Hummer M, et al. Osteoporosis in patients with schizophrenia. *Am J Psychiatry.* 162:162, 2005.

MacKay-Sim A, et al. Schizophrenia, vitamin D, and brain development. *Int Rev Neurobiol.* 59:351, 2004.

Marco CA, Vaughan J. Emergency management of agitation in schizophrenia. *Am J Emerg Med.* 23:767, 2005.

McEvoy JP, et al. Prevalence of the metabolic syndrome in patients with schizophrenia: baseline results from the Clinical Antipsychotic Trials of Intervention Effectiveness (CATIE) schizophrenia trial and comparison with national estimates from NHANES III. *Schizophr Res.* 80:19, 2005.

McGrath J, et al. Vitamin D supplementation during the first year of life and risk of schizophrenia: a Finnish birth cohort study. *Schizophr Res.* 67:237, 2004.

Menza M, et al. Managing atypical antipsychotic-associated weight gain: 12-month data on a multimodal weight control program. *J Clin Psychiatry.* 65:471, 2004.

Messamore E. Relationship between the niacin skin flush response and essential fatty acids in schizophrenia. *Prostaglandins Leukot Essent Fatty Acids.* 69:413, 2003.

Peet M. Diet, diabetes and schizophrenia: review and hypothesis. *Br J Psychiatry Suppl.* 47:S102, 2004.

Reddy RD, Yao JK. Environmental factors and membrane polyunsaturated fatty acids in schizophrenia. *Prostaglandins Leukot Essent Fatty Acids.* 69:385, 2003.

Richardson AJ, et al. Omega-3 and omega-6 fatty acid concentrations in red blood cell membranes relate to schizotypal traits in healthy adults. *Prostaglandins Leukot Essent Fatty Acids.* 69:461, 2003.

Roffman JL, et al. Neuroimaging-genetic paradigms: a new approach to investigate the pathophysiology and treatment of cognitive deficits in schizophrenia. *Harv Rev Psychiatry.* 14:78, 2006.

Smits L, et al. Association between short birth intervals and schizophrenia in the offspring. *Schizophr Res.* 70:49, 2004.
Velakoulis D, et al. Hippocampal and amygdala volumes according to psychosis stage and diagnosis. *Arch Gen Psychiatry.* 63:139, 2006.
Weiss AP, et al. Treatment of cardiac risk factors among patients with schizophrenia and diabetes. *Psychiatr Serv.* 57:1145, 2006.

SUBSTANCE USE DISORDERS

NUTRITIONAL ACUITY RANKING: LEVEL 1 (WITHDRAWAL/REHABILITATION)

DEFINITIONS AND BACKGROUND

Substance use often leads to addiction. Addiction is a brain disorder, a chronic disorder with compulsive and relapsing behavior. Three predisposing factors exist: constitutional lability (biochemical), personality factor (psychological vulnerability), and social factors (environmental conditioning). Sensitivity to reward (STR) seems to play a role in addictions (Davis et al, 2004).

The master "pleasure" molecule of addiction is dopamine (D2 receptor gene). Heroin, amphetamines, marijuana, alcohol, nicotine, and caffeine all trigger the release of dopamine. Abnormalities in the metabolism of dopamine, serotonin, and norepinephrine may contribute to substance dependency. In some cases, use of antidepressant medications alleviate the dependency. See Figure 4-7.

Abuse of chemical substances may be chronic or acute and may involve abuse of alcohol, prescription or over-the-counter drugs, or illicit drugs. Physiological problems that result are definite and are usually specific to the abused substance. Social, emotional, vocational, and legal problems may arise. Persons with substance dependency tend to have type A personalities and are prone to perfectionism and depression. Substance abusers are codependent, neglecting their own feelings and emotions. Table 4-21 lists common addictions and related issues.

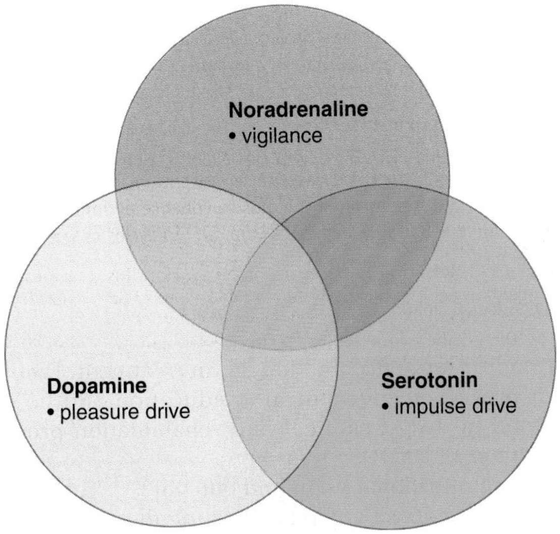

Figure 4-7 Interaction of neurotransmitters.

Eating disorders and substance disorders may represent different expressions of the same underlying problem. Commonalities include cognitive dysfunction, use of food or substance to relieve negative affect (anxiety or depression), secretiveness about the problem, and social isolation.

Studies also suggest that addiction to food may be a reality. Psychomotor stimulant drugs are no longer at the heart of all addictions; brain circuits can also be deranged with natural rewards like food (Davis et al, 2004). Overweight individuals may use food as a reward, just as substance abusers use pharmacological substances for a reward for the dopamine-specific part of the brain.

Alcoholism is a chronic relapsing disease that is frequently unrecognized and untreated; approximately one third of patients remain abstinent, and one third have fully relapsed 1 year after withdrawal from alcohol (Oroszi and Goldman, 2004). Many alcoholics are malnourished, and nutritional interventions are needed to prevent alcoholic liver disease. Use of antioxidants as precursors of the endogenous antioxidant glutathione and new nutritional supplements show promise (Lieber, 2003). Malnutrition is a common finding in chronic alcoholics, and protein–calorie malnutrition (PCM) is predictive of survival in patients with alcoholic liver disease; deficiencies of folate, thiamine, pyridoxine, and vitamin A enhance the likelihood of anemia, altered cognitive states, and night blindness (Halsted, 2004).

Genetics that alter alcoholism-related intermediate phenotypes include common alcohol dehydrogenases, catechol-O-methyltransferase (COMT), opioid receptors, and HTTLPR, which alters serotonin transport—all of which affect the process of addiction and relapse (Oroszi and Goldman, 2004). Other addictions may share some of the same biological pathways. Because polydrug use may alter food intake, taste preferences, and nutrient metabolism and because denial is common, psychotherapy along with substance withdrawal is recommended.

Assertive outreach is effective in engaging and linking persons with substance use disorders to substance abuse treatment services, even when they are homeless (Fisk et al, 2006). Giving up should not be an option.

INTERVENTION: OBJECTIVES

- Protect during withdrawal (e.g., alcohol detoxification may cause tremors, hallucinations, seizures, and delirium tremens). Of persons with delirium tremens, 20% may die, even with therapy; monitor closely.

Table 4-21 Common Addictions and Issues

Substance	Issues
Alcohol	The most consistent predictor of alcohol dependency is alcoholism in a biological parent. Alcoholics have 2.5 times the normal death rate in similar age groups, especially from stroke and cirrhosis. An estimated 3 million children between 14 and 17 years of age are problem drinkers. The earlier the exposure, the more likely dependency will occur. In women who are alcoholics and less than 30 years old, 72% also have an eating disorder. To assess for problems with alcoholism, C-A-G-E questions include: Have you tried to cut back? Has anybody ever annoyed you regarding this behavior? Have you ever felt guilty about it? Have you ever needed an early morning eye opener? With two or more affirmative answers, there is a problem that should be addressed.
Caffeine	Caffeine and nicotine are the most common psychostimulant drugs used worldwide (Dager and Friedman, 2000). Caffeine affects the brain in ways that are similar to cocaine and other stimulants, but it is not as addictive overall.
Chocolate	Chocolate may be used as self-medication for low magnesium levels and to balance low neurotransmitters for mood (serotonin and dopamine). Chocolate cravings are often episodic and related to hormonal swings such as with menses. Chocolate contains methylxanthines, biogenic amines, and cannabinoid-like fatty acids, all of which cause potentially abnormal behaviors and psychological sensations that parallel other addictions (Bruinsma and Taren, 1999). Other attributes are probably more important in determining related self-reports of chocolate cravings and "chocoholism" (Smit et al, 2004).
Club drugs: LSD (acid), MDMA (Ecstasy), GHB, GBL, ketamine (special K), Fentanyl, Rohypnol, amphetamines, and methamphetamine	"Club drug" is a vague term that refers to a wide variety of drugs including MDMA (ecstasy), GHB, Rohypnol, ketamine, methamphetamine, and LSD. Uncertainties about the drug sources, pharmacological agents, chemicals used to manufacture them, and possible contaminants make it difficult to determine toxicity, consequences, and symptoms. Serious health problems may result from their use.
Cocaine	The pure chemical, cocaine hydrochloride, has been an abused substance for more than 100 years, and coca leaves, the source of cocaine, have been ingested for thousands of years. Use has increased, and now over 1.5 million Americans are users. Young adults aged 18–25 are most likely to initiate use. Years later, cocaine use may be linked to Parkinson's disease. A study funded by the National Institutes of Health (NIH) suggests that a common over-the-counter herbal supplement can reduce the cravings associated with chronic cocaine use. N-acetylcysteine (NAC) is a potential agent to modulate the effects of cocaine addiction, heroin addiction, and possibly alcoholism. NAC is available over the counter as an herbal supplement known for its antioxidant effects.
Heroin	Heroin is processed from morphine, a naturally occurring substance extracted from the seedpod of the Asian poppy plant. Heroin usually appears as a white or brown powder. Street names for heroin include smack, H, skag, and junk. Other names may refer to types of heroin produced in a specific geographical area, such as Mexican black tar. Use of heroin may be fatal. Use during pregnancy may cause spontaneous abortion.
Marijuana	Marijuana is the most commonly used illicit drug in the United States. The main active chemical in marijuana is THC (delta-9-tetrahydrocannabinol). The membranes of certain nerve cells in the brain contain protein receptors that bind to THC. Once in place, THC kicks off a series of cellular reactions that ultimately lead to the high that users experience.
Nicotine	Along with directly stimulating the brain's reward system, nicotine stimulates it indirectly by altering the balance of inputs from two types of neurons that help regulate its activity level.
Prescription medications	Pain relievers, tranquilizers, stimulants, and sedatives are very useful treatment tools. When people do not take them as directed, they may become addicted. Inappropriate or nonmedical use of prescription medications is a serious public health concern. Nonmedical use of prescription medications like opioids, central nervous system (CNS) depressants, and stimulants can lead to abuse and addiction, which are characterized by compulsive drug seeking and use.
Steroids, anabolic	Anabolic-androgenic steroids are man-made substances related to male sex hormones. They are available legally only by prescription to treat conditions that occur when the body produces abnormally low amounts of testosterone, such as in delayed puberty and impotence. They are also prescribed to treat body wasting in patients with AIDS and other diseases that result in loss of lean muscle mass. Athletes may abuse anabolic steroids to enhance performance and also to improve physical appearance. Anabolic steroids are taken orally or injected, typically in cycles of weeks or months (referred to as "cycling"), rather than continuously.

Sources: http://www.nida.nih.gov/Drugpages/; Bruinsma and Taren, 1999; Dager and Friedman, 2000; Smit et al, 2004.

- Normalize brain levels of neurotransmitters.
- Correct fluid and electrolyte imbalances or dehydration.
- Modify diet for medical conditions. Alcoholics experience problems such as liver failure, cirrhosis, pancreatitis, GI bleeding, esophageal varices, renal impairment, ascites, and edema. Intravenous drug users are at risk for contracting hepatitis C or HIV infection. See appropriate entries.
- Reorient to reality; develop trusting relationships between patient and care providers.
- Promote abstinence and long-term treatment. Dietitians can provide needed nutrition education and be quite helpful in drug treatment and rehabilitation programs (Grant et al, 2004).
- Improve nutritional status and outcome.
- Prevent or correct any related eating disorders (present in approximately 50% of these individuals). Avoid major changes in food choices and intake during recovery to prevent drastic weight fluctuations.

- The use of motivational interviewing can help work through problems such as resistance and ambivalence for making life changes (Westra, 2004).

INTERVENTION: FOOD AND NUTRITION

- According to intake and output values, adjust fluid intake. Offer beverages that are nonalcoholic favorites. Reductions in the use of caffeine are often suggested.
- Encourage nutrient-dense foods. Fruits, vegetables, whole grains, and fish are important inclusions.
- Adequate intake of protein will be essential.
- Include adequate calories, especially because patients often become hypoglycemic. Feed several times daily to help regulate blood glucose.
- Adequate intake of thiamin and other B-complex vitamins, zinc, protein, vitamin A, and other depleted nutrients will be important during recovery.
- Adjust diet, as appropriate, to reduce excess sweets because many chemical abusers tend to substitute sweets for their dependency drug.
- Adequate fiber intake may be useful to correct or prevent constipation.

CLINICAL INDICATORS

Clinical/History

Height
Weight
BMI
Weight changes
Dietary/intake history
I & O
BP
Tremors, delirium?
Multidimensional Addictions and Personality Profile (MAPP)

Lab Work

Prolactin levels
Serotonin levels
Ca^{++}, Mg^{++}
Na^{+}, K^{+}, Cl^{-}
H & H
Serum Fe
Alb or transthyretin
Gluc
Chol (total profile)
Trig (often very high in alcoholics)
Serum thiamin
Serum folate
Serum B_{12}
Serum homocysteine
CRP
Liver function tests

Common Drugs Used and Potential Side Effects

- Antabuse, when mixed with alcohol, can cause severe nausea, vomiting, low BP, and flushing. Because alcohol abuse causes a deficit of beta-endorphin peptide, scientists are trying to find products that reverse this trend (Boyadjieva et al, 2001).
- Bromocriptine (Parlodel) may also be used for some drug-recovery patients. Nausea, vomiting, or constipation may occur.
- Methadone maintenance therapy continues to be one of the major effective forms of addiction pharmacotherapy and underscores the importance of biological factors in the physiology and treatment of the addictive diseases (Kreek et al, 2004).
- Naltrexone is a drug that decreases pleasurable sensation of alcohol; it is used for narcotic dependency after detoxification. Anorexia, weight loss, nausea, vomiting, and abdominal cramping or pain may occur.
- Subutex/Suboxone (buprenorphine/naloxone) are oral tablets used for the treatment of opiate dependence.
- Stool softeners may be beneficial if constipation results after withdrawal, as with cocaine abuse.
- Tricyclic antidepressants (imipramine, desipramine) are often beneficial with some side effects such as dry mouth.

Herbs, Botanicals, and Supplements

- No studies have been conducted for efficacy of herbs or botanicals in substance abuse patients.
- St. John's wort should not be taken with antidepressants.

INTERVENTION: NUTRITION EDUCATION, COUNSELING, CARE MANAGEMENT

- Help the patient accept responsibility for his or her own actions. Cognitive behavioral therapy and family, group, and self-help therapies are all recommended.
- Treatment should focus on sufficient duration and intensity, family support, after-care and follow-up, self-help groups, collaboration with social services, and a drug-free lifestyle. One of five individuals will be drug free or sober after 5 years. New studies will include new, effective medications and evaluations of the changes that occur in the brain.
- Help to maintain abstinence. Avoid discussion of unanswerable questions such as "why" substances have been abused.
- In recovery, simple guidelines are useful: eat breakfast and regular meals daily; eat a variety of foods; make mealtimes pleasant and unhurried; choose healthy snacks; drink decaffeinated coffee.
- Discuss issues regarding personal "control." Coping skills will be needed to reduce helplessness. Include patient in decision making to increase self-esteem and confidence.

SAMPLE NUTRITION DIAGNOSTIC STATEMENT

Drug Addiction

PES: Inadequate oral food and beverage intake related to inability to manage self-care as evidenced by patient report of no food in last 48 hours.

Assessment Data: Food recall/diet history; assessment of access to food and resources (money, family support, social service agencies, drug counseling or therapy).

Intervention: Provide avenues for acquiring foods and beverages; coordination of social services and referral to rehab if appropriate.

Monitoring and Evaluation: Report of improved food and beverage intake; evaluate intake if patient is in your facility.

- Discuss the dangers of diet pills to control appetite and weight. Assess history of starving to lose weight or being overweight as a child or a teenager.
- Long-term alcohol abuse can specifically target beta cells of the pancreas, increasing risk of diabetes. Heroin use can cause glucose intolerance, but unlike in alcohol abuse, this usually resolves with abstinence.
- Heavy drinkers tend to have higher total and HDL cholesterol levels than controls. Moderate alcohol intake does not seem to be protective against coronary heart disease through lipid reduction alone.
- Sports teams may be important for peer-led education about healthy lifestyles and reduction in disordered eating patterns or substance abuse (Elliott et al, 2004).
- If a person smokes cigarettes, having smoking cessation interventions seems to help long-term sobriety for other addictions (Prochaska et al, 2004).
- Help plan adequate discharge planning, follow-up, and family therapy or other support group interactions. Long-term management of persons with addictions and medical disorders requires integrative care programs involving comprehensive primary and psychiatric care (Wadland and Ferenchick, 2004).

Patient Education—Foodborne Illness

- Careful food handling will be important. The same is true for hand washing.

For More Information

- Alcoholics Anonymous
  http://www.alcoholics-anonymous.org
- American Society of Addiction Medicine
  http://www.asam.org/
- National Clearinghouse for Alcohol and Drug Information
  http://ncadi.samhsa.gov/
- National Council on Alcoholism and Drug Dependence
  http://www.ncadd.org
- National Institute on Drug Abuse (NIDA)
  http://www.nida.nih.gov/NIDAHome1.html
- NIDA Statistics
  http://www.nida.nih.gov/drugpages/stats.html
- Substance Abuse and Mental Health Services
  http://www.samhsa.gov/index.aspx

SUBSTANCE USE DISORDERS—CITED REFERENCES

Boyadjieva N, et al. Chronic ethanol inhibits NK cell cytolytic activity: role of opioid peptide b-endorphin 1. *J Immunology*. 167:5645, 2001.

Bruinsma K, Taren D. Chocolate: food or drug? *J Am Diet Assoc.* 99:1249, 1999.

Dager SR, Friedman SD. Brain imaging and the effects of caffeine and nicotine. *Ann Med.* 32:592, 2000.

Davis C, et al. Sensitivity to reward: implications for overeating and overweight. *Appetite* 42:131, 2004.

Elliott DL, et al. Preventing substance use and disordered eating: initial outcomes of the ATHENA (Athletes Targeting Healthy Exercise and Nutrition Alternatives) program. *Arch Pediatr Adolesc Med.* 158: 1043, 2004.

Fisk D, et al. Assertive outreach: an effective strategy for engaging homeless persons with substance use disorders into treatment. *Am J Drug Alcohol Abuse.* 32:479, 2006.

Grant LP, et al. Nutrition education is positively associated with substance abuse treatment program outcomes. *J Am Diet Assoc.* 104:604, 2004.

Halsted CH. Nutrition and alcoholic liver disease. *Semin Liver Dis.* 24:289, 2004.

Kreek MJ, et al. Evolving perspectives on neurobiological research on the addictions: celebration of the 30th anniversary of NIDA. *Neuropharmacology* 47:324, 2004 (suppl 1).

Lieber CS. Relationships between nutrition, alcohol use, and liver disease. *Alcohol Res Health.* 27:220, 2003.

Oroszi G, Goldman D. Alcoholism: genes and mechanisms. *Pharmacogenomics* 5:1037, 2004.

Prochaska JJ, et al. A meta-analysis of smoking cessation interventions with individuals in substance abuse treatment or recovery. *J Consult Clin Psychol.* 72:1144, 2004.

Smit HJ, et al. Methylxanthines are the psycho-pharmacologically active constituents of chocolate. *Psychopharmacology* 176:412, 2004.

Wadland WC, Ferenchick GS. Medical comorbidity in addictive disorders. *Psychiatr Clin North Am.* 27:675, 2004.

Westra HA. Managing resistance in cognitive behavioural therapy: the application of motivational interviewing in mixed anxiety and depression. *Cogn Behav Ther.* 33:161, 2004.

S E C T I O N 5

Pulmonary Disorders

CHIEF ASSESSMENT FACTORS (SEE FIG. 5-1)

- Cough, Especially with Chest Pain, Hoarseness, Dizziness
- Pain (Chest, Abdominal)
- Wheezing (Whistling, Musical Sound from Obstructed Airways)
- Stridor (Crowing Sound on Inhalation)
- Shortness of Breath (Dyspnea)
- Poor Exercise or Activity Tolerance
- Fever or Chills
- Rapid Breathing, Excessive Perspiration
- Dizziness
- Flaring Nostrils; Red, Swollen Nose
- Cyanosis of Lips, Nail Beds
- Pallor; Ashen or Gray Coloring
- Confusion, Somnolence
- Orthopnea, Tachypnea
- Clubbing of Nail Beds (see Fig. 5-2)
- Engorged Eye Veins
- Altered Respirations
- Anorexia
- Elevated Blood Pressure
- Altered Blood Gases (Decreased Partial Pressure of oxygen [pO_2], Increased Partial Pressure of Carbon Dioxide [pCO_2])
- Restlessness, Irritability
- Hemoptysis (Coughing Up Blood)

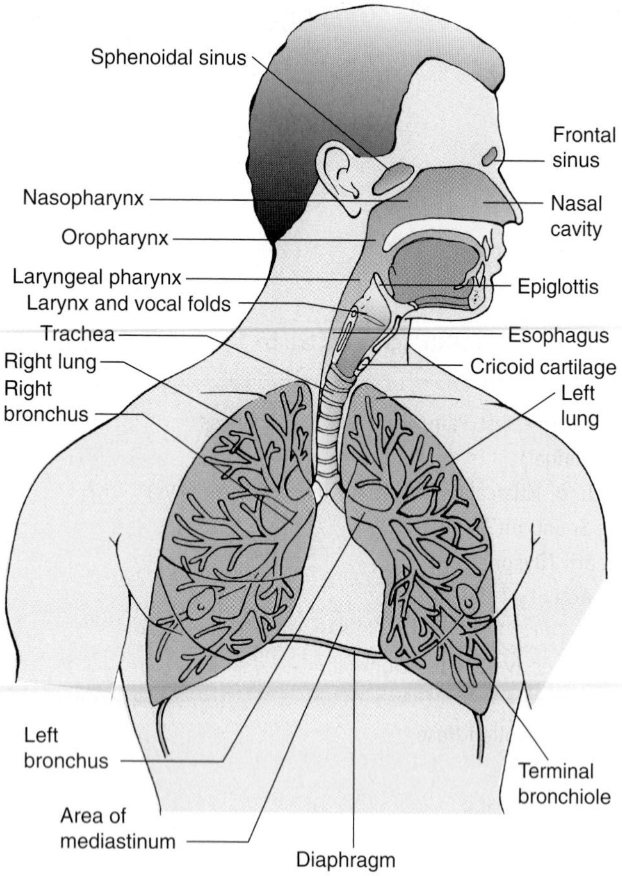

Figure 5-1 The respiratory system. (From Weber J, Kelley J. *Health assessment in nursing*. 2nd ed. Philadelphia: Lippincott Williams & Wilkins; 2003.)

PULMONARY NUTRITION NOTES

Pulmonary surfactant is a complex and highly active material composed of lipids and proteins and is found in the fluid lining the alveolar surface of the lungs. It protects the lungs from injuries and infections caused by inhaled particles and micro-organisms (Wright, 2005a). The role for surfactant was first studied in premature infants with respiratory distress syndrome (RDS), which is now routinely treated with exogenous surfactant replacement (Stevens et al, 2004; Poynter and Levine, 2003). Recombinant forms could be useful therapeutically in attenuating inflammatory processes in neonatal chronic lung disease, cystic fibrosis, and emphysema (Clark and Reid, 2003).

Biochemical surfactant abnormalities have been described in obstructive lung diseases (asthma, bronchiolitis, chronic obstructive pulmonary disease [COPD], and lung transplantation), infectious and suppurative lung diseases (cystic fibrosis, pneumonia, and human immunodeficiency virus), adult respiratory distress syndrome, pulmonary edema, chronic lung disease of prematurity, interstitial lung diseases, pulmonary alveolar proteinosis following cardiopulmonary bypass, and in smokers (Griese, 1999). Surfactant replacement therapy is being tested in several clinical trials; initial outcomes are positive. In acute respiratory syndrome, exogenous surfactant does not improve survival, but patients who received surfactant had a greater improvement in gas exchange during 24-hour treatment, suggesting potential benefits of longer treatment course (Spragg et al, 2004).

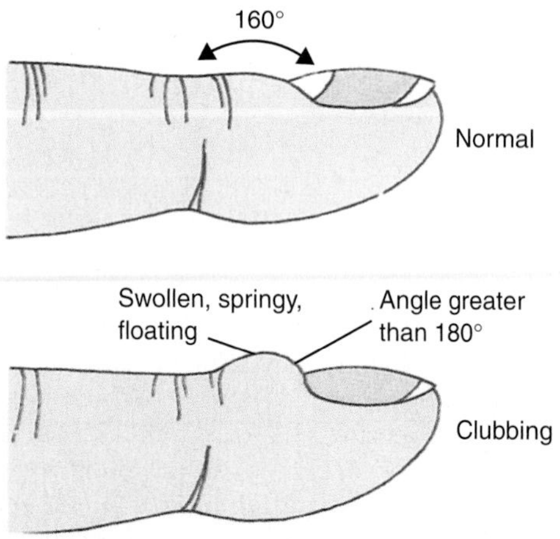

Figure 5-2 Clubbing of fingers. (Reprinted with permission from Taylor C, Lillis C, LeMone P. *Fundamentals of nursing: the art and science of nursing care*. 4th ed. Philadelphia: Lippincott Williams & Wilkins; 2001.)

TABLE 5-1 Causes of Malnutrition in Patients with Pulmonary Disease

Aerophagia and rapid breathing
Anemia (low oxygen-carrying capacity)
Anorexia of chronic illness
Cellular hypoxia
Chronic debility
Decreased lung immunity
Decreased lung surfactant and elasticity
Depression, anxiety with anorexia
Difficulty in eating with continuous dyspnea
Fever
Gastric hypomotility
Hypermetabolism, as in chronic obstructive pulmonary disease (COPD)
Increased mechanical work of breathing
Increased workload of the heart
Inflammation
Lung cancer
Malabsorption, as in cystic fibrosis
Medications causing nausea and anorexia
Pneumonia
Polypharmacy
Poor respiratory muscle strength and endurance
Restricted diet
Right-sided heart failure
Vitamin deficiency, leading to poor epithelial integrity and weak lung muscles

NOTE. Death in patients with COPD is typically due to acute respiratory failure, pneumonia, lung cancer, cardiac disease, or pulmonary embolism.

Adapted from Merck Manual: Chronic obstructive pulmonary disease; accessed January 28, 2006 at http://www.merck.com/mrkshared/mmg/sec10/ch78/ch78a.jsp.

TABLE 5-2 Respiratory Quotient (RQ) and Nutrients

RQ = VO_2/VCO_2
RQ from fat = 0.7
RQ from protein = 0.8
RQ from carbohydrates (CHO) = 1.0

Evidence for a role of diet in pulmonary disease is clear. Associations have been reported between the intake of fruit, fish, antioxidant vitamins, fatty acids, sodium or magnesium, and symptoms of asthma and COPD. Because antioxidant nutrients are positively corrected with lung function, vitamin C, vitamin E, beta-carotene, and selenium are important in the diets of persons with lung disorders (Frei and Higdon, 2003; Hu and Cassano, 2000). Plasma antioxidant capacity increases after drinking cranberry or blueberry juices (Pedersen et al, 2000). Flavonoids, such as quercetin and resveratrol, in apples, onions, oranges, berries, and red wine may be helpful to lung health (Arts and Hollman, 2005; Neuhouser, 2004; Donnelly et al, 2004).

Vitamin D has been found to be helpful in maintaining healthy lung function (Wright, 2005b). It is unclear if increases in 25-hydroxyvitamin D through supplements or dietary intake will actually improve lung function in patients with chronic respiratory diseases.

Vitamin E may be beneficial for staving off upper respiratory infections; 200 IU daily gives better response to vaccines for diseases such as flu, ear infections, pneumonia, bronchitis, sinusitis, and other pathological conditions (Meydani et al, 2004). Otherwise, almonds, mango, sunflower seeds, vegetable oils, and whole grains are helpful to consume often. Omega-3 fatty acids can calm inflamed airways; include salmon, tuna, mackerel, walnuts, and flaxseed oil more often.

Table 5-1 lists factors that contribute to malnutrition with pulmonary disease. Table 5-2 lists the respiratory quotients for fats, protein, and carbohydrates.

CITED REFERENCES

Arts IC, Hollman PC. Polyphenols and disease risk in epidemiologic studies. *Am J Clin Nutr.* 81:317S, 2005.

Clark H, Reid K. The potential of recombinant surfactant protein D therapy to reduce inflammation in neonatal chronic lung disease, cystic fibrosis, and emphysema. *Arch Dis Child.* 88:981, 2003.

Donnelly LE, et al. Anti-inflammatory effects of resveratrol in lung epithelial cells: molecular mechanisms. *Am J Physiol Lung Cell Mol Physiol.* 287:774, 2004.

Frei B, Higdon JV. Antioxidant activity of tea polyphenols in vivo: evidence from animal studies. *J Nutr.* 133:3275S, 2003.

Griese M. Pulmonary surfactant in health and human lung diseases: state of the art. *Eur Respir J.* 13:1455, 1999.

Hu G, Cassano P. Antioxidant nutrients and pulmonary function: the Third National Health and Nutrition Examination Survey. *Am J Epidemiol.* 151:75, 2000.

Meydani SN, et al. Vitamin E and respiratory tract infections in elderly nursing home residents: a randomized controlled trial. *JAMA.* 292:828, 2004.

Neuhouser ML. Dietary flavonoids and cancer risk: evidence from human population studies. *Nutr Cancer.* 50:1, 2004.

Pedersen C, et al. Effects of blueberry and cranberry juice consumption on the plasma antioxidant capacity of healthy female volunteers. *Euro J Clin Nutr.* 54:405, 2000.

Poynter SE, LeVine AM. Surfactant biology and clinical application. *Crit Care Clin.* 19:459, 2003.

Spragg RG, et al. Effect of recombinant surfactant protein C-based surfactant on the acute respiratory distress syndrome. *N Engl J Med.* 351:884, 2004.

Stevens TP, et al. Early surfactant administration with brief ventilation vs selective surfactant and continued mechanical ventilation for preterm infants with or at risk for respiratory distress syndrome. *Cochrane Database Syst Rev.* 3:CD003063, 2004.

Wright JR. Immunoregulatory functions of surfactant proteins. *Nat Rev Immunol.* 5:58, 2005a.

Wright JR. Make no bones about it: increasing epidemiologic evidence links vitamin D to pulmonary function and COPD. *Chest* 128:3781, 2005b.

For More General Information

- American Lung Association
  http://www.lungusa.org/
- Canadian Lung Association
  http://www.lung.ca/
- National Heart, Lung, and Blood Institute
  http://www.nhlbi.nih.gov/
- National Jewish Medical and Research Center
  http://www.njc.org/

ASTHMA

NUTRITIONAL ACUITY RANKING: LEVEL 1

DEFINITIONS AND BACKGROUND

Bronchial asthma involves paroxysmal dyspnea accompanied by wheezing and is caused by spasm of the bronchial tubes or swelling of their mucous membranes. Bronchial asthma differs from wheezing caused by cardiac failure (cardiac asthma), in which an x-ray shows fluid in the lung. Asthma involves inflammation of the lining of the airways, obstruction, and increased sensitivity of the airways.

Between 10 and 15 million Americans are affected by asthma, including about 5% of children. Asthma seems to be inherited in two thirds of cases. Events taking place during pregnancy may well play a role in determining whether or not a genetic susceptibility becomes translated into disease processes (Warner and Warner, 2000).

Signs and symptoms of asthma include respiratory distress, audible wheezing, decreased breath sounds, tachycardia, cyanosis, hypotension, anxiety, pulmonary edema, dehydration, hard and dry cough, and distended neck veins. Two types of bronchial asthma are recognized: allergic (extrinsic) and nonallergic (intrinsic or infectious). Children who are exposed to secondhand smoke may have chronic cough or symptoms of asthma. Table 5-3 provides a checklist for early warning signs of asthma.

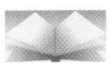

TABLE 5-3 Early Warning Signs of Asthma Checklist

____ Breathing changes	____ Feeling tired
____ Feeling funny in chest	____ Want to be alone
____ Headache	____ Quiet, more than usual
____ Easily upset	____ Feeling weak
____ Eyes look glassy	____ Slowing down
____ Dark circles under eyes	____ Feeling sad
____ More excited than usual	____ Pale
____ Watery eyes	____ Stuffy nose
____ Sweaty	____ Restlessness
____ Feverish	____ Irritability
____ Chin or throat itches	____ Heart beating faster
____ Coughing	____ Sneezing
____ Change in sputum (mucus)	____ Runny nose
____ Dry mouth	____ Trouble sleeping
____ Poor tolerance for exercise	____ A downward trend in peak flow numbers

Adapted from National Jewish Medical and Research Center: http://www.nationaljewish.org/disease-info/diseases/asthma/about/symptoms/checklist.aspx; accessed January 27, 2005.

Chronic poor control can lead to a serious condition, status asthmaticus, which generally requires hospitalization and can be life threatening. Brittle asthma is a rare form of asthma with repeated attacks, either with wide variation from predicted daily peak expiratory flow or with apparent good control of asthma (Baker et al, 2000). A high prevalence of food intolerance has been noted with brittle asthma.

Some studies of children breastfed exclusively for the first 4 months of life show decreased risk for asthma (Oddy, 2004), while other studies suggest that breastfeeding promotes it (Takemura et al, 2001). Longer duration of breastfeeding seems to be more protective (Dell and To, 2001).

Most infants with wheezing have transient conditions that may clear; only a small number have asthma later in life. Among transient cases (i.e., those who possibly had an infection with wheezing at 3–4 years old), day care attendance and early infections reduce the risk of asthma later (Infante-Rivard et al, 2001). For children 2–3 years old, the common cold virus and rhinovirus (RV) continue to be major triggers of wheezing, a pattern that also continues for adults with asthma, especially for allergic patients (Tan, 2005).

Overweight is significantly higher in children with moderate-to-severe asthma than in their healthy peers; overweight promotes severity. The effects of increased BMI on asthma may be mediated by mechanical properties of the respiratory system associated with obesity or by inflammatory mechanisms rather than by allergies (von Mutius et al, 2001). Evidence suggests elevated BMI and dietary patterns, especially intake of excess lipids, contribute to symptoms of asthma (Spector and Surette, 2003).

Nutritional status is important for healthy lungs. Lung function may be better with higher antioxidant levels (Hu and Cassano, 2000). Intravenous treatment with multiple nutrients, including magnesium, may be of considerable benefit; pulmonary function improves progressively with longer treatment (Schrader, 2004). Overall, dietary modification may help patients manage their asthma as well as contribute to their overall health (Spector and Surette, 2003). See Table 5-4 for various nutrients and their potential effects on management of asthma.

INTERVENTION: OBJECTIVES

- Prevent distention of stomach from large meals, resulting in distress and perhaps aggravation of asthma.
- Prevent lung infection and inflammation. Promote improved resistance against infections. Diet affects the pathophysiology of asthma by altered immune or antioxidant activity with consequent effects on airway inflammation.
- For allergic asthma, identify and control allergens in the environment.
- Promote adequate hydration to liquefy secretions.
- Optimize nutritional status. Sufficient vitamins C, B_6, and E, selenium, and magnesium are important. Reduce intake of oleic acid, but increase intake of omega-3 fatty acids if tolerated.
- Encourage a health maintenance program, including physical activity where possible.
- Caffeine relaxes muscles and opens airways of the lung. About 2–3 cups of coffee daily may be useful in adults.

TABLE 5-4 Nutrients and Their Potential Mechanisms in Asthma

Nutrient(s)	Activity and Potential Mechanisms of Effect
Vitamins A (carotenoids), C, and E	Antioxidants for protection against endogenous and exogenous oxidant inflammation (Harik-Kahn et al, 2004; McKeever et al, 2004)
Vitamin C	Prostaglandin inhibition (Harik-Kahn et al, 2004; Mainous, 2000)
Vitamin E	Membrane stabilization, inhibition of immunoglobulin E (IgE) production
Flavones and flavonoids	Antioxidants; mast cell stabilization
Magnesium	Smooth muscle relaxation, mast cell stabilization (Schrader, 2004)
Selenium	Antioxidant cofactor in glutathione peroxidase (Brown and Arthur, 2001)
Copper, zinc	Antioxidant cofactors in superoxide dismutase
Omega-3 fatty acids	Leukotriene substitution, stabilization of inflammatory cell membranes (Wong, 2005; Woods et al, 2000).
Omega-6 polyunsaturated/trans fatty acids	Increased eicosanoid production (Nagel Linseisen, 2005; Huang and Pan, 2001)
Sodium	Increased smooth muscle contraction; reductions can increase airway responsiveness (Mickleborough and Gotshall, 2004)

INTERVENTION: FOOD AND NUTRITION

- Infants should be breastfed to reduce the risk of asthma in susceptible families (Kull et al, 2004). Exclusive breastfeeding is desirable (Oddy et al, 2004).
- Provide balanced, small meals that are nutrient dense (i.e., high-quality protein, vitamins, and minerals), especially to reduce risk of infections and poor state of health. Lose weight by following a lower energy intake if needed (Oddy et al, 2004).
- Encourage extra fluids unless contraindicated. Theobromine in cocoa tends to increase blood flow to the brain and to reduce coughing; use often.
- Use less sodium (Mickleborough and Gotshall, 2004).
- Highlight foods rich in vitamins A and C, magnesium, and zinc (see Table 5-4). Use more broccoli, grapefruit, oranges, sweet peppers, kiwi, tomato juice, and cauliflower for vitamin C. Other nutrients that support immunocompetence should be included. Quercetin in apples, pears, onions, oranges, and berries should be encouraged (5 or more servings per week).
- Omit food allergens as identified; common allergens are milk, eggs, seafood, and fish. Sulfites and salicylates may aggravate asthma in 2% of patients. If tolerated, soy may be useful for some people (Smith et al, 2004) but not others (Woods et al, 2003). If fish is tolerated, consumption of fish 2–3 times weekly has been shown to help reduce leukotriene synthesis (Wong, 2005). If nuts are tolerated, include selenium from Brazil nuts; include vitamin E from nuts, salad dressings, and vegetable oils.
- Saturated and monounsaturated fats may have different effects on airway inflammation; saturated fatty acids (SFAs) may aggravate inflammation and monounsaturated fatty acids (MUFAs) may be inversely related (Huang and Pan, 2001). Omega-3 fatty acids may be useful for those persons without fish allergy; walnuts and flaxseed may be used if tolerated. In addition, oleic acid (from margarine) may contribute to clinical onset of asthma, and use should be low (Nagel and Linseisen, 2005).

CLINICAL INDICATORS

Clinical/History

Height
Weight
Body mass index (BMI)
Diet history
Blood pressure (BP)
Temperature
Intake and output (I & O)
Spirometry test (see Fig. 5-3 for use of peak flow meter)

Lab Work

Glucose (Gluc)
Albumin (Alb)
Hemoglobin and hematocrit (H & H)
Serum Fe
Transferrin
Serum lipids
Uric acid
Bilirubin
Ca^{++}, Mg^{++}
pCO_2, pO_2
Cholesterol (Chol)
Triglycerides (Trig)
C-reactive protein (CRP)
Serum theophylline levels (if needed)

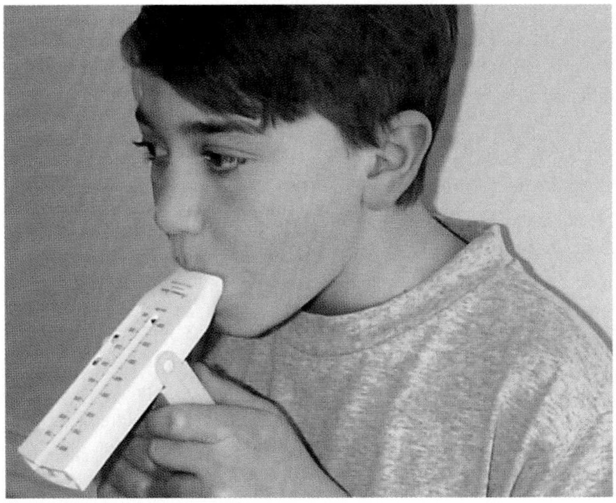

Figure 5-3 Use of peak flow meter. (From Nettina SM. *The Lippincott manual of nursing practice*. 7th ed. Philadelphia: Lippincott, Williams & Wilkins; 2001.)

Common Drugs Used and Potential Side Effects

- See Table 5-5.

Herbs, Botanicals, and Supplements

- Many patients with asthma are attracted to the use of alternative therapies. There might be a possible role for antioxidant dietary supplementation and natural anti-inflammatory and immunomodulatory remedies (Gyorik and Brutsche, 2004).
- In China, a combination of three herbal extracts has been found to be useful; it is identified as ASHMI to indicate its role in antiasthma medical intervention (Wen et al, 2005).
- Dietary fatty acids such as gamma linolenic acid (GLA; borage oil) modulate endogenous inflammatory mediators without side effects and may play a role in asthma (Ziboh et al, 2004).
- Ephedra (ma huang) is an effective bronchodilator, but it increases blood pressure significantly. Problems with blood glucose, arrhythmias, increased heart rate, and central nervous system (CNS) stimulation can also occur. The Food and Drug Administration (FDA) has removed it from the market, but some forms are still available.
- Stinging nettle, licorice, gingko, and anise have been suggested; efficacy and side effects must be evaluated.
- St. John's wort can inhibit theophylline's effectiveness.
- Seaweed may be used to treat asthma in Vietnamese and oriental cultures (Dang and Hoang, 2004).

INTERVENTION: NUTRITION EDUCATION, COUNSELING, CARE MANAGEMENT

- Mild, chronic asthma can be a warning, and, if untreated, it can lead to an acute exacerbation.
- Despite tradition, waiting to introduce solids to an infant does not necessarily protect against onset of asthma and allergy (Zutavern et al, 2004).

TABLE 5-5 Medications Used in Asthma

Medication	Description
Antibiotics	Long-term use can cause diarrhea and other problems. Penicillin should not be taken with fruit juices.
Anticholinergics (Atrovent, Combivent)	Quick-relief asthma medications. Dry mouth is common side effect.
Beta-agonists (Alupent, albuterol Maxair, Proventil)	Relaxes smooth muscle around airways. Side effects include shakiness, rapid heart rate, and nervousness. Metaproterenol (Metaprel, Alupent) may alter taste and cause nausea or vomiting. Albuterol (Ventolin, Proventil) may have cardiac side effects or may cause nausea or diarrhea.
Bronchodilators (theophylline [Theo-Dur, Slo-BID, Slo-Phyllin, Theolair, Uniphyl])	No longer first choice of asthma medication. Nausea, vomiting, and sleeplessness can be a problem. Theophylline metabolism is affected by protein and CHO availability; avoid extreme changes in protein and CHO intake. Because it is a methylxanthine, avoid extreme changes in usual intakes of caffeine-containing foods. Theophylline depresses levels of vitamin B_6. In addition, lipid levels (cholesterol, HDL, and LDL) are higher in children who take theophylline.
Corticosteroids (methylprednisolone [Medrol], Deltasone, Orapred, Prelone)	Many side effects such as fluid retention, low serum potassium, GI distress, retaining excess sodium, causing hyperglycemia, and other problems. Monitor carefully, especially if needed over a long period of time. AeroBid contains an anti-inflammatory steroid and is inhaled; it may cause nausea, vomiting, or diarrhea. Bone mineral density is often decreased after long-term use of inhaled corticosteroids (Sivri and Coplu, 2001). A follow-up of patients with asthma who are taking inhaled corticosteroids is needed to assess bone density, decreases in osteocalcin levels, and dietary intakes of calcium.
Epinephrine	May be required for emergencies. Intravenous (IV) administration of epinephrine results in a prolonged increase in resting energy expenditure (REE) as measured by respiratory quotient (RQ); fuel for this is increased CHO oxidation. Rate of protein oxidation does not change, and REE returns to normal 24 hours after epinephrine infusion stops (Ratheiser et al, 1998).
Expectorants	Potassium iodide may affect existing thyroid problems.
Long-term control medications	Anti-immunoglobulin E: Reduces histamine release; may be useful with allergies.
	Combination therapy (Advair): Combining an inhaled corticosteroid and a long-lasting beta$_2$-agonist seems to provide consistent relief for people with asthma.
	Intal (cromolyn) and Tilade (nedocromil) are inhaled medications that may be useful for asthma triggered by cold weather, exercise, and allergies.
	Inhaled nasal steroids: AeroBid (flunisolide), Azmacort (triamcinolone), Flovent (fluticasone), Pulmicort (budesonide), and Qvar (beclomethasone HFA). These prevent inflammation and reduce swelling inside airways; they also reduce mucus production.
	Leukotriene modifiers: Accolate, Singulair, Zyflo. These work by relaxing smooth muscle around the airway and reducing inflammation.
	The FDA wants warnings added to labels for Serevent Diskus (salmeterol xinafoate inhalation powder), Advair Diskus (fluticasone propionate and salmeterol inhalation powder) and Foradil Aerolizer (formoterol fumarate inhalation powder); these medications can worsen asthma or cause death.
Omega-3 fatty acid supplements	Omega-3 fatty acid supplements (in the form of perilla seed oil, which is rich in ALA) may decrease inflammation and improve lung function in adults with asthma. Omega-6 fatty acids have the opposite effect; they tend to increase inflammation and worsen respiratory function. In a small, well-designed study of 29 children with asthma, those who took fish oil supplements rich in EPA and DHA for 10 months had improvement in their symptoms compared to children who took a placebo pill (Nagakura et al, 2000).

- Avoid early multivitamin-mineral supplementation because it may actually trigger asthma in susceptible children and allergies in exclusively formula-fed children; the exact reasons are under study (Milner et al, 2004). A healthy, nutrient-dense diet should be consumed instead.
- All medications should be taken as directed by the physician.
- Work with the patient/family to avoid precipitating events or triggers. Discuss exercise, rest, and nutrition.
- Massage therapy for children with asthma reveals increased relaxation, decreased anxiety, and better lung function scores.
- Reduction in available triggers will be useful (for example, reducing exposure to pet dander, food allergens, secondhand smoke). Environmental exposures seem to play an important role (Holguin et al, 2005).

Patient Education—Foodborne Illness

- Careful food handling will be important. Hand washing is key as well.

For More Information

- Allergy and Asthma Advocate
  http://www.aaaai.org/

- Allergy and Asthma Network–Mothers of Asthmatics
  http://www.aanma.org/
- Asthma and Allergy
  http://allergy.healthcentersonline.com/allergyasthmabasics/
- Asthma Resource Center
  http://www.emedicine.com/rc/rc/i3/asthma.htm
- Jewish Center for Immunology and Respiratory Disease
  National Asthma Center
  http://asthma.nationaljewish.org/
- National Asthma Education and Prevention Program (NAEPP)
  http://aspe.hhs.gov/sp/asthma/
- Practical Guide for Asthma
  http://www.nhlbi.nih.gov/health/prof/lung/asthma/practgde/practgde.pdf

ASTHMA—CITED REFERENCES

Baker J, et al. Development of a standardized methodology for double-blind, placebo-controlled food challenge in patients with brittle asthma and perceived food intolerance. *J Am Diet Assoc.* 100:1361, 2000.

Brown K, Arthur J. Selenium, selenoproteins, and human health: a review. *Public Health Nutr.* 4:593, 2001.

Dang DH, Hoang TM. Nutritional analysis of Vietnamese seaweeds for food and medicine. *Biofactors* 22:323, 2004.

Dell S, To T. Breastfeeding and asthma in young children: findings from a population-based study. *Arch Pediatr Adolesc Med.* 155:1261, 2001.

Gyorik SA, Brutsche MH. Complementary and alternative medicine for bronchial asthma: is there new evidence? *Curr Opin Pulm Med.* 10:37, 2004.

Harik-Kahn RI, et al. Serum vitamin levels and the risk of asthma in children. *Am J Epidemiol.* 159:351, 2004.

Holguin F, et al. Country of birth as a risk factor for asthma among Mexican Americans. *Am J Respir Crit Care Med.* 171:103, 2005.

Hu G, Cassano P. Antioxidant nutrients and pulmonary function: the Third National Health and Nutrition Examination Survey. *Am J Epidemiol.* 151:975, 2000.

Huang S, Pan W. Dietary fats and asthma in teenagers: analyses of the first Nutrition and Health Survey in Taiwan (NAHSIT). *Clin Exp Allergy.* 31:1875, 2001.

Infante-Rivard C, et al. Family size, day-care attendance, and breastfeeding in relation to the incidence of childhood asthma. *Am J Epidemiol.* 153:653, 2001.

Kull I, et al. Breast-feeding reduces the risk of asthma during the first 4 years of life. *J Allergy Clin Immunol.* 114:755, 2004.

Mainous A, et al. Serum vitamin C levels and use of health care resources for wheezing episodes. *Arch Fam Med.* 9:241, 2000.

McKeever TM, et al. Serum nutrient markers and skin prick testing using data from the Third National Health and Nutrition Examination Survey. *J Allergy Clin Immunol.* 114:1398, 2004.

McKeever TM, Britton J. Diet and asthma. *Am J Respir Crit Care Med.* 170:725, 2004.

Mickleborough T, Gotshall RW. Dietary salt intake as a potential modifier of airway responsiveness in bronchial asthma. *J Altern Complement Med.* 10:633, 2004.

Milner JD, et al. Early infant multivitamin supplementation is associated with increased risk for food allergy and asthma. *Pediatrics* 114:27, 2004.

Nagakura T, et al. Dietary supplementation with fish oil rich in omega-3 polyunsaturated fatty acids in children with bronchial asthma. *Eur Respir J.* 16:861, 2000.

Nagel G, Linseisen J. Dietary intake of fatty acids, antioxidants and selected food groups and asthma in adults. *Eur J Clin Nutr.* 59:8, 2005.

Oddy WH, et al. The relation of breastfeeding and body mass index to asthma and atopy in children: a prospective cohort study to age 6 years. *Am J Public Health.* 94:1531, 2004.

Ratheiser K, et al. Epinephrine produces a prolonged elevation in metabolic rate in humans. *Am J Clin Nutr.* 68:1046, 1998.

Schrader WA Jr. Short and long term treatment of asthma with intravenous nutrients. *Nutr J.* 3:6, 2004.

Sivri A, Coplu L. Effect of the long-term use of inhaled corticosteroids on bone mineral density in asthmatic women. *Respirology* 6:131, 2001.

Smith LJ, et al. Dietary intake of soy genistein is associated with lung function in patients with asthma. *J Asthma.* 41:833, 2004.

Specter SL, Surette ME. Diet and asthma: has the role of dietary lipids been overlooked in the management of asthma? *Ann Allergy Asthma Immunol.* 90:371, 2003.

Takemura Y, et al. Relation between breastfeeding and the prevalence of asthma: the Tokorozawa Childhood Asthma and Pollinosis Study. *Am J Epidemiol.* 154:115, 2001.

Tan WC. Viruses in asthma exacerbations. *Curr Opin Pulm Med.* 11:21, 2005.

von Mutius E, et al. Relation of body mass index to asthma and atopy in children: the National Health and Nutrition Examination Study III. *Thorax* 56:835, 2001.

Warner J, Warner J. Early life events in allergic sensitization. *Br Med Bull.* 56:883, 2000.

Wen MC, et al. Efficacy and tolerability of anti-asthma herbal medicine intervention in adult patients with moderate-severe allergic asthma. *J Allergy Clin Immunol.* 116:517, 2005.

Wong KW. Clinical efficacy of n-3 fatty acid supplementation in patients with asthma. *J Am Diet Assoc.* 105:98, 2005.

Woods R, et al. Dietary marine fatty acids (fish oil) for asthma. *Cochrane Database Syst Rev.* 2:CD001283, 2000.

Woods RK, et al. Food and nutrient intakes and asthma risk in young adults. *Am J Clin Nutr.* 78:414, 2003.

Ziboh VA, et al. Suppression of leukotriene B4 generation by ex-vivo neutrophils isolated from asthma patients on dietary supplementation with gammalinolenic acid-containing borage oil: possible implication in asthma. *Clin Dev Immunol.* 11:13, 2004.

Zutavern A, et al. The introduction of solids in relation to asthma and eczema. *Arch Dis Child.* 89:303, 2004.

BRONCHIECTASIS

NUTRITIONAL ACUITY RANKING: LEVEL 1

DEFINITIONS AND BACKGROUND

Bronchiectasis belongs to the family of chronic obstructive lung diseases, although it is much less common than asthma, chronic bronchitis, or emphysema (Mysliwiec and Pina, 1999). Bronchiectasis is an irreversible widening of portions of the bronchi resulting from damage to the bronchial wall. Chronic dilation of the bronchi (or a bronchus) occurs in this condition.

Bronchiectasis should be suspected in children with recurrent bronchitis or pneumonia and when, despite appropriate therapy, pulmonary infiltrates or atelectasis persist for 3 months or longer (Chang et al, 2002). Chronic cough; profuse, foul, and purulent sputum; and hemoptysis are common. Other symptoms and signs include early morning paroxysmal cough, decreased breath sounds, weight loss, fatigue, anorexia, pneumonia, and fever.

The most common causes are acute respiratory illness in patients with COPD. Other causes include measles, whooping cough, tuberculosis, fungal infection, inhaled object, lung tumor, cystic fibrosis, ciliary dyskinesia, immunoglobulin deficiency syndromes, rheumatoid arthritis, ulcerative colitis, human immunodeficiency virus (HIV) infection, and heroin abuse.

The relapse of bronchiectasis can be controlled with antibiotics, chest physiotherapy, inhaled bronchodilators, proper hydration, and good nutrition (Mysliwiec and Pina, 1999). In rare circumstances, surgical resection or bilateral lung transplantation may be the only option available for improving quality of life. Surgery has few complications and improves symptoms in the great majority of patients, especially when complete resection of the disease is achieved (Prieto et al, 2001). Physiological lung exclusion is sometimes used for control of massive hemoptysis in cases where lung resection is not advised. Lung transplantation may be recommended.

INTERVENTION: OBJECTIVES

- Promote recovery and prevent relapse of symptoms.
- Avoid fatigue associated with mealtimes.
- Prevent or correct dehydration.
- Improve weight status, when necessary.
- Reduce fever and inflammation.
- Support lung function, which is found to be better with higher antioxidant levels (Hu and Cassano, 2000).
- Prevent lung collapse or atelectasis.
- Prepare patient for surgery if needed.

INTERVENTION: FOOD AND NUTRITION

- Use a diet with 1.0–1.25 g protein/kg and sufficient calories to meet elevated metabolic requirements appropriate for age and sex.
- Small, frequent feedings may be better tolerated.
- Fluid intake of 2–3 L daily may be offered, unless contraindicated.
- Intravenous fat emulsions may be indicated (eicosanoids are inflammatory modulators, and thromboxanes and leukotrienes tend to be potent mediators of inflammation). Omega-3 fatty acids should be enhanced in the oral diet by including salmon, tuna, sardines, walnuts, and flaxseed. Supplements may also be useful.
- Adequate antioxidant use with vitamins C and E and selenium may be beneficial. Ensure adequate potassium intake, depending on medications used.

CLINICAL INDICATORS

Clinical/History		
Height	I & O	Coughing up blood
Weight	Respiratory rate	Breath odor
BMI	Shortness of breath	Wheezing
Weight loss?	Fatigue	Chest x-ray
Diet history	Bluish skin or paleness	Sputum culture
BP		

Lab Work		
Transthyretin	Gluc	Serum Fe
Retinol-binding protein (RBP)	Na+, K+	Transferrin
	Ca++, Mg++	Blood urea nitrogen (BUN)
	Chol	pO_2, pCO_2
	Trig	
	H & H	

Common Drugs Used and Potential Side Effects

- Antibiotics are used if the condition is bacterial in origin. Aerosol administration of high-dose tobramycin in non–cystic fibrosis (CF) bronchiectatic patients appears to be safe (Drobnic et al, 2005).
- Analgesics and antipyretics may be used. Monitor side effects according to the specific drugs used.
- Dry powder mannitol has been shown to improve tracheobronchial clearance in bronchiectasis but is not yet available for clinical use.

Herbs, Botanicals, and Supplements

No clinical trials have proven efficacy for use of herbs or botanicals in bronchiectasis.

INTERVENTION: NUTRITION EDUCATION, COUNSELING, CARE MANAGEMENT

- Discuss the role of nutrition in health and recovery; emphasize quality proteins and nutrient-dense foods, especially if the patient is anorexic.
- Emphasize fluid intake, perhaps recommending juices or calorie-containing beverages instead of water.
- Discuss desirable sources of fatty acids, such as omega-3 foods.

Patient Education—Foodborne Illness

- Careful food handling will be important. Hand washing is key as well.

For More Information

- Bronchiectasis
  http://www.lung.ca/diseases/bronchiectasis.html

BRONCHIECTASIS—CITED REFERENCES

Chang AB, et al. Bronchiectasis in indigenous children in remote Australian communities. *Med J Aust.* 177:200, 2002.

Drobnic ME, et al. Inhaled tobramycin in non-cystic fibrosis patients with bronchiectasis and chronic bronchial infection with *Pseudomonas aeruginosa. Ann Pharmacother.* 39:39, 2005.

Hu G, Cassano P. Antioxidant nutrients and pulmonary function: the Third National Health and Nutrition Examination Survey. *Am J Epidemiol.* 151:975, 2000.

Mysliwiec V, Pina J. Bronchiectasis: the 'other' obstructive lung disease. *Postgrad Med.* 106:123, 1999.

Prieto D, et al. Surgery for bronchiectasis. *Eur J Cardiothorac Surg.* 20:19, 2001.

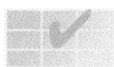

BRONCHITIS (ACUTE)

NUTRITIONAL ACUITY RANKING: LEVEL 1

DEFINITIONS AND BACKGROUND

Bronchitis is caused by inflammation of the air passages. The acute form may follow a cold or other upper respiratory infection, producing hemoptysis, sore throat, nasal discharge, slight fever, cough, and back and muscle pain. Causes include *Mycoplasma pneumoniae* and *Chlamydia* and exposure to strong acids, ammonia or chlorine fumes, air pollution ozone, or nitrogen dioxide. The chronic form, which is believed to be due mostly to cigarette smoking and air pollution, can produce breathing difficulty, wheezing, blueness, fits of coughing, and sputum production. (See Chronic Obstructive Pulmonary Disease entry.)

Risks for acute bronchitis are much higher in smokers. For example, mental patients and homeless persons tend to smoke more than other individuals and are at higher risk for acute bronchitis (Himelhoch et al, 2004; Snyder and Eisner, 2004). In pregnant women who acquire acute bronchitis, there is usually no major concern because it is short term and medications are not required (Lim et al, 2003).

INTERVENTION: OBJECTIVES

- Normalize body temperature when there is fever.
- Replenish nutrients used in respiratory distress.
- Prevent complications such as dehydration and otitis media; avoid further infections.
- Allow ample rest before and after feedings.
- Prevent dehydration. Extra fluids are needed.
- Relieve discomfort.
- Support lung function, which is found to be better with higher antioxidant levels (Hu and Cassano, 2000).

INTERVENTION: FOOD AND NUTRITION

- Provide a regular or high-calorie diet, specific to the patient's needs.
- If milk gives a sensation of thickening mucus secretions, skim milk may be better tolerated and is important for adequate calcium consumption.
- Provide adequate amounts of vitamins C and E, selenium, and potassium.
- Increase the intake of fluids (2–3 L), unless contraindicated.
- Appropriate fatty acid intake may be beneficial to reduce inflammation.
- A low energy intake may be needed after the acute phase to promote weight loss, improve BMI, and promote a healthier level of respiratory functioning (Canoy et al, 2004).

CLINICAL INDICATORS

Clinical/History	Productive cough?	H & H
Height	**Lab Work**	Serum Fe
Weight	Gluc	Alb, transthyretin
BMI	Na+, K+	Total lymphocyte count (TLC)
Diet history	Ca++, Mg++	
I & O		
Edema		

Common Drugs Used and Potential Side Effects

- Bronchodilators can cause gastric irritation. They should be taken with milk, food, or an antacid.
- Theophylline can be toxic if a diet high in carbohydrates and low in protein is used. Avoid large amounts of stimulant beverages, namely, coffee, tea, cocoa, and cola, unless the physician permits.
- Antibiotics may be used. Avoid taking penicillin with fruit juice. Gemifloxacin (a fluoroquinolone) can be used for the treatment of acute bacterial bronchitis and mild community-acquired pneumonia, including pneumonia caused by multidrug-resistant *Streptococcus pneumoniae* (File and Tillotson, 2004).

Herbs, Botanicals, and Supplements

- No clinical trials have proven efficacy for use of herbs or botanicals, such as eucalyptus, mullein, horehound, stinging nettle, or marshmallow.
- Belladonna leaf and root are respiratory antispasmodic agents. They should not be used with tricyclic antidepressants, some antihistamines, phenothiazines, or quinidine. Sedation, dry mouth, and difficult urination may occur.

INTERVENTION: NUTRITION EDUCATION, COUNSELING, CARE MANAGEMENT

- Explain to the patient that adequate hydration is one of the best ways to liquefy secretions.
- Maintain body weight within a healthy range.

Patient Education—Foodborne Illness

- Careful food handling will be important. Hand washing is key as well.

For More Information

- Medline–Bronchitis
  http://www.nlm.nih.gov/medlineplus/bronchitis.html

BRONCHITIS—CITED REFERENCES

Canoy D, et al. Abdominal obesity and respiratory function in men and women in the EPIC-Norfolk Study, United Kingdom. *Am J Epidemiol.* 159:1140, 2004.

File TM Jr, Tillotson GS. Gemifloxacin: a new, potent fluoroquinolone for the therapy of lower respiratory tract infections. *Expert Rev Anti Infect Ther.* 2:831, 2004.

Himelhoch S, et al. Prevalence of chronic obstructive pulmonary disease among those with serious mental illness. *Am J Psychiatry.* 161:2317, 2004.

Hu G, Cassano P. Antioxidant nutrients and pulmonary function: the Third National Health and Nutrition Examination Survey. *Am J Epidemiol.* 151:975, 2000.

Lim WS, et al. Treatment of community-acquired lower respiratory tract infections during pregnancy. *Am J Respir Med.* 2:221, 2003.

Snyder LD, Eisner MD. Obstructive lung disease among the urban homeless. *Chest* 125:1719, 2004.

CHRONIC OBSTRUCTIVE PULMONARY DISEASE

NUTRITIONAL ACUITY RANKING: LEVEL 3

DEFINITIONS AND BACKGROUND

Chronic obstructive pulmonary disease (COPD) may result from a history of emphysema, asthma, or chronic bronchitis with persistent lower airway obstruction. Smoking is the most common cause. According to the Centers for Disease Control and Prevention (CDC) (2003), approximately 440,000 persons die each year of a cigarette smoking–attributable illness in the United States. Other nonsmoking causes of emphysema include alpha-1 antitrypsin deficiency, connective tissue diseases, hypocomplementemic urticarial vasculitis syndrome, intravenous drug use, HIV infection, and several rare metabolic disorders (Lee et al, 2002).

Symptoms and signs of COPD include dyspnea on exertion, frequent hypoxemia, decreased forced expiratory volume in 1 second (FEV_1), and destruction of alveolar capillary bed. In COPD, total air quantity is blown out much sooner. COPD is a leading cause of death in the United States.

The chronic bronchitis ("blue bloater") patient has inflamed bronchial tubes, excess mucus production, chronic cough (for 3 months each year), shortness of breath, and no weight loss. Cardiac enlargement with failure is common. COPD is associated with muscular impairment, nutritional depletion, and systemic inflammation (Gosker et al, 2000).

Emphysema ("pink puffer") patients have weight loss and thinness without heart failure. It is characterized by tissue destruction, distention, and destruction of pulmonary air spaces by smoking and air pollution. Wheezing, shortness of breath (SOB), and chronic mild cough result. Nutritional depletion is significantly greater in patients who have emphysema than in those who have chronic bronchitis. Serious weight loss occurs from anorexia, secondary to significant SOB and gastrointestinal (GI) distress. Lung volume reduction surgery increases the chance of improved exercise capacity but does not confer a survival advantage over medical therapy (Ware, 2003).

Malnutrition and tissue wasting are common (Farber and Mannix, 2000); oxidative stress may play a role (Boots et al, 2003). Approximately 75% of patients with COPD suffer from weight loss, where chronic mouth breathing, dyspnea, aerophagia, certain medications, and depression often act in concert. Low body weight or recent weight loss and, in particular, depleted lean body mass in patients with COPD are predictors of mortality, outcomes after acute exacerbations, hospital admission rates, and need for mechanical ventilation (Mallampalli, 2004). Malnutrition decreases ventilatory muscle strength, exercise tolerance, and immunocompetence; risk of respiratory mortality is high (Thorsdottir et al, 2001).

Elevated resting and activity-related energy expenditure, reduced dietary intake relative to resting energy expenditure, accelerated negative nitrogen balance, medication effects, and an elevated systemic inflammatory response contribute to weight loss (Mallampalli, 2004). Nutritional supplementation may have a role in the management of COPD when provided as part of an integrated rehabilitation program incorporating a structured exercise component as an anabolic stimulus.

The pathological mechanisms of COPD involve neutrophil granulocytes, cytotoxic T cells, macrophages, and mast cells (Ekberg-Jansson et al, 2005). There are cytokine-induced inflammatory markers; interventions aimed at controlling cytokine production may be required to reverse the cachexia syndrome and improve functional status (Thomas, 2002). Starvation (as in anorexia nervosa) can cause emphysema, even without smoking (Coxson et al, 2004). Pulmonary inflammation, loss of skeletal muscle mass, limited exercise capacity, and poor health status all have a negative impact on prognosis (Agusti, 2001).

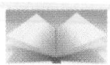

Recommendations for fats, carbohydrates (CHO), proteins, and water must be individualized (Chapman and Winter, 1996). For patients with acute exacerbations of COPD in the intensive care unit (ICU), serum total protein is associated with hospital mortality; therefore, protein intake must be carefully monitored (Yang et al, 2004). A high dietary intake of omega-3 fatty acids may be protective because of anti-inflammatory effects, but studies are not clear (Romieu and Trenga, 2001). High fruit intake can be immune enhancing and protective for COPD patients (Denny et al, 2003). Indeed, fruit and vegetable consumption may explain why some smokers do not develop COPD (Watson et al, 2002).

Underweight subjects with COPD may have significantly higher bitter taste thresholds than normal-weight subjects, which is related to bicarbonate levels and pH (Chapman-Novakofski et al, 1999). Foods such as meats, vegetables, and coffee may be more bland to the patient than he or she remembers; recognition of this may be important in planning meals.

INTERVENTION: OBJECTIVES

- Screen early and correct any malnutrition. Because there is less oxygen available for energy production, the patient is less active, and there is less blood flow to the GI tract and muscles. Malnutrition increases likelihood of infections. Prevent excessive weight loss, especially in underweight patients.
- Promote a nutrient-dense diet. Lung function is found to be better with higher antioxidant levels (Hu and Cassano, 2000).
- Overcome anorexia resulting from slowed peristalsis and digestion. Patient lethargy, poor appetite, and gastric ulceration result from inadequate oxygen to the gut.
- Improve ventilation before meals with intermittent positive-pressure breathing and overall physical conditioning to strengthen respiratory muscles.
- Lessen work efforts by losing weight, if needed.
- Prevent respiratory infections or respiratory acidosis from decreased elimination of CO_2. Decrease excess CO_2 production as well.
- Alleviate difficulty in chewing or swallowing related to SOB.
- Prevent or correct dehydration, which thickens mucus.
- Avoid constipation and straining at stool.
- Avoid distention from large meals or gaseous foods.
- Ensure adequate flavor of foods because appetite is often minimized.

INTERVENTION: FOOD AND NUTRITION

- A high-protein/high-calorie diet is necessary to correct malnutrition. Use 1.2–1.5 g protein/kg and sufficient kcals for anabolism (start with 30–35 kcal/kg, depending on current weight).
- Promote weight loss through a calorie-controlled diet for obese patients. Diets should be 40–55% CHO, 30–40% fat, and 15–20% protein. It is acceptable to start with a weight loss plan of 20–25 kcal/kg with frequent monitoring to prevent rapid weight loss.
- A diet without tough or stringy foods and an antireflux regimen are useful. Gas-forming vegetables may cause discomfort for some patients.
- Increased use of omega-3 fatty acids in foods such as salmon, haddock, mackerel, tuna, and other fish sources may be beneficial (Romieu et al, 2005).
- To enrich the diet with antioxidants, use more citrus fruits, whole grains, and nuts. There is a protective effect of fruit and possibly vitamin E intake; vitamin C, beta-carotene, vegetables, and fish are not as protective but are still encouraged for general nutritional value (Walda et al, 2002).
- Fluid intake should be high, especially if the patient is febrile. Use 1 mL/kcal as a general rule. This may translate to 8 or more cups of fluid daily. For discomfort, consume liquids between meals to increase ability to consume nutrient-dense foods at mealtimes.
- Limit salt intake; too much sodium can cause fluid retention or peripheral edema, which may interfere with breathing.
- Fiber should be increased gradually, perhaps through use of psyllium, crushed bran, prune juice, or extra fruits and vegetables.
- If necessary, moderation in carbohydrate intake is needed to avoid overload (Cai et al, 2003); less than 50% of energy intake may be needed. Pulmonary tube feeding products have a fat ratio that is higher than usual.
- Use small, concentrated feedings at frequent intervals to lessen fatigue. For example, eggnogs and shakes may be helpful between meals. See Tables 5-6 and 5-7 for ways to add extra protein or calories to the diet of COPD patients.

TABLE 5-6 Tips for Adding Calories to a Diet

Food	Tip
Fats	Butter or margarine, cream, sour cream, gravies, salad dressings, and shortening. Mix butter into hot foods such as soups and vegetables, mashed potatoes, cooked cereals, and and rice. Serve hot bread with lots of melted butter. Mayonnaise can be added to salads or sandwiches. Sour cream or yogurt can be used on vegetables such as potatoes, beans, carrots, and squash. Try sour cream or yogurt in gravy or salad dressings for fruit. Whipping cream has 60 kcal per tablespoon; add it to pies, fruits, pudding, hot chocolate, gelatin, eggnog, and other desserts. Fry the entree (e.g., chicken, meat, fish) and sauté vegetables in butter or oil.
Sweets	Spread jelly or honey on toast or cereal; mix honey in tea. Add marshmallows to hot chocolate.
Snacks	Have snacks ready to eat, such as nuts, dried fruits, candy, buttered popcorn, crackers and cheese, granola, ice cream, and popsicles.
Beverages	Drink milk shakes with lots of ice cream added; these will be high in calories and protein. Use sugar-sweetened beverages such as carbonated beverages, coffees with whipped cream and sugar, and sugar-sweetened ades.

TABLE 5-7 Tips for Adding Protein to a Diet[a]

Food	Tip
Meats and meat substitutes	Add diced or ground meat to soups and casseroles. Serve a chef salad that includes chunks of cheese, ham, turkey, and sliced egg. Peanut butter can be spread on crackers, apples, celery, pears, and bananas. Nuts are a good snack with fat and protein.
Dairy products	Add milk powder to hot or cold cereals, scrambled eggs, mashed potatoes, soups, gravies, ground meats (e.g., meat patties, meatballs, meatloaf), casserole dishes, and baked goods. Use milk or half and half instead of water when making soups, cereals, instant puddings, cocoa, and canned soups. Add grated cheese or cheese chunks to sauces, vegetables, soups, casseroles, hot crab dip, and mashed potatoes. Add extra cheese to pizza. Use yogurt as a fruit dip, or add yogurt to sauces and gravies.
Milk powder	Add skim milk powder to the regular amount of milk used in recipes or for a beverage. Or, add 1 cup of dry powder to 1 quart of fluid milk, allow it to sit overnight. This adds 286 kcal and 15 g of protein. This is "double-strength milk."
Beverages	Add protein powder to casseroles, soups, sauces, gravies, milkshakes, and eggnogs. One scoop may have 4 or 5 g of protein, depending on the brand. Some do not stir in as well as others; some dissolve better in hot foods. Buy instant breakfast mixes and use them instead of milk with meals or as snacks; one 8-oz glass provides 280 kcal. Formula products that are high in protein may be useful as supplements with or between meals or with medication pass in an institution.
Desserts	Choose dessert recipes that contain egg such as sponge or angel food cake, egg custard, bread pudding, and rice pudding.

[a] Protein can be added to many foods without having to increase the number of foods eaten.

CLINICAL INDICATORS

Clinical/History

Height
Weight
BMI
Diet history
Temperature
I & O
BP
Chest x-ray
Electrocardiogram (ECG)
Respirations
Ascites
Edema

Pulmonary function tests

Lab Work

Gluc
Na+, K+
Ca++, Mg++
Serum Fe
Hemoglobin
Hct >48% may reflect chronic hypoxemia
TLC
pH
pO_2 <50 mm Hg
$PaCO_2$ >50 mm Hg
Alb, transthyretin
Total protein
BUN
CRP
Chol
Trig

SAMPLE NUTRITION DIAGNOSTIC STATEMENT

COPD

PES: Involuntary weight loss related to early satiety and inadequate intake of calorie-dense foods as evidenced by 20-lb weight loss and fatigue at mealtimes.

Assessment: Food intake records, weight, preferred foods.

Intervention: Frequent small meals of easily digested foods with added fats and calorie-dense oral supplements.

Monitoring and Evaluation: Weight changes, improvement in calorie intake, less fatigue while eating.

Common Drugs Used and Potential Side Effects

- Bronchodilators (Atrovent, Theo-Dur, etc.) are used to liquefy secretions, treat infections, and dilate the bronchi. They can cause gastric irritation and ulceration.
- Antibiotics, steroids, expectorants, antihistamines, diuretics, anticholinergics, and other drugs may be used. Monitor side effects accordingly.
- Treatment of an exacerbation of COPD with oral or parenteral corticosteroids significantly reduces treatment failure and the need for additional medical treatment; adverse drug reactions may occur and should be monitored (Wood-Baker et al, 2005).

Herbs, Botanicals, and Supplements

- No clinical trials have proven efficacy for use of herbs or botanicals, such as mullein, camu-camu, licorice, red pepper, peppermint, and eucalyptus.
- Ephedra (ma huang) is an effective bronchodilator, but it increases blood pressure significantly. Avoid taking with digoxin, hypoglycemic agents for diabetes, monoamine oxidase inhibitor (MAOI) antidepressants, antihypertensive medications, oxytocin, theophylline, caffeine, and dexamethasone steroids. Problems with blood pressure, blood glucose, arrhythmias, increased heart rate, and central nervous system (CNS) stimulation can occur.

INTERVENTION: NUTRITION EDUCATION, COUNSELING, CARE MANAGEMENT

- Early detection, prevention, and early treatment of involuntary weight loss means putting more emphasis on dietary change than on medically prescribed supplementation (Brug et al, 2004). Explain how to concentrate protein and calories in 5–6 small meals a day rather than 3 large ones.

- To conserve energy while preparing meals at home, choose foods that are easy to prepare. Try having the main meal early in the day to have more energy throughout the rest of the day.
- Encourage rest periods before and after meals. Encourage slow eating.
- Encourage the patient to make small, attractive meals. Six small meals will prevent overfilling the stomach and causing more shortness of breath.
- Explain that excessively hot or cold foods may cause coughing spells.
- Limit fluid intake with meals to decrease early satiety and subsequent decreased food intake.
- Schedule treatments to mobilize mucus (postural drainage, aerosol treatment) 1 hour before and after meals to prevent nausea.
- Improve physical conditioning with planned exercises, especially strengthening exercises and dancing. Consumption of an oral supplement may be beneficial to support exercise (Steiner et al, 2003).
- If using oxygen, be sure the cannula is worn during and after meals. Eating and digestion require energy and oxygen.
- Maintain a relaxed atmosphere to make meals attractive and enjoyable.
- Promote good oral hygiene; periodontal disease is common in COPD (Scannapieco and Ho, 2001).
- Persons who have diabetes may also have decreased pulmonary function; they are especially encouraged not to smoke (Walter et al, 2003).
- Exercise is recommended to maintain or increase strength, but sufficient energy intake is needed to prevent nutritional decline (Engelen et al, 2003). If nearing the end of life, exercise is not usually recommended.

Patient Education—Foodborne Illness

- Careful food handling will be important. Hand washing is key as well.

For More Information

- American Thoracic Society
  http://www.thoracic.org/
- COPD
  http://www.aarc.org/patient_education/tips/copd.html
- National Emphysema Treatment Trial (Nett)
  http://www.nhlbi.nih.gov/health/prof/lung/nett/lvrsweb.htm
- Your Lung Health
  http://www.yourlunghealth.org/lung_disease/copd/decrease/index.cfm

CHRONIC OBSTRUCTIVE PULMONARY DISEASE—CITED REFERENCES

Agusti A. Systemic effects of chronic obstructive pulmonary disease. *Novartis Found Symp.* 234:242, 2001.

Boots AW, et al. Oxidant metabolism in chronic obstructive pulmonary disease. *Eur Respir J Suppl.* 46:14s, 2003.

Brug J, et al. Dietary change, nutrition education and chronic obstructive pulmonary disease. *Patient Educ Couns.* 52:249, 2004.

Cai B, et al. Effect of supplementing a high-fat, low-carbohydrate enteral formula in COPD patients. *Nutrition* 19:229, 2003.

Centers for Disease Control and Prevention. Cigarette smoking-attributable morbidity–United States, 2000. *MMWR Morb Mortal Wkly Rep.* 52:842, 2003.

Chapman K, Winter L. COPD: using nutrition to prevent respiratory function decline. *Geriatrics* 51:37, 1996.

Chapman-Novakofski K, et al. Alterations in taste thresholds in men with chronic obstructive pulmonary disease. *J Am Diet Assoc.* 99:1536, 1999.

Coxson HO, et al. Early emphysema in patients with anorexia nervosa. *Am J Respir Crit Care Med.* 170:748, 2004.

Denny SI, et al. Dietary factors in the pathogenesis of asthma and chronic obstructive pulmonary disease. *Curr Allergy Asthma Rep.* 3:130, 2003.

Ekberg-Jansson A, et al. Bronchial mucosal mast cells in asymptomatic smokers relation to structure, lung function and emphysema. *Respir Med.* 99:75, 2005.

Engelen MP, et al. Response of whole-body protein and urea turnover to exercise differs between patients with chronic obstructive pulmonary disease with and without emphysema. *Am J Clin Nutr.* 77:868, 2003.

Farber M, Mannix E. Tissue wasting in patients with chronic obstructive pulmonary disease. *Neurol Clin.* 18:245, 2000.

Gosker H, et al. Skeletal muscle dysfunction in chronic obstructive pulmonary disease and chronic heart failure: underlying mechanisms and therapy perspectives. *Am J Clin Nutri* 71:1033, 2000.

Hu G, Cassano P. Antioxidant nutrients and pulmonary function: the Third National Health and Nutrition Examination Survey. *Am J Epidemiol.* 151:975, 2000.

Lee P, et al. Emphysema in nonsmokers: alpha 1-antitrypsin deficiency and other causes. *Cleve Clin J Med.* 69:928, 2002.

Mallampalli A. Nutritional management of the patient with chronic obstructive pulmonary disease. *Nutr Clin Pract.* 19:550, 2004.

Romieu I, et al. Omega-3 fatty acid prevents heart rate variability reductions associated with particulate matter. *Am J Respir Crit Care Med.* 172:1534, 2005.

Scannapieco F, Ho A. Potential associations between chronic respiratory disease and periodontal disease: analysis of National Health and Nutrition Examination Survey III. *J Periodontol.* 72:50, 2001.

Steiner MC, et al. Nutritional enhancement of exercise performance in chronic obstructive pulmonary disease: a randomised controlled trial. *Thorax* 58:745, 2003.

Thomas DR. Dietary prescription for chronic obstructive pulmonary disease. *Clin Geriatr Med.* 18:835, 2002.

Thorsdottir I, et al. Screening method evaluated by nutritional status measurements can be used to detect malnourishment in chronic obstructive pulmonary disease. *J Am Diet Assoc.* 101:648, 2001.

Walda IC, et al. Diet and 20-year chronic obstructive pulmonary disease mortality in middle-aged men from three European countries. *Eur J Clin Nutr.* 56:638, 2002.

Walter RE, et al. Association between glycemic state and lung function: the Framingham Heart Study. *Am J Respir Crit Care Med.* 167:911, 2003.

Ware JH. The National Emphysema Treatment Trial: how strong is the evidence? *N Engl J Med.* 348:2055, 2003.

Watson L, et al. The association between diet and chronic obstructive pulmonary disease in subjects selected from general practice. *Eur Respir J.* 20:313, 2002.

Wood-Baker RR, et al. Systemic corticosteroids for acute exacerbations of chronic obstructive pulmonary disease. *Cochrane Database Syst Rev.* 1:CD001288, 2005.

Yang S, et al. Acute exacerbation of COPD requiring admission to the intensive care unit. *Respirology* 9:543, 2004.

CHYLOTHORAX

NUTRITIONAL ACUITY RANKING: LEVEL 2–4

DEFINITIONS AND BACKGROUND

Chylothorax involves accumulation of clear lymph (chyle) in the pleural or thoracic space. It may be spontaneous or caused by invasion of the thoracic space. Etiologies may include amyloidosis, congenital chylothorax, coronary artery bypass grafting (CABG), violent vomiting or coughing after heavy meals, cancer (such as lymphoma), complications from neck surgery including a radical dissection, thoracic cage compression after cardiopulmonary resuscitation (CPR), thoracic duct trauma from thoracotomy tubes, thoracic surgery affecting the heart, lungs, or esophagus, and tuberculosis.

Chylous effusions look like milk. Since chyle represents direct absorption of fat from the small intestine lacteals, it is rich in fat, calories, vitamins, and immunoglobulins (Evans et al, 2003). Management of chylothorax may include use of total parenteral nutrition (TPN), low-fat enteral nutrition, thoracentesis to remove the chylous fluid, or surgical ligation of the thoracic duct (Suddaby and Schiller, 2004).

In the congenital form of chylothorax, breast milk and/or regular infant feeding formula should be used before proceeding to medium-chain triglyceride (MCT)–rich formula. Surgery should be considered if conservative management of congenital chylothorax fails after 4–5 weeks (Al-Tawil et al, 2001).

INTERVENTION: OBJECTIVES

- Offer continuous chest-tube drainage to decrease pleural chyle.
- Drainage of chyle from the chest or abdomen results in rapid weight loss and profound cachexia (Evans et al, 2003). Lessen consequences of a nutritional or immunological nature from drainage (e.g., sepsis, protein–calorie malnutrition, decreased lymphocytes, etc.).
- Replace fat, protein, and micronutrient losses from exudates.
- Achieve a positive nitrogen balance.
- Support involvement of a surgical nutrition support team (NST), which is associated with better patient management and a reduction in inappropriate TPN orders (Saalwachter et al, 2004).

INTERVENTION: FOOD AND NUTRITION

- Decrease enteral fat intake for patients who are tube fed. For patients who are fed orally, reduce total fat intake until condition is resolved; also for these patients, a low-fat diet may be used alone or with an elemental product.
- Some patients may be able to tolerate a low long-chain fatty acid formula given as a tube feeding (Cormack et al, 2004).
- For patients without sepsis, TPN may be indicated; care is needed to avoid aggravating the condition.
- Replace exudate losses of nutrients such as vitamin A and zinc. Check serum levels and replace with higher levels of the recommended intakes if necessary.

CLINICAL INDICATORS

Clinical/History	Lab Work	
Height	Alb, transthyretin	Gluc
Weight	RBP	Ca++, Mg++
BMI	H & H	Na+, K+
Weight changes	Transferrin	CRP
Diet history	Chol	BUN, creatinine (Creat)
Temperature	Trig	pCO_2, pO_2
I & O	TLC (decreased)	
Lung x-ray		

Common Drugs Used and Potential Side Effects

- Octreotide (Sandostatin) may be given as conservative medical management (Suver et al, 2004). Nausea, vomiting, abdominal pain, diarrhea, and flatulence can occur. Use with the low-fat diet to decrease GI side effects.
- Medications are given, as appropriate, for the etiology. Monitor side effects accordingly, especially in conditions such as tuberculosis (TB) or cancer in which numerous side effects are created from drug therapies.
- Bronchodilators may be used. Some nausea and vomiting may occur.

Herbs, Botanicals, and Supplements

- No clinical trials have proven efficacy for use of herbs or botanicals in chylothorax.

INTERVENTION: NUTRITION EDUCATION, COUNSELING, CARE MANAGEMENT

- Discuss the importance of adequate nutrition in recovery.
- Discuss interventions that are appropriate for the conditions and diagnoses involved.

Patient Education—Foodborne Illness

- Careful food handling will be important. Hand washing is key as well.

For More Information

- E-medicine
http://www.emedicine.com/med/topic381.htm

CHYLOTHORAX—CITED REFERENCES

Al-Tawil K, et al. Congenital chylothorax. *Am J Perinatol.* 17:121, 2001.

Cormack BE, et al. Use of Monogen for pediatric postoperative chylothorax. *Ann Thorac Surg.* 77:301, 2004.

Evans J, et al. Chylous effusions complicating lymphoma: a serious event with octreotide as a treatment option. *Hematol Oncol.* 21:77, 2003.

Saalwachter AR, et al. A nutrition support team led by general surgeons decreases inappropriate use of total parenteral nutrition on a surgical service. *Am Surg.* 70:1107, 2004.

Suddaby EC, Schiller S. Management of chylothorax in children. *Pediatr Nurs.* 30:290, 2004.

Suver DW, et al. Somatostatin treatment of massive lymphorrhea following excision of a lymphatic malformation. *Int J Pediatr Otorhinolaryngol.* 68:845, 2004.

COR PULMONALE

NUTRITIONAL ACUITY RANKING: LEVEL 2–4

DEFINITIONS AND BACKGROUND

Right ventricular failure (acute cor pulmonale) occurs when relevant increases in pulmonary vascular resistance overwhelm compensatory mechanisms. A heart disease that follows disease of the lung (end-stage emphysema, silicosis, etc.), cor pulmonale strains the right ventricle, creating enlargement (hypertrophy) and eventual failure. Long-term exposure to combustion-related fine particulate air pollution is a risk factor.

Secondary pulmonary hypertension (PH) and cor pulmonale are the major clinical cardiovascular complications affecting prognosis in patients with COPD (Bacakoglu et al, 2003). Children who have Prader-Willi syndrome generally survive into adulthood, but one common cause of death is obesity-related cor pulmonale (Stevenson et al, 2004).

Cor pulmonale may be acute, subacute, or chronic. Signs and symptoms include hypoxia, wheezing, cough, fatigue, weakness, cyanosis, and clubbing of the fingers and toes. The body secretes B-type natriuretic peptide from the cardiac ventricles in response to ventricular stretch and pressure overload; this counteracts vasoconstriction that occurs as a compensatory mechanism (Prahash and Lynch, 2004).

INTERVENTION: OBJECTIVES

- Improve the patient's capacity to eat meals without straining the diaphragm.
- Correct malnourished status. Avoid weight gain, which adds stress on the heart.
- Reduce or prevent fluid retention and edema to lessen cardiac workload.
- Prevent additional damage to cardiac and respiratory tissues.
- Support adequate lung function, which is found to be better with higher antioxidant levels (Hu and Cassano, 2000).

INTERVENTION: FOOD AND NUTRITION

- Recommend small, frequent meals rather than 3 large ones.
- Use a nutrient-dense diet with concentrated protein sources. Double-strength milk, foods with milk powder added to them, high-calorie supplements, and addition of extra gravies or sauces to meals are useful when quantity of food must be kept minimal because of difficulty breathing.
- To reduce fluid retention, intake of fluids may be restricted to 500 mL plus the amount of the previous day's fluid intake. Sodium restriction may also be necessary.
- Use foods that reduce likelihood of gastric irritation and reflux. For example, use low-acidic fruits, vegetables, and juices.
- Provide adequate potassium intake; monitor for high serum levels.
- Include adequate levels of vitamins C and E and selenium for their antioxidant properties.

CLINICAL INDICATORS

Clinical/History		Lab Work
Height	Right upper quadrant (RUQ) pain	Alb
Weight	Hepatomegaly	Na+, K+
BMI	Dyspnea	Ca++, Mg++
Diet history	Distended neck veins	H & H
I & O	Clubbing of fingers and toes	Serum Fe
Edema		BUN, Creat
Chest x-ray		pCO_2 (increased)
Echocardiography		pO_2 (decreased)
BP		CRP

Common Drugs Used and Potential Side Effects

- Corticosteroids can cause sodium retention, negative nitrogen balance, etc. Monitor carefully.
- Diuretics can cause potassium depletion with diuresis.

Herbs, Botanicals, and Supplements

- No clinical trials have proven efficacy for use of herbs or botanicals in cor pulmonale.

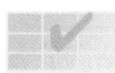

INTERVENTION: NUTRITION EDUCATION, COUNSELING, CARE MANAGEMENT

- Plan small, attractive meals that are nutrient dense. If fluid and sodium must be limited, provide tips.
- Recommend snacks that are high in calories and protein but that do not provide excessive amounts of sodium.
- Emphasize the importance of eating slowly.
- Weight loss may be needed (Olson and Zwillich, 2005).

Patient Education—Foodborne Illness

- Careful food handling will be important. Hand washing is key as well.

For More Information

- Dr. Koop
  http://www.drkoop.com/ency/article/000129.htm

COR PULMONALE—CITED REFERENCES

Bacakoglu F, et al. Plasma and bronchoalveolar lavage fluid levels of endothelin-1 in patients with chronic obstructive pulmonary disease and pulmonary hypertension. *Respiration* 70:594, 2003.

Hu G, Cassano P. Antioxidant nutrients and pulmonary function: the Third National Health and Nutrition Examination Survey. *Am J Epidemiol.* 151:975, 2000.

Olson AL, Zwillich CH. The obesity hypoventilation syndrome. *Am J Med.* 118:948, 2005.

Prahash A, Lynch T. B-type natriuretic peptide: a diagnostic, prognostic, and therapeutic tool in heart failure. *Am J Crit Care.* 13:46, 2004.

Stevenson DA, et al. Unexpected death and critical illness in Prader-Willi syndrome: report of ten individuals. *Am J Med Genet A.* 124:158, 2004.

CYSTIC FIBROSIS

NUTRITIONAL ACUITY RANKING: LEVEL 3

DEFINITIONS AND BACKGROUND

Cystic fibrosis (CF) is a life-limiting, autosomal recessive inherited disease characterized by thick mucus and frequent pulmonary infections. There is general dysfunction of mucus-producing exocrine glands; high levels of sodium and chloride in the saliva, tears, and sweat; and highly viscous secretions in the pancreas, bronchi, bile ducts, and small intestine. Meconium ileus is a classic sign in newborn infants with CF; it is thicker than usual and passes more slowly.

According to the Cystic Fibrosis Foundation, CF affects approximately 30,000 children and adults in the United States. About one in 3200 Caucasians is affected; 2–5% of Caucasians carry the CF gene. The majority of CF patients have been diagnosed by age 3, but about 10% are not diagnosed until age 18 or older. The median life expectancy for CF patients is 33 years. The need to identify the CF gene and its product, CF transmembrane conductance regulator (CFTR), supports newborn screening for CF (Doull, 2001).

The CFTR system controls the efflux of physiologically important anions, such as glutathione (GSH) and bicarbonate, as well as chloride (Hudson, 2004). Interleukin-8 and cytokines also play a role in CF (Augarten et al, 2004). Anti-inflammatory and antioxidant treatments are recommended, including use of omega-3 fatty acids and selenium.

The percentage of CF children who are malnourished depends on whether anthropometric or body composition data are used; weight-based indicators greatly underestimate the extent of malnutrition (McNaughton et al, 2000). Stature is a significant prognostic indicator of CF survival (Beker et al, 2001).

A link has been established between the degree of malnutrition and the severity of the disease. Inadequate intake, malabsorption, and increased energy requirements are common. Body cell mass, which can be quantified by measurement of total body potassium, provides an ideal standard for measurements of energy expenditure (Shepherd et al, 2001). Careful follow-up, better knowledge of energy requirements, dietary counseling, and nutritional intervention help optimize the growth of these patients.

A major goal in the management of CF patients is to maintain a good nutritional status because it improves long-term survival (Munck and Navarro, 2000). Early diagnosis of CF and aggressive nutritional therapy are important to prevent growth failure and malnutrition (Farrell et al, 2005). When appropriate, lung transplantation may be considered.

Pancreatic insufficiency occurs in 80–90% of CF patients; 85% show growth retardation. Intestinal malabsorption is severe in virtually all people who have CF. The main cause is deficiency of pancreatic enzymes, but bicarbonate deficiency, abnormalities of bile salts, mucosal transport and motility, and anatomical structural changes are other factors (Littlewood and Wolfe, 2000). Appropriate pancreatic replacement therapy, combined with pharmacotherapy to address increased acidity of the intestines, achieves near-normal absorption in many patients. Most CF patients who have evidence of fat malabsorption are candidates for enzyme replacement therapy (Littlewood and Wolfe, 2000).

Decreased bone density and increased risk of fractures are seen in patients with CF; osteoporosis is seen more often due to longer life expectancy (Lambert, 2000). Nutrition problems, hypogonadism, inactivity, corticosteroid use, and cytokines may contribute to the low bone mass seen in these patients. Treatment recommendations must be individualized and may include nutrition, vitamin D, bisphosphonates, and exercise.

Diabetes may also occur in persons with CF (more commonly in older individuals), reflecting impairment of beta-cell function, which is probably genetically determined. Onset of CF-related diabetes (CFRD) is often associated with a decline in health and nutritional status. Energy requirements may be higher than usual for patients with CF and CFRD during periods of recovery from mild exercise because of increased work of breathing consistent with higher ventilatory requirements (Ward et al, 1999). Microvascular complications are common in CFRD; microalbuminuria is a sensitive indicator of progression to diabetic nephropathy in non-CF diabetes, but it is less sensitive for CF patients (Dobson et al, 2005).

Some patients are diagnosed in adulthood; patients diagnosed as adults differ distinctly from long-term CF survivors diagnosed as children (Nick and Rodman, 2005). While respiratory symptoms are not as severe and prognosis is more favorable, pancreatitis is more common (Nick and Rodman, 2005).

Research continues to support the potential benefits of gene therapy, in which compacted DNA is used rather than a virus to get healthy genes into CF cells.

Overall, patients with CF who receive optimal nutrition have better growth, maintain better nutritional reserves, and have better pulmonary function than patients with CF who have poor nutrition (Hart et al, 2004; Erdman, 1999). Metabolic and immunological response to infection and the increased work of breathing escalate calorie requirements. Growth hormone helps bring onset of puberty in prepubescent children who have CF (Vanderwel and Hardin, 2006).

Because no single strategy works for every patient, close monitoring of growth, symptoms, and changes in respiratory status must occur. The American Dietetic Association recommends a minimum of 4 medical nutrition therapy visits for patients who have CF.

INTERVENTION: OBJECTIVES

- Determine current level of care needed (Table 5-8). Effective treatment should allow a normal diet, symptom control, malabsorption correction, and attainment of a normal nutritional state and growth.

TABLE 5-8 Nutritional Management for CF

Routine care	Within desired BMI
Anticipatory guidance	At 90–95% desired BMI
Supportive intervention	At 85–90% desired BMI
Rehabilitative care	At 75–85% desired BMI
Resuscitative or palliative care	Below 75% desired BMI

- Achieve or maintain desirable BMI. BMI percentile is a better evaluation than % ideal body weight (IBW) in CF patients; %IBW underestimates the severity of malnutrition in children with short stature and overestimates the severity of malnutrition in children with tall stature (Zhang and Lai, 2004).
- Correct anorexia from respiratory distress.
- Provide optimal amounts of protein for growth, development, and resistance to infection. Increase lean body mass if depleted. Spare protein by providing up to twice the normal amount of calories from CHO and fat as in usual diet plans. Stunting may require extra protein, as from tube feeding (Geukers et al, 2005).
- Decrease electrolyte losses in vomiting and steatorrhea. Replace lost electrolytes.
- Achieve adequate enzyme replacement to bring about near-normal digestion. Reduce excessive nutrient losses from maldigestion and malabsorption.
- Provide essential fatty acids in tolerated form. Reduce arachidonic acid use to lessen inflammatory cascade. Include a sufficient supply of omega-3 fatty acids and antioxidants such as selenium and vitamins C and E. Vitamin E may be especially important in improving cognitive function (Koscik et al, 2004).
- Correct edema, diarrhea, anemia, azotorrhea, and steatorrhea.
- Prevent progressive pulmonary disease or complications such as glucose intolerance, intestinal obstruction, cirrhosis, and pancreatic or cardiac diseases.
- Improve tolerance for therapies and medications.

INTERVENTION: FOOD AND NUTRITION

- Energy expenditure may be as high as 199% of predicted in CF patients. CF patients may need to be given 120–150% more calories than for age-matched and gender-matched controls; this may mean 3000–4000 kcal for teens. Design the plan for 45–65% CHO and 20–30% fat. For persons with acute disease, starch and fat will not be well tolerated unless adequate levels of pancreatic enzymes are provided. Calorie intake should be about 150 kcal/kg for children and 200 kcal/kg for infants. Specific interventions for increasing total energy intake in CF patients are the role of the dietitian (Powers et al, 2004). Many supplements are available at little or no cost to the patient.
- Manage glucose levels if CF diabetes mellitus (CFDM) develops. Intensive insulin therapy and CHO counting will be important.
- Protein should be 10–35% of total calories. This may translate into 4 g/kg for infants, 3 g/kg for children, 2 g/kg for teens, and 1.5 g/kg for adults.
- Increase fat:CHO ratio with respiratory distress. Special respiratory formulas may be useful during those times, or use of MCTs and safflower oil may be beneficial. Be sure to time intake according to the use and type of pancreatic enzymes.
- Encourage intake of omega-3 fatty acids (DHA and EPA) to reduce inflammation.
- Supplement the diet with two times the normal RDAs for fat-soluble vitamins A, D, and E (use water-miscible sources such as "ADEKS" brand). Replace iron, zinc,

copper, and vitamin K as needed; check serum levels regularly. Use extra riboflavin if there is cheilosis, and include the other B-complex vitamins and vitamin C at recommended levels. Be sure to include selenium.

- Use 4–6 g of sodium to replace perspiration losses.
- Lactose intolerance is common. Omit milk during periods of diarrhea if lactose intolerance persists.
- Intolerance for gas-forming foods and concentrated sweets may occur; alter dietary plans accordingly.
- Soft foods may be useful if chewing causes fatigue.
- Fluid intake should be liberal unless contraindicated.
- Salt may be added to commercial baby foods; monitor carefully, especially to prevent cor pulmonale.
- Use of turmeric and cumin in foods may be beneficial for CF patients (Berger et al, 2005). Research is ongoing to determine overall practicality of uses.
- Infants can tolerate most formulas (may need 24 kcal/oz) and commercial products that include some MCT oil. Do not add pancreatic enzymes to formula because desired amounts may not be totally consumed or enzymes may block the opening of the nipple.
- Nocturnal tube feeding may be appropriate with growth failure. If gastroenteritis (GE) reflux occurs, a gastrostomy feeding tube may be well tolerated (Oliver et al, 2004).
- Parenteral nutrition (PN) is not recommended due to high risk of infection in CF patients.

CLINICAL INDICATORS

Clinical/History

Height, weight
Growth chart for height and weight
BMI
Diet history
Fecal fat study
pH
Chest x-ray or computed tomography (CT) scan
Pulmonary function test
Dual-energy x-ray absorptiometry (DEXA) scan for bone density

Lab Work

pCO_2, pO_2
Chol, Trig
Na+, K+, CL−
Alb
H & H
Serum Fe
Pancreatic enzymes (amylase, lipase)
White blood cell count (WBC)
Prothrombin time (PT) or international normalized ratio (INR)
Gluc
Serum carotene levels
Ca++, Mg++
Positive pilocarpine iontophoresis sweat test
Secretin stimulation test
Trypsin or chymotrypsin in stool
Fecal elastase-1 in stool
Serum copper (Cu)

Common Drugs Used and Potential Side Effects

- See Table 5-9.

Herbs, Botanicals, and Supplements

- Interesting studies suggest that curcumin may directly stimulate CFTR Cl− channels (Berger et al, 2005). Additional research is needed, but the use of turmeric and cumin in foods served to this population may have therapeutic benefits.
- Dietary supplement use is prevalent among CF children; it is important to become aware of patients' use of nonprescribed supplements because of the unknown effects of many supplements on growth and development and the potential for adverse drug interactions (Ball et al, 2005).
- The individual with CF should work with the CF nutritionist to maintain a healthy diet before considering adding herbal therapies. Each label on any supplement should be read carefully because there are some ingredients that can be toxic to people with CF but not to people who do not have CF.

INTERVENTION: NUTRITION EDUCATION, COUNSELING, CARE MANAGEMENT

- Diet must be periodically reevaluated to reflect growth and disease process.
- New foods may be introduced gradually.
- A behavioral and nutrition intervention can be used with children to enhance weight and height velocities (Powers et al, 2005).
- To liquefy secretions, adequate fluid intake should be ensured. Discuss signs of dehydration and how to prevent or correct.
- Bronchopulmonary drainage, three times daily, may be required. Plan meals to be 1 hour before or after therapy.
- Ensure that all foods and beverages are nutrient dense.
- If the patient is a teen, discuss issues related to fertility (most males with CF are infertile, but females are not).
- In adults with CF, 40% have some glucose intolerance. Discuss how to manage CF with diabetes in those cases.
- Discuss reimbursement issues for tube feedings and pumps.
- Hypnosis may be useful in reducing the effects of pain from frequent intravenous injections or other treatments.

Patient Education—Foodborne Illness

- Careful food handling will be important. Hand washing is key as well.

For More Information

- Cystic Fibrosis Foundation
  http://www.cff.org/
- Cystic Fibrosis for Children
  http://www.cff.org/UploadedFiles/living_with_cf/Files/Nutrition%20for%20Your%20Child.pdf
- Cystic Fibrosis for Teens
  http://www.cff.org/living_with_cf/teen_focus/
- Cystic Fibrosis Guide for Infants
  http://www.cff.org/UploadedFiles/living_with_cf/Files/Nutrition%20for%20Your%20Infant.pdf
- Cystic Fibrosis Research
  http://www.cfri.org/indexframes.htm
- International Association of Cystic Fibrosis Adults
  http://www.iacfa.org/

TABLE 5-9 Medications Used in Cystic Fibrosis (CF) and Potential Side Effects

Medication	Description and Side Effects
Aerosolized antibiotics	TOBI (tobramycin solution for inhalation) can be delivered in a more concentrated dose directly to the site of CF lung infections and is preservative free.
Antibiotics	Antibiotics are needed during infections. Monitor for magnesium depletion.
Azithromycin	Azithromycin is an antibiotic that is effective in people with CF whose lungs are chronically infected with the common *Pseudomonas aeruginosa* bacteria.
Bisphosphonates	Bisphosphonates may be used to increase bone density
Bronchodilators	Bronchodilators are used to open breathing passages. Monitor for side effects.
Glutathione (GSH)	Buffered GSH has been tested in some CF patients. Nebulized buffered GSH may ameliorate CF disease; longer and larger studies of inhaled GSH are warranted (Bishop et al, 2005).
L-arginine	Oral L-arginine (200 mg) may reduce nitric oxide levels, which can be detrimental (Grasemann et al, 2005). More studies are needed.
Mucolytics	Mucolytics, such as potassium iodide, liquefy secretions.
Pancreatic enzymes (pancrelipase)	Pancreatic granules (Viokase or Cotazym) are used to help improve digestion/absorption. Doses up to 10,000 IU lipase/kg/d help to sustain a normal nutritional state and growth rate (Littlewood and Wolfe, 2000). Enteric preparations (Pancrease) act in the duodenum, so give before meals; for nocturnal feedings, give before, during, and after feedings. Avoid mixing with milk or ice cream. If too much is given, anorexia and constipation may result. Return of a voracious appetite and increase in stool bulk suggest an inadequate dosage. Dosing should be based on stool tests for malabsorption.
Pulmozyme	A mucus-thinning drug shown to reduce the number of lung infections and improve lung function.
Ursodeoxycholic acid	Used for meconium ileus and liver disease associated with CF (Lamireau et al, 2004; Kumar and Tandon, 2001).

NOTE. The need to take up to 40–60 pills daily is common in CF.

CYSTIC FIBROSIS—CITED REFERENCES

Augarten A, et al. Systemic inflammatory mediators and cystic fibrosis genotype. *Clin Exp Med.* 4:99, 2004.

Ball SD, et al. Dietary supplement use is prevalent among children with a chronic illness. *J Am Diet Assoc.* 105:78, 2005.

Beker L, et al. Stature as a prognostic indicator in cystic fibrosis survival. *J Am Diet Assoc.* 101:438, 2001.

Berger AL, et al. Curcumin stimulates CFTR Cl-channel activity. *J Biol Chem.* 280:5221–5226, 2005.

Bishop C, et al. A pilot study of the effect of inhaled buffered reduced glutathione on the clinical status of patients with cystic fibrosis. *Chest* 127:308, 2005.

Dobson L, et al. Microalbuminuria as a screening tool in cystic fibrosis-related diabetes. *Pediatr Pulmonol.* 39:103, 2005.

Doull I. Recent advances in cystic fibrosis. *Arch Dis Child.* 85:62, 2001.

Erdman S. Nutritional imperatives in cystic fibrosis therapy. *Pediatr Ann.* 128:129, 1999.

Farrell PM, et al. Evidence on improved outcomes with early diagnosis of cystic fibrosis through neonatal screening: enough is enough! *J Pediatr.* 147:S30, 2005 (suppl 3).

Geukers VG, et al. Short-term protein intake and stimulation of protein synthesis in stunted children with cystic fibrosis. *Am J Clin Nutr.* 81:605, 2005.

Grasemann H, et al. Oral L-arginine supplementation in cystic fibrosis patients: a placebo-controlled study. *Eur Respir J.* 25:62, 2005.

Hart N, et al. Nutritional status is an important predictor of diaphragm strength in young patients with cystic fibrosis. *Am J Clin Nutr.* 80:1201, 2004.

Hudson VM. New insights into the pathogenesis of cystic fibrosis: pivotal role of glutathione system dysfunction and implications for therapy. *Treat Respir Med.* 3:353, 2004.

Koscik RL, et al. Cognitive function of children with cystic fibrosis: deleterious effect of early malnutrition. *Pediatrics* 113:1549, 2004.

Kumar D, Tandon R. Use of ursodeoxycholic acid in liver diseases. *J Gastroenterol Hepatol.* 16:3, 2001.

Lambert J. Osteoporosis: a new challenge in cystic fibrosis. *Pharmacotherapy* 20:34, 2000.

Lamireau T, et al. Epidemiology of liver disease in cystic fibrosis: a longitudinal study. *J Hepatol.* 41:920, 2004.

Littlewood J, Wolfe S. Control of malabsorption in cystic fibrosis. *Pediatr Drugs.* 2:205, 2000.

McNaughton S, et al. Nutritional status of children with cystic fibrosis measured by total body potassium as a maker of body cell mass: lack of sensitivity of anthropometric measures. *J Pediatr.* 136:188, 2000.

Munck A, Navarro J. Nutritional management of cystic fibrosis in children. *Arch Pediatr.* 7:396, 2000.

Nick JA, Rodman DM. Manifestations of cystic fibrosis diagnosed in adulthood. *Curr Opin Pulm Med.* 11:513, 2005.

Oliver MR, et al. Factors affecting clinical outcome in gastrostomy-fed children with cystic fibrosis. *Pediatr Pulmonol.* 37:324, 2004.

Powers SW, et al. A comparison of food group variety between toddlers with and without cystic fibrosis. *J Hum Nutr Diet.* 17:523, 2004.

Powers SW, et al. Randomized clinical trial of behavioral and nutrition treatment to improve energy intake and growth in toddlers and preschoolers with cystic fibrosis. *Pediatrics* 116:1442, 2005.

Shepherd R, et al. Energy expenditure and the body cell mass in cystic fibrosis. *Nutrition* 17:22, 2001.

Vanderwel M, Hardin DS. Growth hormone normalizes pubertal onset in children with cystic fibrosis. *J Pediatr Endocrinol Metab.* 19:237, 2006.

Ward S, et al. Energy expenditure and substrate utilization in adults with cystic fibrosis and diabetes mellitus. *Am J Clin Nutr.* 69:913, 1999.

Zhang Z, Lai HJ. Comparison of the use of body mass index percentiles and percentage of ideal body weight to screen for malnutrition in children with cystic fibrosis. *Am J Clin Nutr.* 80:982, 2004.

INTERSTITIAL LUNG DISEASE

NUTRITIONAL ACUITY RANKING: LEVEL 1–2

DEFINITIONS AND BACKGROUND

Interstitial lung disease (ILD) is a general term that includes a variety of chronic lung disorders, sometimes also known as "interstitial pulmonary fibrosis." In ILD, the lung tissue is damaged; the walls of the air sacs in the lung become inflamed; and, finally, scarring (fibrosis) occurs in the interstitium (tissue between the air sacs), and the lung becomes stiff. Causes of ILD include environmental exposure to inorganic dust (such as silica) or organic dust (such as animal or bacterial proteins); exposure to gases, fumes, or poisons; or medical conditions such as sarcoidosis, scleroderma, rheumatic arthritis, and lupus. Agricultural workers also can be affected, with moldy hay causing allergic reactions in a disorder known as Farmer's Lung. Figure 5-4 shows silicosis.

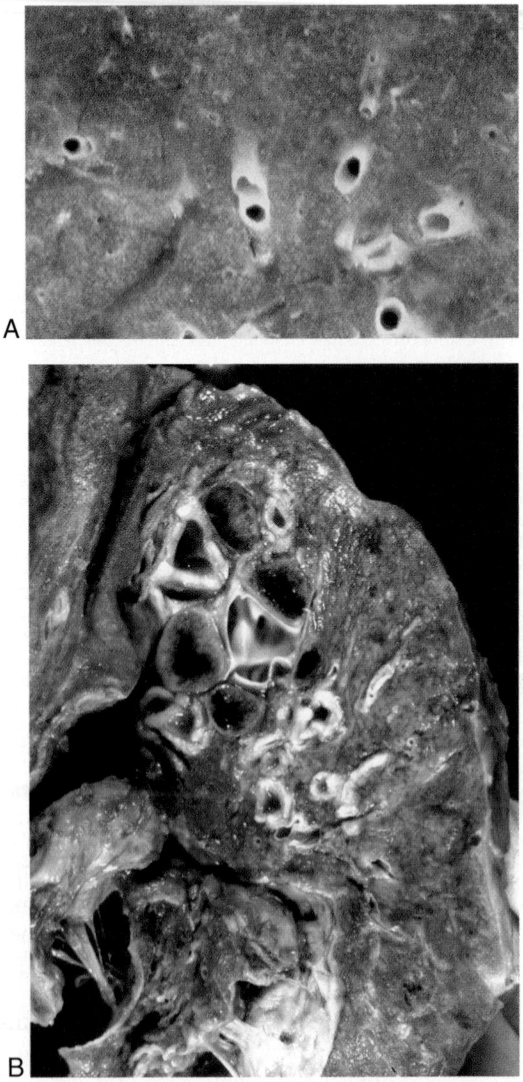

Figure 5-4 Silicosis. (From Cagle PT. *Color atlas and text of pulmonary pathology*. Philadelphia: Lippincott Williams & Wilkins; 2005.)

Breathlessness during exercise and dry cough can be the first symptoms. Other symptoms vary in severity. Further testing is usually recommended to identify the specific type of ILD a person has; some have known causes and some have unknown causes (idiopathic). The course of these diseases is unpredictable.

Some ILDs improve with medication if treated when inflammation occurs. Inflammation of these parts of the lung may heal or may lead to permanent scarring of the lung tissue. Fibrosis results in scarring and permanent loss of that tissue's ability to transport oxygen. The level of disability that a person experiences depends on the amount of scarring of the tissue. Oxygen may be needed; some patients need it all of the time, and others need it only during sleep and exercise.

A pulmonary rehabilitation program is often recommended for education, exercise conditioning, breathing retraining, energy-saving techniques, respiratory therapy, nutritional counseling, and psychosocial support. Lung transplantation has become an option for some patients with advanced-stage ILD (Sulica et al, 2001).

INTERVENTION: OBJECTIVES

- Early identification and aggressive treatment are needed to lessen inflammation and prevent further lung damage.
- Remove the source of the problem, if known.
- Lessen the effect of complications.
- Maintain nutritional immunity as far as possible. Improve poor status.
- Provide nutritional repletion before surgery, if surgery is scheduled.

INTERVENTION: FOOD AND NUTRITION

- If not contraindicated, offer 3–3.5 L fluid daily to liquefy secretions and to help lower temperature.
- A high-calorie, soft diet is recommended, especially if oxygen is used. Frequent, small meals may be beneficial.
- Discuss how to make mealtimes relaxed, especially if oxygen is required at the same time. Plan for longer mealtimes accordingly.
- A multivitamin-mineral supplement may be beneficial, especially for vitamins A, C, and E. Vitamin E reduces the extent of pulmonary damage in some types of ILD (Card et al, 2003).
- Ensure adequate potassium intake, as from fruits and juices.
- When possible, add more fiber to prevent constipation.
- Tube feeding at night may be beneficial if intake is poor during the day.

CLINICAL INDICATORS

Clinical/History		Lab Work
Height, weight	Lung biopsy	pCO_2, pO_2
Growth chart for height and weight	Chest x-ray or CT scan	Chol, Trig
BMI	Pulmonary function test	Na+, K+, Cl−
Diet history	Exercise function test	Alb
Fecal fat study	Clubbing of fingers	H & H
pH	Dry cough	Serum Fe
Bronchoalveolar lavage (BAL)		WBC count
		PT or INR
		Gluc
		Ca++, Mg++

Common Drugs Used and Potential Side Effects

- Oral prednisone or methylprednisone is frequently the first medication used to help decrease inflammation.
- Cyclophosphamide (Cytoxan) may be used if steroid therapy fails or if it is not possible. It reduces inflammation by killing some inflammatory cells and suppressing their function. Response to therapy may require up to 6 months or longer. In some cases, a combination of prednisone and cyclophosphamide is used with good results. Side effects include GI irritation, bladder inflammation, bone marrow suppression, infection, and blood disorders.
- Azathioprine (Imuran) is used if there are problems tolerating the side effects of the above medications. It is not as effective as cyclophosphamide, but side effects are more tolerable. Side effects include fever, skin rash, GI irritation, and blood disorders.

Herbs, Botanicals, and Supplements

- Herbs and botanicals should not be used for ILD because there are no controlled trials to prove efficacy.

INTERVENTION: NUTRITION EDUCATION, COUNSELING, CARE MANAGEMENT

- Discuss how a balanced diet supports overall immunity and health status. Teach principles of the Food Guide Pyramid and the Dietary Guidelines.
- Teach how to incorporate antioxidants and related nutrients in the diet, especially if energy intake is low because of poor appetite.
- Influenza vaccine and pneumococcal pneumonia vaccine are both recommended for people with ILD.
- Rehabilitation and education programs may help some people. Local support groups have benefited people with ILD and their family members and friends.

Patient Education—Foodborne Illness

- Careful food handling will be important. Hand washing is key as well.

For More Information

- Interstitial Lung Disease Program http://www.nationaljewish.org/a4.html

INTERSTITIAL LUNG DISEASE—CITED REFERENCES

Card JW, et al. Attenuation of amiodarone-induced pulmonary fibrosis by vitamin E is associated with suppression of transforming growth factor-beta1 gene expression but not prevention of mitochondrial dysfunction. *J Pharmacol Exp Ther.* 304:277, 2003.

Sulica R, et al. Lung transplantation in interstitial lung disease. *Curr Opin Pulm Med.* 7:314, 2001.

PNEUMONIA

NUTRITIONAL ACUITY RANKING: LEVEL 1–2

DEFINITIONS AND BACKGROUND

Pneumonia involves acute inflammation of the alveolar spaces of the lung. Lung tissue is consolidated as alveoli fill with exudate, usually after a cold or the flu. To protect against pneumonia, dental and oral health care are important. Dental plaque germs may be inhaled and may lead to onset of pneumonia; regular tooth brushing, dental flossing, and dental check-ups are recommended (El-Solh et al, 2004).

Signs and symptoms include difficult, painful respirations, shortness of breath, rales, rhonchi, tachypnea, chills, fever (102–106°F), delirium, anorexia, malaise, abdominal distention, restlessness, cyanosis of nail beds, tachycardia, atelectasis, anxiety, and a productive cough that is painful and incessant (generally with green/yellow sputum that progresses to pink, brown, or rust color).

Pneumonia may be classified as community acquired, hospital acquired, or atypical. The most common form is community-acquired pneumococcal pneumonia (Fig. 5-5). Table 5-10 describes the common types of pneumonia. With treatment, most types of bacterial pneumonia can be cured within 1–2 weeks; viral pneumonia may last longer. Mycoplasmal pneumonia resolves in 4–6 weeks.

Before antibiotics, pneumonia caused many deaths in elderly individuals; it now ranks sixth among causes of death in the United States. In 2002, there were over 60,000 deaths related to pneumonia in the United States (Centers for Disease Control and Prevention [CDC], 2005).

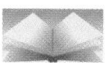

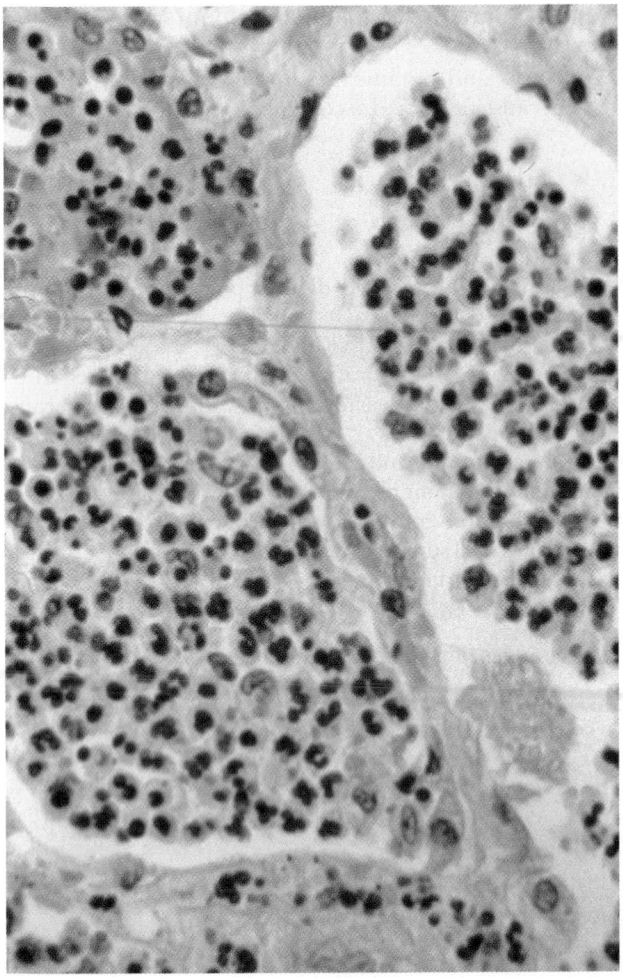

Figure 5-5 Pneumococcal pneumonia. (Image from Rubin E, Farber JL. *Pathology*. 3rd ed. Philadelphia: Lippincott Williams & Wilkins; 1999.)

People at high risk for pneumonia include the elderly; the very young; those with COPD, diabetes mellitus, congestive heart failure, sickle cell anemia, AIDS, or asthma; and people undergoing cancer therapy or organ tranplantation. Nursing home residents have chronic medical conditions that gradually lead to "decompensation" in functional status, nutritional status, and pulmonary clearance; dysphagia and aspiration are common complications, and prevention is essential (Langmore et al, 2002).

Elderly patients with low body weight and hypoalbuminemia are more likely to die from pneumonia than healthy patients. Inflammation may cause low serum albumin levels in many pneumonia patients. Since glutathione is the primary antioxidant that lines alveolar space, higher antioxidant intake may be needed at this time (Hu and Cassano, 2000). Selenium and vitamins E and C may be beneficial. However, supplementation alone will not prevent pneumonia in well-nourished older individuals (Merchant et al, 2004).

Enteral feeding provides nutrients for patients who require endotracheal tubes and mechanical ventilation. There is a presumed increase in the risk of ventilator-associated pneumonia (VAP) with tube feeding, but this is not always true (Kearns et al, 2000). There is no significant difference between the incidence of pneumonia and other parameters such as intensive care length of stay or mortality and placement into the stomach or postpyloric placement (Marek and Zaloga, 2003).

Pneumonia due to immune system suppression and membrane damage induced by oxidative stress suggest that sufficient fatty acid intake may be useful in the nutritional repletion of such patients with pneumonia. The American Dietetic Association previously recommended 3 medical nutrition therapy visits for persons who have pneumonia.

TABLE 5-10 **Types of Pneumonia**

Type	Description
Allergic	From sensitivity to dust or pollen.
Aspiration	From swallowing a foreign substance. The gastric volume predisposing to aspiration is larger than 30 mL (Kalinowski and Kirsch, 2004). It is now standard practice to shorten the time to a few hours with "nothing by mouth" to prepare for surgery because risk of aspiration is lower than previously believed (Brady et al, 2003).
	Ventilator-associated pneumonia (VAP), a common and serious complication in critically ill patients who require a ventilator, results from pneumonia occurring >48 hours after endotracheal intubation (Parker and Heyland, 2004). It is caused by microaspiration of contaminated oropharyngeal or gastrointestinal secretions into the airways (Parker and Heyland, 2004).
Bacterial	From bacteria normally present in mouth/throat. Quick onset with high fever and rapid breathing. Several bacteria may be relevant. *Streptococcus pneumoniae* causes about 25% of bacterial types. *Mycoplasma* causes walking pneumonia, notorious for sore throat and headache in addition to the usual symptoms; causes about 20% of all kinds of pneumonia. When pneumonia is due to pertussis (whooping cough), long coughing spells, turning blue from lack of air, and making a classic "whoop" sound when trying to take a breath will occur. *Haemophilus influenzae* type b (Hib) is America's most common cause of bacterial meningitis; it is also an agent of pneumonia.
Chemical	From accidental inhalation of toxic fumes and chemicals, often in the workplace or when using cleaning agents such as bleach in a closed space.
Hypostatic	In bedridden persons, usually elderly individuals.
Pneumocystis carinii pneumonia (PCP)	Caused by a fungus, primarily in AIDS patients.
Viral	More common; leads to about 50% of pneumonia cases. Symptoms appear more gradually; less severe than bacterial form. Wheezing is common in this type. Adenoviral infections often affect infants and young children. Other viruses that can cause pneumonia include rhinovirus, influenza, respiratory syncytial virus (RSV), and parainfluenza virus (croup).

INTERVENTION: OBJECTIVES

- Prevent or correct dehydration.
- Relieve breathing difficulty and discomfort. Oxygenate all tissues.
- Prevent weight loss from hypermetabolic state.
- Support diet with adequate antioxidants and nutrient-dense foods.
- Avoid additional infections; prevent sepsis and multiple organ dysfunction syndrome.
- In convalescent stage, avoid constipation.

INTERVENTION: FOOD AND NUTRITION

- If not contraindicated, offer 3 L or more of fluid daily to liquefy secretions and to help lower elevated temperature.
- Progress, as tolerated, to a high-calorie diet. If overweight, allow normal calorie intake for age and sex.
- Early enteral nutrition, properly administered, can decrease upper GI intolerance and nosocomial pneumonia (Kompan et al, 2004).
- Frequent, small meals and soft diet may be tolerated better.
- A multivitamin-mineral supplement may be beneficial, especially including selenium and vitamins E and C. Vitamin A is needed to keep mucous membranes healthy.
- When possible, add more fiber to prevent constipation.
- Ensure adequate potassium intake, as from fruits and juices.

CLINICAL INDICATORS

Clinical/History		Lab Work
Height	Respiratory rate (increase)	WBCs (increase)
Weight	I & O	pCO_2, pO_2
BMI	BP	Na+, K+
Diet history	Modified barium swallow study (MBSS) for evaluation of aspiration risk	Ca++, Mg++
Temperature (fever, chills)		Alb, transthyretin
Pleuritic pain		CRP
Bronchoscopy		RBP
Productive cough (purulent, green, or rust)		H & H
		Serum Fe
		Transferrin
		Gluc
		BUN, Creat

Common Drugs Used and Potential Side Effects

- A 7-day course of low-dose hydrocortisone infusion speeds recovery from community-acquired pneumonia and prevents complications due to sepsis (Confalonieri et al, 2005).
- Antibiotics, such as clarithromycin (Biaxin), are used in bacterial pneumonia. Nausea, diarrhea, and abdominal pain can occur.
- Telithromycin (Ketek) is used for the treatment of infections caused by bronchitis, bacterial sinusitis, and community-acquired pneumonia.
- Analgesics are used to reduce pain.
- Antipyretics are used to lower fever.
- Cephalosporins are often useful for nursing home–acquired pneumonia (Muder et al, 2004).

Herbs, Botanicals, and Supplements

- No clinical trials have proven efficacy for use of herbs or botanicals, such as echinacea, honeysuckle, garlic, dandelion, astragalus, and baikal skullcap in pneumonia patients.

INTERVENTION: NUTRITION EDUCATION, COUNSELING, CARE MANAGEMENT

- Discuss the role of diet and fluid intake in recovery.
- In hypostatic pneumonia, suggest greater levels of activity (within restraints of complicating disorders).
- Fruit and vegetable juices add calories, fluid, and sometimes fiber to the diet and can be available at bedside.
- Routine immunizations are available against *Haemophilus influenzae* and pertussis beginning at 2 months of age pertussis immunization is the "P" part of the routine DtaP or DTP.
- Vaccines are now also given against the pneumococcus organism (PCV), a common cause of bacterial pneumonia.
- Flu vaccines are recommended for individuals with chronic illnesses such as heart and lung disorders, including asthma. Premature infants may need protection against respiratory syncytial virus (RSV). Individuals who have HIV infection may need protection against *Pneumocystis carinii.*
- Protect people who have pneumonia from others who have respiratory tract infections, such as the common cold.
- For presurgical patients, there is a shortened fluid fasting requirement to prevent aspiration pneumonia; drinking water preoperatively results in significantly lower gastric volumes, which is actually desirable (Brady et al, 2003).

Patient Education—Foodborne Illness

- Careful food handling will be important.
- Hand washing is key as well, especially after sneezing and coughing and before eating.

For More Information

- American Lung Association–Pneumonia
  http://www.lungusa.org/diseases/lungpneumoni.html
- KidsHealth
  http://kidshealth.org/kid/ill_injure/sick/pneumonia.html

PNEUMONIA—CITED REFERENCES

Brady M, et al. Preoperative fasting for adults to prevent perioperative complications. *Cochrane Database Syst Rev.* 4:CD004423, 2003.

Centers for Disease Control and Prevention. Pneumonia. Accessed February 1, 2005 at http://www.cdc.gov/nchs/fastats/pneumonia.htm.

Confalonieri M, et al. Hydrocortisone infusion for severe community-acquired pneumonia: a preliminary randomized study. *Am J Respir Crit Care Med.* 171:242, 2005.
El-Solh AA, et al. Colonization of dental plaques: a reservoir of respiratory pathogens for hospital-acquired pneumonia in institutionalized elders. *Chest* 126:1575, 2004.
Hu G, Cassano P. Antioxidant nutrients and pulmonary function: the Third National Health and Nutrition Examination Survey. *Am J Epidemiol.* 151:975, 2000.
Kalinowski CP, Kirsch JR. Strategies for prophylaxis and treatment for aspiration. *Best Pract Res Clin Anaesthesiol.* 18:719, 2004.
Kearns P, et al. The incidence of ventilator-associated pneumonia and success in nutrient delivery with gastric versus small intestinal feeding: a randomized clinical trial. *Crit Care Med.* 28:1742, 2000.
Kompan L, et al. Is early enteral nutrition a risk factor for gastric intolerance and pneumonia? *Clin Nutr.* 23:527, 2004.
Langmore SE, et al. Predictors of aspiration pneumonia in nursing home residents. *Dysphagia* 17:298, 2002.
Marek PE, Zaloga GP. Gastric versus post-pyloric feeding: a systematic review. *Crit Care.* 7:46, 2003.
Merchant AT, et al. Vitamin intake is not associated with community-acquired pneumonia in U.S. men. *J Nutr.* 134:439, 2004.
Muder RR, et al. Nursing home-acquired pneumonia: an emergency department treatment algorithm. *Curr Med Res Opin.* 20:1309, 2004.
Parker CM, Heyland DK. Aspiration and the risk of ventilator-associated pneumonia. *Nutr Clin Pract.* 19:597, 2004.

PULMONARY EMBOLISM

NUTRITIONAL ACUITY RANKING: LEVEL 1–2

DEFINITIONS AND BACKGROUND

A pulmonary embolism is caused by a partial or complete occlusion of a pulmonary artery from a blood clot from another part of the body that has found its way to the lung. The condition can be life threatening; it is one of the primary concerns during pregnancy (Stone and Morris, 2005).

Sudden, sharp substernal pain, shortness of breath (SOB), cyanosis, pallor, faintness, fever, hypotension, and wheezing can occur, sometimes followed by right heart failure. See Figure 5-6. Approximately 10% of patients suffer some form of tissue death or pulmonary infarction. Hormone replacement therapy (HRT) is no longer recommended for women after menopause because of the risks of cardiovascular disease (CVD), stroke, pulmonary embolism, and breast cancer (Hillman et al, 2004).

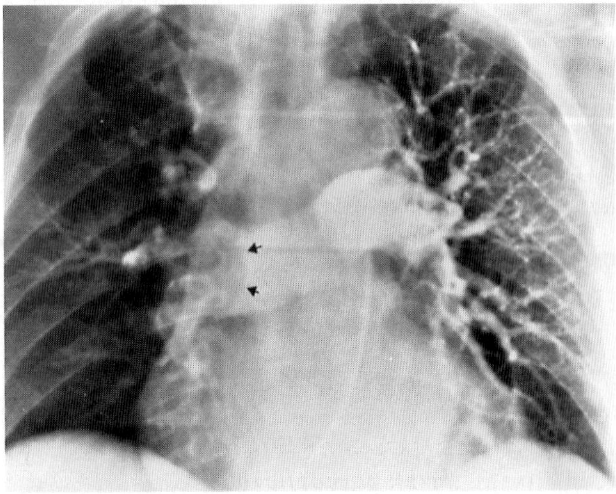

Figure 5-6 Pulmonary embolus. (From Eisenberg RL. *Clinical imaging: an atlas of differential diagnosis.* 4th ed. Philadelphia: Lippincott Williams & Wilkins; 2003.)

INTERVENTION: OBJECTIVES

- Prevent right-sided heart failure, atelectasis, and bleeding.
- Maintain lung function, which is found to be better with higher antioxidant levels (Hu and Cassano, 2000).
- Normalize body temperature if there is fever.
- Replenish nutrients depleted by respiratory distress.
- Stabilize prothrombin time if warfarin (Coumadin) is used.
- Eliminate edema when present.
- Prepare for possible surgery (embolectomy).

INTERVENTION: FOOD AND NUTRITION

- Use a regular or high-calorie diet; use a low-sodium diet for patients with edema.
- Increase fluid intake as tolerated.
- Control vitamin K in diet if prothrombin time is not stabilized.
- Small meals may be needed.
- Provide sufficient antioxidants such as vitamins C and E and selenium.

Common Drugs Used and Potential Side Effects

- Anticoagulants: Warfarin (Coumadin) increases clotting times by thinning the blood. If problems in stabilizing the prothrombin time exist, the diet may need to be controlled concerning vitamin K. Use low to moderate amounts of green leafy vegetables and fish.

CLINICAL INDICATORS

Clinical/History		
Height	Perfusion scans	pCO_2, pO_2
Weight	Pulmonary catheter angiography	PT or INR
BMI	Pulse (NL = 60–100 beats/min)	Lactate dehydrogenase (LDH) (increased)
Diet history	**Lab Work**	WBCs (increased)
Edema	Alb, transthyretin	Bilirubin (increased)
Temperature (fever)	Na+, K+	H & H
I & O	Ca++, Mg++	Serum Fe
Chest x-ray		CRP
ECG		
Echocardiography		

- Antibiotics, cardiotonic drugs, diuretics, or antiarrhythmics may be used.

Herbs, Botanicals, and Supplements

- No clinical trials have proven efficacy for use of herbs or botanicals in pulmonary embolism.

INTERVENTION: NUTRITION EDUCATION, COUNSELING, CARE MANAGEMENT

- Explain sources of vitamin K in the diet. Therapy often continues for 3–6 months.
- Discuss relaxation techniques, especially related to mealtimes.

Patient Education—Foodborne Illness

- Careful food handling will be important. Hand washing is key as well.

For More Information

- E-medicine
  http://www.emedicine.com/EMERG/topic490.htm

PULMONARY EMBOLISM—CITED REFERENCES

Hillman JJ, et al. The impact of the Women's Health Initiative on hormone replacement therapy in a Medicaid program. *J Womens Health (Larchmt).* 13:986, 2004.

Hu G, Cassano P. Antioxidant nutrients and pulmonary function: the Third National Health and Nutrition Examination Survey. *Am J Epidemiol.* 151:975, 2000.

Stone SE, Morris TA. Pulmonary embolism during and after pregnancy. *Crit Care Med.* 33:294S, 2005.

RESPIRATORY DISTRESS SYNDROME

NUTRITIONAL ACUITY RANKING: LEVEL 3–4

DEFINITIONS AND BACKGROUND

Acute respiratory distress syndrome (ARDS) is a secondary lung state that develops within 24–48 hours in patients who have sepsis or who are critically ill, in shock, or severely injured. Other causes include pneumonia, aspiration of food into the lung, several blood transfusions, pulmonary embolism, chest injury, burns, near drowning, cardiopulmonary bypass surgery, pancreatitis, and overdose of drugs such as heroin, methadone, and aspirin.

Patients often have pulmonary edema but have normal left atrial and pulmonary venous pressures. **Respiratory distress syndrome (RDS)** may occur as part of systematic inflammatory response syndrome (SIRS), affecting approximately 70% of patients in the intensive care unit.

In infants, RDS often occurs in low birth weight babies, and the condition may be called **hyaline membrane disease**. Such babies are often born to mothers who have diabetes.

Indirect calorimetry (IC) accurately estimates a patient's energy expenditure, particularly the complex critically ill patient who benefits most from nutritional support; this bedside technique measures variables related to gas exchange and replaces assumptions about physiological stress (McCarthy, 2000). Data are valuable to the health care team when trying to identify reasons for weaning failure.

In sepsis-induced ARDS, a low-carbohydrate, high-fat diet combining the anti-inflammatory and vasodilatory properties of eicosapentaenoic acid (fish oil), gamma linolenic acid (GLA; borage oil), and antioxidants improves lung microvascular permeability, oxygenation, and cardiopulmonary function and reduces proinflammatory eicosanoid synthesis and lung inflammation (Gadek et al, 1999). Specialized enteral formulas may be beneficial adjunctive therapy by reducing lung inflammation and improving oxygenation (Priestley and Helfaer, 2004). Finally, surfactant treatment may be of significant benefit in newborn infants with respiratory compromise secondary to a number of insults (Finer, 2004).

INTERVENTION: OBJECTIVES

- Identify the cause and remove the ongoing insult. Promote rapid recovery and oxygenation of tissues; support ventilator management.
- Prevent relapse. Avoid secondary insults through aggressive immune surveillance, complete nutrition, and adequate oxygen delivery.

- Counteract side effects of medications as ordered.
- Replace essential fatty acids, carnitine, and other nutrients.
- Prevent malnutrition. CNS output for ventilatory drive may be depressed. Starvation decreases desire to breathe, causing abnormal breathing pattern, pneumonia, and atelectasis. Muscle mass (including diaphragm) varies with body weight, and refeeding may take 2–3 weeks.
- Prevent overfeeding (hepatic dysfunction, fatty liver, and CO_2 overproduction) and underfeeding (morbidity, mortality, and decreased response to therapy). Avoid refeeding syndrome.
- Prevent fluid overload.
- Support lung function, which is found to be better with higher antioxidant intake levels (Singer et al, 2006; Hu and Cassano, 2000).

INTERVENTION: FOOD AND NUTRITION

- Provide parenteral fluids as ordered. Progress, when possible, to oral feedings. Use TPN only if GI tract is nonfunctional.
- For calories, use 30–35 kcal/kg. Nonprotein calories should come from 50% glucose and 50% lipid.
- Increased fat may be required to normalize the respiratory quotient (RQ). Fat also adds extra energy intake and palatability to the diet.
- Ensure adequate provision of EFA. Low linoleic acid status in critically ill RDS infants may require IVs with a fat emulsion added.
- Increase intake of omega-3 fatty acids, especially EPA and GLA (Singer et al, 2006). Include antioxidants, such as vitamins C and E and selenium, at slightly higher than RDA levels and fat-soluble vitamins in appropriate forms (water-miscible if necessary).
- Inositol supplementation promotes survival of premature infants with RDS (Howlett and Ohlsson, 2003).
- Be careful with TPN-induced changes in CO_2 production. Do not overfeed.

CLINICAL INDICATORS

Clinical/History	I & O	pCO_2, pO_2
Height	BP	Complete blood count (CBC)
Weight	Temperature	Transthyretin
BMI	Respiratory quotient (RQ)	Na+, K+
Growth profile	**Lab Work**	Ca++, Mg++
Diet history	H & H	Serum phosphorus
Indirect calorimetry (IC)	Serum Fe	BUN, Creat
	Transferrin	

Common Drugs Used and Potential Side Effects

- Heparin or warfarin (Coumadin) may be used as a blood thinner.
- Ventilator-dependent surgical patients receiving oxandrolone have prolonged courses of mechanical ventilation; oxandrolone may enhance collagen deposition and fibrosis in the later stages of ARDS and thus delay recovery (Bulger et al, 2004).

Herbs, Botanicals, and Supplements

- No clinical trials have proven efficacy for use of herbs or botanicals in ARDS or RDS.

INTERVENTION: NUTRITION EDUCATION, COUNSELING, CARE MANAGEMENT

- Discuss the role of fat intake on respiratory requirements. Fat decreases CO_2 production.
- Small, frequent feedings may be beneficial.

Patient Education—Foodborne Illness

- Careful food handling will be important. Hand washing is key as well.

For More Information

- Acute Respiratory Distress Clinical Network http://hedwig.mgh.harvard.edu/ardsnet/
- Respiratory Distress Syndrome http://www.nhlbi.nih.gov/health/dci/Diseases/Ards/Ards_WhatIs.html

RESPIRATORY DISTRESS SYNDROME—CITED REFERENCES

Bulger EM, et al. Oxandrolone does not improve outcome of ventilator dependent surgical patients. *Ann Surg.* 240:472, 2004.

Finer NN. Surfactant use for neonatal lung injury: beyond respiratory distress syndrome. *Paediatr Respir Rev.* 5:S289, 2004.

Gadek J, et al. Effect of enteral feeding with eicosapentaenoic acid, gamma-linolenic acid, and antioxidants in patients with acute respiratory distress syndrome. Enteral Nutrition in ARDS Study Group. *Crit Care Med.* 27:1409, 1999.

Howlette A, Ohlsson A. Inositol for respiratory distress syndrome in preterm infants. *Cochrane Database Syst Rev.* 4:CD000366, 2003.

Hu G, Cassano P. Antioxidant nutrients and pulmonary function: the Third National Health and Nutrition Examination Survey. *Am J Epidemiol.* 151:975, 2000.

McCarthy M. Use of indirect calorimetry to optimize nutrition support and assess physiologic dead space in the mechanically ventilated ICU patient: a case study approach. *AACN Clin Issues.* 11:619, 2000.

Priestley MA, Helfaer MA. Approaches in the management of acute respiratory failure in children. *Curr Opin Pediatr.* 16:293, 2004.

Singer P, et al. Benefit of an enteral diet enriched with eicosapentaenoic acid and gamma-linolenic acid in ventilated patients with acute lung injury. *Crit Care Med.* 34:1033, 2006.

RESPIRATORY FAILURE AND VENTILATOR DEPENDENCY

NUTRITIONAL ACUITY RANKING: LEVEL 4

DEFINITIONS AND BACKGROUND

Respiratory failure involves ineffective gas exchange across the lungs by the respiratory system; arterial blood gas should be used to determine the presence of respiratory failure. Acute respiratory failure (ARF) involves sudden absence of respirations, with confusion or unresponsiveness and failure of pulmonary gas exchange mechanism. Chronic pulmonary disease or an acute injury can cause acute pulmonary failure, which requires mechanical ventilation. Table 5-11 lists common causes of respiratory failure.

Anabolic and catabolic hormones, muscle work, and nutritional status affect skeletal muscle mass and muscle strength. Substrate and muscle work stimulate protein synthesis. Forced vital capacity (FVC) is used to measure ventilatory function; percentage of body fat and fat-free mass can be estimated from skinfold thicknesses. Handgrip strength is positively related to adjusted FVC (Lazarus et al, 1998).

Hypermetabolic patients often have at least a 30% increase in oxygen use. In starvation, respiratory muscles are catabolized to meet energy needs; refeeding helps ventilatory response. Lung function is found to be better with higher antioxidant levels (Hu and Cassano, 2000); use of intravenous fat emulsions may help reduce inflammation.

Daily screening of patients requiring mechanical ventilation, followed by trials of spontaneous breathing, can reduce duration, costs, and complications (Ely et al, 2002). Weaning from a ventilator takes a few days and requires proper refeeding. Table 5-12 identifies ventilator-dependency feeding stages.

The length of ventilator dependency significantly positively correlates with energy and carbohydrate intake (Huang et al, 2000). Indirect calorimetry is confounded by both the presence of oxygen and mechanical ventilation (Branson and Johannigman, 2004).

The use of aggressive immune surveillance, nutritional support, and fluid management is critical to support ventilator management for oxygenation and ventilation (Michaels, 2004). Enteral feedings started within 3 days can reduce length of time on a ventilator and improve outcomes for critically ill patients (Healthcare Benchmarks, 1998). Use of an evidence-based nutrition support protocol improves the likelihood of meeting nutritional requirements (Mackenzie et al, 2005).

Older patients may be harder to wean from the ventilator and are more at risk for having respiratory failure (Sevransky and Haponik, 2003; Ely et al, 2002). Attention must be paid to reversible factors such as electrolytes, infections, anemia, heart failure, and medications; hypothyroidism is another problem (Datta and Scalise, 2004).

High-frequency oscillatory ventilation, airway pressure release ventilation, and partial liquid ventilation are potential protective ventilatory modes for children with ARDS.

TABLE 5-11 Causes of Respiratory Failure

Symptom	Cause
Airway obstruction	Chronic bronchitis, emphysema, bronchiectasis, cystic fibrosis, asthma, bronchiolitis, inhaled particles, subglottic stenosis, tumor, laryngeal edema
Poor breathing	Obesity, sleep apnea, drug intoxication, trauma, hypothyroidism
Neuromuscular disease	Myasthenia gravis, muscular dystrophy, polio, Guillain-Barré syndrome, botulism, polymyositis, stroke, amyotrophic lateral sclerosis, spinal cord injury
Abnormality of lung tissue	Acute respiratory distress, drug reaction, pulmonary fibrosis, fibrosing alveolitis, widespread tumors, radiation therapy, sarcoidosis, burns
Abnormality of chest wall	Kyphoscoliosis, chest wound

TABLE 5-12 Ventilatory-Dependency Feeding Stages

Stage	Action
Acute repletion	Replenish muscle glycogen stores and reverse catabolism.
Preweaning	Maintain positive nitrogen balance, improve visceral protein stores, improve creatinine-height index (CHI), and promote weight gain.
Weaning	Provide energy substrates to cover needs of respiratory muscles that are working harder; minimize CO_2 production. Be careful not to overfeed, which may impair weaning.
Postweaning	Maintain nutrient needs despite anorexia or dysphagia; support anabolism.

Sources: Burns et al, 2000; Irwin and Openbrier, 1985.

INTERVENTION: OBJECTIVES

- Promote normalized nutritional intake despite hypermetabolic status of the patient and the prohibition of oral intake due to endotracheal tubes.
- Oxygenate tissues and relieve breathlessness; decrease CO_2 production.
- Monitor sensations of hunger because patients are unable to communicate their hunger and thirst.
- Prevent respiratory muscle dysfunction by ensuring that the patient is properly nourished. Achieve or maintain weight; not all patients are malnourished.
- Counteract hypotension caused by positive-pressure ventilation, acidosis, or both.
- Provide nutritional substrates that will not greatly increase CO_2 production while maintaining surfactant production and keeping lean body mass (LBM).
- Prevent atelectasis, pulmonary infection, sepsis, glucose or lipid intolerance, multiple organ dysfunction syndrome, and aspiration.

- Protocol-driven weaning reduces use of mechanical ventilation (Dries et al, 2004). Adjust goals as appropriate. Maintain flexible approaches to patient requirements.
- Alleviate GI complications, which are a concern with mechanical ventilation; hypomotility and diarrhea are common. Correct electrolyte abnormalities and avoid medications that impair GI motility (Mutlu et al, 2003).

INTERVENTION: FOOD AND NUTRITION

- Begin nourishing the patient as soon as possible to wean the patient from the ventilator. Start any tube feeding slowly to avoid gastric retention or diarrhea. Some institutions add blue food coloring to feedings to detect problems in tracheal secretions, but this is not recommended. Advance gradually and use continuous administrations unless contraindicated. Tube feedings of low osmolality are needed.
- A diet with 35–50% CHO and 30–50% lipid (high omega-3 fatty acids) is common. Adults need a daily diet of at least 25–35 kcal/kg. Increases from labored breathing will occur; monitor using indirect calorimetry when possible. For some cases, use of specialty products such as Pulmocare or Respalor may be recommended, but they are not always necessary.
- Protein needs may be as high as 1.5–2 g/kg.
- Essential fatty acids are important; 2% of total fat will be required.
- Monitor TPN carefully for complications such as pneumonia, refeeding syndrome from high-calorie loading, and increased CO_2 production.
- Patients with pulmonary edema should have their sodium intake reduced as needed. Include adequate protein in the diet to prevent additional fluid retention because of lowered colloidal osmotic pressure.
- Supplement diet with multivitamins, especially vitamins A and C.
- Phosphorus and magnesium may be needed if stores are depleted.

CLINICAL INDICATORS

Clinical/History	Lab Work	
Height	Gluc	WBC (elevated)
Weight	Urinary Gluc	Chol, Trig
BMI	Transthyretin (decreased)	Transferrin
Resting energy expenditure (REE) from IC	TLC (decreased)	Thyroid tests
Diet history	H & H	CRP
I & O	Serum Fe	Serum phosphorus (decrease can cause acute respiratory failure)
Respiratory rate	Na+, K+	pH (acidemia below 7.4, alkalemia above 7.4)
RQ	Ca++, Mg++	
BP		
Temperature (fever is common)		

Common Drugs Used and Potential Side Effects

- Bronchodilators and corticosteroids may be needed. Monitor side effects related to potassium, etc.
- Antibiotics are often required; monitor specific side effects.
- For diarrhea, treatment depends on the cause. For *Clostridium difficile* infection, antibacterial therapy should be discontinued, if possible, and treatment with oral metronidazole should be initiated (Mutlu et al, 2003).

Herbs, Botanicals, and Supplements

- No clinical trials have proven efficacy for use of herbs or botanicals in respiratory failure.

INTERVENTION: NUTRITION EDUCATION, COUNSELING, CARE MANAGEMENT

- A daily calorie count may be needed to assess the patient's nutritional status.
- The greatest danger in using enteral nutrition is aspiration. Low-osmolarity products are essential, as well as elevation of the head of the bed.
- Discuss early satiety, bloating, fatigue, dyspnea, and so on, as related to food or tube feeding (TF) intake.
- Pressure preset bilevel ventilators are now the dominant form of ventilator; discharge planning is vital for the home ventilator patient (Simonds, 2003).

Patient Education—Foodborne Illness

- Careful food handling will be important. Hand washing is key as well.

For More Information

- Merck Manual–Respiratory Failure
  http://www.merck.com/mmhe/sec04/ch055/ch055a.html
- Respiratory Failure
  http://www.med-help.net/AcuteRespiratoryFailure.html

RESPIRATORY FAILURE AND VENTILATOR DEPENDENCY—CITED REFERENCES

Branson RD, Johannigman JA. The measurement of energy expenditure. *Nutr Clin Pract.* 19:622, 2004.

Burns S, et al. The weaning continuum use of Acute Physiology and Chronic Health Evaluation III, Burns Wean Assessment Program, Therapeutic Intervention Scoring System, and Wean Index scores to establish stages of weaning. *Crit Care Med.* 28:2259, 2000.

Datta D, Scalise P. Hypothyroidism and failure to wean in patients receiving prolonged mechanical ventilation at a regional weaning center. *Chest* 126:1307, 2004.

Dries DJ, et al. Protocol-driven ventilator weaning reduces use of mechanical ventilation, rate of early reintubation, and ventilator-associated pneumonia. *J Trauma.* 56:943, 2004.

Ely E, et al. Recovery rate and prognosis in older persons who develop acute lung injury and the acute respiratory distress syndrome. *Ann Intern Med.* 136:25, 2002.

Healthcare Benchmarks. Nutrition intervention in ICU improves outcomes. *Healthc Benchmarks.* 5:175, 1998.

Hu G, Cassano P. Antioxidant nutrients and pulmonary function: the Third National Health and Nutrition Examination Survey. *Am J Epidemiol.* 151:975, 2000.
Huang Y, et al. Nutritional status of mechanically ventilated critically ill patients: comparison of different types of nutritional support. *Clin Nutr.* 19:101, 2000.
Irwin M, Openbrier D. A delicate balance—strategies for feeding ventilated COPD patients. *Am J Nurs.* 85:274, 1985.
Lazarus R, et al. Effects of body composition and fat distribution on ventilatory function in adults. *Am J Clin Nutr.* 68:35, 1998.
Mackenzie SL, et al. Implementation of a nutrition support protocol increases the proportion of mechanically ventilated patients reaching enteral nutrition targets in the adult intensive care unit. *JPEN J Parenter Enteral Nutr.* 29(2):74, 2005.
Michaels AJ. Management of post traumatic respiratory failure. *Crit Care Clin.* 20:83, 2004.
Mutlu GM, et al. Prevention and treatment of gastrointestinal complications in patients on mechanical ventilation. *Am J Respir Med.* 2:395, 2003.
Priestley MA, Helfaer MA. Approaches in the management of acute respiratory failure in children. *Curr Opin Pediatr.* 16:293, 2004.
Sevransky JE, Haponik EF. Respiratory failure in elderly patients. *Clin Geriatr Med.* 19:205, 2003.
Simonds AK. Home ventilation. *Eur Respir J.* 47:38S, 2003 (suppl).

SARCOIDOSIS

NUTRITIONAL ACUITY RANKING: LEVEL 1–2

DEFINITIONS AND BACKGROUND

Sarcoidosis is a disease of undetermined origin (Alliot, 2000); it is a rare disease in which tiny patches of inflammation (granulomas) occur in almost any organ. Etiology is unknown. Pulmonary effects are most common. It develops most often between ages 20–40 years, more often among women than men, and more commonly among Swedes, Danes, and African Americans. Sarcoidosis is more common among nonsmokers than smokers.

Symptoms and signs may include weight loss, fever, anorexia, weakness, aching joints, abdominal pain, lymphadenopathy, bone cysts in hands and feet, pulmonary hypertension, cor pulmonale, clubbing of fingers, dyspnea, cough, hypoxemia, iritis, glaucoma, blindness, chest pain, shortness of breath, and heart failure. There is a correlation between 1-alpha-hydroxylase gene expression in alveolar macrophages and the activity of sarcoidosis and its associated disturbances in calcium metabolism (Inui et al, 2001).

In children, renal impairment of sarcoidosis usually is caused by either hypercalcemia leading to nephrocalcinosis or interstitial nephritis with or without granulomata (Thumfart et al, 2005). Overall, prognosis is good for most cases, and most sarcoidosis subsides on its own. In 10% of cases, the condition becomes chronic.

INTERVENTION: OBJECTIVES

- Reduce heart failure, bronchiectasis, and related problems.
- Correct weight loss, anorexia, fever, and abdominal pain.
- Improve ability to breathe and eat normally.
- Prevent further deterioration of organ functions with any and all affected organ systems.
- Prevent or correct fluid retention.
- High levels of calcium may accumulate in the blood and urine; control accordingly for related nausea, anorexia, vomiting, thirst, excessive urination, and potential renal failure.

INTERVENTION: FOOD AND NUTRITION

- Restrict salt if necessary for congestive heart failure or for use of corticosteroids. A 2- to 3-g sodium diet may be beneficial.
- Use a diet containing adequate to high potassium (unless medications are used).
- As needed, decrease calcium and vitamin D if bone involvement is suggested; monitor use of supplements accordingly.

CLINICAL INDICATORS

Clinical/History	Lab Work	
Height Weight BMI Diet history BP Chest x-ray Biopsy Gallium scan Tender red lumps, usually on the shins Uveitis TB test to rule out tuberculosis Pulmonary function tests	H & H (anemia common) Serum Fe Alb (decrease common) CRP Alkaline phosphatase (Alk phos) Nitrogen (N) balance Transferrin Globulin (increase common) Serum Ca++ (increased)	Ca++ in urine (increased) Serum level of 1,α-25 vitamin D Na+, K+ Mg++ Uric acid (increased) PO_4 Kveim test Erythrocyte sedimentation rate (ESR)

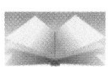

Common Drugs Used and Potential Side Effects

- Glucocorticoids or corticosteroids may be used to suppress severe symptoms such as shortness of breath. Need to watch electrolytes, nitrogen balance, and other changes. Treatment may require several years.
- Isoniazid (INH) may be ordered for pulmonary status. Watch use of vitamin B_6; increase intake accordingly of foods high in vitamin B_6 to prevent neuritis.
- Calcium-chelating agents may be used if hypercalcemia persists.
- Sarcoid granulomatous interstitial nephritis may respond to infliximab therapy (Thumfart et al, 2005). The drug seems to work against tumor necrosis factor (TNF), which may be elevated.

Herbs, Botanicals, and Supplements

- No clinical trials have proven efficacy for use of herbs or botanicals in sarcoidosis.

INTERVENTION: NUTRITION EDUCATION, COUNSELING, CARE MANAGEMENT

- If the patient is using steroids, antacids could also be taken to reduce GI side effects. Check with the doctor.
- Discuss the role of diet in maintaining immunocompetence and in improving tolerance for other therapies.
- Follow closely on the low-calcium intake; avoid vitamin D supplements and exposure to sunlight to avoid hypercalcemia and hypercalciuria.

Patient Education—Foodborne Illness

- Careful food handling will be important. Hand washing is key as well.

For More Information

- National Heart, Lung, and Blood Institute–Sarcoidosis
  http://www.nhlbi.nih.gov/health/public/lung/other/sarcoidosis/index.htm
- National Sarcoidosis Resources Center
  http://www.nsrc-global.net/
- Sarcoidosis Center
  http://www.sarcoidcenter.com/
- Sarcoidosis Family Aid and Research Foundation Hotline
  Phone: 800-223-6429
  http://www.medicinenet.com/sarcoidosis/page10.htm
- Sarcoidosis Research Institute
  http://www.sarcoidcenter.com/sricontents.htm

SARCOIDOSIS—CITED REFERENCES

Alliot C, et al. Neurosarcoidosis associated with Hodgkin's disease; malignancy. *Hematology* 5:285, 2000.

Inui N, et al. Correlation between 25-hydroxyvitamin D3 1-alpha-hydroxylase gene expression in alveolar macrophages and the activity of sarcoidosis. *Am J Med.* 110:687, 2001.

Thumfart J, et al. Isolated sarcoid granulomatous interstitial nephritis responding to infliximab therapy. *Am J Kidney Dis.* 45:411, 2005.

SLEEP APNEA

NUTRITIONAL ACUITY RANKING: LEVEL 2–3

DEFINITIONS AND BACKGROUND

Approximately 4% of middle-aged men and 2% of middle-aged women suffer from obstructive sleep apnea (OSA). OSA affects 12–18 million Americans and is associated with irritability, excessive daytime sleepiness, an inability to concentrate, depression, morning headaches, and decreased job performance in adults. Untreated sleep apnea also can increase an individual's risk of heart attack, high blood pressure, diabetes, stroke, and automobile accidents. OSA is often undiagnosed. A growing body of evidence suggests that OSA is a major contributing factor in the development of essential hypertension (Silverberg et al, 2002).

Sleep apnea occurs in both genders and in all ages, weights, and ethnicities. Certain risk factors are associated with a higher incidence, such as excess weight or obesity (BMI >25); family history of sleep apnea; male sex; large neck (greater than 17 inches in men, greater than 16 inches in women); recessed chin; physical abnormality in the nose, throat, or upper airway structure; older age; smoking; use of alcohol or sleeping pills; ethnicity (African Americans, Pacific Islanders, and Hispanics seem to be at an increased risk); and snoring.

Sleep apnea may develop in any patient who has an endocrine disorder or is receiving certain hormonal therapies; effective assessment and management of OSA may lead to a reduction in insulin resistance and hypertension as well as other markers of vascular risk in patients with metabolic syndrome (Yee et al, 2004). Untreated severe OSA results in elevated CRP levels; this may contribute to cardiovascular risk (Shamsuzzaman et al, 2002).

Clinicians should be aware that OSA may be a risk factor for the development of cardiovascular disease. Both atherosclerosis and OSA are associated with endothelial dysfunction; increased CRP, interleukin-6, fibrinogen, and plasminogen activator inhibitor; and reduced fibrinolytic activity. OSA has also been associated with enhanced platelet activity and aggregation and leukocyte adhesion on endothelial cells (Parish and Somers, 2004).

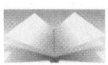

Obstructive sleep–disordered (OSD) breathing is common in children (3–12% of children snore); mild sleep apnea affects 1–10% of children (Chan et al, 2004). Risk factors of children who are more at risk for OSA are physical abnormalities of the face or skull, cerebral palsy, muscular dystrophy, Down syndrome, sickle cell disease, obesity, and mouth breathing. Consequences of untreated OSA include failure to thrive, enuresis, attention-deficit disorder, behavior problems, poor academic performance, and cardiopulmonary disease (Chan et al, 2004). Sleep deprivation and sleep apnea may even be related to some sudden infant death syndrome (SIDS) cases; upper airway obstruction and depressed arousability from sleep may contribute (Franco et al, 2004).

Treatment includes the use of continuous positive airway pressure (CPAP), weight loss in obese children, or adenotonsillectomy. Use of a CPAP device can be worn while sleeping. This device works to keep the airway open by continuously blowing air through the nasal passages at a high pressure. CPAP may help medically treated patients with heart failure and other cardiovascular conditions (Kaneko et al, 2003). See Figure 5-7.

In addition, some dental appliances may reposition the tongue or lower jaw so that the airway remains open while the patient sleeps, thus preventing the apnea. Surgical treatments may also be done, such as septoplasty, tonsillectomy, uvulopalatopharyngoplasty (UPPP, also known as UP3), and laser-assisted uvulopalatopharyngoplasty (LAUP).

INTERVENTION: OBJECTIVES

- If obese, weight loss will be beneficial. A focus on weight control is especially important given the expanding epidemic of overweight and obesity in the United States (Young et al, 2002).
- In children with failure to thrive, medical or surgical treatments may help to alleviate the problem so catch-up growth can occur.
- Manage other medical and health complications that are present in the individual; cardiovascular disease (Jelic et al, 2002), hypertension, or metabolic syndrome may coexist with OSA.

INTERVENTION: FOOD AND NUTRITION

- Lower energy intake to promote weight loss of 1–1.5 pounds weekly if possible.

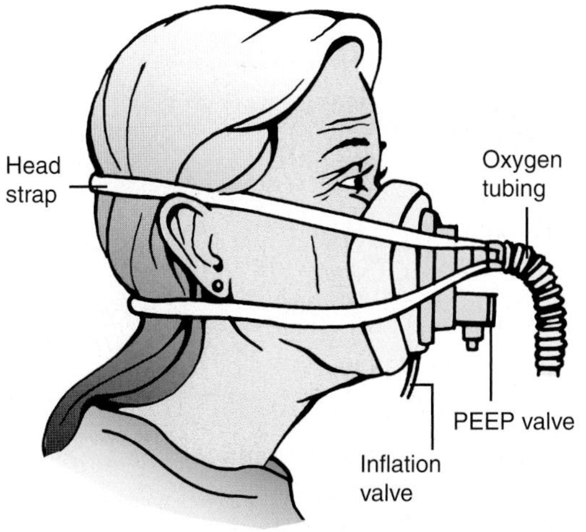

Figure 5-7 Continuous positive airway pressure (CPAP) for sleep apnea. (From Nettina SM. *The Lippincott manual of nursing practice.* 7th ed. Philadelphia: Lippincott, Williams & Wilkins; 2001.)

- Alter diet plan if needed to manage diabetes, sickle cell anemia, or other underlying conditions. The DASH diet or a calorie-controlled diet may be useful.

CLINICAL INDICATORS

Clinical/History

Height
Weight
BMI
Diet history
BP
Chest x-ray
Polysomnography (sleep study)
Hypopnea (less than normal breath)
Apnea–hypopnea index (AHI)
Respiratory disturbance index (RDI)
Epworth Sleepiness Scale (ESS)

Lab Work

Gluc
Serum insulin
CBC
H & H (anemia common)
Serum Fe
CRP
Homocysteine
Alb, transthyretin
Ca++, Mg++
Na+, K+
pCO_2, pO_2

Common Drugs Used and Potential Side Effects

- OSA can be induced, unmasked, or exacerbated by the effects of sedative, analgesic, and anesthetic agents (Jain and Dhand, 2004). Sleeping agents are not generally recommended for sleep apnea.
- Treatment of depression or mood disorders may be needed (Bardwell et al, 2003). In patients who are on chronic neuroleptic drugs for schizophrenia, weight management will be very important (Winkelman, 2001).

Herbs, Botanicals, and Supplements

- No clinical trials have proven efficacy for use of herbs or botanicals in sleep apnea.
- Very limited data are available to support a beneficial effect of nonprescription therapies on snoring; minimal evidence is available to support their use in treating OSA (Meoli et al, 2003).

INTERVENTION: NUTRITION EDUCATION, COUNSELING, CARE MANAGEMENT

- Typically, patients diagnosed with sleep apnea are advised to avoid tobacco, alcohol, sedatives, and medications that relax the airway and/or reduce respiratory function.
- Regular exercise and weight reduction can help some patients with mild or moderate sleep apnea minimize their symptoms. Sleep apnea sufferers are also advised to avoid sleeping on their back, if possible. Using pillows and other devices that help the patient sleep in a side position may help.
- The relationship of OSA with hypertension and cardiovascular disease should be discussed if necessary. There may be a relationship between sleep apnea and stroke, for example (Dyken et al, 1996).

- Patients who have cough, OSA, rhinosinusitis, and esophageal reflux clustered together can be categorized as having CORE syndrome (Arter et al, 2004).

Patient Education—Foodborne Illness

- Careful food handling will be important. Hand washing is key as well.

For More Information

- Narcolepsy Network
  http://www.websciences.org/narnet/
- National Sleep Foundation
  http://www.sleepfoundation.org/
- Sleep Apnea Association
  http://www.sleepapnea.org/

SLEEP APNEA—CITED REFERENCES

Arter JL, et al. Obstructive sleep apnea, inflammation, and cardiopulmonary disease. *Front Biosci.* 9:2892, 2004.

Bardwell WA, et al. Fatigue in obstructive sleep apnea: driven by depressive symptoms instead of apnea severity? *Am J Psychiatry.* 160:350, 2003.

Chan J, et al. Obstructive sleep apnea in children. *Am Fam Physician.* 69:1147, 2004.

Dyken ME, et al. Investigating the relationship between stroke and obstructive sleep apnea. *Stroke* 27:401, 1996.

Franco P, et al. Decreased arousals among healthy infants after short-term sleep deprivation. *Pediatrics* 114:192, 2004.

Jain SS, Dhand R. Perioperative treatment of patients with obstructive sleep apnea. *Curr Opin Pulm Med.* 10:482, 2004.

Jelic S, et al. Arterial stiffness increases during obstructive sleep apneas. *Sleep* 25:850, 2002.

Kaneko Y, et al. Cardiovascular effects of continuous positive airway pressure in patients with heart failure and obstructive sleep apnea. *N Engl J Med.* 348:1233, 2003.

Meoli AL, et al. Nonprescription treatments of snoring or obstructive sleep apnea: an evaluation of products with limited scientific evidence. *Sleep* 26:619, 2003.

Parish JM, Somers VK. Obstructive sleep apnea and cardiovascular disease. *Mayo Clin Proc.* 79:1036, 2004.

Shamsuzzaman AS, et al. Elevated C-reactive protein in patients with obstructive sleep apnea. *Circulation.* 105:2462, 2002.

Silverberg DS, et al. Treating obstructive sleep apnea improves essential hypertension and quality of life. *Am Fam Physician.* 65:229, 2002.

Winkelman JW. Schizophrenia, obesity, and obstructive sleep apnea. *J Clin Psychiatry.* 62:8, 2001.

Yee B, et al. Neuroendocrine changes in sleep apnea. *Curr Opin Pulm Med.* 10:475, 2004.

Young T, et al. Epidemiology of obstructive sleep apnea: a population health perspective. *Am J Respir Crit Care Med.* 65:1217, 2002.

THORACIC EMPYEMA

NUTRITIONAL ACUITY RANKING: LEVEL 2

DEFINITIONS AND BACKGROUND

Thoracic empyema involves accumulation of pus in the pleural cavity. It may be a complication of pneumonia. Signs and symptoms may include dyspnea, orthopnea, constant localized chest pain, productive cough, malaise, fatigue, fever, tachycardia, tachypnea, weight loss, and anorexia. Complications may include septic shock, multiple organ failure, cardiac insufficiency, and end-stage renal failure.

An increase in the incidence of thoracic empyema in children has been noted, and the causative pathogen is often unknown (Saglani et al, 2005). *Staphylococcus aureus* is a common micro-organism isolated from the bacterial cultures, as is *Mycobacterium tuberculosis* (Ozel et al, 2004). With an increasing incidence of *S. aureus*, particularly methicillin-resistant *S. aureus*, the use of video-assisted thoracoscopy (VATS) results in decreased duration of fever and length of hospitalization (Schultz et al, 2004).

INTERVENTION: OBJECTIVES

- Lessen fatigue; promote improved well-being.
- Reduce fever. Prevent sepsis, organ failure, and other complications.
- Correct weight loss.
- Control and reduce anorexia.
- Support the capacity for wound healing if surgery is needed (Michaels et al, 1997).

INTERVENTION: FOOD AND NUTRITION

- Provide diet as ordered. Patient may need high-calorie/high-protein foods served at frequent intervals.
- Two or more liters of fluid may be needed daily, unless contraindicated.
- Meals should be served in an attractive manner to stimulate appetite.
- A multivitamin-mineral supplement may be useful.

CLINICAL INDICATORS

Clinical/History		
Height	I & O	Na+, K+
Weight	CT scan	Ca++, Mg++
BMI	Ultrasound	pO_2 (often decreased)
Diet history	**Lab Work**	pCO_2
BP	Alb, transthyretin	Transferrin
Temperature (fever?)	H & H	CRP
Pleural examination	Serum Fe	
	Gluc	

Common Drugs Used and Potential Side Effects

- Antibiotics (such as streptokinase) are often provided (Cameron and Davies, 2004). Monitor side effects accordingly.
- Monitor effects of other medications as prescribed.

Herbs, Botanicals, and Supplements

- No clinical trials have proven efficacy for use of herbs or botanicals in thoracic empyema.

INTERVENTION: NUTRITION EDUCATION, COUNSELING, CARE MANAGEMENT

- Discuss the role of nutrition in illness and recovery, especially as it relates to immunocompetence.
- With family, discuss signs to observe for future problems or relapses.

Patient Education—Foodborne Illness

- Careful food handling will be important. Hand washing is key as well.

For More Information

- Thoracic Empyema
  http://www.encyclopedia.com/html/e1/empyema.asp

THORACIC EMPYEMA—CITED REFERENCES

Cameron R, Davies HR. Intra-pleural fibrinolytic therapy versus conservative management in the treatment of parapneumonic effusions and empyema. *Cochrane Database Syst Rev.* 2:CD002312, 2004.

Michaels BM, et al. Flap closure of postpneumonectomy empyema. *Plast Reconstr Surg.* 99:437, 1997.

Ozel SK, et al. Conservative treatment of postpneumonic thoracic empyema in children. *Surg Today.* 34:1002, 2004.

Saglani S, et al. Empyema: the use of broad range 16S rDNA PCR for pathogen detection. *Arch Dis Child.* 90:70, 2005.

Schultz KD, et al. The changing face of pleural empyemas in children: epidemiology and management. *Pediatrics* 113:1735, 2004.

TRANSPLANTATION, LUNG

NUTRITIONAL ACUITY RANKING: LEVEL 3–4

DEFINITIONS AND BACKGROUND

Lung transplantation (LTX) is an accepted treatment for end-stage pulmonary parenchymal and vascular diseases. LTX is a well-tolerated, effective therapy for respiratory failure in patients with interstitial lung disease (Sulica et al, 2001), as well as in patients with cystic fibrosis or COPD. The International Society for Heart and Lung Transplantation and the Cystic Fibrosis Foundation have uniform guidelines for transplantation candidate selection. Over 13,000 LTXs have occurred worldwide (Tynan and Hasse, 2004).

Proper nutrition plays a key role in preparing for LTX. Therefore, the LTX dietitian plays an important role and meets with the patient for an initial interview. Weight and weight history, foods typically eaten, and appetite are reviewed. Being at ideal body weight range for height helps assure good physical condition for pretransplantation pulmonary rehabilitation and for the transplantation itself. Certain patients with advanced pulmonary disease are unable to eat enough to maintain ideal body weight because of increased metabolic demands and breathlessness with eating. In such situations, it may be recommended that a percutaneous endoscopic gastrostomy (PEG) feeding tube be placed.

Proper nutrition is critical to maximize the chances of a successful transplantation. Occasionally, listing for transplantation will be delayed until the patient's nutritional status improves. In patients with a low pretransplantation BMI (<17) or high BMI (>27), LTX is more risky (Madill et al, 2001). In a group of underweight patients with lung disease assessed for LTX, it was possible to increase energy intake by an intensified nutritional support to achieve a significant weight gain, compared with the regular nutritional support, during a short hospital stay (Forli et al, 2001). Lean body mass depletion may be associated with more severe hypoxemia, reduced walking distance, and a higher mortality (Schwebel et al, 2000). Both undernutrition and obesity should be carefully managed before surgery.

As with other types of transplantations, graft–host resistance and sepsis are the major concerns after LTX. Infections are the most common cause of morbidity and mortality in LTX recipients; half are bacterial in origin (Speich and van Der Bij, 2001). Immunosuppressive therapy with glucocorticoids contributes to protein degradation. Nitrogen balance after LTX is negative because of high glucocorticoid requirements; aggressive nutritional intervention and increased nitrogen intake are needed to reduce protein losses in these patients. Chronic infection (bronchiolitis obliterans syndrome) is the most common cause of death after transplantation (Quattrucci et al, 2005).

INTERVENTION: OBJECTIVES

Preoperative

- Because nutritional depletion in LTX candidates is highly prevalent, it should be precisely assessed with a special reference to lean body mass since it has specific consequences both before and after LTX (Schwebel et al, 2000). Attempts should be made to increase lean body

mass and reverse cachexia and vitamin and mineral deficiencies before LTX.
- Prepare for surgical procedure. Most patients will require sodium or fluid restrictions; monitor serum potassium as well.
- Allow for mild weight loss with a planned diet if the patient is obese and has time to do this.

Postoperative
- Prevent infection, surgical complications, organ rejection, and organ failure.
- Promote wound healing.
- Support ideal body weight and lean body mass maintenance.
- Reduce protein losses, support nitrogen balance, and correct hypoalbuminemia.
- Prevent aspiration.
- Wean from ventilator or oxygen when possible.
- Treat comorbid conditions such as cardiovascular disease (CVD), osteoporosis, dyslipidemia, diabetes, hyperglycemia, metabolic syndrome, and hyperkalemia (Tynan and Hasse, 2004).

INTERVENTION: FOOD AND NUTRITION

Preoperative
- Prepare patient nutritionally to alleviate malnutrition in advance (Inouye et al, 2004). Home enteral or parenteral nutrition may be useful.
- Promote adequate intake of kcal (25–30 kcal/kg) and protein (1 g/kg body weight).
- Manage coexisting problems such as diabetes, heart disease, and hypertension with an appropriate diet such as the DASH diet.

Postoperative
- Return to oral intake by 48–72 hours postoperatively, when possible. Limit simple carbohydrates when there are signs of hyperglycemia (Tynan and Hasse, 2004).
- Promote adequate intake of kcal (30–35 kcal/kg) and protein of 1.3–1.5 g/kg body weight (Tynan and Hasse, 2004). Use high nitrogen tube feeding when needed, but do not overfeed, and monitor for needed changes in electrolytes according to lab values. Discontinue tube feeding when intake meets >60% of estimated needs (Tynan and Hasse, 2004).
- Parenteral solutions may be used if the gut is nonfunctioning (Tynan and Hasse, 2004).
- Calorie-dense options should be considered if fluid restriction is required. Use caution with high-caloric loads because of respiratory quotient (RQ); maintain sufficient fat intake to prevent excess CO_2 production from a high-CHO intake.
- Restrict sodium and potassium if needed to improve cardiac or renal status.
- Reduce energy intake and increase activity if weight gain or diabetes occurs after long-term corticosteroid use (Tynan and Hasse, 2004).
- Prevent osteoporosis by using adequate calcium and vitamin D. Provide sufficient magnesium and vitamins to heal and promote adequate nutritional status.

CLINICAL INDICATORS

Clinical/History	Lab Work	
Height	Alb, transthyretin	Na+, K+
Weight	CRP	Ca++, Mg++
BMI	Transferrin	PO_4
Weight changes	Chol, Trig	AST, ALT
Diet history	H & H	Lactate
RQ	Serum Fe	TLC
Ventilator support	Gluc	CRP
I & O	BUN, Creat	pCO_2, pO_2

Common Drugs Used and Potential Side Effects

- See Table 5-13.

Herbs, Botanicals, and Supplements

- No clinical trials have proven efficacy for use of herbs or botanicals after LTX.

INTERVENTION: NUTRITION EDUCATION, COUNSELING, CARE MANAGEMENT

- Discuss appropriate calorie and protein levels. Protein helps to heal after surgery.
- Drink plenty of water until restriction is prescribed.
- Decreased saturated fat and cholesterol intakes may be useful to decrease cardiac risks and to prevent unwanted weight gain, which is common. Read food labels and monitor portions carefully. Choose condiments such as mustard rather than mayonnaise or salad dressing. Choose healthy cooking methods. Instead of frying, try baking, grilling, broiling, or steaming foods; instead of oil, use nonstick, fat-free spray or sauces.
- Adequate fiber (from fresh fruits, vegetables, and whole grains) is important.
- A gradual return to activity will be important.
- Eat a minimum amount of salt, processed foods, and snacks. Use herbs and spices to add flavor instead of salt.
- Add calcium by eating calcium-rich foods, such as low-fat dairy products and green, leafy vegetables, or by using calcium supplements.
- Avoid alcohol and do not use drugs that are not prescribed.

Patient Education—Foodborne Illness

- Preventing infection is very important after transplantation surgery. Hand washing is critically important.
- Careful food handling will be important.

For More Information

- Division of Transplantation
  http://www.hrsa.gov/osp/dot/dotmain.htm
- Fast Facts about Transplants
  http://www.ustransplant.org/csr/current/fastfacts.aspx

TABLE 5-13 Medications Used for Lung Transplant Patients

Medication	Description
Azathioprine (Imuran)	May cause leukopenia, thrombocytopenia, oral and esophageal sores, macrocytic anemia, pancreatitis, vomiting, diarrhea, and other side effects that are complex. Folate supplementation and other dietary modifications (liquid or soft diet, use of oral supplements) may be needed. The drug works by lowering the number of T cells; it is often prescribed along with prednisone for conventional immunosuppression.
Corticosteroids (such as prednisone, hydrocortisone)	Used for immunosuppression. Side effects include increased catabolism of proteins, negative nitrogen balance, hyperphagia, ulcers, decreased glucose tolerance, sodium retention, fluid retention, and impaired calcium absorption and osteoporosis. Cushing's syndrome, obesity, muscle wasting, and increased gastric secretion may result. A higher protein intake and lower intake of simple CHOs may be needed.
Cyclosporine	Does not retain sodium as much as corticosteroids do. Intravenous doses are more effective than oral doses. Nausea, vomiting, and diarrhea are common side effects. Hyperlipidemia, hypertension (HPN), and hyperkalemia also may occur; decrease sodium and potassium as necessary. Elevated glucose and lipids may occur. The drug is also nephrotoxic; a controlled renal diet may be beneficial.
Immunosuppressants (muromonab [Orthoclone OKT3] and antithymocyte globulin)	Less nephrotoxic than cyclosporine but can cause nausea, anorexia, diarrhea, and vomiting. Monitor carefully. Fever and stomatitis also may occur; alter diet as needed.
Diuretics	Diuretics such as furosemide may cause hypokalemia. Low-sodium/low-calorie diets may be indicated. If spironolactone is used, it spares potassium.
Tacrolimus (Prograf, FK506)	Suppresses T-cell immunity; it is 100 times more potent than cyclosporine, thus requiring smaller doses. Side effects include GI distress, nausea, vomiting, hyperkalemia, and hyperglycemia. Tacrolimus therapy has aided in success of lung transplantation and has become the primary immunosuppressant agent used (Garrity and Mehra, 2004). A low-potassium diet may be needed to prevent cardiac arrhythmia (Tynan and Hasse, 2004).

- International Society for Heart and Lung Transplantation
  http://www.ishlt.org/
- Lung Transplantation
  http://www.nlm.nih.gov/medlineplus/lungtransplantation.html
- Organ Procurement and Transplantation Network
  http://www.optn.org/
- Transplant Terms
  http://www.transplantliving.org/Community/glossary.aspx
- Trans Web
  http://www.transweb.org/

TRANSPLANTATION, LUNG—CITED REFERENCES

Forli L, et al. Dietary support to underweight patients with end-stage pulmonary disease assessed for lung transplantation. *Respiration* 68:51, 2001.

Garrity ER Jr, Mehra MR. An update on clinical outcomes in heart and lung transplantation. *Transplantation* 77:S68, 2004.

Inouye Y, et al. Benefits of home parenteral nutrition before lung transplantation: report of a case. *Surg Today.* 34:525, 2004.

Madill J, et al. Nutritional assessment of the lung transplant patient: body mass index as a predictor of 90-day mortality following transplantation. *J Heart Lung Transplant.* 20:288, 2001.

Quattrucci S, et al. Lung transplantation for cystic fibrosis: 6-year follow-up. *J Cyst Fibros.* 4:107, 2005.

Schwebel C, et al. Prevalence and consequences of nutritional depletion in lung transplant candidates. *Eur Respir J.* 16:1050, 2000.

Speich R, van Der Bij W. Epidemiology and management of infections after lung transplantation. *Clin Infect Dis.* 33:58S, 2001.

Sulica R, et al. Lung transplantation in interstitial lung disease. *Curr Opin Pulm Med.* 7:314, 2001.

Tynan C, Hasse JM. Current nutrition practices in adult lung transplantation. *Nutr Clin Pract.* 19:587, 2004.

TUBERCULOSIS

NUTRITIONAL ACUITY RANKING: LEVEL 1–2

DEFINITIONS AND BACKGROUND

Tuberculosis (TB) is caused by a tubercle bacillus (*Mycobacterium tuberculosis*) invading the lungs and setting up an inflammatory process. Healing occurs with a calcification of the tubercular cavity. TB causes loss of appetite, constant fatigue, tissue wasting, exhaustion, hemoptysis, cough lasting 3 weeks or longer with occasional blood-tinged sputum, fever or chills, profuse night sweats, and weight loss. The acute form resembles pneumonia; the chronic form causes low-grade fever.

Nearly one third of the world's population is infected with *M. tuberculosis* (Pai et al, 2006). An increase in TB in the United States may be related to inadequate compliance with prescribed drug therapy or to recently acquired or reactivated latent infections. Figure 5-8 shows TB of the lung.

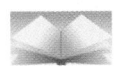

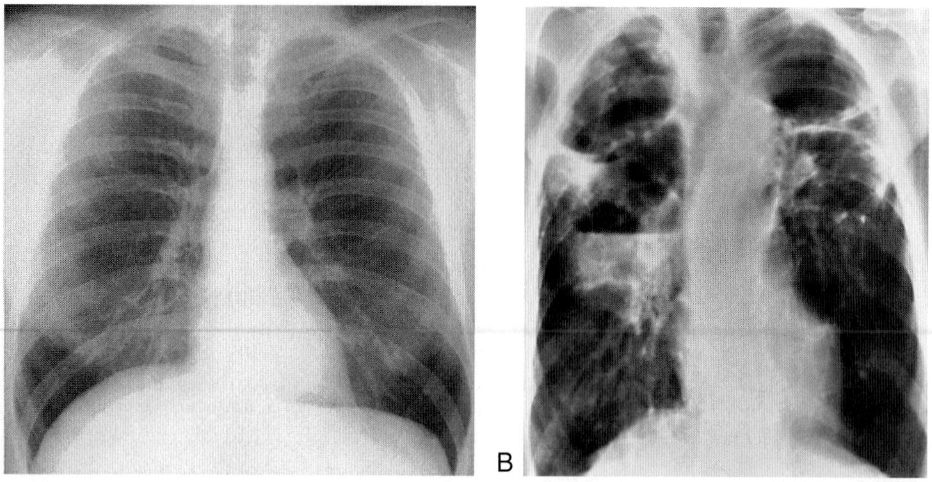

A B

Figure 5-8 Tuberculosis. (**A.** From Kahn GP, Lynch JP. *Pulmonary disease diagnosis and therapy: a practical approach*. Philadelphia: Lippincott Williams & Wilkins; 1997. **B.** From Eisenberg RL. *Clinical imaging: an atlas of differential diagnosis*. 4th ed. Philadelphia: Lippincott Williams & Wilkins; 2003.)

Immunocompromised persons are more vulnerable to the effects of TB, especially those persons who have HIV infection. These patients exhibit altered iron metabolism that leads to increased deposition of this element in the tissues; this may promote increased susceptibility of AIDS patients to mycobacterial infections, namely, by *M. avium* (Gomes et al, 2001). Hypermetabolism appears to play a role in the wasting process in patients infected with both HIV and TB. HIV infection is associated with a significant downregulation of whole-body protein flux, adding to the nutritional decline if TB is also present (Paton et al, 2003).

Active TB begins in the lungs but often spreads through the bloodstream as extrapulmonary TB. Fatigue, abdominal tenderness, painful urination, headache, shortness of breath, arthritis-like symptoms, kidney damage, and pain in the spine and bones can occur. TB meningitis is a very dangerous complication, especially for the elderly.

Because many TB patients have early, unplanned readmission and often need assistance with activities of daily living, ambulatory treatment may not be appropriate for selected patients (Chu et al, 2001). They may have drug complications, the need to use a nonstandard drug regimen, and other illnesses. With a high prevalence of malnutrition, a relatively low utilization rate of nutritional services, and the potential effect of adverse reactions to therapeutic drugs, careful attention is needed for this patient population.

According to the World Health Organization (2005), drug-resistant TB is caused by inconsistent or partial treatment because patients do not take all their medicines regularly for the required period because they start to feel better, because doctors and health workers prescribe the wrong treatment regimens, or because the drug supply is unreliable. Multidrug-resistant TB (MDR-TB) is caused by TB bacilli that are resistant to at least isoniazid and rifampicin, the two most powerful anti-TB drugs.

INTERVENTION: OBJECTIVES

- Maintain weight (or prevent losses). Reduce fever. The basal metabolic rate is 20–30% above normal to counteract fever of 102°F or higher.
- Normalize calcium levels in serum; either hypocalcemia or hypercalcemia may occur.
- Replace nutrient losses from lung hemorrhage, if present.
- Promote healing of the cavity.
- Counteract neuritis from isoniazid (INH) therapy, when used.
- Stimulate appetite, which is generally poor.
- Prevent dehydration.
- Prevent lung inflammation, infections, and complications.

INTERVENTION: FOOD AND NUTRITION

- Use a well-balanced diet containing liberal amounts of protein and adequate calories. It may be useful to calculate needs as 35–45 kcal/kg if weight loss has been significant.
- Use adequate fluids (35 cc/kg or 2 L is a common amount) unless otherwise contraindicated.
- It may be useful to add more omega-3 fatty acids; they may improve food intake, restore normal eating patterns, and prevent body weight loss (Ramos et al, 2004).
- Ensure that the diet provides sufficient calcium without excess; vitamin D is needed in controlled amounts; iron

SAMPLE NUTRITION DIAGNOSTIC STATEMENT

Tuberculosis

PES: Involuntary weight loss related to insufficient intake and frequent coughing spells, medication-related GI symptoms as evidenced by 15-lb weight loss since diagnosis last month.

Assessment Data: Analysis of estimated oral intake below estimated needs.

Intervention: Interventions would include timing of meals and snacks and possible nutrition supplemental intake in relation to medication administration and coughing episodes.

Monitoring and Evaluation: Monitor and evaluate changes in intake and weight.

and vitamin C are needed for proper hemoglobin formation and wound healing; B-complex vitamins, especially vitamin B_6, are needed to counteract INH therapy. Use supplemental vitamin A as carotene if poorly converted.
- Alcohol should not be used as a calorie replacement or appetite enhancer.

CLINICAL INDICATORS

Clinical/History

- Height
- Weight
- BMI
- Diet history
- BP
- TB skin tests—tine or purified protein derivative
- Chest x-rays (irregular white areas on dark background)
- Temperature, fever
- Sputum test for *M. tuberculosis*
- Spinal tap for polymerase chain reaction (PCR)
- I & O

Lab Work

- Alb, transthyretin
- CRP
- RBP
- TLC
- Serum pyridoxine
- H & H
- Serum Fe
- N balance
- Chol (decreased)
- Na+, K+
- Ca++, Mg++
- Serum folate
- Transferrin
- BUN, Creat
- Liver function tests (from medication use)

Common Drugs Used and Potential Side Effects

- See Table 5-14.

Herbs, Botanicals, and Supplements

- No clinical trials have proven efficacy for use of herbs or botanicals in tuberculosis, including eucalyptus, echinacea, garlic, licorice, honeysuckle, or forsythia.

INTERVENTION: NUTRITION EDUCATION, COUNSELING, CARE MANAGEMENT

- Add protein powders or nonfat dry milk to beverages, casseroles, soups, and desserts to increase protein and calcium intake, unless contraindicated.
- Encourage the preparation of appetizing meals.
- Plan rest periods before and after meals. Discuss anxiety related to weight loss, night sweats, loss of strength, high fever, and abnormal chest x-rays.
- Discuss communicability of TB. Family members and those living in proximity should have x-rays and other tests. About 5% of exposures result in TB within 1 year; others may be dormant until another condition sets in such as HIV infection, diabetes, or leukemia.
- Promote adequate rehabilitation if the patient is an alcoholic.
- Promote as much quality of life as possible. This is often overlooked in TB management (Marra et al, 2004).
- A new TB vaccine is being tested through the FDA.

Patient Education—Foodborne Illness

- Careful food handling will be important. Foodservice employees who are exposed to those at risk for active TB should be tested regularly.

TABLE 5-14 Medications Used for Tuberculosis (TB)

Medication	Description
Aminosalicylic acid	Interferes with vitamin B_{12} and folate absorption. Nausea and vomiting are common.
Chemotherapy	Chemotherapy can increase serum calcium levels.
Ethionamide (Trecator-SC)	Requires a vitamin B_6 supplement. It may cause anorexia, metallic taste, nausea, vomiting, diarrhea, weight loss, and hypoglycemia.
Ethambutol (Myambutol)	May cause GI distress, nausea, or anorexia. It should not be used longer than 2 months because it can harm the eyes.
Immunotherapy	According to the Centers for Disease Control and Prevention (2004): TB disease is a potential adverse reaction from treatment with tumor necrosis factor-alpha (TNF-α) antagonists infliximab (Remicade), etanercept (Enbrel), and adalimumab (Humira). These products block TNF-α, an inflammatory cytokine, and are approved for treating rheumatoid arthritis and other selected autoimmune diseases. Blocking TNF-α can allow TB disease to emerge from latent *Mycobacterium tuberculosis* infection. Health care providers should take steps to prevent TB in immunocompromised patients and remain vigilant for TB as a cause of unexplained fever.
Isoniazid (INH)	May cause neuritis by depleting vitamin B_6. Its bad taste can be disguised in pureed fruit or jam to make it palatable, especially for pediatric patients. Niacin, calcium, and vitamin B_{12} are also depleted. Nausea, vomiting, stomach cramping, and dry mouth are common. It must be taken for 9 months to be effective in eradicating the condition completely.
Pyrazinamide (PZA)	May cause anorexia, nausea, and vomiting. It can be hepatotoxic.
Rifampin (Rifadin, Rimactane)	Has side effects such as anorexia and GI distress.
Streptomycin	One of the first drugs used to treat TB. It is given by injection. Use of longer than 3 months can affect balance and hearing.

NOTE. Therapy always involves two or more drugs because of the long-term treatment period required.

- People are at risk and may need to be tested if they are:
  - A person who has symptoms of active TB disease
  - A person who has been exposed to someone (a family member, friend, or coworker) who has active TB disease
  - A person who has HIV infection, diabetes, or chronic kidney failure
  - A person who is taking steroids or other immune-suppressing drugs for chronic medical conditions
  - A person who lives or works in a homeless shelter, prison, hospital, nursing home, or other similar group setting
  - A person who has recently come to the United States from a region with a lot of active TB such as Africa, Asia, the Caribbean, Eastern Europe, and Latin America
  - A student entering the New York City school system for the first time at the secondary school level (intermediate, junior, or middle schools and high schools)
- When preparing food:
  - Separate raw meat from cooked or ready-to-eat foods. Do not use the same chopping board or the same knife for preparing raw meat and cooked or ready-to-eat foods.
  - Do not handle either raw or cooked foods without washing hands in between.
  - Do not place cooked meat back on the same plate or surface it was on before it was cooked.
  - All foods from poultry should be cooked thoroughly, including eggs. Egg yolks should not be runny or liquid. Because influenza viruses are destroyed by heat, the cooking temperature for poultry meat should reach 70°C (158°F).
  - Wash egg shells in soapy water before handling and cooking, and wash hands afterwards.
  - Do not use raw or soft-boiled eggs in foods that will not be cooked.
  - After handling raw poultry or eggs, wash hands and all surfaces and utensils thoroughly with soap and water.
  - Do not eat uncooked or undercooked poultry or poultry products, including food with uncooked poultry blood.

For More Information

- Avian Flu
  http://www.who.int/csr/disease/avian_influenza/en/
- Joint HIV/TB Interventions
  http://www.who.int/hiv/topics/tb/tuberculosis/en/
- National TB Center
  http://www.nationaltbcenter.edu/
- Travelers Health Website
  http://www.cdc.gov/travel
- World Health Organization
  http://www.who.int/tb/en/

TUBERCULOSIS—CITED REFERENCES

Centers for Disease Control and Prevention. Tuberculosis associated with blocking agents against tumor necrosis factor-alpha—California, 2002–2003. *MMWR Morb Mortal Wkly Rep.* 53:683, 2004.

Chu C, et al. Early unplanned readmission of patients with newly diagnosed tuberculosis discharged from acute hospital to ambulatory treatment. *Respirology* 6:145, 2001.

Gomes M, et al. Role of iron in experimental *Mycobacterium avium* infection. *J Clin Virol.* 20:117, 2001.

Marra CA, et al. Factors influencing quality of life in patients with active tuberculosis. *Health Qual Life Outcomes.* 2:58, 2004.

Pai M, et al. New tools and emerging technologies for the diagnosis of tuberculosis. Part I. Latent tuberculosis. *Expert Rev Mol Diagn.* 6:413, 2006.

Paton NI, et al. Effects of tuberculosis and HIV infection on whole-body protein metabolism during feeding, measured by the [15N]glycine method. *Am J Clin Nutr.* 78:319, 2003.

Ramos EJ, et al. Effects of omega-3 fatty acid supplementation on tumor-bearing rats. *J Am Coll Surg.* 199:716, 2004.

World Health Organization. Fact sheet: tuberculosis. Accessed February 4, 2005 at http://www.who.int/mediacentre/factsheets/fs104/en/.

S E C T I O N 6

Cardiovascular Disorders

CHIEF ASSESSMENT FACTORS

- Decreased Cardiac Output: Arrhythmias, Rales, Vertigo, Pallor, Fatigue, Labored Respirations
- Cardiogenic Shock: Tachycardia, Low Systolic Blood Pressure (BP), Cool and Moist Skin, Weak Pulses, Decreased Urinary Output, Pulmonary Edema
- Ascites, Edema
- Chest Pain
- Blood Pressure
- Dietary Pattern Including High Saturated Fat Intake and Related Parameters
- Use of Herbs or Botanical Products
- Cholesterol and Lipid Profiles (for example, higher HDL is more protective, small dense LDL is atherogenic)
- C-Reactive Protein (CRP)
- Serum Homocysteine
- Lactic Acid Dehydrogenase (LDH), Creatine Phosphokinase (CPK) Levels
- Electrolyte Balance
- Age: Males $\geq$ 45 Years of Age and $\geq$ 55 Years of Age in Females
- Women: Contraceptive Use or Menopause
- History of Tobacco Use
- Diabetes
- Exercise Patterns
- Family Hx (Use ATP III Guidelines) and Sibling Cardiovascular Disease
- Type A Personality, Stressful Lifestyle
- Xanthomas, Pancreatitis, Other Complications
- Medications
- Alcohol Use
- Angiograms (see Fig. 6-2), ECG, Echocardiograms
- Obesity
- Low Waist to Hip Ratio (over 0.85 for women and over 0.9 for men indicates greater risk; Mitka, 2005)

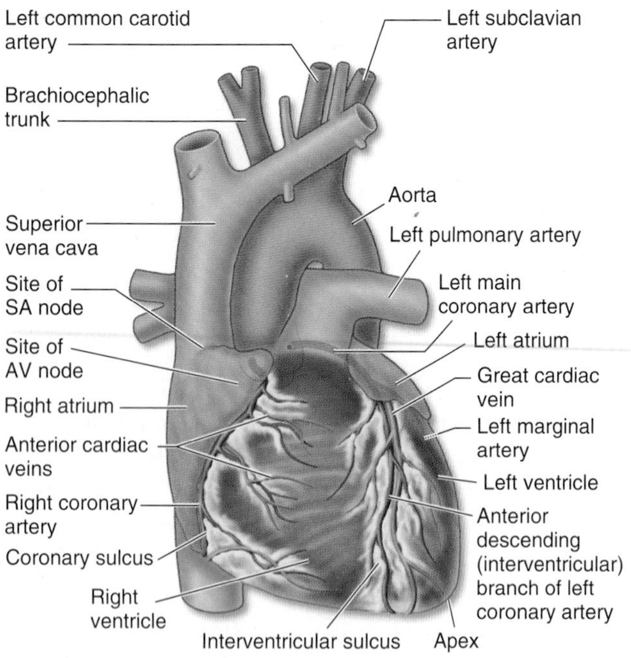

Figure 6-1 Anatomy of the heart. (From McArdle WD, Katch FI, Katch VL. *Essentials of exercise physiology*. 2nd ed. Baltimore: Lippincott Williams and Wilkins, 2000.)

OVERVIEW: DIET IN HEART DISEASES—LIPIDS

Cardiovascular disease (CVD) includes hypertension, coronary heart disease (CHD), heart failure, congenital heart defects, and stroke; CHD accounts for about 700,000 deaths annually (Jonnalagadda, 2005). Despite a dramatic decline in mortality over the past three decades, CHD is the leading cause of death and disability in the United States (Shaw et al, 2006).

CVD accounts for almost 50% of all deaths in industrialized nations, but as much as 70% of CVD can be prevented or delayed with dietary choices and lifestyle modifications (Forman and Bulwer, 2006). The adult treatment panel (ATP III) report is important because there is a greater scientific evidence base than in previous reports (Pasternak, 2003).

The benefits of primary prevention of CVD are greatest for people who have multiple risk factors. Secondary prevention is beneficial for high-risk and low-risk patients. Estimation of heart disease risk, for men or for women, can be accomplished by entering factors in a Framingham Heart Study Prediction Score sheet (see http://www.nhlbi.nih.gov/about/framingham/riskabs.htm). Sibling CVD confers increased risk of future CVD events above and beyond established risk factors and parental CVD in middle-aged adults (Muraabito et al, 2005).

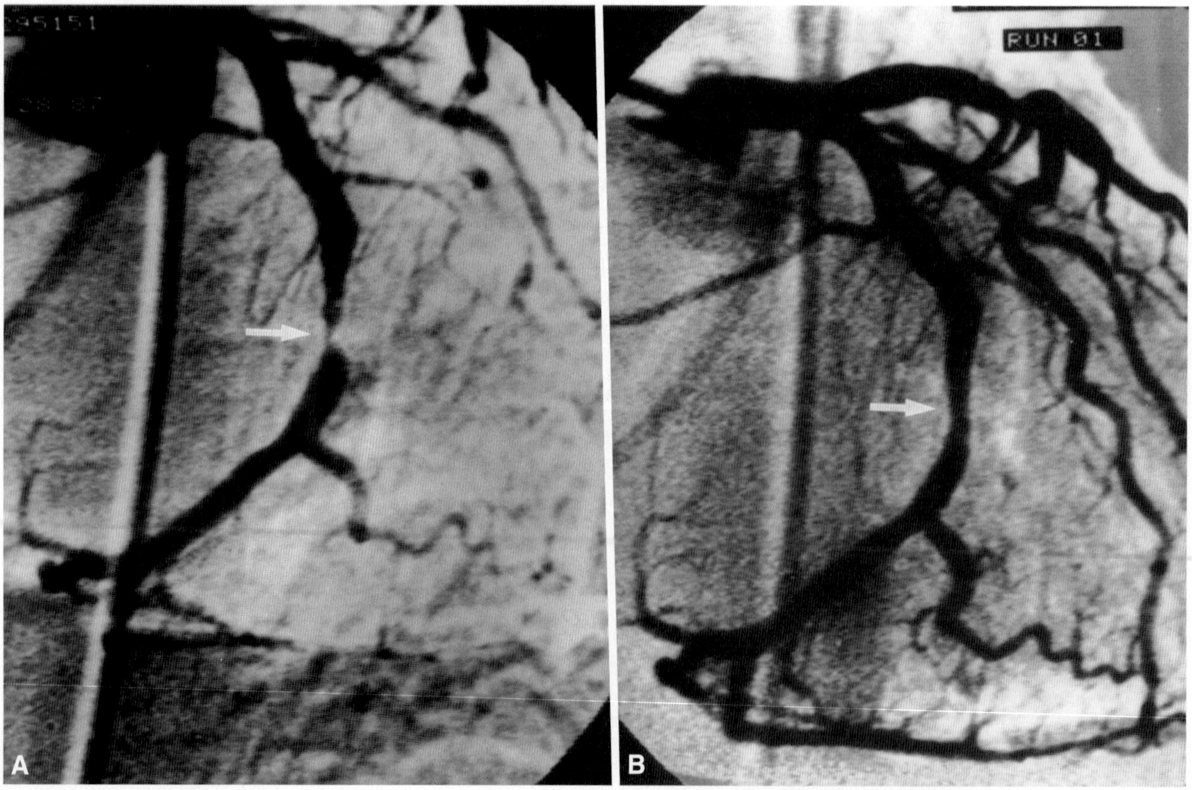

Figure 6-2 Coronary angiogram. Figure on *left* shows narrowing. (From Snell R. *Clinical anatomy*. 7th ed. Baltimore: Lippincott, Williams & Wilkins, 2003.)

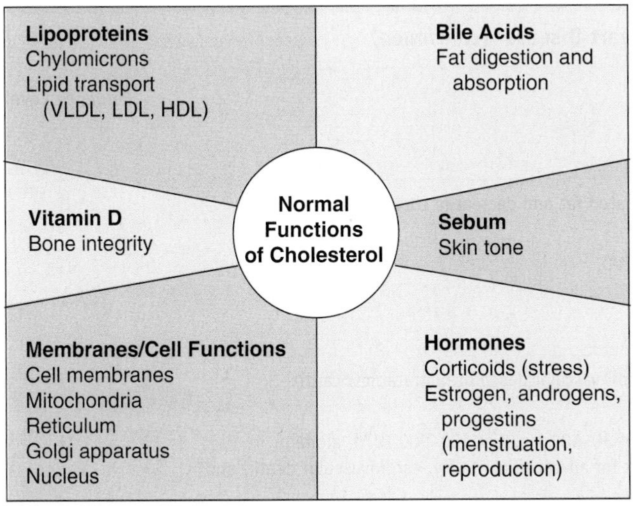

Figure 6-3 Normal functions of cholesterol.

Dyslipidemia is one of the most important modifiable risk factors (Talbert, 2002). While dyslipidemia with small dense low-density lipoprotein (LDL) molecules is more atherogenic (Berneis et al, 2005; Goff et al, 2005), dietary cholesterol is only one of many factors to play a role in the etiology of heart disease. Cholesterol is readily made from acetate in all animal tissues and has many roles in the body (see Fig. 6-3). In children and teens, widespread cholesterol screening is not warranted, except where there is early cardiovascular morbidity and mortality in immediate family members.

Studies show a link between intake of fruit, vegetables, and whole grains and protection against CHD due to fiber, vitamin, mineral, and phytochemical content. There is some weak evidence of protective effects for folate, vitamins B_6, B_{12}, E, and C, flavonoids, phytoestrogens, and a wholesome total dietary pattern (Tucker, 2004).

Many patients with classic CVD risk factors can achieve risk reduction goals without medications in 12 weeks after initiating therapeutic lifestyle changes (TLC) (Gordon et al, 2004). TLC includes exercise training, nutrition counseling, and other appropriate lifestyle interventions based on several well-established behavior change models.

Recent advances in the field of cardiovascular medicine have not led to significant declines in case fatality rates for women when compared to the dramatic declines for men, as noted by the Women's Ischemia Syndrome Evaluation (WISE) study (Shaw et al, 2006).

In a specific analysis of "low-fat" diets, there were no significant effects on the incidence of stroke and CHD, but there were small, statistically significant reductions in LDL and total cholesterol levels, diastolic blood pressure, and factor VIIc levels (Howard et al, 2006). There are indirect benefits of a diet with a lower intake of saturated and trans fats, higher intake of vegetable and fruits, use of specific types of fats including fish oils, as well as fish, and perhaps energy restriction (Anderson, 2006).

Nutrition counseling should receive high priority, both in medical training and in patient care for both men and women (Krummel, 2004). The American Dietetic Association estimates cost savings per cardiovascular case to be nearly $2500 annually with nutrition counseling, thereby reducing the need for many medications. Key components of healthy diet counseling include: (1) reduced caloric intake; (2) reduced total fat, saturated fat, trans fat, and cholesterol with proportional increases in monounsaturated, omega-3, and omega-6 fatty acids; (3) increased dietary fiber, fruit, and vegetables; (4) increased micronutrients (e.g., folate and vitamins B_6 and B_{12}); (5) increased plant protein in lieu of animal protein; (6) reduced portions of highly processed foods; and (7) adopting a more Mediterranean or "prudent" dietary pattern over the prevailing "Western" dietary pattern (Forman and Bulwer, 2006). Other important lifestyle interventions include increased physical activity and smoking cessation (Forman and Bulwer, 2006).

Classic cardiovascular risk factors are consistent and common but largely undertreated and undercontrolled in many regions of the world (Bhatt et al, 2006). See Table 6-1 regarding the strength of evidence related to dietary recommendations in heart disease. Table 6-2 lists other influential factors on lipids as related to heart disease. Table 6-3 highlights key nutrients (folic acid, potassium, magnesium, and calcium) and provide lists of heart healthy food choices based on the Dietary Approaches to Stop Hypertension (DASH) diet principles.

TABLE 6-1 Levels of Evidence in Dietary Recommendations for Heart Disease[a]

Dietary Recommendation	Evidence Level
LDL Cholesterol Reduction	
1. A diet consisting of 25–35% total fat, <7% saturated and trans fat, and <200 mg dietary cholesterol lowers serum total and LDL cholesterol 9–16% and decreases the risk of CHD.	I
2. Isocalorically replacing saturated fatty acids with MUFA and PUFA is associated with reductions in LDL cholesterol.	I
3. Data on the ideal isocaloric substitution of carbohydrate and protein to maximize LDL cholesterol lowering are unavailable.	V
Hypertension	
4. Consuming a diet rich in fruits and vegetables and low-fat dairy products and low in sodium and saturated fat will decrease blood pressure. Reductions have been 4–12 mm Hg in systolic and 1–3 mm Hg in diastolic blood pressure. This dietary pattern is enhanced by weight loss and increased physical activity, which will also have beneficial effects (4–10 mm Hg in systolic pressure and 3-5 mm Hg in diastolic pressure).	I

(continued)

TABLE 6-1 Levels of Evidence in Dietary Recommendations for Heart Disease[a] *(continued)*

Dietary Recommendation	Evidence Level
Nuts	
5. Consumption of 50–113 g (1/2 to 1 cup) of nuts daily with a diet low in saturated fat and decreased total cholesterol by 4–21% and LDL cholesterol by 6–29% when weight was not gained.	II
6. Consumption of 5 ounces of nuts per week is associated with reduced risk of CVD.	II
Antioxidants	
7. Supplemental beta-carotene (60–200 mg/d) does not decrease the risk for cardiovascular death or nonfatal myocardial infarction (MI) in primary and secondary prevention patients.	I
8. Supplemental vitamin E, given in both natural and synthetic forms, in doses of 30–600 mg/d or 400–800 IU/d, alone or in combination with other antioxidants, has not been shown to decrease the risk for all-cause mortality, cardiovascular death, and fatal or nonfatal MI. Doses at this level have not been shown to cause harm.	II
9. Supplemental vitamin E (100–1200 IU/d) alone or in combination with other antioxidants has not been shown to have a favorable or unfavorable effect on serum lipids.	II
10. Supplemental vitamin C (50–1000 mg/d) in combination with other antioxidants (vitamin E, beta-carotene, selenium) has not been shown to have any effect on all-cause mortality, cardiovascular death, and fatal or nonfatal MI.	II
11. Supplemental beta-carotene (60–120 mg/d) is associated with an increase in all-cause mortality and cardiovascular death in patients at increased risk for lung cancer.	II
12. Supplemental vitamins C and E, beta-carotene, and selenium should not be taken with simvastatin–niacin drug combinations because the combination of these antioxidants may lower HDL2 cholesterol, a beneficial subfraction of HDL cholesterol.	II
13. Not enough evidence exists to demonstrate the benefits or harm of supplemental coenzyme Q10 and its use in CVD.	III
14. 3-Hydroxy-3-methylglutaryl coenzyme A (HMG-CoA) reductase inhibitors (a cholesterol-lowering class of medicines, also called statins) have been shown to decrease plasma levels of coenzyme Q10. Levels can be normalized when coenzyme Q10 supplementation is taken at the same time as the statin drugs; however, the clinical significance of this has not been determined.	IV
15. Epidemiological data suggest that intake of foods rich in vitamins E and C and beta carotene (dietary antioxidants) as part of a cardioprotective dietary pattern have been associated with decreased risk for coronary heart disease.	III
Soy Protein and Cholesterol and Triglyceride Levels	
16. Studies varied greatly in their estimation of the effect of diets low in saturated fat and cholesterol containing ~26–50 g of soy protein either as food or as a soy supplement, with 0–165 mg of isoflavones. Studies of individuals with normal and elevated cholesterol (total cholesterol >200 mg/dL) and individuals with diabetes varied, showing: • no effect on total cholesterol to up to 20% lower serum total cholesterol • no effect on triglycerides to up to 22% lower triglycerides • small effect (4%) on LDL to up to 24% lower LDL cholesterol	II
17. A significant dose-response relationship has not been established between level of soy protein and/or isoflavones in the diet needed to achieve significant decreases in total and LDL cholesterol	III
18. Effect of soy protein and/or isoflavones may vary based on initial cholesterol levels.	III
19. There is insufficient evidence supporting the benefit of added isoflavones on improving total and LDL cholesterol.	III
20. Diets containing up to 30 g of soy protein (as supplements) per day were well tolerated.	II
Fiber	
21. Consuming diets high in total fiber (17–30 g/d) and soluble fiber (7–13 g/d) as part of a diet low in saturated fat and cholesterol can further reduced total cholesterol by 2–3% and LDL by up to 7%.	I
22. Consuming diets high in total dietary fiber (>25 g/d) is associated with decreased risk for CHD and CVD.	II
23. Limited research indicates that other risk factors for CHD may be modified by a diet low in saturated fat and cholesterol and high in total and soluble fiber. These risk factors include blood pressure, lipoprotein subclasses and particle sizes, and fasting and postprandial insulin.	III

(continued)

TABLE 6-1 Levels of Evidence in Dietary Recommendations for Heart Disease[a] *(continued)*

Dietary Recommendation	Evidence Level
Statins, Sterols, and Hyperlipidemia	
24. Plant sterols and stanols are potent hypocholesterolemic agents, and a daily consumption of 2–3 g (through margarine, low-fat yogurt, orange juice, breads, and cereals) lowers total cholesterol concentrations in a dose-dependent manner by 4–11% and LDL cholesterol concentrations by 7–15% without changing HDL cholesterol or triacylglycerol concentrations.	I
25. For patients receiving statin therapy, plant stanols further reduce LDL and total cholesterol.	I
26. The total and LDL cholesterol-lowering effects of stanols and sterols are evident even when sterols and stanols are consumed as part of a cholesterol-lowering diet.	I
27. The cholesterol-lowering effects are similarly caused by sterols and stanols. Sterols lowered total cholesterol by 6–11% and LDL cholesterol by 7–15%. Stanols lowered total cholesterol by 4–10% and LDL cholesterol by 7–14%. Although the reductions in total and LDL cholesterol are similar, two high-quality randomized controlled trials in hypercholesterolemic adults report slightly greater, although nonsignificant, effects with consumption of stanols compared to sterols.	II
28. Nonesterified and esterified forms of sterols and stanols are equally effective. Consumption of 2–3 g of nonesterified sterols and stanols reduced total cholesterol by 4–11% and LDL cholesterol by 8–15%, and esterified sterols and stanols reduced total cholesterol by 6–10% and LDL cholesterol by 7–15%.	III
29. An intake of 2–3 g of plant sterols and stanols per day generally appears to be safe.	II
30. Data regarding whether the dose of statins can be reduced by the use of stanols and sterols are needed.	V
31. It is unclear whether there are unintended adverse effects when consuming stanols and sterols. Some studies have observed no significant differences in plasma carotenoid concentrations, including alpha-carotene and lycopene, and vitamins A, D, and E, but other studies have found that alpha-tocopherol and alpha- and beta-carotene plasma concentrations decrease after consumption of sterols and stanols, even after adjusting for changes in plasma lipid levels.	V
32. Preliminary research suggests that consuming one extra carotenoid-rich fruit or vegetable per day can maintain plasma carotenoid levels when also consuming sterol-enriched spreads.	V
Omega-3 Fatty Acids	
33. Randomized clinical trials have shown that approximately 1 g/d of eicosapentaenoic acid (EPA) and docosahexaenoic acid (DHA) from a supplement or fish decreases the risk of death from cardiac events in patients with heart disease.	II
34. Epidemiological studies indicate that regular consumption of an average of two servings of fatty fish per week (about 3.5 oz per serving; high in long-chain omega-3 fatty acids, such as EPA and DHA) is associated with a 30–40% reduced risk of death from cardiac events in subjects without prior disease.	II
35. Increased plasma levels and adipose tissue and cholesterol ester concentrations of alpha linolenic acid, EPA, and DHA have been associated with reduced risk of mortality.	II
36. Epidemiological studies indicate that inclusion of vegetable oils and food sources high in alpha linolenic acid, resulting in a total intake of >1.5 g/d, is associated with a 40–65% reduced risk of death from cardiac events.	III
37. One recent study of moderate quality has shown no protective effect of fish in patients with angina (n = 1109). However, the fish oil-supplemented group with angina in this study (3 g/wk, n = 462) showed significantly higher cardiac death and sudden death ($p < 0.05$). There is insufficient research to indicate whether the harm associated with fish oil supplement intake by angina patients is a result of the difference between fish and supplement intervention or special population characteristics.	III

Source: American Dietetic Association. Evidence analysis library. http://www.adaevidencelibrary.org/default.cfm?auth=1. Summary adapted by Chris Biesemeier, March 23, 2005.

[a] Key: Level I evidence = strong evidence from randomized controlled trials; level II evidence = moderate evidence; level III evidence = less evidence supporting a finding; level IV evidence = consensus of expert opinion.

TABLE 6-2 Key Influences on Lipids and Other Factors in Heart Disease

Influence	Description
Alcohol	Moderate red wine consumption for 4 weeks may be associated with desirable changes in HDL cholesterol and fibrinogen (Hansen et al, 2005). The "French paradox" suggests that wine intake and type of fat consumed are especially protective (Bellisle, 2005; Curtis et al, 2005). The 2005 Dietary Guidelines do not support a beverage-specific effect on risk reduction for heart disease.
Alpha linolenic acid (ALA)	ALA in flaxseed, walnuts, and canola oil may protect against sudden cardiac death. It may prevent cardiac arrhythmias; optimal intake of ALA seems to be about 2 g/d or 0.6–1% of total energy intake (de Lorgeril and Salen, 2004).
Aspirin and salicylates	Aspirin (usually 80 mg/d) and other salicylates inhibit production of enzymes that influence platelet release and aggregation, vasoconstriction, and vasodilation. Salicylates have analgesic, antipyretic, and anti-inflammatory properties. They occur naturally in many foods, including herbs, spices, fruits, and tomatoes. Post-MI patients experience a reduction in the risk of coronary heart disease (CHD) death from a pharmacologic approach (Robinson and Maheshwari, 2005), but since aspirin may cause GI bleeding, it should be used with caution.
Apolipoprotein (Apo) E phenotype	ApoE genotype modifies the serum lipid response to changes in dietary fat and cholesterol intake. Inherited hypercholesterolemias are common disorders characterized by elevated LDL cholesterol levels and premature coronary heart disease; autosomal recessive hypercholesterolemia (ARH) has reduced LDL catabolism (Fellin et al, 2003). People in rural Italy often have very low HDL but live without heart disease; they have ApoA1 genetic mutations.
Carbohydrate	High-glycemic index foods should be studied further for their effects on heart disease (Mozaffarian et al, 2004).
C-reactive protein (CRP)	Laboratory evidence suggests that inflammation is important in atherosclerosis. CRP is one of the acute phase proteins that increase during systemic inflammation (Bickel et al, 2002). Testing CRP levels in the blood may be a way to assess cardiovascular disease risk. A higher intake of fat tends to be associated with lower CRP values among women (Fredrikson et al, 2004); this may reflect the role of fats on inflammatory processes. Irrespective of LDL cholesterol levels, patients who have low CRP levels after statin therapy have more favorable clinical outcomes than those with higher CRP levels (Ridker et al, 2005). Dietary/lifestyle factors that decrease CRP levels are: weight loss (Li et al, 2005), alpha linolenic acid (Zhao et al, 2004), vegetarian diet (Jenkins et al, 2003; Szeto et al, 2004), low glycemic load diet (Pereira et al, 2004), and moderate alcohol consumption (Sierksma et al, 2002).
Cholesterol, total serum	<200 mg/dL is desirable; 200–239 mg/dL is borderline high; >240 mg/dL is high (NHLBI, 2001). Serum total cholesterol shows a positive association with CHD morbidity and mortality in men aged 65 years and older (Anum and Adera, 2004). Age, lifestyle habits (expressed as smoking and body mass index), and serum cholesterol levels are consistently associated with CHD mortality (Pitsavos et al, 2003). The ATP III report found that older persons with established CHD can show benefit from LDL-lowering therapy.
Cholesterol, HDL	Low levels of HDL cholesterol are an independent risk factor for cardiovascular death (NHLBI, 2001). HDL <40 mg/dL is low and not desirable; >60 mg/dL is high and better (NHLBI, 2001). In women, changes in HDL cholesterol and triglyceride levels are better predictors of coronary risk than LDL or total cholesterol (Meagher, 2004; Shai et al, 2004).
Cholesterol, LDL	Initiate therapeutic lifestyle changes (TLC) if LDL is above goal; this is a primary target of therapy. LDL <100 mg/dL is optimal; 100–129 mg/dL is near optimal; 130–159 mg/dL is borderline high; 160–189 mg/dL is high; and >190 mg/dL is very high (NHLBI, 2001). Drugs such as statins may be helpful in lowering LDL cholesterol (Nesto, 2005).
Copper	Elevated serum copper levels appear to be positively correlated with CHD; copper is a strong pro-oxidant (Ford and Giles, 2000). Zinc and copper relationships may also be relevant; larger and less atherogenic LDL particles are associated with a high zinc to copper ratio (Schulpis et al, 2004). However, supplementation with zinc is not recommended at this time because the relationship of these two minerals is complex and excesses of zinc are not desirable.
Dairy products	It may be useful to consume lower fat dairy products, especially because they provide a major source of vitamins and minerals (Ranganathan et al, 2005).
Diabetes	There are many factors that affect cardiovascular disease (CVD) in diabetes. Elevated systolic and diastolic blood pressure, high serum cholesterol level, high body mass index, presence of diabetes, and smoking status are key risks for CHD among women (Daviglus et al, 2004). Among diabetic persons, replacement of saturated fat with monounsaturated fat may be especially important (Tanasescu et al, 2004).
Eggs	Eggs are a source of dietary cholesterol. However, healthy men and women who eat 1 egg daily are unlikely to have a higher risk of coronary artery disease (CAD) or stroke than those who do not (Hu et al, 1999). Persons who eat eggs often may want to limit their intake to no more than 1 whole egg daily, especially if they also have diabetes.
Erythrocyte rate sedimentation and inflammation	Erythrocyte sedimentation rate is a marker of inflammation (Godsland et al, 2004). Whether this signifies an independent marker for heart disease remains to be seen. The relationship between asthma-related inflammation and heart failure is also being studied.
Estrogen	High plasma triglycerides are an independent risk factor for CHD; levels are reduced by androgens (methyltestosterone) combined with esterified estrogen in women (Chiuve et al, 2005). Hormone replacement therapy may protect younger rather than older women.

(continued)

TABLE 6-2 Key Influences on Lipids and Other Factors in Heart Disease *(continued)*

Influence	Description
Exercise	Low fitness in adolescents and adults is common in the U.S. population and is associated with an increased prevalence of CVD risk factors (Carnethon et al, 2005). Increased exercise is associated with a lower waist circumference and higher HDL cholesterol levels (Heim et al, 2000). Physical activity is associated with reduced risk of CVD among women; inactive women would benefit by even slightly increasing activity, such as walking (Oguma and Shinoda-Tagawa, 2004).
Fats, monounsaturated fatty acids (MUFA)	Substitution of virgin olive oil for saturated fats may decrease saturated fatty acids (SFA), increase HDL cholesterol, lower triglycerides, and increase antioxidant polyphenols (Ferrara et al, 2000). Extra virgin olive oil has the most phytochemicals and strongest flavor. Nuts provide a good source of MUFA also.
Fats, saturated	SFA is more important than total cholesterol intake in affecting serum total and LDL cholesterol levels. Intake of fatty red meat versus lean red meat or poultry and fish and high-fat versus low-fat dairy products results in a significant decrease in SFA (Hu et al, 1999). A higher level of energy from SFA intake yields greater risk of CHD, especially in women (Jakobsen et al, 2004).
Fermented milk products	Regular intake of yogurt containing an appropriate strain of *Lactobacillus acidophilus* may reduce risk for CAD and stroke (Anderson et al, 1999). Fermented milk acts like an ACE inhibitor when taken daily (just ½ cup) for several months or longer (Seppo et al, 2003).
Fiber and whole grains	Whole grains and high fiber intakes, particularly from cereals, vegetables, and fruits, are protective against CHD (Lairon et al, 2005). Mechanisms by which fiber may protect against CHD include lowering blood cholesterol (soluble fibers), attenuating blood triglyceride levels (mostly soluble fibers), decreasing hypertension (all fibers), and normalizing postprandial blood glucose levels (all fibers). The total amount of fiber from fiber-containing foods is important, and individuals should not focus on soluble fiber only.
Folic acid	Diets that are low in folate and carotenoids (beta-carotene and lutein/zeaxanthin) contribute to increased coronary risk mortality (Connor et al, 2004).
Glycemic load, high	High glycemic load due to high intake of refined carbohydrates is positively related to CAD risk, independent of other known risk factors (Liu et al, 2000).
Grapefruit juice	Grapefruit juice can alter oral drug pharmacokinetics. Irreversible inactivation of intestinal cytochrome P-450 (CYP) 3A4 is produced by commercial grapefruit juice given as a single normal amount (e.g., 200–300 mL) or by whole fresh fruit segments (Bailey and Dresser, 2004). Avoid use with cardiac medications.
Homocysteine (tHcy)	Elevated plasma or serum tHcy levels are prevalent in the general population and are associated with increased risk of cardiac disease, stroke, and peripheral artery disease (Omland et al, 2000). Simple, inexpensive therapy with 400 μg folic acid and vitamins B_6 and B_{12} (500 μg cyanocobalamin) reduces plasma tHcy levels (Nallamothu et al, 2000). Habitual intake of commercially fortified breakfast cereals that contain 200 μg folic acid can reduce tHcy levels readily (Malinow et al, 2000). The Dietary Approaches to Stop Hypertension (DASH) diet also reduces levels of tHcy; this diet includes high quantities of fruits, vegetables, low-fat dairy products, whole grains, poultry, fish, and nuts. Sources of folate, calcium, potassium, and magnesium are listed in Table 6-3.
Iron	Controversy continues about the role of iron in heart disease. For example, in one study, middle-aged women with a relatively high heme iron intake may have an increased risk of CHD (Van der A et al, 2005). In other studies, anemia may be damaging to the heart (Silverberg et al, 2004). A carefully balanced intake is a safe recommendation.
Mediterranean diet	Long-term adoption of a Mediterranean type of diet, physical activity, and optimism is protective (Pitsavos et al, 2003). Mediterranean diets have a healthier balance between omega-3 and omega-6 fatty acids; many studies have shown that people who follow this diet are less likely to develop heart disease. The Mediterranean diet does not include much meat (higher in omega-6 fatty acids) and emphasizes foods rich in omega-3 fatty acids (e.g., whole grains, fresh fruits and vegetables, fish, olive oil, garlic, and wine).
Metabolic syndrome	Atherogenic dyslipidemia is a common form of dyslipidemia characterized by three lipid abnormalities: elevated triglycerides, small LDL particles, and reduced HDL cholesterol. The constellation of dyslipidemia, elevated blood pressure, impaired glucose tolerance, and central obesity is identified as metabolic syndrome (Deen, 2004). Prevention steps include: (1) correct overweight by reducing the energy density of the habitual diet (i.e., fat intake); and (2) improve insulin sensitivity and associated metabolic abnormalities through a reduction of dietary saturated fat, partially replaced, when appropriate, by monounsaturated and polyunsaturated fats (Riccardi et al, 2004). Alcohol intake is controversial, since mild to moderate intake may be protective (Freiberg et al, 2004) while excessive intake is detrimental (den Boer et al, 2004).
Methionine	Found in red meats. May contribute to fatty plaque buildup by its relationship to homocysteine (Weisberg et al, 2003).
Nicotinic acid	Niacin has a potent effect on HDL cholesterol levels; data on cardiovascular event rate reductions are limited, and more research is needed (Birjhomun et al, 2005).
Nuts and seeds	Nuts provide monounsaturated fat, natural vitamin E, magnesium, and other heart-healthy nutrients (Maguire et al, 2004). Walnuts are rich in alpha linolenic acid and may lower total cholesterol and triglycerides in people with high cholesterol levels. Almonds improve plasma alpha-tocopherol and reduce plasma lipids (Jambazian et al, 2005). Frequent nut and seed consumption lowers risk for CVD and diabetes (Jiang et al, 2006).

(continued)

TABLE 6-2 **Key Influences on Lipids and Other Factors in Heart Disease *(continued)***

Influence	Description
Obesity	For individuals with no cardiovascular risk factors and for individuals with 1 or more risk factors, those who are obese in middle age have a higher risk of hospitalization and mortality from CHD, CVD, and diabetes in older age than those who are normal weight (Yan et al, 2006). A major goal of dietary prevention and treatment of most heart diseases is to attain and maintain weight control at an ideal body weight. Decreasing excess calories, reducing total fat intake, adding fiber, reducing excess intake of refined carbohydrates, and increasing exercise can all help achieve this goal. Of the many weight loss plans (Atkins, Ornish, Weight Watchers, and Zone diets), each diet modestly reduced body weight and several cardiac risk factors after 1 year; increased adherence was associated with greater weight loss and cardiac risk factor reductions for each diet group (Dansinger et al, 2005). Waist to hip ratio is a greater predictor of heart disease than body mass index (BMI) (Mataix et al, 2005; Mitka, 2005).
Omega-3 fatty acids	Both eicosapentaenoic acid (EPA) and docosahexaenoic acid (DHA) in foods decrease production of inflammatory mediators (Mantzioris et al, 2000). DHA supplementation may be of benefit for hyperlipidemic children (Engler et al, 2005). Omega-3 polyunsaturated fatty acids (PUFAs) from both seafood and plant sources may reduce CHD risk, and plant-based omega-3 PUFAs may particularly reduce CHD risk when seafood-based omega-3 PUFA intake is low, which has implications for populations with low intake of fatty fish (Mozaffarian et al, 2005).
Oral health	Poor oral health may be a risk factor for CHD; improvement of periodontal status may influence the related systemic inflammation (Craig et al, 2003).
Phytosterols and stanols	Plant stanol or sterol esters are found in plant foods such as corn, soy, and other vegetable oils; they are derived from plant phytosterols. Plant stanol esters block intestinal absorption of dietary and biliary cholesterol (Hallikainen et al, 2000). Fat-soluble vitamins are not signficantly affected. Evidence is sufficient to promote use of sterols and stanols for lowering LDL cholesterol levels in persons at increased risk for CHD (Patch et al, 2005; Katan et al, 2003). Products such as Benecol Smart Chews require intake of 4 daily to acquire 3.4 g. Sunflower kernels and pistachio nuts have the highest content of phytosterols that are commonly consumed; sesame seeds and wheat germ are also very high in natural content (Phillips et al, 2005).
Plasma lipoprotein (a) [Lp(a)]	Elevated plasma Lp(a) is an independent risk factor of heart disease. Ethnicity-related differences in mean Lp(a) exist among children and adolescents in the United States, and parental history of premature heart attack/angina is significantly associated with levels of Lp(a) in children (Obesisan et al, 2004).
Quercetin, flavonols, and antioxidants in fruits and vegetables	Quercetin protects against CHD, stroke, cataracts, and hypertension (Knekt et al, 2000). Fruit and vegetable intake is also protective against CHD and stroke (Sampson et al, 2002). Risk reduction by 20–40% has been estimated. Flavonoids in red wine, grape juice, grapefruit, tea, onions, and apples are possible risk reducers; cloves, licorice, and sage may also be beneficial (Keevil et al, 2000). Research is ongoing to evaluate how dark chocolate has flavonols that tend to lower serum cholesterol and blood pressure, as well as improve insulin sensitivity. Pomegranate has been found to be especially beneficial in lowering cholesterol synthesis and foam cell production (Fuhrman et al, 2005). The activation of nuclear transcription factor kappa B has been linked with a variety of inflammatory diseases, including atherosclerosis and myocardial infarction; use of spices and herbs can suppress this pathway (Aggarwal and Shishodia, 2004). Vegetables, citrus fruits, seeds, olive oil, tea, and flavonoid spices may be beneficial antioxidant foods to include in the diet (Blomhoff, 2005). Fruits are more protective than vegetables.
Smoking	Both active smoking and secondary exposure are associated with the progression of an index of atherosclerotic heart disease; smoking is of greater concern for persons who also have diabetes mellitus and hypertension (Howard et al, 1998) or who drink alcohol (Ebbert et al, 2005).
Soy protein	The FDA permits labeling of products high in soy protein as helpful in lowering heart disease risk. Products must contain at least 6.25 g per serving. Tofu contains 13 g of soy protein in one 4-oz serving; one soy burger contains 10–12 g of protein; 1/4 cup of soy nuts and 1/2 cup of tempeh contain 19 g of protein each. Dietary intake of soy isoflavones improves the lipid profile of premenopausal women during all phases of the menstrual cycle (Merz-Demlow et al, 2000). Dietary intakes of soy protein (at least 20 g) and isoflavones (at least 80 mg) for 5 weeks are effective in reducing CHD risk among high-risk, middle-aged men (Sagara et al, 2004).
Trans fatty acids (TFAs)	TFAs are strongly associated with systemic inflammation in patients with heart disease; attention to TFA intake may be important for secondary prevention efforts (Mozaffarian et al, 2004). By January 1, 2006, food labels were required to list the amount of TFAs in all products (Eller et al, 2005).
Triglycerides	High level of triglycerides is an independent risk factor of cardiovascular death (NHLBI, 2001). A high-fat triglyceride-lowering diet for patients with only slightly elevated serum triglyceride concentrations may be helpful; however, a lower fat diet is more suitable to lower more elevated triglycerides (Jacobs et al, 2004).
Vitamin C	Vitamin C has a role in cholesterol metabolism and affects levels of LDL cholesterol. Men, smokers, elderly individuals, and persons with diabetes mellitus or hypertension tend to have lower levels of serum ascorbic acid and higher risks for heart disease. Antioxidant therapy with vitamins C and E may restore endothelial function in hyperlipidemic children; early detection and treatment may retard the progression of atherosclerosis (Engler et al, 2003).
Vitamin E	Alpha-tocopherol decreases lipid peroxidation and platelet aggregation and functions as a potent anti-inflammatory agent, but prospective human clinical trials with alpha-tocopherol have not shown effectiveness in lowering CHD risk (Jialal and Devaraj, 2005). Tocotrienols may be more effective in reducing endothelial expression of adhesion molecules in the blood vasculature, which is a critical step in the formation of plaque (Halliwell et al, 2005; Schaffer et al, 2005; Sen et al, 2004).
Vitamin K	Vitamin K influences vascular health. Factor X-a and thrombin relate to smooth muscle cells, and vitamin K–dependent matrix GLA protein is found in many cells, including the vascular smooth muscle cells (Bern, 2004). Studies about the role of vitamin K in heart health are continuing.

TABLE 6-3 Key Sources of Folate, Potassium, Calcium, and Magnesium and DASH Diet Principles

Folate Sources	Micrograms (μg)	Folate Sources	Micrograms (μg)
Breakfast cereals fortified with 100% of the daily value (DV), ¾ cup	400	Avocado, raw, all varieties, sliced, ½ cup sliced	45
Beef liver, cooked, braised, 3 oz	185	Peanuts, all types, dry roasted, 1 ounce	40
Cowpeas (blackeyes), immature, cooked, boiled, ½ cup	105	Lettuce, romaine, shredded, ½ cup	40
Breakfast cereals, fortified with 25% of the DV, ¾ cup	100	Wheat germ, crude, 2 tablespoons	40
Spinach, frozen, cooked, boiled, ½ cup	100	Tomato juice, canned, 6 oz	35
Great Northern beans, boiled, ½ cup	90	Orange juice, chilled, includes concentrate, ¾ cup	35
Asparagus, boiled, 4 spears	85	Turnip greens, frozen, cooked, boiled, ½ cup	30
Rice, white, long-grain, parboiled, enriched, cooked, ½ cup	65	Orange, all commercial varieties, fresh, 1 small	30
Vegetarian baked beans, canned, 1 cup	60	Bread, white, 1 slice	25
Spinach, raw, 1 cup	60	Bread, whole wheat, 1 slice	25
Green peas, frozen, boiled, ½ cup	50	Egg, whole, raw, fresh, 1 large	25
Broccoli, chopped, frozen, cooked, ½cup	50	Cantaloupe, raw, ¼ medium	25
Egg noodles, cooked, enriched, ½ cup	50	Papaya, raw, ½ cup cubes	25
Broccoli, raw, 2 spears (each 5 inches long)	45	Banana, raw, 1 medium	20

From: U.S. Department of Agriculture, Agricultural Research Service. USDA national nutrient database for standard reference, Release 16. 2003. Nutrient Data Laboratory Home Page, accessed at http://www.nal.usda.gov/fnic/cgi-bin/nut_search.pl.

Potassium Sources	Milligrams (mg)	Potassium Sources	Milligrams (mg)
Apricots, 3 medium	272	Orange juice, 8 oz	473
Artichoke, 1 cup, raw	644	Papaya, 1 whole	781
Avocado, Jerusalem, 1 medium	976	Potato, baked with skin, medium	1081
Banana, 1 cup	537	Pumpkin, 1 cup, cooked	564
Beans, canned white, 1 cup	1189	Prunes (dried plums), 1 cup, stewed	796
Beet greens, boiled, ½ cup	653	Prune juice, 1 cup	707
Broccoli, 1 cup chopped	457	Raisins, 1/3 cup	362
Cantaloupe, 1 cup	427	Refried beans, canned, 1 cup	673
Grapefruit juice, sweetened, 1 cup	405	Spinach, 1 cup, cooked	574
Halibut, cooked, ½ fillet	916	Sweet potato, canned, 1 cup	796
Kidney beans, 1 cup	713	Tomato, 1 medium	426
Kiwifruit, 1 medium	252	Tomato juice, 6 oz	417
Lima beans, cooked, 1 cup	955	Tomato puree, ½ cup	1328
Milk, 1 cup, skim	382	Tomato sauce, 1 cup	940
Milk, 1 cup, chocolate	425	Tropical trail mix, 1 cup	993
Milkshake, 16 oz, vanilla	579	Vegetable juice cocktail, 1 cup, canned	467
Nectarine, 1 medium	273	Winter squash, 1 cup	896
Orange, 1 medium	237	Yogurt, 8 oz, low fat	443

For other sources, see http://www.nal.usda.gov/fnic/foodcomp/Data/SR17/wtrank/sr17w306.pdf; accessed March 15, 2005.

Calcium Sources	Milligrams (mg)	Calcium Sources	Milligrams (mg)
Broccoli, cooked, 1 cup	156	Collards, 1 cup, cooked	266
Cheddar cheese, 1 oz	204	Eggnog, 1 cup	330
Cheese sauce, 1 cup	756	Enchilada with cheese, 1	324
Cheese, Swiss, 1 oz	224	Milk, canned evaporated, 1 cup	742
Clam chowder, New England, 1 cup	186	Milk, fluid, 1%, 1 cup	290

(continued)

TABLE 6-3 Key Sources of Folate, Potassium, Calcium, and Magnesium and DASH Diet Principles *(continued)*

Calcium Sources	Milligrams (mg)	Calcium Sources	Milligrams (mg)
Milk, fluid, chocolate, low fat, 1 cup	288	Tofu made with calcium, ¼ block	164
Milkshake, thick, vanilla, 11 oz	457	Total brand cereal, ¾ cup	1104
Molasses, blackstrap, 1 tablespoon	172	Sardines, canned with bones, 3 oz	325
Pudding, chocolate, 4 oz, ready to serve	102	Spinach, canned, 1 cup	272
Ricotta cheese, part skim, 1 cup	669	Turnip greens, frozen, cooked, 1 cup	249
Soybeans, green, cooked, 1 cup	261	Yogurt, low fat with fruit, 1 cup	345

For a more specific list, see http://www.nal.usda.gov/fnic/foodcomp/Data/SR17/wtrank/sr17w301.pdf; accessed March 22, 2005.

Magnesium Sources	Milligrams (mg)	Magnesium Sources	Milligrams (mg)
Barley, pearled, raw 1 cup	158	Okra, cooked, 1 cup	94
Beans, canned white, 1 cup	134	Plantain, raw, 1 medium	66
Broccoli, cooked, 1 cup	33	Seeds, pumpkin or squash seed kernels, 1 oz (142 seeds)	151
Cereal, All-Bran, ½ cup	109	Soybeans, mature, cooked, 1 cup	148
Chocolate candy, semisweet, 1 cup	193	Spinach, cooked, 1 cup	163
Halibut, cooked, ½ fillet	170	Tomato paste, 1 cup	110
Nuts, Brazil, 6–8	107	Trail mix, with chocolate chips, nuts, seeds, 1 cup	235
Oat bran, 1 cup	221	Whole-grain wheat flour, 1 cup	166

For a more specific list, see http://www.nal.usda.gov/fnic/foodcomp/Data/SR17/wtrank/sr17w304.pdf; accessed March 23, 2005.

Food	DASH Diet Principles
Vegetables, choose 4–5 servings daily	Carrots, sweet potatoes, pumpkin, winter squash Green leafy vegetables (broccoli, kale, cabbage, etc.), green beans Tomato salsas, 6-oz servings of tomato juice or other vegetable juices
Fruits, choose 4–5 servings daily	Fresh fruits, including apples, bananas, cantaloupe, melons, berries Red or black grapes; grape juice (1 cup per day) Grapefruit, especially pink (40% more beta-carotene) Dried fruits, especially apricots, dates, prunes Pomegranates and other antioxidant juices (blueberry juice, red wine, orange juice, cranberry juice, green tea)
Protein-rich foods, choose 2 or less	Lean chicken and turkey breast Salmon and other fish Meats that are lean or have fat trimmed away
Low-fat dairy, 2–3 servings daily	Skim milk and yogurt (8 oz) Low-fat cheeses (1–1/2 oz per serving)
Low-fat foods	Tomato sauces with pasta Homemade pizza with low-fat toppings (chicken, vegetables, low-fat cheese)
Grains, choose 7–8 servings daily	Oatmeal, shredded wheat; high-fiber, low-sugar cereals Baked whole-wheat chips and tortillas Whole-grain breads and pastas
Nuts, seeds, and dry beans, 4–5 servings per week	Peanuts, walnuts, almonds, other nuts in moderation Bean and chickpea dishes and dips
Oils, 2–3 servings	Olive oil and canola oil substituted for other oils Salad dressings and dips with nonfat sour cream or homemade yogurt

Note: Most of these foods are recommended in the DASH and Mediterranean diets. For more information, see http://www.nhlbi.nih.gov/health/public/heart/hbp/dash/new_dash.pdf.

CITED REFERENCES

Aggarwal BB, Shishodia S. Suppression of the nuclear factor-kappaB activation pathway by spice-derived phytochemicals: reasoning for seasoning. *Ann N Y Acad Sci.* 1030:434, 2004.

Anderson C. Dietary modification and CVD prevention: a matter of fat. *JAMA.* 295:693, 2006.

Anderson J, et al. Effect of fermented milk (yogurt) containing *Lactobacillus* L1 on serum cholesterol in hypercholesterolemic humans. *J Am Col Nutr.* 18:43, 1999.

Anum EA, Adera T. Hypercholesterolemia and coronary heart disease in the elderly: a meta-analysis. *Ann Epidemiol.* 14:705, 2004.

Bailey DG, Dresser GK. Interactions between grapefruit juice and cardiovascular drugs. *Am J Cardiovasc Drugs.* 4:281, 2004.

Bellisle F. Nutrition and health in France: dissecting a paradox. *J Am Diet Assoc.* 105:1870, 2005.

Bern M. Observations on possible effects of daily vitamin K replacement, especially on warfarin therapy. *JPEN J Parenter Enteral Nutr.* 28:388, 2004.

Berneis K, et al. Low-density lipoprotein size and subclasses are markers of clinically apparent and non-apparent atherosclerosis in type 2 diabetes. *Metabolism* 54:227, 2005.

Bhatt DL, et al. International prevalence, recognition, and treatment of cardiovascular risk factors in outpatients with atherothrombosis. *JAMA.* 295:180, 2006.

Bickel C, et al. Relation of markers of inflammation (C-reactive protein, fibrinogen, von Willebrand factor, and leukocyte count) and statin therapy to long-term mortality in patients with angiographically proven coronary artery disease. *Am J Cardiol.* 89:901, 2002.

Birjhomun RS, et al. Efficacy and safety of high-density lipoprotein cholesterol-increasing compounds: a meta-analysis of randomized controlled trials. *J Am Coll Cardiol.* 45:185, 2005.

Blomhoff R. Dietary antioxidants and cardiovascular disease. *Curr Opin Lipidol.* 16:47, 2005.

Carnethon MR, et al. Prevalence and cardiovascular disease correlates of low cardiorespiratory fitness in adolescents and adults. *JAMA.* 294:2981, 2005.

Chiuve SE, et al. Effect of the combination of methyltestosterone and esterified estrogens compared with esterified estrogens alone on apolipoprotein CIII and other high-density lipoproteins in surgically postmenopausal women. *Obstet Gynecol Surv.* 60:39, 2005.

Connor S, et al. Diets lower in folic acid and carotenoids are associated with the coronary disease epidemic in central and eastern Europe. *J Am Diet Assoc.* 104:1793, 2004.

Craig RG, et al. Relationship of destructive periodontal disease to the acute-phase response. *J Periodontol.* 74:1007, 2003.

Curtis A, et al. Alcohol-free red wine prevents arterial thrombosis in dietary-induced hypercholesterolemic rats: experimental support for the 'French paradox'. *J Thromb Haemost.* 3:346, 2005.

Dansinger ML, et al. Comparison of the Atkins, Ornish, Weight Watchers, and Zone diets for weight loss and heart disease risk reduction: a randomized trial. *JAMA.* 293:43, 2005.

Daviglus ML, et al. Favorable cardiovascular risk profile in young women and long-term risk of cardiovascular and all-cause mortality. *JAMA.* 292:1588, 2004.

Deen D. Metabolic syndrome: time for action. *Am Fam Physician.* 69:2875, 2004.

de Lorgeril M, Salen P. Alpha-linolenic acid and coronary heart disease. *Nutr Metab Cardiovasc Dis.* 14:162, 2004.

den Boer M, et al. Hepatic steatosis: a mediator of the metabolic syndrome. Lessons from animal models. *Arterioscler Thromb Vasc Biol.* 24:644, 2004.

Ebbert J, et al. The association of alcohol consumption with coronary heart disease mortality and cancer incidence varies by smoking history. *J Gen Intern Med.* 20:14, 2005.

Eller FJ, et al. Preparation of spread oils meeting U.S. Food and Drug Administration labeling requirements for trans fatty acids via pressure-controlled hydrogenation. *J Agric Food Chem.* 53:5982, 2005.

Engler MM, et al. Docosahexaenoic acid restores endothelial function in children with hyperlipidemia: results from the EARLY study. *Int J Clin Pharmacol Ther.* 42:672, 2004.

Engler MM, et al. Effect of docosahexaenoic acid on lipoprotein subclasses in hyperlipidemic children (the EARLY study). *Am J Cardiol.* 95:869, 2005.

Fellin R, et al. Clinical and biochemical characterization of patients with autosomal recessive hypercholesterolemia (ARH). *Nutr Metab Cardiovasc Dis.* 13:278, 2003.

Ferrara L, et al. Olive oil and reduced need for antihypertensive medications. *Arch Int Med.* 160:837, 2000.

Ford E, Giles W. Serum vitamins, carotenoids, and angina pectoris: findings from the National Health and Nutrition Examination Survey III. *Ann Epidemiol.* 10:106, 2000.

Forman D, Bulwer BE. Cardiovascular disease: optimal approaches to risk factor modification of diet and lifestyle. *Curr Treat Options Cardiovasc Med.* 8:47, 2006.

Fredrikson GN, et al. Association between diet, lifestyle, metabolic cardiovascular risk factors, and plasma C-reactive protein levels. *Metabolism* 53:1436, 2004.

Freiberg MS, et al. Alcohol consumption and the prevalence of the metabolic syndrome in the U.S. *Diab Care.* 27:2954, 2004.

Fuhrman B, et al. Pomegranate juice inhibits oxidized LDL uptake and cholesterol biosynthesis in macrophages. *J Nutr Biochem.* 16:570, 2005.

Godsland IF, et al. Inflammation markers and erythrocyte sedimentation rate but not metabolic syndrome factor score predict coronary heart disease in high socioeconomic class males: the HDDRISC study. *Int J Cardiol.* 97:543, 2004.

Goff DC, et al. Insulin resistance and adiposity influence lipoprotein size and subclass concentrations. Results from the Insulin Resistance Atherosclerosis Study. *Metabolism* 54:264, 2005.

Gordon NF, et al. Effectiveness of therapeutic lifestyle changes in patients with hypertension, hyperlipidemia, and/or hyperglycemia. *Am J Cardiol.* 94:1558, 2004.

Hallikainen M, et al. Plant stanol esters affect serum cholesterol concentrations of hypercholesterolemic men and women in a dose-dependent manner. *J Nutr.* 130:767, 2000.

Halliwell B, et al. Health promotion by flavonoids, tocopherols, tocotrienols, and other phenols: direct or indirect effects? Antioxidant or not? *Am J Clin Nutr.* 81:268S, 2005.

Hansen AS, et al. Effect of red wine and red grape extract on blood lipids, haemostatic factors, and other risk factors for cardiovascular disease. *Eur J Clin Nutr.* 55:449, 2005.

Heim D, et al. Exercise mitigates the association of abdominal obesity with high-density lipoprotein cholesterol in premenopausal women: results from the third National Health and Nutrition Examination Survey. *J Am Diet Assoc.* 100:1347, 2000.

Howard BV, et al. Low-fat dietary pattern and risk of cardiovascular disease: the Women's Health Initiative Randomized Controlled Dietary Modification Trial. *JAMA.* 295:655, 2006.

Howard G, et al. Cigarette smoking and progression of atherosclerosis. *JAMA.* 279:119, 1998.

Hu F, et al. A prospective study of egg consumption and risk of cardiovascular disease in men and women. *JAMA.* 281:1387, 1999.

Jacobs B, et al. Individual serum triglyceride responses to high-fat and low-fat diets differ in men with modest and severe hypertriglyceridemia. *J Nutr.* 134:1400, 2004.

Jakobsen MU, et al. Dietary fat and risk of coronary heart disease: possible effect modification by gender and age. *Am J Epidemiol.* 160:141, 2004.

Jambazian PR, et al. Almonds in the diet simultaneously improve plasma alpha-tocopherol concentrations and reduce plasma lipids. *J Am Diet Assoc.* 105:449, 2005.

Jiang R, et al. Nut and seed consumption and inflammatory markers in the multi-ethnic study of atherosclerosis. *Am J Epidemiol.* 163:222, 2006.

Jonnalagadda SS. Dietary counseling is an important component of cardiac rehabilitation. *J Am Diet Assoc.* 105:1529, 2005.

Jenkins DJ, et al. Effects of a dietary portfolio of cholesterol-lowering foods vs lovastatin on serum lipids and C-reactive protein. *JAMA.* 290:502, 2003.

Jialal L, Devaraj S. Scientific evidence to support a vitamin E and heart disease health claim: research needs. *J Nutr.* 135:348, 2005.

Katan MB, et al. Efficacy and safety of plant stanols and sterols in the management of blood cholesterol levels. *Mayo Clin Proc.* 78:965, 2003.

Keevil J, et al. Grape juice, but not orange or grapefruit juice, inhibits human platelet aggregation. *J Nutr.* 130:53, 2000.

Knekt P, et al. Quercetin intake and the incidence of cerebrovascular disease. *Euro J Nutr.* 54:415, 2000.

Krummel D. Nutrition in cardiovascular disease. In: Mahan K, Escott-Stump S, eds. *Krause's food, nutrition, and diet therapy.* 11th ed. Philadelphia: WB Saunders, 2004.

Lairon D, et al. Dietary fiber intake and risk factors for cardiovascular disease in French adults. *Am J Clin Nutr.* 82:1185, 2005.

Li Z, et al. Long-term efficacy of soy-based meal replacements vs an individualized diet plan in obese type II DM patients: relative effects on weight loss, metabolic parameters, and C-reactive protein. *Eur J Clin Nutr.* 59:411, 2005.

Liu S, et al. A prospective study of dietary glycemic load, carbohydrate intake, and risk of coronary heart disease in U.S. women. *Am J Clin Nutr.* 71:1455, 2000.

Maguire LS, et al. Fatty acid profile, tocopherol, squalene and phytosterol content of walnuts, almonds, peanuts, hazelnuts and the macadamia nut. *Int J Food Sci Nutr.* 55:171, 2004.

Malinow M, et al. Increased plasma homocystine after withdrawal of ready-to-eat breakfast cereal from the diet: prevention by breakfast cereal providing 200 mg folic acid. *J Am Col Nutr.* 19:452, 2000.

Mantzioris E, et al. Biochemical effects of a diet containing foods enriched with n-3 fatty acids. *Am J Clin Nutr.* 72:42, 2000.

Mataix J, et al. Factors associated with obesity in an adult Mediterranean population: influence on plasma lipid profile. *J Am Coll Nutr.* 24:456, 2005.

Meagher EA. Addressing cardiovascular disease in women: focus on dyslipidemia. *J Am Board Fam Pract.* 17:424, 2004.
Merz-Demlow B, et al. Soy isoflavones improve plasma lipids in normocholesterolemic premenopausal women. *Am J Clin Nutr.* 71:1462, 2000.
Mitka M. Obesity's role in heart disease requires apples and pears comparison. *JAMA.* 294:3071, 2005.
Mozaffarian D, et al. Interplay between different polyunsaturated fatty acids and risk of coronary heart disease in men. *Circulation* 111:157, 2005.
Mozaffarian D, et al. Trans fatty acids and systemic inflammation in heart failure. *Am J Clin Nutr.* 80:1521, 2004.
Mozaffarian D, Rimm EB, Herrington DM. Dietary fats, carbohydrate, and progression of coronary atherosclerosis in postmenopausal women. *Am J Clin Nutr.* 80:1175, 2004.
Murabito JM, et al. Sibling cardiovascular disease as a risk factor for cardiovascular disease in middle-aged adults. *JAMA.* 294:3117, 2005.
Nallamothu B, et al. Potential clinical and economic effects of homocysteine lowering. *Arch Intern Med.* 160:3406, 2000.
National Heart, Lung, and Blood Institute (NHLBI). Third Report of the Expert Panel on Detection, Evaluation, and Treatment of High Blood Cholesterol in Adults (Adult Treatment Panel III). 2001. Accessed at http://www.nhlbi.nih.gov/guidelines/cholesterol/atglance.htm.
Nesto RW. Beyond low-density lipoprotein: addressing the atherogenic lipid triad in type 2 diabetes mellitus and the metabolic syndrome. *Am J Cardiovasc Drugs.* 5:379, 2005.
Nissen SE, et al. Effect of recombinant ApoA-I Milano on coronary atherosclerosis in patients with acute coronary syndromes: a randomized controlled trial. *JAMA.* 290:2292, 2003.
Obesisan TO, et al. Correlates of serum lipoprotein (A) in children and adolescents in the United States. The third National Health Nutrition and Examination Survey (NHANES-III). *Lipids Health Dis.* 3:29, 2004.
Oguma Y, Shinoda-Tagawa T. Physical activity decreases cardiovascular disease risk in women: review and meta-analysis. *Am J Prev Med.* 26:407, 2004.
Omland T, et al. Serum homocysteine concentration as an indicator of survival in patients with acute coronary syndromes. *Arch Intern Med.* 160:1834, 2000.
Pasternak RC. Report of the Adult Treatment Panel III: the 2001 National Cholesterol Education Program guidelines on the detection, evaluation and treatment of elevated cholesterol in adults. *Cardiol Clin.* 21:393, 2003.
Patch CS, et al. Plant sterol/stanol prescription is an effective treatment strategy for managing hypercholesterolemia in outpatient clinical practice. *J Am Diet Assoc.* 105:46, 2005.
Pereira MA, et al. Effects of a low-glycemic load diet on resting energy expenditure and heart disease risk factors during weight loss. *JAMA.* 292:2482, 2004
Phillips KM, et al. Phytosterol composition of nuts and seeds commonly consumed in the United States. *J Agric Food Chem.* 53:9436, 2005.
Pitsavos C, et al. Forty-year follow-up of coronary heart disease mortality and its predictors: the Corfu cohort of the seven countries study. *Prev Cardiol.* 6:155, 2003.
Ranganathan R, et al. The nutritional impact of dairy product consumption on dietary intakes of adults (1995-1996): The Bogalusa Heart Study. *J Am Diet Assoc.* 105:1391, 2005.
Riccardi G, et al. Dietary fat, insulin sensitivity and the metabolic syndrome. *Clin Nutr.* 23:447, 2004.
Ridker PM, et al. C-reactive protein levels and outcomes after statin therapy. *N Engl J Med.* 352:20, 2005.
Robinson JG, Maheshwari N. A "poly-portfolio" for secondary prevention: a strategy to reduce subsequent events by up to 97% over five years. *Am J Cardiol.* 95:373, 2005.
Sagara M, et al. Effects of dietary intake of soy protein and isoflavones on cardiovascular disease risk factors in high risk, middle-aged men in Scotland. *J Am Coll Nutr.* 23:85, 2004.
Sampson L, et al. Flavonol and flavone intakes in US health professionals. *J Am Diet Assoc.* 102:1414, 2002.
Schaffer S, et al. Tocotrienols: constitutional effects in aging and disease. *J Nutr.* 135:151, 2005.
Schulpis KH, et al. The association of serum lipids, lipoproteins and apolipoproteins with selected trace elements and minerals in phenylketonuric patients on diet. *Clin Nutr.* 23:401, 2004.
Sen CK, et al. Tocotrienol: the natural vitamin E to defend the nervous system? *Ann N Y Acad Sci.* 1031:127, 2004.
Seppo L, et al. A fermented milk high in bioactive peptides has a blood pressure-lowering effect in hypertensive subjects. *Am J Clin Nutr.* 77:326, 2003.
Shai I, et al. Multivariate assessment of lipid parameters as predictors of coronary heart disease among postmenopausal women: potential implications for clinical guidelines. *Circulation* 110:2824, 2004.
Shaw LJ, et al. Insights from the NHLBI-Sponsored Women's Ischemia Syndrome Evaluation (WISE) Study. Part I: gender differences in traditional and novel risk factors, symptom evaluation, and gender-optimized diagnostic strategies. *J Am Coll Cardiol.* 47:4S, 2006.
Sierksma A, et al. Moderate alcohol consumption reduces plasma C-reactive protein and fibrinogen levels; a randomized, diet-controlled intervention study. *Eur J Clin Nutr.* 56:1130, 2002
Silverberg DS, et al. The role of anemia in the progression of congestive heart failure. Is there a place for erythropoietin and intravenous iron? *J Nephrol.* 17:749, 2004.
Szeto YT, et al. Effects of a long-term vegetarian diet on biomarkers of antioxidant status and cardiovascular disease risk. *Nutrition* 20:863, 2004
Talbert RL. New therapeutic options in the National Cholesterol Education Program Adult Treatment Panel III. *Am J Manag Care.* 8:S301, 2002.
Tanasescu M, et al. Dietary fat and cholesterol and the risk of cardiovascular disease among women with type 2 diabetes. *Am J Clin Nutr.* 79:999, 2004.
Tucker KL. Dietary intake and coronary heart disease: a variety of nutrients and phytochemicals are important. *Curr Treat Options Cardiovasc Med.* 6:291, 2004.
Van der ADL, et al. Dietary haem iron and coronary heart disease in women. *Eur Heart J.* 26:257, 2005.
Weisberg IS, et al. Investigations of a common genetic variant in betaine-homocysteine methyltransferase (BHMT) in coronary artery disease. *Atherosclerosis* 167:205, 2003.
Yan LL, et al. Midlife body mass index and hospitalization and mortality in older age. *JAMA.* 295:190, 2006.
Zhao G, et al. Dietary alpha-linolenic acid reduces inflammatory and lipid cardiovascular risk factors in hypercholesterolemic men and women. *J Nutr.* 134:2991, 2004.

OVERVIEW: DIET IN HEART DISEASES—SODIUM AND MINERALS

Hypertension increases the risk for coronary artery disease (CAD), myocardial infarction (MI), stroke, and congestive heart failure. Renal failure is also related to sodium intake (Weir and Fink, 2005). Identification of hypertension in premenopausal women is an important CAD risk factor (Gierach et al, 2006). Careful attention to hypertension is essential.

African Americans and Hispanics of Caribbean descent tend to have a high prevalence of hypertension with a worse prognosis than whites (Richardson and Piepho, 2000). A majority of Americans over age 60 have high blood pressure. Shortened life expectancy results.

Vascular biology assumes a pivotal role in hypertension and organ damage (Houston, 2005). Mutations in cardiac Na(+) and K(+) channels can disrupt the balance of ionic currents that support normal cardiac excitation and relaxation; arrhythmogenic phenotypes may lead to syncope, seizures, and sudden cardiac death (Clancy and Kass, 2005). Endothelial activation, oxidative stress, and vascular smooth muscle dysfunction (hypertrophy, hyperplasia, remodeling) are initial events that start hypertension (Houston, 2005).

Because nutrient–gene interactions determine a broad array of conditions including hypertension, the use of optimal nutrition, nutraceuticals, vitamins, antioxidants, and minerals; weight loss; exercise; smoking cessation; and moderate restriction of alcohol and caffeine, in addition to other lifestyle modifications, can prevent, delay onset, reduce severity, treat, and control hypertension in many patients (Houston, 2005).

Plasma tonicity is determined by variations in glucose, sodium, and potassium; it is suspected that plasma hypertonicity is a factor in the progression of elevated plasma glucose to diabetes (Stookey et al, 2005). There are many benefits in reducing sodium intake (McCarron, 2000) while increasing intakes of potassium, calcium, magnesium, and whole grains (Anderson, 2003; Vaskonen, 2003).

The Institute of Medicine of the National Academy of Sciences (2004) issued recommendations for intake of water, sodium, and potassium, and general guidelines for good health that include:

- **CHLORIDE:** 2300 mg daily for adults to replace losses in perspiration.
- **POTASSIUM:** 4700 mg is needed to lower blood pressure and reduce the risk of kidney stones and bone loss for most adults. No upper limit is set. African Americans may benefit. Natural sources are best.
- **SODUM:** 1500 mg for adults aged 19–50; 1300 mg for adults aged 50–70; 1200 mg for adults aged 71 and over. Highly active people may need more. If sodium sensitive, intake may need to be lower. Upper limit (UL) is set at 5800 mg/d, and over 95% of the American public consumes sodium above the UL level.
- **WATER:** 91 oz daily for women, 125 oz daily for men; more in hot climates or with physical activity. Drinking fluids with meals and between meals according to thirst is usually sufficient, although the elderly may lose their awareness of thirst. About 80% of daily intake comes from beverages, and 20% comes from food.

CITED REFERENCES

Anderson JW. Whole grains protect against atherosclerotic cardiovascular disease. *Proc Nutr Soc.* 62:135, 2003.

Clancy CE, Kass RS. Inherited and acquired vulnerability to ventricular arrhythmias: cardiac Na+ and K+ channels. *Physiol Rev.* 85:33, 2005.

Gierach GL, et al. Hypertension, menopause, and coronary artery disease risk in the Women's Ischemia Syndrome Evaluation (WISE) Study. *J Am Coll Cardiol.* 47:50S, 2006.

Houston MC. Nutraceuticals, vitamins, antioxidants, and minerals in the prevention and treatment of hypertension. *Prog Cardiovasc Dis.* 47:396, 2005.

Institute of Medicine. *Dietary Reference Intakes: water, potassium, sodium, chloride, and sulfate.* Washington, DC: National Academies of Science, 2004.

McCarron D. The dietary guideline for sodium: should we shake it up? Yes! *Am J Clin Nutr.* 71:1013, 2000.

Richardson A, Piepho R. Effect of race on hypertension and antihypertensive therapy. *Int J Clin Pharmacol Ther.* 38:75, 2000.

Stookey JD, et al. Hypertonic hyperglycemia progresses to diabetes faster than normotonic hyperglycemia. *Eur J Epidemiol.* 19:935, 2004.

Weir MR, Fink JC. Salt intake and progression of chronic kidney disease: an overlooked modifiable exposure? A commentary. *Am J Kidney Dis.* 45:176, 2005.

Vaskonen T. Dietary minerals and modification of cardiovascular risk factors. *J Nutr Biochem.* 14:492, 2003.

For More Information

- American Association of Cardiovascular Pulmonary Rehabilitation
  http://www.aacvpr.org/
- American Heart Association
  http://www.americanheart.org/
- Patient Videos
  http://www.patientvideo.com/cardiovascular/

ANGINA PECTORIS

NUTRITIONAL ACUITY RANKING: LEVEL 1

DEFINITIONS AND BACKGROUND

Angina pectoris involves retrosternal chest pain or discomfort from decreased blood flow to the myocardium from decreased oxygen supply (often during exertion). Traditional risk factors include tobacco use, hypertension, diabetes mellitus, dyslipidemia, obesity, sedentary lifestyle, and atherogenic diet; more recently identified risk factors in women include high-sensitivity C-reactive protein (hsCRP), lipoprotein (a), and homocysteine (Bello and Mosca, 2004).

Angina can also occur from anemia, hyperthyroidism, aortic stenosis, or vasospasm. In hypertrophic cardiomyopathy, an area of abnormally thick heart muscle impairs the heart's pumping action and causes angina during or shortly after exercise.

Stable (classic) angina occurs after exertion and is relieved by rest and vasodilation; it lasts 3–5 minutes. Intractable (progressive) angina causes chronic chest pain that is not relieved by medical treatment. Variant angina is a mixed condition. In addition to chest pain, signs and symptoms of angina include shortness of breath, sweating, nausea, vertigo, ache in neck or jaw, earache, and numbness or burning sensations. If diagnosed early, the chance of living longer than 10–12 years is at least 50%.

Invasive treatments for chronic stable angina are only needed in a small number of patients (Kirwan at el, 2005). Women often have chest pain and normal angiograms; symptom relief includes tricyclic agents and beta-blockers and aggressive antiatherosclerotic therapy with statins or angiotensin-converting enzyme (ACE) inhibitors (Bugiardini and Bairey Mertz, 2005).

The "ABCDE" approach is effective: "A" for antiplatelet therapy, anticoagulation, ACE inhibition, and angiotensin receptor blockade; "B" for beta-blockade and blood pressure control; "C" for cholesterol treatment and cigarette smoking cessation; "D" for diabetes management and diet; and "E" for exercise (Gluckman et al, 2005). Cardiac rehabilitation helps to improve aerobic exercise capacity, physical functioning, and mental depression.

Some carotenoids decrease the risk for angina pectoris (Ford and Giles, 2000). A very low–fat diet (i.e., 10% fat calories) has a substantial impact (Griel and Kris-Etherton, 2006).

INTERVENTION: OBJECTIVES

- Relieve chest pain. Improve circulation to the heart.
- Increase activity only as tolerated or prescribed. Gradually increase exercise, especially through programs in cardiac rehabilitation.
- Maintain adequate rest periods.

- Maintain weight or lose weight if obese. A conventional dietetic intervention with weight loss helps to reduce atherosclerotic and thrombotic risk and pain frequency in angina patients (Hankey et al, 2002).
- Avoid constipation with straining.
- Control blood pressure and lower elevated serum cholesterol.

INTERVENTION: FOOD AND NUTRITION

- Small, frequent feedings rather than three large meals are indicated.
- Increase fiber as tolerated; include an adequate fluid intake. Increase intake of fruits.
- Restrict saturated fats, dietary cholesterol, and sodium as necessary according to the individual profile. A very low–fat diet can be quite effective (Griel and Kris-Etherton, 2005).
- Limit stimulants such as caffeine to less than 5 cups of coffee or the equivalent daily.
- Promote calorie control if overweight; modify by age and sex.
- If homocysteine levels are high, add more foods with folic acid, vitamins B_6 and B_{12}, and riboflavin to the diet. Supplementation with B-complex vitamins with or without antioxidants reduces total homocysteine levels in men who have mildly elevated levels (Woodside et al, 1998).
- A Mediterranean diet that is rich in alpha linolenic acid is effective (Estruch et al, 2006; Singh et al, 2002). It is prudent to increase intake of olive, soybean, and canola oils and seeds and nuts, including walnuts, almonds, macadamias, pecans, peanuts, and pistachios. Walnuts contain alpha linolenic acid; almonds are a good source of vitamin E. Nuts also contain flavonoids, phenols, phytosterols, saponins, elegiac acid, folic acid, magnesium, copper, potassium, and fiber. Pistachios, sunflower kernels, sesame seeds, and wheat germ are highest in phytosterols; use often.
- Beta-carotene supplements actually seem to increase angina. Dietary sources of carotenoids are a healthier choice.

CLINICAL INDICATORS

Clinical/History		Lab Work
Height	Blood pressure (BP)	Cholesterol (Chol)—LDL, HDL, total
Weight	Intake and output (I & O)	Advanced lipid testing—lipoprotein particle size
Body mass index (BMI)	Electrocardiogram (ECG)	Triglycerides (Trig)
Waist–hip ratio	Radionucleotide imaging	
Recent weight changes (e.g., gain)	Stress test	
Diet history	Coronary angiography	
Pulse (NL = 60–100 beats/min)		

Lactate dehydrogenase (LDH)	Serum Fe	Transferrin
Homocysteine levels	Total iron-binding capacity (TIBC)	Na+, K+
C-reactive protein (CRP)	Aspartate aminotransferase (AST)	Ca++, Mg++
Serum folate	Alanine aminotransferase (ALT)	Alkaline phosphatase (Alk phos)
Glucose (Gluc)		
Hemoglobin and hematocrit (H & H)		

Common Drugs Used and Potential Side Effects

- Antiplatelet therapy, anticoagulation therapy, angiotensin-converting enzyme (ACE) inhibitors, angiotensin receptor blockers, beta-blockers, and blood pressure medications will often be prescribed. Isosorbide (Isordil or Imdur) may cause nausea, vomiting, or dizziness; take on an empty stomach. Nadolol (Corgard) is a beta-blocker; it may cause weakness. Disopyramide (Norpace) may cause abdominal pain, nausea, or constipation.
- Calcium channel blockers (verapamil [Calan], nicardipine, or diltiazem [Cardizem]) are used to dilate coronary arteries and slow down nerve impulses through the heart, thereby increasing blood flow. Nausea, edema, or constipation may be side effects. Take on an empty stomach. These drugs may also cause heart failure or dizziness; avoid taking with aloe, buckthorn bark and berry, cascara, and senna leaf. With nifedipine (Procardia), nausea, weakness, dizziness, and flatulence may occur; take after meals.

Herbs, Botanicals, and Supplements

- The patient should not take herbals and botanicals without discussing with the physician. Evidence of significant harm and fatalities have been observed when certain herbal products are used in excess or in combination with other herbs or prescription drugs (Hermann, 2002).
- Coenzyme Q10 (CoQ10; ubiquinone) should not be used with gemfibrozil, tricyclic antidepressants, or warfarin. CoQ10 may act similarly to vitamin K. Because CoQ10 and statins share a similar pathway, they can be taken simultaneously (Mabuchi et al, 2005; Strey et al, 2005; Silver et al, 2004).
- Danshen may be used for ischemic heart disease. Avoid large amounts with warfarin, aspirin, and other antiplatelet drugs. It can increase risks of bleeding or bruising.
- Garlic should not be taken in large amounts with warfarin, aspirin, and other antiplatelet drugs because of increased risks of bleeding or bruising. It may also increase insulin levels with hypoglycemic results; monitor carefully in patients with diabetes.

- Grapefruit juice decreases drug metabolism in the gut (via P-450–CYP3A4 inhibition) and can affect medications up to 24 hours later. Consistency of use may be more important than total quantity. Avoid taking with alprazolam, buspirone, cisapride, cyclosporine, statins, tacrolimus, and other drugs.
- Niacin (nicotinic acid) should not be taken with statins, antidiabetic medications, or carbamazepine because of potentially serious risks of myopathy and altered glucose control.
- Omega-3 fatty acids in fish oil capsules can cause hypervitaminosis A and D if taken in large doses. Avoid use in pregnant or lactating women. Avoid taking with warfarin, aspirin, and other antiplatelet medications because of the risk of increased bruising or bleeding.
- Vitamin E should not be taken with warfarin because of the possibility of increased bleeding. Avoid doses greater than 400 IU/d.

INTERVENTION: NUTRITION EDUCATION, COUNSELING, CARE MANAGEMENT

- The patient will require stress management, activity, and education about proper eating habits.
- Discuss the role of nutrition in maintenance of wellness and in cardiovascular disease. Discuss in particular: fiber, total fat intake, potassium and sodium, calcium and other nutrients, and caffeine.
- Discuss the importance of weight control in reduction of cardiovascular risks.
- Elevate the head of the bed 30–45° for greater comfort.
- Unstable angina is dangerous and should be treated as a potential emergency; new, worsening, or persistent chest discomfort should be evaluated in a hospital emergency department or "chest pain unit" and monitored carefully for acute myocardial infarction (heart attack), severe cardiac arrhythmia, or cardiac arrest leading to sudden death.

Patient Education—Foodborne Illness

- Careful food handling will be important. Hand washing is key as well.

For More Information

- American Heart Association–Angina http://www.americanheart.org/downloadable/heart/1056719919740HSFacts2003text.pdf

ANGINA PECTORIS—CITED REFERENCES

Bello N, Mosca L. Epidemiology of coronary heart disease in women. *Prog Cardiovasc Dis.* 46:287, 2004.

Bugiardini R, Bairey Mertz CN. Angina with "normal" coronary arteries: a changing philosophy. *JAMA.* 293:477, 2005.

Estruch R, et al. Effects of a Mediterranean-style diet on cardiovascular risk factors: a randomized trial. *Ann Intern Med.* 145:1, 2006.

Ford E, Giles W. Serum vitamins, carotenoids, and angina pectoris: findings from the National Health and Nutrition Examination Survey III. *Ann Epidemiol.* 10:106, 2000.

Gluckman TJ, et al. A simplified approach to the management of non-ST-segment elevation acute coronary syndromes. *JAMA.* 293:349, 2005.

Griel AE, Kris-Etherton PM. Beyond saturated fat: the importance of the dietary fatty acid profile on cardiovascular disease. *Nutr Rev.* 64:257, 2006.

Hankey CR, et al. Effects of moderate weight loss on anginal symptoms and indices of coagulation and fibrinolysis in overweight patients with angina pectoris. *Eur J Clin Nutr.* 56:1039, 2002.

Hermann DD. Naturoceutical agents in the management of cardiovascular disease. *Am J Cardiovasc Drugs.* 2:173, 2002.

Kirwan BA, et al. Treatment of angina pectoris: associations with symptom severity. *Int J Cardiol.* 98:299, 2005.

Mabuchi H, et al. Reduction of serum ubiquinol-10 and ubiquinone-10 levels by atorvastatin in hypercholesterolemic patients. *J Atheroscler Thromb.* 12:111, 2005.

Silver MA, et al. Effect of atorvastatin on left ventricular diastolic function and ability of coenzyme Q10 to reverse that dysfunction. *Am J Cardiol.* 94:1306, 2004.

Singh RB, et al. Effect of an Indo-Mediterranean diet on progression of coronary artery disease in high risk patients (Indo-Mediterranean Diet Heart Study): a randomised single-blind trial. *Lancet* 360:1455, 2002.

Strey CH, et al. Endothelium-ameliorating effects of statin therapy and coenzyme Q10 reductions in chronic heart failure. *Atherosclerosis* 179:201, 2005.

Woodside J, et al. Effect of B-group vitamins and antioxidant vitamins on hyperhomocysteinemia: a double-blind, randomized factorial-design, controlled trial. *Am J Clin Nutr.* 67:858, 1998.

ARTERITIS

NUTRITIONAL ACUITY RANKING: LEVEL 1

DEFINITIONS AND BACKGROUND

Arteritis involves inflammation of artery walls with decreased blood flow. Tumor necrosis factor appears to influence susceptibility and interleukin (IL)-1 receptor antagonist seems to play a role in the pathogenesis. Genetic traits are being studied.

Cranial arteritis (temporal or giant-cell arteritis) yields chronically inflamed temporal arteries with a thickening of the lining and a reduction in blood flow; this condition is linked to polymyalgia rheumatica (PMR). Women older than 55 years of age are twice as likely to have the condition compared with other people. Signs and symptoms include a severe, throbbing headache at the temples or back of the head. The artery may be red, swollen, and painful. Anorexia, weight loss, mild fever, scalp tenderness, dysphagia, hearing problems, vision changes, jaw pain, and muscular aches may be indicators. The greatest danger is permanent blindness or stroke.

Buerger's disease involves an arteritis that causes limb pain and numbness. **Periarteritis nodosa** is an autoimmune disease that can affect any artery in the body. A rare form of arteritis, **Takayasu's arteritis**, affects the mesenteric artery and creates local ischemia; IL-8 may be involved.

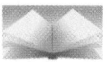

INTERVENTION: OBJECTIVES

- Prevent stroke and blindness, which are potential complications.
- Reduce inflammation.
- Promote increased blood flow through the affected vessels.
- Modify intake according to requirements and coexisting problems such as hypertension.

INTERVENTION: FOOD AND NUTRITION

- Follow usual diet, with increased calories if patient is underweight or decreased calories if the patient is obese.
- Reduce excess sodium and total fat intake; monitor regularly. Increase intake of fruits.
- Patient may need to include carnitine in the diet. Although not yet proven, it may be reasonable to include in the diet more sources of vitamins E, B_6, and B_{12}, riboflavin, and folic acid or to use a multivitamin supplement that includes sufficient amounts.
- With steroids, decreased sodium intake with higher potassium intake may be needed; adequate to high protein may also be necessary. Monitor for glucose intolerance.
- Omega-3 fatty acids may be useful to reduce inflammatory process. Eat more salmon, tuna, mackerel, walnuts, and related foods (Yaqoob and Calder, 2003).
- Treatment with supplements of folic acid and/or vitamin B_{12} reduces elevated homocysteine concentrations, which are common (Martinez-Taboada et al, 2003).

CLINICAL INDICATORS

Clinical/History

Height
Weight
BMI
Waist–hip ratio
Diet history
BP
Temperature
Biopsy
Ultrasonography

Lab Work

White blood cell count (WBC) (increased)
Erythrocyte sedimentation rate (ESR), autoantibodies
CRP
Na+, K+
Ca++, Mg++
Gluc
Albumin (Alb) or transthyretin
Creatinine kinase (CK)
Transferrin
Chol—total, HDL, LDL
Trig
H & H (often decreased)
Serum Fe, ferritin
Homocysteine level
Serum B_{12}
Serum folate

Common Drugs Used and Potential Side Effects

- Glucocorticoids, typically high-dose prednisone, are first-line treatment and successfully control the inflammatory process (Spiera and Spiera, 2004). Most patients can be tapered off steroids within 6 months to 2 years; side effects include elevated glucose and decreased nitrogen levels, especially with long-term use (Spiera and Spiera, 2004).
- Grapefruit juice decreases drug metabolism in the gut (via P-450–CYP3A4 inhibition) and can affect medications up to 24 hours later. Consistency of use may be more important than total quantity. Avoid taking with alprazolam, buspirone, cisapride, cyclosporine, statins, tacrolimus, and many other drugs.

Herbs, Botanicals, and Supplements

- The patient should not take herbals or botanicals without discussing with the physician.
- Coenzyme Q10 (CoQ10; ubiquinone) should not be used with gemfibrozil, tricyclic antidepressants, or warfarin. CoQ10 may act similarly to vitamin K. Because CoQ10 and statins share a similar pathway, they can be taken simultaneously (Mabuchi et al, 2005; Strey et al, 2005; Silver et al, 2004).
- Niacin (nicotinic acid) should not be taken with statins, antidiabetic medications, or carbamazepine because of potentially serious risks of myopathy and altered glucose control.
- Omega-3 fatty acids in fish oil capsules can cause hypervitaminosis A and D if taken in large doses. Avoid use in pregnant or lactating women. Avoid taking with warfarin, aspirin, and other antiplatelet medications because of the risk of increased bruising or bleeding.
- Vitamin E should not be taken with warfarin because of the possibility of increased bleeding. Avoid doses greater than 400 IU/d.

INTERVENTION: NUTRITION EDUCATION, COUNSELING, CARE MANAGEMENT

- Discuss the role of nutrition in the maintenance of health for cardiovascular disease.
- Discuss the effects of medications on nutritional status and appetite.

Patient Education—Foodborne Illness

- Careful food handling will be important. Hand washing is key as well.

For More Information

- American Autoimmune Association
  http://www.aarda.org/
- Journal of Immunology
  http://www.jimmunol.org/
- Takayasu Arteritis Foundation
  http://www.takayasu.org/

ARTERITIS—CITED REFERENCES

Mabuchi H, et al. Reduction of serum ubiquinol-10 and ubiquinone-10 levels by atorvastatin in hypercholesterolemic patients. *J Atheroscler Thromb.* 12:111, 2005.
Martinez-Taboada VM, et al. Homocysteine levels in polymyalgia rheumatica and giant cell arteritis: influence of corticosteroid therapy. *Rheumatology (Oxford)* 42:1055, 2003.
Silver MA, et al. Effect of atorvastatin on left ventricular diastolic function and ability of coenzyme Q10 to reverse that dysfunction. *Am J Cardiol.* 94:1306, 2004.
Spiera R, Spiera H. Inflammatory disease in older adults. Cranial arteritis. *Geriatrics* 59:25, 2004.
Strey CH, et al. Endothelium-ameliorating effects of statin therapy and coenzyme Q10 reductions in chronic heart failure. *Atherosclerosis* 179:201, 2005.
Yaqoob P, Calder PC. N-3 polyunsaturated fatty acids and inflammation in the arterial wall. *Eur J Med Res.* 8:337, 2003.

ATHEROSCLEROSIS, CORONARY ARTERY DISEASE, DYSLIPIDEMIA

NUTRITIONAL ACUITY RANKING: LEVEL 3

DEFINITIONS AND BACKGROUND

Atherosclerosis involves progressive narrowing of the arterial tree, giving rise to collateral vessels. Fat-deposit accumulations occur; the heart, brain, and leg arteries are most often affected. Sagittal abdominal diameter (height of abdomen at the umbilical level measured from exam couch in a supine position with straight legs) is more strongly correlated with cardiovascular risk factors than waist circumference, waist to hip ratio, or BMI (Ohrvall et al, 2000).

According to recently defined criteria, metabolic syndrome is prevalent and is associated with a greater risk of atherosclerosis than any of its individual components; obesity is the key factor that leads to a proinflammatory and prothrombotic state that potentiates atherosclerosis (Moller and Kaufman, 2005). Vascular lipid accumulation and inflammation are hallmarks of atherosclerosis and perpetuate plaque development; mediators such as interleukin (IL)-6 are elevated in patients with acute coronary syndromes and may contribute to the exacerbation of atherosclerosis (Schieffer et al, 2004).

Coronary artery disease (CAD) occurs when the arteries that supply blood to the heart muscle (coronary arteries) become hardened and narrowed. The arteries harden and become narrow due to the buildup of plaque on the inner walls or lining of the arteries (atherosclerosis). Blood flow to the heart is reduced as plaque narrows the coronary arteries, thus diminishing oxygen supply to the heart muscle.

CAD is the most common type of heart disease. While CAD involves plaque buildup in the arteries of the heart, gum disease may actually precede CAD. Because atherosclerosis is an underlying cause of CAD, a reduced rate of progression of atherosclerosis associated with intensive statin treatment is related to reductions in the levels of both atherogenic lipoproteins and CRP (Nissen et al, 2005).

CAD is caused by smoking, high blood pressure, low HDL cholesterol (<40 mg/dL), family history of early coronary heart disease, and age for males over 45 years and females over 55 years. Obesity and elevated serum homocysteine and copper levels are lesser risk factors. Diabetes is a precursor for many individuals. In women who have had more than six pregnancies, CAD may occur as a result of insulin resistance. See Table 6-1 for a long list of dietary and other factors regarding CAD.

Dyslipidemia (hypertriglyceridemia and low levels of high-density lipoprotein cholesterol) indicates that imbalances in individual lipid components contribute to the increased risk of CAD. Serum lipid reductions decrease CAD risk; for each 1% reduction in serum cholesterol, there is a 2% reduction in CAD risk. Cholesterol screening is recommended, even for older adults. When treated, risks decrease by 25–30% for those persons treated for 5 or more years (Hall and Luepker, 2000); therefore, early nutritional intervention is beneficial.

Ischemia is a local and temporary deficiency of blood caused by obstruction, as from thrombosis. Risk of **ischemic heart disease** is lower in subjects with very high fruit and vegetable intakes (Law and Morris, 1998). People with ischemic heart disease benefit from diets high in monounsaturated fatty acids (MUFA), omega-3 fatty acids, whole grains, vitamin E, wine, vegetables, and fruits (Pieke et al, 2000).

Clinical trials have established that secondary prevention of hyperlipidemia in patients after **coronary artery bypass graft (CABG) surgery** prevents progression of atherosclerosis; a multidisciplinary team is needed to promote secondary prevention by prescribing antihyperlipidemic agents, screening for risk factors, and providing education on disease, diet, and medications (Brackbill and Sytsma, 2004). Angioplasty is as safe and effective as bypass surgery.

A therapeutic lifestyle modification program is effective as a nutrition and physical activity intervention and has the potential to dramatically reduce the risks associated with common chronic diseases (Aldana et al, 2005). Dietary counseling and education by a registered dietitian are associated with improved diet-related outcomes, and sufficient time to consult with a dietitian should be planned in cardiac rehabilitation (Locklin Holmes et al, 2005).

INTERVENTION: OBJECTIVES

- Use a team approach to support the best possible outcomes: doctors, nurses, dietitians, and other therapists as needed.

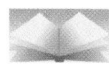

- Improve LDL and HDL cholesterol levels. Prevent formation of new lesions. Lower elevated serum lipids, especially cholesterol levels >200 mg/dL and triglyceride levels >200 mg/dL. Follow the Therapeutic Lifestyle Change diet (National Heart, Lung, and Blood Institute [NHLBI], 2001; Stone and Van Horn, 2002; Aldana et al, 2005; Tucker et al, 2005).
- Initiate and maintain weight loss if overweight. Obesity with a high waist circumference is especially important to correct in both men and women. Physical activity should be encouraged.
- Moderate carbohydrate restriction and weight control are useful for improving atherosclerotic dyslipidemia (Krauss et al, 2006).
- Correct elevated levels of homocysteine by supplementing with B-complex vitamins (Woodside et al, 1998).
- Use more flavonoids, phytochemicals, soy products, and fruits and vegetables.
- Treat elevated triglycerides if over 150 mg/dL (NHLBI, http://www.nhlbi.nih.gov/guidelines/cholesterol/atglance.htm#Step1).
  - Primary aim of therapy is to reach LDL goal.
  - Intensify weight management.
  - Increase physical activity.
  - If triglycerides are ≥200 mg/dL after LDL goal is reached, set secondary goal for non-HDL cholesterol (total – HDL) 30 mg/dL higher than LDL goal.
- Treat metabolic syndrome (NHLBI, 2001). Address underlying causes (overweight/obesity and physical inactivity); intensify weight management, and increase physical activity. Treat lipid and nonlipid risk factors if they persist despite these lifestyle therapies; treat hypertension; use aspirin for CAD patients to reduce prothrombotic state; help lower elevated triglycerides and/or lower HDL through diet first, then drug therapies. See Table 6-4.

TABLE 6-4 Clinical Identification of the Metabolic Syndrome (Any 3 of the Following)

Risk Factor	Defining Level
Abdominal obesity[a]	Waist circumference[b]
Men	>102 cm (>40 in)
Women	>88 cm (>35 in)
Triglycerides	≥50 mg/dL
HDL cholesterol	
Men	<40 mg/dL
Women	<50 mg/dL
Blood pressure	≥130/≥85 mm Hg
Fasting glucose	≥110 mg/dL

[a] Overweight and obesity are associated with insulin resistance and the metabolic syndrome. However, the presence of abdominal obesity is more highly correlated with the metabolic risk factors than is an elevated BMI. Therefore, the simple measure of waist circumference is recommended to identify the body weight component of the metabolic syndrome.

[b] Some male patients can develop multiple metabolic risk factors when the waist circumference is only marginally increased, e.g., 94–102 cm (37–39 in). Such patients may have a strong genetic contribution to insulin resistance. They should benefit from changes in life habits, similar to men with categorical increases in waist circumference.

From: National Heart, Lung, and Blood Institute, http://www.nhlbi.nih.gov/guidelines/cholesterol/atglance.htm#Step1; accessed February 5, 2005.

INTERVENTION: FOOD AND NUTRITION

Despite reports that many types of diet alterations can be effective in lowering elevated lipids, blood pressure, and glucose, there is no "one size fits all" guideline at this time (Chahoud et al, 2004). Diet must be combined with exercise and other lifestyle changes. The Mediterranean diet tends to be quite acceptable to most people and works well in lowering coronary risk factors; it encourages use of olive oil, red wine, fish, fruits, and vegetables.

Evidence Analysis Conclusion Statements (American Dietetic Association) suggest the following recommendations:

- A "Therapeutic Lifestyle" diet consisting of 25–35% total fat, <7% saturated and trans fat, and <200 mg dietary cholesterol (NHLBI, 2001). Keep fat at about 3 g/100 kcal. Examples include:

25% of kcal	30% of kcal	35% of kcal
28 g in 1000 kcals	33 g in 1000 kcals	39 g in 1000 kcals
33 g in 1200 kcals	40 g in 1200 kcals	47 g in 1200 kcals
42 g in 1500 kcals	50 g in 1500 kcals	59 g in 1500 kcals
50 g in 1800 kcals	60 g in 1800 kcals	70 g in 1800 kcals
56 g in 2000 kcals	67 g in 2000 kcals	78 g in 2000 kcals
67 g in 2400 kcals	80 g in 2400 kcals	93 g in 2400 kcals

- Use isocaloric replacement of saturated fatty acids with MUFA and polyunsaturated fatty acids (PUFA). Use of extra virgin olive oil and canola oil in cooking and salad dressings is an easy way to start.
- Consumption of a diet rich in fruits and vegetables and low-fat dairy products and low in sodium and saturated fat decreases blood pressure, an effect that is enhanced by weight loss and increased physical activity.
- Consume one-half cup of nuts daily with a diet low in saturated fat and cholesterol to decrease total cholesterol; include measures to ensure that weight is not gained. Consume 5 oz of nuts per week to reduce risk of CVD. Nuts contain flavonoids, phenols, sterols, saponins, elegiac acid, folic acid, magnesium, copper, potassium, and fiber. Almonds are a very good source of vitamin E; walnuts contain alpha linolenic acid. Nuts are beneficial for cardiac health in general (Zambon et al, 2000; Morgan and Clayshultze, 2000).
- Consume antioxidants from dietary sources. Vitamin E foods include asparagus, spinach, wheat germ, nuts, salad oils, and creamy salad dressings. Vitamin C foods should be consumed in amounts that meet at least DRI levels; use caution with large amounts because they may act as a pro-oxidant (Lee et al, 2004). There does not appear to be benefit to warrant use of supplemental antioxidants alone or in combination with other antioxidants. In fact, there is evidence of potential harm; supplemental beta-carotene (60–120 mg/d) is associated with an increase in all-cause mortality and cardiovascular death in patients at increased risk for lung cancer. And there is evidence of potential nutrient (as supplement)–drug interactions.

- Use flavonoids frequently. Tea, blueberries, yellow onions, red wine, grape juice, apples, cocoa, dark chocolate, products such as CocoaVia, and grapefruit contain phenolic acids and antioxidants. In the Middle East, use of beverages such as pomelo increases antioxidant consumption and lowers LDL cholesterol (Arias and Ramon-Laca, 2005). Use more cinnamon, cloves, licorice, and sage; cinnamon contains proanthocyanidin.
- Consumption of a diet high in total fiber (17–30 g/d) and soluble fiber (7–13 g/d) as part of a diet low in saturated fat and cholesterol reduces further cholesterol and LDL cholesterol. Use of soluble fiber may include oat bran, corn bran, apples, and legumes as good sources.
- Consume of 2–3 g of plant sterols and stanols (through margarine, low-fat yogurt, orange juice, breads, and cereals) daily to lower cholesterol and LDL cholesterol, including patients currently on statins. Stanol-containing margarines may be consumed in 2–3 servings daily; allow at least 3 weeks before results are assessed. Pistachios, sunflower kernels, sesame seeds, and wheat germ are highest in phytosterols; use often.
- Consume one extra carotenoid-rich fruit or vegetable per day to maintain plasma carotenoid levels when also consuming sterol-enriched spreads. The Dietary Approaches to Stop Hypertension (DASH) diet is useful; see Tables 6-2 and 6-3 for foods to include often.
- Intake of approximately 1 g/d of EPA and DHA from a supplement or fish may decrease the risk of death from cardiac events in patients with heart disease. Regular consumption of an average of two servings of fatty fish per week (about 3.5 oz per serving) reduces risk of death from cardiac events in subjects without prior disease.
- Include vegetable oils and food sources high in alpha linolenic acid, resulting in a total intake of more than 1.5 g/d, to reduce risk of death from cardiac events.
- Diets containing soy are well tolerated. However, caution should be used in recommending soy to improve dyslipidemia. Soy use is likely to produce varied results based on initial cholesterol level and condition (e.g., diabetes mellitus). Food labels should now indicate soy content.
- Other useful dietary recommendations include:
  - Use fewer animal proteins and more legumes and vegetable protein sources. Fish and shellfish may be used 3–4 times weekly, especially sources rich in omega-3 fatty acids. Remove chicken skin before cooking or just before serving. Lean beef and chicken are considered to be comparable.
  - Trans fatty acids should be used in limited amounts. Foods such as pound cake, regular microwave popcorn, snack crackers, vegetable shortening, stick margarine, vanilla wafers, snack chips, boxed chocolate chip cookies, French fries, and similar foods may be sources of trans fatty acids. Food labels state content of trans fatty acids as part of total saturated fatty acid amounts as of January 2006.
  - Provide chromium and copper in adequate amounts from food sources. Vitamin K may also play an important role in reducing risks of CHD (Geleijnse et al, 2004). Sufficient folic acid, vitamins B_6 and B_{12}, and choline should be consumed (da Costa et al, 2005).
  - Olestra, a fat substitute, has been associated with a decrease in dietary fat and serum total cholesterol levels; use in moderate amounts only in order to prevent side effects such as diarrhea.

SAMPLE NUTRITION DIAGNOSTIC STATEMENT

Hypercholesterolemia

PES: Inappropriate intake of saturated and trans fats related to food choices at fast food restaurants on most days of the week as evidenced by LDL of 160 mg/dL and total cholesterol of 240 mg/dL.

Assessment Data: Dietary intake records; lipid profile; National Cholesterol Education Program screening data.

Intervention: Education and counseling; serving appropriate meals if in your facility; self-monitoring (food diary, food prep skills, access to wholesome food choices).

Monitoring and Evaluation: Repeat labs in 3–6 months; intake records and food diaries.

CLINICAL INDICATORS

Clinical/History

Height
Weight
BMI
Waist–hip ratio
Diet history
BP
Pancreatitis?
Xanthomas?

Lab Work

CRP
Trig
Total Chol (often increased)
HDL, LDL—ideal: 40% HDL or higher, 60% LDL or lower
Advanced lipid testing—small particle size
Homocysteine: serum and urinary
Serum and urinary folate
Serum and urinary B_{12}
Serum B_6
H & H
Serum Fe
Na^+, K^+
Ca^{++}, Mg^{++}
Gluc
AST, ALT
Serum copper

Common Drugs Used and Potential Side Effects

- "Diet First, Then Drugs": see Table 6-5.
- Anticoagulants (warfarin) may be needed. Limit vitamin K–containing foods to 1 per day; consistency of intake is often more important than quantity. Foods high in vitamin K include mayonnaise, canola and

SAMPLE NUTRITION DIAGNOSTIC STATEMENT

Dyslipidemia

PES: Inappropriate intake of food fats related to food and nutrition-related knowledge deficit as evidenced by daily consumption of butter and ice cream, saturated fat intake of 15% of kcal, and LDL cholesterol of 165 mg/dL and HDL cholesterol of 30 mg/dL.

Assessment Data: Food frequency recall and intake records; computer nutrient analysis.

Intervention: Education, identify alternate sources of fats that are more desirable.

Monitoring and Evaluation: Repeat lab values after 3–6 months; dietary recall.

TABLE 6-5 Drugs Affecting Lipoprotein Metabolism

Drug Class	Agents and Daily Doses	Lipid/Lipoprotein Effects	Side Effects and Comments	Contraindications
Statins—HMG-CoA reductase inhibitors	Lovastatin (20–80 mg) Pravastatin (20–40 mg) Simvastatin (20–80 mg) Fluvastatin (20–80 mg) Atorvastatin (10–80 mg) Cerivastatin (0.4–0.8 mg)	LDL-C, ↓18–55% HDL-C, ↑5–15% TG, ↓7–30%	Muscle pain and tenderness; myopathy Severe cases: rhabdomyolysis and release of myoglobin into the bloodstream Increased liver enzymes	Absolute: Active or chronic liver disease Relative: Concomitant use of certain drugs[a]
Bile acid sequestrant	Cholestyramine (4–16 g) Colestipol (5–20 g) Colesevelam (2.6–3.8 g)	LDL-C, ↓15–30% HDL-C, ↑3–5% TG, No change or increase	GI distress Constipation; use more fiber Decreased absorption of other drugs Add folate and fat-soluble vitamins; mix with liquids	Absolute: Dysbetalipoproteinemia TG >400 mg/dL Relative: TG >200 mg/dL
Nicotinic acid (Nico-Bid, Nico-400)	Immediate-release (crystalline) nicotinic acid (1.5-3 g), extended-release nicotinic acid (Niaspan) (1–2 g), sustained-release nicotinic acid (1–2 g)	LDL-C, ↓5–25% HDL-C, ↑15–35% TG, ↓20–50%	Flushing Hyperglycemia Hyperuricemia (or gout) Upper GI distress Hepatotoxicity or altered LFTs Vomiting, diarrhea	Absolute: Chronic liver disease Severe gout Relative: Diabetes Hyperuricemia Peptic ulcer disease
Fibric acids	Gemfibrozil (600 mg BID) Fenofibrate (200 mg) Clofibrate (1000 mg BID)	LDL-C, ↓5–20% (may be increased in patients with high TG) HDL-C, ↑10–20% TG, ↓20–50%	Dyspepsia Gallstones Myopathy Weight gain Diarrhea, nausea	Absolute: Severe renal disease Severe hepatic disease

HDL-C, high-density lipoprotein cholesterol; LDL-C, low-density lipoprotein cholesterol; TG, triglycerides; LFT, liver function test; GI, gastrointestinal.
[a] Cyclosporine, macrolide antibiotics, various antifungal agents, and cytochrome P-450 inhibitors (fibrates and niacin should be used with appropriate caution).
Adapted from National Heart, Lung, and Blood Institute, 2001, http://www.nhlbi.nih.gov/guidelines/cholesterol/atp3full.pdf; accessed January 25, 2005.

soybean oils, Brussels sprouts, collards, endive, spinach, watercress, red bibb lettuce, cabbage, broccoli, kale, and parsley.

- Aspirin may decrease serum ferritin by increasing occult blood loss (Fleming et al, 2001).
- Digitalis and digoxin (Lanoxin) require the patient to avoid excessive amounts of vitamin D or natural licorice. In addition, a low potassium intake should be avoided because these drugs could become toxic. Avoid taking with high-fiber meals and herbal teas; take drugs 30 minutes before meals. Do not take with Siberian ginseng, milkweed, hawthorn, guar gum, or St. John's wort.
- Garlic: Trials suggest that garlic has short-term benefits on levels of some blood lipids (Ackermann, 2001). Parsley may be used as a breath freshener (Stevinson et al, 2000). Avoid excesses when a patient is on cardiac medications.
- Gemfibrozil (Lopid) is used for elevated triglycerides when there is a risk of pancreatitis; taste changes or abdominal pain may occur. Probucol (Lorelco) may cause vomiting or anorexia.
- Grapefruit juice decreases drug metabolism in the gut (via P-450–CYP3A4 inhibition) and can affect medications up to 24 hours later. Consistency of use may be more important than total quantity. Avoid taking with alprazolam, buspirone, cisapride, cyclosporine, statins, tacrolimus, and many other drugs.
- Psyllium (Metamucil) has been promoted as an effective agent in lowering total and LDL cholesterol levels,

but the evidence is not sufficient (Van Rosendaal et al, 2004).

- Statins reduce cholesterol production by the liver. They are being considered for over-the-counter use. Good nutritional practices should be followed (Kris-Etherton, 2000). Statins may lower coenzyme Q10 to the point of deficiency. Simvastatin may cause constipation; fluvastatin may cause nausea and abdominal cramps; pravastatin can elevate AST and ALT levels or cause nausea, vomiting, and diarrhea. Interestingly, statins may increase bone growth in legs and spine; they may be useful in women taking hormone replacement therapy. Increasing the amount of omega-3 fatty acids in the diet and reducing the omega-6 to omega-3 ratio, may allow statins (such as atorvastatin, lovastatin, and simvastatin), which are cholesterol-lowering medications, to work more effectively.
- Supplemental vitamins C and E, beta-carotene, and selenium should not be taken with simvastatin–niacin drug combinations because the combination of these antioxidants may lower HDL2 cholesterol, a beneficial subfraction of HDL cholesterol.
- Thiazides, propranolol, estrogens, and oral contraceptives may increase lipid levels or may lower folate levels.
- Colesevelam HCl (WelChol) can be used with statins; it is not absorbed into the bloodstream and has few side effects.

Herbs, Botanicals, and Supplements

- Herbs and botanicals such as angelica, hawthorn, canola, cinchona, valerian, willow, grape, pigweed, and chicory have been recommended for managing coronary heart disease, but no clinical trials have proven efficacy.
- Chromium is sometimes used for dyslipidemia. Do not use excesses of chromium with insulin or hypoglycemic agents because chromium may lower glucose levels excessively.
- Coenzyme Q10 (CoQ10; ubiquinone) should not be used with gemfibrozil, tricyclic antidepressants, or warfarin. CoQ10 may act similarly to vitamin K. Because CoQ10 shares a similar pathway as statins, they may be taken together (Mabuchi et al, 2005; Strey et al, 2005; Silver et al, 2004).
- Danshen may be used for ischemic heart disease. Avoid large amounts with warfarin, aspirin, and other antiplatelet drugs. It can increase risks of bleeding or bruising.
- Fenugreek may improve serum lipid levels slightly (Morelli and Zoorob, 2000). Further research is needed. Do not take with diuretics.
- Garlic tablets (0.6% allicin) given 3 times daily have lowered cholesterol levels and LDLs in some studies (Stevinson et al, 2000), but this has not been verified in all cases (Morelli and Zoorob, 2000). Large amounts should not be taken with warfarin, aspirin, and other antiplatelet drugs because of increased risks of bleeding or bruising. Garlic use may increase insulin levels with hypoglycemic results; monitor carefully in diabetes.
- Guggul (yellowish resin from mukul myrrh tree) is used in Indian Ayurveda medicine. It lowers LDL and increases HDL because of its plant sterols; it also stimulates the thyroid and is an anti-inflammatory and an antioxidant. Gugulipid is the safest form, but a high dose is needed. Gastrointestinal (GI) discomfort may occur. Do not take with Inderal or Cardizem, and do not use during pregnancy or lactation.
- Hawthorn should not be taken with digoxin, ACE inhibitors, and other cardiovascular drugs.
- Niacin (nicotinic acid) should not be taken with statins, antidiabetic medications, and carbamazepine because of potentially serious risks of myopathy and altered glucose control.
- Omega-3 fatty acids in fish oil capsules can cause hypervitaminosis A and D if taken in large doses. Avoid use in pregnant or lactating women. Avoid taking with warfarin, aspirin, and other antiplatelet medications because of the risk of increased bruising or bleeding.
- Vitamin E should not be taken with warfarin because of the possibility of increased bleeding. Avoid doses greater than 400 IU/d.

INTERVENTION: NUTRITION EDUCATION, COUNSELING, CARE MANAGEMENT

- Discuss the roles of heredity, exercise, and lifestyle habits. Blood pressure, cholesterol, obesity, and diabetes are affected by dietary patterns; some control is possible.
- There is no cholesterol in foods of plant origin. Encourage use of a plant-based diet.
- Explain which foods are sources of saturated fats and trans fatty acids. Most people eat about 3% of dietary kcal as trans fatty acids; the goal is to eat less than 1% kcal as trans fatty acids. Identify foods that are sources of polyunsaturated fats and monounsaturated fats (olive and peanut oils). An easy first step is changing to skim milk products instead of whole milk.
- Diets low in fat have different tastes and textures. If one changes diet too quickly, the diet may seem dry and unpalatable. Suggest changing gradually. Teach new ideas for moistening foods without adding excess fat (e.g., using applesauce instead of oil in some baked goods). Provide lists of resources such as cookbooks, newsletters, product samples, or coupons.
- Describe food sources of saturated MUFAs and PUFAs and cholesterol; discuss olive, soybean, walnut, and peanut oil uses. Help the patient make suitable substitutions. Although eggs contain cholesterol in the yolk, they can be planned into the diet 3–4 times weekly.
- Fish should be included several times weekly. Omega-3 fatty acids are found in fatter fish such as salmon, herring, tuna, mackerel, and other seafood.
- Teach the sources of soluble fiber (guar gum, pectin), as in apples, legumes, and oat and corn bran. Include other whole-grain foods for insoluble fiber. Both types of fiber are useful in reducing heart disease risk.
- Encourage the reading of food labels, including how to identify various ingredients on the label such as "free, low, reduced" cholesterol.
- Aerobic exercise, weight loss, smoking cessation, and lifestyle changes are needed (Leon et al, 2005). Help the

patient who is following an energy-controlled diet by providing ideas. Discuss coping skills, motivational factors, and environmental factors.

- Sources of vitamin B_6 include eggs, meats, fish, vegetables, yeast, whole-wheat grains, and milk. Sources of vitamin B_{12} include liver, meat, eggs, dairy products, and fish. Folate is found in liver, green vegetables, peas/beans, bread, bananas, and whole-grain cereals. Riboflavin is found primarily in dairy products.
- Have serum lipids and lipoproteins checked regularly. Note that very low cholesterol levels are not necessarily desirable; levels below 150 mg/dL may be associated with increased mortality from stroke, cancer, and other noncardiovascular diseases.
- Discuss low-fat cooking methods, such as baking, broiling, flame cooking, grilling, marinating, poaching, roasting, smoking, or steaming.
- Intensive lifestyle changes maintained for 5 years or longer can result in regression of CAD; more moderate changes are associated with progression of CAD (Ornish et al, 1998). Dr. Ornish's treatment for patients with coronary heart disease is a demanding regimen: a vegetarian diet with less than 10% of calories from fat, with minimal amounts of saturated fat (the "Reversal Diet").
- A combination regimen aimed at increasing HDL cholesterol levels improves cholesterol profiles, helps prevent angiographic progression of coronary stenosis, and may prevent cardiovascular events in some people who exercise regularly and eat low-fat diets (Whitney et al, 2005).

Patient Education—Foodborne Illness

- Careful food handling will be important. Hand washing is key as well.

For More Information

- National Cholesterol Education Program–National Heart, Lung, and Blood Institute
  http://www.nhlbi.nih.gov/guidelines/cholesterol/index.htm
- Your LDL and You
  http://nhlbisupport.com/chd1/treatment.htm

ATHEROSCLEROSIS, CORONARY ARTERY DISEASE, DYSLIPIDEMIA—CITED REFERENCES

Ackermann R, et al. Garlic shows some promise for improving some cardiovascular risk factors. *Arch Intern Med.* 161:813, 2001.

Aldana SG, et al. Effects of an intensive diet and physical activity modification program on the health risks of adults. *J Am Diet Assoc.* 105:371, 2005.

Arias BL, Ramon-Laca L. Pharmacological properties of citrus and their ancient and medieval uses in the Mediterranean region. *J Ethnopharmacol.* 97:89, 2005.

Brackbill ML, Sytsma C. Secondary prevention of hyperlipidemia after coronary artery bypass graft: from acute care to primary care. *Am J Crit Care.* 13:411, 2004.

Chahoud G, et al. Dietary recommendations in the prevention and treatment of coronary heart disease: do we have the ideal diet yet? *Am J Cardiol.* 94:1260, 2004.

da Costa KA, et al. Choline deficiency in mice and humans is associated with increased plasma homocysteine concentration after a methionine load. *Am J Clin Nutr.* 81:440, 2005.

Fleming D, et al. Aspirin intake and the use of serum ferritin as a measure of iron status. *Am J Clin Nutr.* 74:219, 2001.

Geleijnse JM, et al. Dietary intake of menaquinone is associated with a reduced risk of coronary heart disease: the Rotterdam Study. *J Nutr.* 134:3100, 2004.

Hall K, Luepker R. Is hypercholesterolemia a risk factor and should it be treated in the elderly? *Am J Health Promotion.* 14:347, 2000.

Kris-Etherton P. Over-the-counter statin medications: emerging opportunities for RDs. *JAMA.* 100:1126, 2000.

Law M, Morris J. By how much does fruit and vegetable consumption reduce the risk of ischemic heart disease? *Euro J Clin Nutr.* 52:549, 1998.

Lee DH, et al. Does supplemental vitamin C increase cardiovascular disease risk in women with diabetes? *Am J Clin Nutr.* 80:1194, 2004.

Leon AS, et al. Cardiac rehabilitation and secondary prevention of coronary heart disease: an American Heart Association scientific statement from the Council on Clinical Cardiology (Subcommittee on Exercise, Cardiac Rehabilitation, and Prevention) and the Council on Nutrition, Physical Activity, and Metabolism (Subcommittee on Physical Activity), in collaboration with the American Association of Cardiovascular and Pulmonary Rehabilitation. *Circulation* 111:369, 2005.

Locklin Holmes A, et al. Dietitian services are associated with improved patient outcomes and the MEDFICTS dietary assessment questionnaire is a suitable outcome measure in cardiac rehabilitation. *J Am Diet Assoc.* 105:1533, 2005.

Mabuchi H, et al. Reduction of serum ubiquinol-10 and ubiquinone-10 levels by atorvastatin in hypercholesterolemic patients. *J Atheroscler Thromb.* 12:111, 2005.

Moller DE, Kaufman KD. Metabolic syndrome: a clinical and molecular perspective. *Annu Rev Med.* 56:45, 2005.

Morelli V, Zoorob RJ. Alternative therapies. Part II: congestive heart failure and hypercholesterolemia. *Am Fam Physician.* 62:1325, 2000.

Morgan W, Clayshultze B. Pecans lower low-density lipoprotein cholesterol in people with normal lipid levels. *J Am Diet Assoc.* 100:312, 2000.

National Heart, Lung, and Blood Institute (NHLBI). Third Report of the Expert Panel on Detection, Evaluation, and Treatment of High Blood Cholesterol in Adults (Adult Treatment Panel III). 2001. Accessed at http://www.nhlbi.nih.gov/guidelines/cholesterol/atglance.htm.

Nissen SE, et al. Statin therapy, LDL cholesterol, C-reactive protein, and coronary artery disease. *N Engl J Med.* 352:29, 2005.

Ohrvall M, et al. Sagittal abdominal diameter compared with other anthropometric measurements in relation to cardiovascular risk. *Int J Obesity Relat Metab Disord.* 24:497, 2000.

Ornish D, et al. Intensive lifestyle changes for reversal of coronary heart disease. *JAMA.* 280:2001, 1998.

Pieke B, et al. Treatment of hypertriglyceridemia by two diets rich either in unsaturated fatty acids or in carbohydrates: effects on lipoprotein subclasses, lipolytic enzymes, and lipid transfer proteins, insulin and leptin. *Int J Obes Relat Metab Disord.* 24:1286, 2000.

Schieffer B, et al. Impact of interleukin-6 on plaque development and morphology in experimental atherosclerosis. *Circulation* 110:3493, 2004.

Silver MA, et al. Effect of atorvastatin on left ventricular diastolic function and ability of coenzyme Q10 to reverse that dysfunction. *Am J Cardiol.* 94:1306, 2004.

Stevinson C, et al. Garlic for treating hypercholesterolemia: a meta analysis of randomized clinical trials. *Ann Intern Med.* 133:411, 2000.

Stone NJ, Van Horn L. Therapeutic lifestyle change and Adult Treatment Panel III: evidence then and now. *Curr Atheroscler Rep.* 4:433, 2002.

Strey CH, et al. Endothelium-ameliorating effects of statin therapy and coenzyme Q10 reductions in chronic heart failure. *Atherosclerosis* 179:201, 2005.

Tucker KL, et al. The combination of high fruit and vegetable and low saturated fat intakes is more protective against mortality in aging men than is either alone: the Baltimore Longitudinal Study of Aging. *J Nutr.* 135:556, 2005.

Van Rosendaal GM. Effect of time of administration on cholesterol-lowering by psyllium: a randomized cross-over study in normocholesterolemic or slightly hypercholesterolemic subjects. *Nutr J.* 28:17, 2004.

Whitney EJ, et al. randomized trial of a strategy for increasing high-density lipoprotein cholesterol levels: effects on progression of coronary heart disease and clinical events. *Ann Intern Med.* 142:95, 2005.

Woodside J, et al. Effect of B-group vitamins and antioxidant vitamins on hyperhomocystinemia: a double-blind, randomized factorial-design, controlled trial. *Am J Clin Nutr.* 67:858, 1998.

Zambon D, et al. Substituting walnuts for monounsaturated fat improves serum lipid profile of hypercholesterolemic men and women: a randomized cross-over trial. *Ann Intern Med.* 132:538, 2000.

CARDIAC CACHEXIA

NUTRITIONAL ACUITY RANKING: LEVEL 4

DEFINITIONS AND BACKGROUND

Cardiac cachexia is concurrent with heart failure of such severity that patients cannot eat adequately to maintain weight. It involves a loss of more than 10% of lean body mass and can clinically be defined as a body weight loss of 7.5% of previous dry body weight in a period longer than 6 months (Bourdel-Marchasson and Emeriau, 2001).

The condition usually follows heart failure (moderate to severe), with some valvular heart disease. Nutritional insults generally affect the heart muscle severely, and the insult may be significant. Signs and symptoms of cardiac cachexia include increased total body fluid, which occurs in an effort to improve heart function; supraclavicular and temporal muscle wasting; weight loss; anorexia; and malabsorption with steatorrhea or diarrhea.

While the pathophysiological alterations leading to cardiac cachexia are unclear, metabolic, neurohormonal and immune abnormalities may play a role. Cachectic heart failure patients show raised plasma levels of epinephrine, norepinephrine, cortisol, renin, and aldosterone; tumor necrosis factor may also be involved (Anker et al, 2004). The wasting (cardiac cachexia) associated with chronic heart failure is an independent predictor of mortality (Adigun and Ajayi, 2001).

Patients with cardiac cachexia suffer from a general loss of fat tissue, lean tissue, and bone tissue. Left ventricular mass is lost (Florea et al, 2004). Data support findings that lower, rather than higher, cholesterol levels are associated with poor clinical outcome in patients with chronic heart failure. A moderate excess of body fat and elevated blood cholesterol are desirable in these patients (Louis et al, 2001). The ability of all lipoprotein fractions to bind endotoxin and to serve as natural buffer substances may explain the relationship between lower lipoprotein levels, higher cytokine concentrations, and impaired prognosis (Rauchhaus et al, 2000).

INTERVENTION: OBJECTIVES

- Improve hypoxic state and heart functioning.
- Correct malnutrition, wasting, malabsorption, and steatorrhea. Patients with heart failure have symptoms (e.g., breathing difficulties, fatigue, nausea, loss of appetite, early feeling of fullness, and ascites) that tend to decrease intake (Jacobsson et al, 2004).
- Optimize heart function through balance of medications, fluids, and electrolytes.
- Meet hypermetabolic state with adequate energy intake.
- Prevent infection or sepsis, especially if tracheostomy is required.
- Provide gradual repletion to prevent overloading in a severely depleted patient.
- Treat constipation or diarrhea as necessary.

INTERVENTION: FOOD AND NUTRITION

- Energy needs may be calculated at 50% above basic needs.
- Protein should be estimated at a rate of 1.0–1.5 g/kg, increasing or decreasing depending on renal or hepatic status.
- Offer tube feeding or parenteral nutrition if appropriate. Sometimes, tube feedings are not well tolerated because of access to the thoracic cavity and reduced blood flow to the gastrointestinal (GI) tract. High-calorie, low-volume products have a high density of calories; they are appropriate for persons with a fluid limitation but must be monitored with renal or hepatic insufficiency.
- Provide small, frequent meals to prevent overloading with high glucose levels or with rapid fat infusion.
- Provide as many preferred foods as feasible to improve appetite and intake.
- Antioxidants are often used in chronic heart failure, but there is only weak evidence for benefit. Foods containing omega-3 fatty acids can be safely recommended (Berger and Mustafa, 2003). Use more foods such as fish, fruits, cinnamon, cocoa, green tea and foods that contain flavonols, and nuts.
- A diet low in saturated fat may be appropriate to lessen cardiac effects of diet, but the focus is on adequate intake at this time.
- Sodium may need to be restricted to 1–2 g daily; modify potassium intake as appropriate for serum levels. The DASH diet is useful.
- Diet may need to be high in folate, magnesium, zinc, and iron (depending on serum levels). Increasing vitamins E, B_6, and B_{12} may also be beneficial. Thiamin should be included (Blanc and Boussuges, 2000) to alleviate cardiac beri-beri.

CLINICAL INDICATORS

Clinical/History

Height
Weight, current
Dry weight
BMI
Waist–hip ratio
Diet history
Edema
BP

Lab Work

Chol—total, HDL, LDL
Trig
CRP
Gluc
Fecal fat (in steatorrhea)
H & H
Serum Fe
Total lymphocyte count (TLC)
Serum insulin
Alb, transthyretin
Serum thiamin
Retinol-binding protein (RBP)
Transferrin
Na+, K+
Ca++, Mg++
Homocysteine
Serum folate
Serum B_{12}
Blood urea nitrogen (BUN), creatinine (Creat)

Common Drugs Used and Potential Side Effects

- Diuretics: Side effects may include potassium depletion; review types used and alter diet accordingly. Some diuretics spare calcium and protect bone health.
- Insulin may be needed if patient has diabetes or becomes hyperglycemic. Alter mealtimes accordingly.
- Digoxin: Monitor potassium intake or depletion carefully, especially when combining with diuretics. Avoid excessive intakes of fiber and wheat bran. Avoid use with hawthorn, milkweed, guar gum, and St. John's wort.
- Increased subcutaneous fat (increased skinfold thickness) and greater muscle bulk (increased mid-upper arm and thigh circumferences) together with a significant elevation in plasma albumin and the hematocrit will reflect the anabolic state in patients treated with angiotensin-converting enzyme (ACE) inhibitors, digoxin, and diuretic therapy in heart failure (Adigun and Ajayi, 2001).

Herbs, Botanicals, and Supplements

- Danshen may be used for ischemic heart disease. Avoid large amounts with warfarin, aspirin, and other antiplatelet drugs. It can increase risks of bleeding or bruising.
- Garlic should not be taken in large amounts with warfarin, aspirin, and other antiplatelet drugs because of increased risks of bleeding or bruising. It may also increase insulin levels with resulting hypoglycemic results; monitor carefully in patients with diabetes.
- Coenzyme Q10 (CoQ10; ubiquinone) should not be used with gemfibrozil, tricyclic antidepressants, or warfarin. CoQ10 may act similarly to vitamin K. Because CoQ10 shares a similar pathway as statins, they may be taken together (Mabuchi et al, 2005; Strey et al, 2005; Silver et al, 2004).
- Grapefruit juice decreases drug metabolism in the gut (via P-450–CYP3A4 inhibition) and can affect medications up to 24 hours later. Consistency of use may be more important than total quantity. Avoid taking with alprazolam, buspirone, cisapride, cyclosporine, statins, tacrolimus, and other drugs.
- Niacin (nicotinic acid) should not be taken with statins, antidiabetic medications, and carbamazepine because of the potentially serious risks of myopathy and altered glucose control.
- Omega-3 fatty acids in fish oil capsules can cause hypervitaminosis A and D if taken in large doses. Avoid use in pregnant or lactating women. Avoid taking with warfarin, aspirin, and other antiplatelet medications because of the risk of increased bruising or bleeding.
- Vitamin E should not be taken with warfarin because of the possibility of increased bleeding. Avoid doses greater than 400 IU/d.

INTERVENTION: NUTRITION EDUCATION, COUNSELING, CARE MANAGEMENT

- Balance medications, fluid, and electrolytes carefully.
- Supplements may be beneficial between meals to improve total calorie intake (e.g., sherbet shakes).
- The importance of diet in cardiovascular health should be addressed. However, rapid weight loss should be prevented.
- Patients with low BMI are at higher risk after cardiac surgery than obese or severely obese patients. Focusing on avoiding and/or reversing cachexia is more efficacious than reducing obesity in this population (Potapov et al, 2003).
- Exercise, with supervised guidance, can be beneficial (Schulze et al, 2002).

Patient Education—Foodborne Illness

- Careful food handling will be important. Hand washing is key as well.

For More Information

- Cardiac Cachexia
  http://www.gpnotebook.co.uk/cache/-617283577.htm
- Heart Hope
  http://www.hearthope.com/

CARDIAC CACHEXIA—CITED REFERENCES

Adigun A, Ajayi A. The effects of enalapril-digoxin-diuretic combination therapy on nutritional and anthropometric indices in chronic congestive heart failure: preliminary findings in cardiac cachexia. *Eur J Heart Fail.* 3:359, 2001.

Anker SD, et al. Cardiac cachexia. *Ann Med.* 36:518, 2004.

Berger MM, Mustafa I. Metabolic and nutritional support in acute cardiac failure. *Curr Opin Clin Nutr Metab Care.* 6:195, 2003.

Blanc P, Boussuges A. Cardiac beriberi. *Arch Mal Coeur Vaiss.* 93:371, 2000.

Bourdel-Marchasson I, Emeriau JP. Nutritional strategy in the management of heart failure in adults. *Am J Cardiovasc Drugs.* 1:363, 2001.

Florea VG, et al. Wasting of the left ventricle in patients with cardiac cachexia: a cardiovascular magnetic resonance study. *Int J Cardiol.* 97:15, 2004.

Jacobsson A, et al. Emotions, the meaning of food and heart failure: a grounded theory study. *J Adv Nurs.* 46:514, 2004.

Louis A, et al. Clinical Trials Update: CAPRICORN, COPERNICUS, MIRACLE, STAF, RITZ-2, RECOVER and RENAISSANCE and cachexia and cholesterol in heart failure. Highlights of the Scientific Sessions of the American College of Cardiology, 2001. *Eur J Heart Fail.* 3:381, 2001.

Mabuchi H, et al. Reduction of serum ubiquinol-10 and ubiquinone-10 levels by atorvastatin in hypercholesterolemic patients. *J Atheroscler Thromb.* 12:111, 2005.

Potapov EV, et al. Impact of body mass index on outcome in patients after coronary artery bypass grafting with and without valve surgery. *Eur Heart J.* 24:1933, 2003.

Rauchhaus M, et al. Inflammatory cytokines and the possible immunological role for lipoproteins in chronic heart failure. *Int J Cardiol.* 76:125, 2000.

Schulze PC, et al. Chronic heart failure and skeletal muscle catabolism: effects of exercise training. *Int J Cardiol.* 85:141, 2002.

Silver MA, et al. Effect of atorvastatin on left ventricular diastolic function and ability of coenzyme Q10 to reverse that dysfunction. *Am J Cardiol.* 94:1306, 2004.

Strey CH, et al. Endothelium-ameliorating effects of statin therapy and coenzyme Q10 reductions in chronic heart failure. *Atherosclerosis* 179:201, 2005.

CARDIOMYOPATHIES

NUTRITIONAL ACUITY RANKING: LEVEL 3

DEFINITIONS AND BACKGROUND

Cardiomyopathies may be caused by many known diseases or have no specific known cause. They are progressive disorders that impair the structure or function of the muscular wall of the lower chambers of the heart. Echocardiography is useful in demonstrating cardiac abnormalities seen in idiopathic cardiomyopathies, especially to differentiate constrictive pericarditis from restrictive cardiomyopathy (Nakatani and Miyatake, 2000). Figure 6-4 shows how atrial fibrillation differs from the normal heartbeat.

Dilated congestive cardiomyopathy (DCC) is most commonly caused by coronary heart disease in the United States. DCC may also occur from a viral infection such as coxsackievirus B, from diabetes or thyroid disease, or from excessive alcohol, cocaine, or antidepressant use. Rarely, pregnancy or rheumatory arthritis can also trigger DCC. The first symptoms are shortness of breath on exertion and easy fatigability; sometimes, a fever and flu-like symptoms occur if triggered by a virus. In some patients, deficiencies in calcium and potassium regulation have been noted (Olson et al, 2005).

Remaining heart muscle stretches to compensate for lost pumping action, and when the stretching no longer compensates, DCC occurs. Blood may pool in the swollen heart, and clots may form on the chamber walls. Seventy percent of patients with DCC die within 5 years of the beginning of their symptoms, and the prognosis worsens as the walls become thinner and the heart valves begin to leak. Because of this, DCC is the most common cause for heart transplantation.

Hypertrophic cardiomyopathy (HCM) may occur as a birth defect or as a result of acromegaly (excessive growth hormone in the blood), a pheochromocytoma, or a neurofibromatosis. Glycogen storage disease may also present with some cardiomyopathy (Arad et al, 2005). The differences in serum carnitine levels between HCM and hypertensive heart disease reflect altered myocardial fatty acid metabolic impairment, and the levels can help to distinguish between these two diseases (Nakamura, 2000).

Thickening of the heart wall causes high blood pressure, pulmonary hypertension, and chronic shortness of breath. Faintness, chest pain, irregular heartbeats and palpitations, and heart failure with dyspnea will occur. HCM is a possible cause of sudden death; it is largely confined to young people but can occur suddenly at any stage of life. Most patients with mild hypertrophy are at low risk and can be reassured regarding their prognosis (Spirito et al, 2000).

Treatment options for patients with obstructive HCM include medical therapy, pacemaker insertion, percutaneous transluminal septal myocardial ablation, mitral valve replacement, and surgical resection of the obstructing muscle (Meisel et al, 2000). Septal myectomy reduces or abolishes left ventricular outflow tract gradient in these patients and provides long-lasting symptomatic improvement in most patients (Merrill et al, 2000). Nonsurgical septal reduction therapy is also an effective therapy for symptomatic patients

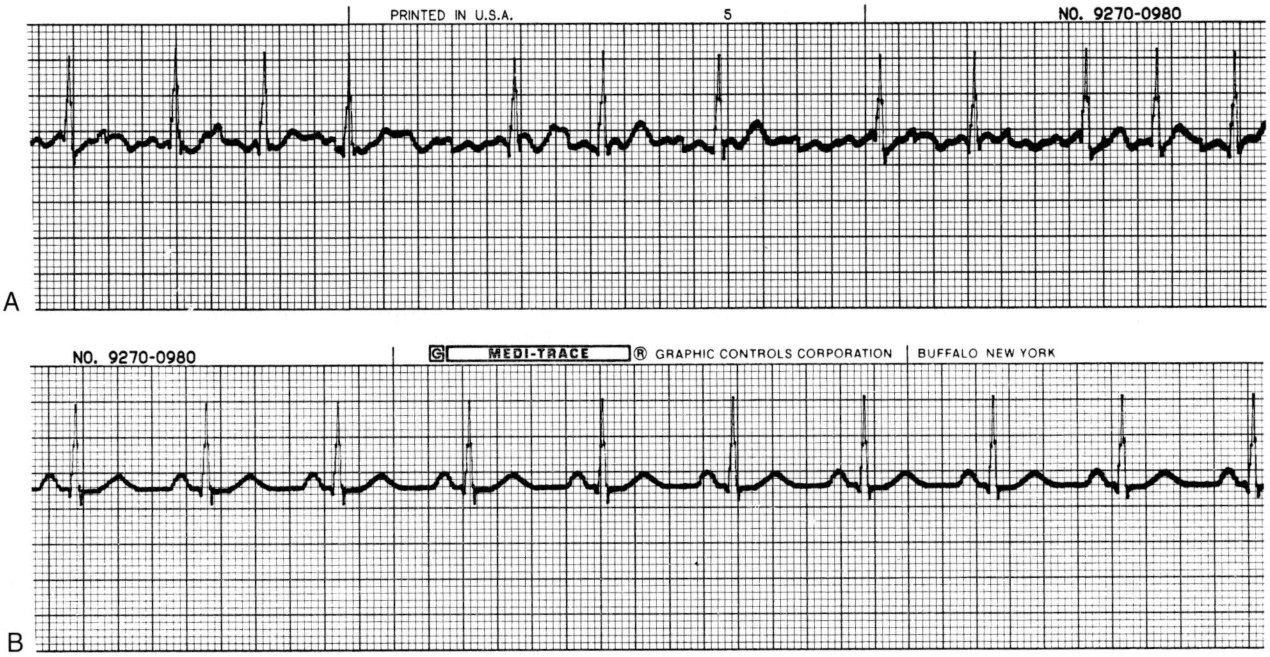

Figure 6-4 Atrial fibrillation. (From Smeltzer SC, Bare BG. *Textbook of medical-surgical nursing*. 9th ed. Philadelphia: Lippincott Williams & Wilkins, 2000.)

with obstructive HCM, with persistence of the favorable outcome up to 1 year after the procedure (Lakkis et al, 2000).

INTERVENTION: OBJECTIVES

- Improve hypoxic state and heart functioning.
- Correct malnutrition, malabsorption, and steatorrhea.
- Optimize heart function through balance of medications, fluids, and electrolytes.
- Meet hypermetabolic state with adequate calories.
- Provide gradual repletion to prevent overloading in a severely depleted patient.
- Treat constipation or diarrhea as necessary.
- Prepare for surgery, if planned.

INTERVENTION: FOOD AND NUTRITION

- Energy intake may be calculated at 50% above usual needs.
- Protein should be calculated at a rate of 1.0–1.5 g/kg, increasing or decreasing depending on renal or hepatic status.
- Provide small, frequent meals to prevent overloading with high glucose or with rapid fat infusion. Provide as many preferred foods as feasible to improve appetite and intake.
- A prudent diet may be appropriate to reduce cardiac effects of diet. Follow therapeutic lifestyle change (TLC) diet interventions. Pistachios, sunflower kernels, sesame seeds, and wheat germ are high in phytosterols; use often.
- The DASH diet is useful. Diet may need to be high in calcium and potassium (Olson et al, 2005); folate, magnesium, zinc, and iron may also be needed, depending on serum levels. Increasing vitamins E, B_6, and B_{12} may be beneficial. Thiamin should also be included (Blanc and Boussuges, 2000) because of likelihood of cardiac beri-beri.
- Sodium may need to be restricted to 2–4 g daily; modify potassium intake as appropriate for serum levels.
- Offer tube feeding or parenteral nutrition if appropriate. Sometimes, tube feedings are not well tolerated because of access to the thoracic cavity and because of reduced blood flow to the GI tract. High-calorie, low-volume products are useful for their high density of calories. They are appropriate for persons with a fluid limitation but must be monitored in patients with renal or hepatic difficulty.

CLINICAL INDICATORS

Clinical/History

Height
Weight, current
Dry weight
BMI
Waist–hip ratio
Diet history
Heart murmur
BP (normal or low)
Edema (common)
Echocardiography
ECG
Cardiac catheterization
Temperature

Lab Work

Chol—total, HDL, LDL
Trig
CRP
Prothrombin time (PT) or international normalized ratio (INR)
Na+, K+
Ca++, Mg++
Gluc
H & H
Serum Fe
Serum insulin
Alb, transthyretin
RBP
Transferrin
BUN, Creat
Homocysteine
Serum folate
Serum B_{12}

Common Drugs Used and Potential Side Effects

- Anticoagulant therapy is needed to prevent clots from causing heart attacks, strokes, and other problems. With warfarin (Coumadin), use a controlled amount of vitamin K; check tube feeding (TF) products and supplements. Limit foods high in vitamin K to 1 serving per day. Foods high in vitamin K include mayonnaise, canola and soybean oils, Brussels sprouts, collards, endive, spinach, watercress, red bibb lettuce, cabbage, broccoli, kale, and parsley.
- Blood-thinning medications: Omega-3 fatty acids may increase the blood-thinning effects of aspirin or warfarin. While the combination of aspirin and omega-3 fatty acids may actually be helpful under certain circumstances (such as heart disease), they should only be taken together under the guidance and supervision of a health care provider. Be wary of using supplements containing vitamins A and C with these drugs; side effects may be detrimental. Vitamin E should not be taken with warfarin because of the possibility of increased bleeding; avoid doses greater than 400 IU/d. Avoid taking with dong quai, fenugreek, feverfew, excessive garlic, ginger, ginkgo, and ginseng because of their effects.
- Beta-blockers and calcium channel blockers may be used to reduce the force of heart contractions.
- Diuretics: Side effects may include potassium depletion; review types used and alter diet accordingly. Some diuretics spare calcium and protect bone health.
- Digoxin: Monitor potassium intake or depletion carefully, especially when combining with diuretics. Avoid excessive intakes of fiber and wheat bran. Avoid use with hawthorn, milkweed, guar gum, and St. John's wort.
- Grapefruit juice decreases drug metabolism in the gut (via P-450–CYP3A4 inhibition) and can affect medications up to 24 hours later. Consistency of use may be more important than total quantity. Avoid taking with alprazolam, buspirone, cisapride, cyclosporine, statins, tacrolimus, and many other drugs.
- Insulin may be needed if patient has diabetes or becomes hyperglycemic. Alter mealtimes accordingly.
- Omega-3 fatty acids in fish oil capsules can cause hypervitaminosis A and D if taken in large doses. Avoid use in pregnant or lactating women. Avoid taking with warfarin, aspirin, and other antiplatelet medications because of the risk of increased bruising or bleeding.

Herbs, Botanicals, and Supplements

- Danshen may be used for ischemic heart disease. Avoid large amounts with warfarin, aspirin, and other antiplatelet drugs. It can increase risks of bleeding or bruising.
- Garlic should not be taken in large amounts with warfarin, aspirin, or other antiplatelet drugs because of increased risks of bleeding or bruising. It may also increase insulin levels with hypoglycemic results; monitor carefully in patients with diabetes.
- Coenzyme Q10 (CoQ10; ubiquinone) should not be used with gemfibrozil, tricyclic antidepressants, or warfarin. CoQ10 may act similarly to vitamin K. Because CoQ10 and statins share a similar pathway, they can be taken simultaneously (Mabuchi et al, 2005; Strey et al, 2005; Silver et al, 2004).
- Niacin (nicotinic acid) should not be taken with statins, antidiabetic medications, or carbamazepine because of potentially serious risks of myopathy and altered glucose control.

INTERVENTION: NUTRITION EDUCATION, COUNSELING, CARE MANAGEMENT

- Adequate rest is essential. Avoidance of stress is also important.
- Balance medications, fluid, and electrolytes carefully.
- Supplements may be beneficial between meals to improve total calorie intake (e.g., sherbet shakes).
- The importance of diet in cardiovascular health should be addressed.
- Because of the high risk for sudden death in HCM patients, they should be advised against participation in competitive sports (DeLuca and Tak, 2000).
- For inherited forms of HCM, genetic counseling may be beneficial if planning a family.

Patient Education—Foodborne Illness

- Careful food handling will be important. Hand washing is key as well.

For More Information

- Cardiomyopathy
  http://www.americanheart.org/presenter.jhtml?identifier=4468
- Hypertrophic cardiomyopathy
  http://www.cardiomyopathy.org/

CARDIOMYOPATHIES—CITED REFERENCES

Arad M, et al. Glycogen storage diseases presenting as hypertrophic cardiomyopathy. *N Engl J Med.* 352:362, 2005.

Blanc P, Boussuges A. Cardiac beriberi. *Arch Mal Coeur Vaiss.* 93:371, 2000.

DeLuca M, Tak T. Hypertrophic cardiomyopathy. Tools for identifying risk and alleviating symptoms. *Postgrad Med.* 107:127, 2000.

Lakkis N, et al. Nonsurgical septal reduction therapy for hypertrophic obstructive cardiomyopathy: one-year follow-up. *J Am Col Cardiol.* 36:852, 2000.

Mabuchi H, et al. Reduction of serum ubiquinol-10 and ubiquinone-10 levels by atorvastatin in hypercholesterolemic patients. *J Atheroscler Thromb.* 12:111, 2005.

Meisel E, et al. Pacemaker therapy of hypertrophic obstructive cardiomyopathy. PIC (Pacing in Cardiomyopathy) Study Group. *Herz.* 25:461, 2000.

Merrill W, et al. Long-lasting improvement after septal myectomy for hypertrophic obstructive cardiomyopathy. *Ann Thorac Surg.* 69:1732, 2000.

Nakamura T, et al. Can serum carnitine levels distinguish hypertrophic cardiomyopathy from hypertensive hearts? *Hypertension.* 36:215, 2000.

Nakatani S, Miyatake K. Echocardiography of idiopathic cardiomyopathies. *Nippon Rinsho.* 58:37, 2000.

Olson TM, et al. Sodium channel mutations and susceptibility to heart failure and atrial fibrillation. *JAMA.* 293:447, 2005.

Silver MA, et al. Effect of atorvastatin on left ventricular diastolic function and ability of coenzyme Q10 to reverse that dysfunction. *Am J Cardiol.* 94:1306, 2004.

Spirito P, et al. Magnitude of left ventricular hypertrophy and risk of sudden death in hypertrophic cardiomyopathy. *N Engl J Med.* 342:1778, 2000.

Strey CH, et al. Endothelium-ameliorating effects of statin therapy and coenzyme Q10 reductions in chronic heart failure. *Atherosclerosis* 179:201, 2005.

HEART FAILURE

NUTRITIONAL ACUITY RANKING: LEVEL 3

DEFINITIONS AND BACKGROUND

Heart failure (HF) is the leading cause of cardiovascular disease and related death. There are nearly 5 million cases of HF in the United States, with more than 500,000 new cases diagnosed each year (American Heart Association, 2005). See Figure 6-5 for a picture of HF, showing backflow of blood into the lung space.

HF results in reduced heart pumping efficiency in the lower two chambers, with less blood circulating to body tissues, congestion in lungs or body circulation, ankle swelling, abdominal pain, ascites, hepatic congestion, jugular vein distention, and breathing difficulty. HF is a common diagnosis in hospitalized patients. Four stages have been identified (Hunt et al, 2005):

Stage A has mild symptoms and no limitation on physical activity, with few signs or symptoms of HF.

Stage B shows structural heart disease but no signs or symptoms of HF.

Stage C demonstrates signs and symptoms of structural HF.

Stage D shows refractory HF requiring specialized interventions.

HF can be caused by coronary heart disease, previous heart attack, history of cardiomyopathy, lung disease such as chronic obstructive pulmonary disease (COPD), severe

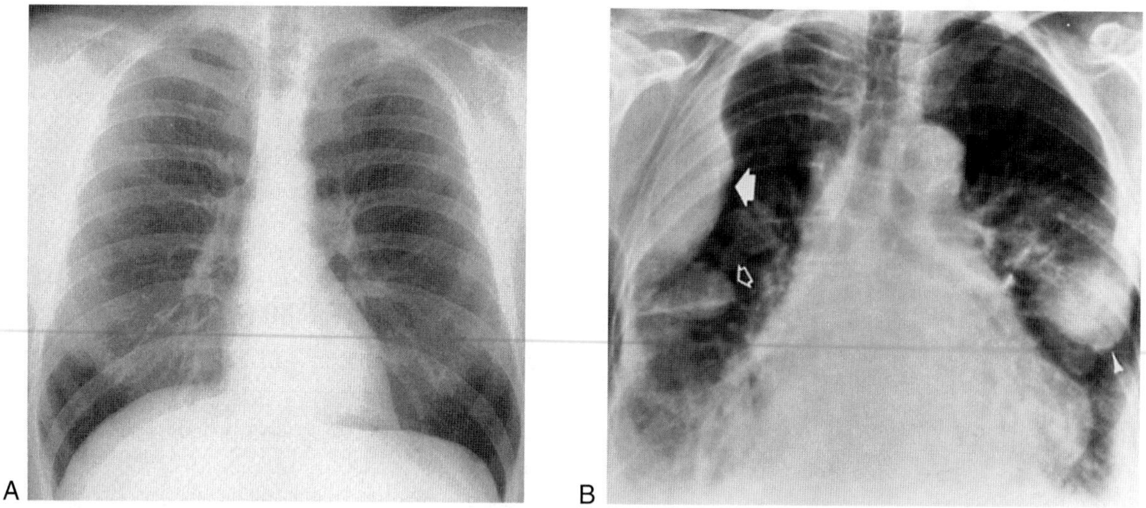

Figure 6-5 Heart failure. (From Kahn GP, Lynch JP. *Pulmonary disease diagnosis and therapy: a practical approach*. Philadelphia: Lippincott Williams & Wilkins, 1997; Eisenberg RL. *Clinical imaging: an atlas of differential diagnosis*. 4th ed. Philadelphia: Lippincott Williams & Wilkins, 2003.)

anemia, excessive alcohol consumption, or low thyroid function. Male sex, lower education, physical inactivity, cigarette smoking, overweight, diabetes, hypertension, valvular heart disease, and coronary heart disease are all independent risk factors, with coronary heart disease being the most likely risk factor (He et al, 2001). Since the leading cause of HF in Western countries is ischemic heart disease, aggressive therapy to halt progression of coronary atherosclerosis can have a major impact on controlling and often curing HF (Futterman and Lemberg, 2003).

Right-sided failure yields pitting edema of extremities and fatigue. Left-sided failure affects the lungs, with pulmonary edema, rales, and dyspnea. Decreased renal flow is common; BUN may be increased. Early adaptations to mild HF show susceptibility to sodium excess. Evidence suggests that advanced HF is a multifactorial metabolic syndrome that can lead to cardiac cachexia, which then carries a very poor prognosis. The mechanisms underlying this association are poorly understood.

Inflammatory cytokines may play a pathogenic role in HF. HF is associated with elevated levels of angiotensin II in the blood, causing vessel contraction and high blood pressure in addition to muscle wasting. Studies are currently reviewing the role of various hormonal factors.

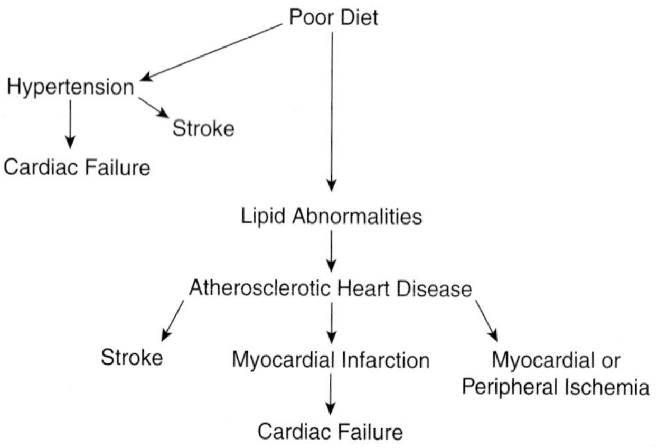

Figure 6-6 Effects of diet on cardiac failure.

Dietary sodium restriction and diuretics are basic requirements in the treatment of congestive HF. Treatment may also include implantation of a pacemaker or cardiac transplantation. Joint efforts of cardiologists, endocrinologists, and immunologists are required to develop therapeutic strategies able to improve the metabolic status of HF patients (Anker and Rauchhaus, 1999).

The relationship between asthma-related inflammation and HF is currently being studied. In addition, in obese patients, HF can lead to cardiac cachexia (anorexia with fat and muscle wasting and edema). In cardiac cachexia, dietary and metabolic factors and levels and activity of cytokines, thyroid hormone, catecholamines, and cortisol may be responsible for causing weight loss. The American Dietetic Association has recommended at least four medical nutrition therapy visits for patients with HF.

INTERVENTION: OBJECTIVES

- Promote rest to lessen demands on the heart. Restore hemodynamic stability; prevent cardiogenic shock or thromboembolism.
- Eliminate or reduce edema.
- Avoid distention and elevation of diaphragm, which reduces vital capacity. Prevent excessive refeeding.
- Attain desirable BMI and waist to hip ratio to decrease oxygen requirements and tissue nutrient demands. Replace lean body mass (LBM), if needed.
- Limit cardiac stimulants.
- Prevent or correct cardiac cachexia, low blood pressure, listlessness, weak pulse from potassium-depleting diuretics, anorexia, nausea and vomiting, and sepsis.
- Correct any nutrient deficits.
- Prevent pressure ulcers from reduced activity levels and poor circulation.
- Long-term, nondrug therapy, including weight reduction, physical activity, and restriction of dietary sodium

and alcohol intake, is an effective strategy for lowering BP; if these measures are not adequate, then the addition of drug therapy is needed to provide gradual BP normalization (Flack and Staffinelo, 1998).

INTERVENTION: FOOD AND NUTRITION

- Limit sodium; 4–6 g of sodium may be satisfactory. Consider use of the DASH diet (see Hypertension entry). The diet should provide adequate potassium and magnesium (Gums, 2004) to replace losses; monitor potassium in medications and salt substitutes. Table 6-6 lists the sodium content of common foods. Table 6-7 provides some alternative tips for lowering sodium in the diet.
- A vegan diet is useful. Provide 5–6 small meals a day, with no more than 3 L fluid per day. Patients with refractory edema may need a limit of 0.5 mL/kcal given. For tube feeding (TF), use a low-sodium product and increase volume gradually.
- Antioxidants such as vitamin E are needed in DRI levels. There is no evidence that more is better, and the pro-odixant effects may actually be detrimental.
- With total parenteral nutrition, ensure adequate intake of all micronutrients as well as macronutrients.
- If patient is obese, a calorie-controlled diet is beneficial.
- Restrict caffeine intake. At first, no caffeine is allowed; later, coffee intake may be limited to 5 cups of regular coffee per day to reduce stimulants.

TABLE 6-6 Sodium Content of Typical Food Items

Food Item	mg	Food Item	mg
Meat, poultry, and fish		**Dairy products**	
Sirloin steak (3 oz)	53	Butter, salted (1 tbsp)	116
Baked salmon (3 oz)	55	Milk (1 cup)	122
Chicken breast (3 oz)	64	Sour cream (1 cup)	123
Ground beef patty (4 oz)	87	Margarine (1 tbsp)	134
Chicken leg, fried (2.5 oz)	194	Chocolate pudding (1 cup)	180
Tuna, canned (3 oz)	468	Baked custard (1 cup)	209
Hot dog (1)	504	Buttermilk (1 cup)	257
Salami (2 slices)	607	Parmesan cheese (1/4 cup)	465
Fast food hamburger (4 oz)	763	Cheddar cheese (1 cup)	701
Corned beef (3 oz)	802	Cottage cheese, creamy (1 cup)	911
Ham, canned (3 oz)	908	Cheese sauce, prepared from recipe (1 cup)	1198
Fast foods, shrimp, breaded and fried (6–8 shrimp)	1446	**Snacks, drinks, condiments, desserts**	
Submarine sandwich (one 6″ roll, cold cuts)	1651	Orange juice (1 cup)	2
Smoked salmon (3 oz)	1700	Peanuts, unsalted (1 cup)	22
Soups, Vegetables, Fruit		Chocolate fudge (1 oz)	54
Apple (1)	0	Diet cola, with saccharin	75
Banana (1)	1	Club soda (12 oz)	78
Mixed vegetables, frozen (1 cup)	64	Potato chips (10)	94
Mixed vegetables, canned (1 cup)	243	Mustard (1 tbsp)	129
Chicken noodle soup, canned (1 cup)	1106	Ketchup (1 tbsp)	156
Tomato sauce, canned (1 cup)	1482	Hard pretzel (1)	258
Sauerkraut (1 cup)	1560	Shortbread cookies (2)	300
Breads and grains		Apple pie (1 slice)	476
Wheat bread (1 slice)	106	Peanuts, salted (1 cup)	626
Oatmeal, cooked (1 cup)	2	Vegetable juice (1 cup)	883
Italian bread (1 slice)	176	Dill pickle (1)	928
Bagel (1)	245	Pretzel twists (10)	966
English muffin (1)	378	Pie crust, 1 shell	976
Bread crumbs (1 cup)	3180	Beef bouillon (1 packet)	1019

Reference: USDA Nutrient Database, http://www.nal.usda.gov/fnic/foodcomp/Data/SR14/wtrank/sr14w307.pdf; accessed February 6, 2006.

TABLE 6-7 Tips for Lowering Sodium in the Diet

Choose More Often:

- Fresh, plain frozen, or canned "with no salt added" vegetables
- Fresh poultry, fish, and lean meat, rather than canned or processed types
- Herbs, spices, and salt-free seasoning blends in cooking and at the table
- Rice, pasta, and hot cereals cooked without salt. Cut back on instant or flavored rice, pasta, and cereal mixes, which usually have added salt.
- "Convenience" foods that are lower in sodium. Cut back on frozen dinners, pizza, packaged mixes, canned soups or broths, and salad dressings; these often have a lot of sodium.
- Canned foods, such as tuna, drained and rinsed to remove some sodium
- Low- or reduced-sodium or no salt added versions of foods
- Ready-to-eat breakfast cereals that are lower in sodium, such as shredded wheat

Choose Less Often:

- Hogmaws, ribs, and chitterlings
- Smoked or cured meats like bacon, bologna, hot dogs, ham, corned beef, luncheon meats, and sausage
- Canned fish like tuna, salmon, sardines, and mackerel
- Buttermilk
- Most cheese spreads and cheeses
- Salty chips, nuts, pretzels, and pork rinds
- Some cold (ready to eat) cereals highest in sodium, instant hot cereals
- Quick cooking rice and instant noodles, boxed mixes like rice, scalloped potatoes, macaroni and cheese, and some frozen dinners, pot pies, and pizza
- Regular canned vegetables
- Pickled foods like herring, pickles, relish, olives, and sauerkraut
- Regular canned soups, instant soups
- Butter, fatback, and salt pork
- Soy sauce, steak sauce, salad dressing, ketchup, barbecue sauce, garlic salt, onion salt, seasoned salts like lemon pepper, bouillon cubes, meat tenderizer, and monosodium glutamate (MSG)*

From: National Heart, Lung, and Blood Institute. Reduce Salt and Sodium in Your Diet; accessed at http://www.nhlbi.nih.gov/hbp/prevent/sodium/sodium.htm.

- Use foods that are not gas forming to reduce heartburn, distention, and flatulence. Beans, cabbage, onions, cauliflower, and Brussels sprouts may cause these problems.
- Use soft textures to reduce the amount of chewing. Add soluble fiber from apples or oat bran if tolerated.
- Ensure adequate intakes of vitamins E, B_6, and B_{12} and folic acid from the diet.
- Thiamin levels also tend to be low and should be supplemented (Blanc and Boussuges, 2000). Those individuals who are alcoholics, malnourished, elderly, or have AIDS are at special risk for thiamin deficiency. Cardiovascular problems associated with beri-beri include peripheral vasodilatation with increased cardiac output, myocardial lesion, sodium and water retention, and biventricular myocardial failure; thiamin administration is the treatment (Blanc and Boussuges, 2000).
- Pistachios, sunflower kernels, sesame seeds, and wheat germ are highest in phytosterols; use often.
- Reduce or eliminate alcohol intake if needed. For women, this means no more than 1 drink per day; for men, this means 2 drinks or less a day.

CLINICAL INDICATORS

Clinical/History

Height
Weight
BMI
Waist–hip ratio
Diet history
BP
Dry, hacking cough
Skin, cyanotic or pale
Abnormal breath sounds
Pulse (NL = 60–100 beats/min)
Temperature
Edema
Glomerular filtration rate (GFR)
Oliguria
I & O
Chest x-ray
Echocardiography
ECG
Cardiac catheterization

Lab Work

CRP
BNP (hormone secreted by ventricles when pressure goes up, signaling heart failure)
Uric acid
Oximetry
Partial pressure of carbon dioxide (pCO_2)
Partial pressure of oxygen (pO_2)
Specific gravity (increased)
Chol–total, HDL, LDL
Trig
Homocysteine
Serum folate
Serum B_{12}
Na+, K+
Ca++, Mg++
Gluc
H & H
Serum Fe
Serum zinc
Alk phos
Alb, transthyretin
BUN, Creat
PT or INR
LDH (increased)
Nitrogen (N) balance
AST, ALT

Common Drugs Used and Potential Side Effects

- See Table 6-8. Note: Most patients with HF require combination therapy that includes a diuretic, an ACE inhibitor, a beta-blocker, and digoxin (Talbert, 2003). Selected patients may benefit from alternative or additional medications, such as anticoagulants for atrial fibrillation.

Herbs, Botanicals, and Supplements

- The patient should not take herbals and botanicals without discussing with the physician. It is important to stress that no supplement or diet can cure HF.
- L-arginine, found in health food stores, needs more formal studies (Schulman et al, 2006). This amino acid appears to reduce endothelin, a protein that causes blood vessel constriction and is found in high amounts in HF patients. It should not be used after a myocardial infarction (Schulman et al, 2006).
- Chromium is sometimes used for dyslipidemia. Do not use excesses with insulin or hypoglycemic agents, because chromium may lower glucose levels excessively.
- Coenzyme Q10 (CoQ10; ubiquinone) should not be used with gemfibrozil, tricyclic antidepressants, or warfarin. CoQ10 may act similarly to vitamin K. Because CoQ10 and statins share a similar pathway, they can be taken simultaneously (Mabuchi et al, 2005; Strey et al, 2005; Silver et al, 2004).
- Grapefruit juice decreases drug metabolism in the gut (via P-450–CYP3A4 inhibition) and can affect medications up to 24 hours later. Consistency of use may be more important than total quantity. Avoid taking with alprazolam, buspirone, cisapride, cyclosporine, statins, tacrolimus, and many other drugs.
- Hawthorn is used in Germany for HF, but no well-designed studies have been completed in the United States (Morelli and Zoorob, 2000).
- Niacin (nicotinic acid) should not be taken with statins, antidiabetic medications, and carbamazepine because of potentially serious risks of myopathy and altered glucose control.
- Omega-3 fatty acids in fish oil capsules can cause hypervitaminosis A and D if taken in large doses. Avoid use in pregnant or lactating women. Avoid taking with warfarin, aspirin, and other antiplatelet medications because of the risk of increased bruising or bleeding.
- Vitamin E should not be taken with warfarin because of the possibility of increased bleeding. Avoid doses greater than 400 IU/d.

INTERVENTION: NUTRITION EDUCATION, COUNSELING, CARE MANAGEMENT

- Identify the appropriate stage of readiness for change in the patient. Behavioral changes that prevent disease progression are just as important as the medications prescribed to treat HF; the most difficult lifestyle changes include smoking cessation, weight loss, and restriction of dietary sodium (Paul and Sneed, 2004). Supervised nutrition intervention is of great importance (Colin Ramirez et al, 2004).
- A congested feeling may cause a poor appetite. Ensure that the patient takes smaller, more appetizing, and more frequent meals. Never force the patient to eat. Allow rest before and after meals. Use high-calorie, low-volume supplements to increase nutrient density when needed.
- Help patient plan fluid intake over waking hours, usually 75% with meals and 25% with medications and for thirst between meals.
- Alcohol should be avoided.

TABLE 6-8 Medications Used in Heart Failure

Medication	Description
ACE Inhibitors Benazepril Captopril Enalapril (Vasotec) Fosinopril Lisinopril (Zestoretic, Zestril) Moexipril Perindopril Quinapril Ramipril Trandolapril	ACE inhibitors block angiotensin II and decrease aldosterone output, thereby decreasing sodium and water retention. Monitor for hyperkalemia, nausea, vomiting, dizziness, and abdominal pain.
Angiotensin Receptor Blockers Candesartan Eprosartan Irbesartan Losartan Olmesartan Telmisartan Valsartan	Common adverse effects include hypotension and dizziness, a concern when there is also blurred vision or worsening renal function.
Aldosterone Blockers Eplerenone Spironolactone	
Anticoagulants Warfarin (Coumadin)	Consume foods high in vitamin K no more than once per day. Foods high in vitamin K include mayonnaise, canola and soybean oils, Brussels sprouts, collards, endive, spinach, watercress, red bibb lettuce, cabbage, broccoli, kale, and parsley. Avoid taking with dong quai, fenugreek, feverfew, ginger, ginkgo, ginseng, or excesses of ginger because of their undesired side effects. Aniseed, celery, cranberry juice, dandelion, licorice, onion, passion flower, or willow bark can increase the effects. Coenzyme Q10, green tea, goldenseal, St. John's wort, and yarrow may decrease the effectiveness of warfarin.
Beta-Blockers Acebutolol Atenolol Betaxolol Bisoprolol Carteolol Carvedilol Labetalol Metoprolol succinate Metoprolol tartrate Nadolol Penbutolol Pindolol Propranolol Timolol	Beta-adrenergic blockers reduce cardiac output in competing for available receptor sites; they decrease sympathetic stimulation of the heart. When first used, they may promote fluid retention and fatigue.
Digitalis Digoxin	Digitalis can deplete potassium, especially when taken with furosemide. Beware of excesses of wheat bran, which can decrease serum drug levels. Anorexia or nausea may occur.
Diuretics:	Avoid use with fenugreek, ginkgo, and yohimbe. Some diuretics spare calcium and protect bone health.
Loop diuretics Bumetanide Furosemide Torsemide	Most loop diuretics deplete potassium and magnesium; calcium levels also decline. Glucose tolerance may be decreased; anorexia, nausea, or vomiting may occur. Use a low-sodium diet.
Thiazide diuretics Chlorothiazide Chlorthalidone Hydrochlorothiazide Indapamide Metolazone	Most thiazide diuretics deplete potassium, which must be replaced, either orally or by medication.
Potassium-sparing diuretics Amiloride Spironolactone Triamterene	Hyperkalemia can occur with use of potassium-sparing diuretics if lab values are not carefully monitored. Avoid use with NSAIDs.
Salt Substitutes	Salt substitutes generally contain KCl, and their use could lead to hyperkalemia if potassium-sparing diuretics such as spironolactone (Aldactone) or triamterene (Dyrenium) are part of treatment.
Statins	Statins may be used if the underlying problem is related to coronary artery disease or dyslipidemia. See Table 6-5.

Reference: Hunt et al, 2005.

- Bed rest may be required in cases of severe congestive HF. To reduce congestion in the lungs, the patient's upper body should be elevated; for most patients, resting in an armchair is better than lying in bed. Relaxing and contracting leg muscles are important exercises to prevent clots. As the patient improves, progressively more activity will be recommended.
- HF is associated with sleep apnea, in which tissues at the back of the throat periodically collapse and become blocked, causing the sleeper to gasp for air. Sleep apnea has been associated with poorer survival in patients with HF. A continuous positive airway pressure (CPAP) device is effective and appears to improve ejection fraction in HF patients. See Section 5 for more details.
- Check the water supply for use of softening agents. Also, have the patients monitor sodium-containing medications, toothpastes, and mouthwashes.
- Discuss spices and seasonings as salt alternatives.
- Teach label reading and tips for easy meal preparation. Choose items that state: sodium free, very low sodium, low sodium, reduced sodium, light in sodium, or unsalted. Avoid excessive use of canned soups, cured or smoked meats, and commercial sauces. Many frozen dinners are high in sodium also; use healthier brands.
- Freeze small meal portions for use when energy levels are low.
- Refer to local congregate meal programs or inquire about home-delivered meals for elderly individuals. Many will provide low-sodium meals upon request.
- Implantation of circulatory assist devices as a permanent alternative to heart transplantation (destination therapy) is used with patients with HF who are not responding to medications. The HeartMate Left Ventricular Assist System is the device the FDA has approved.

Patient Education—Foodborne Illness

- Careful food handling will be important. Hand washing is key as well.

For More Information

- Heart Failure
  http://www.hearthope.com/learn.html
- National Heart, Lung, and Blood Institute
  http://www.nhlbi.nih.gov/hbp/hbp/effect/heart.htm
  http://www.nhlbi.nih.gov/hbp/prevent/h_eating/h_eating.htm
- Spices and Seasonings
  http://www.nhlbi.nih.gov/hbp/prevent/sodium/flavor.htm

HEART FAILURE—CITED REFERENCES

American Heart Association. American Heart Association homepage. Accessed June 3, 2005 at http://www.amhrt.org/.

Anker S, Rauchhaus M. Heart failure as a metabolic problem. *Eur J Heart Fail.* 1:127, 1999.

Blanc P, Boussuges A. Cardiac beriberi. *Arch Mal Coeur Vaiss.* 93:371, 2000.

Colin Ramirez E, et al. Effects of a nutritional intervention on body composition, clinical status, and quality of life in patients with heart failure. *Nutrition* 20:890, 2004.

Flack JM, Staffinelo BA. Therapeutic strategies for hypertension treatment in patients with selected cardiovascular diseases. *Drugs Today* 34:813, 1998.

Futterman LG, Lemberg L. Diuretics, the most critical therapy in heart failure, yet often neglected in the literature. *Am J Crit Care.* 12:376, 2003.

Gums JG. Magnesium in cardiovascular and other disorders. *Am J Health Syst Pharm.* 61:1569, 2004.

He J, et al. Risk factors for congestive heart failure in U.S. men and women: NHANES I epidemiologic follow-up study. *Arch Intern Med.* 161:996, 2001.

Hunt SA, et al. ACC/AHA 2005 guideline update for the diagnosis and management of chronic heart failure in the adult: a report of the American College of Cardiology/American Heart Association Task Force on Practice Guidelines (Writing Committee to Update the 2001 Guidelines for the Evaluation and Management of Heart Failure). *J Am Coll Cardiol.* 46:e-1, 2005.

Mabuchi H, et al. Reduction of serum ubiquinol-10 and ubiquinone-10 levels by atorvastatin in hypercholesterolemic patients. *J Atheroscler Thromb.* 12:111, 2005.

Morelli V, Zoorob RJ. Alternative therapies. Part II: congestive heart failure and hypercholesterolemia. *Am Fam Physician.* 62:1325, 2000.

Paul S, Sneed NV. Strategies for behavior change in patients with heart failure. *Am J Crit Care.* 13:305, 2004.

Schulman SP, et al. L-arginine therapy in acute myocardial infarction: the Vascular Interaction with Age in Myocardial Infarction (VINTAGE MI) randomized clinical trial. *JAMA.* 295:58, 2006.

Silver MA, et al. Effect of atorvastatin on left ventricular diastolic function and ability of coenzyme Q10 to reverse that dysfunction. *Am J Cardiol.* 94:1306, 2004.

Strey CH, et al. Endothelium-ameliorating effects of statin therapy and coenzyme Q10 reductions in chronic heart failure. *Atherosclerosis* 179:201, 2005.

Talbert RL. Treatment of acute and chronic heart failure. *J Am Pharm Assoc.* 43:S18, 2003 (suppl 1).

HEART TRANSPLANTATION OR HEART-LUNG TRANSPLANTATION

NUTRITIONAL ACUITY RANKING: LEVEL 4

DEFINITIONS AND BACKGROUND

Heart transplantation (HTx) is usually performed for terminal heart failure, often with cardiomyopathy. Usually, the transplantation will be a Jarvik-7 or a live donor heart. Screening includes evaluations for chronic, coexisting illness, psychosocial stability, and normal or reversible cardiac status. The best candidates are younger than 55 years of age with normal hepatic and renal functioning and are free of diabetes mellitus and pulmonary problems, peptic ulcers, and peripheral heart disorders.

Survival rates after transplantation are getting better. Pre-HTx diabetes, donor age, and incidences of infection and rejection within 2 years of HTx predict long-term (>10 years) survival (Radovancevic et al, 2005). Main causes of death early after transplantation are rejection, nonspecific graft failure, and right ventricular failure due to pulmonary hypertension (Bauer et al, 2005). Implantation of circulatory assist devices as a permanent alternative to HTx (destination therapy) has become a promising new option for treatment of patients with advanced heart failure who are not candidates for HTx (Lietz and Miller, 2005).

Omega-3 fatty acids lower cholesterol levels and improve endothelial function in HTx recipients and use of 3-hydroxy-3-methylglutaryl coenzyme A (HMG-CoA) reductase inhibitors (statins) may reduce cholesterol levels (Wenke, 2004). Omega-3 fatty acids reduce the risk of sudden death from myocardial infarction, which is believed to occur via the incorporation of eicosapentaenoic acid (EPA) and docosahexaenoic acid (DHA) into the myocardium itself, altering the dynamics of sodium and calcium channel function (Harris et al, 2004).

Heart-lung transplantation is performed rarely, as in complex cases of cystic fibrosis, pulmonary fibrosis, emphysema, Eisenmenger's syndrome, and primary pulmonary hypertension. As with other types of transplantations, graft–host resistance and sepsis are the major concerns.

INTERVENTION: OBJECTIVES

- Promote adequate wound healing; prevent or correct wound dehiscence.
- Normalize heart functioning; prevent morbidity and death.
- Control infection and rejection during the first 2 years after HTx to improve survival.
- Prevent complications such as hypertension, hepatic or renal failure, and diabetes mellitus.
- Control side effects of steroid and immunosuppressive therapy.
- Maintain or improve nutritional status and fluid balance.
- Protect against posttransplantation hyperlipidemia, hypertension, and graft coronary vasculopathy (GCV). GCV is an accelerated form of atherosclerosis in transplanted hearts that is one of the most important late complications of HTx and is the single most limiting factor for long-term survival (Wenke, 2004).

INTERVENTION: FOOD AND NUTRITION

Pretranplantation

- Control calories, protein, sodium, potassium, fat, and cholesterol as appropriate for specific underlying condition (see appropriate sections). Keep in mind the role of nutrients needed for wound healing, including adequate energy intake.
- Fluid overload must be avoided; limit to 1 L daily, using a nutrient-dense product if needed.
- Avoid alcohol, which can aggravate cardiomyopathies.
- Reduce cardiac stimulants (e.g., caffeine) until fully recovered.

Posttransplantation

- Increase diet as tolerated and as appropriate for status. Alter as needed.
- For tube feeding (TF), use a product low in sodium and advance gradually.
- Include appropriate levels of calcium, magnesium, potassium, and fiber. The DASH diet is beneficial.
- Increase use of omega-3 fatty acids from fish and fish oils.
- Increase use of cardioprotective agents such as vitamins E, B_6, and B_{12} and folic acid. It is also prudent to use olive, soybean, and canola oils.
- Nuts contain flavonoids, phenols, sterols, saponins, elegiac acid, folic acid, magnesium, copper, potassium, and fiber. Walnuts contain alpha linolenic acid; almonds are a good source of vitamin E. Macadamias, pecans, and pistachios are also beneficial.

CLINICAL INDICATORS

Clinical/History		
Height	Ultrasound of abdomen and blood vessels	Complete blood cell count (CBC)
Weight	Cardiac catheterization	BUN, Creat
BMI	**Lab Work**	AST, ALT
Waist–hip ratio	Urinary Na+	ECG
Diet history	Na+, K+	pCO_2, pO_2
Edema	Ca++, Mg++	Alb, transthyretin
BP	CRP	Chol—HDL, LDL, total
Stress test	H & H	Trig
Chest x-ray	Serum Fe	Gluc
ECG	Transferrin	Homocysteine
Coronary angiogram		Serum folate and B_{12}
Echocardiogram		
Cardiopulmonary test		

Common Drugs Used and Potential Side Effects

- See Table 6-9.

Herbs, Botanicals, and Supplements

- The patient should not take herbals and botanicals without discussing with the physician.
- Grapefruit juice decreases drug metabolism in the gut (via P-450–CYP3A4 inhibition) and can affect medications up to 24 hours later. Consistency of use may be more important than total quantity. Avoid taking with alprazolam, buspirone, cisapride, cyclosporine, statins, tacrolimus, and many other drugs.
- Niacin (nicotinic acid) should not be taken with statins, antidiabetic medications, or carbamazepine because of potentially serious risks of myopathy and altered glucose control.

TABLE 6-9 Medications Used after Transplantation

Medication	Description
Analgesics	Analgesics are used to reduce pain. Long-term use may affect such nutrients as vitamin C and folacin; monitor carefully for each specific medication.
Cardiac medications	Antihypertensives, antilipemics, diuretics, and potassium supplements may be used. Monitor side effects accordingly. Some diuretics spare calcium and protect bone health.
Azathioprine (Imuran)	Azathioprine may cause leukopenia, thrombocytopenia, oral and esophageal sores, macrocytic anemia, pancreatitis, vomiting, diarrhea, and other complex side effects. Folate supplementation and other dietary modifications (liquid or soft diet, use of oral supplements) may be needed. The drug works by lowering the number of T cells; it is often prescribed along with prednisone for conventional immunosuppression.
Corticosteroids (prednisone, hydrocortisone [Solu-Cortef])	Corticosteroids such as prednisone and hydrocortisone are used for immunosuppression. Side effects include increased catabolism of proteins, negative nitrogen balance, hyperphagia, ulcers, decreased glucose tolerance, sodium retention, fluid retention, and impaired calcium absorption and osteoporosis. Cushing's syndrome, obesity, muscle wasting, and increased gastric secretion may result. A higher protein intake and lower intake of simple CHOs may be needed.
Cyclosporine	Cyclosporine does not retain sodium as much as corticosteroids do. Intravenous doses are more effective than oral doses. Nausea, vomiting, and diarrhea are common side effects. Hyperlipidemia, hypertension, and hyperkalemia may also occur; decrease sodium and potassium as necessary. Elevated glucose and lipids may occur. The drug is also nephrotoxic; a controlled renal diet may be beneficial. Taking omega-3 fatty acids during cyclosporine therapy may reduce the toxic side effects (such as high blood pressure and kidney damage) associated with this medication in transplantation patients (Holm et al, 2001).
Diuretics	Diuretics such as furosemide may cause hypokalemia. Aldactone actually spares potassium; monitor drug changes closely. In general, avoid use with fenugreek, yohimbe, and ginkgo.
Immunosuppressants	Immunosuppressants such as muromonab (Orthoclone OKT3) and antithymocyte globulin (ATG) are less nephrotoxic than cyclosporine but can cause nausea, anorexia, diarrhea, and vomiting. Monitor carefully. Fever and stomatitis also may occur; alter diet as needed.
Statins	Statins may be used to manage coronary artery disease or dyslipidemia. See Table 6-5.
Tacrolimus (Prograf, FK506)	Tacrolimus suppresses T-cell immunity; it is 100 times more potent than cyclosporine, thus requiring smaller doses. Side effects include GI distress, nausea, vomiting, hyperkalemia, and hyperglycemia.

- Omega-3 fatty acids in fish oil capsules can cause hypervitaminosis A and D if taken in large doses. Avoid use in pregnant or lactating women. Avoid taking with warfarin, aspirin, and other antiplatelet medications because of the risk of increased bruising or bleeding.
- Vitamin E should not be taken with warfarin because of the possibility of increased bleeding. Avoid doses greater than 400 IU/d.

INTERVENTION: NUTRITION EDUCATION, COUNSELING, CARE MANAGEMENT

- Discuss the role of nutrition in wound healing, immunocompetence, and cardiovascular health. Specify nutrients that are known to be protective.
- Discuss how exercise affects the use of calories.
- Discuss, as appropriate, fiber intake and sources of fat and cholesterol. Highlight the importance of maintaining an adequate diet to reduce risks of further heart disease and complications. Transplant coronary artery disease (CAD) proceeds at an accelerated rate; the patient must not see this procedure as a permanent cure.
- To improve quality of life in transplantation patients, web-based counseling and support may play a vital role in follow-up care and in patients' and families' adjustment (Dew et al, 2005). This type of support is helpful, especially in rural areas where access to medical nutrition therapy is limited.

Patient Education—Foodborne Illness

- Careful food handling will be important. Hand washing is key as well.

For More Information

- American Heart Association
  http://www.americanheart.org/presenter.jhtml?identifier=4588
- Heart Transplantation
  http://www.pbs.org/wgbh/nova/eheart/transplant.html

HEART TRANSPLANTATION OR HEART-LUNG TRANSPLANTATION—CITED REFERENCES

Bauer J, et al. Perioperative management in pediatric heart transplantation. *Thorac Cardiovasc Surg.* 53:S155, 2005.

Dew MA, et al. An internet-based intervention to improve psychosocial outcomes in heart transplant recipients and family caregivers: development and evaluation. *J Heart Lung Transplant.* 23:745, 2004.

Harris WS, et al. Omega-3 fatty acids in cardiac biopsies from heart transplantation patients: correlation with erythrocytes and response to supplementation. *Circulation* 110:1645, 2004.

Holm T, et al. Omega-3 fatty acids improve blood pressure control and preserve renal function in hypertensive heart transplant recipients. *Eur Heart J.* 22:428, 2001.

Lietz K, Miller LW. Will left-ventricular assist device therapy replace heart transplantation in the foreseeable future? *Curr Opin Cardiol.* 20:132, 2005.

Radovancevic B, et al. Factors predicting 10-year survival after heart transplantation. *J Heart Lung Transplant.* 24:156, 2005.

Wenke K. Management of hyperlipidaemia associated with heart transplantation. *Drugs* 64:1053, 2004.

HEART VALVE DISEASES

NUTRITIONAL ACUITY RANKING: LEVEL 2

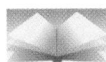

DEFINITIONS AND BACKGROUND

The heart has four valves (tricuspid, pulmonary, aortic, and mitral). Inflammation of any or several of these valves can cause stenosis with thickening (which narrows the opening) or incompetence (with distortion and inability to close fully).

If the mitral valve is not functioning properly, due to injury or disease, blood leaks back into the left atrium (regurgitates) when the left ventricle contracts and backs up into the lungs. Because some of the blood being pumped by the left ventricle flows back into the left atrium, less blood is pumped into the aorta and throughout the body. The heart compensates for this by increasing the size of the left ventricle to increase the amount of blood it is pumping and to maintain an adequate forward flow of blood throughout the body. Unfortunately, compensation eventually leads to impairment of the left ventricle's ability to contract, which leads to further backup of blood into the lungs.

Mitral valve prolapse is a common valvular abnormality and is the most common cause of severe nonischemic mitral regurgitation in the United States; overall prognosis of patients is excellent, but a small subset will develop serious complications, including infective endocarditis, sudden cardiac death, and severe mitral regurgitation (Hayek et al, 2005). Echocardiography is used for diagnosing this condition, and mitral valve repair is the treatment. With advancements in percutaneous coronary interventions (PCIs), some patients requiring coronary revascularization and valve surgery may benefit from a hybrid approach involving initial planned PCI followed by valve surgery, rather than conventional coronary artery bypass graft/valve surgery (Byrne et al, 2005).

Mitral stenosis can cause lung congestion, breathlessness after exercise or while lying down, hemoptysis, bronchial infections, and chest pains. In mitral stenosis, right heart failure can occur; 60% of persons with rheumatic heart disease later have heart valve problems; 75% of these persons have mitral stenosis. **Aortic stenosis** can cause symptoms of angina, vertigo, fainting on exertion, and left heart failure. **Tricuspid stenosis** increases the risk of heart failure. **Pulmonary stenosis** is rare and occurs in only 2% of all valve disorders. Patients at high risk for valvular disease should be screened for hyperhomocysteinemia; for prevention, folic acid and a multivitamin supplement with vitamins B_6 and B_{12} should be taken.

INTERVENTION: OBJECTIVES

- Prevent heart failure (right- or left-sided), bacterial endocarditis, emboli or atrial fibrillation, and sudden death. Prevent stroke; mitral annular calcification is an independent predictor of stroke.
- Prepare, if necessary, for valve replacement surgery.
- Prevent or correct cardiogenic shock with tachycardia and other symptoms.
- Correct or manage atherosclerosis.

INTERVENTION: FOOD AND NUTRITION

- Avoid excesses of calories, sodium, and fluid (as appropriate for the patient). In some patients with vertigo, fluid and sodium restrictions may actually be detrimental (Pappas, 2003).
- If weight loss has taken place, add extra calories and snacks to return to a more desirable body weight.
- Use adequate vitamins E, B_6, and B_{12} and folic acid.
- The DASH diet is useful. Encourage use of flavonoids such as grapefruit, grape juice, apples, onions, tea, and red wine (small amounts) when feasible. Flavonoids may help to reduce blood clot formation. Pomegranate juice, for example, is quite a beneficial choice of fruit juices. See http://www.pomwonderful.com/health_benefits.html.
- Ensure adequate intake of omega-3 fatty acids.

CLINICAL INDICATORS

Clinical/History	Lab Work	
Height	CRP	BUN, Creat
Weight	Alb, transthyretin	Na+, K+
BMI	H & H	Ca++, Mg++
Waist–hip ratio	Serum ferritin	Gluc
Diet history	Cardiac catheterization	Homocysteine
Weight changes	ECG	Serum folate
Pulse	Chol—total, HDL, LDL	Serum B_{12}
Cool, moist skin	Trig	
BP		
Urinary output (decreased)		
I & O		

Common Drugs Used and Potential Side Effects

- Anticoagulants are used commonly. Monitor vitamin K–rich foods carefully; use no more than 1 per day (especially green leafy vegetables). If aspirin is used, monitor for GI side effects; aspirin may also decrease serum ferritin by increasing occult blood loss (Fleming et al, 2001).
- Diuretics may be used if fluid overload occurs. Monitor potassium and sodium intake carefully. Some diuretics spare calcium and protect bone health.

- Fenfluramine-phentermine (Fen-Phen) weight reduction drug therapy is associated with valvular heart disease and pulmonary hypertension (Connolly et al, 1997). Cardiac surgical interventions that were performed found plaque like that found in carcinoid syndrome. These drugs have been removed from the market. Fenfluramine-associated valvular regurgitation is less common than initially reported but was still present in one of eight patients treated for >90 days (Sachdev et al, 2002).
- Digoxin may be needed to strengthen the heart's pumping action after surgery. Monitor potassium intake or depletion carefully, especially when combining with diuretics. Avoid excessive intakes of fiber and wheat bran. Avoid use with hawthorn, milkweed, guar gum, and St. John's wort.
- Statins may be used to manage coronary artery disease or dyslipidemia. See Table 6-5.

Herbs, Botanicals, and Supplements

- Chromium is sometimes used for dyslipidemia. Do not use excesses with insulin or hypoglycemic agents, because chromium may lower glucose levels excessively.
- Coenzyme Q10 (CoQ10; ubiquinone) should not be used with gemfibrozil, tricyclic antidepressants, or warfarin. CoQ10 may act similarly to vitamin K. Because CoQ10 and statins share a similar pathway, they can be taken simultaneously (Mabuchi et al, 2005; Strey et al, 2005; Silver et al, 2004).
- Danshen may be used for ischemic heart disease. Avoid large amounts with warfarin, aspirin, and other antiplatelet drugs. It can increase risks of bleeding or bruising.
- Garlic should not be taken in large amounts with warfarin, aspirin, and other antiplatelet drugs because of increased risks of bleeding or bruising. It may also increase insulin levels with hypoglycemic results; monitor carefully in patients with diabetes.
- Grapefruit juice decreases drug metabolism in the gut (via P-450–CYP3A4 inhibition) and can affect medications up to 24 hours later. Consistency of use may be more important than total quantity. Avoid taking with alprazolam, buspirone, cisapride, cyclosporine, statins, tacrolimus, and many other drugs.
- Niacin (nicotinic acid) should not be taken with statins, antidiabetic medications, or carbamazepine because of potentially serious risks of myopathy and altered glucose control.
- Omega-3 fatty acids in fish oil capsules can cause hypervitaminosis A and D if taken in large doses. Avoid use in pregnant or lactating women. Avoid taking with warfarin, aspirin, and other antiplatelet medications because of the risk of increased bruising or bleeding.
- Vitamin E should not be taken with warfarin because of the possibility of increased bleeding. Avoid doses greater than 400 IU/d.

INTERVENTION: NUTRITION EDUCATION, COUNSELING, CARE MANAGEMENT

- Careful use of all prescribed medications will be essential, with adequate return visits to the physician at appropriate intervals.
- Alternative food preparation methods may be suggested to reduce sodium intake or to alter calorie levels.
- Persons with a history of heart valve abnormalities may require antibiotic therapy to prevent infections, especially before surgery or dental work.
- After surgery, which may involve valvotomy, valvulotomy, balloon valvuloplasty, percutaneous balloon valvuloplasty, valvoplasty, commissurotomy, balloon commissurotomy, or annuloplasty, the patient should receive information about nutrition in wound healing.

Patient Education—Foodborne Illness

- Careful food handling will be important. Hand washing is key as well.

For More Information

- Heart Valve Disorders
  http://www.torrancememorial.org/carvalve.htm

HEART VALVE DISEASES—CITED REFERENCES

Byrne JG, et al. Staged initial percutaneous coronary intervention followed by valve surgery ("hybrid approach") for patients with complex coronary and valve disease. *J Am Coll Cardiol.* 45:14, 2005.

Connolly H, et al. Valvular heart disease associated with fenfluramine-phentermine. *N Engl J Med.* 337:581, 1997.

Fleming D, et al. Aspirin intake and the use of serum ferritin as a measure of iron status. *Am J Clin Nutr.* 74:219, 2001.

Hayek E, et al. Mitral valve prolapse. *Lancet* 365:507, 2005.

Mabuchi H, et al. Reduction of serum ubiquinol-10 and ubiquinone-10 levels by atorvastatin in hypercholesterolemic patients. *J Atheroscler Thromb.* 12:111, 2005.

Pappas DG Jr. Autonomic related vertigo. *Laryngoscope* 113:1658, 2003.

Sachdev M, et al. Effect of fenfluramine-derivative diet pills on cardiac valves: a meta-analysis of observational studies. *Am Heart J.* 144:1065, 2002.

Silver MA, et al. Effect of atorvastatin on left ventricular diastolic function and ability of coenzyme Q10 to reverse that dysfunction. *Am J Cardiol.* 94:1306, 2004.

Strey CH, et al. Endothelium-ameliorating effects of statin therapy and coenzyme Q10 reductions in chronic heart failure. *Atherosclerosis* 179:201, 2005.

HYPERTENSION

NUTRITIONAL ACUITY RANKING: LEVEL 3

DEFINITIONS AND BACKGROUND

Hypertension is defined as having a sustained systolic and diastolic blood pressure (BP) greater than 140 and 90 mm Hg, respectively. It affects about 600 million people worldwide; about 27% of the U.S. adult population is hypertensive. The Seventh Report of the Joint National Committee on Prevention, Detection, Evaluation, and Treatment of High Blood Pressure, also known as the JNC 7 Report (Chobanian et al, 2003), identified issues that have nutritional implications:

- In persons older than age 50, systolic BP of greater than 140 mm Hg is a more important cardiovascular disease (CVD) risk factor than diastolic BP.
- Beginning at 115/75 mm Hg, CVD risk doubles for each increment of 20/10 mm Hg.
- Those who are normotensive at 55 years of age will have a 90% lifetime risk of developing hypertension.
- Prehypertensive individuals (systolic BP of 120–139 mm Hg or diastolic BP of 80–89 mm Hg) require health-promoting lifestyle modifications to prevent the progressive rise in BP and CVD.
- Regardless of therapy or care, hypertension will be controlled only if patients are motivated to stay on their treatment plan.

Hypertension nearly doubles the risk for heart attack, stroke, and heart failure, especially for people over age 65 (National Heart, Lung, and Blood Institute [NHLBI], 2001). BP often increases with age and is highly prevalent in elderly individuals, the most rapidly growing segment of the U.S. population (Schrier, 2001). Symptoms of hypertension include frequent headaches, impaired vision, shortness of breath, nose bleeds, chest pain, dizziness, failing memory, snoring and sleep apnea, and GI distress.

The JNC 7 Report (Chobanian et al, 2003) identified a "prehypertension" level and merged other categories. See Table 6-10.

TABLE 6-10 Categories for Blood Pressure Levels in Adults (Ages 18 years and Older)

	Blood Pressure Level (mm Hg)		
Category	**Systolic**		**Diastolic**
Normal	<120	and	<80
Prehypertension	120–139	or	80–89
High blood pressure:			
Stage 1 hypertension	140–159	or	90–99
Stage 2 hypertension	≥160	or	≥100

From: National Heart, Lung, and Blood Institute; accessed at http://www.nhlbi.nih.gov/hbp/detect/categ.htm.

Identifiable causes of high BP include sleep apnea, drug-related causes, chronic kidney disease, Cushing's syndrome, steroid therapy, pheochromocytoma, primary aldosteronism, thyroid and parathyroid diseases, and renovascular disease. Untreated hypertension can result in stroke, heart failure, renal failure, myocardial infarction (MI), accelerated bone loss and risk of fractures, and long-term memory problems. If dyspnea occurs on exertion, left-sided heart failure must be prevented. If edema of extremities occurs, right-sided heart failure must be prevented.

With inflammation, blood vessels get stiff, and elevated CRP may be a marker. CRP may reduce the production of nitric acid in the cells that line the blood vessels; CRP over 3.5 is considered high and may represent endothelial dysfunction (Streppel et al, 2005). Endothelial dysfunction is one of the earliest events in atherogenesis, with lower availability of vasodilator nitric oxide (Cuevas and Guerlain, 2004).Weight loss is important since abdominal adiposity is a predictor for high CRP levels.

With endothelial dysfunction in hypertension, dyslipidemia, diabetes, smoking, and hyperhomocysteinemia, diet may greatly affect vascular reactivity. Use of fish oil, antioxidants, folic acid, soy protein, and the Mediterranean diet (high consumption of vegetables, fish, and olive oil and moderate wine consumption) may have a positive effect (Cuevas and Guerlain, 2004). Increasing intake of fiber in populations where intake is far below recommended levels may help to prevent hypertension (Streppel et al, 2005).

There is increasing evidence for an association of other nutrients, such as omega-3 polyunsaturated fatty acids, vitamin C, folic acid, and potassium, with decreased BP. The Dietary Approaches to Stop Hypertension (DASH) eating plan is rich in fiber, vegetables, fruit, and nonfat dairy products and significantly lowers BP. The decreases are often comparable to those achieved with BP-lowering medication. Large intakes of folic acid may help to lower high BP (Mason et al, 2004); one study suggests intake of 1000 μg daily (Schutte et al, 2004).

For patients with chronic kidney disease (CKD) who have hypertension; it is critical to control BP to reduce negative consequences. Current JNC 7 and National Kidney Foundation guidelines recommend reducing sodium intake to less than 2.4 g/d; potassium intake should be restricted in patients with a glomerular filtration rate (GFR) of less than 60 mL/min; and calcium intake may have to be limited in low-GFR populations (Lancaster, 2004). Black populations are especially sensitive to the BP-lowering effects of reduced salt intake, increased potassium intake, and the DASH diet (Appel et al, 2006).

Because nutrient–gene interactions determine a broad array of phenotypic consequences such as vascular problems and hypertension, consuming optimal nutrition, nutraceuticals, vitamins, antioxidants, and minerals and moderately restricting alcohol and caffeine may prevent, delay the onset, reduce the severity, treat, or control hypertension in many patients (Houston, 2005). Clinicians are encouraged to work closely with patients to agree on BP goals and develop a treatment plan.

Reduced salt intake, weight loss, moderate alcohol consumption among those who drink, increased potassium intake, and use of the DASH diet are among the most effective strategies (Appel et al, 2006). In addition, inclusion of omega-3 fatty acids, fiber, calcium, magnesium, and vitamin C is associated with lower BP, but supplements are not promoted. The American Dietetic Association recommends at least three medical nutrition therapy visits for patients with hypertension.

INTERVENTION: OBJECTIVES

- Control BP to lessen the likelihood of heart failure or stroke. Lower BP to a safe level. Use diet first and then medications. Induce negative sodium balance in the body only when this is absolutely required. A low-sodium diet (10 mEq) increases vascular and lymphocyte beta-adrenergic responsiveness, thereby lowering BP. Only 20–50% of patients with hypertension are sodium sensitive.
- Assess medical risk factors, comorbidities, and identifiable causes of the hypertension. Lose weight if obese.
- A high-potassium intake helps to maintain normal fluid balance, lowers BP, and reduces likelihood of stroke or MI. Use caution if there is CKD or use of potassium-sparing diuretics.
- If diet does not help within 2 weeks, medications may be needed. For stage 1, thiazide diuretics may suffice; in stage 2, two-drug combinations are used (Chobanian et al, 2003).
- Calcium supplementation may be useful in lowering BP in persons who have low dietary intakes of calcium (Dwyer et al, 1998). Increase magnesium and vitamins D, E, and K, as appropriate.
- Encourage adequate intake of fluids unless contraindicated.
- Moderate intake of alcohol, which may increase blood pressure.
- Increase physical activity to 30 minutes daily most days of the week.

INTERVENTION: FOOD AND NUTRITION

- The DASH diet is effective within 14 days of initiation. This diet is rich in fruits, vegetables, and low-fat dairy foods; it is low in saturated fatty acids (SFA) and total fat, which can reduce high BP (Appel et al, 1997). Adequate amounts of potassium from skim milk, baked potatoes, grapefruit, oranges, bananas, lima beans, and other fruits and vegetables should be planned daily.
- Tips on eating the DASH way: Start small; make gradual changes in eating habits. Organize meals around carbohydrates such as pasta, rice, beans, or vegetables. Carbohydrates such as beans, whole grains, oat bran, and fruits (apples, blueberries) and vegetables should make up 50% of the diet.
- Treat meat as one part of the whole meal, instead of the main focus. Use fruits or low-fat, low-calorie foods such as sugar-free gelatin for desserts and snacks. See Tables 6-2 and 6-3 for more information.
- Increase fruits and vegetables for their flavonoids and phytochemical properties. Besides the DASH diet, Mediterranean and vegetarian diet patterns tend to lower BP and can be beneficial.
- Limit sodium to 2–4 g daily. Patients with essential hypertension (EH) may be more sodium sensitive than some other patients whose conditions are secondary to other disorders (Houben et al, 2005). Table 6-11 lists common salt substitutes and their content.
- Use an energy-controlled diet if weight loss is needed. Aim for a BMI between 18.9 and 24.9; waist to hip ratio should be monitored since values over 0.85 for women and over 0.9 for men indicate greater risk for heart disease (Chobanian et al, 2003).
- Fat intake should be moderate. Olive, soybean, and canola oils can be substituted for some saturated fats in cooking. Pistachios, sunflower kernels, sesame seeds, and wheat germ are good sources of phytosterols; use often.
- Severely restrict alcoholic beverages to one drink or less for women and to two drinks or less for men.
- Use sources of omega-3 fatty acids, such as mackerel, haddock, sardines, and salmon, several times weekly. Tuna should be used less often because its potential mercury content could elevate BP.
- Increase calcium by about 400–500 mg daily; use low-fat dairy products. Higher intake of dairy products seems to reduce serum uric acid levels, and uric acid levels are often correlated with BP and stroke risks (Choi et al, 2005).
- Increase food sources of folic acid and vitamins B_{12} and B_6 for overall cardiovascular health.
- Control intake of caffeine from sugared or diet colas; habitual coffee intake is less problematic (Winkelmayer et al, 2005).

TABLE 6-11 Samples of Salt, Salt Substitutes, and Content of Sodium and Potassium (per 1/2 teaspoon)

Type	mg Sodium	mg Potassium	mEq Potassium
Salt Brand			
Morton's	—	1250	32
Adolph's	—	1205	31
McCormick's	—	1170	30
Diamond Crystal	—	1104	28
Co-Salt	—	987	25
Adolph's Seasoned	—	849	22
Morton's Lite Salt	488	650	16
Other Seasonings			
Salt	969	—	—
Baking soda	410	—	—
Baking powder	170	—	—
Monosodium glutamate (MSG)	246	—	—

SAMPLE NUTRITION DIAGNOSTIC STATEMENT

Hypertension (HTN)

PES: Excessive intake of sodium related to high intake of commercially prepared and packaged foods as evidenced by blood pressure (BP) of 160/105 mm Hg.

Assessment Data (sources of info): Diet history and food records, BP records.

Intervention: Promote use of food diary and BP monitoring records, food choices that are lower in sodium, easy preparation meals made from scratch and recipe alterations, shopping tips, tips for dining away from home.

Monitoring and Evaluation: BP reports, food records.

CLINICAL INDICATORS

Clinical/History	Lab Work	
Height	H & H	Plasma renin
Weight	Serum Fe	Na+, K+
BMI	CRP	Serum Ca++, Mg++
Waist–hip ratio	Alb, transthyretin	Chloride
Diet history	Urinary Alb to Creat ratio (elevated levels may impair arterial dilatory capacity)	Trig
Headache	Chol—HDL, LDL	Parathormone (PTH)
I & O	LDH	AST, ALT
BP pattern	BUN	Alk phos
Renal arteriography	Creat, GFR	PT or INR
Chest x-ray	Uric acid	Gluc
Renal ultrasound		Homocysteine
Intravenous pyelogram		Serum folate
ECG		Serum B_{12}
		Plasma ascorbic acid
		Urinary Ca++
		Urinary cortisol

Common Drugs Used and Potential Side Effects

- See Table 6-12.
- Use of a diuretic is part of the treatment plan in most patients. The guidelines also list other drug classes that have been shown to be effective in reducing hypertension's cardiovascular complications, such as angiotensin-converting enzyme (ACE) inhibitors, angiotensin receptor blockers, beta-blockers, and calcium channel blockers. Use additional drugs for severe hypertension or to lower BP to the desired level; most persons will need multiple medications to lower BP to a desired level.
- In uncomplicated stage 1 hypertension, dietary changes serve as initial treatment before drug therapy; in those hypertensive patients already on drug therapy, lifestyle modifications, particularly a reduced salt intake, can further lower BP (Appel et al, 2006).
- Antihypertensive therapy is challenging in the elderly because of metabolic and physiological alterations, comorbidities, polypharmacy, and biological variability. Drugs with a convenient dosing schedule, minimal side effects, and the ability to impact comorbid conditions are important considerations in the treatment of hypertension in the elderly (Schrier, 2001).
- Note that use of estrogens and oral contraceptives can increase blood pressure.

Herbs, Botanicals, and Supplements

- Danshen may be used for ischemic heart disease. Avoid large amounts with warfarin, aspirin, and other antiplatelet drugs. It can increase risks of bleeding or bruising.
- Coenzyme Q10 (CoQ10; ubiquinone) should not be used with gemfibrozil, tricyclic antidepressants, or warfarin. CoQ10 may act similarly to vitamin K (Mabuchi et al, 2005; Strey et al, 2005; Silver et al, 2004).
- Green coffee bean extract may be beneficial in lowering blood pressure (Kozuma et al, 2005).
- Grapefruit juice decreases drug metabolism in the gut (via P-450–CYP3A4 inhibition) and can affect medications up to 24 hours later. Consistency of use may be more important than total quantity. Avoid taking with alprazolam, buspirone, cisapride, cyclosporine, statins, tacrolimus, and many other drugs.
- Hawthorn should not be taken with digoxin, ACE inhibitors, and other cardiovascular drugs.
- Indian snakeroot should not be taken with digoxin, furosemide, thiazides, monoamine oxidase (MAO) inhibitors, and beta-blockers such as atenolol and propranolol because of increased or decreased sedation and changed effects on BP.
- Niacin (nicotinic acid) should not be taken with statins, antidiabetic medications, and carbamazepine because of potentially serious risks of myopathy and altered glucose control.
- Omega-3 fatty acids in fish oil capsules can cause hypervitaminosis A and D if taken in large doses. Avoid use in pregnant or lactating women. Avoid taking with warfarin, aspirin, and other antiplatelet medications because of the risk of increased bruising or bleeding.
- Tea consumption (oolong and moderate-strength green tea) has been noted to lower BP in the Chinese population (Yang et al, 2004).
- Vitamin E should not be taken with warfarin because of the possibility of increased bleeding. Avoid doses greater than 400 IU/d.
- Yohimbe should not be used with MAO inhibitors, antianxiety medications, appetite suppressants, antihypertensives, clonidine, or phenothiazines because of effects on BP.

INTERVENTION: NUTRITION EDUCATION, COUNSELING, CARE MANAGEMENT

- Encourage patience; it takes 2 weeks to see the results of dietary changes while following the DASH diet. Empathy

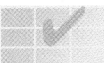

TABLE 6-12 Medications for Hypertension

Medication	Description
Angiotensin-Converting Enzyme (ACE) Inhibitors (quinipril/Accupril, ramipril/Altace, benzepril/Lotensin, lisinopril/Prinivil, monopril/Monopril, enalapril/ Vasotec, captopril/Capoten, perindopril/Aceon)	ACE inhibitors prevent angiotensin I from conversion; they are useful in heart failure. Ramipril has been noted to prevent diabetes in hypertensive patients. Nausea, vomiting, and abdominal pain may occur; do not take with potassium supplements. Captopril (Capoten) can alter BUN/creatinine; take 1 hour before meals and reduce calories and sodium. Loss of taste can occur. Patients who take captopril and enalapril may develop zinc deficiency (Golik et al, 1998).
Angiotensin II Receptor Antagonists (candesartan/Atacand, eprosartan/Teveten, irbesartan/Avapro, olmesatran/Benicar, valsatran/Diovan)	Use with low-sodium, low-calorie diet. GI distress can occur. Some are mixed with thiazide diuretics; monitor for potassium depletion.
Beta-Blockers (atenolol/Tenormin, pindolol/Visken, propranolol/Inderal, acebutolol/Sectral, bisoprolol/Zebeta, metoprolol/Lopressor, timolol/Blocadren, prazosin/Minipress)	Beta-blockers decrease the force and rate of heart contractions, thereby decreasing blood pressure. Dizziness and nausea are common side effects. Low-calorie, low-sodium diet may be useful. Metoprolol (Lopressor) should be taken with a low-calorie, low-sodium diet. Diarrhea, nausea, vomiting, or abdominal cramps may occur. Prazosin (Minipress) may cause nausea, weight gain, anorexia, diarrhea, or constipation.
Calcium Channel Blockers (amlodipine/Norvasc; diltiazem/Cardizem; felodipine/Plendil)	Use with low-sodium, low-calorie diet. Avoid natural licorice.
Central Adrenergic Inhibitors (terazosin/Hytrin and clonidine/Catapres)	Central adrenergic inhibitors require a low-sodium, low-calorie diet. Dry mouth, vomiting, nausea, constipation, or edema can occur. Avoid taking with kava, ma huang, yohimbe, fenugreek, or licorice.
Diuretics	Spironolactone (Aldactone, Aldactazide) is potassium-sparing. Thiazides (e.g., bumetanide [Bumex], furosemide [Lasix], chlorothiazide [Diuril], indapamide [Lozol]) deplete potassium and may require supplementation; diarrhea or GI bleeding can occur. Avoid natural licorice. Acetazolamide (Diamox) may cause GI distress; take with food and include extra potassium. Chlorthalidone (Hygroton) may alter blood glucose or potassium levels; it may cause anorexia, vomiting, constipation, and nausea. In general, avoid use with fenugreek, yohimbe, and ginkgo.
Diuretic-Antihypertensives (amiloride/Moduretic)	A low-calorie, low-sodium diet is important. Potassium loss is minimized. Avoid use with alcohol.
Melatonin	The nocturnal decline of blood pressure (BP) coincides with the elevation of melatonin, which may exert vasodilatating and hypotensive effects; prolonged administration of melatonin may improve the day–night rhythm of BP, particularly in women (Cagnacci et al, 2005). More studies are needed.

encourages trust and motivation, as well as adherence to therapy (Chobanian et al, 2003).

- Encourage the adequate intake of fruits and vegetables; a plant-based diet can be quite effective in lowering BP (Leitzmann, 2005).
- Remove the salt shaker from the table. Have the patient taste food before salting. Avoid excesses of processed and canned foods. The normal adult needs only 1/2 teaspoon of sodium (200 mg) per day. Greater amounts of salt are required only in hot, humid conditions, during lactation, or with other salt-losing states. In such conditions, 2000 mg of salt is sufficient.
- Interesting food flavors are often hidden by salt. Discuss use of other seasonings and recipes. Monitor potassium in salt substitutes and medications to prevent either hypokalemia or hyperkalemia. Read all labels carefully.
- Where there is metabolic syndrome, obesity leads to a proinflammatory and prothrombotic state that potentiates hypertension (Moller and Kaufman, 2005). Work on a weight loss program if needed.
- Increase physical activity when possible; walk briskly 30–45 minutes 5 times weekly. Enhanced pedometer feedback in conjunction with nutritional counseling is feasible and results in significant weight loss and increased walking among individuals at high risk for cardiovascular disease (Richardson et al, 2005).
- Omit or reduce alcohol intake severely, if needed.

Patient Education—Foodborne Illness

- Careful food handling will be important. Hand washing is key as well.

For More Information

- DASH Diet
  http://www.nih.gov/news/pr/apr97/Dash.htm

- JNC 7
  http://www.nhlbi.nih.gov/guidelines/hypertension/jnc7full.htm
- National High Blood Pressure Education Program
  http://www.nhlbi.nih.gov/about/nhbpep/index.htm
  http://www.nhlbi.nih.gov/hbp/index.html
  http://www.nhlbi.nih.gov/health/public/heart/index.htm
- World Hypertension League
  http://www.mco.edu/whl/

HYPERTENSION—CITED REFERENCES

Appel L, et al. A clinical trial of the effects of dietary patterns on blood pressure: DASH Collaborative Research Group. *N Engl J Med.* 336:1117, 1997.

Appel LJ, et al. Dietary approaches to prevent and treat hypertension: a scientific statement from the American Heart Association. *Hypertension* 47:296, 2006.

Cagnacci A, et al. Prolonged melatonin administration decreases nocturnal blood pressure in women. *Am J Hypertens.* 18:1614, 2005.

Chobanian AV, et al. Seventh report of the Joint National Committee on Prevention, Detection, Evaluation, and Treatment of High Blood Pressure. *Hypertension* 42:1206, 2003.

Choi HK, et al. Intake of purine-rich foods, protein, and dairy products and relationship to serum levels of uric acid: the Third National Health and Nutrition Examination Survey. *Arthritis Rheum.* 52:283, 2005.

Cuevas AM, Guerlain AM. Diet and endothelial function. *Biol Res.* 37:225, 2004.

Dwyer J, et al. Dietary calcium, calcium supplementation and blood pressure in African American adolescents. *Am J Clin Nutri.* 68:648, 1998.

Golik A, et al. Effects of captopril and enalapril on zinc metabolism in hypertensive patients. *J Am Col Nutr.* 17:75, 1998.

Houben AJ, et al. Microvascular adaptation to changes in dietary sodium is disturbed in patients with essential hypertension. *J Hypertens.* 23:127, 2005.

Kozuma K, et al. Antihypertensive effect of green coffee bean extract on mildly hypertensive subjects. *Hypertens Res.* 28:711, 2005.

Lancaster KJ. Dietary treatment of blood pressure in kidney disease. *Adv Chronic Kidney Dis.* 11:217, 2004.

Leitzmann C. Vegetarian diets: what are the advantages? *Forum Nutr.* 57:147, 2005.

Mabuchi H, et al. Reduction of serum ubiquinol-10 and ubiquinone-10 levels by atorvastatin in hypercholesterolemic patients. *J Atheroscler Thromb.* 12:111, 2005.

Mason PJ, et al. Blood pressure and risk of secondary cardiovascular events in women: the Women's Antioxidant Cardiovascular Study (WACS). *Circulation* 109:1623, 2004.

Moller DE, Kaufman KD. Metabolic syndrome: a clinical and molecular perspective. *Annu Rev Med.* 56:45, 2005.

National Heart, Lung, and Blood Institute (NHLBI). Third Report of the Expert Panel on Detection, Evaluation, and Treatment of High Blood Cholesterol in Adults (Adult Treatment Panel III). 2001. Accessed at http://www.nhlbi.nih.gov/guidelines/cholesterol/atglance.htm.

Richardson CR, et al. Feasibility of adding enhanced pedometer feedback to nutritional counseling for weight loss. *J Med Internet Res.* 7:e56, 2005.

Schrier R. Treating hypertension in the elderly. *Am J Geriatr Cardiol.* 10:355, 2001.

Schutte AE, et al. Cardiovascular effects of oral supplementation of vitamin C, E and folic acid in young healthy males. *Int J Vitam Nutr Res.* 74:285, 2004.

Silver MA, et al. Effect of atorvastatin on left ventricular diastolic function and ability of coenzyme Q10 to reverse that dysfunction. *Am J Cardiol.* 94:1306, 2004.

Streppel MT, et al. Dietary fiber and blood pressure: a meta-analysis of randomized placebo-controlled trials. *Arch Intern Med.* 165:150, 2005.

Strey CH, et al. Endothelium-ameliorating effects of statin therapy and coenzyme Q10 reductions in chronic heart failure. *Atherosclerosis* 179:201, 2005.

Winkelmayer WC, et al. Habitual caffeine intake and the risk of hypertension in women. *JAMA.* 294:2330, 2005.

Yang YC, et al. The protective effect of habitual tea consumption on hypertension. *Arch Intern Med.* 164:1534, 2004.

MYOCARDIAL INFARCTION

NUTRITIONAL ACUITY RANKING: LEVEL 3

DEFINITIONS AND BACKGROUND

Myocardial infarction (MI) is necrosis in the heart muscle caused by prolonged inadequate blood supply or oxygen deficit. A **coronary occlusion** (heart attack) is the closing of a coronary artery feeding heart muscle by fatty deposits or a blood clot; it manifests with heavy squeezing pain radiating to the jaw or back, nausea, vomiting, diaphoresis, anxiety, and weakness.

Abnormal lipids, smoking, hypertension, diabetes, abdominal obesity, psychosocial factors, inadequate consumption of fruits and vegetables, alcohol consumption, and lack of regular physical activity account for most of the risk factors for MI worldwide in both sexes and at all ages in all regions (Yusuf et al, 2004). Table 6-13 provides a list of risk factors for an MI.

Women have symptoms of an MI that often differ from men (Legato, 2000). Women with acute MI may be treated less vigorously than men, especially concerning the use of drugs such as thrombolytic therapy (Mallik and Vaccarino, 2004). Prodromal symptoms include unusual fatigue, shortness of breath, and pain in the shoulder blade/upper back; medical practitioners must develop an awareness of and a more comprehensive approach to treating women at risk for coronary heart disease (CHD) (McSweeney et al, 2001).

Stages after an MI include critical (first 48 hours), acute (3–14 days), and convalescent (15–90 days). Treatment with cholesterol-lowering medications and antioxidants may decrease MI and may reduce adverse coronary events. Table 6-14 lists potential complications after an MI.

Controlled trials and evidence are lacking for use of vitamin C and folic acid supplements, but fruit and vegetable intake should be encouraged (Joshipura et al, 2001). Platelet aggregation is central in acute coronary syndromes, including MI and unstable angina. Effects of flavonoids on endothelial and platelet function might explain the protective benefits on cardiac risk (Vita, 2005). Studies relate wine/resveratrol with reduction in myocardial damage during ischemia-reperfusion, modulation of vascular cell functions, inhibition of LDL oxidation, and suppression of platelet aggregation (Wu et al, 2001).

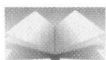

An **arrhythmia** is a variation from normal heartbeat rhythm. Among its many forms is a slowing of the heartbeat to less than 60 beats per minute (bradycardia), a speedup to more than 100 beats per minute (tachycardia), and prema-

TABLE 6-13 Risk Factors for Myocardial Infarction

- Family history of heart disease
- Patient history of heart disease
- Diabetes or elevated blood glucose, even in nondiabetics
- Hypertension
- Advanced age
- High lipoprotein (a) lipids
- African American ethnicity
- Stress, smoking, sedentary lifestyle, compulsive personality
- Poor diet (high sodium, high fat, high intake of alcohol; low intake of B-complex vitamins, calcium, magnesium, and potassium; low intake of fruits and vegetables)
- Obesity

ture or "skipped" beats. Post-MI patients will need to monitor themselves for arrhythmias.

INTERVENTION: OBJECTIVES

- Promote rest to reduce heart strain. Avoid the distention of heavy meals.
- Prevent arrhythmias by serving food at body temperature.
- Avoid both constipation and flatulence.
- Avoid excessive heart stimulation from caffeine.
- Reduce elevated levels of lipids: keep cholesterol below 200 mg/dL, triglycerides below 200 mg/dL, HDL between 40–60 mg/dL, and LDL between 100–129 mg/dL.
- Decrease energy required to chew, prepare meals, etc.
- Initiate healing and promote convalescence.
- Decrease excess weight to reduce stress on the heart.
- Identify modifiable risk factors and complications; reduce when possible (see Tables 6-13 and 6-14).
- Consume more fish, which may reduce the risk of sudden cardiac death in men if eaten weekly (Albert, 1998). Similarly, people who eat a diet rich in alpha linolenic acid (ALA) are less likely to suffer a fatal heart attack.

TABLE 6-14 Complications After Myocardial Infarction

- Arrhythmias with risk of sudden death
- Cardiogenic shock
- Cardiac tamponade
- Cholesterol emboli due to cardiac catheterization or during CABG
- Heart failure with pulmonary edema
- Left ventricular free wall rupture
- Pericarditis
- Re-infarction
- Renal failure
- Splenic infarction with fever, tachycardia, left upper quadrant abdominal pain
- Thrombosis or CVA with ischemic bowel or renal infarct
- Valve insufficiency
- Ventricular septal defect

Sources: O'Keefe JH Jr, et al. Thromboembolic splenic infarction. *Mayo Clin Proc.* 61:967, 1986; Puletti M, et al. Incidence of systemic thromboembolic lesions in acute myocardial infarction. *Clin Cardiol.* 9:331, 1986; Prieto A, et al. Nonarrhythmic complications of acute MI. *Emerg Med Clin North Am.* 19:397, 2001.

INTERVENTION: FOOD AND NUTRITION

- Initially, use clear to full liquids to promote rest while reducing the dangers of aspiration or vomiting. Reduce fluid and caffeine intake to that recommended by the physician.
- As treatment progresses, diet should include soft, easily digested foods that are low in saturated fats and cholesterol. Diet should exclude gas-forming foods. Limit diet to 2 g of sodium, or remove salt from the table. Schedule 3–6 small meals daily. Avoid stimulants such as caffeine.
- If needed, use an energy-controlled diet to reduce the heart's workload.
- The DASH diet and Mediterranean diet are useful. Increase intake of fish, whole grains, and olive oil. Onions, tea, apples, grape juice, and grapefruit, which contain flavonoids, should be used often; red wine is recommended, if approved by the physician.
- Adequate calcium and potassium will be needed. Avoid excessive amounts; no consistent data suggest that consuming micronutrients at levels exceeding those provided by a dietary pattern consistent with American Heart Association (AHA) Dietary Guidelines will confer additional benefit with regard to CVD risk reduction (Kris-Etherton et al, 2004). Magnesium is also essential; a DRI level of magnesium supplement may be helpful when patients are deficient (Gums, 2004).
- Decrease intake of whole-milk products, red meats, visible fat on meat/poultry, and commercial baked goods. Limit egg yolks to 4–5 weekly if lipids are elevated.
- Increase food sources of vitamin E, folic acid, and vitamins B_6 and B_{12}. Vitamin K may also be an important nutrient in the diet (Geleijnse et al, 2004).
- Fiber is especially important; choose vegetables, fruits, and cereal grains.
- Include judicious use of nuts, such as walnuts, almonds, macadamias, pecans, and pistachios. Walnuts contain alpha linolenic acid; almonds are a good source of vitamin E. Nuts also contain flavonoids, phenols, sterols,

SAMPLE NUTRITION DIAGNOSTIC STATEMENT

Myocardial Infarction (MI)

PES: Inappropriate intake of types of food fats due to nutrition-related knowledge deficit as evidenced by LDL cholesterol of 155 mg/dL and use of large meat portions at lunch and dinner meals.

Assessment Data (sources of info): Diet history and food records, lipid profile, review of current and previous medications used for heart disease.

Intervention: Easy meal preparation and recipe adaptations, shopping and dining away from home tips, one-on-one counseling and goal setting for making changes in choices of food fats.

Monitoring and Evaluation: Lipid profile, food diary and records, goal achievement.

saponins, elegiac acid, folic acid, magnesium, copper, potassium, and fiber. Pistachios, sunflower kernels, sesame seeds, and wheat germ are highest in phytosterols; use often.

CLINICAL INDICATORS

Clinical/History	Lab Work	
Height	CRP	PT or INR
Weight	Gluc (elevated levels will increase risk)	CPK increase
BMI	AST	Chol—total, HDL, LDL
Waist–hip ratio	Serum Cu (increased)	Trig (often increased)
Diet history	LDH (increased)	CBC
Temperature (elevated?)	Sedimentation rate	BUN
Pulse (NL = 60–100 beats/min)	WBC count (increased)	Creat, GFR
BP	Na+, K+	Homocysteine
I & O	Ca++, Mg++	Serum folate
Radionucleotide imaging	pCO_2, pO_2	Serum B_{12}
Echocardiography		H & H
ECG		Serum Fe

Common Drugs Used and Potential Side Effects

- Appropriate drugs are provided according to needs established by the profile (elevated blood pressure, serum cholesterol, etc.). Review specific drugs given to the patients and treat accordingly; nitrates, beta-blockers, and calcium channel blockers are commonly used.
- Anticoagulant therapy: Warfarin (Coumadin) or heparin may be given in some cases (e.g., when bleeding tendencies do not exist). Limit to one food per day that is high in vitamin K (green leafy vegetables such as kale, broccoli, spinach, and turnip greens). Avoid taking with dong quai, fenugreek, feverfew, excessive garlic, ginger, ginkgo, and ginseng.
- Aspirin is often recommended later to prevent recurrent MIs. Watch for GI bleeding or other side effects; aspirin may decrease serum ferritin by increasing occult blood loss (Fleming et al., 2001).
- Mexiletine (Mexitil) and propafenone (Rythmol) are used to treat arrhythmias. Nausea, vomiting, or constipation may occur. Procainamide (Procan) is also used commonly; it may result in a bitter taste, nausea, anorexia, or diarrhea.
- Morphine is used for relief of pain and should be given in minimal amounts to prevent hypotension.
- Statins, hypertensive medications, and related drugs will be needed according to the cause and risk factors of the patient.

Herbs, Botanicals, and Supplements

- At this time, the scientific data do not justify the use of antioxidant vitamin supplements for CVD risk reduction (Kris-Etherton et al, 2004).
- Chromium is sometimes used for dyslipidemia. Do not use excesses with insulin or hypoglycemic agents, because chromium may lower glucose levels excessively.
- Coenzyme Q10 (CoQ10; ubiquinone) should not be used with gemfibrozil, tricyclic antidepressants, or warfarin. CoQ10 may act similarly to vitamin K. Because CoQ10 and statins share a similar pathway, they can be taken simultaneously (Mabuchi et al, 2005; Strey et al, 2005; Silver et al, 2004).
- Danshen may be used for ischemic heart disease. Avoid large amounts with warfarin, aspirin, and other antiplatelet drugs. It can increase risks of bleeding or bruising.
- Garlic tablets (0.6% allicin) given 3 times daily have lowered cholesterol and LDL levels greatly (Stevinson et al., 2000). Large amounts should not be taken with warfarin, aspirin, and other antiplatelet drugs because of increased risks of bleeding or bruising. Garlic may also increase insulin levels with hypoglycemic results; monitor carefully in patients with diabetes.
- Gingko biloba should not be taken with warfarin and other anticoagulant drugs.
- Hawthorn should not be taken with digoxin, ACE inhibitors, and other cardiovascular drugs.
- L-arginine does not improve vascular stiffness measurements or ejection fraction and may be associated with higher postinfarction mortality; it should not be recommended following acute MI (Schulman et al, 2006).
- Niacin (nicotinic acid) should not be taken with statins, antidiabetic medications, or carbamazepine because of potentially serious risks of myopathy and altered glucose control.
- Omega-3 fatty acids in fish oil capsules can cause hypervitaminosis A and D if taken in large doses. Avoid use in pregnant or lactating women. Avoid taking with warfarin, aspirin, and other antiplatelet medications because of the risk of increased bruising or bleeding.
- Vitamin E should not be taken with warfarin because of the possibility of increased bleeding. Avoid doses greater than 400 IU/d.

INTERVENTION: NUTRITION EDUCATION, COUNSELING, CARE MANAGEMENT

- Position patient and arrange utensils to avoid or lessen fatigue. Encourage relaxation, especially at mealtimes.
- If needed, use a weight-control diet.
- Discuss roles of fats, cholesterol, sodium, potassium, calcium, magnesium, and fiber in the diet. Encourage use of the DASH or Mediterranean diets (see Table 6-3). Monitor for changes in renal status because even mild renal disease (with estimated GFR) should be considered a major risk factor for cardiovascular complications after an MI (Anavekar et al, 2004).
- Avoid excesses of carbohydrate and alcohol, especially with diabetes or elevated blood pressure.

- Individuals who undergo cardiac surgery continue to have multiple risk factors for CAD that place them at high risk for future events. Other steps, such as stopping smoking, following the recommended diet, and managing other risk factors, must be taken. Discuss convalescence regarding progression of atherosclerosis and preventing heart failure. A positive attitude toward the modified diet is essential for changing food behaviors.
- Discuss activity (gradual increase). Cardiac rehabilitation programs are very helpful (Lisspers et al, 2005). Aerobic physical activities, such as exercise or walking at work, seem to reduce the risk of MI, whereas anaerobic activities, such as heavy lifting at work, may increase risk of MI (Fransson et al, 2004).
- A comprehensive management plan can be assembled through an "ABCDE" approach: "A" for antiplatelet therapy, anticoagulation, ACE inhibition, and angiotensin receptor blockade; "B" for beta-blockade and blood pressure control; "C" for cholesterol treatment and cigarette smoking cessation; "D" for diabetes management and diet; and "E" for exercise (Gluckman et al, 2005).

Patient Education—Foodborne Illness

- Careful food handling will be important. Hand washing is key as well.

For More Information

- Myocardial Infarction
  http://www-medlib.med.utah.edu/WebPath/TUTORIAL/MYOCARD/MYOCARD.html

MYOCARDIAL INFARCTION—CITED REFERENCES

Albert C, et al. Fish consumption and risk of sudden cardiac death. *JAMA.* 279:23, 1998.

Anavekar NS, et al. Relation between renal dysfunction and cardiovascular outcomes after myocardial infarction. *N Engl J Med.* 351:1285, 2004.

Fleming D, et al. Aspirin intake and the use of serum ferritin as a measure of iron status. *Am J Clin Nutr.* 74:219, 2001.

Fransson E, et al. The risk of acute myocardial infarction: interactions of types of physical activity. *Epidemiology* 15:573, 2004.

Geleijnse JM, et al. Dietary intake of menaquinone is associated with a reduced risk of coronary heart disease: the Rotterdam Study. *J Nutr.* 134:3100, 2004.

Gluckman TJ, et al. A simplified approach to the management of non-ST-segment elevation acute coronary syndromes. *JAMA.* 293:349, 2005.

Gums JG. Magnesium in cardiovascular and other disorders. *Am J Health Syst Pharm.* 61:1569, 2004.

Joshipura K, et al. The effect of fruit and vegetable intake on risk for coronary heart disease. *Ann Intern Med.* 134:1106, 2001.

Kris-Etherton PM, et al. Antioxidant vitamin supplements and cardiovascular disease. *Circulation.* 110:637, 2004.

Legato MJ. Dyslipidemia, gender, and the role of high-density lipoprotein cholesterol: implications for therapy. *Am J Cardiol.* 86:15, 2000.

Lisspers J, et al. Long-term effects of lifestyle behavior change in coronary artery disease: effects on recurrent coronary events after percutaneous coronary intervention. *Health Psychol.* 24:41, 2005.

Mabuchi H, et al. Reduction of serum ubiquinol-10 and ubiquinone-10 levels by atorvastatin in hypercholesterolemic patients. *J Atheroscler Thromb.* 12:111, 2005.

Mallik S, Vaccarino V. Outcomes of thrombolytic therapy for acute myocardial infarction in women. *Prog Cardiovasc Dis.* 47:58, 2004.

McSweeney JC, et al. Do you know them when you see them? Women's prodromal and acute symptoms of myocardial infarction. *J Cardiovasc Nurs.* 15:26, 2001.

Schulman SP, et al. L-arginine therapy in acute myocardial infarction: the Vascular Interaction with Age in Myocardial Infarction (VINTAGE MI) randomized clinical trial. *JAMA.* 295:58, 2006.

Silver MA, et al. Effect of atorvastatin on left ventricular diastolic function and ability of coenzyme Q10 to reverse that dysfunction. *Am J Cardiol.* 94:1306, 2004.

Stevinson C, et al. Garlic for treating hypercholesterolemia: a meta analysis of randomized clinical trials. *Ann Intern Med.* 133:411, 2000.

Strey CH, et al. Endothelium-ameliorating effects of statin therapy and coenzyme Q10 reductions in chronic heart failure. *Atherosclerosis* 179:201, 2005.

Vita JA. Polyphenols and cardiovascular disease: effects on endothelial and platelet function. *J Clin Nutr.* 81:292S, 2005.

Wu J, et al. Mechanism of cardioprotection by resveratrol, a phenolic antioxidant present in red wine. *Int J Mol Med.* 8:3, 2001.

Yusuf S, et al. Effect of potentially modifiable risk factors associated with myocardial infarction in 52 countries (the INTERHEART study): case-control study. *Lancet* 364:937, 2004.

PERICARDITIS AND CARDIAC TAMPONADE

NUTRITIONAL ACUITY RANKING: LEVEL 2

DEFINITIONS AND BACKGROUND

Pericarditis is inflammation of the pericardium due to human immunodeficiency virus (HIV)/acquired immunodeficiency syndrome (AIDS), myocardial infarction, rheumatic diseases, radiation treatment, viral infection, trauma, neoplasm, chronic renal failure, or lupus. Substernal chest pain that is severe, dyspnea, shortness of breath, fever, chills, diaphoresis, nausea, fatigue, and anxiety are common symptoms of the acute stage.

Bacterial pericarditis occurs by direct infection during trauma, thoracic surgery, or catheter drainage, by spread from other causes; *Staphylococcus, Streptococcus, Haemophilus,* and *Mycobacterium tuberculosis* are common causes (Pankuweit et al, 2005).

The chronic stage of pericarditis often results from tuberculosis and may involve ascites, edema of the extremities, heart failure, and shrinkage of the pericardium. Shortness of breath, coughing, fatigue, ascites, and leg edema may result.

Although pericarditis usually is not a life-threatening condition, other life-threatening conditions may cause chest pain and should be ruled out. These include myocardial infarction, dissection of the aorta, pulmonary embolus, collapsed lung, and perforation or rupture of parts of the esophagus or stomach. Control of symptoms through diuretics is the usual treatment.

The most serious complication is **cardiac tamponade**. Cardiac tamponade involves an accumulation of fluid or blood within the pericardial sac. If uncontrolled, this condition may lead to heart failure, arrest, or shock (Meltzer and Karia, 2005). Decreased heart sounds, distended neck veins with inspiratory rise in venous pressure (Kussmaul's sign), decreased blood pressure, and abdominal pain may occur. In children, cases of cardiac tamponade have occurred as a complication of malignancies, cardiac surgery, trauma, infections, central venous catheter placement, and rheumatologic and autoimmune diseases (Cousineau and Savitsky, 2005).

INTERVENTION: OBJECTIVES

- It is critical for anyone who experiences chest pain to seek immediate medical attention to determine the cause and receive prompt, appropriate treatment to improve cardiac functioning.
- Maintain bed rest during acute stages.
- Prevent sepsis, heart failure, and shock, especially if cardiac tamponade occurs.
- Decrease fever and inflammation, which may last 10–14 days in the acute form.
- Reduce nausea and anorexia.

INTERVENTION: FOOD AND NUTRITION

- Maintain an adequate diet as needed for any underlying conditions; increase protein and calories if tolerated and if needed to prevent loss of lean body mass.
- Alter sodium and fluids if necessary.
- Small, frequent feedings to reduce nausea may be indicated.
- Monitor diet and supplements adequately. Thiamin for the heart muscle and potassium may be especially necessary; vitamins B_6 and B_{12} and folic acid may be needed if homocysteine levels are elevated. It may also be prudent to increase vitamin E levels.
- The DASH diet, therapeutic lifestyle change (TLC) diet, and Mediterranean diet are good choices.

CLINICAL INDICATORS

Clinical/History

Height
Weight
Weight changes
BMI
Waist–hip ratio
Diet history
Temperature
ECG
Cardiac catheterization
Magnetic resonance imaging (MRI) or computed tomography (CT) scan
I & O
Ascites or hepatomegaly?
Tachypnea, dyspnea
Cyanosis?

Lab Work

CRP
Gluc
Alb, transthyretin
BP
BUN, Creat, GFR
H & H
Serum Fe
Transferrin
Na+, K+
Ca++, Mg++
WBC
Homocysteine
Serum folate
Serum B_{12}

Common Drugs Used and Potential Side Effects

- Analgesics or nonsteroidal anti-inflammatory drugs (NSAIDs) may be used to relieve pain. Monitor for specific side effects.
- Antibiotics are needed for bacterial infections. Intravenous antibacterial therapy, such as vancomycin, ceftriaxone, or ciprofloxacin, is used in purulent pericarditis (Pankuweit et al, 2005). Monitor for side effects.
- Diuretics may be used. If a potassium-depleting diuretic is chosen, monitor serum potassium levels closely and manage dietary changes if needed.
- Treatment of tuberculous pericarditis includes isoniazid, rifampin, pyrazinamide, and ethambutol (Pankuweit et al, 2005). Prednisone is given and then progressively reduced in 6–8 weeks; GI distress, hyperglycemia, and calcium and nitrogen depletion may result.
- Some medications can trigger an immune response that causes pericarditis. These medications include isoniazid (Nydrazid), hydralazine (Apresoline), penicillin, antiarrhythmic agents such as procainamide (Procanbid or Pronestyl), and seizure medications such as phenytoin (Dilantin).

Herbs, Botanicals, and Supplements

- Coenzyme Q10 (CoQ10; ubiquinone) should not be used with gemfibrozil, tricyclic antidepressants, or warfarin. CoQ10 may act similarly to vitamin K. Because CoQ10 and statins share a similar pathway, they can be taken simultaneously (Mabuchi et al, 2005; Strey et al, 2005; Silver et al, 2004).
- Danshen may be used for ischemic heart disease. Avoid large amounts with warfarin, aspirin, and other antiplatelet drugs. It can increase risks of bleeding or bruising.
- Garlic tablets (0.6% allicin) given 2 times daily have lowered cholesterol and LDL levels greatly (Stevinson et al, 2000). Large amounts should not be taken with warfarin, aspirin, and other antiplatelet drugs because of increased risks of bleeding or bruising. Garlic also may increase insulin levels with hypoglycemic results; monitor carefully in patients with diabetes.
- Hawthorn should not be taken with digoxin, ACE inhibitors, and other cardiovascular drugs.
- Omega-3 fatty acids in fish oil capsules can cause hypervitaminosis A and D if taken in large doses. Avoid use in pregnant or lactating women. Avoid taking with warfarin, aspirin, and other antiplatelet medications because of the risk of increased bruising or bleeding.

- Niacin (nicotinic acid) should not be taken with statins, antidiabetic medications, or carbamazepine because of potentially serious risks of myopathy and altered glucose control.
- Vitamin E should not be taken with warfarin because of the possibility of increased bleeding. Avoid doses greater than 400 IU/d.

INTERVENTION: NUTRITION EDUCATION, COUNSELING, CARE MANAGEMENT

- Discuss the importance of avoiding fatigue.
- The patient should plan rest periods before and after activities and meals.
- Highlight the importance of nutrition in immunocompetence.

Patient Education—Foodborne Illness

- Careful food handling will be important. Hand washing is key as well.

For More Information

- Merck Manual–Pericarditis
  http://www.merck.com/mrkshared/mmanual/section16/chapter209/209b.jsp
- Pericarditis
  http://cardiologychannel.com/pericarditis/
  http://www.mssm.edu/cvi/pericarditis.shtml
- Pericarditis and Cardiac Tamponade
  http://www.emedicine.com/emerg/topic412.htm

PERICARDITIS AND CARDIAC TAMPONADE—CITED REFERENCES

Cousineau A, Savitsky E. Cardiac tamponade presenting as an apparent life-threatening event. *Pediatr Emerg Care.* 21:104, 2005.

Mabuchi H, et al. Reduction of serum ubiquinol-10 and ubiquinone-10 levels by atorvastatin in hypercholesterolemic patients. *J Atheroscler Thromb.* 12:111, 2005.

Meltzer H, Karia VG. Cardiac tamponade. *Catheter Cardiovasc Interv.* 64:245, 2005.

Pankuweit S, et al. Bacterial pericarditis: diagnosis and management. *Am J Cardiovasc Drugs.* 5:103, 2005.

Silver MA, et al. Effect of atorvastatin on left ventricular diastolic function and ability of coenzyme Q10 to reverse that dysfunction. *Am J Cardiol.* 94:1306, 2004.

Stevinson C, et al. Garlic for treating hypercholesterolemia: a meta-analysis of randomized clinical trials. *Ann Intern Med.* 133:411, 2000.

Strey CH, et al. Endothelium-ameliorating effects of statin therapy and coenzyme Q10 reductions in chronic heart failure. *Atherosclerosis* 179:201, 2005.

PERIPHERAL ARTERY DISEASE

NUTRITIONAL ACUITY RANKING: LEVEL 2

DEFINITIONS AND BACKGROUND

Peripheral vascular disease (PVD) can affect the arteries, the veins, or the lymph vessels. The most common and important type of PVD is **peripheral artery disease (PAD)**. PAD affects more than 5 million adults (Selvin and Erlinger, 2004). PAD prevalence increases dramatically with age; by age 70, about 20% of the population has PAD. PAD disproportionately affects Mexican Americans and nonhispanic blacks (Gregg et al, 2004). It is associated with significant morbidity and mortality (Selvin and Erlinger, 2004); people with PAD face a 6 to 7 times higher risk of heart attack or stroke.

PAD is caused by occlusion of an artery by a clot or by plaque buildup in the extremities, such as the hands and feet. Symptoms can include numbness, tingling in lower extremities, pain, and difficult ambulation. Gangrene with potential amputation can occur. See Table 6-15 and Figure 6-7.

Causes of PAD include heavy smoking, arterial embolism, obesity, diabetes mellitus, poor circulation, and atherosclerosis. Exposure to metals may also be related. Urinary cadmium, tungsten, and possibly antimony have been associated with PAD in a representative sample of the U.S. population (Navas-Acien et al, 2005). Finally, there is a high prevalence of PAD among patients with renal insufficiency (O'Hare et al, 2004).

Buerger's disease is the obstruction of small- and medium-sized arteries by inflammation triggered by smoking and is usually found among men aged 20–40 years. Skin ulcers or gangrene may result if smoking is not discontinued. Walking is important, unless the person has gangrene, sores, or pain at rest.

Raynaud's syndrome allows small arterioles in the fingers and toes to go into spasm, and the skin turns pale or patchy red to blue. Sometimes the underlying cause is not known. Approximately 60–90% of cases occur in young women. Scleroderma, rheumatoid arthritis, atherosclerosis, nerve disorders, hypothyroidism, injury, and reactions to certain drugs are causes. Some people also have migraine headaches and pulmonary hypertension. These individuals must protect their extremities from the cold or take mild sedatives.

The interaction between neutrophils and platelets is an important component of proinflammatory activity seen in peripheral blood of stable and unstable forms of coronary artery disease (Nijm et al, 2005). Elevated levels of fibrinogen and CRP may occur, which indicates that there is

TABLE 6-15 Sites Where Peripheral Arterial Disease (PAD) Produces Symptoms

1. Arteries supplying blood to the brain: Cerebrovascular disease (including carotid artery disease) is the number one cause of stroke and disability in the United States.
2. Arteries supplying blood to the kidneys: PAD of the renal arteries (renal artery stenosis) is one of the causes of high blood pressure and renal failure.
3. Arteries supplying blood to the legs: PAD of the lower extremities is a major cause of diminished ability to walk, and advanced cases can lead to leg amputation.
4. Arteries supplying blood to the intestines: PAD of the mesenteric arteries (mesenteric arterial disease) is less frequent but can cause severe pain, weight loss, and death from intestinal gangrene.

From Heart Center Online. Peripheral arterial disease, http://www.heartcenteronline.com/myheartdr/common/articles.cfm?ARTID=449; accessed February 24, 2005.

inflammation in the blood vessels (Selvin and Erlinger, 2004). There may be a role for vitamin C as an antioxidant; excesses are not warranted because these supplements may function as pro-oxidants. Fish oils alter vascularity favorably and may protect arterial walls.

Modifiable risk factors such as cessation of cigarette smoking and control of dyslipidemia, hypertension, and diabetes should be treated (Aronow, 2005). Angioplasty may be needed to clear obstruction, relieve symptoms, heal ulcers, and prevent amputation. Indications for lower extremity angioplasty, preferably with stenting, or bypass surgery are (1) incapacitating claudication in persons that interferes with work or lifestyle; (2) limb salvage in persons with limb-threatening ischemia as manifested by rest pain, nonhealing ulcers, and/or infection or gangrene; and (3) vasculogenic impotence (Aronow, 2005). If the limb cannot be salvaged, amputation would be needed.

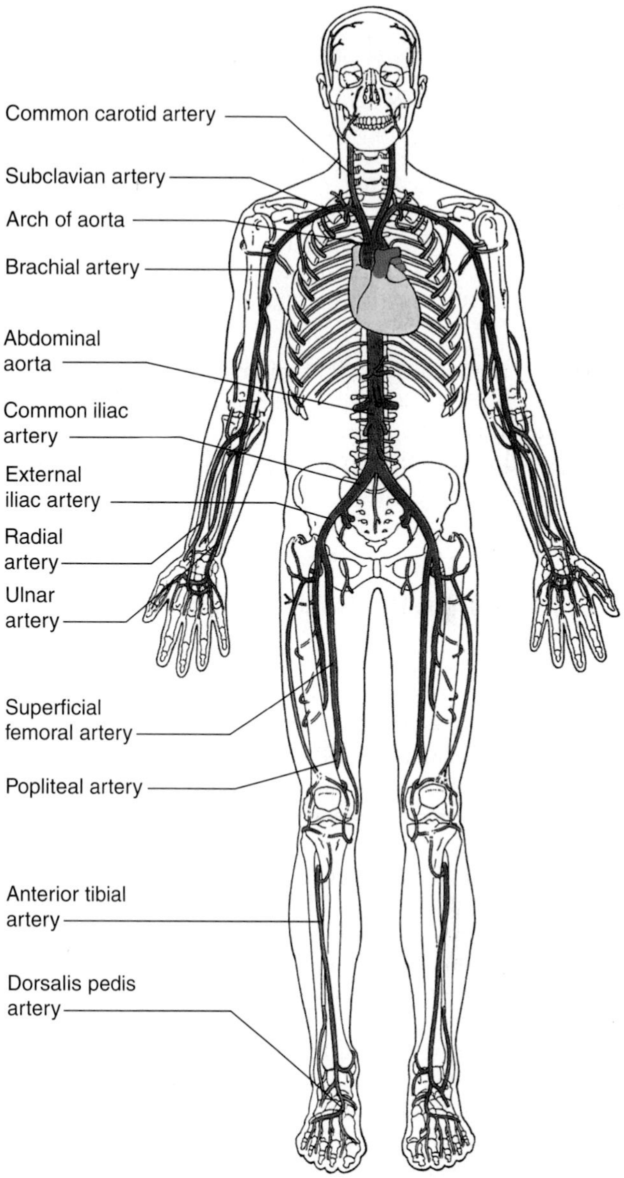

Figure 6-7 Sites of peripheral artery disease. (From Moore KL, Agur A. *Essential clinical anatomy*. 2nd ed. Philadelphia: Lippincott Williams & Wilkins, 2002.)

INTERVENTION: OBJECTIVES

- Reduce symptoms and complications such as severe leg cramps on walking, angina, heart failure, heart attack, stroke, renal failure, ulcerative disease, gangrene of lower extremities or toes, slow-healing foot ulcers, cold extremities, and paresthesia.
- Prevent sepsis, pressure ulcers, and other complications, including the need for amputation.
- Correct high levels of homocysteine.
- Attain desired body weight if obese.

INTERVENTION: FOOD AND NUTRITION

- If patient is obese, use a low-calorie diet. Use a low-fat, high–soluble fiber diet.
- Diet should provide adequate intake for wound healing when ulcers exist or after surgery. Diet should provide adequate protein.
- Vitamin E also is suggested. Almonds, filberts, avocados, sunflower seeds, vegetable oils, margarine, mayonnaise, and wheat germ are the best dietary sources.
- Pistachios, sunflower kernels, sesame seeds, and wheat germ are highest in phytosterols; use often.
- Increase folic acid, riboflavin, and vitamins B_6 and B_{12} if serum homocysteine levels are elevated.
- The DASH, therapeutic lifestyle change (TLC), and Mediterranean diet patterns are useful. Olive oil consumption along with a dietary supplement of fish oil may be helpful in the nutritional management of PVD by increasing plasma omega-3 long-chain PUFA and by decreasing susceptibility to LDL oxidation (Ramirez-Tortosa et al, 1999). The use of butter increases the risk of PAD even in patients who regularly consume olive oil, and thus, its use should be discouraged (Ciccarone et al, 2003).

CLINICAL INDICATORS

Clinical/History		
Height	Gangrene	BUN, Creat
Weight	ECG	Uric acid
BMI	Cardiac catheterization	Homocysteine
Waist–hip ratio	MRI or CT scan	Serum folate
Diet history		Serum B_{12}
BP	**Lab Work**	Gluc
Smoking history	CRP	Serum insulin
Exercise tolerance, stress testing	Chol—total, HDL, LDL	Na+, K+
Ulcerations	Trig	Ca++, Mg++

Common Drugs Used and Potential Side Effects

- Antiplatelet drugs such as aspirin or clopidogrel may be helpful; beta-blockers should be given if CAD is present (Aronow, 2005).
- Antibiotics may be used to control infections.
- Evidence from randomized controlled clinical trials has demonstrated the effectiveness of ACE inhibitors as an important risk reduction therapy for patients with PAD (Al-Omran et al, 2005).
- Anticoagulants such as warfarin may be used. Use no more than one high–vitamin K food source daily. Avoid taking with dong quai, fenugreek, feverfew, excessive garlic, ginger, ginkgo, or ginseng because of their effects.
- Isoxsuprine (Vasodilan) may be used to dilate the vessels. In some cases, niacin may be used as a vasodilator; do not use large doses without monitoring by a physician.
- Pentoxifylline (Trental) improves blood flow. GI distress, nausea, and anorexia may occur; take with meals.
- Statins reduce the incidence of intermittent claudication and improve exercise duration until the onset of intermittent claudication in persons with PAD and hypercholesterolemia (Aronow, 2005).

Herbs, Botanicals, and Supplements

- Herbs and botanicals such as ginger, purslane, and gingko have been recommended for PAD, but no clinical trials have proven efficacy.
- Chromium is sometimes used for dyslipidemia. Do not use excesses with insulin or hypoglycemic agents, because chromium may lower glucose levels excessively.
- Coenzyme Q10 (CoQ10; ubiquinone) should not be used with gemfibrozil, tricyclic antidepressants, or warfarin. CoQ10 may act similarly to vitamin K. Because CoQ10 and statins share a similar pathway, they can be taken simultaneously (Mabuchi et al, 2005; Silver et al, 2004).
- Danshen may be used for ischemic heart disease. Avoid large amounts with warfarin, aspirin, and other antiplatelet drugs. It can increase risks of bleeding or bruising.
- Garlic tablets (0.6% allicin) given 3 times daily have lowered cholesterol and LDL levels greatly (Stevinson et al, 2000). Large amounts should not be taken with warfarin, aspirin, and other antiplatelet drugs because of increased risks of bleeding or bruising. Garlic may also increase insulin levels with hypoglycemic results; monitor carefully in patients with diabetes.
- Hawthorn should not be taken with digoxin, ACE inhibitors, and other cardiovascular drugs.
- Niacin (nicotinic acid) should not be taken with statins, antidiabetic medications, or carbamazepine because of potentially serious risks of myopathy and altered glucose control.
- Omega-3 fatty acids in fish oil capsules can cause hypervitaminosis A and D if taken in large doses. Avoid use in pregnant or lactating women. Avoid taking with warfarin, aspirin, and other antiplatelet medications because of the risk of increased bruising or bleeding.
- Vitamin E should not be taken with warfarin because of the possibility of increased bleeding. Avoid doses greater than 400 IU/d.

INTERVENTION: NUTRITION EDUCATION, COUNSELING, CARE MANAGEMENT

- Emphasize the importance of weight control and exercise.
- Reduce alcohol consumption, especially if triglycerides are elevated.
- Fish and meatless meals should be used 3–4 times weekly.
- Hyperbaric oxygen treatments may be needed to heal lesions. Oxygen permeates the flesh, and anaerobic bacteria cannot survive.
- Encourage a smoking cessation program.

Patient Education—Foodborne Illness

- Careful food handling will be important. Hand washing is key as well.

For More Information

- Heart Center Online
  http://www.heartcenteronline.com/myheartdr/common/articles.cfm?ARTID=449
- National Institutes of Health–Peripheral Artery Disease Research
  http://patientrecruitment.nhlbi.nih.gov/HeartDiseases.aspx#18

PERIPHERAL ARTERY DISEASE—CITED REFERENCES

Al-Omran M, et al. Should all patients with peripheral arterial disease be treated with an angiotensin-converting enzyme inhibitor? *Can J Cardiol.* 21:189, 2005.

Aronow WS. Management of peripheral arterial disease. *Cardiol Rev.* 13:61, 2005.

Ciccarone E, et al. A high-score Mediterranean dietary pattern is associated with a reduced risk of peripheral arterial disease in Italian patients with type 2 diabetes. *J Thromb Haemost.* 1:1744, 2003.

Gregg EW, et al. Prevalence of lower-extremity disease in the US adult population ≥40 years of age with and without diabetes: 1999-2000 national health and nutrition examination survey. *Diabetes Care.* 27:1591, 2004.

Mabuchi H, et al. Reduction of serum ubiquinol-10 and ubiquinone-10 levels by atorvastatin in hypercholesterolemic patients. *J Atheroscler Thromb.* 12:111, 2005.
Navas-Acien A, et al. Metals in urine and peripheral arterial disease. *Environ Health Perspect.* 113:164, 2005.
Nijm J, et al. Circulating levels of proinflammatory cytokines and neutrophil-platelet aggregates in patients with coronary artery disease. *Am J Cardiol.* 95:452, 2005.
O'Hare AM, et al. High prevalence of peripheral arterial disease in persons with renal insufficiency: results from the National Health and Nutrition Examination Survey 1999-2000. *Circulation* 109:320, 2004.
Ramirez-Tortosa M, et al. Extra virgin olive oil increases the resistance of LDL to oxidation more than refined olive oil in free-living men with peripheral vascular disease. *J Nutr.* 129:2177, 1999.
Selvin E, Erlinger TP. Prevalence of and risk factors for peripheral arterial disease in the United States: results from the National Health and Nutrition Examination Survey, 1999-2000. *Circulation* 110:738, 2004.
Silver MA, et al. Effect of atorvastatin on left ventricular diastolic function and ability of coenzyme Q10 to reverse that dysfunction. *Am J Cardiol.* 94:1306, 2004.
Stevinson C, et al. Garlic for treating hypercholesterolemia: a meta-analysis of randomized clinical trials. *Ann Intern Med.* 133:411, 2000.

THROMBOPHLEBITIS

NUTRITIONAL ACUITY RANKING: LEVEL 1

DEFINITIONS AND BACKGROUND

Phlebitis is inflammation of a vein that usually is caused by infection or injury. Blood flow may be disturbed, with blood clots (thrombi) adhering to the wall of the inflamed vein. This condition usually occurs in leg veins, especially in varicose veins. Blood clots in the thigh veins are usually more serious than those in the lower leg and are usually deep vein thromboses (DVTs). Signs and symptoms of thrombophlebitis include pain, redness, warmth, tenderness, itching, and hard or cord-like swelling along the affected vein.

Fatty acids have been implicated in the etiology of thrombophlebitis, but there is no clearly demonstrated and plausible mechanism. Blood homocysteine levels are an important, independent, and frequent risk factor for venous thrombosis. Venous thromboembolism (VTE) is a major cause of morbidity and mortality worldwide, and the annual incidence of VTE is 1 per 1000 (Bramlage et al, 2005). Table 6-16 lists common causes of thrombophlebitis. See also Figure 6-8.

INTERVENTION: OBJECTIVES

- Stop the clot from getting bigger.
- Reduce inflammation and swelling.
- Prevent septicemia, pulmonary embolism (with chest pain and shortness of breath), and related complications.

INTERVENTION: FOOD AND NUTRITION

- Weight control diet may be needed if the patient is obese. The DASH, therapeutic lifestyle change (TLC), and Mediterranean diets may be beneficial (De Lorgeril et al, 1996).
- Sodium restriction may be beneficial for persons with a generally high salt or sodium intake. Monitor carefully.
- For general cardiovascular health, adequate vitamins B_6 and B_{12} and folic acid intakes should be included. Intake of B vitamins through diet, supplementation, and fortified foods effectively reduces homocysteine concentration and thus may reduce the risk.
- Thiamin and vitamin E are also beneficial for heart health at levels meeting but not exceeding daily requirements.
- Encourage use of omega-3 fatty acids from fish and other foods.
- Pistachios, sunflower kernels, sesame seeds, and wheat germ are high in phytosterols; use often.
- Flavonoids (including tannins, quercetin, and phenols) in grapes, strawberries, blueberries, apples, kale, broccoli, onions, garlic tea, beer, and red wine may reduce platelet activity and prevent clots.
- Foods that contain vitamin K can change how well warfarin (Coumadin) will work. Monitor intake of green leafy vegetables and in canola and soybean oils. Eat a balanced diet that does not vary in usual content of

TABLE 6-16 Causes of Thrombophlebitis

- Age: Over age 60 is more common, but it can occur any time
- Cancer and its treatment; especially in recently diagnosed patients, patients with cancer that has spread to distant sites (metastases), and those with certain genetic mutations (Blom et al, 2005)
- Central venous catheters
- Inherited conditions that cause increased risk for clotting; factor V Leiden, the genetic defect underlying resistance to activated protein C, is one factor that causes inherited thrombophilia
- Low blood flow in a deep vein due to injury, surgery, or immobilization
- Obesity or overweight
- Oral contraceptives or hormone replacement therapy; both estrogen and progesterone affect the condition
- Pregnancy, especially the first 6 weeks after giving birth
- Sitting for a long period of time (long trips in a car or airplane)
- Varicose veins, which are enlarged, twisted, painful superficial veins resulting from poorly functioning valves, usually in the legs. They affect women more commonly than men. See Figure 6-8.

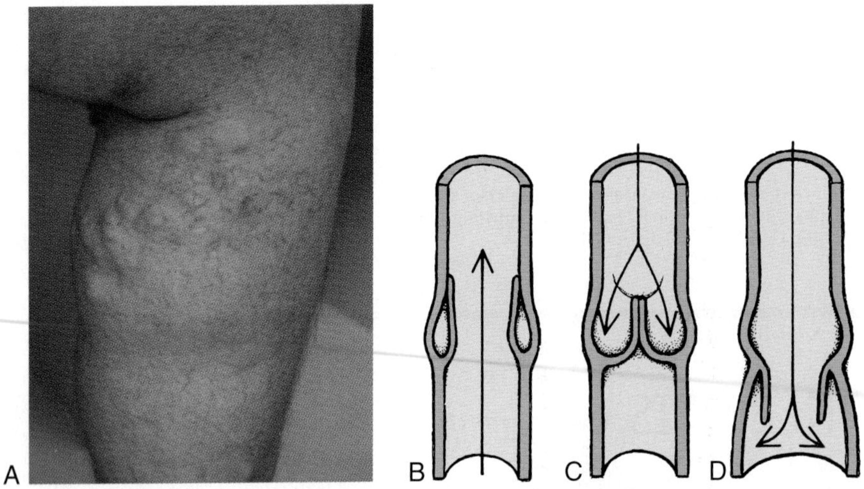

Figure 6-8 Varicose veins. (**A**, Image provided by Stedman's; **B–D**, images provided by Neil O. Hardy, Westpoint, CT.)

these vitamin K–rich foods so that the medication can be regulated.

CLINICAL INDICATORS

Clinical/History

Height
Weight
BMI
Waist–hip ratio
Diet history
Recent weight changes
Temperature
I & O
BP
Venography
Duplex ultrasound
Doppler study
Ankle BP measurements

Lab Work

CRP
Factor V Leiden kit
Alb, transthyretin
Chol—total, HDL, LDL
Trig
BUN, Creat
Uric acid
WBC
H & H
Gluc
TLC
Na+, K+
Ca++, Mg++
Homocysteine
Serum folate and B_{12}
Sex hormone–binding globulin (SHBG)—for oral contraceptive users

Common Drugs Used and Potential Side Effects

- The anticoagulant warfarin (Coumadin) may be used, with side effects that alter use of vitamin K. Monitor intake carefully. Avoid supplements that are high in vitamins E, C, or A during use. Avoid taking with dong quai, fenugreek, feverfew, excessive garlic, ginger, ginkgo, and ginseng because of their effects.
- Another anticoagulant drug, ximelagatran (Exanta), may be useful as well (O'Brien and Gage, 2005). It is an oral direct thrombin inhibitor (DTI) that binds noncovalently and reversibly to both fibrin-bound and freely circulating thrombin (Petersen, 2005).
- Antibiotics are used in bacterial infections.
- Aspirin or acetaminophen may be used to reduce fever or pain. Aspirin may decrease serum ferritin by increasing occult blood loss (Fleming et al, 2001).
- Thrombolytics may be given to quickly dissolve blood clots that cause symptoms during life-threatening situations. Thrombin inhibitors may be used to interfere with the clotting process.

Herbs, Botanicals, and Supplements

- Chromium is sometimes used for dyslipidemia. Do not use excesses with insulin or hypoglycemic agents, because chromium may lower glucose levels excessively.
- Coenzyme Q10 (CoQ10; ubiquinone) should not be used with gemfibrozil, tricyclic antidepressants, or warfarin. CoQ10 may act similarly to vitamin K. Because CoQ10 and statins share a similar pathway, they can be taken simultaneously (Mabuchi et al, 2005; Silver et al, 2004).
- Danshen may be used for ischemic heart disease. Avoid large amounts with warfarin, aspirin, and other antiplatelet drugs. It can increase risks of bleeding or bruising.
- Garlic tablets (0.6% allicin) given 3 times daily have lowered cholesterol and LDL levels greatly (Stevinson et al, 2000). Large amounts should not be taken with warfarin, aspirin, and other antiplatelet drugs because of increased risks of bleeding or bruising. It may also increase insulin levels with hypoglycemic results; monitor carefully in patients with diabetes.
- Hawthorn should not be taken with digoxin, ACE inhibitors, and other cardiovascular drugs.
- Niacin (nicotinic acid) should not be taken with statins, antidiabetic medications, or carbamazepine because of potentially serious risks of myopathy and altered glucose control.
- Omega-3 fatty acids in fish oil capsules can cause hypervitaminosis A and D if taken in large doses. Avoid use in pregnant or lactating women. Avoid taking with

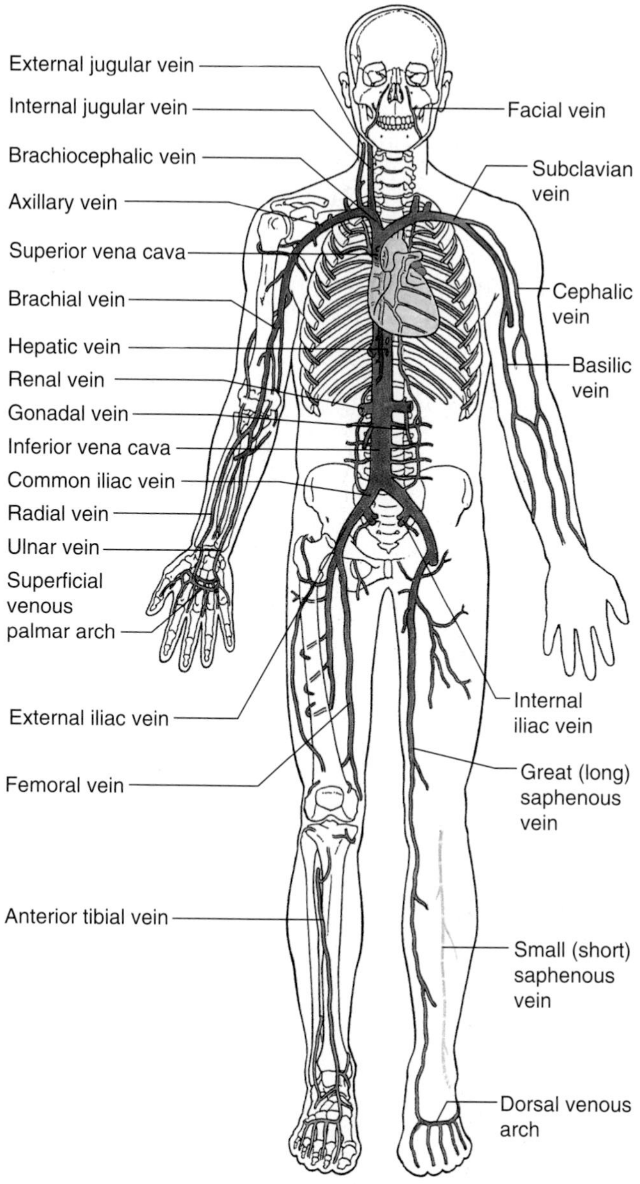

Figure 6-9 Venous blood system. (From Moore KL, Agur A. *Essential clinical anatomy*. 2nd ed. Philadelphia: Lippincott Williams & Wilkins, 2002.)

warfarin, aspirin, and other antiplatelet medications because of the risk of increased bruising or bleeding.

- Vitamin E should not be taken with warfarin because of the possibility of increased bleeding. Avoid doses greater than 400 IU/d.

INTERVENTION: NUTRITION EDUCATION, COUNSELING, CARE MANAGEMENT

- Bed rest may be important during acute stages of DVT. Leg and foot elevation may be required. Monitor side effects of immobility if patient will be immobilized for a long period of time.
- Zinc ointment may relieve itching.
- The DASH diet plan should be taught. Discuss flavonoids and other nutrients.
- For overall improvement of venous health, encourage patient to stop smoking, increase exercise, lower elevated lipids, and wear compression stockings if needed. See Figure 6-9.

Patient Education—Foodborne Illness

- Careful food handling will be important. Hand washing is key as well.

For More Information

- Coumadin–Interactive Tutorial
  http://www.nlm.nih.gov/medlineplus/tutorials/coumadinintroduction/htm/index.htm
- National Institutes of Health—Thrombophlebitis
  http://www.nlm.nih.gov/medlineplus/thrombophlebitis.html
- Vein Disease
  http://www.sirweb.org/patPub/vascularDiagnosis.shtml

THROMBOPHLEBITIS—CITED REFERENCES

Blom JW, et al. Malignancies, prothrombotic mutations, and the risk of venous thrombosis. *JAMA.* 293:715, 2005.

Bramlage P, et al. Current concepts for the prevention of venous thromboembolism. *Eur J Clin Invest.* 35:4S, 2005.

De Lorgeril M, et al. Effect of a Mediterranean type of diet on the rate of cardiovascular complications in patients with coronary artery disease. Insights into the cardioprotective effect of certain nutriments. *J Am Coll Cardiol.* 28:1103, 1996.

Fleming D, et al. Aspirin intake and the use of serum ferritin as a measure of iron status. *Am J Clin Nutr.* 74:219, 2001.

Mabuchi H, et al. Reduction of serum ubiquinol-10 and ubiquinone-10 levels by atorvastatin in hypercholesterolemic patients. *J Atheroscler Thromb.* 12:111, 2005.

O'Brien CL, Gage BF. Costs and effectiveness of ximelagatran for stroke prophylaxis in chronic atrial fibrillation. *JAMA.* 293:699, 2005.

Petersen P. Ximelagatran: a promising new drug in thromboembolic disorders. *Curr Pharm Des.* 11:527, 2005.

Silver MA, et al. Effect of atorvastatin on left ventricular diastolic function and ability of coenzyme Q10 to reverse that dysfunction. *Am J Cardiol.* 94:1306, 2004.

Stevinson C, et al. Garlic for treating hypercholesterolemia: a meta analysis of randomized clinical trials. *Ann Intern Med.* 133:411, 2000.

SECTION 7

Gastrointestinal Disorders

CHIEF ASSESSMENT FACTORS

- Dentition
- Painful Oral Tissues, Tongue
- Dysphagia
- Appetite, Anorexia, Weight Loss
- Indigestion, Heartburn
- Bezoars (Undigested Foreign Matter, Usually in Stomach)
- Nausea, Vomiting, Reflux, Regurgitation
- Abdominal Pain or Distention
- Ascites, Jaundice
- Painful or Cramping Abdomen, Flatulence
- Easy Fatigue
- Change in Eating or Bowel Habits
- Change in Stools, Consistency and Frequency; Fecal Incontinence
- Edema of Extremities
- Constipation, Diarrhea
- Hemorrhoids, Rectal Bleeding, Polyps
- Use of Gastrointestinal Medications—Antacids, Stool Softeners, Diuretics, Laxatives, Histamine Blockers
- Feeding Modality Related to Digestion or Absorption Problems (see Table 7-1)

TABLE 7-1 Digestion and Absorption Issues

Digestion: Processes that physically and chemically break down food in preparation for absorption. Digestion begins with mastication and mixing of food with salivary fluid and enzymes (oral phase). In the gastric phase, pepsin and gastric acid begin to work. Chyme is then delivered to the small intestine for mixing with pancreatic and biliary juices; the pancreatic phase involves pancreatic amylase and lipase, proteases, and phospholipase; the intestinal phase involves disaccharidases (maltase, lactase, and sucrase), peptidases, and cholecystokinin for bile salts. Maldigestion involves the interference at any of these stages, including abnormal emptying of the stomach and pancreatic insufficiency. The entire process of digestion/absorption takes about 24 hours, with large variations among individuals. Table 7-2 describes gastrointestinal (GI) conditions that may lead to malnutrition. Table 7-3 gives more information about the role of enteral nutrition, prebiotics, probiotics, and synbiotics in GI health.

Absorption: Passage of molecular nutrients into the bloodstream from the intestinal cells, mostly starting in the duodenum, with monosaccharides, amino acids and small peptides, monoglycerides, and free fatty acids. Water is also absorbed to maintain isotonicity of blood and cells. Bile and fat are needed to absorb fat-soluble vitamins A, D, E, and K. Water-soluble vitamins C and B-complex are usually absorbed in the intestinal mucosa with some storage in the liver. Malabsorption can result from dysfunction from any of the above steps.

Small intestine: Approximately 3.8 cm in diameter and 4.8 m long, covered with villi projections to increase absorptive surface. Villi cells have a rapid turnover rate of 2–5 days. Fecal fat is a valuable test of lipid digestion/absorption.

Large intestine: Approximately 5 cm in diameter and 1.5 m long, with two sections (colon and rectum) forming a frame around a highly convoluted small intestine. A diet high in whole and unrefined foods (whole grains, dark green and yellow/orange vegetables and fruits, legumes, nuts, and seeds) is high in antioxidant phenolic compounds, fibers, and other phytochemicals, all of which are beneficial.

Rectum: Approximately 12 cm long. The area is susceptible to polyps and tumors.

TABLE 7-2 Gastrointestinal Conditions That May Lead to Malnutrition

Malabsorption:	*Conditions that May Cause Fear of Eating:*
Celiac disease	Aspiration risk
Disaccharidase deficiencies	Bloating/obstruction/distension/pain (e.g., in a patient with inflammatory bowel disease and a stricture)
Pancreatic insufficiency	Cholelithiasis and other biliary diseases
Dumping syndrome	Crohn's disease
Short bowel syndrome	Dental disease
Crohn's disease	Diarrhea
Ulcerative colitis	Diverticulitis
HIV infection or AIDS	Dumping syndrome
Mechanical Function:	Dysphagia
Esophageal stricture	Esophageal spasm
Esophageal obstruction	Flatulence
Achalasia or esophageal hypomotility	Food allergies
Tracheoesophageal fistula	Gastritis
Pyloric stenosis	Ill-fitting dentures
Adynamic ileus	Irritable bowel syndrome
Bowel obstruction	Lactose intolerance
Hirschsprung's disease	Pancreatitis (acute or chronic)
Infantile achalasia	Peptic ulcer
Bezoar formation, especially after gastric surgery	Proctitis
	Rectal fissures
	Reflux esophagitis
	Ulcerative colitis

TABLE 7-3 Role of Enteral Nutrition, Prebiotics, Probiotics, and Synbiotics in Gastrointestinal (GI) Tract Function

When an oral diet is not feasible, **enteral nutrition (EN)** is needed to avoid prolonged starvation, to prevent deterioration of intestinal integrity, and to avoid translocation of gut bacteria. One or two basic formulas can meet most patients' needs. Glutamine (an amino acid needed in stress/sepsis) requires GI processing to become effective; the same is likely true for other nutrients. Therefore, it is beneficial to employ a nutrition support team (NST) in facilities where patients have need for EN until their oral dietary intake is sufficient again or to manage those cases where oral diet will not be possible again. The right product and the right ingredients can make a difference. See Table 7-5 for the role of the dietitian in GI disorders.

Prebiotics: Low-digestible carbohydrates that are not digested in the upper GI tract become fermented in the large intestine. They have physiological benefits similar to those of dietary fiber (Murphy, 2001). Short-chain fatty acids (SCFAs) are produced from fermentation of fiber; the SCFAs are fuel for mucosal cells, so they benefit the gut tissue. Fermentation leads to the selective stimulation and growth of beneficial gut bacteria such as bifidobacteria (prebiotics). Carbohydrates that offer desirable physiological properties are resistant starch (RS), oligofructose, and polydextrose. These functional benefits have been used for the development of new "healthy" products (Murphy, 2001).

Probiotics are live microbial food supplements that support balance in the intestinal tract (Kopp-Hoolihan, 2001). Probiotics have been studied as a result of reports indicating they have the ability to modify gut pH, antagonize pathogens, produce lactase, and stimulate immunomodulatory cells. Functional foods such as yogurt with live cultures may provide these probiotics (Beyer, 2004). These products may help to decrease the incidence of cancer, allergic reactions, and lactose intolerance. Probiotics also have immunomodulating properties and enhance the mucosal barrier in inflammatory bowel disease, pancreatitis, liver transplantation, and diarrhea (Jenkins et al, 2005).

Synbiotics are combinations of prebiotics and probiotics. By combining specific prebiotics and plant fibers into multifiber synbiotics, immunosupportive effects are possible (Bengmark and Martindale, 2005). In intensive care patients, the use of these products may become common practice. In the GI unit, these products may also be helpful. Crohn's disease and ulcerative colitis are caused by overly aggressive immune responses to a nonpathogenic enteric bacteria in genetically predisposed individuals (Sartor, 2004). While antibiotics can decrease tissue invasion and eliminate aggressive bacteria, administration of probiotics, poorly absorbed dietary oligosaccharides (prebiotics), or synbiotics can restore a predominance of beneficial *Lactobacillus* and *Bifidobacterium* (Sartor, 2004). Diets that contain prebiotics, probiotics, or synbiotics may be beneficial in many GI disorders and can be especially protective against colon cancer (Pool-Zobel, 2005).

TABLE 7-4 Conditions That May Benefit from Use of Intestinal Fuels

Glutamine, short-chain fatty acids, soy, fermentable fiber, prebiotics, probiotics, and fiber may be useful for:
Dumping syndrome
Inflammatory bowel disease
Bowel resection
Constipation
Diarrhea
Diverticulosis
Irritable bowel syndrome
Radiation/chemotherapy damage to the GI tract
Total parenteral nutrition (TPN)–induced bowel atrophy
Tube feeding

TABLE 7-5 Knowledge and Skills of Dietetics Practitioners for Gastrointestinal (GI) Disorders

The dietetics practitioner:
Recognizes extremes of dietary intake and the effects of diet on GI function and symptoms
Knows normal secretion, digestion, and absorption of foods
Knows sites of digestion and absorption of foods as well as macronutrients and micronutrients
Understands how GI dysfunction, surgical resections, and diseases affect nutrition
Understands how other diseases and conditions can affect GI function, such as diabetes and gastroparesis, postanesthetic ileus, neurological injury, and hormonal changes
Understands consequences of eating patterns in healthy persons and in those with GI disease
Can identify screening factors for persons with GI disease
Can explain relative strength of association between diet and other therapies in treating GI disorders
Knows value and limitations of enteral and parenteral nutrition formulas and common functional food ingredients
A team approach and the assistance of a registered dietitian are extremely valuable in managing the GI and liver manifestations of cystic fibrosis and related disorders.

From: Beyer, 1998; Mascarenhas, 2003.

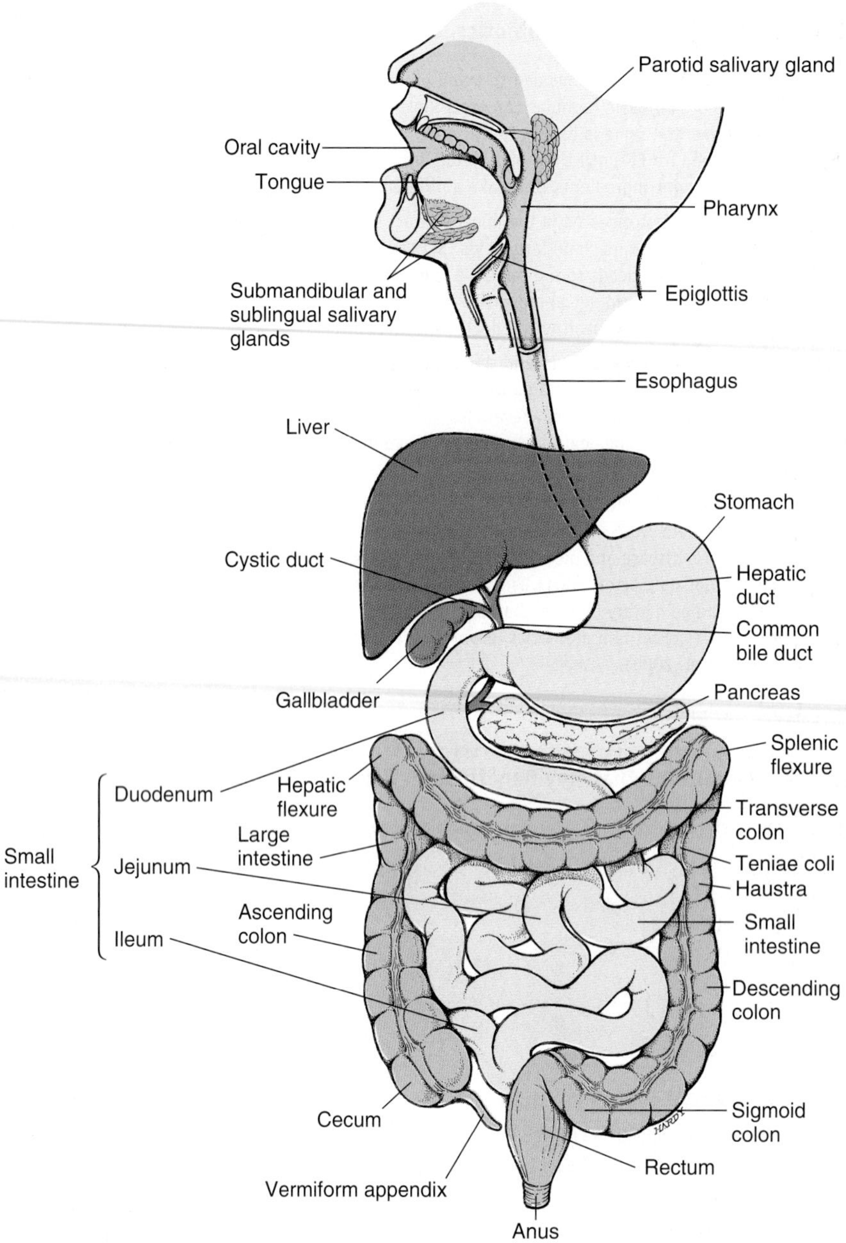

Figure 7-1 The digestive system: absorption sites. (From *Stedman's medical dictionary*. 27th ed. Baltimore: Lippincott Williams & Wilkins, 2000.)

CITED REFERENCES

Bengmark S, Martindale R. Prebiotics and synbiotics in clinical medicine. *Nutr Clin Pract.* 20:244, 2005.

Beyer P. Nutritional care and the lower GI system. In: Mahan K, Escott-Stump S, eds. *Krause's food, nutrition, and diet therapy.* 11th ed. Philadelphia: WB Saunders, 2004.

Beyer P. Role of the dietitian in gastrointestinal disorders. *J Am Diet Assoc.* 98:108, 1998.

Jenkins B, et al. Probiotics: a practical review of their role in specific clinical scenarios. *Nutr Clin Pract.* 20:262, 2005.

Kopp-Hoolihan L. Prophylactic and therapeutic uses of probiotics: a review. *J Am Diet Assoc.* 101:229, 2001.

Mascarenhas MR. Treatment of gastrointestinal problems in cystic fibrosis. *Curr Treat Options Gastroenterol.* 6:427, 2003

Murphy O. Nonpolyol low-digestible carbohydrates: food applications and functional benefits. *Br J Nutr.* 85:47S, 2001.

Pool-Zobel BL. Inulin-type fructans and reduction in colon cancer risk: review of experimental and human data. *Br J Nutr.* 93:S73, 2005.

Sartor RB. Therapeutic manipulation of the enteric microflora in inflammatory bowel diseases: antibiotics, probiotics, and prebiotics. *Gastroenterology* 126:1620, 2004.

For More Information

- American College of Gastroenterology
  http://www.acg.gi.org/
- American Digestive Health Foundation
  http://www.fdhn.org/
- American Gastroenterological Association
  http://www.gastro.org
- American Society of Gastrointestinal Endoscopy
  http://www.asge.org
- Atlas of Gastroenterology and Hepatology
  http://www.arsmedica.com/cu/cu-gah02.html
- Cleveland Clinic Foundation
  http://www.clevelandclinic.org/gastro/
- Colon and Rectal Cancer (see Section 13)
  http://www.patientcenters.com/colon

- Digestive Disorders Foundation
  http://www.digestivedisorders.org.uk
- Gastrolab
  http://gastrolab.net
- Gutfeelings
  http://www.gutfeelings.com
- Jackson's Gastroenterology–Images
  http://www.gicare.com/pated/eieg0001.htm
- National Institute of Diabetes and Digestive and Kidney Diseases (NIDDK)
  http://www.niddk.nih.gov/
- North American Society for Pediatric Gastroenterology and Nutrition
  http://www.naspgn.org
- Society of American Gastrointestinal Endoscopic Surgeons
  http://www.sages.org
- Society of Gastroenterology Nurses and Associates
  http://www.sgna.org
- World Organization for Digestive Endoscopy
  http://www.omed.org

Upper GI: Esophagus

DYSPHAGIA

NUTRITIONAL ACUITY RANKING: LEVEL 3–4

DEFINITIONS AND BACKGROUND

Anatomic or physiological swallowing problems of dysphagia create a disturbance in the normal transfer of food from the oral cavity to the stomach. Swallowing requires 5–10 seconds and three phases for completion—oral phase, pharyngeal phase, and esophageal phase. All must be adequate to prevent choking and/or aspiration into the lung. Common causes of dysphagia are found in Table 7-6.

TABLE 7-6 Common Causes of Dysphagia

Achalasia	Head or neck cancer
Aging	Head trauma
Alzheimer's disease, dementia	Hiatal hernia
Amyotrophic lateral sclerosis	Huntington's disease
Anoxia	Lung cancer
Cerebral palsy	Meningitis
Cerebrovascular accident (stroke)	Multiple sclerosis
Chronic obstructive lung disease	Muscular dystrophy
Cleft lip or palate	Myasthenia gravis
Closed head injury	Myotonic dystonia
Dehydration from medications	Parkinson's disease
Dermatomyositis	Pneumonia with aspiration history
Diabetes, type 1 (long term)	Poliomyelitis
Encephalopathy	Prematurity
Esophageal inflammation	Pulmonary disorders
Esophageal fistula	Radiation treatment to head/neck
Esophageal obstruction	Sjögren's disease
Esophageal stricture	Spinal cord injury
Esophageal trauma	Throat cancer or injury
Gastroparesis	Tongue cancer
Gastroesophageal reflux	Tracheoesophageal fistula
Goiter	Zenker's diverticulum
Guillain-Barré syndrome	

Watch for signs such as coughing, choking, drooling, and pocketing of foods. Consult speech therapist for a full evaluation; progression of diet is made when possible, under guidance of the therapist. A barium swallow may reveal silent aspiration. Inadequate dietary intake, weight loss, nutrient deficiencies, protein–energy malnutrition, and dehydration may result from prolonged dysphagia.

A structured approach is needed. Detection of aspiration by bedside examination may be clinically inadequate when compared with videofluoroscopy (VF) as the gold standard for identification (Shaw et al, 2004). Oral health status assessment is an important measure of nutritional health in older individuals especially. Lower intakes of vitamin A and vitamin B_6 and impaired intake of certain foods and nutrients can be associated with persistent oral health problems (Bailey et al, 2004).

In children with developmental disabilities, diagnosis-specific treatment of feeding disorders results in significantly improved energy consumption and nutritional status. These data also indicate that decreased morbidity and a lower acute-care hospitalization rate may be related, at least in part, to successful management of feeding problems (Schwarz et al, 2001).

INTERVENTION: OBJECTIVES

- Prevent choking and aspiration of foods and beverages.
- Provide foods that stimulate the swallowing reflex.
- Promote weight maintenance or gain if losses have occurred.
- Individualize diet based on patient needs and preferences. Refer to speech therapist, who will help to determine the level of consistency that is required (e.g., nectar or syrup, honey, pudding). Monitor for pocketing of food.
- For some patients, thin liquids may be needed. Modify levels of dysphagia diets as impairment level changes; upgrade when and if safe for the patient.
- Support independence in eating whenever possible.

- Provide moistened foods or thickened beverages for adequate hydration.
- Correct any nutrient deficits.
- Prevent pressure ulcers from poor nutritional status and weight loss, if relevant.
- For persons who have viscous oral secretions or dry mouth, liquefy foods before serving by adding broth, juice, or water.

INTERVENTION: FOOD AND NUTRITION

- The patient may be fed enterally if needed. Results from the FOOD (Feed or Ordinary Food) Collaboration Trials showed that nasogastric tube feeding was favored over percutaneous endoscopic gastrostomy as the early route of feeding in dysphagic stroke patients (Prosser-Loose and Paterson, 2006). If needed, jejunostomy feedings may be more appropriate for the patient's condition. Home tube feeding may be needed, depending on medical condition and cause of dysphagia. If total parenteral nutrition (TPN) is needed, monitor closely for ability to progress back to tube feeding or oral diet.
- Following a protocol may be beneficial. Research has indicated that implementing clinical guidelines and algorithms improves dysphagia management and patient outcomes (Runions et al, 2004).
- Calculate needs at approximately 30–35 kcal/kg. Use a 1- to 1.5-g protein intake per kg to assure adequacy and to prevent loss of lean body mass; monitor cardiac, hepatic, and renal status accordingly.
- Prevent aspiration by careful selection of foods, such as thick, soft, pureed foods instead of thin liquids. Thickening may be at honey, nectar, or pudding consistency; the label on the thickener will indicate the amount required for the differing levels. When a thickened liquid diet is ordered, foods such as gelatin should not be used because they liquefy at body temperature. Thicken foods and beverages with special products such as Thick-It, Thicken-Up, and Thick 'n Easy; these products use thickeners to make semisolids out of coffee, soup, beverages, juices, and shakes. It is possible to use mashed potato flakes to thicken some meat and casserole dishes. Baby rice cereal is an inexpensive thickener as well. Fruit purees are also helpful in thickening juices and some desserts.
- Progress over time to a soft diet. Avoid alcoholic beverages, extremely hot liquids and beverages, caffeine, and spicy foods. Avoid foods that cause choking or that are hard to manage, including tart juices and foods, dry or crisp foods such as crackers, bony fish, fibrous or chewy meats such as steak, peanut butter, bananas, thinly pureed foods that are easily aspirated, foods with varying consistency, excessively sweet drinks or fruits that aggravate drooling, and carbonated beverages that may cause choking.
- For decreased saliva production, moisten foods with small amounts of liquid. Extra fats, mild sauces, and gravies may be useful as well.
- Monitor for deficiencies in fiber and vitamins A and C if whole grains, fruits, and vegetables are not consumed.
- Avoid foods that are easily aspirated such as popcorn, bran cereals, nuts, dry mashed potatoes, cottage cheese, fruits with skins, corn, celery, pineapple, and other fruits or vegetables with fibrous pulp. Sometimes dry bread in sandwiches can also be a problem. Chewy meats such as steak, crumbly foods like crackers or cake, dry foods like chips, or sticky foods such as peanut butter or bananas should also be avoided at this time.
- Where there is reduced oral sensation, position food in the most sensitive area and use colder foods.
- To form a more cohesive bolus of food in the mouth, serve semisolid consistencies.
- For a severely sore mouth, avoid acidic foods and use soft foods at moderate temperatures.
- For delayed or absent swallowing reflex, use of temperature extremes and spicy foods may help excite the nerves necessary to function better. Some thickening of liquids may actually be beneficial. Use of cohesive foods that do not fall apart is also recommended.
- Crushed bran on cereal or high-fiber tube-feeding products can help alleviate constipation. It is possible as well to use powdered fiber products in the same way.

CLINICAL INDICATORS

Clinical/History

Height
Weight
Body mass index (BMI)
Weight changes
BMI and waist–hip ratio
Diet history
Swallowing problems—current, history, duration
Fiberoptic endoscopic evaluation of swallowing (FEES)
Videofluoroscopic swallowing study
Esophagoscopy
Barium swallow
Cookie swallow test
Pocketing of food under tongue or in cheeks
Spitting food out of mouth
Facial weakness
Slow oral transit time
Choking
Coughing before, during, or after swallowing
Excessive eating time
Wet, gurgly voice after drinking or eating
Slurred speech
Poor tongue control or excessive movement
Hoarseness, breathy voice
Recurrent pneumonia
Mealtime resistance—clenching teeth or throat
Regurgitation of food through nose or mouth
Edema
Presence of upper gastrointestinal (GI) bleeding
Blood pressure (BP)

Lab Work

Hemoglobin and hematocrit (H & H)
Blood urea nitrogen (BUN)
Albumin (Alb)
C-reactive protein (CRP)
$Na+$, $K+$, $Cl-$
$Ca++$, $Mg++$
Transferrin
Prothrombin time (PT) or international normalized ratio (INR)
Total lymphocyte count (TLC)

Common Drugs Used and Potential Side Effects

- For thick saliva and gagging, artificial saliva such as lemon glycerin may be useful.
- Papain or citrus juices may be useful for thinning secretions.

Herbs, Botanicals, and Supplements

- Herbs and botanical supplements should not be used without discussing with the physician.
- It is important to stress that no supplement or diet can cure dysphagia.

INTERVENTION: NUTRITION EDUCATION, COUNSELING, CARE MANAGEMENT

- Follow meals by brushing teeth to reduce dental caries; encourage optimal mouth care.
- Offer suggestions for specific changes in food preparation (e.g., adding moistening sauces, gravies, etc.) and cutting or mincing foods to increase control of the swallowing process.
- Encourage regular review of changes in swallowing abilities to identify early decline or to lessen restrictions when possible.
- Monitor for quality of life factors and adjust where possible. The presence of aspiration is associated with substantial weight loss, advanced initial tumor stage, diminished oropharyngeal swallowing efficiency, and lower scores on quality-of-life scales (Campbell et al, 2004).

For More Information

- Dysphagia Resource Center
http://dysphagia.com/

DYSPHAGIA—CITED REFERENCES

Bailey RL, et al. Persistent oral health problems associated with comorbidity and impaired diet quality in older adults. *J Am Diet Assoc.* 104:1273, 2004.

Campbell BH, et al. Aspiration, weight loss, and quality of life in head and neck cancer survivors. *Arch Otolaryngol Head Neck Surg.* 130:1100, 2004.

Prosser-Loose EJ, Paterson PG. The FOOD Trial Collaboration: nutritional supplementation strategies and acute stroke outcome. *Nutr Rev.* 64:289, 2006.

Runions S, et al. Practice on an acute stroke unit after implementation of a decision-making algorithm for dietary management of dysphagia. *J Neurosci Nurs.* 36:200, 2004.

Schwarz S, et al. Diagnosis and treatment of feeding disorders in children with developmental disabilities. *Pediatrics* 108:671, 2001.

Shaw JL, et al. Bronchial auscultation: an effective adjunct to speech and language therapy bedside assessment when detecting dysphagia and aspiration? *Dysphagia* 19:211, 2004.

ESOPHAGEAL STRICTURE OR SPASM, ACHALASIA, AND ZENKER'S DIVERTICULUM

NUTRITIONAL ACUITY RANKING: LEVEL 3 (STRICTURE/SPASM); LEVEL 2 (ACHALASIA)

DEFINITIONS AND BACKGROUND

Esophageal stricture is normally caused by chemical ingestion, sliding hiatal hernia, neoplasm, or reflux esophagitis. Balloon dilation without fluoroscopy is an effective treatment for esophageal strictures less than 8 cm in length; predilation diameter and stricture length are factors (Chiu et al, 2004). There are many causes of esophageal stricture, including lye burns, reflux, radiation, and several mucocutaneous diseases. Another cause is eosinophilic esophagitis, a distinct disease entity in both pediatric and adult gastroenterology with solid food dysphagia on presentation (Arora and Yamazaki, 2004).

In **esophageal spasm**, segmented, concentric contractions occur simultaneously in the lower two thirds of the esophagus. Barium and manometric studies are useful in the evaluation of patients with diffuse esophageal spasm (Prabhakar et al, 2004). Achalasia and diffuse esophageal spasm are associated with hypertrophy of circular and longitudinal muscle layers (Mittal et al, 2005). Chemical denervation with *Clostridium botulinum* toxin (Botox) is effective in relieving pharyngeal constrictor spasm, and more studies are needed (Chao et al, 2004).

Achalasia is failure of the cardiac sphincter to relax, with obstruction of food passage into the stomach. In addition, the esophagus does not demonstrate normal waves of contraction after swallowing. The mechanisms are poorly understood, but problems with nerve cell signaling may be relevant (Kraichely and Farrugia, 2006). Signs and symptoms include dysphagia, substernal pain after meals, weight loss, regurgitation, and halitosis. Esophageal dilatation or surgical myotomy may be required. In addition, botulinum toxin has been increasingly used in the interventional treatment of disorders characterized by excessive or inappropriate muscle contractions, including achalasia (Maria et al, 2005).

Zenker's diverticulum (pharyngeal pouch) generally presents after 60 years of age, but patients may have years of symptoms. Regurgitation of undigested food when patient bends over or lies down may occur and may lead to aspiration pneumonia. Diagnosis is by barium swallow, and treatment is surgical resection. Esophagodiverticulostomy has been used for many patients (Thaler et al, 2001). With recognition of the central role of the cricopharyngeus muscle in the pathogenesis of pouch formation, the emphasis on treatment has shifted, and minimally invasive (endoscopic stapling) devices are now often used (Aly et al, 2004; Chang et al, 2003).

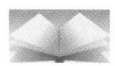

INTERVENTION: OBJECTIVES

- **Esophageal stricture:** Avoid large boluses of food. Provide adequate nutrition. Prevent weight loss. Remove cause or dilate, if necessary.
- **Esophageal spasm:** Avoid either very cold or very hot foods or beverages. Monitor dysphagia.
- **Achalasia:** Individualize diet according to patient tolerances and preferences. Monitor chronic dysphagia. Avoid aspiration.

INTERVENTION: FOOD AND NUTRITION

- **Esophageal stricture:** Begin with liquid diet and progress to soft diet as tolerance increases. Adequate calories are needed. Gastrostomy may be needed. Antireflux regimen (no alcohol, weight loss) may be helpful. Avoid sticky and dry foods. Use thin liquids and pureed or soft foods.
- **Esophageal spasm:** Use diet as tolerated with modified temperatures for foods and beverages.
- **Achalasia:** Provide large volumes of fluids with each meal, unless dysphagia prevents appropriate swallowing of liquids. Tube feed if needed; may need to use gastrostomy tube feeding.

CLINICAL INDICATORS

Clinical/History		Lab Work
Height	Heartburn	Glucose (Gluc)
Weight	Specific symptoms	Alb
Weight changes	Upper GI examination	CRP
BMI	Esophagoscopy	Gastrin
Diet history	Cine esophagography	H & H
Abdominal adiposity	BP	Na+, K+, Cl−
Ascites		Ca++, Mg++
Intake and output (I & O)		

Common Drugs Used and Potential Side Effects

- Antacids: Check the label for aluminum, calcium, magnesium, or sodium if other medical problems exist. Beware of long-term side effects.
- Nitroglycerin often helps spasm. Headache is one possible side effect.
- Isosorbide dinitrate and calcium channel blockers such as nifedipine may be needed 30 minutes before meals.

Herbs, Botanicals, and Supplements

- Herbs and botanical supplements should not be used without discussing with the physician.

INTERVENTION: NUTRITION EDUCATION, COUNSELING, CARE MANAGEMENT

- Emphasize the importance of spacing meals and achieving relaxation. Recommend intake of food at moderate temperature only.
- Elevate head of bed for 30–45 minutes after meals and at bedtime.
- Encourage fluids at mealtimes.
- Avoid foods that aggravate dysphagia.
- Bland foods are not clearly beneficial and not required.

For More Information

- Achalasia
  http://www.medicinenet.com/achalasia/article.htm
- Esophagitis
  http://chorus.rad.mcw.edu/doc/00858.html

ESOPHAGEAL STRICTURE OR SPASM, ACHALASIA, AND ZENKER'S DIVERTICULUM—CITED REFERENCES

Aly A, et al. Evolution of surgical treatment for pharyngeal pouch. *Br J Surg.* 91:657, 2004.

Arora AS, Yamazaki K. Eosinophilic esophagitis: asthma of the esophagus? *Clin Gastroenterol Hepatol.* 2:523, 2004.

Chang CY, et al. Endoscopic staple diverticulostomy for Zenker's diverticulum: review of literature and experience in 159 consecutive cases. *Laryngoscope* 113:957, 2003.

Chao SS, et al. Management of pharyngoesophageal spasm with Botox. *Otolaryngol Clin North Am.* 37:559, 2004.

Chiu YC, et al. Factors influencing clinical applications of endoscopic balloon dilation for benign esophageal strictures. *Endoscopy* 36:595, 2004.

Kraichely RE, Farrugia G. Achalasia: physiology and etiopathogenesis. *Dis Esophagus.* 19:213, 2006.

Maria G, et al. Management of bladder, prostatic and pelvic floor disorders with botulinum neurotoxin. *Curr Med Chem.* 12:247, 2005.

Mittal RK, et al. Sensory and motor function of the esophagus: lessons from ultrasound imaging. *Gastroenterology* 128:487, 2005.

Prabhakar A, et al. Relationship between diffuse esophageal spasm and lower esophageal sphincter dysfunction on barium studies and manometry in 14 patients. *Am J Roentgenol.* 183:409, 2004.

Thaler E, et al. Feasibility and outcome of endoscopic staple-assisted esophagodiverticulostomy for Zenker's diverticulum. *Laryngoscope* 111:1506, 2001.

ESOPHAGEAL TRAUMA

NUTRITIONAL ACUITY RANKING: LEVEL 3–4

DEFINITIONS AND BACKGROUND

Esophageal trauma is a major traumatic condition that affects the esophagus; it is often caused by chemical burns, ingestion of foreign bodies, or injury. Signs and symptoms include nausea, vomiting, loss of consciousness, dysphagia, respiratory distress, shock, and esophageal perforation. Following trauma, patients may be at increased risk for developing achalasia, possibly from neuropathic dysfunction due to vagal nerve damage (Shah et al, 2004).

Boerhaave syndrome involves complete laceration of the esophagus, sometimes spontaneously from alcohol abuse with retching or secondary to endoscopy or vagotomy. **Mallory-Weiss syndrome** involves a mucosal gastric tear that can occur at the gastroesophageal (GE) junction or proximal stomach; it is also associated with retching or alcohol abuse.

INTERVENTION: OBJECTIVES

- Emergency care, such as adequate ventilation or shock therapy, is given as needed.
- Allow the esophagus to rest and heal.
- Prepare for esophageal surgery, as necessary.
- Keep the patient adequately hydrated.
- Improve swallowing capacity as rapidly as possible; prevent aspiration.
- Prevent malnutrition, weight loss, sepsis, constipation, fluid loss from exudates, and other complications.
- For serious injuries with permanent damage, it may be necessary for a gastrostomy tube feeding to be used.

INTERVENTION: FOOD AND NUTRITION

- NPO as needed. Provide TPN, gastrostomy, or jejunostomy feedings as appropriate for the patient's condition. Home tube feeding may be needed, for which a gastrostomy or jejunostomy will be important.
- Calculate needs with extra protein, if applicable. Monitor cardiac, hepatic, and renal status.
- Progress over time to a soft diet. Avoid alcoholic beverages, extremely hot liquids and beverages, caffeine, and spicy foods.
- Force fluids unless overhydration is a problem or unless dysphagia prevents use of thin liquids.
- If the patient has dysphagia, use appropriately thick liquids or pureed foods until swallowing ability improves. Work with a speech therapist for proper consistency evaluations.

CLINICAL INDICATORS

Clinical/History	Dysphagia	TLC
Height	Temperature	H & H
Weight		Serum Fe
BMI	**Lab Work**	Alb or transthyretin
Diet history	Gluc	Transferrin
Weight changes	BUN, creatinine (Creat)	Ca++, Mg++
Barium swallow	Na+, K+	
I & O		

Common Drugs Used and Potential Side Effects

- Liquid topical anesthetizing agents (such as lidocaine) may be used before meals to reduce pain.
- Antibiotics may be used in bacterial infections.

Herbs, Botanicals, and Supplements

- Herbs and botanical supplements should not be used without discussing with the physician.

INTERVENTION: NUTRITION EDUCATION, COUNSELING, CARE MANAGEMENT

- When the patient can swallow, discuss the need to chew well and swallow carefully. The patient should also learn to eat slowly to prevent aspiration.
- Discuss the appropriate food textures for different stages of progress. This plan will be developed in accordance with the speech therapist and the physician.

For More Information

- Esophageal trauma
  http://chorus.rad.mcw.edu/doc/00150.html

ESOPHAGEAL TRAUMA—CITED REFERENCES

Shah RN, et al. Achalasia presenting after operative and nonoperative trauma. *Dig Dis Sci.* 49:1818, 2004.

ESOPHAGEAL VARICES

NUTRITIONAL ACUITY RANKING: LEVEL 2–3

DEFINITIONS AND BACKGROUND

Acute bleeding from esophageal varices due to portal hypertension is a frequent and severe complication of liver cirrhosis (Lata et al, 2006). In esophageal varices, small esophageal veins become distended and may rupture due to increased pressure in the portal system. This condition is usually caused by cirrhosis with portal hypertension. Signs and symptoms include respiratory distress, aspiration of emesis, shock, hemorrhage, confusion, abdominal distention, melena, jaundice, and hepatic coma. Thrombocytopenia and splenomegaly are independent predictors of large esophageal varices.

All cirrhotic patients without a history of variceal hemorrhage should undergo endoscopic screening to detect large varices (Madhotra et al, 2002; Zaman et al, 2001). Severe fibrosis and esophageal varices may be diagnosed through a prothrombin index of less than 60%, alkaline phosphatase activity greater than 110 IU/L, and hyaluronate greater than 100 g/L in alcoholic patients (Vanbiervliet et al, 2005). Maintenance of good renal function should be considered in these patients (Lata et al, 2006).

With the advent of variceal band ligation and transjugular intrahepatic portosystemic shunt, almost every acute variceal bleed can be controlled; great strides have been made because of noninvasive imaging and pressure measurement (Miller and Abdalla, 2003). Mortality has been substantially reduced. Band ligation is the first-line endoscopic treatment; vasoactive agents such as somatostatin analog and terlipressin are safe and effective pharmacological treatments of esophageal variceal hemorrhage (Wu and Chan, 2004).

INTERVENTION: OBJECTIVES

- Promote healing and recovery. Prevent worsening of symptoms.
- Prevent constipation and straining with stool.
- Prevent or correct hepatic encephalopathy or coma. (See appropriate disorder sections, such as Hepatic Cirrhosis and Hepatic Failure, Encephalopathy, and Coma in Section 8.)

INTERVENTION: FOOD AND NUTRITION

- Generally, unless comatose, the patient can tolerate 5–6 small meals of soft foods. Avoid foods such as tacos, tortilla chips, or large pieces of raw fruits and vegetables.
- Alter carbohydrate, protein, and fat intake according to hepatic function and state of consciousness. Monitor micronutrient needs, such as iron if patient is anemic.
- Provide adequate fluid as allowed or controlled.
- To prevent constipation and straining, foods such as prune juice or formulas with fiber added can help normalize bowel function.

CLINICAL INDICATORS

Clinical/History	Lab Work	
Height	H & H	Platelet count (<200,000/mm^3)
Weight	Ammonia (NH_3)	Prothrombin index (<60%)
BMI	BUN	Hyaluronate (>100 g/L)
Diet history	Alb (<40 g/L)	Alkaline phosphatase (Alk phos) (>110 IU/L)
Weight changes	Ascites	
Esophagoscopy	Na+, K+, Cl−	
Edema	Ca++, Mg++	
Melena	Transferrin	
Upper GI bleeding	Bilirubin (>20 mg/dL)	
BP		

Common Drugs Used and Potential Side Effects

- Antacids may be beneficial to buffer gastric acidity. Extended use can cause problems with pH, altered mineral and nutrient use, and other imbalances.
- Beta-blockers are important. Empiric prophylaxis with beta-blockers may be viable in comparison with endoscopic screening in patients with cirrhosis (Suzuki et al, 2005). Propranolol therapy reduces risk of bleeding, especially in patients with cirrhosis (Abraczinskas et al, 2001).
- Vasoactive agents, such as somatostatin analog and terlipressin, are useful (Wu and Chan, 2004).
- Vitamin K may be needed to help with adequate clotting.

Herbs, Botanicals, and Supplements

- Herbs and botanical supplements should not be used without discussing with the physician.

INTERVENTION: NUTRITION EDUCATION, COUNSELING, CARE MANAGEMENT

- The role of alcohol in contributing to the disease process should be discussed with the patient and family.
- The importance of good nutrition with adequate consistency should be addressed.
- Teach the patient to avoid rough or crunchy foods that are fibrous or sharp and to chew all foods well before swallowing.
- If gastrostomy is needed, discuss how to manage the feeding process.
- Advise the patient to avoid mouthwashes, cough syrups, and other products that contain alcohol.

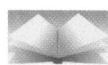

For More Information

- Esophageal Varices
  http://www.nlm.nih.gov/medlineplus/ency/article/000268.htm

ESOPHAGEAL VARICES—CITED REFERENCES

Abraczinskas D, et al. Propranolol for the prevention of first esophageal variceal hemorrhage: a lifetime commitment? *Hepatology* 34:1096, 2001.

Lata J, et al. Factors participating in the development and mortality of variceal bleeding in portal hypertension—possible effects of the kidney damage and malnutrition. *Hepatogastroenterology* 53:420, 2006.

Madhotra R, et al. Prediction of esophageal varices in patients with cirrhosis. *J Clin Gastroenterol.* 34:81, 2002.

Miller L, Abdalla A. The role of endoscopy in the treatment of esophageal varices, 2002–2003. *Curr Opin Gastroenterol.* 19:483, 2003.

Suzuki A, et al. Diagnostic model of esophageal varices in alcoholic liver disease. *Eur J Gastroenterol Hepatol.* 17:307, 2005.

Vanbiervliet G, et al. Serum fibrosis markers can detect large oesophageal varices with a high accuracy. *Eur J Gastroenterol Hepatol.* 17:333, 2005.

Wu JC, Chan FK. Esophageal bleeding disorders. *Curr Opin Gastroenterol.* 20:386, 2004.

Zaman A, et al. Risk factors for the presence of varices in cirrhotic patients without a history of variceal hemorrhage. *Arch Intern Med.* 26:2564, 2001.

HIATAL HERNIA, ESOPHAGITIS, AND GASTROESOPHAGEAL REFLUX DISEASE

NUTRITIONAL ACUITY RANKING: LEVEL 2–3

DEFINITIONS AND BACKGROUND

Hiatal hernia is caused by protrusion of part of the stomach through the diaphragm muscle, which separates the chest from the abdomen. This causes an enlarged diaphragm opening (hiatus) through which the esophagus passes to join the stomach. Hiatal hernia may show no symptoms or may contribute to heartburn, swallowing difficulty, reflux, or vomiting of blood. Hiatal hernia surgery has evolved from anatomic repair to physiological restoration (Stylopoulous and Rattner, 2005).

Esophagitis results from gastric juice being forced into the esophagus from the stomach; persons who take nonsteroidal anti-inflammatory drugs (NSAIDs) risk developing esophagitis. Proton pump inhibitors (PPIs) are recommended in the healing of erosive esophagitis (Lowe and Wolfe, 2004). **Eosinophilic esophagitis (EoE)** is a disorder characterized by a severe, isolated eosinophilic infiltration of the esophagus that is unresponsive to aggressive acid blockade but responsive to the removal of dietary antigens or dietary elimination using an amino acid–based formula (Liacouras et al, 2005).

Barrett's esophagus is a condition that affects men more then women, and length of impact is greater in men than in women (Falk et al, 2005). It is also more common in Caucasians and in persons older than age 50. Symptoms are similar to gastroesophageal reflux disease (GERD), but Barrett's esophagus is more likely to precede esophageal cancer. Barrett's esophagus is a major risk factor for esophageal adenocarcinoma; upper endoscopy and surveillance biopsies may be needed (Liu and Saltzman, 2006).

GERD and peptic ulcer disease are seen more commonly in elderly individuals than in other age groups. GERD affects approximately 19 million Americans; the prevalence is as high as 80% among asthma patients. Most patients with symptomatic GERD do not have erosive reflux disease; transient lower esophageal sphincter relaxations and hiatal hernias have emerged as major and interacting factors in GERD (Triadafilopoulos, 2004). Most patients with GERD also have hiatal hernias. Distal esophageal cancer is associated with symptomatic gastrointestinal (GI) reflux disease and Barrett's esophagus; surveillance programs are identifying patients with early, curable esophageal adenocarcinoma (Demeester, 2006).

GERD is a frequent phenomenon in infants and children. In infants, GERD usually resolves by 6–12 months of age. Management involves thickened feedings and positioning (Jung, 2001). The recommended approach for infants with uncomplicated regurgitation is the reassurance of the parents about the physiological nature of excessive regurgitation and dietary recommendations for formula feeding. Symptoms of pediatric GERD include colic, inconsolable crying, frequent spitting up or vomiting, food refusal, failure to thrive, heartburn, stomach pains, chronic sore throat, chronic respiratory problems, asthma, and apnea. GERD diagnosis in older children warrants review for upper GI tract disorders, cow's milk allergy, or metabolic, infectious, renal, or central nervous system diseases. Intractable disease may require minor surgery to strengthen a weak sphincter.

Treatment guidelines address lifestyle changes, patient-directed (over the counter) therapy, acid suppression, promotility therapy, maintenance therapy, antireflux surgery, and endoscopic therapy (DeVault and Castell, 2005). Up to 70% of patients with typical symptoms of GERD have nonerosive reflux disease (NERD), also termed endoscopy-negative reflux disease. In life-threatening situations or in patients who are resistant to or dependent on acid-suppressive medication, surgery is considered (Vandenplas, 2000). Laparoscopic antireflux surgery is highly effective as a long-term treatment for severe GERD.

INTERVENTION: OBJECTIVES

- Eliminate heartburn and reflux into the esophagus. Neutralize gastric acidity, when possible. Alcoholic beverages,

soft drinks, coffee, and tea are often associated with heartburn, especially if consumed before bedtime.
- Achieve and maintain desirable body weight to improve mechanical and postural states. There seems to be a dose-response relationship between increasing weight and GERD.
- Avoid large meals that increase gastric pressure and alter pressure on the lower esophageal sphincter (LES), thereby allowing reflux to occur. The LES limits aspiration of gastric contents when functioning properly.
- Provide an individual diet reflecting patient needs. Assess intake of fat, alcohol, spices, and caffeine.
- Patients should avoid garments that fit tightly around the abdomen.

INTERVENTION: FOOD AND NUTRITION

- If needed, a reduced-energy diet should be used to promote weight loss. BMI may be associated with symptomatic gastroesophageal reflux independent of diet and exercise (Nandurkar et al, 2004).
- During acute episodes, provide small, frequent feedings of soft foods. Instruct the patient to remain upright for 2 hours after meals and avoid intake of food (especially fatty foods) for several hours before bedtime. If needed, elevate the head of the bed.
- Diet should be high in protein to stimulate gastrin secretion and to increase LES pressure. Avoid foods that decrease LES pressure, including chocolate, peppermint, onions, garlic, and spearmint. Instruct patients to limit or stop smoking and reduce their use of salt; tobacco smoking and table salt intake seem to be risk factors for GERD symptoms (Nilsson et al, 2004). Avoid carbonated beverages as well.
- Diet should be low in fat (Sifrim and Zhang, 2004). Use fewer fried foods, cream sauces, gravies, fatty meats, pastries, nuts, potato chips, butter, and margarine.
- Dietary fiber and physical exercise may be protective, whereas alcohol, coffee, and tea are only mild risk factors (Nilsson et al, 2004).

SAMPLE NUTRITION DIAGNOSTIC STATEMENT

Gastroesophageal Reflux Disease (GERD)

PES: Undesirable food choices related to lack of knowledge regarding role of diet in GERD symptoms and complications as evidenced by frequent consumption of large, high-fat meals and alcoholic beverages and subsequent upper GI disorders.

Assessment: Knowledge about the role of diet in GERD; food diary; timing of meals and related symptoms.

Intervention: Teach/counsel about dietary changes that will alleviate GERD symptoms and possibly prevent complications; address physical/behavioral changes, such as weight loss, tight restrictive clothing, and posture during and after eating.

Monitoring and Evaluation: Report of relief from symptoms and no report of complications from GERD; reduction in need for medication.

- Avoid foods that may irritate the esophagus, such as citrus juices, tomatoes, and tomato sauce. Other spicy foods are to be eliminated according to individual experience. If there is EoE, it may be helpful to try a dietary elimination diet and add back foods one at a time to identify potential allergens (Liacouras et al, 2005).
- Fluids can be taken between meals if consumption with meals causes abdominal distention and discomfort.

CLINICAL INDICATORS

Clinical/History

- Height
- Weight
- BMI
- Diet history
- Weight changes
- Upper GI endoscopy
- Esophagoscopy
- PillCAM (noninvasive visualization)
- Manometry
- Feeding difficulties in children
- Recurrent vomiting
- Reactive airway disease and nocturnal asthma
- Choking attacks
- Dental erosion or caries

Lab Work

- H & H
- Mean cell volume (MCV)
- Na+, K+
- Ca++, Mg++
- Gluc
- Gastrin
- Alb, transthyretin
- CRP
- *Helicobacter pylori* infection?
- Cholesterol (Chol)
- Triglycerides (Trig)
- Transferrin
- Total iron-binding capacity (TIBC)
- Bernstein test: HCl solution is dripped into the distal esophagus; positive test mimics patient symptoms

Common Drugs Used and Potential Side Effects

- Antacids are used to neutralize gastric contents; antacids destroy thiamin and may provide excess sodium for the body. Check labels carefully. If the antacid contains calcium (e.g., Tums, which contains calcium carbonate), excess calcium may cause decreased levels of magnesium and phosphorus. Aluminum hydroxide (Maalox) depletes phosphorus, which is acceptable for patients with certain types of renal diseases, but otherwise phosphorus levels must be observed. When used as an antacid, sodium bicarbonate can decrease iron absorption and causes sodium retention; use with caution.
- Pill-induced esophageal injury may occur from use of aspirin, tetracycline, vitamin C, ferrous sulfate, potassium chloride, or NSAIDs. Take these with plenty of liquid.
- Calcium glycerophosphate (Prelief) is somewhat useful for relief of heartburn by neutralizing the acid in foods; it is available over the counter.
- Proton pump inhibitors (PPIs), such as lansoprazole (Prevacid), omeprazole (Prilosec), and esomeprazole (Nexium), are popular treatments (Thomson, 2001).

When clarithromycin-resistant *Helicobacter pylori* (CRHP) occur, PPIs tend to inhibit the growth and motility of CRHP. Omeprazole is useful for refractory reflux esophagitis.

- Acid-suppressive drugs, such as PPIs and H_2-receptor antagonists (H2RAs), may increase patients' risk of developing community-acquired pneumonia (Laheij et al, 2004). Reduction of gastric acid secretion by acid-suppressive therapy allows pathogen colonization from the upper GI tract; bacteria and viruses in the contaminated stomach have been identified as species from the oral cavity (Laheij et al, 2004).
- Metoclopramide (Reglan) may be used. Nausea or diarrhea may occur.

Herbs, Botanicals, and Supplements

- Herbs and botanical supplements should not be used without discussing with the physician.
- Chamomile, peppermint, fennel, cardamom, cinnamon, dill, and licorice have been recommended for this condition, but no clinical trials have proven efficacy.

INTERVENTION: NUTRITION EDUCATION, COUNSELING, CARE MANAGEMENT

- Encourage the patient to avoid late evening meals and snacks and to avoid lying down or sleeping or swimming soon after a meal to guard against reflux.
- Teach the proper measures for controlling weight, including small, frequent feedings.
- Instruct the patient to maintain an upright position for 2 hours after eating. Elevating the head of the bed at night may also be beneficial. Patients with heartburn probably should not sleep in a waterbed.
- Stop smoking to reduce reflux.
- Chewing sugarless gum after meals may reduce reflux somewhat because of the saliva production.

Patient Education—Foodborne Illness

- Careful food handling and washing hands before eating are useful recommendations.

For More Information

- AstraZenica–GERD
http://www.gerd.com
- International Foundation for Gastrointestinal Disorders
http://www.aboutgerd.org/
- Heartburn and Regurgitation Algorithm
http://www.uwgi.org/guidelines/ch_03/ch03.htm
- National Institute of Diabetes and Digestive and Kidney Diseases (NIDDK)
http://digestive.niddk.nih.gov/ddiseases/pubs/gerd/
- Pediatric and Adolescent Gastroesophageal Reflux Association
http://www.reflux.org/
- Prelief
http://www.akpharma.com/prelief/preliefindex.html

HIATAL HERNIA, ESOPHAGITIS, AND GASTROESOPHAGEAL REFLUX DISEASE—CITED REFERENCES

Demeester SR. Adenocarcinoma of the esophagus and cardia: a review of the disease and its treatment. *Ann Surg Oncol.* 13:12, 2006.
DeVault K, Castell D. Updated guidelines for the diagnosis and treatment of gastroesophageal reflux disease. *Am J Gastroenterol.* 100:190, 2005.
Falk GW, et al. Barrett's esophagus in women: demographic features and progression to high-grade dysplasia and cancer. *Clin Gastroenterol Hepatol.* 3:1089, 2005.
Jung A. Gastroesophageal reflux in infants and children. *Am Fam Physician.* 64:1853, 2001.
Laheij RJ, et al. Risk of community-acquired pneumonia and use of gastric acid-suppressive drugs. *JAMA.* 292:1955, 2004.
Liacouras CA, et al. Eosinophilic esophagitis: a 10-year experience in 381 children. *Clin Gastroenterol Hepatol.* 3:1198, 2005.
Liu JJ, Saltzman JR. Management of gastroesophageal reflux disease. *South Med J.* 99:735, 2006.
Lowe RC, Wolfe MM. The pharmacological management of gastroesophageal reflux disease. *Minerva Gastroenterol Dietol.* 50:227, 2004.
Nandurkar S, et al. Relationship between body mass index, diet, exercise and gastro-oesophageal reflux symptoms in a community. *Aliment Pharmacol Ther.* 20:497, 2004.
Nilsson M, et al. Lifestyle related risk factors in the aetiology of gastroesophageal reflux. *Gut* 53:1730, 2004.
Sifrim D, Zhang X. Pathophysiology of GERD in China: the same factors at a lower scale. *Am J Gastroenterol.* 99:2094, 2004.
Stylopoulos N, Rattner DW. The history of hiatal hernia surgery: from Bowditch to laparoscopy. *Ann Surg.* 241:185, 2005.
Thomson A. Gastro-oesophageal reflux in the elderly: role of drug therapy in management. *Drugs Aging.* 18:409, 2001.
Triadafilopoulos G. Gastroesophageal reflux. *Curr Opin Gastroenterol.* 20:369, 2004.
Vandenplas Y. Diagnosis and treatment of gastroesophageal reflux disease in infants and children. *Can J Gastroenterol.* 14:26D, 2000.

STOMACH

DYSPEPSIA/INDIGESTION

NUTRITIONAL ACUITY RANKING: LEVEL 1–2

DEFINITIONS AND BACKGROUND

Indigestion (dyspepsia) may be secondary to other systemic disorders such as atherosclerotic heart disease, hypertension, liver disease, or renal disease. It may have psychogenic causes as well, such as during periods of anxiety. Signs and symptoms of dyspepsia include burning sensation in the stomach, bloating, heartburn, nausea, burping, vomiting, early satiety, postprandial fullness, and epigastric soreness. Symptoms may be graded from mild to severe for the individual patient.

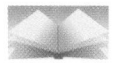

The concept of gastric hypersensitivity is an important factor in the pathophysiology of functional dyspepsia (FD) (Rhee et al, 2000). While basal tone, gastric compliance, and postprandial receptive relaxation are similar in controls and patients, abdominal discomfort is more common in FD patients than in controls. Hypnotherapy may be a preferred treatment over pharmacotherapy (Kleibeuker and Thijs, 2004).

In rare cases, a patient may exhibit signs of **bezoar formation**, such as after gastric surgery or chronic use of medications that do not dissolve easily for that individual. A bezoar (foreign matter accumulation) may be made of plant material, medications, or swallowed foreign objects. The patient complains of vague abdominal pain or indigestion and may experience nausea or vomiting. An x-ray of the GI tract may be useful for a clarifying diagnosis.

INTERVENTION: OBJECTIVES

- Determine whether the problem is psychogenic or organic in etiology. Do not oversimplify the patient's discomfort.
- As appropriate, review and discuss irritable bowel syndrome symptoms as well; they are often related.

INTERVENTION: FOOD AND NUTRITION

- Diet should make use of well-cooked foods that are adequate in amount but not overly seasoned.
- Evaluate for any undetected food allergies and manage accordingly.
- A relaxed atmosphere is helpful, and small meals may be better tolerated.
- If the dyspepsia is organic in etiology, a soft, low-fat diet may be helpful. If there is irritable bowel as well, discuss fiber (especially fruits and vegetables; bran is not always well tolerated; see Irritable Bowel Syndrome entry).
- If the patient has an obstruction or bezoar, a liquid diet may be useful until resolved.

CLINICAL INDICATORS

Clinical/History		
Height	Epigastric pain or burning	H & H
Weight	Postprandial fullness, early satiation	Serum Fe
Weight changes	Stool consistency	MCV
BMI	I & O	Alb, transthyretin
Diet history	**Lab Work**	CRP
Anorexia	*Helicobacter pylori* infection	Gluc
Gastric barostat tests		BUN, Creat
Endoscopy		Na+, K+
Nausea or vomiting		Ca++, Mg++

Common Drugs Used and Potential Side Effects

- Antacids: Beware of nutritional side effects resulting from chronic use or dependency.
- Antisecretory drugs are useful (Suzuki et al, 2006). Proton pump inhibitors may be used, especially if reflux also exists (Kleibeuker and Thijs, 2004; Ligumsky et al, 2001). Lansoprazole (Prevacid), omeprazole (Prilosec), and esomeprazole (Nexium) are commonly used.
- Avoid anti-inflammatory medicines like ibuprofen, aspirin, and naproxen (Aleve), which can irritate the stomach. Acetaminophen (Tylenol) is a better choice for pain.
- Nonsteroidal anti-inflammatory drugs (NSAIDs) are nonselective cyclooxygenase-1 (COX-1) and COX-2 inhibitors and may be associated with dyspepsia (Watson et al, 2004).

Herbs, Botanicals, and Supplements

- Herbs and botanical supplements should not be used without discussing with the physician.
- Ginger is often used as an antinauseant. Do not use large doses with warfarin, aspirin, other antiplatelet drugs, antihypertensive drugs, and hypoglycemic drugs. Additive effects can cause unpredictable changes in blood pressure and decreases in blood glucose levels and may decrease platelet aggregation and thus increase bleeding. Ginger ale has few side effects.
- Chamomile, peppermint, red pepper, angelica, and coriander have been recommended, but no clinical trials have proven efficacy.

INTERVENTION: NUTRITION EDUCATION, COUNSELING, CARE MANAGEMENT

- Encourage the patient to eat in a relaxed atmosphere.
- Yoga and other stress-relieving lifestyle changes may be beneficial.
- Discuss the role of fiber in maintaining bowel regularity.

Patient Education—Food Safety

- Careful food handling and hand washing are important to prevent introduction of foodborne pathogens to the diet of the individual. Preparation and storage techniques are also essential.

For More Information

- Dyspepsia
  http://familydoctor.org/474.xml
- Dyspepsia Algorithm
  http://www.uwgi.org/guidelines/ch_02/ch02.htm

DYSPEPSIA/INDIGESTION—CITED REFERENCES

Kleibeuker JH, Thijs JC. Functional dyspepsia. *Curr Opin Gastroenterol.* 20:546, 2004.

Ligumsky M, et al. Effect of long-term, continuous versus alternate-day omeprazole therapy on serum gastrin in patients treated for reflux esophagitis. *J Clin Gastroenterol.* 33:32, 2001.

Rhee P, et al. Evaluation of individual symptoms cannot predict presence of gastric hypersensitivity in functional dyspepsia. *Dig Dis Sci.* 45:1680, 2000.
Suzuki H, et al. Therapeutic strategies for functional dyspepsia and the introduction of the Rome III classification. *J Gastroenterol.* 41:513, 2006.
Watson DJ, et al. Use of gastroprotective agents and discontinuations due to dyspepsia with the selective cyclooxygenase-2 inhibitor etoricoxib compared with non-selective NSAIDs. *Curr Med Res Opin.* 20:1899, 2004.

GASTRECTOMY AND VAGOTOMY

NUTRITIONAL ACUITY RANKING: LEVEL 3–4

DEFINITIONS AND BACKGROUND

Gastrectomy and **vagotomy** are surgical procedures that are used for gastric cancer or when medical management for peptic ulcer has failed. Perforation is one of the main reasons why the surgery is done. The frequency with which elective gastric surgeries are performed has decreased in the past 20 years as drugs have become increasingly effective in treating ulcers. Billroth I (gastroduodenostomy) is an anastomosis between the stomach and duodenum after removal of the distal portion of the stomach. Billroth II (gastrojejunostomy) is an anastomosis between the stomach and jejunum after removal of two thirds to three fourths of the stomach; iron loss can occur. Laparoscopic-assisted gastrectomy is an increasingly common procedure for gastric cancer, with fewer side effects (Mochiki et al, 2005). See Figure 7-2.

Vagotomy is a procedure in which the vagus nerve is cut to reduce pain. Much less nutritional intervention is required for the vagotomy than for the other two procedures. However, gastrectomy or vagotomy may result in reactive hypoglycemia, which may reduce the plasma glucose levels to as low as 30–40 mg/dL due to rapid digestion and absorption of food, especially carbohydrates.

Partial gastrectomy usually leads to fast emptying, but if performed after vagotomy, it may lead to gastric stasis (Mistiaen, 2001). Gastric emptying rate for solids may increase in some patients. In most of them, however, there is a normal to decreased emptying rate. When vagotomy precedes the resective procedure, the gastric emptying rate decreases significantly (Mistiaen et al, 2001).

INTERVENTION: OBJECTIVES

Preoperative

- Empty the stomach and upper intestines.
- Ensure high-calorie intake for glycogen stores and weight maintenance or weight gain if needed. Ensure adequate nutrient storage to promote postoperative wound healing.
- Maintain normal fluid and electrolyte balance.

Postoperative

- Prevent distention and pain. Reduce the likelihood of the dumping syndrome: nausea, vomiting, abdominal distention, diarrhea, malaise, profuse sweating, hypoglycemia,

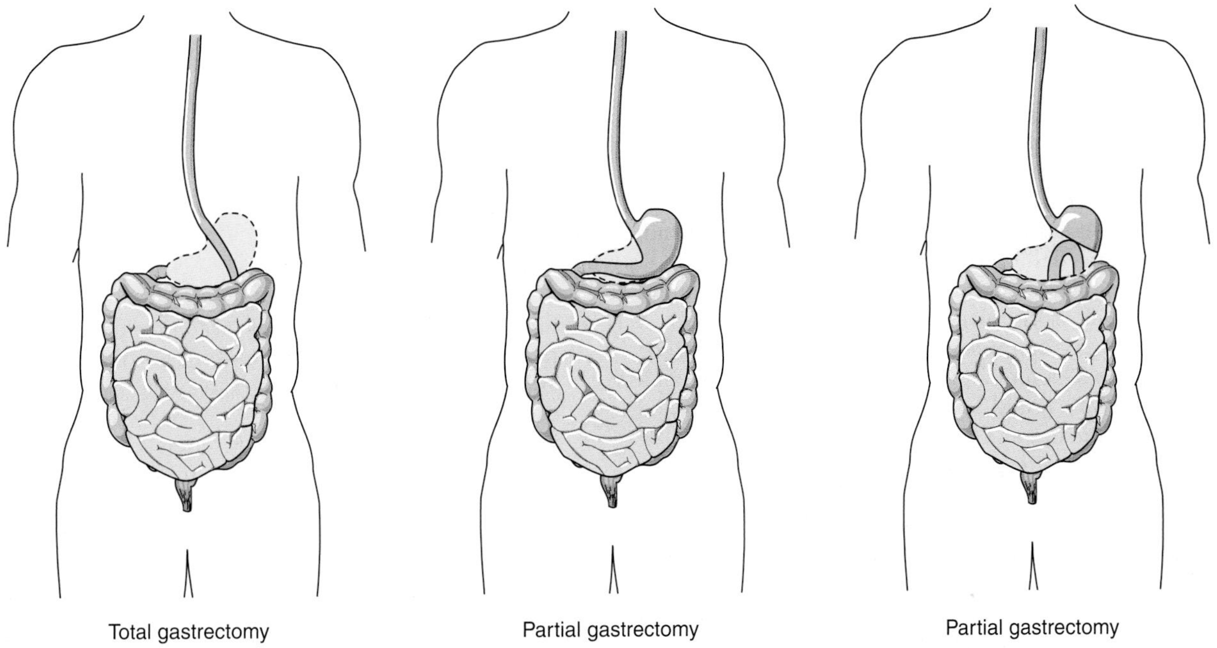

Figure 7-2 Gastrectomy procedures.

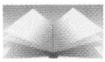

hypotension, increased bowel sounds, and vertigo. Additional use of soy and fermentable fiber may be useful; liquid pectin may prolong gastric emptying time and reduce the onset of dumping.
- Compensate for loss of storage/holding space and lessen dumping of large amounts of chyme into the duodenum/jejunum at one time. Overcome effects of decreased hormonal output (secretin, pancreozymin, and cholecystokinin).
- Overcome negative nitrogen balance after surgery; restore healthy nutritional status.
- Prevent or correct iron malabsorption; steatorrhea, calcium malabsorption, and vitamin B_{12} or folacin anemias.
- Prevent or treat metabolic bone disease, which can occur over time.
- Prevent or treat problems such as bezoars, gastric stasis, or gastroparesis.

INTERVENTION: FOOD AND NUTRITION

Preoperative

- Use a soft diet that is high in calories with adequate protein and vitamins C and K.
- Regress to soft diet with full liquids and then NPO about 8 hours before surgery.

Postoperative

- Within a total quantity limit, intake of complex carbohydrates such as bread, rice, and vegetables should be liberal (50–60%). To lessen the hyperosmolar load, use only 0–15% of diet from foods made with sucrose, fructose, and glucose. Initial diet may need to be 20 mL of liquid nutritional supplement every few hours, progressing as tolerated. Gastrectomy patients will be limited by the size of the remaining stomach as well.
- A protein-rich food should be consumed with each meal. Foods such as eggs, cheese, dried beans or peas, tender meat or poultry, boneless fish, yogurt, peanut butter, nuts, tofu, and cottage cheese are good choices.
- Lactose intolerance is common in patients with these conditions; use less milk or omit if needed. Monitor calcium intake carefully.
- Use a moderate fat intake (about one third of energy intake). If needed, medium-chain triglycerides may be beneficial with fat maldigestion, and pancreatic enzymes may also be needed in some cases.
- The diet should also provide adequate chromium, vitamin B_{12}, riboflavin, iron, folacin, calcium, and vitamin D. A liquid multivitamin-mineral supplement may be needed.
- If weight loss becomes a problem, a liquid supplemental beverage may be useful between meals and can be sipped throughout the day and evening.
- Diet should provide a moderate sodium intake; excess salt draws fluid into the duodenum. If there is diarrhea, losses of sodium in the stool may occur.
- Fluids should be taken 1 hour before or after meals, rather than with meals; assure adequate fluid intake overall.
- Sit upright while eating. Encourage slow eating and adequate chewing for all meals and snacks.
- Diet should provide frequent, small meals. Avoid extremes in food temperature.

CLINICAL INDICATORS

Clinical/History	Lab Work	
Height	H & H	BUN
Weight	Serum Fe	Alb, transthyretin
BMI	Serum ferritin	Retinol-binding protein (RBP)
Diet history	Gluc	Serum amylase
BP	Chol, Trig	Transferrin
Temperature, fever	PT or INR	Serum B_{12}
Electrogastrogram (EGG)	$Na+$, $K+$, $Cl-$	$Ca++$, $Mg++$
Dual-energy x-ray absorptiometry (DEXA) scan (over time)	Glucose tolerance test (GTT)	Serum folate
	Blood guaiac	TIBC
	Urine acetone	
	White blood cell count (WBC)	

Common Drugs Used and Potential Side Effects

- Antibiotics may be used to control bacterial overgrowth.
- Antidiarrheals such as Kaopectate and loperamide may be useful. Dry mouth, nausea, vomiting, and bloating may occur. Use plenty of fluids.
- For reactive hypoglycemia, use of an alpha-glucosidase inhibitor, acarbose, may be beneficial. GI side effects are common.
- Pancreatic enzymes may be useful; the usual dose provides 2–3 capsules with meals.
- If vitamin B_{12} deficiency occurs, shots may be needed.
- If bone density loss occurs, the use of calcium, vitamin D, or bisphosphonates may be prescribed, and these should be taken as directed.

Herbs, Botanicals, and Supplements

- Herbs and botanical supplements should not be used without discussing with the physician.

INTERVENTION: NUTRITION EDUCATION, COUNSELING, CARE MANAGEMENT

- Stress the importance of self-care and optimal functioning—what to do for illness, episodes of vomiting, eating away from home, and how to read labels for carbohydrate (CHO) content.
- Discuss the use of artificial sweeteners.
- Instruct the patient to eat slowly in an upright position and to remain upright for awhile after meals.
- Help the patient to overcome reluctance and the fear of eating. Discuss the dumping syndrome and its effects on nutrient absorption if untreated.

For More Information

- Gastrectomy
  http://www.shands.org/health/surgeries/100022.html#

- Vagotomy
http://www.healthatoz.com/healthatoz/Atoz/ency/vagotomy.jsp

GASTRECTOMY AND VAGOTOMY—CITED REFERENCES

Mistiaen W, et al. Gastric emptying rate for solid and for liquid test meals in patients with dyspeptic symptoms after partial gastrectomy and after vagotomy followed by partial gastrectomy. *Hepatogastroenterology* 48:299, 2001.
Mochiki E, et al. Laparoscopic assisted distal gastrectomy for early gastric cancer: Five years' experience. *Surgery* 137:317, 2005.

GASTRITIS AND GASTROENTERITIS

NUTRITIONAL ACUITY RANKING: LEVEL 3

DEFINITIONS AND BACKGROUND

Gastritis involves inflammation of the stomach. Types of gastritis include bacterial (from *Helicobacter pylori*), autoimmune gastritis with pernicious anemia, erosive gastritis (from aspirin or NSAID use), alcohol-induced gastritis, hypertrophic gastritis, granulomatous gastritis, and atrophic gastritis. See Figure 7-3.

The treatment of gastritis will depend on its cause; reduction of stomach acid by medication is often most helpful. **Hemorrhagic gastritis** may result from chronic intake of alcohol or medications, Crohn's disease, human immunodeficiency virus (HIV) infection, or other causes.

Atrophic gastritis is chronic inflammation of the gastric mucosa without erosion but with hypochlorhydria or achlorhydria; it is important to monitor vitamin B_{12}, calcium, and ferric iron intake. People who get their vitamin B_{12} from dairy products, fortified cereals, and supplements are better protected than those who eat mostly meats.

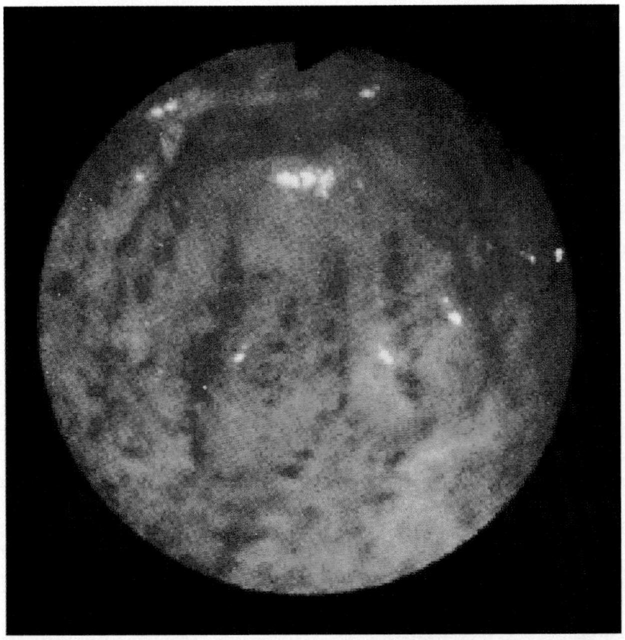

Figure 7-3 Gastritis. (From Porth C. *Pathophysiology: concepts of altered health states*. 5th ed. Philadelphia: Lippincott Williams & Wilkins, 1998.)

Gastroenteritis is an inflammation of the stomach and intestinal lining. Eating chemical toxins in food (such as seafood, mushrooms, arsenic, and lead), drinking excessive alcohol, food allergies, foodborne illness, intestinal viruses, cathartics, and other drugs can cause gastroenteritis. Norovirus infection is associated with approximately 90% of nonbacterial acute gastroenteritis (Sala et al, 2005). Gastroenteritis produces malaise, nausea, vomiting, intestinal rumbles, diarrhea with or without blood and mucus, and sometimes fever and prostration. In the past century, more than 79% of gastroenteritis cases caused by contaminated shellfish were due to an unknown agent; raw oysters are a major contributor (Graczyk and Schwab, 2000).

Hemorrhagic colitis may result from eating undercooked beef or drinking unpasteurized milk. *Escherichia coli* O157:H7 is the causative agent and may cause diarrhea for 1–8 days, slight fever; 5% of patients develop hemolytic-uremic syndrome, seizures, and strokes and may even die. *E. coli* O157:H7 pathogenesis is linked to several potential virulent factors such as Shiga-like toxins (LeBlanc, 2003). In this century, with the globalization of sushi, other raw fish may contribute to this problem.

INTERVENTION: OBJECTIVES

- Prevent or correct dehydration, shock, hypokalemia, and hyponatremia. If hemorrhage occurs, it is a medical emergency.
- Allow the stomach and GI tract to rest, but relieve thirst with water and tolerated fluids.
- Empty stomach to permit mucous lining to heal.
- Omit lactose if not tolerated during bouts of gastroenteritis.

INTERVENTION: FOOD AND NUTRITION

- **Gastritis:** Omit foods that are poorly tolerated. Provide adequate hydration. If chronic, mucosal atrophy can lead to nutritional deficits (e.g., pernicious anemia, achlorhydria). Alter diet accordingly.

- **Acute gastroenteritis:** Patient will be NPO or on partial parenteral nutrition (PPN) for the first 24–48 hours to rest stomach. Use crushed ice to relieve thirst. Oral rehydration therapy may be useful. Progress to a soft diet, if desired. Alcohol is prohibited. Omit lactose if needed. Gradually add fiber-containing foods as tolerance improves. Rehydration solutions may be effective.
- **Chronic gastroenteritis:** Use small, frequent feedings of easily tolerated foods. Progress with larger amounts and greater variety of foods, as tolerated. Restrict fat intake, which depresses food motility, and alcohol intake. Monitor lactose intolerance. Add fiber-containing foods as tolerated.

CLINICAL INDICATORS

Clinical/History		
Height	Upper GI endoscopy	Ferritin
Weight	Gastric biopsy	Folate
BMI	Blood in stool?	Serum B_{12}
Diet history		Gluc
I & O	**Lab Work**	Alb, transthyretin
Esophageal manometry	Na+, K+, Cl−	Ca++, Mg++
Barium swallow study	H & H	Hydrogen breath test
	Serum Fe	BUN
	MCV	

Common Drugs Used and Potential Side Effects

- Antacids: Watch for constipation caused by aluminum and calcium agents. Watch for diarrhea caused by magnesium agents.
- Antibiotics are used for infection. If used in excess over a long period of time, they may cause or aggravate gastroenteritis. Monitor carefully and suggest use of probiotics such as yogurt with active cultures.
- Sucralfate may be useful. Take separately from calcium or magnesium supplements by 30 minutes. Constipation may occur.
- Early postoperative medication with a proton pump inhibitor was shown to be effective in preventing gastritis after open heart surgery (Hata et al, 2005). Lansoprazole (Prevacid), omeprazole (Prilosec), and esomeprazole (Nexium) are commonly used.
- Eliminate use of aspirin and other agents that may aggravate gastritis.

Herbs, Botanicals, and Supplements

- Herbs and botanical supplements should not be used without discussing with the physician. Products such as ginger and ginger ale may alleviate some nausea.
- A potential new probiotic from a Polynesian traditional food is poi, a starchy paste made from taro plants (Brown et al, 2005). Green bananas or plantains, which are boiled and eaten in the Caribbean and South America as starches in a meal, can also fulfill this role (Phillips et al, 1995).

INTERVENTION: NUTRITION EDUCATION, COUNSELING, CARE MANAGEMENT

- Omit offenders in chronic conditions: alcohol, caffeine, and aspirin.
- Patients with chronic gastritis should be assessed for folate and vitamin B_{12} status. Atrophy of the stomach and intestinal lining interferes with folate and vitamin B_{12} absorption.
- Discuss calcium and riboflavin sources if dairy products must be omitted.
- Discuss the role of fiber in achieving or maintaining bowel integrity.
- Discuss foodborne illness and its prevention (e.g., avoiding raw shellfish).
- Oral rehydration therapy (ORT) is recommended as first-line therapy for both mildly and moderately dehydrated children with gastroenteritis (Spandorfer et al, 2005).

Patient Education—Foodborne Illness

- Careful food handling will be important. To prevent gastroenteritis, cook all foods to proper temperatures; wash all produce before cutting or eating; use careful hand washing. See Section 2.

For More Information

- Gastritis
  http://www.gicare.com/pated/ecdgs46.htm
  http://www.mayoclinic.com/invoke.cfm?id=DS00488
- Gastroenteritis
  http://www.cdc.gov/ncidod/dvrd/revb/gastro/faq.htm

GASTRITIS AND GASTROENTERITIS—CITED REFERENCES

Brown AC, et al. A non-dairy probiotic's (poi) influence on changing the gastrointestinal tract's microflora environment. *Altern Ther Health Med.* 11:58, 2005.

Graczyk T, Schwab K. Foodborne infections vectored by molluscan shellfish. *Curr Gastroenterol Rep.* 2:305, 2000.

Hata M, et al. Prospective randomized trial for optimal prophylactic treatment of the upper gastrointestinal complications after open heart surgery. *Circ J.* 69:331, 2005.

LeBlanc JJ. Implication of virulence factors in *Escherichia coil* O157:H7 pathogenesis. *Crit Rev Microbiol.* 29:277, 2003.

Phillips J, et al. Effect of resistant starch on fecal bulk and fermentation-dependent events in humans. *Am J Clin Nutr.* 62:121, 1995.

Sala MR, et al. An outbreak of food poisoning due to a genogroup I norovirus. *Epidemiol Infect.* 133:187, 2005.

Spandorfer PR, et al. Oral versus intravenous rehydration of moderately dehydrated children: a randomized, controlled trial. *Pediatrics* 115:295, 2005.

GASTROPARESIS AND GASTRIC RETENTION

NUTRITIONAL ACUITY RANKING: LEVEL 2–3

DEFINITIONS AND BACKGROUND

Gastric retention is caused by partial obstruction at the outlet of the stomach into the small bowel. **Gastroparesis** is a condition in which stomach emptying is prolonged because the nerves are damaged or have stopped working. Gastric retention or gastroparesis may result from diabetes, vagal autonomic neuropathy, scleroderma, Parkinson's disease, hypothyroidism, postviral syndromes, surgery on the stomach or the vagus nerve, prolonged hyperglycemia, or vascular insufficiencies. Vagal function and regulation of ghrelin levels are impaired in diabetic gastroparesis (Gaddipati et al, 2006). Ghrelin is produced by enteroendocrine cells in the gastric mucosa and increases gastric emptying in patients with gastroparesis (Levin et al, 2006).

Gastroparesis is often a complication of end-stage liver disease; portal hypertension interferes with the neuromuscular functions of the stomach (Ramkumar and Schultze, 2003). In addition, idiopathic gastroparesis is characterized by severely delayed gastric emptying of solids without obvious underlying organic cause (Karamanolis et al, 2006).

Signs and symptoms of gastroparesis include heartburn, nausea, abdominal pain, vomiting, early satiety, weight loss, belching, bloating, gastroesophageal reflux, and constipation. Complications from gastroparesis include ketoacidosis, infection, and bezoar formation (Feigenbaum, 2006). Bezoars allow formation of food into solid masses that further obstruct the flow from the stomach to the small intestine.

Phases of normal digestion include: phase I (45–60 minutes of inactivity); phase II (30–45 minutes of intermittent peristaltic contractions); phase III (10 minutes of intense, regular contractions); and phase IV (brief transition between cycles). With gastroparesis, any of these phases may be prolonged.

Treatment of gastroparesis may include clonidine, sildenafil, and intrapyloric botulinum toxin (Ramkumar and Schultze, 2003). A new treatment option is gastric electrical stimulation (GES) with an implantable device (Monnikes and van der Voort, 2006).

INTERVENTION: OBJECTIVES

- Decrease volume of meals served. Use liquids or foods that liquefy at body temperature so they are able to pass by a partial obstruction before or during digestion. Bypass or correct obstruction or other causes of retention.
- If diabetes is also a problem, manage blood glucose levels to ensure that control is maintained. Differentiate from ketoacidosis, which has similar symptoms of nausea and vomiting.
- Correct dehydration and electrolyte abnormalities.
- Reduce or control pain, diarrhea, and constipation.
- Ensure adequate intake of diet as prescribed to prevent weight loss and control malnutrition.
- Prevent or correct bezoar formation of indigestible solids.
- Pernicious vomiting may occur; distinguish from bulimia.
- Monitor use of, or avoid where possible, medications that cause gastric stasis (see Common Drugs Used and Potential Side Effects).

INTERVENTION: FOOD AND NUTRITION

- A soft-to-liquid diet lower in fat may be useful to prevent delay in gastric emptying. Isotonic liquids empty more quickly than hypertonic liquids. Six small meals may be better tolerated than large meals.
- Calculate protein and energy requirements according to underlying medical condition(s).
- Alter fiber intake according to needs (more to alleviate diarrhea, constipation; less with a history of bezoar formation).
- If patient complains of dry mouth, add extra fluids and moisten foods with broth or allowed sauces or gravies.
- For patients with a lesser obstruction of the stomach, progress to a mechanical soft diet. For patients with greater obstruction of the stomach, use a low-fiber diet or tube feed, checking residuals frequently.
- For persistent problems, a jejunostomy tube feeding may be indicated. It can be used temporarily if needed to correct malnutrition. Consider if there is a history of significant weight loss, cyclical nausea and vomiting, or repeated hospitalizations for gastroparesis.
- Ensure that the patient sits upright during meals.

CLINICAL INDICATORS

Clinical/History

Height
Weight
Weight changes
BMI
Diet history
I & O
Gastric x-rays–EGG
Changes in appetite
Heartburn
Abdominal pain or nausea after eating
Early satiety
Gastric emptying test with slow emptying of liquids and/or solids

Lab Work

H & H
BUN, Creat
Alb, transthyretin
CRP
Gluc (poorly controlled, over 200 mg/dL)
Gastrin
Ghrelin levels
Na+, K+, Cl−
Ca++, Mg++
Serum B_{12}

Common Drugs Used and Potential Side Effects

- Ghrelin receptor agonists may be developed in the future to have a role as prokinetic agents (Levin et al, 2006).
- If there is hyperglycemia, oral agents and insulin may be needed.
- Metoclopramide (Reglan) may be given 30 minutes before meals to increase gastric contractions and to relax pyloric sphincter. Dry mouth, sleepiness, anxiety, and nausea can be side effects. Monitor for nausea.
- Medications that may cause or aggravate gastric emptying include: alcohol, antacids containing aluminum, anticholinergics, calcitonin, calcium channel blockers, glucagon, interleukin-1, levodopa, lithium, octreotide, narcotics, nicotine, potassium salts, progesterone, sucralfate, tricyclic antidepressants, selective serotonin reuptake inhibitors (SSRIs) including Celexa, Paxil, Prozac, and Zoloft.
- Botulinum toxin has gained widespread acceptance as a treatment option, but more studies are needed (Vittal and Pasricha, 2006).

Herbs, Botanicals, and Supplements

- Herbs and botanical supplements should not be used without discussing with the physician. Products such as ginger and ginger ale may alleviate some nausea. Use of herbal remedies is common in the Hispanic population; dyspepsia is a common reason for herb use (Dole et al, 2000).
- In Japan, Gorei-san (TJ-17) is composed of five herbs (*Alismatis rhizoma, Atractylodes lanceae rhizoma, Polyporus, Hoelen*, and *Cinnamomi cortex*) and is an herbal medicine that has been used to treat nausea, dry mouth, edema, headache, and dizziness (Yamada et al, 2003).
- *Cuminum cyminum* is widely used in Ayurvedic medicine for the treatment of dyspepsia, diarrhea, and jaundice (Dhandapani et al, 2002). More trials are needed.

INTERVENTION: NUTRITION EDUCATION, COUNSELING, CARE MANAGEMENT

- Help the patient determine a specific dietary regimen.
- Discuss methods for liquefying foods as needed.
- Bezoar formation may occur after eating oranges, coconuts, green beans, apples, figs, potato skins, Brussels sprouts, broccoli, and sauerkraut.

For More Information

- Association of Gastrointestinal Motility Disorders, Inc.
  http://www.agmd-gimotility.org
- Cyclic Vomiting Association
  http://www.cvsaonline.org
- GastroLab
  http://www.gastrolab.net/lc1.htm
- Gastroparesis and Dysmotilities Association
  http://gpda.net
- International Foundation for Functional Gastrointestinal Disorders
  http://www.iffgd.org

GASTROPARESIS AND GASTRIC RETENTION—CITED REFERENCES

Dhandapani S, et al. Hypolipidemic effect of *Cuminum cyminum* L. on alloxan-induced diabetic rats. *Pharmacol Res.* 46:251, 2002.

Dole EJ, et al. The influence of ethnicity on use of herbal remedies in elderly Hispanics and non-Hispanic whites. *J Am Pharm Assoc (Wash).* 40:359, 2000.

Feigenbaum K. Update on gastroparesis. *Gastroenterol Nurs.* 29:239, 2006.

Gaddipati KV, et al. Abnormal ghrelin and pancreatic polypeptide responses in gastroparesis. *Dig Dis Sci.* 51:1339, 2006.

Karamanolis G, et al. Determinants of symptom pattern in idiopathic severely delayed gastric emptying: gastric emptying rate of proximal stomach dysfunction. *Gut* 2006. In press.

Levin F, et al. Ghrelin stimulates gastric emptying and hunger in normal weight humans. *J Clin Endocrinol Metab.* 2006. In press.

Monnikes H, van der Voort IR. Gastric electrical stimulation in gastroparesis: where do we stand? *Dig Dis.* 24:260, 2006.

Ramkumar D, Schultze KS. Gastroduodenal motility. *Curr Opin Gastroenterol.* 19:540, 2003.

Vittal H, Pasricha PF. Botulinum toxin for gastrointestinal disorders: therapy and mechanisms. *Neurotox Res.* 9:149, 2006.

Yamada K, et al. Effectiveness of Gorei-san (TJ-17) for treatment of SSRI-induced nausea and dyspepsia: preliminary observations. *Clin Neuropharmacol.* 26:112, 2003.

GIANT HYPERTROPHIC GASTRITIS AND MÉNÉTRIER'S DISEASE

NUTRITIONAL ACUITY RANKING: LEVEL 3

DEFINITIONS AND BACKGROUND

Giant hypertrophic gastritis (GHG) is a pathological condition with increased loss of plasma proteins, resulting in hydrolysis by the proteolytic enzymes of the gut. The hydrolyzed proteins are then reabsorbed as amino acids. Ascites or edema may occur if the liver cannot produce sufficient albumin rapidly enough. The condition may precede stomach cancer. The disease is rare and diagnosed in patients with giant gastric folds, dyspeptic symptoms, and hypoalbuminemia due to gastrointestinal protein loss. Protein-losing gastropathy with hypertrophic gastric folds (PLGH) may occur with acute infection with cytomegalovirus (Suter et al, 2000).

Ménétrier's disease is classified as a form of hyperplastic gastropathy and not really a form of gastritis because inflammation is minimal; GHG and Ménétrier's disease may be variants of the same disorder (National Organization for Rare Disorders, 2005). Ménétrier's disease is often associated with *Helicobacter pylori* infection (Yoshimura et al, 2003). Complete normalization of the gastric mucosa and gastrointestinal protein loss follows eradication therapy (Madsen et al, 2000). Gastric resection is one way to achieve permanent relief where *H. pylori* bacteria are not found.

INTERVENTION: OBJECTIVES

- Replace protein; maintain adequate nitrogen balance.
- Reduce edema.
- Spare protein for tissue synthesis and repair.
- Promote normal dietary intake with a return to wellness. Delay or prevent onset of stomach cancer if possible.
- Gastric juice ascorbic acid is lower in individuals with *H. pylori* infections (Fraser and Woollard, 1999); increase intake.

INTERVENTION: FOOD AND NUTRITION

- Use a high-protein/high-calorie diet. The protein level should be approximately 20% total kcal unless contraindicated for renal or hepatic problems.
- Omit any food intolerances.
- Include adequate sources of vitamin C in the diet; a supplement may be warranted.

CLINICAL INDICATORS

Clinical/History		
Height	Generalized edema	Ca++, Mg++
Weight	**Lab Work**	Nitrogen (N) balance
BMI	Alb, transthyretin	Transferrin
Diet history	RBP	Pepsin levels
Weight changes	Globulin	H & H
Gastroscopy	A:G ratio	Serum Fe
Gastric biopsy	CRP	Serum folate
Abdominal ultrasound	Gluc	Serum B_{12}
Fecal occult blood test	Na+, K+	BUN, Creat

Common Drugs Used and Potential Side Effects

- Treatment with a monoclonal antibody against epidermal growth factor receptors can reduce the frequency of nausea and vomiting, improve serum albumin concentration, and improve abnormalities of the stomach. More studies are being conducted.
- For eradication of *H. pylori*, 2 weeks of treatment with an acid-suppressing drug (one time daily), Pepto-Bismol (four times daily), and antibiotics (3–4 times daily) are prescribed. This therapy often must be used more than once. Other combinations may include the antibiotics omeprazole, clarithromycin, and ranitidine bismuth (Tritec).
- Lansoprazole (Prevacid), omeprazole (Prilosec), and esomeprazole (Nexium) may be prescribed.

Herbs, Botanicals, and Supplements

- Herbs and botanical supplements should not be used without discussing with the physician.

INTERVENTION: NUTRITION EDUCATION, COUNSELING, CARE MANAGEMENT

- Elimination of aggravating foods specific to the patient is warranted.
- Teach the patient about use of high–biological value (HBV) proteins to replenish serum protein levels.
- During recovery, the use of probiotics such as yogurt with active cultures may be helpful.

For More Information

- Hypertrophic Gastritis
http://www.medterms.com/script/main/art.asp?articlekey=30848

GIANT HYPERTROPHIC GASTRITIS AND MÉNÉTRIER'S DISEASE—CITED REFERENCES

Fraser A, Woollard G. Gastric juice ascorbic acid is related to *Helicobacter pylori* infection but not ethnicity. *J Gastroenterol Hepatol.* 14:1070, 1999.

Madsen L, et al. Menetrier's disease. Another *Helicobacter pylori* associated disease. *Ugeskr Laeger.* 162:4250, 2000.

National Organization of Rare Diseases. Gastritis, giant hypertrophic. Accessed March 5, 2005 at http://www.rarediseases.org/search/rdbdetail_abstract.html?disname=Gastritis%2C+Giant+Hypertrophic.

Suter W, et al. Cytomegalovirus-induced transient protein-losing hypertrophic gastropathy in an immunocompetent adult. *Digestion.* 62:276, 2000.

Yoshimura M, et al. Remission of severe anemia persisting for over 20 years after eradication of *Helicobacter pylori* in cases of Ménétrier's disease and atrophic gastritis: *Helicobacter pylori* as a pathogenic factor in iron-deficiency anemia. *Intern Med.* 42:971, 2003.

PEPTIC ULCER DISEASE

NUTRITIONAL ACUITY RANKING: LEVEL 2

DEFINITIONS AND BACKGROUND

A peptic ulcer is an area of the GI tract that is eroded by gastric acid and pepsin, leaving exposed nerves. Peptic ulcer disease, however complicated, involves perforation and damage to adjacent viscera. Signs and symptoms of a peptic ulcer may include burning or gnawing pain that improves after eating but returns later, nausea, vomiting, frequent bloating, weight and appetite changes, black or tarry stools, and sharp and sudden abdominal pain.

Fifteen percent of peptic ulcers are gastric (often later correlated with stomach cancer), and 85% are duodenal, usually in the first 25–30 cm. *Helicobacter pylori* bacteria play a role in the etiology of most ulcers. One out of 10 Americans suffers from peptic ulcer disease. While the main cause of duodenal ulcer is *H. pylori,* only 20% of *H. pylori*–infected people develop an ulcer. Poor hand washing (as per fecal–oral route) may be another concern; *H. pylori* can be transmitted from person to person through close contact and exposure to vomit. See Figure 7-4.

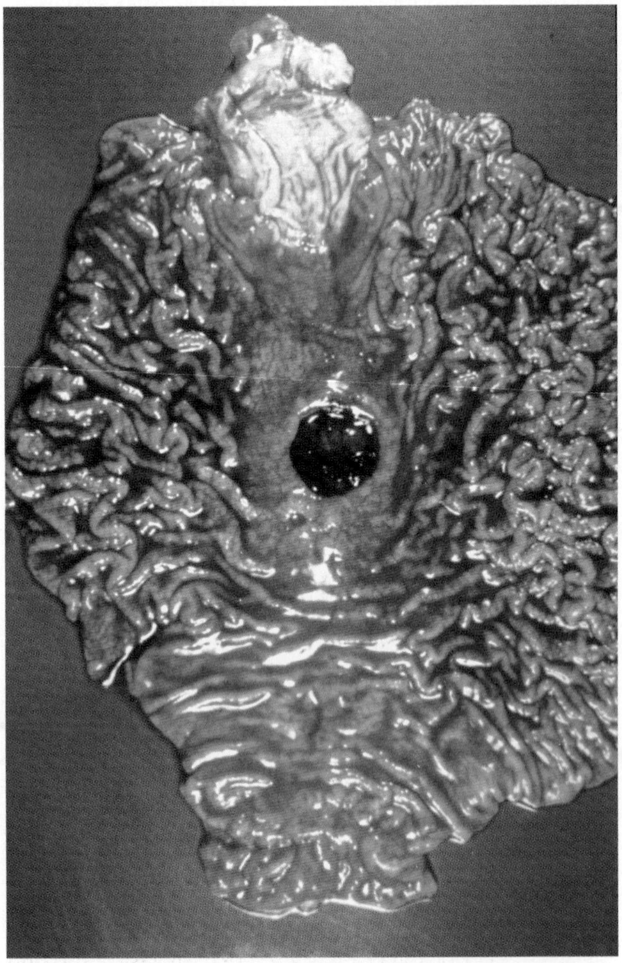

Figure 7-4 Peptic ulcer disease. (From Rubin E, Farber JL. *Pathology.* 3rd ed. Philadelphia: Lippincott Williams & Wilkins, 1999.)

Diets and stress are not specific causative factors. No evidence exists that bland diets affect the healing of an ulcer or cause a decrease in gastric acid secretion. Vitamin B_{12} tends to be lower in patients who have peptic ulcers; anemias may result. Monitor for vitamin B_{12} deficiency where *H. pylori* have been found.

Drug therapy is most effective in preventing ulcer recurrence and primarily consists of antibiotics and antacids. The decline in duodenal ulcer disease and the established relation of peptic ulcer to *H. pylori* have eliminated the need for elective ulcer surgery (von Holstein, 2000). Peptic ulcer disease is declining in prevalence but increasing in virulence, perhaps because of the overall aging of the population (Louw and Marks, 2004). Studies are under way to create a vaccine to prevent *H. pylori* infection.

INTERVENTION: OBJECTIVES

- Eradicate any *H. pylori* infection.
- Take medications as directed. Rest during healing stages.
- Reduce pain. Avoid distention from large meals.
- Dilute stomach contents and provide buffering action.
- Correct anemia, if present. Vitamin B_{12} deficiency is often corrected after effective *H. pylori* treatment.
- Monitor steatorrhea, bone disease, dumping syndrome, and other complications such as perforation and obstruction.

INTERVENTION: FOOD AND NUTRITION

- Use small feedings, frequently if preferred. Include some high-protein foods and vitamin C to speed healing.
- Avoid personal intolerances. Citrus juices may cause pain during exacerbations.
- Use fewer saturated fats and more polyunsaturated fats if increased lipid levels are found. Arachidonic acid metabolites may play a role in peptic ulcer disease.
- Limit gastric stimulants if not tolerated, such as caffeine, alcohol, peppermint, black pepper, garlic, cloves, and chili powder (a "liberal bland" diet). If a particular food bothers an individual, it should be avoided. See Table 7-7 regarding caffeine in beverages and medications.

TABLE 7-7 Typical Caffeine Content of Beverages and Medications

Beverages/Medications	Caffeine (mg)
5 oz coffee, brewed	65–120 (average, 85)
5 oz coffee, instant	60–85 (average, 75)
8 oz Starbucks Coffee Frappucino	83
1 oz espresso coffee	30–50 (average, 40)
5 oz decaffeinated coffee	2–4
5 oz black tea, brewed (most U.S. brands)	20–50
5 oz black tea, brewed (imported)	25–60
6 oz tea, instant	28–30
12 oz cola drinks	36–47
8 oz Ovaltine	0
12 oz Mountain Dew	54
8 oz cocoa beverage	3–32 (average, 6)
8 oz chocolate milk	2–7 (average, 5)
4 oz coffee ice cream	28
1 oz milk chocolate	1–15 (average, 6)
1 oz dark chocolate	5–35 (average, 20)
1 oz baker's chocolate	26
1 oz chocolate syrup	4
1 tablet cold preparation	30
1 tablet analgesic	30–66
12 oz 7-Up or Sprite	0

Data from Leonard T, et al. The effects of caffeine on various body systems: a review. *J Am Diet Assoc.* 87:1048, 1987; and the International Food Information Council.

CLINICAL INDICATORS

Clinical/History

- Height
- Weight
- BMI
- Diet history
- GI bleeding?
- Stool test for *H. pylori*
- Endoscopy
- Chronic idiopathic urticaria or atopic dermatitis

Lab Work

- Red blood cell count (RBC)
- Blood test for *H. pylori* (anti-*H. pylori* immunoglobulin G antibody titer)
- C-Urea breath test for *H. pylori*
- Chol, Trig
- BUN, Creat
- Alb, transthyretin
- Alanine aminotransferase (ALT), aspartate aminotransferase (AST)
- Blood guaiac
- Amylase (if ulcer is perforated, this is increased)
- H & H
- Serum Fe
- Serum folate
- PT or INR
- Transferrin
- Ca++, Mg++
- Serum B_{12}
- Alk phos (increased)
- TIBC
- Na+, K+, Cl−
- Serum gastrin (increased)
- Ca++, Mg++

SAMPLE NUTRITION DIAGNOSTIC STATEMENT

Peptic Ulcer Disease

PES: Undesirable food choices related to not ready for diet/lifestyle change as evidenced by alcohol intake (beer and wine, 10 drinks per week) and complaints of abdominal discomfort/pain.

Assessment: Food diary.

Intervention: Teach and counsel about role of alcohol in GI mucosal damage.

Monitoring and Evaluation: Report of decreased alcohol consumption and less GI discomfort and pain.

Common Drugs Used and Potential Side Effects (see Table 7-8)

- Analgesics and corticosteroids, when taken over a long time, may cause GI bleeding and ulceration and should be taken with food.
- High doses of Advil or Motrin (ibuprofen), even for a few days, can significantly increase the risk of GI bleeding. A combination of aspirin and the proton pump inhibitor esomeprazole (Nexium) may actually prevent recurrent ulcer bleeding. However, aspirin may exacerbate GI bleeding especially in those taking it on a regular basis as prophylaxis
- For eradication of *H. pylori*, 2 weeks of treatment with an acid-suppressing drug (one time daily), Pepto-Bismol (four times daily), and antibiotics (3–4 times daily) are prescribed. A 1- to 2-week course of *H. pylori* eradication therapy is an effective treatment (Ford et al, 2006); triple therapy often must be used more than once. Quadruple therapy is also being tested (Feng et al, 2005). Some FDA-approved combinations include the antibiotics omeprazole, clarithromycin, and ranitidine bismuth (Tritec). Other antibiotics include amoxicillin, metronidazole, and tetracycline. Suggest use of probiotics, such as yogurt with active cultures, with antibiotic therapy.

Herbs, Botanicals, and Supplements

- Herbs and botanical supplements should not be used without discussing with the physician.
- Ginger may be used as an antinauseant. Do not use large doses with warfarin, aspirin, or other antiplatelet drugs, antihypertensive drugs, and hypoglycemic drugs. Additive effects can cause unpredictable changes in blood pressure and decreases in blood glucose levels and may decrease platelet aggregation and thus increase bleeding. Ginger ale is commonly used with few side effects.
- Licorice root may be recommended for gastric and duodenal ulcers. Do not take with digoxin, because it may cause potassium loss and digoxin toxicity. Licorice root

TABLE 7-8 Medications Used in Peptic Ulcer Disease

Medication Type	Description	Specific Drugs
Antacids	Aluminum-containing and magnesium-containing antacids can be helpful in relieving symptoms of gastritis by neutralizing gastric acids. These agents are inexpensive and safe. Aluminum ions inhibit smooth muscle contraction, thus inhibiting gastric emptying. Use aluminum-containing antacids cautiously with upper GI hemorrhage. Magnesium and aluminum antacid mixtures are used to avoid bowel function changes.	Gaviscon contains magnesium as well as aluminum and may decrease absorption of thiamine, phosphate, and vitamin A. Gelusil contains magnesium, aluminum, and simethicone; it may have side effects similar to those of Gaviscon. Mylanta and Amphogel (aluminum hydroxide) may cause nausea, vomiting, and lowered vitamin A, calcium, and phosphate absorption. Take between meals, followed by water. Milk of magnesia (magnesium hydroxide) is a laxative–antacid and can deplete phosphorus and calcium over time. Magaldrate (Riopan) decreases serum vitamin A but can be used on a low-sodium diet.
H_2-receptor antagonists	These drugs inhibit the action of histamine on the parietal cell, which inhibits acid secretion. The drugs in this class are all equally effective and are available over the counter in half prescription strength for heartburn treatment. Histamine H_2 blockers should be taken with food. Since acid secretion and ulcer pain are most prevalent at night, taking Zantac or Tagamet before bed may be helpful. These drugs can elevate AST/ALT and creatinine, cause confusion in elderly individuals, and cause diarrhea, constipation, or urticaria.	Cimetidine (Tagamet) inhibits histamine at H_2receptors of the gastric parietal cells, resulting in reduced gastric acid secretion, gastric volume, and hydrogen ion concentrations. Famotidine (Pepcid) competitively inhibits histamine at the H_2 receptor of the gastric parietal cells, resulting in reduced gastric acid secretion, gastric volume, and reduced hydrogen concentrations. Nizatidine (Axid) competitively inhibits histamine at H_2 receptors of gastric parietal cells, resulting in reduced gastric acid secretion, gastric volume, and reduced hydrogen concentrations. Ranitidine (Zantac) competitively inhibits histamine at the H_2 receptors of gastric parietal cells, resulting in reduced gastric acid secretion, gastric volume, and hydrogen concentrations. Ranitidine can cause nausea, constipation, and vitamin B_{12} malabsorption; may alter serum levels of serum iron.
Proton pump inhibitors (PPIs)	PPIs bind to the proton pump of parietal cell, inhibiting secretion of hydrogen ions into gastric lumen. PPIs relieve pain and heal peptic ulcers more rapidly than H_2 antagonists do. Drugs in this class are equally effective. All PPIs decrease serum concentrations of drugs that require gastric acidity for absorption, such as ketoconazole or itraconazole. PPIs are used for up to 4 weeks to treat and relieve symptoms of active duodenal ulcers. Physicians may prescribe for up to 8 weeks to treat all grades of erosive esophagitis.	Lansoprazole (Prevacid) decreases gastric acid secretion by inhibiting the parietal cell $H+/K+$ ATP pump. Omeprazole (Prilosec) decreases gastric acid secretion by inhibiting the parietal cell $H+/K+$ ATP pump. Omeprazole will soon go off patent and be available as a generic. Esomeprazole (Nexium) is the S-isomer of omeprazole. It decreases gastric acid secretion by inhibiting the parietal cell $H+/K+$ ATP pump. May increase absorption of digoxin; may decrease absorption of iron. Rabeprazole (Aciphex) decreases gastric acid secretion by inhibiting the parietal cell $H+/K+$ ATP pump. It is used for short-term (4–8 weeks) treatment and symptomatic relief of gastritis. Pantoprazole (Protonix) decreases gastric acid secretion by inhibiting the parietal cell $H+/K+$ ATP pump. It is used for short-term (4–8 weeks) treatment and symptomatic relief of gastritis.
Gastrointestinal agents	These agents are effective in the treatment of peptic ulcers and in preventing relapse. Their mechanism of action is not clear. Multiple doses are required, and they are not as effective as the other options.	Sucralfate (Carafate) binds with positively charged proteins in exudates and forms a viscous adhesive substance that protects the GI lining against pepsin, peptic acid, and bile salts. Used for short-term management of ulcers. Sucralfate may cause constipation as one side effect.
Stomach acid protector	Bismuth subsalicylate	Bismuth is a component of Pepto-Bismol and is used to protect the stomach lining from acid; it kills *Helicobacter pylori*.

Adapted from: Shayne P. Gastritis and peptic ulcer disease. Accessed February 28, 2005 at http://www.emedicine.com/emerg/topic820.htm.

may potentiate the effects of steroids, especially hydrocortisone, progesterone, and estrogens. Also avoid taking with thiazide diuretics and antihypertensive medications because of increased sodium and water retention, along with potential hypokalemia; spironolactone is especially antagonized by licorice root.

- Banana, garlic, cabbage, and yellow root have been recommended for this condition, but no clinical trials have proven efficacy.

INTERVENTION: NUTRITION EDUCATION, COUNSELING, CARE MANAGEMENT

- As needed by the individual, offer guidance about dietary alterations that may be useful.
- Discuss the need to complete treatments for eradication of *H. pylori* bacteria, where present. One treatment is usually not sufficient.
- Reduce intake of alcoholic beverages; stop smoking; and monitor any family history of ulcer disease to address it as quickly as possible.

Patient Education—Foodborne Illness

- Careful food handling will be important. Hand washing is important to reduce the spread of *H. pylori*. Always wash hands after using the bathroom and before eating.

For More Information

- American College of Gastroenterology
  http://www.acg.gi.org
- Centers for Disease Control and Prevention–Peptic Ulcer
  http://www.cdc.gov/ulcer/md.htm
- Foundation for Digestive Health
  http://www.fdhn.org/html/education/ulcer/facts.html
- Helicobacter Foundation
  http://www.helico.com/
- Medline–Peptic Ulcer
  http://www.nlm.nih.gov/medlineplus/pepticulcer.html
- National Institute of Diabetes and Digestive and Kidney Diseases (NIDDK)
  http://digestive.niddk.nih.gov/ddiseases/pubs/pepticulcers_ez/index.htm
  http://digestive.niddk.nih.gov/ddiseases/pubs/hpylori/

PEPTIC ULCER DISEASE—CITED REFERENCES

Feng LY, et al. Effects of killing *Helicobacter pylori* quadruple therapy on peptic ulcer: a randomized double-blind clinical trial. *World J Gastroenterol.* 11:1083, 2005.

Ford AC, et al. Eradication therapy for peptic ulcer disease in *Helicobacter pylori* positive patients. *Cochrane Database Syst Rev.* 2:CD003840, 2006.

Louw JA, Marks IN. Peptic ulcer disease. *Curr Opin Gastroenterol.* 20:533, 2004.

von Holstein C. Long-term prognosis after partial gastrectomy for gastroduodenal ulcer. *World J Surg.* 24:307, 2000.

VOMITING, PERNICIOUS

NUTRITIONAL ACUITY RANKING: LEVEL 3 (LONGER THAN 7 DAYS)

DEFINITIONS AND BACKGROUND

Pernicious (uncontrolled) vomiting may occur in any of several disorders, including concussion or brain trauma, meningitis or encephalitis, intestinal blockage, migraine headaches, brain tumor or other forms of cancer, foodborne illness, gastroparesis, and pregnancy (hyperemesis gravidarum, see Pregnancy entry in Section 1). Hyperemesis gravidarum involves pregnancy-induced hormonal changes associated with concurrent gastrointestinal dysmotility and possible *Helicobacter pylori* infection (Eliakim et al, 2000).

The presence of symptoms or signs such as weight loss, gastrointestinal bleeding, persistent fever, chronic severe diarrhea, and significant vomiting is associated with a higher prevalence of organic disease in children and should be carefully assessed (American Academy of Pediatrics, 2005).

The biggest immediate risk with pernicious vomiting is dehydration, where losses of water, potassium, and sodium can affect the brain, kidneys, and heart. Watch for signs such as dry mouth membranes, dry lips, sunken eyes, rapid but weak pulse, rapid breathing, cold hands and feet, and confusion and difficulty with arousal. Nutritional deficits are possible when the vomiting is prolonged.

INTERVENTION: OBJECTIVES

- Correct electrolyte and fluid imbalances.
- Eliminate oral intake until vomiting ends.
- Prevent weight loss.
- Distinguish symptoms that could be related to bulimia.
- If there is hyperglycemia or diabetes, return to normal blood glucose levels as quickly as possible; insulin may be needed.

INTERVENTION: FOOD AND NUTRITION

- For patients with an acute condition, NPO for 24 hours with intravenous glucose is common. Oral rehydration solution may be needed. (See Diarrhea entry.)
- When tolerated, gastrostomy tube feeding or jejunostomy may be warranted. An isotonic formula is desirable to reduce imbalances between solute and solvent. TPN may also be a consideration if the condition is prolonged.
- As the patient progresses to an oral diet, clear liquids such as cranberry juice or boullion may be helpful. Gradually

SAMPLE NUTRITION DIAGNOSTIC STATEMENT

Nausea and Vomiting

PES: Inadequate food and beverage intake related to intolerance to oral diet and chemotherapy treatment as evidenced by nausea and vomiting after meals and weight loss of 5 lb over past month.

Assessment Data (sources of info): Food records, I & O reports, chemotherapy schedule and frequency.

Intervention: Alter meal pattern according to chemotherapy medications and timing, review timing of fluid intake related to meals.

Monitoring and Evaluation: Food records, I & O reports, weight records, no patient complaints about nausea and vomiting after meals.

add toast, crackers, jelly, and simple carbohydrates in small, frequent meals. Give fluids between meals (a "dry diet"). Avoid acidic fruit and vegetable juices if not tolerated. Consider avoiding foods that delay gastric emptying (high-fat, hypertonic, or highly fibrous foods).

- Gradually have the patient resume a normal diet, but decrease fats if not tolerated.

CLINICAL INDICATORS

Clinical/History	Lab Work	
Height	Na+, K+, Cl−	Serum Fe
Weight	Ca++, Mg++	Serum folate
Weight changes	Alb, transthyretin	Serum B_{12}
BMI	BUN, Creat	Gastric emptying tests
Diet history	N balance	
Temperature (fever?)	Gluc	
Dehydration?	H & H	

Common Drugs Used and Potential Side Effects

- Antiemetic agents may be indicated for some conditions. Meclizine or cyclizine may be prescribed; they are antihistamines and powerful antinausea agents. Selective serotonin 5-hydroxytryptamine-3 (5-HT3) receptor antagonists have proven to be safe and effective for postoperative nausea and vomiting; these include dolasetron, granisetron, ondansetron, and tropisetron, which bind to 5-HT3 receptors, blocking serotonin binding at vagal afferents in the gut and in the regions of the CNS involved in emesis (Gan, 2005).
- Insulin or oral agents may be needed if diabetes is also present. Peristaltic agents may be used for cases of gastroparesis.
- Chronic use of cannabinoids can lead to hyperemesis (Allen et al, 2004). This includes oral use of marijuana for cancer, multiple sclerosis, and other medical conditions as well as social use.

Herbs, Botanicals, and Supplements

- Herbs and botanical supplements should not be used without discussing with the physician.
- Ginger is often used as an antinauseant. Do not use large doses with warfarin, aspirin, other antiplatelet drugs, antihypertensive drugs, and hypoglycemic drugs. Additive effects can cause unpredictable changes in blood pressure and decreases in blood glucose levels and may decrease platelet aggregation and thus increase bleeding. Ginger ale is commonly used and generally has few side effects.

INTERVENTION: NUTRITION EDUCATION, COUNSELING, CARE MANAGEMENT

- Explain why fluids should be taken between meals. Identify adequate amounts of fluids to be consumed every day
- Discuss the role of carbohydrates and fiber in maintaining blood glucose levels.
- Share the ingredients for oral rehydration solution, if it needs to be made at home. There are many suitable products available from a pharmacy as well; discuss appropriate products with the pharmacist.
- Do not force eating. Eat and drink slowly; stop when full. Make up lost calories at another time.
- Eat meals in a well-ventilated area free from odors.
- Do not lie down for 2 hours after eating. Do not overeat.

Patient Education—Food Safety

- Careful food handling and hand washing are important to prevent introduction of foodborne pathogens to the diet of the individual.

For More Information

- Nausea and Vomiting Algorithm
  http://www.uwgi.org/guidelines/ch_01/ch01txt.htm
- Pernicious Vomiting of Pregnancy
  http://www.medterms.com/script/main/art.asp?articlekey=8619

VOMITING, PERNICIOUS—CITED REFERENCES

Allen JH, et al. Cannabinoid hyperemesis: cyclical hyperemesis in association with chronic cannabis abuse. *Gut* 53:1566, 2004.

American Academy of Pediatrics. Subcommittee on Chronic Abdominal Pain; North American Society for Pediatric Gastroenterology Hepatology, and Nutrition. Chronic abdominal pain in children. *Pediatrics* 115:370, 2005.

Gan TJ. Selective serotonin 5-HT(3) receptor antagonists for postoperative nausea and vomiting: are they all the same? *CNS Drugs.* 19:225, 2005.

Eliakim R, et al. Hyperemesis gravidarum: a current review. *Am J Perinatol.* 17:207, 2000.

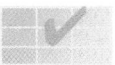

Lower GI: Intestinal Disorders

CARCINOID SYNDROME

NUTRITIONAL ACUITY RANKING: LEVEL 3

DEFINITIONS AND BACKGROUND

A rare neuroendocrine growth that develops in the wall of the intestine, carcinoid syndrome, is usually discovered in x-rays or during surgery performed for other reasons. Gastrointestinal carcinoid tumors are difficult to diagnose (Gore et al, 2005). Sometimes, the growth occurs in the appendix area. The incidence of carcinoid tumors is approximately 1.5 per 100,000 of the population (Bell et al, 2005).

The growths can become large enough to cause intestinal obstruction. Some of these growths metastasize to the liver, creating hormone-producing tumors that have signs that include flushing of the head and neck (usually triggered by alcohol or exercise). Survival ranges from 3 to 20 years.

Flushing symptoms can last for several hours. These symptoms are caused by the release of vasoactive substances, such as serotonin, histamine, and prostaglandins. The patient may have swollen and watery eyes, explosive diarrhea and abdominal cramps, wheezing as in asthma, breathlessness, and symptoms similar to heart failure.

Despite medical and therapeutic advances that have alleviated symptoms and prolonged life, a substantial subset of patients develops mesenteric and small bowel carcinoid fibrosis (Modlin et al, 2004). Cardiac valvular lesions are seen; tricuspid valvular disease is especially common, and advanced valvular involvement is associated with poor long-term survival. Liver involvement can also occur, and liver resection or transplantation may be needed (Ahlman et al, 2004; Fenwick et al, 2004).

Diversion of tryptophan to 5-hydroxytryptamine (5-HT) synthesis occurs, resulting in less tryptophan for protein and nicotinamide synthesis. Pellagra and psychiatric symptoms can occur due to a depletion of tryptophan, which is consumed by the carcinoid tumor for serotonin synthesis (van der Horst-Schrivers et al, 2004). Psychiatric symptoms should be evaluated carefully; impulse control disorders are prevalent in patients with carcinoid syndrome (Russo et al, 2004).

Severe clinical indicators are the malignant carcinoid syndrome, carcinoid heart disease, and high concentrations of the tumor markers urinary 5-hydroxyindoleacetic acid (5-HIAA) and plasma chromogranin A (Rorstad, 2005). The malignant carcinoid syndrome, which is caused by circulating neuroendocrine mediators produced by the tumor, occurs in less than 10% of patients (Bell et al, 2005).

In patients with this syndrome, surgery is combined with continuous biotherapy with long-acting somatostatin analogs and interferon, which may alleviate symptoms and cause stable disease with slow progression (Akerstrom et al, 2005). Active surgical and medical therapy of the tumor disease reduces the hormonal secretion and makes right ventricular heart failure a rare cause of death these days (Westberg et al, 2001). Because insulin-like growth factor I (IGF-I) is an autocrine regulator of carcinoid tumors, blockade of IGF-I signaling has been proposed as a therapeutic target (Van Gompel and Chen, 2004).

INTERVENTION: OBJECTIVES

- Ease symptoms of secretory diarrhea and reduce any pain.
- Slow progression of the disease, which is not curable through surgery.
- Control side effects of medications.
- Replenish electrolyte and fluid losses.
- Correct pellagra-like rash.

INTERVENTION: FOOD AND NUTRITION

- Decrease fiber intake during acute stages of diarrhea. Add pectin and ensure adequate fluid intake during those periods.
- Avoid alcoholic beverages. Limit caffeine intake to a controlled amount.
- During testing, omit foods that contain 5-HIAA. Several days of a diet free from intake of avocados, pineapple, bananas, kiwi fruit, plums, eggplant, walnuts, hickory nuts, and pecans will be needed.
- Omega-3 fatty acids may useful in this condition for their role in reduction of inflammation; include fish such as salmon, sardines, tuna, and herring often.

CLINICAL INDICATORS

Clinical/History

Height
Weight
BMI
Diet history
Wheezing
Explosive diarrhea
Number of stools, consistency
Biopsy
Endoscopy
X-rays of GI tract
Skin changes (scleroderma, pellagra)?
Psychiatric symptoms?
Magnetic resonance imaging (MRI) for carcinoid heart disease

Lab Work

Alb, transthyretin
Transferrin
5-HIAA test (urine S-HIAA)
TLC
H & H
Serum Fe
Na+, K+
Ca++, Mg++
Serum histamine
Serum serotonin

Common Drugs Used and Potential Side Effects

- The standard treatment involves subcutaneous injections of the somatostatin analog octreotide; this is expensive, and treatment may be for many years. Newer somatostatin analogs (such as lanreotide) are being tested. Other vasoconstricting, interleukin, or cytotoxic drugs may be used to control side effects.
- Kaolin (Kaopectate) and other medications may be used to control diarrhea. Constipation is a possible side effect.
- Bronchodilators may be used to control wheezing. Check the specific type of drug to evaluate potential side effects.

Herbs, Botanicals, and Supplements

- Herbs and botanical supplements should not be used without discussing with the physician.

INTERVENTION: NUTRITION EDUCATION, COUNSELING, CARE MANAGEMENT

- Discuss measures specifically designed for the patient's status and tolerance levels.
- Suggest ways to make meals more appetizing if appetite is poor.
- Describe techniques for management of diarrhea, abdominal pain, or cramping by reducing fiber and fat intake during that time.
- Probiotics such as acidophilus milk and yogurt with live cultures may be useful in the diet.

For More Information

- Carcinoid Syndrome
  http://www.oncologychannel.com/cancermalignancy/
  http://www.merck.com/mrkshared/mmanual/section2/chapter17/17b.jsp
  http://www.emedicine.com/med/topic2649.htm

CARCINOID SYNDROME—CITED REFERENCES

Ahlman H, et al. Interventional treatment of the carcinoid syndrome. *Neuroendocrinology* 80:67S, 2004.

Akerstrom G, et al. Management of midgut carcinoids. *J Surg Oncol.* 89:161, 2005.

Bell HK, et al. Cutaneous manifestations of the malignant carcinoid syndrome. *Br J Dermatol.* 152:71, 2005.

Fenwick SW, et al. Hepatic resection and transplantation for primary carcinoid tumors of the liver. *Ann Surg.* 239:210, 2004.

Gore RM et al. GI carcinoid tumours: appearance of the primary and detecting metastases. *Best Pract Res Clin Endocrinol Metab.* 19:245, 2005.

Modlin IM, et al. Carcinoid tumors and fibrosis: an association with no explanation. *Am J Gastroenterol.* 99:2466, 2004.

Rorstad O. Prognostic indicators for carcinoid neuroendocrine tumors of the gastrointestinal tract. *J Surg Oncol.* 89:151, 2005.

Russo S, et al. Patients with carcinoid syndrome exhibit symptoms of aggressive impulse dysregulation. *Psychosom Med.* 66:422, 2004.

van der Horst-Schrivers AN, et al. Complications of midgut carcinoid tumors and carcinoid syndrome. *Neuroendocrinology* 80:28S, 2004.

Van Gompel JJ, Chen H. Insulin-like growth factor 1 signaling in human gastrointestinal carcinoid tumor cells. *Surgery* 136:1297, 2004.

Westberg G, et al. Prediction of prognosis by echocardiography in patients with midgut carcinoid syndrome. *Br J Surg.* 88:865, 2001

CELIAC DISEASE

NUTRITIONAL ACUITY RANKING: LEVEL 4

DEFINITIONS AND BACKGROUND

Celiac disease is a common, lifelong, genetically based autoimmune disorder that causes inflammation of the proximal small intestine (See and Murray, 2006). It is characterized by an immune response to ingested wheat gluten and related proteins of rye and barley that leads to inflammation, villous atrophy, and crypt hyperplasia in the small intestine (Alaedini and Green, 2005). A major consensus panel determined that 1% of white populations (or upwards of 3 million people) may have celiac disease, many of whom remain undiagnosed (See and Murray, 2006; National Institutes of Health, 2004). New screening tests are demonstrating that 1 in 125–300 people may have it; patients often present as adults.

Celiac disease results from an inappropriate T-cell–mediated immune response against ingested gluten in genetically predisposed people (Farrell and Kelly, 2002). The disease is closely associated with genes that code for human leukocyte antigens DQ2 and DQ8, and transglutaminase 2 appears to be an important component of the disease (Alaedini and Green, 2005). Other names for this disorder include celiac sprue, gluten enteropathy, or nontropical sprue.

Celiac disease involves mucosal malabsorption. Intestinal villi are decreased in number, with less absorptive surface and fewer enzymes in the damaged cells; crypts are markedly elongated. Symptoms and signs include frequent, strong-smelling stools that are pale and foamy, diarrhea, irritability, a distended abdomen, easy fatigue, pallor, weight loss, vomiting, and anemia.

According to a consensus panel (Thompson, 2005), all persons with gastrointestinal (GI) symptoms should be tested for celiac disease, as should individuals with unexplained iron deficiency anemia, elevated levels of transaminases, short stature, delayed puberty, fetal loss, and infertility. Diagnosis can occur at any age (infancy through old age) and often occurs after stress, pregnancy, or viral infections. Infants may present with impaired growth, diarrhea, abdominal distention, pallor, edema, or vomiting (Farrell and Kelly, 2002). Pica and growth failure often precede diagnosis in infants or children.

A new technology, capsule endoscopy, is a useful tool for examining the lumen of the GI tract (Petroniene et al, 2005). Tissue transglutaminase is the main antigen for the antiendomysial antibodies used for diagnosis of celiac disease. False-negative test results can occur in children under age 2 years or in patients who have followed a gluten-free diet for a month or longer. Screening should occur in relatives of patients who have celiac disease, in patients with type 1 diabetes, and in patients who have unexplained anemia.

Early diagnosis is important because duration of exposure to gluten can increase the risk of other autoimmune diseases, including non-Hodgkin's or intestinal lymphoma, squamous cell cancer of the esophagus, type 1 diabetes, autoimmune thyroid disease, Addison's disease, lupus, primary biliary cirrhosis, osteoporosis, psoriasis, Sjogren's syndrome, and rheumatoid arthritis (National Institutes of Health, 2004). It is harder to normalize body composition when celiac disease is diagnosed in adulthood (Barera et al, 2000).

Dermatitis herpetiformis (DH) is the skin manifestation of celiac disease. DH is characterized by intensely pruritic papulovesicular lesions that occur over the surface of the elbows, knees, legs, buttocks, trunk, neck, or scalp (Farrell and Kelly, 2002). Abnormal biopsy is evident, but GI symptoms may not be present. There may be immunoglobulin (IgA) deposits around the lesions, and large intake of iodine may trigger flares of DH.

Careful attention to health will be essential. Because of decreased absorptive surface area for calcium in celiac patients, bone fractures may be more common (Farrell and Kelly, 2002). Celiac disease should be considered in patients, even older patients, who have unexplained metabolic bone disease or hypocalcemia. Screening for celiac disease in patients who have otherwise unexplained osteopenia or osteoporosis is warranted (Stenson et al, 2005).

Monitor closely for thyroid disorders in this population (Hakanen, 2001). In pregnant women, severe anemia may persist; other adults may have episodic or nocturnal diarrhea, flatulence, intestinal bloating that mimics irritable bowel syndrome, steatorrhea, weight loss, recurrent aphthous stomatitis, or anemias (Farrell and Kelly, 2002). Neurological complications are estimated to occur in 10% of affected patients, with ataxia and peripheral neuropathy being common (Chin et al, 2003).

When wheat, rye, and barley grains are consumed, they damage the mucosa of the small intestine, eventually leading to nutrient malabsorption. Moderate amounts of oats can be consumed (Peraaho et al, 2004; Hogberg et al, 2004). However, much of the commercially available oat flour may be contaminated with wheat gluten and caution is advised for new patients. One day, it may be possible to breed wheat species with low or absent levels of harmful gluten proteins (Molberg et al, 2005).

Gastroenterologists should follow patients with celiac disease, a form of inflammatory bowel disease, to reduce morbidity and mortality (Abdulkarim and Murray, 2002). The North American Society for Pediatric Gastroenterology, Hepatology, and Nutrition recommends that children and adolescents with symptoms of or an increased risk for celiac disease have a blood test for antibody to tissue transglutaminase (TTG), that those with an elevated TTG be referred to a pediatric gastroenterologist for an intestinal biopsy, and that those with the intestinal histopathology be treated with a strict gluten-free diet (Hill et al, 2005).

Since the defect is permanent, the gluten-free (GF) diet is curative and must be a permanent change. In celiac patients who follow a strict diet, there are eventually few or no symptoms. The National Institutes of Health (NIH) consensus panel stresses that consultation with a dietetics professional knowledgeable in celiac disease is essential and that this professional should be the primary source of nutritional information (National Institutes of Health, 2004). An individualized, team approach is best, including the person with CD and his or her family, physician, dietitian, and celiac support group (Case, 2005).

INTERVENTION: OBJECTIVES

The consensus panel identified six elements required for the management of this disease (Thompson, 2005):

1. Consult a skilled dietetics professional.
2. Educate about the disease.
3. Adhere to a gluten-free diet. Remove the offending protein (gliadin fraction) from the diet; glutenin is harmless. Improvement is noted within 4–5 days.
4. Identify and treat nutritional deficiencies. Deficiencies of iron, folate, calcium, and vitamin D may be found in patients with untreated disease (Farrell and Kelly, 2002). Replace nutrients lost from diarrhea and steatorrhea. Reverse bone demineralization, hypoalbuminemia, and hypoprothrombinemia where present. Whole-body protein breakdown is common in celiac disease, contributing to a high level of protein–calorie malnutrition. Glutamine is an important fuel for the health of intestinal epithelial cells.
5. Provide access to an advocacy group. A local celiac support chapter is most helpful.
6. Provide continuous long-term follow-up care by a multidisciplinary team.

INTERVENTION: FOOD AND NUTRITION

- A gluten-free diet excludes wheat, buckwheat, rye, and barley. Avoid products such as breading, stuffing, croutons, graham, bulgur, matzo, broth, breading or coating mixes, communion wafers, pastas, cracked wheat, semolina, farina, malt, malt flavoring, brown rice syrup, commercial soups, imitation bacon, imitation seafood, marinades, processed meats, roux, sauces, seasonings, self-basting poultry, soups and soup bases, thickeners, vegetarian meat substitutes, and commercial potato and rice mixes. Soy sauce, white and nonmalt vinegars, and wheat starch must be pure; read labels. Plan a diet that includes grains and starches that may be used freely. See Table 7-9.
- Since oats do not damage the small intestinal mucosa, include small-to-moderate amounts without adverse effects. However, oats are sometimes contaminated with wheat during processing and should be avoided in initial stages of treatment (Farrell and Kelly, 2002).

TABLE 7-9 Grains and Starches to Use Freely in Celiac Disease

Amaranth
Arrowroot
Beans (black, garbanzo, kidney, northern, pinto)
Black-eyed peas, lentils, split peas
Buckwheat
Cassava
Corn, corn bran, hasa marina
Gluten-free bread
Hominy, grits
Indian rice grass
Montina
Nut flours
Quinoa
Poha flakes
Potato, potato starch, potato flour
Rice
Sorghum
Soy
Tapioca
Tef
Wild rice

- For infants with diarrhea, provide fluids, electrolytes, and a formula that is not high in fat content.
- Diet for adults should provide 1–2 g of protein/kg body weight from fresh meat, fresh fish, milk, cheese, and eggs. Examine processed items carefully since there is often gluten added.
- Diet should provide 35–40 kcal/kg body weight for adults.
- During bouts of diarrhea, infants may tolerate banana powder; adults and children may do well with starchy-type carbohydrates, bananas, leans meats, and fish. Rehydrate with oral rehydration solution or other fluids.
- Initially, the diet should include low amounts of fiber because of flattening of the mucosal villi. Intake can be increased as tolerated. Fruits and vegetables are naturally low in gluten.
- If tube feeding is used, a glutamine-enriched product may be useful. Monitor ingredients and avoid gluten.
- Watch for lactose intolerance that is either temporary or permanent. Initially, dairy products (primarily milk and products made with milk) should be avoided because these patients often have secondary lactase deficiency; after 3–6 months of treatment, dairy products may be gradually reintroduced (Farrell and Kelly, 2002).
- The diet and gluten-free products are often low in B vitamins, calcium, vitamin D, iron, zinc, magnesium, and fiber; few gluten-free products are enriched or fortified, adding to the risk of nutrient deficiencies (Kupper, 2005; Thompson, 2000). Correction of vitamin and mineral deficiencies is important (Murray, 1999; Abdulkarim and Murray, 2002). Supplements to the diet should include water-miscible vitamins A, D, E, and K, iron, calcium, folic acid, vitamin B_{12}, thiamine, and other B-complex vitamins.
- Products containing medium-chain triglycerides (MCTs) often are used when fat malabsorption is present, especially in adults.
- Foods that often are not allowed include cream soups, creamed vegetables, ice cream (labels should be checked for thickening agents), oatmeal (tolerated by some people; check with the physician before using), cakes, cookies, and breads (unless made with rice, corn, or potato flours). For toddlers, mixed infant dinners and junior dinners that contain flour thickeners, spaghetti, macaroni, and other pastas should not be used.

CLINICAL INDICATORS

Clinical/History

Height
Weight
BMI
Diet history
Growth pattern (child)
Failure to thrive?
Aphthous stomatitis
Fatigue, lassitude, depression
Recurrent abdominal pain, bloating
Steatorrhea, chronic diarrhea
Dermatitis herpetiformis
Enamel defects of permanent teeth
Osteopenia, bone pain?
Infertility, frequent miscarriages?
Short stature?
Small bowel biopsy with flat villi (multiple biopsies needed)
Abdominal computed tomography (CT) or MRI scan
Capsule endoscopy

Lab Work

Anti-tissue transglutaminase antibodies (tTG)—IgA and IgG (95–100% sensitive and specific)
Antigliadin IgA and IgG (IgA is specific; IgG is 100% sensitive)
Antiendomysial antibodies (EMA)—IgA
Antireticulum antibodies—IgA
HLA-DQ2 and HLA-DQ8 haplotype
Serum carotene
H & H
Serum Fe and ferritin (anemia is common)
Macrocytic anemia (low vitamin B_{12} or folate)
Na^+, K^+
Ca^{++} (often low)
Mg^{++}
Serum phosphorus (PO_4) (decreased)
Alb, transthyretin
CRP
Transferrin, TIBC
Serum copper (decreased)
Lactic acid dehydrogenase (LDH) (increased)
Xylose absorption
DEXA scan
Fecal chymotrypsin level
Fecal fat study
Liver function tests (mildly abnormal)

Common Drugs Used and Potential Side Effects

- No drug therapy has been proven to suppress the disease (Abdulkarim and Murray, 2002).
- Check all labels *each time* for gluten-containing ingredients. Gluten-free laxatives include psyllium seed laxatives (Metamucil, Naturacil), docusate sodium (Surfak), and

bisacodyl (Dulcolax). Gliadins are often impurities in medications, including acetaminophen; check carefully.
- Corticosteroids may be used with numerous side effects. Take with food. Weight gain is common. Monitor for negative nitrogen or calcium balances.

Herbs, Botanicals, and Supplements

- Herbs and botanical supplements should not be used without discussing with the physician.
- With use of bisacodyl, avoid aloe, cascara, senna, and yellow dock because of enhancing effects.

INTERVENTION: NUTRITION EDUCATION, COUNSELING, CARE MANAGEMENT

- **Strict lifelong elimination of gluten** and dietary adherence are essential for those persons with diagnosis of celiac disease (Chand and Mihas, 2006). If strictly followed, improvement will occur in most patients within 2 weeks. If results are not seen after 6–9 months of diet therapy, a new diagnosis should be sought.
- The execution and maintenance of the "theoretically simple" exclusion of gluten are difficult; patient education and motivation are crucial to a successful outcome (Abdulkarim and Murray, 2002). An effective gluten-free diet requires extensive, repeated counseling and instruction of the patient by the physician and dietitian (Farrell and Kelly, 2002).
- Instruct the patient to read food labels *each time* for cereal, starch, flour, thickening agents, emulsifiers, gluten, stabilizers, hydrolyzed vegetable proteins, semolina, durum, triticale, bulgur, farina, couscous, broth, and related gluten ingredients. "Wheat free" is not gluten free because products may contain rye or barley. Wheat starch is acceptable because the gliadin/gluten has been removed. Caramel coloring and monosodium glutamate (MSG) may not be tolerated. A gluten-free symbol is used widely by food manufacturers in Europe but, unfortunately, less so in the United States (Farrell and Kelly, 2002). Contact the manufacturer if there are questionable ingredients.
- Carefully check the ingredients of all recipes.
- Because of possible contamination with wheat, oats should be avoided in all patients with newly diagnosed celiac until remission is achieved through the use of a gluten-free diet; then, up to 2 oz of oats from a reliable source can be eaten every day, if the patient has no ill effects (Farrell and Kelly, 2002).
- Toothpaste, mouthwash, lipstick or chapstick, glue on envelopes or teabags, boxed candy, chewing gum wrappers, utensils in buffet lines, toasters, bulk food bins, jars used for various purposes, and other related items should be checked carefully and avoided if gluten is present.

Patient Education—Foodborne Illness

- Careful food handling and hand washing are important to prevent introduction of foodborne pathogens to this individual who may be experiencing diarrhea and related discomfort.

For More Information

- American Dietetic Association (ADA)
  Dietitians in Gluten Intolerance Disease, subunit of Dietitians in General Clinical Practice (DGCP); contact ADA at
  http://www.eatright.org
  Celiac Disease Nutrition Guide: www.eatright.org
  Nutrition Care Manual: Web-based manual: www.nutritioncare-manual.org.
- Celiac Disease and Gluten-Free Diet Support Group
  http://www.celiac.com/
- Celiac Disease Foundation
  http://www.celiac.org
- Celiac Sprue Association
  http://www.csaceliacs.org/
- Freeda Vitamins
  http://www.freedavitamins.com
- Gluten-Free Diet by Shelley Case
  http://www.glutenfreediet.ca
- Gluten-Free Medications
  http://www.glutenfreedrugs.com
- Gluten-Free Pantry
  http://www.glutenfree.com/
- Gluten Intolerance Group of North America
  http://www.gluten.net/
- Guidelines for a Gluten-Free Lifestyle
  http://www.celiac.org/newsEvents.php
- National Celiac-Sprue Society
  http://www.csaceliacs.org
- Scott Adams' Celiac Page
  http://www.celiac.com

CELIAC DISEASE—CITED REFERENCES

Abdulkarim A, Murray J. Celiac disease. *Curr Treat Options Gastroenterol.* 5:27, 2002.
Alaedini A, Green PH. Narrative review: celiac disease: understanding a complex autoimmune disorder. *Ann Intern Med.* 142:289, 2005.
Barera G, et al. Body composition in children with celiac disease and the effects of a gluten-free diet: a prospective, case-control study. *Am J Clin Nutr.* 72:71, 2000.
Case S. The gluten-free diet: how to provide effective education and resources. *Gastroenterology* 128:S128, 2005.
Chand N, Mihas AA. Celiac disease: current concepts in diagnosis and treatment. *J Clin Gastroenterol.* 40:3, 2006.
Chin RL, et al. Celiac neuropathy. *Neurology* 60:1581, 2003.
Farrell R, Kelly C. Celiac sprue. *N Engl J Med.* 346:180, 2002.
Hakanen M. Clinical and subclinical autoimmune thyroid disease in adult celiac disease. *Dig Dis Sci.* 46:2631, 2001.
Hill ID, et al. Guideline for the diagnosis and treatment of celiac disease in children: recommendations of the North American Society for Pediatric Gastroenterology, Hepatology and Nutrition. *J Pediatr Gastroenterol Nutr.* 40:1, 2005.
Hogberg L, et al. Oats to children with newly diagnosed celiac disease: a randomised double blind study. *Gut* 53:649, 2004.
Kupper C. Dietary guidelines and implementation for celiac disease. *Gastroenterology* 128(suppl 1):S121, 2005.
Molberg O, et al. Mapping of gluten T-cell epitopes in the bread wheat ancestors: implications for celiac disease. *Gastroenterology* 128:393, 2005.
Murray JA. The widening spectrum of celiac disease. *Am J Clin Nutr.* 69:354, 1999.
National Institutes of Health. National Institutes of Health Consensus Development Conference Statement: Celiac disease, 2004. Accessed December 2, 2004 at http://consensus.nih.gov/2004/2004CeliacDisease118html.htm.
Peraaho M, et al. Oats can diversify a gluten-free diet in celiac disease and dermatitis herpetiformis. *J Am Diet Assoc.* 104:1148, 2004.

Petroniene R, et al. Given capsule endoscopy in celiac disease: evaluation of diagnostic accuracy and interobserver agreement. *Am J Gastroenterol.* 100:685, 2005.
See J, Murray JA. Gluten-free diet: the medical and nutrition management of celiac disease. *Nutr Clin Pract.* 21:1, 2006.
Stenson WF, et al. Increased prevalence of celiac disease and need for routine screening among patients with osteoporosis. *Arch Intern Med.* 165:393, 2005.
Thompson T. Folate, iron, and dietary fiber contents of the gluten-free diet. *J Am Diet Assoc.* 100:1389, 2000.
Thompson T. National Institutes of Health consensus statement on celiac disease. *J Am Diet Assoc.* 105:194, 2005.

CONSTIPATION

NUTRITIONAL ACUITY RANKING: LEVEL 1–2

DEFINITIONS AND BACKGROUND

Constipation occurs when the fecal mass remains in the colon longer than the normal 24–72 hours after meal ingestion or when the patient strains to defecate. Stool type and frequency could be used to determine another problem, such as irritable bowel syndrome. Constipation and fecal incontinence are common symptoms in patients with cerebral palsy, traumatic spinal cord injuries, spina bifida, multiple sclerosis, diabetic polyneuropathy, Parkinson's disease, and stroke.

Spastic constipation entails increased narrowing of the colon with small, ribbon-like stools caused by inactivity, immobility, or obstruction; increasing physical activity may be useful. Atonic constipation ("lazy bowel") occurs when musculature of the bowel no longer functions properly, sometimes from laxative overuse or poor bowel habits. Tube feeding constipation occurs with use of low-fiber products, medications, or other products. In infants and children, chronic constipation is a concern, with encopresis from poor bowel habits and poor fiber intake. There may be food allergies, such as to milk or wheat, that should also be addressed.

Increasing physical activity may be helpful (Muller-Lissner et al, 2005). Treatment modalities for constipation include prokinetic agents, enemas administered through the enema continence catheter, and biofeedback. For chronic problems, bowel retraining may be necessary.

Some patients may be helped by a fiber-rich diet, but patients with more severe constipation may get increased symptoms of bloating and distention when increasing dietary fiber intake, and there is limited evidence that constipation can successfully be treated by increasing fluid intake unless there is evidence of dehydration (Muller-Lissner et al, 2005). In contrast, water-soluble fiber (e.g., pectins, gums, mucilages, and some hemicelluloses) delays intestinal transit, and lignin, cellulose, and hemicelluloses accelerate intestinal transit, thereby increasing fecal weight.

INTERVENTION: OBJECTIVES

- **Atonic constipation ("lazy bowel"):** Stimulate peristalsis, provide bulk, and retain water in the feces.
- **Spastic constipation:** Undue distention and stimulation of the bowel should be prevented during exacerbations. After the patient is well, fiber should be increased.
- **Tube feeding constipation:** Check for obstruction (nausea, vomiting, distention, and dehydration). Record intake and output, along with activity levels.
- **Pediatric constipation and encopresis:** Provide laxatives and lubricants initially, followed by improved fiber and fluid intakes.

INTERVENTION: FOOD AND NUTRITION

- In general, it may be helpful to consume more fruits and vegetables and more servings from the bread/cereal group each day, especially whole grains, root vegetables such as carrots or potatoes, stewed dried fruit, and cabbage. Gradually increase fiber, maintain adequate fluid intake, and exercise regularly.
- **Atonic constipation:** The diet should contain 20–35 g of fiber, with liberal use of whole grains, fruits, and vegetables. Adding a few carrots and some whole-grain cereal to the diet may be an easy solution. Use adequate fluid (30–35 cc/kg).
- **Spastic constipation:** The diet should be decreased in fiber during painful episodes. Then, increase use of prune juice, dried fruits, raw fruits and vegetables, nuts, and whole grains. If wheat allergy is a concern for a patient, do not promote use of bran.
- **Tube feeding constipation:** Use a fiber-containing formula if appropriate. Use adequate flushes.
- **Pediatric constipation and encopresis:** Add more fruits and vegetables to the diet; increase whole-grain fiber and fluid intake.

CLINICAL INDICATORS

Clinical/History
Height
Weight
Recent weight changes
BMI
Diet history
Bowel habits
Stool color and number
I & O
BP
Headaches
Abdominal distention

Lab Work
Alb, transthyretin
BUN, Creat
H & H
Serum Fe
Ferritin
Gluc
Na+, K+
Ca++, Mg++
Stool guaiac

SAMPLE NUTRITION DIAGNOSTIC STATEMENT

Constipation

PES: Altered GI function related to very low fluid intake and use of constipating medications as evidenced by patient complaints of hard, dry, infrequent stools.

Assessment Data (sources of info): Fluid intake records (I & O), medication history and recent changes, stool patterns and frequency.

Intervention: Counseling about fluid sources and ways to incorporate more fluids into meals and nourishments, discussion of fluid tracking with staff or family as well as patient, discuss need for stool softener with doctor or nursing staff.

Monitoring and Evaluation: Fluid intake records, stool patterns and frequency records, review of medication changes or addition of stool softener.

Common Drugs Used and Potential Side Effects (see Table 7-10)

- There is limited evidence about efficacy of treatments used for constipation. Good evidence (grade A) was found to support the use of polyethylene glycol (PEG) and tegaserod; moderate evidence (Grade B) was found to support the use of psyllium and lactulose; limited-quality data were found regarding many commonly used agents including milk of magnesia, senna, bisacodyl, and stool softeners (Kamm et al, 2005; Ramkumar and Rao, 2005).
- Antacids containing iron, aluminum, or calcium often cause problems with constipation. In addition, narcotics (codeine and morphine), NSAIDs (such as ibuprofen), verapamil, monoamine oxidase (MAO) inhibitors and tricyclic antidepressant agents (Nardil, Elavil, Endep), phenobarbital, Benadryl, clonidine (Catapres), vincristine (Oncovin), Artane, Cogentin, Haldol, Thorazine, Questran, Colestid, furosemide (Lasix), and iron preparations (ferrous fumarate, gluconate, or sulfate) may be constipating. Changes in bowel motility and tone, bloating, and sensations of "fullness" often occur.

Herbs, Botanicals, and Supplements

- Herbs and botanical supplements should not be used without discussing with the physician.
- Flax, aloe (anthraquinones), fenugreek, and rhubarb have been recommended for constipation, but no clinical trials have proven efficacy.
- With use of bisacodyl, avoid aloe, cascara, senna, and yellow dock because of enhancing effects.

INTERVENTION: NUTRITION EDUCATION, COUNSELING, CARE MANAGEMENT

- Explain that proper diet can produce relief but cannot cure the condition. A normal bowel routine is needed, but daily fecal evacuation is not needed for everyone.
- Specifically identify foods that have a laxative effect for the patient. Explain that fiber may be increased on a gradual basis only and that prune juice may help. For every gram of cereal fiber, stool weight increases by 3–9 g. For some, a cup of hot prune juice may be useful.
- Have the patient drink 8–10 glasses of water daily, as permitted. Warm fluids are especially useful.
- Exercise may be beneficial in maintaining regularity, especially abdominal-strengthening exercises.
- Discuss overuse of laxatives and cathartics.
- Discuss foods that have caused constipation, flatus, and GI distress in the past. Offer relevant suggestions.

TABLE 7-10 Medications for Constipation

Medication	Description
Bulking agents Psyllium (Metamucil, Effersyllium, Perdiem Fiber), Benefiber (with guar gum), methylcellulose (Citrucel), calcium polycarbophil (FiberCon)	Bulking agents contain fiber-based ingredients that retain water and are safe choices. Take with plenty of water or juice (8 oz per teaspoonful). Results may require 1–4 teaspoons of the product.
Lactulose (Chronulac)	Lactulose treats constipation by increasing the number and frequency of stools. Cramping, flatulence, nausea, vomiting, and potassium losses may occur. Lactulose contains galactose; avoid use of this product with a galactose-free diet.
Golitely (PEG 3350 or Transipeg: polyethylene glycol with electrolytes)	Safe and effective in pediatrics and pregnancy.
Lubricant laxatives (Fleet Mineral Oil)	Lubricant laxatives coat the intestinal lining to allow easier passage of stool but may also interfere with absorption of calcium and fat—soluble vitamins.
Prebiotics and probiotics	Use of probiotics such as yogurt with active cultures, lactobacilli and bifidobacteria, and prebiotics (nondigestible oligosaccharides) may be beneficial for gut integrity.
Stimulant laxatives Bisacodyl (Fleet Stimulant Laxative, Correctol, Dulcolax) Ex-Lax or Senokot (with senna) Herbal Authority Aloe Vera	Stimulant laxatives may irritate the intestine, causing bowel contractions. They can cause severe cramping, diarrhea, nausea, and electrolyte imbalances. Avoid using bisacodyl (Dulcolax) with dairy products; take with a high-fiber diet. Generally not recommended.
Stool softeners Docusate sodium (Colace, Fleet Sof-lax, Peri-Colace)	Stool softeners are short-term solutions; they allow more water to penetrate stool and to facilitate elimination. Docusate sodium (Colace) should be taken with milk or juice.
Tegaserod (a serotonin-4 receptor agonist)	Tegaserod is a prokinetic agent that speeds small bowel transit and right colon transit in irritable bowel syndrome, reducing symptoms of constipation (Mertz, 2005).

- Discuss the need for medical assistance for diarrhea, bleeding, infection, and changes in bowel habits.
- Bowel retraining programs may be helpful and may include increasing exercise, including more fiber in the diet, drinking more liquids, and setting aside 15 minutes to spend on the toilet after breakfast. Regular practices may help reestablish a healthy pattern.
- In a pediatric population, dietary changes, corn syrup, or both may resolve constipation in 25% of children; laxatives such as milk of magnesia and polyethylene glycol are efficient and safe for almost all cases (Loening-Baucke, 2005).

For More Information

- Constipation
  http://digestive.niddk.nih.gov/ddiseases/pubs/constipation/
  http://www.vh.org/adult/patient/internalmedicine/constipation/
  http://www.medinfo.co.uk/conditions/constipation.html
  http://www.emedicine.com/med/topic2833.htm
- Constipation Algorithm
  http://www.uwgi.org/guidelines/ch_05/AlgA.htm
- International Foundation for Functional Gastrointestinal Disorders
  http://www.aboutconstipation.org/
- Jackson Gastroenterology
  http://www.gicare.com/pated/ecdgs07.htm

CONSTIPATION—CITED REFERENCES

Kamm MA, et al. Tegaserod for the treatment of chronic constipation: a randomized, double-blind, placebo-controlled multinational study. *Am J Gastroenterol.* 100:362, 2005.
Loening-Baucke V. Prevalence, symptoms and outcome of constipation in infants and toddlers. *J Pediatr.* 146:359, 2005.
Mertz H. Psychotherapeutics and serotonin agonists and antagonists. *J Clin Gastroenterol.* 39:S247, 2005.
Muller-Lissner SA, et al. Myths and misconceptions about chronic constipation. *Am J Gastroenterol.* 100:232, 2005.
Ramkumar D, Rao SS. Efficacy and safety of traditional medical therapies for chronic constipation: systematic review. *Am J Gastroenterol.* 100:936, 2005.

DIARRHEA, DYSENTERY, AND TRAVELER'S DIARRHEA

NUTRITIONAL ACUITY RANKING: LEVEL 2

DEFINITIONS AND BACKGROUND

Diarrhea (acute enteritis) is a symptom of many disorders in which there is usually an increased peristalsis with decreased transit time through the GI tract. Reduced reabsorption of water and watery stools result. In Table 7-11, etiologies and comments related to diarrhea are given.

Chronic diarrhea is the production of loose stools with or without increased frequency for more than 4 weeks; it affects 3–5% of the U.S. population (American Gastroenterology Association, 1999). While diet is often blamed for diarrhea, an individualized approach, knowledge of gastrointestinal physiology, and awareness of the physiological effects of foods or medications are best used to design an effective dietary plan (Schiller, 2006).

Dehydration is a common problem; watch for decreased skin turgor, dry mucous membranes, thirst, 2% weight loss or more, low blood pressure, postural hypotension, increased BUN and hematocrit, and decreased urinary output.

Early childhood diarrhea can come from or lead to malnutrition (Ochoa et al, 2004; Guerrant et al, 2000). Diarrhea is the leading cause of death in children younger than 5 years of age; persistent diarrhea accounts for 30–50% of these deaths in developing countries (Ochoa et al, 2004). Early rehydration may prevent many deaths in high-risk infants if mothers seek medical attention and offer proper rehydration solutions as soon as diarrhea begins. Oral rehydration solutions (ORS) are well tolerated and shorten illness and decrease fluid losses. Diarrhea can be prevented by breastfeeding, by immunizing all children against measles, by keeping food safe and water clean, and by washing hands before touching food.

Clostridium difficile **colitis and diarrhea** can be caused by use of most antibiotics. There may be profuse watery diarrhea that may be foul smelling; abdominal pain, cramping, and tenderness; stools that may be guaiac positive and grossly bloody; and fever or white blood cell count of 12,000–20,000/µL. In severe cases, toxic megacolon, colonic perforation, peritonitis, hypovolemic shock, sepsis, and hemorrhage might occur. Symptoms may develop within a few days or even 6–10 weeks after antibiotic therapy is completed. Because *C. difficile* may be a normal bowel organism (especially in children), simply culturing the organism does not mean that diarrhea is caused by *C. difficile*. In mild cases, symptoms will usually resolve spontaneously once the causative antibiotic is withdrawn. More severe cases warrant therapy with oral antibiotic therapy. Both vancomycin and metronidazole for 10 days are effective treatments. See Section 15 for more information about this infection.

For **traveler's diarrhea (TD)**, high-risk destinations include most countries in Latin America, Africa, the Middle East, and Asia. Both cooked and uncooked foods are a concern if they have been improperly handled; risky foods include raw or undercooked meat and seafood and raw fruits and vegetables. Tap water, ice, and unpasteurized milk and dairy products can be associated with increased risk. Daily doses of rifaximin (Xifaxan) appear to significantly decrease the incidence of TD from *Escherichia coli.*

TABLE 7-11 Diarrhea: Etiologies and Comments

Diarrhea Type	Cause	Comments
Functional	From irritation or stress	Often resolves on its own
Organic	From intestinal lesion	May require further medical evaluation
Osmotic	From carbohydrate intolerance	Lactose, fructose, or sorbitol malabsorption may be a cause (Johlin et al, 2004).
Antibiotic-induced	*Clostridium difficile* is the gram-positive anaerobic bacterium most often responsible.	Clindamycin or cephalosporin often causes diarrhea.
Secretory	From bacteria, viruses, bile acids, laxatives, or hormones	This is typically a more serious condition.
		Rotavirus and *Norwalk virus* commonly affect infants and school-aged children; vomiting and watery diarrhea may occur. Some stool specimens from nursing home residents, who become ill during outbreaks of gastroenteritis, are positive for Norwalk-like viruses (Green et al, 2002).
Chronic diarrhea	From celiac disease, cow's milk allergy, bacterial and parasitic factors, cystic fibrosis, and postinfectious gastroenteritis	Manage the underlying condition and often the diarrhea resolves. Celiac disease is more common than previously identified. Food allergy should also be considered (Sicherer, 2005).
Traveler's diarrhea (TD) and dysentery	TD is from contaminated food or water. Dysentery is from poor sanitation; causes range from contact with feces to contamination by houseflies.	TD is usually caused by enterotoxic bacteria (*Escherichia coli*, *Campylobacter*, *Shigella*, *Salmonella*, or *Yersinia*) or viruses or protozoa (Juckett 1999); *Giardia* is less common. Dysentery may involve diarrhea, with blood and mucus, intestinal rumbling, cramps, fever, and pus in stools.

INTERVENTION: OBJECTIVES

- Determine causation; apply an appropriate treatment.
- Prevent or alleviate dehydration, electrolyte imbalances, anemia, weight loss, and hypoglycemia. Avoid cautious refeeding or use of TPN, which may lead to reduction in nutrient intake and atrophy of the gut.
- Restore normal bowel motility. Alter stool consistency and quantity; up to 200 g of stool per day is normal.
- Avoid extremes in food and beverage temperatures, which may stimulate extra colonic activity.
- Correct intolerances for CHO and protein. Ensure adequate fat intake. Short-chain fatty acids enhance sodium reabsorption; include adequate fiber as well.
- Probiotic foods may be useful, with live active cultures that help deter further diarrhea. For example, yogurt may be recommended.

INTERVENTION: FOOD AND NUTRITION

- It may be useful to hold food for 12 hours with use of intravenous fluids and electrolytes. Start oral fluids as soon as allowed. Oral rehydration therapy (ORT) (Table 7-12) or prepared products, such as CeraLyte, should be used. The addition of resistant starch to a standard ORT solution reduces fecal fluid loss and shortens duration of diarrhea in patients with cholera (Ramakrishna et al, 2000).
- **Adults:** Start with broth, tea, and toast, and gradually add foods to a normal diet as tolerance progresses. Three to four small meals may be better tolerated. Products such as Gatorade may be useful. Banana flakes may be a safe, cost-effective treatment for diarrhea in critically ill patients on tube feedings (TF), even while waiting for results of *C. difficile* testing (Emery et al, 1997). Use products containing probiotics, such as yogurt with live cultures. For potassium, include bananas, orange juice, fruits, and vegetables in the diet. Cocoa beans contain a large amount of flavonoids; dark chocolate may offer mild relief from diarrhea (Schuier et al, 2005).
- **Infants:** Use rehydration solutions if allowed. Breastfeeding may be continued, or return to lactose-containing formula when feasible. Cut back on use of sorbitol (as in apple juice).
- If TF is being used, check tube placement and medications, presence of bloody stools, and endoscopic exams. Treatment includes changing medications, decreasing rate of feeding, changing formula, antibiotic therapy, and using antidiarrheal medications (Williams et al, 1998). High-fiber products are recommended in many cases. A jejunal placement may be too far for some patients and may actually cause some diarrhea.
- Use TPN only for intractable diarrhea. Osmotic diarrhea abates with NPO. Short-chain fatty acids from high-fiber sources may be useful.
- Multivitamin-mineral supplements may be needed to replace vitamins A and C, zinc, iron, and other nutrients.

TABLE 7-12 UNICEF/WHO Oral Rehydration Therapy

Sodium chloride 3.5 g
Sodium bicarbonate 2.5 g
Potassium chloride 1.5 g
Glucose 20 g to be dissolved in 1 L of clean drinking water

From: Rehydration Project. Oral rehydration therapy: how it works. 2006. Accessed at http://www.rehydrate.org/ors/ort_how_it_works.htm.

SAMPLE NUTRITION DIAGNOSTIC STATEMENT

Diarrhea

PES: Altered GI function related to excessive intake of poorly absorbed CHOs as evidenced by frequent intake of apple juice and sorbitol-containing dietetic products with cramping and loose stools.

Assessment: Food diary, bowel patterns.

Intervention: Educate about impact of poorly absorbed CHO on bowel function.

Monitoring/Evaluation: Reports of less abdominal cramping and loose stools.

CLINICAL INDICATORS

Clinical/History	Lab Work	
Height	Na+ (decreased)	Serum copper
Weight	K+, Cl−	N balance
Weight changes	Ca++, Mg++	Transferrin
BMI	Stool culture such as for *C. difficile*	H & H
Diet history	BUN:Creat ratio	Serum Fe
Stool consistency	Gluc	Lactose tolerance test
BP	Alb, transthyretin	Hydrogen breath test
I & O; dehydration?	CRP	
Temperature		
Abdominal pain		

Common Drugs Used and Potential Side Effects

- Antibiotics are used if shigellae or amoebae are causing the problem. Suggest use of probiotics, such as yogurt with active cultures, with antibiotic therapy. Intestinal flora modifiers (e.g., *Lactobacillus acidophilus*, Lactinex, Bacid) also help recolonize normal intestinal flora in people on antibiotics. A common prescription is 3–4 packages every day for 3 days in adults. They may be mixed with water for tube-fed patients.
- Antidiarrheal drugs are used to slow peristalsis or thicken stools. Kaolin (Kaopectate) has no major side effects but is not useful with infants. Lomotil should be taken with food; it may cause bloating, constipation, dry mouth, swollen gums, dizziness, nausea, and vomiting. Avoid using it with alcohol. Psyllium ingestion reduces stool looseness.
- Cholestyramine (Questran) may be used for bile acid diarrhea. Nausea, belching, or constipation may result. Replace fat-soluble vitamins.
- Ciprofloxacin is used for TD; one dose is often sufficient. It is a quinolone-class antibiotic. Avoid milk or yogurt. Nausea is one side effect.
- Vancomycin is used for treating *C. difficile*. Anorexia, GI distress, diarrhea, and nausea may result.
- Daily doses of rifaximin (Xifaxan) may significantly decrease TD from *Escherichia coli*. It is not known yet if this same treatment is effective against TD from *Salmonella* and other bacteria.
- Every patient should receive a careful medication review. Magnesium-containing antacids, digoxin, broad-spectrum antibiotics, antifungal agents, colchicine, thiazide diuretics and other antihypertensives, Azulfidine, methotrexate and other anticancer agents, cholinergic stimulants, antiemetics such as metoclopramide, and laxatives such as mineral oil or methylcellulose may cause drug-induced diarrhea. Sorbitol may cause diarrhea; it is found in many medications. Megadoses of vitamin C (>1 g daily) may cause diarrhea.

Herbs, Botanicals, and Supplements

- Herbs and botanical supplements should not be used without discussing with the physician. Apple, carrot, blackberry, carob, bilberry, and tea have been recommended, but no clinical trials have proven efficacy.
- Probiotic medications may be helpful: for children, *Lactobacillus* GG or Culturelle; and for adults, *Saccharomyces boulardii*. Probiotics in foods can help to maintain good bacteria in the GI tract of those taking antibiotics. Yogurt may help to reculture the GI tract; check labels for active cultures. Acidophilus milk is also useful.

INTERVENTION: NUTRITION EDUCATION, COUNSELING, CARE MANAGEMENT

- Describe the effects of pectin as a thickening agent (as in apples and bananas), and inform about yogurt or acidophilus milk or other specific probiotic foods/supplements.
- Avoid sweetened carbonated beverages because their electrolyte content is low and osmolality is high. Caffeine, apple juice, and milk can aggravate diarrhea; omit until resolved.
- Limit fruit juice to 6 oz daily in children.
- Partially hydrolyzed guar gum (Benefiber) added to a diet ferments in the colon and produces short-chain fatty acids. This improves intestinal function, including colonic salt and water absorption (Alam et al, 2005). It may be a useful addition until diarrhea resolves.

Patient Education—Foodborne Illness (see Table 7-13)

The World Health Organization (2005) states the following:

- 1.8 million people die every year from diarrheal diseases (including cholera); 90% are children under 5, and most live in developing countries.
- 88% of diarrheal disease is attributed to unsafe water supply and inadequate sanitation and hygiene.
- Improved water supply reduces diarrhea morbidity by 21%.
- Improved sanitation reduces diarrhea morbidity by 37.5%.
- The simple act of washing hands at critical times can reduce the number of diarrheal cases by up to 35%.

TABLE 7-13 Guidelines for Preventing Traveler's Diarrhea

- Use safe, bottled water for drinking and brushing teeth.
- Wash hands before eating, using antiseptic gel or hand wipes.
- Avoid ice in drinks.
- Do not eat raw vegetables or salads, raw fruits, or unpasteurized dairy products.
- Avoid swimming in streams and lakes.
- Use only cooked foods and bottled beverages (e.g., water, juices, beer, etc.).
- Brush teeth with bottled water only.
- Use caution with fresh foods that may have been washed in contaminated water and foods prepared with unheated water (e.g., jello) or ice cubes made with contaminated water.
- If symptoms persist, medical attention should be sought.

- Additional improvement of drinking water quality, such as point of use disinfection, would lead to a reduction of diarrheal episodes of 45%.

For More Information

- CeraLyte
  http://www.ceralyte.com
- Centers for Disease Control and Prevention (CDC) Division of Parasitic Diseases
  http://www.cdc.gov/ncidod/dpd/
- Diarrhea
  http://digestive.niddk.nih.gov/ddiseases/pubs/diarrhea/
  http://www.medicinenet.com/diarrhea/article.htm
- Diarrhea Algorithm
  http://www.uwgi.org/guidelines/ch_04/ch04.htm
- Giardiasis
  http://www.cdc.gov/ncidod/dpd/parasites/giardiasis/factsht_giardia.htm
- Rehydration Formula
  http://www.rehydrate.org/
  http://www.rehydrate.org/ors/ort_how_it_works.htm
- Travelers' Health (CDC)
  http://www.cdc.gov/travel/diarrhea.htm
- World Health Organization–Dysentery
  http://www.who.int/topics/dysentery/en/

DIARRHEA, DYSENTERY, AND TRAVELER'S DIARRHEA—CITED REFERENCES

Alam NH, et al. Partially hydrolysed guar gum supplemented comminuted chicken diet in persistent diarrhoea: a randomised controlled trial. *Arch Dis Child.* 90:195, 2005.

American Gastroenterology Association. Medical position statement: guidelines for the evaluation and management of chronic diarrhea. Clinical Practice and Practice Economics Committee. *Gastroenterology.* 116:1461, 1999.

Emery E, et al. Banana flakes control diarrhea in enterally fed patients. *Nutr Clin Pract.* 12:72, 1997.

Green K, et al. A predominant role for Norwalk-like viruses as agents of epidemic gastroenteritis in Maryland nursing homes for the elderly. *J Infect Dis.* 185:133, 2002.

Guerrant R, et al. Micronutrients and infection: interactions and implications with enteric and other infections and future priorities. *J Infect Dis.* 182:S134, 2000.

Johlin FC Jr, et al. Dietary fructose intolerance: diet modification can impact self-rated health and symptom control. *Nutr Clin Care.* 7:92, 2004.

Juckett G. Prevention and treatment of traveler's diarrhea. *Am Fam Physician.* 60:119, 1999.

Ochoa TJ, et al. Management of children with infection-associated persistent diarrhea. *Semin Pediatr Infect Dis.* 15:229, 2004.

Ramakrishna B, et al. Amylase-resistant starch plus oral rehydration solution for cholera. *N Engl J Med.* 343:308, 2000.

Schiller LR. Nutrition management of chronic diarrhea and malabsorption. *Nutr Clin Pract.* 21:34, 2006.

Schuier M, et al. Cocoa-related flavonoids inhibit CFTR-mediated chloride transport across T84 human colon epithelia. *J Nutr.* 135:2320, 2005.

Sicherer SH. Food protein-induced enterocolitis syndrome: case presentations and management lessons. *J Allergy Clin Immunol.* 115:149, 2005.

Williams M, et al. Diarrhea management in enterally fed patients. *Nutr Clin Pract.* 13:225, 1998.

World Health Organization. Rehydration Project. Accessed March 5, 2005 at http://rehydrate.org/diarrhoea/index.html.

DIVERTICULAR DISEASES

NUTRITIONAL ACUITY RANKING: LEVEL 2–3

DEFINITIONS AND BACKGROUND

Diverticular disease results from formation of small pouches (diverticula) in the colon wall and lining due to chronic constipation. Diverticular disease occurs in Westernized countries because of low-fiber diets but is rare in societies that subscribe to high-fiber, low–total fat and low–red meat dietary patterns (Aldoori and Ryan-Harshman, 2002).

These disorders may be classified as asymptomatic, atypical, acute or uncomplicated, and complicated (Wolff and Devine, 2000). Lower gastrointestinal bleeding is one of the most common gastrointestinal indications for hospital admission, particularly in the elderly, and diverticulosis accounts for up to 50% of cases (Strate, 2005).

Diverticulitis (inflammation) develops when bacteria or other irritants are trapped in the pouches, causing spasm and pain in the lower left side of the abdomen, as well as distention, nausea, vomiting, constipation or diarrhea, chills, and fever. See Figure 7-5.

Epidemiological and anatomic evidence indicates that approximately 60% of humans of Westernized societies living into the sixth decade will develop diverticulosis (Floch and Bina, 2004). More than half of individuals older than 70 years of age are affected, with sigmoid involvement a common site. Bowel cancer has been associated with the presence of diverticular disease.

Medical management is usually sufficient for acute or uncomplicated diverticulitis, but complicated diverticulitis is

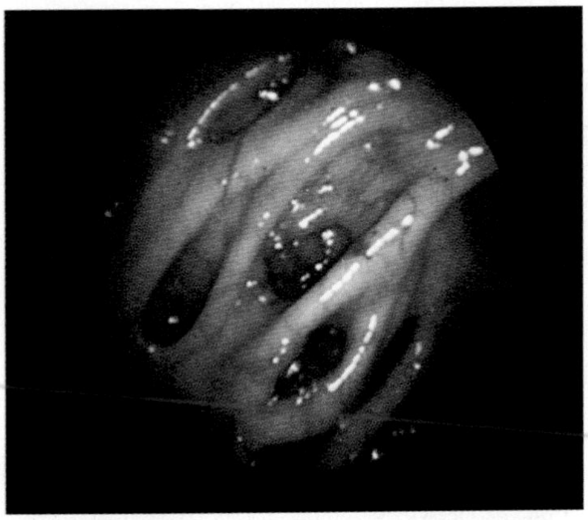

Figure 7-5 Diverticulitis.

generally managed promptly with sigmoid resection with a high success rate (Wolff and Devine, 2000). Probiotics and prebiotics are being tested for their role in relief of pain and inflammation. Otherwise, a high-fiber diet is the mainstay of management for diverticulosis (Steel, 2004); see Table 7-14.

INTERVENTION: OBJECTIVES

Diverticulosis (Convalescent State)

- Improve stool quality and increase volume, mostly from fiber (see Table 7-14). Relieve intraluminal pressure; decrease the contractions of colonic circular smooth muscle.
- Distend the bowel wall to prevent development of high-pressure segments.
- Prevent inflammation.

Diverticulitis (Inflamed State)

- Allow complete bowel rest to prevent perforation by avoiding the laxative effect of excess fiber.
- Eliminate food particles that accumulate in sacs. These food particles are capable of causing bacterial contamination.
- Prevent peritonitis and abscess.
- Correct any GI bleeding, hypoalbuminemia, or anemia.

TABLE 7-14 How to Eat More Fiber

- To get adequate fiber in the diet, follow the U.S. Department of Agriculture Food Guidance System (MyPyramid), which recommends eating 2–4 servings of fruit, 3–5 servings of vegetables, and 6–11 servings of cereal and grain foods each day.
- Begin the day by eating a whole-grain cereal that contains at least 5 g of fiber per serving; ½ cup of bran cereal contains 10 g of fiber.
- Eat vegetables raw as much as possible because cooking may reduce fiber content. A baked potato with skin is a great choice, as are broccoli, shredded carrots, and cauliflower when added to salads.
- Try not to peel fruits (such as apples and pears) and vegetables because much of the fiber is found in the skin.
- Add beans to soups, stews, and salads. Beans, peas, and lentils contain 6–9 g per ½ cup portion.
- Eat fresh and dried fruits as snacks. Pears, apples, oranges, strawberries, other berries, prunes, bananas, and figs are all good choices for fiber.
- Read food labels for fiber content. Select foods that contain fiber whenever possible.

Sources: U.S. Department of Agriculture Nutrient Database, Release 17, 2004; and Medline Plus. Dietary fiber. 2006. Accessed at http://www.nlm.nih.gov/medlineplus/dietaryfiber.html.

INTERVENTION: FOOD AND NUTRITION

Diverticulosis (Convalescent State)

- Diet should be high in fiber; 25–35 g/d is desirable. See Table 7-14. Avoid excessive fiber since it might interfere with micronutrient absorption, especially minerals. Whole grains, stewed or dried fruits, potato skins, raw carrots, or celery may also be used. Increase fiber gradually. Popcorn, seeds, and nuts may not be tolerated. Adequate fluid is recommended.
- A vegetarian, plant-based diet would be beneficial (Leitzmann, 2005).
- A low-fat diet may also be indicated to reduce intracolonic pressure.

Diverticulitis (Inflamed State)

- As treatment begins, use a soft diet with low fiber. Avoid nuts, seeds, popcorn, and fibrous vegetables. Gradually add fiber as inflammation and pain decrease.
- Ensure adequate intake of protein and iron sources.
- A low-fat diet may be beneficial.

CLINICAL INDICATORS

Clinical/History

Height
Weight
BMI
Diet history
Stool number, frequency
BP
Sigmoidoscopy
CT scan
Barium enema

Lab Work

H & H
Serum Fe
Transferrin, TIBC
CRP
Erythrocyte sedimentation rate (ESR) (increased)
Alb, transthyretin
Na+, K+
Ca++, Mg++
WBC (increased)

SAMPLE NUTRITION DIAGNOSTIC STATEMENT

Diverticular Conditions

PES: Inadequate fiber intake related to food- and nutrition-related knowledge deficit as evidenced by inability to list 5 foods high in fiber and average daily fiber intake less than 3 g/d.

Assessment Data (sources of info): Dietary recall of food intake with calculation of average fiber intake based on 24-hour recall and food frequency.

Intervention: Provide list of high-fiber foods for inclusion in the diet, discuss the importance of fiber in diverticulosis, discuss foods to avoid when there is discomfort.

Monitoring and Evaluation: Reassess dietary intake of fiber at next visit in 3 months; goal is to increase intake to 25–35 g/d.

Common Drugs Used and Potential Side Effects

- Antibiotics: For patients with severe and complicated diverticulitis, ampicillin, gentamicin, metronidazole, piperacillin, and tazobactam are used; ciprofloxacin, metronidazole, and rifaximin are used for uncomplicated diverticular disease (Tursi, 2004). Side effects may include nausea, vomiting, stomatitis, and other GI effects.
- Mesalazine (5-ASA) and an antibiotic improve the severity of symptoms and bowel habits (Tursi, 2004).
- Overusing laxatives may result in dependence on them.
- Probiotics also seem to be effective in preventing recurrence of the disease, especially if used with salicylates (Tursi, 2004).

Herbs, Botanicals, and Supplements

- Herbs and botanical supplements should not be used without discussing with the physician.
- Flax, wheat, wild yam, slippery elm, and chamomile have been recommended for this condition, but no clinical trials have proven efficacy.

INTERVENTION: NUTRITION EDUCATION, COUNSELING, CARE MANAGEMENT

- Instruct patient concerning dietary fiber. Some ingested plant material is not digested by GI enzymes, including cellulose, pectin, lignin, and hemicelluloses. Some dietary fibers (whole grains) resist intestinal disintegration, whereas others (fruits and vegetables) are more or less disintegrated. In general, increased fiber increases stool volume, frequency, and transit rate and decreases intracolonic pressure. Increased stool volume and decreased intracolonic pressure improve transit time.
- Instruct patient to chew slowly and to avoid constipation and straining.
- Fluid intake should be adequate.
- If flatulence is a problem, advise the individual that approximately 6 weeks will be needed to allow bacterial flora to adapt to increased fiber intakes.
- Adequate activity and exercise are beneficial.

Patient Education—Foodborne Illness

- Careful food handling and hand washing are important to prevent introduction of foodborne pathogens to the individual who may be experiencing diarrhea and related discomfort.

For More Information

- Diverticular Diseases
  http://www.fascrs.org/displaycommon.cfm?an=1&subarticlenbr=10
  http://www.emedicine.com/EMERG/topic152.htm
  http://www.clevelandclinicmeded.com/diseasemanagement/gastro/colonic/colonic.htm
  http://patients.uptodate.com/topic.asp?file=digestiv/6237

DIVERTICULAR DISEASES—CITED REFERENCES

Aldoori W, Ryan-Harshman M. Preventing diverticular disease. Review of recent evidence on high-fiber diets. *Can Fam Physician*. 48:1632, 2002.

Floch MH, Bina I. The natural history of diverticulitis: fact and theory. *J Clin Gastroenterol*. 38:2S, 2004.

Leitzmann C. Vegetarian diets: what are the advantages? *Forum Nutr*. 57:147, 2005.

Steel M. Colonic diverticular disease. *Aust Fam Physician*. 33:983, 2004.

Strate LL. Lower GI bleeding: epidemiology and diagnosis. *Gastroenterol Clin North Am*. 34:643, 2005.

Tursi A. Acute diverticulitis of the colon—current medical therapeutic management. *Expert Opin Pharmacother*. 5:55, 2004.

Wolff B, Devine R. Surgical management of diverticulitis. *Am Surg*. 66:153, 2000.

FAT MALABSORPTION SYNDROME

NUTRITIONAL ACUITY RANKING: LEVEL 3

DEFINITIONS AND BACKGROUND

Fat malabsorption syndrome is caused by functional or organic causes. Symptoms and signs include fatigue, weight changes, steatorrhea, abdominal distention with cramps and gas, explosive diarrhea with foul-smelling stools, malnutrition and weight loss, and biochemical abnormalities. Exocrine pancreatic insufficiency is the principal disorder that leads to severe fat malabsorption. Other causes may include: GI tract—postgastrectomy, blind loop syndrome, Crohn's disease, or small bowel resection; pancreas—cystic fibrosis, chronic pancreatitis, pancreatic cancer, or pancreatectomy; biliary—biliary atresia or steatorrhea; other causes—celiac disease, lipoprotein deficiency, or HIV infection.

The individual with malabsorption syndrome must be monitored for dehydration (dry tongue, mouth, and skin; increased thirst; low, concentrated urine output; feeling weak or dizzy when standing). Signs of nutrient depletion should be evaluated, including nausea or vomiting, fissures at corner of mouth, fatigue or weakness, and dry, pluckable hair.

Long-term nutritional monitoring is necessary after operations for morbid obesity, which can lead to fat malabsorption and vitamin deficiencies for vitamins A, D, and K (Malinowski, 2006). Malabsorption can also have severe clinical consequences; altered calcium metabolism can lead to a decline in bone health. Finally, malabsorption of dietary and biliary phosphatidylcholine may result in choline deficiency (Chen and Innis, 2004).

Individuals who have inflammatory bowel disease have an increased risk of nephrolithiasis; enteric hyperoxaluria is the major risk factor with fat malabsorptive states, and use of

TABLE 7-15 Altered Stools and Related Disorders

Characteristic	Disorder
Yellow or silver color	Fat malabsorption
Pale, foamy, mushy, or floating	Pan malabsorption
Formed in morning	Diarrhea
Formed in evening	Bile salt malabsorption

probiotics to decrease calcium oxalate levels is being studied (Lieske et al, 2005).

To avoid nutritional deterioration, early screening for fat malabsorption should be recommended, using the acid steatocrit, a reliable and inexpensive test (Dumasy et al, 2004). Intake of 40 g of olestra can cause false-positive results on tests for steatorrhea and can lead to an erroneous diagnosis of malabsorption syndrome (Balasekaran et al, 2000). Low total cholesterol (<120 mg/dL) or low serum carotene levels may be typical of fat malabsorption but are not necessarily diagnostic. Altered stools characterize different types of malabsorption (see Table 7-15); a fecal fat study may be useful (see Table 7-16).

INTERVENTION: OBJECTIVES

- Monitor for malabsorption of fat-soluble vitamins (A, D, E and K). Long-term consequences of vitamin deficiency may result if the fat malabsorption is not corrected.
- Prevent calcium oxalate stone formation, or correct where present.
- Correct all other nutrient deficiencies.
- Alleviate steatorrhea and reduce intake of fat sources that are not tolerated. Medium-chain triglycerides (MCT) are useful. See Table 7-17.

INTERVENTION: FOOD AND NUTRITION

- Initial treatment should consist of parenteral solutions or liquid formulas that contain MCT. MCTs alleviate steatorrhea in some cases; start with 20–60 g and increase gradually in an adult.

TABLE 7-16 Fecal Fat Study

Fat absorption is tested by quantitative measurement of total fat in the stool.

Preparation:	Consume 100 g of long-chain triglycerides (LCT) over 3 days
Normal excretion:	Less than 7 g (5% of a 60–100 g intake)
Mild malabsorption:	7–25 g (defects in micelle formation)
Moderate malabsorption:	25–30 g (intestinal mucosal disease)
Severe malabsorption:	More than 40 g (massive ileal resection or pancreatic disease)

Adapted from Hermann-Zaidins M. Malabsorption. *J Am Diet Assoc.* 86:1171, 1986.

TABLE 7-17 Medium-Chain Triglycerides (MCTs)

- MCTs use portal (albumin-free fatty acids) rather than lymphatic system transport and absorption (using less lipase and bile).
- MCTs have an 8- to 10-carbon source of fat and are useful when longer chain fatty acids (16–18 carbons) cannot be efficiently digested or absorbed.
- MCTs have concentrated calories made from coconut oil for adjunct therapy.
- MCT oil has 230 kcal/30 mL (6–7 kcal/g). Use instead of vegetable oil in recipes.
- Many products now contain MCTs as the primary fat source.

- For mild cases, oral feeding is preferred because it stimulates brush-border activity. For moderate to severe cases, tube feed if necessary (50 mL/hr full strength initially; advance gradually).
- Dietary fat may be limited to one egg and 4–6 oz of meat, poultry, or fish. Gradually check tolerance for long-chain triglycerides (LCTs) and work up to 30–40 g.
- Increase intake of protein, which may be in the form of skim milk, egg white, cereals, or legumes.
- Complex carbohydrates may be better tolerated than simple sugars. Lactose may not be tolerated.
- A multivitamin-mineral supplement may be necessary to offset fecal losses of nutrients, vitamins, and water in patients with malabsorption syndromes—especially zinc, folate, vitamin B_{12}, calcium, magnesium, iron, and fat-soluble vitamins (A, D, E, and K).
- Monitor or decrease dietary oxalate intake to prevent renal stones. Use of probiotics may be helpful.

CLINICAL INDICATORS

Clinical/History

Height
Weight
BMI
Diet history
BP (may be low)
Signs of dehydration?
Failure to thrive in children
Perianal itching or soreness
Frequent, foul-smelling stools
Small intestine biopsy
CT scan or MRI
Barium enema or x-rays

Lab Work

Chol (may be decreased)
Trig
H & H
Serum Fe
Gluc
Serum cholesterol
Na+, K+, Cl− (may be low from diarrhea)
Ca++, Mg++ (may be low)
Tryptophan load test for vitamin B_6
Fecal Ca++
Acid steatocrit
Fecal fat study: 72-hour stool collection
Labeled carbon breath test
Sudan stain test
Serum carotene, vitamin A (may be low)
D-xylose test (decreased excretion?)
Serum vitamin E
Schilling test for vitamin B_{12}
PO_4
Alb, transthyretin (may be low)
CRP

Common Drugs Used and Potential Side Effects

- Antibiotics are used for bacterial overgrowth. Suggest use of yogurt with active cultures with antibiotic therapy. Intestinal flora modifiers (e.g., *Lactobacillus acidophilus*, Lactinex, Bacid) also help recolonize normal intestinal flora, perhaps 3–4 packages every day for 3 days in adults. They may be mixed with water for tube feedings.
- Antidiarrheals may be used, such as kaolin (Kaopectate). Cholestyramine may be needed for bile salt diarrhea; fat-soluble vitamins can be depleted.
- Cholylsarcosine (CS) is a semisynthetic bile salt replacement. If used properly, no side effects persist.
- Orlistat inhibits pancreatic lipase and blocks the absorption of 30% of ingested fat in patients seeking weight loss. By its nature, it has the potential to create fat malabsorption syndrome, and use should be carefully monitored to assure that nutrient deficiencies do not occur.
- Pancreatic enzymes may be needed if there is pancreatic insufficiency.

Herbs, Botanicals, and Supplements

- Herbs and botanical supplements should not be used without discussing with the physician.

INTERVENTION: NUTRITION EDUCATION, COUNSELING, CARE MANAGEMENT

- Caution the patient about rapid consumption of MCTs; if they are consumed too rapidly, hyperosmolar diarrhea may result. Abdominal discomfort, flatulence, diarrhea, or steatorrhea may indicate continued malabsorption; the physician should be contacted.
- Remember that a source of essential fatty acids may be needed if MCTs are used with a low-fat diet.
- Encourage several small, frequent meals throughout the day, avoiding fluids and foods that promote diarrhea. Monitor intake and output of fluids, along with the number, color, and consistency of stools.

Patient Education—Foodborne Illness

- Careful food handling and hand washing are important to prevent introduction of foodborne pathogens to this individual who may be experiencing diarrhea and related discomfort.

For More Information

- Fat Malabsorption Syndrome
  http://www.emedicine.com/PED/topic1356.htm
  http://www.merck.com/mrkshared/mmanual/section3/chapter30/30a.jsp
  http://www.healthatoz.com/healthatoz/Atoz/ency/malabsorption_syndrome.jsp

FAT MALABSORPTION SYNDROME—CITED REFERENCES

Balasekaran R, et al. Positive results on tests for steatorrhea in persons consuming olestra potato chips. *Ann Intern Med.* 132:279, 2000.
Chen A, Innis S. Assessment of phospholipid malabsorption by quantification of fecal phospholipid. *J Pediatr Gastroenterol Nutr.* 39:85, 2004.
Dumasy V, et al. Fat malabsorption screening in chronic pancreatitis. *Am J Gastroenterol.* 99:1350, 2004.
Malinowski SS. Nutritional and metabolic complications of bariatric surgery. *Am J Med Sci.* 331:219, 2006.

INFLAMMATORY BOWEL DISEASE: CROHN'S DISEASE

NUTRITIONAL ACUITY RANKING: LEVEL 3–4

DEFINITIONS AND BACKGROUND

Crohn's disease involves acute and chronic granulomatous, inflammatory bowel disease (IBD) with a cobblestone effect (usually of the terminal ileum and cecum). Onset is generally between 15 and 30 years of age. Crohn's disease differs from ulcerative colitis (UC) by affecting the GI tract from oral cavity to rectum; UC involves the mucosal tissue of the colon and rectum. As many as 1.4 million persons in the United States and 2.2 million persons in Europe suffer from these diseases (Loftus, 2004).

The activation of nuclear transcription factor-κB has been linked with a variety of inflammatory diseases, including Crohn's disease; use of spices and herbs can suppress this pathway (Aggarwal and Shishodia, 2004). Phytochemicals from turmeric (curcumin), red pepper (capsaicin), cloves (eugenol), ginger (gingerol), cumin, anise, and fennel (anethol), basil and rosemary (ursolic acid), garlic (diallyl sulfide, *S*-allylmercaptocysteine, ajoene), and pomegranate (ellagic acid) may be protective (Aggarwal and Shishodia, 2004).

In Crohn's disease, the intestinal lumen decreases; peristalsis from food intake causes cramping pain, especially in the right lower quadrant. Other symptoms include fever, weight loss, debility, nausea, mouth sores, anal fissures, vomiting, abdominal pain, intestinal bleeding, and sporadic flare-ups. See Figure 7-6. Chronic watery diarrhea results from edema, bile salt malabsorption, bacterial overgrowth, and ulceration. Stricture may precipitate bowel obstruction. Arthritis, iritis or uveitis, conjunctivitis, jaundice, or pruritus may also be present.

Only 25% of Crohn's disease cases present with the classic triad of abdominal pain, weight loss, and diarrhea (Beattie et al, 2006). Approximately one third of children present with growth failure; their symptoms may not be of GI origin but may

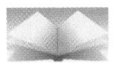

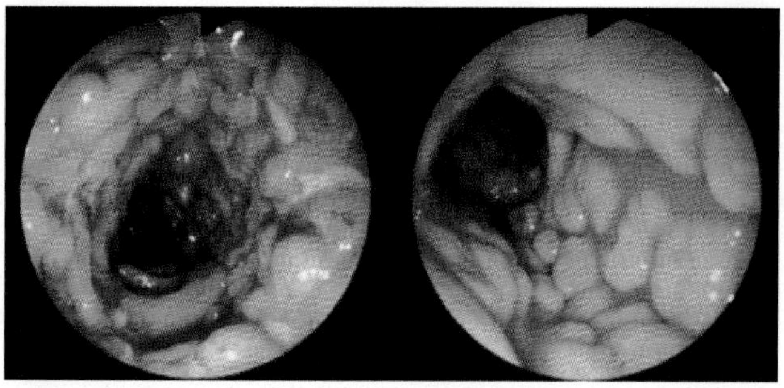

Figure 7-6 Crohn's disease erosions. (From Yamada T, et al. *Atlas of gastroenterology*. 3rd ed. Philadelphia: Lippincott Williams & Wilkins, 2003.)

include inflammation, fever, pallor, and anemia. Elevated plasma homocysteine is a consequence of IBD in children, probably mediated by poor folate status associated with diet or the pathophysiology of the disease (Nakano et al, 2003). Nutritional therapy is an important adjunctive treatment.

One million people suffer from this disorder. In one third of cases, only the ileum is involved; in 45%, both the ileum and the large intestine are affected. Only 25% of cases ever go into remission. Persons with Crohn's disease are at increased risk for colon cancer, obstruction, anorectal fistulas, and abscesses.

Total enteral nutrition may be the preferred therapy for children with specific problems; the ideal candidate is an adolescent with newly diagnosed Crohn's disease and terminal ileitis complicated by growth failure and delayed maturation (Ruemmele et al, 2000). In other cases with short bowel syndrome, TPN may be essential.

Epidemiological, clinical, and experimental evidence support an association between IBD and a large number of seemingly unrelated environmental factors; smoking and enteric bacterial flora have the most evidence; northern geographic location and allergic and autoimmune disease processes may also be related (Danese et al, 2004). Crohn's disease is associated with multiple genetic mutations; evidence suggests that the disease involves abnormal immune responses to gut microbial flora (James, 2005). Anti–tumor necrosis factor alpha (anti-TNFα) therapies have been used to treat patients with Crohn's disease with good success (Brown and Abreu, 2005).

If medical management fails, surgery may be indicated. Surgery may be needed when there is continuous bleeding; recurrent ileus, abscesses, or fistulae; and failed pharmacological treatment such as resistance to steroids. Patients after total proctocolectomy have less morbidity and are more likely to be weaned off all Crohn's-related medications (Fichera et al, 2005).

INTERVENTION: OBJECTIVES

- Replace fluid and electrolytes lost through diarrhea and vomiting. Lessen mechanical irritation and promote rest, especially with diarrhea.
- Replenish nutrient reserves; correct malabsorption or anemia. Wasting in patients with Crohn's disease is a consequence of malnutrition and not of hypermetabolism (Schneeweiss et al, 1999). Poor nutritional status may be related to decreased intake from anorexia, nausea or vomiting, abdominal pain, restrictive diets, side effects of medications, protein losses from ulcerated mucosal lesions, blood loss or wound healing requirements, bacterial overgrowth, and malabsorption.
- Monitor lactose and gluten intolerances, which may be present.
- Promote healing; rest bowel from offending agents but feed to prevent loss of critical protein mass. Provide foods that contain short-chain fatty acids and glutamine to promote healing.
- Prevent peritonitis, obstruction, renal calculi, and fistulas.
- Promote weight gain or prevent losses from exudates or inadequate intake.
- Prepare for surgery if necessary (perhaps from failed medical management, obstruction, fistula, or peritonitis). A total colectomy or a right-sided ileocolectomy may be necessary.
- In a child, promote growth. Growth spurts follow sustained weight gain.
- When controlled, fish oil intake may reduce severity of symptoms.
- Monitor mineral and trace element levels carefully to ensure adequacy. Iron tends to be low (Lomer et al, 2004). Antioxidant intake should be increased.
- Prevent or correct metabolic bone disease (e.g., osteopenia, arthropathies) caused by disease itself, nutrient malabsorption, side effects of medications, or lifestyle factors.

INTERVENTION: FOOD AND NUTRITION

- For adult energy requirements, estimate needs according to current BMI. A low BMI (<15) may require 35–45 kcal/kg; a BMI of 15–19 may require 30–35 kcal/kg; a BMI of 20–29 may require 25–30 kcal/kg; and a high BMI (>30) may only require 15–25 kcal/kg. Estimate needs at the high end of normal for growth and repair in infants or children.
- With strictures or fistulas, use a low-fiber diet that is high in energy with a high protein content of 1–1.5 g/kg.
- For some patients, tube feeding with added glutamine may be useful. Polymeric formulas are acceptable, and elemental products are not required. Randomized controlled trials show that enteral nutrition is effective in >50% of the cases in this population (Dray and Marteau, 2005).
- Perioperative parenteral nutrition may ameliorate humoral immunity, reverse malnutrition, and facilitate rehabilitation (Yao et al, 2005). If TPN is needed after total colectomy, use indirect calorimetry to estimate needs (Cormier et al, 2005).
- A diet relatively high in fat may improve energy balance (Mingrone et al, 1999). Limit fat intake only if steatorrhea is present, in which case MCTs may be better tolerated.
- Use of omega-3 fatty acids may be indicated. Use of oleic acid in the diet of Crohn's patients and increased intake of a diet rich in antioxidants could decrease inflammatory activity in Crohn's disease (Alzoghaibi et al, 2003).
- Supplement the diet with multivitamins and minerals, especially thiamine, folacin, vitamin B_{12}, vitamin E, zinc, vitamin D, calcium, magnesium, and iron. Vitamins A and K should be given every other day. With resection

SAMPLE NUTRITION DIAGNOSTIC STATEMENT

Crohn's Disease

PES: Inadequate food and beverage intake related to GI stricture and abdominal distention and discomfort as evidenced by 1/3 normal intake for past 5 days and complaints of abdominal discomfort and radiological evidence of 12-cm narrowed segment.

Assessment: Food diary, x-ray report.

Intervention: Alter diet (liquids, TF, or TPN if needed); education.

Monitoring and Evaluation: Improved intake and type of foods; symptoms resolved or improved.

greater than 200 cm, selenium may become deficient; monitor carefully.

- Reduce lactose intake if not tolerated. Check for wheat and gluten tolerances.
- Monitor progress carefully; patients may be finicky. Small, frequent meals may be better tolerated.

CLINICAL INDICATORS

Clinical/History

Height
Weight
BMI
Diet history
BP
Temperature
Number of bowel movements, frequency
Sigmoidoscopy
X-rays, endoscopy
Barium enema, barium swallow
Crohn's disease activity factor (CDAI)

Lab Work

CRP
H & H
Serum Fe (decreased)
Na+, K+
Alb, transthyretin (low)
RBP
Transferrin, TIBC
Serum homocysteine
Serum folate
N balance
Schilling test (for B_{12})
Ca++, Mg++
Serum B_{12}
Total protein
BUN, Creat
Serum carotene
Serum zinc (decreased)
TLC
Serum Cu
WBC, ESR (increased)
Hydrogen breath test
Fecal fat analysis

Common Drugs Used and Potential Side Effects

- Antibiotics work well for fistulas; vitamin K may be needed. Metronidazole and/or ciprofloxacin are quite effective (Sartor, 2004). Metronidazole may be used when there is anal involvement; nausea, vomiting, anorexia, or diarrhea may occur. Mesalamine or olsalazine may be used if sulfasalazine causes allergic reactions; nausea or vomiting may occur.
- Antidiarrheal agents: Sulfasalazine (Azulfidine) decreases inflammation but also decreases folate levels; the patient may need folate supplements. Fever, hair loss, bone marrow suppression, or nephrotoxicity can occur. Extra fluid will be needed.
- Anti-TNFα therapy is beneficial. Infliximab infusions provide relief. Infliximab blocks TNFα and reduces its resulting inflammation.
- Corticosteroids commonly cause electrolyte imbalance; they are more effective for colon involvement. The patient may then need a diet that provides sodium restriction, with extra protein, calcium, and potassium for increased losses. A new locally active medication, budesonide (Entocort), reduces episodes of acne and facial swelling.
- The use of cannabis-derived drugs as an adjunct in treating IBD is under study; a CB1 receptor is present in colonic epithelial and smooth muscle cells, while a CB2 receptor is part of the immune system cells, including macrophages and plasma cells.
- Methotrexate may be useful in reducing the need for steroids and for improving symptoms. Stomatitis, gingivitis, nausea, and diarrhea may occur.
- Probiotics may be beneficial; clinical studies are needed to verify the specific bacteria to be recommended (Brown and Valiere, 2004). Studies have been performed with antioxidants, glutamine, short-chain fatty acids, prebiotics, probiotics, low-microparticle diets, and transforming growth factor beta 2–enriched products (Dray and Marteau, 2005).
- Monthly injections of an investigational biological medication for Crohn's disease offer relief from symptoms and may induce remission. Use of 400 mg certolizumab pegol (Cimzia), a humanized anti-TNF agent, is awaiting FDA approval for use with Crohn's disease.

Herbs, Botanicals, and Supplements

- Use of complementary medicine is common in this population (Langhorst et al, 2005). Onion, valerian, and tea have been recommended for IBD, but no clinical trials have proven efficacy.
- Carrageenan, a seaweed soluble-fiber extract used as a food additive in many manufactured food products to alter texture, replace fat, and prevent syneresis, might be harmful to individuals with preexisting intestinal lesions (Shah and Huffman, 2003).
- Omega-3 fatty acids may help to reduce symptoms of Crohn's disease; studies to investigate this finding are under way. Alpha linoleic acid (ALA) works better at decreasing bowel inflammation than EPA and DHA. Fish oil supplements can cause side effects such as flatulence and diarrhea.

INTERVENTION: NUTRITION EDUCATION, COUNSELING, CARE MANAGEMENT

- Encourage patient to eat. Alleviate fears associated with mealtimes. Discuss fiber, fluid, and supplements.
- Periodic assistance or reevaluation by a dietitian may be helpful regarding dietary intake.
- Ensure that sources of potassium are increased during periods of diarrhea.

- Instruct patient to chew foods well and avoid swallowing air.
- Highlight calcium and vitamin D in their roles in bone mineralization; discuss alternate sources when milk cannot be used. Bone density should be monitored yearly. Promote exercise as well.
- Nocturnal tube feedings have been useful to regain weight or for growth. Total enteral nutrition with a liquid formula can suppress gut inflammation and induce remission in active Crohn's disease (Johnson et al, 2006; Newby et al, 2005).

Patient Education—Foodborne Illness

- Careful food handling and hand washing are important to prevent introduction of foodborne pathogens to the individual who may be experiencing diarrhea and related discomfort.

For More Information

- Colon Cancer Screening
  http://www.uwgi.org/guidelines/ch_08/ch08txt.htm
- Crohn's Disease
  http://digestive.niddk.nih.gov/ddiseases/pubs/crohns/
- Crohn's and Colitis Foundation of America
  http://www.ccfa.org/
- HealingWell Crohn's Disease Resource Center
  http://www.healingwell.com/ibd/
- National Association for Colitis and Crohn's Disease
  http://www.nacc.org.uk/content/home.asp

INFLAMMATORY BOWEL DISEASE: CROHN'S DISEASE–CITED REFERENCES

Aggarwal BB, Shishodia S. Suppression of the nuclear factor-kappaB activation pathway by spice-derived phytochemicals: reasoning for seasoning. *Ann N Y Acad Sci.* 1030:434, 2004.

Alzoghaibi MA, et al. Linoleic acid, but not oleic acid, upregulates the production of interleukin-8 by human intestinal smooth muscle cells isolated from patients with Crohn's disease. *Clin Nutr.* 22:529, 2003.

Beattie RM, et al. Inflammatory bowel disease. *Arch Dis Child.* 91:426, 2006.

Brown AC, Valiere A. Probiotics and medical nutrition therapy. *Nutr Clin Care.* 7:56, 2004.

Brown SJ, Abreu MT. Antibodies to tumor necrosis factor-alpha in the treatment of Crohn's disease. *Curr Opin Drug Discov Dev.* 8:160, 2005.

Cormier K, et al. Resting energy expenditure in the parenterally fed pediatric population with Crohn's disease. *J Parenter Enteral Nutr.* 29:102, 2005.

Danese S, et al. Inflammatory bowel disease: the role of environmental factors. *Autoimmun Rev.* 3:394, 2004.

Dray X, Marteau P. The use of enteral nutrition in the management of Crohn's disease in adults. *J Parenter Enteral Nutr.* 29:S166, 2005.

Fichera A, et al. Long-term outcome of surgically treated Crohn's colitis: a prospective study. *Dis Colon Rectum.* 48:963, 2005.

James SP. Prototypic disorders of gastrointestinal mucosal immune function: celiac disease and Crohn's disease. *J Allergy Clin Immunol.* 115:25, 2005.

Johnson T, et al. Treatment of active Crohn's disease in children using partial enteral nutrition with liquid formula: a randomised controlled trial. *Gut* 55:356, 2006.

Langhorst J, et al. Amount of systemic steroid medication is a strong predictor for the use of complementary and alternative medicine in patients with inflammatory bowel disease: results from a German national survey. *Inflamm Bowel Dis.* 11:287, 2005.

Loftus EV Jr. Clinical epidemiology of inflammatory bowel disease: incidence, prevalence, and environmental influences. *Gastroenterology* 126:1504, 2004.

Lomer MC, et al. Intake of dietary iron is low in patients with Crohn's disease: a case-control study. *Br J Nutr.* 91:141, 2004.

Mingrone G, et al. Elevated diet-induced thermogenesis and lipid oxidation rate in Crohn's disease. *Am J Clin Nutr.* 69:325, 1999.

Nakano E, et al. Hyperhomocysteinemia in children with inflammatory bowel disease. *J Pediatr Gastroenterol Nutr.* 37(5):586, 2003.

Newby EA et al. Interventions for growth failure in childhood Crohn's disease. *Cochrane Database Syst Rev.* 3:CD003873, 2005.

Ruemmele F, et al. Nutrition as primary therapy in pediatric Crohn's disease: fact or fantasy? *J Pediatr.* 136:285, 2000.

Sartor RB. Therapeutic manipulation of the enteric microflora in inflammatory bowel diseases: antibiotics, probiotics, and prebiotics. *Gastroenterology* 126:1620, 2004.

Schneeweiss B, et al. Energy and substrate metabolism in patients with active Crohn's disease. *J Nutr.* 129:844, 1999.

Shah ZC, Huffman FG. Current availability and consumption of carrageenan-containing foods. *Ecol Food Nutr.* 42:357, 2003.

Yao GX, et al. Role of perioperative parenteral nutrition in severely malnourished patients with Crohn's disease. *World J Gastroenterol.* 11:5732, 2005.

INFLAMMATORY BOWEL DISEASE: ULCERATIVE COLITIS

NUTRITIONAL ACUITY RANKING: LEVEL 4

DEFINITIONS AND BACKGROUND

Ulcerative colitis (UC) is a chronic inflammatory disease of the colon. Ulceration of the mucosa occurs and causes crampy abdominal pain, explosive or bloody diarrhea, pus or mucus discharged between stools, anemia, fatigue, and anorexia. Complications can include arthritis, severe skin rashes, endocarditis, cirrhosis, splenomegaly, and stomatitis.

Although the incidence and prevalence of UC is beginning to stabilize in high-incidence areas such as northern Europe and North America, it continues to rise in low-incidence areas such as southern Europe, Asia, and much of the developing world (Loftus, 2004).

UC usually begins in the rectum or sigmoid colon. When UC affects only the rectum, it is called **ulcerative proctitis**. If the disease affects only the left side of the colon, it is called **distal colitis**; and if it permeates the entire colon, it is termed **pancolitis**. The condition is often a relentless, continuous lesion of the colon with some involvement of the terminal ileum. It does not affect full thickness of the intestine and never affects the small intestine. UC may be acute, mild, or chronic. See Figure 7-7.

The pathogenesis of inflammatory bowel disease (IBD) is complex and involves environmental, genetic, microbial, and immune factors (Danese et al, 2004). Viruses or bacteria, diet, smoking, stress, infections, and antibiotic use have been implicated. Higher consumption of sweets, alcoholic beverages, and red meats with low intake of vitamin C may be causative, but further studies are needed (Jowett et al, 2004; Sakamoto et al, 2005). Evidence for a major role of the diet in

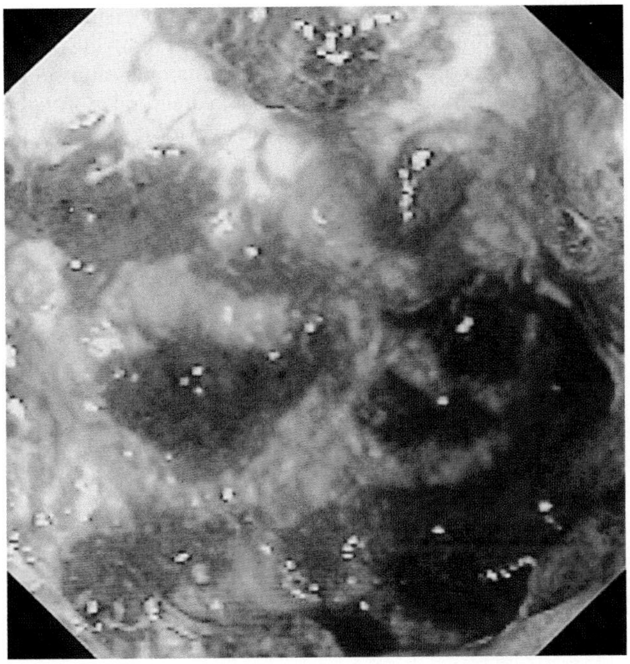

Figure 7-7 Ulcerative colitis. (From Yamada T, et al. *Atlas of gastroenterology*. 3rd ed. Philadelphia: Lippincott Williams & Wilkins, 2003.)

inducing or modifying IBD is limited, whereas the evidence for inflammation is more convincing (Danese et al, 2004).

Onset of UC is usually between 15 and 35 years of age. There is a second, lesser peak of onset at ages 50–70 years. Children who present with UC may have growth failure. Blood in the stool is the most common symptom (Beattie et al, 2006).

Flares often involve non-GI symptoms such as arthritis, uveitis, and ankylosing spondylitis. Remissions are common, and there may be long periods between exacerbations. Increased risk of colon cancer exists for the more extensive disease, especially a decade after onset.

Treatment to reduce inflammation is needed. The use of probiotics seems to be quite beneficial. Probiotic bacterial mixtures provide relief in mild to moderate UC by reducing the number of "bad" bacteria, reducing the amount of inflammation, increasing the mucus layer of the gut, and increasing the number of anti-inflammatory molecules in the intestine (Bibiolni et al, 2005).

If medical management fails, surgery is considered (Kornbluth and Sachar, 2004). Colectomy to remove the large intestine and rectum is curative. The ileocecal valve should be preserved, if possible. Temporary or permanent ileostomy is a common procedure after colorectal surgery.

INTERVENTION: OBJECTIVES

- In acute stages, allow the bowel to heal and use products that include short-chain fatty acids and glutamine to prevent a decline in nutritional status.
- Correct fluid and electrolyte imbalance. Induce or support periods of remission.
- Replenish depleted stores and correct poor nutritional status. Poor nutritional status may be related to decreased intake from anorexia, nausea or vomiting, abdominal pain, restrictive diets, side effects of medications, protein losses from ulcerated mucosal lesions, blood loss or wound healing requirements, bacterial overgrowth, or malabsorption.
- Avoid further irritation of the bowel by managing fiber intake. Large fecal volume distends the bowel and could create obstruction. Correct for diarrhea, steatorrhea, obstruction, and related anemias.
- Provide sufficient dietary antioxidants and omega-3 fatty acids, which play a role in inflammatory processes. Ulcerative colitis patients may be able to reduce steroid doses and achieve good symptom control by drinking a nutritionally balanced cocktail of fish oil, soluble fiber, and antioxidants daily.
- Prolonged use of corticosteroids, calcium and vitamin D deficiency, and a low BMI are some of the possible contributing factors to bone disease in patients with IBD (Lopez and Buchman, 2000). Replenish as needed.

INTERVENTION: FOOD AND NUTRITION

- For adult energy requirements, estimate needs according to current BMI. A low BMI (<15) may require 35–45 kcal/kg; a BMI of 15–19 may require 30–35 kcal/kg; a BMI of 20–29 may require 25–30 kcal/kg; and a high BMI (>30) may only require 15–25 kcal/kg. Estimate needs at the high end of normal for growth and tissue repair in infants or children.
- To treat the condition in its acute state, a low-fiber diet is needed to minimize fecal volume. A nutritional supplement that contains fish oil, soluble fiber, and antioxidants reduces reliance on traditional therapies and lessens the need to start on corticosteroid therapy (Seidner et al, 2005).
- Dietary changes that have been suggested include use of less red meat, dairy products, artificial sweeteners, and caffeine. Controlled trials are needed to confirm efficacy of these changes.
- TPN is useful when needed, often for 2 weeks or longer during acute stages or long term when there is short-gut syndrome.
- As the patient progresses, a high-protein diet (1–1.5 g/kg) with high energy intake, given in six small feedings, is recommended. Protein may have to be restricted in patients with renal disease.
- Diet should exclude nuts, seeds, legumes, and coarse whole grains. Fresh fruits and vegetables may not be tolerated if they are highly fibrous; monitor carefully. A low-residue diet may be useful during exacerbations.
- Persons with this condition often have lactose, wheat, or gluten intolerance. Alter diet accordingly.
- Vitamin-mineral supplementation may be needed. Supplement the diet with multivitamins and minerals, especially thiamine, folacin, vitamin B_{12}, vitamin E, zinc, vitamin D, calcium, magnesium, and iron. Vitamins A and K should be given every other day. With resection greater than 200 cm, selenium may become deficient; monitor carefully.
- MCTs may be helpful. Use more omega-3 fatty acid sources, such as salmon, mackerel, and tuna; supplements also may be beneficial.

- **After colectomy with ileostomy:** Intravenous feeding should continue for 1–2 days. Diet should progress slowly to a low-fiber, high-protein regimen with high energy, vitamins, and minerals (especially sodium and potassium). The patient will need vitamin B_{12} injections and adequate fluid. TPN may be needed if progress is slow. Once liberalized, foods are added one at a time. Avoid gas-forming foods that may cause increased peristalsis; products to reduce flatulence may be helpful.

CLINICAL INDICATORS

Clinical/History

Height
Weight
BMI
Diet history
Temperature
Stool sample
Biopsy
Sigmoidoscopy
Colonoscopy

Lab Work

CRP
ESR
Perinuclear antineutrophilic cytoplasmic antibody (pANCA)
Anti–*Saccharomyces cerevisiae* antibody (ASCA)
Bilirubin
Chol, Trig
Na+, K+, Cl
BUN, Creat
Alb, RBP
Ca++, Mg++
Serum phosphorus, Alk phos
PT or INR
Transferrin, TIBC
N balance
Schilling test (B_{12})
Serum B_{12}
H & H
Serum Fe
Serum folate
Gluc
Complete blood count (CBC), ESR
WBC
Hydrogen breath test
Fecal fat study

Common Drugs Used and Potential Side Effects

- Aminosalicylates (mesalamine, olsalazine, and sulfasalazine) contain 5-aminosalicylic acid (5-ASA) and reduce inflammation. Aminosalicylates are effective in treating mild to moderate episodes of UC and are also useful in preventing relapses of this disease. Extra fluid intake is needed to avoid renal stone formation. Anorexia, nausea, vomiting, and GI distress may occur. Folic acid supplements also may be required.
- Antibiotics such as metronidazole and ciprofloxacin help control IBD by reducing the intestinal bacteria and by directly suppressing the intestine's immune system.
- Corticosteroids (prednisone, methylprednisolone, and budesonide) are used for patients with moderate to severe disease to reduce inflammation also. Although steroids can be quite effective for short-term control of acute episodes of colitis (flare-ups), they are not recommended for long-term use due to side effects. Negative nitrogen and calcium balances may result. Monitor the need for extra vitamins and minerals.
- Immunomodulatory medicines including azathioprine, 6-mercaptopurine (6-MP), 6-thioguanine (6-TG), and cyclosporine alter the immune cell interaction with the inflammatory process. They are used for patients when aminosalicylates and corticosteroids have been ineffective. Azathioprine and 6-MP may be useful in reducing dependence on corticosteroids and in maintaining remission in some patients. These medications take several months before their beneficial effects begin to work.
- Psyllium laxatives (Metamucil) can help with constipation and diarrhea. Long-term use alters electrolytes. Flatulence or steatorrhea may occur.
- TNF-neutralizing agent infliximab (Remicade) appears to be an effective option for patients with UC not responding to conventional treatment
- Therapies under investigation include tacrolimus (FK506) and mycophenolate mofetil, now being tested in IBD. Tacrolimus seems to work in patients with IBD who do not respond to steroids.

Herbs, Botanicals, and Supplements

- Probiotics may be beneficial; studies are needed to verify the specific bacteria to be recommended (Brown and Valiere, 2004). Inulin and oligofructose have been suggested to increase the number of natural intestinal flora.
- Use of complementary medicine is common in this population (Langhorst et al, 2005). For example, further study is needed to evaluate whether glutathione or coenzyme Q10 affects prevention or treatment of IBD (Liu et al, 2004).
- Herbs and botanical supplements should not be used without discussing with the physician. Onion, cat's claw, boswellia, honeysuckle, peppermint, valerian, and tea have been recommended for this condition, but no clinical trials have proven efficacy.
- Omega-3 fatty acids may help to reduce symptoms of UC; studies to investigate this finding are under way. ALA works better at decreasing bowel inflammation than EPA and DHA. Fish oil supplements can cause side effects such as flatulence and diarrhea.

INTERVENTION: NUTRITION EDUCATION, COUNSELING, CARE MANAGEMENT

- Ensure that the patient avoids foods that are known to cause diarrhea. Avoid extremes in food or beverage temperatures.
- Pleasant mealtimes are an important part of treatment. Frequent, small meals may increase the total nutritional intake.
- Avoid iced or carbonated beverages, which may stimulate peristalsis in times of discomfort.
- Instruct the patient to eat slowly and chew foods well. Discuss fears related to eating.
- Frequent counseling by a dietitian may be helpful.
- Stop eating 2–3 hours before bedtime.

Patient Education—Foodborne Illness

- Careful food handling and hand washing are important to prevent introduction of foodborne pathogens to this individual who may be experiencing diarrhea and related discomfort. Do not use hand sanitizers excessively.

For More Information

- Colon Cancer Screening
  http://www.uwgi.org/guidelines/ch_08/ch08txt.htm
- Crohn's and Colitis Foundation of America
  http://www.ccfa.org/research/info/aboutcd
- HealingWell.com
  http://www.healingwell.com/ibd/
- National Institute of Diabetes and Digestive and Kidney Diseases (NIDDK)
  http://digestive.niddk.nih.gov/ddiseases/pubs/colitis/index.htm
- National Institutes of Health–Ulcerative Colitis
  http://www.nlm.nih.gov/medlineplus/ulcerativecolitis.html

INFLAMMATORY BOWEL DISEASE: ULCERATIVE COLITIS—CITED REFERENCES

Beattie RM, et al. Inflammatory bowel disease. *Arch Dis Child.* 91:426, 2006.

Bibiolni R, et al. VSL#3 probiotic-mixture induces remission in patients with active ulcerative colitis. *Am J Gastroenterol.* 100:1539, 2005.

Brown AC, Valiere A. Probiotics and medical nutrition therapy. *Nutr Clin Care.* 7:56, 2004.

Danese S, et al. Inflammatory bowel disease: the role of environmental factors. *Autoimmun Rev.* 3:394, 2004.

Jowett SL, et al. Influence of dietary factors on the clinical course of ulcerative colitis: a prospective cohort study. *Gut* 53:1479, 2004.

Kornbluth A, Sachar DB. Ulcerative colitis practice guidelines in adults (update): American College of Gastroenterology, Practice Parameters Committee. *Am J Gastroenterol.* 99:1371, 2004.

Langhorst J, et al. Amount of systemic steroid medication is a strong predictor for the use of complementary and alternative medicine in patients with inflammatory bowel disease: results from a German national survey. *Inflamm Bowel Dis.* 11:287, 2005.

Liu C, et al. The effect of dietary glutathione and coenzyme Q10 on the prevention and treatment of inflammatory bowel disease in mice. *Int J Vitam Nutr Res.* 74:74, 2004.

Loftus EV Jr. Clinical epidemiology of inflammatory bowel disease: incidence, prevalence, and environmental influences. *Gastroenterology* 126:1504, 2004.

Lopez I, Buchman A. Metabolic bone disease in IBD. *Gastroenterology* 2:317, 2000.

Sakamoto N, et al. Dietary risk factors for inflammatory bowel disease: a multicenter case-control study in Japan. *Inflamm Bowel Dis.* 11:154, 2005.

Seidner DL, et al. An oral supplement enriched with fish oil, soluble fiber, and antioxidants for corticosteroid sparing in ulcerative colitis: a randomized, controlled trial. *Clin Gastroenterol Hepatol.* 3:358, 2005.

INTESTINAL FISTULA

NUTRITIONAL ACUITY RANKING: LEVEL 4

DEFINITIONS AND BACKGROUND

An intestinal fistula is an unwanted pathway from intestines to other organs (e.g., the bladder). External fistulas are between the small intestine and the outside (e.g., skin). Internal fistulas are between two internal organs. Most fistulas occur secondary to abdominal surgery, and a high proportion occurs in association with inflammatory bowel disease (Hollington et al, 2004). Other causes may include intestinal cancer or trauma. In patients with a suspected fistula, computed tomography (CT) followed by a colonoscopy helps to rule out malignancy.

Enterocutaneous fistula has traditionally been associated with substantial morbidity and mortality, which are related to fluid, electrolyte, and metabolic disturbance, sepsis, and malnutrition (Hollington et al, 2004). Persistent perineal sinus is a common and serious cause of morbidity after proctectomy for Crohn's disease (Yamamoto et al, 2001). Laparoscopic surgery may be a safe and effective procedure in many cases (Laurent et al, 2005), but usually surgery is performed only after about 6 months of medical therapy (Hollington et al, 2004).

INTERVENTION: OBJECTIVES

- Promote rest and healing, minimize drainage from fistula, and prevent organ failure from sepsis.
- Monitor the type of dietary regimen according to the location of the fistula and surgical or medical treatment. Surgery may be performed to drain infection, to establish a stoma, or to repair the fistula if possible.
- Replace fluid and electrolyte imbalances.
- Decrease malnutrition and infections through aggressive nutritional support. Promote positive nitrogen balance. Nutrition support may help to allow spontaneous fistula closure (Hollington et al, 2004).

INTERVENTION: FOOD AND NUTRITION

- Use TPN or elemental diet at first; use TPN especially for jejunal fistulas. A jejunostomy may help a duodenal fistula. A higher protein intake than usual may be needed.
- Use of an elemental formula diet also may be beneficial for an extended period of time to support GI tract recovery.
- Progress to a low-residue, soft or normal diet as tolerated.

CLINICAL INDICATORS

Clinical/History		
Height	CT scan	Serum folate
Weight	Colonoscopy	N balance
Weight loss	Endosonography	Alb, transthyretin
BMI	**Lab Work**	RBP
Diet history	H & H	BUN, Creat
Temperature	Serum Fe	$Na+$, $K+$, $Cl-$
I & O		Transferrin
		$Ca++$, $Mg++$

Common Drugs Used and Potential Side Effects

- Antibiotics commonly are used. Metronidazole and ciprofloxacin are useful for perianal fistulae (Sartor, 2004). Probiotic and prebiotic therapy may be used in the future, and research is under way.
- Octreotide (somatostatin analog) inhibits endocrine/exocrine secretions and excessive GI motility. It is only used parenterally and can cause nausea, vomiting, abdominal pain, diarrhea, or flatulence.

Herbs, Botanicals, and Supplements

- Herbs and botanical supplements should not be used without discussing with the physician.

INTERVENTION: NUTRITION EDUCATION, COUNSELING, CARE MANAGEMENT

- Defined formula diets can help support spontaneous closure in approximately 4–6 weeks. If closure has not occurred, surgery is aided by better nutritional status.
- Instruct the patient regarding the fiber content of foods. Discuss how much to include during periods of flare-up and how to gradually increase fiber to achieve the goal set individually for that person.

Patient Education—Foodborne Illness

- Careful food handling and hand washing are important to prevent introduction of foodborne pathogens to this individual.

For More Information

- Intestinal Fistula
  http://www.medicinenet.com/inflammatory-bowel-disease

INTESTINAL FISTULA—CITED REFERENCES

Hollington P, et al. An 11-year experience of enterocutaneous fistula. *Br J Surg.* 91:1646, 2004.

Laurent SR, et al. Laparoscopic sigmoidectomy for fistulized diverticulitis. *Dis Colon Rectum.* 48:148, 2005.

Sartor RB. Therapeutic manipulation of the enteric microflora in inflammatory bowel diseases: antibiotics, probiotics, and prebiotics. *Gastroenterology* 126:1620, 2004.

Yamamoto T, et al. Omentoplasty for persistent perineal sinus after proctectomy for Crohn's disease. *Am J Surg.* 181:265, 2001.

INTESTINAL LYMPHANGIECTASIA

NUTRITIONAL ACUITY RANKING: LEVEL 3

DEFINITIONS AND BACKGROUND

Intestinal lymphangiectasia, which can be classified as primary or secondary, is an unusual cause of protein-losing enteropathy (Makhija et al, 2004). Increased intestinal lymphatic pressure with vessel dilatation occurs, discharging fluid into the bowel lumen. The fluid is then digested by intestinal enzymes and is reabsorbed. Massive fluid retention occurs from obstructed lymph vessels, especially in the abdomen and pleural cavities. While malabsorption and protein-losing enteropathy occur, only marginal loss of protein occurs in most cases.

The main clinical features of this disorder include edema, fat malabsorption, lymphopenia, and hypoalbuminemia (Makhija et al, 2004). Nausea, vomiting, diarrhea, and abdominal pain result. Clinical management generally includes a low-fat diet and supplementation with medium-chain triglycerides (MCTs) (Makhija et al, 2004).

INTERVENTION: OBJECTIVES

- Identify and correct the cause (e.g., constrictive pericarditis).
- Decrease symptoms and promote recovery.
- Decrease ingested fat because it stimulates lymphatic flow into the gut.
- Meet all nutritional needs for age and sex. Monitor absorption of fat-soluble vitamins; ensure adequacy from dietary or supplemental sources.

INTERVENTION: FOOD AND NUTRITION

- A formula or low-fat diet using a high concentration of MCTs is useful (Alfano et al, 2000; Makhija et al, 2004).
- Adequate protein and calories are needed, according to the individual's needs.
- Fat-soluble vitamins may be required in water-miscible form for adequate absorption.

CLINICAL INDICATORS

Clinical/History		
Height	Midarm circumference (MAC)	Steatorrhea
Weight	Midarm muscle circumference (MAMC)	Peripheral edema
BMI		
Diet history		
Triceps skinfold (TSF)		

Lab Work		
BUN, Creat	Chol, Trig	Fecal concentration of alpha-1 antitrypsin
Serum Alb, transthyretin	H & H	Jejunal biopsy (dilated lymphatic lacteal vessels)
Alb (decreased)	Serum Fe	
Na+, K+	Transferrin (decreased)	
RBP	TLC	
	Gluc	
	Ca++, Mg++	

Common Drugs Used and Potential Side Effects

- A small number of recent reports advocate the use of octreotide in intestinal lymphangiectasia (Makhija et al, 2004; Filik et al, 2004).

Herbs, Botanicals, and Supplements

- Herbs and botanical supplements should not be used without discussing with the physician.

INTERVENTION: NUTRITION EDUCATION, COUNSELING, CARE MANAGEMENT

- Discuss the role of fat in digestion, along with the need for MCT oils in the daily diet.
- Discuss fat-soluble vitamins and their sources in the diet.

For More Information

- Intestinal Lymphangiectasia
  http://www.emedicine.com/med/topic1178.htm
  http://www.merck.com/mmhe/sec09/ch125/ch125f.html

INTESTINAL LYMPHANGIECTASIA—CITED REFERENCES

Alfano V, et al. Stable reversal of pathologic signs of primitive intestinal lymphangiectasia with a hypolipidic, MCT-enriched diet. *Nutrition* 16:303, 2000.
Filik L, et al. A case with intestinal lymphangiectasia successfully treated with slow-release octreotide. *Dig Liver Dis.* 36:687, 2004.
Makhija S, et al. Octreotide in intestinal lymphangiectasia: lack of a clinical response and failure to alter lymphatic function in a guinea pig model. *Can J Gastroenterol.* 18:681, 2004.

INTESTINAL TRANSPLANTATION

NUTRITIONAL ACUITY RANKING: LEVEL 4

DEFINITIONS AND BACKGROUND

Transplantation is an effective therapy for the treatment of patients with end-stage intestine failure who cannot tolerate parenteral nutrition (PN) (Grant et al, 2005). Life-threatening complications warranting consideration of intestinal transplantation include PN-associated liver disease, recurrent sepsis, and threatened loss of central venous access (Kaufman et al., 2001). Short bowel syndrome, cancers, and other major intestinal diseases may also warrant intestinal transplantation.

Transplantation of the small bowel restores quality of life for recipients who have functioning grafts (DiMartini et al, 1998; Silver et al, 2000). Intestinal transplantations should be considered early in intestinal failure patients who develop liver injury to prevent irreversible liver disease that would mandate a simultaneous liver transplantation (Fryer, 2005).

Medicare pays for intestinal transplantation in patients who fail PN therapy (Buchman et al, 2003), which implies impending liver failure, frequent catheter-related sepsis, repeated bouts of dehydration despite PN and intravenous supplementation, and thrombosis of two or more major central veins, which prevents PN access.

Morbidity and mortality following intestinal transplantation are greater than that following liver or kidney transplantation, but long-term survival is improving (Kaufman et al, 2001). Infectious enteritis can occur in recipients after intestinal transplantation; viral agents are the cause in most cases (Ziring et al, 2005). With newer immune-suppressive protocols, 1-year graft and patient survival rates approach the results of liver transplantation (Grant et al, 2005). Because survival rates have increased, there has been a growing trend toward shortened hospitalizations with earlier discharge (Snell and Randolph, 2004).

Surgery and high-dose immunosuppression must be managed. Radiation to the small bowel before transplanting the organ, then administration of donor's bone marrow stem cells may reduce organ rejection. An organized multidisciplinary approach to the patient with short bowel syndrome is recommended (Sudan et al, 2005). Patients with intestinal transplantation require regular expert follow-up care and careful attention to even the smallest medical problem for years following transplantation (Andersen and Horslen, 2004).

INTERVENTION: OBJECTIVES

- Timely nutrition assessment and intervention may improve outcomes; a pretransplantation nutrition assessment should be very thorough (Hasse, 2001). Recovery of normal motility and absorptive capacity are the goals after surgery.
- Prevent infection and promote wound healing.
- Replenish lost nutrient stores. Malnutrition compromises posttransplantation survival; prolonged waiting times worsen outcomes when patients are already malnourished (Hasse, 2001).

- Meet metabolic demands and support recovery.
- Control complications. Diarrhea and high stomal output are common problems and can lead to nutrient deficits, especially electrolytes.

INTERVENTION: FOOD AND NUTRITION

- PN is rarely needed before transplantation except in cases of intestinal failure (Hasse, 2001).
- After transplantation, progress from clear liquids to solids as quickly as possible. Monitor fluid status and adjust as needed.
- Daily intake of protein should be appropriate for age and sex; 1.5 g/kg while on steroids may be recommended. Calories should be calculated as 30–35 kcal/kg.
- Control CHO intake and encourage use of whole grains, vegetables, and fruits in cases of hyperglycemia.
- Plan fat intake to be 30–35% of total kcal; encourage monounsaturated fats and omega-3 fatty acids. Low saturated fat intake may be needed for prevention and treatment of dyslipidemia.
- Daily intake of sodium should be 2–4 g until the drug regimen is reduced. Adjust potassium levels as needed.
- Daily intake of calcium should be 1–1.5 times the DRI levels to offset poor absorption. Children especially need adequate calcium for growth. Daily intake of phosphorus should be equal to calcium intake.
- Supplement diet with vitamin D, magnesium, and thiamine if needed.
- Reduce gastric irritants as necessary if GI distress or reflux occurs.
- The special diet may be discontinued when drug therapy is reduced to maintenance levels. Encourage exercise and a weight control plan thereafter.

CLINICAL INDICATORS

Clinical/History

Height
Dry weight, present weight
BMI
Diet history
BP
I & O
Temperature
Wireless capsule endoscopy (CE)
Colonoscopy
CT scan to monitor for fistula or obstruction

Lab Work

Alb, transthyretin
CRP
Ca++, Mg++
Na+, K+
H & H
Serum Fe
Serum folacin
BUN, Creat
Glomerular filtration rate (GFR)
WBC, TLC
Gluc
Chol, Trig
N balance
Alk phos, phosphorus
AST, ALT
Bilirubin

Common Drugs Used and Potential Side Effects

- See Table 7-18.

Herbs, Botanicals, and Supplements

- Herbs and botanical supplements should not be used without discussing with the physician.
- Grapefruit juice decreases drug metabolism in the gut (via P-450–CYP3A4 inhibition). One glass can affect medications up to 24 hours later. Avoid taking with alprazolam, buspirone, cisapride, cyclosporine, statins, tacrolimus, and many other drugs.

INTERVENTION: NUTRITION EDUCATION, COUNSELING, CARE MANAGEMENT

- Indicate which foods are sources of protein, calcium, and other key nutrients in the diet.
- If the patient does not drink milk or use dairy products, discuss other sources of calcium.
- Alcohol should be avoided unless permitted by the doctor.
- Discuss control of hyperglycemia when appropriate.
- Discuss long-term problems such as obesity and hypercholesterolemia. Patients should learn when to seek medical attention.
- Encourage moderation in diet; promote adequate exercise.
- Financial constraints can be a burden. With length of stay over 100 days and a lifetime of posttransplantation outpatient follow-up care, it is beneficial to have a fundraising program to assist patients (Chaney, 2004).
- Home care has evolved during this same period, with development of the resources, training, and processes required for in-home management of patients with multiple complex needs (Snell and Randolph, 2004).

Patient Education—Foodborne Illness

- Careful food handling and hand washing are important to prevent introduction of foodborne pathogens to the individual who may be experiencing graft–host rejection.
- Prevent infections from foodborne illness; patients who have undergone transplantation may be prone to increased risk more than other individuals.

For More Information

- Intestinal Transplantation
  http://www.emedicine.com/ped/topic2845.htm
- Medicare Guidelines–Intestinal Transplantation
  http://www.cms.hhs.gov/mcd/viewdecisionmemo.asp?id=168

INTESTINAL TRANSPLANTATION—CITED REFERENCES

Andersen DA, Horslen S. An analysis of the long-term complications of intestine transplant recipients. *Prog Transplant.* 14:277, 2004.

Buchman A, et al. AGA technical review on short bowel syndrome and intestinal transplantation. *Gastroenterology* 124:1105, 2003.

Chaney M. Financial considerations insurance and coverage issues in intestinal transplantation. *Prog Transplant.* 4:312, 2004.

DiMartini A, et al. Quality of life after small intestine transplantation and among home parenteral nutrition patients *Parenter Enter Nutr.* 22:357, 1998.

Fryer JP. Intestinal transplantation: an update. *Curr Opin Gastroenterol.* 21:162, 2005.

Grant D, et al. 2003 Report of the Intestine Transplant Registry: a new era has dawned. *Ann Surg.* 241:607, 2005.

TABLE 7-18 **Medications Used after Intestinal Transplantation**

Medication	Description
Analgesics	Analgesics are used to reduce pain. Long-term use may affect such nutrients as vitamin C and folacin; monitor carefully for each specific medication.
Azathioprine (Imuran)	Azathioprine may cause leukopenia, thrombocytopenia, oral and esophageal sores, macrocytic anemia, pancreatitis, vomiting, diarrhea, and other complex side effects. Folate supplementation and other dietary modifications (liquid or soft diet, use of oral supplements) may be needed. The drug works by lowering the number of T cells; it is often prescribed along with prednisone for conventional immunosuppression.
Corticosteroids (prednisone or Solu-Cortef)	Corticosteroids such as prednisone and Solu-Cortef are used for immunosuppression. Side effects include increased catabolism of proteins, negative nitrogen balance, hyperphagia, ulcers, decreased glucose tolerance, sodium retention, fluid retention, and impaired calcium absorption and osteoporosis. Cushing's syndrome, obesity, muscle wasting, and increased gastric secretion may result. A higher protein intake and lower intake of simple CHOs may be needed.
Cyclosporine	Cyclosporine does not retain sodium as much as corticosteroids do. Intravenous doses are more effective than oral doses. Nausea, vomiting, and diarrhea are common side effects. Hyperlipidemia, hypertension, and hyperkalemia may also occur; decrease sodium and potassium as necessary. Elevated glucose and lipids may occur. The drug is also nephrotoxic; a controlled renal diet may be beneficial. Taking omega-3 fatty acids during cyclosporine therapy may reduce the toxic side effects (such as high blood pressure and kidney damage) associated with this medication in transplantation patients.
Diuretics	Diuretics such as furosemide (Lasix) may cause hypokalemia. Aldactone actually spares potassium; monitor drug changes closely. In general, avoid use with fenugreek, yohimbe, and ginkgo.
Immunosuppressants	Immunosuppressants such as muromonab (Orthoclone OKT3) and antithymocyte globulin (ATG) are less nephrotoxic than cyclosporine but can cause nausea, anorexia, diarrhea, and vomiting. Monitor carefully. Fever and stomatitis also may occur; alter diet as needed.
Probiotics and Prebiotics	Although research is still preliminary, the use of probiotics and prebiotics may become common practice in the future.
Tacrolimus (Prograf, FK506)	Tacrolimus suppresses T-cell immunity; it is 100 times more potent than cyclosporine, thus requiring smaller doses. Side effects include GI distress, nausea, vomiting, hyperkalemia, and hyperglycemia.

Hasse J. Nutrition assessment and support of organ transplant recipients. *J Parenter Enteral Nutr.* 25:120, 2001.
Kaufman S, et al. Indications for pediatric intestinal transplantation: a position paper of the American Society of Transplantation. *Pediatr Transplant.* 5:80, 2001.
Silver H, et al. Nutritional complications and management of intestinal transplant. *J Am Diet Assoc.* 100:680, 2000.
Snell L, Randolph S. Home care management of intestinal transplant recipients. *Prog Transplant.* 14:299, 2004.
Sudan D, et al. A multidisciplinary approach to the treatment of intestinal failure. *J Gastrointest Surg.* 9:165, 2005.
Ziring D, et al. Infectious enteritis after intestinal transplantation: incidence, timing, and outcome. *Transplantation* 79:702, 2005.

IRRITABLE BOWEL SYNDROME

NUTRITIONAL ACUITY RANKING: LEVEL 3

DEFINITIONS AND BACKGROUND

Irritable bowel syndrome (IBS) is found in 10–15% of the U.S. population (Hadley and Gaardner, 2005). IBS is one of the most common "functional" gastrointestinal (GI) disorders, representing 3% of all primary care consultations, with a strong female predominance (Spiller, 2005a). Approximately 58 million individuals suffer from IBS (American College of Gastroenterology, 2005).

Bacterial gastroenteritis may be followed by the development of IBS in 5–10% of patients, depending on the severity of initial illness and prior anxiety or depression (Spiller, 2005a). Signs and symptoms of IBS include chronic abdominal pain, belching, flatulence, heartburn, mucus in the stool, constipation alternating with diarrhea, and nausea. Having a first-degree relative with abdominal pain or bowel problems is significantly associated with reporting of IBS (Locke et al, 2000).

Diagnostic criteria for IBS include at least 3 months of continuous or recurrent symptoms of abdominal pain or discomfort relieved with defecation or associated with change in frequency of stool or changed consistency of stool. There are several subgroups of IBS. One IBS subgroup is IBS with alternating bowel habits (IBS-A), another is constipation-predominant IBS (IBS-C), and the last is diarrhea-predominant IBS (IBS-D). Signs that IBS patients may require medical attention include anemia, fever, persistent diarrhea, rectal bleeding, weight loss, and nocturnal symptoms. Any of these symptoms requires further diagnostic work-up.

IBS patients have elevated food-specific immunoglobulin IgG4 antibodies to common foods such as wheat, beef, pork, lamb, and soya bean, suggesting that food hypersensitivities play a role in the pathophysiology of IBS; this is consistent for all three subgroups of IBS (Zar et al, 2005). Whereas the prevalence of food hypersensitivities in the general population is estimated at about 5%, up to 65% of IBS patients attribute their symptoms to food allergies (Zar et al, 2005). Because dietary intolerances, dietary allergies, and other food metabolites may trigger and aggravate the symptoms of IBS, a food diary may be useful (Floch, 2005). Symptoms and specific foods or practices that cause problems should be noted.

Therapies should focus on specific GI dysfunctions (e.g., constipation, diarrhea, pain), and medications only should be used when nonprescription remedies do not work or when symptoms are severe (Hadley and Gaardner, 2005). In some IBS patients, there is *Helicobacter pylori* infection (Su et al, 2000). Correcting that infection with appropriate antibiotics may relieve symptoms. Symptoms may also be improved by diets supplemented with hydrolyzed guar gum (Hadley and Gaardner, 2005).

Carbohydrate malabsorption of lactose, fructose, or sorbitol has also been described; dietary restriction of the offending sugar(s) should be implemented before drug therapy (Goldstein et al, 2000). Others who have prominent anxiety and/or depression may respond to psychotherapy or antidepressants.

Functional GI disorders are associated with a reduction in quality of life (Lacy and Lee, 2005). Present therapies for functional GI disorders are symptomatic. Therapies focus on nerve–gut communication dysfunction (5-hydroxytryptamine-3 [5-HT3] antagonists and 5-hydroxytryptamine-4 [5-HT4] agonists) and antibiotics. Probiotics are another important therapy (Floch, 2005; Spiller, 2005a). The American Dietetic Association has recommended three medical nutrition therapy visits for patients who have IBS.

INTERVENTION: OBJECTIVES

- Encourage regular eating patterns, regular bowel hygiene, adequate rest, and relaxation.
- Avoid constipation by increasing physical activity and consuming adequate fluids and fiber.
- Monitor for lactose intolerance, food allergies (chocolate, dairy products, wheat, yeast, and eggs have been cited), or gluten intolerance, and omit offending agents.
- Individualize diet management to the patient's symptoms. Alleviate pain, symptoms, and flatulence. Production of colonic gas, especially hydrogen, may be uncomfortable.

INTERVENTION: FOOD AND NUTRITION

- In acute phases, a low-fiber diet may be better tolerated. As treatment progresses, use adequate but not excessive fiber and ensure adequate fluid intake (30–35 cc/kg). Avoid high-fat foods, which may increase cholecystokinin release. Avoid high sugar intake, which increases osmolarity.
- Liberal amounts of fruits and vegetables are useful. Omit spicy foods or gas-forming oligosaccharides (beans, barley, Brussels sprouts, cabbage, nuts, figs, and soybeans), if not tolerated.
- Omit milk, if lactose is not tolerated. Add calcium in other forms. Some patients benefit from exclusion of wheat, beef, lamb, and pork (Zar et al, 2005).
- In patients with celiac disease, omit gluten. Be aware that supplementation of B-complex vitamins may be needed.

CLINICAL INDICATORS

Clinical/History	Lower GI x-rays	H & H
Height	Colonoscopy	Serum Fe
Weight	**Lab Work**	Alb, transthyretin
Weight changes	Serum IgG4 antibody titers to wheat, beef, pork, and lamb (elevated)	CRP
BMI	CRP	Gluc
Diet history		Na+, K+
Stool consistency and number		Ca++, Mg++
Abdominal pain		Hydrogen breath test
Urgency for defecation		

SAMPLE NUTRITION DIAGNOSTIC STATEMENT

Irritable Bowel Syndrome

PES: Altered GI function (constipation) related to undesirable food choices as evidenced by inadequate fiber and fluid intake and excessive intake of refined CHOs.

Assessment Data: Diet history with nutrient analysis of fiber, fluid, and CHOs; family history and medication/food allergies; bowel patterns.

Intervention: Educate about self-monitoring, role of fiber and fluid, probiotics, prebiotics, bioactive substances.

Monitoring and Evaluation: Dietary and fluid intake changes; changes in bowel patterns.

Common Drugs Used and Potential Side Effects

- Moderately severe diarrheal symptoms respond to loperamide (Imodium) and 5-HT3 receptor antagonists (Hadley and Gaardner, 2005; Spiller, 2005a). Cilansetron is a novel serotonin 5-HT3 receptor antagonist currently being evaluated for IBS diarrhea (Chey and Cash, 2005).
- Constipation responds to serotonin-4 receptor (5-HT4) agonists (Spiller, 2005a). Tegaserod (Zelnorm) given as 6 mg twice daily appears to be safe, well tolerated, and effective in the treatment of non–IBS-D over 8 weeks (Fried et al, 2005). Diarrhea is one side effect.
- Antispasmodics may have limited benefit in treating pain (Spiller, 2005a). Anticholinergic and other side effects limit their use in some patients (Hadley and Gaardner, 2005).
- Antidepressants have been shown to relieve pain and may be effective in low doses (Hadley and Gaardner, 2005).
- Low-dose tricyclic antidepressants are helpful in alleviating anxiety (Spiller, 2005a; Jackson et al, 2000; Olden and Drossman, 2000). If antianxiety medications such as Xanax are used, abdominal pain, nausea and vomiting, and weight changes may result.
- Methylcellulose (Metamucil) and other bulking agents always must be taken with large amounts of water. Generally, 1 tablespoon is sufficient per day. Increased peristalsis occurs.
- Probiotics such as acidophilus and yogurt in the diet may be useful. A double-blind, randomized, placebo-controlled study identified that *Bifidobacterium infantis* provides relief from IBS (Spiller, 2005b).
- Speculative therapeutic approaches include anti-inflammatory agents, antibiotics, antagonists of CCK1 receptors, tachykinins, and other novel neuronal receptors (Farthing, 2004).
- Naltrexone may also be helpful.

Herbs, Botanicals, and Supplements

- Herbs and botanical supplements should not be used without discussing with the physician.
- Herbal therapies such as peppermint oil also may be effective in the treatment of IBS (Hadley and Gaardner, 2005).
- Yogurt and other cultured foods may not be as effective as specific probiotics with high concentrations of microbes, but they may be well tolerated and are good sources of nutrients.

INTERVENTION: NUTRITION EDUCATION, COUNSELING, CARE MANAGEMENT

- Slowly increase dietary fiber to prevent discomfort. Large servings of bran may aggravate IBS; assess individually.
- Explain that regular times for bowel evacuation should be planned.
- Ensure the patient has adequate food intake and is not afraid to eat because of potential pain.
- Refer the patient for stress management, if needed. Patients with rapidly cycling symptoms may need further psychological evaluation (Tillisch et al, 2005).
- A food diary may help to identify any food sensitivities.
- Regular exercise is important.
- To prevent intestinal gas from forming, try Beano and other products available on the market.

Patient Education—Foodborne Illness

- Careful food handling and hand washing are important to prevent introduction of foodborne pathogens to the individual who may be experiencing diarrhea and related discomfort.

For More Information

- American College of Gastroenterology–IBS
  http://www.acg.gi.org/patients/ibsrelief/
- National Digestive Diseases Information Clearinghouse
  http://digestive.niddk.nih.gov/ddiseases/pubs/ibs_ez/
  http://digestive.niddk.nih.gov/ddiseases/pubs/ibs_ez/IBS.pdf

IRRITABLE BOWEL SYNDROME—CITED REFERENCES

American College of Gastroenterology. Irritable bowel syndrome resource center. Accessed October 31, 2005 at http://www.acg.gi.org/patients/ibsrelief/.

Chey WD, Cash BD. Cilansetron: a new serotonergic agent for the irritable bowel syndrome with diarrhoea. *Expert Opin Investig Drugs.* 14:185, 2005.

Farthing MJ. Treatment options in irritable bowel syndrome. *Best Pract Res Clin Gastroenterol.* 18:773, 2004.

Floch MH. Use of diet and probiotic therapy in the irritable bowel syndrome: analysis of the literature. *J Clin Gastroenterol.* 39:243S, 2005.

Fried M, et al. Tegaserod is safe, well tolerated and effective in the treatment of patients with non-diarrhoea irritable bowel syndrome. *Eur J Gastroenterol Hepatol.* 17:421, 2005.

Goldstein R, et al. Carbohydrate malabsorption and the effect of dietary restriction on symptoms of irritable bowel syndrome and functional bowel complaints. *Isr Med Assoc.* 2:583, 2000.

Hadley SK, Gaardner SM. Treatment of irritable bowel syndrome. *Am Fam Physician.* 72:2501, 2005.

Jackson J, et al. Treatment of functional gastrointestinal disorders with antidepressant medications: a meta-analysis. *Am J Med.* 108:65, 2000.

Lacy BE, Lee RD. Irritable bowel syndrome: a syndrome in evolution. *J Clin Gastroenterol.* 39:S230, 2005.

Locke G, et al. Familial association in adults with functional gastrointestinal disorders. *Mayo Clin Proc.* 75:907, 2000.

Olden K, Drossman D. Psychologic and psychiatric aspects of gastrointestinal disease. *Med Clin North Am.* 84:131, 2000.

Spiller RC. Irritable bowel syndrome. *Br Med Bull.* 72:15, 2005a.

Spiller RC. Probiotics: an ideal anti-inflammatory treatment for IBS? *Gastroenterology* 128:783, 2005b.

Su Y, et al. The association between *Helicobacter pylori* infection and functional dyspepsia in patients with irritable bowel syndrome. *Am J Gastroenterol.* 95:1900, 2000.

Tillisch K, et al. Characterization of the alternating bowel habit subtype in patients with irritable bowel syndrome. *Am J Gastroenterol.* 100:896, 2005.

Zar S, et al. Food-specific serum IgG4 and IgE titers to common food antigens in irritable bowel syndrome. *Am J Gastroenterol.* 100:1550, 2005.

LACTOSE MALABSORPTION (LACTASE DEFICIENCY)

NUTRITIONAL ACUITY RANKING: LEVEL 2–3

DEFINITIONS AND BACKGROUND

Lactose is a disaccharide (glucose-l galactose) found in milk. If lactase enzyme is missing, lactose passes into the colon, where it is fermented to gases and organic acids by colonic bacteria, resulting in bloating, cramping, nausea, or diarrhea.

Lactase "nonpersistence" is common. A staggering 4000 million people cannot digest lactose properly (Campbell et al, 2005). As many as 75% of all African American, Jewish, Native American, and Mexican American adults and 90% of Asian American adults are lactose intolerant; it is least common among people of northern European descent (American Gastrointestinal Association, 2005).

Symptoms caused by lactose maldigestion need not hinder ingestion of a diet rich in dairy products that supplies around 1500 mg calcium daily (i.e., 2 cups of milk, 1 cup of yogurt, and several ounces of cheese). Bloating, abdominal pain, diarrhea, and overall symptom severity are often tolerable. Decreases in breath hydrogen suggest that colonic adaptation to the high-lactose diet occurs over several weeks of intakes of 1200 mg calcium and 33 g lactose (Pribela et al, 2000).

Celiac disease can lead to lactase deficiency and is more common than previously recognized (Ojetti et al, 2005). An increased prevalence of lactose intolerance is often seen in patients with irritable bowel syndrome, but this may be related to small intestinal bacterial overgrowth more than actual lactose intolerance (Pimentel et al, 2003). In addition, fructose intolerance may be unrecognized, and testing should clarify which disaccharide is poorly tolerated rather than assuming it is always lactose (Choi et al, 2003).

Lactose maldigestion should not be a contradiction in developing adequate-calcium diets in susceptible populations. Pregnant women who are lactose intolerant, for example, are not better able to tolerate lactose during gestation and should be given appropriate counseling about intake of calcium from nonlactose sources (Paige et al, 2003).

Individuals who are self-described as lactose intolerant may restrict dairy and calcium intake and are at greater risk of osteoporosis and bone fractures (Savaiano, 2003). Lactose maldigesters can consume up to 1 cup (8 oz) of milk without experiencing symptoms; tolerance can be improved by consuming the milk with a meal, choosing yogurt or hard cheeses, or using products that aid in the digestion of lactose such as lactase supplements or lactose-reduced milks (Byers and Savaiano, 2005). The American Dietetic Association recommends at least three medical nutrition therapy visits for adults who have lactose maldigestion; Table 7-19 describes the various types of this condition.

INTERVENTION: OBJECTIVES

- Manage pain and discomfort related to lactose ingestion that is caused by flatulence and bloating or diarrhea. Control lactose intake, which composes 10% of the carbohydrate found in the American diet.
- Regular consumption of milk by lactase-deficient persons may improve colonic tolerance. Check for actual tolerance by monitoring intake. Most people can tolerate 1/2 cup milk (6 g of lactose) with a meal over time, if not immediately. Whole milk may be better tolerated than skim because it slows gastric emptying more effectively.
- Offer calcium and riboflavin from other foods and sources besides lactose-containing dairy products.

INTERVENTION: FOOD AND NUTRITION

- Most people can tolerate up to 6 g of lactose, which is found in 4 oz of milk. If small amounts are gradually added over approximately 3 months, most adults can ultimately adapt to 121 g/d, equal to one 8-oz glass of regular milk.
- Dairy foods contain approximately 1–8% lactose by weight (milk, 4–5%; yogurt, 4%; ice cream, 3–4%; milk chocolate, 8%; cottage cheese, 1–2%). Because symptoms are related to dose, consume no more than 8 oz of lactose-containing milk at a time after other foods have been consumed to slow down transit time. See Table 7-20.
- Lactase supplements (e.g., Lactaid, Lactrase, Dairy Ease) may be taken 30 minutes before the consumption of a lactose-containing product. Two capsules provide enough lactase to hydrolyze the lactose in an 8-oz glass of whole milk. Lactose-hydrolyzed milk is generally tolerated for other meals. Note that not all preparations are equally effective.

TABLE 7-19 Types of Lactose Malabsorption

Type	Description	Incidence
Congenital, primary, or genetic	Rare, present at birth	Low incidence in children
Lactase "nonpersistence" or hypolactasia	Lactase decline, often to about 10% of neonatal values	Occurs after weaning; more common in adults
Secondary or acquired	From gastrointestinal disease, food allergy, antibiotics, or intestinal trauma	May occur in children after diarrhea, giardiasis, or HIV infection; more than one third of pediatric patients with inflammatory bowel disease have lactase deficiency (Pfefferkorn et al, 2002)

TABLE 7-20 Lactose in Common Foods

Food and Portion	Lactose (g)
Milk, reduced fat, 1 cup	11–14
Buttermilk, 1 cup	10
Yogurt, whole milk, 1 cup	10–12
Ice cream, ½ cup	5–6
Yogurt, plain, low fat, 1 cup	5–19
Sour cream, ½ cup	4
Cottage cheese, ½ cup	3–4
Swiss cheese, 1 oz	1
Cream cheese, 1 oz	1

- Persons on a lactose-free diet can use lactate, casein (curds), lactalbumin, and calcium. If the patient is highly sensitive, check labels of foods for fillers, whey protein, milk, whey solids, and milk solids; most people can tolerate small amounts in mashed potatoes, breads, and medications. Processed cheese or cheese foods may have nonfat dry milk solids; use in moderate amounts.
- If tolerated, fermented products (buttermilk, natural or aged cheese, yogurt with active cultures, cottage cheese, or sour cream) can be used. Yogurt with active cultures may be better tolerated than milk by many individuals. Frozen yogurt has little or no lactase activity.
- For infants with the condition, try milk-free formulas; gradually introduce foods that contain milk or lactose to test for tolerance.

CLINICAL INDICATORS

Clinical/History	Lab Work	
Height	Alb, transthyretin	H & H
Weight	BUN, Creat	Serum Fe
BMI	Ca++ (better absorption can occur over time)	Na+, K+
Weight changes	Mg++	Hydrogen breath test (3–5 hours)
Lactose challenge test	Alk phos	Stool acidity test
Genetic test of C/T(-13910) polymorphism	Gluc	

Common Drugs Used and Potential Side Effects

- Many drugs contain lactose but seldom over 500 mg. Most should be well tolerated.

Herbs, Botanicals, and Supplements

- Probiotics (such as lactobacilli and bifidobacteria) and prebiotics (nondigestible oligosaccharides) assist in alleviating lactose intolerance and improving calcium absorption (Doron and Gorbach, 2006; Hamilton-Miller, 2004).
- Herbs and botanical supplements should not be used without discussing with the physician.

SAMPLE NUTRITION DIAGNOSTIC STATEMENT

Lactose Intolerance

PES: Undesirable food choices related to limited adherence to nutrition-related recommendations as evidenced by recent use of dairy products and complaints of abdominal pain and diarrhea.

Assessment Data (sources of info): Food diary and records with analysis of grams of lactose consumed on average day, stool frequency, and GI complaint reports.

Intervention: Counseling on lactose-restricted diet, use of LactAid and lactose-reduced products in meals and in cooking.

Monitoring and Evaluation: Food records and reports of GI distress or diarrhea after diet alterations have been implemented consistently for at least 7 days.

INTERVENTION: NUTRITION EDUCATION, COUNSELING, CARE MANAGEMENT

- Identify foods that are lactose free and foods that are lactose-free sources of calcium. Reading labels will be helpful. Store-bought cookies, cakes, bread, baked goods, cereals, instant potatoes, soups, margarine, lunch meat, salad dressings, pancakes, biscuits, and candy may contain lactose.
- The patient must become a label reader looking for and avoiding "milk" and "lactose." In addition, foods that contain butter, cheese, cream, milk or milk solids, powdered milk, and whey will contain lactose.
- Home-cooked meals and recipes may be useful. Recipes are available for use of lactose-free formulas in products such as meat loaf.
- Pregnant women who are lactose intolerant should take a calcium supplement.
- Advise that heating of milk does not change lactose.
- Kosher foods are often acceptable if they are pareve (nonmilk, nonmeat).
- Discuss how to use LactAid drops to allow the enzyme to hydrolyze the lactose.
- Drink milk with meals rather than alone to decrease symptoms.

Patient Education—Foodborne Illness

- Careful food handling and hand washing are important to prevent introduction of foodborne pathogens to the individual who may be experiencing diarrhea and related discomfort.

For More Information

- Dairy-Ease
  http://www.dairyease.com/

- Lactose-Free Diet
  http://www.gicare.com/pated/edtgs05.htm
- Lactose Intolerance
  http://digestive.niddk.nih.gov/ddiseases/pubs/lactoseintolerance/
  http://www.lactose.co.uk/
  http://www.gicare.com/pated/ecdgs24.htm
- LactAid (McNeil Consumer Products)
  http://www.lactaid.com/
- National Institute of Diabetes and Digestive and Kidney Diseases (NIDDK)
  http://digestive.niddk.nih.gov/ddiseases/pubs/lactoseintolerance_ez/#food

LACTOSE MALABSORPTION—CITED REFERENCES

American Gastrointestinal Association. Lactose intolerance. Accessed March 25, 2005 at http://www.gastro.org/wmspage.cfm?parm1=854.

Byers KG, Savaiano DA. The myth of increased lactose intolerance in African-Americans. *J Am Coll Nutr.* 24:569S, 2005.

Campbell AK, et al. The molecular basis of lactose intolerance. *Sci Prog.* 88:157, 2005.

Choi YK, et al. Fructose intolerance: an under-recognized problem. *Am J Gastroenterol.* 98:1348, 2003.

Doron S, Gorbach SL. Probiotics: their role in the treatment and prevention of disease. *Expert Rev Anti Infect Ther.* 4:261, 2006.

Hamilton-Miller JM. Probiotics and prebiotics in the elderly. *Postgrad Med J.* 80:447, 2004.

Ojetti V, et al. High prevalence of celiac disease in patients with lactose intolerance. *Digestion* 71:106, 2005.

Paige DM, et al. Lactose digestion in pregnant African-Americans. *Public Health Nutr.* 6:801, 2003.

Pfefferkorn MD, et al. Lactase deficiency: not more common in pediatric patients with inflammatory bowel disease than in patients with chronic abdominal pain. *J Pediatr Gastroenterol Nutr.* 35:339, 2002.

Pimentel M, et al. Breath testing to evaluate lactose intolerance in irritable bowel syndrome correlates with lactulose testing and may not reflect true lactose malabsorption. *Am J Gastroenterol.* 98:2700, 2003.

Pribela B, et al. Improved lactose digestion and intolerance among African-American adolescent girls fed a dairy-rich diet. *J Am Diet Assoc.* 100:524, 2000.

Savaiano D. Lactose intolerance: a self-fulfilling prophecy leading to osteoporosis? *Nutr Rev.* 61:221, 2003.

MEGACOLON

NUTRITIONAL ACUITY RANKING: LEVEL 3

DEFINITIONS AND BACKGROUND

Acquired megacolon is a chronic disease associated with constipation and malnutrition and possibly surgical intervention (Vieira et al, 1996). The enlarged bowel results from an abnormal colonic dilatation often reaching 8–10 cm in diameter. It is often present in elderly persons who have a long history of elimination problems created by laxative abuse or constipation. Persons with diabetes, hypothyroidism, scleroderma, multiple sclerosis, electrolyte imbalances, tumor, strictures, and other conditions may be affected. Family physicians must be alert for the presence of uncommon but serious causes of constipation, such as megacolon (Biggs and Dery, 2006).

Signs and symptoms of megacolon involve abdominal distention, flatus, absence of stool, smearing or bowel incontinence, nausea, anorexia, fatigue, and headache. Note that the colon provides reabsorption of water and electrolytes as well as elimination of waste and regulation of bacterial homeostasis; motility is crucial for these roles. Normal urges to defecate are affected by physical activity, neurological status, chemical/drug use, and bowel condition. Normal reflexes are needed for muscular and sphincter control.

Nitric oxide production modulates cholinergic nerve-mediated contractions in normal colonic circular muscle; acquired megacolon is associated with altered release of this neurochemical, and the reasons are not clear (Koch et al, 2000). For toxic megacolon, subtotal colectomy with ileostomy remains the procedure of choice (Ausch et al, 2006; Gladman et al, 2005).

INTERVENTION: OBJECTIVES

- Prevent complications such as lung atelectasis from distention, sepsis, ulceration with hemorrhage or perforation, or sigmoid volvulus.
- Normalize bowel function as much as possible. Evaluate bowel pattern by history and at present, including drug use and abuse (laxatives, etc.).
- Identify and correct any nutrient deficiencies, electrolyte imbalances, or protein–energy malnutrition.

INTERVENTION: FOOD AND NUTRITION

- Use adequate fluid and fiber, pending status and other conditions (such as heart failure). Prune juice added to hot cereal may help normalize bowel function. If raw fruits and vegetables are not tolerated at first, add over time.
- Avoid excesses of refined foods and concentrated sweets to the exclusion of desirable foods.
- Tube feeding deserves consideration in selected patients. Nutritional status tends to improve after surgery, with normalization of bowel function (Vieira et al, 1996).

CLINICAL INDICATORS

Clinical/History		
Height	Barium x-rays	Serum Fe
Weight	Abdominal girth	Na+, K+, Cl−
BMI	Stool consistency	Ca++, Mg++
Diet history	**Lab Work**	Thyroid function
Stool pattern	BUN, Creat	Stool guaiac
BP	Gluc	
I & O	H & H	
Endoscopy		

Common Drugs Used and Potential Side Effects

- Anticholinergics, opiates, and antidepressants may increase or aggravate constipation. Watch use carefully.
- Suppositories and stool softeners may be used or may have been used excessively. Monitor specific medications accordingly and their side effects.

Herbs, Botanicals, and Supplements

- Herbs and botanical supplements should not be used without discussing with the physician.

INTERVENTION: NUTRITION EDUCATION, COUNSELING, CARE MANAGEMENT

- Discuss the role of exercise in maintaining normal bowel function.
- Discuss the role of fluid and fiber in bowel regularity. For example, drinking a cup of hot prune juice may be effective for some patients.
- Inclusion of probiotic foods such as yogurt with active cultures, lactobacilli and bifidobacteria, and prebiotics (nondigestible oligosaccharides) may be beneficial for gut integrity.

For More Information

- Acquired Megacolon
  http://www.emedicine.com/med/byname/megacolon-chronic.htm

MEGACOLON—CITED REFERENCES

Ausch C, et al. Aetiology and surgical management of toxic megacolon. *Colorectal Dis.* 8:195, 2006.

Biggs WS, Dery WH. Evaluation and treatment of constipation in infants and children. *Am Fam Physician.* 73:469, 2006.

Gladman MA, et al. Systematic review of surgical options for idiopathic megarectum and megacolon. *Ann Surg.* 241:562, 2005.

Koch TR, et al. Nitric oxide production is diminished in colonic circular muscle from acquired megacolon. *Dis Colon Rectum.* 43:821, 2000.

Vieira M, et al. Preoperative assessment in cases of adult megacolon suffering from moderate malnutrition. *Nutrition* 12:491, 1996.

OSTOMY: COLOSTOMY

NUTRITIONAL ACUITY RANKING: LEVEL 2–3

DEFINITIONS AND BACKGROUND

The colon functions primarily to absorb water and sodium and to excrete potassium and bicarbonate. A colostomy is an artificial outlet for intestinal wastes created surgically by bringing a portion of the colon through the abdominal wall, resulting in a stoma.

Colostomy can be permanent or temporary. It may be indicated for intestinal cancer, diverticulitis, perforated bowel, radiation enteritis, obstruction, and Hirschsprung's disease. While abdominoperineal resection, with iliac colostomy, remains the gold standard treatment for rectal cancer, it definitely alters quality of life, and new procedures are continually being sought (Portier et al, 2005). With proper patient selection, laparoscopic colorectal surgery can be performed without undue morbidity and mortality (Geisler et al, 2004). Figure 7-8 shows the colostomy procedure. Table 7-21 describes the common types of colostomies.

Colostomy output is generally more formed than ileostomy output. Some colostomates can "irrigate," using a procedure similar to an enema to clean stool directly out of the colon through the stoma. This requires special irrigation appliances: an irrigation bag and a connecting tube (or catheter), a stoma cone, and an irrigation sleeve. A special lubricant is sometimes used on the stoma in preparation for irrigation. Following irrigation, some colostomates can use a stoma cap, a one- or two-piece system that simply covers and protects the stoma. This procedure is usually done to avoid the need to wear an appliance.

INTERVENTION: OBJECTIVES

- To avoid major problems of blockage, increased flatulence, and problems with certain foods, preoperative teaching and postoperative follow-up must include anticipatory guidance on food selection (Floruta, 2001).

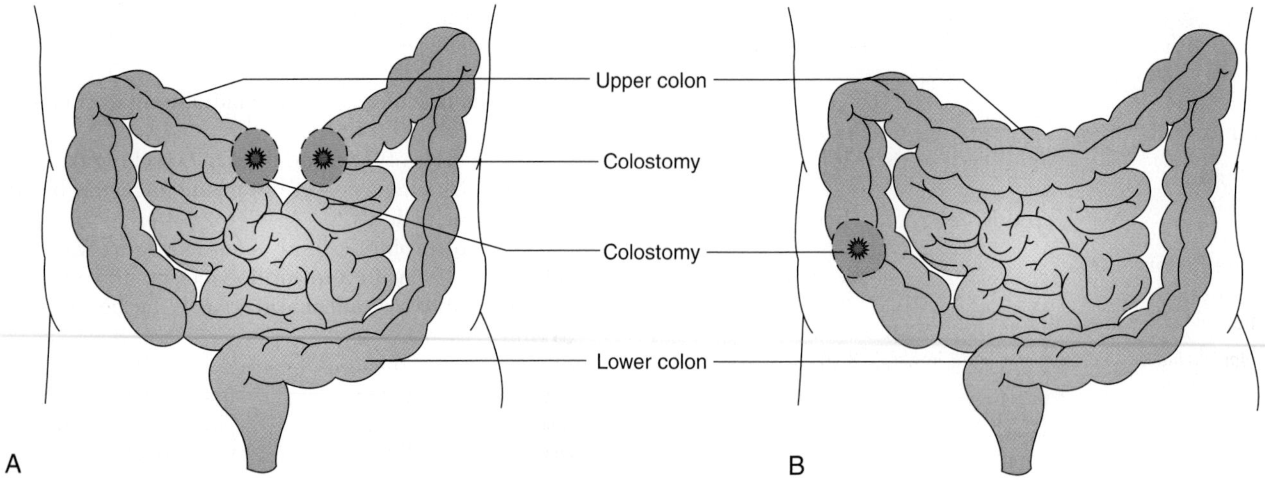

Figure 7-8 Colostomy. (From Pillitteri A. *Maternal and child nursing*. 4th ed. Philadelphia: Lippincott Williams & Wilkins, 2003.)

- Speed wound healing and recovery.
- Prevent weight loss. Correct malnutrition from GI blood loss, anemia, protein malabsorption, and steatorrhea.
- Prevent watery or unscheduled bowel movements. Correct or prevent dehydration.
- Individualize the diet: Eat regularly, avoid odor-causing foods, and monitor food preferences. Normalize the patient's lifestyle as much as possible.
- Avoid infection and skin irritants.

TABLE 7-21 Common Types of Colostomies

Colostomy Type	Description
Temporary Colostomy	Allows the lower portion of the colon to rest or heal. It may have one or two openings (if two, one will discharge only mucus).
Permanent Colostomy	Usually involves the loss of part of the colon, most commonly the rectum. The end of the remaining portion of the colon is brought out to the abdominal wall to form the stoma.
Sigmoid or Descending Colostomy	The most common type of ostomy surgery, in which the end of the descending or sigmoid colon is brought to the surface of the abdomen. It is usually located on the lower left side of the abdomen.
Transverse Colostomy	The surgical opening created in the transverse colon resulting in one or two openings. It is located in the upper abdomen, middle or right side.
Loop Colostomy	Usually created in the transverse colon. This is one stoma with two openings; one discharges stool, the second discharges mucus.
Ascending Colostomy	A relatively rare opening in the ascending portion of the colon. It is located on the right side of the abdomen.

Source: United Ostomy Association, Inc. What is ostomy? Accessed March 31, 2005 at http://www.uoa.org/ostomy_main.htm.

INTERVENTION: FOOD AND NUTRITION

- Early oral feeding in the patients undergoing colorectostomy is feasible, safe, and associated with reduced postoperative discomfort; it can accelerate the return of bowel function and improve rehabilitation (Zhou et al, 2006). Progress from a liquid to a low-residue diet. To speed healing, the formula or diet should also be high in protein, energy, vitamins, and minerals.
- Diet should provide normal or increased salt intake. One to two quarts of fluid, taken between meals, should be ingested daily.
- Gradually introduce new foods; if done slowly, offending foods can be identified and obstruction can be controlled or prevented.
  - **Foods that may cause loose stools or diarrhea:** apple juice, prune juice, dried beans, chocolate, green beans, raw fruits and raw vegetables, fried foods, highly spiced foods, broccoli, and leafy green vegetables. **Foods that thicken stool:** applesauce, bananas, marshmallows, rice, pasta, peanut butter, tapioca, and yogurt.
  - **Odor-causing foods** include alcohol (beer), beans, onions, cabbage, broccoli, cauliflower, Brussels sprouts, fish, eggs, asparagus, and garlic. Fresh parsley is a natural deodorizer. Foods that cause **urinary odor** include asparagus and seafood. Beets and red gelatin can cause abnormal stool coloration.
  - **Gas-forming foods** include beans, beer, Brussels sprouts, broccoli, cabbage, corn, cucumbers, cauliflower, radishes, and spinach. Special products are on the market that can reduce flatulence.
- Progress to a high-fiber diet with short-fibered foods; avoid granola, bean sprouts, bamboo shoots, bran, whole-kernel corn, mushrooms, celery, nuts, pineapple, popcorn, coleslaw, apple skins, seeds, or coconut. Foods most often avoided because of an ostomy include fresh fruits and vegetables such as cabbage, beans, and onions (Floruta, 2001). Hot dogs and meats with casings may be a problem also.

SAMPLE NUTRITION DIAGNOSTIC STATEMENT

Ileostomy/Colostomy

PES: Inadequate fluid intake related to self-monitoring deficit as evidenced by output of 2 L/d via ileostomy and intake of only 1.5 L/d and hypernatremia.

Assessment Data: I & O records or food diary; lab values (Na+), weight fluctuations, hemoglobin.

Intervention: Educate about how to meet estimated fluid needs; how to track I & O; goals on fluid intake.

Monitoring and Evaluation: Fluid intake (I & O); weights, labs.

- If calcium oxalate stones develop after the colostomy, diet should provide a high-fluid intake. Restrict intake of oxalates from spinach, rhubarb, wild greens, coffee and tea, and chocolate.
- Signs of blockage include: almost constant spurt of highly watery stool, bloating, cramping, swelling around stoma, strong odor of stool, nausea, vomiting, and pain. Avoid eating solid food, and do not take any laxatives or stool softeners. Drink a hot, caffeinated beverage; try a hot bath; gently massage the abdomen; and apply a pouch that has a larger opening.

CLINICAL INDICATORS

Clinical/History

Height
Weight
BMI
Diet history
I & O, hydration status
Diarrhea or constipation
Renal stones?

Lab Work

H & H
Serum Fe
Na+, K+
Gluc
Alb, transthyretin
Ca++, Mg++
Chol, Trig
Transferrin, TIBC
Serum B_{12}
Serum folate
PT or INR

Common Drugs Used and Potential Side Effects

- Polyethylene glycol solution may be used for colostomy irrigation; it seems to be better than use of water alone (O'Bichere et al, 2004).
- Probiotics and prebiotics may be useful for return of gut immunity.
- Prednisone: Restrict excessive sodium intake. Monitor nitrogen, calcium, and potassium losses when used over a long period of time.
- Lomotil is a stool thickener and deodorizer; use plenty of fluids.
- Bulk-forming agents such psyllium (Metamucil) may be useful. Increased peristalsis occurs.

Herbs, Botanicals, and Supplements

- Herbs and botanical supplements should not be used without discussing with the physician.

INTERVENTION: NUTRITION EDUCATION, COUNSELING, CARE MANAGEMENT

- Approximately 6 weeks are required to acclimate the bowel to new procedures of irrigation. Enemas are used to wash the bowel up to the ileocecal valve (with 1000 mL of tap water). Constipation can occur with dehydration; therefore, adequate intake of fluid and fiber is important.
- Use of a commercial deodorant in the colostomy bag is preferred to eliminating highly flavored or nutrient-dense foods.
- Instruct the patient to eat slowly, chew foods well, and avoid swallowing air.
- Irrigations should not be performed when there is vomiting or diarrhea. Working with an enterostomal therapist can be helpful for more suggestions.
- Regular mealtimes should be encouraged.
- Reassurance is needed, without misleading the patient.
- Patients should limit intake of aspirin, NSAIDs, red meat, poultry, fish, some raw vegetables, and vitamin C prior to lab testing (American College of Physicians, 1997).

Patient Education—Foodborne Illness

- Careful food handling and hand washing are important to prevent introduction of foodborne pathogens to the individual who may be experiencing diarrhea and related discomfort.

For More Information

- British Colostomy Association
  http://www.bcass.org.uk/
- Colostomy
  http://www.shands.org/health/surgeries/100011.html#
- Colostomy for Cancer Treatments
  http://www.cancer.org/docroot/MIT/content/MIT_7_2X_Special_Aspects_Of_Some_Cancer_Treatments_Men.asp
- United Ostomy Association (UOA)
  http://www.uoa.org/ostomy_main.htm

OSTOMY: COLOSTOMY—CITED REFERENCES

American College of Physicians. Clinical guideline: Part 1. Suggested technique for fecal occult blood testing and interpretation in colorectal cancer screening. *Ann Intern Med.* 126:808, 1997.

Floruta C. Dietary choices of people with ostomies. *J Wound Ostomy Continence Nurs.* 28:28, 2001.

Geisler D, et al. Laparoscopic colorectal surgery in the irradiated pelvis. *Am J Surg.* 188:267, 2004.

O'Bichere A, et al. Randomized cross-over trial of polyethylene glycol electrolyte solution and water for colostomy irrigation. *Dis Colon Rectum.* 47:1506, 2004.

Portier G, et al. Use of malone antegrade continence enema in patients with perineal colostomy after rectal resection. *Dis Colon Rectum.* 48:499, 2005.

Zhou T, et al. Early removing gastrointestinal decompression and early oral feeding improve patients' rehabilitation after colorectostomy. *World J Gastroenterol.* 2:2459, 2006.

OSTOMY: ILEOSTOMY

NUTRITIONAL ACUITY RANKING: LEVEL 3

DEFINITIONS AND BACKGROUND

Used to treat intractable cases of ulcerative disease, Crohn's disease, polyposis, and colon cancer, an ileostomy is a surgical procedure (stoma/opening formation) that brings the ileum through the abdominal wall. It may be temporary or permanent. This procedure causes a decrease in fat, bile acid, and vitamin B_{12} absorption, as well as greater losses of sodium and potassium.

Patients will be incontinent of gas and stool. Ideally, the ileocecal valve can be kept to decrease bacterial influx into the small intestine. Of these patients, 50–70% will have recurrent disease. Effective ostomy management is important and involves establishment of an effective system for managing altered dietary and fluid intake, maintaining fluid and electrolyte balance, and preventing food blockage (Doughty, 2005).

Subtotal colectomy with ileostomy remains a safe and effective treatment for patients requiring urgent surgery (Hyman et al, 2005). Interval ileal pouch–anal anastomosis reconstruction without a stoma after colectomy equals the more traditional protocol in terms of clinical outcome but yields lower hospital costs and probably a shorter length of hospital stay (Swenson et al, 2005). Table 7-22 describes the procedures for ileostomy.

TABLE 7-22 Ileostomy Procedures

Procedure	Description
Ileoanal Anastomosis	This is now the most common alternative to the conventional ileostomy. Technically, it is not an ostomy since there is no stoma. In this procedure, the colon and most of the rectum are surgically removed, and an internal pouch is formed out of the terminal portion of the ileum. An opening at the bottom of this pouch is attached to the anus such that the existing anal sphincter muscles can be used for continence. This procedure should only be performed on patients with ulcerative colitis or familial polyposis and who have not previously lost their rectum or anus. It is also called J-pouch, pull-thru, endorectal pullthrough, pelvic pouch, or a combination of these terms.
Continent Ileostomy	This surgical variation of the ileostomy is also called a **Kock pouch**. A reservoir pouch is created inside the abdomen with a portion of the terminal ileum. A valve is constructed in the pouch, and a stoma is brought through the abdominal wall. A catheter or tube is inserted into the pouch several times a day to drain feces from the reservoir. This procedure has generally been replaced in popularity by the ileoanal pouch (Regimbeau et al, 2001). A modified version of this procedure called the Barnett continent ileal reservoir is performed at a limited number of facilities.

Source: United Ostomy Association, Inc. What is ostomy? Accessed March 31, 2005 at http://www.uoa.org/ostomy_main.htm.

INTERVENTION: OBJECTIVES

- Modify the diet to counteract malabsorption of nutrients secondary to diarrhea, protein and fluid losses, negative nitrogen balance from nutrient loss, and anorexia.
- Correct anemia caused by inadequate intake or blood losses.
- Counteract weakness and muscle cramping from potassium losses.
- Counteract increased energy requirements if there is fever or infection.
- Replenish calcium to reverse losses caused by steatorrhea and the bone density loss as side effects of steroid therapy.
- Prevent gallstones, renal oxalate stones, bacterial overgrowth, and fatty acid malabsorption.

INTERVENTION: FOOD AND NUTRITION

- **Preoperatively:** Fiber and lactose intolerances are common; alter diet accordingly. With strictures, avoid popcorn, nuts, seeds, mushrooms, celery, fruit skins, and vegetable skins. Have the patient chew thoroughly.
- **Postoperatively:** Provide a high-energy, high-protein diet for wound healing that is low in excess insoluble fiber. Avoid the high-fiber foods suggested for preoperative care for about 4 weeks. Pectin in apples and oligosaccharides in oatmeal may be beneficial to add back first. Spinach or parsley are natural intestinal deodorizers, but beware of excesses of oxalate-rich foods.
- The patient needs an adequate intake of protein (provided by low-fat sources such as lean meats and egg white), vitamin B_{12} (provided by liver, fish, and eggs), folacin, calcium, magnesium, iron, sodium, vitamin C, and potassium. Add salt as needed to the diet.
- Diet should provide an adequate amount of fluids, especially in hot weather.
- Since obesity can cause more discomfort, a long-range weight management plan may be useful.

CLINICAL INDICATORS

Clinical/History	Lab Work	
Height	H & H	TIBC
Weight	Serum Fe	Gluc
BMI	BUN, Creat	WBC
Diet history	Na+, K+	Ca++, Mg++
Stool (occult blood)	Alb, transthyretin	Serum B_{12}
BP	Transferrin	Schilling test if needed
		Serum folate

Common Drugs Used and Potential Side Effects

- Corticosteroids: With prednisone, restrict excessive sodium intake and monitor nitrogen and calcium losses. The corticosteroid budesonide (Entocort) may be administered to increase the absorptive capacity of the intestinal mucosa in patients with ileostomies (Ecker et al, 2005). Side effects may include increased appetite and weight gain, hypokalemia, and elevated CRP.
- Lomotil: This drug is a stool thickener and deodorizer. Plenty of fluids should be used.
- Use of probiotics and prebiotics may be useful to help with recovery of gut immunity.
- Psyllium (Metamucil) is used as a bulk-forming agent. Increased peristalsis will occur.

Herbs, Botanicals, and Supplements

- Herbs and botanical supplements should not be used without discussing with the physician.

INTERVENTION: NUTRITION EDUCATION, COUNSELING, CARE MANAGEMENT

- Explain which foods are common sources of the needed nutrients in a diet or suggest supplementation with multivitamins and minerals.
- Monitor individual tolerance to offending foods such as gas-forming or fried foods, highly seasoned foods, nuts, raisins, and pineapple. Patients may prefer to avoid odor-causing foods such as legumes, cheese, onions, eggs, fish, cabbage, and cruciferous vegetables. Gas-forming foods may include dried beans and peas, carbonated beverages, cabbage, onions, cucumbers, spinach, and broccoli. Foods that may cause rapid intestinal transit or discomfort may include dried fruits, prune juice, fresh strawberries or peaches, coconut, nuts, seeds, cabbage, celery, bamboo shoots, corn, and milk.
- An enterostomal therapist may be of assistance.
- Discuss replacement of fluid and sodium, especially during hot weather.
- Eating before bedtime should be avoided to lessen discomfort.

Patient Education—Foodborne Illness

- Careful food handling and hand washing are important to prevent introduction of foodborne pathogens to the individual who may be experiencing diarrhea and related discomfort.

For More Information

- Ileostomy
  http://digestive.niddk.nih.gov/ddiseases/pubs/ileostomy/
  http://www.uoa.org/ostomy_facts_ileostomy.htm
  http://www.gicare.com/pated/ecdgs11.htm
- Probiotics
  http://www.about-probiotics.org
- United Ostomy Association (UOA)
  http://www.uoa.org/

OSTOMY: ILEOSTOMY—CITED REFERENCES

Doughty D. Principles of ostomy management in the oncology patient. *J Support Oncol.* 3:59, 2005.
Ecker KW, et al. Long-term treatment of high intestinal output syndrome with budesonide in patients with Crohn's disease and ileostomy. *Dis Colon Rectum.* 48:237, 2005.
Hyman NH, et al. Urgent subtotal colectomy for severe inflammatory bowel disease. *Dis Colon Rectum.* 48:70, 2005.
Regimbeau J, et al. Long-term results of ileal pouch-anal anastomosis for colorectal Crohn's disease. *Dis Colon Rectum.* 44:769, 2001.
Swenson BR, et al. Modified two-stage ileal pouch-anal anastomosis: equivalent outcomes with less resource utilization. *Dis Colon Rectum.* 48:256, 2005.

PERITONITIS

NUTRITIONAL ACUITY RANKING: LEVEL 2

DEFINITIONS AND BACKGROUND

In peritonitis, inflammation of the peritoneal cavity due to infiltration of intestinal contents occurs. Contents from such conditions as ruptured appendix, gastric or intestinal perforation, trauma, fistula, anastomotic leaks, or failure in peritoneal dialysis may initiate the problem.

Spontaneous bacterial peritonitis is a common illness in patients with cirrhosis and ascites that occurs related to bacterial translocation; the gut is a major source of these bacteria (Ramachandran and Balasubramanian, 2001). Sclerosing peritonitis (SP) is a manifestation of chronic allograft failure in liver transplantation; its presence may suggest chronic rejection (Macedo et al, 2005).

INTERVENTION: OBJECTIVES

- Provide bowel rest and recovery.
- Improve nutritional status, especially if patient has been malnourished over a period of time or if there is anorexia or ileus.
- Correct dehydration and fluid/electrolyte imbalances when present.

INTERVENTION: FOOD AND NUTRITION

- Patient generally is NPO with intravenous feedings for at least 24 hours. Progress as tolerated to a soft or general diet appropriate for the condition that caused the peritonitis originally.
- Increase protein intake to correct catabolic state. Increase calories because basal energy expenditure is generally elevated by 10–17%.

CLINICAL INDICATORS

Clinical/History		
Height	X-rays	Gluc
Weight	Laparoscopy	Alb, transthyretin
BMI	**Lab Work**	CRP
Diet history	H & H	Na+, K+
Temperature	Serum Fe	Ca++, Mg++
BP	WBC	TLC
I & O	BUN, Creat	

Common Drugs Used and Potential Side Effects

- Ciprofloxacin is effective in the treatment of serious, non–self-limiting intra-abdominal infections and peritonitis from continuous ambulatory peritoneal dialysis (CAPD) (Finch, 2000).
- Other antibiotics are used for bacterial peritonitis. Monitor for specific side effects. Probiotics may be useful; research continues in this area.

Herbs, Botanicals, and Supplements

- Herbs and botanical supplements should not be used without discussing with the physician.

INTERVENTION: NUTRITION EDUCATION, COUNSELING, CARE MANAGEMENT

- With patients on CAPD, diet may need to be altered similar to the diet typical for renal patients.
- Discuss diet appropriate for the illness of origin (such as diabetes, hypertension, toxemia, or renal disease).

Patient Education—Foodborne Illness

- Careful food handling and hand washing are important to prevent introduction of foodborne pathogens to the individual.

For More Information

- Peritonitis
  http://www.nlm.nih.gov/medlineplus/ency/article/001335.htm
  http://en.wikipedia.org/wiki/Peritonitis

PERITONITIS—CITED REFERENCES

Finch R. Ciprofloxacin: efficacy and indications. *J Chemother.* 12:5S, 2000.

Macedo C, et al. Sclerosing peritonitis after intestinal transplantation in children. *Pediatr Transplant.* 9:187, 2005.

Ramachandran A, Balasubramanian K. Intestinal dysfunction in liver cirrhosis: its role in spontaneous bacterial peritonitis. *J Gastroenterol Hepatol.* 16:607, 2001.

SHORT BOWEL SYNDROME

NUTRITIONAL ACUITY RANKING: LEVEL 4

DEFINITIONS AND BACKGROUND

Short bowel syndrome (SBS) is the predominant cause of intestinal failure and is associated with a high degree of morbidity and mortality (Jackson and Buchman, 2004). Intestinal failure involves reduction of gut mass below the minimal amount needed for nutrient absorption. SBS involves surgical resection of a portion of the small bowel, compromising the absorptive surface and resulting in malabsorption (especially if more than 50% of the small intestine has been removed).

Malnutrition from maldigestion, malabsorption diarrhea, and steatorrhea may result. A bowel resection that results in SBS may be due to Crohn's disease, intestinal cancer, scleroderma, or fistula in adults; or it may be due to necrotizing enterocolitis, intestinal atresia, or mesentery artery occlusion in infants. See Table 7-23 regarding the implications of bowel resections.

If only 30% of the small intestine remains in an adult (or <30 cm in infants), the resulting malabsorption may be life threatening. Problems are significant when more than 70% of the bowel is resected, unless the terminal ileum and ileocecal valve remain. Every attempt should be made to keep the ileocecal valve to prevent contamination of the small intestine.

Normal bowel length is about 600 cm. SBS generally leaves less than 150 cm of small intestine; 100 cm is necessary to completely absorb bile salts; 50–70 cm of jejunum-ileum maintains minimal intestinal autonomy. The minimal length of functional bowel needed for enteral feeding is over 100 cm in the absence of an intact colon and over 60 cm in continuity with the colon (Johnson, 2000).

TABLE 7-23 Implications of Bowel Resections

Loss of jejunum. Ileum undergoes hyperplasia; length and absorption per cm increases.

Loss of ileum. This is more serious than loss of jejunum because vitamin B_{12} and bile salts will be reabsorbed poorly as a result. The ileocecal valve keeps colonic bacteria out of the small intestine and regulates chyme flow. Some colonic adaptation occurs during the next 2–5 years.

Loss of colon. Overall, with removal of the colon versus the small intestine, fewer malabsorption problems occur. Loss of electrolyte and water-absorbing capacity occurs, as well as loss of salvage absorption of CHO and other nutrients. Most oxalate absorption occurs here.

In short bowel syndrome (SBS), short-chain triglycerides have a precursor in pectin; oligosaccharides increase O_2 uptake in the colon, thereby maintaining gut integrity. Early refeeding (i.e., free fatty acids, sugars, proteins) stimulates mucosal growth. Hyperphagia can increase enterocyte production. Adaptation requires adequate nutrition, intraluminal nutrients, and bile and pancreatic secretions. Enhancers of the adaptive process seem to include gastrin, glutamine, growth hormone, insulin, short-chain fatty acids, fats, some dietary fibers, cholecystokinin (CCK), glucagon, insulin-like growth factor I, neurotensin, and glucose.

Patients with SBS require long-term parenteral nutrition (PN) support. After massive intestinal resection, the intestine undergoes adaptation, and nutritional autonomy may be obtained if the adaptive process is supported by both nutritive and nonnutritive factors (Weale et al, 2005). Length of small intestine remaining after resection is the best predictor of final success in terminating PN. Home PN may cost between \$250 and \$400 a day, and most insurance companies cover up to \$1 million, or about 10 years of reimbursement.

Early and aggressive nutritional intervention is necessary for resolution of nutritional deficits and recovery of health. Early oral feeding after colorectal surgery is safe (Hartsell et al, 1997). There are three postresection phases (see Objectives) (Johnson, 2000). Bowel adaptation takes about 1 year. Use of growth hormone, insulin-like growth factor-I (IGF-I), and glutamine may help enhance this process (Ladd et al, 2005).

Transplantation of the small bowel restores quality of life for recipients who have functioning grafts (DiMartini et al, 1998). Advances in transplantation hold promise as an alternative to intestinal failure and chronic dependence on TPN (Silver et al, 2000). Surgery and high-dose immunosuppression are a problem. Recovery of normal motility and absorptive capacity are the goals.

Diarrhea and high stomal output are common problems and can lead to nutrient deficits, especially electrolytes. Other effects of SBS include dehydration; hypokalemia; deficiencies of calcium, magnesium, and zinc; carbohydrate and lactose malabsorption; protein malabsorption; renal oxalate stone formation; cholesterol biliary stones; gastric acid hypersecretion; vitamin B_{12} or iron deficiency; fat-soluble vitamin deficiency; and diarrhea. See Table 7-24 for malabsorption concerns in SBS. Figure 7-9 indicates where nutrients are absorbed and how important it is to know which parts have been resected and which remain.

Patient education and motivation are key factors in successful PN weaning (DiBaise et al, 2006). The use of trophic substances may increase the absorptive function of the remaining gut (DiBaise et al, 2004). Assessment of hydration

TABLE 7-24 Malabsorption Concerns in Short Bowel Syndrome

Decreased bile acid concentration (with loss of ileum and bacterial overgrowth)

Decreased surface area and lessened fluid reabsorption

Maladaptive remaining small bowel, especially from original bowel disease, lactase deficiency

Dumping syndrome from rapid transit and reduced bowel length

Bacterial overgrowth, if ileocecal valve is absent

Gastric acid oversecretion with resulting damage to duodenal cells and altered pH, thus affecting pancreatic enzyme and bile activity

Decreased pancreatic enzyme activity in duodenum, with malnutrition

and nutritional status must include oral intake, stool and urine output, serum electrolytes and visceral proteins, and body weight (DiBaise et al, 2006).

INTERVENTION: OBJECTIVES

- Provide step-wise management of care (Jeejeeboy, 2002). Determine the location and amount of the intestine that was resected to predict likelihood of diarrhea, malabsorption, and malnutrition (see Table 7-24). Provide nutrient replacements, dependent on area of resection (proximal jejunum—calcium, iron, magnesium, protein, CHO, and fat; terminal ileum—bile acids and intrinsic factor-bound vitamin B_{12}).
- Manage the three phases after surgery.
  - Phase 1: 1–3 months, massive diarrhea and limited absorption.
  - Phase 2: 4–12 months, weight gain begins and absorption improves.

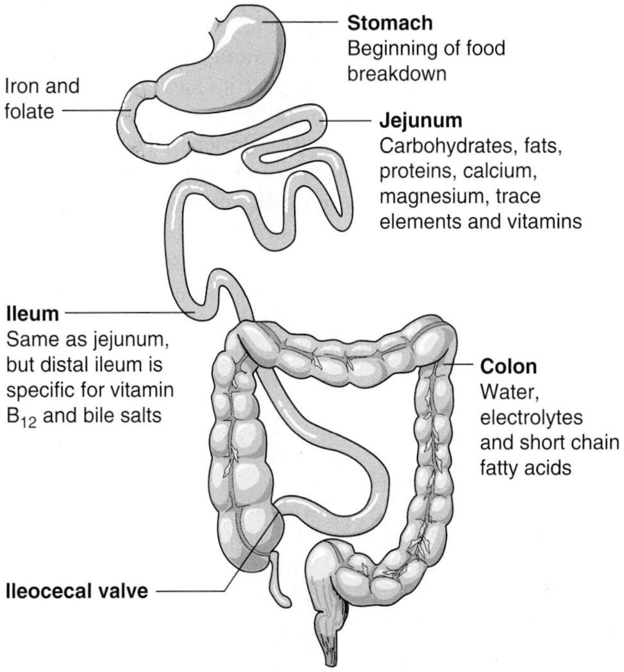

Figure 7-9 Nutrients and short bowel syndrome.

- Phase 3: 18–24 months, maximal adaptation with possible discontinuation of parenteral nutrition when intake of fluid is up to 7 L daily and when energy intake is sufficient for desired weight goal. Support hyperphagia, in which the amount of protein absorbed increases relative to the amount of remnant small bowel length (Crenn et al, 2004). It is best to try weaning off PN without trophic factors; if this is unsuccessful, a recombinant human growth hormone (r-hGH) regimen or investigational studies using other trophic factors should be attempted (Steiger et al, 2006).

- Prevent and correct fluid and electrolyte imbalances and dehydration. Oral intake could aggravate already massive losses of fluid (3–10 L/d is common). Immediately postoperatively, NPO with intravenous fluid replacement is likely. Eventually switch to oral intake as tolerated.
- Use remaining bowel surface and maximize efficacy. Prevent atrophy of small bowel mucosa, catheter sepsis, metabolic bone disease, and liver disease with long-term use of TPN. Carefully monitor for signs and symptoms of these problems and manage accordingly.
- Correct symptoms of deficiency and malabsorption, when possible, for vitamins B_{12}, A, D, E, and K and for the minerals zinc, potassium, and magnesium.
- Decrease weight loss (approximately 10 lb monthly until adaptation occurs). Maximize energy intake from fats and carbohydrates without worsening the diarrhea, and maximize nitrogen content (Jeejeeboy, 2002).
- Omit lactose if not tolerated; provide adequate calcium replacements.
- Decrease oxalate from the diet to reduce renal stone formation. Excess bile in the colon from decreased ileal absorption enhances absorption of free oxalate (normally only 10–15% is absorbed). In addition, therapeutic doses of vitamin C increase urinary oxalate excretion, potentially predisposing susceptible individuals to nephrolithiasis; consider this for patients receiving home TPN (Pena de la Vega et al, 2004).
- Control or prevent gallstone formation (increased risk of 2–3 times normal), anemia, protein-losing enteropathy, peptic ulcer from increased gastric acid secretion, and liver disease (often in home TPN).
- Allow remaining intestine to compensate over time by hypertrophy of villi and increased diameter. Less than 100 cm yields more severe problems; less than 60 cm of remaining intestine may require long-term TPN. Home TPN is expensive but can be lifesaving for months to years.
- Transitional feedings may be needed over several months from PN to oral diet. For care of colostomy or ileostomy, see appropriate entries.

INTERVENTION: FOOD AND NUTRITION

- **First Postoperative Phase:** Intravenous (IV) nutrition or TPN may be appropriate immediately before and approximately 5 days after surgery to allow rest. Determine whether the patient has problems with bloating. The first phase involves extensive diarrhea greater than 2 L daily; TPN is used, advancing slowly to avoid refeeding syndrome. At the end of this time, if diarrhea continues to be greater than 2 L, TPN may be lifelong.
- **Second Postoperative Phase:** Diarrhea is lessened and intestinal adaptation begins; TPN may be slowly reduced and tube feeding (TF) started at a slow, continuous rate according to stomal output or stool output. Need 40–60 kcal/kg and 1.2–1.5 g protein/kg. If weight loss is greater than 1 kg/wk or if diarrhea is greater than 600 g/d, TPN may need to be restarted (Johnson, 2000). When TF is used, polymeric solutions may be beneficial. Providing patients with enteral nutrition, glutamine, dietary fiber, and r-hGH during bowel rehabilitation therapy allows weaning from TPN in a significant number of patients (Weiming et al, 2004). Nocturnal enteral rehydration is an intervention using oral rehydration solutions through percutaneous endoscopic gastrostomy tubes at night; this allows for earlier discontinuation of TPN and improved fluid absorption (Nauth et al, 2004).
- **Third Postoperative Phase:** Complete bowel adaptation begins as TF is tolerated and oral diet is slowly resumed (from 2 months to 1 year). Six small feedings that are high CHO and low fat may be tolerated (60% CHO, 20% protein, 20% fat, with limit in MCT of 40 g/d). With no colon, the diet may need to be 30–40% fat, 20% protein, and 40–50% CHO; jejunostomy feedings may be needed, and oxalates need not be restricted (Johnson, 2000). PN reductions can be made by either decreasing the days of PN infusion per week or decreasing the PN infusion volume equally across all days of the week (DiBiase et al, 2006).
- Adequate zinc, potassium, liquid magnesium, oral calcium (600–1000 mg), manganese, iron, vitamin C, selenium, B-complex vitamins (especially folic acid), and other nutrients may be needed as supplements; determine needs based on site of resection and signs of malnutrition. With antibiotic use, the patient will need extra vitamin K. Monitor for needs for vitamins A, E, and D. Water-miscible forms of the fat-soluble vitamins may be useful.
- Lactose-restricted and oxalate-restricted diets may be needed for an extended period of time. Rhubarb, spinach, beets, cocoa and chocolate, sweet potatoes, strawberries, celery, and peanuts are high-oxalate foods; nuts and nut butters, berries, Concord grapes, sweet potatoes and potatoes, and most vegetables have smaller amounts.
- Omit alcoholic beverages and caffeine unless physician permits small quantities.
- Taking fluids between instead of with meals may be helpful in reducing dumping. Restrict at first to 1500 mL; progress as tolerated.
- With osmotic diarrhea, a reduction in simple carbohydrates and an increase in complex carbohydrates may be needed. Sorbitol, mannitol, and xylitol are usually poorly absorbed.
- Restricted foods such as lactose may be attempted and added back to the diet if they are tolerated. Bowel adaptation occurs over time and may eventually lead the patient back to an unrestricted diet.

CLINICAL INDICATORS

Clinical/History

Height
Weight
BMI
Diet history
Weight changes
I & O
Steatorrhea
DEXA bone density scan

Lab Work

H & H
Serum Fe
Transferrin
CRP, ESR
D-xylose absorption
Serum gastrin (increased)
Ca++, Mg++
25-hydroxyvitamin D level
Alk phos
Na+ (serum, urine, stool)
K+ (serum, urine, stool)
Fecal nitrogen
GTT
Gluc
RBP
N balance
Serum oxalate
Alb, transthyretin
Barium follow-through (BaFT) examination
Schilling test
Serum B_{12}
Serum amylase, lipase
Serum copper
Bile acid breath test
Lactose tolerance test
Hydrogen breath test
Fecal fat test

Common Drugs Used and Potential Side Effects (see Table 7-25)

- **Note: Most oral medications are poorly tolerated in this condition!** Accelerated intestinal luminal transit time causes a reduction in absorption of certain antimicrobial agents, digoxin, hydrochlorothiazide, cyclosporine, cimetidine, mesalazine (5-aminosalicylic acid), oral contraceptives, and levothyroxine (Severijnen et al, 2004).
- Pharmacological advances, including the use of antibacterial drugs, antimotility drugs, and hormonal therapies, have had a significant impact on SBS (Vanderhoof et al, 2003). Antidiarrheal agents, H_2 antagonists and proton pump inhibitors, pancreatic enzymes, somatostatin analogs, antimicrobials, and trophic factors have been quite helpful in addition to nutritional therapy (Matarese and Steiger, 2006).
- Use of r-hGH, with or without glutamine, may play a role in facilitating the PN weaning process (DiBaise et al, 2006).

TABLE 7-25 Medications Used in Short Bowel Syndrome

Medication	Description
Antibiotics	Tetracycline, Flagyl, Septra, or Cipro may be needed for bacterial overgrowth. Monitor hydrogen breath tests (especially with blind loop).
Antidiarrheals	Antidiarrheals such as Lomotil, Imodium, and codeine are useful. Liquid preparations often are better tolerated. If dehydration-occurs, use oral rehydration therapy but not sports drinks, which do not have the adequate electrolyte replacements.
Bile salt replacements	Cholylsarcosine (CS) is a semisynthetic bile salt that may be useful in bile salt replacement therapy of short bowel syndrome (Furst et al, 2005).
Calcium supplements	Oral calcium supplements (OsCal or Tums four times daily) often are used to bind oxalate excesses and to decrease diarrhea. Do not take with a bulk-forming laxative or with an iron supplement. Increase water intake.
Cholestyramine	Cholestyramine may be used for choleraic diarrhea when less than 100 cm is resected and when the colon is in continuity; prevent excessive use. Take before meals. Nausea, vomiting, or constipation may occur.
Cimetidine or omeprazole	Cimetidine and omeprazole may be needed to decrease gastric hypersecretion; parenteral administration may be needed (Kato et al, 2004). Serum gastrin levels should be monitored. A dose 2–3 times higher than normal may be needed because of gastric hypersecretion; lack of sufficient time with intestinal mucosa leads to insufficient absorption (Severijnen et al, 2004). Vitamin B_{12} absorption decreases with use of these medications.
Clonidine	Clonidine can effectively reduce intestinal fluid and electrolyte losses and should be considered in patients with short bowel syndrome (McDoniel et al, 2004).
Growth hormone	Growth hormone increases water/sodium transport. It is useful in combination with glutamine and a modified diet (Matarese et al, 2004), but results have been mixed.
Minerals	Liquid potassium and intravenous or intramuscular magnesium may be needed.
Pancreatic enzymes	Pancrelipase may improve fat and protein absorption after jejunal resection; results are variable.
Peptides	Glucagon-like peptide-2 (GLP-2) is an enteroendocrine peptide that is released in response to luminal nutrients; it seems to help support the adaptive response to resection (Martin et al, 2005).
Probiotics and prebiotics (synbiotics)	This type of therapy might be a potent modulator of intestinal flora and a promising strategy to treat short bowel patients with enterocolitis (Kanamori et al, 2004).
Vitamins	Vitamins that are chewable or in liquid form may be better tolerated. Parenteral vitamin B_{12} may be necessary. Add extra fat-soluble vitamins A, E, D, and K if deficiency occurs. Do not use vitamin C in excessively large quantities; some links with oxalate stones have been noted (Pena de la Vega et al, 2004).

Herbs, Botanicals, and Supplements

- Herbs and botanical supplements should not be used without discussing with the physician.
- Probiotics and foods such as acidophilus or yogurt are useful aids in bowel adaptation phases. Not all probiotic bacteria have similar therapeutic effects; controlled clinical trials are under way to test which strains are most useful (Fedorak and Madsen, 2004).

INTERVENTION: NUTRITION EDUCATION, COUNSELING, CARE MANAGEMENT

- Importance of adequate nutrition and supplementation must be discussed to prevent or correct malnutrition and malabsorption. After adaptation, some people will require significant energy intakes to maintain desired weight.
- Recipes and food preparation tips will be needed to support the specific dietary regimen and to evaluate tolerances over time.
- Progression in diet is allowed when the small intestine adapts over several months. Use of yogurt with live active cultures is useful.
- Discuss the need for free water.
- The use of home TPN is beneficial in many cases. Judicious use of home TPN in this setting requires careful clinical assessment on a patient-by-patient basis (Hoda et al, 2005). A supportive attitude from family and caregivers is essential.
- There are potential benefits of having a multidisciplinary intestinal rehabilitation program involved in the care of these patients (DiBaise et al, 2004). Interventions can help decrease incidence and economic impact of intestinal failure; education of patients and families are needed for managing intestinal rehabilitation, and education of medical staff about basic nutrition and nutritional rehabilitation will be needed (Kocoshis et al, 2004).
- In children, the need for long-term PN does not preclude achieving productive adulthood (Quiros-Tejeira et al, 2004).

Patient Education—Foodborne Illness

- Careful food handling and hand washing are important to prevent introduction of foodborne pathogens to the individual who may be experiencing diarrhea and related discomfort.

For More Information

- Short Bowel Syndrome
  http://digestive.niddk.nih.gov/ddiseases/pubs/shortbowel/
  http://www.emedicine.com/ped/topic2088.htm
- Short Bowel Syndrome–Pediatrics
  http://depts.washington.edu/growing/Assess/SBS.htm

SHORT BOWEL SYNDROME—CITED REFERENCES

Crenn P, et al. Net digestive absorption and adaptive hyperphagia in adult short bowel patients. *Gut* 53:1279, 2004.

DiBaise JK, et al. Intestinal rehabilitation and the short bowel syndrome: part 2. *Am J Gastroenterol.* 99:1823, 2004.

DiBaise JK, et al. Strategies for parenteral nutrition weaning in adult patients with short bowel syndrome. *J Clin Gastroenterol.* 40:S94, 2006.

DiMartini A, et al. Quality of life after small intestine transplantation and among home parenteral nutrition patients *Parenter Enter Nutr.* 22:357, 1998.

Fedorak RN, Madsen KL. Probiotics and the management of inflammatory bowel disease. *Inflamm Bowel Dis.* 10:286, 2004.

Furst T, et al. Enteric-coated cholylsarcosine microgranules for the treatment of short bowel syndrome. *J Pharm Pharmacol.* 57:53, 2005.

Hartsell P, et al. Early postoperative feeding after elective colorectal surgery. *Arch Surg.* 132:518, 1997.

Hoda D, et al. Should patients with advanced, incurable cancers ever be sent home with total parenteral nutrition? A single institution's 20-year experience. *Cancer* 103:863, 2005.

Jackson CA, Buchman AL. The nutritional management of short bowel syndrome. *Nutr Clin Care.* 7:114, 2004.

Jeejeeboy KN. Short bowel syndrome: a nutritional and medical approach. *CMAJ.* 166:1297, 2002.

Johnson M. Management of short bowel syndrome—a review. *Support Line* 22:11, 2000.

Kanamori Y, et al. Experience of long-term synbiotic therapy in seven short bowel patients with refractory enterocolitis. *J Pediatr Surg.* 39:1686, 2004.

Kato J, et al. A prospective within-patient comparison clinical trial on the effect of parenteral cimetidine for improvement of fluid secretion and electrolyte balance in patients with short bowel syndrome. *Hepatogastroenterology* 51:1742, 2004.

Kocoshis SA, et al. Intestinal failure and small bowel transplantation, including clinical nutrition: Working Group Report of the Second World Congress of Pediatric Gastroenterology, Hepatology, and Nutrition. *J Pediatr Gastroenterol Nutr.* 39:655S2, 2004.

Ladd AP, et al. The effect of growth hormone supplementation on late nutritional independence in pediatric patients with short bowel syndrome. *J Pediatr Surg.* 40:442, 2005.

Martin GR, et al. Nutrient-stimulated GLP-2 release and crypt cell proliferation in experimental short bowel syndrome. *Am J Physiol Gastrointest Liver Physiol.* 288:431, 2005.

Matarese L, Steiger E. Dietary and medical management of short bowel syndrome in adult patients. *J Clin Gastroenterol.* 40:S85S, 2006.

Matarese LR, et al. Growth hormone, glutamine, and modified diet for intestinal adaptation. *J Am Diet Assoc.* 104:1265, 2004.

McDoniel K, et al. Use of clonidine to decrease intestinal fluid losses in patients with high-output short-bowel syndrome. *J Parenter Enteral Nutr.* 28:265, 2004.

Nauth J, et al. A therapeutic approach to wean total parenteral nutrition in the management of short bowel syndrome: three cases using nocturnal enteral rehydration. *Nutr Rev.* 62:221, 2004.

Pena de la Vega L, et al. Urinary oxalate excretion increases in home parenteral nutrition patients on a higher intravenous ascorbic acid dose. *J Parenter Enteral Nutr.* 28:435, 2004.

Quiros-Tejeira RE, et al. Long-term parenteral nutritional support and intestinal adaptation in children with short bowel syndrome: a 25-year experience. *J Pediatr.* 145:157, 2004.

Severijnen R, et al. Enteral drug absorption in patients with short small bowel: a review. *Clin Pharmacokinet.* 43:951, 2004.

Silver H, et al. Nutritional complications and management of intestinal transplant. *J Am Diet Assoc.* 100:680, 2000.

Steiger E, et al. Indications and recommendations for the use of recombinant human growth hormone in adult short bowel syndrome patients dependent on parenteral nutrition. *J Clin Gastroenterol.* 40:S99S, 2006.

Vanderhoof JA, et al. New and emerging therapies for short bowel syndrome in children. *Paediatr Drugs.* 5:525, 2003.

Weale AR, et al. Intestinal adaptation after massive intestinal resection. *Postgrad Med J.* 81:178, 2005.

Weiming Z, et al. Effect of recombinant human growth hormone and enteral nutrition on short bowel syndrome. *J Parenter Enteral Nutr.* 28:377, 2004.

TROPICAL SPRUE

NUTRITIONAL ACUITY RANKING: LEVEL 4

DEFINITIONS AND BACKGROUND

Tropical sprue is an acquired disorder that presents with chronic diarrhea, anorexia, weight loss, megaloblastic anemia (folic acid deficiency), light-colored stools, diarrhea, weight loss, pallor, sore tongue (vitamin B_{12} deficiency), and easy bruising (vitamin K deficiency). Etiology is often bacterial, viral, or parasitic infection or toxins in spoiled food. The most common cause is an intestinal infection with small intestinal protozoa including *Giardia intestinalis, Cryptosporidium parvum, Isospora belli, Cyclospora cayetanensis,* and the microsporidia (Farthing, 2002). Tropical sprue may occur after traveling to tropical areas such as the Caribbean, southern India, and Southeast Asia.

Tropical sprue is a disease that causes progressive villus atrophy in the small intestine, similar to celiac disease (which is also called "nontropical" sprue) (Westergaard, 2004; Morales et al, 2001). Villi of the small intestinal mucosa become scalloped in appearance, blunted, or obliterated (Shah et al, 2000). Treatment of tropical sprue with folic acid replacement has become standard medical treatment, and vitamin B_{12} replacement is usually added if there is evidence of deficiency or malabsorption (Westergaard, 2004). However, even prolonged treatment with these vitamins fails to resolve villus atrophy, and malabsorption remains a problem (Westergaard, 2004).

Tropical sprue is less common than it was 20–30 years ago (Farthing, 2002). However, research about microbial factors, pathogenesis, immunogenetics, and hormonal and immune regulation is needed to settle some of the unanswered issues and open new venues for diagnosis, prevention, and treatment (Nath, 2005).

INTERVENTION: OBJECTIVES

- Differentiate between tropical and celiac disease. Control diarrhea, which could lead to malabsorption and malnutrition over time.
- Improve or correct folic acid, vitamin B_{12}, and vitamin K deficiencies, among others. Treatment of tropical sprue with folate and vitamin B_{12} cures the macrocytic anemia and the accompanying glossitis and often results in increased appetite and weight gain (Westergaard, 2004).

INTERVENTION: FOOD AND NUTRITION

- Use a regular diet with supplements of vitamin B_{12} and folic acid. Good sources of folacin include liver, kidney, yeast, leafy greens, lean beef, and eggs. Good sources of vitamin B_{12} include meat, poultry, fish, dairy products, and eggs.
- Diet should provide sufficient amounts of energy intake, protein, calcium, iron, and vitamins.
- Extra fluid may be needed for dehydration, but no gluten restriction is needed.

CLINICAL INDICATORS

Clinical/History	Lab Work	
Height	Gluc	Ca^{++} (decreased)
Weight	Na^+, K^+	Mg^{++}
BMI	H & H, serum Fe (decreased)	PT or INR (altered)
Diet history	Alb, transthyretin (decreased)	
Weight loss?	Serum B_{12} (decreased)	
Anorexia	Serum folate (decreased)	
I & O; dehydration?		
Malabsorption, especially for xylose		
Glossitis		

Common Drugs Used and Potential Side Effects

- Tetracycline may be used; do not take within 2 hours of a calcium-containing supplement or meal because calcium makes the drug less effective.
- Vitamin supplements are required, especially for vitamin B_{12}, folate, and vitamin K. Calcium may also be needed. Avoid excesses of any single nutrient for an extended time period.
- Suggest use of probiotics such as yogurt with active cultures with antibiotic therapy. Intestinal flora modifiers (e.g., *Lactobacillus acidophilus,* Lactinex, Bacid) also help recolonize normal intestinal flora in people on antibiotics. A common order is 3–4 packages every day for 3 days in adults. They may be mixed with water for tube feedings.

Herbs, Botanicals, and Supplements

- Herbs and botanical supplements should not be used without discussing with the physician.

INTERVENTION: NUTRITION EDUCATION, COUNSELING, CARE MANAGEMENT

- Explain to the patient which foods are good sources of folic acid and vitamin B_{12}.
- Describe good sources of protein and calories from the diet.
- Describe how to follow a low-fat diet and how to use MCT oil, etc.

Patient Education—Foodborne Illness

- Careful food handling and hand washing are important to prevent introduction of foodborne pathogens to the individual who may be experiencing diarrhea and related discomfort.

For More Information

- Tropical Sprue
  http://www.intelihealth.com/IH/ihtIH/WSIHW000/9339/10902.html
  http://health.allrefer.com/health/tropical-sprue-info.html

TROPICAL SPRUE—CITED REFERENCES

Farthing MJ. Tropical malabsorption. *Semin Gastrointest Dis.* 13:221, 2002.
Morales M, et al. Exocrine pancreatic insufficiency in tropical sprue. *Digestion* 63:30, 2001.
Nath SK. Tropical sprue. *Curr Gastroenterol Rep.* 7:343, 2005.
Shah V, et al. All that scallops is not celiac disease. *Gastrointest Endosc.* 51:717, 2000.
Westergaard H. Tropical sprue. *Curr Treat Options Gastroenterol.* 7:7, 2004.

WHIPPLE'S DISEASE (INTESTINAL LIPODYSTROPHY)

NUTRITIONAL ACUITY RANKING: LEVEL 3–4

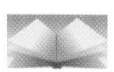

DEFINITIONS AND BACKGROUND

Whipple's disease is a rare systemic disorder classically presenting with weight loss, arthralgias, and diarrhea that involves infiltration of the small intestine with glycoprotein-laden macrophages and some rod-shaped bacilli (*Tropheryma whippelii*) in varying body tissues (Muller et al, 2005).

Altered immune functions play a role in the manifestation of the disease (Mahnel and Marth, 2004). Host susceptibility may be exacerbated by iron loading, altered levels of interferon-gamma and interleukin-4, as well as serum ferritin (Weinberg, 2001).

Endocarditis and heart murmur are common. Patients may also have arthralgias for years before diarrhea occurs (Dobbins, 1995). Other signs and symptoms include malabsorption and cholestasis, fever of unknown origin, anemia, hypoproteinemia, gray to brown skin pigmentation, lymphadenopathy, edema, wasting, and sarcoidosis-like illness. Infection may spread to the central nervous system, which may lead to loss of memory, confusion, or disturbed gait (Mahnel and Marth, 2004). While untreated disease may be lethal, treatment is often able to eradicate the organism through antibiotic therapy (Mahnel and Marth, 2004).

INTERVENTION: OBJECTIVES

- Reduce fever and inflammatory processes.
- Correct malnutrition and malabsorption; intestinal involvement occurs with abdominal pain and diarrhea, which leads to weight loss, malnutrition, and anemia (Mahnel and Marth, 2004).
- Correct anemia, iron overloading, or hypoproteinemia when present.
- Prevent or correct dehydration and electrolyte imbalances.

INTERVENTION: FOOD AND NUTRITION

- Use a high-protein/high-calorie diet appropriate for the patient's age and sex.
- Ensure that the diet includes sufficient vitamins and minerals, especially for vitamin D and calcium, when steatorrhea is a problem. Vitamins A, B-complex, and K may also be needed.
- Provide adequate fluid intake to reduce fever and replenish tissues. If edema is a problem, control excess sodium.

CLINICAL INDICATORS

Clinical/History	Lab Work	
Height	Alk phos	H & H (decreased)
Weight	Na+, K+	Serum Fe, serum ferritin
BMI	Ca++, Mg++	Transferrin
Diet history	Alb (decreased)	RBP
Temperature	CRP	PT
I & O		Macrophages

Common Drugs Used and Potential Side Effects

- Antibiotic treatment is mandatory and leads to a rapid clinical improvement and remission in most patients: 2-week parenteral cephalosporins followed by long-term therapy with trimethoprim-sulfamethoxazole

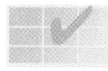

(Bai et al, 2004). Trimethoprim-sulfamethoxazole (Bactrim) combinations may have numerous side effects; monitor closely for anorexia, nausea, vomiting, and diarrhea. Use probiotic or prebiotic foods when possible to replenish "good" gut bacteria.

Herbs, Botanicals, and Supplements

- Herbs and botanical supplements should not be used without discussing with the physician.

INTERVENTION: NUTRITION EDUCATION, COUNSELING, CARE MANAGEMENT

- Discuss inclusion of high-quality proteins in the diet. Frequent snacks may be beneficial if large meals are not tolerated.
- Provide lists for nutrient-dense foods rich in specific and needed nutrients (e.g., iron, calcium, etc.).

Patient Education—Foodborne Illness

- Careful food handling and hand washing are important to prevent introduction of foodborne pathogens to the individual.

For More Information

- Whipple's Disease
  http://www.whipplesdisease.net/
  http://www.nlm.nih.gov/medlineplus/ency/article/000209.htm
- Whipple's Disease Info
  http://www.whipplesdisease.info/

WHIPPLE'S DISEASE—CITED REFERENCES

Bai JC, et al. Whipple's disease. *Clin Gastroenterol Hepatol.* 2:849, 2004.

Dobbins W. The diagnosis of Whipple's disease. *N Engl J Med.* 332:390, 1995.

Mahnel R, Marth T. Progress, problems, and perspectives in diagnosis and treatment of Whipple's disease. *Clin Exp Med.* 4:39, 2004.

Muller SA, et al. Deadly carousel or difficult interpretation of new diagnostic tools for Whipple's disease: case report and review of the literature. *Infection* 33:39, 2005.

Weinberg E. Iron loading: a risk factor for Whipple's disease? *Med Hypotheses.* 57:59, 2001.

RECTAL DISORDERS

FECAL INCONTINENCE

NUTRITIONAL ACUITY RANKING: LEVEL 1

DEFINITIONS AND BACKGROUND

Fecal incontinence is the inability to control bowel movements, and stool may leak from the rectum unexpectedly (Rao and American College of Gastroenterology Practice Parameters Committee, 2004). More than 5.5 million Americans have fecal incontinence, affecting both children and adults. Fecal incontinence is more common in women than in men (Novi and Mulvihill, 2005) and is more common in older adults (see Table 7-26).

Bowel training helps some people relearn how to control their bowels. In some cases, it involves strengthening muscles; in others, it means training the bowels to empty at a specific time of day. Biofeedback helps strengthen and coordinate the muscles; Kegel exercises may be used to strengthen the muscles in the pelvic floor, including those involved in controlling stool.

This condition is often correlated with the presence of certain conditions (e.g., stroke and diabetes) and use of certain psychoactive medications (Quander et al, 2005). Treatment depends on the cause and severity of fecal incontinence; it may include dietary changes, medication, bowel training, and/or surgery.

Surgery may be needed if fecal incontinence occurs in severe cases where injury has taken place. People who have severe fecal incontinence may decide to have a colostomy (see appropriate entry). Sacral nerve stimulation should be considered for patients with ongoing fecal incontinence following rectal prolapse repair if conservative treatment does not work (Jarrett et al, 2005).

INTERVENTION: OBJECTIVES

- Timely nutrition assessment and intervention are needed to manage constipation and incontinence of stool. Maintain a food diary to determine when incontinence occurs and to identify changes that may be helpful.
- Prepare for surgery if needed.
- Establish a bowel training regimen to develop a regular pattern of bowel movements; some people train themselves to have bowel movements at specific times during the day, such as after every meal.

INTERVENTION: FOOD AND NUTRITION

- Daily intake of protein should be appropriate for age and sex. Calories should be calculated as 30–35 kcal/kg.
- Foods that may make the problem worse are drinks containing caffeine, like coffee, tea, and chocolate, which relax the internal anal sphincter muscle. Other foods that have been implicated are cured or smoked meats like sausage, ham, or turkey; spicy foods; alcohol; dairy products like milk, cheese, and ice cream; fruits like apples, peaches, or

TABLE 7-26 Fecal Incontinence: Causes and Comments

Cause	Comments
Constipation	One of the most common causes of fecal incontinence, constipation causes large, hard stools to become lodged in the rectum. Watery stool can then leak out around the hardened stool. Constipation also causes the muscles of the rectum to stretch, which weakens the muscles so they can't hold stool in the rectum long enough for a person to reach a bathroom. In children, early toilet training or some developmental disorders can cause or aggravate constipation. Consult the doctor for specific management techniques.
Damage to the anal sphincter muscles	Fecal incontinence can be caused by injury to one or both of the ring-like muscles at the end of the rectum called the anal internal and/or external sphincters. The sphincters keep stool inside. When damaged, the muscles are not strong enough to do their job, and stool can leak out. In women, the damage often happens when giving birth. The risk of injury is greatest if the doctor uses forceps to help deliver the baby or does an episiotomy, which is a cut in the vaginal area to prevent it from tearing during birth. Hemorrhoid surgery can damage the sphincters as well.
Damage to the nerves of the anal sphincter muscles or the rectum	Fecal incontinence can also be caused by damage to the nerves that control the anal sphincters or to the nerves that sense stool in the rectum. If the nerves that control the sphincters are injured, the muscle does not work properly, and incontinence can occur. If the sensory nerves are damaged, they do not sense that stool is in the rectum. The individual will not feel the need to use the bathroom until stool has leaked out. Nerve damage can be caused by childbirth, a long-term habit of straining to pass stool, stroke, and diseases that affect the nerves, such as diabetes and multiple sclerosis.
Loss of storage capacity in the rectum	Normally, the rectum stretches to hold stool until a person can get to a bathroom. But rectal surgery, radiation treatment, and inflammatory bowel disease can cause scarring that makes the walls of the rectum stiff and less elastic. The rectum then cannot stretch as much and cannot hold stool, and fecal incontinence results. Inflam matory bowel disease also can make rectal walls very irritated and thereby unable to contain stool.
Diarrhea	Diarrhea, or loose stool, is more difficult to control than solid stool that is formed. Even people who do not have fecal incontinence can have an accident when they have diarrhea.
Pelvic floor dysfunction	Abnormalities of the pelvic floor can lead to fecal incontinence. Examples of some abnormalities are decreased perception of rectal sensation, decreased anal canal pressures, decreased squeeze pressure of the anal canal, impaired anal sensation, a dropping down of the rectum (rectal prolapse), protrusion of the rectum through the vagina (rectocele), and/or generalized weakness and sagging of the pelvic floor. Often the cause of pelvic floor dysfunction is childbirth, and incontinence does not show up until the midforties or later (Bharucha et al, 2005).

pears; fatty and greasy foods; sweeteners, like sorbitol, xylitol, mannitol, and fructose, which are found in diet drinks, sugarless gum and candy, chocolate, and fruit juices.

- Serve smaller meals more frequently. Since liquid helps move food through the digestive system, drink half an hour before or after meals.
- Foods that contain soluble, or digestible, fiber slow the emptying of the bowels. Bananas, rice, tapioca, bread, potatoes, applesauce, cheese, smooth peanut butter, yogurt, pasta, and oatmeal may be helpful.
- High-fiber foods will add bulk and make stool easier to control. Fiber is found in fruits, vegetables, and grains; 20–30 g of fiber a day is needed, but add it slowly. Too much fiber all at once can cause bloating, gas, or even diarrhea. If fiber intake makes diarrhea worse, cut back to two servings each of fruits and vegetables and remove skins and seeds. Increase fluid intake when fiber intake is increased to prevent fecal obstruction.

CLINICAL INDICATORS

Clinical/History

Height
Weight
BMI
Diet history
I & O
BP
History of diarrhea
Constipation
Anal manometry
Anorectal ultrasonography
Proctography
Proctosigmoidoscopy
Anal electromyography tests for nerve damage

Lab Work

H & H
Serum Fe
BUN
Transferrin, TIBC
PT
Alb, transthyretin
Stool (occult blood)
Na+, K+
Ca++, Mg++

Common Drugs Used and Potential Side Effects

- If diarrhea is causing the incontinence, medication may help. Sometimes doctors recommend using bulk laxatives to help people develop a more regular bowel pattern. Antidiarrheal medicines, such as loperamide or diphenoxylate, may be used to slow down the bowel activity.
- Use of probiotic or prebiotic therapy is under study for this condition.

Herbs, Botanicals, and Supplements

- Herbs and botanical supplements should not be used without discussing with the physician.

TABLE 7-27 Foods That Have Fiber

Food	Fiber Content (g)
Breads, cereals, and beans	
1/2 cup of black-eyed peas, cooked	4
1/2 cup of kidney beans, cooked	5.7
1/2 cup of lima beans, cooked	4.5
Whole-grain cereal, cold	
• 1/2 cup of All-Bran	9.6
• 3/4 cup of Total	2.4
• 3/4 cup of Post Bran Flakes	5.3
1 packet of whole-grain cereal, hot (oatmeal, Wheatena)	3
1 slice of whole-wheat or multigrain bread	1.7
Fruits	
1 medium apple	3.3
1 medium peach	1.8
1/2 cup of raspberries	4
1 medium tangerine	1.9
Vegetables	
1 cup of acorn squash, raw	2.1
1 medium stalk of broccoli, raw	3.9
5 Brussels sprouts, raw	3.6
1 cup of cabbage, raw	2
1 medium carrot, raw	1.8
1 cup of cauliflower, raw	2.5
1 cup of spinach, cooked	4.3
1 cup of zucchini, raw	1.4

Source: U.S. Department of Agriculture. USDA/ARS Nutrient Data Laboratory. Accessed March 31, 2005 at http://www.ars.usda.gov/main/site_main.htm?modecode=12354500.

INTERVENTION: NUTRITION EDUCATION, COUNSELING, CARE MANAGEMENT

- The skin around the anus is delicate and sensitive. Constipation and diarrhea or contact between skin and stool can cause pain or itching. To relieve discomfort, wash the area with water, but not soap, after a bowel movement; wash in the shower with lukewarm water or use a sitz bath. Premoistened, alcohol-free towelettes are a better choice than toilet paper. Let the area air dry after washing. Use a moisture-barrier cream. Wear cotton underwear and loose clothing.
- Ensure that the patient adequately exercises, rests, and maintains regular bowel habits.
- Indicate which foods are sources of fiber and other key nutrients in the diet. See Table 7-27.

Patient Education—Food Safety

- Careful food handling and hand washing are important to prevent introduction of foodborne pathogens to the individual.

For More Information

- International Foundation for Functional Gastrointestinal Disorders http://www.iffgd.org

FECAL INCONTINENCE—CITED REFERENCES

Bharucha AE, et al. Relationship between symptoms and disordered continence mechanisms in women with idiopathic faecal incontinence. *Gut* 54:546, 2005.

Jarrett ME, et al. Sacral nerve stimulation for fecal incontinence following surgery for rectal prolapse repair: a multicenter study. *Dis Colon Rectum.* 48:1243, 2005.

Novi JM, Mulvihill BH. Fecal incontinence in women: a review of evaluation and management. *Obstet Gynecol Surv.* 60:261, 2005.

Quander CR, et al. Prevalence of and factors associated with fecal incontinence in a large community study of older individuals. *Am J Gastroenterol.* 100:905, 2005.

Rao SS, American College of Gastroenterology Practice Parameters Committee. Diagnosis and management of fecal incontinence. *Am J Gastroenterol.* 99:1585, 2004.

HEMORRHOIDS

NUTRITIONAL ACUITY RANKING: LEVEL 1

DEFINITIONS AND BACKGROUND

Chronic constipation is believed to be the main cause of hemorrhoids. The disorder is common in Americans (50% of Americans older than 50 years of age will have suffered at least once, especially if obese). Causes include increased abdominal pressure secondary to straining during bowel movements, heavy lifting, childbirth, and benign prostatic hypertrophy.

The theory of a sliding anal canal lining and the knowledge that hemorrhoidal cushions are a normal part of the anal anatomy should encourage symptom control rather than radical removal of tissue (Hulme-Moir and Bartolo, 2001). Internal hemorrhoids are normal anatomical structures and rarely are painful (they may only bleed). External hemorrhoids are usually from excessive diarrhea or from constipation; they are tender, painful, bluish, localized swellings of varicose veins at the anal margin.

Bleeding, pain, soiling, and prolapse are the classic symptoms in hemorrhoid disease, but the patients sometimes report a variety of other symptoms (Johannsson et al, 2005). Although some patients fear that rectal bleeding signifies colorectal cancer, most patients with the primary diagnosis of symptomatic hemorrhoids do not need further investigative procedures (Tang et al, 2005).

Techniques that fix the cushions back in position can be performed in outpatients with reasonable success rates. If required, surgery should be aimed at symptomatic hemorrhoids; sutureless closed hemorrhoidectomy is well received (Sayfan et al, 2001). Stapled hemorrhoidopexy is a safe and effective procedure; patients have reduced pain, shorter length of stay, and earlier resumption to work (Chung et al, 2005; Hulme-Moir and Bartolo, 2001).

INTERVENTION: OBJECTIVES

- Provide comfort. Prevent prolapse and thrombosis.
- Avoid constipation, infection, and anemia.
- Reduce possible irritation from too much roughage.
- Avoid irritants such as laxatives.
- After surgery, reduce irritation while patient heals. Promote rapid healing. Prevent future recurrence.

INTERVENTION: FOOD AND NUTRITION

- Diet should be low in fiber only when the patient is in pain. Otherwise, a high-fiber diet (25–35 g) should be used.
- Fluids should be increased to 8–10 glasses daily.
- After surgery, a low-fiber/soft diet should be used until full recovery occurs. Eventually, adequate fiber (25–35 g) should be taken.
- Omit lactose and highly seasoned foods only if not tolerated by the individual.

CLINICAL INDICATORS

Clinical/History		
Height	History of diarrhea	Transferrin, TIBC
Weight	Constipation	PT
BMI		Alb, transthyretin
Diet history	**Lab Work**	Stool (occult blood)
I & O	H & H	Na+, K+
BP	Serum Fe	Ca++, Mg++
	BUN	

Common Drugs Used and Potential Side Effects

- Laxatives and enemas may have caused faulty bowel function. Avoid use unless prescribed by the doctor.
- Troxerutin and carbazochrome are new medications often used as combination therapy. Monitor for any untoward side effects.
- Lubrication with glycerin suppositories may help to reduce symptoms.
- Medicated suppositories such as Anusol HC (contains hydrocortisone) may help to decrease inflammation. Limit steroid-containing medications to less than 2 weeks of continuous use to avoid atrophy of anal tissues.
- Psyllium laxatives (Metamucil) can help with constipation; long-term use alters electrolytes. Flatulence or steatorrhea may occur.

Herbs, Botanicals, and Supplements

- Herbs and botanical supplements should not be used without discussing with the physician.
- Comfrey, plantain, butcher's broom, horse chestnut, and witch hazel have been recommended for this condition, but no clinical trials have proven efficacy.

INTERVENTION: NUTRITION EDUCATION, COUNSELING, CARE MANAGEMENT

- Ensure that the patient adequately exercises, rests, and maintains regular bowel habits.
- Teach the patient about the role of fiber in the diet.
- Persistent or recurrent bleeding requires medical attention, especially to monitor vitamin K, iron, and B-complex vitamin levels and to prevent additional losses.
- It is important to keep the anal skin area dry.
- Over-the-counter products may aggravate an allergic response.
- Warm sitz baths may help to reduce symptoms.

Patient Education—Foodborne Illness

- Careful food handling and hand washing are important to prevent introduction of foodborne pathogens to the individual.

For More Information

- Ano-Rectal Algorithm
  http://www.uwgi.org/guidelines/ch_10/ch10.htm
- Hemorrhoids
  http://digestive.niddk.nih.gov/ddiseases/pubs/hemorrhoids/

HEMORRHOIDS—CITED REFERENCES

Chung CC, et al. Stapled hemorrhoidopexy vs. harmonic scalpel hemorrhoidectomy: a randomized trial. *Dis Colon Rectum.* 48:1213, 2005.
Hulme-Moir M, Bartolo D. Hemorrhoids. *Gastroenterol Clin North Am.* 30:183, 2001.
Johannsson HO, et al. Bowel habits in hemorrhoid patients and normal subjects. *Am J Gastroenterol.* 100:401, 2005.
Sayfan J, et al. Sutureless closed hemorrhoidectomy: a new technique. *Ann Surg.* 234:21, 2001.
Tang T, et al. An approach to haemorrhoids. *Colorectal Dis.* 7:143, 2005.

PROCTITIS

NUTRITIONAL ACUITY RANKING: LEVEL 1

DEFINITIONS AND BACKGROUND

Proctitis is inflammation of the lining of the rectal mucosa. It can be acute or chronic. Proctitis may be a side effect of medical treatments like radiation therapy or antibiotics, or it may be caused by ulcerative colitis, Crohn's disease, sexually transmitted diseases, rectal injury, bacterial infection, allergies, and malfunction of the nerves in the rectum. Symptoms include frequent or continuous urge to defecate, constipation, rectal fullness, left-sided abdominal pain, passage of mucus through the rectum, rectal bleeding, and pain.

Treatment depends on the cause of proctitis; antibiotics will be used for proctitis caused by bacterial infection. If the inflammation is caused by Crohn's disease or ulcerative colitis, 5-aminosalicyclic acid (5-ASA) or corticosteroids may be applied directly to the area or taken in pill form.

INTERVENTION: OBJECTIVES

- Manage symptoms and alleviate pain.
- Reduce inflammation and promote healing.

INTERVENTION: FOOD AND NUTRITION

- Diet therapy depends on the cause of proctitis. Identify appropriate etiology and review entries in this text for dietary management.
- Some patients find that avoidance of caffeine, red meat, dairy products, and artificial sweeteners can be beneficial.
- Use of omega-3 fatty acids may be helpful to reduce inflammation.

CLINICAL INDICATORS

Clinical/History	Lab Work	
Height	Stool (occult blood)	Alb, transthyretin
Weight	H & H	CRP
BMI	Serum Fe	Na+, K+
Diet history	Gluc	Ca++, Mg++
I & O	BUN, Creat	Serum folate
BP	Transferrin, TIBC	Serum B_{12}
Proctoscopy		
Sigmoidoscopy		

Common Drugs Used and Potential Side Effects

- Ulcerative proctitis patients with more frequent relapses may need a longer duration of topical therapy; prolonged oral mesalazine treatment period protects against the proximal spread of rectal inflammation (Pica et al, 2004).
- 5-ASA or corticosteroids may be needed if inflammatory bowel disease is the cause. Monitor for numerous side effects.

Herbs, Botanicals, and Supplements

- Herbs and botanical supplements should not be used without discussing with the physician.

INTERVENTION: NUTRITION EDUCATION, COUNSELING, CARE MANAGEMENT

- Teach the patient about the role of fiber in the diet.
- It is important to keep the anal skin area dry. Over-the-counter products may aggravate an allergic response.

Patient Education—Foodborne Illness

- Careful food handling and hand washing are important to prevent introduction of foodborne pathogens to the individual who may be experiencing discomfort.

For More Information

- Ano-Rectal Algorithm
  http://www.uwgi.org/guidelines/ch_10/ch10.htm
- Proctitis
  http://digestive.niddk.nih.gov/ddiseases/pubs/proctitis/

PROCTITIS—CITED REFERENCES

Pica R, et al. Oral mesalazine (5-ASA) treatment may protect against proximal extension of mucosal inflammation in ulcerative proctitis. *Inflamm Bowel Dis.* 10:731, 2004.

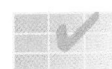

SECTION 8

Hepatic, Pancreatic, and Biliary Disorders

CHIEF ASSESSMENT FACTORS

Clinical Factors:

- Abdominal or Radiating Pain
- Hepatomegaly or Shrunken Liver (in cirrhosis)
- Ascites, Large Abdominal Girth, Edema
- Abnormal Liver MRI, Ultrasound, or Biopsy
- Varices, Gastrointestinal (GI) Bleeding, Encephalopathy?
- Diarrhea, Steatorrhea
- Vomiting, Nausea
- Anorexia, Malaise, Fatigue
- Diabetes, Hyperglycemia, Hypoglycemia
- Jaundice
- Malnutrition, Subjective Global Assessment (SGA) Score (see Figure 8-1)

Laboratory Assessment:

- Altered Serum Bilirubin (total or indirect)
- Abnormal Liver Enzymes: Alanine Aminotransferase (ALT), Aspartate Aminotransferase (AST), Lactic Acid Dehydrogenase (LDH)
- Abnormal Cholestasis Tests: Serum Alkaline Phosphatase (Alk Phos), Gamma-Glutamyltransferase (GGT)
- Markers of Specific Liver Disease: Serum Ferritin, Ceruloplasmin, Alpha-Fetoprotein, Alpha-1 Antitrypsin
- Viral Hepatitis Tests (hepatitis A, B, and C serologies)
- Altered Serum Proteins: Prothrombin Time (PT), International Normalized Ratio (INR), Partial Thromboplastin Time (PTT), Albumin, Globulin, Mitochondrial Antibodies, Antinuclear and Smooth Muscle Antibodies
- Elevated Serum Ammonia
- Altered Pancreatic Enzyme Levels
- Altered Bleeding/Clotting Times (prothrombin time, international normalized ratio)

Patient's Name: ____________________________

SGA Score

A	B	C

Part 1: Medical History

1. Weight Change

A. Overall change in past 6 months: __________ kgs. or lbs.

B. Percent change: _____ gain-< 5% loss
_____ 5-10% loss
_____ > 10% loss

C. Change in past 2 weeks: _____ increase
_____ no change
_____ decrease

2. Dietary Intake

A. Overall change: _____ no change
_____ change

B. Duration: _____ weeks

C. Type of change:
_____ suboptimal solid diet _____ full liquid diet
_____ hypocaloric liquid _____ starvation

3. Gastrointestinal Symptoms (persisting for > 2 weeks)

_____ none _____ nausea _____ vomiting _____ diarrhea _____anorexia

4. Functional Impairment (nutritionally related)

A. Overall impairment: __________ none
__________ moderate
__________ severe

B. Change in past 2 weeks: __________ improved
__________ no change
__________ regressed

Part 2: Physical Examination

SGA

Score

5. Evidence of:

	Normal	Mild	Moderate	Severe
Loss of subcutaneous fat				
Muscle wasting				
Edema				
Ascites (hemo only)				

Part 3: SGA Rating Well-Nourished Mildly-Moderately Malnourished Severely malnourished

Figure 8-1 Subjective global assessment scoring sheet (liver disease).

LIVER FACTS

Nutrition and the liver are interrelated since everything is refined and detoxified by the liver. The liver is the largest organ in the body, and it performs many complex and essential functions (see Table 8-1). As the body's internal chemical power plant, one cannot live without a liver. Mild elevations in liver chemistries such as alanine aminotransferase (ALT) and aspartate aminotransferase (AST) can reveal serious underlying conditions, such as viral hepatitis, alcohol use, medication use, steatosis or steatohepatitis (nonalcoholic fatty liver disease or nonalcoholic steatohepatitis), and cirrhosis, or more chronic health conditions, such as diabetes, heart disease, and thyroid disease (Giboney, 2005). Evaluate use of medications, vitamins, herbs, drugs, and alcohol; family history; and history of blood product transfusions in the population (Giboney, 2005).

Malnutrition is common in this set of diseases. Enteral nutrition (EN) with oral nutritional supplements (ONS) and tube feeding (TF) can increase or ensure nutrient

TABLE 8-1 Liver, Gallbladder, and Pancreatic Functions

Liver

The largest single organ of the body; it is the central biochemical organ of the body. Functionally, it:

1. Converts galactose and fructose to glucose; makes glycogen; degrades glycogen upon demand.
2. Converts proteins into glucose; synthesizes albumin, globulin, fibrinogen, prothrombin, and transferrin; removes nitrogenous wastes (ammonia); provides transamination; synthesizes purines and pyrimidines; forms amines by decarboxylation.
3. Synthesizes triglycerides; forms very low-density lipoproteins (VLDLs); oxidizes fatty acids for energy and ketones.
4. Synthesizes cholesterol from acetate; makes high-density lipoproteins (HDLs).
5. Stores vitamins A, D, E, and K and some vitamin B_{12} and C.
6. Hydroxylates vitamin D for renal activation; activates folic acid to tetrahydrofolic acid (THFA).
7. Stores minerals (e.g., iron, copper, zinc, magnesium).
8. Detoxifies drugs.
9. Produces bile.

Gallbladder

Stores bile, which helps counteract stomach acidity and aids in fat digestion through emulsification

Pancreas

1. Produces pancreatic juice when stimulated by secretin. Pancreatic juice contains bicarbonate, which helps neutralize acid chyme.
2. Secretes insulin and glucagon hormones.
3. Secretes metabolic/digestive enzymes involved in protein, carbohydrate, and fat metabolism. Pancreatic secretion has gastric, cephalic, and intestinal phases. The islets secrete insulin (b) and glucagon (a). The acini secrete lipase, amylase, trypsin, chymotrypsin, ribonuclease, and carboxypolypeptidase. The pancreas secretes enzymes (trypsin, lipase, and amylase) into the collecting duct as stimulated by cholecystokinin (also called pancreozymin), which is produced by the duodenum.

intake in case of insufficient oral food intake (Plauth et al, 2006), as follows:

- ONS improve nutritional status and survival in severely malnourished patients with alcoholic hepatitis.
- In patients with cirrhosis, TF improves nutritional status and liver function, reduces the rate of complications, and prolongs survival.
- In acute liver failure, TF is feasible and used in the majority of patients.
- TF commenced early after liver transplantation can reduce complication rate and cost and is preferable to parenteral nutrition.

PANCREAS AND GALLBLADDER FACTS

In the United States, acute pancreatitis, chronic pancreatitis, and pancreatic cancer are the most common pancreatic disease states. Pancreatic cancer is responsible for nearly 30,000 deaths annually, and gallstone disease is strongly associated with obesity. Excessive consumption of alcohol is the major risk factor for pancreatic disease, and smoking causes pancreatic cancer (Lowenfels et al, 2005). Therefore, to reduce the burden of pancreatic disease, focus on the control of three lifestyle factors: smoking, drinking, and obesity.

CITED REFERENCES

Giboney PT. Mildly elevated liver transaminase levels in the asymptomatic patient. *Am Fam Physician.* 1:1105, 2005.
Lowenfels AB, et al. The epidemiology and impact of pancreatic diseases in the United States. *Curr Gastroenterol Rep.* 7:90, 2005.

For More Information

- Abnormal Liver Function Test Algorithm
  http://www.uwgi.org/guidelines/ch_09/ch09txt.htm
- American Association for the Study of Liver Diseases
  http://www.aasld.org/
- American Liver Foundation
  http://www.liverfoundation.org/
- National Digestive Diseases Information Clearinghouse
  http://digestive.niddk.nih.gov/

LIVER DISORDERS

ALCOHOLIC LIVER DISEASE

NUTRITIONAL ACUITY RANKING: LEVEL 3

DEFINITIONS AND BACKGROUND

Alcoholic liver disease is a major cause of illness and death in the United States (Purohit et al, 2004). Alcohol is a hepatotoxin and is also ulcerogenic, especially to the esophagus. Alcohol may increase resting energy expenditure, nitrogen excretion, and appetite and can lead to cirrhosis of the liver; it affects most organs (Falck-Ytter & McCullough, 2000). Alcohol cannot be stored and is used preferentially over other energy fuels. Alcoholic liver disease affects about 2 million people in the United States.

Signs and symptoms of alcoholism include restlessness, agitation, spider angiomas on the face or back or belly, insomnia, anorexia, weight loss, GI cramping, malnutrition, delirium tremens, and hand tremors. In men, altered hair distribution and gynecomastia may occur. See Substance Abuse in Section 4 and Table 8-2 for stages of the effects of alcoholism.

Cerebellar deficits may play a causal role in the addiction process (Manzardo et al, 2005). People with a genetic deficit of beta-endorphin peptide are susceptible to alcoholism (Zalewska-Kaszubska and Czarnecka, 2005). The molecular side of the disease may eventually help identify appropriate therapies for treatment.

Alcoholics are more often malnourished than are individuals with nonalcoholic liver disease; this is true either because they eat poorly (e.g., carbohydrates, proteins, and vitamins) or because alcohol and its metabolism prevent the body from properly absorbing, digesting, and using those nutrients, particularly vitamin A (Plauth et al, 2006; Lieber, 2003). Classic effects of malnutrition from alcoholism include Wernicke's encephalopathy, Korsakoff's psychosis, muscle wasting, weight loss, and liver disease. Alcoholics may replace as much as 30% of their daily energy requirements from alcohol; alcoholic beverages account for about 6% of total energy consumed in the United States. A balanced diet will be needed to prevent or alleviate malnutrition (Lieber, 2003).

Most tissues of the body contain enzymes capable of ethanol metabolism, but significant activity occurs only in the liver and stomach (Lieber, 2005). Alcohol dehydrogenase is made with zinc. Alcohol decreases absorption of fats, fat-soluble vitamins, thiamine, folic acid, vitamin B_{12}, and zinc. Nicotine adenine dinucleotide (NADH) is significant in alcohol metabolism; through reduction of pyruvate, elevated NADH increases lactate and promotes steatosis (Lieber, 2004). The hepatotoxicity of alcohol generates oxidative stress despite an adequate diet through microsomal cytochrome P-450 2E1 and the resulting production of toxic acetaldehyde (Purohit et al, 2004; Lieber, 2000). Methionine metabolism, which needs to be activated to *S*-adenosylmethionine (SAMe), is also impaired in liver disease.

Prolonged exposure to alcohol depletes polyunsaturated fatty acids in the liver (Pawlosky and Salem, 2004). Alcohol-induced liver injury is a reflection of the immunological response of the liver to this stimulus; alcoholic fatty liver disease, necrosis, and cirrhosis are promoted by neutrophils that are damaging liver cells through cytotoxicity (Leevy and Elbeshbeshy, 2005). While there is controversy at this time about the best fatty acids to consume for protection of the liver (Purohit et al, 2004; Lakshman, 2004), sufficient intake of dietary fatty acids seems to be important.

Men and women metabolize alcohol differently. Alcohol adversely affects skeletal muscle, which is 40% of body mass and in higher proportion in men (Preedy et al, 2001). It takes less time and lower doses of alcohol exposure to cause liver damage in females than in males because there are two potential pathways (Kovacs and Messingham, 2002). See Figure 8-2.

TABLE 8-2 Stages of Alcoholism-Related Effects

Stage	Effects
I. Fatty Liver (steatosis, nonalcoholic fatty liver disease)	Reversible. Cytochrome P-450 2E1 induction, free radical generation, lipid peroxidation, and increased transcription of proinflammatory mediators, including tumor necrosis factor alpha. Acetaldehyde promotes hepatic fat accumulation. Hepatomegaly, hypertriglyceridemia, and hypoalbuminemia can occur.
II. Alcoholic Hepatitis	Fibrosis begins. Fever with tachycardia; liver enlargement is mild, and tenderness can occur.
III. Cirrhosis	Not reversible. Diffuse necrosis and regeneration of fibrous tissue leading to loss of normal hepatic function.
IV. Encephalopathy or Coma	May lead to death if not treated. Clinical syndrome characterized by impaired mentation, altered neuromuscular function, and altered consciousness.

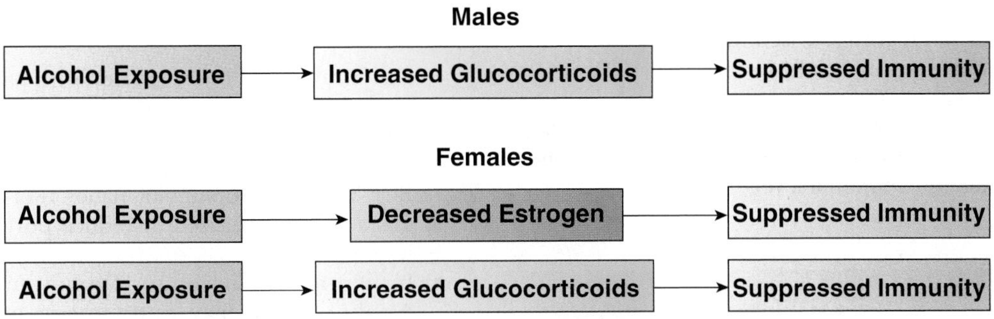

Figure 8-2 Effects of alcohol immunity in males and females. (From Kovacs EJ, Messingham KA. Influence of alcohol and gender on immune response. *Alcohol Res Health*. 26:257, 2002.)

Plasma homocysteine levels are altered in actively drinking patients with alcoholism; there may be a pathogenetic role of increased plasma homocysteine levels in alcohol-related disorders such as brain atrophy and alcohol withdrawal seizures (Bleich et al, 2005). Community-dwelling heavy drinkers who are not in alcoholism treatment have dose-related gray matter volume losses (Cardenas et al, 2005).

Treatment strategies for alcoholic liver disease include lifestyle changes to reduce alcohol consumption, cigarette smoking, and obesity; nutrition therapy; and medications (Marsano et al, 2003). Nutritional therapy either enterally or parenterally improves various aspects of malnutrition and survival (Stickel et al, 2003).

INTERVENTION: OBJECTIVES

- Remove alcohol to allow the disabled liver to function more effectively while protecting it from metabolic stress.
- Prevent hypoglycemia from blocked gluconeogenesis. Correct comorbid states, such as the metabolic syndrome with hyperglycemia, hypertension, and hypertriglyceridemia.
- Repair hepatic damage from fatty liver and diminished bile salt synthesis.
- Repair neural damage from malnutrition and malabsorption.
- Help liver tissue regenerate and replenish plasma proteins that are lost from increased nitrogen excretion.
- Correct fluid and electrolyte imbalances, nutritional deficits (such as iron deficiency anemia from chronic blood loss in varices, ulcers), and vomiting.
- Manage hypertension and other complications.
- Improve skeletal muscle synthesis.
- Improve health of liver so it can synthesize albumin and other serum proteins.
- Be honest and direct in approach. Gently confront conflicting information when stated by the patient.

INTERVENTION: FOOD AND NUTRITION

- Malnourished alcoholics should be administered a diet rich in carbohydrate and protein calories preferentially via the oral or enteral route (Stickel et al, 2003). Diet should provide protein as 1.5 g/kg body weight if malnourished or less if not malnourished. Plan adequate amounts of carbohydrates and fat to spare protein, but monitor carbohydrate and fat intake carefully in cases of hyperglycemia and dyslipidemia.
- In hypertensive patients, obesity is often of greater importance. A weight loss diet may be planned that provides a sufficient mixture of nutrients without aggravating liver disease; fasting and very low–calorie diets should be avoided.
- Monitor the type of fat selected, since amount and type seem to affect hepatic steatosis, fibrosis, and cirrhosis (Pawlosky and Salem, 2004). The diet should include a mix of fat from omega-3 (fish oils) and omega-6 fatty acids. Medium-chain fatty acids may also be well tolerated.
- Micronutrient deficiencies typically encountered in alcoholics, such as thiamin and folate, require supplementation (Stickel et al, 2003). Supplement the diet with B-complex vitamins; synthetic folacin is needed because the patient is less able to use what is provided by diet because of liver damage. Avoid excesses of supplemental vitamins A and D, which may not be well tolerated by the liver.
- Oral diet should provide adequate amounts of vitamins E and K, as well as phosphorus, potassium, selenium, magnesium, zinc, and calcium. Include fruits and vegetables or supplement with vitamin C if dietary intake is low.
- Provision of small frequent meals may be necessary to prevent hypoglycemia due to limited glycogen storage.
- Monitor iron intake carefully and avoid excesses from diet or supplements, especially if there is the possibility of iron storage disease (Swanson, 2003).

SAMPLE NUTRITION DIAGNOSTIC STATEMENT

Alcoholism

PES: Inadequate protein intake to meet needs in alcoholic liver disease related to inadequate oral food and beverage intake as evidenced by dietary intake of $<$30 g protein/d.

Assessment Data: Dietary intake records; estimate protein and energy requirements for age/gender.

Intervention: Intervention would address intake of protein foods or supplements; education/counseling about protein sources and requirements.

Monitoring and Evaluation: Track food intake (food diary or history).

- Make meals appetizing to stimulate the appetite.
- Avoid alcohol in all forms. Discontinuation allows the liver to begin healing, especially in early stages (DiCecco and Francisco-Ziller, 2006).
- If tube feeding (TF) or total parenteral nutrition (TPN) is needed, do not use a glutamine-enriched formula, which may increase ammonia levels.

CLINICAL INDICATORS

Clinical/History

Height
Weight
Body mass index (BMI)
Usual body weight (UBW)
Diet history
Blood pressure (BP)
Intake and output (I & O)
Ultrasound of abdomen
Abdominal computed tomography (CT) scan
Liver biopsy
Ascites (mild, moderate, or severe)
Fatigue
CAGE test (Cut down, Annoyed, Guilty, Eye opener)
Alcohol Use Disorders Identification Test (AUDIT)
Scurvy—ecchymoses, hemorrhagic gingivitis, perifollicular hemorrhages, leg edema, poor wound healing
Dual-energy x-ray absorptiometry (DEXA) bone scan
Diet history: level of protein, sodium, fat, and kcal intake
Food intolerances, allergies, taste aversions, anorexia
Nausea, vomiting, diarrhea
Intake of nutritional supplements (vitamins, minerals, herbs)
Nutrient/medication interactions

Lab Work

Glucose (Gluc) (increased or decreased)
AST (increased)
Glucose tolerance test (GGT) (sensitive and reliable)
ALT (normal or only mildly elevated)
Prothrombin time (PT) or international normalized ratio (INR)
Bilirubin (often elevated)
Serum ammonia (may be elevated)
Blood urea nitrogen (BUN) (may be low)
Albumin (Alb), transthyretin (often low)
C-reactive protein (CRP)
Triglycerides (Trig) (increased)
Cholesterol (Chol) (increased or decreased)
White blood cell count (WBC)
Serum B_{12}
Serum folate
Plasma homocysteine (high?)
Na+ (hyponatremia is common)
K+
Hemoglobin and hematocrit (H & H) (decreased)
Ferritin
Transferrin
Total iron-binding capacity (TIBC)
Uric acid (increased)
Globulin
Alkaline phosphatase (Alk phos) (mildly elevated)
Mg++ (decreased)
Ca++
Serum phosphorus (decreased)

Common Drugs Used and Potential Side Effects

- Disulfiram (Antabuse) is given with patient's consent. It causes the patient to vomit after ingesting alcohol and can be dangerous. Avoid alcohol in vinegar, sauces, and cough syrup.
- Beta-blockers (propranolol, nadolol) or octreotide (Sandostatin) may be used to reduce portal hypertension if varices occur.
- Insulin may be necessary. Do not mix with alcohol. Alcohol intake may cause severe hypoglycemia in patients taking insulin (Pedersen-Bjergaard et al, 2005).
- Methylprednisolone may be used in alcoholic hepatitis, with improved ability to produce albumin and to normalize PT and bilirubin levels. As a steroid, there are many possible side effects (i.e., negative nitrogen or calcium balance, hyperglycemia, etc.).
- Metformin should be avoided in patients with liver disease.
- Naltrexone may be ineffective when used alone in the treatment of chronic alcohol dependence (Krystal et al, 2001). Consideration of biological susceptibility and other factors should be considered because it is more effective in some individuals than in others (Rubio et al, 2005).

Herbs, Botanicals, and Supplements

- Antioxidants are increasingly used in liver disease, especially agents involved in methionine metabolism; SAMe and betaine have shown efficacy in animal models of alcoholic liver disease (Krueger et al, 2004).
- Milk thistle (*Silybum marianum*) may have some therapeutic effect in liver disease, but controlled trials are necessary before patients with alcoholic liver disease are advised to use it (Luper, 1998; Bass, 1999).
- *Curcuma longa* (turmeric) and *Glycyrrhiza glabra* (licorice) have been studied for their potential effects in alcoholic liver disease (Luper, 1998; Luper, 1999).
- Tea polyphenols, especially green tea, may alleviate liver damage from alcohol intake (Zhang et al, 2005; Arteel et al, 2002).
- Polyenylphosphatidylcholine was thought to prevent liver injury by downregulating cytochrome P-450 2E1 activity, but clinical trials have not proven efficacy (Purohit et al, 2004; Stickel et al, 2003).
- Herbs and botanical supplements should not be used without discussing with the physician. Chaparral is especially toxic to the liver and should be avoided; severe hepatitis or liver failure may result (Sheikh et al, 1997).
- Aloe vera has been suggested to regenerate liver cells, but evidence is not clear.

INTERVENTION: NUTRITION EDUCATION, COUNSELING, CARE MANAGEMENT

- Help patient in the planning or preparation of appetizing, nutrient-dense meals.
- Instruct patient in the sources of necessary nutrients in the diet and use of the prescribed multivitamins.

- Explain that alcohol is metabolized readily by the liver but cannot be used for muscular activity. Other nutrients are required for energy production.
- General multivitamin-mineral supplementation may improve a poor appetite.
- Discuss chemical addiction as a disease. Self-help programs and follow-up can reduce dependency.
- Obesity, diabetes, and hyperinsulinemia play a role in the development of hepatic steatosis; weight loss remains a critical part of protecting the liver against damage (Neuschwander-Tetri, 2001).
- Identify sources of assistance for persons who need help with meal preparation or with access to meals.

For More Information

- Alcoholics Anonymous (AA) World Services
  http://www.alcoholics-anonymous.org/
- Alcoholic Hepatitis
  http://www.emedicine.com/med/topic101.htm
- International Society for Biomedical Research on Alcoholism
  http://www.isbra.com/
- National Council on Alcoholism and Drug Dependence
  http://www.ncadd.org/
  http://www.ncadd.org/links/index.html
- National Institute on Alcohol Abuse and Alcoholism (NIAAA)
  http://www.niaaa.nih.gov/
- International Research Society on Alcoholism
  http://www.rsoa.org/
- Substance Abuse and Mental Health Administration (DHHS)
  http://www.samhsa.gov/

ALCOHOLIC LIVER DISEASE—CITED REFERENCES

Arteel GE, et al. Green tea extract protects against early alcohol-induced liver injury in rats. *Biol Chem.* 383:663, 2002.

Bass N. Is there any use for nontraditional or alternative therapies in patients with chronic liver disease? *Curr Gastroenterol Rep.* 1:50, 1999.

Bleich S, et al. Evidence of increased homocysteine levels in alcoholism: the Franconian Alcoholism Research Studies (FARS). *Alcohol Clin Exp Res.* 29:334, 2005.

Cardenas VA, et al. Chronic active heavy drinking and family history of problem drinking modulate regional brain tissue volumes. *Psychiatry Res.* 138:115, 2005.

DiCecco SR, Francisco-Ziller N. Nutrition in alcoholic liver disease. *Nutr Clin Pract.* 21:245, 2006.

Falck-Ytter Y, McCullough A. Nutritional effects of alcoholism. *Gastroenterology* 2:331, 2000.

Kovacs EJ, Messingham KA. Influence of alcohol and gender on immune response. *Alcohol Res Health.* 26:257, 2002.

Krueger KJ, et al. Nutritional supplements and alternative medicine. *Curr Opin Gastroenterol.* 20:130, 2004.

Krystal JH, et al. Naltrexone in the treatment of alcohol dependence. *N Engl J Med.* 345:1734, 2001.

Lakshman MR. Some novel insights into the pathogenesis of alcoholic steatosis. *Alcohol* 34:45, 2004.

Leevy CB, Elbeshbeshy HA. Immunology of alcoholic liver disease. *Clin Liver Dis.* 9:55, 2005.

Lieber CS. Alcoholic fatty liver: its pathogenesis and mechanism of progression to inflammation and fibrosis. *Alcohol* 34:9, 2004.

Lieber CS. Alcohol: its metabolism and interaction with nutrients. *Annu Rev Nutr.* 20:395, 2000.

Lieber CS. Metabolism of alcohol. *Clin Liver Dis.* 9:1, 2005.

Lieber CS. Relationships between nutrition, alcohol use, and liver disease. *Alcohol Res Health.* 27:220, 2003.

Luper S. A review of plants used in the treatment of liver disease: part 1. *Altern Med Rev.* 3:410, 1998.

Luper S. A review of plants used in the treatment of liver disease: part 2. *Altern Med Rev.* 4:178, 1999.

Manzardo AM, et al. Developmental differences in childhood motor coordination predict adult alcohol dependence: proposed role for the cerebellum in alcoholism. *Alcohol Clin Exp Res.* 29:353, 2005.

Marsano LS, et al. Diagnosis and treatment of alcoholic liver disease and its complications. *Alcohol Res Health.* 27:247, 2003.

Neuschwander-Tetri B. Fatty liver and nonalcoholic steatohepatitis. *Clin Cornerstone.* 3:47, 2001.

Pawlosky JR, Salem N Jr. Perspectives on alcohol consumption: liver polyunsaturated fatty acids and essential fatty acid metabolism. *Alcohol* 34:27, 2004.

Pedersen-Bjergaard U, et al. Psychoactive drugs, alcohol, and severe hypoglycemia in insulin-treated diabetes: analysis of 141 cases. *Am J Med.* 118:307, 2005.

Plauth M, et al. ESPEN Guidelines on Enteral Nutrition: liver disease. *Clin Nutr.* 25:285, 2006.

Preedy V, et al. Alcoholic skeletal muscle myopathy: definitions, features, contribution of neuropathy, impact, and diagnosis. *Eur J Neurol.* 8:677, 2001.

Purohit V, et al. Role of fatty liver, dietary fatty acid supplements, and obesity in the progression of alcoholic liver disease: introduction and summary of the symposium. *Alcohol* 34:3, 2004.

Rubio G, et al. Clinical predictors of response to naltrexone in alcoholic patients: who benefits most from treatment with naltrexone? *Alcohol Alcohol.* 40:227, 2005.

Sheikh NM, et al. Chaparral-associated hepatotoxicity. *Arch Intern Med.* 157:913, 1997.

Stickel F, et al. Review article: nutritional therapy in alcoholic liver disease. *Aliment Pharmacol Ther.* 18:357, 2003.

Swanson CA. Iron intake and regulation: implications for iron deficiency and iron overload. *Alcohol* 30:99, 2003.

Zalewska-Kaszubska J, Czarnecka E. Deficit in beta-endorphin peptide and tendency to alcohol abuse. *Peptides* 26:701, 2005.

Zhang Y, et al. Effect of tea polyphenols on alcoholic liver injury. *Zhonghua Gan Zang Bing Za Zhi.* 13:125, 2005.

ASCITES AND CHYLOUS ASCITES

NUTRITIONAL ACUITY RANKING: LEVEL 2

DEFINITIONS AND BACKGROUND

Ascites is defined as pathological fluid in the peritoneal cavity caused by portal hypertension. Low serum proteins or sodium retention may contribute. It is seen in patients with hepatic cirrhosis, cardiac failure, or renal insufficiency and may result from fluid loss from cells because of osmolar imbalances. A distended abdomen results.

Although weight is not used for nutritional assessment here, it does help determine fluid balance. The goal of diuretic therapy in ascites is to promote weight loss of 1–3 kg/d. Sodium restriction is needed with ascites. Renal compromise may occur with aggressive diuretic therapy. Paracentesis can complement diuretic therapy; intravenous (IV) albumin often follows this procedure. Paracentesis improves patient comfort and reduces intra-abdominal pressure and secondary renal dysfunction, but it also carries risk for peritonitis. Spontaneous bacterial peritonitis (SBP), renal failure, and hepatic cancer are the most serious complications (Sargent, 2006). Liver transplantation is the only way to improve survival in refractory ascites (Sandhu and Sanyal, 2005).

Nutrient depletion can occur if left untreated; fat, proteins, fat-soluble vitamins, and electrolytes may be lost (Cardillo, 2001). An oral diet devoid of long-chain triglycerides (LCTs) but that includes medium-chain triglycerides (MCTs) may be used in mild cases.

Chylous ascites is a rare form of ascites. This condition results from increased hydrostatic pressure and lymphatic blockade, with accumulation of LCT dense chyle in the peritoneum. Chylous ascites may result from trauma, cancer, or fistula; it is sometimes associated with a poor outcome when it is secondary to neoplasms (Laterre et al, 2000). Any source of large fluid volume losses, lymph vessel obstruction, or leakage may cause chylous effusions in the peritoneal cavities. Most chylous effusions heal spontaneously, but early and full treatment will reduce morbidity and mortality (Laterre et al, 2000). Total parenteral nutrition along with somatostatin can relieve the symptoms in patients with chylous ascites rapidly (Huang et al, 2004).

INTERVENTION: OBJECTIVES

- Reduce fluid retention, usually by diuretics. Mild ascites may present with fluid excess of 3–5 kg; moderate ascites may present with excess of 7–9 kg; and severe ascites may present with excess of 14–15 kg above usual weight.
- Prevent electrolyte imbalances.
- Prevent further pain, fatigue, loss of lean body mass (LBM), and anorexia.
- If possible, prevent hepatorenal syndrome, which can occur in patients with severe liver disease. If severe, it may require transplantation.
- Individualize diet as needs change.
- For **chylous ascites**, treatment of the underlying cause will be essential to decrease production of the chylous fluid. Malnutrition is a common result if left untreated; essential fatty acid deficiency must be avoided. Fluid and electrolyte replacement may be needed.

INTERVENTION: FOOD AND NUTRITION

- Energy needs are often as high as 1.5 times normal, and protein needs are often 1.5 g/kg of body weight (Hasse and Matarese, 2004; Riley and Bhatti, 2001). Smaller, more frequent meals are often better tolerated.
- If TF or TPN is needed, a nutrient-dense formula may help. No glutamine-enriched formulas should be used because they may increase ammonia production.
- Ensure that intake of vitamins and minerals is adequate. Water-soluble forms of vitamins may be needed; zinc and magnesium may be needed since levels are often low after diuretic therapy (Hasse and Matarese, 2004). Monitor for signs of malnutrition.
- Fluid restriction may be necessary (1–1.5 L/d), with two thirds with meals and one third for thirst/medicines.
- Restrict patient's intake of sodium to 2 g/d (Hasse and Matarese, 2004).
- Often, patients take spironolactone (Aldactone) or have renal insufficiency, which may increase potassium retention. Diet should be altered in potassium if serum levels so indicate. Other diuretics may cause potassium losses.
- For **chylous ascites,** a low-fat diet or enteral feeding is needed with MCTs as the preferred fat source; the addition of essential fatty acids (EFAs) will be needed. Adequate protein and calories are also needed since there may be significant losses. If oral diet fails, TPN may be needed, with extra water-miscible forms of fat-soluble vitamins. Assure adequate replacement of fluid and electrolytes.

CLINICAL INDICATORS

Clinical/History

- Height
- Weight
- Dry weight or estimated dry weight
- BMI
- Diet history
- BP
- I & O
- Temperature
- Abdominal ascites (mild = 3–5 kg; moderate = 7–8 kg; severe = 13–15 kg)
- Ultrasonography

Lab Work

- Serum ascites-albumin gradient (>1.1 g/dL = portal hypertension)
- Alb (decreased)
- Transthyretin
- CRP
- Na+, K+
- Ca++, Mg++
- BUN, creatinine (Creat)
- ALT
- AST
- H & H (high in hemochromatosis)
- Serum ferritin
- TIBC, % saturation
- Gluc
- Chol, Trig

Common Drugs Used and Potential Side Effects

- Diuretics are the most important treatment (Rosner et al, 2006). Check whether the specific drug retains or spares potassium. Furosemide (Lasix) is not very effective. Use of spironolactone requires monitoring of serum potassium levels closely because it spares potassium.
- Albumin replacement, while costly, may help to maintain oncotic pressure.
- Somatostatin analogs have been demonstrated to be effective (Huang et al, 2004; Laterre et al, 2000).
- With bacterial peritonitis, antibiotic therapy is needed. Monitor for specific side effects.

Herbs, Botanicals, and Supplements

- Herbs and botanical supplements should not be used without discussing with physician.

- Milk thistle may have some therapeutic effects in liver disease, but no controlled trials have shown efficacy for ascites at this time.

INTERVENTION: NUTRITION EDUCATION, COUNSELING, CARE MANAGEMENT

- Instruct patient concerning good sources of key nutrients to include and which nutrients to limit. Instruct patient to follow high-energy, high-protein diet to prevent wasting
- Ensure that the patient follows a 2-g, low-sodium diet. Explain which foods have hidden sources of sodium, and share recipes if needed.
- For chylous ascites, treatment is generally managed through a hospital stay.

ASCITES AND CHYLOUS ASCITES—CITED REFERENCES

Cardillo K. Nutrition interventions for chylous effusions. *Support Line.* 23:18, 2001.
Hasse J, Matarese L. Medical nutrition therapy for liver, biliary system, and exocrine pancreas disorders. In: Mahan L, Escott-Stump S. *Krause's food nutrition and diet therapy.* 11th ed. Philadelphia: WB Saunders Co., 2004.
Huang Q, et al. Chylous ascites: treated with total parenteral nutrition and somatostatin. *World J Gastroenterol.* 10:2588, 2004.
Laterre P, et al. Chylous ascites: diagnosis, causes, and treatment. *Acta Gastroenterol Belg.* 63:260, 2000.
Riley TR 3rd, Bhatti AM. Preventive strategies in chronic liver disease: part II. Cirrhosis. *Am Fam Physician.* 64:1735, 2001.
Rosner MH, et al. Management of cirrhotic ascites: physiological basis of diuretic action. *Eur J Intern Med.* 17:8, 2006.
Sandhu BS, Sanyal AJ. Management of ascites in cirrhosis. *Clin Liver Dis.* 9:715, 2005.
Sargent S. The management and nursing care of cirrhotic ascites. *Br J Nurs.* 15:212, 2006.

HEPATITIS

NUTRITIONAL ACUITY RANKING: LEVEL 2

DEFINITIONS AND BACKGROUND

Hepatitis is defined as liver inflammation resulting from alcohol use, toxic materials (carbon tetrachloride), or viral infection (transmitted in food, liquids, or blood transfusions). There is also an autoimmune hepatitis and a nonalcoholic steatohepatitis (NASH).

Acute viral hepatitis is a widespread inflammation of the liver and is caused by hepatitis viruses A, B, C, D, and E (Hasse and Matarese, 2004). Hepatitis causes nausea, fever, liver tenderness and enlargement, jaundice, pale stools, and anorexia. The first stage of viral hepatitis is preicteric/prodromal (with flu-like symptoms); the second stage is icteric (with jaundice, dark urine, and light stools); and the third stage is posticteric/convalescent. Fifty percent of hepatitis cases are due to hepatitis A virus (HAV), which is transmitted by fecal–oral route. Signs may include severe nausea, vomiting, right upper quadrant abdominal pain, dark urine, and jaundice (Hasse and Matarese, 2004). See Figure 8-3.

Hepatitis B virus (HBV) is considered a sexually transmitted disease. Of persons with HBV, 20% develop some form of chronic liver disease.

Hepatitis C virus (HCV) infection is a complex and challenging medical condition among injection drug users (Edlin et al, 2005). Many persons with HCV develop chronic disease. Nearly 20% of Americans test positive for HCV. A higher risk of liver cancer occurs with HCV; it can lead to cirrhosis and liver failure.

Hepatitis D virus (HDV) is an incomplete virus found accompanying HBV. Hepatitis E virus (HEV) is rare in the United States but may be transmitted by water and tends to be acute (Hasse and Matarese, 2004). See Table 8-3 for various types and symptoms or treatments for the many forms of hepatitis.

With chronic active hepatitis, inflamed liver cells continue for years, which is usually an autoimmune response. Metabolic diseases, such as Wilson's disease, hemochromatosis, and alpha-1 antitrypsin deficiency, and use of some drugs, such as methyldopa, nitrofurantoin, papaverine,

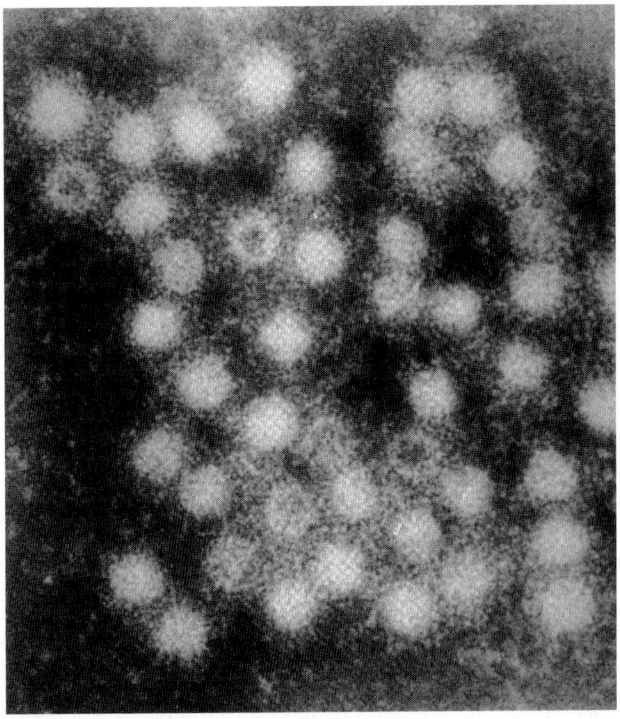

Figure 8-3 Hepatitis A. (Image from Rubin E, Farber JL. *Pathology.* 3rd ed. Philadelphia: Lippincott Williams & Wilkins, 1999.)

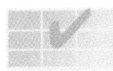

TABLE 8-3 Hepatitis Symptoms, Transmission, and Treatment

Type	Incubation	Symptoms	Transmission	Treatment
Hepatitis A Infectious HAV	30 days	Flu-like illness, jaundice, nausea, fatigue, abdominal pain, anorexia, diarrhea, fever	Ingestion of items contaminated with infected feces, drinking water or ice contaminated with raw sewage, eating fruits, vegetables, or uncooked food contaminated during handling. Risk factors: overseas travel, anal sex, IV drug use, living in poor sanitation.	Immunoglobulin 2–3 months before or 2 weeks after exposure. Vaccine is available.
Hepatitis B Serum HBV	Can survive 7 days outside of the body	Flu-like illness, jaundice, nausea, fatigue, vomiting, fever, often no symptoms	Contact with contaminated body fluids, exposure to sharp instruments that contain contaminated blood, human bites, blood transfusion before 1975. Risk factors: IV drug use, multiple sex partners, travel or work in developing countries, transfusion before 1975.	Interferon alfa and lamivudine. HBV immunoglobulin (HBIG) within 14 days of exposure. There are safe and effective vaccines. Ribavirin is under study.
Hepatitis C HCV	Average 7–9 weeks; can live 28 weeks	Often no symptoms until liver damage occurs, flu-like illness, fatigue, nausea, headaches, abdominal pain	Blood-to-blood contact, especially IV drug use and shared needles. Exposure to items with contaminated blood, such as needles (tattoo, body piercing, acupuncture), razors, nail files, toothbrushes, scissors, tampons. Sexually transmitted disease with rashes or sores. Blood transfusions before July 1992. At risk: IV drug use, had a blood transfusion or organ transplantation before July 1992, snorts cocaine. Widespread—affects 4 million people. Silent. Leading cause of cirrhosis in the U.S.	Interferon or combination drug treatments. Liver transplantation for end-stage. There are no vaccines. Treatment takes minimum of 1 year. Ribavirin is under study.
Hepatitis D HDV	Occurs only with HBV infection, cannot survive on own	Flu-like illness, jaundice, nausea, fatigue, vomiting, fever, often no symptoms	Sexual contact with HBV-infected person. Exposure to sharp instruments contaminated with HBV. At risk: IV drug use.	Interferon alpha for chronic cases. Vaccination against HBV provides protection against type D.
Hepatitis E HEV	2–9 weeks	Malaise, loss of appetite, abdominal pain, joint pain, fever	Fecal transmission, often through contaminated water. At risk: pregnant women, those who travel in developing countries.	No specific treatment.
Hepatitis G HGV	Average 7–9 weeks; can live up to 28 weeks	Often no symptoms until liver damage occurs, flu-like illness, fatigue, nausea, headaches, abdominal pain	Transmitted through blood.	No proven treatment.

dantrolene, clometacine, and ticrynafen, can cause chronic hepatitis (Hasse and Matarese, 2004).

INTERVENTION: OBJECTIVES

- Promote liver regeneration. Prevent further injury. Promote rest.
- Prevent or correct weight loss, which often results from a poor appetite, nausea, and vomiting.
- Spare protein by providing a diet high in carbohydrates.
- Force fluids to prevent dehydration, unless contraindicated.
- Prevent the spread to others. Encourage hand washing and other safe hygiene practices.

INTERVENTION: FOOD AND NUTRITION

- For patients with all forms of hepatitis, provide a complete and balanced diet. If nutritional support is necessary, consider tube feeding. Progress to a diet of small, frequent feedings of regular or soft foods. Use TPN only if necessary because of ileus or obstruction, and avoid products containing glutamine.
- Diet should provide 30–35 kcal/kg body weight. Provide sufficient carbohydrate to replenish liver stores of glycogen; include 50–55% total energy as carbohydrate.
- Intake of protein should be 1–1.2 g/kg body weight for acute hepatitis. Well-nourished or chronic active hepatitis patients may need levels that just meet DRI.
- Fat intake should be moderate to liberal, depending on tolerance. Cut back if diarrhea or other signs of malabsorption occur.
- Supplement diet with B-complex vitamins (especially thiamine, folate, and vitamin B_{12}), vitamin K (to normalize bleeding tendency), vitamin C, and zinc for anorexia and to improve encephalopathy.
- Extra fluid should be encouraged, unless contraindicated. Coffee intake may actually reduce onset of hepatocellular cancer and can be encouraged (Inouye et al, 2005).

SAMPLE NUTRITION DIAGNOSTIC STATEMENT

Hepatitis

PES: Inadequate food and beverage intake related to loss of appetite as evidenced by 10-lb weight loss in 1 month.

Assessment Data: Weight and diet history.

Intervention: Interventions would address high-protein, high-calorie diet in frequent small meals.

Monitoring and Evaluation: Plan would include scheduling patient for clinic visit in 1 month and plan to evaluate weight and diet history.

CLINICAL INDICATORS

Clinical/History

Height
Weight
BMI
Diet history
Joint pain
Upper gastrointestinal (GI) pain
Jaundice
I & O
Temperature, fever

Lab Work

Globulin
Bilirubin (increased)
AST (increased)
ALT
Alk phos (increased)
Chol
Lactate dehydrogenase (LDH) (increased)
Alb, transthyretin
CRP
BUN
Serum ammonia
Lipase
Amylase (increased)
PT or INR
Gluc
Transferrin (increased in acute stage)
H & H, ferritin
WBC
GGT
Antigen and antibody tests
Na+, K+
Ca++, Mg++

Common Drugs Used and Potential Side Effects

- A combined HAV and HBV vaccine, Twinrix, is available in many parts of the world.
- Chronic HBV and HCV are risk factors for antiretroviral-induced liver injury in patients coinfected with human immunodeficiency virus (HIV) and in patients receiving antituberculosis therapy (Novak and Lewis, 2003).
- Analgesics are used for pain in many conditions. Acetaminophen is the most common cause of acute drug-induced liver failure in many countries (Novak and Lewis, 2003).
- Avoid excessive fat-soluble vitamin intake (vitamins A and D). Vitamin A toxicity is possible in compromised liver function; monitor all supplements carefully. Beta-carotene is much less toxic and may offer reasonable antioxidant protection (Gumpricht et al, 2004).
- Interferon-α2b (Intron-A) shows promise for HBV and HCV. Dry mouth, stomatitis, nausea, vomiting, and calcium depletion can occur.
- The current gold standard of efficacy for new patients with chronic HCV is the combination of pegylated interferon and ribavirin (Camma et al, 2005). There are hemolytic side effects, possible depression, and weight and lipid changes. Etanercept as adjuvant therapy to interferon and ribavirin improves response and has decreased adverse effects (Zein and Enteracept Study Group, 2005).
- Steroids may cause side effects (i.e., sodium retention, nitrogen depletion, or hyperglycemia).

Herbs, Botanicals, and Supplements

- Herbs and botanical supplements should not be used without discussing with the physician. Carrot, schisandra, dandelion, Indian almond, and licorice have been recommended for this condition, but there are no clinical trials to prove efficacy.

- Chaparral is especially toxic to the liver and should be avoided; severe hepatitis or liver failure may result (Sheikh et al, 1997). Kava kava may also be toxic.
- *Silybum marianum* (milk thistle) has been shown to have clinical applications in the treatment of toxic hepatitis and viral hepatitis via its antioxidative, antilipid peroxidative, antifibrotic, anti-inflammatory, immunomodulating, and liver-regenerating effects (Luper, 1998). Further studies are under way.
- Oregano, sage, peppermint, garden thyme, lemon balm, clove, allspice, and cinnamon as well as the Chinese medicinal herbs *Cinnamomi cortex* and *Scutellariae radix* contain very high concentrations of antioxidants. In a normal diet, intake of herbs contributes significantly to the total intake of plant antioxidants and can be an even better source of dietary antioxidants than many other food groups such as fruits, berries, cereals, and vegetables.
- An herbal glycyrrhizin preparation used as an intravenous injection for the treatment of chronic hepatitis boosts total antioxidant intake (Dragland et al, 2003).

INTERVENTION: NUTRITION EDUCATION, COUNSELING, CARE MANAGEMENT

- Help patient make attractive, appetizing meals. Encourage frequent, small meals.
- Educate patient about how to increase calorie, protein, and vitamin intakes. Discuss pros and cons of supplemental products.
- Ensure patient abstains from use of alcohol and drugs that are hepatotoxic.

Patient Education—Food Safety

- Teach safe personal hygiene in regard to hand washing and use of disinfectants, especially when traveling overseas.
- Discuss other principles of food safety.

For More Information

- Centers for Disease Control and Prevention (CDC) Information
  http://www.cdc.gov/ncidod/diseases/hepatitis/
- Hepatitis Information Network
  http://www.hepnet.com/
  Slide Presentations: http://www.hepnet.com/pres/present.html
- Hepatitis Information
  http://www.hepatitis.org
- Hepatitis B Foundation
  http://www.hepb.org/
- Hepatitis C Central
  http://www.hepatitis-central.com/
- Hepatitis D Info Center
  http://www.hepnet.com/hepd.html

HEPATITIS—CITED REFERENCES

Camma C, et al. Treatment of hepatitis C: critical appraisal of the evidence. *Expert Opin Pharmacother.* 6:399, 2005.
Dragland S, et al. Several culinary and medicinal herbs are important sources of dietary antioxidants. *J Nutr.* 133:1286, 2003.
Edlin BR, et al. Overcoming barriers to prevention, care, and treatment of hepatitis C in illicit drug users. *Clin Infect Dis.* 40:S276, 2005.
Gumpricht E, et al. Beta-carotene prevents bile acid-induced cytotoxicity in the rat hepatocyte: evidence for an antioxidant and anti-apoptotic role of beta-carotene in vitro. *Pediatr Res.* 55:814, 2004.
Hasse J, Matarese L. Medical nutrition therapy for liver, biliary system, and exocrine pancreas disorders. In: Mahan L, Escott-Stump S. *Krause's food nutrition and diet therapy.* 11th ed. Philadelphia: WB Saunders Co., 2004.
Inouye M, et al. Influence of coffee drinking on subsequent risk of hepatocellular carcinoma: a prospective study in Japan. *J Natl Cancer Inst.* 97:293, 2005.
Luper S. A review of plants used in the treatment of liver disease: part 1. *Altern Med Rev.* 3:410, 1998.
Novak D, Lewis JH. Drug-induced liver disease. *Curr Opin Gastroenterol.* 19:203, 2003.
Sheikh NM, et al. Chaparral-associated hepatotoxicity. *Arch Intern Med.* 157:913, 1997.
Zein NN, Enteracept Study Group. Etanercept as an adjuvant to interferon and ribavirin in treatment-naive patients with chronic hepatitis C virus infection: a phase 2 randomized, double-blind, placebo-controlled study. *J Hepatol.* 42:315, 2005.

HEPATIC CIRRHOSIS

NUTRITIONAL ACUITY RANKING: LEVEL 2–3

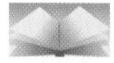

DEFINITIONS AND BACKGROUND

Hepatic cirrhosis is caused by chronic degeneration of the parenchymal liver cells and thickening of the surrounding tissue. Symptoms and signs may include fatigue, weight loss, lowered immune resistance, jaundice, and GI disturbances. It may result from alcoholic liver disease, viral hepatitis, cystic fibrosis, biliary stenosis, hemochromatosis, Wilson's disease, and other diseases; alcoholism and hepatitis C are the most common causes.

In 2001, cirrhosis was the 12th leading cause of death in the United States. Alcoholic cirrhosis is also called Laennec's cirrhosis. The Veterans Administration Cooperative Studies reported that patients with cirrhosis and alcoholic hepatitis had a 4-year mortality rate of >60% (Arteel et al, 2003). Figure 8-4 shows the cirrhotic liver.

Malnutrition plays a significant role in the pathogenesis of liver injury and should be carefully managed (Donaghy, 2002). Cirrhosis is a disease of accelerated use of alternative fuels, such as fat, since the liver stores of glycogen tend to be de-

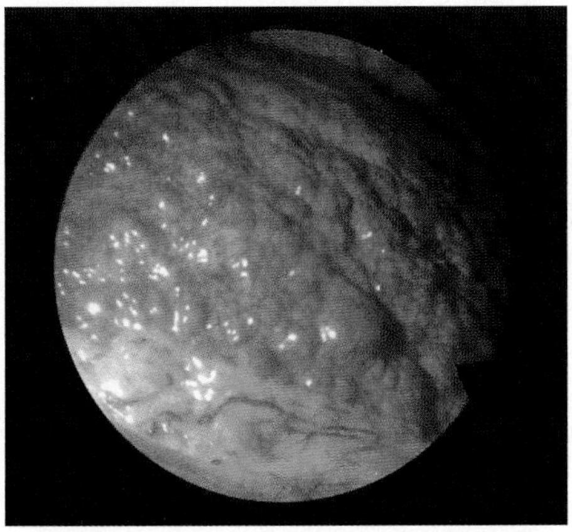

Figure 8-4 Cirrhotic liver. (From Moore KL, Agur A. *Essential clinical anatomy*. 2nd ed. Philadelphia: Lippincott Williams & Wilkins, 2002.)

pleted after an overnight fast. About half of kilocalories should be consumed from carbohydrate to minimize use of fat stores or use of protein for energy. Glucose intolerance, insulin resistance, and higher circulating glucagon may cause early satiety, hypophagia, and depleted nutrient stores (Richardson et al, 1999; Hasse et al, 1997). The deficient hepatic and muscle glycogen stores that occur with cirrhosis cause accelerated rate of starvation (Wei-Kuo et al, 1997; Crawford, 1995). Table 8-4 lists the related forms of malnutrition related to cirrhosis.

There is a high incidence of muscle wasting, weight loss, and malnutrition with cirrhosis. Decrease in caloric intake is an independent risk factor of short-term mortality (Campillo et al, 2003). Exercise and protein-rich nutrition at the early stage of liver cirrhosis can help to maintain or increase muscular volume (Kotoh et al, 2005). Nutritionally depleted

TABLE 8-4 Causes of Malnutrition in Cirrhosis

Decrease Oral Intake

- Anorexia
- Ascites
- Altered mental status or encephalopathy
- Delayed gastric emptying
- Early satiety
- Medications causing GI distress or taste changes
- Nausea
- Restrictive diets or NPO for several days

Maldigestion and Malabsorption

- Accelerated intestinal transit
- Anemia from impaired GI and liver function
- Bacterial overgrowth
- Biliary flow changes
- Decreased hepatic production and storate of nutrients
- Diuresis, paracentesis, and micronutrient losses
- Increased urinary and fecal losses
- Lactulose use
- Pancreatic insufficiency
- Villi damaged by alcohol
- Vomiting

Sources: Gottschlich MM. *The science and practice of nutrition support: a case-based core curriculum*. Gaithersburg, MD: Aspen, 2001, p 541; Stockslager JL, et al. *Nutrition made incredibly easy*. Baltimore: Lippincott Williams & Wilkins, 2003, p 242.

patients may need 1.5 g protein/kg—as much as possible without inducing encephalopathy (Hasse et al, 1997). Both enteral and parenteral nutritional support can improve the general nutrition condition of these patients, but enteral nutritional support leads to fewer complications, including bacterial translocation and intensive care unit (ICU) length of stay (Zhang et al, 2005).

Plasma aromatic amino acid (AAA) concentrations (phenylalanine, tyrosine, and tryptophan) tend to increase from rapid muscle proteolysis, decreased synthesis of proteins, and decreased liver clearance (Hasse et al, 1997). Branched-chain amino acid (BCAA) levels increase; BCAAs are leucine, isoleucine, and valine.

The imbalance in BCAA to AAA ratio seems to be an etiological factor in hepatic encephalopathy; when AAAs are high, BCAAs are limited in cerebral uptake. A higher BCAA intake helps to improve cognitive status (Charlton, 2006; Bianchi et al, 2005). Long-term BCAA supplementation is associated with decreased frequency of hepatic failure and overall complication frequency, along with improved nutritional status, as demonstrated in a large clinical trial of over 600 patients (Charlton, 2006).

Severe cirrhosis may lead to decreases in all serum lipids (Hasse et al, 1997). A low respiratory quotient (RQ) indicates reduced glucose and increased lipid oxidation and may be a useful marker for assessment of possible dietary changes that can be made (Scolapio et al, 2000). While standard IV lipid emulsions fail to improve dietary-induced steatotic injury to the liver, omega-3 fatty acids in enteral supplementation completely protect the liver, and IV sources provide partial protection (Alwayn et al, 2005).

Treatment with fermentable fiber is an alternative to lactulose for the management of minimal hepatic encephalopathy in patients with cirrhosis (Liu et al, 2004). Liver damage from cirrhosis cannot be reversed, but treatment can stop or delay further progression and reduce complications. Treatment will depend on the cause of cirrhosis and any related complications.

When end-stage liver disease results in **portal hypertension** with increased collateral flow, it causes varices in parts of the GI tract. Varices are veins that become distended near the mucosa of the GI tract due to portal hypertension and may cause pain and bleeding. Esophageal varices are the most serious complication of cirrhosis. While the pathogenesis of portal-systemic hepatic encephalopathy probably is multifactorial, serum ammonia levels may be high. Splenorenal shunting is performed when flow is diverted from the liver by anastomosis of the splenic vein to the renal vein; this is performed when the portal vein is obstructed. Portacaval blood flow is diverted from the liver by anastomosing the portal vein to the inferior vena cava. The shunt procedure called transjugular intrahepatic portosystemic shunt (TIPS) has resulted in positive outcomes in most cases.

Liver transplantation may be used for the treatment of end-stage cirrhosis, when encephalopathy, ascites, or bleeding varices are uncontrollable.

INTERVENTION: OBJECTIVES

- Support residual liver function.
- Provide supportive treatment for ascites, edema, muscle wasting, weight loss, esophageal varices, and portal hypertension.

- Monitor steatorrhea; offer suggestions for managing.
- Correct nutritional deficiencies, which are common.
- Drowsiness and disorientation are potential signs of hepatic encephalopathy; monitor closely.
- Provide adequate glucose for brain metabolism but beware of glucose intolerance, especially with alcoholic cirrhosis.
- Prevent bone disease, hyperkalemia or hypokalemia, hyponatremia, renal problems, and anemia.

INTERVENTION: FOOD AND NUTRITION

- Increased energy is needed. Calculate energy at 50–75% above usual requirements if malabsorption is present or if repletion is needed. Use ideal or estimated dry weight; fat is the preferred fuel in cirrhosis, and frequent small meals are needed (Hasse et al, 1997).
- Diet should provide 1–1.5 g of high-quality protein/kg body weight with adequate carbohydrates to spare protein. Meat has a high level of AAAs; vegetable proteins and casein may be better tolerated by some patients.
- Ensure that fat intake is sufficient; omega-3 fatty acids should be included (Alwayn et al, 2005). Malabsorption occurs from diminished lipase output. With steatorrhea, decrease LCTs, but carefully monitor use of MCTs because they may cause diarrhea or acidosis.
- Supplement diet with B-complex vitamins, vitamins C and K, zinc, and magnesium through foods or supplements. Monitor need for vitamins A and D; do not use excesses in liver disease. Liquid form may be needed for patients with esophageal varices.
- Check use of tube feedings. Tube feeding can be used with esophageal varices (Hasse and Matarese, 2004). Glutamine is not generally recommended in liver disease.
- Avoid alcoholic beverages.
- Control total carbohydrate intake with signs of hyperglycemia or with diabetes.
- Low sodium intake (2–4 g) is recommended with ascites.
- Decrease fluid in hyponatremia.
- Enhance nutrient density of food choices if malnourished.

CLINICAL INDICATORS

Clinical/History	Lab Work	
Height	BUN	Globulin
Weight	Triceps skinfold (TSF)	Somatomedin C
BMI	Alb, transthyretin (not valid in cirrhosis)	Total protein
Diet history	Retinol-binding protein (RBP)	Uric acid (UA)
Bowel changes		Gluc (increased or decreased)
BP		PT (prolonged); INR
I & O		Na+, K+
CT scan		Ca++, Mg++
Liver biopsy		Transferrin
Ascites		

H & H (decreased)	Alk phos (increased)	Copper, ceruloplasmin (increased)
Serum ammonia	WBC	Folate
ALT	Trig (increased)	GGT
AST (increased)	Chol	
Bilirubin (increased)	LDH (increased)	

Common Drugs Used and Potential Side Effects

- See Table 8-5.

Herbs, Botanicals, and Supplements

- Herbs and botanical supplements should not be used without discussing with the physician. Some herbal tea preparations may be harmful (such as Comfrey tea) and should be avoided.
- Chaparral is an herbal product used for antioxidant properties; severe hepatitis or liver failure may result (Stickel et al, 2005).
- *Silybum marianum* (milk thistle) has been shown to have clinical applications in the treatment of cirrhosis through its antioxidative, antilipid peroxidative, antifibrotic, anti-inflammatory, immunomodulating, and liver-regenerating effects (Arteel et al, 2003; Luper, 1998).
- *S*-adenosylmethionine (SAMe) may be effective in alcoholic cirrhosis (Arteel et al, 2003).

INTERVENTION: NUTRITION EDUCATION, COUNSELING, CARE MANAGEMENT

- A better appetite at certain meals may be common. Identify if breakfast or another meal is best tolerated. Some patients sleep late with a sleep reversal pattern.
- Discuss use of nutrient-dense foods and higher intakes of vegetable and dairy sources of protein if intolerant to meat.
- Dietary intake must be adjusted according to the changing status of the patient. Large meals increase portal pressure; recommend use of smaller meals throughout the day.
- Avoid skipping meals. Discuss proper menu planning.
- Avoid high doses of vitamins A and D, which may be toxic to the diseased liver.

For More Information

- CDC–Cirrhosis
  http://www.cdc.gov/nchs/fastats/liverdis.htm
- Deaths from Cirrhosis of the Liver
  http://www.niaaa.nih.gov/Resources/DatabaseResources/QuickFacts/Liver
- Family Doctor
  http://familydoctor.org/188.xml
- Liver Diseases
  http://cpmcnet.columbia.edu/dept/gi/other.html
- National Institutes of Health—Cirrhosis
  http://www.nlm.nih.gov/medlineplus/cirrhosis.html

TABLE 8-5 Medications Used in Cirrhosis

Medication	Description
Antibiotics: tetracycline (Achromycin V), ampicillin (Polycillin), trimethoprim-sulfamethoxazole (Bactrim, Septra)	Antibiotics kill the bacteria that cause infections, a common complication of cirrhosis. Possible side effects include nausea and vomiting, poor appetite, diarrhea, sore mouth or tongue, and increased sensitivity to sunlight (tetracycline).
Antiviral Medications: interferon-alpha (Alferon N, Roferon-A, Intron A), ribavirin (Virazole), lamivudine (Epivir, Epivir-HBV), baraclude (Entecavir)	These may be used if viral hepatitis B or C is the cause of cirrhosis. Treatment usually lasts for 4 months. Ribavirin is an oral antiviral agent that is given twice a day. Lamivudine is used to treat hepatitis B infection. Sometimes lamivudine is combined with interferon. Side effects may include severe GI pain, feeling of fullness, nausea, tingling, burning, numbness, or pain in the hands, arms, feet, or legs.
Anti-Inflammatory Medications (corticosteroids): prednisone, azathioprine (Imuran)	Corticosteroids reduce liver inflammation and prevent the progression of cirrhosis. High doses given long term are associated with an increase in serious side effects. Lower doses of prednisone may be used when combined with azathioprine. Possible side effects include: hypertension, glucose intolerance, and bone thinning.
Antihypertensives (beta-blockers): atenolol (Tenormin), metoprolol (Lopressor), nadolol (Corgard), propranolol (Inderal), timolol (Blocadren)	Beta-blockers are used to reduce venous blood pressure in the abdomen (portal hypertension) to reduce the risk of esophageal variceal bleeding and other complications. Possible side effects associated with beta-blocker use include: drowsiness, dizziness, cold sensitivity, and sleep disorders.
Diuretics: "Loop" diuretics: bumetanide (Bumex), furosemide (Lasix); thiazide diuretics: hydrochlorothiazide (HydroDIURIL, Esidrix), chlorothiazide (Diuril); potassium-sparing diuretics: amiloride (Midamor), triamterene (Dyrenium)	Diuretics are used to treat the buildup of excess fluid in the body that occurs with cirrhosis (as well as other diseases). These drugs act on the kidneys to increase urine output, which reduces the amount of fluid in the bloodstream. This can help to reduce portal vein hypertension and help alleviate some of the symptoms of cirrhosis, such as fluid accumulation in the abdomen and legs. Possible side effects associated with diuretic use include: loss of appetite, nausea and vomiting, dizziness, headache, lethargy, and altered blood potassium level.
Insulin	If insulin is needed, monitor carefully for hypoglycemic episodes.
Laxatives: beta-galactosidofructose (lactulose [Cephulac] and kristalose [Chronulac])	In cirrhosis, laxatives such as beta-galactosidofructose (lactulose) can help to absorb or bind toxins, such as ammonia, in the intestine and remove them from the body. Possible side effects associated with laxative use include: diarrhea, abdominal cramping, flatulence and bloating, dehydration, and weakness. Take with food or milk.
Metal Chelating Agents: penicillamine (Cuprimine, Depen), trientine (Syprine), deferoxamine (Desferal)	Metal chelating agents draw toxic metals from the bloodstream so that the body can excrete them. Chelating agents are used to rid the body of excess copper in Wilson's disease or excess iron in hemochromatosis. Both of these rare inherited diseases can produce liver damage resulting in cirrhosis. Possible side effects include: fever; joint pain; lesions on the face, neck, scalp, and/or trunk; rash, hives, or itching; swollen glands; sores or white spots on lips or in mouth; cyanosis; blurred vision; convulsions; wheezing or fast breathing; tachycardia; flushing of skin; nausea, vomiting or diarrhea; and blood in the urine.
Vitamin K: phytonadione (AquaMEPHYTON, Mephyton)	Bleeding abnormalities are common in cirrhosis. Vitamin K helps prevent excessive bleeding. Possible side effects include: flushing of the face and unusual taste.

HEPATIC CIRRHOSIS—CITED REFERENCES

Alwayn IP, et al. Omega-3 fatty acid supplementation prevents hepatic steatosis in a murine model of nonalcoholic fatty liver disease. *Pediatr Res.* 57:445, 2005.

Arteel G, et al. Advances in alcoholic liver disease. *Best Pract Res Clin Gastroenterol.* 17:625, 2003.

Bianchi G, et al. Update on branched-chain amino acid supplementation in liver diseases. *Curr Opin Gastroenterol.* 21:197, 2005.

Campillo B, et al. Evaluation of nutritional practice in hospitalized cirrhotic patients: results of a prospective study. *Nutrition* 19:515, 2003.

Charlton M. Branched-chain amino acid enriched supplements as therapy for liver disease. *J Nutr.* 136:295S, 2006.

Crawford D. Recent advances in malnutrition and liver disease. *What's New in Gastroenterology* 48:1, 1995.

Donaghy A. Issues of malnutrition and bone disease in patients with cirrhosis. *J Gastroenterol Hepatol.* 17:462, 2002.

Hasse J, et al. Nutrition therapy for end-stage liver disease: a practical approach. *Support Line* XIX:8, 1997.

Hasse J, Matarese L. Medical nutrition therapy for liver, biliary system, and exocrine pancreas disorders. In: Mahan L, Escott-Stump S. *Krause's food nutrition and diet therapy.* 11th ed. Philadelphia: WB Saunders Co., 2004.

Kotoh K, et al. High relative fat-free mass is important for maintaining serum albumin levels in patients with compensated liver cirrhosis. *World J Gastroenterol.* 11:1356, 2005.

Liu Q, et al. Synbiotic modulation of gut flora: effect on minimal hepatic encephalopathy in patients with cirrhosis. *Hepatology* 39:1441, 2004.

Luper S. A review of plants used in the treatment of liver disease: part 1. *Altern Med Rev.* 3:410, 1998.

Richardson R, et al. Influence of the metabolic sequelae of liver cirrhosis on nutritional intake. *Am J Clin Nutr.* 69:331, 1999.

Scolapio J, et al. Substrate oxidation in patients with cirrhosis: comparison with other nutritional markers. *J Parenter Enteral Nutr.* 24:150, 2000.

Stickel F, et al. Herbal hepatotoxicity. *J Hepatol.* 43:901, 2005.

Wei-Kuo C, et al. Effects of extra-carbohydrate supplementation in the late evening on energy expenditure and substrate oxidation in patients with liver cirrhosis. *J Parenter Enteral Nutr.* 21:96, 1997.

Zhang K, et al. Early enteral and parenteral nutritional support in patients with cirrhotic portal hypertension after pericardial devascularization. *Hepatobiliary Pancreat Dis Int.* 4:55, 2005.

HEPATIC FAILURE, ENCEPHALOPATHY, AND COMA

NUTRITIONAL ACUITY RANKING: LEVEL 3–4

DEFINITIONS AND BACKGROUND

Hepatic failure is common in critical illnesses. Acetaminophen overdosing is the leading cause of acute hepatic failure. Typical nutrition assessment measures may not reflect the severity of malnutrition because ascites can mask loss of lean body mass. Blood levels of lactate appear to be good markers for predicting which patients in fulminant hepatic failure can be managed medically and which need a transplantation (MacQuillan et al, 2005). Hallmarks of acute liver failure are coagulopathy, usually an international normalized ratio (INR) of 1.5 or more, and encephalopathy.

With liver failure, renal insufficiency and hepatorenal syndrome may occur. Hemodialysis may be needed until an appropriate donor is available. Creatinine measures are not useful here; glomerular filtration rate (GFR) is more relevant.

Hepatic encephalopathy (HE) is a recognized clinical complication of chronic liver disease. It can be precipitated by GI bleeding, abnormal electrolytes, renal failure, infection, diuretic therapy, use of sedatives or medications that affect the central nervous system, and constipation. HE can be induced by portacaval shunting. The spectrum of HE ranges from minimal cerebral functional deficits, which can only be found by sensitive tests, to coma with signs of decerebration (Gerber and Schomerus, 2000). Acute forms may be reversible, while chronic forms may worsen or lead to coma.

The pathogenesis of HE is multifactorial. The basis of neurotoxicity of ammonia, gamma-aminobutyric acid (GABA), or other agents implicated in this condition is not clear. Astrocytes are the most abundant cell type in the brain; they buffer extracellular $K(+)$, regulate neurotransmitter release, form the blood–brain barrier, release growth factors, and regulate the brain immune response (Gee and Keller, 2005). Acute exposure of the astrocytes to ammonia results in alkalinization, with calcium-dependent glutamate release and dysfunction (Rose et al, 2005). Glutamine, a byproduct of ammonia detoxification, is found elevated in brain in HE (Rama Rao et al, 2005).

Encephalopathy is usually not caused by altered protein in the diet (Shawcross and Jalan, 2005). Protein restriction is only necessary in rare patients with refractory encephalopathy. Other causes of hyperammonemia include GI bleed, muscle catabolism, infection, dehydration, noncompliance with lactulose/neomycin, and constipation. Decreased dopamine and elevated serotonin can occur, as well as decreased BCAAs and increased AAAs. The use of BCAA solutions is not fully supported by the literature. The effects of BCAA supplements are basically related to the severity of liver damage, and further investigations are required to determine if they are really beneficial (Suzuki et al, 2004).

Because oxidative stress is a possible trigger in the progression of chronic liver disease, antioxidant vitamins A, E, and C and carotenes may be useful to prevent the progression of chronic liver disease (Okita, 2004). In addition, because omega-3 polyunsaturated fatty acids (PUFA) modulate lymphocyte proliferation and eicosapentaenoic acid (EPA) upregulates the metabolic action of insulin, fat intake needs to be adequate (Okita, 2004).

Zinc depression occurs in advanced liver disease, and it reduces taste and immune function (Okita, 2004). Zinc deficiency may be involved in the pathogenesis of encephalopathy because it is a cofactor in ornithine transcarbamylase (OTC) activity and also influences ammonia production from aspartate (Hasse et al, 1997). Zinc supplementation improves neurological symptoms and signs of malnutrition in this population (Grungrieff and Reinhold, 2005). Measuring nutritional status can be a challenge in this population. Handgrip strength is a technique that predicts a significant incidence of major complications in undernourished cirrhotic patients (Alvares da Silva and Reverbel da Silveira, 2005). Subjective global assessment and other techniques are not quite as effective.

See Table 8-6 for stages of HE. Therapy includes timely recognition and correction of precipitating factors.

Intrahepatic portal-systemic venous shunt is a rare, spontaneous communication between the portal and the systemic-venous circulation, measuring more than 1 mm in diameter and at least partially located inside the liver (Pocha and Maliakkal, 2004). These shunts may be congenital or acquired.

Patients who have been given a **portacaval shunt (transjugular intrahepatic portosystemic shunt)** are at increased risk of encephalopathy and may benefit from mild protein restriction (Plauth et al, 2000). Gradually, their nutritional status will improve after the shunt.

Hepatic coma is a potentially serious complication of advanced liver disease; signs of impending coma are noted in

TABLE 8-6 Stages of Hepatic Encephalopathy

- Grade 0: Clinically normal mental status but minimal changes in memory, concentration, intellectual function, and coordination
- Grade 1: Mild confusion, euphoria, or depression; decreased attention; slowing of ability to perform mental tasks; irritability; and disordered sleep pattern, such as inverted sleep cycle
- Grade 2: Drowsiness, lethargy, gross deficits in ability to perform mental tasks, obvious personality changes, inappropriate behavior, and intermittent disorientation, usually regarding time
- Grade 3: Somnolent but can be aroused, unable to perform mental tasks, disorientation about time and place, marked confusion, amnesia, occasional fits of rage, and present but incomprehensible speech
- Grade 4: Coma with or without response to painful stimuli

Adapted from: Hasse J, Matarese L. Medical nutrition therapy for liver, biliary system, and exocrine pancreas disorders. In: Mahan L, Escott-Stump S. *Krause's food nutrition and diet therapy*. 11th edi. Philadelphia: WB Saunders Co., 2004; and Emedicine. Encephalopathy, hepatic. Accessed April 8, 2005 at http://www.emedicine.com/med/topic3185.htm.

TABLE 8-7 Signs of Impending Hepatic Coma

1. Irritability, change in mentation
2. Disorientation to time and place
3. Asterixis or metabolic flap (involuntary jerky movements, especially of hands)
4. Constructional apraxia (inability to draw simple diagrams)
5. Difficulty in writing
6. Ascites, edema, and fetor hepaticus (sweet, musty odor of the breath)
7. Bleeding

Table 8-7. These patients have increased intracranial pressure and brain edema with a deleterious clinical course and poor prognosis unless liver transplantation is available. Increased intracellular glutamine may be a contributory cause of brain edema in hyperammonemia; lowering of brain ammonia can include the use of L-ornithine-L-aspartate (Butterworth, 2002).

INTERVENTION: OBJECTIVES

According to the Practice Parameters Committee of the American College of Gastroenterology (Blei and Cordoba, 2001):

- **For acute encephalopathy in cirrhosis**, correct the precipitating factor. Withhold oral intake for 24–48 hours, and provide intravenous glucose until improvement is noted. Tube feeding can be started if the patient appears unable to eat after this period. Protein intake begins at a dose of 0.5 g/kg/d with added BCAAs (Okita, 2004). Progressively increase to 1–1.5 g/kg/d.
- **For chronic encephalopathy in cirrhosis**, avoid and prevent precipitating factors. Focus protein intake on dairy products and vegetable-based diets. Consider oral BCAAs for individuals intolerant of all protein.
- **For problematic encephalopathy** (nonresponsive to therapy), consider the combination of lactulose and neomycin, oral zinc, and invasive approaches such as surgical shunts.

OTHER OBJECTIVES

- Avoid skeletal muscle catabolism from protein–energy malnutrition and severely restricted diets or NPO status; decrease ammonia and toxin production. Normalize serum amino acid patterns.
- Avoid daytime or nocturnal fasting by using frequent meals and late evening snacks (Okita, 2004).
- Provide nutrition support because of elevated catabolic hormone levels.
- Promote regeneration of liver tissue.
- Support other systems (respiratory, neurological, GI, circulatory) while the liver regenerates.
- Prevent hypokalemia, sepsis, starvation, and acute crises.
- Reduce circulating amines and lessen shunting of blood around the liver.
- Control hemorrhage and blood loss into the gut.

TABLE 8-8 Nutrient Relationships in Hepatic Failure and Hepatic Encephalopathy

Increased sodium and fluid—Fluid retention

Decreased protein—Swollen belly (ascites) from decreased albumin production

Decreased protein and fat with malabsorption—Somnolence, euphoria, asterixis, coma

Decreased vitamin A—Increased respiratory infections

Decreased vitamins C and K—Hemorrhage, scurvy

Decreased magnesium, niacin, thiamin—Hallucinations, delirium, beri-beri, pellagra

Decreased B-complex vitamins, iron, and protein—Glossitis, anemias

Decreased thiamin—Amnesia, confabulation, Korsakoff's psychosis

Decreased niacin—Memory loss

Decreased folacin—Degeneration of spinal cord

Decreased vitamin K—Muscle weakness

Decreased magnesium—Marked anxiety, hyperirritability, confusion, seizures, tremor

Decreased zinc—Poor taste acuity, impaired wound healing

- Prevent progression to hepatic cancer and improve quality of life.
- Correct anemia, zinc deficiency, and other nutritional deficits such as deficiencies in magnesium, thiamin, and folate (see Table 8-8).

INTERVENTION: FOOD AND NUTRITION

- For the patient with coma, use tube feeding with 0.5–0.6 g protein/kg body weight; advance to 1–1.5 g/kg euvolemic weight. Higher intake of BCAAs in specialty hepatic products does not always give an advantage. Avoid glutamine-enriched products (Butterworth, 2002).
- Glucose is needed to reduce likelihood or presence of hypoglycemia. It may be best to start feeding slowly to prevent refeeding syndrome and then to progress to desired level of intake in the malnourished patient. It is prudent to start with 15–20 kcal/kg and progress as tolerated over several days.
- Management by protein restriction has been abandoned in recent years (Cordoba et al, 2004). For the patient who is not comatose, diet should provide moderate to high levels of protein (Shawcross and Jalan, 2005).
- Use enteral nutrition if needed to correct protein–energy malnutrition (Kato and Suzuki, 2004). A calorie-dense product is desirable. A nasogastric tube placement may be better tolerated than a gastrostomy or jejunostomy if there is ascites.
- To minimize muscle catabolism, diet should provide extra energy when tolerance is evident. Adequate intake of carbohydrates and fats is needed. Use 30 kcal/kg to maintain and 35 kcal/kg body weight to replete tissue. Use indirect calorimetry whenever possible to measure actual needs. Fats should be 30–35% of kcal, using MCT if needed.

- Parenteral solutions are to be used less often because of the risks of infection and metabolic complications. When needed, administer PN with 50% of energy as nonprotein kilocalories. Because PN does not use the gut, where bacteria would otherwise produce ammonia, parenteral protein is well tolerated and may be given as 1.0–1.5 g/kg in most cases.
- Ensure adequate intake of fluids and electrolytes as monitoring determines. Often, sodium is limited to aid diuresis. Restrict fluid only with dilutional hyponatremia (usually 1000–1500 mL).
- Vitamin-mineral supplements may be needed (niacin, thiamine, folate, phosphate, and zinc). Calcium or magnesium may be supplemented as needed. Monitor fat-soluble vitamin intake (vitamins A, D, E, and K) carefully and avoid excesses. Avoid copper and manganese at this time, and do not give iron supplements randomly.
- When oral diet is tolerated, use of a bedtime snack to avoid hypoglycemia is often desirable. Small meals and snacks throughout the day can be helpful to increase intake; oral liquid supplements can be readily available. Avoid any dietary restrictions that are severe (e.g., protein, sodium, fluid). Avoid excesses of fiber, which can slow down gastric emptying. Liquids are often better tolerated than bulky meals.

CLINICAL INDICATORS

Clinical/History

Height
Weight
Euvolemic (dry) weight
BMI
Diet history
I & O
BP
Subjective global assessment
Electroencephalogram (EEG)
Muscle stiffness or rigidity
Changes in mentation or personality
Decreased self-care
Dysfunctional movements
Flapping tremor (positive Babinski reflex)
Jaundice
Ascites
Early satiety?
Musty odor of breath and urine
Handgrip strength

Lab Work

Serum lactate levels
BUN (decreased)
Creatinine (not a valid measure in many cases)
Bilirubin (increased)
Alk phos (increased)
AST (increased)
Tumor necrosis factor (elevated)
ALT
GGT
Ca^{++}, Mg^{++}
H & H (decreased)
Ferritin and serum iron
Na^{+}, K^{+}
Chol, Trig
UA
Ammonia
Alb (decreased)
Transthyretin, RBP
CRP
PT or INR
Transferrin
Nitrogen (N) balance
Gluc (decreased)
Globulin (decreased)
Plasma amino acids (isoleucine, leucine, valine, tryptophan, phenylalanine, tyrosine)
Serum insulin, epinephrine, adrenocortical, steroids, thyroxine

Common Drugs Used and Potential Side Effects

- See Table 8-9.

Herbs, Botanicals, and Supplements

- Herbs and botanical supplements should not be used without discussing with physician. For example, chaparral is an herbal product used for antioxidant properties; severe hepatitis or liver failure may result (Sheikh et al, 1997).
- *Silybum marianum* (milk thistle) has been shown to have clinical applications in the treatment of liver disease, but it is not proven to have a therapeutic role in management of liver failure.
- Probiotics for use in HE or hepatic failure are being studied (Solga, 2003). It is suggested that probiotic, CO_2-producing lactobacilli are preferred in the treatment of HE (Bongaerts et al, 2005). Probiotics have multiple mechanisms of action that can disrupt the pathogenesis of HE (Solga, 2003).

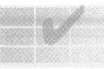

INTERVENTION: NUTRITION EDUCATION, COUNSELING, CARE MANAGEMENT

- Milk and eggs tend to produce less ammonia than meats or poultry. It is not necessary to use vegetable protein to lessen production of ammonia (Bianchi et al, 1993).
- Discuss the importance of refraining from use of alcoholic beverages.
- A better appetite at certain meals may be common. Identify if breakfast or another meal is best tolerated. Some patients sleep late with a sleep reversal pattern.
- Dietary intake must be adjusted according to the changing status of the patient.
- Large meals increase portal pressure. Recommend use of smaller meals more frequently.
- Avoid skipping meals. Discuss proper menu planning.
- Avoid high doses of vitamins A and D, which may be toxic to the diseased liver.

For More Information

- Dr. Koop–Hepatic Encephalopathy
  http://www.drkoop.com/encyclopedia/43/368.html
- Hepatic Encephalopathy
  http://www.nlm.nih.gov/medlineplus/ency/article/000302.htm
- Jackson Gastroenterology
  http://www.gicare.com/pated/ecdlv14.htm
- Medline
  http://www.nlm.nih.gov/medlineplus/print/ency/article/000302.htm

HEPATIC FAILURE, ENCEPHALOPATHY, AND COMA—CITED REFERENCES

Alvares da Silva MR, Reverbel da Silveira T. Comparison between handgrip strength, subjective global assessment, and prognostic nutritional index in assessing malnutrition and predicting clinical outcome in cirrhotic outpatients. *Nutrition* 21:113, 2005.

TABLE 8-9 Medications Used for Hepatic Encephalopathy (HE)

Medication	Description
Laxatives: lactulose (Chronulac, Duphalac)	Constipation must be avoided. One or two bowel movements a day are needed. Take lactulose with juice. It may cause abdominal bloating or gas. Lactulose, branched-chain amino acids, and ornithine aspartate are effective and can be applied for long-term use in patients with lower grades of HE (Gerber and Schomerus, 2000). Be careful not to miss doses, but also avoid excesses, which can cause or aggravate diarrhea.
Antibiotics: neomycin, metronidazole (Flagyl)	Orally administered antibiotics kill some of the bacteria present within the intestines that produce the dangerous toxins. Nonabsorbable antibiotics (aminoglycosides) have adverse effects and are limited to higher grades of HE. Be careful not to miss doses.
Medications to avoid: sedative drugs (Valium, Ativan, Xanax), pain medications (Darvocet, codeine, Vicodin, Percocet, Demerol), antinausea agents (Phenergan, Compazine), and antihistamines (Benadryl)	Certain medications can increase the brain's sensitivity to ammonia and other toxins and should not be taken.
Dietary supplements	Vitamin D and calcium may be needed if osteopenia occurs. Zinc sulfate or acetate may be needed. Other vitamins and minerals will be important, but fat-soluble forms have to be monitored, and excesses should be avoided since the liver is damaged.
Octreotide	A brief infusion induces an inhibitory effect on renin aldosterone secretion, which may yield beneficial effects on sodium excretion.
Cholestyramine or ursodeoxycholic acid	For itching.

Bianchi GP, et al. Vegetable versus animal protein diet in cirrhotic patients with chronic encephalopathy. A randomized cross-over comparison. *J Intern Med.* 233:385, 1993.

Blei A, Cordoba J. Hepatic encephalopathy. *Am J Gastroenterol.* 96:1968, 2001.

Bongaerts G, et al. Effect of antibiotics, prebiotics and probiotics in treatment for hepatic encephalopathy. *Med Hypotheses.* 64:64, 2005.

Butterworth RF. Pathophysiology of hepatic encephalopathy: a new look at ammonia. *Metab Brain Dis.* 17:221, 2002.

Cordoba J, et al. Normal protein diet for episodic hepatic encephalopathy: results of a randomized study. *J Hepatol.* 41:38, 2004.

Gee JR, Keller JN. Astrocytes: regulation of brain homeostasis via apolipoprotein E. *Int J Biochem Cell Biol.* 37:1145, 2005.

Gerber T, Schomerus H. Hepatic encephalopathy in liver cirrhosis: pathogenesis, diagnosis and management. *Drugs* 60:1353, 2000.

Grungrieff K, Reinhold D. Liver cirrhosis and "liver" diabetes mellitus are linked by zinc deficiency. *Med Hypotheses.* 64:316, 2005.

Hasse J, Matarese L. Medical nutrition therapy for liver, biliary system and exocrine pancreas disorders. In: Mahan L, Escott-Stump S. *Krause's food nutrition and diet therapy.* 11th ed. Philadelphia: WB Saunders Co., 2004.

Hasse J, et al. Nutrition therapy for end-stage liver disease: a practical approach. *Support Line* XIX:8, 1997.

Kato A, Suzuki K. How to select BCAA preparations. *Hepatol Res.* 30: 30S, 2004.

Macquillan GC, et al. Blood lactate but not serum phosphate levels can predict patient outcome in fulminant hepatic failure. *Liver Transpl.* 11:1073, 2005.

Okita M. Chronic hepatic disease and dietary instruction. *Hepatol Res.* 30:92S 2004.

Plauth M, et al. Post-feeding hyperammonaemia in patients with transjugular intrahepatic portosystemic shunt and liver cirrhosis: role of small intestinal ammonia release and route of nutrient administration. *Gut* 46:849, 2000.

Pocha C, Maliakkal B. Spontaneous intrahepatic portal-systemic venous shunt in the adult: case report and review of the literature. *Dig Dis Sci.* 49:1201, 2004.

Rama Rao KV, et al. Differential response of glutamine in cultured neurons and astrocytes. *J Neurosci Res.* 79:193, 2005.

Rose C, et al. Acute insult of ammonia leads to calcium-dependent glutamate release from cultured astrocytes: an effect of pH. *J Biol Chem.* 280:20937, 2005.

Shawcross D, Jalan R. Dispelling myths in the treatment of hepatic encephalopathy. *Lancet* 365:431, 2005.

Sheikh NM, et al. Chaparral-associated hepatotoxicity. *Arch Intern Med.* 157:913, 1997.

Solga SF. Probiotics can treat hepatic encephalopathy. *Med Hypotheses.* 61:307, 2003.

Suzuki K, et al. Branched-chain amino acid treatment in patients with liver cirrhosis. *Hepatol Res.* 30:25S, 2004.

JAUNDICE

NUTRITIONAL ACUITY RANKING: LEVEL 1

DEFINITIONS AND BACKGROUND

A yellowish discoloration of the skin, mucous membranes, and some body fluids, jaundice results from accumulation of bile or bilirubin. It is a sign, not a disease. Causes of jaundice include excessive red blood cell (RBC) destruction and biliary obstruction from gallstones, tumors, or parasites.

Jaundice is classified as *hemolytic* (from excess bilirubin production), *hepatic* (from an immature liver or from damage), or *obstructive* (from obstructed biliary ducts). Prehepatic causes of jaundice include hemolysis and hematoma resorption, which lead to elevated levels of unconjugated (indirect) bilirubin (Roche and Kobos, 2004). In intrahepatic disorders, bilirubin levels are elevated by alcohol, infectious hepatitis,

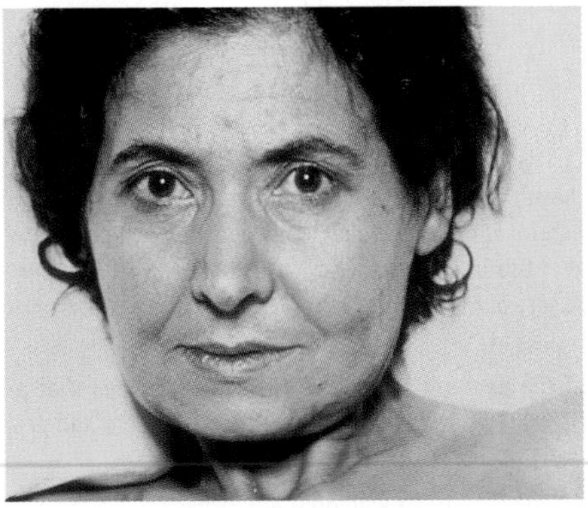

Figure 8-5 Signs of jaundice. (From Smith DS. *Field guide to bedside diagnosis*. Philadelphia: Lippincott Williams & Wilkins, 1999.)

drug reactions, and autoimmune disorders (Roche and Kobos, 2004). Posthepatic disorders that cause jaundice may include gallstone formation, biliary tract infection, pancreatitis, and malignancies (Roche and Kobos, 2004). See Figure 8-5.

In the obstructive type of jaundice, no bile pigment is present, and the stool becomes pale and clay colored, indicating fat maldigestion or malabsorption. Anorexia is a frequent finding in patients with biliary obstruction. Decreased food intake may be related to the degree of obstruction and increases in cholecystokinin levels; biliary drainage improves biochemical and food intake (Padillo et al, 2001). Plastic stents are placed in cases of malignant jaundice but can be complicated by recurrent obstruction; use of ciprofloxacin may help to maintain patency (Chan et al, 2005).

Obstructive jaundice leads to bacterial translocation (BT) by disruption of the gut barrier, intestinal microecology, and impaired host immune defense. Oral administration of an arginine, omega-3 fatty acids, glutamine, and an RNA-supplemented enteral diet for immunonutrition has been recommended but has not been widely accepted yet (Kuru et al, 2004; Zulfikaroglu et al, 2003).

In neonatal jaundice, there is a somewhat normal pattern of hyperbilirubinemia that is not detrimental. The challenge to clinicians is to distinguish the features of normalcy from abnormal conditions that place the infant at risk (Gartner and Herschel, 2001).

INTERVENTION: OBJECTIVES

- Correct underlying cause of jaundice.
- Correct fat malabsorption.
- Prevent osteopenia.
- Correct anorexia and poor intake from the underlying disease or condition.

INTERVENTION: FOOD AND NUTRITION

- Use a diet according to etiology of the jaundice and current weight status. If weight loss has occurred, a high-energy diet may be needed. If tube feeding is needed, products containing arginine and glutamine may be beneficial (Kuru et al, 2004).
- Include rich dietary sources of calcium, vitamin K, vitamin D, and other nutrients.
- Exclude alcoholic beverages from the diet.

CLINICAL INDICATORS

Clinical/History	Lab Work	
Height	Serum bilirubin	CRP
Weight	Urine test for bilirubin	BUN
BMI	ALT	Amylase
Diet history	AST	Trig
Ultrasonography	GGT	Alk phos
Biopsy if necessary	Serum lipase	H & H
Yellowing of skin and eyes	Chol (increased if obstructive)	Carotenoids (increased/ decreased)
	Alb	Gluc
		Na+, K+
		Ca++, Mg++

Common Drugs Used and Potential Side Effects

- Bile salts may be used to correct faulty fat absorption if that is related.
- Avoid excesses of vitamins A and D because liver function is abnormal and toxicity may occur.

Herbs, Botanicals, and Supplements

- Herbs and botanical supplements should not be used without discussing with physician. Herbal and dietary supplements are potential hepatotoxins in a high proportion of patients with jaundice and hepatic failure (Estes et al, 2003).
- Milk thistle may have some role in liver disease but has not been proven to be efficacious in jaundice through controlled clinical trials.
- Yin Zhi Huang, a decoction of *Artemisia capillaris* and three other herbs, is widely used in Asia to prevent and treat neonatal jaundice; more studies are needed (Huang et al, 2004).

INTERVENTION: NUTRITION EDUCATION, COUNSELING, CARE MANAGEMENT

- Show the patient how to make meals that are appetizing and balanced in all key nutrients.
- Discuss the role of organs in digestion and absorption. Jaundice does not always involve fat malabsorption, although this may occur in the obstructive form.

JAUNDICE—CITED REFERENCES

Chan G, et al. The role of ciprofloxacin in prolonging polyethylene biliary stent patency: a multicenter, double-blinded effectiveness study. *J Gastrointest Surg.* 9:481, 2005.

Estes JD, et al. High prevalence of potentially hepatotoxic herbal supplement use in patients with fulminant hepatic failure. *Arch Surg.* 138:852, 2003.
Gartner L, Herschel M. Jaundice and breastfeeding. *Pediatr Clin North Am.* 48:389, 2001.
Huang W, et al. A traditional herbal medicine enhances bilirubin clearance by activating the nuclear receptor CAR. *J Clin Invest.* 113:137, 2004.
Kuru B, et al. Effect of different enteral nutrients on bacterial translocation in experimental obstructive jaundice. *Eur Surg Res.* 36:45, 2004.
Padillo F, et al. Anorexia and the effect of internal biliary drainage on food intake in patients with obstructive jaundice. *J Am Col Surg.* 192:584, 2001.
Roche SP, Kobos R. Jaundice in the adult patient. *Am Fam Physician.* 69:299, 2004.
Zulfikaroglu B, et al. The effect of immunonutrition on bacterial translocation, and intestinal villus atrophy in experimental obstructive jaundice. *Clin Nutr.* 22:277, 2003.

LIVER TRANSPLANTATION

NUTRITIONAL ACUITY RANKING: LEVEL 4

DEFINITIONS AND BACKGROUND

Liver transplantation is now a viable alternative for patients with end-stage hepatic failure due to cirrhosis, viral hepatitis, chronic active liver disease, alpha-1 antitrypsin deficiency, primary sclerosing cirrhosis, cholangiocarcinoma, hemochromatosis, autoimmune hepatitis, Budd-Chiari syndrome, hepatoma, or primary biliary cirrhosis. In addition, cystic fibrosis patients may suffer from the consequences of liver disease, and without liver transplantation, variceal hemorrhage, malnutrition, or end-stage liver disease can lead to death (Molmenti et al, 2003).

Nutritional depletion occurs in this population before surgery. Muscle wasting, cachexia, and decreased fat stores are common. Supportive care for all patients with acute liver failure includes adequate enteral nutrition, aggressive screening and treatment of infection, prophylactic broad-spectrum antibiotics, and antifungal agents (Hay, 2004). Alcohol is a major contributor to cirrhosis and the need for transplantation. Nonalcoholic steatohepatitis (NASH) is a precursor to cirrhosis; obesity, diabetes, and hyperinsulinism play a role in the 1–2% of liver transplantations performed for NASH (Neuschwander-Tetri, 2001).

Patients are screened carefully for other underlying conditions; many will not be suitable for transplantation. Symptoms and signs leading to the need for transplantation include ascites, jaundice, edema, CNS dysfunction, and cachexia. In living donor liver transplantation (LDLT), a healthy, living person donates a portion of his or her liver to another person.

Preoperative and early postoperative nutrition may speed recovery, lessen time in the intensive care unit, and promote fewer infections. Subjective global assessment (SGA) is often useful because lab work varies so much in liver disease. SGA includes physical signs and symptoms, dietary changes and intolerances, medical/surgical history, GI symptoms and complaints, history of weight loss, and functional capacity (see Fig. 8-1). Transthyretin (transthyretin) may be a reliable test when the inflammatory process resolves (Raguso et al, 2002).

In general, enteral nutrition is effective in maintaining nutritional status after transplantation. Nutritional supplementation after liver transplantation quickly restores protein synthesis in the allograft (Geevarghese et al, 1999).

Patients with end-stage liver disease are prone to develop osteopenia and osteoporosis, and additional bone loss may occur with the use of immunosuppression agents after orthotopic liver transplant (OLT) (Scolapio et al, 2003). Bone loss occurs early after OLT in all liver transplantation recipients and leads to postoperative fractures, especially in patients with the lowest bone mass (Guichelaar et al, 2004). Bone mineral density after the first year from a successful pediatric liver transplantation can be normal if care is taken to provide adequate nutrition and lower doses of corticosteroids (D'Antiga et al, 2004). Calcium and vitamin D intake must be a priority.

Primary cancer of the liver has the lowest long-term survival rate (50–60%) after transplantation, and some other causes have survival rates of over 90% (Jackson Gastroenterology, 2005). In patients who have received a transplantation because of hepatitis C, it is important to monitor carefully for recurrence of the underlying disorder to prevent allograft rejection (Testa et al, 2000).

INTERVENTION: OBJECTIVES

Pretransplantation

- Correct malnutrition; lessen edema and ascites.
- Treat hyponatremia and electrolyte imbalances, depending on medications and renal function.
- Prevent or correct catabolic wasting of muscle mass from increased hormonal levels (insulin, glucagon, epinephrine, and cortisol may be elevated).
- Provide nutritional support in an appropriate mode of feeding (considering nausea, vomiting, etc.) to provide a normalized nitrogen balance and other normalized laboratory values.
- Normalize blood glucose levels and prevent hypoglycemia; diabetes is common.
- Correct fat malabsorption, with or without steatorrhea and diarrhea.
- Correct abnormal amino acid metabolism and neural accumulation of amino acids that are precursors for dopamine, serotonin, and norepinephrine. Normalize serum ammonia.

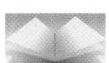

Posttransplantation

- Promote normalized protein synthesis in the liver (i.e., albumin, globulins, clotting factors, etc.). Monitoring nutritional parameters will not be a simple process, and many usual measurements are not useful markers of nutritional decline (Shahid et al, 2005).
- Prevent or correct hyperglycemia, fasting hypoglycemia, and abnormal glucagon storage. Diabetes is a common complication. Transplantation patients are at risk of glucose intolerance from use of prednisone, cyclosporine, and tacrolimus (Hasse et al, 1995).
- Prevent hypophosphatemia (Burak et al, 2004).
- Support wound healing.
- Prevent infection and rejection, the most common complications.
- Manage long-term hypercholesterolemia, hypertension, and obesity. Protect against osteopenia and bone fractures.

INTERVENTION: FOOD AND NUTRITION (SEE TABLE 8-10)

Pretransplantation

- Energy should be 35–45 kcal/kg dry weight for malnourished patients and 30–35 kcal/kg dry weight to maintain (Hasse, 2005). Sufficient carbohydrate and fat to meet energy needs will be needed; use carbohydrate counting for persons who have hyperglycemia or diabetes.
- Protein needs will vary: 0.8–1.0 g/kg dry weight in compensated liver disease; 1.5–2.0 g/kg dry weight in decompensated liver disease; and 0.6–1.0 g/kg dry weight for hepatic encephalopathy; consider use of BCAA-enriched formulas (Hasse, 2005).
- Modify for fluid, sodium, potassium, and other electrolytes depending on lab values and renal status. Sodium restriction may require 2- to 4-g limit. Fluid may require 1000- to 1500-mL daily limit with edema (Hasse, 2005).
- If tube feeding (TF), use a low-volume, diluting concentration as needed. Avoid glutamine-enriched solutions if ammonia levels are a concern.
- Beware of excess vitamins and minerals because of liver functioning; use levels that meet recommended daily allowances. Fat malabsorption is common; use water-miscible forms of vitamins A, D, E, and K with steatorrhea. B-complex vitamins may be depleted, and stores of calcium, magnesium, potassium, phosphorus, manganese, copper, and zinc are often low (Hasse, 2005).

CLINICAL INDICATORS

Clinical/History
- Height
- Weight—usual
- Present weight
- BMI
- Diet history
- Edema
- Nausea and vomiting
- I & O
- BP
- SGA
- Ascites?
- Early satiety?
- DEXA

Lab Work
- Serum lactate levels
- BUN, Creat
- Alb
- Transthyretin
- N balance
- Amino acid profiles
- Na+, K+
- CRP
- Alk phos
- Bilirubin
- Serum ammonia
- Cerebrospinal fluid (CSF)
- Ca++, Mg++
- H & H
- Serum Fe
- Transferrin
- Urea
- Chol, Trig
- Carotenoids
- AST, ALT
- GGT
- Gluc
- PT or INR

TABLE 8-10 Post–Liver Transplantation Nutrition Guidelines

Nutrient	Short-Term Recommendations	Long-Term Recommendations
Calories	120–130% of BEE or measure REE; increase for weight gain	Maintenance: 120–130% of BEE depending on activity level
Protein	1.3–2 g/kg/d	1 g/kg/day
Carbohydrate	50–70% of calories	50–70% of calories; restrict simple sugars
Fat	30% of calories	<30% of total calories
	Up to 50% of calories with severe hyperglycemia	<10% of calories as saturated fat
Calcium	800–1200 mg/d	1000–1500 mg/d (consider the need for estrogen or vitamin D supplements)
Sodium	2–4 g/d	3–4 g/d
Magnesium and Phosphorus	Encourage intake of foods high in these nutrients	Encourage intake of foods high in these nutrients
	Supplement as needed	Supplement as needed
Potassium	Supplement or restrict based on serum potassium levels	Supplement or restrict based on serum potassium levels
Other Vitamins and Minerals	Multivitamin-mineral: supplement to DRI or RDA levels	Adequate vitamin D will be needed to prevent deficiency; multivitamin-mineral: supplement to DRI or RDA levels

BEE, basal energy expenditure; REE, resting energy expenditure.

Source: Hasse, 2005; Segal et al, 2003.

TABLE 8-11 Medications Used after Liver Transplantation

Medication	Description
Analgesics	Analgesics are used to reduce pain. Long-term use may affect such nutrients as vitamin C and folacin; monitor carefully for each specific medication.
Azathioprine (Imuran)	Azathioprine may cause anorexia, leukopenia, thrombocytopenia, oral and esophageal sores, macrocytic anemia, pancreatitis, vomiting, diarrhea, and altered taste acuity. Folate supplementation and other dietary modifications (liquid or soft diet, use of oral supplements, and flavor enhancements) may be needed. The drug works by lowering the number of T cells; it is often prescribed along with prednisone for conventional immunosuppression.
Corticosteroids (prednisone or Solu-Cortef)	Corticosteroids such as prednisone and Solu-Cortef are used for immunosuppression. Side effects include increased catabolism of proteins, negative nitrogen balance, hyperphagia, ulcers, decreased glucose tolerance, sodium retention, fluid retention, and impaired calcium absorption and osteoporosis. Cushing's syndrome, obesity, muscle wasting, and increased gastric secretion may result. A higher protein intake and lower intake of carbohydrate and sodium may be needed.
Cyclosporine	Cyclosporine does not retain sodium as much as corticosteroids do. Intravenous doses are more effective than oral doses. Nausea, vomiting, and diarrhea are common side effects. Hyperlipidemia, hyperglycemia, and hyperkalemia may also occur; decrease fat intake as well as sodium and potassium if necessary. Magnesium may need to be replaced. The drug is also nephrotoxic; a controlled renal diet may be beneficial. Taking omega-3 fatty acids during cyclosporine therapy may reduce toxic side effects (such as high blood pressure and kidney damage) associated with this medication in transplantation patients (Tsipas and Morphake, 2003). Avoid use with St. John's wort.
Diuretics	Diuretics such as furosemide (Lasix) may cause hypokalemia. Aldactone actually spares potassium; monitor drug changes closely. In general, avoid use with fenugreek, yohimbe, and ginkgo.
Immunosuppressants	Immunosuppressants such as muromonab (Orthoclone OKT3) and antithymocyte globulin (ATG) are less nephrotoxic than cyclosporine but can cause nausea, anorexia, diarrhea, and vomiting. Monitor carefully. Fever and stomatitis also may occur; alter diet as needed.
Insulin	Insulin may be necessary during periods of hyperglycemia. Monitor for hypoglycemic symptoms during use.
Mycophenolate mofetil	Diarrhea is common. Extra fluids will be needed.
Muromonab (Orthoclone OKT3)	This drug can lead to nausea, vomiting, diarrhea, and anorexia, and meal adjustments may be needed.
Tacrolimus (Prograf, FK506)	Tacrolimus suppresses T-cell immunity; it is 100 times more potent than cyclosporine, thus requiring smaller doses (McAlister, 2001). Side effects include GI distress, nausea, vomiting, hyperkalemia, and hyperglycemia; adjust diet accordingly by reducing carbohydrate or elevating potassium intake. Maternal therapy with tacrolimus for liver transplantation may be compatible with breastfeeding (French et al, 2003).

Common Drugs Used and Potential Side Effects

- See Table 8-11.

Herbs, Botanicals, and Supplements

- Use of probiotics may be quite helpful in this population. A synbiotic composition in an enteral feeding, consisting of one lactic acid bacteria (LAB) and one fiber, greatly reduces incidence of postoperative bacterial infections (Rayes et al, 2005).
- Herbs and botanical supplements should not be used without discussing with physician. Chaparral is an herbal product used for antioxidant properties; severe hepatitis or liver failure may result, and it should be avoided after transplantation (Sheikh et al, 1997).
- In one study, 50% of liver transplantation patients admitted to using vitamins after surgery, and 19% used herbal remedies combined with vitamins, mostly silymarin (Neff et al, 2004). *Silybum marianum* (milk thistle) has been shown to have clinical applications in the treatment of liver disease.
- St. John's wort interferes with the metabolism of cyclosporine and should not be used after transplantation (Karliova et al., 2000).

INTERVENTION: NUTRITION EDUCATION, COUNSELING, CARE MANAGEMENT (POSTTRANSPLANTATION)

- Discuss the role of diet in wound healing, graft retention, and improvement in health status.
- Provide patient or family with recipes for no-added-salt and sugar-free foods as needed.
- Obesity can occur unless energy intakes are controlled. This is often the most significant long-term concern.
- Discuss sources of foods that contain calcium and magnesium and other specific nutrients. Individualize to patient preferences and needs.
- Discuss the need for alcohol rehabilitation, family counseling, or other available services. Ethanol/ethyl alcohol (ETOH) abuse affects such key nutrients as niacin, folate, vitamin B_{12}, zinc, phosphorus, and magnesium.
- Maintaining good diet and physical activity is to be recommended to support bone density.

Patient Education—Foodborne Illness

- Careful food handling and hand washing are important to prevent introduction of foodborne pathogens to the transplantation individual who may be experiencing graft–host rejection.

- Prevent infections from foodborne illness; patients who have undergone transplantation may be prone to increased risk more than other individuals.

For More Information

- American Society of Transplantation
  http://www.a-s-t.org/about/bylaws/bylaws_article-lll.htm
- Biliary Atresia and Liver Transplant Network
  http://www.transweb.org/people/recips/resources/support/oldbilitree.html
- Columbia University–Transplantation
  http://cpmcnet.columbia.edu/dept/gi/transplant.html
- Jackson Gastroenterology
  http://www.gicare.com/pated/epdlv44.htm
- Liver Foundation–Transplant
  http://www.liverfoundation.org/db/articles/1016
- Medicine Net
  http://www.medicinenet.com/liver_transplant/article.htm
- National Institute of Diabetes and Digestive and Kidney Diseases (NIDDK)–Liver Transplant
  http://digestive.niddk.nih.gov/ddiseases/pubs/livertransplant/
- United Network for Organ Sharing
  http://www.unos.org/
- USC Liver Transplant Guide
  http://www.surgery.usc.edu/divisions/hep/patientguide/

LIVER TRANSPLANTATION—CITED REFERENCES

Burak KW, et al. Hypophosphatemia after right hepatectomy for living donor liver transplantation. *Can J Gastroenterol.* 18:729, 2004.

DiAntiga L, et al. Long-term outcome of bone mineral density in children who underwent a successful liver transplantation. *Transplantation* 78:899, 2004.

French AE, et al. Milk transfer and neonatal safety of tacrolimus. *Ann Pharmacother.* 37:815, 2003.

Geevarghese S, et al. The effect of nutritional and hormonal supplementation on protein synthesis immediately after liver transplantation. *J Surg Res.* 81:196, 1999.

Guichelaar MM, et al. Immunosuppressive and postoperative effects of orthotopic liver transplantation on bone metabolism. *Liver Transpl.* 10:638, 2004.

Hasse J. Liver transplantation. Accessed May 1, 2006 at http://www.center-span.org/pubs/liver/hasse1.htm#acute.

Hasse J, et al. Early enteral nutrition support in patients undergoing liver transplantation. *J Parenter Enteral Nutr.* 19:437, 1995.

Hay JE. Acute liver failure. *Curr Treat Options Gastroenterol.* 7:459, 2004.

Jackson Gastroenterology. Liver transplant. Accessed April 9, 2005 at http://www.gicare.com/pated/epdlv44.htm.

Karliova M, et al. Interaction of *Hypericum perforatum* (St John's wort) with cyclosporin A metabolism in a patient after liver transplantation. *J Hepatol.* 33:853, 2000.

McAlister V, et al. Orthotopic liver transplantation using low-dose tacrolimus and sirolimus. *Liver Transpl.* 7:701, 2001.

Molmenti EP, et al. Liver transplantation for cholestasis associated with cystic fibrosis in the pediatric population. *Pediatr Transplant.* 7:93, 2003.

Neff GW, et al. Consumption of dietary supplements in a liver transplant population. *Liver Transpl.* 10:881, 2004.

Neuschwander-Tetri B. Fatty liver and nonalcoholic steatohepatitis. *Clin Cornerstone.* 3:47, 2001.

Raguso CA, et al. Assessment of nutritional status in organ transplant: is transthyretin a reliable indicator? *Clin Chem Lab Med.* 40:1325, 2002.

Rayes N, et al. Supply of pre- and probiotics reduces bacterial infection rates after liver transplantation—a randomized, double-blind trial. *Am J Transplant.* 5:125, 2005.

Scolapio JS, et al. Influence of tacrolimus and short-duration prednisone on bone mineral density following liver transplantation. *J Parenter Enteral Nutr.* 27:427, 2003.

Segal E, et al. Predominant factors associated with bone loss in liver transplant patients after prolonged post-transplantation period. *Clin Transplant.* 17:13, 2003.

Shahid M, et al. Nutritional markers in liver allograft recipients. *Transplantation* 79:359, 2005.

Sheikh NM, et al. Chaparral-associated hepatotoxicity. *Arch Intern Med.* 157:913, 1997.

Testa G, et al. Liver transplantation for hepatitis C: recurrence and disease progression in 300 patients. *Liver Transpl.* 6:553, 2000.

Tsipas G, Morphake P. Beneficial effects of a diet rich in a mixture of n-6/n-3 essential fatty acids and of their metabolites on cyclosporine nephrotoxicity. *J Nutr Biochem.* 14:626, 2003.

PANCREATIC DISORDERS

PANCREATITIS, ACUTE

NUTRITIONAL ACUITY RANKING: LEVEL 3–4

DEFINITIONS AND BACKGROUND

Acute pancreatitis (AP) is an inflammatory process that involves the pancreas or other organs (Khokhar and Seidner, 2004). The exocrine pancreas secretes proteolytic, lipolytic, and amylolytic enzymes for nutrient digestion in the intestines. AP is initiated inside acinar cells by premature activation of digestive enzymes and disturbances of intracellular calcium (Adler, 2004). AP can range from a mild, self-limited course requiring only brief hospitalization to a rapidly progressive, fulminant illness resulting in multiple organ dysfunction or sepsis (Nathens et al, 2004).

Inflammation with edema, fat necrosis, and cellular exudate occur. Enzymes become activated in the pancreas instead of the duodenum. AP is common in men between the ages of 35 and 45 years, primarily from alcohol abuse and secondarily from gallstones (cholelithiasis). It is difficult to differentiate between pancreatitis and acute cholecystitis; but a correct diagnosis is important because the treatments are very different. Besides alcohol abuse and gallstones, other causes of AP include end-stage renal disease, lupus, biliary tract disease, abdominal trauma, certain dyslipidemias (especially triglycerides >1000 mg/dL), acquired immunodeficiency syndrome (AIDS), and pancreatic cancer. Evaluation for a susceptible genotype may become important (Balog et al, 2005).

Symptoms of AP include sudden, severe abdominal pain, nausea, vomiting, and diarrhea. It is possible to use magnetic resonance imaging (MRI) and computed tomography (CT) in staging (Kwon and Brugge, 2005).

Complications include sepsis, acute renal failure, hypovolemia, circulatory shock, and pancreatic necrosis. Abdominal pain can be constant and disabling, causing some patients to become addicted to pain medications. About 25% of persons with AP go on to have chronic pancreatitis. Surgery for AP may include necrosectomy, pancreaticoduodenectomy, or sphincterotomy.

Oxygen free radical–mediated tissue damage is well established in the pathogenesis of AP, and use of antioxidants may be beneficial. Cytokines involved in the systemic inflammatory response in AP include lipid mediators (prostanoids, thromboxanes, and leukotrienes) generated from arachidonic acid (AA) and eicosapentaenoic acid (EPA) (Foitzik et al, 2002).

The role of the gut in maintaining immune system integrity is widely recognized. Therefore, nutrition support by the enteral route is now the preferred modality in patients with severe AP. Nasojejunal feeding tube and a low-molecular diet provide clear advantages compared to parenteral nutrition, such as fewer infectious complications, shorter length of hospital stay, lower cost, and less need for surgery (Meier and Beglinger, 2006; Lasztity et al, 2005; McClave, 2004; Weimann et al, 2004).

Parenteral nutrition (PN) is used when full nutritional requirements cannot be met enterally so that body composition is preserved (Chandrasegaram et al, 2005). Failure to use the gut in AP results in increased gut permeability and increased systemic bacterial challenge, so use of PN should be short term (McClave, 2004).

INTERVENTION: OBJECTIVES

- Reduce pain. Achieve pancreatic rest simultaneously with gut use (McClave, 2004). Failure to use the GI tract in AP may exacerbate the stress response and disease severity (McClave et al, 2006).
- Avoid pancreatic irritants, especially alcohol and caffeine. Monitor for increased need for pancreatic enzymes with the use of tube feeding.
- Avoid overfeeding. The exact volume of feedings that can reduce gut permeability and modulate the stress response has yet to be determined (McClave, 2004).
- Correct fluid and electrolyte imbalances and malnutrition. Acid–base imbalance is common with nasogastric suctioning, fistula losses, renal failure, nausea, and vomiting.
- Reduce fever; prevent shock and hypovolemia, hypermetabolism, sepsis, and compression of the stomach or colon. Avoid or control other complications (cardiovascular, pulmonary, hematological, renal, neurological, or metabolic); prevent organ failure. Extensive necrosis and infection are associated with the development of organ failure (Garg et al, 2005).
- Use TPN if abdominal pain is refractory. TPN use can promote positive nitrogen balance (Chandrasegaram et al, 2005).

INTERVENTION: FOOD AND NUTRITION

- Enteral products containing MCT are useful for tube feeding, especially when there is steatorrhea. Omega-3 fatty acids are helpful (Lasztity et al, 2005). Transition to jejunostomy can be considered when pain is refractory, using a standard formula and needle catheter jejunostomy.

SAMPLE NUTRITION DIAGNOSTIC STATEMENT

Pancreatitis, Chronic

PES: Impaired nutrient utilization related to pancreatic enzyme deficiency as evidenced by steatorrhea and report of medication noncompliance.

Assessment Data: Patient statement of not taking medication, report of frequent diarrhea after eating.

Intervention: Interventions would address the appropriate dose and frequency of medication intake.

Monitoring and Evaluation: Plan would include asking patient time of next clinic visit and plan to evaluate change in steatorrhea and improvement in medication compliance.

- Progress to a diet given in six daily feedings used with pancreatic enzymes for all meals and snacks.
- Alcoholic beverages and nicotine are prohibited. Limit gastric stimulants, such as peppermint and black pepper, if not tolerated.
- Diet should include adequate amounts of vitamin C, B-complex vitamins, and folic acid for water-soluble vitamin needs. Vitamin B_{12} deficiency can occur in AP because intrinsic factor is prevented from binding with vitamin B_{12} (Khokhar and Seidner, 2004). Fat-soluble vitamins in water-miscible form may be needed.
- Antioxidants including selenium may be needed (Musil et al, 2005). Adequate calcium, magnesium, and zinc supplementation should also be provided.

CLINICAL INDICATORS

Clinical/History

Height
Weight
BMI (obese?)
Diet history
BP (low)
Left upper quadrant abdominal pain
Vomiting
Temperature
Chvostek's sign
Steatorrhea
Multiple Organ System Score (MOSS)
CT scan showing interstitial pancreatic edema

Lab Work

CRP (used to measure severity in AP)
Lipase (>110; more sensitive than amylase)
Amylase (>250)
K+ (decreased)
Na+ (decreased)
PT or INR
Bilirubin (elevated)
Ca++ (decreased)
Gluc (increased, >200)
Chol (LDL up, or total decreased)
Trig (increased)
Mg++ (decreased)
LDH (>700)
ALT (elevated)
AST (>250)
WBC (>10,000 cells/mm^3)
Alb (low)
RBP
Partial pressure of carbon dioxide (pCO_2) (increased)
Partial pressure of oxygen (pO_2) (decreased)
BUN
H & H
Serum folate
Alk phos (increased)
CT scan for necrosis
Ultrasound
Fecal fat study

TABLE 8-12 Medications Used in Acute Pancreatitis

Medication	Description
Antibiotics	Antibiotics may be needed to manage necrosis and systemic complications.
Bile salts	Bile salts or water-miscible forms of fat-soluble vitamins may be needed.
Diuretics	Diuretics such as acetazolamide (Diamox) may be needed to control fluid retention. Nausea, vomiting, and diarrhea may result.
Insulin	Insulin may be necessary. Monitor for hypoglycemia during use.
Octreotide	Octreotide may have a beneficial role in the management of acute pancreatitis.
Opiates	Opiates may be prescribed for pain.
Pancreatic enzymes	30,000 IU per meal may be needed to reduce steatorrhea to less than 20 g/d. Enteric coating is necessary to prevent destruction by enzymes. Capsules or tablets should be swallowed whole. Take enteric-coated enzymes with cimetidine, food, or antacids.

Note: Medications sometimes associated with causing acute pancreatitis include acetaminophen, azathioprine, estrogens, furosemide, methyldopa, nitrofurantoin, steroids, thiazides, cimetidine, erythromycin, salicylates, sulfonamides, and tetracyclines.

Common Drugs Used and Potential Side Effects

- See Table 8-12.

Herbs, Botanicals, and Supplements

- Herbs and botanical supplements should not be used without discussing with physician.
- Combinations of traditional Chinese and Western medicines with an early short-term use of somatostatin may improve severe AP (Xia et al, 2005). Further study is needed.
- Both *S*-adenosylmethionine and betaine have shown efficacy in animal models of alcoholic liver disease; there is great interest in these complementary and alternative medicine agents in both alcoholic liver disease and nonalcoholic steatohepatitis, but more research is needed (Krueger et al, 2004).

INTERVENTION: NUTRITION EDUCATION, COUNSELING, CARE MANAGEMENT

- Instruct patient to watch for signs and symptoms of diabetes, tetany, peritonitis, acute respiratory distress syndrome, and pleural effusion. These patients are best managed by a multidisciplinary team approach, especially children (Stringer et al, 2005).
- Discuss omission of alcohol from the typical diet.
- Discuss tips for handling nausea and vomiting (e.g., dry meals, taking liquids a few hours before or after meals, use of ice chips, sipping beverages, asking physician about available antiemetics, etc.).
- Coffee, tea, and gas-forming foods may need to be omitted.
- Home enteral nutrition may be needed for awhile. Teach appropriate management methods. Teach use of a low-fat, high-protein, high-calorie oral diet when and if appropriate.

For More Information

- American Gastroenterological Association
  http://www.gastro.org/clinicalRes/brochures/pancreatitis.html
- Childhood Pancreatitis
  http://www.aafp.org/afp/990501ap/2507.html

PANCREATITIS, ACUTE—CITED REFERENCES

Adler G. Has the biology and treatment of pancreatic diseases evolved? *Best Pract Res Clin Gastroenterol.* 18:83S, 2004.

Balog A, et al. Polymorphism of the TNF-alpha, HSP70-2, and CD14 genes increases susceptibility to severe acute pancreatitis. *Pancreas* 30:46, 2005.

Chandrasegaram MD, et al, The impact of parenteral nutrition on the body composition of patients with acute pancreatitis. *J Parenter Enteral Nutr.* 29:65, 2005.

Foitzik T, et al. Omega-3 fatty acid supplementation increases anti-inflammatory cytokines and attenuates systemic disease sequelae in experimental pancreatitis. *J Parenter Enteral Nutr.* 26:351, 2002.

Garg PK, et al. Association of extent and infection of pancreatic necrosis with organ failure and death in acute necrotizing pancreatitis. *Clin Gastroenterol Hepatol.* 3:159, 2005.

Khokhar AS, Seidner DL. The pathophysiology of pancreatitis. *Nutr Clin Pract.* 19:5, 2004.

Krueger KJ, et al. Nutritional supplements and alternative medicine. *Curr Opin Gastroenterol.* 20:130, 2004.

Kwon RS, Brugge WR. New advances in pancreatic imaging. *Curr Opin Gastroenterol.* 21:561, 2005.

Lasztity N, et al. Effect of enterally administered n-3 polyunsaturated fatty acids in acute pancreatitis—a prospective randomized clinical trial. *Clin Nutr.* 24:198, 2005.

McClave SA. Defining the new gold standard for nutrition support in acute pancreatitis. *Nutr Clin Pract.* 19:1, 2004.

McClave SA, et al. Nutrition support in acute pancreatitis: a systematic review of the literature. *J Parenter Enteral Nutr.* 30:143, 2006.

Meier RF, Beglinger C. Nutrition in pancreatic diseases. Nutrition in pancreatic diseases. *Best Pract Res Clin Gastroenterol.* 20:507, 2006.

Musil F, et al. Dynamics of antioxidants in patients with acute pancreatitis and in patients operated for colorectal cancer: a clinical study. *Nutrition* 21:118, 2005.

Nathens AB, et al. Management of the critically ill patient with severe acute pancreatitis. *Crit Care Med.* 32:2524, 2004.

Russell MK. Acute pancreatitis: a review of pathophysiology and nutrition management. *Nutr Clin Pract.* 19:16, 2004.

Stringer MD, et al. Multidisciplinary management of surgical disorders of the pancreas in childhood. *J Pediatr Gastroenterol Nutr.* 40:363, 2005.

Weimann A, et al. Feasibility and safety of needle catheter jejunostomy for enteral nutrition in surgically treated severe acute pancreatitis. *J Parenter Enteral Nutr.* 28:324, 2004.

Xia Q, et al. Comparison of integrated Chinese and Western medicine with and without somatostatin supplement in the treatment of severe acute pancreatitis. *World J Gastroenterol.* 11:1073, 2005.

PANCREATITIS, CHRONIC

NUTRITIONAL ACUITY RANKING: LEVEL 3

DEFINITIONS AND BACKGROUND

Chronic pancreatitis (CP) is an inflammatory disorder that results in permanent impairment of the glandular anatomy of the pancreas (Giger et al, 2004). CP also involves edema, fat necrosis, and cellular exudate. As a fibrotic, necrotic disease state, CP involves decreased enzymatic processes with abdominal pain, nausea, vomiting, and diarrhea. See Figure 8-6.

The most common cause of CP is chronic alcohol abuse (60–90% of cases). The development of CP is proportional to the dose and duration of alcohol consumption (a minimum of 6–12 years of approximately 80 g of alcohol per day) (Dufour and Adamson, 2003). The factors determining which alcoholic will develop alcoholic CP involve genetic factors, dietary factors, and susceptibility to pancreatic injury from trauma, gallstones, or viruses (Oruc and Whitcomb, 2004). Pancreatic fibrosis is activated by ethanol and its metabolites and by growth factors, cytokines, and oxidant stress; potential antifibrotic strategies such as antioxidants and cytokine inhibition are being evaluated (Apte and Wilson, 2004).

Approximately 5% of persons with acute pancreatitis go on to have CP. Other causes of CP include hyperparathyroidism, hyperlipidemia, pancreatic carcinoma, hypercalcemia, cystic fibrosis, pancreatic fistulae, trypsinogen-enterokinase deficiency, and lipase deficiency. Genetic and environmental factors also play a role in the process of this disease. Although an autoimmune process affecting the exocrine pancreas was suspected many years ago, only recently has autoimmunity been recognized as a distinct entity (Lara and Chari, 2005).

Signs and symptoms include severe upper abdominal pain that is often worsened by eating or drinking, unintentional weight loss, and diarrhea with pale, fatty stools. Analysis of pancreatograms and textural changes of the parenchyma may prove helpful in diagnosing CP (Kwon and Brugge, 2005). See Table 8-13 for a more complete list of signs and complications.

To avoid nutritional deterioration, early screening for fat malabsorption should be recommended in CP, regardless of etiology (Dumasy et al, 2004). Many patients will progress to having insulin-dependent diabetes, and they have a higher risk for pancreatic cancer. There appears to be a gradual decrease in antioxidant enzyme expression in pancreatic cells from normal pancreas to CP to pancreatic cancer (Cullen et al, 2003).

Abstinence from alcohol, dietary modifications, use of oral supplements, and pancreatic enzyme supplementation will be sufficient in over 80% of patients with CP (Meier and Beglinger, 2006). Enteral nutrition may be necessary for the other 20% in whom weight loss continues; long-term use of a percutaneous endoscopic gastrostomy (PEG) tube or jejunostomy feeding may be needed (Stanga et al, 2005). Parenteral nutrition is very seldom used in patients with CP.

Duct obstruction with increased pressure within the duct causes pain in these patients (Gabbrielli et al, 2005). This abdominal pain can be constant and disabling, causing some patients to become dependent on pain medications. Supportive treatments, inhibition of gastric acid secretion, nerve blocks, reduction of oxidative stress, and endoscopic and surgical treatments are all possibilities for treating CP patients.

Some patients will have surgery, such as pancreatic head excision combined with longitudinal pancreaticojejunostomy. Distal pancreatectomy achieves pain relief and good quality of life in a large percentage (80%) of patients (Sakorafas et al, 2001). Endoscopic retrograde cholangiopancreatography and

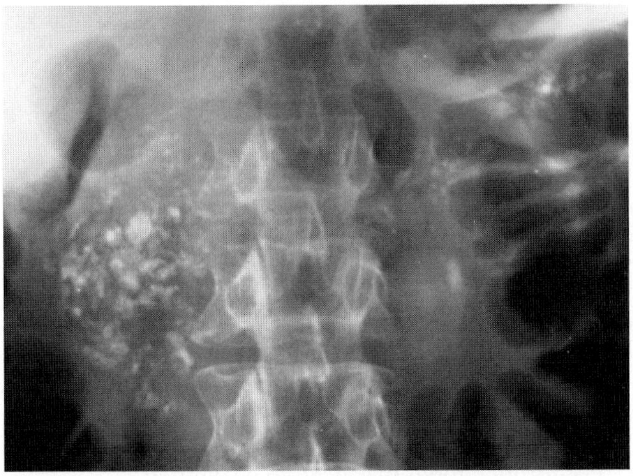

Figure 8-6 Chronic pancreatitis. (From Eisenberg RL. *Clinical imaging: an atlas of differential diagnosis*. 4th ed. Philadelphia: Lippincott Williams & Wilkins, 2003.)

TABLE 8-13 Clinical Signs and Complications of Chronic Pancreatitis

Pain
Weight loss
Jaundice
Hypoalbuminemia
Pancreatic pseudocysts or calcification
Splenic vein thrombosis
Bile duct or duodenal obstruction
Loss of exocrine function with malabsorption and steatorrhea
Loss of endocrine function, leading to diabetes

Source: Giger et al, 2004.

stent placement are relatively new alternatives to surgery in this population (Vitale et al, 2004).

INTERVENTION: OBJECTIVES

- Provide optimal nutrition support and allow weight gain to occur. Weight loss is common in the late course of CP (Stanga et al, 2005).
- Decrease pain.
- Avoid alcohol.
- Correct fluid and electrolyte imbalances and malnutrition; avoid overfeeding. Acid–base imbalance is common with nasogastric (NG) suctioning, fistula losses, renal failure, nausea, and vomiting.
- Alleviate fat malabsorption (steatorrhea), and decrease number of stools per day. Diarrhea usually indicates the presence of steatorrhea (Giger et al, 2004).
- With diabetes, it may be better to have glucose elevated slightly (200 mg/dL) than to allow prolonged hypoglycemia to occur.
- Avoid or control complications (cardiovascular, pulmonary, hematological, renal, neurological, or metabolic); prevent multiple organ dysfunction.
- If tube fed, monitor for abdominal pain or discomfort, and offer pain medication as needed. Administer pancreatic enzymes with meals or tube feeding (Dominguez-Munoz et al, 2005; Stanga et al, 2005).
- TPN may be needed for resistant cases where pain does not subside.

CLINICAL INDICATORS

Clinical/History	Lab Work
Height	CRP and WBC (elevated)
Weight	K+ (decreased)
BMI	Na+ (decreased)
Diet history	Ca++ (decreased)
Left upper quadrant abdominal pain	Gluc (often increased)
Vomiting	2-Hour postprandial glucose test
Steatorrhea	Lipase (increased)
Temperature	Bicarbonate levels (decreased)
I & O	Serum trypsinogen (low)
Chvostek's sign	Fecal chymotrypsin
CT scan or endoscopic ultrasound	Urinary *p*-aminobenzoic acid (bentiromide test)
Exploratory laparotomy	Fecal fat studies
Endoscopic retrograde cholangiopancreatography (ERCP)	Chol (LDL up, or total decreased)
	Trig (increased)
	Mg++ (decreased)
	LDH (>700)
	AST (>250)
	WBC (>200)
	Amylase (>200)
	Alk phos (increased)
	pCO_2 (increased) and pO_2 (decreased)
	Alb, RBP
	BUN
	H & H
	Serum folate
	PT or INR
	Bilirubin

INTERVENTION: FOOD AND NUTRITION

- If tolerated, use a diet with low to moderate fat, moderate protein (1 g with renal or liver failure, 2 g/kg for repletion), and high carbohydrates; calculate needs accordingly. Diet should be low in fiber with six small meals a day.
- Diet should include adequate amounts of antioxidants and vitamin C, B-complex vitamins, and folic acid. Fat-soluble vitamins (A, D, E, and K) in water-miscible form may be better tolerated. Adequate calcium, magnesium, selenium, and zinc supplementation should be provided.
- Treat steatorrhea with a high-calorie, high-protein, and low-fat diet to minimize symptoms of the underlying disease and to promote weight retention or gain (Giger et al, 2004). Medium-chain triglycerides can be helpful. Pancreatic replacement therapy is used to combat maldigestion and malabsorption (Stanga et al, 2005). Monitor for hyperglycemia with high-carbohydrate diet.
- High-energy, standard feeding is desirable in most cases. Needle catheter jejunostomy may be used safely in many cases (Stanga et al, 2005). Jejunal feeding versus gastric placement seems to be beneficial.
- If TPN is needed, estimate needs according to similar parameters as for oral diet. The benefits of BCAAs and glutamine are not clear. If intravenous lipids are used, do not use more than 1.5 g/kg for adults. Provide no more than 5 mg/kg/min of glucose.
- Alcoholic beverages are absolutely prohibited.

Common Drugs Used and Potential Side Effects

- See Table 8-14.

Herbs, Botanicals, and Supplements

- Herbs and botanical supplements should not be used without discussing with physician.
- The combination of pre- and probiotics ("synbiotics") may be useful in this population. Longer trials are needed.

INTERVENTION: NUTRITION EDUCATION, COUNSELING, CARE MANAGEMENT

- Instruct patient to watch for signs and symptoms of diabetes, tetany, peritonitis, acute respiratory distress syndrome, and pleural effusion.
- Discuss omission of alcohol from the typical diet.
- Discuss tips for handling nausea and vomiting (e.g., dry meals, taking liquids a few hours before or after meals, use of ice chips, sipping beverages, asking physician about available antiemetics, etc.).
- Gas-forming foods may need to be omitted.
- To prevent onset of pancreatic cancer, avoiding tobacco smoking (Vimalachandran et al, 2004).
- Teach high-calorie, high-protein, low-fat diet and small frequent meal pattern.

TABLE 8-14 Medications Used in Chronic Pancreatitis

Medication	Description
Pancreatic enzymes	Take during or after meals for greatest effect (Dominguez-Munoz et al, 2005). 30,000 IU per meal may be needed to reduce steatorrhea to less than 20 g/d. Enteric coating is necessary to prevent destruction by enzymes. Capsules or tablets should be swallowed whole. Take enteric-coated enzymes with cimetidine, food, or antacids.
Antibiotics	Antibiotics may be needed to manage necrosis and systemic complications.
Bile salts	Bile salts or water-miscible forms of fat-soluble vitamins may be needed.
Diuretics	Diuretics such as acetazolamide (Diamox) may be needed to control fluid retention. Nausea, vomiting, and diarrhea may result.
H_2-receptor antagonists (cimetidine or ranitidine)	Cimetidine may deplete vitamin B_{12}, especially among the elderly. Histamine H_2-receptor antagonists or proton pump inhibitors can improve fat malabsorption and steatorrhea.
Insulin	Insulin may be necessary in hyperglycemia. Monitor for hypoglycemia during use.
Pain killers	Pain control requires the use of morphine-like drugs (pethidine, morphine, and diamorphine), which have the risk of addiction, particularly if their use is not controlled.

For More Information

- Medline Plus
  http://www.nlm.nih.gov/medlineplus/ency/article/000221.htm
- Merck Manual
  http://www.merck.com/mrkshared/mmanual/section3/chapter26/26c.jsp

PANCREATITIS, CHRONIC—CITED REFERENCES

Apte MV, Wilson JS. Mechanisms of pancreatic fibrosis. *Dig Dis.* 22:273, 2004.

Cullen JJ, et al. Expression of antioxidant enzymes in diseases of the human pancreas: another link between chronic pancreatitis and pancreatic cancer. *Pancreas* 26:23, 2003.

Dominguez-Munoz JE, et al. Effect of the administration schedule on the therapeutic efficacy of oral pancreatic enzyme supplements in patients with exocrine pancreatic insufficiency: a randomized, three-way crossover study. *Aliment Pharmacol Ther.* 21:993, 2005.

Dufour MC, Adamson MD. The epidemiology of alcohol-induced pancreatitis. *Pancreas* 27:286, 2003.

Dumasy V, et al. Fat malabsorption screening in chronic pancreatitis. *Am J Gastroenterol.* 99:1350, 2004.

Gabbrielli A, et al. Efficacy of main pancreatic-duct endoscopic drainage in patients with chronic pancreatitis, continuous pain, and dilated duct. *Gastrointest Endosc.* 61:576, 2005.

Giger U, et al. Management of chronic pancreatitis. *Nutr Clin Pract.* 19:37, 2004.

Kwon RS, Brugge WR. New advances in pancreatic imaging. New advances in pancreatic imaging. *Curr Opin Gastroenterol.* 21:561, 2005.

Lara LP, Chari ST. Autoimmune pancreatitis. *Curr Gastroenterol Rep.* 7:101, 2005.

Meier R, et al. ESPEN Guidelines on Enteral Nutrition: pancreas. *Clin Nutr.* 25:275, 2006.

Oruc N, Whitcomb DC. Theories, mechanisms, and models of alcoholic chronic pancreatitis. *Gastroenterol Clin North Am.* 33:733, 2004.

Sakorafas G, et al. Postobstructive chronic pancreatitis: results with distal resection. *Arch Surg.* 136:643, 2001.

Stanga Z, et al. Effect of jejunal long-term feeding on chronic pancreatitis. *J Parenter Enteral Nutr.* 29:12, 2005.

Vimalachandran D, et al. Genetics and prevention of pancreatic cancer. *Cancer Control.* 11:6, 2004.

Vitale GC, et al. Role of pancreatic duct stenting in the treatment of chronic pancreatitis. *Surg Endosc.* 18:143, 2004.

PANCREATIC INSUFFICIENCY

NUTRITIONAL ACUITY RANKING: LEVEL 2–3

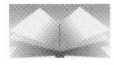

DEFINITIONS AND BACKGROUND

Pancreatic insufficiency is caused by decreased secretion of lipase, often from cystic fibrosis, protein–calorie malnutrition, congenital problems, pancreatic cancer, or pancreatitis.

In cystic fibrosis, there may be recurrent problems with management of fatty acid abnormalities. There seems to be increased levels of arachidonic acid and decreased levels of docosahexaenoic acid (DHA) (Freedman et al, 2004). Children with residual fecal elastase (FE) had greater fat absorption and improved growth and nutritional status; FE assessment should be used to verify pancreatic status in patients with cystic fibrosis (Cohen et al, 2005). Pancreatitis can be the first manifestation of cystic fibrosis (DeBoeck et al, 2005).

Lipase is the key enzyme for breaking down triglycerides. Patients often have mild to moderate fat malabsorption with pancreatic insufficiency. Oral pancreatic enzyme supplements should be properly administered to ensure an adequate gastric mixing with the food and simultaneous gastric emptying with the chyme (Dominguez-Munoz et al, 2005).

INTERVENTION: OBJECTIVES

- Maintain BMI >19 or >90% ideal body weight (IBW).
- Prevent essential fatty acid deficiency.
- Correct fatty acid abnormalities, maldigestion, diarrhea, and steatorrhea.

- Provide adequate energy intake while lowering intake of fats.
- Provide missing fat-soluble vitamins, if needed, from malabsorption.
- Prevent overloading of minerals such as iron.

INTERVENTION: FOOD AND NUTRITION

- Use a moderate- to low-fat diet. MCTs also may be tolerated because they do not require lipase. They may be taken with simple sugars, jelly, and jams in mixed dishes.
- Use tender meats and low-fiber fruits and vegetables.
- Alcoholic beverages are prohibited.
- Zinc may be needed in supplemental form or from an elemental diet.
- Tube feed in severe cases.
- Increase use of omega-3 fatty acids from tuna, mackerel, salmon, and other fatty fish, as well as flaxseed.
- For cystic fibrosis, encourage high-calorie, high-fat intake to maintain body weight. Dose pancreatic enzyme replacement to minimize fat malabsorption.
- If diabetes is present due to insulin insufficiency, emphasis should be on mealtime and carbohydrate spacing to prevent hyperglycemia.

CLINICAL INDICATORS

Clinical/History	CRP	Gluc
Height	Serum carotene	Na+, K+
Weight	CT scan or ultrasound	Chol
BMI	Fecal elastase (FE) 1 levels (indicates lipase activity)	Alk phos
Diet history	Ca++, Mg++	Lipase
I & O	Trig	H & H
Stool weight	PT or INR	
Steatorrhea	Bicarbonate	
Lab Work		
Amylase (increased)		

Common Drugs Used and Potential Side Effects

- FDA monitors pancreatic extract preparations containing pancreatin and pancrelipase; both ingredients are extracted mainly from animal pancreata and contain principally amylase, protease, and lipase. Pancreatic enzymes (pancreatin or pancrelipase [Cotazym]) should be taken with food. Take enteric-coated tablets with cimetidine or antacids.
- Fat-soluble vitamins should be taken in water-miscible form and taken with pancreatic enzymes.

Herbs, Botanicals, and Supplements

- Herbs and botanical supplements should not be used without discussing with physician.

INTERVENTION: NUTRITION EDUCATION, COUNSELING, CARE MANAGEMENT

- Instruct patient in the role of the pancreas in digestion.
- Discuss how pancreatic enzymes should be taken with meals or afterward for best results.
- Discuss appropriate measures for recovery and control.
- Share menu planning tips for altered-fat diets and how to include desired nutrients.

For More Information

- Food and Drug Administration (FDA)
  http://www.fda.gov/cder/drug/infopage/pancreatic_drugs/default.htm

PANCREATIC INSUFFICIENCY—CITED REFERENCES

Cohen JR, et al. Fecal elastase: pancreatic status verification and influence on nutritional status in children with cystic fibrosis. *J Pediatr Gastroenterol Nutr.* 40:438, 2005.

DeBoeck K, et al. Pancreatitis among patients with cystic fibrosis: correlation with pancreatic status and genotype. *Pediatrics* 115:e463, 2005.

Dominguez-Munoz JE, et al. Effect of the administration schedule on the therapeutic efficacy of oral pancreatic enzyme supplements in patients with exocrine pancreatic insufficiency: a randomized, three-way crossover study. *Aliment Pharmacol Ther.* 21:993, 2005.

Freedman SD, et al. Association of cystic fibrosis with abnormalities in fatty acid metabolism. *N Engl J Med.* 350:560, 2004.

PANCREATIC TRANSPLANTATION

NUTRITIONAL ACUITY RANKING: LEVEL 4

DEFINITIONS AND BACKGROUND

Pancreatic transplantation may be a viable option for brittle type 1 diabetes mellitus. It helps to decrease nephropathy, early or mild retinopathy, and neuropathy. It does not improve gastroparesis (Cashion et al, 2004). Pancreas transplantation alone (PTA) involves transplanting a pancreas from a cadaver to a patient whose kidneys have not been damaged by diabetes.

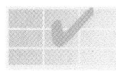

Simultaneous pancreas and kidney (SPK) transplantation involves kidney and pancreas being transplanted at the same time from a cadaver, often leading to freedom from both dialysis and insulin dependency. Pancreas after kidney (PAK) surgery is another option, as is islet cell or isolated beta-cell transplantation.

Pancreatic transplantation is major surgery, with risk of bleeding, infection, and reactions to anesthesia. Antirejection medicines, which have many side effects, have to be taken for a long time.

INTERVENTION: OBJECTIVES

- **Preoperatively:** Meet nutritional needs; improve visceral protein stores; maintain lean tissue.
- **Postoperatively:** Support graft survival. Promote wound healing. Improve or maintain nutritional status.
- Most transplantation patients can be weaned off TPN within the first year, and optimal nutritional status can be achieved (Rovera et al, 2003).
- **Long Term:** Prevent weight gain. Prevent complications such as gastroparesis, hypertension, hyperlipidemia, hyperglycemia, and osteoporosis. Beta-cell function tends to decline in these patients despite the transplantation (Robertson, 2004).

INTERVENTION: FOOD AND NUTRITION (SEE TABLE 8-15)

- **Preoperatively:** Meet nutritional needs; improve visceral protein stores; maintain lean tissue. Control of carbohydrates will be important if there is diabetes or hyperglycemia. Manage diet carefully to prevent hypoglycemia in patients who are given insulin.

CLINICAL INDICATORS

Clinical/History		
Height	I & O	H & H
Weight, dry	BP	Serum Fe
BMI	Temperature	Serum amylase
Diet history		Urinary amylase (only if bladder drained)
Weight changes and goals	**Lab Work**	Na+, K+
	Gluc	Ca++, Mg++
	BUN, Creat	

Common Drugs Used and Potential Side Effects

- See Table 8-16.

Herbs, Botanicals, and Supplements

- Herbs and botanical supplements should not be used without discussing with physician.
- St. John's wort interferes with the metabolism of cyclosporine and should not be used after transplantation (Karliova et al, 2000).

INTERVENTION: NUTRITION EDUCATION, COUNSELING, CARE MANAGEMENT

- Encourage activity to prevent excessive weight gain; 14–30 pounds may be a common gain.

TABLE 8-15 Post–Pancreatic Transplantation Nutrition Guidelines

Nutrient	Short-Term Recommendations	Long-Term Recommendations
Energy	20–30% above normal or measure through indirect calorimetry; increase for weight gain	Maintenance: 30–35 kcal/kg depending on activity level
Protein	1.3–2 g/kg/d	1 g/kg/d
Carbohydrate	45–55% of kcals; use CHO counting to manage blood glucose levels	45–55% of kcals; use CHO counting to manage blood glucose levels
Fat	25–35% of total calories depending on lipid levels Up to 50% of calories with severe hyperglycemia	25–35% of total calories depending on lipid levels <10% of calories as saturated fat
Calcium	800–1200 mg/d	1000–1500 mg/d (consider the need for estrogen or vitamin D supplements)
Sodium	2–4 g/d	3–4 g/d
Magnesium and Phosphorus	Encourage intake of foods high in these nutrients Supplement as needed	Encourage intake of foods high in these nutrients Supplement as needed
Potassium	Supplement or restrict based on serum potassium levels	Supplement or restrict based on serum potassium levels
Other Vitamins and Minerals	Multivitamin-mineral: supplement to RDA levels	Multivitamin/mineral: supplement to RDA levels

Adapted from: Hasse, 2005.

TABLE 8-16 Medications Used after Pancreatic Transplantation

Medication	Description
Analgesics	Analgesics are used to reduce pain. Long-term use may affect such nutrients as vitamin C and folacin; monitor carefully for each specific medication.
Azathioprine (Imuran)	Azathioprine may cause leukopenia, thrombocytopenia, oral and esophageal sores, macrocytic anemia, pancreatitis, vomiting, diarrhea, and other complex side effects. Folate supplementation and other dietary modifications (liquid or soft diet, use of oral supplements) may be needed. The drug works by lowering the number of T cells; it is often prescribed along with prednisone for conventional immunosuppression.
Corticosteroids (prednisone or Solu-Cortef)	Corticosteroids such as prednisone and Solu-Cortef are used for immunosuppression. Side effects include increased catabolism of proteins, negative nitrogen balance, hyperphagia, ulcers, decreased glucose tolerance, sodium retention, fluid retention, and impaired calcium absorption and osteoporosis. Cushing's syndrome, obesity, muscle wasting, and increased gastric secretion may result. A higher protein intake and lower intake of carbohydrate and sodium may be needed.
Cyclosporine	Cyclosporine does not retain sodium as much as corticosteroids do. Intravenous doses are more effective than oral doses. Nausea, vomiting, and diarrhea are common side effects. Hyperlipidemia, hyperglycemia, and hyperkalemia may also occur; decrease fat intake as well as sodium and potassium if necessary. Magnesium may need to be replaced. The drug is also nephrotoxic; a controlled renal diet may be beneficial. Taking omega-3 fatty acids during cyclosporine therapy may reduce toxic side effects (such as high blood pressure and kidney damage) associated with this medication in transplantation patients (Tsipas and Morphake, 2003). Avoid use with St. John's wort.
Diuretics	Diuretics such as furosemide (Lasix) may cause hypokalemia. Aldactone actually spares potassium; monitor drug changes closely. In general, avoid use with fenugreek, yohimbe, and ginkgo.
Immunosuppressants	Immunosuppressants such as muromonab (Orthoclone OKT3) and antithymocyte globulin (ATG) are less nephrotoxic than cyclosporine but can cause nausea, anorexia, diarrhea, and vomiting. Monitor carefully. Fever and stomatitis also may occur; alter diet as needed.
Insulin	Insulin may be necessary during periods of hyperglycemia. Monitor for hypoglycemic symptoms during use; teach patient self-management tips.
Pancreatic Enzymes	Pancreatic enzymes may be needed if pancreatitis occurs again after transplantation.
Tacrolimus (Prograf, FK506)	Tacrolimus suppresses T-cell immunity; it is 100 times more potent than cyclosporine, thus requiring smaller doses. Side effects include GI distress, nausea, vomiting, hyperkalemia, and hyperglycemia; adjust diet accordingly by controlling carbohydrate and enhancing potassium intake. Maternal therapy with tacrolimus for liver transplantation may be compatible with breastfeeding (French et al, 2003). The drug is also useful for uremic patients with simultaneous pancreatic-kidney transplantation (Bechstein et al, 2004).

- Discuss surgical stress. Encourage positive protein balance in the short term to promote anabolism and wound healing.
- Over the long term, follow a low-cholesterol and low–saturated fatty acid dietary plan.
- Sudden abdominal pain, fever, and increased amylase and glucose can occur and are signs of pancreatitis even after transplantation. Report these warning signs immediately to the physician.
- Problems after transplantation include diabetic complications, bone loss, and failure of the pancreas graft. A multidisciplinary team is required to maximize long-term quality of life (Larsen, 2004).

For More Information

- Insulin
  http://www.insulin-free.org/
- National Institute of Diabetes and Digestive and Kidney Diseases (NIDDK)
  http://diabetes.niddk.nih.gov/dm/pubs/pancreaticislet/
- USC Pancreatic Transplant Program
  http://www.pancreastransplant.org/

PANCREATIC TRANSPLANTATION—CITED REFERENCES

Bechstein WO, et al. Efficacy and safety of tacrolimus compared with cyclosporine microemulsion in primary simultaneous pancreas-kidney transplantation: 1-year results of a large multicenter trial. *Transplantation* 77:1221, 2004.

Cashion AK, et al. Gastroparesis following kidney/pancreas transplant. *Clin Transplant.* 18:306, 2004.

French AE, et al. Milk transfer and neonatal safety of tacrolimus. *Ann Pharmacother.* 37:815, 2003.

Hasse J. Liver transplantation. Accessed April 12, 2005 at http://www.centerspan.org/pubs/liver/hasse1.htm#acute.

Karliova M, et al. Interaction of *Hypericum perforatum* (St John's wort) with cyclosporin A metabolism in a patient after liver transplantation. *J Hepatol.* 33:853, 2000.

Larsen JL. Pancreas transplantation: indications and consequences. *Endocr Rev.* 25:919, 2004.

Robertson RP. Consequences on beta-cell function and reserve after long-term pancreas transplantation. *Diabetes* 53:633, 2004.

Rovera G, et al. Intestinal and multivisceral transplantation: dynamics of nutritional management and functional autonomy. *J Parenter Enteral Nutr.* 27:252, 2003.

Tsipas G, Morphake P. Beneficial effects of a diet rich in a mixture of n-6/n-3 essential fatty acids and of their metabolites on cyclosporine nephrotoxicity. *J Nutr Biochem.* 14:626, 2003.

ZOLLINGER-ELLISON SYNDROME

NUTRITIONAL ACUITY RANKING: LEVEL 3

DEFINITIONS AND BACKGROUND

Zollinger-Ellison syndrome (ZES) is a severe form of peptic ulcer disease with ulceratogenic tumor (gastrinoma) of the delta-cells of the pancreatic islets of Langerhans. Almost every patient with ZES has marked gastric acid hypersecretion and fulminating ulceration of the esophagus, stomach, duodenum, and jejunum (Gibril and Jensen, 2004).

Gastrinomas producing ZES are the most frequent symptomatic, malignant pancreatic endocrine tumor syndromes (Gibril and Jensen, 2005). They frequently are accompanied by secretory diarrhea. Interestingly, insulin production is often increased in the beta-cells. Of all cases, 60% occur in males; two thirds of cases are malignant. Widespread metastasis indicates a poor prognosis.

Gastric carcinoids are occurring with increasing frequency in patients with pernicious anemia (Jordan et al, 2004). Gastric carcinoid tumors in patients with longstanding ZES may be symptomatic and aggressive and may metastasize to the liver; they require long-term medical treatment (Norton et al, 2004). Curing gastrinoma or appropriately inhibiting gastric acid hypersecretion in ZES patients prevents death and favors long-term survival (Quatrini et al, 2005). Total gastrectomy is reserved for patients with extensive tumor involvement of the gastric wall or for patients with emergency bleeding (Jordan et al, 2004).

INTERVENTION: OBJECTIVES

- Overcome malabsorption.
- Decrease steatorrhea with losses of nitrogen, fat, sodium, and potassium.
- Lessen diarrhea.
- Eliminate gastric acid secretion, usually with medications or, less often, surgery (gastrectomy).
- Where existing, lessen problems with dysphagia and reflux.

INTERVENTION: FOOD AND NUTRITION

- Diet should provide low to moderate fat (50–70 g).
- According to the patient's stool losses, modify calories, fat, protein, and electrolytes as needed.
- Modify fiber, seasonings, and textures as necessary.
- Alter feeding modality to TF or TPN if needed.

CLINICAL INDICATORS

Clinical/History		
Height	BMI	Stool volume
Weight	Diet history	BP
	Steatorrhea	I & O

Lab Work		
N balance	Alb	Serum gastrin
Na+	H & H	Trig, Chol
Ca++ (usually increased)	K+ (decreased)	Gluc
	Mg++	Gastrin radioimmunoassay
	BUN	CT scan
	Serum insulin	

Common Drugs Used and Potential Side Effects

- Histamine H_2-receptor antagonists (ranitidine or cimetidine) can reduce hypergastric acid secretion. Vitamin B_{12} may be depleted, especially in elderly persons.
- The proton pump inhibitors (PPIs) are used for the treatment of acid-related disorders, including ZES. Take omeprazole, esomeprazole, or lansoprazole before meals. Iron and vitamin B_{12} levels may become depleted. Overall outcome with use of these medications can prevent the need for surgery (Hirschowitz et al, 2005).
- Pancreatic enzymes may be needed if steatorrhea is excessive.

Herbs, Botanicals, and Supplements

- Herbs and botanical supplements should not be used without discussing with physician.

INTERVENTION: NUTRITION EDUCATION, COUNSELING, CARE MANAGEMENT

- Explain which modifications of fiber in the diet are appropriate.
- Explain how malabsorption compromises nutritional status.
- Discuss limiting fat intake, as appropriate for the patient.

ZOLLINGER-ELLISON SYNDROME—CITED REFERENCES

Gibril F, Jensen JT. Advances in evaluation and management of gastrinoma in patients with Zollinger-Ellison syndrome. *Curr Gastroenterol Rep.* 7:114, 2005.

Gibril F, Jensen JT. Zollinger-Ellison syndrome revisited: diagnosis, biologic markers, associated inherited disorders, and acid hypersecretion. *Curr Gastroenterol Rep.* 6:454, 2004.

Hirschowitz BI, et al. Clinical outcome using lansoprazole in acid hypersecretors with and without Zollinger-Ellison syndrome: a 13-year prospective study. *Clin Gastroenterol Hepatol.* 3:39, 2005.

Jordan PH Jr, et al. Gastric carcinoids in patients with hypergastrinemia. *J Am Coll Surg.* 199:552, 2004.

Norton JA, et al. Gastric carcinoid tumors in multiple endocrine neoplasia-1 patients with Zollinger-Ellison syndrome can be symptomatic, demonstrate aggressive growth, and require surgical treatment. *Surgery* 136:1267, 2004.

Quatrini M, et al. Follow-up study of patients with Zollinger-Ellison syndrome in the period 1966–2002: effects of surgical and medical treatments on long-term survival. *J Clin Gastroenterol.* 39:376, 2005.

BILIARY DISORDERS

GALLBLADDER DISEASE

NUTRITIONAL ACUITY RANKING: LEVEL 2

DEFINITIONS AND BACKGROUND

The **gallbladder**, located under the liver, collects and stores bile, which is made up of bile salts, electrolytes, bilirubin, cholesterol, and other fats. Bile helps the small intestine digest fats and remove waste products, especially through bilirubin. It passes from the liver's bile duct into the duodenum through the common bile duct. See the gallbladder in Figure 8-7.

If the gallbladder is removed, fat absorption still occurs, but it is less efficient because bile is not as concentrated. Table 8-17 lists common causes of gallbladder disease.

Cholelithiasis is defined as the presence of gallstones. In developed countries, at least 10% of white adults harbor cholesterol gallstones; women have twice the risk, and age further increases the prevalence in both sexes (Shaffer, 2005). There is also prevalence among persons who have hepatitis C (Bini and McGready, 2005). Incidence also increases with diabetes, obesity, pregnancy, and use of estrogens; prepregnancy obesity is a strong risk factor (Ko et al, 2005), and there is an increase in risk of biliary tract disease among postmenopausal women using estrogen therapy (Cirillo et al, 2005). Gallstone disease is increasing among East Asian countries where overall daily energy intake has increased (Tsunoda et al, 2004).

Gallstones form if the gallbladder does not contract completely or often enough to empty bile; this can occur after eating too little or after periods of starvation. Preventive measures include a controlled weight loss rate, reduction of the length of overnight fast, and maintenance of a small amount of fat in the diet (Erlinger, 2000). High intake of refined sugars and saturated fatty acids may lead to gallstone formation. Eating nuts, vegetable protein, beans, and soy may be protective. Finally, people who are more active are less likely to develop gallstones.

Some gallbladders can concentrate bile normally but cannot acidify it. The result is that calcium may be less soluble in bile and precipitates out. Gallstones contain primarily cholesterol, bilirubin, and calcium salts. There are two forms of stones: cholesterol and pigment stones. Cholesterol precipitates as gallstones whenever cholesterol is greater than bile acids and phospholipids. Cholesterol is the primary component of stones in Western society. While prevalence of total gallbladder disease is relatively unrelated to coffee consumption, increased intake of coffee seems to reduce symptoms in some women who have the condition (Ruhl and Everhart, 2000). Further studies on the role of caffeine on gallstones are warranted.

Symptoms of gallstones may include steady pain in the upper abdomen that increases rapidly and lasts from 30 minutes

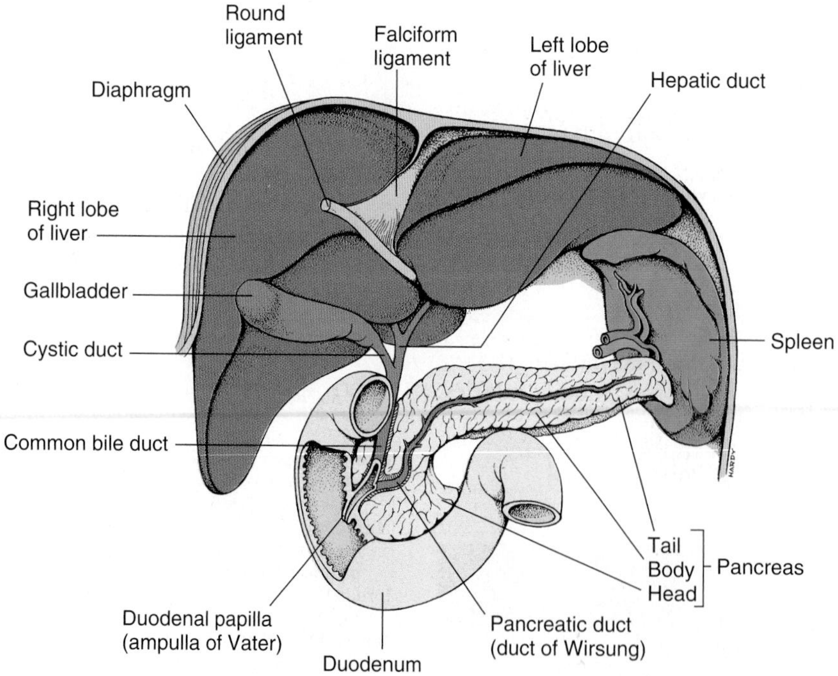

Figure 8-7 Gallbladder. (From *Stedman's medical dictionary*. 27th ed. Baltimore: Lippincott Williams & Wilkins, 2000.)

TABLE 8-17 Risk Factors for Gallbladder Disease

Age: Advanced age (especially after age 65)

Diet: Western diet with high-energy, high-fat, high–refined carbohydrate, low-fiber intake

Enzyme defects: Such as sickle cell anemia and some other genetic alterations

Ethnicity: Being Hispanic or Native American

Gender: Female

Hormonal imbalance: Such as in pregnancy or diabetes

Medications: Estrogens, insulin, oral contraceptives, cholestyramine

Obesity: Especially with the highest BMI (Dittrick et al, 2005; Erlinger, 2000)

Weight loss: Rapid weight loss, fasting, or crash dieting

to several hours, pain in the back between the shoulder blades or under the right shoulder, nausea, vomiting, abdominal bloating, intolerance for fatty foods, belching, and indigestion.

Cholecystitis is inflammation of the gallbladder that is almost always caused by gallstones. Surgery is needed to remove gallstones unless the condition subsides as a result of medical therapy. Extracorporeal shock wave lithotripsy (ESWL) is effective in the treatment of symptomatic cholecystolithiasis and preserves the organ in patients who are carefully chosen (Adamek et al, 2004).

Gallstone disease is common and costly, resulting in over 700,000 cholecystectomies annually in the United States alone (Shaffer, 2005). Laparoscopic cholecystectomy (LC) reduces the length of hospital stay and can be performed on patients who are morbidly obese (Simopoulos et al, 2005).

Surgical management of symptomatic cholelithiasis is safe, decreases days in hospital, and reduces the rate of preterm deliveries in pregnant women (Lu et al, 2004). Cholecystectomy is also frequently done within the first year postpartum (Ko et al, 2005).

Chronic cholecystitis involves prolonged presence of gallstones and low-grade inflammation. Scarring causes the gallbladder to become stiff and thick; nausea and abdominal discomfort are common. Endoscopic stent placement in the gallbladder is safe and effective for patients with gallbladder disease who are poor surgical candidates (Conway et al, 2005).

Gallbladder cancer is not common but is more prevalent in women who have had gallstones for many years. Jaundice, pain above the stomach, lumps in the abdomen, and fever should be addressed in patients who have gallstones. Gallbladder cancer is usually associated with late diagnosis, unsatisfactory treatment, and poor prognosis.

INTERVENTION: OBJECTIVES

- Lose excess weight, if needed. Avoid rapid weight loss, which can lead to gallstone formation.
- Limit foods that cause pain or flatulence.
- For the patient with cholelithiasis, overcome fat malabsorption caused by obstruction and prevent stagnation in a sluggish gallbladder, which may be caused by decreased bile secretion, bile stasis, bacteria, hormones, or fungi. Bacterial overgrowth alters bile acids so that they can no longer emulsify fats.
- Prevent biliary obstruction, cancer, and pancreatitis.
- Provide fat-soluble vitamins, if needed in cases of steatorrhea.
- Ascorbic acid affects the catabolism of cholesterol to bile acids and the development of gallbladder disease (Simon and Hudes, 2000); supplement the diet if needed.

INTERVENTION: FOOD AND NUTRITION

- Provide a calorie-controlled, balanced diet. Use NPO during an acute attack.
- For the patient with **acute cholecystitis**, use a low-fat diet. Progress to a diet with fewer condiments and gas-forming vegetables, which cause distention, increased peristalsis, and irritation.
- For the patient with **chronic cholecystitis**, use a fat/calorie-controlled diet to promote drainage of the gallbladder without excessive pain. Patient should consume adequate amounts of CHO, especially fiber (such as pectin, which binds excess bile acids).
- For the patient with **cholelithiasis**, encourage a diet that is high in fiber and, when needed, low in calories.
- Fat-soluble vitamins may need to be replaced in water-miscible forms.
- Increase dietary intake of sources of vitamin C such as citrus fruits and juices. Use supplemental forms if needed.
- To prevent gallbladder cancer, it may be useful to consume a diet that includes sufficient amounts of selenium, zinc, and vitamin E (Shukla et al, 2003).

CLINICAL INDICATORS

Clinical/History

Height
Weight
BMI
Diet history
WBC
Jaundice
Nausea
I & O
Temperature
CT scan or endoscopic ultrasound
Magnetic resonance cholangiography (MRC)
Hepatobiliary iminodiacetic acid (HIDA) scan (cholescintigraphy)
Endoscopic retrograde cholangiopancreatography (ERCP)
Cholecochoscopy

Lab Work

Alb, transthyretin
Bilirubin (increased)
Gamma-glutamyl transpeptidase (GGTP) (increased)
Lipase (often increased)
Chol, Trig
AST
PT
H & H
LDH
Na+, K+
Amylase
Ca++, Mg++
Alk phos

Common Drugs Used and Potential Side Effects

- Oral dissolution therapy: drugs made from bile acid help dissolve the stones. These drugs, ursodiol (Actigall) and chenodiol (Chenix), work best for small cholesterol stones over months or years. Both drugs cause mild diarrhea. Chenodiol may elevate blood cholesterol and the liver enzyme transaminase. Take with food or milk. Ursodiol can lead to metallic taste, abdominal pain, or vomiting. Ursodeoxycholic acid decreases cholesterol saturation of bile and gallstone incidence during weight loss and may help to prevent gallstone formation (Erlinger, 2000); use of orlistat is another option (Trouillot et al, 2001).
- Contact dissolution therapy involves an experimental injection of methyl tertbutyl ether directly into the gallbladder to dissolve stones. The drug can dissolve some stones in 1–3 days and is being tested in patients with symptomatic, noncalcified cholesterol stones.
- Antibiotics may be used to counteract any infection. Evaluate the need to take with food or milk or with other specific liquids.
- Analgesics (Demerol, meperidine) may be used to relieve pain. Nausea, vomiting, constipation, and GI distress can occur.
- Oral contraceptives and estrogens may increase the risk of gallstones, especially after prolonged use. Use of thiazide diuretics has also been linked with gallstones (Leitzmann et al, 2005).

Herbs, Botanicals, and Supplements

- Herbs and botanical supplements should not be used without discussing with physician. Herbal medicine such as turmeric, Oregon grape, bupleurum, and coin grass may reduce gallbladder inflammation and relieve liver congestion (Moga, 2003). Celandine, peppermint, couch grass, and goldenrod have been recommended for gallbladder disease, but no clinical trials have proven efficacy at this time.

INTERVENTION: NUTRITION EDUCATION, COUNSELING, CARE MANAGEMENT

- After a cholecystectomy, fat intake should be limited for several months to allow the liver to compensate for the gallbladder's absence. Fats should be introduced gradually; excessive amounts of fat at one meal should be avoided. If diarrhea persists after surgery, try using antidiarrheal medications, such as loperamide (Imodium) and a high-fiber diet for more bulk.
- Avoid fasting and rapid weight loss schemes.
- People who have had their gallbladders removed should have their cholesterol levels checked periodically, as should every adult.
- To prevent new gallstones from forming, maintain a healthy weight. Dietary changes that lower plasma insulin levels, such as a change in dietary fats and substitution of unrefined carbohydrates for refined carbohydrates, may be helpful (Moga, 2003).
- Regular aerobic exercise has a beneficial effect on hyperinsulinemia, which is frequently associated with gallbladder disease (Moga, 2003).

For More Information

- American College of Surgeons–Cholecystectomy
  http://www.facs.org/public_info/operation/cholesys.pdf
- Bile Duct Diseases
  http://www.nlm.nih.gov/medlineplus/bileductdiseases.html
- Gallbladder Disease Information
  http://www.nlm.nih.gov/medlineplus/gallbladderandbileduct-diseases.html
- Liver Foundation
  http://www.liverfoundation.org/db/articles/1047
- National Institute of Diabetes and Digestive and Kidney Diseases (NIDDK)–Gallstones
  http://digestive.niddk.nih.gov/ddiseases/pubs/gallstones/index.htm

GALLBLADDER DISEASE—CITED REFERENCES

Adamek HE, et al. Predictions and associations of cholecystectomy in patients with cholecystolithiasis treated with extracorporeal shock wave lithotripsy. *Dig Dis Sci.* 49:1938, 2004.

Bini EJ, McGready J. Prevalence of gallbladder disease among persons with hepatitis C virus infection in the United States. *Hepatology* 41:1029, 2005.

Cirillo DJ, et al. Effect of estrogen therapy on gallbladder disease. *JAMA.* 293:330, 2005.

Conway JD, et al. Endoscopic stent insertion into the gallbladder for symptomatic gallbladder disease in patients with end-stage liver disease. *Gastrointest Endosc.* 61:32, 2005.

Dittrick GW, et al. Gallbladder pathology in morbid obesity. *Obes Surg.* 15:238, 2005.

Erlinger S. Gallstones in obesity and weight loss. *Eur J Gastroenterol Hepatol.* 12:1347, 2000.

Ko CW, et al. Incidence, natural history, and risk factors for biliary sludge and stones during pregnancy. *Hepatology* 41:359, 2005.

Leitzmann MF, et al. Thiazide diuretics and the risk of gallbladder disease requiring surgery in women. *Arch Intern Med.* 165:567, 2005.

Lu EJ, et al. Medical versus surgical management of biliary tract disease in pregnancy. *Am J Surg.* 188:755, 2004.

Moga MM. Alternative treatment of gallbladder disease. *Med Hypotheses.* 60:143, 2003.

Ruhl CE, Everhart JE. Association of coffee consumption with gallbladder disease. *Am J Epidemiol.* 152:1034, 2000.

Shaffer EA. Epidemiology and risk factors for gallstone disease: has the paradigm changed in the 21st century? *Curr Gastroenterol Rep.* 7:132, 2005.

Shukla VK, et al. Micronutrients, antioxidants, and carcinoma of the gallbladder. *J Surg Oncol.* 84:31, 2003.

Simon JA, Hudes ES. Serum ascorbic acid and gallbladder disease prevalence among US adults: the Third National Health and Nutrition Examination Survey (NHANES III). *Arch Intern Med.* 160:931, 2000.

Simopoulos C, et al. Laparoscopic cholecystectomy in obese patients. *Obes Surg.* 15:243, 2005.

Trouillot T, et al. Orlistat maintains biliary lipid composition and hepatobiliary function in obese subjects undergoing moderate weight loss. *Am J Gastroenterol.* 96:1888, 2001.

Tsunoda K, et al. Prevalence of cholesterol gallstones positively correlates with per capita daily calorie intake. *Hepatogastroenterology* 51:1271, 2004.

BILIARY CIRRHOSIS

NUTRITIONAL ACUITY RANKING: LEVEL 2

DEFINITIONS AND BACKGROUND

Biliary atresia is the result of an inflammatory process that affects the intrahepatic and extrahepatic bile ducts, leading to fibrosis and obliteration of the biliary tract with the development of **biliary cirrhosis** in infants (Tang et al, 2005). Biliary cirrhosis is also called cholangiolitic hepatitis (obstructive jaundice). There is a prevalence of between 2 and 5 cases per 100,000 worldwide. Symptoms include pruritus, jaundice, and portal hypertension. See Figure 8-8.

Primary biliary cirrhosis (PBC) is a chronic cholestatic liver disease that predominantly affects middle-aged women. Environmental or autoimmune factors may act to trigger the disease in genetically susceptible hosts. Sjögren's syndrome, Raynaud's syndrome, a high rate of urinary tract infection (UTI), and a history of smoking have been reported (Parikh-Patel et al, 2001). Testing for celiac disease may also be important because there is often a relationship (Duggan and Duggan, 2005). Dietary treatment may prevent progression to hepatic failure in patients with celiac disease (Kaukinen et al, 2002).

Antinuclear antibodies (ANA) are highly specific in this condition (Muratori et al, 2005; Rigopoulou et al, 2005). Osteoporosis is more prevalent in women with PBC than in the general population (Guanabens et al, 2005).

Homocysteine, an intermediate in methionine metabolism, has been proposed to be involved in hepatic fibrogenesis (Ebrahimkhani et al, 2005). PBC slowly progresses and may lead to liver failure.

In symptomatic patients, advanced age, elevated serum bilirubin levels, and decreased serum albumin levels lead to shortened survival (Nishio et al, 2001). Transplantation is the only effective therapy in the end-stage liver disease.

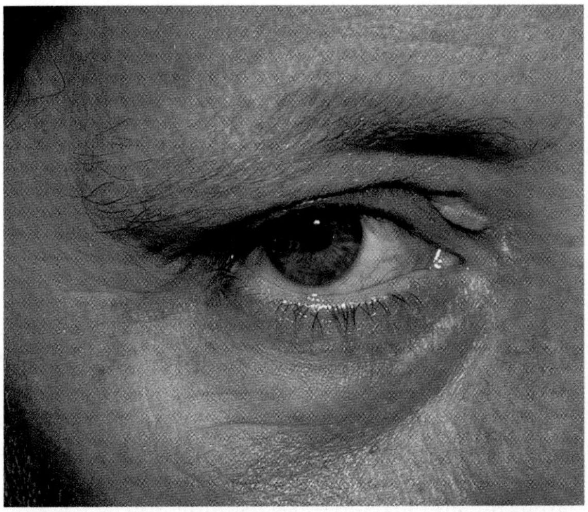

Figure 8-8 Xanthomas in biliary cirrhosis. (From Gold DH, Weingeist TA. *Color atlas of the eye in systemic disease*. Baltimore: Lippincott Williams & Wilkins, 2001.)

INTERVENTION: OBJECTIVES

- Correct diarrhea, steatorrhea, malnutrition, and osteomalacia. Up to 50% of adults with primary biliary cirrhosis are deficient in vitamin D (Phillips et al, 1991); prevention of bone density loss is important.
- Limit or control symptoms. Prevent progression to end-stage liver disease when possible.
- Prevent or correct zinc and vitamin deficiencies.
- Manage related disorders (such as Sjögren's syndrome or celiac disease).

INTERVENTION: FOOD AND NUTRITION

- Increase vitamin D and calcium intake to protect against osteopenia. Vitamin K may also play an important role in protection of bone health and may be supplemented in this condition (Plaza and Lamson, 2005).
- Use water-miscible sources of vitamins A, D, E, and K with steatorrhea.
- Reduce cholesterol and saturated fats in hypercholesterolemia.
- Ensure adequate intake of zinc from diet.
- To lower elevated homocysteine levels, which seem to aggravate hepatic fibrogenesis, be sure the diet contains adequate amounts of folic acid and vitamins B_6 and B_{12} (Ebrahimkhani et al, 2005).
- If the patient also has celiac disease, omit gluten from the diet (e.g., wheat, rye, barley). Initiation of a gluten-free diet may help to resolve iron deficiency anemia, pruritus, and elevated serum liver biochemistries (Sedlack et al, 2002). See appropriate entry.
- Control carbohydrate intake if there is hyperglycemia.

CLINICAL INDICATORS

Clinical/History

Height
Weight
BMI
Diet history
Jaundice
Xanthomas

Lab Work

Alb, transthyretin
Antinuclear antibodies (ANA)
PT (decreased)
Serum homocysteine
Transferrin
Tissue transglutaminase (for celiac disease)
Globulin
Bilirubin (increased)
Gluc
Alk phos (increased)
Ca++, Mg++
Na+, K+
Chol (increased)
Ceruloplasmin
ALT/AST
GGT

Common Drugs Used and Potential Side Effects

- Prolonged administration of ursodeoxycholic acid (UDCA) in patients with PBC is associated with survival benefit and a delaying of liver transplantation; it might even prevent progression of the histological stage of PBC (Kumar and Tandon, 2001). Studies with UDCA and immunosuppressants such as prednisone, budesonide, and azathioprine have shown that, in selected patients, combination therapy may be superior to UDCA monotherapy (Holtmeier and Leuschner, 2001).
- Budesonide is a glucocorticoid that may be helpful when given with UDCA to improve liver status; more studies are needed (Rautiainen et al, 2005). Weight gain and increased appetite often result.
- Bezafibrate, a hypolipidemic drug, has been shown to benefit patients with PBC in some studies (Akbar et al, 2005). Cholestyramine may be used to decrease bile acids; belching or constipation may occur.
- Antiretroviral therapies have been tested with some promising results, but larger placebo-controlled trials are required (Mason et al, 2004).

Herbs, Botanicals, and Supplements

- Herbs and botanical supplements should not be used without discussing with physician.
- High doses of vitamin E (tocopherol) will elevate transaminases; lab results improve with discontinuation (Neff et al, 2004).

INTERVENTION: NUTRITION EDUCATION, COUNSELING, CARE MANAGEMENT

- Discuss the role of bile salts in fat and fat-soluble vitamin absorption. If supplements are used, water-miscible forms may be needed.
- Protection of bone mineral density will be important. Discuss the role of medications, calcium, and vitamin D on bone health (Di Bisceglie et al, 2004; Plaza and Lamson, 2005).

BILIARY CIRRHOSIS—CITED REFERENCES

Akbar SM, et al. Therapeutic efficacy of decreased nitrite production by bezafibrate in patients with primary biliary cirrhosis. *J Gastroenterol.* 40:157, 2005.

Di Bisceglie AM, et al. Long term follow up of bone mineral density in patients with primary biliary cirrhosis. *Minerva Med.* 95:529, 2004.

Duggan JM, Duggan AE. Systematic review: the liver in celiac disease. *Aliment Pharmacol Ther.* 21:515, 2005.

Ebrahimkhani MR, et al. Homocysteine alterations in experimental cholestasis and its subsequent cirrhosis. *Life Sci.* 76:2497, 2005.

Guanabens N, et al. Severity of cholestasis and advanced histological stage but not menopausal status are the major risk factors for osteoporosis in primary biliary cirrhosis. *J Hepatol.* 42:573, 2005.

Holtmeier J, Leuschner U. Medical treatment of primary biliary cirrhosis and primary sclerosing cholangitis. *Digestion* 64:137, 2001.

Kaukinen K, et al. Celiac disease in patients with severe liver disease: gluten-free diet may reverse hepatic failure. *Gastroenterology* 122:881, 2002.

Kumar D, Tandon R. Use of ursodeoxycholic acid in liver diseases. *J Gastroenterol Hepatol.* 16:3, 2001.

Mason AL, et al. Pilot studies of single and combination antiretroviral therapy in patients with primary biliary cirrhosis. *Am J Gastroenterol.* 99:2348, 2004.

Muratori L, et al. The Western immunoblotting pattern of anti-mitochondrial antibodies is independent of the clinical expression of primary biliary cirrhosis. *Dig Liver Dis.* 37:108, 2005.

Neff GW, et al. Consumption of dietary supplements in a liver transplant population. *Liver Transpl.* 10:881, 2004.

Nishio A, et al. Primary biliary cirrhosis: from induction to destruction. *Semin Gastrointest Dis.* 12:89, 2001.

Parikh-Patel A, et al. Risk factors for primary biliary cirrhosis in a cohort of patients from the United States. *Hepatology.* 33:16, 2001.

Phillips JR, et al. Fat-soluble vitamin levels in patients with primary biliary cirrhosis. *Am J Gastroenterol.* 96:2745, 2001.

Plaza SM, Lamson DW. Vitamin K2 in bone metabolism and osteoporosis. *Altern Med Rev.* 10:24, 2005.

Rautiainen H, et al. Budesonide combined with UDCA to improve liver histology in primary biliary cirrhosis: a three-year randomized trial. *Hepatology* 41:747, 2005.

Rigopoulou EI, et al. Prevalence and clinical significance of isotype specific antinuclear antibodies in primary biliary cirrhosis. *Gut* 54:528, 2005.

Sedlack RE, et al. Celiac disease-associated autoimmune cholangitis. *Am J Gastroenterol.* 97:3196, 2002.

Tang ST, et al. Diagnosis and treatment of biliary atresia: a retrospective study. *Hepatobiliary Pancreat Dis Int.* 4:108, 2005.

CHOLESTATIC LIVER DISEASE (CHOLESTASIS)

NUTRITIONAL ACUITY RANKING: LEVEL 2–3

DEFINITIONS AND BACKGROUND

Cholestatic liver disease (cholestasis) involves any liver disease with bilirubin over 2.0 mg/dL. Disturbance of the flow of bile leads to intracellular retention of biliary constituents. In the sequence of events that leads to liver injury, the cytotoxic action of bile salts is pivotal to all forms of cholestasis (Kullak-Ublick and Meier, 2000).

Common hepatic causes of cholestasis include viral hepatitis, alcoholic liver disease, hemochromatosis, and autoimmune hepatitis. Biliary causes include primary sclerosing cholangitis (in which the intrahepatic and/or extrahepatic bile ducts undergo inflammation and fibrosis), choledocholithiasis, primary biliary cirrhosis, and biliary atresia. It can also occur with inflammatory bowel disease (Huang and Lichtenstein, 2005). Prolonged parenteral nutrition may be needed in the absence of GI tract stimulation.

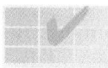

Cholestasis interferes with excretion of the bile salts required for emulsification and absorption of dietary fat. Reduced bile secretion impairs micelle formation, which is needed for digestion of fat by pancreatic enzymes, and this in turn affects fat-soluble vitamin utilization. Vitamin and mineral deficiencies and alterations are common, especially if cholestasis is significant. Zinc, magnesium, and calcium may be deficient because they are albumin-bound and the liver is not working properly. Deficiency of fat-soluble vitamins A, D, E, and K may occur. Of particular concern is vitamin E, which tends to be low in this condition; vitamin E circulates in the blood almost exclusively attached to the lipoprotein fractions.

In chronic cholestasis with biliary obstruction, hyperlipidemia and accumulation of copper result, and manganese can accumulate in the brain; avoid overfeeding with copper or manganese. Hepatic copper overload in TPN patients occurs through chronic cholestasis in TPN-associated liver disease regardless of duration (Blaszyck et al, 2005).

Chronic total parenteral nutrition may induce fatty liver and inflammation, especially in patients with short bowel syndrome. Deficiency of choline in parenteral solutions has been proposed as the mechanism for liver disease. With TPN, cholestatic jaundice may occur from a lack of enteral nutrition and failure of biliary stimulation. In patients receiving home PN, prevalence of liver disease increases with duration (Cavicchi et al, 2000).

Signs and symptoms of cholestasis can include glossitis from B-complex vitamin deficiency, protein and iron deficiency, hemorrhagic tendencies due to vitamin C or K inadequacy, and flatulence. Patients with steatorrhea may benefit from a low-fat diet or from use of MCTs. Intrahepatic cholestatic syndromes cause a decrease in bile flow with no overt bile duct obstruction; bile constituents accumulate in the liver and blood. Treatment of extrahepatic manifestations of cholestatic liver disease such as pruritus, fatigue, osteoporosis, and steatorrhea can be problematic and time consuming (Holtmeier and Leuschner, 2001).

The central role of bile salts in the pathogenesis of cholestasis has become evident from the improvement of many cholestatic syndromes with oral bile salt therapy (Kullak-Ublick and Meier, 2000). Ursodeoxycholic acid and adequate nutritional support are the usual treatments, with liver transplantation being performed in severe cases only (Huang and Lichtenstein, 2005).

Depending on the cause (such as medication effects, postoperative jaundice, sepsis, TPN, or acalculous cholecystitis), treatment includes removal of offending drugs, supportive care, broad-spectrum antibiotic agents with drainage of infected fluids, TPN adjustment, including cycling and limiting carbohydrates, and cholecystectomy (Faust and Reddy, 2004).

INTERVENTION: OBJECTIVES

- Promote return of normal liver function and bile flow.
- Treat fat malabsorption and deficiency of any nutrients.
- Correct steatorrhea, GI bleeding, and copper overloading when present.
- Prevent or correct for liver failure, osteomalacia, or osteoporosis.
- Correct nutrient excesses (e.g., manganese).
- Prepare for surgery when indicated.

INTERVENTION: FOOD AND NUTRITION

- In chronic cases, 10–20% added kilocalories may be needed. Infants need more kilocalories, and adults tend to use CHO poorly. In acute stages, use IV glucose to prevent hypoglycemia and protein catabolism.
- In acute stages, infants will need 1.0–1.5 g/kg protein. Children, teens, and adults need 0.5–1.2 g protein/kg; highlight branched-chain amino acid sources. In chronic cases, use 3 g protein/d for infants and 1–1.5 g protein/kg in adults.
- Supplement with vitamins and minerals, especially fat-soluble vitamins. Vitamin D and calcium will be needed if osteopenia is present (Sharma et al, 2004; Hay, 1998).
- Small, frequent feedings and snacks may be better tolerated than large meals.
- Use enteral nutrition (where possible), if TPN has caused cholestasis (Krawinkel, 2004). If TPN is required, early use of cyclic TPN may be useful (Hwang et al, 2000). Avoid excesses of copper (Blaszyk et al, 2005) in the solutions, but do include it (Zambrano et al, 2004).
- Zinc and selenium may be needed.

CLINICAL INDICATORS

Clinical/History

Height
Weight
BMI
Diet history
Ascites
Edema
I & O
Nausea

Lab Work

Chol, Trig (increased)
PT (prolonged)
AST, ALT (increased)
Bilirubin (increased, >2 mg/dL)
Somatomedin C
Alk phos (increased)
RBP
Bun, Creat
H & H
Serum Fe
Alb, transthyretin
Serum carotene (increased or decreased)
Transferrin
Globulin
GGT
Amylase, lipase
Serum manganese
Serum zinc
Na+, K+
Ca++, Mg++

Common Drugs Used and Potential Side Effects

- Ursodeoxycholic acid is currently the most promising pharmacological treatment option for slowing disease progression and should be used in relatively high doses (20–30 mg/kg/d) (Huang and Lichtenstein, 2005). It has cytoprotective, antiapoptotic, membrane-stabilizing, antioxidative, and immunomodulatory effects (Kumar and Tandon, 2001).
- Treatment of pruritus due to cholestasis is with bile acid–binding exchange resins such as cholestyramine or colestipol (Huang and Lichtenstein, 2005). Use with a low-fat diet and increase fluids and fiber. Constipation, nausea, or vomiting may be a side effect.

- Water-miscible forms of fat-soluble vitamins A, D, E, and K may be needed in cholestasis. Sample amounts of vitamin A may be given at 25,000–50,000 IU/d as Aquasol A; vitamin D may be given as 12,000–50,000 IU/d over a month; and vitamin E may be given as 10–25 IU/kg/d. Once nutrient stores are repleted and cholestasis is resolved, the supplementation can stop.
- Medications known to cause cholestasis include estrogens and anabolic steroids, chlorpromazine, erythromycin, and the oxypenicillins (Chitturi and Farrell, 2001).

Herbs, Botanicals, and Supplements

- Herbs and botanical supplements should not be used without discussing with physician. Cholestatic liver injury may occur from some herbal remedies, such as greater celandine, glycyrrhizin, chaparral (Chitturi and Farrell, 2001).

INTERVENTION: NUTRITION EDUCATION, COUNSELING, CARE MANAGEMENT

- Discuss the role of fat in normal metabolic processes; simplify explanation in correlation to absorption of fat-soluble vitamins and other nutrients affected by the liver.
- Discuss ways to increase satiety from the diet with appetizing recipes.
- Discuss use of over-the-counter (OTC) vitamin and mineral supplements, especially regarding possible toxicity if taken in large doses with liver disease.
- Liver transplantation works best in a well-nourished patient. Promote good tolerance and intake.

CHOLESTATIC LIVER DISEASE—CITED REFERENCES

Blaszyck H, et al. Hepatic copper in patients receiving long-term total parenteral nutrition. *J Clin Gastroenterol.* 39:318, 2005.

Cavicchi M, et al. Prevalence of liver disease and contributing factors in patients receiving home parenteral nutrition for permanent intestinal failure. *Ann Intern Med.* 132:525, 2000.

Chitturi S, Farrell GC. Drug-induced cholestasis. *Semin Gastrointest Dis.* 12:113, 2001.

Faust TW, Reddy KR. Postoperative jaundice. *Clin Liver Dis.* 8:151, 2004.

Hay JE. Osteoporosis. *Clin Liver Dis.* 2:407, 1998.

Holtmeier J, Leuschner U. Medical treatment of primary biliary cirrhosis and primary sclerosing cholangitis. *Digestion* 64:137, 2001.

Huang CS, Lichtenstein DR. Treatment of biliary problems in inflammatory bowel disease. *Curr Treat Options Gastroenterol.* 8:117, 2005.

Hwang T, et al. Early use of cyclic TPN prevents further deterioration of liver functions for the TPN patients with impaired liver function. *Hepatogastroenterology* 47:1347, 2000.

Krawinkel MB. Parenteral nutrition-associated cholestasis—what do we know, what can we do? *Eur J Pediatr Surg.* 14:230, 2004.

Kullak-Ublick G, Meier P. Mechanisms of cholestasis. *Clin Liver Dis.* 4:357, 2000.

Kumar D, Tandon R. Use of ursodeoxycholic acid in liver diseases. *J Gastroenterol Hepatol.* 16:3, 2001.

Sharma N, et al. Vitamin supplementation: what the gastroenterologist needs to know. *J Clin Gastroenterol.* 38:844, 2004.

Zambrano E, et al. Total parenteral nutrition induced liver pathology: an autopsy series of 24 newborn cases. *Pediatr Dev Pathol.* 7:425, 2004.

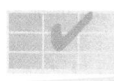

S E C T I O N 9

Endocrine Disorders

CHIEF ASSESSMENT FACTORS

For Diabetes (American Diabetes Association, 2006)

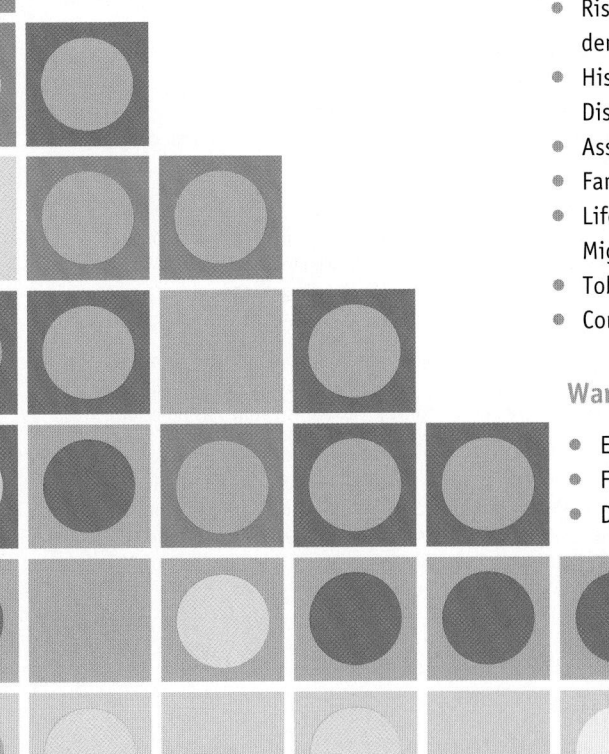

- Symptoms, Results of Laboratory Tests, and Special Examination Results Related to the Diagnosis of Diabetes
- Prior HbA1c Records
- Eating Patterns, Nutritional Status, and Weight History; Growth and Development in Children and Adolescents
- Details of Previous Treatment Programs, Including Nutrition and Diabetes Self-Management Education, Attitudes, and Health Beliefs
- Current Treatment of Diabetes, Including Medications, Meal Plan, and Results of Glucose Monitoring and Patients' Use of Data
- Exercise History
- Frequency, Severity, and Cause of Acute Complications Such as Ketoacidosis and Hypoglycemia
- Prior or Current Infections, Particularly Skin, Foot, Dental, and Genitourinary Infections
- Symptoms and Treatment of Chronic Eye; Kidney; Nerve; Genitourinary (Including Sexual), Bladder, and Gastrointestinal Function (Including Symptoms of Celiac Disease in Type 1 Diabetic Patients); Heart; Peripheral Vascular; Foot; and Cerebrovascular Complications Associated with Diabetes
- Other Medications That May Affect Blood Glucose Levels
- Risk Factors for Atherosclerosis: Smoking, Hypertension, Obesity, Dyslipidemia, and Family History
- History and Treatment of Other Conditions, Including Endocrine and Eating Disorders
- Assessment for Mood Disorder
- Family History of Diabetes and Other Endocrine Disorders
- Lifestyle, Cultural, Psychosocial, Educational, and Economic Factors That Might Influence the Management of Diabetes
- Tobacco, Alcohol, and/or Controlled Substance Use
- Contraception and Reproductive and Sexual History

Warning Signs of Type 1 Diabetes:

- Extreme Thirst
- Frequent Urination
- Drowsiness, Lethargy, Blurred Vision
- Glucose or Ketones in Urine
- Increased Appetite
- Sudden Weight Loss
- Fruity, Sweet, or Wine-Like Odor on Breath
- Heavy, Labored Breathing
- Stupor, Unconsciousness

Risk Factors for Type 2 Diabetes:

- Age ≥ 45 Years
- Family History (Parents or Siblings with DM)
- Obesity with Body Mass Index ≥ 25 kg/m^2
- History of Impaired Fasting Glucose (IFG) or Impaired Glucose Tolerance (IGT)
- High-Density Lipoprotein Cholesterol Level ≤ 35 mg/dL and Triglyceride Level ≥ 250 mg/dL
- History of Gestational Diabetes Mellitus (GDM) or Women Delivering Babies Weighing >9 Pounds
- Hypertension (Blood Pressure ≥ 140/90 mm Hg)
- Ethnicity—African American, Hispanic American, Native American, Asian American, Pacific Islander

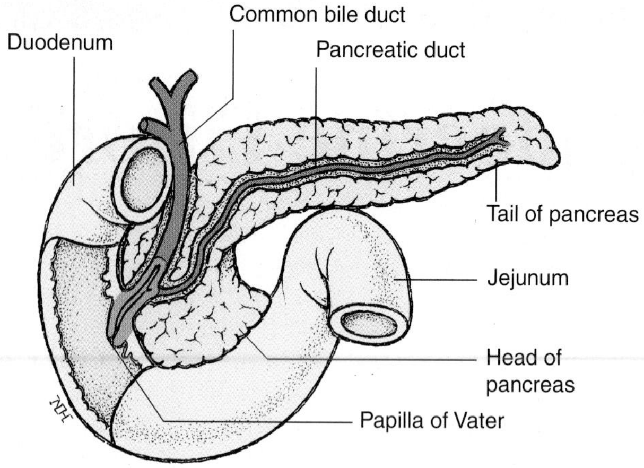

Figure 9-1 The pancreas and its nearby relationships. (Courtesy of Neil O. Hardy, Westpoint, CT.)

Assessment of Other Endocrine Conditions:

- Hormone Imbalances (Excess or Deficiency)
- Numbness, Tingling, Paresthesia
- Bone Pain
- Headache, Seizures, Syncope
- Anorexia, Nausea, Abdominal Pain, Malabsorption, Gastroparesis
- Hyperglycemia, Hypoglycemia
- Weight Changes
- Shortness of Breath, Hoarseness
- Decreased Libido, Erectile Dysfunction
- Dysuria
- Pruritus, Dryness of Skin or Hair
- Altered Consciousness
- Hormone Therapy: Anabolic Hormones—Growth Hormones, Androgens, Sex Hormones; Catabolic Hormones—Stress Hormones (Causing Gluconeogenesis from Protein) Such as Catecholamines (Epinephrine, Norepinephrine), Glucocorticoids (Cortisone, Cortisol), and Glucagon
- Goiter; Exophthalmos; Intolerance to Heat, Cold
- Adult Changes in Size of Head, Hands, Feet
- Postural Hypotension, Weakness
- Diagnosis of Thyroid Disease or Other Endocrine Disorder

CRITERIA FOR SCREENING AND DIAGNOSIS OF DIABETES (AMERICAN DIABETES ASSOCIATION, 2006)

Screen for prediabetes and diabetes in high-risk, asymptomatic, undiagnosed adults and children within the health care setting. An oral glucose tolerance test (OGTT) may be considered in patients with impaired fasting glucose (IFG) to better define the risk of diabetes.

Testing for diabetes should be considered in all individuals at age 45 years and above, particularly in those with a BMI of 25 kg/m^2, and if normal, testing should be repeated at 3-year intervals.

Testing should be considered at a younger age or be carried out more frequently in individuals who are overweight (BMI ≥25 kg/m^2) and have additional risk factors:

- are habitually physically inactive
- have a first-degree relative with diabetes
- are members of a high-risk ethnic population (e.g., African American, Latino, Native American, Asian American, Pacific Islander)
- have delivered a baby weighing >9 lb or have been diagnosed with gestational diabetes mellitus
- are hypertensive (≥140/90 mm Hg)
- have a high-density lipoprotein cholesterol level <35 mg/dL (0.90 mmol/L) and/or a triglyceride level >250 mg/dL (2.82 mmol/L)
- have polycystic ovarian syndrome or other clinical conditions associated with insulin resistance
- have a history of vascular disease
- on previous testing, had impaired glucose tolerance (IGT) or IFG

1. Symptoms of diabetes and a casual plasma glucose of 200 mg/dL (11.1 mmol/L). Casual is defined as any time of day without regard to time since last meal. The classic symptoms of diabetes include polyuria, polydipsia, and unexplained weight loss.

OR

2. To screen for diabetes/prediabetes, a fasting plasma glucose (FPG) test, a 2-hour OGTT (75-g glucose load), or both are appropriate. FPG ≥126 mg/dL (7.0 mmol/L). Fasting is defined as no caloric intake for at least 8 hours.

OR

3. 2-Hour plasma glucose of 200 mg/dL (11.1 mmol/L) during an OGTT. The test should be performed as described by the World Health Organization, using a glucose load containing the equivalent of 75 g anhydrous glucose dissolved in water.

Source: American Diabetes Association. Standards of Medical Care in Diabetes–2006. *Diabetes Care* 29:4S, 2006.

OVERVIEW OF DIABETES MELLITUS

Diabetes mellitus is a group of metabolic diseases characterized by hyperglycemia resulting from defects in insulin secretion, insulin action, or both. Hyperglycemia of diabetes is associated with long-term damage, dysfunction, and failure of various organs, especially the eyes, kidneys, nerves, heart, and blood vessels. Diabetes affects 18.5 million Americans, with 13.3 million who have been diagnosed and about 5.2 million who are unaware of their diagnosis; another 41 million Americans may have prediabetes (Kulkarni et al, 2005).

Diabetes is divided into distinct types: type 1, type 2, prediabetes, gestational diabetes mellitus (GDM), and other types (see Table 9-1). Type 2 diabetes, composing 90% of diabetes cases, is especially affected by both genetic and environmental factors. Types of diabetes affecting children and teens are listed in Table 9-2. Assessment of diabetes patients is outlined in Table 9-3; complications are listed in Table 9-4.

Medical nutrition therapy (MNT) has replaced the words "diet therapy," and there is no single "diabetic" or "ADA" diet; the recommended diet is a nutrition prescription based on assessment and treatment goals and outcomes. MNT for people with diabetes should be individualized, with consideration given to usual eating habits and other lifestyle factors. Strategic patient counseling should ask questions that highlight strengths and benefits (self-efficacy), obstacles (weaknesses), threats, and lifestyle changes the patient is willing and able to make; this will help reach and maintain successful outcomes. Using open-ended discussion and counseling encourages the client to assess and determine a realistic self-management plan.

MNT may be offered in phases, according to patient comprehension and readiness to learn basic principles and

TABLE 9-1 Etiologic Classification of Diabetes Mellitus

I. Type 1 diabetes (results from beta-cell destruction, usually leading to absolute insulin deficiency).

II. Type 2 diabetes (results from a progressive insulin secretory defect on the background of insulin resistance).

III. Other specific types of diabetes due to other causes, e.g., genetic defects in beta-cell function, genetic defects in insulin action, diseases of the exocrine pancreas (such as cystic fibrosis), or drug- or chemical-induced diabetes (such as in the treatment of AIDS or after organ transplantation).

- A. Genetic defects of beta-cell function
  1. Maturity-onset diabetes of youth (MODY)
  2. Mitochondrial DNA
- B. Genetic defects in insulin action
  1. Type A insulin resistance
  2. Leprechaunism
  3. Rabson-Mendenhall syndrome
  4. Lipoatrophic diabetes
- C. Diseases of the exocrine pancreas
  1. Pancreatitis
  2. Trauma/pancreatectomy
  3. Neoplasia
  4. Cystic fibrosis
  5. Hemochromatosis
  6. Fibrocalculous pancreatopathy
- D. Endocrinopathies
  1. Acromegaly
  2. Cushing's syndrome
  3. Glucagonoma
  4. Pheochromocytoma
  5. Hyperthyroidism
  6. Somatostatinoma
  7. Aldosteronoma
- E. Drug- or chemical-induced
  1. Vacor
  2. Pentamidine
  3. Nicotinic acid
  4. Glucocorticoids
  5. Thyroid hormone
  6. Diazoxide
  7. Beta-adrenergic agonists
  8. Thiazides
  9. Dilantin
  10. Alpha-interferon
- F. Infections
  1. Congenital rubella
  2. Cytomegalovirus
- G. Uncommon forms of immune-mediated diabetes
  1. "Stiff-person" syndrome
  2. Anti-insulin receptor antibodies
- H. Other genetic syndromes sometimes associated with diabetes
  1. Down's syndrome
  2. Klinefelter's syndrome
  3. Turner's syndrome
  4. Wolfram's syndrome
  5. Friedreich's ataxia
  6. Huntington's chorea
  7. Laurence-Moon-Biedl syndrome
  8. Myotonic dystrophy
  9. Porphyria
  10. Prader-Willi syndrome

IV. Gestational diabetes mellitus (GDM) (diagnosed during pregnancy).

Adapted from the following resources: American Diabetes Association. Diagnosis and classification of diabetes mellitus. *Diabetes Care* 27:S5, 2004; and American Diabetes Association. Standards of Medical Care in Diabetes–2006. *Diabetes Care* 29:4S, 2006.

TABLE 9-2 Types of Diabetes in Children and Teens

Type 1 Diabetes (Immune-Mediated)

- Usually not obese; often recent weight loss.
- Short duration of symptoms (thirst and frequent urination).
- Presence of ketones at diagnosis, with about 35% presenting with ketoacidosis.
- Often a honeymoon period after blood sugars are in control during which the need for insulin diminishes for awhile. Usually kept on low dose of long-acting insulin, such as glargine (Lantus), which may prolong the honeymoon phase.
- Ultimate complete destruction of the insulin-producing cells needing exogenous insulin for survival.
- Ongoing risk of ketoacidosis.
- Only about 5% with a family history (in first- or second-degree relatives) of diabetes.

Type 2 Diabetes (Insulin-Resistant)

- Usually overweight at diagnosis; little or no weight loss.
- Usually have sugar in the urine but no ketones.
- As many as 30% will have some ketones in the urine at diagnosis.
- About 5% will have ketoacidosis at diagnosis.
- Often little or no thirst and minimal increased urination.
- Strong family history of diabetes.
- 45–80% have at least one parent with diabetes.
- Diabetes may span many generations of family members.
- 74–100% have a first- or second-degree relative with diabetes.
- Typically from African, Hispanic, Asian, or American Indian origin.
- Disorders likely to cause insulin resistance are common.
- About 90% of children with type 2 diabetes have dark shiny patches on the skin (acanthosis nigricans), which are most often found between the fingers and between the toes, on the back of the neck ("dirty neck"), and in axillary creases.
- Polycystic ovarian syndrome (PCOS).

Maturity-Onset Diabetes of the Young (MODY)

- Rare form of diabetes; several varieties exist.
- Early age of onset (ages 9–25 years) with autosomal dominant inheritability.
- Results from defects to insulin-producing cells caused by a genetic defect in the pancreatic beta-cell function.
- Symptoms run the gamut from mild elevation in blood sugar to a severe disturbance.
- MODY can occur in all ethnic groups.
- Gene abnormalities are rare and can only be identified through testing that is currently available only in research laboratories.
- Not usually obese.
- Environmental stressors, such as illness or puberty, may unmask the genetically limited insulin secretory reserve of patients with undiagnosed MODY.
- Unlike type 1 diabetes, MODY does not cause polyuria, thirst, or extreme hunger. The primary goal is euglycemia.
- Fasting insulin and C-peptide levels are usually normal or elevated slightly.

in-depth self-management guidance. Formal nutrition care process steps include assessment, nutrition diagnosis, and intervention, followed by monitoring and evaluation. Nutrition management includes monitoring of blood glucose, medications, physical activity, education, behavior modification, and evaluation of cardiovascular and renal status. The activation of nuclear transcription factor-κB has been linked with a variety of inflammatory diseases, including diabetes; use of spices and herbs may be able to suppress this pathway and may be part of the teaching process (Aggarwal and Shishodia, 2004).

A diabetes educator is defined as a health professional who has mastered the core knowledge and skills, communication, counseling, and education. The credentials of certified diabetes educators (CDE) designate professionals who have at least 1000 hours of direct diabetes teaching and who have successfully completed an examination. An advanced credential has been developed for registered dietitians, nurses, and pharmacists who have advanced degrees and meet experiential requirements; this credential is cited as BC-ADM (Daly et al, 2001).

Collaborative, multidisciplinary teams are best suited to provide such care for people with chronic conditions like diabetes and to empower patients' performance of appropriate self-management (American Diabetes Association, 2006). The National Diabetes Education Program launched a new online resource to help health care professionals better organize their diabetes care; the Better Diabetes Care website (www.betterdiabetescare.nih.gov) should help users design and implement more effective health care delivery systems for those with diabetes (American Diabetes Association, 2006). Table 9-5 describes evidence for diabetes counseling.

TABLE 9-3 Evaluation of the Patient with Diabetes

Evaluation Component	History: Patient/Family	Physical Examination	Laboratory
Blood glucose (BG)	Home glucose monitoring records Hyperglycemia Ketoacidosis Hypoglycemia Lifestyle Nutrition Current and past medications Weight history Diet history Exercise history Dieting history Substance use Contraception in women History of depression/eating disorders Cultural, psychosocial, and economic factors affecting diabetes management Secondary etiologies, such as Cushing's disease, acromegaly, and hemochromatosis	Weight Height Body mass index (BMI) Examination for acanthosis Insulin injection sites Sexual maturation in children and teens Thyroid palpitation	HbA1c Fasting glucose Pre- and post-meal BG values Fructosamine (used for sickle cell patients and hemoglobinopathies)
Coronary and peripheral arterial disease/ hyperlipidemia	Atherosclerotic disease: • Myocardial infarction (MI)/angina • Stroke • Transient ischemic attack (TIA) • Claudication • Surgical history of revascularization Atherosclerotic risks other than diabetes: • Smoking history • Family history • Previous diagnosis of hyperlipidemia Current and previous medications: • Aspirin • Estrogen therapy • Hypolipidemics Nutrition history: • Lipids, Sodium	Cardiac examination: • Heart • Peripheral circulation including pulses and bruits • Cutaneous or tendinous xanthomata	Electrocardiogram (ECG) Fasting lipid profile if not done within last year C-reactive protein Serum homocysteine Triglycerides
Eye	Changes in vision Laser treatment Glaucoma Dilated retinal exam by eye care provider within last year	Visual acuity, if changes in vision are reported	N/A
Foot	Symptoms of neuropathy (pain, paresthesia) Symptoms of peripheral vascular disease Symptoms of systemic or local infection	Visual inspection, including: Nails Web spaces	N/A

(continued)

TABLE 9-3 Evaluation of the Patient with Diabetes *(continued)*

Evaluation Component	History: Patient/Family	Physical Examination	Laboratory
	Previous episodes of foot complications: • Foot deformity • Skin breakdown • Ulcers • Amputations	Ulcers Calluses Deformities	
Hypertension	Previous diagnosis of hypertension Current and previous medications	Blood pressure	N/A
Kidney	Known history of diabetes Family history of hypertension and renal disease	Edema	Routine urinalysis Test for microalbuminuria and serum creatinine level if indicated

Adapted from Department of Veterans Affairs. Veterans Health Administration diabetes program. Accessed April 24, 2005 at http://www1.va.gov/health/diabetes/.

TABLE 9-4 Potential Complications of Diabetes

Degree of Complication	Complication	Description
ACUTE	**Hyperglycemia**	Patients with hyperglycemia fall into three categories when hospitalized (American Diabetes Association, 2006). (1) History of diabetes: diabetes has been previously diagnosed and acknowledged by the patient's treating physician. (2) Unrecognized diabetes: hyperglycemia (fasting blood glucose of 126 mg/dL or random blood glucose of 200 mg/dL) occurring during hospitalization and confirmed as diabetes after hospitalization by standard diagnostic criteria but unrecognized as diabetes by the treating physician during hospitalization. (3) Hospital-related hyperglycemia: hyperglycemia (fasting blood glucose of 126 mg/dL or random blood glucose of ≥200 mg/dL) occurring during the hospitalization that reverts to normal after hospital discharge. Symptoms include polyphagia, polydipsia, polyuria, dehydration, weight loss, weakness, muscle wasting, recurrent or persistent infections, hypovolemia, ketonemia, glycosuria, blurred or changed vision, fatigue, muscle cramps, and dry mouth. Blood glucose >250 mg/dL should be evaluated; monitor blood or urine ketones to check for diabetic ketoacidosis (DKA).
	DKA or nonketotic hyperosmolar state	The stress of illness, trauma, and/or surgery frequently aggravates glycemic control and may precipitate DKA or nonketotic hyperosmolar state (American Diabetes Association, 2006). A vomiting illness accompanied by ketosis may indicate DKA, a life-threatening condition that requires immediate medical care to prevent complications and death; the possibility of DKA should always be considered (American Diabetes Association, 2006). Cerebral edema can occur. Early consultation with an endocrinologist is needed.
	Hypoglycemia	Symptoms include shakiness, confusion, diplopia, irritability, hunger, weakness, headache, rapid and shallow breathing, numbness of mouth/lips/tongue, pulse normal or abnormal, convulsions, lack of coordination, dizziness, staggering gait, pallor, slurred speech, tingling, diaphoresis, nausea, sweating, tremors, and nightmares. Treat when blood glucose level is <70 mg/dL with 15 g of liquid or fat-free sources of glucose or carbohydrates (CHO); wait 15 minutes and retest, then treat with another 15 g of CHO if still <70 mg/dL. Blood glucose should be evaluated again in approximately 60 minutes because additional treatment may be necessary. Continue to monitor until next meal. Adding protein to carbohydrate does not affect the glycemic response and does not prevent subsequent hypoglycemia, but adding fat may retard and then prolong the acute glycemic response (American Diabetes Association, 2006).

(continued)

TABLE 9-4 **Potential Complications of Diabetes** ***(continued)***

Degree of Complication	Complication	Description
		In rare, severe hypoglycemia (when the individual requires the assistance of another person and cannot be treated with oral carbohydrate), emergency glucagon kits may be used; these require a prescription and they can expire over time (American Diabetes Association, 2006).
	Somogyi effect	This involves hormonal rebounding effects of blood glucose levels. Hypoglycemia triggers counterregulatory hormones, which can cause hepatic glucose release, and rebound hyperglycemia results.
	Acute illness or infection	Any condition leading to deterioration in glycemic control necessitates more frequent monitoring of blood glucose and urine or blood ketones (American Diabetes Association, 2006). Insulin may be needed. Aggressive glycemic management with insulin may reduce morbidity in patients with severe acute illness (American Diabetes Association, 2006). The risk for DKA is higher during this time; test blood glucose, drink adequate amounts of fluid, ingest CHO (50 g CHO every 3–4 hours) if blood glucose levels are low, and adjust medications to keep glucose in desired range and to prevent starvation ketosis (Franz et al, 2002). Marked hyperglycemia requires temporary adjustment of the treatment program and, if accompanied by ketosis, frequent interaction with the diabetes care team (American Diabetes Association, 2006). Infection or dehydration is more likely to necessitate hospitalization of the person with diabetes than the person without diabetes (American Diabetes Association, 2006). Annually provide an influenza vaccine to all diabetic patients ≥6 months of age; provide at least one lifetime pneumococcal vaccine for adults with diabetes (American Diabetes Association, 2006). Persons who have diabetes tend to be at higher than normal risk for bacterial forms of pneumonia.
	Critical illness	In critically ill patients, blood glucose levels should be kept as close to 110 mg/dL (6.1 mmol/L) as possible and generally <180 mg/dL (10 mmol/L); intravenous insulin is usually needed (American Diabetes Association, 2006). Scheduled prandial insulin doses should be given in relation to meals and should be adjusted according to point-of-care glucose levels; traditional sliding-scale insulin regimens may be ineffective and are not useful (American Diabetes Association, 2006).
INTERMEDIATE	**Children with type 1 diabetes**	Children's growth and development may be impaired with diabetes; adequate protein and energy must be provided. Children may be picky eaters. Blood glucose goals are less strict. Target range for normal blood glucose (90–130 mg/dL before eating for 13–19 year olds; 90–180 mg/dL for 6–12 year olds; and 100–180 mg/dL for 0–5 year olds) may be altered according to the health care provider's evaluation. Near normalization of blood glucose levels is seldom attainable in children and adolescents after the honeymoon (remission) period (American Diabetes Association, 2006). The A1c goals also vary in children. Most children under 6 or 7 years of age have a form of "hypoglycemic unawareness," and young children lack the cognitive capacity to recognize and respond to hypoglycemic symptoms (American Diabetes Association, 2006). The goal of therapy is a low-density lipoprotein (LDL) value <100 mg/dL (American Diabetes Association, 2006). Children with diabetes differ from adults in many ways, including insulin sensitivity related to sexual maturity, physical growth, ability to provide self-care, vulnerability to hypoglycemia, differing family dynamics, developmental stages, and physiological differences (American Diabetes Association, 2006). It is important to work with the family and school system to plan for emergencies such as low or high blood glucose levels.
	Children with type 2 diabetes	Distinction between type 1 and type 2 diabetes in children can be difficult because autoantigens and ketosis may be present in a substantial number of patients with otherwise straightforward type 2 diabetes, including obesity and acanthosis nigricans (American Diabetes Association, 2006). Children with type 2 diabetes are usually overweight or obese and present with glycosuria with or without ketonuria, absent or mild polyuria and polydipsia, and little or no weight loss. Up to 33% have ketonuria at diagnosis, and some may have ketoacidosis without any associated stress, other illness, or infection.

(continued)

TABLE 9-4 **Potential Complications of Diabetes** ***(continued)***

Degree of Complication	Complication	Description
		Because DKA is associated with high morbidity and mortality in children and cerebral edema can occur, early consultation and referral to pediatric or adolescent endocrinologists is important.
	Preconception	All women with diabetes and childbearing potential should be educated about the need for good glucose control before pregnancy, the need for family planning, and need for early treatment for diabetic retinopathy, nephropathy, neuropathy, and cardiovascular disease (CVD) (American Diabetes Association, 2006). A1c levels should be normal or as close to normal as possible (<1% above the upper limits of normal) in an individual patient before conception is attempted (American Diabetes Association, 2006).
	Pregnancy	Infant mortality rates are approximately twice as high for babies born to women with uncontrolled diabetes compared with babies born to women without diabetes. To reduce the risk of fetal malformations and maternal or fetal complications, pregnant women and women planning to become pregnant require excellent blood glucose control. These women need to be seen frequently by a multidisciplinary team. Specialized laboratory and diagnostic tests may be needed; these women must be trained in self-monitoring of blood glucose (SMBG). Nutrition recommendations for women with preexisting diabetes must be based on a thorough assessment. Monitoring blood glucose levels, blood or urine ketones, appetite, and weight gain is needed to develop an individualized nutrition prescription and to make adjustments to the meal plan. Plasma glucose should be maintained at 65–100 mg/dL before meals and in fasting; 110–135 mg/dL 1 hour after meals; and <120 mg/dL 2 hours after meals. Use an extra 300 kcal daily during the second and third trimester. Needs are: 1 g/kg/d or an additional 25 g/d of protein; a minimum of 175 g/d of CHO, and 600 μg folic acid (Franz et al, 2002). Added iron and calcium may also be required depending on the usual and current dietary intake patterns. For gestational diabetes, see the entry later in this chapter.
	Lactation	Extra kilocalories, protein, calcium, and folic acid will be needed. Monitoring of blood glucose is recommended, but hypoglycemia should be avoided. Lactation may have a positive effect on glycemia in women with diabetes (Reader and Franz, 2004). Breastfeeding lowers blood glucose and may require women to eat a CHO-containing snack either before or during breastfeeding; overall, an extra 330–400 kcal meets the needs of most lactating mothers (Reader and Franz, 2004).
	Older adults	There is little research on the aging individual who has diabetes, and therefore, typical signs such as unexplained weight loss should be viewed as a symptom of a problem (Franz et al, 2002). Diabetes is an important health condition for the aging population; at least 20% of patients over the age of 65 years have diabetes, and these patients tend to have higher rates of premature death, functional disability, and coexisting illnesses such as hypertension, coronary heart disease (CHD), and stroke than those without diabetes (American Diabetes Association, 2006). New-onset diabetes in adults over the age of 50 may signal underlying pancreatic cancer, which should be investigated. Strict diets in long-term care are not warranted and may lead to dehydration and malnutrition; specialized diabetic diets are not required, and a balanced diet with consistent timing of CHO is to be recommended (Franz et al, 2002). Modify medications, rather than diet, as needed. Lower hypertension gradually; implement the DASH diet whenever possible. A multivitamin-mineral supplement may be beneficial for this population. Diabetes educators and health care providers should consider involving the entire family in the management of older patients with type 2 diabetes (Wen et al, 2004).
CHRONIC	**General guidance**	Achieve and maintain normal blood glucose (BG) and lipids. Intensive therapy (IT) helps reduce onset or progression of vascular problems. Maintain hemoglobin A1c levels <7%. Monitor: A1c level of 5 = BG 100 A1c level of 6 = BG 135 A1c level of 7 = BG 170 A1c level of 8 = BG 205 A1c level of 9 = BG 240 A1c level of 10 = BG 275 A1c level of 11 = BG 310

(continued)

TABLE 9-4 Potential Complications of Diabetes *(continued)*

Degree of Complication	Complication	Description
	Microvascular	Microvascular complications include retinopathy and ocular abnormalities, nephropathy, neuropathy (sensory or motor conditions, which may lead to ulceration or even limb amputation, orthostatic hypotension, intractable nausea and vomiting, and diabetic gastroenteropathy), diabetic cystopathy, and chronic diarrhea.
	Retinopathy	Retinopathy from diabetes accounts for 12,000–24,000 cases of blindness each year. Optimal glycemic and blood pressure control can substantially reduce the risk and progression of diabetic retinopathy (American Diabetes Association, 2006). In the presence of proliferative diabetic retinopathy (PDR) or severe nonproliferative diabetic retinopathy (NPDR), vigorous aerobic or resistance exercise may be contraindicated because of the risk of triggering vitreous hemorrhage or retinal detachment (American Diabetes Association, 2006). Pregnancy in type 1 diabetic patients may aggravate retinopathy; laser photocoagulation surgery can minimize this risk (American Diabetes Association, 2006).
	Microalbuminuria and nephropathy	Nephropathy is preceded by microalbuminuria for several years. Early signs of nephropathy include hyperfiltration, renal hypertrophy, and microalbuminuria (loss of 30–300 μg/mg creatinine in the urine); protein losses at a rate of >300 μg/mg creatinine may indicate advancement toward chronic kidney disease (CKD). To reduce the risk and/or slow the progression of nephropathy, optimize glucose and blood pressure control (American Diabetes Association, 2006). The onset of end-stage renal disease is about 5 years after onset of microalbuminuria. For diabetic nephropathy, liberalize CHO intake and control insulin levels accordingly. There is some evidence that controlled protein intake will slow down progression of nephropathy. Adults need <0.8–1 g protein/kg daily (American Diabetes Association, 2006). Protein restriction is of benefit in slowing the progression of albuminuria, glomerular filtration rate (GFR) decline, and occurrence of end-stage renal disease (ESRD); protein restriction should be considered, particularly in patients whose nephropathy seems to be progressing despite optimal glucose and blood pressure control and use of angiotensin-converting enzyme (ACE) inhibitors and/or angiotensin receptor blockers (ARBs) (American Diabetes Association, 2006). Phosphorus should be controlled at 8–12 mg/kg/d; some people may need phosphate binders and calcium supplements. Diabetes is now the leading cause of CKD, especially among blacks, Mexican Americans, and Native Americans. Diabetic nephropathy occurs in 20–40% of patients with diabetes and is the single leading cause of ESRD (American Diabetes Association, 2006). Creatinine and GFR should be assessed annually in this population. Microalbuminuria (30–299 mg/24 h) and macroalbuminuria ($\geq$300 mg/24 h) should be carefully monitored (American Diabetes Association, 2006). Intensive diabetes management with the goal of achieving near normoglycemia has been shown in large prospective randomized studies to delay the onset of microalbuminuria and the progression of micro- to macroalbuminuria in patients with type 1 and type 2 diabetes (American Diabetes Association, 2006). Refer to a physician experienced in the care of diabetic renal disease when the estimated GFR has fallen to <60 mL/min or if difficulties occur in the management of hypertension or hyperkalemia (American Diabetes Association, 2006). While physical activity can acutely increase urinary protein excretion, there is no evidence that vigorous exercise increases the rate of progression of diabetic kidney disease (American Diabetes Association, 2006). ACE inhibitors are almost always prescribed to decrease progression.
	Neuropathy	About 70% of persons who have diabetes have some degree of neuropathy, including impaired sensation in the hands and feet, slowed digestion, or carpal tunnel syndrome. Autonomic neuropathy can decrease cardiac responsiveness to exercise, causing postural hypotension, impaired thermoregulation, impaired skin blood flow and sweating, impaired night vision, impaired thirst, risk of dehydration, and gastroparesis with unpredictable food delivery (American Diabetes Association, 2006). Autonomic neuropathy is strongly associated with CVD in people with diabetes; cardiac investigation before beginning physical activity is important (American Diabetes Association, 2006). Neuropathy may be delayed with careful blood glucose management. Lower extremity amputations are painful and disabling; prevention is desirable in all cases. Neuropathy is more common in obese patients; weight loss may be beneficial. Decreased pain sensation in the extremities may result in increased risk of skin breakdown and infection and of joint destruction; it may be best to encourage non–weight-bearing activities such as swimming, bicycling, or arm exercises (American Diabetes Association, 2006).

(continued)

TABLE 9-4 Potential Complications of Diabetes *(continued)*

Degree of Complication	Complication	Description
		Diabetic autonomic neuropathy is associated with recurrent genitourinary tract disturbances or bladder and/or sexual dysfunction; amputation and foot ulceration are the most common consequences of diabetic neuropathy and the major causes of morbidity and disability in people with diabetes (American Diabetes Association, 2006). Major clinical manifestations of cardiac neuropathy in diabetes include resting tachycardia, exercise intolerance, orthostatic hypotension, constipation, gastroparesis, erectile dysfunction, sudomotor dysfunction, impaired neurovascular function, "brittle diabetes," and hypoglycemic autonomic failure (American Diabetes Association, 2006). Gastrointestinal (GI) disturbances (esophageal enteropathy, gastroparesis, constipation, diarrhea, and fecal incontinence) are common, and any section of the GI tract may be affected; gastroparesis should be suspected in individuals with erratic glucose control (American Diabetes Association, 2006).
	Macrovascular Coronary artery disease and arterial vascular disease	CVD is a major cause of mortality and also a major contributor to morbidity in diabetics; about 80% of people who have diabetes die of CVD. Type 2 diabetes is an independent risk factor for macrovascular disease (American Diabetes Association, 2006). Other risk factors include insulin resistance, hyperglycemia, hypertension, dyslipidemia, and smoking. Smoking is related to the premature development of microvascular complications of diabetes and may have a role in the development of type 2 diabetes (American Diabetes Association, 2006). Advise all patients not to smoke; include smoking cessation counseling and other forms of treatment as a routine component of diabetes care (American Diabetes Association, 2006).
	Dyslipidemia	Lifestyle modification focusing on the reduction of saturated fat and cholesterol intake, weight loss (if indicated), and increased physical activity has been shown to improve the lipid profile in patients with diabetes (American Diabetes Association, 2006). Guidelines promote LDL cholesterol levels of <100 mg/dL as optimal for all patients and lowering of triglyceride levels when >150 mg/dL. Statins may be helpful. Elevate high-density lipoprotein (HDL) to levels >40 mg/dL. If HDL is <40 mg/dL and LDL is between 100 and 129 mg/dL, a fibric acid derivative or niacin might be used. Niacin is the most effective drug for raising HDL but can significantly increase blood glucose at high doses (American Diabetes Association, 2006). Use aspirin therapy (75–162 mg/d) as a secondary prevention strategy in those with diabetes with a history of CVD (American Diabetes Association, 2006). Nutrition intervention should be tailored according to each patient's age, type of diabetes, pharmacological treatment, lipid levels, and other medical conditions and should focus on the reduction of saturated fat, cholesterol, and trans fat intake (American Diabetes Association, 2006). Monitoring of homocysteine levels and related actions should be taken. Adequate insulin therapy often returns lipids to normal in type 1 diabetes (Franz et al, 2002). Elevated levels in type 2 diabetes require use of rigorous management guidelines; limit saturated fat to 7–10% of total calories. The rate of heart disease is about 2–4 times higher in adults who have diabetes; it is the leading cause of diabetes-related deaths. Since people with diabetes tend to have high triglyceride and low HDL levels, omega-3 fatty acids from DHA and EPA (fish and marine oils) can help. See entries for coronary heart disease.
	Hypertension	Hypertension is common in diabetics. Over 70% of adults with diabetes also have hypertension; this means that 2.5 million people have both. Control of hypertension in diabetes has been linked to reduction in the progression of both microvascular and macrovascular disease. In type 1 diabetes, hypertension is often the result of underlying nephropathy, whereas in type 2 diabetes, it may be present as part of the metabolic syndrome (American Diabetes Association, 2006). Patients with hypertension (systolic blood pressure ≥140 mm Hg or diastolic blood pressure ≥90 mm Hg) should receive drug therapy in addition to lifestyle and behavioral therapy (American Diabetes Association, 2006). Blood pressure should be measured at every routine diabetes visit; patients with diabetes should be treated to reach a systolic blood pressure <130 mm Hg and a diastolic blood pressure <80 mm Hg (American Diabetes Association, 2006). In patients with type 1 diabetes with hypertension and any degree of albuminuria, ACE inhibitors have been shown to delay the progression of nephropathy; with type 2 diabetes, hypertension, and microalbuminuria, ACE inhibitors and ARBs have been shown to delay the progression to macroalbuminuria (American Diabetes Association, 2006).

(continued)

TABLE 9-4 Potential Complications of Diabetes *(continued)*

Degree of Complication	Complication	Description
		Modest weight loss is helpful; prevent hypokalemia, which can blunt insulin release; control glucose; limit alcohol and smoking; and add exercise. Use of the DASH diet is often effective because it increases intake of calcium, magnesium, and potassium while lowering alcohol and excess weight (Franz et al, 2002).
	Hypertension in pregnancy	Pregnancy-induced hypertension is 2–4 times more common in women with type 1 diabetes than in the general population.
		In pregnant patients with diabetes and chronic hypertension, blood pressure target goals of 110–129/65–79 mm Hg are suggested; avoid lower blood pressure because fetal growth may be impaired (American Diabetes Association, 2006). ACE inhibitors and ARBs are contraindicated during pregnancy (American Diabetes Association, 2006). Screen for microalbuminuria because this condition in the absence of urinary tract infection is a strong predictor of preeclampsia (American Diabetes Association, 2006).
	Stroke	Stroke risk is 2–4 times higher among persons with diabetes, and high blood pressure should be carefully controlled.
Other Complications	**Catabolic illness**	Catabolic illness (such as HIV infection, AIDS, or cancer) changes body compartments, with increased extracellular fluid and shrinkage of body fat and body cell mass (Franz et al, 2002). Monitor unexplained weight losses carefully, especially 10% or more of usual weight.
		Standard tube feedings are usually well tolerated in persons with diabetes (50% CHO or lower); monitor fluid status, weight, plasma glucose and electrolytes, and acid–base balance (Franz et al, 2002). Overfeeding is to be avoided; start with 25–35 kcal/kg of body weight. Protein needs may be 1 g/kg up to 1.5 g/kg in stressed individuals, and pressure ulcers may require a higher level of protein and calories than normal for healing; addition of insulin may be needed at this time. Oral glucose-lowering medications need to be adjusted to achieve adequate control of glycemia.

Additional data from: American Diabetes Association, 2006; Centers for Disease Control and Prevention, 2005; and Franz and Wheeler, 2003.

TABLE 9-5 Evidence for Nutrient Guidelines in Diabetes

Nutrient	Grade of Evidence	Guideline
Carbohydrate	**A**	Include whole grains, fruits, vegetables, and low-fat milk for their essential nutrients in a healthy diet. Control the total amount of carbohydrate; the source or type is less important. Sucrose-containing foods do not have to be excluded but should be substituted for other carbohydrate-containing foods. Nonnutritive sweeteners are safe when consumed within acceptable daily intakes established by the Food and Drug Administration (FDA).
		2006 Guidelines recommend 45–65% intake from CHO.
Protein	**B**	Ingested protein does not increase plasma glucose concentration in persons with controlled diabetes.
		2006 Guidelines recommend 10–35% intake from protein.
Fat	A	Decreasing intake of saturated fats to <10% of total fat intake is important, and when low-density lipoprotein (LDL) cholesterol levels are >100 mg/dL, lower even further to <7%. Dietary cholesterol intake should be <300 mg/d, or lower in those persons whose LDL levels are elevated.
		2006 Guidelines recommend 20–35% intake from fat.
Micronutrients	B	There is no clear evidence of benefit from supplements or antioxidants in individuals who have no underlying deficiencies. Folate is needed for prevention of birth defects, and calcium is needed for prevention of osteoporosis.
Alcohol	B	If individuals choose to drink, intake should be the same as for persons who do not have diabetes. One drink for women and two for men is the recommended limit daily. Persons who take insulin or insulin secretagogues should consume alcohol with food.

Key: "A" grade is indicated where there is considerable evidence; "B" grade indicates intermediate support.
Derived from: American Diabetes Association grading system. *Diabetes Care* 25:550, 2002; American Diabetes Association, Standards of Medical Care in Diabetes–2006. *Diabetes Care* 29:4S, 2006.

Medical nutrition therapy provided by registered dietitians to patients with type 1 and type 2 diabetes has been shown to improve glycemic outcomes (Pastors et al, 2003). The Lewin Group documented a 9.5% reduction in hospital utilization and 23.5% reduction in physician visits when a specialized MNT was provided to persons with diabetes mellitus (Johnson, 1999).

Community-based education that incorporates Social Cognitive Theory and Stages of Change Theory, with three group sessions focused on meal planning with cooking demonstrations, is effective; the education successfully promotes use of herbs in place of salt, use of olive or canola oils, use of artificial sweeteners in baking, knowledge of diabetes and nutrition, and self-efficacy (Chapman-Novakofski and Karduck, 2005). Key concepts in setting glycemic goals with patients include the following:

- A1c is the primary target for glycemic control.
- Goals should be individualized.
- Certain populations (children, pregnant women, and elderly) require special considerations.
- More stringent glycemic goals (i.e., a usual A1c, <6%) may further reduce complications at the cost of increased risk of hypoglycemia.
- Less intensive glycemic goals may be indicated in patients with severe or frequent hypoglycemia.
- Postprandial glucose may be targeted if A1c goals are not met despite reaching preprandial glucose goals.

The specific guidelines are as follows:

1. **Glucose control**
   a. Research studies in the United States and abroad have found that improved glycemic control benefits people with either type 1 or type 2 diabetes. In general, for every 1% reduction in results of A1c blood tests (e.g., from 8.0% to 7.0%), the risk of developing microvascular diabetic complications (eye, kidney, and nerve disease) is reduced by 40%. Glucose goals:

Glycemic Control (Adults)

A1c	<7.0%
Preprandial capillary plasma glucose	90–130 mg/dL (5.0–7.2 mmol/L)
Peak postprandial capillary plasma glucose	<180 mg/dL (<10.0 mmol/L); 1–2 hours after beginning of meal

Plasma Blood Glucose and A1c Goals for Type 1 Diabetes by Age Group

	Plasma Blood Glucose Goal Range (mg/dL)			
Values by Age (years)	**Before Meals**	**Bedtime/ Overnight**	**A1c**	**Rationale**
Toddlers and preschoolers (0–6)	100–180	110–200	<8.5% (but >7.5%)	High risk and vulnerability to hypoglycemia
School age (6–12)	90–180	100–180	<8%	Risks of hypoglycemia and relatively low risk of complications prior to puberty
Adolescents and young adults (13–19)	90–130	90–150	<7%	Risk of severe hypoglycemia; developmental and psychological issues; a lower goal (<7.0%) is reasonable if it can be achieved without excessive hypoglycemia

Key concepts in setting glycemic goals:

- Goals should be individualized, and lower goals may be reasonable based on benefit-risk assessment.
- Blood glucose goals should be higher than those listed above in children with frequent hypoglycemia or hypoglycemia unawareness.
- Postprandial blood glucose values should be measured when there is a disparity between preprandial blood glucose values and A1c levels.

2. **Blood pressure control**
   a. Blood pressure control can reduce cardiovascular disease (heart disease and stroke) by approximately 33–50% and can reduce microvascular disease (eye, kidney, and nerve disease) by approximately 33%.
   b. In general, for every 10-mm Hg reduction in systolic blood pressure, the risk for any complication related to diabetes is reduced by 12%.
   c. Restriction of sodium to 2400 mg/d or possibly, for some, to 2000 mg/d assists in the control of hypertension (Franz and Wheeler, 2003).
   d. Goal: blood pressure <130/80 mm Hg.
3. **Control of blood lipids**
   a. Improved control of cholesterol or blood lipids (for example, high-density lipoprotein [HDL], low-density lipoprotein [LDL], and triglycerides) can reduce cardiovascular complications by 20–50%.
   b. Lipid Goals:

Lipids	Current NCEP/ATP III guidelines suggest that in patients with triglycerides ≥200 mg/dL, the "non-HDL cholesterol" (total cholesterol minus HDL) should be used. The goal is ≤130 mg/dL.
LDL	<100 mg/dL (<2.6 mmol/L)
Triglycerides	<150 mg/dL (<1.7 mmol/L)
HDL	>40 mg/dL (>1.1 mmol/L); 10% higher in women

4. Preventive care practices for eyes and feet

a. Detecting and treating diabetic eye disease with laser therapy can reduce the development of severe vision loss by an estimated 50–60%.

b. Comprehensive foot care programs can reduce amputation rates by 45–85%.

5. Preventive care for kidneys

a. Detecting and treating early diabetic kidney disease by lowering blood pressure can reduce the decline in kidney function by 30–70%. Treatment with angiotensin-converting enzyme (ACE) inhibitors and angiotensin receptor blockers (ARBs) is more effective in reducing the decline in kidney function than other blood pressure–lowering drugs.

b. With protein intakes greater than 20% of energy intake, there is an association with increased albumin excretion rate. Once albuminuria is present, reduction of protein to 0.8–1.0 g/kg/d with microalbuminuria and to 0.8 g/kg/d with macroalbuminuria is recommended (Franz and Wheeler, 2003).

c. In macroalbuminuria, there may be additional benefits in lowering phosphorus intake to 500–1000 mg/d (Franz and Wheeler, 2003).

d. There is no strong evidence to suggest benefit from vegetable or plant proteins over animal protein, but there is evidence for benefit on renal function, glucose, lipids, and blood pressure from weight-maintaining diets meeting guidelines for a healthy diet (Franz and Wheeler, 2003).

CITED REFERENCES

Aggarwal BB, Shishodia S. Suppression of the nuclear factor-kappaB activation pathway by spice-derived phytochemicals: reasoning for seasoning. *Ann N Y Acad Sci.* 1030:434, 2004.

American Diabetes Association. Standards of Medical Care in Diabetes–2006. *Diabetes Care* 29:4S, 2006.

Centers for Disease Control and Prevention (CDC). National diabetes fact sheet. Accessed April 24, 2005 at http://www.cdc.gov/diabetes/pubs/general.htm#impaired.

Chapman-Novakofski K, Karduck J. Improvement in knowledge, social cognitive theory variables, and movement through stages of change after a community-based diabetes education program. *J Am Diet Assoc.* 105:1613, 2005.

Daly A, et al. The new credential: advanced diabetes management. *J Am Diet Assoc.* 101:940, 2001.

Franz MJ, Wheeler ML. Nutrition therapy for diabetic nephropathy. *Curr Diab Rep.* 3:412, 2003.

Franz MJ, et al. American Diabetes Association Position Statement: evidence-based nutrition principles and recommendations for the treatment and prevention of diabetes and related conditions. *J Am Diet Assoc.* 102:109, 2002.

Johnson R. The Lewin Group Study: what does it tell us, and why does it matter? *J Am Diet Assoc.* 99:426, 1999.

Kulkarni K, et al. American Dietetic Association: standards of practice and standards of professional performance for registered dietitians (generalist, specialty and advanced) in diabetes care. *J Am Diet Assoc.* 105:819, 2005.

Pastors JG, et al. How effective is medical nutrition therapy in diabetes care? *J Am Diet Assoc.* 103:108, 2003.

Reader D, Franz MJ. Lactation, diabetes, and nutrition recommendations. *Curr Diab Rep.* 4370, 2004.

Wen LK, et al. Family support, diet, and exercise among older Mexican Americans with type 2 diabetes. *Diabetes Educ.* 30:980, 2004.

For More Information

- American Association of Diabetes Educators
  http://www.aadenet.org/
- American Diabetes Association
  http://www.diabetes.org/
- American Diabetes Association Youth Zone
  http://www.diabetes.org/youthzone/youth-zone.jsp
- American Dietetic Association–Diabetes Protocols
  http://www.eatright.org/cps/rde/xchg/ada/hs.xsl/index.html
- Calorie and Nutrient Information
  http://www.calorieking.com
- Canadian Diabetes Association
  http://www.diabetes.ca/
- Centers for Disease Control and Prevention (CDC) Diabetes Public Health Resources
  http://www.cdc.gov/diabetes/index.htm
- CDC Division of Diabetes
  http://www.cdc.gov/diabetes
  http://www.cdc.gov/diabetes/statistics/maps/map1.htm
- Centers for Medicare and Medicaid Services Diabetes Guidelines
  http://www.cms.hhs.gov/DiabetesScreening/
- Children with Diabetes
  http://www.childrenwithdiabetes.com
- Diabetes Care and Dietetic Practice Group
  http://www.dce.org/
- Diabetic Gourmet Magazine
  http://diabeticgourmet.com/dgarchiv2.shtml
- Diabetes Information
  http://www.diabetes123.com
- Diabetes Monitoring
  http://www.diabetesmonitor.com
- Diabetes Research Institute Foundation
  http://www.drinet.org/
- Functional Foods and Nutraceuticals in Endocrinology
  http://www.aace.com/clin/guidelines/Nutraceuticals2003.pdf
- International Diabetes Federation
  http://www.idf.org
- Joslin Diabetes Center, Boston, MA
  http://www.joslin.org/
- Juvenile Diabetes Research Foundation International
  http://www.jdrf.org
- Low Literacy Information
  http://www.learningaboutdiabetes.com
- National Diabetes Education Program
  http://www.ndep.nih.gov/
- National Institute of Diabetes and Digestive and Kidney Diseases (NIDDK)
  http://diabetes.niddk.nih.gov/
- Park Nicollet–International Diabetes Center
  http://www.Parknicollet.com/diabetes

- Professional Resources
  http://www.diabetes.org/for-health-professionals-and-scientists/resources.jsp
- School Guidelines
  http://www.ndep.nih.gov/diabetes/pubs/Youth_NDEPSchoolGuide.pdf
- Taking Control of Your Diabetes
  http://www.tcoyd.org
- Upskilling Credentials
  CDE Credential: http://www.dce.org/professional/upskilling1.htm
  BC-ADM Credential: http://www.dce.org/professional/upskilling1.htm
- Veterans Administration Diabetes Program
  http://www1.va.gov/health/diabetes/

DIABETES MELLITUS, COMPLICATIONS, AND RELATED CONDITIONS

TYPE 1 DIABETES MELLITUS

NUTRITIONAL ACUITY RANKING: LEVEL 4

DEFINITIONS AND BACKGROUND

Type 1 diabetes mellitus (T1DM) is absolute insulin deficiency with total failure to produce insulin. Type 1 involves autoimmune destruction of the pancreatic beta-cells (the islets of Langerhans). It usually starts in children or young adults but can arise at any age. The extent of beta-cell damage is more severe in patients diagnosed with type 1 diabetes before puberty. Type 1 accounts for 10% of all cases of diabetes mellitus.

Previously used terms include "type I," "insulin-dependent diabetes mellitus (IDDM)," "juvenile," "brittle," or "ketosis-prone" diabetes. Onset often follows viral infection such as mumps. Signs and symptoms of diabetes include polyuria (frequent urination, including frequent bedwetting in otherwise trained children), polydipsia (excessive thirst), polyphagia (extreme hunger), weakness, fatigue, irritability, and sudden weight loss.

Glucose enters cells by way of two different types of membrane-associated carrier proteins, the Na+-coupled glucose transporters (SGLT) and glucose transporter facilitators, GLUT (Scheepers et al, 2004). For diagnosis of diabetes, a fasting plasma glucose (FPG) test or an oral glucose tolerance test (OGTT) can be used to identify either prediabetes or diabetes. The FPG is the preferred method. With this test, a fasting blood glucose level of 100–125 mg/dL represents prediabetes, and a level of 126 mg/dL or higher is considered to be diabetes. With the OGTT, blood glucose is measured after fasting and 2 hours after drinking a glucose beverage; results between 140 and 199 mg/dL are considered to be indicative of prediabetes, and a level of 200 mg/dL represents diabetes. Hemoglobin A1c test (HbA1c) is not recommended for diagnosis; finger-prick tests are also not valid.

Serious complications begin earlier than previously thought. Glucose control really matters, as proven by the results of the Diabetes Control and Complications Trial (DCCT) and other trials. More than 65% of people with diabetes die from heart disease or stroke (American Diabetes Association, 2005). Diabetes is the chief cause of blindness, renal failure, and amputations and is a leading cause of birth defects.

Intensive therapy to achieve near-normal glucose levels results in lower onset and progression of complications. Caution is needed to prevent hypoglycemia, especially in the very young (<6 years old) and those with vision loss or kidney disease.

Protein and nutrient metabolism are affected by insulin availability. The long-term effects of diets high in protein and low in carbohydrate (CHO) are unknown at this time (Franz et al, 2002). Vitamin and mineral intakes are being studied for their various impacts on blood glucose levels. In addition, it is important to note that antioxidant foods and spices may be helpful in lowering blood glucose levels; fenugreek is one example that is under study (Shekelle et al, 2005).

Medical costs for patients with diabetes account for a significant percentage of all health care costs. National Standards for Diabetes Self-Management have been written to support a team approach to patient care; they include the registered dietitian (RD) as an essential team member. Ongoing nutrition self-management education includes assessment, care plans, treatment goals, desired outcomes, and monitoring metabolic parameters such as blood glucose, lipids, A1c, and related lab values. The use of evidence-based medical nutrition therapy (MNT) leads to effective lifestyle changes that help to manage diabetes effectively (Franz, 2004). See Table 9-5.

A program called Dose Adjustment for Normal Eating (DAFNE) was implemented in Great Britain. Persons with type 1 diabetes were taught by dietitians to adjust their insulin injections based on the amount of carbohydrate they planned to eat, instead of organizing their meals around their prescribed insulin injections. At 6 months, A1c levels were 1 unit lower (1%) compared with persons who continued the traditional treatment program. Furthermore, quality of life was also significantly improved with no increased incidence of severe hypoglycemia, weight gain, or changes in lipids (DAFNE Training Group, 2002).

The SEARCH for Diabetes in Youth is a multicenter study of diabetes in youth aged 10–22 years. In this study, only 6.5% of the cohort met American Diabetes Association recommendations of <10% of energy from saturated fat; less than 50% met recommendations for total fat, vitamin E, fiber, fruits, vegetables, and grains, although a majority met

TABLE 9-6 American Dietetic Association: Recommended Medical Nutrition Therapy Visits for Type 1 Diabetes

Encounter	Length of Contact	Time between Encounters
1	60–90 minutes	2–4 weeks
2, 3	30–45 minutes	2–4 weeks
4, 5	30–45 minutes	6–12 months
6, 7, 8	30–45 minutes	As indicated by clinical data and/or changes in medication

From: National Guideline Clearinghouse. Nutrition practice guidelines for type 1 and type 2 diabetes mellitus. Accessed April 24, 2005 at http://guidelines.gov/summary/summary.aspx?doc_id=3296&nbr=2522.

recommendations for vitamin C, calcium, and iron (Mayer-Davis et al, 2006).

Multidisciplinary team interventions are suggested to help improve patients' A1c levels and to reduce complications, hospital readmissions, and hospital stays. The American Dietetic Association recommends a specific number of MNT visits to promote the desired outcome (see Table 9-6). Use of technology to track quarterly weight and lab values is an effective way to help patients with their self-management goals (Chima et al, 2005).

INTERVENTION: OBJECTIVES

- Medical nutrition intervention in patients with diabetes should address the metabolic abnormalities of glucose, lipids, and blood pressure (Kulkarni, 2006).
- Meet the specific needs of the patient; modify drug therapy to enhance outcomes and quality of life. Early referral for lifestyle changes and advice will yield the most benefit (Kulkarni, 2006).
- Regularly evaluate food/nutrition history, physical exercise, and activity patterns. Control weight gain.
- Develop food/meal planning with client; share plan with medical team so an insulin regimen can be integrated into the client's usual lifestyle. In hospital settings, avoid use of specific and restrictive diets (Schafer et al, 2004). People with diabetes should receive individualized MNT as needed to achieve treatment goals, preferably provided by a registered dietitian familiar with the components of diabetes MNT (American Diabetes Association, 2006).
- Promote lifestyle changes according to client readiness, educational, and skill level. The primary approach for weight loss (where needed) is therapeutic lifestyle change, which includes a moderate decrease in energy balance (500–1000 kcal/d) for a slow but progressive weight loss of 1–2 lb/wk (American Diabetes Association, 2006).
- Plan meal plan, exercise, and medication to achieve blood glucose and lipid goals. For example, decrease intake of trans fatty acids, and saturated fat intake should be <7% of total calories (American Diabetes Association 2006).
- Prevent early onset of complications by controlling glucose, lipids, and blood pressure. If there are complications, prevent serious consequences as much as possible (such as amputation, blindness, and renal failure).
- Both the amount (grams) of carbohydrate as well as the type of carbohydrate in a food influence blood glucose level; monitoring total grams of carbohydrate, whether by use of exchanges or carbohydrate counting, remains a key strategy in achieving glycemic control (American Diabetes Association, 2006).
- Teach individuals how to use carbohydrate counting and how to adjust insulin doses based on planned carbohydrate intake. For example, active young women may need 2500 kcal, equal to 312 g CHO (or about 75–90 g/meal). A young man who needs 3000 kcal per day would need 375 g/d CHO, spaced out between meals and snacks.
- Choose a variety of foods, including an average of 5 servings of fruits and vegetables, 6 servings of grains (3 whole grain), and 2 servings of low-fat dairy. Foods in the meat and fat groups do not directly affect blood glucose. Make heart healthy choices for optimal health.
- Promote self-monitoring of blood glucose between 4 and 7 times per day and more often during illness.

INTERVENTION: FOOD AND NUTRITION

- A meal plan based on the individual's usual food intake should be used as the basis for integrating insulin therapy into the usual eating and exercise patterns (American Diabetes Association, 2006). Individuals using insulin should eat at consistent times synchronized with the time-action of the insulin preparation used, monitor their blood glucose levels, and determine their required insulin doses for the amount of food usually eaten. Intensified insulin therapy, including multiple daily injections, continuous subcutaneous insulin infusion with an insulin pump, and rapid-acting insulin, allows for more flexibility in the timing of meals and snacks, as well as in the amount of food eaten.
- Discourage meal skipping.
- Determine appropriate energy intake for age, with pregnant and growing individuals receiving more: sedentary, 25 kcal/kg; normal, 30 kcal/kg; undernourished or active, 45–50 kcal/kg. Reassess as activity changes.
- Monounsaturated fatty acids and carbohydrates combined should provide 60–70% of daily energy intake, with individual flexibility in the respective proportions, whereas intake of saturated fats is limited to <10% of energy intake (Kelley, 2003). Ketosis can be prevented by including at least 45% kcal as carbohydrate every day. Use a plan that includes CHO at 45–65% of total energy intake each day (American Diabetes Association, 2006).
- Apply **carbohydrate** counting, dietary guidelines, or MyPyramid food guidance principles. With CHO counting, focus on carbohydrates more than total energy or source of carbohydrate (Franz et al, 2002). Provide consistent carbohydrate with each meal and snack for those on set doses of insulin. Determine insulin to carbohydrate ratios for each individual. One CHO unit equals 15 g CHO (standard starch, fruit, sweet, or milk servings are based on 15 g CHO).

- Each of the following portions is one carbohydrate choice (15 g CHO):
  - Grains, breads, cereals: 1 oz bread (1 slice bread, 1/4 large bagel, 6″ tortilla); 1/2 cup cooked dried beans; 1/3 cup pasta or rice; 1 cup soup; 3/4 cup cold cereal; 1/2 cup cooked cereal.
  - Milk and yogurt: 1 cup milk; 2/3 cup unsweetened yogurt (6 oz) or sweetened with noncaloric sweetener.
  - Fruits: 1 small fresh fruit; 1/2 cup fruit; 1 cup melon or berries; 1/2 cup fruit juice; 1/4 cup dried fruit.
  - Sweets and snack foods: 3/4 oz snack food (pretzels, chips, 4–6 crackers); 1 oz sweet snack (2 small sandwich cookies, 5 vanilla wafers); 1 tbsp sugar or honey; 1/2 cup ice cream.
  - Vegetables: 1/2 cup potato, peas, or corn; 3 cups raw vegetables; 1 1/2 cups cooked vegetables; small portions of nonstarchy vegetables.
- Most women need about 3–4 carbohydrate choices (45–60 g CHO) at each meal. Men generally need about 4–5 carbohydrate choices (60–75 g CHO) at each meal. With snacks, use of 1–2 carbohydrate choices (15–30 g CHO) is reasonable. Body size and activity level will determine the number of choices needed.
- The use of the glycemic index/glycemic load may provide an additional benefit over that observed when total carbohydrate is considered alone (American Diabetes Association, 2006).
- Include plenty of fiber from rice, beans, vegetables, barley, oat bran, fruits, and vegetables. Whole grains are good sources of vitamin E, fiber, and magnesium.
- Maintain protein intake at 15–20% of daily energy intake if renal function is normal. To reduce the risk of nephropathy, protein intake should be limited to the recommended dietary allowance (0.8 g/kg is typical) in those adults with any degree of chronic kidney disease (American Diabetes Association, 2006). If there is microalbuminuria, a more controlled protein intake may be required.
- Maintain diet at 25–35% kcals from total fat (American Diabetes Association, 2006). Diet should provide no more than 7–10% of fat as saturated form; and trans fatty acids should be limited. This may include cutting down or eliminating fried and creamed foods. Include omega-3 fatty acids (as from salmon, mackerel, tuna, walnuts, and canola oil) for control of blood lipids and reduced inflammatory processes. Finally, a high–monounsaturated fat diet seems to have a favorable effect on fasting lipoprotein profile in people with diabetes (Strychar et al, 2003).
- For minerals, assess for adequacy of intake. Routine supplementation is not advised at this time (Franz et al, 2002). Replenish potassium and magnesium, if needed. Adequate calcium is important: 500 mg in 1–3 year olds, 800 mg in 4–8 year olds, 1300 mg in 9–18 year olds, and 1000 mg in adults should be attained daily. Sodium intake should be limited to 2400 mg daily or less.
- For vitamins, assess for adequate intake. Routine supplementation with antioxidants, such as vitamins E and C and beta-carotene, is not advised because of lack of evidence of efficacy and concern related to long-term safety (American Diabetes Association, 2006; Franz et al, 2002). Folate is important in women of childbearing ages (Franz et al, 2002); acquire 400 μg prepregnancy and 600 μg during pregnancy.
- If adults with diabetes choose to use alcohol, daily intake should be limited to a moderate amount (1 drink per day or less for adult women and 2 drinks per day or less for adult men); 1 drink is defined as 12 oz beer, 5 oz wine, or 1.5 oz distilled spirits (American Diabetes Association, 2006). To avoid hypoglycemia, alcohol should be consumed with a carbohydrate-containing food. Abstention is recommended for pregnant women and for those persons who have pancreatitis, advanced neuropathy, extremely elevated triglycerides, or a history of alcohol abuse (Franz et al, 2002).
- Nonnutritive sweeteners are safe when consumed within the acceptable daily intake levels established by the Food and Drug Administration (FDA) (American Diabetes Association, 2006). The FDA has approved use of saccharin, aspartame, acesulfame potassium, neotame, and sucralose. See Table 9-7.
- Adequate carbohydrate replacement during and after exercise seems to be important to prevent hypoglycemia. Adjusting rapid-acting insulin doses during the physical activity is usually recommended; a decrease from 30–50% is reasonable (Grimm et al, 2004; Rabasa-Lhoret et al, 2001), and frequent blood glucose monitoring will elucidate insulin adjustment requirements.
- In critical illness, blood glucose management is a challenge, and enteral feeding is generally preferred (Charney and Hertzler, 2004). Special formulas are not usually required, but regular blood glucose monitoring and insulin replacement may be needed.
- If parenteral nutrition is needed, strict blood glucose control is essential (McMahon, 2004). Hyperglycemia reflects illness severity and results in deleterious conse-

Dietary Reference Intakes for Fiber

Age	Fiber (g/d)
Children	
1–3 years	19
4–8 years	25
Males	
9–13 years	31
14–18 years	38
19–50 years	38
51+ years	30
Females	
9–13 years	26
14–18 years	26
19–50 years	25
51+ years	21
Pregnancy	
≤18 years	28
18+ years	28
Lactation	
≤18 years	29
18+ years	29

TABLE 9-7 Sugar and Sweetener Facts

The percentage of calories from carbohydrate (CHO) in the diet for diabetes will vary; it is individualized based on eating habits and glucose and lipid goals.

Glycemic load = glycemic index [GI] × available CHO amount. Although various starches do have different glycemic responses, first priority should be given to the total amount of CHO consumed rather than the source of the CHO. Fruits and milk have been shown to have a lower glycemic response than most starches, and sucrose produces a glycemic response similar to that of bread, rice, and potatoes.

Sucrose: The use of sucrose as part of total CHO of the diet does not impair blood glucose control in individuals with type 1 or type 2 diabetes, but sucrose and sucrose-containing foods should be substituted for other CHO sources gram for gram. The nutrient content of concentrated sweets and sucrose-containing foods, as well as the presence of other nutrients such as fat, must be considered. Current diabetes guidelines do not specifically restrict intake of sugars (Kelley, 2003).

Sugar (sucrose): 16 kcal/tsp (4 g CHO)

Sugar found in common foods includes:

Item	Equivalent Sugar Content (tsp)
Soft drink, 12 oz	10
Chocolate candy bar, 1 1/2 oz	5 1/2
Cake with icing	4 1/2
Fruit loop-type cereal, 1 cup	3 1/2
Sweet pickle, 1 oz	2 1/4
Catsup, 1 tbsp	1
Barbecued chips, 1 oz	1/2
Unsweetened cereal, 1 cup	1/3

Other nutritive sweeteners: Sweeteners include corn syrup, honey, molasses, dextrose, and maltose. There is no evidence that foods sweetened with these sweeteners have any significant advantage or disadvantage over foods sweetened with sucrose in decreasing total calories or CHO content of the diet or in improving overall diabetes control.

Fructose: Although dietary fructose produces a smaller rise in plasma glucose than equal amounts of sucrose and most starches, it is not to replace more than 20% of calories in adults because of its potential adverse effects on lipids, especially triglycerides. There is no reason to recommend that people with diabetes avoid consumption of fruits and vegetables, in which fructose occurs naturally. In children, fructose works well as a substitute in baked goods because their lipids are not yet a problem and fructose has little impact on blood glucose levels.

Fructose: 11 kcal/tsp (3 g CHO)

Sugar alcohols: Sugar alcohols produce a lower postprandial glucose response than sucrose or glucose and have lower available energy. Sugar alcohols contain, on average, approximately 2 kcal/g (one half of the calories of other sweeteners such as sucrose). With foods containing sugar alcohols, subtraction of one half of sugar alcohol grams from total CHO grams is appropriate, particularly when using the CHO counting method for meal planning. There is no evidence that the amounts of sugar alcohol likely to be consumed will result in significant reduction in energy intake or long-term improvement in glycemia. The use of sugar alcohols appears to be safe. Excessive amounts of polyols may have a laxative effect. The calories and CHO content from all nutritive sweeteners must be accounted for in the meal plan and have the potential to affect blood glucose levels.

Sorbitol: 50% as sweet as sucrose

Xylitol: 16 kcal/tsp (4 g CHO)

Nonnutritive sweeteners: The Food and Drug Administration has approved five nonnutritive sweeteners for use in the United States: acesulfame potassium, aspartame, neotame, saccharin, and sucralose. All have undergone rigorous scrutiny and have been shown to be safe when consumed by the public, including people with diabetes and women who are pregnant.

Acesulfame potassium (Sunette): 200 times sweeter than sugar; use in baking

Aspartame: 180 times sweeter than sugar; 4 kcal/tsp

Neotame: 6000 times sweeter than sugar

Saccharin: 300–400 times sweeter than sugar

Sources: American Diabetes Association, 2006; Franz et al, 2002.

SAMPLE NUTRITION DIAGNOSTIC STATEMENT

Type 1 Diabetes

PES: Altered nutrition-related lab values related to wrong dose of insulin as evidenced by blood glucose readings consistently >250 mg/dL before lunch.

Assessment Data: Blood glucose log and food history.

Intervention: Interventions should address appropriate timing of food and insulin dose; CHO counting.

Monitoring and Evaluation: Ask patient to fax blood glucose logs for next 3 days.

quences; in surgical intensive care, normalization of morning glucose values using insulin infusions decreases mortality (McCowen and Bistrian, 2004). Plan 30% of nutrient intake as fat, 50% as CHO, and 15–20% as protein unless other disease states require alternative therapy.

CLINICAL INDICATORS

Clinical/History	Lab Work	
Height	HbA1c (goal <7%)	Cholesterol (Chol)
Weight	Fasting plasma glucose (FBG) (goal 90–130 mg/dL)	High-density lipoprotein (HDL)
Weight:height percentiles	OGTT results	Low-density lipoprotein (LDL)
Body mass index (BMI)	Urine glucose	Triglycerides (Trig)
Diet history	Blood urea nitrogen (BUN)	Blood or urinary ketones
Waist circumference	Creatinine (Creat)	Na+, K+
Waist–hip ratio	Microalbuminuria	Ca++, Mg++
Visual acuity	C-reactive protein (CRP)	Serum phosphorous (PO_4)
Blood pressure (BP)		Thyroid-stimulating hormone (TSH)
Intake and output (I & O)		

Common Drugs Used and Potential Side Effects

Insulin/diet correlation is essential. Persons with type 1 diabetes are dependent on insulin for life. The primary potential effect is hypoglycemia. Sources of insulin must be noted because they affect the peak times and duration of effect, and some affect the speed of absorption. Human insulin is produced synthetically from *Escherichia coli* or yeast with identical amino acid sequence to the human insulin. See Table 9-8 for insulin onset, peak, and duration times.

TABLE 9-8 Insulin Onset, Peaks, and Duration

Insulin	Onset	Peak	Duration
Bolus Insulin (mealtime or rapid-acting insulins)			
Rapid-acting:			
Lispro (Humalog)	<15 minutes	0.5–1.5 hours	3–5 hours
Aspart (Novolog)	<15 minutes	0.5–1.5 hours	3–5 hours
Glulisine (Apidra)	<15 minutes	0.5–1.5 hours	3–5 hours
Short-acting:			
Regular insulin (Novolin R, Humulin R)	30–60 minutes	1–2 hours	4–6 hours
Basal Insulin			
Intermediate-acting:			
NPH Insulin or Lente	1–2 hours	4–8 hours	10–16 hours; Lente, slightly longer
Ultralente insulin (extended insulin zinc suspension)	4–6 hours	10–16 hours	18–20 hours
Long-acting:			
Glargine (Lantus)	~1 hour	No peak; flat action throughout duration	21–24 hours
Detemir	1–2 hours	No peak	~6–24 hours; dose-dependent increases in duration
Inhaled agents (none is currently approved by Food and Drug Administration for marketing)	1 mg reaches peak of 3 U SQ insulin		Large dose needed because of inefficient absorption

From: Bennet J. Trends in insulin therapy: an update. *On the Cutting Edge* 25:28, 2004.

Insulin pumps (continuous subcutaneous insulin infusion [CSII]) may be good to maintain glucose levels. If a pump is used, meal schedules are not as strict but should not be abused. With multiple daily insulin injections (MDI), test blood glucose before meals to determine insulin doses for injections. There are now insulin pens available that are convenient for insulin dosing.

New insulin analogs are preferred for most patients because they match postprandial blood glucose excursions better than traditional insulin. Bolus analogs are used for more rapid onset to cover meal CHO and to correct hyperglycemia. Basal agents release at a more constant rate to cover between-meal glucose needs or the body's basal insulin needs. Premixed insulins are discouraged except when patients are not able to be compliant with MDI.

Adverse effects include the potential for hypoglycemia, especially when HbA1c is less than 7%. Analog insulins are less likely to lead to hypoglycemia, especially overnight hypoglycemia. Weight gain with use of insulin can be counteracted with attention to food intake and physical activity.

Herbs, Botanicals, and Supplements

- Herbs and botanical supplements should not be used without discussing with the physician. Beans, peanuts, onion, garlic, and bitter gourd have been recommended, but no clinical trials have proven efficacy. There is still insufficient evidence to draw definitive conclusions about the efficacy of individual herbs and supplements for diabetes (Yeh et al, 2003).
- Alpha lipoic acid (thioctic acid) may have some potential benefits. It is found in the mitochondria and seems to have antioxidant properties that protect vitamin C, vitamin E, and glutathione. Natural sources include red meat, yeast, potatoes, and spinach. Supplementation may provide protection against cataracts and neuropathy in diabetes; it may also improve glucose uptake by the heart, but studies are inconclusive.
- Bilberry contains anthocyanosides that counteract cellular damage to the retina. Mild drowsiness and skin rashes have been noted.
- Chromium enhances use of insulin. Skin allergies, renal toxicity, and altered iron and zinc absorption can occur. Use only with deficiency because there are no proven benefits if a patient is not deficient (American Diabetes Association, 2006).
- *Coccinia indica* and American ginseng show promise (Vuksan et al, 2000); positive results are also seen with *Gymnema sylvestre*, aloe vera, vanadium, *Momordica charantia*, and nopal (Yeh et al, 2003).
- Evening primrose oil may prevent or limit neuropathy due to gamma linoleic acid, an essential fatty acid. It can cause headache and gastrointestinal (GI) distress in susceptible individuals.
- Fenugreek may lower glucose levels due to psyllium content. It is part of the peanut family and may cause allergic reactions. Do not take with monoamine oxidase (MAO) inhibitors for depression. It has the potential for drug interactions with other medications as well.
- Garlic may lower blood glucose levels if used in large amounts; more studies are needed.
- Gingko biloba may help control neuropathy by maintaining integrity of blood vessels and reducing stickiness of blood and clotting. It has some antioxidant properties. Avoid taking with warfarin, aspirin, and other anticoagulant drugs because it functions as a blood thinner. Headache and interactions with other drugs can occur.
- Ginseng may lower blood glucose levels. It increases energy and activity levels, which may lead to better glucose control. Avoid with warfarin, aspirin, MAO inhibitors, caffeine, antipsychotics, insulin, and oral hypoglycemics because of fluctuations in blood glucose levels, bleeding and platelet functioning, and changes in blood pressure and heart rate. Avoid taking with steroids because it functions as a steroidal herb. Headache, insomnia, nausea, and occasional menstrual difficulties can occur. Take with a meal.
- *Gymnema sylvestre* is a hypoglycemic herb. It is highly potent and should be used only under doctor's supervision because it may change insulin requirements.
- Peanut products and vinegar are complementary foods that can help reduce postprandial glycemia (Johnston and Buller, 2005).
- Vanadium may lower glucose levels. It has been associated with cancer cell growth and can be toxic at therapeutic levels.
- Zinc should not be used with immunosuppressants, tetracycline, ciprofloxacin, or levofloxacin because of potential antagonist effects.

INTERVENTION: NUTRITION EDUCATION, COUNSELING, CARE MANAGEMENT

- Diabetes self-management education (DSME) is an essential element of diabetes care, and national standards have been based on evidence for its benefits; DSME helps patients optimize metabolic control, prevent and manage complications, and maximize quality of life in a cost-effective manner (American Diabetes Association, 2006). Participation in weekly problem-based, self-management support intervention can yield diabetes-related health benefits (Tang et al, 2005). Table 9-9 provides a detailed list of roles of dietitians in diabetes management.
- Teach patient about the importance of careful control, self-care, and optimal functioning and about the role of carbohydrate intake and physical activity in maintaining metabolic control. Blood glucose testing is essential (see Fig. 9-2). Insulin injections must be given at planned, regular intervals for persons with type 1 diabetes.

TABLE 9-9 Standards of Practice for the Registered Dietitian (RD) in Diabetes Care Management

Nutrition assessment: The RD obtains adequate information in order to identify nutrition-related problems.

Nutrition diagnosis: The RD determines which nutrition problems are most important for immediate and long-range care.

Nutrition intervention: The RD provides the appropriate nutrition care treatments, education, counseling, and referrals for the individual client or patient.

Monitoring and evaluation: The RD in diabetes care monitors and evaluates outcomes directly related to the nutrition diagnosis and goals established in the intervention plan to determine the degree to which progress is being made and that goals or desired outcomes of nutrition care are being met.

For more details, see: Kulkarni K, et al. American Dietetic Association: standards of practice and standards of professional performance for registered dietitians (generalist, specialty and advanced) in diabetes care. *J Am Diet Assoc.* 105:819, 2005.

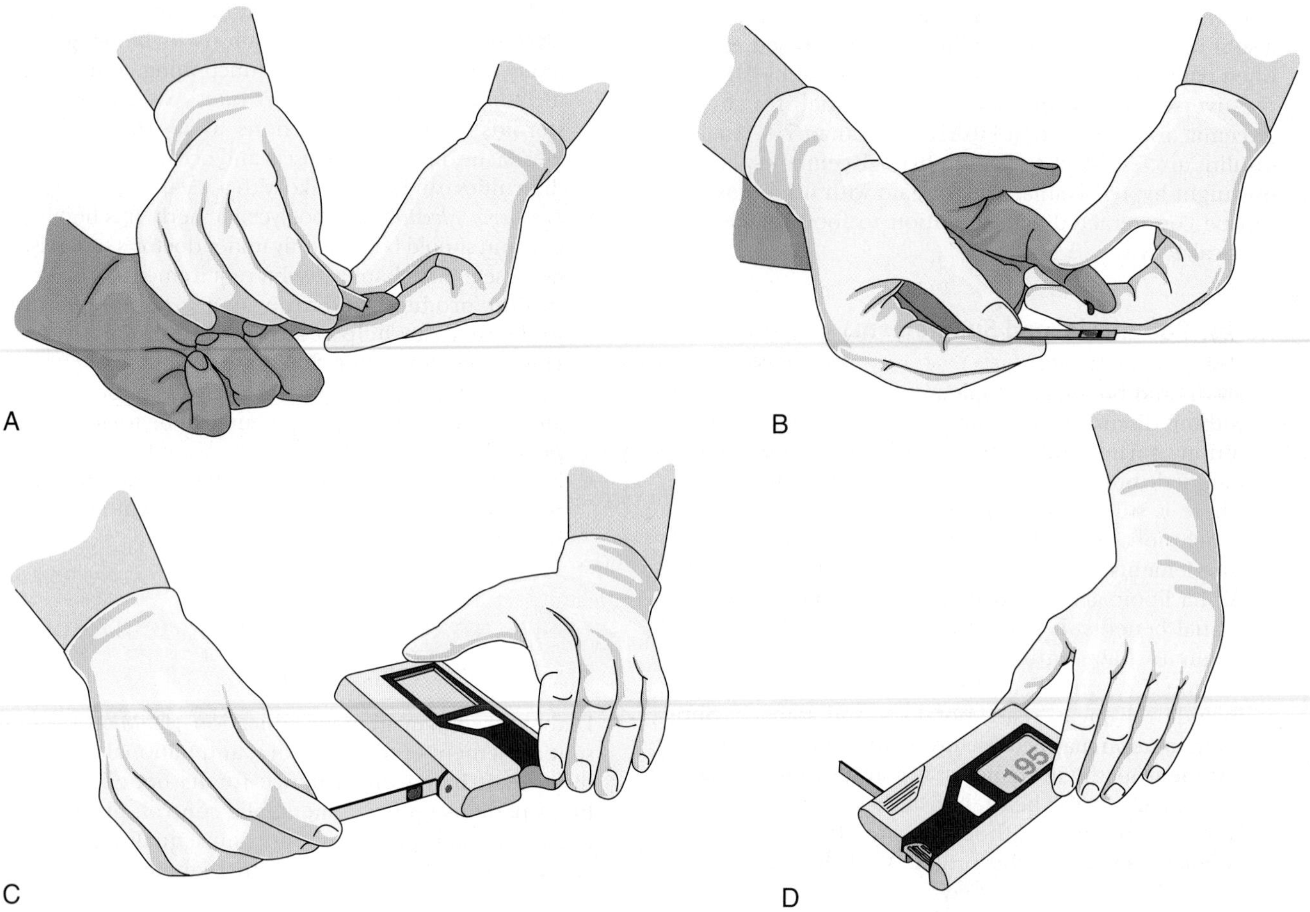

Figure 9-2 Blood glucose testing. (LifeART image. Copyright © 2006 Lippincott Williams & Wilkins. All rights reserved.)

- Identify potential or real obstacles and discuss options. Resisting temptations, dining away from home, feeling deprived, time pressures, temptations to relapse, food offers from others, competing priorities, handling social events, family or social support, and food intolerances should be discussed.
- Encourage regular mealtimes and snacks. Children and teens in particular may need planned snacks.
- Discuss visual assessment of portions. Practice with measuring cups, spoons, and scales.
- Teach patient how to read labels and how to identify carbohydrates in processed foods.
- Empowerment is important; help patients to gain mastery over their affairs and to effect change (Funnell et al, 2005). Discuss emotional eating, such as from boredom, anger, frustration, loneliness, and depression; alternative choices should be designed from the client perspective.
- Discuss the possibility of weight gain that occurs with intensive insulin therapy and improved glucose control.
- Low-carbohydrate diets are not recommended in the management of diabetes (American Diabetes Association, 2006).
- Eating disorders often occur in young women with diabetes; refer for psychotherapy.
- A nondiet approach to diabetes management encourages regular eating according to actual hunger and making gradual changes for healthier eating.
- For sick days: Patients may require more insulin when ill. Liquid diets should provide 200 g CHO in equally divided amounts at mealtime and snacks; liquids should not be sugar free (American Diabetes Association, 2004).
- For surgery: Blood glucose should be in good control; perioperative hyperglycemia can be managed with doses of short-acting insulin. Correct abnormalities before surgery when possible.
- Discuss the risks for cardiovascular disease (American Diabetes Association, 2006; Giesler et al, 2004).
- Discuss the glycemic index (see Table 9-10) and exercise, aiming for 30 min/d to burn a minimum of 1500 kcal/wk (see Table 9-11).

For More Information

- American Dietetic Association
  Type 1 Diabetes Evidence-Based Guidelines for Practice
  http://www.eatright.org

TABLE 9-10 Glycemic Index and Glycemic Load

Glycemic index (GI) is a measure of serum glucose response to a food relative to a reference food that contains equal amounts of carbohydrate. It does not refer directly to quantified food exchanges. **Glycemic load = GI × available carbohydrate amount.**

A mixed diet yields varying results on blood glucose levels. The use of diets with a low GI in the management of diabetes is controversial; it seems that choosing low-GI foods in place of conventional or high-GI foods has a small, clinically useful effect on medium-term glycemic control in patients with diabetes (Brand-Miller et al, 2003). Within a few hours after consumption of carbohydrates with high GIs and high glycemic loads, blood sugar levels begin to decline rapidly due to an exaggerated increase in insulin secretion, and profound hunger is created (Bell and Sears, 2003).

Carbohydrate Choices

Choose low-GI carbohydrates most often because they digest slower and will be less likely to elevate blood glucose. Each choice = 15 g of carbohydrate. Choose desired number of carbohydrate choices per meal or as needed by the individual. Children and teens, as well as young adults and athletes, will need much more per meal than sedentary adults.

Glycemic Index	Grain or Bean Choices	Fruit Choices	Vegetable Choices
Low (best choice)	Barley, 1/3 cup Beans (kidney, pinto, etc.), 1/2 cup cooked Lima beans, 2/3 cup Muesli, 1/4 cup Oat bran, 1/3 cup	Apple, orange, or pear Cherries, 12 Grapes, 17 Grapefruit, 1/2 Cantaloupe, 1 cup Berries (blueberries, raspberries, etc.), 1 cup	Corn, 1/2 cup Squash, acorn, 1 cup cooked Peas, green or lentils, 1/2 cup cooked 1 1/2 cups cooked or 3 cups raw vegetables, including asparagus, beets, broccoli, carrots, cucumbers, mushrooms, onions, peppers, tomatoes, zucchini, and others
Medium (choose less often)	Baked beans, 1/4 cup Bran flakes, 1/2 cup Bread, 100% whole wheat, 1 slice English muffin, whole wheat, 1/2 Granola, low sugar, 1/4 cup Hamburger or hot dog bun, 1/2 bun Oatmeal, old fashioned, 1/2 cup Pasta, 1/3 cup cooked Raisin bran, 1/3 cup Rice, converted or wild, 1/3 cup cooked Special K, 3/4 cup Tortilla, 6″	Banana, 1 small Canned fruit, drained, 1/2 cup Dried fruit, 1/4 cup Watermelon, 1 1/4 cups Raisins, 2 tbsp Orange juice, 1/2 cup Apple juice, 1/2 cup Grape juice, 1/3 cup	Potato, small, "new," 1/2 cup Sweet potato, 1/2 cup cooked
High (choose rarely)	Bagel, large, 1/4 bagel Bread, white, 1 slice Cream of wheat, 1/2 cup cooked Cheerios, 3/4 cup Corn flakes, 3/4 cup Instant oatmeal, 1/2 cup cooked Pancake, 4″ Rice Krispies, 3/4 cup Rice, white, 1/3 cup cooked Shredded wheat, 1/3 cup Waffle, 4″		Potato, small russet, 3″ diameter Potato, mashed, 1/2 cup
Glycemic Index	**Combination Foods**	**Sweets/Snacks**	**Milk/Yogurt/Milk Substitutes**
Low	Soup, cream, low fat, 1 cup Chili, low fat, 1/2 cup	Ice cream, low fat, 1/2 cup Pudding, sugar free, 1/2 cup Chocolate candy, 15 kisses or 1-oz bar	Milk, skim or low fat (1%), 1 cup Yogurt, low fat, artificially sweetened, 1 cup Soy milk, low fat or nonfat, 1 cup
Medium	Burrito, bean, flour tortilla, 7″ long (= 3 carb choices) Pasta dish, 1/2 cup	Popcorn, microwave light, popped, 3 cups Cookie, 3″ across, 1 Muffin, small, 1/2	Yogurt, low fat, sweetened, with fruit, 1/3 cup
High	Pizza, thin crust, medium, 1 slice (= 2 carb choices) Pizza, thick crust, medium, 1 slice (= 3 carb choices)	Pretzel twists, mini, 15 pieces Brownie or cake, no frosting, 2″ square Doughnut, 3″, 1/2 doughnut Granola bar, 1 Potato or tortilla chips, 15 chips Syrup, 1 tbsp	

Sources: Brand-Miller et al, 2003; Bell and Sears, 2003.

TABLE 9-11 American Diabetes Association General Guidelines for Regulating Exercise

1. **Metabolic control before exercise**
   - Avoid exercise if ketosis is present. Use caution if glucose levels are >300 mg/dL without ketosis.
   - Ingest added carbohydrate if glucose levels are <100 mg/dL.
2. **Blood glucose monitoring before and after exercise**
   - Identify when changes in insulin or carbohydrate are necessary.
   - Learn the glycemic response to different exercise conditions.
3. **Food intake**
   - Consume added carbohydrate, as needed, to avoid hypoglycemia. Carbodydrate-based foods should be readily available during and after exercise.

TYPE 1 DIABETES MELLITUS—CITED REFERENCES

American Diabetes Association. Diabetes: heart disease and stroke. Accessed April 24, 2005 at http://www.diabetes.org/diabetes-heart-disease-stroke.jsp.

American Diabetes Association. Nutrition principles and recommendation in diabetes (Position Statement). *Diabetes Care* 27:S36, 2004 (suppl 1).

American Diabetes Association. Standards of Medical Care in Diabetes–2006. *Diabetes Care* 29:4S, 2006.

Bell SJ, Sears B. Low-glycemic-load diets: impact on obesity and chronic diseases. *Crit Rev Food Sci Nutr.* 43:357, 2003.

Bennet J. Trends in insulin therapy: an update. *On the Cutting Edge* 25:28, 2004.

Brand-Miller J, et al. Low-glycemic index diets in the management of diabetes: a meta-analysis of randomized controlled trials. *Diabetes Care* 26:2261, 2003.

Charney P, Hertzler SR. Management of blood glucose and diabetes in the critically ill patient receiving enteral feeding. *Nutr Clin Pract.* 19:129, 2004.

Chima CS, et al. Use of technology to track program outcomes in a diabetes self-management program. *J Am Diet Assoc.* 105:1933, 2005.

Dose Adjustment for Normal Eating Training Group. Training in flexible, intensive insulin management to enable dietary freedom in people with type 1 diabetes: Dose Adjustment for Normal Eating (DAFNE) randomised controlled trial. *BMJ.* 325:746, 2002.

Franz M, et al. Evidence-based nutrition principles and recommendations for the treatment and prevention of diabetes and related conditions. *Diabetes Care* 25:148, 2002.

Franz MJ. Evidence-based medical nutrition therapy for diabetes. *Nutr Clin Pract.* 19:137, 2004.

Funnell MM, et al. Implementing an empowerment-based diabetes self-management education program. *Diabetes Educ.* 31:53, 2005.

Giesler PD, et al. Cardiovascular risk reduction and diabetes education: what are we telling our patients? *Diabetes Educ.* 30:994, 2004.

Grimm JJ, et al. A new table for prevention of hypoglycaemia during physical activity in type 1 diabetic patients. *Diabetes Metab.* 30:465, 2004.

Johnston CS, Buller AJ. Vinegar and peanut products as complementary foods to reduce postprandial glycemia. *J Am Diet Assoc.* 105:1939, 2005.

Kelley DE. Sugars and starch in the nutritional management of diabetes mellitus. *Am J Clin Nutr.* 78:858S, 2003.

Kulkarni K. Diets do not fail: the success of medical nutrition therapy in patients with diabetes. *Endocr Pract.* 12:121S, 2006.

Kulkarni K, et al. American Dietetic Association: standards of practice and standards of professional performance for registered dietitians (generalist, specialty and advanced) in diabetes care. *J Am Diet Assoc.* 105:819, 2005.

Mayer-Davis EJ, et al. Dietary intake among youth with diabetes: the SEARCH for Diabetes in Youth Study. *J Am Diet Assoc.* 106:689, 2006.

McCowen KC, Bistrian BR. Hyperglycemia and nutrition support: theory and practice. *Nutr Clin Pract.* 19:235, 2004.

McMahon MM. Management of parenteral nutrition in acutely ill patients with hyperglycemia. *Nutr Clin Pract.* 19:120, 2004.

Rabasa-Lhoret R, et al. Guidelines for premeal insulin dose reduction for postprandial exercise of different intensities and durations in type 1 diabetic subjects treated intensively with a basal-bolus insulin regimen (Ultralente-Lispro). *Diabetes Care* 24:625, 2001.

Schafer RG, et al. Diabetes nutrition recommendations for health care institutions. *Diabetes Care* 27:55S, 2004.

Scheepers A, et al. The glucose transporter families SGLT and GLUT: molecular basis of normal and aberrant function. *J Parenter Enteral Nutr.* 28:364, 2004.

Shekelle PG, et al. Are Ayurvedic herbs for diabetes effective? *J Fam Pract.* 54:876, 2005.

Strychar I, et al. Impact of a high-monounsaturated-fat diet on lipid profile in subjects with type 1 diabetes. *J Am Diet Assoc.* 103:467, 2003.

Tang TS, et al. Developing a new generation of ongoing diabetes self-management support interventions: a preliminary report. *Diabetes Educ.* 31:91, 2005.

Vuksan V, et al. American ginseng (*Panax quinquefolius* L) reduces postprandial glycemia in nondiabetic subjects and subjects with type 2 diabetes mellitus. *Arch Intern Med.* 160:1009, 2000.

Yeh GY, et al. Systematic review of herbs and dietary supplements for glycemic control in diabetes. *Diabetes Care.* 26:1277, 2003.

PANCREAS OR ISLET CELL TRANSPLANTATION

NUTRITIONAL ACUITY RANKING: LEVEL 4

DEFINITIONS AND BACKGROUND

Pancreas transplantation is the most common form of insulin replacement therapy that is accomplished with transplantation. It is most commonly used in patients with type 1 diabetes who are already going to receive a kidney transplantation.

Islet cell transplantation has also become available; it can lead to insulin independence with excellent metabolic control (Shapiro et al, 2000). Islet transplantation can require more than one donor pancreas to achieve insulin independence (Rickels et al, 2005). This transplantation is not yet common.

Drugs are needed to prevent rejection. The acute posttransplantation phase lasts up to 2 months; the chronic phase starts after 2 months. Islet cell programs try to avoid using large doses of glucocorticoids. Most protocols are designed to use tacrolimus and sirolimus so that high-dose glucocorticoids would not have to be used.

During the acute period of care, there is the issue that patients are variably managed with insulin therapy to allow for recovery of the islets after they have been placed into their new and not totally adequate environment in the liver. Most centers treat patients for up to a month, and treating hypoglycemia during this time is a concern.

Long-term complications may include osteoporosis and hyperlipidemia.

INTERVENTION: OBJECTIVES

- Meet the specific needs of the patient; modify drug therapy to enhance outcomes and quality of life.
- Prevent infection and promote healing.
- Monitor for abnormal electrolyte levels.
- Monitor CHO intolerance but make sure that diet provides enough CHO to spare proteins. Treatment goals should reflect those of the American Diabetes Association and be adjusted as new evidence suggests.
- Alleviate rejection episodes. Control infections, especially during the acute phase. Support protein intake to prevent additional infections.
- Force fluids unless contraindicated, as in retention. Match fluid output.
- Help patient adjust to a lifelong medical regimen during chronic phase. Improve survival rate by supporting immune response.
- Correct or manage complications that occur.
- Control weight gain in the first year after transplantation.

INTERVENTION: FOOD AND NUTRITION

- Progress solids as quickly as possibly postoperatively. Monitor fluid status, and adjust as needed.
- Daily intake of protein should be appropriate for age and sex; 1.5 g/kg while on steroids may be recommended. Energy needs should be calculated as 30–35 kcal/kg.
- Daily intake of sodium should be 2–4 g until the drug regimen is reduced. Adjust potassium levels as needed.
- Daily intake of calcium should be 1–1.5 times the daily requirements to offset poor absorption. Children especially need adequate calcium for growth. Daily intake of phosphorus should be equal to calcium intake.
- Supplement diet with vitamin D, magnesium, and thiamin as needed. Adequate vitamin intake will be essential to maintain immunity and to support wound healing.
- Control CHO intake with hyperglycemia (45–50% total kcal); encourage healthy food sources of carbohydrate. Transplantation patients are at risk of further glucose intolerance from multiple medications.
- Plan fats at 25–35% of total kcal (encourage monounsaturated fats and omega-3 fatty acids). Low saturated fats and cholesterol may be needed. A controlled fat intake is recommended for prevention and treatment of hyperlipidemia.
- Reduce gastric irritants as necessary if GI distress or reflux occurs.
- Monitor electrolytes carefully; hyperkalemia is common with cyclosporine or tacrolimus.
- Special diets may be discontinued when drug therapy is reduced to maintenance levels. Encourage exercise and a weight control plan thereafter.

CLINICAL INDICATORS

Clinical/History

Height
Dry weight, present weight
BMI
Diet history
I & O
BP
Temperature

Lab Work

Albumin (Alb), transthyretin
HbA1c
Na+, K+
Hemoglobin and hematocrit (H & H)
Serum Fe
Serum folacin
BUN, Creat
Ca++, Mg++
White blood cell count (WBC)
Total lymphocyte count (TLC)
Glucose (Gluc)
Chol, Trig
CRP
Nitrogen (N) balance
Glomerular filtration rate (GFR)
Alkaline phosphatase (Alk phos)
Aspartate aminotransferase (AST)
Alanine aminotransferase (ALT)
Bilirubin

Common Drugs Used and Potential Side Effects

- See Table 9-12.

Herbs, Botanicals, and Supplements

- Herbals should be discouraged after transplantation. Those who self-medicate with herbals are taking a chance that their use of an herbal may interact with their immunosuppressive drugs and either cause higher or lower than desired drug levels of these agents.
- Chaparral is an herbal product that may cause severe hepatitis or liver failure; St. John's wort interferes with the metabolism of immunosuppressants and should not be used after transplantation.

INTERVENTION: NUTRITION EDUCATION, COUNSELING, CARE MANAGEMENT

- Indicate which foods are sources of key nutrients such as protein in the diet. If patient does not prefer milk, show how other sources of calcium may be used in the diet.
- Alcohol should be avoided unless permitted by the doctor.
- Patients should know when to seek medical attention.
- Discuss problems with long-term obesity and hypercholesterolemia.
- Encourage moderation in diet; promote adequate exercise.

TABLE 9-12 Medications Used after Islet Cell Transplantation

Medication	Description
Cyclosporine	Cyclosporine does not cause retention of sodium as much as corticosteroids do. Intravenous doses are more effective than oral doses. Nausea, vomiting, and diarrhea are common side effects. Hyperlipidemia, hyperglycemia, and hyperkalemia may also occur; decrease fat intake as well as sodium and potassium if necessary. Magnesium may need to be replaced. The drug is also nephrotoxic; a controlled renal diet may be beneficial. Taking omega-3 fatty acids during cyclosporine therapy may reduce toxic side effects (such as high blood pressure and kidney damage) associated with this medication in transplantation patients (Tsipas and Morphake, 2003). Avoid use with St. John's wort.
Diuretics	Diuretics such as furosemide (Lasix) may cause hypokalemia. Aldactone actually spares potassium; monitor drug changes closely. In general, avoid use with fenugreek, yohimbe, and ginkgo.
Immunosuppressants	Immunosuppressants such as muromonab (Orthoclone OKT3) and antithymocyte globulin (ATG) are less nephrotoxic than cyclosporine but can cause nausea, anorexia, diarrhea, and vomiting. Monitor carefully. Fever and stomatitis also may occur; alter diet as needed.
Insulin	Insulin may be necessary during periods of hyperglycemia. Monitor for hypoglycemic symptoms during use; teach patient self-management tips.
Pancreatic enzymes	Pancreatic enzymes may be needed if pancreatitis occurs again after transplantation.
Tacrolimus (Prograf, FK506)	Tacrolimus suppresses T-cell immunity; it is 100 times more potent than cyclosporine, thus requiring smaller doses. Side effects include gastrointestinal distress, nausea, vomiting, hyperkalemia, and hyperglycemia; adjust diet accordingly by controlling carbohydrate and enhancing potassium intake.
Tetranectin	Tetranectin binds plasminogen and may have a role in regulating pericellular proteolysis and in the survival of islets in the liver after islet transplantation (Hermann et al, 2005).

For More Information

- American Diabetes Association–Islet Cell Transplantation
  http://www.diabetes.org/type-1-diabetes/islet-transplants.jsp
- Immune Tolerance Network (ITN)
  http://www.immunetolerance.org
- Insulin-Free
  http://www.insulin-free.org/
- National Institute of Diabetes and Digestive and Kidney Diseases (NIDDK)–Islet Cell Transplantation
  http://diabetes.niddk.nih.gov/dm/pubs/pancreaticislet/

PANCREAS OR ISLET CELL TRANSPLANTATION—CITED REFERENCES

Hermann M, et al. In the search of potential human islet stem cells: is tetranectin showing us the way? *Transplant Proc.* 37:1322, 2005.

Rickels MR, et al. Beta-cell function following human islet transplantation for type 1 diabetes. *Diabetes* 54:100, 2005.

Shapiro A, et al. Islet transplantation in seven patients with type 1 diabetes mellitus using a glucocorticoid-free immunosuppressive regimen. *N Engl J Med.* 343:230, 2000.

Tsipas G, Morphake P. Beneficial effects of a diet rich in a mixture of n-6/n-3 essential fatty acids and of their metabolites on cyclosporine nephrotoxicity. *J Nutr Biochem.* 14:626, 2003.

METABOLIC SYNDROME

NUTRITIONAL ACUITY RANKING: LEVEL 3–4

DEFINITIONS AND BACKGROUND

The metabolic syndrome (formerly called insulin resistance syndrome or syndrome X) has simultaneous clustering of low levels of high-density lipoprotein cholesterol, hyperglycemia, high waist circumference, hypertension, and elevated triglycerides; is associated with cardiovascular disease (Ellison et al, 2005); and often leads to type 2 diabetes. This condition affects some young people but usually affects persons aged 55 years and older. More than 64 million Americans have metabolic syndrome, including roughly one in four adults and 40% of adults aged 40 years and older, which is an increase of 60% over the last decade. See Figure 9-3.

Genes that increase birth weight can also worsen the metabolic syndrome (Stern et al, 2000). Excessive calorie consumption, physical inactivity, excess weight, and smoking also contribute. Finally, inflammation in cardiovascular disease and hypertension may contribute to the onset of the syndrome.

Individuals who are obese and insulin resistant are particularly prone to this syndrome. An "apple" shaped figure (high waist circumference) is riskier because fat cells located in the abdomen release fat into the blood more easily

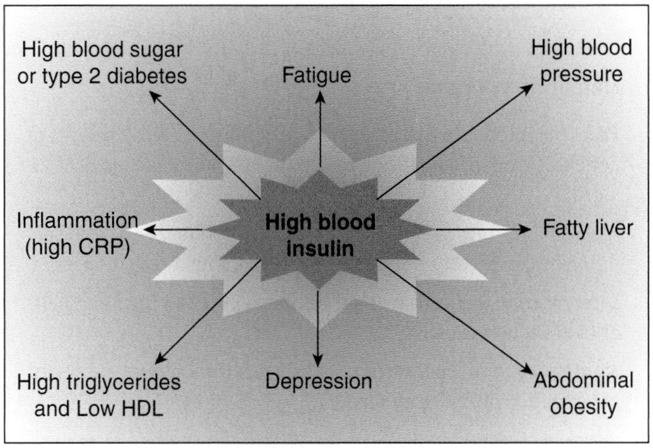

Any 3 of 5 Criteria Constitute Diagnosis of Metabolic Syndrome:

- Elevated waist circumference*
  ≥102 cm in men or >40"
  ≥88 cm in women or >35"
- Elevated TG ≥150 mg/dL (1.7 mmol/L)
  Or Drug treatment for elevated TG
- Reduced HDL-C
  ≤40 mg/dL (0.9 mmol/L) in men
  ≤50 mg/dL (1.1 mmol/L) in women
  Or Drug treatment for reduced HDL-C
- Elevated BP
  ≥130 mmHg systolic BP or ≥85 mmHg diastolic BP
  Or Drug treatment for hypertension
- Elevated fasting glucose ≥100 mg/dL
  Or Drug treatment for elevated glucose

* To measure waist circumference, locate top of right iliac crest. Place a measuring tape in a horizontal plane around the abdomen at level of iliac crest. Before reading tape measure, ensure that tape is snug but does not compress the skin and is parallel to the floor. Measurement is made at end of normal expiration.

Figure 9-3 The metabolic syndrome: symptoms and diagnostic criteria.

than fat cells found elsewhere. Obesity should be addressed, especially central obesity, which is associated with insulin resistance.

Although alcohol binges may contribute to this syndrome, mild to moderate alcohol consumption is associated with a lower prevalence of the metabolic syndrome (Dejousse et al, 2004), with a favorable influence on lipids, waist circumference, and fasting insulin (Freiberg et al, 2004). Drinking patterns should be evaluated, with early onset, heavy total volume/lifetime, total number of drinking days, and intensity (drinks per drinking day) playing a part in the onset of metabolic syndrome.

Management of patients with metabolic syndrome should focus on lifestyle modifications (e.g., weight loss and physical activity) with two major components: behavioral change to reduce caloric intake and increased physical activity (Deedwania and Volkova, 2005). It may be beneficial to include phytochemicals, antioxidant foods, and spices such as allspice, cloves, turmeric, cumin, bay leaf, nutmeg, and cinnamon (Anderson et al, 2004).

Any 3 of the following 5 criteria constitute diagnosis of metabolic syndrome (Grundy et al, 2005):

- Elevated waist circumference: 40″ or 102 cm in men; 35″ or 88 cm in women
- Elevated triglycerides (TG) ≥150 mg/dL or drug treatment for elevated TG
- Reduced HDL cholesterol: <40 mg/dL in men and 50 mg/dL in women or drug treatment for low HDL cholesterol levels
- Elevated BP: >130 mm Hg systolic blood pressure (BP) or 85 mm Hg diastolic BP or drug treatment for hypertension
- Elevated fasting glucose: >100 mg/dL or drug treatment for elevated glucose

INTERVENTION: OBJECTIVES

- Achieve improved body weight; maintain it to lessen abdominal obesity in particular. A realistic goal for weight reduction should be 7–10% over 6–12 months (Bestermann et al, 2005).
- Physical activity is associated with successful weight reduction, and therapeutic lifestyle changes (including diet) can reduce by half the progression to new-onset diabetes in patients with metabolic syndrome (Bestermann et al, 2005).
- Achieve and maintain cholesterol, blood glucose, and BP at levels indicated by the most recent American Heart Association Statement, as follows (Grundy et al, 2005):

For Atherogenic Dyslipidemia

- For elevated LDL cholesterol: Give priority to reduction of LDL cholesterol over other lipid parameters. Achieve LDL cholesterol goals based on patient's risk category.
- LDL cholesterol goals for different risk categories are:
  High risk: seek 70–100 mg/dL
  Moderately high risk: seek 100–130 mg/dL
  Moderate risk: seek 130 mg/dL
  Lower risk: 160 mg/dL is acceptable
- If TG is >200 mg/dL, then goal for non-HDL cholesterol for each risk category is 30 mg/dL higher than for LDL cholesterol. If TG is >200 mg/dL after achieving LDL cholesterol goal, consider additional therapies to attain non-HDL cholesterol goal.
- If HDL cholesterol is <40 mg/dL in men or <50 mg/dL in women, raise HDL cholesterol to extent possible with standard therapies for atherogenic dyslipidemia. Either lifestyle therapy can be intensified or drug therapy can be used for raising HDL cholesterol levels, depending on patient's risk category.

For Elevated BP

- Reduce BP to at least achieve BP of <140/90 mm Hg (or <130/80 mm Hg if diabetes is present). Reduce BP further to extent possible through lifestyle changes.
- For BP >120/80 mm Hg: Initiate or maintain lifestyle modification via weight control, increased physical activity, alcohol moderation, sodium reduction, and emphasis on increased consumption of fresh fruits, vegetables,

and low-fat dairy products in all patients with metabolic syndrome.

- For BP >140/90 mm Hg (or >130/80 mm Hg if diabetes is present), add BP medication as needed to achieve goal BP.

For Elevated Glucose

- For impaired fasting glucose (IFG), delay progression to type 2 diabetes mellitus. Encourage weight reduction and increased physical activity.
- In diabetes, for hemoglobin A1c at or above 7.0%, lifestyle therapy and pharmacotherapy, if necessary, should be used. Modify other risk factors and behaviors (e.g., abdominal obesity, physical inactivity, elevated BP, or lipid abnormalities).

For Prothrombotic State

- Reduce thrombotic and fibrinolytic risk factors. Low-dose aspirin therapy or prophylaxis is recommended.

For Proinflammatory State

- There are no specific therapies beyond lifestyle changes.

INTERVENTION: FOOD AND NUTRITION

- The general dietary recommendations include low intake of saturated fats, trans fats, and cholesterol and diets with low glycemic index (Bestermann et al, 2005). Use of 35% kcal from total fat is acceptable, but lower levels will work even faster. Increase use of omega-3 and omega-6 fatty acids, and keep saturated fatty acids (SFA) down to 5–10%. The Mediterranean diet plan has been useful (Maki and Kurlandsky, 2001).
- Plan a diet using more fiber and starches, especially whole grains, raw fruits, and vegetables. There is ultra-grain white bread available now for those who prefer the taste of white bread over whole wheat. A low-fat, plant-based diet may be useful (Barnard et al, 2005).
- A diet with 45–50% CHO levels has been suggested; monitor blood glucose levels accordingly.
- Protein should be maintained at 15% of kcal. Encourage soy protein as a meat substitute several times a week. Soy protein could be beneficial in weight reduction and correction of dyslipidemia (Bestermann et al, 2005).
- Ensure adequate intake of vitamins such as folate and vitamins B_6, B_{12}, C, and E, preferably from food.
- Follow a diet with 3–4 g sodium; include good sources of potassium, calcium, and magnesium as from the DASH diet. Dark chocolate in small amounts regularly may help lower blood pressure, improve cholesterol, and help with insulin sensitivity; more studies are under way. Consumption of skim milk may be helpful because it offers calcium and potassium in an easily consumed beverage.
- There may be advantages to spreading nutrient load by eating smaller meals or foods with lower glycemic index (Maki and Kurlandsky, 2001).
- In addition to diet, counselors should promote physical activity. Recommendations should include practical, regular, and moderated regimens of exercise, with a daily minimum of 30–60 minutes and equal balance between aerobic and strength training (Bestermann et al, 2005).

SAMPLE NUTRITION DIAGNOSTIC STATEMENT

Metabolic Syndrome

PES: Inappropriate intake of types of CHO related to knowledge deficit as evidenced by triglycerides of 300 mg/dL and HDL of 25 mg/dL.

Assessment Data: Food intake records; refined CHO and soft drink intake; dietary fiber. Physical activity history.

Intervention: Education about desirable CHO and fiber and benefits of regular exercise.

Monitoring and Evaluation: Labs in 3–6 months; reports of physical activity; dietary records.

CLINICAL INDICATORS

Clinical/History

- Height
- Weight
- Weight pattern history
- BMI
- Diet history
- Waist circumference (40″ or 102 cm in men; 35″ or 88 cm in women)
- BP (≥130/85 mm Hg)

Lab Work

- Gluc (>100 mg/dL)
- HbA1c
- HDL Chol (<40 mg/dL for men, <50 mg/dL for women)
- LDL Chol
- Trig (>150 mg/dL)
- Na+, K+
- Serum insulin
- Serum uric acid (elevated?)
- CRP (elevated)
- Prothrombotic state (e.g., high fibrinogen or plasminogen activator inhibitor [–1] in the blood)
- Prothrombin time (PT) or international normalized ratio (INR)

Common Drugs Used and Potential Side Effects

- Glucose-lowering medications must be carefully prescribed and monitored. Metformin may be indicated for type 2 diabetes (Bestermann et al, 2005; Orchard et al, 2005).
- Blood pressure medications may be prescribed; monitor for necessary restrictions of sodium and/or higher need for potassium. Starting with an angiotensin-converting enzyme inhibitor or an angiotensin receptor blocker is typical (Bestermann et al, 2005).
- Medications that diminish insulin resistance and directly alter lipoproteins are also necessary; combination therapy is often required to optimize attainment of treatment goals (Bestermann et al, 2005; Cohn et al, 2001).
- To lower lipids, a statin should be used initially unless contraindicated (Bestermann et al, 2005).
- If patients with metabolic syndrome also have elevations in fibrinogen and other coagulation factors leading to prothrombotic state, aspirin may be beneficial

for primary prevention in these patients (Deedwania and Volkova, 2005).

- Low-dose aspirin is not generally a problem, but it might be taken with a meal or snack to prevent any potential for GI bleeding.

Herbs, Botanicals, and Supplements

- Herbs and botanical supplements should not be used without discussing with physician.
- Essential oils such as fenugreek, cinnamon, cumin, and oregano may enhance insulin sensitivity (Talpur et al, 2005). Studies are ongoing.

INTERVENTION: NUTRITION EDUCATION, COUNSELING, CARE MANAGEMENT

- Widespread screening is recommended to slow the growth of this syndrome, and prevention should start in childhood with healthy nutrition, daily physical activity, and annual measurement of weight, height, and blood pressure beginning at 3 years of age (Bestermann, 2005).
- Discuss role of nutrition and weight control in managing or controlling this syndrome. Obesity is a major contributor to the problem, so weight loss (even 10 pounds) can help improve health status.
- Exercise daily. Aerobic and strength training exercises are especially helpful. Reduce sedentary activities, including watching television and sitting in front of the computer (Ford et al, 2005). Regular physical activity can help to lower elevated blood cholesterol levels and blood pressure. Walking, or an exercise that is pleasant to the individual, is the best one to select.
- Smoking cessation measures should be taken where needed. Offer guidance on how not to gain weight after quitting.
- Limit consumption of alcoholic beverages, which may elevate triglycerides.

For More Information

- American Diabetes Association–Metabolic Syndrome
  http://www.diabetes.org/diabetes-research/summaries/ekelund-metabolic.jsp
- American Heart Association–Metabolic Syndrome
  http://www.americanheart.org/presenter.jhtml?identifier=4756
- Heart Center Online
  http://heart.healthcentersonline.com/riskfactor/metabolicsyndromex.cfm
- Pritikin Longevity Center
  http://www.pritikin.com

METABOLIC SYNDROME—CITED REFERENCES

Anderson RA, et al. Isolation and characterization of polyphenol type-A polymers from cinnamon with insulin-like biological activity. *J Agric Food Chem.* 52:65, 2004.

Barnard ND, et al. The effects of a low-fat, plant-based dietary intervention on body weight, metabolism, and insulin sensitivity. *Am J Med.* 118:991, 2005.

Bestermann G, et al. Addressing the global cardiovascular risk of hypertension, dyslipidemia, diabetes mellitus, and the metabolic syndrome in the southeastern United States, part II: treatment recommendations for management of the global cardiovascular risk of hypertension, dyslipidemia, diabetes mellitus, and the metabolic syndrome. *Am J Med Sci.* 329:292, 2005.

Cohn G, et al. Pathophysiology and treatment of the dyslipidemia of insulin resistance. *Curr Cardiol Rep.* 3:416, 2001.

Deedwania PC, Volkova N. Current treatment options for the metabolic syndrome. *Curr Treat Options Cardiovasc Med.* 7:61, 2005.

Dejousse L, et al. Alcohol consumption and metabolic syndrome: does the type of beverage matter? *Obes Res.* 12:1375, 2004.

Ellison RC, et al. Relation of the metabolic syndrome to calcified atherosclerotic plaque in the coronary arteries and aorta. *Am J Cardiol.* 95:1180, 2005.

Ford ES, et al. Sedentary behavior, physical activity, and the metabolic syndrome among U.S. adults. *Obes Res.* 13:608, 2005.

Freiberg MA, et al. Alcohol consumption and the prevalence of the metabolic syndrome in the US: a cross-sectional analysis of data from the Third National Health and Nutrition Examination Survey. *Diabetes Care* 27:2954, 2004.

Grundy S, et al. Diagnosis and management of the metabolic syndrome. *Circulation* 112:105, 2005.

Maki K, Kurlandsky S. Syndrome X: A tangled web of risk factors for coronary heart disease and diabetes mellitus. *Top Clin Nutr.* 16:32, 2001.

Orchard TJ, et al. The effect of metformin and intensive lifestyle intervention on the metabolic syndrome: the Diabetes Prevention Program randomized trial. *Ann Intern Med.* 142:611, 2005.

Stern M, et al. Birth weight and the metabolic syndrome: thrifty phenotype or thrifty genotype? *Diabetes Metab Res Rev.* 6:88, 2000.

Talpur N, et al. Effects of a novel formulation of essential oils on glucose-insulin metabolism in diabetic and hypertensive rats: a pilot study. *Diabetes Obes Metab.* 7:193, 2005.

PREDIABETES

NUTRITIONAL ACUITY RANKING: LEVEL 3–4

DEFINITIONS AND BACKGROUND

Prediabetes is a term used to distinguish people who are at increased risk of developing diabetes. People with prediabetes have impaired fasting glucose (IFG) or impaired glucose tolerance (IGT); some people may have both conditions. More than 16 million Americans are affected. A combination of genes, obesity, and physical inactivity is related.

People who have prediabetes may have a family history of heart disease and apple-shaped (intra-abdominal) obesity. Dyslipidemia includes elevated triglycerides and low HDL cholesterol as a risk factor for type 2 diabetes (Zacharova et al, 2005).

Under recent criteria, a normal blood glucose level is <100 mg/dL. IFG is a condition in which the fasting blood glucose level is elevated (100–125 mg/dL) after an overnight fast but is not high enough to be classified as diabetes. IGT is a condition in which the blood glucose level is elevated (140–199 mg/dL) after a 2-hour oral glucose tolerance test (OGTT) but is not high enough to be classified as diabetes.

According to the American Diabetes Association, studies suggest that most people with prediabetes go on to develop type 2 diabetes within 10 years unless they make lifestyle changes (e.g., food/nutrition and physical activity) to reduce the risk of diabetes. Research studies have evaluated interventions among people with IGT and risks for developing diabetes.

The Diabetes Prevention Program (DPP) was a large prevention study of people at high risk for diabetes (American Diabetes Association, 2006). Metabolic syndrome affected approximately half of the participants in the program at baseline; lifestyle intervention and metformin therapy reduced the development of the syndrome in the remaining participants (Orchard et al, 2005).

Lifestyle modification was nearly twice as effective in preventing diabetes as the use of drugs in the DPP; the benefits of weight loss and physical activity strongly suggest that lifestyle modification should be the first choice to prevent or delay diabetes (American Diabetes Association, 2006). Lifestyle interventions included modest weight loss resulting from a low-calorie, low-fat diet and increases in moderate-intensity physical activity (such as walking for 2 1/2 hours each week).

People treated with an intensive lifestyle intervention reduced their risk of developing diabetes by 58% over 4 years, whereas people treated with the drug metformin reduced their risk by 31% (American Diabetes Association, 2006). In this same study, metformin was most effective among younger, heavier people (those 25–40 years of age who were 50–80 pounds overweight) and less effective among older people and people who were not as overweight. In the Study to Prevent Non–Insulin-Dependent Diabetes Mellitus (STOP-NIDDM) Trial, treatment of people with IGT with the drug acarbose reduced the risk of developing diabetes by 25% over 3 years.

INTERVENTION: OBJECTIVES

- Both lifestyle changes and medication have also been shown to increase the probability of reverting from IGT to normal glucose tolerance. Lifestyle interventions in all age groups are more cost effective than medications.
- Prevent further insulin resistance, hyperglycemia, and progression to diabetes.
- Modest weight loss and increased physical activity among people with prediabetes prevent or delay diabetes and may return blood glucose levels to normal. Modest weight loss (5–10% of body weight) and modest physical activity (30 min daily) are the recommended goals (American Diabetes Association, 2006).
- Prevent or delay heart and kidney diseases, stroke, and other undesirable conditions.
- Encourage activity up to 150 min/wk; walking is beneficial.

INTERVENTION: FOOD AND NUTRITION

- Control CHO intake with hyperglycemia (about 50% of total kcal), and limit excess added sugars; encourage less processed carbohydrate and fiber food sources. Individualize according to lab work, body mass index, and other risk reduction requirements.
- Maintain protein at about 15–20% of total energy.
- Plan fats at 25–35% of total kcal (encourage monounsaturated fats and omega-3 fatty acids). Low saturated fats and cholesterol may be needed. A controlled fat intake is recommended for prevention and treatment of hyperlipidemia.
- A moderate reduction in total energy intake is important for weight management. Modest weight loss of 5–7% of body weight may be recommended.
- Sufficient intake of minerals such as magnesium may be protective against diabetes. Include more almonds, whole wheat, cooked spinach, baked potatoes, and other magnesium-rich foods.
- Excesses of iron should be avoided; some studies suggest that high intakes cause deposits in the internal organs, including the pancreas. Further studies are needed.
- Include adequate intake of fiber.
- Essential oils such as fenugreek, cinnamon, cumin, and oregano enhance insulin sensitivity (Talpur et al, 2005). Cinnamon may improve blood sugar and lipid levels in diabetes mellitus (1/2 teaspoon daily). It can lower blood glucose, cholesterol, and triglycerides and improve insulin sensitivity (Kahn et al, 2003; Anderson et al, 2004).

CLINICAL INDICATORS

Clinical/History	Lab Work	
Height	Gluc	H & H
Weight	HbA1c	Serum Fe
Waist circumference	Chol, HDL and LDL profiles	Serum folacin
BMI	Trig	BUN, Creat
Diet history	CRP	Ca++, Mg++
I & O	Alb, transthyretin	GFR
BP	Na+, K+	
Temperature		

Common Drugs Used and Potential Side Effects

- Acarbose: The STOP-NIDDM Trial has shown that acarbose treatment in IGT subjects decreased the risk of progression to diabetes by 36% (Delorme and Chiasson, 2005).
- Metformin reduces risk of developing diabetes by 31% over 3 years; it is most effective among younger, heavier people such as those 25–40 years of age who are 50–80 pounds overweight (Herman et al, 2005). It is less effective among older people and people who were not as overweight.

INTERVENTION: NUTRITION EDUCATION, COUNSELING, CARE MANAGEMENT

- Indicate which foods and meal patterns will be most helpful to reduce risk factors for the individual client (for example, controlled carbohydrate, total energy intake). Weight loss is generally needed (Norris et al, 2005). Address total fat intake, including type of fat and control of lipids.
- Promote physical activity that matches client interest and ability. Accumulating 150 minutes or more of physical activity, such as walking, each week is a good plan.

For More Information

- American Diabetes Association–Prediabetes
http://www.diabetes.org/diabetes-prevention/pre-diabetes.jsp
- National Institute of Diabetes and Digestive and Kidney Diseases (NIDDK)–Prediabetes and Insulin Resistance
http://diabetes.niddk.nih.gov/dm/pubs/insulinresistance/
- Prediabetes
http://my.webmd.com/content/Article/75/89896.htm

PREDIABETES—CITED REFERENCES

American Diabetes Association. Standards of Medical Care in Diabetes–2006. *Diabetes Care* 29:4S, 2006.

Anderson RA, et al. Isolation and characterization of polyphenol type-A polymers from cinnamon with insulin-like biological activity. *J Agric Food Chem.* 52:65, 2004.

Delorme S, Chiasson JL. Acarbose in the prevention of cardiovascular disease in subjects with impaired glucose tolerance and type 2 diabetes mellitus. *Curr Opin Pharmacol.* 5:184, 2005.

Herman WH, et al. Diabetes Prevention Program Research Group. The cost-effectiveness of lifestyle modification or metformin in preventing type 2 diabetes in adults with impaired glucose tolerance. *Ann Intern Med.* 142:323, 2005.

Kahn A, et al. Cinnamon improves glucose and lipids of people with type 2 diabetes. *Diabetes Care* 26:3215, 2003.

Norris SL, et al. Long-term effectiveness of weight loss interventions in adults with pre-diabetes. A review. *Am J Prev Med.* 28:126, 2005.

Orchard TJ, et al. The effect of metformin and intensive lifestyle intervention on the metabolic syndrome: the Diabetes Prevention Program randomized trial. *Ann Intern Med.* 142:61, 2005.

Talpur N, et al. Effects of a novel formulation of essential oils on glucose-insulin metabolism in diabetic and hypertensive rats: a pilot study. *Diabetes Obes Metab.* 7:193, 2005.

Zacharova J, et al. The common polymorphisms (single nucleotide polymorphism [SNP] +45 and SNP +276) of the adiponectin gene predict the conversion from impaired glucose tolerance to type 2 diabetes: the STOP-NIDDM trial. *Diabetes* 54:893, 2005.

TYPE 2 DIABETES IN ADULTS

NUTRITIONAL ACUITY RANKING: LEVEL 4

DEFINITIONS AND BACKGROUND

Type 2 diabetes (T2DM) arises because of insulin resistance, when there is failure to use insulin properly combined with relative insulin deficiency. Increased and unrestrained hepatic glucose production as well as diminished glucose uptake and utilization results from insulin resistance occurring in the cells of the liver and other peripheral tissue, especially skeletal muscle; the mechanism is hypothesized to be related to defects in the binding of insulin receptors, decreases in the number of insulin receptors themselves, or the reduced insulin action of postreceptors (Chan and Abrahamson, 2003).

Previous names for type 2 diabetes include "non–insulin-dependent diabetes (NIDDM)," "adult-onset," "type II," "maturity-onset," and "ketosis-resistant" diabetes. Americans with type 2 diabetes account for 90% of all persons with diabetes. A significant percentage (about one third) of individuals who have type 2 diabetes are unaware of their diagnosis. Because type 2 diabetes is progressive, most type 2 diabetic patients will have already lost at least 50% of beta-cell function at the time of diagnosis.

The American Diabetes Association recommends diagnostic screening at 3-year intervals beginning at the age of 45, especially in individuals who have a body mass index (BMI) greater than 25 kg/m^2 (overweight). Risk factors include genetics, obesity, age, history of gestational diabetes, sedentary lifestyle, and smoking. Smith et al (2005) concluded that smoking cessation, decreasing BMI, and decreasing blood pressure (BP) are major modifiable risk factors that are also major determinants of acquiring type 2 diabetes.

For reducing BP, numerous clinical trials and experts support reduction of sodium intake; modest weight loss (4.5 kg); increased physical activity; a low-fat diet that includes fruits, vegetables, and low-fat dairy products; and moderate alcohol intake (Chobanian et al, 2003; Whitworth-Chalmers, 2004).

Randomized controlled trials and outcome studies of medical nutrition therapy (MNT) primarily from registered dietitians in the treatment of type 2 diabetes report improved glycemic outcomes with a decrease in A1c of approximately 1–2%, depending of the duration of diabetes (American Diabetes Association, 2006; Franz et al, 1995; UK Prospective Diabetes Study Group, 1990). Early referral for lifestyle changes and advice will yield the most benefit in prevention of development of type 2 diabetes or minimization of progression of known disease (Kulkarni, 2006).

Patients should be educated about the progressive nature of type 2 diabetes and the importance of glycemic control with appropriate food choices and physical activity in conjunction with antidiabetes medication (Kulkarni, 2006). Maintain focus on lifestyle strategies that will improve blood

TABLE 9-13 Number of Medical Nutrition Therapy Visits Recommended for Type 2 Diabetes

Encounter	Length of Contact	Time between Encounters
1	60–90 minutes	2–4 weeks
2, 3	30–45 minutes	2–4 weeks
4, 5	30–45 minutes	6–12 months

From: National Guideline Clearinghouse. Nutrition practice guidelines for type 1 and type 2 diabetes mellitus. Accessed August 1, 2006 at http://guidelines.gov/summary/summary.aspx?doc_id=3296&nbr=2522.

glucose, BP, and lipids. Diabetes self-management training (DSMT), consisting of a 4-hour class, followed by individual dietitian consults and monthly support meetings can lower A1c at a very low cost when compared with medical interventions (Banister et al, 2004).

The American Dietetic Association recommends 4 MNT visits initially, then 1 visit every 6–12 months for type 2 diabetes (see Table 9-13). Referral to a dietitian within the first month after diagnosis is important. Lifestyle counseling will be needed, especially for special concerns, as in pregnancy. Encouragement for weight management and exercise is especially helpful for managing type 2 diabetes.

INTERVENTION: OBJECTIVES

- Primary care providers should: provide persons with diabetes initial basic nutrition messages; refer patients to a registered dietitian for medical nutrition therapy; follow-up on the person's progress with nutrition intervention; and provide continued education and support (Pastors, 2003).
- Maintain as near normal blood glucose levels as possible by balancing food intake with insulin (either endogenous or exogenous) or oral glucose-lowering medications and activity levels. Improvement with MNT, if successful, is usually seen within 6 weeks and up to a maximum of 6 months; medication may be needed if blood glucose levels are not under control (Pastors, 2003).
- Maintain glycosylated A1c levels <7%, preprandial capillary plasma glucose levels between 90 and 130 mg/dL, and peak postprandial capillary plasma glucose levels <180 mg/dL (American Diabetes Association, 2005). The target goal range for the patient may vary by age and underlying disorders.
- Protect beta-cell function by controlling hyperglycemia. A1c tests should be done at least 2 times a year in patients who are meeting treatment goals and quarterly in patients whose therapy has changes or who are not meeting glycemic goals. NHANES III showed that only 50% of diabetics have been able to achieve an HbA1c level that is <7% (Albu and Raja-Khan, 2003).
- Achieve optimal serum lipid levels to reduce the risk for macrovascular disease. Dyslipidemia is a central component of insulin resistance in all ethnic groups (Howard et al, 1998).
- Emphasis of MNT is on lifestyle strategies to reduce glycemia, dyslipidemia, and BP. Because most patients with type 2 diabetes are overweight and insulin resistant, lifestyle strategies that result in reduced energy intake, usually through reducing the fat content of the diet, and increased energy expenditure through physical activity are recommended (Franz et al, 2002).
- Prevent and treat the acute complications of insulin-treated diabetes such as hypoglycemia, short-term illnesses, and exercise-related problems. Also prevent and treat the long-term complications of diabetes such as renal disease, autonomic neuropathy, hypertension, and cardiovascular disease (see Table 9-2). Consensus about protein currently suggests maintaining usual intake levels (15–20% of total energy intake) and lowering to 0.8 g/kg with early signs of nephropathy.
- Improve overall health through optimal nutrition and physical activity. Dietary Guidelines for Americans and the MyPyramid food guide illustrate nutritional guidelines and nutrient needs for all healthy Americans and can be used by people with diabetes.
- Encourage regular mealtimes. Maintain lifestyle changes through behavior modification, education, and problem-solving strategies.
- Address individual needs according to culture, ethnicity, and lifestyle, while respecting willingness to change. For older adults, provide for nutritional and psychosocial needs. For pregnant or lactating women, provide adequate energy and nutrients for optimal outcomes. Encourage therapeutic lifestyle changes (TLC), considering client's readiness, skills, resources, and current needs.
- Maintain BP levels that reduce risk for vascular disease. Elevated BP has a major impact on renal function.
- Manage problems related to compulsive or binge eating. Patients often report deliberate omission of insulin or oral hypoglycemic agents (OHA) to lose weight (Herpertz et al, 1998).
- Manage children with type 2 diabetes or maturity-onset diabetes of youth (MODY) differently than children who have type 1 diabetes. See the appropriate entries.

INTERVENTION: FOOD AND NUTRITION

- The dietitian should calculate CHO and fat requirements individually according to lipid and glucose levels. Assess dietary history, physical exercise, and activity patterns. Studies support the importance of including food containing CHO from whole grains, fruits, vegetables, and low-fat milk in the diet (American Diabetes Association, 2004).
- Weight control is helpful. A moderate caloric restriction (250–500 calories less than average daily intake as calculated from a food history) and a nutritionally adequate meal plan should be recommended. Moderate weight loss in an obese patient (5–10% of starting weight) may reduce hyperglycemia, dyslipidemia, and hypertension. Extremely low–calorie diets for adults should be performed only in a hospital setting. Restricting calories is important, and people who have a high insulin level lose more weight when they eat a diet with a low glycemic index (Pittas et al, 2005).

- Low-fat, plant-based dietary interventions allow weight loss in overweight individuals, which promotes improved insulin sensitivity and glycemic control (Barnard et al, 2005).
- In morbidly obese patients, gastric bypass surgery is used with favorable results (Pories and Albrecht, 2001). For the severely obese diabetic patient, bariatric surgery may be the only effective treatment; gastric bypass produces significant weight loss and improved glycemic control on a long-term basis (Albu and Raja-Khan, 2003). There are risks from surgery and anesthesia, but the benefits are important as well.
- Spacing of meals (spreading nutrient intake, particularly carbohydrate, throughout the day) and eating breakfast has beneficial effects on fasting lipid and postprandial insulin sensitivity (Farshchi et al, 2005a, 2005b). Meal skipping should be discouraged. Individualize meal plan according to patient preferences.
- Carbohydrate should be calculated as 45–65% of energy intake. Consistency is important.
- Protein should be calculated at 15–20% of daily energy intake with normal renal function and control at 0.8–1.0 g/kg with renal disease. Where weight loss is needed, use of a diet slightly higher in protein may help to enhance insulin sensitivity (Sargrad et al, 2005), but the ADA guidelines do not promote high-protein diets because CHO is an important source of energy, vitamins, minerals, and fiber.
- Fat should be 25–35% of energy intake, with 7–10% of kcal from saturated fats, 10% from polyunsaturated fats, and 10–15% from monounsaturated fats. Limit intake of cholesterol to <200–300 mg/d.
- A vegetarian diet provides natural products and foods that benefit both the carbohydrate and lipid abnormalities in diabetes; whole grains, nuts, soluble fibers (oats, barley), soy proteins, and plant sterols should be consumed often (Jenkins et al, 2003).
- Recommendations for people with diabetes are the same as for the general population concerning fiber. Use more rice, beans, vegetables, oat bran, legumes, barley, produce with skins, apples, oranges, and other produce.
- As part of a healthy lifestyle and to manage hypertension, teach the principles of the DASH diet; 2300 mg/d of sodium is recommended.
- For vitamins and minerals, ensure that patient has adequate dietary intakes. Higher levels of magnesium, chromium, and potassium have been recommended when serum levels are low. There is no need for daily supplements of any singular nutrient; a multivitamin-mineral supplement may be useful.
- Discuss usefulness of artificial sweeteners and food diaries.
- Cinnamon may help to improve blood sugar and lipid levels; 1/2 teaspoon daily can lower blood glucose, cholesterol, and triglycerides and improve insulin sensitivity (Kahn et al, 2003; Anderson et al, 2004). Other essential oils may also improve insulin sensitivity and are being evaluated (Talpur et al, 2005).
- Discuss use of alcohol; to avoid hypoglycemia, alcohol should be consumed with food and limited to 1 drink daily for women and 2 for men (Franz et al, 2002). Light to moderate amounts of alcohol do not increase triglyceride or BP levels, and in a systematic review, moderate alcohol consumption was associated with a decreased incidence of diabetes and a decreased incidence of heart disease in persons with diabetes (Howard et al, 2004); this is likely because alcohol has been reported to increase insulin sensitivity and raise HDL cholesterol levels. Alcoholic beverages should be considered an addition to the regular food/meal plan, and no food needs to be omitted. If consumed daily, calories from alcohol are calculated into the total caloric intake (American Diabetes Association, 2004).
- Abstention from alcohol is recommended for pregnant women and for those persons who have pancreatitis,

Dietary Reference Intakes for Fiber

Age	Fiber (g/d)
Children	
1–3 years	19
4–8 years	25
Males	
9–13 years	31
14–18 years	38
19–50 years	38
51+ years	30
Females	
9–13 years	26
14–18 years	26
19–50 years	25
51+ years	21
Pregnancy	
≤18 years	28
18+ years	28
Lactation	
≤18 years	29
18+ years	29

SAMPLE NUTRITION DIAGNOSTIC STATEMENT

Type 2 Diabetes Mellitus

PES: Self-monitoring knowledge deficit related to lack of understanding how to record food and beverage intake as evidenced by incomplete food records at last two clinic visits and lab of HbA1c = 8.5 mg/dL.

Assessment Data (sources of info): Blood glucose self-monitoring records, food diary worksheets and meal records, blood glucose levels (fasting, 2-hour postprandial and/or HbA1c levels).

Intervention: Teaching patient and family member(s) about use of simple blood glucose self-monitoring records (recording of timing, amount, blood glucose levels) and meal records.

Monitoring and Evaluation: HbA1c levels (goal <7 mg/dL); other glucose labs, food diary and records, discussion about complications of using the records.

advanced neuropathy, severe hypertriglyceridemia, or a history of alcohol abuse (Franz et al, 2002).

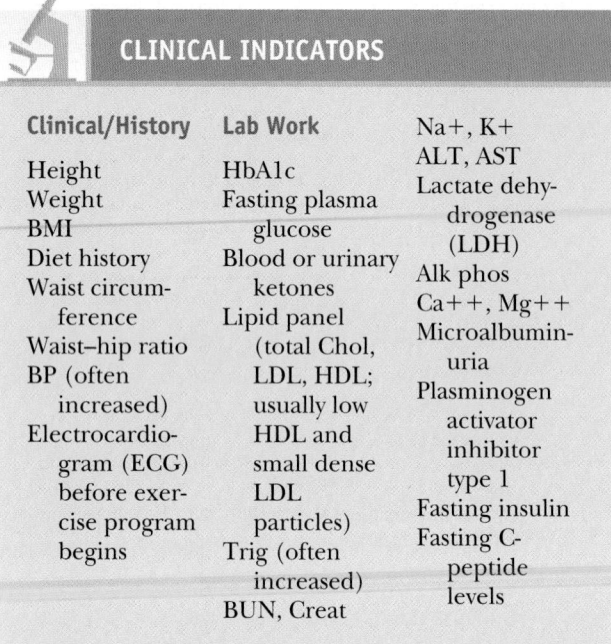

CLINICAL INDICATORS

Clinical/History	Lab Work	
Height	HbA1c	Na+, K+
Weight	Fasting plasma glucose	ALT, AST
BMI	Blood or urinary ketones	Lactate dehydrogenase (LDH)
Diet history	Lipid panel (total Chol, LDL, HDL; usually low HDL and small dense LDL particles)	Alk phos
Waist circumference	Trig (often increased)	Ca++, Mg++
Waist–hip ratio	BUN, Creat	Microalbuminuria
BP (often increased)		Plasminogen activator inhibitor type 1
Electrocardiogram (ECG) before exercise program begins		Fasting insulin
		Fasting C-peptide levels

Common Drugs Used and Potential Side Effects (see Table 9-14)

- Type 2 diabetes is a progressive disease. Medications will need to be combined with lifestyle strategies. Insulin may be used in combination with oral therapy or alone. If oral glucose-lowering medications do not achieve normoglycemia, combined oral therapies (drugs from two or more classes) can be initiated. If combination oral therapy does not work, insulin is needed.
- When insulin therapy is required in the treatment of the obese diabetic patient, combinations with oral agents that have been shown to minimize the amount of exogenous insulin that is required may minimize weight gain (Albu and Raja-Khan, 2003). Insulin may also be needed for refractory hyperglycemia, diabetic ketoacidosis, stress, infection, or pregnancy.
- Multiple drug therapy is generally required to achieve BP targets. Angiotensin-converting enzyme (ACE) inhibitors, angiotensin receptor blockers (ARBs), beta-blockers, diuretics, and calcium channel blockers may all be helpful in managing high BP.
- Aspirin therapy (75–162 mg/d) is recommended as a primary prevention strategy to protect against cardiovascular events and as a secondary prevention strategy in those with a history of cardiovascular disease.
- In individuals with diabetes over the age of 40 years and without overt cardiovascular disease (CVD), statin therapy to achieve an LDL <100 mg/dL is recommended. For people with diabetes and overt CVD, an LDL cholesterol goal of <70 mg/dL is recommended. Lifestyle modifications focusing on reducing saturated fat and cholesterol and increasing physical activity are also important.
- Antipsychotic agents may contribute to the development of the metabolic syndrome and increase the risk for type 2 diabetes and heart disease (Newcomer, 2004). More research is needed in this area.
- Metformin improves insulin sensitivity in patients with IGT (Diabetes Prevention Program Research Group, 2002; Polonsky et al, 2003).
- Medications such as steroids, beta-blockers, and diuretics may cause hyperglycemia in some patients.
- Vitamin C may cause false-positive urinary glucose levels when given in large doses.
- Xenical (fat blocker) may help cut heart risk in patients with type 2 diabetes. The obese diabetic patient who is poorly controlled with maximum oral hypoglycemic therapy may benefit from weight-reducing agents, such as sibutramine or orlistat (Albu and Raja-Khan, 2003).

Herbs, Botanicals, and Supplements

- Herbs and botanical supplements should not be used without discussing with physician. There is insufficient evidence to draw definitive conclusions about the efficacy of individual herbs and supplements for diabetes, and several supplements may warrant further study (Yeh et al, 2003).
- Bilberry contains anthocyanosides that counteract cellular damage to the retina. Mild drowsiness and skin rashes have been noted.
- Chromium has been widely studied for its enhancement of insulin utilization (Yeh et al, 2003). Skin allergies, renal toxicity, and altered iron and zinc absorption can occur. Use only with noted deficiency levels. A randomized, double-blind, placebo-controlled study found no beneficial effects of chromium supplementation (800 μg/d) in people with IGT despite increases in serum chromium levels (Gunton et al, 2005).
- Evening primrose oil may prevent or limit neuropathy due to gamma linoleic acid, an essential fatty acid. It can cause headache and GI distress in susceptible individuals.
- Fenugreek may lower glucose levels due to psyllium content. It is part of the peanut family and may cause allergic reactions. Do not take with MAO inhibitors for depression. It has the potential for drug interactions with other medications as well.
- Garlic may lower blood glucose levels if used in large amounts. Evidence is preliminary.
- Gingko biloba may help control neuropathy by maintaining integrity of blood vessels and reducing stickiness of blood and clotting. It has some antioxidant properties. Avoid taking with warfarin, aspirin, and other anticoagulant drugs because it functions as a blood thinner. Headache and interactions with other drugs can occur
- Ginseng (American) may lower blood glucose levels (Yeh et al, 2003). It increases energy and activity levels, which may lead to better glucose control. Do not take with warfarin, aspirin, MAO inhibitors, caffeine, antipsychotics, insulin, and oral hypoglycemics because of fluctuations in blood glucose levels, bleed-

TABLE 9-14 Drugs Used for Type 2 Diabetes

Combination therapy rather than monotherapy is typically used to achieve glucose control in patients who are not at glycemic goals (Chipkin, 2005). In pediatrics, current management involves lifestyle modification (nutritional and exercise) along with pharmacological agents, such as insulin (Gungor and Arslanian, 2002).

Drugs	Action	How to Take	Potential Effects	Other
Secretagogues				
Sulfonylureas	Lower blood glucose by augmenting insulin secretion.	30–60 minutes before eating	Weight gain and hypoglycemia can occur.	Never give to a patient who is fasting for any reason. Avoid taking with alcohol to avoid flushing, altered heart rate.
Long-acting: Glyburide (DiaBeta, Micronase); glipizide (Glucotrol); glimepiride (Amaryl)		Take with breakfast or a main meal, 1–2 times daily.	Nausea, GI distress, diarrhea, and heartburn may occur. With glimepiride, elevated liver enzymes may occur; hypoalbuminemia can increase effects.	
Short-acting: Repaglinide (Prandin); senaglinide (Starlix)	Action on insulin secretions is more rapid and shorter than that of sulfonylureas. Offers better control of postprandial hyperglycemia and is associated with a lower risk of delayed hypoglycemic episodes.	Take within 30 minutes before meals.		
Sensitizers				
Metformin (Glucophage)	Inhibit glucose release by liver. Hepatic glucose output inhibited. Enhances weight loss.	Take with food. Increase dose slowly over 2 weeks.	Diarrhea, abdominal pain, flatulence	Avoid with IBD, DKA.
Alpha-Glucosidase Inhibitors				
Acarbose (Precose); miglitol (Glyset)	Starch blockers that delay intestinal glucose absorption.	Take with first bite of food.	GI intolerance may occur.	Exercise enhances effectiveness. Not usually given alone. If taking this medication with insulin or sulfonylurea, treat hypoglycemia with glucose because breakdown of other sources of CHO is delayed.
Thiazolidinediones: Rosiglitazone (Avandia); pioglitazone (Actos)	Increase tissue glucose utilization, mostly in peripheral tissue such as muscle.	Take with or without food.	Liver damage is possible.	Should not take with significant heart disease because of potential fluid retention or heart failure. May lead to weight gain.

IBD, inflammatory bowel disease; DKA, diabetic ketoacidosis.

ing and platelet functioning, or changes in BP and heart rate. Avoid taking with steroids because ginseng functions as a steroidal herb. Headache, insomnia, nausea, and occasional menstrual difficulties can occur. Take with a meal to avoid unintentional hypoglycemia.

- *Gymnema sylvestre* is a hypoglycemic herb. It is highly potent and should be used only under doctor's supervision because it may change insulin requirements. It warrants further study (Yeh et al, 2003).
- Pancreas tonic, an Ayurvedic herbal supplement, given as 2 capsules 3 times per day for 3 months, significantly improved glucose control in type 2 diabetic patients with HbA1c levels between 10.0% and 12.0% in a properly designed, prospective intervention trial (Hsia et al, 2004).
- Turmeric, the rhizome of *Curcuma,* may decrease blood glucose levels.
- Vanadium can lower serum glucose levels. It has been associated with cancer cell growth and can be toxic at therapeutic levels. It shows potential (Yeh et al, 2003).

INTERVENTION: NUTRITION EDUCATION, COUNSELING, CARE MANAGEMENT

- Medical nutrition intervention in patients with diabetes should address the metabolic abnormalities of glucose, lipids, and BP (Kulkarni, 2006). To meet the specific needs of the patient, adapt drug therapy to enhance outcomes and quality of life.

- Diabetes self-management education (DSME) is an essential element of diabetes care, and national standards have been based on evidence for its benefits; DSME helps patients optimize metabolic control, prevent and manage complications, and maximize quality of life in a cost-effective manner (American Diabetes Association, 2006). Health care providers should refer newly diagnosed patients to a dietitian. The dietitian should then regularly reassess patients who have diabetes over time for modification of medications and food intake patterns.
- Emphasize the importance of regular mealtimes, use of medications, and balanced activity (Diabetes Prevention Program Research Group, 2004).
- Emphasize the importance of self-care and optimal functioning. Include instructions on how to handle illness, stress, dining out, exercise, and label reading and how to use sucrose or fructose and sugar alcohols.
- To improve glycemic control, assist with weight maintenance, and reduce risk of CVD, at least 150 min/wk of moderate-intensity aerobic physical activity (50–70% of maximum heart rate) is recommended and/or at least 90 min/wk of vigorous aerobic exercise (>70% of maximum heart rate); activity should be distributed over at least 3 d/wk, with no more than 2 consecutive days without physical activity (American Diabetes Association, 2006). Another easy guideline for physical activity is to exercise for 30 min/d (American Diabetes Association, 2006; Church et al, 2004; Kriska et al, 2003).
- High-intensity exercise may be beneficial, even in older adults; start gradually and increase to desired intensity and duration (Dunstan et al, 2002). However, high-intensity exercise and resistance training may be harmful for those persons with complications such as neuropathy, coronary heart disease, and retinopathy.
- In the absence of contraindications, people with type 2 diabetes should be encouraged to perform resistance exercise 3 times a week, targeting all major muscle groups and progressing to 3 sets of 8–10 repetitions at a weight that cannot be lifted more than 8–10 times (American Diabetes Association, 2006).
- Identify potential or real obstacles and discuss options (e.g., negative emotions, resisting temptations, dining away from home, feeling deprived, time pressures, temptations, competing priorities, social events, family support, food refusal, and lack of support from friends should be discussed).
- Food and nutrition labeling should be explained. Shopping education may also be beneficial.
- Encourage group support, behavior modification, and nutritional counseling for overweight persons. Intensive weight loss and physical activity interventions are designed to achieve and maintain weight loss in overweight type 2 diabetic patients in the Look AHEAD clinical trial (Ryan et al, 2003).
- Small changes lead to greater self-esteem than continued failures at change. Sequential rather than simultaneous dietary changes work well for most people and can improve a sense of self-efficacy.
- A comprehensive lifestyle self-management program (Mediterranean low–saturated fat diet, stress management training, exercise, group support, and smoking cessation) can reduce cardiovascular risk factors in postmenopausal women with type 2 diabetes (Toobert et al, 2003). Discuss foods that have a low glycemic index such as salads with oil and vinegar dressing, high-fat granola cereal, and most fresh fruits and vegetables (Pittas et al, 2005).
- MNT is effective; a healthy meal plan or a low-literacy tool can be useful in teaching key changes for those who need it (Ziemer et al, 2003).
- Campaigns to reduce the risk of obesity and type 2 diabetes should promote not only increasing exercise levels but also decreasing sedentary behaviors, especially prolonged TV watching (Hu, 2003).
- Before any type of surgery, blood glucose should be maintained in a range between 100 and 200 mg/dL. Perioperative hyperglycemia may be managed with doses of rapid-acting insulin. Correct abnormalities before surgery, when possible.
- In critically ill hospitalized patients, blood glucose levels should be kept as close to 110 mg/dL as possible and generally <180 mg/dL. These patients will usually require intravenous insulin. In non–critically ill hospitalized patients, premeal blood glucose should be kept as close to 90–130 mg/dL as possible, with a postprandial blood glucose <180 mg/dL, and insulin should be used as necessary (American Diabetes Association, 2005).

For More Information

- American Diabetes Association
  GENNID Resource
  http://www.diabetes.org/
- American Diabetes Association–Medicare Policy and Benefits
  http://www.diabetes.org/for-health-professionals-and-scientists/recognition/dsmt-mntfaqs.jsp
- American Diabetes Association–Type 2 Diabetes
  http://www.diabetes.org/type-2-diabetes.jsp
- American Dietetic Association: Type 2 Diabetes Practice Guidelines
  http://www.eatright.org/cps/rde/xchg/ada/hs.xsl/index.html

TYPE 2 DIABETES IN ADULTS—CITED REFERENCES

Albu J, Raja-Khan N. The management of the obese diabetic patient. *Prim Care.* 30:465, 2003.

American Diabetes Association. Nutrition principles and recommendations in diabetes. *Diabetes Care* 27:S36, 2004 (suppl 1).

American Diabetes Association. Standards of Medical Care in Diabetes. *Diabetes Care* 28:S4, 2005 (suppl 1).

American Diabetes Association. Standards of Medical Care in Diabetes–2006. *Diabetes Care* 29:4S, 2006.

Anderson RA, et al. Isolation and characterization of polyphenol type-A polymers from cinnamon with insulin-like biological activity. *J Agric Food Chem.* 52:65, 2004.

Banister NA, et al. Diabetes self-management training program in a community clinic improves patient outcomes at modest cost. *J Am Diet Assoc* 104:807, 2004.

Barnard ND, et al. The effects of a low-fat, plant-based dietary intervention on body weight, metabolism, and insulin sensitivity. *Am J Med.* 118:991, 2005.

Chan JL, Abrahamson MJ. Pharmacological management of type 2 diabetes mellitus: rationale for rational use of insulin. *Mayo Clin Proc.* 78:459, 2003.

Chipkin SR. How to select and combine oral agents for patients with type 2 diabetes mellitus. *Am J Med.* 118:4S, 2005.

Chobanian AV, et al. National Heart, Lung, and Blood Institute Joint National Committee on Prevention, Detection, Evaluation, and Treatment of High Blood Pressure. The Seventh Report of the Joint National Committee on Prevention, Detection, Evaluation, and Treatment of High Blood Pressure: the JNC 7 report. *JAMA.* 289:2560, 2003.

Church TS, et al. Exercise capacity and body composition as predictors of mortality among men with diabetes. *Diabetes Care* 27:83, 2004.
Diabetes Prevention Program Research Group. Achieving weight and activity goals among diabetes prevention program lifestyle participants. *Obes Res.* 12:1426, 2004.
Diabetes Prevention Program Research Group. Reduction in the incidence of type 2 diabetes with lifestyle intervention or metformin. *N Engl J Med.* 346:393, 2002.
Dunstan DW, et al. High-intensity resistance training improves glycemic control in older patients with type 2 diabetes. *Diabetes Care* 25:1729, 2002.
Farshchi HR, Taylor MA, Macdonald IA. Beneficial metabolic effects of regular meal frequency on dietary thermogenesis, insulin sensitivity, and fasting lipid profiles in healthy obese women. *Am J Clin Nutr.* 81:16, 2005a.
Farshchi HR, Taylor MA, Macdonald IA. Deleterious effect of omitting breakfast on insulin sensitivity and fasting lipid profiles in healthy lean women. *Am J Clin Nutr.* 81:388, 2005b.
Franz M, et al. American Diabetes Association Position Statement: evidence-based nutrition principles and recommendations for the treatment and prevention of diabetes and related conditions. *J Am Diet Assoc.* 102:109, 2002.
Franz MJ, et al. Effectiveness of medical nutrition therapy provided by dietitians in the management of non-insulin-dependent diabetes mellitus: a randomized, controlled clinical trial. *J Am Diet Assoc.* 95:1009, 1995.
Gungor N, Arslanian S. Pathophysiology of type 2 diabetes mellitus in children and adolescents: treatment implications. *Treat Endocrinol.* 1:359, 2002.
Gunton JE, et al. Chromium supplementation does not improve glucose tolerance, insulin sensitivity, or lipid profile. *Diabetes Care* 28:712, 2005.
Herpertz S, et al. Comorbidity of diabetes and eating disorders: does diabetes control reflect disturbed eating behavior? *Diabetes Care* 21:1110, 1998.
Howard AA, Amsten JH, Gourevitch MN. Effect of alcohol consumption on diabetes mellitus. A systematic review. *Ann Intern Med.* 140:211, 2004.
Howard B, et al. Relationship between insulin resistance and lipoproteins in nondiabetic African Americans, Hispanics, and non-Hispanic whites: The Insulin Resistance Atherosclerosis Study. *Metabolism* 47:1174, 1998.
Hsia SH, et al. Effect of pancreas tonic (an ayurvedic herbal supplement) in type 2 diabetes mellitus. *Metabolism* 53:1166, 2004.
Hu FB. Sedentary lifestyle and risk of obesity and type 2 diabetes. *Lipids* 38:103, 2003.
Jenkins DJ, et al. Type 2 diabetes and the vegetarian diet. *Am J Clin Nutr.* 78:610S, 2003.
Kahn A, et al. Cinnamon improves glucose and lipids of people with type 2 diabetes. *Diabetes Care* 26:3215, 2003.
Kriska AM, et al. Physical activity, obesity, and the incidence of type 2 diabetes in a high-risk population. *Am J Epidemiol.* 158:669, 2003.
Kulkarni K. Diets do not fail: the success of medical nutrition therapy in patients with diabetes. *Endocr Pract.* 12:121S, 2006.
Newcomer JL. Metabolic risk during antipsychotic treatment. *Clin Ther.* 26:1936, 2004.
Pastors JG. Medications or lifestyle change with medical nutrition therapy. *Curr Diabetes Rep.* 3:386, 2003.
Pittas AG, et al. A low-glycemic load diet facilitates greater weight loss in overweight adults with high insulin secretion but not in overweight adults with low insulin secretion in the CALERIE Trial. *Diabetes Care* 28:2939, 2005.
Polonsky WH, et al. Integrating medical management with diabetes self-management training. A randomized control trial of the Diabetes Outpatient Intensive Treatment program. *Diabetes Care* 26:3048, 2003.
Pories W, Albrecht R. Etiology of type II diabetes mellitus: role of the foregut. *World J Surg.* 25:527, 2001.
Ryan DH, et al. Look AHEAD (Action for Health in Diabetes): design and methods for a clinical trial of weight loss for the prevention of cardiovascular disease in type 2 diabetes. *Control Clin Trials.* 24:610, 2003.
Sargrad KR, et al. Effect of high protein vs high carbohydrate intake on insulin sensitivity, body weight, hemoglobin A1c, and blood pressure in patients with type 2 diabetes. *J Am Diet Assoc.* 105:573, 2005.
Smith GD, et al. Incidence of type 2 diabetes in the randomized multiple risk factor intervention trial. *Ann Intern Med.* 142:313, 2005.
Talpur N, et al. Effects of a novel formulation of essential oils on glucose-insulin metabolism in diabetic and hypertensive rats: a pilot study. *Diabetes Obes Metab.* 7:193, 2005.
Toobert DJ, et al. Biologic and quality-of-life outcomes from the Mediterranean Lifestyle Program: a randomized clinical trial. *Diabetes Care* 26:2288, 2003.
UK Prospective Diabetes Study Group. Response of fasting plasma glucose to diet therapy in newly presenting type II diabetic patients (UKPDS 7). *Metabolism* 39:905, 1990.
Whitworth JA, Chalmers J. World Health Organization-International Society of Hypertension (WHO/ISH) hypertension guidelines. *Clin Exp Hypertens* 26:747, 2004.
Yeh GY, et al. Systematic review of herbs and dietary supplements for glycemic control in diabetes. *Diabetes Care* 26:1277, 2003.
Ziemer DC, et al. A simple meal plan emphasizing healthy food choices is as effective as an exchange-based meal plan for urban African Americans with type 2 diabetes. *Diabetes Care* 26:1719, 2003.

TYPE 2 DIABETES IN CHILDREN AND TEENS

NUTRITIONAL ACUITY RANKING: LEVEL 4

DEFINITIONS AND BACKGROUND

Type 2 diabetes (T2DM) arises because of insulin resistance, when there is failure to use insulin properly combined with relative insulin deficiency. Increased and unrestrained hepatic glucose production as well as diminished glucose uptake and utilization results from insulin resistance occurring in the cells of the liver and other peripheral tissue, especially skeletal muscle; the mechanism is hypothesized to be related to defects in the binding of insulin receptors, decreases in the number of insulin receptors themselves, or the reduced insulin action of postreceptors (Chan and Abrahamson, 2003).

In children, puberty often unmasks type 2 diabetes in genetically susceptible individuals. Obesity is another factor. For example, the emergence of type 2 diabetes mellitus in the American Indian/Alaskan Native pediatric populations presents a new challenge for pediatricians and other health care professionals; preventive efforts, early diagnosis, and collaborative care of the patient and family are essential (Gahagan et al, 2003).

Childhood obesity and type 2 diabetes can be prevented. Breastfeeding, reduced television and sedentary lifestyles, teaching healthy eating principles early in life, family-based approaches, and screening are all important in managing this epidemic. Screening should be available for children whose BMI is greater than the 85th percentile at puberty or at age 10 plus any two of the following risk factors: family history, increased risk by ethnicity, or signs of insulin resistance such as polycystic ovary syndrome (PCOS), hypertension, dyslipidemia, or acanthosis. Weight greater than 120% of ideal for height also warrants screening.

Fasting blood glucose levels should be checked at least every 2 years in high-risk children. Type 2 diabetes in childhood can lead to end-stage renal disease and mortality in middle age; long duration is more detrimental (Pavkov et al, 2006).

INTERVENTION: OBJECTIVES

- Maintain as near normal blood glucose levels as possible by balancing food intake with insulin (either endogenous or exogenous) or oral glucose-lowering medications and activity levels.
- Try to maintain glycosylated A1c levels <7%. Target goal range for the patient may vary by age and underlying disorders: <6 years old, 7.5–8.5%; 6–12 years old, <8%; 13–19 years old, <7.5%. Preprandial capillary plasma glucose levels should be kept between 90 and 130 mg/dL.
- Protect beta-cell function by controlling hyperglycemia. A1c tests should be done at least twice a year in patients who are meeting treatment goals and quarterly in patients who are not meeting glycemic goals.
- Achieve optimal serum lipid levels to reduce the risk for macrovascular disease.
- Emphasis of medical nutrition therapy (MNT) is on lifestyle strategies to reduce hyperglycemica, dyslipidemia, and blood pressure (BP).
- Prevent and treat acute complications, short-term illnesses, and exercise-related problems and the long-term complications of renal disease, autonomic neuropathy, hypertension, and cardiovascular disease.
- Maintain BP levels that reduce risk for vascular disease. Elevated BP has a major impact on renal function.
- Improve overall health through optimal nutrition and physical activity. Dietary Guidelines for Americans and the MyPyramid food guidance system illustrate nutritional guidelines and can be used by young people with diabetes.
- Encourage regular mealtimes. Maintain lifestyle changes through behavior modification, education, and problem-solving strategies.
- Working with the whole family is important. Promote family and individualized psychosocial counseling to handle depression and emotions.
- Address individual needs according to culture, ethnicity, and lifestyle, while respecting willingness to change. Encourage therapeutic lifestyle changes (TLC), considering the child's needs and family circumstances.
- Manage problems related to compulsive or binge eating. Patients often report deliberate omission of medication in order to lose weight.

INTERVENTION: FOOD AND NUTRITION

- The dietitian should calculate CHO and fat requirements individually according to age and to serum lipid and glucose levels. Assess dietary history, physical exercise, and activity patterns. Studies support the importance of carbohydrate from whole grains, fruits, vegetables, and low-fat milk (American Diabetes Association, 2004).
- Moderate weight loss in an obese patient (5–10% of starting weight) may reduce hyperglycemia, dyslipidemia, and hypertension. A moderate caloric restriction (250–500 calories less than average daily intake as calculated from a food history) and a nutritionally adequate meal plan should be recommended.
- For teen boys over age 15, it may be useful to calculate caloric needs as 18 kcal/lb for usual activity and 16 kcal/lb if sedentary; teen girls over age 15 have needs that are estimated the same as for an adult. Extremely low–calorie diets are not recommended for children or teens. In morbidly obese children, gastric bypass surgery should be the last option.
- Spacing of meals (spreading nutrient intake, particularly carbohydrate, throughout the day) and eating breakfast have beneficial effects on fasting lipid and postprandial insulin sensitivity (Farshchi et al, 2005). Meal skipping should be discouraged. Individualize meal plan according to patient preferences.
- Carbohydrate should be calculated as 45–65% of energy intake. Consistency is important.
- Protein should be calculated at 15–20% of daily energy intake with normal renal function, and control at 0.8–1.0 g/kg with renal disease.
- Fat should be 25–35% of energy intake, with 7–10% of kcal from saturated fats, 10% from polyunsaturated fats, and 10–15% from monounsaturated fats. Limit intake of cholesterol to 200–300 mg/d.
- Recommendations for fiber include rice, beans, vegetables, oat bran, legumes, barley, produce with skins, apples, oranges, and other produce. The guideline for fiber suggests 19–38 g/d.
- As part of a healthy lifestyle and to manage hypertension, teach the principles of the DASH diet; 2300 mg/d of sodium is recommended.
- For vitamins and minerals, ensure that patient has adequate dietary intakes. Higher levels of magnesium, chromium, and potassium have been recommended when serum levels are low. There is no need for daily supplements of any singular nutrient; a multivitamin-mineral supplement may be useful.
- Include phytochemicals and antioxidants in the diet, such as cinnamon (Anderson et al, 2004) and fenugreek (Talpur et al, 2005). Although studies have been performed in adults, there may be benefit for children and teens as well.
- Discuss usefulness of artificial sweeteners and food diaries.
- Discuss menu options at school or fast food choices that are lower in total fat.
- Discuss exercise benefits and goals.
- Discuss the need for adequate fluid intake.

CLINICAL INDICATORS

Clinical/History		
Height	BMI	Waist–hip ratio
Weight	Diet history	BP (often increased)
	Waist circumference	

Lab Work	Plasminogen activator inhibitor type 1	Trig (often increased)
Fasting plasma glucose	Total Chol, LDL, HDL (usually low HDL and small dense LDL particles)	BUN, Creat
HbA1c		Na+, K+
CRP		ALT, AST
Blood or urinary ketones		LDH
Urinary microalbuminuria		Alk phos
		Ca++, Mg++
		Alb

Common Drugs Used and Potential Side Effects (see Table 9-14; Children with Diabetes, 2005)

- Oral agents may be used when blood glucose and other treatment goals are not met through diet and exercise alone. Glucophage should be the first oral agent used because it works as well as the sulfonylureas in controlling blood sugar levels and carries little risk of low blood sugar reactions. Glucophage should not be used in children with known liver and kidney disease, low oxygen problems, or severe infections. Other oral agents such as a sulfonylurea or meglitinide can be added if control does not improve after 3–6 months.
- The thiazolidinediones probably should not be used in children.
- Insulin therapy should be started in children with severely elevated blood sugar levels or children with intense thirst and frequent urination. There are a wide variety of insulin regimens that can be used. The regimens range anywhere from bedtime alone to multiple daily injections. Once blood sugars are under control, glucophage can be added while decreasing insulin dosage.
- Pharmacologic options for weight loss, including metformin, orlistat, and sibutramine, are being studied (Miller and Silverstein, 2006).

Herbs, Botanicals, and Supplements

- Herbs and botanical supplements should not be used in children and teens. In addition, there is insufficient evidence to draw definitive conclusions about the efficacy of individual herbs and supplements for diabetes (Yeh et al, 2003).

INTERVENTION: NUTRITION EDUCATION, COUNSELING, CARE MANAGEMENT

- Health care providers are encouraged to refer newly diagnosed patients to a dietitian. The dietitian should regularly reassess children and teens for overall growth and health status.
- Stress the importance of parental supervision and support.
- Children with diabetes often benefit from attending diabetes camps for youth and support groups for family counseling.
- Children with type 2 diabetes and their significant others should participate in a diabetes self-management education, where self-monitoring of blood glucose, medications and their use, exercise, and meal planning are taught (Children with Diabetes, 2005).
- Emphasize the importance of regular mealtimes, use of medications, and balanced activity (Diabetes Prevention Program Research Group, 2004). Home blood glucose monitoring records and food/exercise records are important to maintain.
- Emphasize the importance of self-care and optimal functioning. Include instructions on how to handle illness, stress, dining out, exercise, and label reading and how to use sucrose or fructose and sugar alcohols.
- Identify potential or real obstacles and discuss options (e.g., negative emotions, resisting temptations, dining away from home, feeling deprived, time pressures, competing priorities, social events, family support, food refusal, and lack of support from friends should be discussed).
- Food and nutrition labeling should be explained.
- Encourage group support, behavior modification, and nutritional counseling for overweight persons. Small changes lead to greater self-esteem than continued failures at change. Sequential rather than simultaneous dietary changes work best and can improve a sense of self-efficacy.
- Suggested guidelines for physical activity: 3–4 times a week, exercise for 30–60 min/d (Church et al, 2004; Kriska et al, 2003).

For More Information

- Centers for Disease Control and Prevention (CDC) Diabetes Projects
  http://www.cdc.gov/diabetes/projects/cda2.htm
- CDC Reference Documents
  http://www.cdc.gov/diabetes/projects/ref.htm
- Children with Diabetes
  http://www.childrenwithdiabetes.com/d_0n_d00.htm

TYPE 2 DIABETES IN CHILDREN AND TEENS—CITED REFERENCES

American Diabetes Association. Nutrition principles and recommendations in diabetes. *Diabetes Care* 27:S36, 2004 (suppl 1).

Anderson RA, et al. Isolation and characterization of polyphenol type-A polymers from cinnamon with insulin-like biological activity. *J Agric Food Chem.* 52:65, 2004.

Chan JL, Abrahamson MJ. Pharmacological management of type 2 diabetes mellitus: rationale for rational use of insulin. *Mayo Clin Proc.* 78:459, 2003.

Children with Diabetes. Type 2 diabetes in children. 2005. Available at http://www.childrenwithdiabetes.com/d_0n_d00.htm.

Church TS, et al. Exercise capacity and body composition as predictors of mortality among men with diabetes. *Diabetes Care* 27:83, 2004.

Diabetes Prevention Program Research Group. Achieving weight and activity goals among diabetes prevention program lifestyle participants. *Obes Res.* 12:1426, 2004.

Farshchi HR, Taylor MA, Macdonald IA. Beneficial metabolic effects of regular meal frequency on dietary thermogenesis, insulin sensitivity, and fasting lipid profiles in healthy obese women. *Am J Clin Nutr.* 81:16, 2005.

Gahagan S, et al. Prevention and treatment of type 2 diabetes mellitus in children, with special emphasis on American Indian and Alaska Native children. American Academy of Pediatrics Committee on Native American Child Health. *Pediatrics* 112:e328, 2003.

Herpertz S, et al. Comorbidity of diabetes and eating disorders: does diabetes control reflect disturbed eating behavior? *Diabetes Care* 21:1110, 1998.

Kriska AM, et al. Physical activity, obesity, and the incidence of type 2 diabetes in a high-risk population. *Am J Epidemiol.* 158:669, 2003.

Miller JL, Silverstein JH. The treatment of type 2 diabetes mellitus in youth: which therapies? *Treat Endocrinol.* 5:201, 2006.
Pavkov ME, et al. Effect of youth-onset type 2 diabetes mellitus on incidence of end-stage renal disease and mortality in young and middle-aged Pima Indians. *JAMA.* 296:421, 2006.
Talpur N, et al. Effects of a novel formulation of essential oils on glucose-insulin metabolism in diabetic and hypertensive rats: a pilot study. *Diabetes Obes Metab.* 7:193, 2005.
Yeh GY, et al. Systematic review of herbs and dietary supplements for glycemic control in diabetes. *Diabetes Care* 26:1277, 2003.

GESTATIONAL DIABETES

NUTRITIONAL ACUITY RANKING: LEVEL 4

DEFINITIONS AND BACKGROUND

Gestational diabetes mellitus (GDM) involves any level of glucose intolerance with the first onset or recognition during pregnancy. It affects 7% of all pregnancies. While pregnancy itself is a metabolic stress test, increased insulin resistance occurs because gestational hormones such as human placental lactogen (HPL) interfere with insulin action. GDM is also associated with increased anti–human leukocyte antigen (HLA) class II antibodies in the maternal circulation (Steinborn, 2006).

Obesity and other factors that promote insulin resistance appear to enhance the risk of type 2 diabetes after GDM, whereas markers of islet cell–directed autoimmunity are associated with an increase in the risk of type 1 diabetes (American Diabetes Association, 2004). About half of women who have GDM will proceed to have type 2 diabetes later and are mostly the same women who were at risk for type 2 diabetes before pregnancy. Offspring of women with GDM are at increased risk of obesity, glucose intolerance, and diabetes in late adolescence and young adulthood (American Diabetes Association, 2004).

High-risk individuals should undergo glucose testing as soon as feasible; obesity, previous history of GDM, and strong family history of diabetes are risks that should be evaluated early in pregnancy.

Inflammation is associated with the development of GDM (Wolf et al, 2004). Prepregnancy weight is strongly associated with GDM, whereas weight gain during pregnancy is associated with impaired glucose tolerance only among overweight women (Saldana et al, 2006). During the first half of pregnancy, transfer of maternal glucose to the fetus occurs; during the second half of pregnancy, diabetogenic action of placental hormones outweighs glucose transfer, and average insulin requirement typically doubles. Table 9-15 lists the risk factors for GDM.

Diabetes in pregnancy poses many complications and risks. Poor glucose control in pregnancy can lead to problems for the infant such as macrosomia, shoulder dystocia, neural tube defects, hypocalcemia, hypomagnesemia, hyperbilirubinemia, birth trauma, prematurity syndrome, neonatal hypoglycemia, and an increased risk for obesity and diabetes in the future (Preece and Jovanovic, 2002). Daily self-monitoring of blood glucose (SMBG) is important; the risk for fetal demise is higher when fasting glucose levels exceed 105 mg/dL or pregnancy progresses past term (American Diabetes Association, 2004).

For the mother with GDM, there is a higher risk of hypertension, preeclampsia, urinary tract infections, cesarean section, and future diabetes. Excellent blood glucose control with diet and, when necessary, insulin will result in improved perinatal outcome (Gabbe and Graves, 2003).

Despite the potential for increased morbidity in GDM, corrected perinatal outcomes are usually quite good (Lucas, 2001). Use of family planning, early screening for fetal abnormalities, compliance, glycemic and blood pressure control during pregnancy, and improved neonatal care make a big difference. While GDM is not itself an indication for cesarean delivery or for delivery before 38 weeks of gestation, prolonged gestation past 38 weeks increases the risk of fetal macrosomia (American Diabetes Association, 2004).

Nutrition recommendations for women with GDM should be based on a thorough nutrition assessment, especially for height and weight. Monitoring blood glucose levels, urine ketones, appetite, and weight gain guides the individualized nutrition prescription and meal plan. Adjustments should be made to the meal plan throughout pregnancy to ensure desired outcomes. See Table 9-16.

TABLE 9-15 Risk for Developing Gestational Diabetes Mellitus (GDM) (one or more of the following factors)

- Obesity in the woman; body mass index >29.
- Family history of diabetes in a first-degree relative (parents or siblings).
- Gestational diabetes or presence of a birth defect in a previous pregnancy.
- Older maternal age (>25 years old).
- Previous stillbirth or spontaneous miscarriage.
- Previous birth of a large baby (>9 lb).
- A history of pregnancy-induced high blood pressure, urinary tract infections, or hydramnios (extra amniotic fluid).
- History of abnormal glucose tolerance.
- Hispanic American, African American, Asian, Pacific Islander, American Indian background.

GDM often presents with hyperglycemia and glycosuria. Selective screening at 24–28 weeks of pregnancy is generally recommended, with a glucose challenge test and 1-hour assessment using either a 100-g or 75-g oral glucose load. Two or more of the venous plasma glucose concentrations must be met or exceeded for a positive diagnosis. The test should be done in the morning after an overnight fast. American Diabetes Association criteria for GDM are noted in Table 9-16.

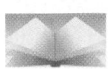

TABLE 9-16 Glucose Testing for Gestational Diabetes Mellitus (GDM)

One-Step Approach

Perform a diagnostic oral glucose tolerance test (OGTT) without prior plasma or serum glucose screening. The one-step approach may be cost effective in high-risk patients or populations.

Two-Step Approach

Perform an initial screening by measuring the plasma or serum glucose concentration 1 hour after a 50-g oral glucose load (glucose challenge test [GCT]), and perform a diagnostic OGTT on the subset of women exceeding the glucose threshold value on the GCT. When the two-step approach is used, a glucose threshold value >140 mg/dL (>7.8 mmol/L) identifies approximately 80% of women with GDM, and the yield is further increased to 90% by using a cutoff of >130 mg/dL (>7.2 mmol/L).

Glucose Load	Glucose (mg/dL)
Glucose load, 100 g	
Fasting	95
1 hour	180
2 hours	155
3 hours	140
Glucose load, 75 g (not as well validated)	
Fasting	95
1 hour	180
2 hours	155
Glucose load, 50 g	
1 hour	130–140

Sources: National Institutes of Health. Diagnosis of gestational diabetes. Available at http://www.ncbi.nih.gov/books/bv.fcgi?rid=diabetes.table.986; and American Diabetes Association. Standards of Medical Care in Diabetes–2006. *Diabetes Care* 29:4S, 2006.

Cost effectiveness of nutritional interventions in GDM saves thousands of dollars per case. Multidisciplinary prenatal care must include nutritional education, counseling, and support. All women with GDM should receive nutritional counseling by a registered dietitian, including individualized therapy according to maternal weight and height (American Diabetes Association, 2004).

The American Dietetic Association recommends three medical nutrition therapy (MNT) visits over the first few months, then one visit every 2–3 weeks during treatment for GDM until delivery. MNT for GDM includes a carbohydrate-controlled meal plan with adequate intake to keep weight gain appropriate while preventing glycemic shifts or ketonuria. After delivery, a review of glucose tolerance and postpartum nutrition is suggested at 6–12 weeks.

INTERVENTION: OBJECTIVES

- Lower the glucose level to a normoglycemic level to prevent complications.
- Prevent perinatal morbidity and mortality by normalizing the levels of glycemia and other metabolites (i.e., lipids and amino acids) to the levels of nondiabetic pregnant individuals.
- Optimize growth and development of the fetus. Desirable maternal weight gain will vary according to prepregnancy and current weight. Optimal weight gain is generally as follows: first trimester 0.5–1 kg (1–2 lb); second and third trimester 0.2–0.5 kg/wk (0.5–1 lb/wk). Prevent weight loss; avoid excessive weight gain in obese women.
- Prevent complications of diabetes and fetal problems, including infections. Minimize morbidity and prevent death of mother or infant. For example, the risk of spontaneous preterm birth increases with increasing levels of pregnancy glycemia, independent of perinatal complications that could trigger early delivery (Hedderson et al, 2003).
- Control blood pressure.
- Maintain normoglycemia. Avoid incidents of starvation ketosis (where glucose is needed) and diabetic acidosis (where insulin and potassium are needed) by regular preprandial and postprandial self-monitoring of blood glucose levels.
- Use insulin when necessary, based on measures of maternal glycemia with or without assessment of fetal growth. Insulin therapy is recommended when nutrition intervention fails to maintain fasting whole-blood glucose at desired levels.
- Prevent hypoglycemic episodes, urinary tract infections, and candidiasis.
- Promote healthy lifestyle changes for the mother that will last long after delivery (Gabbe and Graves, 2003).
- Exercise, especially after meals, can help to maintain blood glucose control. Avoid vigorous exercise when there is ketosis (American Diabetes Association, 2006).
- Women with GDM should be encouraged to breastfeed.

INTERVENTION: FOOD AND NUTRITION

- Diet should match age and weight goals. Provide adequate calories and nutrients to meet the needs of pregnancy, and diet should be consistent with the maternal blood glucose goals that have been established (American Diabetes Association, 2004). The typical diet may include 30–35 kcal/kg. A common diet plan includes 20% total calories as protein, 40–45% as CHO, and 35–40% as fat.
- Select CHO from more whole grains, 1 fruit portion, or 1 milk portion at a time; do not include juices, sweets, or desserts. Sufficient CHO intake is needed (175 g at minimum).
- For obese women (BMI >30), a calorie restriction (to ~25 kcal/kg actual weight/d) has been shown to reduce hyperglycemia and plasma triglycerides with no increase in ketonuria; restriction of carbohydrates to 35–40% of calories has been shown to decrease maternal glucose levels and improve maternal and fetal outcomes (American Diabetes Association, 2004).
- Maintain an adequate intake of polyunsaturated fats; keep saturated fats to 10% of total fat or less.

- Most women require 3 meals and 2 to 4 snacks; snacks are eaten at least 2–3 hours between feedings and should contain carbohydrate. Smaller, more frequent meals and snacks will be beneficial because of the insulin resistance. Working closely with a dietitian is helpful to establish the best pattern according to typical blood glucose levels of the individual mother.
- For obese women with BMI >30, reduce calories by about one third. For many women, this translates to an energy intake around 1700–1800 kcal. Artificial sweeteners may be used, but not saccharin.
- DASH diet principles may be helpful if blood pressure is elevated. Include regular use of antioxidant foods and spices in the diet, such as cinnamon (Talpur et al, 2005).
- Ensure intake of a prenatal vitamin-mineral supplement (especially containing 600 μg folic acid, 30–60 mg iron, vitamin C, and adequate calcium). Include adequate chromium intake from diet (as in yeast breads).
- Carefully spaced meals and snacks, especially before bedtime, are needed. Four to six small meals may be helpful, and a snack upon arising may be important to prevent hypoglycemia.
- No meals should be skipped. Many women with GDM undereat out of fear of needing insulin; interval weight loss may indicate presence of fasting ketones. The required amount of CHO should be consumed (175 g), and insulin should be given when blood glucose is elevated.
- Tube feeding with CHO-controlled specialty products may be useful in patients who cannot be fed orally.

CLINICAL INDICATORS

Clinical/History

- Height
- Pregravid weight
- Pregravid BMI
- Current weight
- Goal weight
- Weight gain pattern
- Diet history
- Expected date of confinement (EDC)
- BP
- Edema
- Ultrasonography for fetal growth
- Periodontal disease (Xiong et al, 2006)

Lab Work

- Ketones, fasting
- H & H
- Serum Gluc (>105 mg/100 mL fasting, start insulin)
- 1-Hour postprandial glucose (>155 mg/100mL, start insulin)
- Na+, K+
- BUN
- Creat (often elevated)
- Alb, transthyretin
- Microalbuminuria
- Ca++, Mg++
- TSH (altered?)
- OGTT
- HbA1c is not useful in GDM
- CRP

Common Drugs Used and Potential Side Effects

- Insulin may be required to control blood glucose if diet and exercise do not help. Careful physician monitoring will be needed. Self-monitoring may be important for glucose and insulin control. Insulin lispro is associated with fewer hypoglycemic events.
- Oral glucose-lowering agents are not yet recommended during pregnancy. There are studies currently under way evaluating use of metformin and glyburide during pregnancy.
- Insulin therapy is recommended when MNT fails to maintain self-monitored glucose at the following levels:
  Fasting plasma glucose ≤105 mg/dL (5.8 mmol/L)
  or
  1-Hour postprandial plasma glucose ≤155 mg/dL (8.6 mmol/L)
  or
  2-Hour postprandial plasma glucose ≤130 mg/dL (7.2 mmol/L)
- Prenatal vitamin-mineral supplements should be used as prescribed. Be aware that excessive doses of vitamin C may show false-positive urinary glucose levels; more than 200 mg/d probably is not needed.
- Low-dose estrogen-progesterone oral contraceptives may be used after GDM, if no medical contraindications exist. However, medications that worsen insulin resistance (e.g., glucocorticoids, nicotinic acid) should be avoided if possible.

Herbs, Botanicals, and Supplements

- In general, pregnant women should not take any herbs and botanical products. They should discuss any previous use with their physician.

INTERVENTION: NUTRITION EDUCATION, COUNSELING, CARE MANAGEMENT

- Communicate the importance of meal spacing, timing, adequacy, and consistency (i.e., patient should not skip meals).
- Careful instructions on what to eat and what to avoid will be important.
- Carrying a snack at all times is helpful (e.g., fruit, milk, crackers).
- Regular aerobic exercise may be beneficial (Franz et al, 2002). Exercise after meals may help to control blood sugar, but do not exercise until short of breath. Walking is often recommended. Upper body exercises are also beneficial. Do not exercise while lying on back because it decreases blood flow (weight of fetus presses on main artery), and avoid exercises that increase the risk of falling.
- Encourage breastfeeding.
- Babies born to women who have GDM may have low levels of lipids such as arachidonic acid and docosahexaenoic acid (DHA); further studies are needed to identify the impact of these altered lipids on growth and development of the infant (Bitsanis, 2006).
- Counseling regarding risk for diabetes should be provided. For example, a person with GDM may continue to be hyperglycemic after delivery, and 50% will go on to develop type 2 diabetes.
- According to the American Diabetes Association, if glucose levels are normal postpartum, reassessment of glycemia should be undertaken at a minimum of 3-year intervals and more frequently for women with impaired

fasting glucose or impaired glucose tolerance in the postpartum period. Long-term lifestyle modifications that lessen insulin resistance, including maintenance of normal body weight through MNT and physical activity, should be discussed.

- The need for family planning exists to ensure optimal glucose regulation from the start of subsequent pregnancies.
- Discuss the potential impact on offspring, who are at increased risk of obesity, glucose intolerance, and diabetes in late adolescence or adulthood.

For More Information

- American Diabetes Association
  http://www.diabetes.org/gestational-diabetes.jsp
- March of Dimes
  http://www.marchofdimes.com/

GESTATIONAL DIABETES—CITED REFERENCES

American Diabetes Association. Position statement: gestational diabetes mellitus. *Diabetes Care* 27:88S, 2004.

American Diabetes Association. Standards of Medical Care in Diabetes–2006. *Diabetes Care* 29:4S, 2006.

Bitsanis D, et al. Gestational diabetes mellitus enhances arachidonic and docosahexaenoic acids in placental phospholipids. *Lipids* 41:341, 2006.

Franz M, et al. American Diabetes Association Position Statement: evidence-based nutrition principles and recommendations for the treatment and prevention of diabetes and related conditions. *J Am Diet Assoc.* 102:109, 2002.

Gabbe SG, Graves CR. Management of diabetes mellitus complicating pregnancy. *Obstet Gynecol.* 102:857, 2003

Hedderson MM, et al. Gestational diabetes mellitus and lesser degrees of pregnancy hyperglycemia: association with increased risk of spontaneous preterm birth. *Obstet Gynecol.* 102:850, 2003.

Lucas M. Diabetes complicating pregnancy. *Obstet Gynecol Clin North Am.* 28:513, 2001.

Preece R, Jovanovic L. New and future diabetes therapies: are they safe during pregnancy? *J Matern Fetal Neonatal Med.* 12:365, 2002.

Saldana TM, et al. The relationship between pregnancy weight gain and glucose tolerance status among black and white women in central North Carolina. *Am J Obstet Gynecol.* 2006. In press.

Steinborn A, et al. The presence of gestational diabetes is associated with increased detection of anti-HLA-class II antibodies in the maternal circulation. *Am J Reprod Immunol.* 56:124, 2006.

Talpur N, et al. Effects of a novel formulation of essential oils on glucose-insulin metabolism in diabetic and hypertensive rats: a pilot study. *Diabetes Obes Metab.* 7:193, 2005.

Wolf M, et al. Inflammation and glucose intolerance: a prospective study of gestational diabetes mellitus. *Diabetes Care* 27:21, 2004.

Xiong X, et al. Periodontal disease and gestational diabetes mellitus. *Am J Obstet Gynecol.* 2006. In press.

PREGNANCY-INDUCED HYPERTENSION AND PREECLAMPSIA

NUTRITIONAL ACUITY RANKING: LEVEL 2

DEFINITIONS AND BACKGROUND

Preeclampsia, often called toxemia or pregnancy-induced hypertension (PIH), is a syndrome of edema, proteinuria, and hypertension (EPH-gestosis) that occurs during the second half of pregnancy (usually after week 20). It is more common in primigravidas and in patients with multiple gestation, malnutrition, hydatidiform mole, positive family history of PIH, or underlying vascular disease.

Taking vitamin supplements before pregnancy or in early pregnancy does not prevent miscarriage or stillbirth, but women taking vitamin supplements may be less likely to develop preeclampsia (Rumbold et al, 2005). Vitamins C and E have been studied in PIH, and large trials are under way (Beazley et al, 2005; Poston et al, 2004; Raijmakers et al, 2004).

Because African American women have an increased risk of preeclampsia compared with white women and because plasma homocysteine is increased in preeclampsia, evaluation of the differences in diet, adherence to folic acid supplementation, and interactions of nutritional and maternal factors warrant further study by race and pregnancy status (Patrick et al, 2004). Sufficient intakes of folic acid and vitamins B_{12} and B_6 are recommended (Mignini et al, 2005; Hermann et al, 2004; Williams et al, 2004).

Antioxidant protection may be important in PIH. Abnormal lipid and carnitine metabolism may play a role in the pathophysiology (Thiele et al, 2004). More research is needed.

PIH occurs in approximately 6–10% of all pregnancies. The condition is often found in women with high body mass index (BMI), chronic hypertension, diabetes, or chronic renal disease. Women with type 1 diabetes have a PIH rate 2–4 times higher than other women (Holmes et al, 2004). Early sonogram is recommended for PIH, and many women will have to have total bed rest. Delivery of the fetus is the only cure; women who are 34 weeks pregnant will be induced immediately.

Preeclampsia is either mild or severe. Criteria for **mild preeclampsia** include hypertension as defined at 140/90 to 159/109 mm Hg; proteinuria >300 mg/24 h; mild edema with weight gain >2 lb/wk or >6 lb/month; and urine output >500 mL/24 h. Signs and symptoms include increased blood pressure (BP), proteinuria, facial edema, pretibial pitting edema, irritability, nausea and vomiting, nervousness, headache, altered states of consciousness, epigastric pain, and oliguria.

Criteria for **severe preeclampsia** include: BP >160/110 mm Hg on two occasions with patient on bed rest; systolic BP rise >60 mm Hg over baseline; diastolic BP increase of >30 mm Hg over baseline; proteinuria >5 g/24 h or 3+ or 4+ on a urine dipstick; massive edema; and oliguria <400 mL/24 h. Symptoms include pulmonary edema, severe headaches, visual changes, right upper quadrant pain, elevated liver enzymes, and thrombocytopenia in addition to the symptoms listed for mild preeclampsia.

In **eclampsia,** a seizure occurs. Eclamptic seizures and symptoms of the HELLP syndrome (hemolysis, elevated liver function tests, low platelet count) occur. In severe cases, there may also be hepatic rupture, pulmonary edema, acute renal failure, placental abruption, elevated creatinine, intrauterine growth restriction, cerebral hemorrhage, cortical blindness, and retinal detachment. Maternal mortality rate is 8–36%.

INTERVENTION: OBJECTIVES

- Preeclampsia is a leading cause of maternal and neonatal mortality and morbidity. In pregnant patients with diabetes and chronic hypertension, BP target goals of 110–129/65–79 mm Hg are suggested; avoid lower BP because fetal growth may be impaired (American Diabetes Association, 2006).
- Lessen edema when present. Screen for microalbuminuria because this condition in the absence of urinary tract infection is a strong predictor of preeclampsia (American Diabetes Association, 2006).
- Correct any underlying malnutrition or micronutrient deficiencies.
- Monitor any sudden weight gains (>1 kg/wk) that are unexplained by food intake.
- Prevent, if possible, chronic hypertension and metabolic syndrome (Forest et al, 2005) after delivery.

INTERVENTION: FOOD AND NUTRITION

- Maintain diet as ordered for age and pregnancy stage (generally 300 kcal more than prepregnancy diet). Use extra fruits and vegetables and less sucrose.
- Supplement with prenatal vitamins, folic acid, and calcium as needed. Inadequate micronutrient intakes have been implicated (Rumbold et al, 2005). Assure adequate intakes of calcium, folic acid, other B-complex vitamins, protein, selenium (Rayman et al, 2003), magnesium, and potassium from diet. The role of vitamins C and E is still being defined.
- Sodium intake may need to be controlled to 2 g/d if edema is severe. Diuretics generally are not used.
- Linoleic and arachidonic acids have been used to serve as vasodilators under careful medical supervision. There may be some merit for including a sufficient intake of omega-3 fatty acids from salmon, tuna, walnuts, and flaxseed oil.

SAMPLE NUTRITION DIAGNOSTIC STATEMENT

Preeclampsia and Eclampsia

PES: Disordered eating pattern related to harmful beliefs about diet in pregnancy as evidenced by elevated blood pressure and diet records indicating low intake of calcium, magnesium, and vitamins and daily skipping of meals.

Assessment Data: Food records, weight records.

Intervention: Education and counseling about appropriate dietary intake and meal frequency during pregnancy; dangers of skipping meals related to ketosis.

Monitoring and Evaluation: Weight and prenatal growth charts; successful outcome for infant and mother; lab reports and blood pressure records.

CLINICAL INDICATORS

Clinical/History

Height
Weight
Prepregnancy BMI
Weight gain pattern
Diet history
Edema, especially in lower extremities
BP (mild, ≥140/90 mm Hg; severe, >160/110 mm Hg)
Decreased urine output
Confusion, apprehension
Shortness of breath
Right upper quadrant abdominal pain
Dizziness
Visual changes (blurring, double vision)
Excessive nausea
Severe headaches

Lab Work

GFR
Alb, transthyretin (often low)
Proteinuria (>300 mg/d is mild; >500 mg/d is severe)
H & H
Serum Fe
Chol, Trig (elevated?)
Gluc
Ca++, Mg++
Na+, K+
Uric acid (elevated)
BUN
Creat (may be elevated)
Homocysteine
CRP
Coagulation series (PT, partial thromboplastin time [PTT], fibrinogen degradation)
HELLP syndrome (decreased platelets, abnormal liver function tests)
Liver function tests (AST, ALT, LDH)

Common Drugs Used and Potential Side Effects

- Magnesium sulfate and corticosteroids are often used to prevent seizures.
- Some studies suggest that calcium supplementation may reduce PIH (Ritchie and King, 2000). More studies are needed.
- During pregnancy, many typical diuretics and cardiac drugs are not used. Intravenous hydralazine may be administered. Angiotensin-converting enzyme (ACE) inhibitors and angiotensin receptor blockers (ARBs) are contraindicated during pregnancy (American Diabetes Association, 2006).
- Some doctors will prescribe low-dose acetylsalicylic acid (ASA) to alter levels of vasodilation and vasoconstriction to the placenta.
- Because there is an abnormally low plasma vitamin C concentration in preeclampsia, a combination of vitamins C and E is a prophylactic strategy for prevention of preeclampsia; several multicenter randomized clinical trials have been initiated (Raijmakers et al, 2004).

Herbs, Botanicals, and Supplements

- Herbs and botanical supplements should not be used in pregnancy.
- Evening primrose has been suggested for this condition. Coenzyme Q10 and alpha-tocopherol are potent antioxidants and should not be used until larger trials prove efficacy (Palan et al, 2004).

INTERVENTION: NUTRITION EDUCATION, COUNSELING, CARE MANAGEMENT

- Rest is essential during this time. Biofeedback, yoga, meditation, and other forms of stress reduction are often beneficial.
- Meal skipping should be avoided at all costs.
- Discuss adequate sources of calcium from the diet, especially if dairy products are not tolerated or preferred.
- Good sources of potassium and magnesium include fruits and vegetables. The DASH diet is an excellent diet to continue, even after pregnancy.

For More Information

- Diabetes and Preeclampsia
  http://diabetes.healthcentersonline.com/womensdiabetes/preeclampsia.cfm
- Pregnancy and Preeclampsia
  http://familydoctor.org/064.xml

PREGNANCY-INDUCED HYPERTENSION AND PREECLAMPSIA—CITED REFERENCES

American Diabetes Association. Standards of Medical Care in Diabetes–2006. *Diabetes Care* 29:4S, 2006.

Beazley D, et al. Vitamin C and E supplementation in women at high risk for preeclampsia: a double-blind, placebo-controlled trial. *Am J Obstet Gynecol.* 192:520, 2005.

Forest JC, et al. Early occurrence of metabolic syndrome after hypertension in pregnancy. *Obstet Gynecol.* 105:1373, 2005.

Hermann W, et al. Alteration of homocysteine catabolism in pre-eclampsia, HELLP syndrome and placental insufficiency. *Clin Chem Lab Med.* 42:1109, 2004.

Holmes VA, et al. The Diabetes and Pre-eclampsia Intervention Trial. *Int J Gynaecol Obstet.* 87:66, 2004.

Mignini LE, et al. Mapping the theories of preeclampsia: the role of homocysteine. *Obstet Gynecol.* 105:411, 2005.

Palan PR, et al. Lipid-soluble antioxidants and pregnancy: maternal serum levels of coenzyme Q10, alpha-tocopherol and gamma-tocopherol in preeclampsia and normal pregnancy. *Gynecol Obstet Invest.* 58:8, 2004.

Patrick TE, et al. Homocysteine and folic acid are inversely related in black women with preeclampsia. *Hypertension* 43:1279, 2004.

Poston L, et al. Vitamin E in preeclampsia. *Ann N Y Acad Sci.* 1031:242, 2004.

Raijmakers MT, et al. Oxidative stress and preeclampsia: rationale for antioxidant clinical trials. *Hypertension* 44:374, 2004.

Rayman MP, et al. Low selenium status is associated with the occurrence of the pregnancy disease preeclampsia in women from the United Kingdom. *Am J Obstet Gynecol.* 189:1343, 2003.

Ritchie LD, King JC. Dietary calcium and pregnancy-induced hypertension: is there a relation? *Am J Clin Nutr.* 71:1371S, 2000.

Rumbold A, et al. Vitamin supplementation for preventing miscarriage. *Cochrane Database Syst Rev.* 2:CD004073, 2005.

Thiele IG, et al. Increased plasma carnitine concentrations in preeclampsia. *Obstet Gynecol.* 103:876, 2004.

Williams MA, et al. Methylenetetrahydrofolate reductase 677 C→T polymorphism and plasma folate in relation to pre-eclampsia risk among Peruvian women. *J Matern Fetal Neonatal Med.* 15:337, 2004.

DIABETIC GASTROPARESIS

NUTRITIONAL ACUITY RANKING: LEVEL 3–4

DEFINITIONS AND BACKGROUND

Gastroparesis occurs in approximately 50% of all cases of diabetes (Aring et al, 2005), with delayed gastric emptying in the absence of mechanical obstruction. Gastroparesis is the result of ongoing damage to the nerves that are responsible for peristalsis and normal motility

The key problem is that foods digest abnormally slowly or peristalsis is diminished so that it is difficult to match insulin action to digestion and absorption of the meals. Hypoglycemia can occur if insulin is working and if food remains in the stomach. Later, insulin action is diminished and food finally digests, causing hyperglycemia.

Signs and symptoms include recent changes in appetite; heartburn, abdominal pain or bloating, or nausea after eating; early fullness after eating small amounts of food; constipation or diarrhea; poor blood glucose control; and weight loss. Other symptoms may include vomiting of undigested food, gastroesophageal reflux, and spasms of the stomach wall. Diabetic patients with nausea and vomiting need evaluation to determine symptom etiology (Jones, 2004).

Problems occur more often in type 1 than in type 2 diabetes. Strict glycemic control is key for preventing this complication (Aring et al, 2005). A gastrostomy is rarely indicated, but a jejunostomy may be helpful in maintaining nutrition, and parenteral nutrition should generally be avoided because of high complication rates (Jones, 2004).

Intrasphincteric injection of botulinum toxin A represents a novel technique to treat gastroparesis; in refractory cases, the use of a gastric electric stimulator has been shown to be beneficial (Blank et al, 2004; van der Voort et al, 2005). Prokinetic agents are the best treatment option, whereas surgical intervention cannot be recommended (Jones, 2004). See Section 7 for more details on management of gastroparesis.

INTERVENTION: OBJECTIVES

- Correct the fluctuating blood glucose levels through careful food provision and insulin management. Frequent blood glucose checks and monitoring records are important.

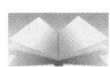

- Correct dehydration and electrolyte abnormalities.
- Treatment focuses on effectively relieving symptoms while maintaining adequate nutritional status; therapy for patients with nausea and vomiting consists of restoring volume and glycemic and electrolyte status and providing antiemetics generously (Jones, 2004).
- Reduce or control pain, diarrhea, and constipation.
- Ensure adequate intake of diet as prescribed to prevent weight loss and control malnutrition.
- Differentiate from ketoacidosis, which has similar symptoms of nausea and vomiting.
- Prevent bezoar formation of indigestible solids.
- Pernicious vomiting may occur; distinguish from bulimia.

INTERVENTION: FOOD AND NUTRITION

- Monitor intake carefully; blood glucose fluctuations are common in gastroparesis.
- Soft-to-liquid diet may be useful to prevent delay in gastric emptying. Six small meals may be better tolerated than large meals.
- Use a low-fat diet to improve digestion and to improve stomach emptying.
- Decrease overall fiber intake.
- If patient complains of dry mouth, add extra fluids and moisten foods with broth or allowed sauces or gravies.
- In severe problems, a jejunostomy tube feeding may be indicated. It can be used temporarily if needed to correct malnutrition.

CLINICAL INDICATORS

Clinical/History

Height
Weight
BMI
Diet history
Abdominal pain
Diarrhea or constipation
Vomiting, nausea
Gastro-esophageal reflux disease (GERD)
I & O
Upper endoscopy
Barium x-ray
Gastric emptying scan
Gastric manometry

Lab Work

HbA1c
H & H
Serum Fe
Gastrin
Gluc (fasting and 30 minutes after meals)
Na+, K+
Alb, transthyretin
CRP
Chol, Trig

Common Drugs Used and Potential Side Effects

- Prokinetics such as metoclopramide (Reglan) may be given 30 minutes before meals to increase gastric contractions and to relax pyloric sphincter. Dry mouth, sleepiness, anxiety, or nausea can be side effects. Emitasol is a nasal spray form of this medication. Metoclopramide prophylaxis to reduce gastric volumes before elective surgery is unnecessary unless the patient has a prolonged history of poor blood glucose control (Jellish et al, 2005).
- Rapid-acting insulin should be injected with or after meals. Use self-monitoring of blood glucose (SMBG) to monitor delayed absorption and glucose changes. Insulin lispro (Humalog) is quite effective because it starts working shortly after injection. To control blood glucose, it may be necessary to take insulin more often, to take insulin after eating instead of before, and to check blood glucose often after eating.
- Insulin pumps may be beneficial because insulin delivery rates can be programmed to the patient's individual needs.
- Antiemetics may be used for vomiting. Monitor for specific side effects.
- Erythromycin improves stomach emptying by increasing the contractions that move food through the stomach. Side effects are nausea, vomiting, and abdominal cramps.
- Domperidone has been used elsewhere in the world to treat gastroparesis. It is a promotility agent like metoclopramide and helps with nausea. The FDA is reviewing it for use in the United States.
- Some researchers have treated diabetic gastroparesis with botulinum toxin injection of the pylorus with positive results (Lacey et al, 2004).

Herbs, Botanicals, and Supplements

- Herbs and botanical supplements should not be used without discussing with physician.

INTERVENTION: NUTRITION EDUCATION, COUNSELING, CARE MANAGEMENT

- Discuss delayed digestion and absorption of food.
- Discuss role of diet in maintaining weight and controlling discomfort. Emphasize nutrient-dense foods if intake has been poor.
- Bezoar formation may occur after eating oranges, coconuts, green beans, apples, figs, potato skins, Brussels sprouts, broccoli, sauerkraut, and other high-fiber foods.
- Discuss management of insulin dosing, as appropriate. Include information about SMBG and meal spacing.

For More Information

- Diabetic Gastroparesis
http://digestive.niddk.nih.gov/ddiseases/pubs/gastroparesis/

DIABETIC GASTROPARESIS—CITED REFERENCES

Aring AM, et al. Evaluation and prevention of diabetic neuropathy. *Am Fam Physician.* 71:2123, 2005.

Blank C, et al. Pediatric gastric and duodenal disorders. *Curr Opin Gastroenterol.* 20:551, 2004.

Jellish WS, et al. Effect of metoclopramide on gastric fluid volumes in diabetic patients who have fasted before elective surgery. *Anesthesiology* 102:904, 2005.

Jones MP. Management of diabetic gastroparesis. *Nutr Clin Pract.* 19:145, 2004.

Lacy BE, et al. The treatment of diabetic gastroparesis with botulinum toxin injection of the pylorus. *Diabetes Care* 27:2341, 2004.

van der Voort IR, et al. Gastric electrical stimulation results in improved metabolic control in diabetic patients suffering from gastroparesis. *Exp Clin Endocrinol Diabetes.* 113:38, 2005.

DIABETIC KETOACIDOSIS

NUTRITIONAL ACUITY RANKING: LEVEL 3–4

DEFINITIONS AND BACKGROUND

Ketones in the urine mean that the body is burning fat to get energy. Large amounts in the serum and urine can be dangerous. Diabetic ketoacidosis (DKA) is classic metabolic acidosis, a medical emergency that accounts for more than 100,000 hospital admissions yearly in the United States and 4–9% of hospital discharges for patients who have diabetes (Umpierrez and Kitabchi, 2003). Table 9-17 indicates causes of DKA.

The triad of uncontrolled hyperglycemia, metabolic acidosis, and increased total body ketone concentration characterizes DKA; these metabolic derangements result from the combination of absolute or relative insulin deficiency and increased levels of the counterregulatory hormones of glucagon, catecholamines, cortisol, and growth hormone (Umpierrez and Kitabchi, 2003).

Preceding diabetic coma, symptoms and signs of DKA include intense thirst, nausea and vomiting, dim vision, labored breathing, sweet acetone breath, pruritus, polyuria, hot or dry and flushed skin, cramping, seizures, and drowsiness. Diagnosis of DKA requires the patient's plasma glucose concentration to be >250 mg/dL, pH level to be <7.30, and bicarbonate level to be ≤18 mEq/L; beta-hydroxybutyrate is a better measurement of the degree of ketosis than serum ketones (Trachtenbarg, 2005). Table 9-18 provides defining characteristics for DKA.

DKA is seen primarily in patients with type 1 diabetes, with about 3% of type 1 diabetic patients presenting with DKA on initial diagnosis. In children, DKA is a leading cause of hospitalization and is a cause of cerebral edema, which may lead to death if untreated. DKA can also occur in type 2 diabetic patients, usually from urinary tract infections, trauma, stress, pregnancy, surgery, or myocardial infarction.

Recent studies suggest that inflammatory processes may play a role in DKA. Both DKA and its treatment produce varying degrees of immunological stress during the time of acute complications (Jerath et al, 2005). Use of standardized written guidelines for therapy have demonstrated a mortality rate of less than 5%, with higher mortality rates observed in elderly patients and those with other illnesses (Umpierrez and Kitabchi, 2003).

INTERVENTION: OBJECTIVES

- Decrease hyperglycemia and ketosis; provide fluids and sufficient insulin to achieve euglycemia. Frequent blood glucose and ketone monitoring is necessary. Note that urine ketones lag behind serum ketones because it takes time to the empty bladder, where they have accumulated and been stored.
- Correct hypovolemia and fluid or electrolyte imbalances.
- Promote return to wellness; patient most likely has been in poor health for several days preceding acidosis. Monitor frequently to prevent recurrence.
- Evaluate precipitating factors such as surgery, myocardial infarction, or trauma.
- Prevent complications such as shock, arterial thrombosis, and cerebral edema (CEDKA). CEDKA remains a significant problem with a high mortality rate (Lawrence et al, 2005).
- For chronically high fasting glucose levels, adjust evening intermediate- or long-acting insulin doses or timing. If obese, lose weight to reduce insulin resistance.

TABLE 9-17 Causes of Ketoacidosis

- Not getting enough insulin from missed injections.
- Alkaline reserves may be depleted by too little insulin, flu or colds, fever, pregnancy, stress, trauma, or myocardial infarction.
- Worldwide, infection is the leading cause of diabetic ketoacidosis; urinary tract infections and pneumonia are often involved (Umpierrez and Kitabchi, 2003).

INTERVENTION: FOOD AND NUTRITION

- If patient is in a coma, intravenous insulin, electrolytes, and fluids are used. A nasogastric tube may be placed to prevent aspiration during feeding. If patient is alert and oriented, offer plenty of fluids orally.
- As treatment progresses, a 5% glucose solution is usually given as glucosuria and hyperglycemia subside. If glucosuria and hyperglycemia do not decrease, try tea and salty broth. Later, fruit juices and liquids high in potassium may be given.
- Eventually, return to usual diet. Monitor closely.
- A weight loss plan may be needed in obesity.

CLINICAL INDICATORS

Clinical/History

Height
Weight
BMI
Diet history
Nausea
Vomiting
BP (often low)
Tachycardia
Flushed face
Temperature
I & O
Diarrhea

Lab Work

Gluc (>250 mg/dL)
Blood pH (<7.3)
Bicarbonate (≤18 mEq/L)
Ketones in urine (increased); test when glucose is >240 mg/dL
Serum ketones
CRP
BUN (increased)
Creat
Na+ (decreased)
K+
Cl− (decreased)
HbA1c
Amylase (increased)
WBC (elevated with infections)
Partial pressure of carbon dioxide (pCO_2) (decreased); partial pressure of oxygen (pO_2)
Uric acid (increased)
AST (decreased)

TABLE 9-18 Diagnostic Criteria for Diabetic Ketoacidosis (DKA) and Hyperosmolar Hyperglycemic State (HHS)

	DKA			
Criteria	**Mild**	**Moderate**	**Severe**	**HHS**
Plasma glucose (mg/dL)	>250	>250	>250	>600
Arterial pH	7.25–7.30	7.00–7.24	<7.00	>7.30
Serum bicarbonate (mEq/L)	15–18	10–<15	<10	>15
Urine ketones	Positive	Positive	Positive	Small
Serum ketones	Positive	Positive	Positive	Small
Effective serum osmolality (mOsm/kg)	Variable	Variable	Variable	>320
Altered mental status	Alert	Alert/drowsy	Stupor/coma	Stupor/coma

Adapted from: Kitabchi AE, et al. Hyperglycemic crises in diabetes. *Diabetes Care* 27:S94, 2004.

ALT, LDH, creatine kinase (CK) (increased)	Phosphate (often decreased)	Chol (increased)
	Mg++ (often decreased)	Trig
		Ca++

Common Drugs Used and Potential Side Effects

- Insulin and fluid are usually given intravenously. The goal is to decrease blood glucose by 50–75 mg/dL/h.
- Dextrose in saline is often given once plasma glucose decreases to prevent accidental hypoglycemia.
- Potassium deficit is common, as are deficits of phosphate and magnesium. Bicarbonate therapy is needed only rarely (Trachtenbarg, 2005).

Diabetes Record										**Week Starting** ________
	Other Blood Glucose	Breakfast Blood Glucose	Medicine	Lunch Blood Glucose	Medicine	Dinner Blood Glucose	Medicine	Bedtime Blood Glucose	Medicine	Notes: (Special events, sick days, exercise)
Monday										
Tuesday										
Wednesday										
Thursday										
Friday										
Saturday										
Sunday										

Figure 9-4 Diabetes record. (Source: National Institute of Diabetes and Digestive and Kidney Diseases, http://www2.niddk.nih.gov/.)

- Intravenous antibiotic therapy will be needed for sepsis.
- Atypical antipsychotics (AAP) have been widely used for the management of patients with schizophrenia; hyperglycemia and DKA may result if the patient is not carefully monitored (Jin et al, 2004).

Herbs, Botanicals, and Supplements

- Herbs and botanical supplements should not be used without discussing with physician.

INTERVENTION: NUTRITION EDUCATION, COUNSELING, CARE MANAGEMENT

- Explain demand for more insulin during illness and infection. Use of a diabetes record may be useful if episodes of high blood glucose are frequent; see Figure 9-4.
- Never exercise when there are ketones present.
- Because every episode of DKA implies breakdown in clinical communication, appropriate diabetes education should be reinforced. Address more specific sick-day guidelines and when to contact the physician (Trachtenbarg, 2005).
- Novel approaches to patient education incorporating a variety of health care beliefs and socioeconomic issues will support a more effective prevention program (Umpierrez and Kitabchi, 2003).
- When strict control of diabetes through insulin is administered, weight gain is common. Insulin omission and reduction, which are eating disorder symptoms unique to diabetes mellitus, are associated with an increased risk of DKA and with other complications of diabetes mellitus (Goebel-Fabbri et al, 2002). Attention to this disorder is important in overall treatment planning and management.
- The biggest risk of insulin pump therapy is DKA since no long-acting insulin is used. Any interruption to insulin delivery or pump malfunctioning can cause DKA. To prevent this reaction, monitor blood glucose regularly.

For More Information

- American Diabetes Association
  http://www.diabetes.org/type-1-diabetes/ketoacidosis.jsp
- National Institute of Diabetes and Digestive and Kidney Diseases (NIDDK)–Diabetic Ketoacidosis
  http://diabetes.niddk.nih.gov/dm/pubs/america/pdf/chapter13.pdf

DIABETIC KETOACIDOSIS—CITED REFERENCES

Goebel-Fabbri AE, et al. Identification and treatment of eating disorders in women with type 1 diabetes mellitus. *Treat Endocrinol.* 1:155, 2002.
Jerath RS, et al. Complement activation in diabetic ketoacidosis and its treatment. *Clin Immunol.* 116:11, 2005.
Jin H, et al. Atypical antipsychotics and glucose dysregulation: a systematic review. *Schizophr Res.* 71:195, 2004.
Lawrence SE, et al. Population-based study of incidence and risk factors for cerebral edema in pediatric diabetic ketoacidosis. *J Pediatr.* 146:688, 2005.
Trachtenbarg DE. Diabetic ketoacidosis. *Am Fam Physician.* 71:1705, 2005.
Umpierrez GE, Kitabchi AE. Diabetic ketoacidosis: risk factors and management strategies. *Treat Endocrinol.* 2:95, 2003.

HYPEROSMOLAR HYPERGLYCEMIC STATE

NUTRITIONAL ACUITY RANKING: LEVEL 3–4

DEFINITIONS AND BACKGROUND

Diabetic hyperosmolar hyperglycemic state (HHS) is a life-threatening emergency with marked elevation of blood glucose, hyperosmolarity, and minimal or no ketosis (Stoner, 2005). The condition occurs in elderly patients with type 2 diabetes. HHS is preventable if blood glucose is monitored regularly in order to notice and correct elevating levels before problems occur.

Signs and symptoms include polydipsia, polyuria, nausea and vomiting, diarrhea, fever, respirations that are abnormal, profound dehydration, lethargy, confusion, grand mal seizures, tachycardia, hypotension, and oliguria. Coma may occur in about 10% of cases. Other names for this syndrome include hyperosmolar hyperglycemic nonketotic syndrome (HHNS) or hyperosmolar coma. Table 9-18 provides diagnostic criteria.

Predisposing factors for this syndrome include long-term uncontrolled hyperglycemia, pancreatic disease, infections or sepsis, stroke, surgery, extensive burns, renal or cardiovascular disease, corticosteroid use, diuretics, excessive total parenteral nutrition (TPN), dialysis, and excessive tube feeding. Underlying infections and substance abuse are the most common causes.

Identification and treatment of the underlying and precipitating causes of HHS are absolutely essential. If recognized early, hyperglycemia can frequently be treated in the outpatient setting if the patient can take fluids; monitor blood glucose frequently, and follow standard sick-day rules (Gaglia et al, 2004).

INTERVENTION: OBJECTIVES

- Correct dehydration, shock, and cardiac arrhythmias. Prevent death.
- Monitor fluid status and replace deficits, which may be 10–20% of total body weight. It may require up to 9 L in 48 hours (Stoner, 2005).

- Reduce elevated blood glucose levels, generally, with isotonic saline and then hypotonic saline along with insulin.
- Prevent future crises by appropriate diabetes self-management education and regular monitoring of blood glucose.
- Prevent acute renal failure, which may result from prolonged hypovolemia.

INTERVENTION: FOOD AND NUTRITION

- Offer fluid replacement, often 1 L/h until volume is restored; 9–12 L may be needed.
- Patient is likely to NPO during a crisis or perhaps tube fed during a comatose state. As appropriate, intake may be progressed gradually to a balanced diet, controlling calories as needed.
- Correct electrolyte deficits. Potassium or magnesium may be needed.
- A renal diet plan may be needed if renal failure is identified.

CLINICAL INDICATORS

Clinical/History

Height
Weight
BMI
Diet history
Absence of ketonemia
BP
I & O
Signs of dehydration
Fever (>101°F)
Excessive thirst and urination
Dry, parched mouth
Warm, dry skin with no sweating
Weakness
Leg cramps
Sleepiness or confusion
Rapid pulse
Convulsions or coma

Lab Work

Gluc (>600 mg/dL)
Na+, K+
Bicarbonate
Hyperosmolality (usually >320 mOsm)
BUN, Creat
Alb
H & H
PO_4
Chol
Trig
CRP
Ketones and pH (to distinguish between diabetic ketoacidosis [DKA] and HHS)

Common Drugs Used and Potential Side Effects

- Insulin is needed to normalize blood glucose levels. Infusions will be needed until full rehydration is complete. DKA and HHS are associated with elevation of proinflammatory cytokines; insulin therapy provides a strong anti-inflammatory effect (Stentz et al, 2004).
- Potassium replacements may be needed. Monitor carefully.
- Antibiotic therapy may be needed in cases of underlying infections.

Herbs, Botanicals, and Supplements

- Herbs and botanical supplements should not be used without discussing with physician.

INTERVENTION: NUTRITION EDUCATION, COUNSELING, CARE MANAGEMENT

- Discuss, where possible, predisposing factors, how to avoid future incidents, and blood glucose monitoring.
- Calorie-controlled diets may be beneficial if patient can comprehend. Family intervention may be required.

For More Information

- Diabetic Hyperosmolar Hyperglycemic State
  http://www.diabetes.org/type-2-diabetes/treatment-conditions/hhns.jsp
- E-medicine
  http://www.emedicine.com/emerg/topic264.htm
- National Guideline Clearinghouse
  http://www.guideline.gov/summary/summary.aspx?doc_id=4694

HYPEROSMOLAR HYPERGLYCEMIC STATE—CITED REFERENCES

Gaglia JL, et al. Acute hyperglycemic crisis in the elderly. *Med Clin North Am.* 88:1063, 2004.
Stentz FB, et al. Proinflammatory cytokines, markers of cardiovascular risks, oxidative stress, and lipid peroxidation in patients with hyperglycemic crises. *Diabetes* 53:2079, 2004.
Stoner GD. Hyperosmolar hyperglycemic state. *Am Fam Physician.* 71:1723, 2005.

HYPOGLYCEMIA

NUTRITIONAL ACUITY RANKING: LEVEL 3

DEFINITIONS AND BACKGROUND

Hypoglycemia occurs primarily in patients with type 1 diabetes mellitus (Dagogo-Jack, 2004). Except in diabetic patients receiving insulin or sulfonylureas, hypoglycemia is a rare disorder. True low blood sugar (70 mg/100 dL or lower) releases hormones such as catecholamines, which produce hunger, trembling, headache, dizziness, weakness, and palpitations.

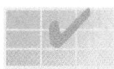

Sources of bodily glucose are dietary intake, glycogenolysis, and gluconeogenesis. The metabolism of glucose involves oxidation and storage as glycogen or fat. The body makes great effort to supply glucose for the CNS and red blood cells. Glycogenolysis is stimulated by secretion of glucagon from the alpha-cells of the pancreas; when this is impaired in patients with type 1 diabetes, it contributes to defective glucose counterregulation (Cersosimo et al, 2001).

Many different causes can stimulate hypoglycemia, and treatments through dietary means will differ accordingly. Skipped or insufficient meals, errors in insulin dosing, taking too much insulin, alcohol consumption, or extra physical exertion can lead to hypoglycemic episodes.

Recurrent episodes of iatrogenic hypoglycemia induce a state of hypoglycemia unawareness and defective counterregulation, which defines the syndrome of hypoglycemia-associated autonomic failure (HAAF). It is essential to manage the episodes carefully.

Approaches to the prevention of hypoglycemia include glucose monitoring, patient education, meal planning, and medication adjustment. Adequate carbohydrate replacement during and after exercise seems to be an important measure to prevent hypoglycemia; insulin dosage adjustment with a decrease from 20–30% is needed only for exercise duration over an hour (Grimm et al, 2004).

INTERVENTION: OBJECTIVES

- Normalize blood glucose levels. If the problem is recurrent, stabilize blood glucose levels through normal mealtimes, meal and CHO consistency, insulin dose adjustments, and blood glucose self-monitoring. For those individuals on insulin, appropriate insulin timing with food and possible use of CHO to insulin ratio are important factors to consider.
- Minimize length of time between meals.
- Prevent seizures and coma, with precipitating symptoms such as neuroglycopenia with confusion, light headaches, and aberrant behavior.
- Determine frequency, symptoms of hypoglycemia, activity levels, and exercise for the individual.
- Delayed hypoglycemia after strenuous or prolonged exercise may occur up to 24 hours after exercise and is related to increased insulin sensitivity from exercise as well as repletion of glycogen stores. Plan appropriately by increasing carbohydrate, decreasing insulin for periods of activity, and increasing frequency of blood glucose monitoring.
- Always recheck blood glucose 15–20 minutes after treatment to make sure problem is resolved. Very low blood glucose levels (<50 g/dL) may take 30 g CHO or more to resolve, especially after exercise.

INTERVENTION: FOOD AND NUTRITION

- For insulin-induced hypoglycemia, use a normal diet with adequate CHO content. Consider a possible reduction of medication if the hypoglycemia is recurrent.
- Have patient ingest fruit juice when needed and carry candy as a corrective measure.
- If there are symptoms of hypoglycemia (blood glucose <70 g/dL), use quick sources of glucose (see Table 9-19). Fat is not as effective as CHO in normalizing blood glucose.
- In most cases, mild hypoglycemia can be handled with use of readily available CHOs, including milk, fruit, and crackers. Balanced, regular mealtimes are also useful. Frequent feedings may also be beneficial.
- For hypoglycemia at night that is caused by excessive insulin or insufficient dinner meal or evening snack, evening and bedtime doses of insulin should be adjusted. A slightly larger dinner or snack containing CHO may be needed as well.

TABLE 9-19 Quick Sources of Glucose

1 cup skim milk (12 g CHO)
4 oz orange, apple, pineapple, grapefruit juice (12–15 g CHO)
4 oz grape, cranberry, or prune juice (19 g CHO)
4 oz regular soft drink (13 g CHO)
1 tbsp sugar, dissolved in water (13 g CHO)
1 tbsp corn syrup, jam, or jelly (15 g CHO)
5 Lifesavers candies (15 g CHO)
4 Starburst candies or 15 Skittles
1 tbsp honey (17 g CHO)
1/2 cup sweetened gelatin (17 g CHO)
3–4 glucose tablets (4–5 g CHO each)
8 oz (1 cup) of milk (12 g CHO)

CLINICAL INDICATORS

Clinical/History		Lab Work
Height Weight BMI Diet history I & O Temperature BP Trembling Headache Dizziness, weakness Palpitations Seizures or coma	Blood glucose and insulin regimen records Exercise history and habits History of hypoglycemia unawareness Type and duration of diabetes	Serum Gluc (≤70 mg/dL) HbA1c Serum insulin Na+, K+ Alb CRP Chol, Trig Ca++ Mg++ OGTT results using 1 g glucose/kg

Common Drugs Used and Potential Side Effects

- Glucagon may be given before paramedics arrive; vomiting is one side effect. Intravenous dextrose is administered by medical professionals.
- Insulin and other glucose-lowering medications must be carefully prescribed and monitored. Careful use of sliding scales of insulin is an important goal for preventing hypoglycemia (Smith et al, 2005).
- Chemotherapy (e.g., streptozocin, fluorouracil) can be nephrotoxic; these drugs are often used for insulinomas. Monitor GI side effects.
- Glucose tablets have 4–5 g CHO per tablet. Patients should receive instructions regarding their use including quantity, when to use, and when not to use. Most

people will need 3–4 tablets to treat low blood glucose levels.
- If the individual passes out from hypoglycemia and uses insulin on a daily basis, it may be necessary to give a glucagon shot and call for emergency assistance.

Herbs, Botanicals, and Supplements

- Herbs and botanical supplements should not be used without discussing with physician.

INTERVENTION: NUTRITION EDUCATION, COUNSELING, CARE MANAGEMENT

- Teach benefits of frequent blood glucose monitoring. Explain signs, symptoms, and treatment of hypoglycemia.
- Review appropriate timing of meals, snacks, and medications. Promote regular mealtimes, meal spacing, and planned exercise.
- Teach routine blood glucose before and after exercise
- Encourage patients to obtain and carry diabetes identification.
- Teach patients to carry a quick source of glucose.
- Discuss observations that require medical attention. Teach when to contact physician for medication adjustment.
- Discuss use of alcoholic beverages and potential effects. Excess alcohol increases the risk of hypoglycemia. Alcohol is processed in the liver to acetaldehyde at a time when the liver cannot do gluconeogenesis because nicotinamide adenine dinucleotide (NAD) is used up; so hypoglycemia occurs. The biggest risk occurs when a patient drinks without carbohydrates being available, such as 4 hours or longer after the last meal. One drink takes 1–1.5 hours to process in the liver. Women should stick to one alcoholic beverage a day; men should limit their intake to two per day, and all should consume carbohydrate with their drinks.
- In the elderly who are monitoring blood glucose levels closely, the benefits of intensive therapy in an effort to lower A1c must be weighed against the greater risk of unpredictable hypoglycemia (Alam et al, 2005).

For More Information

- National Institute of Diabetes and Digestive and Kidney Diseases (NIDDK)–Hypoglycemia in Diabetes http://diabetes.niddk.nih.gov/dm/pubs/hypoglycemia/

HYPOGLYCEMIA—CITED REFERENCES

Alam T, et al. What is the proper use of hemoglobin A1c monitoring in the elderly? *J Am Med Dir Assoc.* 6:200, 2005.

Cersosimo E, et al. Abnormal glucose handling by the kidney in response to hypoglycemia in type 1 diabetes. *Diabetes* 50:2087, 2001.

Dagogo-Jack S. Hypoglycemia in type 1 diabetes mellitus: pathophysiology and prevention. *Treat Endocrinol.* 3:91, 2004.

Grimm JJ, et al. A new table for prevention of hypoglycaemia during physical activity in type 1 diabetic patients. *Diabetes Metab.* 30:465, 2004.

Smith WD, et al. Causes of hyperglycemia and hypoglycemia in adult inpatients. *Am J Health Syst Pharm.* 62:714, 2005.

HYPERINSULINISM AND SPONTANEOUS HYPOGLYCEMIA

NUTRITIONAL ACUITY RANKING: LEVEL 3–4

DEFINITIONS AND BACKGROUND

Spontaneous hypoglycemia is not a diagnosis but an underlying symptom of some other disease process. It is unrelated to diabetes. It may occur in conditions such as intrauterine growth retardation (Russell-Silver syndrome), where regular feedings are needed to correct the hypoglycemic episodes (Azcona and Stanhope, 2006).

Fasting and postprandial hypoglycemia are categorized as two spontaneous forms. In **fasting hypoglycemia,** the body is not able to maintain adequate levels of sugar in the blood after a period without food. Prolonged fasting or strenuous exercise, even after fasting, seldom causes hypoglycemia in otherwise healthy people. However, heavy drinkers who do not eat; people with viral hepatitis, cirrhosis, or liver cancer; and children with carbohydrate metabolic disorders may have fasting hypoglycemia. Islet cell tumors may also lead to fasting hypoglycemia (Virally and Guillausseau, 1999).

Congenital hyperinsulinism (CHI) is characterized by profound hypoglycemia because of excessive insulin secretion. One form, from a beta-cell tumor, may be cured by partial pancreatectomy (Fournet et al, 2001).

In **postprandial or alimentary hypoglycemia,** excessive amounts of insulin are secreted after 1.5–5 hours in response to carbohydrate-rich foods. Postprandial hypoglycemia is generally caused by excessive insulin effect, often after gastric surgery, and is rarely seen in early diabetes mellitus (Pourmotabbed and Kitabchi, 2001). This type of hypoglycemia may occur in very lean people, in people after massive weight reduction, and in women with moderate lower body overweight and may be influenced by a patient's eating habits (e.g., high-carbohydrate/low-fat diet, alcohol intake). Problems with digestion of some sugars (fructose and galactose) and amino acids (leucine) may cause reactive hypoglycemia. An uncommon form of reactive hypoglycemia can occur after drinking alcohol in combination with sugar.

Symptoms resemble those of the dumping syndrome and include weakness and agitation 2–4 hours after meals, perspiration, nervousness, and mental confusion. Postprandial hypoglycemia can result from: (1) an exaggerated insulin response, either related to insulin resistance or to increased glucagon-like peptide 1; (2) renal glycosuria; (3) defects in glucagon response; or (4) high insulin sensitivity, which is probably the cause in 50–70% of cases (Brun et al, 2000).

Diet remains the main treatment, although alpha-glucosidase inhibitors and some other drugs may be helpful.

INTERVENTION: OBJECTIVES

- Reduce intake of concentrated CHO to a level that does not overstimulate the pancreas to secrete inappropriately large amounts of insulin, which may cause blood sugar to drop to 40 mg/dL or lower.
- Monitor patient carefully because this condition can precede diabetes or can be related to mild overt diabetes.
- If required, ensure that patient loses weight gradually.
- Reduce counterregulatory hormone responses to excessive insulin.

INTERVENTION: FOOD AND NUTRITION

- Individualize CHO intake. Simple sugars and dried fruits are allowed in limited amounts.
- Maintain protein intake at RDA levels because protein may stimulate insulin secretion. Fat furnishes the remainder of calories.
- Diet should include frequent small meals and at least a well-balanced diet.

CLINICAL INDICATORS

Clinical/History	Lab Work	
Height	Gluc	Trig
Weight	Serum insulin	HgA1c
BMI	Serum glucagon	Ca++, Mg++
Diet history	Growth hormone levels	Acetone
Recent weight losses	Chol	PO_4
BP	Trig	CRP
Seizures, confusion	Na+, K+	
Palpitations		

Common Drugs Used and Potential Side Effects

- Alpha-glucosidase inhibitors may be useful for postprandial hypoglycemia, but this requires further study.
- Monitor all medications for their potential hypoglycemic effects.

Herbs, Botanicals, and Supplements

- Herbs and botanical supplements should not be used without discussing with physician.

INTERVENTION: NUTRITION EDUCATION, COUNSELING, CARE MANAGEMENT

- Explain that alcohol blocks gluconeogenesis and should be avoided.
- Ensure that patient keeps snacks available such as cheese and crackers. More frequent feedings are needed.
- Emphasize that meals should not be skipped and that large meals should not be taken. Meals should be eaten on time.
- Avoid any one meal that is unbalanced or especially high in carbohydrates.
- Control caffeine intake and use of other stimulants, which may aggravate condition.

For More Information

- National Institute of Diabetes and Digestive and Kidney Diseases (NIDDK)–Hypoglycemia (Nondiabetes) http://diabetes.niddk.nih.gov/dm/pubs/hypoglycemia/#nodiabetes

HYPERINSULINISM AND SPONTANEOUS HYPOGLYCEMIA—CITED REFERENCES

Azcona C, Stanhope R. Hypoglycaemia and Russell-Silver syndrome. *J Pediatr Endocrinol Metab.* 18:663, 2005.
Brun J, et al. Postprandial reactive hypoglycemia. *Diabetes Metab.* 26:337, 2000.
Fournet J, et al. Unbalanced expression of 11p15 imprinted genes in focal forms of congenital hyperinsulinism: association with a reduction to homozygosity of a mutation in ABCC8 or KCNJ11. *Am J Pathol.* 158:2177, 2001.
Pourmotabbed G, Kitabchi A. Hypoglycemia. *Obstet Gynecol Clin North Am.* 28:383, 2001.
Virally M, Guillausseau P. Hypoglycemia in adults. *Diabetes Metab.* 25:477, 1999.

OTHER ENDOCRINE DISORDERS

Hormones can be separated into three categories: **amines,** these are simple molecules, **proteins and peptides,** which are made from chains of amino acids, and **steroids,** which are derived from cholesterol. **Glands** discharge hormones directly into the bloodstream, and they have feedback mechanisms that maintain a proper balance of hormones and prevent excess secretion. See Figure 9-5.

Endocrine disorders require varying levels of nutritional intervention. If medications are taken appropriately, many conditions can be readily managed. See Table 9-20.

For More Information on Other Endocrine Conditions

- American Association of Clinical Endocrinologists http://www.aace.com/
- American Medical Association http://www.ama-assn.org/ama/pub/category/7157.html
- Endocrine Society http://www.aace.com/
- The Hormone Foundation http://www.hormone.org/
- National Institutes of Health–Endocrine Disorders http://www.niddk.nih.gov/health/endo/endo.htm

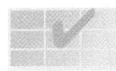

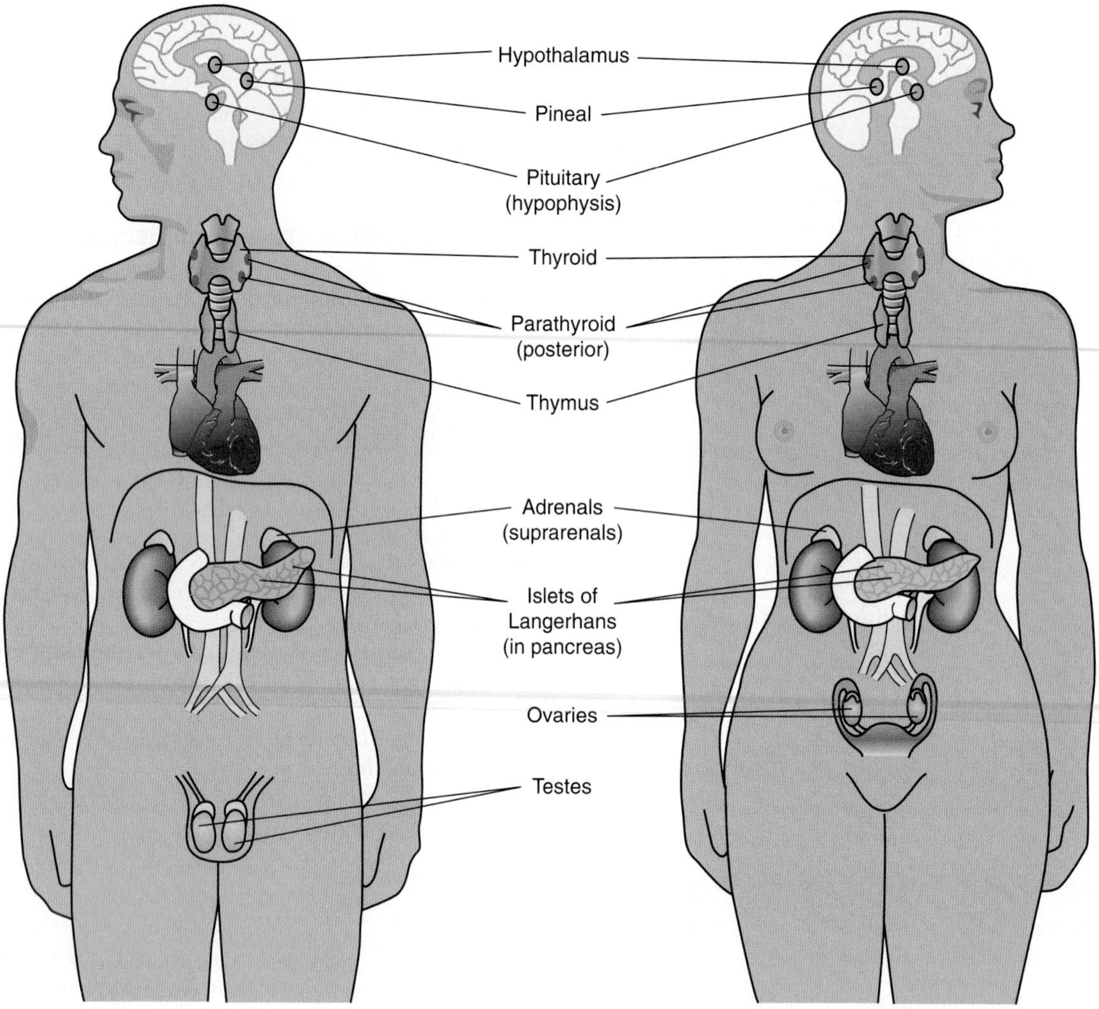

Figure 9-5 Major endocrine glands. (From Smeltzer SC, Bare BG. *Textbook of medical-surgical nursing.* 9th ed. Philadelphia: Lippincott Williams & Wilkins, 2000.)

TABLE 9-20 Other Endocrine Conditions

There are many other disorders of endocrine function besides those affecting the pancreas that require some level of nutritional intervention. Listed below are essential hormones and functions of the endocrine glands.

Gland	Hormones	Functions
Pancreas	Glucagon (from alpha-cells)	Alpha-cells in the pancreatic islets secrete the hormone glucagon in response to a low concentration of glucose in the blood.
	Insulin (from beta-cells)	Beta-cells in the pancreatic islets secrete insulin in response to high blood glucose concentrations. See diabetes section.
Gastric mucosa	Gastrin	Stimulates production of hydrochloric acid and the enzyme pepsin, used in digestive processes.
Small intestinal mucosa	Secretin Cholecystokinin	Stimulates the pancreas to produce bicarbonate-rich fluid to neutralize stomach acid. Stimulates contraction of the gallbladder to release bile after a meal containing fat. Also stimulates the pancreas to secrete digestive enzymes.
Placenta	Human chorionic gonadotropin	Signals the mother's ovaries to secrete hormones to maintain the uterine lining during pregnancy.
Hypothalamus	Gonadotropin-releasing hormone (GnRH) and other releasing hormones	Hunger and thirst; emotional and sexual responses of the limbic system; heart rate and blood pressure; circadian cycles; body temperature; bladder function; moods. Hypothalamus links the nervous system by synthesizing and secreting neurohormones that stimulate release of hormones from the anterior pituitary gland.

(continued)

TABLE 9-20 Other Endocrine Conditions *(continued)*

Gland	Hormones	Functions
Pituitary (anterior)	Adrenocorticotropic hormone (ACTH)	Reacts with receptor sites in the cortex of the adrenal gland to stimulate the secretion of cortical hormones, particularly cortisol.
	Human growth hormone (hGH or somatotropin hormone)	Growth of bones, muscles, and other organs by promoting protein synthesis; influences height.
	Thyroid-stimulating hormone (TSH or thyrotropin)	Causes thyroid to secrete thyroid hormone.
	Gonadotropins (follicle-stimulating hormone [FSH]; luteinizing hormone [LH])	React with gonads to regulate growth and function of these organs. In females, FSH stimulates egg production; in males, it stimulates sperm production. In females, LH causes ovulation; in males, it causes the testes to secrete testosterone.
	Prolactin (PRL)	Promotes development of glandular tissue in the female breast during pregnancy and stimulates milk production after the birth of the infant.
Pituitary (posterior)	Oxytocin (OT)	Causes contraction of the smooth muscle in the wall of the uterus. It also stimulates the ejection of milk from the lactating breast.
	Vasopressin (antidiuretic hormone [ADH])	ADH promotes the reabsorption of water by the kidney tubules; less water is lost as urine to conserve water for the body. Insufficient amounts of ADH cause excessive water loss in the urine.
Pineal gland	Melatonin (5-methoxy-*N*-acetyltryptamine)	Reproductive development and daily sleep–wake cycles; skin blanching. Derived from tryptophan. Production is stimulated by darkness and inhibited by light. Beta-blockers decrease release of melatonin.
Adrenal cortex		Adrenal cortex has control of 28 hormones, all of which are steroids.
	Mineralocorticoids (such as aldosterone)	Aldosterone conserves sodium ions and water.
	Glucocorticoids (such as cortisol)	Cortisol increases blood glucose levels.
	Gonadocorticoids (sex hormones: androgens and estrogens)	Normal reproductive functioning.
Adrenal medulla	Epinephrine (adrenalin) and norepinephrine (noradrenalin)	These two hormones are secreted in response to stimulation by the sympathetic nerve, particularly during stressful situations. They cause faster heartbeat and increased blood glucose levels.
		A lack of hormones from the adrenal medulla produces no significant effects. Hypersecretion, usually from a tumor, causes prolonged or continual sympathetic responses.
Thyroid	Thyroid hormones: thyroxine (95%) and triiodothyronine (5%)	Growth and development, metabolism. Thyroid hormones need iodine.
	Calcitonin	Calcitonin is secreted by the parafollicular cells of the thyroid gland. This hormone opposes the action of the parathyroid glands by reducing the calcium level in the blood. If blood calcium becomes too high, calcitonin is secreted until calcium ion levels decrease to normal.
Thymus	Thymosin	Immunity; T cells; lymphocytes. Currently being studied for its possible role in AIDS and hepatitis.
Parathyroid glands	Parathyroid hormone (PTH)	Regulation of calcium and phosphorus; secreted in response to low blood calcium levels in order to increase those levels. PTH mobilizes calcium by increasing calcium resorption from bone and by raising calcium reabsorption in the proximal kidney tubule.
Gonads (testes and ovaries)	Androgens (testosterone)	Growth and development of the male reproductive structures; increased skeletal and muscular growth; enlargement of the larynx accompanied by voice changes; growth and distribution of body hair; increased male sexual drive.
	Estrogen and progesterone	Development of the breasts; distribution of fat evidenced in the hips, legs, and breasts; maturation of reproductive organs such as the uterus and vagina. Progesterone causes the uterine lining to thicken in preparation for pregnancy. Together, progesterone and estrogens are responsible for the changes that occur in the uterus during the female menstrual cycle.

Sources: Surveillance, Epidemiology, and End Results. Endocrine glands and their functions. Accessed July 1, 2005 at http://training.seer.cancer.gov/module_anatomy/unit6_3_endo_glnds.html; and Cotterill S. The endocrine system (hormones). Accessed July 1, 2005 at http://www.cancerindex.org/medterm/medtm12.htm#function.

PITUITARY GLAND

HYPOPITUITARISM

NUTRITIONAL ACUITY RANKING: LEVEL 1

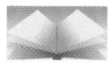

DEFINITIONS AND BACKGROUND

Hypopituitarism is an underactive pituitary gland. A deficiency in production of pituitary hormones may be caused by tumor, trauma, radiation to the brain, aneurysm, infarction, or surgery. The pituitary hormones include adrenocorticotropic hormone (ACTH), human growth hormone (hGH), luteinizing hormone (LH), follicle-stimulating hormone (FSH), prolactin, oxytocin (OT), and antidiuretic hormone (ADH). Table 9-21 lists symptoms of a pituitary disorder.

Symptoms of hypopituitarism will depend on which hormones are not being produced at sufficient levels. It may take years for an accurate diagnosis to be made. Patients with hypopituitarism caused by a craniopharyngioma (CP) or its treatment have a higher mortality rate than patients with other etiologies (Velherst et al, 2005).

If all of the pituitary hormones are missing, this is called panhypopituitarism. The condition is relatively rare.

If GH is deficient in children, short stature results; the condition causes 10% of all dwarfism. Weight gain occurs, with greater subcutaneous fat deposition and decreased muscle mass. Low libido, weakness, sleep disturbances, fatigue, and mental confusion are also symptoms of GH deficiency (GHD). Vascular abnormalities are common (Kearney et al, 2001). GHD in the adult has now been fully recognized, and symptoms include abnormal body composition, osteopenia, impaired quality of life, cardiac dysfunction, and an adverse lipid profile (Verhelst and Abs, 2002).

If ACTH is missing, depression, fatigue, low blood pressure, nausea and diarrhea, dizziness, pale skin, weakness, and weight loss are signs and symptoms. A shortage of cortisol occurs, and this can be life threatening.

If ADH is deficient, severe thirst and excessive urination occur. Diabetes insipidus may occur. In rare instances, ADH deficiency may occur after an event, such as after brain surgery.

If gonadotropin (FSH, LH) deficiency occurs, men and women will lose interest in sex and can experience fatigue and weakness, loss of body hair, impotence in men, and loss of menstruation in women. Prolactin deficiency is rare but can stop milk production in women.

If thyroid-stimulating hormone (TSH) is deficient, this can lead to an underactive thyroid (hypothyroidism). Cold intolerance, constipation, weight gain, and pale and waxy or dry skin can occur.

TABLE 9-21 Symptoms of a Pituitary Disorder

Headaches	Eating disorders:	High blood pressure
Depression	Anorexia	Diabetes
Mood/emotion swings	Obesity	Infertility
Anger	Bulimia	Impotence
Loss of memory	Weight gain	Irregular menses
Loss of sleep	Lethargy	Lactating
Sexual dysfunction	Weakness in limbs	Unusual hair growth

Source: Pituitary Network Association. Available at http://www.pituitary.org/.

INTERVENTION: OBJECTIVES

- Replenish missing hormones.
- Prevent dehydration, hypoglycemia, and related problems.
- Improve lean muscle mass stores.
- Monitor serum levels of cholesterol and triglycerides; prevent vascular complications.

INTERVENTION: FOOD AND NUTRITION

- Dietary alterations may be needed, such as higher or lower energy intake, until hormone levels are normalized. A modified fat, cholesterol, and carbohydrate intake may be needed. Assure sufficient intake of protein.
- Six small feedings may be better tolerated than larger meals.
- Increase fluids unless contraindicated.
- Ensure adequate intake of all vitamins and minerals. Calcium and vitamin D should be taken in sufficient amounts to prevent osteoporosis.

CLINICAL INDICATORS

Clinical/History

Height
Weight
BMI
Diet history
BP
Dual-energy x-ray absorptiometry (DEXA) scan

Lab Work

Thyroxine (T4) (decreased?)
Triiodothyronine (T3)
FSH, LH, TSH (decreased?)
Protein-bound iodine (PBI) uptake (decreased?)
Gluc, glucose tolerance test (GTT)
Chol, Trig
Homocysteine
CRP
Alb
Complete blood count (CBC)
Osmolarity
Na+, K+
Ca++, Mg++
Serum Gluc
Uric acid
H & H
Serum ferritin
Transferrin

Common Drugs Used and Potential Side Effects

Hormone replacement therapy may include any of all of the following:

1. Corticosteroids (hydrocortisone [Cortef], cortisol) are often used and can alter glucose, calcium, and phosphate tolerance. Potassium and folacin must be increased; sodium must be decreased. Monitor for signs of hyperglycemia.
2. Thyroid preparations (levothyroxine) may be needed.
3. GH (somatotropin) requires no specific dietary interventions. It may help alleviate elevated triglycerides. Long-term GH replacement therapy in adults can be safely used, and GH replacement should be considered as a possible lifelong therapy in order to maintain its benefits (Velherst and Abs, 2002).
4. Estrogen, progesterone, or testosterone replacement should be monitored for side effects related to heart disease and elevated lipids.
5. Cortisone may be needed during periods of stress or illness if ACTH is deficient.

Herbs, Botanicals, and Supplements

- Herbs and botanical supplements should not be used without discussing with physician.

INTERVENTION: NUTRITION EDUCATION, COUNSELING, CARE MANAGEMENT

- Have patient avoid fasting and stress.
- Discuss the need to use small, frequent meals instead of large meals.
- Discuss the possibility of hyperglycemia and how to manage.
- Hormone replacement is usually permanent, so doctor visits will be needed to check for diabetes and signs of osteoporosis.

For More Information

- Hormone Foundation–Pituitary Hormone
  http://www.hormone.org/public/pituitary.cfm
- Pituitary Disorders Network
  http://www.pituitarydisorder.net/
- The Pituitary Society
  http://www.pituitarysociety.org/

HYPOPITUITARISM—CITED REFERENCES

Kearney T, et al. Hypopituitarism is associated with triglyceride enrichment of very low-density lipoprotein. *J Clin Endocrinol Metab.* 86:3900, 2001.

Verhelst J, et al. Baseline characteristics and response to 2 years of growth hormone replacement of hypopituitary patients with growth hormone deficiency due to adult-onset craniopharyngioma in comparison to patients with non-functioning pituitary adenoma: data from KIMS. *J Clin Endocrinol Metab.* 90:4636, 2005.

Verhelst J, Abs R. Long-term growth hormone replacement therapy in hypopituitary adults. *Drugs* 62:2399, 2002.

PITUITARY GLAND (ANTERIOR)

ACROMEGALY

NUTRITIONAL ACUITY RANKING: LEVEL 1

DEFINITIONS AND BACKGROUND

Acromegaly is a hormonal disorder caused by overproduction of human growth hormone (hGH or GH) by the pituitary gland. Incidence is rare, with 50–70 cases per million in the U.S. population. Diagnosis commonly is made about a decade after oversecretion of GH begins.

GH (somatotropin) affects the growth of almost all cells and tissues and has direct and indirect effects. Direct effects of GH include hyperinsulinism, lipolysis, insulin resistance in peripheral tissues, ketogenesis, hyperglycemia, and sodium and water retention. Elevated insulin-like growth factor I (IGF-I) also occurs in acromegaly, resulting in greater protein synthesis, amino acid transportation, muscle and bone growth, DNA and RNA synthesis, and cell proliferation.

Symptoms and signs of acromegaly include enlarged extremities with disproportionate growth of nose, lips, brow, lower jaw, tongue, hands, and feet; increased coarse body hair; coarse, leathery skin; excessive diaphoresis and oily skin; skin tags; impaired vision; osteoarthritis; carpal tunnel syndrome; deepening voice; headaches; and moderate weight gain. The serious side effects include heart failure, colon polyps that become cancerous, and diabetes. Surgical removal of the pituitary gland may help; it can provide a 50–70% chance of cure (Vance and Laws, 2005). Otherwise, premature death may result if left untreated.

In over 90% of acromegaly patients, the overproduction of GH is related to a benign tumor. If GH-producing tumors occur in children, the disease is called gigantism rather than acromegaly. In a few patients, acromegaly is caused by tumors of the pancreas, lungs, or adrenal glands.

Somatostatin analogs have been key in medical therapy for acromegaly. Pegvisomant, a GH-receptor antagonist, competitively binds to the GH receptor, blocking IGF-I production and allowing for better control of cardiac disorders and glucose metabolism (Vance and Lawes, 2005).

INTERVENTION: OBJECTIVES

- Control weight and metabolic rate, which may be increased.
- Control diabetes and heart disease when involved.

- Prevent osteoporosis with calcium balance (often negative in acromegaly).
- Monitor for complications such as colon polyps, which may lead to cancer.
- Goal for GH levels should be 1–2 μg/L as a therapeutic target (Sheppard, 2005).

INTERVENTION: FOOD AND NUTRITION

- A diet with controlled calories (higher or lower) may be needed to control weight.
- Extra fluid intake may be needed.
- Control sodium and fluid intake if needed for heart failure.
- Offer sufficient intake of calcium and vitamin D; a multivitamin-mineral supplement may be useful.

CLINICAL INDICATORS

Clinical/History	Lab Work	
Height	GH (may be 5× higher than normal)	Ca++ (decreased)
Weight	N balance	Phosphorus (P) (may be increased)
BMI	BUN	Alb
Diet history	Serum Creat (increased)	GTT
BP (increased)	Urine sugar	Na+, K+
I & O	Gluc, HbA1c	H & H
Syndrome of inappropriate antidiuretic hormone (SIADH) or fluid retention	Serum insulin	
	IGF-I levels	

Common Drugs Used and Potential Side Effects

- Bromocriptine (Parlodel) reduces GH secretion from some pituitary tumors. Side effects include gastrointestinal upset, nausea, vomiting, light-headedness when standing, and nasal congestion. Take with food.
- Octreotide (Sandostatin) injection may be used as a synthetic form of somatostatin. Side effects include diarrhea, nausea, gallstones, and loose stools.
- Insulin may be needed if diabetes is also present. Be wary of excess doses; hypoglycemia is a dangerous side effect.
- Cardiac medications may be needed; monitor for specific side effects accordingly. Atorvastatin treatment is safe, well tolerated, and effective in improving the atherogenic lipoprotein profile in acromegaly (Mishra et al, 2005).
- Pegvisomant, a treatment for acromegaly, was approved for clinical use in the United States to normalize circulating levels of IGF-I, the principal mediator of GH action (Drake and Trainer, 2003).

Herbs, Botanicals, and Supplements

- Herbs and botanical supplements should not be used without discussing with physician.

INTERVENTION: NUTRITION EDUCATION, COUNSELING, CARE MANAGEMENT

- Discuss body changes and self-image alterations.
- Teach patient about control of diabetes or heart failure, where present.
- After surgery, potential complications include cerebrospinal fluid leaks, meningitis, and damage to the surrounding normal pituitary tissue, requiring lifelong pituitary hormone replacement.
- Exercise can help to improve physical functioning and quality of life (Woodhouse et al, 2006).

For More Information

- National Institute of Diabetes and Digestive and Kidney Diseases (NIDDK)–Acromegaly
  http://www.niddk.nih.gov/health/endo/pubs/acro/acro.htm
- Pituitary Network Association
  http://www.pituitary.com/
- Skull Base Institute
  http://www.skullbaseinstitute.com/acromegaly_gigantism.htm

ACROMEGALY—CITED REFERENCES

Drake WM, Trainer PJ. Clinical use of pegvisomant for the treatment of acromegaly. *Treat Endocrinol.* 2:369, 2003.

Mishra M, et al. The effect of atorvastatin on serum lipoproteins in acromegaly. *Clin Endocrinol.* 62:650, 2005.

Sheppard MC. GH and mortality in acromegaly. *J Endocrinol Invest.* 28:75S, 2005.

Vance ML, Laws ER Jr. Role of medical therapy in the management of acromegaly. *Neurosurgery* 56:877, 2005.

Woodhouse LJ, et al. The influence of growth hormone status on physical impairments, functional limitations, and health-related quality of life in adults. *Endocr Rev.* 27:287, 2006.

PITUITARY GLAND (ANTERIOR)

CUSHING'S SYNDROME

NUTRITIONAL ACUITY RANKING: LEVEL 1–2

DEFINITIONS AND BACKGROUND

Cushing's syndrome is a disease caused by an excess of cortisol production or excess use of cortisol or other similar steroid (glucocorticoid) hormones. It can be caused by extrinsic and excessive hormonal stimulation of the adrenal cortex by tumor of the anterior pituitary gland, adrenal hyperplasia, or exogenous cortisol use. Differential diagnosis is not simple. No existing test is accurate when used alone; focused imaging, including computed tomography (CT), magnetic resonance imaging (MRI), and nuclear imaging modalities, can provide a diagnosis (Lindsay and Nieman, 2005).

Pituitary Cushing's syndrome occurs after puberty with equal frequency in boys and girls. In adults, it has a greater frequency in women than men, with most diagnosed between ages 20 and 50 years. The total incidence is about 10–15 million people per year. It is a disorder characterized by virilism, upper body obesity with thin arms and legs, hyperglycemia, glucosuria, hypertension, red moon face, vertigo, emotional lability, buffalo hump, purple striae over obese areas, acne, female balding or hirsutism, blurry vision, and pitting ankle edema. In some cases, osteoporosis and severe depression may also be present.

If left untreated, Cushing's syndrome can be fatal. Treatments differ according to the cause: adrenocorticotropic hormone (ACTH) dependent (pituitary or ectopic) or independent (an adrenal tumor) or iatrogenic (from excessive steroid hormone use). If iatrogenic, depletion of steroid hormones will be needed. If pituitary, the gland may need to be removed.

Cushing's syndrome caused by ACTH production from solid tumors can result in life-threatening hypercortisolemia (Uecker and Janzow, 2005). Radiation, chemotherapy, or surgery may be needed. After surgical removal of the adrenal glands, most symptoms of Cushing's syndrome disappear, but psychological impairment could persist despite successful treatment (Iacabone et al, 2005).

The fact that obesity is a prominent feature of hypercortisolism (Cushing's syndrome) has stimulated investigation that hypercortisolism is a feature of obesity; studies are inconsistent, and whether the enzymatic overactivity is a cause or a result of obesity is still unclear (Salehi et al, 2005). Figure 9-6 is a photograph of a person with Cushing's syndrome.

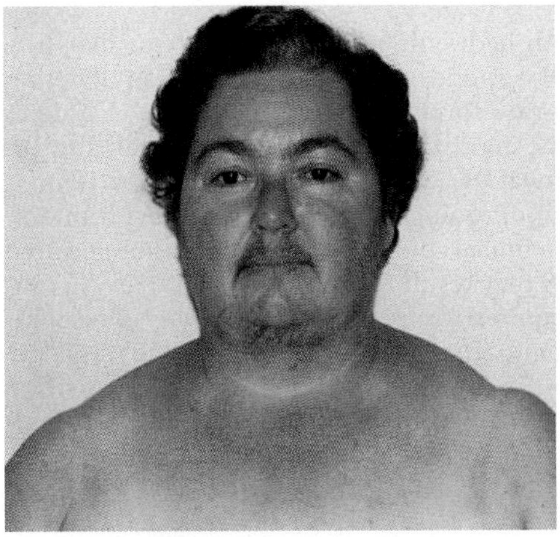

Figure 9-6 Patient with Cushing's syndrome. (From Rubin E, Farber JL. *Pathology*. 3rd ed. Philadelphia: Lippincott Williams & Wilkins, 1999.)

INTERVENTION: OBJECTIVES

- Chronic cortisol hypersecretion causes central obesity, hypertension, insulin resistance, dyslipidemia, and prothrombotic state, which are manifestations that form a metabolic syndrome in all patients with Cushing's syndrome (Arnaldi et al, 2004). Control symptoms of elevated blood glucose; manage diabetes and cardiovascular disease.
- Promote weight loss if needed. Control patient's weight while increasing lean body mass.
- Control hypertension.
- Prevent vertebral collapse and other side effects such as congestive heart failure, bone demineralization, osteoporosis, and hypokalemia.
- Control side effects of corticosteroid therapy.

INTERVENTION: FOOD AND NUTRITION

- Restrict sodium if steroids are used.
- Use a calorie-controlled diet, if needed. Calculate diet according to patient's desirable body weight. Control glucose levels when elevated; carbohydrate counting can be useful.
- Ensure adequate intake of calcium and potassium.
- Ensure adequate intake of protein if losses are excessive (e.g., 1 g protein/kg or more).

CLINICAL INDICATORS

Clinical/History		Lab Work
Height Weight BMI Diet history BP (increased) Edema	Computed tomography (CT) or magnetic resonance imaging (MRI) (checking for tumors) DEXA scan	24-Hour urinary free cortisol level (>50–100 μg/d) Dexamethasone suppression test

Corticotropin-releasing hormone (CRH) stimulation test for ACTH levels (altered depending on cause)	Urinary Gluc (increased) Gluc (increased) HbA1c Ca++, Mg++ Urinary Ca+ Lipid profile, Chol, Trig K+ (decreased)	Na+ (increased) Alb, N balance CRP pCO_2 (increased), pO_2 WBC, TLC (decreased)

Common Drugs Used and Potential Side Effects

- With glucocorticoid therapy, osteoporosis and hypercalciuria are common side effects. Withdrawal of these medications after autoimmune or cancer management may cause iatrogenic Cushing's syndrome. Adrenal insufficiency or steroid withdrawal symptoms may occur (Hopkins and Leinung, 2005).
- Large doses of vitamin D may be necessary; do not use for extended periods of time because toxicity may occur.

Herbs, Botanicals, and Supplements

- Herbs and botanical supplements should not be used without discussing with physician.

INTERVENTION: NUTRITION EDUCATION, COUNSELING, CARE MANAGEMENT

- Help patient control weight as needed.
- Explain which foods are good sources of calcium in the diet.
- Explain how to control elevated blood sugars through balanced dietary intake.
- Manage symptoms of metabolic syndrome through dietary changes and exercise.

For More Information

- Cushing's Support and Research Foundation
  http://csrf.net/
- National Institute of Diabetes and Digestive and Kidney Diseases (NIDDK)–Cushing's Syndrome
  http://www.niddk.nih.gov/health/endo/pubs/cushings/cushings.htm

CUSHING'S SYNDROME—CITED REFERENCES

Arnaldi G, et al. Cardiovascular risk in Cushing's syndrome. *Pituitary* 7:253, 2004.
Hopkins RL, Leinung MC. Exogenous Cushing's syndrome and glucocorticoid withdrawal. *Endocrinol Metab Clin North Am.* 34:371, 2005.
Iacabone M, et al. Results and long-term follow-up after unilateral adrenalectomy for ACTH-independent hypercortisolism in a series of fifty patients. *J Endocrinol Invest.* 28:327, 2005.
Lindsay JR, Nieman LK. Differential diagnosis and imaging in Cushing's syndrome. *Endocrinol Metab Clin North Am.* 34:403, 2005.
Salehi M, et al. Obesity and cortisol status. *Horm Metab Res.* 37:193, 2005.
Uecker JM, Janzow MT. A case of Cushing syndrome secondary to ectopic adrenocorticotropic hormone producing carcinoid of the duodenum. *Am Surg.* 71:445, 2005.

PITUITARY GLAND (POSTERIOR)

DIABETES INSIPIDUS

NUTRITIONAL ACUITY RANKING: LEVEL 3

DEFINITIONS AND BACKGROUND

Diabetes insipidus (DI) can be caused by two fundamentally different defects: inadequate or impaired secretion of antidiuretic hormone (ADH) from the posterior pituitary gland (neurogenic or central DI) or impaired or insufficient renal response to ADH (nephrogenic DI); distinction is essential for effective treatment (Makaryus and MacFarlane, 2006). DI may be primary (congenital) or secondary (acquired after trauma, surgery, tumor, or infection). DI is marked by excessive thirst and drinking, copious urination, and dry skin; there is potential for dehydration and weakness. Urine output may be 5–10 L/24 hours.

Nephrogenic DI is a kidney disorder characterized by the kidney's inability to respond to the ADH, arginine vasopressin (AVP). Nephrogenic DI requires monitoring of body chemistry and adequate hydration.

Neurogenic (primary) DI is more common in males. Children with DI may be irritable or listless and may have problems with bedwetting, fever, vomiting, or diarrhea. Neurogenic DI responds to nasal administration of desmopressin.

Very rare forms of DI occur because of a defect in the thirst mechanism (**dipsogenic DI**) or during pregnancy (**gestational DI**). Sometimes, the exact cause is unknown. Patients undergoing surgery for pituitary tumors present unique clinical, biochemical, and pathological considerations; DI may result (Dumont et al, 2005).

In **acquired** forms, the kidneys' ability to respond to ADH can be impaired by drugs (like lithium) and by chronic disorders including polycystic kidney disease, sickle cell disease, kidney failure, partial blockage of the ureters, and inherited genetic disorders.

INTERVENTION: OBJECTIVES

- **Nephrogenic DI:** reduce urine osmolality, increase electrolyte-free water excretion, and raise serum sodium con-

centration. It is important to avoid fluid overload and rapid fluctuations in sodium concentration, especially in persons who cannot control their fluid intake themselves (Toumba and Stanhope, 2006).
- Check patient's weight three times weekly to determine fluid retention and effectiveness of drug therapy.
- Reduce excess workload for the kidney. Prevent stone formation.

INTERVENTION: FOOD AND NUTRITION

- Adjust fluid, sodium, and potassium intakes according to the cause.
- A low-sodium diet and diuretics may also be needed to minimize workload of the kidney.
- Sometimes a controlled-protein diet is needed to protect renal function.

CLINICAL INDICATORS

Clinical/History

Height
Weight
BMI
Diet history
BP
Excessive thirst and urination
I & O
Brain MRI

Lab Work

Arginine vasopressin (AVP) in serum, urine (neurogenic DI can be clearly diagnosed from the relative deficiency of AVP)
Osmolality (may be <300 mOsm/kg)
Fluid deprivation test to detect neurogenic vs. nephrogenic causes
Urinary specific gravity (decreased)
Uric acid (increased in adults)
BUN
Creat
Na+ (increased)
K+ (altered?)
Alb

Common Drugs Used and Potential Side Effects

- Desmopressin (DDAVP) may cause abdominal pain, headaches, gastrointestinal distress, and weakness. It is administered parenterally, by pill, or by nasal spray. Patients should drink fluids or water only when thirsty, but be aware that a low urine volume is a risk factor for kidney stone formation (Mehandru and Goldfarb, 2005). Hyponatremic hypervolemia leading to seizures is a rare but potentially life-threatening side effect.
- If diuretics such as thiazides or amiloride are used, monitor for side effects. Potassium may be needed if a supplement is not used.

Herbs, Botanicals, and Supplements

- Herbs and botanical supplements should not be used without discussing with physician.

INTERVENTION: NUTRITION EDUCATION, COUNSELING, CARE MANAGEMENT

- Fluid adjustments will be made according to the type of DI. Caution patients not to limit fluid intake in an effort to lessen urine output.
- Cold water may be preferred.
- Select low-calorie beverages to prevent excessive weight gain.
- Avoid stimulant/diuretic-type beverages (e.g., coffee, tea, alcohol).

For More Information

- Diabetes Insipidus Foundation, Inc.
  http://diabetesinsipidus.com
- Nephrogenic Diabetes Insipidus Foundation
  http://www.ndif.org/

DIABETES INSIPIDUS—CITED REFERENCES

Dumont AS, et al. Postoperative care following pituitary surgery. *J Intensive Care Med.* 20:127, 2005.
Makaryus AN, MacFarlane SI. Diabetes insipidus: diagnosis and treatment of a complex disease. *Cleve Clin J Med.* 73:65, 2006.
Mehandru S, Goldfarb DS. Nephrolithiasis complicating treatment of diabetes insipidus. *Urol Res.* 33:244, 2005.
Toumba M, Stanhope R. Morbidity and mortality associated with vasopressin analogue treatment. *J Pediatr Endocrinol Metab.* 19:197, 2006.

PITUITARY GLAND

SYNDROME OF INAPPROPRIATE ANTIDIURETIC HORMONE (SIADH)

NUTRITIONAL ACUITY RANKING: LEVEL 2

DEFINITIONS AND BACKGROUND

Syndrome of inappropriate antidiuretic hormone (SIADH) involves water intoxication with hyponatremia and hyperosmolarity of urine. Normal renal and adrenal functioning with abnormal elevation of plasma vasopressin occurs (inappropriate for serum osmolality). Hyponatremia can occur among elderly long-term care patients with febrile illness;

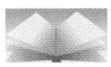

TABLE 9-22 Causes of Syndrome of Inappropriate Antidiuretic Hormone

Head injury
Acute leukemia
Lung cancer (especially small-cell lung cancer)
Brain abscess or other central nervous system disorders, including stroke or meningitis
Pneumonia
Lung abscess
Myxedema
Temporal arteritis, polyarteritis nodosa
Sarcoidosis
Rocky Mountain spotted fever
Carcinoma of the cervix
Olfactory neuroblastoma
Herpes zoster infection of the chest wall
Drugs: chlorpropamide, cyclophosphamide, carbamazepine

SIADH is common (Arinzon et al, 2005). Other causes of SIADH are listed in Table 9-22.

Hyponatremia may be the first symptom. In severe hyponatremia, convulsions or coma can occur. Other signs and symptoms include irritability, lethargy, seizures, and confusion. A systematic approach by clinicians, using a detailed history, physical examination, and relevant diagnostic tests, will assist in efficient management (Vachharajani et al, 2003).

Hyponatremia is a frequent occurrence after pituitary surgery, produced by SIADH or by the cerebral salt-wasting syndrome (CSWS); differential diagnosis can be difficult (Casulari et al, 2004). SIADH syndrome often requires sodium replacement (Johnson and Criddle, 2004). Loop diuretics are useful in managing chronic SIADH (Goh, 2004).

INTERVENTION: OBJECTIVES

- Restrict water intake.
- Replace electrolytes as appropriate. Usually intravenous saline is provided.
- Normalize hormone secretion through drug therapy.

INTERVENTION: FOOD AND NUTRITION

- Restrict fluid intake, usually 1 L/d.
- Alter dietary sodium and potassium, as deemed appropriate for the condition. This will vary by patient condition and medications used.
- When enteral feeding is needed, select a formula that is fluid restricted, such as those that are 2 kcal/mL. Monitor carefully for signs of dehydration. Check content of formula for sodium and potassium; select according to patient status and needs.

CLINICAL INDICATORS

Clinical/History

- Height
- Current weight
- Edema-free weight
- BMI
- Diet history
- I & O
- Temperature
- Edema
- Irritability
- Lethargy, confusion
- Low urine volume

Lab Work

- Serum Na+ (<135 mmol/L)
- Osmolality (<280 mOsm/kg)
- Serum AVP (elevated)
- BUN (low, <10 mg/dL)
- Creat
- K+
- Ca++, Mg++
- Bicarbonate (normal)
- Uric acid (may be low)
- GFR (increased)

Common Drugs Used and Potential Side Effects

- Demeclocycline (Declomycin) may be used with side effects like those of tetracycline. Avoid taking with calcium or dairy products.
- Conivaptan is a new agent available for use to antagonize the effects of vasopressin, especially in heart failure patients (Schwarz and Sanghi, 2006).
- Hyponatremia as a result of SIADH is a relatively common serious side effect of the use of selective serotonin reuptake inhibitors (SSRIs) in (mostly elderly) adults (Vanhaesebrouk et al, 2005).

Herbs, Botanicals, and Supplements

- Herbs and botanical supplements should not be used without discussing with physician.

INTERVENTION: NUTRITION EDUCATION, COUNSELING, CARE MANAGEMENT

- Provide counseling regarding water and fluid restrictions, as ordered.
- Discuss any underlying conditions that may have caused the syndrome; highlight needed dietary alterations.

For More Information

- E-medicine
  http://www.emedicine.com/ped/topic2190.htm
- National Library of Medicine–Dilutional Hyponatremia
  http://www.nlm.nih.gov/medlineplus/ency/article/000394.htm

SYNDROME OF INAPPROPRIATE ANTIDIURETIC HORMONE—CITED REFERENCES

Arinzon Z, et al. Water and sodium disturbances predict prognosis of acute disease in long term cared frail elderly. *Arch Gerontol Geriatr.* 40:317, 2005.

Casulari LA, et al. Differential diagnosis and treatment of hyponatremia following pituitary surgery. *J Neurosurg Sci.* 48:11, 2004.
Goh KP. Management of hyponatremia. *Am Fam Physician.* 69:2387, 2004.
Johnson AL, Criddle LM. Pass the salt: indications for and implications of using hypertonic saline. *Crit Care Nurse.* 24:36, 2004.
Schwarz ER, Sanghi P. Conivaptan: a selective vasopressin antagonist for the treatment of heart failure. *Expert Rev Cardiovasc Ther.* 4:17, 2006.
Vachharajani TJ, et al. Hyponatremia in critically ill patients. *J Intensive Care Med.* 18:3, 2003.
Vanhaesebrouk P, et al. Phototherapy-mediated syndrome of inappropriate secretion of antidiuretic hormone in an in utero selective serotonin reuptake inhibitor-exposed newborn infant. *Pediatrics* 115:508, 2005.

OVARY

POLYCYSTIC OVARIAN DISEASE

NUTRITIONAL ACUITY RANKING: LEVEL 2

DEFINITIONS AND BACKGROUND

Polycystic ovarian disease (PCOD; or polycystic ovarian syndrome [PCOS]) is an endocrine disorder characterized by hyperandrogenism, bilaterally enlarged polycystic ovaries, and insulin resistance. This syndrome affects about 6–10% of women of childbearing age (Barbieri, 2000). There is a lack of consensus between endocrinologists and gynecologists in the definition, diagnosis, and treatment of PCOD (Cussons et al, 2005).

PCOD is currently considered as possibly the most frequent cause of female infertility; it is also closely associated with the metabolic syndrome (Gleicher and Barad, 2006).

Hyperandrogenism, insulin resistance, and acanthosis nigricans (HAIR-AN syndrome) cause presentation of the insulin-resistant syndrome PCOD (Barbieri, 2000). Insulin resistance and hyperandrogenism are caused by both genetic and environmental factors. Acanthosis nigricans is a dark, velvety patch of skin that indicates insulin resistance (Scalzo and McKittrick, 2000). Women of Caribbean-Hispanic or African American descent seem to be more prone to this condition.

Women with PCOD may have had a history of gestational diabetes mellitus (GDM). Many adolescents present with hirsutism and irregular menses. In PCOD, elevated luteinizing hormone (LH) to follicle-stimulating hormone (FSH) ratio, hirsutism, acne, oily skin, male pattern baldness, menstrual irregularity, oligomenorrhea, and obesity can occur. Abnormally elevated levels of testosterone and LH disrupt the normal maturation process for ovulation. Immature cysts remain on the ovaries, giving the appearance of a "string of pearls."

Girls tested for anorexia nervosa (AN) may also have PCOD, with menstrual irregularities before weight loss and elevated LH and estrogen compared with individuals who have AN alone (Pinhas-Hamiel et al, 2006). In PCOD, biochemical abnormalities include hyperandrogenism, acyclic estrogen production, LH hypersecretion, decreased levels of steroid hormone–binding globulin (SHBG), and hyperinsulinemia (Mascitelli and Pezzetta, 2005). Infertility, hypertension, uterine cancer, diabetes, coronary heart disease, and endometrial carcinoma often follow (Legro, 2001). See Figure 9-7.

INTERVENTION: OBJECTIVES

- Lose weight or maintain a normal weight for height; obesity occurs in 50% of this population.
- Prevent heart problems, stroke, and heart attack. Improve lipid profile.
- Reduce serum androgens and improve menstrual regularity.
- Decrease risk for endometrial cancer.
- Alleviate glucose intolerance and insulin resistance.
- Improve anxiety, moods, and quality of life.

INTERVENTION: FOOD AND NUTRITION

- Offer a weight-control and exercise plan to meet weight goals. Loss of 5–10 lb may reduce symptoms.
- Lower elevated blood glucose and lipids. Eat 5–6 small meals per day.

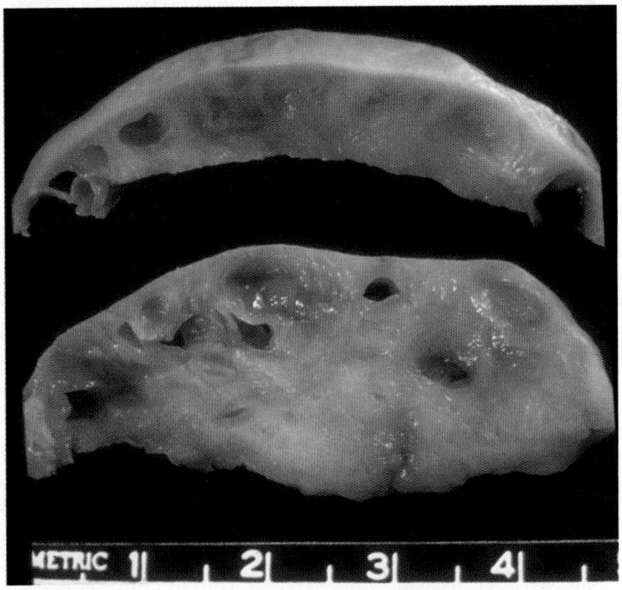

Figure 9-7 Polycystic ovary syndrome. (From Rubin E, Farber JL. *Pathology*. 3rd ed. Philadelphia: Lippincott Williams & Wilkins, 1999.)

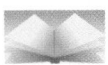

- The DASH diet may be helpful to lower blood pressure. Include low-fat dairy products and more fruits and vegetables.
- Avoid low-fat, high-CHO diets, which promote extra insulin secretion (McKittrick, 2002). A diet of 30–40% fat, 45–50% complex CHOs, and 15–20% protein may be useful.
- Include sufficient fiber (20–35 g/d).
- Include sources of omega-3 fatty acids (fish, walnuts, and flaxseed).
- Dietary or supplemental chromium should be included.

CLINICAL INDICATORS

Clinical/History	Lab Work
Height	Glucose
Weight	CRP
BMI	Chol, Trig (elevated?)
Diet history	Homocysteine
Weight gain pattern	Fasting serum insulin (elevated)
History (Hx) of GDM	C-peptide levels for insulin secretion
Irregular menses	Serum estrogen
Amenorrhea	Serum testosterone
Hirsutism	LH
Infertility	LH:FSH ratio (elevated)
Acne	Plasminogen activator inhibitor-1 (PAI-1) (shows abnormal clotting)
Male pattern baldness	H & H
Acanthosis nigricans (dark, velvety patches on skin)	Alb
Vaginal ultrasound with enlarged ovaries	BUN, Creat
Recurrent pregnancy loss?	ALT
	BP (elevated)

Common Drugs Used and Potential Side Effects

- Symptoms may be managed by antiandrogen medication (e.g., birth control pills, spironolactone, flutamide, or finasteride).
- Insulin-sensitizing drugs improve ovulation and hirsutism in PCOD (Azziz et al, 2001). Metformin (glucophage) allows for improved insulin sensitivity and reduced LH and testosterone. Metformin induces ovulation, has some marginal benefit in improving aspects of the metabolic syndrome, improves objective measures of hirsutism, and seems to be effective in both obese and lean individuals (Lord and Wilkin, 2004). Do not use with heart failure, chronic obstructive pulmonary disease, or chronic kidney disease. Take with food; monitor for minor gastrointestinal side effects such as nausea, diarrhea, and flatulence. Hypoglycemia does not usually occur.
- Rosiglitazone (Avandia) and pioglitazone (Actos) pose minimal risk of hepatotoxicity compared with older medications.

Herbs, Botanicals, and Supplements

- Herbs and botanical supplements should not be used without discussing with physician.
- Chromium picolinate (1000 μg) may be useful as an insulin sensitizer in the treatment of PCOD (Lydic et al, 2006).

INTERVENTION: NUTRITION EDUCATION, COUNSELING, CARE MANAGEMENT

- Counsel about weight loss and nutrition. Regular mealtimes and snacks may help control cravings and overeating.
- Encourage regular exercise and reduced sedentary lifestyle.
- Explain relationship of insulin resistance and increased risk for type 2 diabetes.
- Medical treatments may be needed to support reproduction. Some women will need in vitro fertilization (IVF) treatments.

For More Information

- E-medicine: PCOS
  http://www.emedicine.com/med/topic2173.htm
- Polycystic Ovarian Syndrome Association, Inc.
  http://www.pcosupport.org

POLYCYSTIC OVARIAN DISEASE—CITED REFERENCES

Azziz R, et al. Troglitazone improves ovulation and hirsutism in the polycystic ovary syndrome: a multicenter, double blind, and placebo-controlled trial. *J Clin Endocrinol Metab.* 86:1626, 2001.

Barbieri R. Induction of ovulation in infertile women with hyperandrogenism and insulin resistance. *Am J Obstet Gynecol.* 183:1412, 2000.

Cussons AJ, et al. Polycystic ovarian syndrome: marked differences between endocrinologists and gynaecologists in diagnosis and management. *Clin Endocrinol.* 62:289, 2005.

Essah PA, Nestler JE. The metabolic syndrome in polycystic ovary syndrome. *J Endocrinol Invest.* 29:270, 2006.

Gleicher N, Barad D. An evolutionary concept of polycystic ovarian disease: does evolution favor reproductive success over survival? *Reprod Biomed Online.* 12:587, 2006.

Legro R. Diabetes prevalence and risk factors in polycystic ovary syndrome. *Obstet Gynecol Clin North Am.* 28:99, 2001.

Lord J, Wilkin T. Metformin in polycystic ovary syndrome. *Curr Opin Obstet Gynecol.* 16:481, 2004.

Lydic ML, et al. Chromium picolinate improves insulin sensitivity in obese subjects with polycystic ovary syndrome. *Fertil Steril.* 86:243, 2006.

Mascitelli L, Pezzetta F. Polycystic ovary syndrome. *N Engl J Med.* 352:2756, 2005.

McKittrick M. Diet and polycystic syndrome. *Nutr Today.* 37:63, 2002.

Pinhas-Hamiel O, et al. Clinical and laboratory characteristics of adolescents with both polycystic ovary disease and anorexia nervosa. *Fertil Steril.* 85:1849, 2006.

Scalzo K, McKittrick M. Case problem: dietary recommendations to combat obesity, insulin resistance, and other concerns related to polycystic ovary syndrome. *J Am Diet Assoc.* 100:955, 2000.

ADRENAL GLAND (CORTEX)

ADRENOCORTICAL INSUFFICIENCY AND ADDISON'S DISEASE

NUTRITIONAL ACUITY RANKING: LEVEL 1–2

DEFINITIONS AND BACKGROUND

In adrenocortical insufficiency, the adrenal cortex atrophies with loss of hormones (aldosterone, cortisol, and androgens). Primary adrenal insufficiency in the pediatric population (0–18 years) is most commonly attributed to congenital adrenal hyperplasia, which occurs in about 1 in 15,000 births, followed by Addison's disease, with a likely autoimmune etiology (Perry et al, 2005). Secondary forms often result from tuberculosis, cancer, or surgery in which the adrenal glands are destroyed or damaged. Of patients with adrenocortical insufficiency, 33% also have diabetes. With type 1 diabetes, the expression of organ-specific autoantibodies is very high (Barker et al, 2005), and this suggests a need for careful screening in both of these conditions.

Cortisol, a glucocorticoid, affects almost every organ and tissue in the body. Cortisol helps the body respond to stress. Among other tasks, cortisol helps to maintain blood pressure and cardiac functioning, the immune system's inflammatory response, the effects of insulin in breaking down sugar for energy through metabolism of macronutrients, and proper arousal and well-being.

Aldosterone functions to conserve sodium and excrete potassium. When aldosterone is no longer secreted, the following events occur: excretion of sodium takes place, and the body's store of water decreases, which leads to dehydration, hypotension, and decreased cardiac output. The heart becomes slower due to reduced workload. Increased serum potassium can lead to arrhythmias, arrest, and even death.

In **primary adrenal insufficiency,** known as polyendocrine deficiency syndrome, type I occurs in children with underactive parathyroid glands, pernicious anemia, chronic *Candida* infections, chronic active hepatitis, and slow sexual development. Autoimmune thyroid diseases are often associated with type 1 diabetes mellitus and Addison's disease, characterizing the autoimmune polyendocrine syndrome (Silva et al, 2003). Type II primary adrenal insufficiency (Schmidt's syndrome) affects young adults and presents with underactive thyroid gland, slow sexual development, diabetes, vitiligo, and loss of skin pigmentation. Primary adrenal insufficiency causes abdominal pain, vomiting, weakness, fatigue, weight loss, dehydration, nausea, diarrhea, hyperpigmented (tan or bronze) skin, hypotension, low serum sodium, high serum potassium, and low corticosteroid levels. It may be temporary or may become a chronic insufficiency. Salt cravings can occur.

In the **secondary form** of adrenal insufficiency, which is much more common than the primary form, insufficiency can be traced to a lack of adrenocorticotropic hormone (ACTH). Production of cortisol drops but not production of aldosterone. A temporary form of secondary adrenal insufficiency may occur when a person who has been receiving a glucocorticoid hormone such as prednisone for a long time abruptly stops or interrupts taking the medication. Glucocorticoid hormones, which are often used to treat inflammatory illnesses like rheumatoid arthritis, asthma, or ulcerative colitis, block the release of both corticotropin-releasing hormone (CRH) and ACTH. Normally, CRH instructs the pituitary gland to release ACTH. If CRH levels drop, the pituitary is not stimulated to release ACTH, and the adrenals then fail to secrete sufficient levels of cortisol. In secondary adrenal insufficiency, darkening of the skin does not occur, and GI symptoms are less common. Hypoglycemia, anxiety, nausea, and palpitations can occur.

Addison's disease is a strict insufficiency state of adrenal hormones, including cortisol and aldosterone. It affects about 1 in 100,000 people. An Addisonian crisis can be precipitated by acute infection, trauma, surgery, or excessive body salt loss. Adrenalectomy may require steroid replacement therapy, a 2-g sodium diet, and control of carbohydrate to prevent hyperglycemia. A normal lifespan is possible if daily medications are taken as prescribed.

INTERVENTION: OBJECTIVES

- Relieve symptoms of hormone deficiency by taking synthetic hormones (but not to excess).
- Prevent hypoglycemia; avoid fasting.
- Prevent weight loss. Improve appetite and strength.
- Modify sodium according to drug therapy. Prevent hyponatremia, especially in warm weather when sodium losses from perspiration are higher than usual.
- Prevent dehydration and shock.
- Correct diarrhea, hyperkalemia, nausea, and drug overdosage.
- If hyperglycemia occurs, insulin may be needed.

INTERVENTION: FOOD AND NUTRITION

- During an Addisonian crisis, low blood pressure, low blood glucose, and high levels of potassium can be life threatening. Intravenous injections of hydrocortisone, saline, and dextrose are given by the medical team.
- Use a high-protein, moderate-carbohydrate diet. Snacks may be needed.
- Ensure intake of sodium is adequate according to medications given. Monitor potassium intake according to serum testing.
- Control carbohydrate amount and frequency to prevent either hypoglycemia or hyperglycemia.
- Force fluids (2–3 L) if allowed.

CLINICAL INDICATORS

Clinical/History	Lab Work	
Height	Gluc	ACTH stimulation test
Weight	K+ (increased)	BUN (increased)
BMI	N balance	Cortisol (decreased)
Diet history	Na+ (decreased)	CRH stimulation test
BP (decreased)	Ca++ (increased)	Alb
I & O	Cl_2 (decreased)	Mg++ (increased)
Abdominal x-rays	WBC (decreased)	HbA1c
Skin changes	ACTH (increased)	

Common Drugs Used and Potential Side Effects

- If aldosterone is missing, fludrocortisone (Florinef) is used as an oral, synthetic, sodium-retaining hormone. Be wary about overdosing, with potential side effects of hypertension and ankle edema. Postural hypotension can occur with a dose that is too low. Extra may be needed when exercising or in hot weather.
- Long-acting synthetic glucocorticoids, such as oral dexamethasone or prednisone, are given for replacement. Side effects can include loss of calcium and decreased bone density or risk of osteoporosis.
- To decrease gastric irritation, take hormones with milk or an antacid.
- Signs of insufficient amounts of cortisol replacement include feeling weak and tired all the time, getting sick or vomiting, and anorexia. Weight loss can occur.

Herbs, Botanicals, and Supplements

- Herbs and botanical supplements should not be used without discussing with physician.

INTERVENTION: NUTRITION EDUCATION, COUNSELING, CARE MANAGEMENT

- Help patient individualize diet according to symptoms. During illness or injury, the body normally makes up to 10 times more cortisol than usual. Be prepared to avoid a crisis by prompt treatment.
- Ensure patient does not skip meals. Instruct patient to carry cheese or cracker snack to prevent hypoglycemia.
- Discuss simple meal preparation to lessen fatigue.
- Discuss food sources of sodium and potassium according to the medical plan.
- Use of Medic-Alert identification is recommended. Patients with this condition may need to carry a syringe prefilled with dexamethasone.
- Pregnancy is possible but must be managed with additional replacement medication.

For More Information

- Adrenal Gland Disorders
http://www.nlm.nih.gov/medlineplus/adrenalglanddisorders.html
- National Adrenal Diseases Foundation
http://www.medhelp.org/nadf/
- National Institutes of Health
http://www.cc.nih.gov/ccc/patient_education/pepubs/mngadrins.pdf

ADRENOCORTICAL INSUFFICIENCY AND ADDISON'S DISEASE—CITED REFERENCES

Barker JM, et al. Autoantibody "subspecificity" in type 1 diabetes: risk for organ-specific autoimmunity clusters in distinct groups. *Diabetes Care* 28:850, 2005.

Perry R, et al. Primary adrenal insufficiency in children: twenty years experience at the Sainte-Justine Hospital, Montreal. *J Clin Endocrinol Metab.* 90:3243, 2005.

Silva RC, et al. Autoantibodies against glutamic acid decarboxylase and 21-hydroxylase in Brazilian patients with type 1 diabetes or autoimmune thyroid diseases. *Diabetes Nutr Metab.* 16:160, 2003.

ADRENAL GLAND (CORTEX)

HYPERALDOSTERONISM

NUTRITIONAL ACUITY RANKING: LEVEL 1–2

DEFINITIONS AND BACKGROUND

Hyperaldosteronism is an increased production of aldosterone by the adrenal cortex. It may be primary (usually from adenoma) or secondary (as a result of cancer, heart failure, hyperplasia, malignant hypertension, pregnancy, estrogen use, or cirrhosis). Primary aldosteronism (PA) involves hypertension, hypokalemia, and low plasma renin. Successful finding of specific DNA mutations has emphasized the role of molecular genetics in hypertension (New et al, 2005). PA is a diagnosis that should be considered in refractory hypertension.

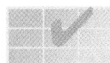

Familial hyperaldosteronism type I (FH-I) represents about 1% of cases of primary hyperaldosteronism. It may be detected in asymptomatic individuals when screening the offspring of affected individuals, or patients may present in infancy with hypertension, weakness, and failure to thrive due to hypokalemia. It is inherited in an autosomal dominant manner and has a low frequency of new mutations

Signs and symptoms of hyperaldosteronism include hypertension, headache, hypokalemia, intermittent paresthesia, fatigue, and numbness. Conn's syndrome is a benign tumor in one adrenal gland that can cause this condition. Urine 18-hydroxycortisol (18-OHF) measurements are sometimes used to detect Conn's syndrome with adrenal adenoma or to identify cases of glucocorticoid-suppressible hyperaldosteronism (Reynolds et al, 2005).

Aldosterone controls water and electrolyte balance by acting on mineralocorticoid receptors in the kidney; recent studies identified these classic receptors also in the vascular system (Oberliethner, 2005). Hyperaldosteronism causes endothelial dysfunction regardless of high blood pressure. Patients may be quite vulnerable to cardiac events, including stroke (Milliez et al, 2005).

Endothelial dysfunction precedes and predicts the development of hypertension in postmenopausal women; oral treatment with L-arginine improves endothelial dysfunction in hypertensives and lowers the blood pressure (Bolad and Delafontaine, 2005).

INTERVENTION: OBJECTIVES

- Hydrate adequately.
- Alter diet as needed (sodium, potassium).
- Correct hypokalemia and hypertension.
- Prepare for surgery if a tumor is involved. Laparoscopic adrenalectomy (LA) is quite successful.

INTERVENTION: FOOD AND NUTRITION

- Provide adequate fluid intake (unless contraindicated for other reasons).
- A sodium-restricted diet may be needed.
- A high potassium intake may be required, depending on the medical or surgical treatment used.
- Small, frequent feedings may be needed.

CLINICAL INDICATORS

Clinical/History	ECG with abnormalities from low K+ levels	Plasma aldosterone levels (elevated)
Height	**Lab Work**	Urinary aldosterone (elevated)
Weight	Sodium load test (6 g common)	Aldosterone: renin ratio
BMI	Plasma renin (low)	Urine sodium (altered)
Diet history	Urine 18-hydroxycortisol (18-OHF)	K+ (low)
I & O	Na+ (altered)	Urine potassium (altered)
BP (high)	Ca++	pCO_2 (altered)
Abdominal CT scan for adrenal mass	Mg++ (altered)	H & H
		Serum Fe

Common Drugs Used and Potential Side Effects

- Antihypertensives may be used; monitor side effects specifically for the medications prescribed. Aldosterone antagonists have been available for many decades; spironolactone may be used alone or with angiotensin-converting enzyme (ACE) inhibitors or angiotensin receptor blockers (ARBs).
- Eplerenone, a selective aldosterone antagonist, avoids the androgen and progesterone receptor–related adverse events that sometimes occur with spironolactone, such as breast tenderness, gynecomastia, sexual dysfunction, and menstrual irregularities (Pratt-Ubunama et al, 2005).
- Digitalis may be used. Avoid herbal teas, high-fiber intakes, and excessive amounts of vitamin D. Include adequate amounts of potassium. Take the drug 30 minutes before meals.

Herbs, Botanicals, and Supplements

- Herbs and botanical supplements should not be used without discussing with physician.
- Products containing natural licorice should be avoided in this condition.

INTERVENTION: NUTRITION EDUCATION, COUNSELING, CARE MANAGEMENT

- Explain altered sodium and potassium requirements, as appropriate.
- Have patient avoid fasting, skipping meals, and fad dieting.
- Provide recipe suggestions.

For More Information

- Medline
  http://www.nlm.nih.gov/medlineplus/ency/article/000330.htm

HYPERALDOSTERONISM—CITED REFERENCES

Bolad I, Delafontaine P. Endothelial dysfunction: its role in hypertensive coronary disease. *Curr Opin Cardiol.* 20:270, 2005.

Milliez P, et al. Evidence for an increased rate of cardiovascular events in patients with primary aldosteronism. *J Am Coll Cardiol.* 45:1243, 2005.

New MI, et al. Monogenic low renin hypertension. *Trends Endocrinol Metab.* 16:92, 2005.

Oberleithner H. Aldosterone makes human endothelium stiff and vulnerable. *Kidney Int.* 67:1680, 2005.

Pratt-Ubunama MN, et al. Aldosterone antagonism: an emerging strategy for effective blood pressure lowering. *Curr Hypertens Rep.* 7:186, 2005.

Reynolds RM, et al. The utility of three different methods for measuring urinary 18-hydroxycortisol in the differential diagnosis of suspected primary hyperaldosteronism. *Eur J Endocrinol.* 152:903, 2005.

ADRENAL GLAND (MEDULLA)

PHEOCHROMOCYTOMA

NUTRITIONAL ACUITY RANKING: LEVEL 1

DEFINITIONS AND BACKGROUND

Pheochromocytoma is a rare tumor of the chromaffin cells most commonly arising from the adrenal medulla, resulting in increased secretion of the hormones epinephrine and norepinephrine. It is slightly more common in males and may be transmitted as an autosomal dominant trait. At least five different genes have been described that, when mutated, can cause pheochromocytoma (Luft, 2003). Hereditary pheochromocytomas are typically intra-adrenal and bilateral, and patients typically present at younger ages compared with sporadic pheochromocytoma (Dluhy, 2002).

Pheochromocytoma may occur as a single tumor or as multiple growths. Symptoms and signs include very high blood pressure, headache, excessive diaphoresis, and palpitations. Less common symptoms are anxiety, chest pain, fatigue, weight loss, abdominal pain, and nervousness. About 10% of these tumors are malignant and can spread. Persons who have difficult-to-treat hypertension, have onset before age 35 or after age 60, or are taking four or more blood pressure medicines may need to be tested for pheochromocytoma.

Diagnosis often involves measurement of urinary catecholamines or their metabolites, vanillylmandelic acid, and total metanephrines. The urinary metanephrines provide a highly sensitive clue to the presence of pheochromocytoma. See Table 9-23.

Treatment usually involves surgical removal of the tumor. Before surgery, alpha-adrenergic blockers may be used. After surgery, about one quarter of patients will still suffer from hypertension and require lifelong management.

INTERVENTION: OBJECTIVES

- Avoid overstimulation (even slight exercise, cold stress, or emotional upsets).
- Correct nausea, vomiting, and anorexia.
- Prepare for surgery to remove tumor, if feasible.
- Manage long-term hypertension and prevent hypertensive crisis (which could cause sudden blindness or stroke).

INTERVENTION: FOOD AND NUTRITION

- Increase fluids but avoid caffeinated beverages.
- Six small feedings may be better tolerated than large meals.
- Increase protein and calories if patient is having surgery. Postoperatively, provide adequate vitamins and minerals for wound healing.
- Reexpansion of plasma volume may be accomplished by liberal salt or fluid intake with use of alpha-1 adrenergic receptor antagonists.
- In recurrent cases, long-term drug therapy will be needed. Monitor for specific dietary changes and side effects.

CLINICAL INDICATORS

Clinical/History	Lab Work (see Table 9-23)	
Height	Urinary epinephrine and norepinephrine (increased)	Gluc
Weight	Urinary catecholamine metabolites (vanillylmandelic acid and metanephrines)	Na+, K+
BMI		Alb
Diet history		CRP
BP (very elevated)		H & H
Orthostatic hypotension		Glucagon test (positive)
CT scan, MRI		T3, T4
Metaiodobenzylguanidine (MIBG) scanning		

TABLE 9-23 Catecholamines

Dopamine is a neurotransmitter (a chemical used to transmit impulses between nerve cells) found mainly in the brain. Norepinephrine is the primary neurotransmitter in the sympathetic nervous system (controls the "fight or flight" reaction) and is also found in the brain. Epinephrine is not only a brain neurotransmitter, but is also a major hormone in the body. Epinephrine is secreted from the adrenal medulla in response to low blood glucose, exercise, and various forms of stress where the brain stimulates release of the hormone. Epinephrine causes a breakdown of glycogen to glucose in liver and muscle, the release of fatty acids from adipose tissue, vasodilation of small arteries within muscle tissue, and increases in the rate and strength of the heartbeat. All of the catecholamines are metabolized by their target tissues or by the liver to become inactive substances that appear in the urine:

- Dopamine becomes homovanillic acid.
- Norepinephrine becomes normetanephrine and vanillylmandelic acid (VMA).
- Epinephrine becomes metanephrine and VMA.

Normal Values

- VMA: 2–7 mg/24 h (For testing, a VMA-restricted diet may be required for lab results; omit chocolate, vanilla extract, and citrus. Check with diagnostic personnel.)
- Epinephrine: 0.5–20 μg/24 h
- Norepinephrine: 15–80 μg/24 h
- Dopamine: 65–400 μg/24 h
- Metanephrine: 24–96 μg/24 h
- Normetanephrine: 75–375 μg/24 h
- Total urine catecholamines: 14–110 μg/24 h

Source: Medline Plus. Catecholamines–urine. Accessed July 4, 2005 at http://www.nlm.nih.gov/medlineplus/ency/article/003613.htm.

Common Drugs Used and Potential Side Effects

- Pharmacological treatment of catecholamine excess is mandatory.
- Phenoxybenzamine (or an alpha-1 adrenergic receptor antagonist such as prazosin) is needed to block alpha-adrenergic activity. Diuretics should not be used.
- Low doses of a beta-blocker such as propranolol are used to control blood pressure and cardiac tachyarrhythmias but only after alpha blockade is established.
- Labetalol, an alpha- and beta-adrenergic blocker, has also been shown to be effective in the control of blood pressure and symptoms of pheochromocytoma.

Herbs, Botanicals, and Supplements

- Herbs and botanical supplements should not be used without discussing with physician.

INTERVENTION: NUTRITION EDUCATION, COUNSELING, CARE MANAGEMENT

- Discuss avoidance of caffeinated foods and beverages (e.g., coffee, tea, and chocolate).
- Maintain a calm atmosphere for patient; prevent undue stress.
- Exercise should be limited until condition is under control.

For More Information

- Endocrine Web
  http://www.endocrineweb.com/pheo.html
- Medline
  http://www.nlm.nih.gov/medlineplus/ency/article/000340.htm
- Merck Manual
  http://www.merck.com/mrkshared/mmanual/section2/chapter9/9d.jsp
- National Cancer Institute
  http://www.cancer.gov/cancerinfo/pdq/treatment/pheochromocytoma/patient
- National Library of Medicine
  http://www.nlm.nih.gov/medlineplus/pheochromocytoma.html
- Urology Health
  http://www.urologyhealth.org

PHEOCHROMOCYTOMA—CITED REFERENCES

Dluhy RG. Screening for genetic causes of hypertension. *Curr Hypertens Rep.* 4:439, 2002.
Luft FC. Mendelian forms of human hypertension and mechanisms of disease. *Clin Med Res.* 1:291, 2003.

THYROID GLAND

HYPERTHYROIDISM

NUTRITIONAL ACUITY RANKING: LEVEL 1

DEFINITIONS AND BACKGROUND

Hyperthyroidism results from oversecretion of the thyroid hormones, thyroxine and/or triiodothyronine. Most often, the entire gland is overproducing thyroid hormone; rarely, a single nodule is responsible for the excess hormone secretion. An elevated metabolic rate, tissue wasting, diaphoresis, tremor, tachycardia, goiter, heat intolerance, cold insensitivity, nervousness, increased appetite, exophthalmos, and loss of glycogen stores can occur. If left untreated, atrial fibrillation and osteoporosis can result. Figure 9-8 shows the placement of the thyroid glands at the base of the throat.

Graves' disease (diffuse toxic goiter) is the most common form; **thyrotoxicosis** is more severe. Clinical thyrotoxicosis in Graves' disease patients is caused by thyrotropin receptor (TSHR)-stimulating autoantibodies (Schott et al, 2005). Most people who develop Graves' ophthalmopathy have one or more of the following symptoms: dry and itchy eyes, a staring or bug-eyed look (exophthalmos), sensitivity to light, excessive tearing, a feeling of pressure around the eyes, difficulty closing the eyes completely, and double vision, especially when looking to the sides. Fifty percent of persons suffering from Graves' disease have had relatives with altered thyroid functioning; an underlying hereditary condition may exist.

Persons who smoke or who have autoimmune disorders such as type 1 diabetes, celiac disease, or Addison's disease seem to be at higher risk for hyperthyroidism. It is also important to screen for thyroid problems in patients with mood and psychotic disorders; further investigation is needed on the nature of the relationship between thyroid function and bipolar disorder (Stowell and Barnhill, 2005). Finally, it is important to recognize the role of thyroid hormone on kidney function. Renal function improves significantly during treatment of hypothyroidism and decreases during treatment of hyperthyroidism (den Hollander et al, 2005).

Thyroidectomy may be needed. With thyroidectomy, often subtotal (up to 90%), the patient may require a high-calorie, high-protein diet preoperatively. Antithyroid agents and iodine are often given 4–6 weeks before surgery to minimize risk of thyroid crisis. Evaluate needs postoperatively with the doctor's care plan.

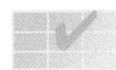

Thyroid storm (thyroid crisis) is a potentially life-threatening condition that develops in a person with hyperthy-

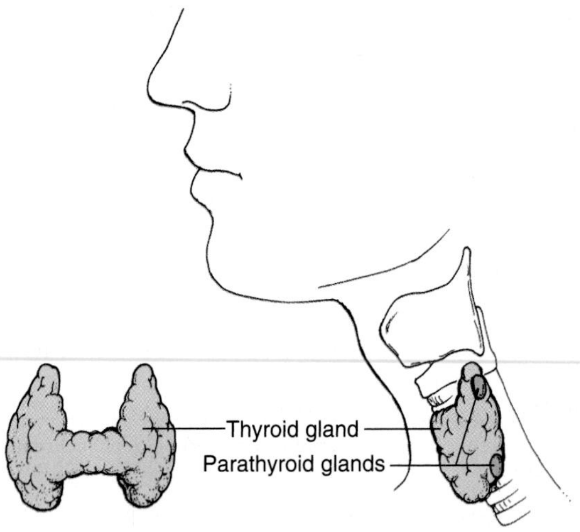

Figure 9-8 Thyroid glands. (LifeART image. Copyright © 2006 Lippincott Williams & Wilkins. All rights reserved.)

roidism; the gland suddenly releases large amounts of thyroid hormone in a short period of time. Signs of thyroid storm include extreme irritability, high systolic blood pressure, low diastolic blood pressure, tachycardia, nausea, vomiting, diarrhea, high fever, confusion, and sleepiness. Shock, delirium, shortness of breath, fatigue, coma, heart failure, and death can result if not treated immediately. Emergency medical treatment is always needed for this condition.

INTERVENTION: OBJECTIVES

- Prevent or treat complications accompanying high metabolic rate, including bone demineralization. This seems to be a greater problem in older women than in adolescents (Poomthavorn et al, 2005).
- Replenish glycogen stores. Replace lost weight (usually 10–20 lb).
- Correct negative nitrogen balance.
- Replace fluid losses from diarrhea, diaphoresis, and increased respirations.
- Exophthalmos, which is caused by increased accumulation of extracellular fluid in the eyes, may require fluid and salt restriction.
- Monitor for fat intolerance and steatorrhea.

INTERVENTION: FOOD AND NUTRITION

- Use a high-calorie diet (start with 40 kcal/kg). The patient's caloric needs may be increased by 50–60% in this condition (or 10–30% in mild cases). Ensure high intake of carbohydrates; use protein in the range of 1–1.75 g/kg body weight.
- Fluid intake should be 3–4 L/d, unless contraindicated by renal or cardiac problems.
- Diet should include 1 quart of milk or equivalent daily to supply adequate calcium, phosphorus, and vitamin D.
- Caffeine stimulants should be excluded from diet because they aggravate excitability and nervousness.
- Supplement diet with vitamins A and C, as well as the B-complex vitamins, especially thiamin, riboflavin, B_6, and B_{12}. A general multivitamin-mineral supplement may be beneficial; monitor for iodine content.
- Be aware of iodine in any supplements used. Chronic iodine intakes greater than 500 μg/L are associated with adverse effects (Zimmermann et al, 2005). Indeed, subclinical hyperthyroidism is more prevalent in the iodine-deficient area than in the severe iodine-excessive area (Yang et al, 2002)
- Be cautious regarding use of raw natural goitrogens (i.e., cabbage, Brussels sprouts, kale, cauliflower, soybeans, peanuts) concomitant with antithyroid medications because these substances can increase side effects of the drugs. Cooking reduces this effect.

CLINICAL INDICATORS

Clinical/History	Lab Work	
Height	T3 (increased)	(decreased)
Weight	T4 (increased)	Na^+, K^+
BMI	TSH (normal or low)	H & H
Diet history	Protein-bound iodine (PBI)	Serum ferritin
Temperature	Gluc (increased)	Chol, Trig (decreased)
BP	Alb, transthyretin	BUN, Creat
I & O	Ca^{++}	N balance
Thyroid scan	Mg^{++}	Alk phos (increased)
Goiter (enlarged thyroid gland)		

Common Drugs Used and Potential Side Effects

- The goal of drug therapy is to prevent the thyroid from producing excess hormones. Antithyroid drugs, also called thionamides, such as methimazole (Tapazole) and propylthiouracil (PTU), can cause nausea, vomiting, altered taste sensation, and gastrointestinal distress. They should be taken with food. Avoid use of natural goitrogens in raw form with these drugs; cooked forms are not a problem.
- Thionamides represent the treatment of choice in pregnant women, during lactation, in children and adolescents, and in preparation for radioiodine therapy or thyroidectomy (Bartelena et al, 2005).
- Radioactive iodine may be used to damage or destroy some of the thyroid cells. It can cause a temporary burning sensation in the throat. Hydrochlorothiazide (HCTZ) may be used to improve radioiodine uptake in hyperthyroid patients; side effects include hypokalemia if potassium is not replaced.
- Some drugs can affect the thyroid glands. Amiodarone is a potent antiarrhythmic drug that also possesses beta-blocking properties; a 100-mg tablet contains an amount of iodine that is 250 times the recommended daily iodine

requirement. Amiodarone-induced thyrotoxicosis is a difficult condition to diagnose and treat; its use should be carefully monitored (Basaria and Cooper, 2005).

Herbs, Botanicals, and Supplements

- Herbs and botanical supplements should not be used without discussing with physician.
- Bugleweed, verbena, lemon balm, kelp, and broccoli have been recommended, but no clinical trials prove efficacy.
- In Japan, where large quantities of iodine-rich seaweed such as kombu (*Laminaria japonica*) are consumed, patients who have hyperthyroidism should be counseled to limit use (Nishiyama et al, 2004).

INTERVENTION: NUTRITION EDUCATION, COUNSELING, CARE MANAGEMENT

- Encourage quiet, pleasant mealtimes.
- Exclude use of alcohol, which may cause a hypoglycemic state.
- To avoid obesity, adjust patient's diet as condition corrects itself.
- Beware of hyperglycemia after carbohydrate-rich meals.
- Frequent snacks may be needed.

For More Information

- American Thyroid Association
  http://www.thyroid.org/
- Endocrine Web–Hyperthyroidism
  http://www.endocrineweb.com/hyper1.html
- European Thyroid Society
  http://www.eurothyroid.com/
- Latin American Thyroid Society
  http://www.lats.org/
- Merck Thyro-Link
  http://www.thyrolink.com/
- National Graves Disease Foundation
  http://www.ngdf.org/
- The Thyroid Foundation
  http://www.tsh.org/
- University of Maryland Medical Center
  http://www.umm.edu/endocrin/hypert.htm

HYPERTHYROIDISM—CITED REFERENCES

Bartelena L, et al. An update on the pharmacological management of hyperthyroidism due to Graves' disease. *Expert Opin Pharmacother.* 6:851, 2005.

Basaria S, Cooper DS. Amiodarone and the thyroid. *Am J Med.* 118:706, 2005.

den Hollander JG, et al. Correlation between severity of thyroid dysfunction and renal function. *Clin Endocrinol.* 62:423, 2005.

Nishiyama S, et al. Transient hypothyroidism or persistent hyperthyrotropinemia in neonates born to mothers with excessive iodine intake. *Thyroid* 14:1077, 2004.

Poomthavorn P, et al. Exogenous subclinical hyperthyroidism during adolescence: effect on peak bone mass. *J Pediatr Endocrinol Metab.* 18:463, 2005.

Schott M, et al. Thyrotropin receptor autoantibodies in Graves' disease. *Trends Endocrinol Metab.* 16:243, 2005.

Stowell CP, Barnhill JW. Acute mania in the setting of severe hypothyroidism. *Psychosomatics* 46:259, 2005.

Yang F, et al. Epidemiological survey on the relationship between different iodine intakes and the prevalence of hyperthyroidism. *Eur J Endocrinol.* 146:613, 2002.

Zimmermann MB, et al. High thyroid volume in children with excess dietary iodine intakes. *Am J Clin Nutr.* 81:840, 2005.

THYROID GLAND

HYPOTHYROIDISM

NUTRITIONAL ACUITY RANKING: LEVEL 1

DEFINITIONS AND BACKGROUND

Hypothyroidism is caused by the underfunctioning of the thyroid gland. It can be classified as primary (thyroid failure), secondary (from pituitary thyroid-stimulating hormone deficit), or tertiary (from hypothalamic deficiency of thyrotropin-releasing hormone) or result from peripheral resistance to the action of thyroid hormones.

Primary hypothyroidism causes about 95% of all cases. The most common cause of thyroid gland failure is **Hashimoto's thyroiditis,** which is inflammation caused by the patient's own antibodies (as in pernicious anemia, lupus, rheumatoid arthritis, diabetes, or chronic hepatitis). The second major cause of thyroid gland failure is from various medical treatments that affect the thyroid gland (e.g., surgery, chronic medication use). Hypothyroidism affects 2% of adult women, usually middle-aged and older women. Women may experience menstrual irregularities or difficulty conceiving. Triiodothyronine (T3) and thyroxine (T4) are elevated during pregnancy and with oral contraceptive and estrogen use.

Physicians must treat hypothyroidism to avoid long-term complications. Untreated hypothyroidism can lead to depression and other symptoms that mimic other conditions. Patients with subclinical hypothyroidism may also be at increased risk for cardiovascular disease; risk decreases if thyroid hormones are taken as directed.

Congenital deficiency of thyroid hormone is rare; incidence is 1 in 4000 births. Screening for this type of hypothyroidism is now quite widespread (Lanting et al, 2005). Treatment involves replacement of thyroid hormones and iodine. Cretinism can occur in areas where soil content of iodine is

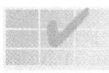

TABLE 9-24 Symptoms of Hypothyroidism

Infants	
Respiratory difficulty	Impaired mental development
Cyanosis	Short stature
Persistent jaundice	Coarse features with protruding tongue
Poor feeding	Broad flat nose
Hoarse cry	Widely set eyes
Constipation	Sparse hair and dry skin
Somnolence	Retarded bone age
Umbilical hernia	Delayed dentition
Marked retardation of bone maturation	
Developmental delay	
Children	
Retarded growth with shortness of stature	
Evidence of mental retardation	
Poor performance at school	
Adults	
Easy fatigue	Constipation from slowed peristalsis
Weakness	Depression or irritability
Weight gain	Memory loss
Increased difficulty losing weight	Low reflexes
Coarse, dry hair	Abnormal menstrual cycles
Dry, rough pale skin	Decreased libido
Yellow skin hue (reduced conversion of carotene to vitamin A)	Brittle nails
Hair loss	Hoarse, husky voice
Cold intolerance	Puffy hands and face
Muscle cramps and frequent muscle aches	

low. Signs and symptoms of hypothyroidism are listed in Table 9-24 for different life stages of onset.

Thyroid autoimmunity is common and may contribute to miscarriages as well as to hypothyroidism; infants are totally dependent on T4 from the mother during the first trimester for normal neurological development (Smallridge et al, 2005). Hypothyroidism from autoimmune disease or suboptimal iodine intake occurs in 2.5% of pregnant women; postpartum thyroid dysfunction (PPTD) occurs in 5–9% of women (Lazarus and Premawardhana, 2005). Because of the potential problems for mother and baby (including neuropsychological and developmental issues), screening, diagnosis, and treatment of thyroid problems among pregnant women should be a priority (Hollowell et al, 2005).

Several minerals and trace elements are essential for normal thyroid hormone metabolism, namely iodine, iron, selenium, and zinc; coexisting deficiencies of these elements can impair thyroid function (Zimmermann and Kohrle, 2002). Iron deficiency impairs thyroid hormone synthesis by reducing activity of heme-dependent thyroid peroxidase; therefore, iron supplementation improves the efficacy of iodine supplementation (Zimmermann and Kohrle, 2002). Anemia is a major manifestation in hypothyroidism not only because of impaired hemoglobin synthesis, but also because of iron deficiency from increased iron loss with menorrhagia, impaired intestinal absorption of iron, folate deficiency due to impaired intestinal absorption of folic acid, and pernicious anemia with vitamin B_{12} deficiency.

Selenium deficiency and disturbed thyroid hormone economy may develop under conditions of long-term total parenteral nutrition, phenylketonuria diet, cystic fibrosis, or poor nutrition in children, elderly people, or sick patients (Zimmermann and Kohrle, 2002). In parts of the world where iodine and selenium are both deficient, dual supplementation may be advisable to optimize glutathione peroxidase (GPx) and iodothyronine deiodinase activity (Chanoine, 2003).

Endemic goiter is an enlargement of the thyroid gland with swelling in front of the neck, resulting from iodine deficiency due to inadequate dietary intake or drug effects. Over 3 billion people in the world are on iodine supplementation programs; the optimal level of iodine intake to prevent thyroid disease may be a relatively narrow range around the recommended daily iodine intake of 150 μg (Bulow Pedersen et al, 2002).

Myxedema is a nonpitting edema that can occur in adults with hypothyroidism; hydrophilic mucopolysaccharide accumulates in the skin and muscles. **Myxedema coma** is the end stage of untreated hypothyroidism where there is progressive weakness, stupor, hypothermia, hypoventilation, hypoglycemia, hyponatremia, water intoxication, shock, and even death. It occurs most often in older patients with underlying pulmonary and vascular disease. Finally, because reduced glomerular filtration rate is often found with hypothyroidism, evaluation is needed in persons with chronic kidney disease to rule out or treat cases that are otherwise hidden (Lo et al, 2005).

INTERVENTION: OBJECTIVES

- Control weight gain that results from a 15–40% slower metabolic rate, especially in the untreated patient. Measure weight frequently to detect losses or fluid retention.
- Correct reasons for imbalance, which can be due to inadequate intake of iodine or congenital deficiency. Hormone replacement will be given.
- Correct vitamin B_{12}, folic acid, and iron deficiency anemias when present.
- Improve energy levels; reduce fatigue.
- Improve cardiac, neurological, and renal functioning.
- Screen for thyroid problems in pregnant or postpartum women, and provide hormone replacement as needed.

INTERVENTION: FOOD AND NUTRITION

- Use a calorie-controlled diet adjusted for age, sex, and height.
- A multivitamin-mineral supplement formula may be beneficial, especially to replace nutrients that have been poorly absorbed.

- Ensure an adequate supply of fiber and laxative foods as well as fluid.
- In diets for pregnant women or children, check to make sure that adequate amounts of iodine are consumed.
- Natural goitrogens in cabbage, turnips, rapeseeds, peanuts, cassava, cauliflower, broccoli, and soybeans may block uptake of iodine by body cells; they are inactivated by heating and cooking.
- To make the thyroid function properly, zinc, copper, and tyrosine are needed.

CLINICAL INDICATORS

Clinical/History

- Height
- Weight
- BMI
- Diet history
- Temperature
- BP

Lab Work

- T4 (decreased)
- T3 (decreased)
- TSH (elevated)
- PBI
- Ca++
- Mg++ (increased)
- H & H (decreased)
- Serum ferritin
- Chol, Trig (increased)
- Gluc
- Alk phos (decreased)
- Serum copper (decreased)
- Na+ (decreased)
- K+ (decreased)
- Serum B_{12} (low)
- Folic acid (low)
- Creatine phosphokinase (CPK)
- GFR (may be decreased)
- Thyrotropin
- Somatomedin C (increased)
- Uric acid (increased)
- Carotenoids (increased)
- Thyroglobulin (useful measure after introducing iodized salt)

Common Drugs Used and Potential Side Effects

- Thyroid hormones (liotrix, sodium levothyroxine, or Synthroid) are used. Use caution with use of soy protein products since they can decrease effectiveness of the hormones. Thyroid hormones elevate glucose and decrease cholesterol; monitor persons who have diabetes carefully. Monitor for weight changes and fluid shifts. If rapid weight loss, sweating, or other symptoms of hyperthyroidism occur, the doctor should be contacted for immediate follow-up.
- Lithium treatment for bipolar disorder has been associated with the development of goiter. Monitor patients closely.

Herbs, Botanicals, and Supplements

- Herbs and botanical supplements should not be used without discussing with physician.
- Avoid kelp tablets and "thyroid support" supplements.
- Kelp, gentian, walnut, mustard, radish, and St. John's wort have been recommended, but no clinical trials have proven efficacy.
- In Japan, large quantities of iodine-rich seaweed such as kombu (*Laminaria japonica*) are consumed (Nishiyama et al, 2004). Their use should be monitored in patients who take thyroid replacement hormones.

INTERVENTION: NUTRITION EDUCATION, COUNSELING, CARE MANAGEMENT

- Discuss goitrogens in cabbage and *Brassica* vegetables, turnips, rapeseeds, peanuts, cassava, and soybeans; they are inactivated by heating and cooking.
- Encourage use of iodized salt, as permitted. Avoid self-medication with iodine supplements.
- Encourage adequate fluid intake.
- Women who are considering pregnancy may want to be screened to rule out thyroid problems.
- In many developing countries, children are at high risk of goiter, vitamin A deficiency, and iron deficiency anemia; selecting the proper supplement can help to eliminate this problem (Zimmermann et al, 2004).

For More Information

- American Thyroid Association
  http://www.thyroid.org/
- Endocrine Web
  http://www.endocrineweb.com/hypo1.html
- Hypothyroidism Booklet
  http://www.thyroid.org/patients/brochures/Hypothyroidism%20_web_booklet.pdf
- Network for Sustained Elimination of Iodine Deficiency
  http://www.sph.emory.edu/PAMM/index.htm
- Synthroid Information
  http://www.synthroid.com/

HYPOTHYROIDISM—CITED REFERENCES

Bulow Pedersen I, et al. Large differences in incidences of overt hyper- and hypothyroidism associated with a small difference in iodine intake: a prospective comparative register-based population survey. *J Clin Endocrinol Metab.* 87:4462, 2002.

Chanoine JP. Selenium and thyroid function in infants, children and adolescents. *Biofactors* 19:137, 2003.

Hollowell JG, et al. 2004 where do we go from here? Summary of working group discussions on thyroid function and gestational outcomes. *Thyroid* 15:72, 2005.

Lanting CI, et al. Clinical effectiveness and cost-effectiveness of the use of the thyroxine/thyroxine-binding globulin ratio to detect congenital hypothyroidism of thyroidal and central origin in a neonatal screening program. *Pediatrics* 116:168, 2005.

Lazarus JH, Premawardhana LD. Screening for thyroid disease in pregnancy. *J Clin Pathol.* 58:449, 2005.

Lo JC, et al. Increased prevalence of subclinical and clinical hypothyroidism in persons with chronic kidney disease. *Kidney Int.* 67:1047, 2005.

Nishiyama S, et al. Transient hypothyroidism or persistent hyperthyrotropinemia in neonates born to mothers with excessive iodine intake. *Thyroid* 14:1077, 2004.

Smallridge RC, et al. Thyroid function inside and outside of pregnancy: what do we know and what don't we know? *Thyroid* 15:54, 2005.

Zimmermann MB, Kohrle J. The impact of iron and selenium deficiencies on iodine and thyroid metabolism: biochemistry and relevance to public health. *Thyroid* 12:867, 2002.

Zimmermann MB, et al. Triple fortification of salt with microcapsules of iodine, iron, and vitamin A. *Am J Clin Nutr.* 80:1283, 2004.

PARATHYROID GLANDS

HYPOPARATHYROIDISM AND HYPOCALCEMIA

NUTRITIONAL ACUITY RANKING: LEVEL 2

DEFINITIONS AND BACKGROUND

Parathyroid hormone (PTH) works with vitamin D to regulate total body calcium. The body secretes PTH in response to hypocalcemia or hypomagnesemia; the hormone then stimulates osteoclasts to increase bone resorption. PTH also stimulates adenyl cyclase to increase renal tubular calcium resorption and phosphate excretion. PTH also activates the conversion of 25-hydroxyvitamin D to 1,25-dihydroxyvitamin D, the active form of vitamin D that stimulates calcium and phosphate absorption from the gastrointestinal (GI) tract. Calcitonin, in contrast to PTH, decreases serum calcium levels and is secreted by the thyroid gland.

Hypoparathyroidism results from a deficiency of PTH from biologically ineffective hormones, damage or accidental removal of the glands, or impaired skeletal or renal response. In the hereditary form, parathyroid glands are either absent or not functioning properly; symptoms appear before age 10. Other causes include magnesium deficiency or neonatal immaturity. If untreated, hypoparathyroidism-retardation-dysmorphism (HRD) may result.

Hypoparathyroidism with hypocalcemia is one of the most common results of damage to parathyroid glands during surgery; in fact, it may be diagnosed during a workup for hypocalcemia. Signs and symptoms include muscle cramps and tetany, tingling of the lips or fingers, hair loss, dry skin, dental hypoplasia, chronic cutaneous moniliasis, hypocalcemia, hyperphosphatemia, and low PTH.

Vitamin D levels may also be deficient. Intraoperative PTH levels are used widely during parathyroidectomy as an indicator of parathyroid gland function; vitamin D supplementation after surgery may be given to anticipate decreased parathyroid gland function and to avoid symptomatic hypocalcemia (Quiros et al, 2005).

Hypoparathyroidism is a chronic (long-lasting) condition that requires lifelong treatment with large doses of calcium and vitamin D supplements. Episodes of tetany are treated with calcium given intravenously to provide quick relief of symptoms. Controlled release of physiological concentrations of PTH can be achieved using a surgically implantable controlled-release delivery system (Anthony et al, 2005).

INTERVENTION: OBJECTIVES

- Normalize serum and urinary levels of calcium, phosphorus, and vitamin D.
- Prevent long-term complications such as cataracts, pernicious anemia, Parkinson's disease, and bone disease.
- Prevent mental retardation or malformed teeth in affected children.
- Decrease symptoms of tetany and improve overall health status.

INTERVENTION: FOOD AND NUTRITION

- Use a high-calcium diet; increase dairy products, nuts, salmon, peanut butter, and green leafy vegetables.
- Oral supplements high in calcium should be used, such as calcium carbonate.
- Reduce excess use of meats, phytates (whole grains), and oxalic acid (spinach, chard, and rhubarb) if the diet contains large amounts.
- If tolerated, lactose should be included in the diet for better absorption of calcium.
- Intake of vitamin D and protein should be adequate, at least meeting recommended levels.

CLINICAL INDICATORS

Clinical/History

Height
Weight
BMI
Diet history
Weakness, fatigue
Tetany
Hyperreflexia—Chvostek's sign (positive to tapping of facial muscles)
Irritability or psychosis
Seizures
Abnormal heart rhythms on ECG

Lab Work

PTH (low)
Ca++ (serum levels <2.5–3 mg/dL)
Urinary Ca++ (altered)
Mg++ (may be low)
Na+, K+
Serum phosphorus (high)
Alk phos

Common Drugs Used and Potential Side Effects

- Calcium lactate (8–12 g) may be used. Ergocalciferol (Calciferol) is a vitamin D analog that is used with calcium supplements in this condition. Calcitriol (Rocaltrol) also may be useful.
- Diuretics sometimes are given to prevent too much calcium from being lost through the urine, which is a problem that can lead to kidney stones. Taking diuretics also reduces the amount of calcium and vitamin D supplements needed.
- Overuse of steroids may cause hypocalcemia, with resulting severe muscle spasms and convulsions.

Herbs, Botanicals, and Supplements

- Herbs and botanical supplements should not be used without discussing with physician.

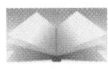

INTERVENTION: NUTRITION EDUCATION, COUNSELING, CARE MANAGEMENT

- Indicate which foods are sources of calcium, phosphorus, and vitamin D.
- Indicate which foods are sources of phytates and oxalates, if dietary intake is a concern.
- Discuss role of sunlight exposure in vitamin D formation and how it relates to the individual patient needs.

For More Information

- American Society for Bone and Mineral Research
  http://www.asbmr.org/
- Hypoparathyroidism Association
  http://www.hypoparathyroidism.org/
- Medline
  http://www.nlm.nih.gov/medlineplus/ency/article/000385.htm
- National Institutes of Health–Osteoporosis and Related Bone Diseases
  http://www.osteo.org/
- Office of Rare Diseases
  http://rarediseases.info.nih.gov/

HYPOPARATHYROIDISM AND HYPOCALCEMIA—CITED REFERENCES

Anthony T, et al. Development of a parathyroid hormone-controlled release system as a potential surgical treatment for hypoparathyroidism. *J Pediatr Surg.* 40:81, 2005.

Quiros RM, et al. Intraoperative parathyroid hormone levels in thyroid surgery are predictive of postoperative hypoparathyroidism and need for vitamin D supplementation. *Am J Surg.* 189:306, 2005.

HYPERPARATHYROIDISM AND HYPERCALCEMIA

NUTRITIONAL ACUITY RANKING: LEVEL 2

DEFINITIONS AND BACKGROUND

The parathyroid glands have an overall regulatory role with action as a thermostat in the systemic calcium homeostasis to ensure tight regulation of serum calcium concentrations and appropriate skeletal mineralization (Akerstrom et al, 2005). Parathyroid hormone (PTH) affects calcium, phosphorus, and vitamin D metabolism by removing calcium from bone to raise serum levels; it promotes hydroxylation of vitamin D to its active form. Calcitonin, in contrast to PTH, decreases serum calcium levels; it is secreted by the thyroid gland.

Primary hyperparathyroidism (pHPT) results from parathyroid adenoma in up to 80% of cases, hyperplasia of the parathyroid glands in 10–20% of cases, or cancer. Double parathyroid adenomas occur in 2–15% of pHPT cases (Abboud et al, 2005). pHPT has been associated with premature death in cardiovascular diseases and should, therefore, be quickly managed (Nilsson et al, 2005).

Secondary hyperparathyroidism occurs in renal failure or even after renal transplantation. Calcitriol deficiency and phosphorus retention are involved in the pathogenesis of renal hyperparathyroidism. Parathyroid gland hyperplasia develops in azotemic patients, producing hypercalcemia and hyperphosphatemia. Secondary hyperparathyroidism in chronic kidney disease is stimulated by dietary phosphate loading and ameliorated by dietary phosphate restriction (Martin et al, 2005). Alterations in dietary protein can profoundly affect intestinal calcium absorption; a moderate protein intake should be administered accordingly (Kerstetter et al, 2003).

Postmenopausal women after Roux-en-Y gastric bypass may show evidence of secondary hyperparathyroidism, elevated bone resorption, and patterns of bone loss (reduced femoral neck and higher lumbar spine) similar to other subjects with hyperparathyroidism (Goode et al, 2004). The impact of this surgery needs further study to determine if specific supplements are needed.

Signs and symptoms of hyperparathyroidism include weakness, fatigue, anorexia, constipation, weight loss, hypercalcemia and hypercalciuria, altered serum phosphorus, and dehydration. In children with renal failure, growth can be impaired. About 28 in 100,000 people have hyperparathyroidism in the United States.

Minimal invasive surgery can be used for parathyroidectomy. Parathyroidectomy can induce long-lasting improvement in regulation of blood pressure, left ventricular diastolic function, and other signs of myocardial ischemia, with improved life expectancy (Nilsson et al, 2005). More than 95% of patients with pHPT will be cured by this operation (Caron et al, 2004).

INTERVENTION: OBJECTIVES

- Lower elevated serum calcium and urinary calcium levels.
- Normalize serum phosphate levels.
- Prepare for surgery if parathyroidectomy is necessary.
- Alleviate constipation, anorexia, weight loss, and weakness.
- Prevent rickets and growth delay in children (Sabbagh et al, 2005).

INTERVENTION: FOOD AND NUTRITION

- Use a low-calcium diet, with fewer dairy products, nuts, salmon, peanut butter, and green leafy vegetables.

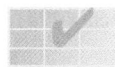

- Extra fluid is useful to prevent dehydration, which can elevate serum calcium levels.
- Limit phosphorus-containing foods, such as milk and meats, if hyperphosphatemia is present.
- Increased dietary protein significantly increases intestinal calcium absorption; dietary protein intakes at and below 0.8 g/kg may be associated with a reduction in intestinal calcium absorption sufficient to cause secondary hyperparathyroidism (Kerstetter et al, 2003). Maintain a balanced intake of protein.

CLINICAL INDICATORS

Clinical/History	Lab Work	
Height	PTH (>60 pg/mL)	Mg++
Weight	Serum Ca++ (>11 mg/dL)	Na+, K+
BMI	Urinary Ca++ (elevated)	Alb, BUN
Diet history	Serum phosphorus (often high)	Creatinine
Weight loss		H & H
Weakness, fatigue		Serum ferritin
BP		Gluc
Constipation		
Growth delay or rickets in children		

Common Drugs Used and Potential Side Effects

- Treatment with active vitamin D from newly developed analogs can increase vitamin D receptor expression, inhibit growth of parathyroid tumors, and reduce PTH levels in patients with hyperparathyroidism (Akerstrom et al, 2005).
- Phosphate-binding agents that do not contain calcium, new vitamin D analogs, and calcimimetic compounds offer therapeutic alternatives for managing renal osteodystrophy (Goodman, 2003). For many practicing dietitians, paricalcitol is the most widely used form of intravenous vitamin D in renal patients (Martin and Reams, 2003).
- Once-yearly intramuscular cholecalciferol injections (600,000 IU) have been used to correct vitamin D deficiency, but controlled trials are needed.
- Beware of overdosing on vitamins A or D (e.g., 10,000 of vitamin A or 50,000 of vitamin D); either may cause hypercalcemia.
- Some antacids may contain high levels of calcium and should be carefully monitored.
- Sevelamer, a relatively new phosphorus binder, lowers serum phosphorus and PTH levels without inducing hypercalcemia (Lorenzo Sellares and Torres Ramirez, 2004). Frequently prescribed phosphate binders may include calcium acetate, sevelamer hydrochloride, and calcium carbonate (Martin and Reams, 2003); standard protocols are recommended.
- Fluid repletion and combination calcitonin and bisphosphonate treatment may be of value when rapid reduction of serum calcium is warranted (Pecherstorfer et al, 2003).

Herbs, Botanicals, and Supplements

- Herbs and botanical supplements should not be used without discussing with physician.
- Conjugated linoleic acid (CLA) reduces prostaglandin E_2 synthesis, which is required for PTH release; its use in humans needs to be studied (Weiler et al, 2004).

INTERVENTION: NUTRITION EDUCATION, COUNSELING, CARE MANAGEMENT

- Discuss foods that are sources of calcium, phosphorus, and vitamin D.
- Indicate which foods are sources of phytates and oxalates, if dietary intake is a concern.
- Discuss role of sunlight exposure in vitamin D formation and how it relates to the individual patient needs.
- In renal patients, there is a need for focused counseling to clarify misunderstanding of simple dietary facts (Poduval et al, 2003). For example, patients who have kidney transplantations might still present with persistent hyperparathyroidism and hypercalcemia because of the role that the parathyroid glands play in maintaining calcium-sensing receptors and vitamin D receptors (Lewin, 2003).

For More Information

- American Society for Bone and Mineral Research
  http://www.asbmr.org/
- Hypoparathyroidism Association
  http://www.hypoparathyroidism.org/
- National Institutes of Health–Osteoporosis and Related Bone Diseases
  http://www.osteo.org/
- Office of Rare Diseases
  http://rarediseases.info.nih.gov/

HYPERPARATHYROIDISM AND HYPERCALCEMIA—CITED REFERENCES

Abboud B, et al. Existence and anatomic distribution of double parathyroid adenoma. *Laryngoscope* 115:1128, 2005.

Akerstrom G, et al. Parathyroid glands in calcium regulation and human disease. *Ann N Y Acad Sci.* 1040:53, 2005.

Caron NR, et al. Persistent and recurrent hyperparathyroidism. *Curr Treat Options Oncol.* 5:335, 2004.

Goode LR, et al. Bone and gastric bypass surgery: effects of dietary calcium and vitamin D. *Obes Res.* 12:40, 2004.

Goodman WG. Medical management of secondary hyperparathyroidism in chronic renal failure. *Nephrol Dial Transplant.* 18:iii2, 2003 (suppl 3).

Kerstetter JE, et al. Dietary protein, calcium metabolism, and skeletal homeostasis revisited. *Am J Clin Nutr.* 78:584S, 2003.

Lewin E. Involution of the parathyroid glands after renal transplantation. *Curr Opin Nephrol Hypertens.* 12:363, 2003

Lorenzo Sellares V, Torres Ramirez A. Management of hyperphosphataemia in dialysis patients: role of phosphate binders in the elderly. *Drugs Aging.* 21:153, 2004.

Martin CJ, Reams SM. The renal dietitian's role in managing hyperphosphatemia and secondary hyperparathyroidism in dialysis patients: a national survey. *J Ren Nutr.* 13:133, 2003.

Martin DR, et al. Acute regulation of parathyroid hormone by dietary phosphate. *Am J Physiol Endocrinol Metab.* 289:E729, 2005.

Nilsson IL, et al. Maintained normalization of cardiovascular dysfunction 5 years after parathyroidectomy in primary hyperparathyroidism. *Surgery* 137:632, 2005.

Pecherstorfer M, et al. Current management strategies for hypercalcemia. *Treat Endocrinol.* 2:273, 2003.

Poduval RD, et al. Hyperphosphatemia in dialysis patients: is there a role for focused counseling? *J Ren Nutr.* 13:219, 2003.

Sabbagh Y, et al. Hypophosphatemia leads to rickets by impairing caspase-mediated apoptosis of hypertrophic chondrocytes. *Proc Natl Acad Sci U S A.* 102:9637, 2005.

Weiler H, et al. Conjugated linoleic acid reduces parathyroid hormone in health and in polycystic kidney disease in rats. *Am J Clin Nutr.* 79:1186S, 2004.

SECTION 10

Weight Management, Undernutrition, and Malnutrition

CHIEF ASSESSMENT FACTORS

- Height
- Weight History, Present Weight, Usual Body Weight
- Reference or Healthy Body Weight
- Body Mass Index (BMI)
- Goal Weight
- Percentage of Goal Body Weight
- Recent Weight Changes (Such as 10% Change in Usual Body Weight in 6 Months)
- Triceps Skinfold (TSF) Measurements; Arm Muscle Circumference (AMC) Measurements—Comparing Individual Against Own Values Over Time
- Frame Size—Small, Medium, Large
- Waist Circumference
- Laboratory Values—Glucose, Blood Urea Nitrogen (BUN), Albumin/Transthyretin, Hemoglobin and Hematocrit (H & H), Cholesterol (Chol), Triglycerides (Trig), Total Lymphocyte Count, C-Reactive Protein (CRP)—As Needed to Determine Nutritional Decline or Improvement
- Sleep Apnea, Altered Lung Function
- Anorexia, Nausea, Vomiting, Diarrhea—Frequency, Length of Time
- Blood Pressure with Elevated or Very Low Levels
- Level of Physical Activity
- History of Eating Disorders (Anorexia Nervosa, Bulimia, Binge Eating, Night Eating Syndrome)
- History of Cancer, Smoking, Use of Alcohol, Other Conditions or Disease States
- History of Menstrual or Reproductive Problems (Women)

TYPES OF MALNUTRITION

The definition of malnutrition in the published standards of the American Society of Parenteral and Enteral Nutrition (ASPEN) is any derangement in the normal nutrition status including under- and overnutrition and obesity (Shikora, 2005).

Undernutrition may be *primary*, from insufficient intake, or *secondary*, from impaired utilization.

- Intrauterine and early neonatal life is a period during which environmental influences may produce long-term effects and disease risk in adulthood (Buckley et al, 2005). Undernutrition in critical periods impairs the development and differentiation of a normal immune system, leading to more chronic and frequent infections (Cunningham-Rundles et al, 2005).
- Children who are undernourished may not reach their potential in many aspects of development. Stunting represents growth failure resulting from poor nutrition and health during the pre- and postnatal periods (Milman et al, 2005). Lack of adequate macronutrients or selected micronutrients (zinc, selenium, iron, and the antioxidant vitamins) can lead to clinically significant immune deficiency and infections in children (Cunningham-Rundles et al, 2005).
- High levels of undernutrition in adult women tend to be associated with high levels of undernutrition in children; this may reflect overall nutritional and food insecurity (Nube, 2005). Prenatal exposure to famine can lead to low birth weight, and low birth weight is associated with cardiovascular disease in adulthood (Painter et al, 2005). A woman with a low body mass index (BMI) may have difficulty becoming pregnant, and preconceptional undernutrition shortens gestation in those women who do become pregnant (Ryaco-Solon et al, 2005).
- Nutritional risk is associated with the length of stay in hospitals (Kyle et al, 2005). In hospitalized patients, undernutrition is associated with increased resting energy expenditure (REE; kcal/kg/d); reduced respiratory quotient (RQ) and protein synthesis (g/kg/d) occur in patients with coexistent disease, and refeeding normalizes this process (Winter et al, 2005). **Recent weight loss** appears to be the most important single indicator of nutritional status; both muscle mass depletion and excess body fat are significantly associated with increased length of stay (Kyle et al, 2005). Malnutrition in pediatric hospitals ranges from 15–30% of patients, with an impact on growth, morbidity, and mortality; nutrition support team intervention can help (Agostoni et al, 2005).
- Among elderly patients, malnutrition may come from the "11 Ds": disease, drinking alcohol, drugs, deficits (sensory), desertion/isolation, dementia, delirium, dysphagia, depression, destitution, and despair. If a person has a BMI that is too low (see Tables 10-1 to 10-5), there is an increased risk for nutrition-related complications such as infections, poor wound healing, and pressure ulcer development. Up to 65% of older adults are protein–calorie undernourished at admission or acquire nutritional deficits while hospitalized; nutritional screening and assessment should be more routine (Pepersack, 2005).
- About 25–50% of hospital patients have been found to be malnourished. With current clinical practices, only 50% of malnourished patients are identified by the medical and nursing staff (Kruizenga et al, 2005). Use of Subjective Global Assessment and the Mini Nutritional Assessment tools are used to detect patients who need preventive nutritional measures (Kyle et al, 2005). A simple short nutritional assessment questionnaire (SNAQ) can be used to screen for **appetite changes,** an important factor leading to undernutrition and its consequences (Wilson et al, 2005).
- Outcome measures to assess improvements in undernutrition should include weight change, use of supplemental drinks and snacks between meals, use of tube feeding, use of parenteral nutrition, number of consultations by the hospital dietitian, and decreased length of hospital stay (Kruizenga et al, 2005). Dementia, falls and mobility disorders, malnutrition, end-of-life issues, pressure ulcers, and urinary incontinence have all been identified as important quality measures among older adults residing in nursing homes (Saliba et al, 2005).

Overnutrition is caused from excessive calorie intake and/or inadequate activity.

- Obesity caused by excess nutrition or excess storage of fat relative to energy expenditure is a form of malnutrition that is increasingly seen in children (Cunningham-Rundles et al, 2005). Leptin is a cytokine-like immune regulator that has complex effects in both overnutrition and in the inflammatory response in malnutrition.
- BMI over 30 is the initial calculated measure used to determine obesity. If a person has too high a BMI, he or she is at increased risk for high blood pressure, high blood cholesterol, diabetes, orthopedic problems, gallstones, gout, osteoarthritis, sleep apnea, and cancers such as breast, colon, and gallbladder.
- Critical factors that may put a person at risk for obesity, as they accumulate and interact over an individual's life span, include rapid weight gain in infancy and childhood, early puberty, and excessive weight gain in pregnancy (Johnson et al, 2006).
- Obesity in women can lead to several health challenges. An obese woman may have problems with her menstrual cycle and may have difficulty becoming pregnant. Epidemiological evidence shows that being overweight contributes to menstrual disorders, infertility, miscarriage, poor pregnancy outcome, impaired fetal well-being, and diabetes mellitus. Changes in sensitivity to insulin may occur. Pregnant women who are obese are more at risk for pregnancy-induced hypertension and preeclampsia.
- Weight management programs should include a strong component of nutrition education (Klohe-Lehman et al, 2006).
- Obesity in older adults is increasing in prevalence, along with related macro- and micronutrient deficiencies (Flood and Carr, 2004). Individualized programs with the goal of achieving modest weight reduction in obese patients are likely to result in immediate (e.g., alleviation of arthritic pains and reduction of glucose intolerance) and possibly long-term (e.g., reduction in cardiovascular risk) health care benefits (Horani and Mooradian, 2002). Lifestyle modifications may be best. Diets based on complex carbohydrates, fibers, red wine, fresh fruit and vegetables, and nonanimal fat may protect against age-related cognitive impairment and dementia (Flood and Carr, 2004).

TABLE 10-1 Important Weight Calculations and Body Mass Index (BMI) Guidelines

Metropolitan Life Insurance height–weight charts are no longer used because BMI more often correctly predicts risks for chronic disease or malnutrition. Calculation of percent usual body weight = (actual weight/usual weight) × 100. Calculation of percent weight change = (usual weight minus actual weight/usual weight) × 100.

Waist measurements: Evidence from epidemiological studies indicates that waist circumference is a better marker of abdominal fat content than waist to hip ratio (WHR) and that it is the most practical anthropometric measurement for assessing a patient's abdominal fat content before and during weight loss treatment. Computed tomography (CT) and magnetic resonance imaging (MRI) are both more accurate but impractical for routine clinical use. Waist circumference correlates with intra-abdominal adipose tissue. Upper body obesity is defined as a waist circumference of greater than 40 inches for men and greater than 35 inches for women. This is the "apple shape." If more of the weight is around the hips, this is called "pear shape," and metabolic risks are lower.

Calculation of lean body mass: Body composition is often measured using dual-energy x-ray absorptiometry (DEXA) or electrical impedance absorptiometry. Underestimation of body fat percentage measured by bioelectrical impedance analysis compared to DEXA is a concern (Eisenkolbl et al, 2001).

Calculation for BMI: (Weight [lb] ÷ Height [in]^2) × 705 (from Stensland and Margolis, 1990)

There are many websites that make it easy to calculate BMI, which may be downloaded to a hand-held device, including http://www.cdc.gov/nccdphp/dnpa/bmi/calc-bmi.htm and http://www.nhlbisupport.com/bmi/.

NHLBI Clinical Guidelines for BMI (http://www.nhlbi.nih.gov/guidelines/obesity/ob_home.htm)

<18.5	Underweight
18.5–24.9	Normal
25–29.9	Overweight
30–34.9	Mildly obese (class I obesity)
35–39.9	Moderately obese (class II obesity)
≥40	Extremely obese (class III obesity)

Using these standards, 55% of American adults are overweight or obese (Strawbridge et al, 2000).

Lowest BMI for Mortality (Stevens, 2000)

Ages 20–29	BMI: Men 21.4; Women 19.5
Ages 30–39	BMI: Men 21.6; Women 23.4
Ages 40–49	BMI: Men 22.9; Women 23.2
Ages 50–59	BMI: Men 25.8; Women 25.2
Ages 60–69	BMI: Men 26.6; Women 27.3

BMIs for Pregnant Women

The amount of weight a woman should gain during her pregnancy depends on her prepregnant BMI. The woman wants to gain enough weight to have a healthy baby but not too much weight to avoid complications and long-term health risks. For twins, ideal weight gain is about 35–45 pounds (National Academy of Sciences, http://books.nap.edu/books/0309041384/html/220.html#pagetop)

Prepregnant BMI	Weight Gain During Pregnancy (lb)
≤19.5	28–40
19.6–26	25–35
27–29	15–25
≥30	~13

BMIs for Children (See also Section 3, Childhood Obesity)

Growth charts are used for children to watch the pattern of their growth. Charts cannot be used to diagnose obesity or malnutrition; if a child is over the 85th percentile or lower than the 5th percentile on the charts, the child should see a doctor.

The curves on the growth chart show the pattern of growth. Growth charts for infants and children are calculated the same as for adults but interpreted differently based on BMI. Children are not just small adults; as they grow, their BMI will change. For example, it may be healthy for a 2-year-old child to have a BMI of 16.1 and for that same child to have a BMI of 15.5 at age 6 years and then a BMI of 20 at age 15 years. Growth charts can be found at http://www.cdc.gov/growthcharts. Children under the 5th percentile should be examined to see if they are normal but small children or if they have a problem that prevents normal growth rate.

(continued)

TABLE 10-1 Important Weight Calculations and Body Mass Index (BMI) Guidelines *(continued)*

BMIs for Adolescents

An expert consensus panel suggests that a BMI of 95% for age and gender should define obesity. BMI charts are used for the specific age and sex of the adolescent. Over the 95th percentile on this chart is "overweight;" 85th to 95th percentiles are "at risk of overweight." Most often, guidance for teens is similar to that for adults.

Estimation of Calorie Requirements in Obese Adults: Mifflin-St. Jeor Equation (Mifflin et al, 1990)

Females: Resting energy expenditure (REE) = 10 × weight (kg) + 6.25 × height (cm) - 5 × age (years) − 161

Males: Resting energy expenditure (REE) = 10 × weight (kg) + 6.25 × height (cm) - 5 × age (years) + 5

TABLE 10-2 Calculations of Ideal Body Weight Range

It is suggested that body mass index (BMI) be used whenever possible.

Estimated Ideal Body Weight (Hamwi, 1974) (Note: this is not an evidence-based calculation)

Medium-frame women: allow 100 lb for first 5 ft of height, plus 5 lb for each additional inch

Medium-frame men: allow 106 lb for first 5 ft of height plus 6 lb for each additional inch

Small/large frame: subtract/add 10%

Adjustment for Disability (O'Brien, 1990)

Paraplegic: subtract 5–10% from ideal body weight

Quadriplegic: subtract 10–15% from ideal body weight

Adjustment of BMI for Amputation (Himes, 1995)

$Wt_E = Wt_O/1 - P$

(Key: Wt_E = estimate of total body weight; Wt_O = observed body weight; P = proportion of total body weight represented by missing limb)

Adjustment for Obese Patients (Frankenfield et al, 2005)

Predictive equations for resting metabolic rates (RMR) have many flaws. The Mifflin-St. Jeor equation is the most reliable, predicting RMR within 10% of that measured by indirect calorimetry, which is the standard. The Mifflin-St. Jeor Equation is noted in Table 10-1 and here:

Men: RMR = 9.99 × weight + 6.25 × height − 4.92 × age + 5

Women: RMR = 9.99 × weight + 6.25 × height − 4.92 × age − 161

Adjustment for Critically Ill Patients (Ireton-Jones and Jones, 1998)

Obese Patients

According to Ireton-Jones and Jones, indirect calorimetry is the "gold standard" for determining energy requirements in the obese patient, or equations can be used; 21 kcal/kg actual weight may be useful in clinical settings. The Harris-Benedict Equation may lead to overfeeding, and common use of formulas for adjusted body weight for obesity [(actual body weight − ideal body weight) × 0.25 + ideal body weight] have not been validated.

Critically Ill, Spontaneously Breathing Patient

Estimated energy expenditure = 629 − 11(A) + 25(W) − 609(O)

Ventilator-Dependent Patient

Estimated energy expenditure = 1784 − 11(A) + 5(W) + 244(G) + 239(T) + 804(B)

Key: A = age in years; W = weight in kg; O = obesity (>130% ideal body weight); G = gender (female = 0, male = 1); T = diagnosis of trauma (absent = 0, present = 1); B = diagnosis of burn (absent = 0, present = 1).

TABLE 10-3 Body Mass Index (BMI) Table for Adults

Height in Inches	58	59	60	61	62	63	64	65	66	67	68	69	70	71	72	73	74	75	76
Height (feet, inches)	4′10″	4′11″	5′0″	5′1″	5′2″	5′3″	5′4″	5′5″	5′6″	5′7″	5′8″	5′9″	5′10″	5′11″	6′0″	6′1″	6′2″	6′3″	6′4″
Weight in Pounds																			
100	21	20	20	19	18	18	17	17	16	16	15	15	14	14	14	13	13	13	12
105	22	21	21	20	19	19	18	18	17	16	16	16	15	15	14	14	14	13	13
110	23	22	22	21	20	20	19	18	18	17	17	16	16	15	15	15	14	14	13
115	24	23	23	22	21	20	20	19	19	18	18	17	17	16	16	15	15	14	14
120	25	24	23	23	22	21	21	20	19	19	18	18	17	17	16	16	15	15	15
125	26	25	24	24	23	22	22	21	20	20	19	18	18	17	17	17	16	16	15
130	27	26	25	25	24	23	22	22	21	20	20	19	19	18	18	17	17	16	16
135	28	27	26	26	25	24	23	23	22	21	21	20	19	19	18	18	17	17	16
140	29	28	27	27	26	25	24	23	23	22	21	21	20	20	19	19	18	18	17
145	30	29	28	27	27	26	25	24	23	23	22	21	21	20	20	19	19	18	18
150	31	30	29	28	27	27	26	25	24	24	23	22	22	21	20	20	19	19	18
155	32	31	30	29	28	28	27	26	25	24	24	23	22	22	21	20	20	19	19
160	34	32	31	30	29	28	28	27	26	25	24	24	23	22	22	21	21	20	20
165	35	33	32	31	30	29	28	28	27	26	25	24	24	23	22	22	21	21	20
170	36	34	33	32	31	30	29	28	27	27	26	25	24	24	23	22	22	21	21
175	37	35	34	33	32	31	30	29	28	27	27	26	25	24	24	23	23	22	21
180	38	36	35	34	33	32	31	30	29	28	27	27	26	25	24	24	23	23	22
185	39	37	36	35	34	33	32	31	30	29	28	27	27	26	25	24	24	23	23

(continued)

TABLE 10-3 Body Mass Index (BMI) Table for Adults *(continued)*

Height in Inches	58	59	60	61	62	63	64	65	66	67	68	69	70	71	72	73	74	75	76
Height (feet, inches)	4′10″	4′11″	5′0″	5′1″	5′2″	5′3″	5′4″	5′5″	5′6″	5′7″	5′8″	5′9″	5′10″	5′11″	6′0″	6′1″	6′2″	6′3″	6′4″
190	40	38	37	36	35	34	33	32	31	30	29	28	27	27	26	25	24	24	23
195	41	39	38	37	36	35	34	33	32	31	30	29	28	27	27	26	25	24	24
200	42	40	39	38	37	36	34	33	32	31	30	30	29	28	27	26	26	25	24
205	43	41	40	39	38	36	35	34	33	32	31	30	29	29	28	27	26	26	25
210	44	43	41	40	38	37	36	35	34	33	32	31	30	29	29	28	27	26	26
215	45	44	42	41	39	38	37	36	35	34	33	32	31	30	29	28	28	27	26
220	46	45	43	42	40	39	38	37	36	35	34	33	32	31	30	29	28	28	27
225	47	46	44	43	41	40	39	38	36	35	34	33	32	31	31	30	29	28	27
230	48	47	45	44	42	41	40	38	37	36	35	34	33	32	31	30	30	29	28
235	49	48	46	44	42	42	40	39	38	37	36	35	34	33	32	31	30	29	29
240	50	49	47	45	44	43	41	40	39	38	37	36	35	34	33	32	31	30	29
245	51	50	48	46	45	43	42	41	40	38	37	36	35	34	33	32	32	31	30
250	52	51	49	47	46	44	43	42	40	39	38	37	36	35	34	33	32	31	30
255	53	52	50	48	47	45	44	43	41	40	39	38	37	36	35	34	33	32	31
260	54	53	51	49	48	46	45	43	42	41	40	38	37	36	35	34	33	33	32
265	56	54	52	50	49	47	46	44	43	42	40	39	38	37	36	35	34	33	32
270	57	55	53	51	49	48	46	45	44	42	41	40	39	38	37	36	35	34	33
275	58	56	54	52	50	49													

Note. A person with larger muscle mass may have a greater BMI; evaluate these cases separately from standard tables.

Key: BMI $<$ 20 is underweight; BMI 20–25 is normal weight; BMI 25–30 is overweight; BMI of 30–39 is obesity; and BMI of $\geq$ 40 is extreme obesity.

To use this table, find the weight in the left hand column and height in the column at the top of the table. BMI numbers are found in the corresponding box. For more information, see http://www.nhlbi.nih.gov/guidelines/obesity/bmi_tbl.htm.

TABLE 10-4 Short Methods for Calculating Energy Needs (kcal)

	Level of Activity or Illness		
Goal	**Low**	**Moderate**	**High**
Lose weight	15 kcal/kg	20 kcal/kg	25 kcal/kg
Maintain weight	20 kcal/kg	25 kcal/kg	30 kcal/kg
Gain weight	25 kcal/kg	30 kcal/kg	35 kcal/kg

Calorie Needs Based on Gender for Adults

There is a simple equation that can be used that may give a calorie level for gender and activity level. To calculate the number of calories an adult needs, select the appropriate number and multiply it times the person's current weight.

Group	Calories Needed for Each lb Body Weight
Men, active women	15
Most women, sedentary men, and adults over 55 years	13
Sedentary women, obese adults	10
Pregnant women	
1st trimester	13–15
2nd and 3rd trimester	16–17
Lactating women	15–17

Calorie Needs Based on Age for Children

There is a general decline in the calories needed per pound as a child gets older. Calculate the calorie needs using the information in the table. These figures are not accurate for obese children.

Age	Calories Needed for Each lb Body Weight
0–12 months	55
1–10 years	45–36
11–15 years–young women	17
11–15 years–young men	30
16–20 years–young women	15
16–20 years–young men	18

TABLE 10-5 Weight and Height Conversion Factors

1 kg = 2.2 lb	1 cm = 0.39 in
1 lb = 0.453 kg	1 m = 39.37 in
1 ft = 30.48 cm	1 fluid oz = 29.57 mL
1 in = 2.54 cm	1 oz = 28 g

CITED REFERENCES

Agostoni C, et al. The need for nutrition support teams in pediatric units: a commentary by the ESPGHAN Committee on Nutrition. *J Pediatr Gastroenterol Nutr.* 41:8, 2005.

Boudville A, Bruce DG. Lack of meal intake compensation following nutritional supplements in hospitalised elderly women. *Br J Nutr.* 93:879, 2005.

Buckley AJ, et al. Nutritional programming of adult disease. *Cell Tissue Res.* 322:73, 2005.

Cunningham-Rundles S, et al. Mechanisms of nutrient modulation of the immune response. *J Allergy Clin Immunol.* 115:1119, 2005.

Eisenkolbl J, et al. Underestimation of percentage fat mass measured by bioelectrical impedance analysis compared to dual energy X-ray absorptiometry method in obese children. *Eur J Clin Nutr.* 55:423, 2001.

Flood KL, Carr DB. Nutrition in the elderly. *Curr Opin Gastroenterol.* 20:125, 2004.

Frankenfield D, et al. Comparison of predictive equations for resting metabolic rate in healthy nonobese and obese adults: a systematic review. *J Am Diet Assoc.* 105:775, 2005.

Hamwi GJ. Therapy: changing dietary concepts. In: Danowski TS, ed. *Diabetes mellitus: diagnosis and treatment.* New York: American Diabetes Federation, 1974, pp. 612-623.

Himes JH. New equation to estimate body mass index in amputees. *J Am Diet Assoc.* 95:646, 1995.

Horani MH, Mooradian ADS. Management of obesity in the elderly: special considerations. *Treat Endocrinol.* 1:387, 2002.

Ireton-Jones CS, Jones JD. Should predictive equations or indirect calorimetry be used to design nutrition support regimens? Predictive equations should be used. *Nutr Clin Pract.* 13:141, 1998.

Johnson DB, et al. Preventing obesity: a life cycle perspective. *J Am Diet Assoc.* 106:97, 2006.

Klohe-Lehman DM, et al. Nutrition knowledge is associated with greater weight loss in obese and overweight low-income mothers. *J Am Diet Assoc.* 106:65, 2006.

Kruizenga HM, et al. Effectiveness and cost-effectiveness of early screening and treatment of malnourished patients. *Am J Clin Nutr.* 82:1082, 2005.

Kyle UG, et al. Hospital length of stay and nutritional status. *Curr Opin Clin Nutr Metab Care.* 8:397, 2005.

Mifflin MD, et al. A new predictive equation for resting energy expenditure in healthy individuals. *Am J Clin Nutr.* 51:241, 1990.

Milman A, et al. Differential improvement among countries in child stunting is associated with long-term development and specific interventions. *J Nutr.* 135:1415, 2005.

Nube M. Relationships between undernutrition prevalence among children and adult women at national and subnational level. *Eur J Clin Nutr.* 59: 1112, 2005.

O'Brien RY. Spinal cord injury. In: Gines DJ, ed. *Nutrition management in rehabilitation.* Rockville, MD: Aspen Publishers, Inc., 1990, p. 165.

Painter RC, et al. Prenatal exposure to the Dutch famine and disease in later life: an overview. *Reprod Toxicol.* 20:345, 2005.

Pepersack T. Outcomes of continuous process improvement of nutritional care program among geriatric units. *J Gerontol A Biol Sci Med Sci.* 60:787, 2005.

Rayco-Solon P, et al. Maternal preconceptional weight and gestational length. *Am J Obstet Gynecol.* 192:1133, 2005.

Saliba D, et al. Feasibility of quality indicators for the management of geriatric syndromes in nursing home residents. *J Am Med Dir Assoc.* 6:50S, 2005.

Shikora SA. Severe obesity: a growing health concern ASPEN should not ignore. *J Parenter Enteral Nutr.* 29:288, 2005.

Stensland SH, Margolis S. Simplifying the calculation of body mass index for quick reference. *J Am Diet Assoc.* 90:856, 1990.

Stevens J. Impact of age on associations between weight and mortality. *Nutr Rev.* 58:129, 2000.

Strawbridge W, et al. New NHBI clinical guidelines for obesity and overweight: will they promote health? *Am J Pub Health.* 90:340, 2000.

Wilson MM, et al. Appetite assessment: simple appetite questionnaire predicts weight loss in community-dwelling adults and nursing home residents. *Am J Clin Nutr.* 82:1074, 2005.

Winter TA, et al. The effect of severe undernutrition and subsequent refeeding on whole-body metabolism and protein synthesis in human subjects. *J Parenter Enteral Nutr.* 29:221, 2005.

OVERWEIGHT

OVERWEIGHT AND OBESITY

NUTRITIONAL ACUITY RANKING: LEVEL 3–4

DEFINITIONS AND BACKGROUND

Obesity is the most common form of disturbed nutrition in the United States; micronutrients are often consumed at lower than desirable levels, while macronutrients are eaten in large amounts. Body mass index (BMI) standards are used to determine weight status. BMI correlates well with body fat and is, therefore, a good predictor of chronic disease and mortality, except in highly trained athletes. Overweight is defined as a BMI of 25–29; obesity is defined as a BMI of 30 or more. The prevalence of overweight (BMI >25) and obesity (BMI >30) has steadily increased over the past decade. Obesity is present in 31% of the population, and 34% of the population is overweight (Pi-Sunyer and Kris-Etherton, 2005). About 59 million American adults are obese, and approximately 9 million children or teens aged 6–19 years are overweight (American Dietetic Association, 2005). This trend is occurring throughout the world in both developed and less developed countries (Pi-Sunyer and Kris-Etherton, 2005).

Obesity is a complex multifactorial chronic disease that develops from an interaction of social, behavioral, cultural, physiological, metabolic, and genetic factors (National Heart, Lung, and Blood Institute [NHLBI], 2005). The condition of obesity is chronic, relapsing, and neurochemical and involves interactions between host and environment (Bray and Champagne, 2005). The need for permanent lifestyle changes supercedes the patient's desire for quick weight loss (Bray and Champagne, 2005).

Genetics account for 30–40% of the variations in weight between individuals (Pi-Sunyer and Kris-Etherton, 2005). For instance, the "perilipin gene" controls breakdown of fat in our cells; resistance to loss of body weight from low-energy diets occurs in persons whose genes have this polymorphism (Corella et al, 2005). Environmental factors include physical activity and dietary intake. Environmental causes of obesity are often related to smoking cessation, overconsumption of high-fat foods, or a decrease in activity.

Overweight and obesity increase risks of chronic diseases, secondary symptoms, and impaired quality of life. According to the summary of the NHLBI (2005), the top evidence-based recommendations suggest that *weight loss is recommended (a) to lower elevated blood pressure in overweight and obese persons with high blood pressure; (b) to lower elevated levels of total cholesterol, low-density lipoprotein (LDL) cholesterol, and triglycerides, and to raise low levels of high-density lipoprotein (HDL) cholesterol in overweight and obese persons with dyslipidemia; and (c) to lower elevated blood glucose levels in overweight and obese persons with type 2 diabetes.* Waist circumference is a predictor of mortality and chronic disease, along with BMI (Folsom et al, 2000).

When a patient reaches the overweight stage, he or she should be given guidance on how to avoid obesity. Morbid obesity (BMI >40) is a strong predictor of premature death. Hypertension is common in persons with central-type obesity and weight cycling patterns (Guagnano et al, 2000). In addition, women who have a BMI over 30 may have problems with fertility (Bolumar et al, 2000).

Reimbursement for obesity counseling and management is a complicated issue. Health care professionals should stay informed about the disease and should advocate for patients who need formal assistance (Stern et al, 2005). Not everyone loses weight easily or steadily, and there are many indirect costs (such as pain and suffering) to consider. BMI can help predict who may benefit from weight loss counseling (see Table 10-6). Changes within a neighborhood or community are a good place to start (Booth et al, 2005; Blackburn and Waltman, 2005).

There are varied options for the management of overweight and obese patients, including dietary approaches, altered physical activity patterns, behavior therapy techniques, pharmacotherapy, surgery, and combinations of these techniques. Studies have shown that small changes in weight and increases in physical activity can make significant improvements in health (Pi-Sunyer and Kris-Etherton, 2005). However, starvation diets are not the solution. Orthostatic hypotension may complicate very low–calorie diets (VLCD)

TABLE 10-6 Overweight and Obesity: Suggested Weights for Counseling Initiation

Height (in)	Overweight (BMI = 25) (lb)	Obese (BMI = 30) (lb)
58	119	143
59	124	148
60	128	153
61	132	158
62	136	164
63	141	169
64	145	174
65	150	180
66	155	186
67	159	191
68	164	197
69	169	203
70	174	207
71	179	215
72	184	221
73	189	227
74	194	233
75	200	240
76	205	246

Derived from: National Heart, Lung, and Blood Institute. Body mass index table. Accessed August, 8, 2005 at http://www.nhlbi.nih.gov/guidelines/obesity/bmi_tbl.pdf.

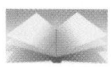

TABLE 10-7 Calculation of Fat Grams

An easy way to calculate number of grams of fat needed is to divide desired body weight by 2. Examples:

120 lb/2 = 60 g

140 lb/2 = 70 g

150 lb/2 = 75 g

170 lb/2 = 85 g

200 lb/2 = 100 g

because of sodium depletion and depressed sympathetic nervous system activity. It is more desirable to calculate basal energy requirements for the individual and determine a reasonable energy intake accordingly.

Avoidance of consuming large portions, energy-dense foods and snacks, high-calorie beverages, and foods with empty calories are important messages for the public (Pi-Sunyer and Kris-Etherton, 2005). Despite numerous diet plans suggesting that macronutrients must be adjusted one way or another, current evidence suggests that hypocaloric weight loss diets should include moderate carbohydrate (35–50% of energy), moderate fat (25–35% of energy), and higher than usual protein (25–35% of energy) (Schoeller and Buchholz, 2005). Reducing fat intake by 10% yields a reduction of about 238 kcal/d (American Dietetic Association, 2005); use of appropriate types of fat is important to protect the heart by causing less of a drop in HDL levels. To estimate the percentage of fat calories in a food, the formula in Table 10-7 is useful, and fat substitutes (such as Olestra) are useful as well.

Dietary influences on hormones that regulate energy intake may become a key way to manage obesity (Orr and Davy, 2005). The hormone leptin, which is produced by adipocytes (fat cells), acts as a lipostat. As the amount of fat stored in adipocytes rises, leptin is released into the blood and signals to the brain that the body has enough to eat. Most overweight people have altered levels of leptin in their bloodstream. Leptin is produced within white adipose tissue, brown fat, the placenta, and fetal heart, bone, and cartilage.

Obesity markedly influences serum insulin, leptin, growth hormone (GH) secretion, and free fatty acid (FFA) levels (Heptulla et al, 2001). Studies have found other hormones that play a role in managing weight. The enterohormones ghrelin, peptide YY-3-36, and cholecystokinin are influenced by macronutrient intake (Orr and Davy, 2005). Preliminary evidence suggests that a low-fat, carbohydrate-rich diet that is also high in fiber tends to modify the hormones related to intake and weight management (Orr and Davy, 2005).

Elevated inflammatory markers, such as tumor necrosis factor (TNF) alpha, soluble TNF receptor II (sTNF-RII), interleukin-6 (IL-6), and C-reactive protein (CRP), are characteristically found in the serum in obese patients; in the morbidly obese, IL-6 may be secreted in an endocrine manner in proportion to the expansion of fat mass, particularly in the abdominal region, with a corresponding increase in hepatic production of CRP (Khaodhiar et al, 2004). The full implications of the role of inflammation have yet to be determined.

Calcium has been implicated as protective against obesity (Zemel, 2002). However, intake of a very high–fat, high-energy diet tends to overwhelm the antiobesity effects of calcium (Venti et al, 2005).

Binge eating disorder (BED) is associated with earlier and more severe onset of obesity (Stunkard and Allison, 2003). Traditional weight management programs can be helpful in binge eating cases.

Night eating syndrome (NES) is another condition that is affected by disordered neuroendocrine functioning (Stunkard and Allison, 2003). Hormone levels of melatonin, leptin, and cortisol are affected. NES consists of morning anorexia, evening hyperphagia, and insomnia. Night eaters awaken more often during the night than others and have a lower nocturnal rise in plasma melatonin and leptin levels, with significantly higher circadian levels of plasma cortisol than controls (Birketvedt et al, 1999). Breakfast is often delayed for several hours after awakening. Men tend to be more affected by NES (Aronoff et al, 2001). See Table 10-8.

Sustained modest weight loss by obese adults can result in substantial health and economic benefits. The American Dietetic Association has recommended eight medical nutrition therapy visits for adult weight management. Self-esteem, body image, self-efficacy, locus of control, motivation, stress management, problem solving and decision making, and assertiveness are important considerations.

TABLE 10-8 Night Eating Syndrome Indicators and Questionnaire

Night eating syndrome (NES) is a special condition that affects 1–2% of the general population (see Table 4-16 also). It is likely that 25% of all morbidly obese individuals have this condition. Psychotherapy is recommended, and self-help groups such as Overeaters Anonymous or group therapy can help. Sertraline, a selective serotonin reuptake inhibitor, may be beneficial in the treatment of NES (O'Reardon et al, 2004). Primary signs include:

1. Not feeling hungry in the morning
2. Overeating in the evening
3. Difficulty falling asleep
4. Waking at night and eating
5. Feeling depressed

Night Eating Questionnaire (adapted from Allison et al, 2004).

1. How hungry are you usually in the morning?
2. When do you usually eat for the first time?
3. Do you have cravings or urges to eat snacks after supper but before bedtime?
4. How much control do you have over your eating between supper and bedtime?
5. How much of your daily food intake do you consume after suppertime?
6. Are you currently feeling blue or down in the dumps?
7. When you are feeling blue, when is your mood lower?
8. How often do you have trouble getting to sleep?
9. Other than using the bathroom, how often do you get up in the middle of the night?
10. Do you have cravings or urges to eat snacks when you wake up at night?
11. Do you eat in order to get back to sleep when you awake at night?
12. When you get up in the middle of the night, how often do you snack?
13. If you snack in the middle of the night, how aware are you of your eating?
14. How much control do you have over your nighttime eating?

INTERVENTION: OBJECTIVES

The Clinical Guidelines on the Identification, Evaluation, and Treatment of Overweight and Obesity in Adults, printed in 2000, provide an excellent summary of evidence and recommendations, as follows (NHLBI, 2005):

Goals for Weight Loss

The general goals of weight loss and management are to reduce body weight, to maintain a lower body weight over the long term, and to prevent further weight gain. Evidence indicates that a moderate weight loss can be maintained over time if some form of therapy continues. It is better to maintain a moderate weight loss over a prolonged period than to regain from a marked weight loss.

1. **Initial Goal of Weight Loss from Baseline**

   The initial goal of weight loss therapy should be to reduce body weight by approximately 10% from baseline. With success, further weight loss can be attempted if indicated through further assessment.

2. **Amount of Weight Loss**

   Weight loss should be about 1–2 lb/wk for a period of 6 months, with the subsequent strategy based on the amount of weight lost. Evidence Category B.

Achievement of Weight Loss

1. **Diet Therapy**

   Low-calorie diets (LCDs) are recommended for weight loss in overweight and obese persons. Reducing fat as part of an LCD is a practical way to reduce calories. Reducing dietary fat alone without reducing calories is not sufficient for weight loss. However, reducing dietary fat, along with reducing dietary carbohydrates, can facilitate caloric reduction. A diet that is individually planned to help create a deficit of 500–1000 kcal/d should be an integral part of any program aimed at achieving a weight loss of 1–2 lb/wk.

2. **Physical Activity**

   The combination of a reduced-calorie diet and increased physical activity is recommended since it produces weight loss that may also result in decreases in abdominal fat and increases in cardiorespiratory fitness (Evidence Category A).

   Physical activity is recommended as part of a comprehensive weight loss therapy and weight control program because it: (1) modestly contributes to weight loss in overweight and obese adults (Evidence Category A), (2) may decrease abdominal fat (Evidence Category B), and (3) increases cardiorespiratory fitness (Evidence Category A).

   Physical activity should be an integral part of weight loss therapy and weight maintenance. Initially, moderate levels of physical activity for 30–45 minutes, 3–5 days a week, should be encouraged. All adults should set a long-term goal to accumulate at least 30 minutes or more of moderate-intensity physical activity on most, and preferably all, days of the week. Evidence Category B.

3. **Behavior Therapy**

   Behavior therapy is a useful adjunct when incorporated into treatment for weight loss and weight maintenance. Evidence Category B.

   Practitioners need to assess the patient's motivation to enter weight loss therapy; assess the readiness of the patient to implement the plan, and then take appropriate steps to motivate the patient for treatment. Evidence Category D.

4. **Summary of Lifestyle Therapy**

   Weight loss and weight maintenance therapy should employ the combination of LCD, increased physical activity, and behavior therapy. Evidence Category A.

5. **Pharmacotherapy**

   Weight loss drugs approved by the Food and Drug Administration (FDA) may be used as part of a comprehensive weight loss program, including dietary therapy and physical activity for patients with a BMI of ≥30 with no concomitant obesity-related risk factors or diseases, and for patients with a BMI of ≥27 with concomitant obesity-related risk factors or diseases. Weight loss drugs should never be used without additional lifestyle modifications. Continual assessment of drug therapy for efficacy and safety is necessary. If the drug is efficacious in helping the patient to lose and/or maintain weight loss and there are no serious adverse effects, it can be continued; if not, it should be discontinued. Evidence Category B.

6. **Weight Loss Surgery**

   Weight loss surgery is an option for carefully selected patients with clinically severe obesity (BMI ≥40 or ≥35 with comorbid conditions) when less invasive methods of weight loss have failed and the patient is at high risk for obesity-associated morbidity or mortality. Evidence Category B.

Goals for Weight Loss Maintenance

1. **Weight Maintenance Phase**

   After successful weight loss, the likelihood of weight loss maintenance is enhanced by a program consisting of dietary therapy, physical activity, and behavior therapy, which should be continued indefinitely. Drug therapy can also be used. However, drug safety and efficacy beyond 1 year of total treatment have not been established. Evidence Category B.

   A weight maintenance program should be a priority after the initial 6 months of weight loss therapy. Evidence Category B.

   The literature suggests that weight loss and weight maintenance therapies that provide a greater frequency of contacts between the patient and the practitioner and are provided over the long term should be used whenever possible. This can lead to more successful weight loss and weight maintenance. Evidence Category C.

Goals for Special Treatment Groups

1. **Smokers**

   All smokers, regardless of their weight status, should quit smoking (Evidence Category A). Prevention of weight gain should be encouraged, and if weight gain does occur, it should be treated through dietary therapy, physical activity, and behavior therapy, maintaining the primary emphasis on the importance of abstinence from smoking. (See Table 10-14 for more information.)

2. **Older Adults**
   Restrictions on overall food intake due to dieting could result in inadequate intake of protein or essential vitamins or minerals, and involuntary weight loss indicative of occult disease might be mistaken for success in voluntary weight reduction. These concerns can be alleviated by providing proper nutritional counseling and regular body weight monitoring in older persons for whom weight reduction is prescribed. Age alone should not preclude treatment for obesity in adult men and women; there is evidence that weight reduction has similar effects in improving cardiovascular disease risk factors in older and younger adults.
3. **Diverse Patient Populations**
   Standard obesity treatment approaches should be tailored to the needs of various patients or patient groups.

Other Advice

- Each pound of body fat contains approximately 3500 kcal. Thus, reducing intake by 500 kcal/d should allow a loss of 1 lb in 7 days.
- Have the patient set own goal. Self-monitoring is important for maintaining calorie, fat gram, and physical activity goals (Berkel et al, 2005).
- Use the "Five A's Approach" to promote physical activity (Estabrooks et al, 2003):
  - **Assess** current level of activity and physical abilities.
  - **Advise** about the health benefits and risks of various activities.
  - **Agree** to work collaboratively for a personalized plan and reasonable goals.
  - **Assist** the individual with strategies to overcome barriers.
  - **Arrange** for follow-up assessments through visits, phone calls, and mailed reminders.
- It is essential to provide a nutritionally balanced, individualized diet pattern.
- Maintain a normal or slightly higher protein intake to maintain nitrogen balance, especially with energy-restricted diets (Schoeller and Buchholz, 2005).
- Weigh weekly on the same scale with the same clothing at about the same time of day. After reaching desired weight, daily weighing often helps maintain motivation for continuing effective lifestyle changes.
- Avoid or correct disordered eating (e.g., abnormal eating, diet cheating, compulsive eating, addictive or manipulative habits, eating disorders, NES). Healthy eating patterns, not constant evaluation of body fat, are the desired end.
- Use water-dense foods, including more fruits and vegetables. Intake of foods high in water content reduces subsequent energy intake more effectively than does intake of water with food (Rolls et al, 2005). The DASH diet works well because it encourages intake of more fruits and vegetables.
- Prevent or improve symptoms of the metabolic syndrome where present (see Section 9).
- When surgery is indicated for patients who are morbidly obese, regular follow-up by a dietitian who can offer advice on diet quality and symptom management is helpful. Use of vitamin-mineral supplements for more than a year after surgery is important. See Section 14.
- Persons who participate only in Internet counseling should be encouraged to seek in-person programs as well because weight regain may be greater (Berkel et al, 2005). Electronic feedback and one-on-one advice from a nutrition counselor are helpful in maintaining positive momentum for weight management.

INTERVENTION: FOOD AND NUTRITION

- Plan a diet with moderate carbohydrate (35–50% of energy), moderate fat (25–35% of energy), and higher than usual protein (25–35% of energy) (Schoeller and Buchholz, 2005). Perceived hunger tends to be lower among those who consume higher protein while dieting (Nickols-Richardson et al, 2005).
- A lower glycemic load is helpful for some people; foods that have a low glycemic index include salads with oil and vinegar dressing, high-fat granola cereal, and most fresh fruits and vegetables (Pittas et al, 2005). **Glycemic load = glycemic index × available carbohydrate amount.**
- Fiber-rich foods take longer to chew, are low in calories, and increase satiety. High-fiber cereal at breakfast seems to curb appetite at lunch slightly. Encourage 25–35 g of fiber per day.
- Eating a handful of walnuts (4–6) before meals seems to curb appetite and intake.
- Schedule 6–8 small meals at frequent intervals to prevent cheating and overeating. Breakfast is a crucial meal to prevent overeating later by many individuals.
- The American Dietetic Association supports a "total diet approach," where the overall food pattern is more important than one food or meal. If food is consumed in moderation with appropriate portion size and regular activity, a more positive approach to food makes the client feel less anxious and guilty (American Dietetic Association, 2002).
- The importance of breakfast should be emphasized (Song et al, 2005); cereal consumption may play a role in helping to maintain a healthful BMI (Barton et al, 2005).
- Diet should provide adequate fluid intake to excrete metabolic wastes. Beverages with meals increase the sensation of fullness. Rule of thumb is to use 1 mL water per 1 kcal, or 30 cc/kg of body weight, whichever is greater for the individual.
- Decrease overall salt intake if fluid retention is a concern.
- With elevated triglycerides, decrease concentrated sweets and sugars, fats, and alcohol. The latest NHLBI guidelines recommend use of 35% kcal from fat, with more from monounsaturated sources and less from saturated fats.
- Teach patient to splurge by plan and not by impulse. Work with friends to be accountable and not give in to temptation to overeat.
- For a modified fast, a meal replacement product for 1–2 meals per day can get the patient started. This method is not recommended for the long term unless sufficient fiber is available from other meals.
- Sweetened sodas, alcoholic beverages, juices, and other high-calorie drinks should be monitored carefully because the calories add up quickly.
- Fat substitutes, when used in moderation, can be safe to lower total energy intake (American Dietetic Association, 2005). Olestra decreases serum carotenoid and other fat-

SAMPLE NUTRITION DIAGNOSTIC STATEMENT

Obesity

PES: Not ready for diet/lifestyle change related to excessive oral food/beverage intake as evidenced by increased weight gain after four individualized counseling sessions.

Assessment: Diet, weight, and physical activity histories and psychosocial issues.

Intervention: Address motivation to get to next stage of change.

Monitoring and Evaluation: Ask patient to return in 1 month to assess changes in motivation.

soluble vitamin absorption mildly, without detrimental biological health effects (Allgood et al, 2001). Overall, there have been positive impacts on dietary fat intakes and serum cholesterol levels among consumers who use olestra-containing foods (Patterson, 2000).

- To calculate needs of the obese patient in hospitals or critical care, estimating needs may be inaccurate. Indirect calorimetry is the gold standard, and hypocaloric nutrition support is generally recommended to prevent overfeeding (Breen and Ireton-Jones, 2004; Dickerson, 2004). While most medical intensive care unit (ICU) patients can be given an estimated 25 kcal/kg, greater energy requirements may be needed in burn or major trauma patients (Breen and Ireton-Jones, 2004).

CLINICAL INDICATORS

Clinical/History

Height
Weight
BMI
Desirable BMI
Weight changes
Percentage of excess weight
Percentage of body fat
Diet history
Blood pressure (BP)
Skinfold thickness
Waist circumference
Sleep apnea?

Lab Work

CRP (elevated from comorbidities?)
Ca++, Mg++
Na+, K+
Uric acid
Triiodothyronine (T3), thyroxine (T4)
Glucose (Gluc)
Cholesterol (Chol)
Triglycerides (Trig)
Hypoxemia?
Plasma cortisol

Common Drugs Used and Potential Side Effects

- Lack of efficacy, undesirable side effects, and safety concerns have given many weight loss medicines a poor track record (Greenway, 2005). Phenylpropanolamine (PPA) produces dose-related, life-threatening cardiovascular and central nervous toxicity from adrenergic overstimulation. Because of these effects and the risk of hemorrhagic stroke, the FDA stopped use of PPA in cold medicines and prescription diet aids.
- Pharmacotherapy is generally not enough; behavior modification must be taught for long-term success (Moyers, 2005). Medications that have been studied in depth include:
  1. **Appetite suppressants** (anorectic agents) may cause excitability, gastrointestinal (GI) distress, and other problems. This is especially true of drugs containing amphetamine. If an anorexiant has been prescribed, avoid using excesses of caffeine; this is not necessary if using a lipase inhibitor. Phentermine (Fastin, Adipex-X, Pro-Fast, Oby-Trim) is a stimulant-like amphetamine; dry mouth can occur. Diethylpropion (Tenuate) suppresses appetite also; dry mouth and GI upset can occur, so short-term use is recommended. Rimonabant (Acomplia) suppresses appetite, but dizziness, diarrhea, and nausea can occur, and FDA approval is pending; see below.
  2. **Orlistat (Xenical)** decreases pancreatic lipase and decreases fat absorption. Soft stools and anal leakage may occur, especially if a diet high in fat (>90 g) is consumed. Orlistat helps minimize weight regain after weight loss and appears to be well tolerated for the long term. HDL levels are much higher, overall total cholesterol levels drop, and vitamin E and beta-carotene levels are significantly higher in orlistat users (Finer et al, 2000). Fat-soluble vitamins may be required during chronic therapy because absorption may be decreased. Patients on orlistat should have a BMI over 27 with risk factors or a BMI over 30 without risk factors; the drug is not for everyone. Be sure to teach the patient about fat intake, or its side effects may cause failure of the plan. Weight loss is about 6 lb in 1 year.
  3. **Sibutramine (Meridia)** increases energy expenditure and satiety, which may contribute to weight-reducing properties. It acts via the central nervous system (CNS) as serotonergic and noradrenergic reuptake inhibitor. It can be used long term. Plasma epinephrine, plasma glucose, and blood pressure are all significantly elevated. Weight loss is about 10 lb in 1 year.
  4. **Acomplia (rimonabant)** is a selective CB1 endocannabinoid receptor antagonist, blocking endogenous cannabinoid binding to neuronal CB1 receptors; it is expected to have potential for use in smoking cessation.
  5. **Drugs under study** for weight management include topiramate, Axokine, and oleoylestrone; their effectiveness and safety will determine whether they are approved by the FDA for obesity management (Greenway, 2005).

Herbs, Botanicals, and Supplements

- Herbs and botanical supplements should not be used without discussing with physician.
- Dietary supplements are often used for providing nutrients that may be inadequate in low-energy diets and stimulating weight loss (Dwyer et al, 2005). Dietitians

TABLE 10-9 Medications That Cause Weight Gain

Medications that affect the central nervous system can cause clinically relevant resting metabolic rate (RMR) effects (from 262–680 kcal/d), and this can occur in all age groups (Dickerson and Roth-Yousey, 2005a). Sedation or analgesia may produce temporary reductions in RMR (Dickerson and Roth-Yousey, 2005a). Medications that can cause weight gain follow.

Medication	Description
Benzodiazepine Antianxiety Agents (alprazolam [Xanax], chlordiazepoxide [Librium])	Psychotropic drugs can cause weight gain.
Antidepressants, Selective Serotonin Reuptake Inhibitors (SSRIs) (Prozac, Zoloft, Paxil, Luvox, Celexa)	SSRIs cause weight loss at first and then weight gain later. Paxil causes the most weight change. Prozac is often used for patients with bulimia nervosa; it may cause headaches, dry mouth, nausea, diarrhea, and hyperglycemia.
Antidepressants, Tricyclic (TCAs) (Elavil, Asendin, Aventyl, Pamelor, Adaptin, Sinequan, Tofranil, Norpramin, Anafranil, and Vivactil)	TCAs can cause much weight gain from slowed metabolism and increased carbohydrate cravings.
Antidepressants, Monoamine Oxidase Inhibitors (MAOIs) (isocarboxazid [Marplan],phenelzine sulfate [Nardil], tranylcypromine sulfate [Parnate])	MAOIs cause more weight gain (i.e., nonselective reversibles, or Marplan, Nardil, Parnate). MAOI selective reversible drugs (RIMAs), such as Manerix or Humoryl, are not as weight enhancing.
Mood Stabilizers and Antipsychotics (lithium; Moban, Clozaril, Serlect, and Zeldox)	Mood stabilizers made with lithium can cause weight gain. Antipsychotics may also cause weight gain.
Antipsychotics (haloperidol [Haldol], perphenazine [Trilafon], thiothixene [Navane], thioridazine HCl (Mellaril])	
Antipsychotics, Atypical (olanzapine [Zyprexa], quetiapine fumarate [Seroquel], risperidone [Risperdal])	
Anticonvulsants (divalproex/valproic acid [Depakote/Depakene], gabapentin [Neurontin], Tegretol, Lamictal, Topamax)	These medications can increase appetite and insulin levels.
Cardiovascular Agents (propranolol, atenolol, carvedilol, bisoprolol)	These medications can reduce RMR by 4–12% over time (Dickerson and Roth-Yousey, 2005a).
Chemotherapy	Chemotherapy can decrease metabolic rate by 6–11%, especially in patients with leukemia, breast cancer, and some solid tumors (Dickerson and Roth-Yousey, 2005b). It is not known if this persists over time since the treatment is short term.
Insulin and Antidiabetic Agents	Side effects include weight gain. For example, glipizide can reduce RMR by 3.5%, while metformin does not (Dickerson and Roth-Yousey, 2005b).
Hormones (corticosteroids [cortisone, methylprednisolone, prednisolone], human growth hormone, somatotropin [Serostim], medroxyprogesterone acetate [Provera, Depo-Provera], oxymetholone [Anadrol-50], testosterone [Androderm, Testoderm])	Prednisone, oral contraceptives (such as Depo-Provera), and other hormones can cause weight gain if taken over time.

should regularly check for information on efficacy and safety (www.cfsan.fda.gov; www.ods.od.nih.gov).

- Bitter orange has no evidence showing efficacy; few data are available (Dwyer et al, 2005).
- Calcium claims for weight loss have not been consistent in weight loss results (Dwyer et al, 2005). Larger studies are needed.
- Chitosan is a major ingredient in many over-the-counter (OTC) products that claim to reduce excess body weight by reducing fat absorption. Little evidence supports its use, and there may be undesirable GI side effects (Dwyer et al, 2005).
- Chromium picolinate has been reported to improve glucose and lipid metabolism. There is little evidence for benefit, but there are few adverse effects (Dwyer et al, 2005).
- Conjugated linoleic acid (CLA) has no documented efficacy (Dwyer et al, 2005).
- Ephedra (ma huang) contains ephedrine and works as an anorexiant. The FDA has removed it from the market because it elevates blood pressure and can cause significant problems.
- Green tea contains polyphenols and catechins, which may help promote weight loss (Nagao et al, 2005).
- Hydroxycitric acid and garcinia are not effective for treatment of obesity (Morelli and Zoorob, 2000). Garcinia has cytotoxic effects and has been demonstrated to have a toxic effect in animals.

- Stanols (Take Control) and sterols (Benacol) do not affect weight but are often used by overweight individuals. They are safely used as directed to lower elevated cholesterol levels.

INTERVENTION: NUTRITION EDUCATION, COUNSELING, CARE MANAGEMENT

- A multidimensional program is best for weight management, including formulation of reasonable goals, prevention of unnecessary weight loss or gain, weight loss when necessary, prevention of relapse, and acceptance of physique. "Health at every size" is a good message to share (Bacon et al, 2005).
- Individualize according to psychosocial, behavioral, and biological factors. Obesity is a chronic condition that requires chronic care with varying levels of intensity (Foster and Nonas, 2004).
- Identify the mind–body connection. Teach patient about physical hunger and how to identify true hunger from emotional "hunger." Practical advice and a Hunger Rating Scale are available in Figure 10-1. Steps to normalize eating include awareness training, changing thoughts and beliefs about food, handling issues of deprivation and guilt, and refocusing on areas other than food and weight. Self-efficacy is especially important; adjusting beliefs toward "I can do this" in the client seems to be quite beneficial (Wamsteker et al, 2005). Table 10-10 further describes the role of the dietitian in weight and obesity management.
- Low-energy diets tend to be higher in nutritional value if carefully planned using water-rich fruits, vegetables, cooked grains, and soups (Rolls et al, 2005). Noncalorie sweeteners and chewing sugarless gum are useful in weight management. Chewing gum may help fight cravings for sweets and suppress the appetite.
- One goal is to develop reduced-calorie eating plans that meet personal food preferences and also provide satisfying food portions (Rolls et al, 2005).
- Instruct the patient how to plan menus and use recipes. Recipe modifications are useful for replacing fat in recipes (e.g., use applesauce or pear puree in muffins or sponge cake; prune or black bean puree in brownies or spice cake or chocolate cake; or white bean puree in cookies).
- Providing guidance on how to eat at parties and away from home will be important. Low-calorie snacking and selection of lower calorie food preparation methods may be needed. Avoid buffets when possible.
- Teach portion control. Sometimes measuring and weighing foods can be useful. Table 10-11 provides a handy portion adjustment guide using everyday objects
- Behavior therapy may be helpful in self-monitoring (food diaries, weights, activity). Teach stimulus control of cues, family intervention, slowing down while eating, and monitoring of intake while at parties and during work breaks.
- To delay automatic eating, drink a glass of water and wait 20 minutes. If the sensation persists, it is probably hunger. Make meals last 20 minutes or longer. Eat slowly; chew well. The best diet is "don't buy it."
- Physical activity is an integral part of weight loss maintenance. Encourage moderate levels of physical activity for 30–60 minutes daily whenever possible. It is reasonable to encourage expenditure of 1000 kcal/wk in some type of physical activity (Berkel et al, 2005). Resistance training increases muscle mass, and aerobic exercise should be directed at 70% of maximal oxygen consumption. See Table 10-12.
- Avoid bizarre fad dieting, skipping meals, or emphasis on any one dietary component. The American Heart Association has a "no fad diet" available that encourages healthy eating patterns.
- Use of meal replacements for one meal a day can be beneficial for improving cholesterol levels, plasma glucose, and diastolic blood pressure (Berkel et al, 2005).
- Avoid an energy level that is too low, which causes hypophagia; sudden death syndrome may occur. Caloric intake less than 1200 kcal for women or 1500 kcal for men requires an additional multivitamin supplement.
- Encourage adequate sleep. Sleep deprivation increases a hunger hormone that can trigger overeating (Spiegel et al, 2004). Further research is needed.
- Cultural emphasis on thinness may lead to unhealthy weight loss efforts (Katzmarzyk and Davis, 2001). Enhancement of self-esteem is important (McArthur and Howard, 2001).
- Phone and mail follow-up contacts are quite helpful interventions (Berkel et al, 2005). The real challenge involves keeping weight off after it has been lost (Hill et al, 2005).
- Special considerations exist with obesity counseling in different life stages. Pediatric and geriatric patients require special assessments and interventions (Kushner and Blatner, 2005). Women may need attention during childbearing years because they should not assume that menstrual cycle weight gain is permanent weight gain; premenstrual weight gain may vary from 2–5 lb of fluid.
- Group counseling may be useful. Corporate wellness programs are often quite effective (Ferko-Adams, 2005).
- Table 10-13 describes cases and suggestions for managing sleep apnea and Pickwickian syndrome.
- Smoking cessation can lead to weight gain if not carefully managed; see Table 10-14 for specific tips.
- Table 10-15 provides a chart with several popular fad diets. In general, permanent lifestyle changes may be associated with maintenance of weight loss to a greater extent than popular diets or trends.

For More Information

- After the Diet
  http://www.afterthediet.com/
- American Dietetic Association–Weight Management Protocol
  http://www.eatright.org/Public/
- Beyond Dieting
  http://www.beyonddieting.com/
- California Adolescent Nutrition and Fitness Program
  http://www.canfit.org/
- Canadian Physical Activity Guide
  http://www.csep.ca/
- Centers for Disease Control and Prevention, National Center for Chronic Disease Prevention and Health Promotion—Report of the Surgeon General on Physical Fitness
  http://www.cdc.gov/nccdphp/sgr/summ.htm
- Cooper Institute–Weight Management Centers
  http://www.cooperinst.org/wtmgmt.asp

Figure 10-1 Dieting: Practical Advice

1. **Finding Balance in a Binge Lifestyle:** A binge lifestyle promotes a lack of balance. Usually it entails overwork, overeating, and overplay with excessive eating, drinking, exercise, shopping, or other negative health behaviors. Treating these behaviors is complex, time-intensive, and requires a team effort.

Identifying Binge Lifestyle Behavior: Clues to look for:	***Potential Strategies for working with this individual include:***
• Lacks effective relaxation strategies or time for relaxation.	• Educate and skill build relaxation strategies (recommend classes in yoga, meditation, suggest "alone" time, etc.).
• Uses food for gratification, relaxation, entertainment, pleasure, and reward.	• Work to find other avenues to pleasure and reward.
• Works excessive hours and subsequently does not have enough time to exercise or procure healthy foods.	• Time management skills, organizing time, setting schedules, dedicating time to exercise/healthy cooking/eating, work to change attitudes towards time for self-care/lifestyle change.
• May be too tired to be motivated to change lifestyle.	• Work with setting time for relaxation, stress management principles, time for play, difference between physical and emotional tiredness.
• Has intensive weekend exercise patterns (the "weekend warrior"), which can lead to injury.	• Set regular exercise schedule, teach basic principles of healthy exercise, emphasize training effects.
• Uses substances or activities to numb, rather than soothe, in order to relax.	• Discuss the difference between numbing and true relaxation, identify the intention behind the behavior.
• Overeating ("compulsive eating")	• Work with awareness of eating, being in the present moment, learning to truly enjoy food, eating when physically hungry.
• Alcohol or drug use	• Refer for help, define "moderation" with alcohol, goal for use of substances (i.e. relaxation, reward, etc.), stress management skill training.
• Excessive, repetitive exercise or self-starvation (as in Anorexia)	• Explore purpose behind behaviors, work towards setting healthy behaviors.
• Obsessive thoughts or organizing behavior	• Set time aside to "worry" (compartmentalizing), work on ability to be spontaneous and flexible.
• Self-Numbing vs. Self-Soothing	• Teach self-soothing strategies

2. **Setting limits – Caloric Intake:**

Too Few	***Too Many***	***"Just Right"****
Weight loss >1-2% body weight per week, caloric intake close to RMR (RMR often between 1200-1500 calories), unreasonable to maintain restrictions for long periods of time.	Weight gains occur, person is routinely eating until stuffed and uncomfortable, health risks increasing.	After age 4: 1800 Kcal/d Women: ~2000 Kcal/d Men: ~2500-2900 Kcal/d Appropriate rate of weight loss is 0.5-2 lb/wk or <1-2% body weight per week. If weight loss desired, a 300-500 calorie/day deficit (200-300 food and 200-300 exercise).

Exercise:

Goal	***Too Little****	***Too Much***	***"Just Right"****
Health Maintenance	None to sporadic exercise, weekend only exercise, sedentary lifestyle.	>60-90 minutes/day, same exercise pattern and muscle use, daily with no rest days planned.	1 hour/day on average max, 5-6 days per week max recommended 2 days of rest per week, listen to body cues of pain, injury or tightness, incorporates active lifestyle & daily movement.
Reduction of risk of CVD	None to sporadic exercise, weekend only exercise, sedentary lifestyle.	>60-90 minutes/day, same exercise pattern and muscle use, daily with no rest days planned.	20-30 minutes per day @ 3-4x/week; 10 minute discontinuous bouts acceptable, listen to body cues of pain, injury or tightness, incorporates active lifestyle & daily movement.
Weight Management	None to sporadic exercise, weekend only exercise, sedentary lifestyle.	>90-120+ min/day, same exercise pattern and muscle use, daily with no rest days planned.	45-90 minutes @ 5-6 x per week, listen to body cues of pain, injury, tightness, and shortness of breath, incorporates active lifestyle & daily movement. 10 minute discontinuous bouts encouraged, especially when unable to get in a full exercise session.

*Actual amounts vary based on body size, age, and activity level.
**Depends on health status (cardiac function, bone density status), mobility issues.

Hunger Rating Scale. (Courtesy of Claudia S. P. Fernandez, MS, RD, LDN.)

3. Using the Mind Body connection: separating physical from emotional hungers

PHYSICAL HUNGER-SATISFACTION RATING SCALE

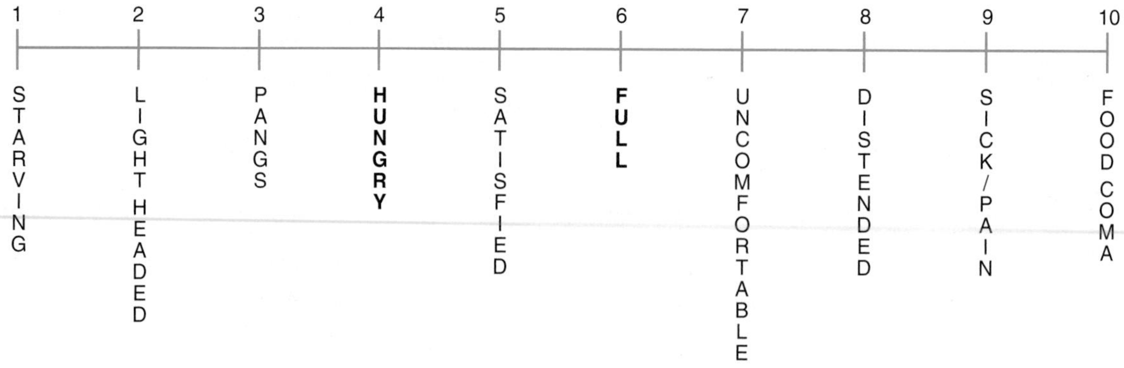

EMOTIONAL "HUNGER" RATING SCALE

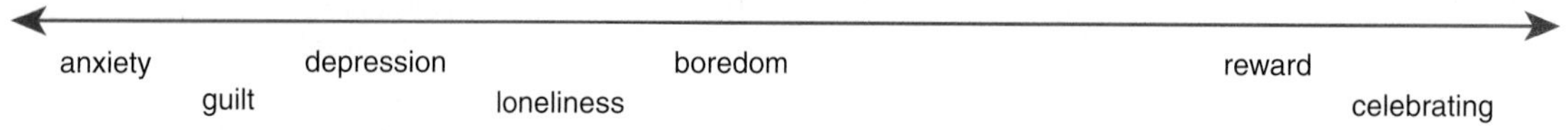

4. Clearing up Myths: working with the self-labeled food addict

What the client says:	What to do:
• My body is different from everyone else's body.	Educate client how a normal human body works, why plateaus happen, the effects of starvation.
• I should (or do) feel guilty about feeding my body.	Legalize foods: no good foods, no bad foods. *Don't* encourage guilt.
• I have to exercise more than other people to get the same benefit.	Educate client about the effects of exercise and the reasons to exercise.
• I have to eat less than other people to get the same benefit.	Educate client about the effects of starvation and the impact of one-time overeating.
• Confusing "fat" with feelings, prejudices, and attitudes (cultural).	Have the patient use other words to describe his or her feelings or beliefs.
• Food as nurturance, stress relief, reward, emotional numbing.	Help client separate emotional from physical hungers (see scale) and develop strategies to answer non-physical needs.
• Myth: I just need more discipline and willpower or I have no discipline or willpower.	EMPOWER! EMPOWER! EMPOWER! Help your client to gain a sense of control and peace with food and exercise issues.

5. Start from where your patient is but don't do the work for him or her.

- Provide some structure if needed, but avoid going too far.
- Work to help your clients think, analyze, decide, and apply their knowledge and skills.
- Don't do the work for them (i.e., creating a week's worth of menus is a different service than helping them with their disordered eating or eating disorder. Work with them to help them develop the skills to do this. Set up a template *with* them, teach them, but have them create the specifics).
- Assess knowledge and skills. No one can implement healthy eating until they know *how* to do it:
  - how to get nutritious food (in restaurants, on the road, in the grocery store, on a budget)
  - how to "be in the present moment" when eating (eating exercises, taste perception analysis)
  - how to interpret and understand their body signals, and separate those from emotional/habitual ones.
  - how to include fun foods (cookies, cheesecake) within a healthy diet.
- What is their underlying issue? Knowledge deficit? Habits? Emotional issues? Beliefs? Relationship (Significant Other) issues?

Figure 10-1 *(continued)*

6. People are complex: use the three domains of learning and focus on tasks that fall under each

Cognitive Domain: working with thinking, understanding, and beliefs (The traditional focus of health care)	• Teach them new knowledge (*traditional*: portions, fat grams and new *paradigm*: non-dieting strategies, lifestyle change) • Clarify myths and misunderstandings • Be a translator: make the technical accessible
Behavioral Domain: working with actions, automatic actions, lack of awareness, and skills	• How to communicate: practice and role play to deal with sabotage and getting needs met • Slow eating and enjoying foods • Reading labels before buying • Acting with intention, not reacting without awareness • Teach them new behaviors • Work with client awareness: people underestimate what they eat by ~50%
Affective Domain: working with feelings and attitudes around food, fitness, and eating	• Exercise resistance • Lack of motivation • Poor self-image • Perception of competence and confidence • Ability to self-soothe and self-nurture • Empower your client!

7. Connecting to other allied health professionals

Nutritionists/Nutrition Therapists/Registered Dietitians, Psychologists (counseling), Social workers, Psychiatrists (medical management), Exercise specialists/Personal Trainers, Physicians/Physician Assistants are the team. Get help if your client has eating disorder or disordered eating issues and work within a team context.

Figure 10-1 *(continued)*

TABLE 10-10 Role of the Dietitian in Weight Management and Obesity

Dietitians should play a role in achieving the goals of the Healthy Weight 2010 Objectives.

- Improve quality of life by reducing diseases and disability associated with obesity.
- Increase quantity of life by reducing premature death associated with obesity.
- Reduce disparities and social stigma related to obesity.
- Promote healthy behaviors for weight control and weight management. Prevent weight gain that may lead to or exacerbate obesity and its comorbidities.
- Educate public about health risks associated with obesity and its comorbidities.
- Increase access to appropriate medical evaluation and treatment of obesity.
- Improve health communication dealing with weight control between health professionals, managed care organizations and patients, and providers of weight control–related services and consumers.
- Form partnerships with organizations, businesses, and governmental health agencies (local, state, and federal) to improve data collection and increase research funding with regard to obesity.

Steps for Helping Clients Lose Weight

1. Measure height and weight to estimate body mass index.
2. Measure waist circumference.
3. Assess health history and potential risk factors or comorbidities.
4. Design a treatment plan.
5. Evaluate readiness, including reasons and motivation for weight loss, previous attempts at weight loss, support expected from family and friends, understanding of risks and benefits, attitudes toward physical activity, time constraints, and potential barriers to the patient's adoption of change. Assessment of the individual's readiness to change stage will be most important in the initial visit (Snetselaar, 2000).
6. Select a diet plan or the nondiet approach. Diets containing less than 1800 kcal for men and 1500 kcal for women should provide a daily multivitamin-mineral supplement. Flexible and creative ways of staying in touch with participants are essential for maintaining weight loss. The Mayo Clinic Healthy Weight Pyramid is a useful tool; it suggests unlimited use of fruits and vegetables; 4–8 servings of grains; 3–7 servings of lean meat, fish, beans, and low-fat dairy; 3–5 servings of nuts, canola or olive oil, or avocados; and up to 75 kcal from candy and other processed sweets.
7. Discuss a physical activity goal. Use the Guide to Physical Activity or other tools to help the client select desirable activities that can be maintained.
8. Review the Weekly Food and Activity Diary. Maintaining food and activity records are very helpful for persons trying to lose weight and keep it off.
9. Give the patient copies of the dietary information. Discuss food eaten away from home. Increased intake of food away from home, especially fast food, often contributes to the increasing prevalence of obesity (Binkley et al, 2000).
10. Enter the patient's information and the targeted goals in weight and goal records at each visit.
11. Encourage other health care providers to talk about weight management with their clients. Health care providers rarely advise patients to lose weight when they are just overweight (Sciamanna et al, 2000).
12. Include discussions about psychological well-being, especially feelings about food and body image (Chapman et al, 2005). Set achievable goals (Nonas and Foster, 2005). Individualized approaches to goal setting, information gathering, and giving advice are key factors in success (Chapman et al, 2005).
13. A behaviorally focused intervention can improve overall diet quality, especially if delivered through small group meetings (Carpenter et al, 2004).

TABLE 10-11 Portion Adjustments Using Everyday Objects

Bread, Cereal, Rice, Pasta

1 cup potatoes, rice, or pasta = 1 tennis ball or 1 ice cream scoop or a fist

1 pancake = 1 compact disc (CD)

½ cup cooked rice = a cupcake wrapper full

1 piece cornbread = bar of soap

1 slice bread = audiocassette tape

2 oz of pretzels = 2 handfuls

Vegetables

1 cup green salad = 1 baseball or a fist

1 baked potato = a fist

1 cup of vegetables = a fist

½ cup tomato juice = small Styrofoam cup

½ cup broccoli = 1 scoop ice cream or one light bulb

½ cup serving = 6 asparagus spears, 7–8 baby carrots, or 1 ear of corn on the cob

Fruit

½ cup grapes (15) = a light bulb

½ cup fresh fruit = 7 cotton balls

1 medium size fruit = a tennis ball or a fist

1 cup cut-up fruit = a fist

½ cup raisins = 1 large egg

Milk, Yogurt, Cheese

1½ oz cheese = one 9-volt battery or 3 dominos

1 oz cheese = pair of dice or your thumb

1 cup ice cream = 1 large scoop the size of a baseball

Meat, Poultry, Fish, Dry Beans, Eggs, Nuts

2 tbsp peanut butter = ping pong ball

1 tsp peanut butter = fingertip

1 tbsp peanut butter = thumb tip

3 oz cooked meat, poultry, fish = your palm; a deck of cards

3 oz grilled or baked fish = a checkbook

3 oz cooked chicken = one chicken leg, thigh, or breast

1 oz of nuts = 1 handful

1 oz of cheese = your index finger

Fats, Oils

1 tsp butter or margarine = size of a stamp, the thickness of your finger or thumb tip

2 tbsp salad dressing = 1 ping pong ball

Adapted from: Oregon State University Extension; used with permission.

TABLE 10-12 Physical Activity Equivalents

People who have lost weight and kept it off limit their intake to about 1800 kcal daily and walk about 4 miles a day (National Weight Control Registry). Other beneficial activities that burn kcal include the following:

Warm Weather	Calories/hour	Cold Weather
Jogging 6 mph	450	Jumping rope
Hiking on steep hills	400	Indoor rappelling
Aerobics (low impact)	400	Snow shoveling, light
Rowing	400	Rowing machine
Swimming	400	Skiing cross-country
Tennis, singles	390	Racquetball
Cycling 10 mph	300	Stationary bike 10 mph
Golf with walking	300	Splitting logs
Gardening	280	Window cleaning
Mowing lawn	275	Mopping floors
Tennis, doubles	235	Indoor basketball
Badminton	250	Indoor volleyball
Walking 3 mph	250	Mall walking

TABLE 10-13 Weight Management for Sleep Apnea and Pickwickian Syndrome

Obstructive sleep apnea (OSA) is characterized by short-duration (<1 minute), repetitive episodes of impaired breathing during sleep. It occurs in 3% of adults in the United States, 70% of whom are obese, which contributes to pharyngeal obstruction. OSA acutely impacts the cardiovascular system (Caples et al, 2005). Cardiovascular morbidity or mortality may be increased. Continuous positive airway pressure (CPAP) is a primary treatment used at night to keep the pharynx from collapsing. Morbid obesity can be associated with excessive daytime sleepiness even in the absence of sleep apnea (Resta et al, 2001). More details can be found in Section 5.

A patient with **Pickwickian syndrome** (obesity-hypoventilation) is obese and hypersomnolent with cor pulmonale, polycythemia, nocturnal enuresis, and personality changes. Even mild obesity can affect lung function, especially in men. Weight loss can decrease symptoms and is a desired intervention.

TABLE 10-14 Weight Control and Smoking Cessation

Nicotine addiction is a chronic relapsing condition that is difficult to treat (Jorenby, 2002). Smoking is often associated with higher energy, fat, and ethanol intakes. Past smokers are more likely to be obese than current smokers. Smoking cessation can lead to weight gain because of increased caloric consumption and changes in activity levels. Smoking increases the basal metabolic rate, so when smoking is stopped, the basal metabolic rate decreases, making weight loss more difficult.

High frequency of weight gain among adults who quit smoking demonstrates the need for interventions that address weight control. Moderate to heavy smokers who attempt to quit may need to reduce intake by 100–200 kcal/d just to maintain weight. Fruit often helps relieve the craving for sweets. Behavioral weight control counseling helps to slow the rate of weight gain after smoking cessation (Spring et al, 2004).

Smoking cessation lowers cardiovascular and cancer risks even when compensating for possible weight gain. Among both boys and girls, contemplation of and experimentation with smoking is often related to weight concerns. Women who quit smoking typically gain 6–12 lb in the first year after quitting; they fear weight gain more than men.

Sustained-release bupropion (bupropion SR) was the first nonnicotine pharmacological treatment approved for smoking cessation (Jorenby, 2002). Smoking cessation lengthens life by several years and is worth the effort.

TABLE 10-15 Fad Diets and Diet Programs: How They Compare

Eating Plan	Premise	Author's Background	Dietary Recommendations	Caloric Guidelines	Low/Missing Nutrients	Negative Health Implications	Scientific Evidence
Atkins Diet	A throwback to the 70's high-protein, low-carbohydrate (CHO) diets. Says CHOs make you fat. Claims diet works fast and keeps you satisfied.	Dr. Atkins was a medical doctor; no formal training in nutrition.	As much meat and fat as you want.	800 kcal	CHO, vitamins, minerals, fiber	May increase risk for heart disease and puts added work on the kidneys. May also experience fatigue, weakness, and irritability due to caloric restriction.	It has not been proven scientifically and is supported by testimonials.
Eat for Your Blood Type	Claims that people absorb nutrients and "react" to foods differently depending on blood type, which is based on our prehistoric ancestors.	Peter D'Adamo is a naturopathic physician.	Type O = eat mostly meats; type A = eat mostly fruits, vegetables, and grains; type B = eat oat and rice flours, bananas, and other prescribed foods; type AB = eat foods like tofu, sardines, oats, and rice.	1200 kcal or less	Depending on blood type, whole food groups are eliminate; vitamins; minerals	By eliminating entire food groups, some essential nutrients are deficient or absent.	No scientific evidence for using blood type as an eating guide to lose weight. No data showing that prehistoric people with any particular blood type ate this way.
Protein Power	A high-protein, low-CHO diet; the book claims the body has no need for CHO, and therefore, they should be avoided.	Authors Michael and Mary Eades are medical doctors with no formal training in nutrition.	30–50% fat, 30–45% protein, 15–35% CHO.	No guidelines are provided, but they warn against eating less than 850–1000 kcal/d.	CHO, vitamins, minerals, fiber	May add stress to kidneys and increase risk for heart disease. May also experience fatigue, weakness, and irritability.	Claims success through testimonials and book sales.
South Beach Diet	Uses the glycemic index to identify good versus bad CHO. Restricts CHO intake to "cure cravings" and promotes weight loss.	Dr. Agatston is a cardiologist.	Modified CHO diet	1200 kcal; too severe for most men and women	Many fruits and vegetables are eliminated as "bad" choices.	It emphasizes a higher intake of animal protein and saturated fat by reducing CHO. Risky for heart patients and those who may be prone to heart disease; risky for persons with chronic renal disease.	It does encourage fruits, vegetables, legumes, and whole-wheat breads and brown rice, which are better for weight loss and health. Lowering of triglycerides and weight loss can be better than from Atkins.

(continued)

TABLE 10-15 Fad Diets and Diet Programs: How They Compare *(continued)*

Eating Plan	Premise	Author's Background	Dietary Recommendations	Caloric Guidelines	Low/Missing Nutrients	Negative Health Implications	Scientific Evidence
Sugar Busters!	Recommends no sugar in the diet. The authors say sugar is toxic to the body, causing it to release insulin and store excess sugar as body fat.	The authors are a corporate CEO and 3 medical doctors.	No firm guidelines. Advises against CHO, especially simple/refined CHO (which would eliminate some grains, fruits, and vegetables). Focuses more on protein and fat.	800–1200 kcal	CHO, vitamins, minerals, fiber	Long-term effects may include increased risk for heart disease and kidney and liver damage; short-term effects may include fatigue, weakness, and irritability.	Testimonial claims support it. Evidence is based on opinions, and not on proven scientific facts.
Zone Diet	Claims CHOs make you fat. It says most of our bodies overproduce insulin when we eat CHO. Does promote exercise.	Author Barry Sears has a Ph.D. in biochemistry and no formal training in nutrition.	40% CHO, 30% protein, 30% fat	800–1200 kcal; restricts foods that have a high glycemic index	CHO, vitamins, minerals, fiber	Takes pleasure out of eating by regarding food as a medicine prescription. Also, may experience fatigue, weakness, and irritability.	It has not been proven scientifically and is supported by testimonials and poorly conducted studies.

Other Diet Programs	Description	Web Address	Pros/Cons
Diet Center	Personal counseling	http://www.dietcenter.com	Consider "Exclusively You" option
eDiets.com	Online dieting	http://www.ediets.com	Bargain; self-motivation needed
Jenny Craig	Personal counseling; at home	http://www.jennycraig.com	Expensive but well structured
LA Weight Loss	Personal counseling	http://www.laweightloss.com	Good exercise centers; costly foods
NutriSystem	Online dieting	http://www.nutrisystem.com	Healthy choices; good structure
Overeaters Anon	Group support	http://www.oa.org	Physical, emotional, spiritual support
Registered Dietitian	Expert personal counseling	http://www.eatright.org	Most flexible; personalized concerns
Take Off Pounds Sensibly	Group or online support	http://www.tops.org	Inexpensive but not personalized
Weight Watchers	Group or online support	http://www.weightwatchers.com	Comprehensive and sound principles

Adapted from: Wheat Food Council and Washington State Dairy Council and Environmental Nutrition; used with permission.
Note. Low-carbohydrate diets are based on an alternative theory of obesity where dietary carbohydrate (particularly unprocessed sugars) causes hyperinsulinemia, leading to insulin resistance, obesity, and cardiovascular disease, but there is no evidence for their physiological claims (Kushner, 2005).

- Dads and Daughters
  http://www.dadsanddaughters.org/
- DASH Diet in Weight Management
  http://www.nhlbi.nih.gov/hbp/prevent/h_weight/h_weight.htm
- Genome Studies of Obesity
  http://www.ncbi.nlm.nih.gov/disease/Obesity.html
- Hugs, International
  http://www.hugs.com/
- Largesse: The Network for Size Esteem
  http://www.uwyo.edu/winwyoming/guiding_principles.htm
- Meridia (Abbott)
  http://www.meridia.net/
- National Association to Advance Fat Acceptance (NAAFA)
  http://www.naafa.org/
- National Heart, Lung, and Blood Institute (NHLBI) Cholesterol and Metabolic Syndrome Guidelines
  http://www.nhlbi.nih.gov/guidelines/cholesterol/index.htm
- National Weight Control Registry
  http://www.nwcr.ws/
- NHLBI Obesity Education Initiative and Evidence Guidelines
  http://www.nhlbi.nih.gov
  http://www.nhlbi.nih.gov/guidelines/obesity/ob_gdlns.htm
- Partners in Nutrition, LLC
  http://www.partnersinnutrition.com/sportsnutrition.html
- Penn Medicine
  http://www.med.upenn.edu/weight/foster.shtml
- Recovery from Eating Disorders
  http://www.soberrecovery.com/links/eatingdisordertreatment.html

- RE-AIM Research on Efficacy
  http://www.re-aim.org/2003/researchers/efficacy_res.html
- Shape Up America
  http://www.shapeup.org/
- Something Fishy
  http://www.something-fishy.org
- Surgeon General
  http://www.surgeongeneral.gov/topics/obesity/
- Weight Watchers International
  http://www.weightwatchers.com/
- Win Wyoming
  http://www.uwyo.edu/winwyoming/guiding_principles.htm
- Women's Sports Foundation
  www.womenssportsfoundation.org
- Xenical—Roche Laboratories
  http://www.xenical.com/

OVERWEIGHT AND OBESITY—CITED REFERENCES

Allgood G, et al. Postmarketing surveillance of new food ingredients: results from the program with the fat replacer olestra. *Regul Toxicol Pharmacol.* 33:224, 2001.

Allison KC, et al. *Overcoming night-eating syndrome.* Oakland, CA: New Harbinger Publications, Inc., 2004.

American Dietetic Association. Position of the American Dietetic Association: fat replacers. *J Am Diet Assoc.* 105:266, 2005.

American Dietetic Association. Position of the American Dietetic Association: total diet approach to communicating food and nutrition information. *J Am Diet Assoc.* 102:100, 2002.

Aronoff N, et al. Gender and body mass index as related to night eating syndrome in obese patients. *J Am Diet Assoc.* 101:102, 2001.

Bacon L, et al. Size acceptance and intuitive eating improve health for obese, female chronic dieters. *J Am Diet Assoc.* 105:929, 2005.

Barton BA, et al. The relationship of breakfast and cereal consumption to nutrient intake and body mass index: the National Heart, Lung, and Blood Institute Growth and Health Study. *J Am Diet Assoc.* 105:1383, 2005.

Berkel LA, et al. Behavioral interventions for obesity. *J Am Diet Assoc.* 105: 35S, 2005.

Binkley JK, et al. The relation between dietary change and rising U.S. obesity. *Int J Obes Relat Metab Disord.* 24:1032, 2000.

Birketvedt G, et al. Behavioral and neuroendocrine characteristics of the night-eating syndrome. *J Am Med Assoc.* 282:657, 1999.

Blackburn GL, Waltman BA. Expanding the limits of treatment—new strategic initiatives. *J Am Diet Assoc.* 105:131S, 2005.

Bolumar F, et al. Body mass index and delayed conception: a European multicenter study on infertility and subfecundity. *Am J Epidemiol.* 151:1072, 2000.

Booth KM, et al. Obesity and the built environment. *J Am Diet Assoc.* 105:110S, 2005.

Bray GA, Champagne CM. Beyond energy balance: there is more to obesity than kilocalories. *J Am Diet Assoc.* 105:17S, 2005.

Breen HB, Ireton-Jones CS. Predicting energy needs in obese patients. *Nutr Clin Pract.* 19:284, 2004.

Caples SM, et al. Cardiopulmonary consequences of obstructive sleep apnea. *Semin Respir Crit Care Med.* 26:25, 2005.

Carpenter RA, et al. Pilot test of a behavioral skill building intervention to improve overall diet quality. *J Nutr Educ Behav.* 36:20, 2004.

Chapman GE, et al. Canadian dietitians' approaches to counseling adult clients seeking weight-management advice. *J Am Diet Assoc.* 105:1275, 2005.

Corella D, et al. Obese subjects carrying the 11482G>A polymorphism at the perilipin locus are resistant to weight loss following dietary energy restriction. *J Clin Endocrinol Metab.* 90:5121, 2005.

Dickerson RN. Specialized nutrition support in the hospitalized obese patient. *Nutr Clin Pract.* 19:245, 2004.

Dickerson RN, Roth-Yousey L. Medication effects on metabolic rate: a systematic review (part 1). *J Am Diet Assoc.* 105:835, 2005a.

Dickerson RN, Roth-Yousey L. Medication effects on metabolic rate: a systematic review (part 2). *J Am Diet Assoc.* 105:835, 2005b.

Dwyer JT, et al. Dietary supplements in weight reduction. *J Am Diet Assoc.* 105:S80, 2005.

Estabrooks PA, et al. Physical activity promotion through primary care. *JAMA.* 289:2913, 2003.

Ferko-Adams D. *A dietitian's guide to corporate health promotion.* Nazareth, PA: Wellness Press, 2005.

Finer N, et al. One-year treatment of obesity: a randomized, double-blind, placebo controlled, multicenter study of orlistat, a gastrointestinal lipase. *Int J Obes Relat Metab Disord.* 24:306, 2000.

Folsom A, et al. Associations of general and abdominal obesity with multiple health outcomes in older women: the Iowa Women's Health Study. *Arch Int Med.* 160:2117, 2000.

Foster GD, Nonas CA. *Managing obesity: a clinical guide.* Chicago: American Dietetic Association, 2004.

Greenway F. Another type of intervention: treating obesity with medication. *J Am Diet Assoc.* 105:895, 2005.

Guagnano M, et al. Risk factors for hypertension in obese women: the role of weight cycling. *Euro J Clin Nutr.* 54:356, 2000.

Heptulla R, et al. Temporal patterns of circulating leptin levels in lean and obese adolescents: relationships to insulin, growth hormone, and free fatty acids rhythmicity. *J Clin Endocrinol Metab.* 86:90, 2001.

Hill JO, et al. Weight maintenance: what's missing? *J Am Diet Assoc.* 105:63S, 2005.

Jorenby D. Clinical efficacy of bupropion in the management of smoking cessation. *Drugs* 62:25S, 2002.

Katzmarzyk PT, Davis C. Thinness and body shape of Playboy centerfolds from 1978 to 1998. *Int J Obes Relat Metab Disord.* 25:590, 2001.

Khaodhiar L, et al. Serum levels of interleukin-6 and C-reactive protein correlate with body mass index across the broad range of obesity. *J Parenter Enteral Nutr.* 28:410, 2004.

Kushner RF. Low-carbohydrate diets, con: the mythical phoenix or credible science? *Nutr Clin Pract.* 20:13, 2005.

Kushner RF, Blatner DJ. Risk assessment of the overweight and obese patient. *J Am Diet Assoc.* 105:53S, 2005.

McArthur L, Howard A. Dietetics majors' weight reduction beliefs, behaviors, and information sources. *J Am Coll Health.* 49:175, 2001.

Morelli V, Zoorob R. Alternative therapies: part 1. Depression, diabetes, obesity. *Am Fam Physician.* 62:1051, 2000.

Moyers SB. Medications as adjunct therapy for weight loss: approved and off-label agents in use. *J Am Diet Assoc.* 105:948, 2005.

Nagao T, et al. Ingestion of a tea rich in catechins leads to a reduction in body fat and malondialdehyde-modified LDL in men. *Am J Clin Nutr.* 81:122, 2005.

National Heart, Lung, and Blood Institute (NHLBI). Clinical Guidelines on the Identification, Evaluation, and Treatment of Overweight and Obesity in Adults–Executive Summary. Accessed August 8, 2005 at http://www.nhlbi.nih.gov/guidelines/obesity/sum_rec.htm.

National Heart, Blood, and Lung Institute (NHBLI). Healthy People 2010. Accessed in 2005 at http://hp2010.nhlbihin.net/.

Nickols-Richardson SM, et al. Perceived hunger is lower and weight loss is greater in overweight premenopausal women consuming a low-carbohydrate/high-protein vs high-carbohydrate/low-fat diet. *J Am Diet Assoc.* 105:1433, 2005.

Nonas CA, Foster GD. Setting achievable goals for weight loss. *J Am Diet Assoc.* 105:118S, 2005.

O'Reardon JP, et al. Clinical trial of sertraline in the treatment of night eating syndrome. *Int J Eat Disord.* 35:16, 2004.

Orr J, Davy B. Dietary influences on peripheral hormones regulating energy intake: potential applications for weight management. *J Am Diet Assoc.* 105:1115, 2005.

Patterson R. Changes in diet, weight, and serum lipid levels associated with Olestra consumption. *Arch Intern Med.* 160:2600, 2000.

Pi-Sunyer X, Kris-Etherton PM. Improving health outcomes: future directions in the field. *J Am Diet Assoc.* 105:14S, 2005.

Pittas AG, et al. A low-glycemic load diet facilitates greater weight loss in overweight adults with high insulin secretion but not in overweight adults with low insulin secretion in the CALERIE Trial. *Diabetes Care* 28:2939, 2005.

Resta O, et al. Sleep-related breathing disorders, loud snoring and excessive daytime sleepiness in obese subjects. *Int J Obes Relat Metab Disord.* 25:669, 2001.

Rolls BJ, et al. Changing the energy density of the diet as a strategy for weight management. *J Am Diet Assoc.* 105:98S, 2005.

Schoeller DA, Buchholz AC. Energetics of obesity and weight control: does diet composition matter? *J Am Diet Assoc.* 105:24S, 2005.

Sciamanna C, et al. Who reports receiving advice to lose weight? *Arch Intern Med.* 160:2334, 2000.

Snetselaar L. Counseling for change. In: Mahan K, Escott-Stump S, eds. *Krause's food, nutrition, and diet therapy.* 10th ed. Philadelphia: WB Saunders, 2000.

Song WO, et al. Is consumption of breakfast associated with body mass index in US adults? *J Am Diet Assoc.* 105:1373, 2005.

Spiegel K, et al. Brief communication: sleep curtailment in healthy young men is associated with decreased leptin levels, elevated ghrelin levels and increased hunger and appetite. *Ann Intern Med.* 14:846, 2004.

Spring B, et al. Randomized controlled trial for behavioral smoking and weight control treatment: effect of concurrent versus sequential intervention. *J Consult Clin Psychol.* 72:785, 2004.

Stern JS, et al. Future and implications of reimbursement for obesity treatment. *J Am Diet Assoc.* 105:104S, 2005.

Stunkard AJ, Allison KC. Two forms of disordered eating in obesity: binge eating and night eating. *Int J Obes Relat Metab Disord.* 27:1, 2003.
Venti CA, et al. Lack of relationship between calcium intake and body size in an obesity-prone population. *J Am Diet Assoc.* 105:1401, 2005.
Wamsteker EW, et al. Obesity-related beliefs predict weight loss after an 8-week low-calorie diet. *J Am Diet Assoc.* 105:441, 2005.
Zemel MB. Regulation of adiposity and obesity risk by dietary calcium: mechanisms and implications. *J Am Coll Nutr.* 21:146S, 2002.

UNDERWEIGHT AND PROTEIN–CALORIE MALNUTRITION

UNDERWEIGHT AND UNINTENTIONAL WEIGHT LOSS

NUTRITIONAL ACUITY RANKING: LEVEL 3–4

DEFINITIONS AND BACKGROUND

Being underweight is defined as having a BMI below 18.5; about 8–9% of the population is underweight. Weight gain may be difficult for some healthy individuals because of genetic tendency toward leanness, excessive activity, or usual eating patterns. Being underweight may or may not be associated with pathology. There are serious health risks associated with low weight and efforts to maintain an unrealistically lean body mass (Strawbridge et al, 2000). Identification and treatment of any related disordered eating can be important for improving the health status of underweight individuals at any age. See Section 4 for eating disorder guidelines.

Body storage of glycogen is approximately 1100 kcal or about a 12- to 16-hour supply. Body storage of protein equals about 40,000 kcal of muscle tissue; loss of 30–50% of lean body mass is incompatible with survival. Body fat is the remainder of calories in fuel storage; it varies depending on the weight of the individual compared with BMI tables for height and sex and by level of physical fitness. The Ancel Keys studies (Keys et al, 1950) demonstrated that starvation results in food preoccupation, unusual eating habits, increased use of caffeine and tea, binge eating, depression, anxiety, social withdrawal, poor judgment, apathy, egocentrism, edema, sleep disturbances, hypothermia, gastrointestinal (GI) disturbances, and lowered basal metabolism. Death related to starvation is often from decreased respiratory muscle function and terminal pneumonia. In addition, patients who have chronic obstructive pulmonary disease (COPD) are more likely to have additional exacerbations when weight loss and poor intake occur (Hallin et al, 2006).

Low BMI is a significant predictor of mortality among young as well as older hospitalized patients (Flegal et al, 2005; Sergi et al, 2005; Landi et al, 2000). A BMI value of 20 kg/m^2 seems to be a reliable threshold for defining underweight in older adults at high risk for short-term mortality (Sergi et al, 2005). The Women's Health Initiative Observational Study evaluated 40,657 women aged 65–79 years at baseline and measured frailty including muscle weakness, impaired walking, exhaustion, low physical activity, and unintended weight loss; death, hip fractures, activities of daily living disability, and hospitalizations were also tracked (Fugate Woods et al, 2005). This study found that underweight is related to frailty and poor outcomes, along with smoking and depression.

Debility, cachexia with unintentional weight loss and loss of lean body mass, implies some undesirable condition or pathology, especially among chronically ill or institutionalized individuals. Malnutrition in older adults is characterized by faulty or inadequate nutritional status, undernourishment with insufficient dietary intake, poor appetite, muscle wasting, and weight loss (Chen et al, 2001).

Blunted responsiveness to neuropeptide Y (NPY), a feeding stimulant, occurs concurrently with age-related anorexia and hypophagia (Pu et al, 2000). In addition, special populations at risk for weight loss and poor intake should be monitored; for instance, persons with chronic renal insufficiency may be at risk (Shlipak et al, 2004).

Nutritional frailty includes sarcopenia (Bales and Ritchie, 2002), and this leads to failure to thrive and functional disability. Cytokines contribute to lipolysis, anorexia, muscle protein breakdown, and nitrogen loss (Bales and Ritchie, 2002). Patients with cardiac cachexia or COPD are often debilitated if they have lost weight fairly rapidly. In older adults, micronutrient deficiency is a common result and should be addressed. Table 10-16 provides tips for helping debilitated persons strengthen their muscles.

It is appropriate to carefully monitor unintentional weight loss in adults following their admission into residential health care facilities using medical nutrition therapy (MNT) protocols that emphasize thorough assessment; interventions including weighing frequency; communication

TABLE 10-16 National Institute on Aging: Strengthening Tips

Patients with wasting conditions who can and will comply with a proper exercise program gain muscle protein mass, strength, and endurance and are often more capable of performing activities of daily living (Zinna and Yarasheski, 2003).

1. Start with a weight that can be lifted 5 times without too much effort.
2. When that is easy, rest a few minutes, and do it again (2 sets).
3. Increase to 3 sets.
4. Lift weight 10 times in each set.
5. Lift weight 15 times in each set.
6. Slowly increase weight and sets.

Source: National Institute on Aging. Exercise: a guide from the National Institute on Aging. Available at http://www.niapublications.org/exercisebook/ExerciseGuideComplete.pdf#search='Exercise%3A%20A%20Guide%20from%20the%20National%20Institute%20on%20Aging'; phone: 1-800-222-2225.

with staff, medical doctor, family, and resident; and reassessment (Splett et al, 2003). The American Dietetic Association has recommended at least three MNT visits for adults who have had unintentional weight loss.

INTERVENTION: OBJECTIVES

- Increase body weight gradually if desired or indicated.
- Encourage weight gain of approximately 1 lb weekly.
- In the case of recent acute illness or general chronic disease, provide diet as tolerated to improve nutritional status. Progress slowly; it may take several days to stimulate the patient's appetite.
- If confusion is present, dehydration may be a factor. Evaluate hydration status carefully and rehydrate if appropriate.
- Try anabolic agents, exercise/physical activity, and cytokine inhibition (Wallace and Schwartz, 2002).

INTERVENTION: FOOD AND NUTRITION

- Calculate patient's goal weight: basal energy requirements plus kilocalories according to activity or stress factors. See Table 10-1.
- Each pound of fat requires 3500 kcal; therefore, diet should be increased by 500 kcal/d to promote a weight gain of 1 lb/wk. Use a high-protein and high-energy diet with frequent feedings. The diet should provide adequate micronutrients, or a supplement may be beneficial.
- Plan meals and snacks according to appetite and preferences; encourage a small snack about every 2–3 hours. Patients who have cancer or other chronic illnesses may not want to eat large meals.
- Provide enteral feeding if needed and appropriate.

CLINICAL INDICATORS

Clinical/History

Height
Weight
Usual weight
Recent weight changes
BMI
Desirable BMI
Diet history
BP
Intake and output (I & O)
Triceps skinfold (TSF)
Midarm circumference (MAC)
Midarm muscle circumference (MAMC)
Exercise tolerance

Lab Work

Hemoglobin and hematocrit (H & H)
Serum ferritin, if anemia is suspected
CRP (elevated?)
Albumin (Alb), transthyretin
Chol (may be low)
Trig
Blood urea nitrogen (BUN)
Creatinine (Creat)
Nitrogen (N) balance
Na+, K+
Alkaline phosphatase (Alk phos)
Ca++, Mg++

SAMPLE NUTRITION DIAGNOSTIC STATEMENT

Underweight

PES: Inadequate nutrient intake related to mismatch of energy intake and expenditure as evidenced by 6-lb loss in 1 month with no change in oral intake.

Assessment Data: Diet, weight, and physical activity histories.

Intervention: Address appropriate matching of energy intake and physical activity.

Monitoring and Evaluation: Ask patient to return in 2 weeks, to assess weight and review diet and activity logs.

Common Drugs Used and Potential Side Effects

- Appetite may be stimulated through use of medications such as oxandrolone, but not everyone responds positively with an increased appetite and weight gain.
- Antidepressants may be warranted when a qualified professional has documented depression. Monitor for dry mouth and other side effects specific to ordered medication.

Herbs, Botanicals, and Supplements

- Herbs and botanical supplements should not be used without discussing with physician.

INTERVENTION: NUTRITION EDUCATION, COUNSELING, CARE MANAGEMENT

- Help patient make meals in a simple manner, using attractive foods.
- Identify spices, seasonings, and other flavor enhancements to stimulate the senses.
- Use of high–caloric density foods may be useful in programs where the patient refuses to eat or to take supplements. Adding or "hiding" calories and extra protein in food also may be feasible (e.g., use of dry milk powder in soups or mashed potatoes).
- Offer tips on weight gain such as eating a small snack every 2–3 hours. A high-calorie bedtime snack is often beneficial (for example, a milkshake or sandwich).
- Malnutrition often presents with loss, loneliness, dependency, and chronic illness, and it impacts morbidity, mortality, and quality of life (Chen et al, 2001). Assist with referrals, such as home-delivered meals.
- Promote lean body mass development through strength training where appropriate (see Table 10-16). Increased physical activity appropriate for the clinical condition can help to improve appetite and intake in many cases. Exercise training has been successful for the treatment of wasting associated with sarcopenia, cancer, chronic renal insufficiency, rheumatoid arthritis, osteoarthritis, and human immunodeficiency virus (HIV) (Zinna and Yarasheski, 2003).

For More Information

- American Dietetic Association–Unintentional Weight Loss Prevention Protocol
  http://www.eatright.org

UNDERWEIGHT AND UNINTENTIONAL WEIGHT LOSS—CITED REFERENCES

Bales CW, Ritchie CS. Sarcopenia, weight loss and nutritional frailty in the elderly. *Annu Rev Nutr* 22:309, 2002.

Chen CCH, et al. A concept analysis of malnutrition in the elderly. *J Adv Nurs.* 36:131, 2001.

Flegal KM, et al. Excess deaths associated with underweight, overweight, and obesity. *JAMA.* 293:1861, 2005.

Fugate Woods N, et al. Frailty: emergence and consequences in women aged 65 and older in the Women's Health Initiative Observational Study. *J Am Geriat Soc.* 53:1321, 2005.

Hallin R, et al. Nutritional status, dietary energy intake and the risk of exacerbations in patients with chronic obstructive pulmonary disease (COPD). *Respir Med.* 100:561, 2006.

Keys A, et al. *The biology of human starvation.* Vol. 1. Minneapolis: University of Minnesota Press, 1950.

Landi F, et al. Body mass index and mortality among hospitalized patients. *Arch Intern Med.* 160:2641, 2000.

Pu S, et al. Neuropeptide Y counteracts the anorectic and weight reducing effects of ciliary neurotropic factor. *J Neuroendocrinol.* 12:827, 2000.

Sergi G, et al. An adequate threshold for body mass index to detect underweight condition in elderly persons: The Italian Longitudinal Study on Aging (ILSA). *J Gerontol A Biol Sci Med Sci.* 60:866, 2005.

Shlipak MG, et al. The presence of frailty in elderly persons with chronic renal insufficiency. *Am J Kidney Dis.* 43:861, 2004.

Splett PL, et al. Medical nutrition therapy for the prevention and treatment of unintentional weight loss in residential healthcare facilities. *J Am Diet Assoc.* 103:352, 2003.

Strawbridge W, et al. New NHBI clinical guidelines for obesity and overweight: will they promote health? *Am J Pub Health.* 90:340, 2000.

Wallace, JI, Schwartz RS. Epidemiology of weight loss in humans with special reference to wasting in the elderly. *Int J Cardiol.* 85:15, 2002.

Zinna EM, Yarasheski KE. Exercise treatment to counteract protein wasting of chronic diseases. *Curr Opin Clin Nutr Metab Care.* 6:87, 2003.

PROTEIN–CALORIE MALNUTRITION

NUTRITIONAL ACUITY RANKING: LEVEL 3–4

DEFINITIONS AND BACKGROUND

Protein–calorie malnutrition (PCM) decreases cardiac output, blood pressure, oxygen consumption, total lymphocyte count (TLC), number of T cells, and glomerular filtration rate (GFR). Malnutrition is associated with increased infection rates; incidence of emphysema, pneumonia, and anemia; GI tract atrophy; intestinal bacterial overgrowth; and hepatic mass losses (Table 10-17). Another name for PCM is protein–energy malnutrition (PEM), and the terms are used interchangeably. Physical assessment and thorough clinical history are essential in determining etiology and appropriate interventions.

PCM is the leading cause of death among children in developing countries. Clinically, in children, PCM has three forms: dry (thin, desiccated), wet (edematous, swollen), or a combination; grading is mild, moderate, or severe. Grade is determined by calculating weight as a percentage of expected weight for length using international standards (normal, 90–110%; mild PCM, 85–90%; moderate PCM, 75–85%; severe PCM, <75%). The dry form, **marasmus,** results from near starvation with deficiency of protein and nonprotein nutrients. The wet form is called **kwashiorkor,** an African word meaning "first child-second child," because the first child often develops PCM after the second child arrives and nutrient-poor foods replace breast milk. The combined form of PCM is called **marasmic kwashiorkor;** these children have some edema and more body fat than those with marasmus. See Figure 10-2.

In adult patients admitted for acute illnesses, the prevalence of PCM is high, especially related to age and metabolic stress (Martinez Olmos et al, 2005). Of patients admitted to hospitals, 35–55% are malnourished on admission; 25–30% more become malnourished during stay. PCM is common in gastrointestinal (GI) patients, especially patients with

TABLE 10-17 Complicating Effects of Chronic Protein–Calorie Malnutrition on Body Systems

Digestive Tract—Frequent, chronic, or even fatal diarrhea; bacterial translocation in gut; low HCl production in stomach; progressive weight loss; gastrointestinal (GI) mucosal or villi atrophy.

Nervous System—Irritability, weakness, and apathy even if intellect remains intact.

Muscular System—Decreased activity; delayed physical rehabilitation; decreased muscle size and strength; delayed hospital discharge and ability to perform work.

Skin and Skeleton—Pale, thin, dry inelastic skin; pressure ulcers; decreased subcutaneous fat; loss of bone density.

Immune System—Depressed cell-mediated immunity; increased infection, particularly gram-negative sepsis; impaired wound healing; more wound infections or disruption; impaired ability to fight infections; delayed response to cancer chemotherapy or radiation therapy.

Pulmonary System—Depressed ventilatory response to hypoxia; decreased lung capacity; slow breathing; pneumonia and eventually respiratory failure.

Cardiac and Hematological System—Anemia; altered clotting time; decreased heart size; decreased amount of blood pumped; slow heart rate; decreased blood pressure; heart failure; decreased number of blood cells.

Renal System—Fluid, electrolyte, and acid–base malfunctioning; increased frequency of urinary tract infections; elevated blood urea nitrogen from muscle and tissue breakdown; decreased glomerular filtration rate.

Endocrine System—Decreased body temperature (hypothermia); fluid accumulation in skin from lower subcutaneous fat and decreased albumin; vitamin and mineral deficiencies.

Reproductive System—Decreased size of ovaries or testes; decreased libido; cessation of menstruation.

Quality of Life—Increased and prolonged use of hospitals, critical care units, and expensive drugs; excessive requirements of hospital support.

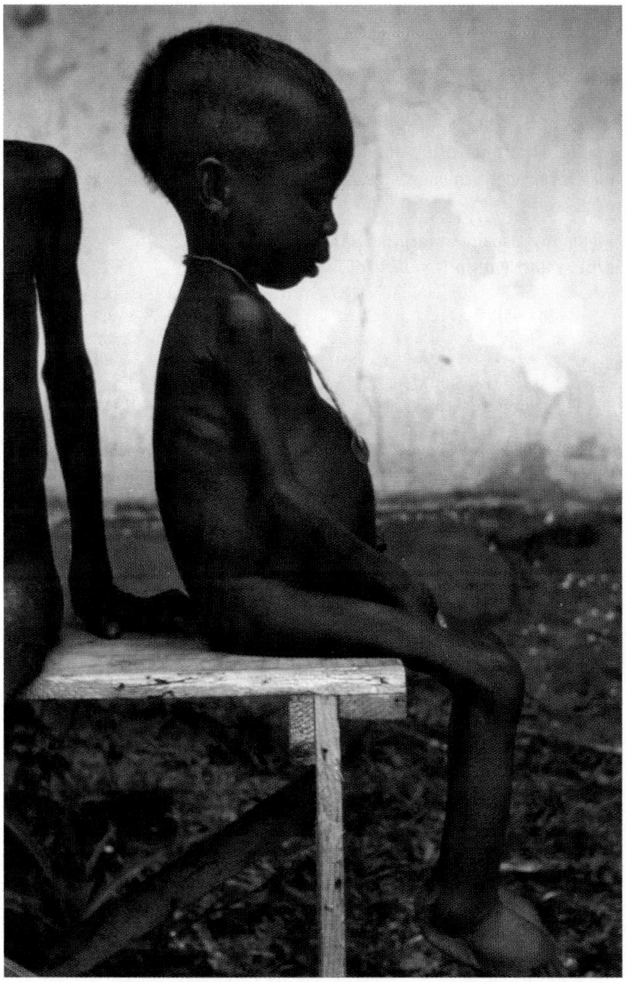
A

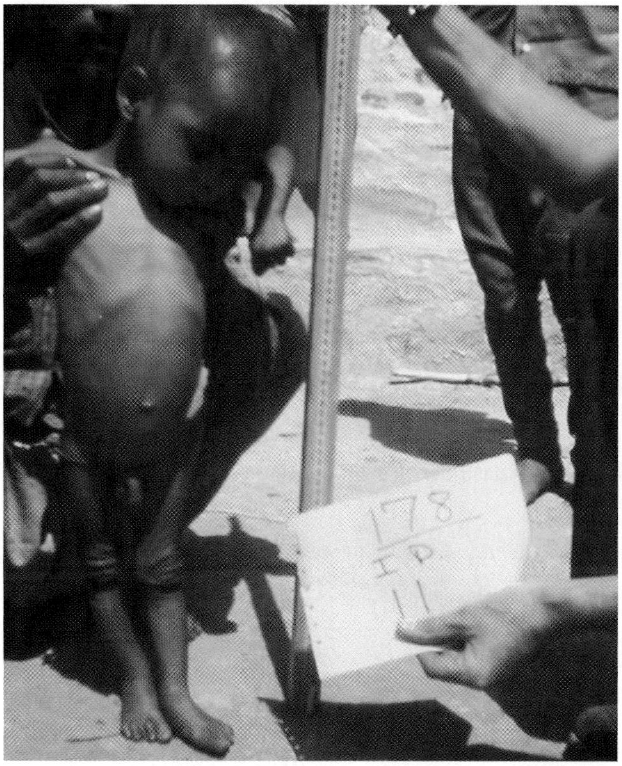

B

Figure 10-2 Children with **(A)** kwashiorkor and **(B)** marasmus. (Images courtesy of the Centers for Disease Control Image Library.)

inflammatory bowel disease (IBD); ventilator, radiation, or chemotherapy patients; burn and surgical patients; and patients with renal failure. Even with dialysis, renal patients are at high risk for PCM (Kopple, 2005). In fact, maintenance hemodialysis (MHD) patients often die within 5 years of commencing dialysis treatment, mostly from cardiovascular disease with markers of PCM and inflammation, the malnutrition–inflammation complex syndrome (Colman et al, 2005).

Tissue catabolism usually begins with lowered plasma proteins, red blood cells, and leukocytes; later, wasting of organs, skeletal muscle, bone, skin, and subcutaneous tissue will occur. Chronic undernutrition (protein and calories) and micronutrient deficiency (especially zinc) will compromise cytokine response and affect immune cell functioning; nutrients act as antioxidants and as cofactors in cytokine regulation (Cunningham-Rundles et al, 2005). The central nervous system is the last system to be catabolized, and magnetic resonance imaging (MRI) scans taken of children who have moderate to severe malnutrition show cerebral atrophy (Odabas et al, 2005). Total starvation is fatal in 8–12 weeks.

Certain types of surgery can lead to PCM if feeding is delayed. Pancreatic surgery is one specific example (Schnelldorfer and Adams, 2005). Other types of stress can be problematic as well. Because PCM and involuntary weight loss is a common problem in the older population, there is a significant increase in infection rate, a decrease in the rate of healing, and an increase in length of stay in older, malnourished burn patients when compared with those who are well nourished (Demling, 2005).

Subjective Global Assessment and other nutritional risk indices can be used to assess nutritional status. Common causes of malnutrition in the elderly involve decreased appetite, dependency on help for eating, impaired cognition and/or communication, poor positioning, frequent acute illnesses with GI losses, medications that decrease appetite or increase nutrient losses, polypharmacy, decreased thirst response, decreased ability to concentrate urine, intentional fluid restriction because of fear of incontinence or choking if dysphagic, psychosocial factors such as isolation and depression, monotony of diet, and higher nutrient density requirements, along with the demands of age, illness, and disease on the body (Harris and Fraser, 2004).

Poor nutritional state may be associated with an increase in postoperative complication rate; low serum albumin levels can be reflected by a higher rate of infectious complications as well as increased intensive care unit (ICU) stay (Schnelldorfer and Adams, 2005). It is helpful to use the designated International Classification of Diagnoses codes in the medical record so that proper care for malnutrition is given. Table 10-18 describes several types of undernutrition that are common in hospitals. Table 10-19 describes a malnutrition evaluation tool for scoring nutritional risks, the "MUST" tool.

TABLE 10-18 Protein–Calorie Malnutrition (PCM) Indicators

Condition	Patient Appearance	Protein Status[a]	Other Lab Values
Stress-Related Protein Malnutrition (ICD.9 code 260)	Patient appears well nourished or even overnourished. Weight may be >90% of standard for height. Triceps skinfold (TSF) and weight for height are often normal. Pitting edema leads to a "wet" PCM. Patient may have easily pluckable hair. This takes place over a few weeks to months.	Had recent stress with protein intake insufficient to maintain visceral stores. Albumin is usually lower than 3.0 g/dL, transthyretin is <17 g/dL.	Depressed cellular immunity also exists. Total lymphocyte count, blood urea nitrogen, and creatinine are low. Delayed wound healing.
Compensated Malnutrition (ICD.9 code 261)	Weight <80% of standard for height. Patient looks chronically starved. Decreased anthropometric values (midarm muscle circumference, TSF, etc.) are produced by chronically inadequate diets and a moderate catabolic illness. This is a "dry," dehydrated PCM in most cases. Absence of subcutaneous fat is common; TSF and weight for height are low. Muscle wasting. This occurs over months or years from low-calorie intake: 10% weight loss in 6 months; 7.5% loss in 3 months; 5% loss in 1 month; or 2% loss in 1 week can be an indicator.	May have normal albumin and transferrin levels. Serum albumin usually >3.0 g/dL.	Glucose and cholesterol may be low. Other labs will vary.

Note. Slow fetal growth and fetal malformation (ICD.9 code 764) and low birth weight due to short gestation (ICD.9 code 765) can be used to code malnutrition in the neonatal population.

[a] Be aware that serum albumin levels drop when there is inflammation; when inflammation is corrected, levels may rise again regardless of nutritional intake. Use albumin as a marker of severity of illness, not as a marker of protein nutriture.

INTERVENTION: OBJECTIVES

- Correct weight loss, weakness, apathy, infections, and poor wound healing.
- Provide adequate macronutrients and micronutrients.
- Avoid hazards of refeeding (hypophosphatemia and low magnesium and potassium). Fluid administration must be monitored carefully. Prevent sepsis, overfeeding, hyperglycemia, heart failure, or other organ failure by refeeding slowly.
- Correct complications, which can include dehydration, electrolyte imbalances, infections, vitamin-mineral deficiencies, and other biochemical changes (Table 10-20).
- Establish nutritional plan according to patient prognosis (Table 10-21).
- Allow normal growth of brain and prevent permanent IQ deficits in children.

INTERVENTION: FOOD AND NUTRITION

- Monitor physical exam and clinical status to determine needed dietary changes.
- **Mild PCM:** Provide sufficient calories and protein, gradually increasing to meet needs. Diet should provide adequate carbohydrate (CHO) and caloric intake to spare protein and correct weight loss. Use tube feeding (TF) or total parenteral nutrition (TPN), if appropriate (see Section 17). Vitamin-mineral supplementation is needed if diet or feeding does not provide all micronutrients.
- **Severe PCM with cachexia:** Start treatment with intravenous glucose. Gradually add lactose-treated milk and soft, easily tolerated solids. Provide high–biologic value proteins with sufficient calories adequate to use nitrogen effectively. Avoid overfeeding (use 20–25 kcal/kg,

TABLE 10-19 Malnutrition Universal Screening Tool (MUST)

MUST is a 5-step screening tool to identify adults who are malnourished, at risk of malnutrition (undernutrition), or obese. It also includes management guidelines that can be used to develop a care plan. It is used in hospitals and community care settings and other care settings and can be used by all care workers. It was established by the British Association for Enteral and Parenteral Nutrition (BASPEN). The guide contains:

- A flow chart showing 5 steps to use for screening and management
- BMI chart
- Weight loss tables
- Alternative measurements when BMI cannot be obtained by measuring weight and height

A more detailed MUST Explanatory Booklet should be used for procedures when weight and height cannot be measured and when screening with more interpretation is needed (e.g., those with fluid disturbances, plaster casts, amputations, or critical illness, or pregnant or lactating women). The 5 MUST Steps are as follows.

Step 1: Measure height and weight to get a BMI score using chart provided.

If height cannot be measured: use recently documented or self-reported height (if reliable and realistic). If the subject does not know or is unable to report their height, use one of the alternative measurements to estimate height (ulna, knee height, or arm span).

If height and weight cannot be obtained: use mid upper arm circumference (MUAC) measurement to estimate BMI category.

If BMI cannot be determined: use subjective clinical impression—thin, acceptable weight, overweight. Obvious wasting (very thin) and obesity (very overweight) can also be noted.

BMI	Score
>20 (>30 Obese)	= 0
18.5–20	= 1
<18.5	= 2
BMI score = ________	

Alternative procedures are available from the guide http://www.baspen.org.uk/the-must.htm.

Step 2: Note percentage of unplanned weight loss, and score using tables in the screening tool.

If recent weight loss cannot be calculated: use self-reported weight loss (if reliable and realistic).

Unplanned weight loss: clothes and/or jewelry have become loose fitting (weight loss); history of decreased food intake, reduced appetite or swallowing problems over 3–6 months; underlying disease or psychosocial/physical disabilities likely to cause weight loss.

Record presence of obesity. Control underlying conditions before treating obesity.

% of Unplanned weight loss in past 3–6 months	Score
<5%	= 0
5–10%	= 1
>10%	= 2
Weight loss score = __________	

Step 3: Establish acute disease effect and score.

No nutritional intake or likelihood of no intake for more than 5 days = score 2.

Acute disease effect score = ________

Step 4: Add scores from steps 1, 2, and 3 together to obtain overall risk of malnutrition.

0 = Low Risk

1 = Medium Risk

≥2 = High Risk

(continued)

TABLE 10-19 Malnutrition Universal Screening Tool (MUST) ***(continued)***

Step 5: Develop care plan and treat.

Observe and document dietary intake for 3 days if patient is in hospital or long-term care (LTC) facility.

If improved or adequate intake—little clinical concern.

If no improvement—clinical concern; follow local policy.

Repeat screening: Hospital, weekly; LTC facility, at least monthly; community, at least every 2–3 months.

Treat (unless detrimental or no benefit expected from nutritional support, e.g., imminent death):

Record need for special diets and follow local policy.

Record malnutrition risk category; as needed, refer to dietitian or nutritional support team or implement local policy.

Treat underlying condition and provide help and advice on food choices, eating, and drinking when necessary.

Improve and increase overall nutritional intake.

Monitor and review care plan: hospital, weekly; LTC facility, monthly; community, monthly.

TABLE 10-20 Selected Biochemical Changes Observed in Severe Protein–Calorie Malnutrition (PCM)

Body Composition	Energy Malnutrition	Protein Malnutrition/ Edema
Total body water	High	High
Extracellular water	High	Higher
Total body potassium	Low	Lower
Total body protein	Low	Low
Serum or plasma		
Transport proteins (transferrin, ceruloplasmin, retinol-, cortisol-, and thyroxine-binding proteins, beta-lipoproteins)[a]	Normal or low	Low
Enzymes such as amylase, alkaline phosphatase	Normal	Low
Transaminase	Normal or high	High
C-reactive protein	Varies by condition	Varies
Liver		
Glycogen	Normal or low	Normal or low
Urea cycle enzymes and other enzymes	Low	Lower
Amino acid synthesizing enzymes	High	Not as high

[a] Note. Inflammatory processes and their effects on hepatic protein metabolism (albumin, transferrin, and transthyretin) have been identified recently; serum hepatic protein levels correlate with *severity* of illness but do not accurately measure effectiveness of nutritional repletion (Fuhrman et al, 2004). Evaluate their value cautiously.

Data from: Torun B, Viteri F. Protein-energy malnutrition. In: Warren K, Mahmood A, eds. *Tropical and geographical medicine.* 2nd ed. New York: McGraw-Hill, 1990.

TABLE 10-21 Poor Prognosis in Protein–Calorie Malnutrition (PCM) and Consequences of Not Feeding a Patient

Clinical manifestations of PCM relate to length of time, extent of nutritional deprivation, and prior health status; there are serious detrimental effects on every organ. "When maintained on a prolonged semi-starvation diet, otherwise healthy individuals experience a **loss of heart tissue** that parallels their loss of body mass. Respiratory rate, vital capacity and minute volume of ventilation also decrease. These **changes in pulmonary function** are thought to result from reduced basal metabolic rate that accompanies starvation. In addition, **liver function declines, kidney filtration rates decline, and nearly every aspect of the immune system is compromised.** Defective ability to fight bacterial and viral infections occurs. Starvation therefore leads to **increased susceptibility to infection, delayed wound healing, reduced rate of drug metabolism, and impairment of both physical and cognitive function.** If starvation is prolonged, complications develop, **leading eventually to death**" (Sullivan, 1995).

Other consequences of not feeding an individual who *will not* or *cannot* eat orally in sufficient amounts include:

- Possibility of **dehydration** with increased risk of urinary tract infections, fever, swollen tongue, sunken eyeballs, decreased urine output, constipation, nausea and vomiting, decreased blood pressure, mental confusion, and electrolyte disturbances.
- **Decreased awareness** of environment from decreased glucose availability for the brain.
- **Development of new or additional pressure ulcers** over bony prominences from lack of sufficient protein, calorie, vitamin, and mineral intakes and decreased body fat.
- **Decreased ability to participate in activities of daily living** (self-feeding, dressing, bathing, toileting).
- **Low body weight or rapid, involuntary weight loss,** which are highly predictive of illness and imminent death. (Note: the elderly are especially unable to regain weight after a stress situation).

Poor prognosis with PCM may be seen among the following kinds of patients:

Age <6 months

Deficit in weight for height >30% or in weight for age >40%

Signs of circulatory collapse: cold hands and feet, weak radial pulse, diminished consciousness

Stupor, coma, or other alterations in awareness

Infections, particularly bronchopneumonia or measles

Petechiae or hemorrhagic tendencies (purpura is usually associated with septicemia or a viral infection)

Dehydration and electrolyte disturbances, particularly hypokalemia and severe acidosis

Persistent tachycardia, signs of heart failure, or respiratory difficulty

Severe anemia with clinical signs of hypoxia

Clinical jaundice or elevated serum bilirubin level

Extensive exudative or exfoliative cutaneous lesions or deep pressure ulcers

Hypoglycemia

Hypothermia

Cachexia from chronic renal failure[a]

[a] Cachexia is characterized by maladaptive responses such as anorexia, elevated basic metabolic rate, wasting of lean body tissue, and underutilization of fat tissue for energy (Mak and Cheung, 2006); inflammation secondary to cytokines (such as leptin) may play a significant role (Mak and Cheung, 2006).

progressing gradually to 35–40 kcal/kg). Add a vitamin-mineral supplement, if necessary, including thiamin. Provide enteral feeding, if needed; start with continuous versus intermittent or bolus feedings at a slow rate until serum electrolyte levels are stable.

- Practical suggestions for improving intake in debilitated patients include liberalizing previous diet restrictions where safe and appropriate, addressing impairments to dentition and swallowing, addressing physical and cognitive deficits, encouraging family and friends to provide favorite foods, addressing poor consumption of specific foods, and providing appropriate nutrient supplements (Harris and Fraser, 2004).
- Oral nutritional supplementation during hospitalization is feasible in nutritionally depleted patients (Vermeeren et al, 2004).

CLINICAL INDICATORS

Clinical/History

Height, arm length, or knee length
Weight
BMI
Recent weight; weight changes
Usual weight
Desirable BMI
Diet history—poor appetite
I & O
BP
Edema
Muscle wasting
TSF
MAMC, MAC

Lab Work

CRP
Alb, transthyretin (may be altered)
Chol, Trig (decreased)
Serum Fe
Alk phos (decreased)
Gluc
H & H
Urine acetone

T3, T4	(decreased)	(<250 mg/dL)
Ca++, Mg++	Na+, K+, Cl−	Serum B_{12}
BUN (decreased)	Total iron-binding capacity (TIBC)	Serum folacin
Creat		Oxygen saturation levels
White blood cell count (WBC)		

Common Drugs Used and Potential Side Effects

- Medications that are often used to increase intake by stimulating appetite include: oxandrolone (Oxandrin), megestrol acetate (Megace), cyproheptadine HCl (Periactin), and Dronabinol (Marinol).
- Comparing oxandrolone, strength training, and nutrition alone for wasting, strength training is most cost effective and improves quality of life more than nutrition alone or oxandrolone (Shevitz et al, 2005).

Herbs, Botanicals, and Supplements

- Herbs and botanical supplements should not be used without discussing with physician.

INTERVENTION: NUTRITION EDUCATION, COUNSELING, CARE MANAGEMENT

- Emphasize importance of gradual refeeding.
- Discuss complicating effects of PCM. Unless nutritional therapy is aggressive, infection and sepsis are major risks, and surgery becomes life threatening. PCM can increase fistula formation, reduce recovery and wound healing after surgery, and lead to pneumonia or poor drug tolerance.
- Allow patients to participate in feeding decisions. Set goals and help plan together with family.

For More Information

- Medical Library
  http://www.chclibrary.org/micromed/00062340.html
- World Health Organization
  http://www.wpro.who.int/health_topics/protein_energy/

PROTEIN-CALORIE MALNUTRITION—CITED REFERENCES

Colman S, et al. The Nutritional and Inflammatory Evaluation in Dialysis Patients (NIED) study: overview of the NIED study and the role of dietitians. *J Ren Nutr.* 15:231, 2005.

Cunningham-Rundles S, et al. Mechanisms of nutrient modulation of the immune response. Mechanisms of nutrient modulation of the immune response. *J Allergy Clin Immunol.* 115:1119, 2005.

Demling RH. The incidence and impact of pre-existing protein energy malnutrition on outcome in the elderly burn patient population. *J Burn Care Rehabil.* 26:94, 2005.

Fuhrman MP, et al. Hepatic proteins and nutrition assessment. *J Am Diet Assoc.* 104:1258, 2004.

Harris CL, Fraser C. Malnutrition in the institutionalized elderly: the effects on wound healing. *Ostomy Wound Manage.* 50:54, 2004.

Kopple JD. The phenomenon of altered risk factor patterns or reverse epidemiology in persons with advanced chronic kidney failure. *Am J Clin Nutr.* 81:1257, 2005.

Mak RH, Cheung W. Energy homeostasis and cachexia in chronic kidney disease. *Pediatr Nephrol.* 2006. In press.

Martinez Olmos MA, et al. Nutritional status study of inpatients in hospitals of Galicia. *Eur J Clin Nutr.* 59:938, 2005.

Odabas D, et al. Cranial MRI findings in children with protein energy malnutrition. *Int J Neurosci.* 115:829, 2005.

Schnelldorfer T, Adams DB. The effect of malnutrition on morbidity after surgery for chronic pancreatitis. *Am Surg.* 71:466, 2005.

Shevitz AH, et al. A comparison of the clinical and cost-effectiveness of 3 intervention strategies for AIDS wasting. *J Acquir Immune Defic Syndr.* 38:399, 2005.

Shils M, et al. *Modern nutrition in health and disease.* 9th ed. Baltimore: Williams & Wilkins, 1998.

Sullivan D. The role of nutrition in increased morbidity and mortality. *Clin Geriatr Med.* 11:663, 1995.

Vermeeren MA, et al. Nutritional support in patients with chronic obstructive pulmonary disease during hospitalization for an acute exacerbation; a randomized controlled feasibility trial. *Clin Nutr.* 23:1184, 2004.

REFEEDING SYNDROME

NUTRITIONAL ACUITY RANKING: LEVEL 4

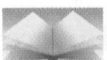

DEFINITIONS AND BACKGROUND

Refeeding syndrome refers to various metabolic abnormalities that may complicate carbohydrate administration in subnourished patients (Marinella, 2005). Aggressive refeeding after a period of starvation can lead to cardiac failure. Refeeding syndrome is marked hypophosphatemia with hypokalemia and (to a lesser extent) hypomagnesemia. Conditions that can lead to refeeding syndrome can be found in Table 10-22.

The metabolic adaptation of semistarvation, as in conditions such as anorexia nervosa, is impaired during refeeding

TABLE 10-22 Risk Factors That Can Lead to Refeeding Syndrome

Feeding after:
Alcoholism
Anorexia nervosa
Chronic underfeeding
Morbid obesity with massive weight loss and fasting
Protein–calorie malnutrition
Prolonged fasting
Prolonged parenteral nutrition

(Melchior, 1998). Patients in inpatient rehabilitation units may have underlying medical disorders and are at risk for poor oral intake, compounded by dysphagia and anorexia (Marinella, 2004). Reinstitution of nutrition by any route in an undernourished patient may lead to the refeeding syndrome.

Abnormal metabolism results in refeeding syndrome, with a shift from body fat to carbohydrate as metabolic fuel sources change. Insulin secretion increases while glucagon decreases, leading to reduced gluconeogenesis, glycogenolysis, and fatty acid mobilization. Glucose is taken up rapidly into the cells, and phosphorus is driven inside the cells, resulting in dangerous hypophosphatemia. Adenosine triphosphate (ATP) levels decrease as a result, with major effects on the cardiac, pulmonary, CNS, hematological, and muscular systems.

Signs of hypophosphatemia include anorexia, bone pain, dizziness, muscle weakness, respiratory failure, and myocardial dysfunction. This phenomenon usually occurs within 4 days of starting to feed again. Respiratory muscle, reduced in mass and ATP content by malnutrition, is unable to respond to the increased workload imposed by aggressive nutrition support, and this may lead to respiratory failure.

Other problems encountered in refeeding syndrome include sodium derangements, possibly leading to heart failure; potassium shifts into cells with resulting hypokalemia and arrhythmias; and magnesium shifts intracellularly with tetany and seizures. Thiamin deficiency is noted with refeeding because it is a cofactor in carbohydrate metabolism. Spontaneous diarrhea may occur at some time (Faintuch et al, 2001).

INTERVENTION: OBJECTIVES

- Gradually correct starvation without overloading the system with nutrients of any type. Use less than full levels of calorie and fluid requirements.
- Advance calories and volume with careful monitoring of cardiac and respiratory side effects.
- Correct vitamin and mineral deficiencies, especially with symptoms.
- Nutrition support in patients at risk should be increased slowly while assuring adequate amounts of vitamins and minerals.
- Organ function, fluid balance, and serum electrolytes (phosphorus, potassium, and magnesium) need to be monitored daily during the first week and less frequently after that time.
- Monitor for neurological, hematological, and metabolic complications of hypokalemia, hypophosphatemia, and hyperglycemia.
- Prevent sudden death (Crook et al, 2001).

INTERVENTION: FOOD AND NUTRITION

- Cautiously initiate feeding, perhaps 20 kcal/kg for the first 3 days, progressing slowly to 25 kcal/kg. Feeding can gradually be increased and be up to desired levels by day 7.
- Protein should be started slowly and increased gradually to protect and restore some lean body mass.
- At first, restrict carbohydrate (CHO) intake to 150–200 g/d to prevent a rapid insulin surge. CHO in parenteral nutrition (PN) should be initiated at 2 mg/kg/min (about 150–200 mg/d).
- Fat calories should make up the difference.
- Maintain fluid balance; adjust when edema exists (e.g., fluid restriction according to I & O, tachycardia, peripheral edema).
- Adjust for sodium and potassium intakes depending on laboratory values until normal.
- Supplement with thiamin and other vitamins and minerals as needed. Excesses are not required.

CLINICAL INDICATORS

Clinical/History	Tachycardia	H & H
Height	Temperature	Serum Fe
Weight	Rhabdomyolysis	Red blood cell dysfunction
BMI	Respiratory insufficiency	Ca++
Desirable BMI		BUN, Creat
Percentage of usual weight	**Lab Work**	Partial pressure of carbon dioxide (pCO_2)
History of weight changes	Alk phos (low)	Partial pressure of oxygen (pO_2)
Diet history	Mg++ (low?)	
I & O	K+ (low?)	
Edema	Gluc	
	Na+	
	Chol, Trig	

Common Drugs Used and Potential Side Effects

- Replacement of phosphorus, potassium, and magnesium may be needed if serum levels are depleted. Monitor specific medications used and their side effects (e.g., gastrointestinal distress).
- Insulin is often used to correct hyperglycemia levels. Monitor blood glucose levels as refeeding occurs.

Herbs, Botanicals, and Supplements

- Herbs and botanical supplements should not be used without discussing with physician.

INTERVENTION: NUTRITION EDUCATION, COUNSELING, CARE MANAGEMENT

- Provide nutrition education to focus on adequate nutrient intake. Consider referral if food insecurity is a concern.
- Offer guidelines according to discharge intervention plan for use at home or elsewhere. Physician may suggest long-term medication use or therapies.

For More Information

- Refeeding Syndrome
  http://www.ccmtutorials.com/misc/phosphate/page_07.htm

REFEEDING SYNDROME—CITED REFERENCES

Crook MA, et al. The importance of the refeeding syndrome. *Nutrition* 17:632, 2001.

Faintuch J, et al. Refeeding procedures after 43 days of total fasting. *Nutrition* 17:100, 2001.

Marinella MA. Refeeding syndrome: implications for the inpatient rehabilitation unit. *Am J Phys Med Rehabil.* 83:65, 2004.

Marinella MA. Refeeding syndrome and hypophosphatemia. *J Intensive Care Med.* 20:155, 2005.

Melchior J. From malnutrition to refeeding during anorexia nervosa. *Curr Opin Clin Nutr Metab Care.* 1:481, 1998.

SECTION 11

Musculoskeletal and Collagen Disorders

CHIEF ASSESSMENT FACTORS

- Actual Height, Measured Annually for Height Loss
- Use of Bone-Wasting Medications
- Bone Density Assessment
- Pain in Muscles, Joints, Bones, Spine
- Edema
- Extremity Weakness
- Movement Problems, Stiffness
- Weight Loss, Anorexia, Depression, Insomnia
- Easy Fatigue
- Unsteady Gait and Propensity to Fall
- Contractures
- Inflammation of Joints
- Psoriasis
- Arthritis—Warning Signs: Early Morning Stiffness; Swelling in One or More Joints; Obvious Redness and Warmth in a Joint; Unexplained Weight Loss, Fever, or Weakness Combined with Joint Pain; Symptoms Such as These That Last More Than 2 Weeks

OVERVIEW—RHEUMATIC DISORDERS

Rheumatic disorders include osteoarthritis, rheumatoid arthritis, juvenile rheumatoid arthritis, spondyloarthropathies, infectious arthritis, polymyositis, bursitis, tendonitis, psoriatic arthritis, systemic lupus erythematosus, scleroderma, polymyalgia rheumatica, polyarthritis nodosa, giant cell arteritis, gout, and fibromyalgia. See Table 11-1.

The cytokine, tumor necrosis factor alpha (TNFα), plays a key role in the pathogenesis of many chronic inflammatory and rheumatic diseases, including rheumatoid arthritis, ankylosing spondylitis, and psoriatic arthritis; TNF inhibitors (etanercept, infliximab, and adalimumab) significantly reduce symptoms and signs and improve function and quality of life (Braun et al, 2006; Nash and Florin, 2005). Gene expression profiling has become common practice for managing rheumatic conditions, especially in pediatric populations (Jarvis, 2005).

The National Arthritis Data Workgroup reviewed data from available surveys and found that over 15% (40 million) of Americans have some form of arthritis. *Spondylosis* is osteoarthritis of the spine. *Infectious arthritis* is caused by bacterial invasion spread from nearby joints following chickenpox, rubella, or mumps. Autoimmune disorders, Crohn's disease, and psoriasis may be the cause of *seronegative arthritis*. *Psoriatic arthritis (PsA)* is managed by use of nonsteroidal anti-inflammatory drugs (NSAIDs) and TNFα antagonists (Manadan et al, 2006). There is also a "*mixed connective tissue disease*" with the features of rheumatoid arthritis, cutaneous systemic sclerosis, and inflammatory myopathies where Raynaud's syndrome is an early sign (Aringer et al, 2005; Grader-Beck and Wigley, 2005).

Early recognition and treatment of these disorders are important. Rheumatoid arthritis, juvenile idiopathic arthritis, the seronegative spondyloarthropathies including PsA, and lupus may have skeletal pathology (Walsh et al, 2005). Atherosclerosis has inflammatory properties and may be present in lupus, rheumatoid arthritis, giant-cell arteritis, and ankylosing spondylitis (Solomon and Goodson, 2005; Hall and Dalbeth, 2005). New treatment of immune-mediated inflammatory disorders is available with anticytokine therapy, including TNFα antagonists and interleukin-1 receptor antagonists (e.g., anakinra) (Efthimiou and Markenson, 2005). A multidisciplinary, multipronged approach is best to manage these complex conditions.

TABLE 11-1 Autoimmunity and Rheumatic Disorders

When the immune system doesn't work right, the immune cells can mistake the body's own cells as invaders and attack them; these are called autoimmune diseases. The following is a sample list of body systems affected by rheumatic diseases:

Blood and blood vessels	**Kidneys**
Polyarteritis nodosa	Gout
Systemic lupus erythematosus	Systemic lupus erythematosus
Digestive tract (including the mouth)	**Lungs**
Scleroderma	Rheumatoid arthritis
Sjögren's syndrome	Scleroderma
Eyes	Systemic lupus erythematosus
Sjögren's syndrome	**Muscles**
Uveitis	Polymyositis
Heart	**Nerves and brain**
Ankylosing spondylitis	Systemic lupus erythematosus
Rheumatic fever	**Skin**
Scleroderma	Scleroderma
Systemic lupus erythematosus	Systemic lupus erythematosus
Joints	
Ankylosing spondylitis	
Osteoarthritis	
Rheumatoid arthritis	
Systemic lupus erythematosus	

Adapted from: National Institutes of Health (NIH). NIH Publication No. 02-4858. Available at http://www.niams.nih.gov/hi/topics/autoimmune/autoimmunity.htm.

Complementary and Alternative Medicine (CAM) Therapies

Controlled scientific studies of many patients can prove that a particular treatment is beneficial or that an apparent improvement is incidental. The important consideration is that treatment should do no harm. Some studies have been done in alternative therapies, particularly diet in the treatment of arthritis, but none have shown any real long-term benefit. Patients often do benefit from complementary therapies, either because the treatment truly works or because of psychological (placebo) effects.

There is preliminary evidence of benefit for vitamin C, vitamin D, and nutraceuticals such as glucosamine, chondroitin, *S*-adenosylmethionine, ginger, and avocado/soybean unsaponifiables (McAlindon, 2006). Specific diets and use of herbal or botanical products should only be undertaken with medical consultation.

Role of Total Diet

A recent prospective study investigated dietary factors for gout and confirmed some of the long-standing suspicions (red meats, seafood, beer, and liquor), exonerated others (total protein, wine, and purine-rich vegetables), and also identified protective factors in dairy products (Choi, 2005).

Higher intakes of meat and total protein as well as lower intakes of fruits, vegetables, and vitamin C are associated with an increased risk of inflammatory polyarthritis or rheumatoid arthritis (Choi, 2005). While flavonoids and some vitamins (especially vitamin C) are effective antioxidants against many chronic diseases (Knekt et al, 2002; Knekt et al, 2004), recent studies suggest that vitamin E, beta-carotene, and retinol do not halt the progression of osteoarthritis, as previously thought (Choi, 2005).

Vitamin D is needed for strong bones and muscles and for a healthy immune system. Rheumatoid arthritis may be aggravated by low intakes of vitamin D. Older individuals may be at risk because their diets tend to be low in vitamin D and they may have limited exposure to sunshine. Supplementation may be needed for these individuals.

Phytochemicals known for their ability to protect tissue also appear to block the activity of an enzyme that triggers inflammation in joints. Phytochemicals in cruciferous plants (e.g., broccoli, cauliflower, cabbage) boost production of phase 2 enzymes. In addition, components of the Mediterranean diet may protect against the development or severity of rheumatoid arthritis (Choi, 2005).

The activation of nuclear transcription factor-κB is linked with inflammatory diseases, including arthritis, osteoporosis, and psoriasis. The pathway that activates this transcription factor can be interrupted by phytochemicals derived from spices such as turmeric (curcumin); red pepper (capsaicin); cloves (eugenol); ginger (gingerol); cumin, anise, and fennel (anethol); basil and rosemary (ursolic acid); garlic (diallyl sulfide, *S*-allylmercaptocysteine, and ajoene); and pomegranate (ellagic acid) (Aggarwal and Shishodia, 2004).

Role of Omega-3 Fatty Acids

Excessive and inappropriate inflammation contributes to acute and chronic human diseases; it is characterized by the production of inflammatory cytokines, arachidonic acid–derived eicosanoids (prostaglandins, thromboxanes, leukotrienes, and other oxidized derivatives), other inflammatory agents (e.g., reactive oxygen species), and adhesion molecules (Calder, 2006). Three major types of omega-3 fatty acids are ingested in foods: alpha linolenic acid (ALA), eicosapentaenoic acid (EPA), and docosahexaenoic acid (DHA). The body converts ALA to EPA and DHA, which are readily used by the body. Omega-3 fatty acids help reduce inflammation, while omega-6 fatty acids tend to promote inflammation; precursor ALA does not appear to exert anti-inflammatory effects at achievable intakes (Calder, 2006).

A balance between omega-3 and omega-6 fatty acids in the diet is needed. The proper balance helps maintain and even improve health; one to four times more omega-6 fatty acids than omega-3 fatty acids is desirable, yet people who follow a Western diet consume much more omega-6 fatty acids than they should. Long-chain omega-3 polyunsaturated fatty acids (PUFAs) act by replacing arachidonic acid as an eicosanoid substrate, inhibiting arachidonic acid metabolism; by altering the expression of inflammatory genes through effects on transcription factor activation; and by leading to anti-inflammatory mediators termed resolvins (Calder, 2006).

RHEUMATIC DISORDERS—CITED REFERENCES

Aggarwal BB, Shishodia S. Suppression of the nuclear factor-kappa B activation pathway by spice-derived phytochemicals: reasoning for seasoning. *Ann N Y Acad Sci.* 1030:434, 2004.

Aringer M, et al. Does mixed connective tissue disease exist? Yes. *Rheum Dis Clin North Am.* 31:411, 2005.

Braun J, et al. First update of the international ASAS consensus statement for the use of anti-TNF agents in patients with ankylosing spondylitis. *Ann Rheum Dis.* 65:316, 2006.

Calder PC. Omega-3 polyunsaturated fatty acids, inflammation, and inflammatory diseases. *Am J Clin Nutr.* 83:1505S, 2006.

Choi HK. Dietary risk factors for rheumatic diseases. *Curr Opin Rheumatol.* 17:141, 2005.

Efthimiou P, Markenson JA. Role of biological agents in immune-mediated inflammatory diseases. *South Med J.* 98:192, 2005.

Grader-Beck T, Wigley FM. Raynaud's phenomenon in mixed connective tissue disease. *Rheum Dis Clin North Am.* 31:465, 2005.

Hall FC, Dalbeth N. Disease modification and cardiovascular risk reduction: two sides of the same coin? *Rheumatology (Oxford)* 44:1473, 2005.

Jarvis JN. Gene expression profiling in pediatric rheumatic disease: what have we learned? What can we learn? *Curr Opin Rheumatol.* 17:606, 2005.

Knekt P, et al. Antioxidant vitamins and coronary heart disease risk: a pooled analysis of 9 cohorts. *Am J Clin Nutr.* 80:1508, 2004.

Knekt P, et al. Flavonoid intake and risk of chronic diseases. *Am J Clin Nutr.* 76:560, 2002.

Manadan AM, et al. The treatment of psoriatic arthritis. *Am J Ther.* 13:72, 2006.

McAlindon TE. Nutraceuticals: do they work and when should we use them? *Best Pract Res Clin Rheumatol.* 20:99, 2006.

Nash PT, Florin TH. Tumour necrosis factor inhibitors. *Med J Aust.* 183:205, 2005.

Solomon DH, Goodson NJ. The cardiovascular system in rheumatic disease: the newest "extraarticular" manifestation? *J Rheumatol.* 32:1415, 2005.

Walsh NC, et al. Rheumatic diseases: the effects of inflammation on bone. *Immunol Rev.* 208:228, 2005.

OVERVIEW—BONE DISORDERS

Bone strength is derived from bone quantity, which consists of density and size, and bone quality, which consists of structure, consistency, and turnover. Adequate provision of nutrients composing the bone matrix and regulating bone metabolism should be provided from birth to achieve maximal bone mass, which is dependent upon individual genetic background, and to prevent osteoporosis later in life (Branca and Vatuena, 2001). Minerals and trace elements (calcium and phosphorus) are involved in skeletal growth; some are matrix constituents (magnesium and fluoride), and others are components of enzymatic systems involved in matrix turnover (zinc, copper, and manganese). Studies at Tufts University indicate that a sufficient protein intake, along with adequate calcium, supports stronger bone density. This contradicts the past suggestion that a high-protein diet would deplete bone strength.

Changes in bone turnover markers may become accurate predictors of fracture risk. Assessing risk factors for low bone mass may be important in monitoring the etiology of fracture of the tibia or fibula in older individuals (Kelsey et al, 2006). In general, women's bone health has been studied more extensively than that of men. More studies on the predictors of fractures in men are needed, such as bone architecture, morphology, biochemical markers of bone turnover, and hormonal levels (Szulc et al, 2005).

Vitamin D plays a role in calcium metabolism; vitamins C and K are cofactors of key enzymes for skeletal metabolism (Branca and Vatuena, 2001). Iron is a bone-promoting nutrient (18 mg is most protective for women) because it promotes production of collagen in bone structure. Mineral balance is also critical; for example, too much iron versus calcium throws off the needed balance.

Studies also suggest that omega-3 fatty acids such as EPA help increase levels of calcium in the body, deposit calcium in the bones, and improve bone strength. Studies also suggest that people who are deficient in certain essential fatty acids (EPA and gamma linolenic acid [GLA], an omega-6 fatty acid) are more likely to suffer from bone loss than those with normal levels of these fatty acids.

Intake of silicon in the form of choline-stabilized orthosilicic acid (BioSil is one brand), which is a more bioavailable form of the mineral than other dietary sources, may prove to be more effective in enhancing bone density than supplementation with calcium and vitamin D_3 alone (Reffitt et al, 2003). Antioxidant nutrients, including vitamins A and

C and selenium, may play a role in maintaining adequate bone health. Further studies are indicated.

Another indicator of bone health is heart health. Evidence indicates that there are similar pathophysiological mechanisms underlying cardiovascular disease (such as dyslipidemia, oxidative stress, inflammation, hyperhomocysteinemia, hypertension, and diabetes) and low bone mineral density (McFarlane et al, 2004). Whether folic acid and vitamins B_6 and B_{12} can help improve bone health remains to be tested.

In a landmark report, the U.S. Surgeon General Richard H. Carmona (2005) warned that, by 2020, half of all American citizens older than 50 will be at risk for fractures from osteoporosis and low bone mass if immediate action is delayed by individuals at risk, doctors, health systems, and policymakers. This report states that 10 million Americans over the age of 50 have osteoporosis, another 34 million are at risk for developing osteoporosis, and roughly 1.5 million people suffer a bone fracture related to osteoporosis. About 20% of senior citizens who suffer a hip fracture die within a year of fracture; 20% of individuals with a hip fracture end up in a nursing home within a year; and hip fractures account for 300,000 hospitalizations each year. While direct care costs for osteoporotic fractures are up to $18 billion each year, that number will increase if preventive measures are not taken. Recommendations to prevent osteoporosis include the following:

- Get the recommended amounts of calcium and vitamin D for age and sex. If diet is not adequate, supplements should be used.
- Maintain a healthy weight and be physically active for at least 30 minutes a day for adults and 60 minutes a day for children, including weight-bearing activities to improve strength and balance.
- Minimize the risk of falls by removing items that might cause tripping, improving lighting, and encouraging regular exercise and vision tests to improve balance and coordination.
- Risks for patients of all ages should be evaluated by health care professionals, and bone density tests for women over the age of 65 and for any man or woman who suffers even a minor fracture after the age of 50 should be recommended. "Red flags" indicate that someone is at risk (i.e., people with a history of multiple fractures, those who take certain medications, and those who have a disease that can lead to bone loss).
- Bone mineral density (BMD) tests can measure bone density in various sites of the body. See Figure 11-1 for the dual-energy x-ray absorptiometry (DEXA) test.
- Bone density is an important determinant of fracture risk even in nursing home patients. A BMD test is used to:
  - Detect osteoporosis before fractures occur
  - Predict chances of future fractures
  - Determine rate of bone loss and monitor the effects of treatment
- Note that a normal BMD is within 1 standard deviation (SD) of a "young normal" adult. Low bone mass (osteopenia): BMD is between 1 and 2.5 SD below that of a "young normal" adult. Osteoporosis: BMD is 2.5 SD or more below that of a "young normal" adult.

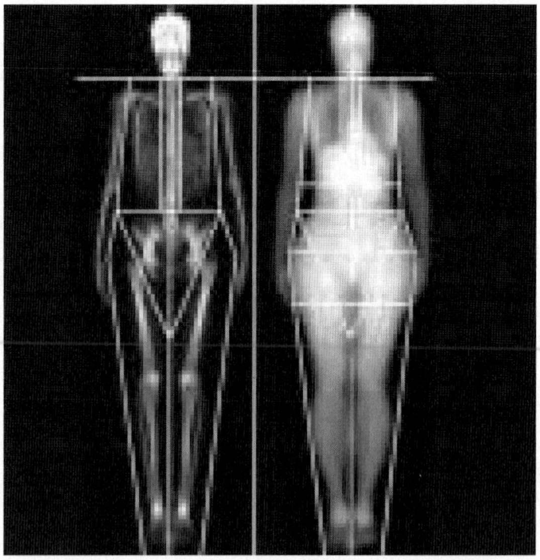

Figure 11-1 Dual-energy x-ray absorptiometry (DEXA) scan. (From Kaminsky LA, et al. *ACSM's resource manual for guidelines for exercise testing and prescription.* 5th ed. Philadelphia: Lippincott Williams & Wilkins, 2005.)

BONE DISORDERS—CITED REFERENCES

Branca F, Vatuena S. Calcium, physical activity and bone health—building bones for a stronger future. *Public Health Nutr.* 4:117, 2001.

Carmona RH. Bone health and osteoporosis: A report of the Surgeon General. Accessed August 3, 2005 at http://www.surgeongeneral.gov/library/bonehealth/.

Kelsey JL, et al. Risk factors for fracture of the shafts of the tibia and fibula in older individuals. *Osteoporos Int.* 17:143, 2006.

McFarlane SI, et al. Osteoporosis and cardiovascular disease: brittle bones and boned arteries, is there a link? *Endocrine* 23:1, 2004.

Reffitt DM, et al. Orthosilicic acid stimulates collagen type 1 synthesis and osteoblastic differentiation in human osteoblast-like cells in vitro. *Bone* 32:127, 2003.

Szulc P, et al. Bone mineral density predicts osteoporotic fractures in elderly men: the MINOS study. *Osteoporos Int.* 16:1184, 2005.

For More Information

- American Academy of Orthopaedic Surgeons
  http://www.aaos.org/
- American Academy of Physical Medicine and Rehabilitation
  http://www.aapmr.org
- American Autoimmune-Related Diseases Association (AARDA)
  http://www.aarda.org/
- American College of Rheumatology
  http://www.rheumatology.org/
- American Osteopathic Association
  http://www.do-online.osteotech.org/
- American Pain Foundation
  http://www.painfoundation.org/
- American Society for Bone and Mineral Research
  http://www.asbmr.org/
- Arthritis Foundation
  http://www.arthritis.org/
- Autoimmunity Resources
  http://www.aarda.org/links.php

- CAM Therapy Resources
  http://nccam.nih.gov/health/bydisease.htm
- Clinical Trials Research Trials
  http://www.aarda.org/links.php
- Drug List
  http://www.rxlist.com/alternative.htm
- Immune-Related Disorder Resources
  http://immune.best.vwh.net/resources/
- Journal of Immunology
  http://www.jimmunol.org/
- National Institute of Arthritis and Musculoskeletal and Skin Disorders
  http://www.niams.nih.gov/hi/index.htm
- National Institutes of Health
  http://www.osteo.org/links.html
- National Osteoporosis Foundation
  http://www.nof.org/
  Powerful Bones Campaign for Girls: http://www.nof.org/powerfulbones/index.htm
- Nutrition Screening Initiative–Physician's Guide to Nutrition in Chronic Disease Management
  http://www.aafp.org/PreBuilt/NSI_newbookletSMALLER.pdf
- Patient Information
  http://www.patientinform.org
- Quack Watch for Unproven Remedies
  http://www.quackwatch.com/
  http://www.chsourcebook.com/about/contents.html
- Rheumatic Diseases Internet Journal
  http://www.rheuma21st.com/
- Rheumatological Links
  http://www.rheuma21st.com/links_index.html

ANKYLOSING SPONDYLITIS (SPINAL ARTHRITIS)

NUTRITIONAL ACUITY RANKING: LEVEL 1

DEFINITIONS AND BACKGROUND

Among the 100 different rheumatic diseases that affect the joints and muscles is a group of five called **spondyloarthropathies.** These include ankylosing spondylitis, reactive arthritis (Reiter's syndrome), psoriatic arthritis or spondylitis, spondylitis of inflammatory bowel disease, and undifferentiated spondyloarthropathy.

Spondylitis is inflammation of the joints linking the vertebrae (a fused spine is not uncommon). Spondylitis affects about 300,000 Americans and is more common in Caucasians than in African Americans. The condition is most common in men aged 16–35 years and may run in families. Genetic marker HLA-B27 can be detected in these individuals.

In **ankylosing spondylitis,** inflammation of connective tissue recedes but leaves hardened and damaged joints that fuse together the bones of the spinal column; etiology is unknown. The sacroiliac joints generally are affected first. Symptoms and signs include chronic lower back pain, early morning stiffness in the lower back where the lower spine is joined to pelvis, vague chest pains, tender heels, weight loss, anemia, anorexia, slight fever, and recurring iritis or reddened eyes. Valvular heart disease may also occur. Pain may occasionally start in the knees and shoulders.

Elevated tumor necrosis factor alpha (TNFα) is believed to be one of the causes of inflammation and bone destruction in this condition (Braun et al, 2005). Therefore, anti-TNF therapy is effective in the treatment of ankylosing spondylitis (Barkham et al, 2005).

Surgery to replace a joint, when needed, may relieve pain. Exercise to strengthen muscles that tend to cause pain on stooping or bending may be useful and may relieve lower back pain. Attention to good posture will reduce some types of pain.

INTERVENTION: OBJECTIVES

- Reduce pain, inflammation, and disease activity; support improved functioning and ability to work or to maintain quality of life.
- Correct anorexia, nausea, poor intake or weight loss, anemia, or fever where present.
- Improve ability to participate in physical activities of choice to maintain lean body mass.

INTERVENTION: FOOD AND NUTRITION

- A normal diet is useful. Support gradual weight loss, if needed, to normalize weight. Some patients claim relief while using a vegetarian diet with less red meat.
- Preferred foods should be offered to stimulate appetite.
- It is prudent to increase dietary intake of foods rich in antioxidants such as vitamins E and C, selenium, and fish oils and rich sources of omega-3 fatty acids.
- Sufficient calcium and vitamin D are also a prudent suggestion (Lange et al, 2001; Akkus et al, 2001).
- Include phytochemicals derived from spices such as turmeric (curcumin); red pepper (capsaicin); cloves (eugenol); ginger (gingerol); cumin, anise, and fennel

(anethol); basil and rosemary (ursolic acid); garlic (diallyl sulfide, S-allylmercaptocysteine, ajoene); and pomegranate (ellagic acid) (Aggarwal and Shishodia, 2004).

CLINICAL INDICATORS

Clinical/History	Lab Work	
Height Weight Body mass index (BMI) Weight changes Anorexia Temperature Lower back pain Pain in knees or shoulders Iritis or reddened eyes X-rays	HLA-B27 gene test (found in 90%) Erythrocyte sedimentation rate (ESR) (high) C-reactive protein (CRP) Ca++, Mg++ Na+, K+ Alkaline phosphatase (Alk phos) Blood urea nitrogen (BUN)	Creatinine (Creat) Phosphorus (P) Hemoglobin and hematocrit (H & H) Aspartate aminotransferase (AST) Alanine aminotransferase (ALT) Serum folate Serum B_{12} Homocysteine levels

Common Drugs Used and Potential Side Effects

- Etanercept (Enbrel), an anti-TNF therapy, which has been used to treat rheumatoid arthritis, may cause significant improvement in pain and mobility (Braun et al, 2006; Temel et al, 2005). Quality of life also improves (Davis et al, 2005). Etanercept blocks TNFα.
- Infliximab (Remicade), another monoclonal antibody, also targets TNFα and provides clinical improvement. Upper respiratory infections, psoriatic rashes, and allergic reactions can occur with these medications.

Herbs, Botanicals, and Supplements

- Herbs and botanical supplements should not be used without discussing with physician. Ginger, corn, pineapple, pigweed, and vegetarianism have been recommended; no clinical trials prove efficacy.
- Alterations in the bowel flora and its activities are now believed to be contributing factors to ankylosing spondylitis and other rheumatic conditions (Hawrelak and Myers, 2004).

INTERVENTION: NUTRITION EDUCATION, COUNSELING, CARE MANAGEMENT

- Exercise is crucial, especially swimming, to relieve back pain.
- Patient should practice deep breathing exercises for pain relief. Stretching and strengthening exercises also are important.
- Patient should be sleeping on a hard bed, supine.
- Discuss role of energy intake for weight control.

For More Information

- Ankylosing Spondylitis International Federation
  http://www.asif.rheumanet.org/
- National Ankylosing Spondylitis Society (NASS)–United Kingdom
  http://www.nass.co.uk/
- Spondylitis Association of America
  http://www.spondylitis.org

ANKYLOSING SPONDYLITIS—CITED REFERENCES

Aggarwal BB, Shishodia S. Suppression of the nuclear factor-kappa B activation pathway by spice-derived phytochemicals: reasoning for seasoning. *Ann N Y Acad Sci.* 1030:434, 2004.

Akkus S, et al. A case of osteomalacia mimicking ankylosing spondylitis. *Rheumatol Int.* 20:239, 2001.

Barkham N, et al. The unmet need for anti-tumour necrosis factor (anti-TNF) therapy in ankylosing spondylitis. *Rheumatology (Oxford)* 44:1277, 2005.

Braun J, et al. First update of the International ASAS Consensus Statement for the use of anti-TNF agents in patients with ankylosing spondylitis. *Ann Rheum Dis.* 65:316, 2006.

Davis JC, et al. Reductions in health-related quality of life in patients with ankylosing spondylitis and improvements with etanercept therapy. *Arthritis Rheum.* 53:494, 2005.

Hawrelak JA, Myers SP. The causes of intestinal dysbiosis: a review. *Altern Med Rev.* 9:180, 2004.

Lange U, et al. Relationship between disease activity and serum levels of vitamin D metabolites and parathyroid hormone in ankylosing spondylitis. *Osteoporos Int.* 12:1031, 2001.

Temel M, et al. A major subset of patients with ankylosing spondylitis followed up in tertiary clinical care require anti-tumour necrosis factor alpha biological treatments according to the current guidelines. *Ann Rheum Dis.* 64:1383, 2005.

GOUT

NUTRITIONAL ACUITY RANKING: LEVEL 2

DEFINITIONS AND BACKGROUND

Gout is a disorder of sudden and recurring attacks of painful arthritis, caused by abnormal metabolism of purines, with inflamed joints (usually the big toe, ankle, knees, and feet). Uric acid is the end product of purine nucleotide metabolism in humans.

Gout affects more than 1% of adults in the United States, and it is the most common form of inflammatory arthritis among men (Saag and Choi, 2006). In gout, hyperuricemia

TABLE 11-2 Acquired Causes of Hyperuricemia

Cause	Description
Increased urate production	
Nutritional	Excess purine, ethanol, fructose consumption
Hematological	Myeloproliferative and lymphoproliferative disorders, polycythemia
Drugs	Ethanol, cytotoxic drugs, vitamin B_{12} (treatment of pernicious anemia)
Miscellaneous	Obesity, psoriasis, hypertriglyceridemia
Decreased renal excretion of urate	
Drugs	Ethanol, cyclosporine (Sandimmune), thiazides, furosemide (Lasix) and other loop diuretics, ethambutol (Myambutol), pyrazinamide, aspirin (low-dose), levodopa (Larodopa), nicotinic acid (Nicolar)
Renal	Hypertension, polycystic kidney disease, chronic renal failure (any etiology)
Metabolic/endocrine	Dehydration, lactic acidosis, ketosis, hypothyroidism, hyperparathyroidism
Miscellaneous	Obesity, sarcoidosis, toxemia of pregnancy

Source: Harris M, et al. Gout and hyperuricemia. *Am Fam Physician.* 59:925, 1999.

results, with deposition of monosodium urate crystals in the joints and tendons. Gout prevalence increases in direct association with age, with metabolic syndrome and hypertension, and with use of thiazide diuretics for hypertension (Saag and Choi, 2006). There is increased incidence in postmenopausal women, with polyarticular onset and hand involvement and early development of tophi (Ene-Stroescu and Gorbien, 2005).

The disease tends to affect men between the ages of 30 and 50 years and is sometimes hereditary. Acquired causes of hyperuricemia are found in Table 11-2. Gout is part of a clinical spectrum of conditions (obesity, diabetes mellitus, hyperlipidemia, and coronary artery disease) that necessitates better education (Ene-Stroescu and Gorbien, 2005).

Risk factors for gout include high alcohol intake, high levels of uric acid (this may be genetic), some hypertensive drugs, obesity, and high intake of purines. The disease may be triggered by injury; starvation; intake of large amounts of alcohol or seafood, beef, pork, and lamb (Choi et al, 2005); emotional stress; or illnesses such as diabetes, sickle cell anemia, or chronic renal disease. Westernization and increased intake of red meat is associated with a marked increase in serum uric acid levels (Johnson et al, 2005).

Acute attacks may be caused by drinking too much alcohol, surgery, sudden and severe illness, fasting, chemotherapy, or joint injury. Severe pain usually occurs, more so at night. The joint swells, and skin turns warm, red, purplish, and shiny. Acute gout most commonly affects the first metatarsal joint of the foot, but other joints may also be involved.

The acute and the chronic phases are treated differently. Gout progresses through four phases: asymptomatic hyperuricemia, acute gouty arthritis, intercritical gout (intervals between acute attacks), and chronic tophaceous gout (Harris, 1999).

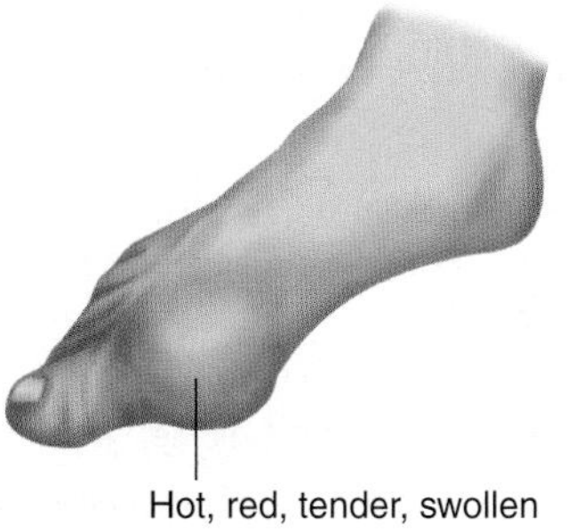

Figure 11-2 Gout in the big toe. (From Bickley LS, Szilagyi P. *Bates' guide to physical examination and history taking.* 8th ed. Philadelphia: Lippincott Williams & Wilkins, 2003.)

After several years, tophi may develop if the condition goes untreated. Tophi are hard lumps of urate crystals that are deposited under the skin around the joints and may be permanent. Although attacks of gout can subside in a few days, repeated attacks can cause permanent joint damage, and the disease often results in substantial disability and frequent medical care. See Figure 11-2.

Treatment includes the pain-relieving nonsteroidal anti-inflammatory drugs (NSAIDs) and, for more serious outbreaks, corticosteroids such as prednisone. Most patients with gout eventually require long-term treatment with medications that lower blood uric acid levels. Patients with asymptomatic hyperuricemia should lower their urate levels by changes in diet or lifestyle.

INTERVENTION: OBJECTIVES

- Promote gradual weight loss. In the obese, controlled weight management has the potential to lower serum urate (Schlesinger, 2005).
- Increase excretion of urates where desirable.
- Force fluid intake to prevent uric acid kidney stones.
- Correct any existing dyslipidemia.
- Prevent complications such as renal disease, hypertension, and stroke.
- Encourage lifestyle changes, if needed (e.g., reduction in energy intake, weight, alcohol intake, red meat intake).

INTERVENTION: FOOD AND NUTRITION

- A high-carbohydrate (CHO) diet increases excretion of urates, as does a low-fat intake; increase CHO ingestion and decrease fat ingestion. Purine-rich vegetables, which include peas, beans, mushrooms, cauliflower, and spinach, yield a protective effect (Choi, 2005). Balance this within a weight loss plan if needed.
- Avoid excessive intake of meat purines by limiting ingestion of anchovies, sardines, liver, caviar, and herring. Beef, pork, and lamb should be used infrequently.
- Diet should exclude alcoholic beverages (Schlesinger, 2005).
- Ensure a high-fluid intake.
- Nonfat milk, low-fat yogurt, dairy products, fruits such as cherries (Jacob, 2003), and high intakes of vegetable protein may reduce serum urate (Schlesinger, 2005).

SAMPLE NUTRITION DIAGNOSTIC STATEMENT

Gout

PES: Excessive protein intake related to history of consuming large meat portions as evidenced by recent painful flare of gout with hyperuricemia.

Assessment Data (sources of info): Diet history and food records, medication history, fluid intake.

Intervention: Discuss role of diet, fluid intake, and medications in managing gout

Monitoring and Evaluation: Evaluation of diet history and food records, improvement in symptoms of gout.

CLINICAL INDICATORS

Clinical/History	Lab Work	
Height	CRP	Triglycerides (Trig) (increased?)
Weight	Uric acid (increased)	Ca++, Mg++
BMI	Birefringent crystals in the synovial fluid	Na+, K+
Obesity	BUN (increased)	Albumin (Alb)
Urate crystals in urine	Cholesterol (Chol)	Creat
Use of alcoholic beverages		Glucose (Gluc)
Use of thiazide diuretics		AST, ALT

Common Drugs Used and Potential Side Effects

- Uricosuric drugs: Probenecid (Benemid) and sulfinpyrazone (Anturane) block renal absorption of urates. Adequate intake of fluid is needed. Anorexia, nausea, vomiting, and sore gums may result.
- Xanthine oxidase inhibitors: Allopurinol (Aloprim) blocks uric acid formation. Adequate intake of fluid is needed. Mild gastrointestinal (GI) upset, taste changes, or diarrhea can occur; take after meals. Febuxostat is even more effective than allopurinol; side effects are transient (Schumacher, 2005). For more serious outbreaks, corticosteroid drugs like prednisone can be prescribed.
- Fenofibrate has a rapid and reversible urate-lowering effect in patients with hyperuricemia and gout on established allopurinol prophylaxis; this may be a potential treatment for prevention of gout when hyperlipidemia is also present (Feher et al, 2003).
- Medications that can increase uric acid levels include hydrochlorothiazide (a diuretic) and some transplantation medications (cyclosporine and tacrolimus) (see Table 11-2).

Herbs, Botanicals, and Supplements

- Herbs and botanical supplements should not be used without discussing with physician.
- Celery, avocado, turmeric, cat's claw, chiso, and devil's claw have been recommended; there are no clinical trials that prove efficacy.

INTERVENTION: NUTRITION EDUCATION, COUNSELING, CARE MANAGEMENT

- Advise patient that alcohol, beef, and pork may precipitate a gouty attack (Choi et al, 2004).
- Weight loss may be helpful, but have patient avoid fasting. Instruct patient to lose weight gradually if obese to prevent release of increased purines.
- The inflammatory response may be suppressed by an increase in omega-3 fatty acids, as found in fatty fish (mackerel, herring, and salmon) and from walnuts, flaxseed, and cherries. Use these foods several times a week.
- Discuss the importance of adequate fluid ingestion.

For More Information

- American College of Rheumatology
  http://www.rheumatology.org/
- Arthritis–Gout
  http://www.arthritis.org/conditions/diseasecenter/gout.asp

GOUT—CITED REFERENCES

Choi HK. Dietary risk factors for rheumatic diseases. *Curr Opin Rheumatol.* 17:141, 2005.

Choi HK, et al. Intake of purine-rich foods, protein, and dairy products and relationship to serum levels of uric acid: the Third National Health and Nutrition Examination Survey. *Arthritis Rheum.* 52:283, 2005.

Choi HK, et al. Purine-rich foods, dairy and protein intake, and the risk of gout in men. *N Engl J Med.* 350:1093, 2004.

Ene-Stroescu D, Gorbien MJ. Gouty arthritis. A primer on late-onset gout. *Geriatrics* 60:24, 2005.

Feher MD, et al. Fenofibrate enhances urate reduction in men treated with allopurinol for hyperuricaemia and gout. *Rheumatology (Oxford)* 42:321, 2003.

Harris M, et al. Gout and hyperuricemia. *Am Fam Physician.* 59:925, 1999.

Jacob RA, et al. Consumption of cherries lowers plasma urate in healthy women. *J Nutr.* 133:1826, 2003.

Johnson RJ, et al. Uric acid, evolution and primitive cultures. *Semin Nephrol.* 25:3, 2005.

Saag KG, Choi H. Epidemiology, risk factors, and lifestyle modifications for gout. *Arthritis Res Ther.* 8:2S, 2006

Schlesinger N. Dietary factors and hyperuricaemia. *Curr Pharm Des.* 11:4133, 2005.

Schumacher HR Jr. Febuxostat: a non-purine, selective inhibitor of xanthine oxidase for the management of hyperuricaemia in patients with gout. *Expert Opin Invest Drugs.* 14:893, 2005.

IMMOBILIZATION

NUTRITIONAL ACUITY RANKING: LEVEL 1–2

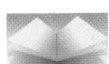

DEFINITIONS AND BACKGROUND

Extended periods of immobilization, for various reasons, may be nutritionally depleting. Patients with orthopedic injuries may lose 15–20 lb from stress, immobilization, trauma, and bed rest. Prolonged immobilization and nonuse of lower and upper limb muscles cause atrophy (Lameu et al, 2004). Immobilization hypercalcemia involves nausea, vomiting, abdominal cramps, constipation, headache, and lethargy.

Nitrogen depletion can be extensive. A large nitrogen loss and high protein oxidation can be related to extensive injury and elevated energy expenditure in many cases (Weekes and Elia, 1996). The adductor pollicis muscle has a positive correlation with estimation of muscle mass but not fat mass; this measurement is now being evaluated as an anthropometric parameter in clinical studies (Lameu et al, 2004).

Unloading of weight-bearing bones as induced by immobilization also has significant impacts on calcium and bone metabolism. With careful attention to functional capacity enhancements, bone mass can be restored (Rittweger et al, 2005). This is important since loss of bone mineral density precedes osteoarthritis (Rittweger et al, 2005).

Persons with physical disabilities frequently are nonambulatory and have bone loss due to immobility. Prevention of osteoporosis and related fractures in this population includes calcium and vitamin D supplementation and risk-based screening procedures (Schrager, 2004).

In old age, sarcopenia is the result of excessive loss of muscle mass and strength, loss of mobility, neuromuscular impairment, and balance failure. Falls and fractures can lead to immobilization, which induces more loss of muscle mass.

INTERVENTION: OBJECTIVES

- Correct negative nitrogen balance from increased losses (perhaps up to 2–3 g of nitrogen per day) to prevent pressure ulcers and infections.
- Prevent deossification and osteoporosis of bones. Prevent hypercalcemia from low serum levels of albumin, which normally binds calcium.
- Prevent kidney and bladder stones.
- Provide adequate fluid intake to aid excretion of nutrients.
- Prevent constipation, impactions, and obstruction.
- Prevent anemias that result from inadequate nitrogen balance.
- Prevent venous thrombosis.

INTERVENTION: FOOD AND NUTRITION

- Diet should provide adequate intake of high–biological value proteins to correct nitrogen balance. An intake of 1.2 g protein/kg body weight is often recommended. Provide adequate energy to spare protein; use sufficient carbohydrates and fats, including 1–2% total kcal as essential fatty acids (EFAs).
- Increased intake of phosphorus during the first few weeks may be useful.
- Encourage adequate intake of calcium since a high-protein diet raises the body's calcium requirements.
- Diet should provide a high-fluid intake.
- Intake of vitamin C and zinc should be adequate to protect against skin breakdown.
- Diet should provide adequate amounts of fiber to prevent constipation. Avoid overuse of fiber in cases where there is impaction.

CLINICAL INDICATORS

Clinical/History

- Height or arm length/knee length
- Weight
- BMI
- Weight changes
- Triceps skinfold (TSF)
- Midarm muscle circumference (MAMC)
- Midarm circumference (MAC)
- Dual-energy x-ray absorptiometry (DEXA)

Lab Work

- H & H
- Alb
- Transthyretin, retinol-binding protein (RBP)
- CRP
- Nitrogen (N) balance
- Ca++ (increased)
- Parathormone (PTH)
- Urinary Ca++
- Alk phos
- Mg++
- Red blood cell count (RBC)
- BUN, Creat
- Na+, K+

Common Drugs Used and Potential Side Effects

- Medications may be used to treat underlying conditions; they may have side effects that contribute to nutrient losses.
- Immobilization-induced hypercalcemia affects bone metabolism in Parkinson's disease; this inhibits secretion of PTH, which in turn suppresses 1,25-dihydroxyvitamin D production (Sato et al, 2005). These abnormalities may be corrected by the suppression of bone resorption with bisphosphonate, and supplementations of calcium and vitamin D should be avoided in these patients (Sato et al, 2005).

Herbs, Botanicals, and Supplements

- Herbs and botanical supplements should not be used without discussing with physician.

INTERVENTION: NUTRITION EDUCATION, COUNSELING, CARE MANAGEMENT

- Explain to patient that early ambulation is the best treatment possible.
- Explain that calcium and nutrient intakes will have to be monitored for patients who will be tube fed or on a liquid diet for extended periods of time.
- Explain need for adequate fiber and fluid intake to prevent constipation, urinary tract infections, and so on.

IMMOBILIZATION—CITED REFERENCES

Lameu EB, et al. The thickness of the adductor pollicis muscle reflects the muscle compartment and may be used as a new anthropometric parameter for nutritional assessment. *Curr Opin Clin Nutr Metab Care.* 7:293, 2004.

Rittweger J, et al. Reconstruction of the anterior cruciate ligament with a patella-tendon-bone graft may lead to a permanent loss of bone mineral content due to decreased patellar tendon stiffness. *Med Hypotheses.* 64:1166, 2005.

Sato Y, et al. Abnormal bone and calcium metabolism in immobilized Parkinson's disease patients. *Mov Disord.* 20:1598, 2005.

Schrager S. Osteoporosis in women with disabilities. *J Womens Health (Larchmt).* 13:431, 2004.

Weekes E, Elia M. Observations on the patterns of 24-hour energy expenditure changes in body composition and gastric emptying in head-injured patients receiving nasogastric tube feeding. *J Parenter Enteral Nutr.* 20:31, 1996.

MUSCULAR DYSTROPHY

NUTRITIONAL ACUITY RANKING: LEVEL 2

DEFINITIONS AND BACKGROUND

Actually a group of nine disorders, muscular dystrophy (MD) involves a hereditary condition with progressive degenerative changes in the muscle fibers, leading to weakness and atrophy. Muscular biopsy is required for the definitive diagnosis of the specific congenital type. Most of the disorders are described in Table 11-3.

Body mass index should be used with caution for the evaluation of the nutritional status of patients with Duchenne MD (DMD); indices that incorporate the assessment of the compartmental distribution of muscle and fat are more sensitive (Pessolano et al, 2003). While extremely elevated serum creatine kinase (CK) levels may indicate muscle disease, muscle biopsy confirms diagnoses of MD in patients with unexplained elevations of AST, ALT, and lactate dehydrogenase (LDH) (Korones et al, 2001).

Vitamin E, selenium, and calcium have been studied for possible roles in the onset of these disorders. In addition, poor intakes should be monitored. Patients with MD may be prone to nutrient deficiency due to mobility limitations or oropharyngeal weakness (Motlagh et al, 2005). Many patients demonstrate inadequate nutrient intake of protein, energy, vitamins, and minerals (calcium and magnesium), and significant correlations exist between measures of strength and copper and water-soluble vitamins (Motlagh et al, 2005).

The prognosis of MD varies according to type and progression. Some cases may be mild and very slowly progressive, with a normal lifespan, while other cases may have more marked progression of muscle weakness, functional disability, and loss of ambulation. Life expectancy may depend on the degree of progression and late respiratory deficit; in DMD, death usually occurs in the late teens to early twenties. Myoblast transfer therapy is under investigation as a possible treatment.

INTERVENTION: OBJECTIVES

- Encourage patient to lead a relatively active life; exercise programs can help prevent contractures.
- Prevent obesity, which may result from inactivity. Obesity complicates physical therapy.
- Avoid constipation because fecal impaction is frequent.
- Encourage activities other than eating to prevent dependency on food as a source of pleasure.
- Adapt to feeding difficulties.
- Malnutrition is a serious threat to patients with muscular disease, especially if there is also respiratory muscle weakness. Monitor nutritional intake and deficits on a regular basis. Prevent aspiration pneumonia or nasal regurgitation.
- Prevent osteoporosis and fractures, which can occur in this population. Peak bone mass is seldom attained in children who have a disability (Apkon, 2002).

INTERVENTION: FOOD AND NUTRITION

- Work with the MyPyramid food guidance system as a basic guide. Use a low-energy diet if necessary to control or lessen obesity. Check patient's BMI and adjust intake accordingly. Some patients' requirements may be 30% lower than normal (Munn et al, 2005).
- Use foods that are easy to chew and swallow for DMD. Use pureed or blenderized foods when needed. Tube feed only if necessary.
- Provide adequate fiber (prune juice, bran and other whole grains, fruits, and vegetables) if constipation becomes a problem.

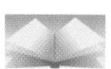

TABLE 11-3 Types of Muscular Dystrophy and Nutritional Implications

Type	Comments	Nutritional Implications
Congenital muscular dystrophy (CMD)	Caused by genetic mutations affecting some of the proteins necessary for muscles and some proteins related to the eyes and/or brain. Onset is at or near time of birth. Indicators include generalized muscle weakness with possible joint stiffness or looseness. Depending on the type, CMD may involve spinal curvature, respiratory insufficiency, mental retardation or learning disabilities, eye defects, and seizures.	
Distal muscular dystrophy (DD)	DD (Miyoshi form) first shows signs between ages 40–60 years, with weakness and muscle wasting of the hands, forearms, and lower legs. It progresses slowly. It is caused by a mutation in any of at least seven genes that affect proteins necessary to the function of muscles. DD is usually passed on as an autosomal dominant trait, or the faulty gene may be inherited from just one parent (autosomal recessive).	Weakness and muscle wasting of the hands and forearms make make self-feeding difficult.
Duchenne muscular dystrophy (DMD)	X-linked recessive; DMD primarily affects boys, who inherit the disease through their mothers. Caused by absence of dystrophin, a protein that helps keep muscle cells intact. Aggressive forms appear in males aged 2–6 years, with frequent falls and difficulty in climbing. Generalized weakness and muscle wasting affect hip, thigh, shoulder, and trunk muscles first; calves are often enlarged. Also called pseudohypertrophic. Survival is rare after the late twenties. Becker muscular dystrophy (BMD) is very similar to DMD, but onset is later (adolescence or adulthood), and patients live longer.	Facial muscles are involved, and the patient cannot suck, close lips, bite, chew, or swallow. DMD eventually affects all voluntary muscles and the heart and breathing muscles.
Emery-Dreyfus muscular dystrophy (EDMD)	EDMD is caused by gene mutations that produce emerin, lamin A, or lamin C, which are proteins in the membrane that surrounds the nucleus of each muscle cell. EDMD has an onset in childhood, usually by age 10. Weakness and wasting of shoulder, upper arm, and shin muscles and joint deformities are common. Disease usually progresses slowly. Frequent cardiac complications are common, and a pacemaker may be needed.	Self-feeding becomes difficult.
Fascioscapulohumeral muscular dystrophy (FSHMD)	FSHMD (also called Landouzy-Dejerine) begins in childhood to early adulthood, with facial muscle weakness and weakness and wasting of the shoulders and upper arms. Caused by a missing piece of DNA on chromosome 4, it progresses slowly with some periods of rapid deterioration. Usually evident by age 20, it may span many decades. Inheritance is autosomal dominant, which means it can be passed on by either parent.	Self-feeding becomes difficult; loss of skeletal muscle occurs. Abdominal muscles are affected.
Limb-girdle muscular dystrophy (LGMD)	LGMD is caused by a mutation in any of at least 15 different genes that affect proteins necessary for muscle function. LGMD has an onset in late childhood to middle age. Weakness and wasting affects shoulder and pelvic girdles first. Progression is slow, with cardiopulmonary complications often occurring in later stages of the disease. It is inherited as an autosomal recessive, autosomal dominant trait.	Self-feeding becomes difficult.
Myotonic dystrophy (MyD)	MyD (Steinert's disease) has onset anywhere from birth to middle age. Generalized weakness and muscle wasting affect the face, feet, hands, and neck first. Delayed relaxation of muscles after contraction. Congenital myotonic form is more severe. Progression is slow, sometimes spanning 50–60 years. Inheritance is autosomal dominant; there is a repeated section of DNA on either chromosome 19 or chromosome 3. Individuals with MyD have long faces and drooping eyelids; men have frontal baldness.	Progression is slow. Often complicated by diabetes (Perseghin et al, 2003). Prone to nutritional deficiencies from associated dysmotility of the entire gastrointestinal tract; handgrip is significantly lower and knee extension is higher compared to other dystrophies (Motlagh et al, 2005).
Oculopharyngeal muscular dystrophy (OPMD)	OPMD has onset in early adulthood to middle age. It affects muscles of eyelids (causing droopy eyelids) and throat and slowly progresses, with swallowing problems common as disease progresses. Inheritance is autosomal dominant, and onset is usually in the 4th or 5th decade. The gene that is defective in OPMD is called the *poly(A) binding protein 2 (PAPB2)* gene; extra amino acids in the protein made from a defective *PABP2* gene cause the protein to clump together in the muscle cell nuclei, interfering with cell function. The disease can often be diagnosed with a DNA test.	Swallowing difficulty is common; tube feeding should be considered before wasting occurs.

- Ensure adequate intake of fluid to prevent fecal impaction, dehydration, and related effects.
- Adequate sodium chloride is important (Yoshida et al, 2006).

CLINICAL INDICATORS

Clinical/History	DEXA	Muscle biopsy
Height	**Lab Work**	BUN
Weight		N balance
BMI (use with other parameters only)	Creatine kinase (CK) (increased)	Alb, transthyretin
MAC, MAMC, TSF	Lactate dehydrogenase (LDH) (increased)	CRP
Ability to swallow	Creat (often decreased)	H & H
Ability to chew		Serum P
Hand-to-mouth coordination		Gluc
		AST
		ALT
		Ca++, Mg++
		Na+, K+

Common Drugs Used and Potential Side Effects

- The myotonia (delayed relaxation of a muscle after a strong contraction) may be treated with medications such as phenytoin or quinine. Side effects can include folic acid depletion.
- It may be useful to try beta$_2$-adrenergic agonists, which can increase muscle mass. Albuterol may be needed for some individuals with forms of MD prior to exercise and strength training (van der Kooi et al, 2004; Kissel et al, 2001).

Herbs, Botanicals, and Supplements

- Herbs and botanical supplements should not be used without discussing with physician.
- While not studied extensively in humans, green tea extract may improve muscle health by reducing or delaying necrosis by an antioxidant mechanism (Dorchies et al, 2006; Buetler et al, 2002).
- Traditional Chinese medicine has been advocated for treatment of types of MD, but there is no evidence of benefit (Urtizberea et al, 2003). Some of the effects may be related to the presence of corticosteroids.
- Some studies are being conducted using creatine supplements; further research is needed.

INTERVENTION: NUTRITION EDUCATION, COUNSELING, CARE MANAGEMENT

- Provide low-calorie snack tips for patients who are obese.
- Help patient modify food textures to meet needs.
- Discuss problems related to inactivity or weight gain.
- Discuss the importance of adequate fluid intake.
- Discuss methods to prevent aspiration and pneumonia (Bulat and Orlando, 2005).

TABLE 11-4 Levels of Dysfunction

Impairment: disturbance at level of organ or limb	Disability: disturbance in function at level of person	Handicap: disturbance in the relationship between person and society as result of disability

Originally adapted from: World Health Organization. *International classification of impairments, disabilities, and handicaps.* Geneva: World Health Organization, 1980. From the Muscular Dystrophy Association. Skill for the job of living. Accessed August 27, 2005 at http://www.mdausa.org/publications/Quest/q65occup.html.

- Work with the occupational therapist and other therapists to maintain optimal levels of function. Table 11-4 describes classifications of dysfunction.

For More Information

- Facioscapulohumeral Dystrophy (FSHD) Society
  http://www.fshsociety.org
- Muscular Dystrophy Association (MDA)
  http://www.mdausa.org/
- Muscular Dystrophy Association of Canada
  http://www.mdac.ca/
- Muscular Dystrophy Family Foundation
  http://www.mdff.org/
- National Institute of Neurological Disorders and Stroke
  http://www.ninds.nih.gov/health_and_medical/disorders/md.htm
- Neuromuscular Disorders in the MDA Foundation
  http://www.mdausa.org/disease/
- Parent Project for Muscular Dystrophy Research
  http://www.parentprojectmd.org
- Rare Muscular Dystrophy types
  http://www.mdausa.org/publications/fa-rareMD.html#dd

MUSCULAR DYSTROPHY—CITED REFERENCES

Apkon SD. Osteoporosis in children who have disabilities. *Phys Med Rehabil Clin N Am.* 13:839, 2002.

Buetler TM, et al. Green tea extract decreases muscle necrosis in mdx mice and protects against reactive oxygen species. *Am J Clin Nutr.* 75:749, 2002.

Bulat RS, Orlando RC. Oropharyngeal dysphagia. *Curr Treat Options Gastroenterol.* 8:269, 2005.

Dorchies OM, et al. Green tea extract and its major polyphenol (-)-epigallocatechin gallate improve muscle function in a mouse model for Duchenne muscular dystrophy. *Am J Physiol Cell Physiol.* 290:C616, 2006.

Kissel JT, et al. Randomized, double-blind, placebo-controlled trial of albuterol in facioscapulohumeral dystrophy. *Neurology* 57:1434, 2001.

Korones D, et al. "Liver function tests" are not always tests of liver function. *Am J Hematol.* 66:46, 2001.

Motlagh B, et al. Nutritional inadequacy in adults with muscular dystrophy. *Muscle Nerve.* 31:713, 2005.

Munn MW. Estimate of daily calorie needs for a neuromuscular disease patient receiving noninvasive ventilation. *Am J Phys Med Rehabil.* 84:639, 2005.

Perseghin G, et al. Contribution of abnormal insulin secretion and insulin resistance to the pathogenesis of type 2 diabetes in myotonic dystrophy. *Diabetes Care* 26:2112, 2003.

Pessolano FA, et al. Nutritional assessment of patients with neuromuscular diseases. *Am J Phys Med Rehabil.* 82:182, 2003.

Urtizberea JA, et al. Looking under every rock: Duchenne muscular dystrophy and traditional Chinese medicine. *Neuromuscul Disord.* 13:705, 2003.

van der Kooi EL, et al. Strength training and albuterol in facioscapulohumeral muscular dystrophy. *Neurology.* 63:702, 2004.

Yoshida M, et al. Dietary NaCl supplementation prevents muscle necrosis in a mouse model of Duchenne muscular dystrophy. *Am J Physiol Regul Integr Comp Physiol.* 290:R449, 2006.

MYOFASCIAL PAIN SYNDROMES: FIBROMYALGIA AND POLYMYALGIA RHEUMATICA

NUTRITIONAL ACUITY RANKING: LEVEL 1–2

DEFINITIONS AND BACKGROUND

Myofascial pain syndromes are a group of disorders characterized by achy pain and stiffness in soft tissues, including muscles, tendons, and ligaments. In the United States, **fibromyalgia syndrome (FMS)** is estimated to occur in 2% of adults (Mease, 2005). Diagnosis is difficult, and the etiology is not clear. Corticotropin-releasing hormone (CRH) and substance P (SP) are found in increased levels in the cerebral spinal fluid (CSF) of FMS patients, and increased interleukin (IL)-6 and IL-8 are found in the serum; FMS may be a neuroimmunoendocrine disorder where these increased levels trigger local mast cells to release proinflammatory and neurosensitizing molecules (Lucas et al, 2006). This supports the hypothesis that FMS results from central nervous system oversensitization (Mease, 2005).

FMS causes widespread pain and stiffness throughout the body, or the pain and stiffness may be localized along the spine. Persistent symptoms may be disruptive but are not life threatening. Symptoms include sleep disturbance, depression, fatigue, headaches, irritable bowel syndrome, numbness in the hands and feet, and mood disorders. Acupuncture may offer relief (Martin et al, 2006).

Polymyalgia rheumatica (PMR) affects people over age 70 years, usually women. It causes aching, severe muscle stiffness and pain. Symptoms start suddenly and may affect several areas in the neck, shoulders, upper arms, lower back, hips, and/or thighs. It usually goes away with treatment but may reoccur. Symptoms include mild joint stiffness and swelling, depression, night sweats, fatigue, mild fever, and anorexia. Many people with PMR also have giant-cell arteritis with symptoms of double vision, severe headaches, or vision loss. The cause of PMR is not known but may be related to aging. Diagnosis is difficult.

Treatment of myofascial pain disorders may include exercise, medications such as glucocorticoids and nonsteroidal anti-inflammatory drugs (NSAIDs), a healthy diet rich in antioxidants, and adequate rest. Nonpharmaceutical treatments, including massage and cognitive behavioral therapy, are helpful (Mease, 2005). It is useful to work with a multidisciplinary team including a rheumatologist, physical therapist, exercise therapist, dietitian, and massage therapist (Lemstra and Olszynski, 2005).

Use of a "living food (LF) diet" results in a decrease in joint stiffness and pain as well as an improvement in self-reported quality of life (Hanninen et al, 2000). Plant foods are rich natural sources of antioxidants (quercetin, myristin, and kaempherol) in addition to fiber and other nutrients. Use of an uncooked vegan diet shows highly increased serum levels of beta- and alpha-carotenes, lycopene, lutein, and vitamins C and E (Hanninen et al, 2000).

INTERVENTION: OBJECTIVES

- Relieve pain. Acupuncture and exercise may be recommended (Assefi et al, 2005).
- Lose weight, if obese.
- Correct underlying problems such as hypertension.
- Support lifestyle changes, including stress reduction, relaxation techniques, and exercise.
- Prevent blindness in PMR when there is giant-cell arteritis.

INTERVENTION: FOOD AND NUTRITION

- An uncooked vegan (LF) diet may be beneficial (Hanninen et al, 2000). The diet includes berries, fruits, vegetables, roots, nuts, germinated seeds, and sprouts. The MyPyramid food guidance system is another useful tool for planning a healthy diet.
- A weight loss plan may be needed.
- Increased intake of omega-3 fatty acids may help to reduce inflammation and relieve pain in some individuals. Increase intake of fatty fish, walnuts, and flaxseed.
- Include phytochemicals derived from spices such as turmeric (curcumin); red pepper (capsaicin); cloves (eugenol); ginger (gingerol); cumin, anise, and fennel (anethol); basil and rosemary (ursolic acid); garlic (diallyl sulfide, *S*-allylmercaptocysteine, and ajoene); and pomegranate (ellagic acid) (Aggarwal and Shishodia, 2004).
- Dietary quercetin should be encouraged (Lucas et al, 2006).

CLINICAL INDICATORS

Clinical/History

- Height
- Weight
- BMI
- Tender areas, back pain
- Headache
- Fibromyalgia Impact Questionnaire (FIQ)
- Pain in shoulders, pelvis, and hips (pain in 11/18 trigger points)
- Carpal tunnel syndrome (in PMR)

Lab Work

- ESR (may be high)
- Plasma adrenomedullin (high in PMR)
- CRP
- Trig
- Chol
- Alb, transthyretin
- BUN
- Creat
- Ca++, Mg++
- Na+, K+
- Gluc
- Alk phos

Common Drugs Used and Potential Side Effects

- Medications that decrease pain and improve sleep may be prescribed. Low doses of tricyclic antidepressants and the serotonin-3 receptor antagonist tropisetron may be helpful (Lucas et al, 2006). Opioids, NSAIDs, sedatives, muscle relaxants, and antiepileptics have been used to treat FMS (Mease, 2005).
- Analgesics may be used; monitor for vitamin C depletion. A tramadol/acetaminophen combination tablet is effective for the treatment of FMS pain without serious adverse effects (Bennett et al, 2003).
- Pramipexole is used to treat Parkinson's disease; it stimulates dopamine production by binding to dopamine receptor sites and is thought to inhibit sensory nerve–mediated responses. It is being tested for FMS.
- Low-dose corticosteroids usually alleviate the symptoms of PMR. Methotrexate plus prednisone may allow use of lower doses for a shorter time (Caporali et al, 2004).

Herbs, Botanicals, and Supplements

- Herbs and botanical supplements should not be used without discussing with physician.
- Complementary and alternative medicine (CAM) is popular for musculoskeletal conditions. Some CAM modalities show significant promise, such as acupuncture (Martin et al, 2006), diets, herbal medicine, homoeopathy, massage, and supplements, but none of the treatments are totally devoid of risks (Ernst, 2004). Excellent resources are available on the Internet from the National Center for Complementary and Alternative Medicine (http://nccam.nih.gov).
- The sulfur-containing amino acids (SAAs) include methionine, cysteine, cystine, homocysteine, homocystine, and taurine; sulfur intake increases synthesis of *S*-adenosylmethionine (SAMe), glutathione (GSH), taurine, and *N*-acetylcysteine (Parcell, 2002). Magnesium; sulfur compounds such as SAMe, dimethylsulfoxide (DMSO), taurine, glucosamine, and chondroitin sulfate; and reduced GSH may have clinical applications in the treatment of FMS; controlled trials are needed (Holdcraft et al, 2003).

✔ INTERVENTION: NUTRITION EDUCATION, COUNSELING, CARE MANAGEMENT

- Discuss weight management goals such as weight loss for obesity.
- Daily exercise will be important for strengthening weak muscles. Exercise adherence is important and can help reduce the need for pain medications; positive health-related outcomes can be obtained with a low-cost, group multidisciplinary intervention (Lemstra and Olszynski, 2005).
- Discuss the role of omega-3 fatty acids in reduction of inflammation.

For More Information

- American Fibromyalgia Syndrome Association, Inc.
  http://www.afsafund.org/
- Fibromyalgia Network
  http://www.fmnetnews.com/
- Myositis Association
  http://www.myositis.org/
- National Fibromyalgia Partnership, Inc.
  http://www.fmpartnership.org/FMPartnership.htm
- National Institute of Arthritis and Musculoskeletal and Skin Diseases
  http://www.niams.nih.gov/hi/topics/fibromyalgia/fibrofs.htm

MYOFASCIAL PAIN SYNDROMES: FIBROMYALGIA AND POLYMYALGIA RHEUMATICA—CITED REFERENCES

Aggarwal BB, Shishodia S. Suppression of the nuclear factor-kappa B activation pathway by spice-derived phytochemicals: reasoning for seasoning. *Ann N Y Acad Sci.* 1030:434, 2004.

Assefi NP, et al. A randomized clinical trial of acupuncture compared with sham acupuncture in fibromyalgia. *Ann Intern Med.* 143:10, 2005.

Bennett RM, et al. Tramadol and acetaminophen combination tablets in the treatment of fibromyalgia pain: a double-blind, randomized, placebo-controlled study. *Am J Med.* 114:537, 2003.

Caporali R, et al. Prednisone plus methotrexate for polymyalgia rheumatica: a randomized, double-blind, placebo-controlled trial. *Ann Intern Med.* 141:493, 2004.

Ernst E. Musculoskeletal conditions and complementary/alternative medicine. *Best Pract Res Clin Rheumatol.* 18:539, 2004.

Hanninen O, et al. Antioxidants in vegan diet and rheumatic disorders. *Toxicology* 155:45, 2000.

Holdcraft LC, et al. Complementary and alternative medicine in fibromyalgia and related syndromes. *Best Pract Res Clin Rheumatol.* 17:667, 2003.

Lemstra M, Olszynski WP. The effectiveness of multidisciplinary rehabilitation in the treatment of fibromyalgia: a randomized controlled trial. *Clin J Pain.* 21:166, 2005.

Lucas HJ, et al. Fibromyalgia—new concepts of pathogenesis and treatment. *Int J Immunopathol Pharmacol.* 19:5, 2006.

Martin DP, et al. Improvement in fibromyalgia symptoms with acupuncture: results of a randomized controlled trial. *Mayo Clin Proc.* 81:749, 2006.

Mease P. Fibromyalgia syndrome: review of clinical presentation, pathogenesis, outcome measures, and treatment. *J Rheumatol.* 75:6S, 2005.

Parcell S. Sulfur in human nutrition and applications in medicine. *Altern Med Rev.* 7:22, 2002.

OSTEOARTHRITIS AND DEGENERATIVE JOINT DISEASE

NUTRITIONAL ACUITY RANKING: LEVEL 1–2

DEFINITIONS AND BACKGROUND

Osteoarthritis (OA) is a common health problem in populations over age 40 years, and it is a leading cause of pain and disability in the United States (Barnes and Edwards, 2005). OA may be primary (in elderly individuals) or may follow an injury or disease involving the articular surfaces of synovial joints; it is technically "osteoarthrosis." An estimated 43 million Americans report having arthritis, and 8 million people report that arthritis limits their daily activities, according to the Centers for Disease Control and Prevention. Symptoms include pain, swelling, and synovial joint stiffness. Serum concentrations of tumor necrosis factors are significantly associated with lower physical function and more symptoms of pain, stiffness, and physical disability (Penninx et al, 2004).

Treatments for OA combine nonpharmacological modalities, pharmacological agents, and surgical procedures (Barnes and Edwards, 2005). Weight loss is a primary treatment for OA. Surgery is reserved for those persons for whom other treatments have been unsuccessful.

Many individuals with OA are obese. Overweight causes strain on joints and should be managed early by health professionals to protect the joints (Gasbarrini and Piscaglia, 2005). As part of a long-term study of the effects of diet and exercise on knee OA, researchers have found that an average weight loss of 5% in overweight and obese older patients brings an 18% gain in overall function (Messier et al, 2005), and a 10% weight loss improves function by 28% (Christensen et al, 2005).

While vitamins A, C, D, and E have major roles in modulating oxidative stress, immune responses, and cell differentiation, recent controlled trials with these vitamins did not halt progression of knee OA (Choi, 2005). Diets rich in omega-3 fatty acids and low in omega-6 fatty acids may benefit people with OA by reducing joint stiffness and pain, increasing grip strength, and enhancing walking pace. Pomegranate fruit extracts can block interleukin-1β (IL-1β) enzymes that contribute to cartilage destruction and OA, according to a Case Western Reserve University School of Medicine study.

INTERVENTION: OBJECTIVES

- If patient is obese, lessen pressure on weight-bearing joints by losing weight.
- Encourage patient (especially if elderly) to consume adequate amounts of protein and calcium from a healthy diet.
- Joint replacement may be necessary; prepare for surgery accordingly. Weight loss may be beneficial.
- Maintain integrity of cartilage in affected joints; omega-3 fatty acids may reduce the activity of enzymes that destroy cartilage. Include fish oils and certain plant seed oils that impact immune and inflammatory responses as precursors of eicosanoids.

INTERVENTION: FOOD AND NUTRITION

- Use a calorie-controlled diet if obesity is present. Use of a meal replacement may help to promote weight loss, even among those who have low incomes (Huerta et al, 2004).
- The inflammatory response may be suppressed by an increase in omega-3 fatty acids, as found in fatty fish (mackerel, herring, and salmon) and from walnuts and flaxseed. Use these foods several times a week.
- Milk, fatty fish such as salmon, eggs, some fortified cereals, and multivitamin supplements may be used under supervision to provide vitamin D.
- Include plenty of fruits and vegetables for their phytochemicals. Pomegranates, for example, are especially protective because of their content of ellagic acid. Include spices such as turmeric (curcumin); red pepper (capsaicin); cloves (eugenol); ginger (gingerol); cumin, anise, and fennel (anethol); basil and rosemary (ursolic acid); and garlic (diallyl sulfide, *S*-allylmercaptocysteine, and ajoene) (Aggarwal and Shishodia, 2004).

CLINICAL INDICATORS

Clinical/History	Lab Work	
Height	Antistreptolysin titer (ASO)	Antirheumatoid factor
Weight	Antinuclear antibodies (ANA) (to rule out other conditions)	BUN, Creat
BMI	Lupus erythematosus (LE) prep (to rule out other conditions)	Sedimentation rate
Obesity		CRP
X-rays; DEXA		Gluc
Osteoarthritis Index for pain, physical function, and stiffness		Alk phos
		Uric acid
		Ca++, Mg++
		Na+, K+
		Serum folate
		Serum B_{12}

SAMPLE NUTRITION DIAGNOSTIC STATEMENT

Osteoarthritis

PES: Overweight related to eating double portions at lunch and dinner meals as evidenced by increased pain in weight-bearing joints with diagnosis of osteoarthritis.

Assessment Data (sources of info): Food intake records, weight records, symptoms diary.

Intervention: Counseling about dietary weight management tips, tips for dining out or snacking, referral to physical therapy for acceptable exercises to reduce pain in affected joints.

Monitoring and Evaluation: Weight changes, food intake records, symptoms diary.

Common Drugs Used and Potential Side Effects (see Table 11-5)

- Pharmacological measures should be examined carefully by the physician and the patient, evaluating risks and benefits (Barnes and Edwards, 2005). A useful online drug information guide is available at http:// www.arthritis.org/ conditions/DrugGuide/drug_index.asp.

Herbs, Botanicals, and Supplements

- See Table 11-6.

INTERVENTION: NUTRITION EDUCATION, COUNSELING, CARE MANAGEMENT

- Encourage patient to avoid fad diets for "arthritis cure." Ensure that the patient's diet is balanced and includes all nutrients.
- Physical and occupational therapies, diet, and exercise play an extremely important role; thus significant patient education is important (Barnes and Edwards, 2005). The Arthritis, Diet, and Activity Promotion Trial (ADAPT) was a randomized, single-blind clinical trial designed to determine whether long-term exercise and dietary weight loss are more effective than usual care in obese adults with knee OA; diet plus exercise yielded significant improvements in physical function, walking distance, stair-climb time, and knee pain (Messier et al, 2004).
- Weight loss to alleviate stress on the joints is important where needed (Nicklas et al, 2004). Pharmacological and behavioral techniques, such as self-monitoring, should be included (Berkel et al, 2005).
- OA has no life-threatening risks but does allow muscles around the joints to become weak when there is disuse. Exercise and stretching should be suggested for daily application to maintain flexibility. Long-term weight training and aerobic walking programs significantly improve balance in older adults.
- Acupuncture may relieve pain. Tai Chi can help balance and protect bones.

For More Information

- American Juvenile Arthritis Foundation
  http://arthritis.about.com/gi/dynamic/offsite.htm?zi=1/XJ&sdn=arthritis&zu=http%3A%2F%2Fwww.arthritis.org%2F

TABLE 11-5 Medications Commonly Used for Osteoarthritis

Medication	Comments	Side Effects
Aspirin	Can be taken with meals to reduce gastric distress.	Prolonged use can cause gastrointestinal (GI) bleeding; intake of folate should be increased.
Nonsteroidal anti-inflammatory drugs (NSAIDs)	COX-2 selective agents (Vioxx, Celebrex, and Bextra) may be associated with an increased risk of serious cardiovascular events (heart attack and stroke); FDA has removed Vioxx from the market. Long-term use of a nonselective NSAID, naproxen (sold as Aleve, Naprosyn, and other trade name and generic products), may be associated with an increased cardiovascular risk compared to placebo. Take NSAIDs with food; anorexia, flatulence, and GI distress may result otherwise. Add extra folic acid and vitamin B_{12} to diet.	Indomethacin (Indocin) and sulindac (Clinoril) may cause nausea, renal failure, or diarrhea. Etodolac (Lodine) may cause renal failure or abdominal pain. Naprosyn can cause abdominal pain, nausea, or heartburn. Tolmetin (Tolectin) causes abdominal pain, nausea and vomiting, and GI upset. Ibuprofen (Advil/Motrin) may cause nausea and vomiting. Choline magnesium trisalicylate (Trilisate) may cause constipation, diarrhea, and nausea and vomiting.
Misoprostol (Cytotec)	Misoprostol reduces stomach acid if NSAIDs are used	Abdominal cramps may occur.
Glucosamine sulfate and chondroitin	Glucosamine reduces cartilage damage and decreases pain associated with osteoarthritis; with chondroitin, it may help relieve symptoms of osteoarthritis (McAlindon et al, 2000). X-rays have shown that cartilage thickness is somewhat protected. Sulfate may be a key factor (Hoffer et al, 2001). Some pills do not contain sufficient levels to be effective; check brand with www.consumerlab.com to assure that the choice is best.	Glucosamine can increase blood glucose levels and aggravate shellfish allergy because it is made from these shells. Chondroitin may alter blood clotting activity in a manner similar to that of aspirin.
Omega-3 fatty acids	Supplementation specifically with omega-3 fatty acids causes a decrease in both degradative and inflammatory aspects of chondrocyte metabolism. Data provide evidence of the beneficial effect of slowing and reducing inflammation in the pathogenesis of degenerative joint diseases (Curtis et al, 2002).	May increase effects of blood-thinning drugs and herbs.
Corticosteroids	Steroids may cause sodium retention; calcium, nitrogen, and potassium depletion; truncal obesity; and hyperglycemia.	Corticosteroids may have a short-term effect in osteoarthritis (Bellamy et al, 2005).

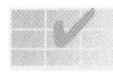

TABLE 11-6 Side Effects of Common Herbs Used for Arthritis

Bromelain: May increase effects of blood-thinning drugs and tetracycline antibiotics.

Echinacea: Might counteract immunosuppressant drugs, such as glucocorticoids, taken for lupus and rheumatoid arthritis; might increase side effects of methotrexate.

Evening primrose oil: Can counteract the effects of anticonvulsant drugs.

Folic acid: Interferes with methotrexate.

Gamma linoleic acid (GLA): May increase effects of blood-thinning drugs and herbs.

Garlic: Can increase effects of blood-thinning drugs and herbs.

Ginger: Can increase nonsteroidal anti-inflammatory drug (NSAID) side effects and effects of blood-thinning drugs and herbs.

Ginkgo: May increase effects of blood-thinning drugs and herbs.

Ginseng: May increase effects of blood-thinning drugs, estrogens, and glucocorticoids; shouldn't be used by those with diabetes; may interact with monoamine oxidase (MAO) inhibitors.

Kava: Can increase effects of alcohol, sedatives, and tranquilizers.

Magnesium: May interact with blood pressure medications.

***S*-adenosylmethionine (SAMe):** SAMe is being studied for its role in rebuilding eroded joint cartilage; it is also useful for mild depression. Enteric coating is needed because of gastrointestinal (GI) side effects.

Soy: Soy and avocado extracts have been approved for use in France for several years for their antioxidant effects in reducing the symptoms of osteoarthritis.

St. John's wort: May enhance effects of narcotics, alcohol, and antidepressants; increases risk of sunburn; interferes with iron absorption.

Valerian: Can increase the effects of sedatives and tranquilizers.

Vitamin E: Gamma-tocopherol may worsen osteoarthritis; alpha-tocopherol is better. A double-blind study in Australia found no relief of symptomatic pain (Brand et al, 2001).

Zinc: Can interfere with glucocorticoids and other immunosuppressive drugs.

Note: Herbs and botanical supplements should not be used without discussing with physician. Excerpted from the Arthritis Foundation. The Arthritis Foundation's guide to alternative therapies. Available at http://www.arthritis.org.

- Arthritis Resource Center at Healingwell
  http://www.healingwell.com/arthritis
- Information on Osteoarthritis
  http://www.niams.nih.gov/hi/topics/arthritis/oahandout.htm
- Johns Hopkins Arthritis Center
  http://www.hopkins-arthritis.som.jhmi.edu/

OSTEOARTHRITIS AND DEGENERATIVE JOINT DISEASE—CITED REFERENCES

Aggarwal BB, Shishodia S. Suppression of the nuclear factor-kappa B activation pathway by spice-derived phytochemicals: reasoning for seasoning. *Ann N Y Acad Sci.* 1030:434, 2004.

Barnes EV, Edwards NL. Treatment of osteoarthritis. *South Med J.* 98:205, 2005.

Bellamy N, et al. Intraarticular corticosteroid for treatment of osteoarthritis of the knee. *Cochrane Database Syst Rev.* 2:CD005328, 2005.

Berkel LA, et al. Behavioral interventions for obesity. *J Am Diet Assoc.* 105:35S, 2005.

Brand C, et al. Vitamin E is ineffective for symptomatic relief of knee osteoarthritis: a 6-month double-blind, randomized, placebo-controlled study. *Ann Rheum Dis.* 60:946, 2001.

Choi HK. Dietary risk factors for rheumatic diseases. *Curr Opin Rheumatol.* 17:141, 2005.

Christensen R, et al. Weight loss: the treatment of choice for knee osteoarthritis? A randomized trial. *Osteoarthritis Cartilage* 13:20, 2005.

Curtis CL, et al. Effects of n-3 fatty acids on cartilage metabolism. *Proc Nutr Soc.* 61:381, 2002.

Gasbarrini A, Piscaglia AC. A natural diet versus modern Western diets? A new approach to prevent "well-being syndromes." *Dig Dis Sci.* 50:1, 2005.

Hoffer L, et al. Sulfate could mediate the therapeutic effect of glucosamine sulfate. *Metabolism* 50:767, 2001.

Huerta S, et al. Feasibility of a partial meal replacement plan for weight loss in low-income patients. *Int J Obes Relat Metab Disord.* 28:1575, 2004.

McAlindon T, et al. Glucosamine and chondroitin for treatment of osteoarthritis: a systematic quality assessment and meta-analysis. *JAMA.* 283:1469, 2000.

Messier SP, et al. Exercise and dietary weight loss in overweight and obese older adults with knee osteoarthritis: the Arthritis, Diet, and Activity Promotion Trial. *Arthritis Rheum.* 50:1501, 2004.

Messier SP, et al. Weight loss reduces knee-joint loads in overweight and obese older adults with knee osteoarthritis. *Arthritis Rheum.* 52:2026, 2005.

Nicklas BJ, et al. Diet-induced weight loss, exercise, and chronic inflammation in older, obese adults: a randomized controlled clinical trial. *Am J Clin Nutr.* 79:544, 2004.

Penninx BW, et al. Inflammatory markers and physical function among older adults with knee osteoarthritis. *J Rheumatol.* 31:1004, 2004.

OSTEOMYELITIS

NUTRITIONAL ACUITY RANKING: LEVEL 1–2

DEFINITIONS AND BACKGROUND

Acute osteomyelitis may be caused by localized infection of the long bones or injury to bone and surrounding soft tissue. *Staphylococcus aureus* is implicated in most patients with acute hematogenous osteomyelitis; *S. epidermidis, S. aureus, Pseudomonas aeruginosa, Serratia marcescens,* and *Escherichia coli* are commonly isolated in patients with chronic osteomyelitis (Carek et al, 2001). See Figure 11-3.

When a bone is infected, the bone marrow swells and compresses against the rigid outer wall of bone, and blood vessels may be compressed or die; abscesses may form. Symptoms and signs include sudden, acute pain (often in the joint nearest the site of infection), fever, chills, tachycardia, diaphoresis, nausea and vomiting, dehydration, electrolyte imbalance, contractures in affected extremities, and pressure ulcers.

Some diseases predispose patients to osteomyelitis, including diabetes mellitus, sickle cell disease, acquired immunodeficiency virus (AIDS), intravenous drug abuse, alcoholism, chronic steroid use, immunosuppression, and chronic joint disease. Use of prosthetic orthopedic devices

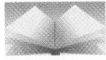

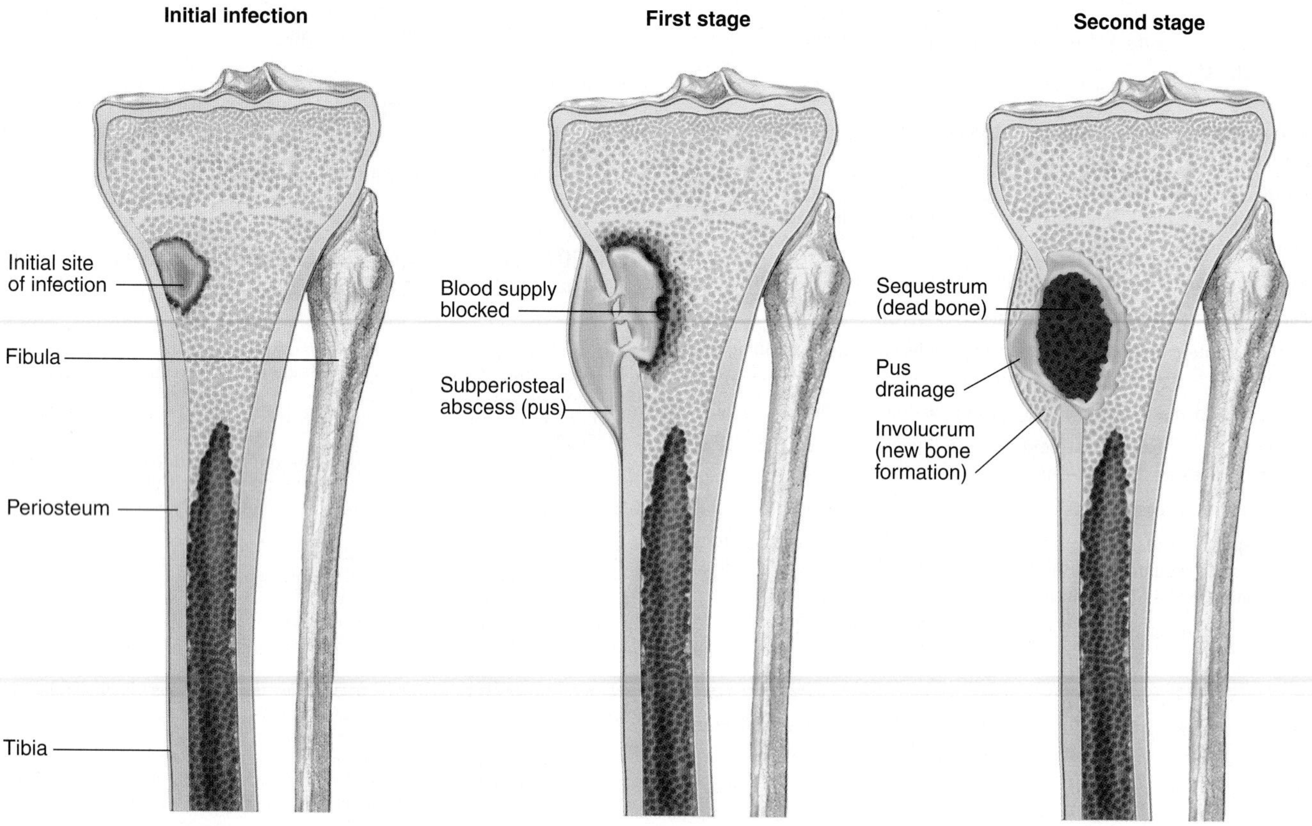

Figure 11-3 Osteomyelitis. (Image provided by Anatomical Chart Co.)

and recent orthopedic surgery or open fracture may also place a patient at risk for osteomyelitis.

Patients with diabetes mellitus with poor glucose control may experience infections of the lower extremities, from superficial cellulitis to deep soft tissue infections and osteomyelitis (Clay et al, 2004). Because osteomyelitis is prevalent after diabetic foot ulcers, careful treatment is crucial to avoid amputation (Schinabeck and Johnson, 2005).

In children, serious musculoskeletal infections include osteomyelitis, septic arthritis, pyomyositis, and necrotizing fasciitis (Frank et al, 2005). Prompt treatment is important. If not treated properly, the condition may become chronic. The chronic form has a poor prognosis.

Treatment generally involves evaluation, staging, determination of etiology, antimicrobial therapy, and debridement or stabilization of bone (Carek et al, 2001).

INTERVENTION: OBJECTIVES

- Characterize and treat the infection. Prevent further infection, dehydration, and other complications.
- Promote recovery and healing; reduce fever.
- Correct defective blood flow to allow nutrients and oxygen to reach all tissues.
- Control hyperglycemia.
- Correct nausea and vomiting where present.

INTERVENTION: FOOD AND NUTRITION

- Encourage adequate fluid intake.
- Maintain a normal to high calorie and protein intake, with adequate amounts of vitamins and minerals included (e.g., zinc, vitamin A, and vitamin C).
- With diabetes, control carbohydrate to promote more effective healing.

CLINICAL INDICATORS

Clinical/History

Height
Weight
BMI
Intake and output (I & O)
Temperature
Blood pressure (BP)
Magnetic resonance imaging (MRI) or bone densitometry
Bone x-rays
Skin lesions with a sinus tract

Lab Work

CRP and ESR (increased)
Gluc
Alb, transthyretin
BUN, Creat
Alk phos
AST, ALT
Ca++, Mg++
Na+, K+
White blood cell count (WBC) (increased)

Common Drugs Used and Potential Side Effects

- Antibiotics are needed to correct infections that are present; vancomycin or amphotericin B may be used. Monitor for specific side effects and timing of meals. For optimal results, antibiotic therapy must be started early, with antimicrobial agents administered parenterally for at least 4–6 weeks (Carek et al, 2001).
- Analgesics may be used for pain. Gastrointestinal distress is a common side effect. Extra vitamin C may be needed.
- Metronidazole/ceftriaxone (MTZ/CTX) given once daily plus ticarcillin/clavulanate potassium (T/C) given every 6 hours in hospitalized older males with diabetic lower extremity infections may reduce institutional costs (Clay et al, 2004).

Herbs, Botanicals, and Supplements

- Herbs and botanical supplements should not be used without discussing with physician.

INTERVENTION: NUTRITION EDUCATION, COUNSELING, CARE MANAGEMENT

- Discuss role of nutrition in wound healing, immunity, and other conditions related to this disorder.
- Discuss signs that may indicate reversal of status or recovery.

For More Information

- National Institutes of Health–Osteomyelitis
  http://www.nlm.nih.gov/medlineplus/ency/article/000437.htm

OSTEOMYELITIS—CITED REFERENCES

Carek P, et al. Diagnosis and management of osteomyelitis. *Am Fam Physician.* 63:2413, 2001.

Clay PG, et al. Clinical efficacy, tolerability, and cost savings associated with the use of open-label metronidazole plus ceftriaxone once daily compared with ticarcillin/clavulanate every 6 hours as empiric treatment for diabetic lower-extremity infections in older males. *Am J Geriatr Pharmacother.* 2:181, 2004.

Frank G, et al. Musculoskeletal infections in children. *Pediatr Clin North Am.* 52:1083, 2005.

Schinabeck MK, Johnson JL. Osteomyelitis in diabetic foot ulcers. Prompt diagnosis can avert amputation. *Postgrad Med.* 118:11, 2005.

OSTEOMALACIA

NUTRITIONAL ACUITY RANKING: LEVEL 2

DEFINITIONS AND BACKGROUND

Osteomalacia, adult rickets, causes demineralization of the bone from deficiency of vitamin D. Osteomalacia may occur in conjunction with bone loss and hip fractures but more commonly results from vitamin D deficiency that occurs with Crohn's disease, colon resection, chronic renal failure, cystic fibrosis, celiac disease, or chronic use of anticonvulsants.

Severe vitamin D deficiency leads to secondary hyperparathyroidism, increased bone turnover and loss, and osteomalacia; deficiency is common in elderly people, especially the institutionalized (Lips et al, 2001). Dark-skinned individuals are also at risk, especially in northern states and latitudes.

In osteomalacia, bones become softened and deformed. Other symptoms include muscular weakness, listlessness, and aches.

INTERVENTION: OBJECTIVES

- Provide correct amount of calcium, phosphorus, and vitamin D. Because vitamins K and B_{12} and folic acid have been found to support bone health, include them in sufficient amounts to meet DRI levels.
- Prevent or reverse, if possible, bone density loss resulting from calcium loss in the bone matrix.

INTERVENTION: FOOD AND NUTRITION

- Diets should be high in calcium; adults will need 1200–1500 mg.
- If patient is lactose intolerant, try Lactaid or other forms of lactose-free milk, broccoli, greens, and other sources of calcium.
- Potassium, magnesium, and fruit and vegetable intake may contribute to maintenance of bone mineral density (Tucker et al, 1999). Include micronutrients vitamin C and vitamin K and other potentially important nutrients.
- Vitamin D treatment is now administered at higher levels because of reduced concerns about toxicity.

CLINICAL INDICATORS

Clinical/History

Height
Weight
BMI
Bone pain

Bone densitometry, DEXA

Lab Work

Serum P (decreased)
Serum Ca++ (decreased)
Urinary Ca++
Serum 25-hydroxyvitamin D (25-OHD) to

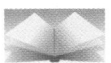

evaluate deficiency levels	Na+, K+	transthyretin
PTH	Alk phos (increased)	CRP
Mg++	Alb,	BUN
		Creat

Common Drugs Used and Potential Side Effects

- Treatment with calcium salts should be monitored frequently to prevent hypercalcemia; use with plenty of liquids. Avoid taking with iron supplements or bulk-forming laxatives. High-calcium diets may reduce zinc absorption and balance and may, therefore, increase zinc requirements (Wood and Zheng, 1997).
- Anticonvulsant therapy, tranquilizers, sedatives, muscle relaxants, and oral diabetic agents may deplete vitamin D. Phosphate binders with aluminum may precipitate osteomalacia; calcium carbonate may be useful, but do not take it with whole grains, bran, high-oxalate foods, or iron tablets.
- Drugs that inhibit calcium absorption include neomycin, thyroid hormone, triamterene, heparin, steroids, and cholestyramine.

Herbs, Botanicals, and Supplements

- Herbs and botanical supplements should not be used without discussing with physician.

INTERVENTION: NUTRITION EDUCATION, COUNSELING, CARE MANAGEMENT

- Explain which foods are good sources of calcium, phosphorus, and vitamin D. Encourage patient to spend time in the sun for skin synthesis of vitamin D; avoid sunburn.
- Explain that fortified margarine and milk are dietary sources of vitamin D.
- Vegetarians who avoid dairy products may be at risk for calcium and vitamin D depletion; discuss alternative sources from diet or from necessary supplementation.

For More Information

- Osteomalacia
  http://www.nlm.nih.gov/medlineplus/ency/article/000376.htm#Definition

OSTEOMALACIA—CITED REFERENCES

Lips P, et al. A global study of vitamin D status and parathyroid function in postmenopausal women with osteoporosis: baseline data from the multiple outcomes of raloxifene evaluation clinical trial. *J Clin Endocrinol Metab.* 86:1212, 2001.

Tucker K, et al. Potassium, magnesium, and fruit and vegetable intakes are associated with greater bone mineral density in elderly men and women. *Am J Clin Nutr.* 69:727, 1999.

Wood R, Zheng J. High dietary calcium intakes reduce zinc absorption and balance in humans. *Am J Clin Nutr.* 65:1803, 1997.

OSTEOPENIA AND OSTEOPOROSIS

NUTRITIONAL ACUITY RANKING: LEVEL 2

DEFINITIONS AND BACKGROUND

Osteopenia is a decrease in the amount of calcium and phosphorus in the bones. It is identified by a decrease in bone density, which is evident through a dual-energy x-ray absorptiometry (DEXA) scan. It can occur in premature infants or in adults as a result of long-term inflammatory bowel disease, especially Crohn's disease, or from factors such as low body mass index (BMI).

Nutrient intake is important. Plasma 25-hydroxyvitamin D (25-OHD) is the most sensitive clinical index of vitamin D status and is related to bone mineral density (BMD) in middle-aged and elderly women (Budak et al, 2004). Intake of biologically active silicon, orthosilicic acid, may be more effective in enhancing bone density than use of calcium and vitamin D_3 alone (Reffitt et al, 2003). In addition, protein intake above current recommendations may be needed in elderly women to preserve bone mass (Devine et al, 2005; Dawson-Hughes and Harris, 2002).

Osteoporosis is the most common bone disease in humans, especially in Western society. It is characterized by low bone mass, structural deterioration, and decreased bone strength. In the whole population, more than 7.8 million people have osteoporosis; about 2 million men are affected. The aging population is highly affected.

Seven percent of non-Hispanic white and Asian men aged 50 and older are estimated to have osteoporosis, and 35% are estimated to have low bone mass. Men are especially vulnerable when they have renal failure, smoke, or take medications on a regular basis, such as anticonvulsants, corticosteroids, or barbiturates.

Osteoporosis can be a silent disease until a fragility fracture occurs at the hip and proximal humerus, when significant physical disability may result. One out of every two white women will experience an osteoporotic fracture at some point in time. Osteoporosis is responsible for more than 1.5 million fractures annually, including 300,000 hip fractures, 700,000 vertebral fractures, 250,000 wrist fractures, and more than 300,000 fractures at other sites (National Institutes of Health, 2000). Fractures of the hip and spine are most common (see Fig. 11-4).

The National Osteoporosis Foundation (NOF, 2005) estimates that 20% of postmenopausal white women in the United States have osteoporosis and an additional 52% have

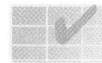

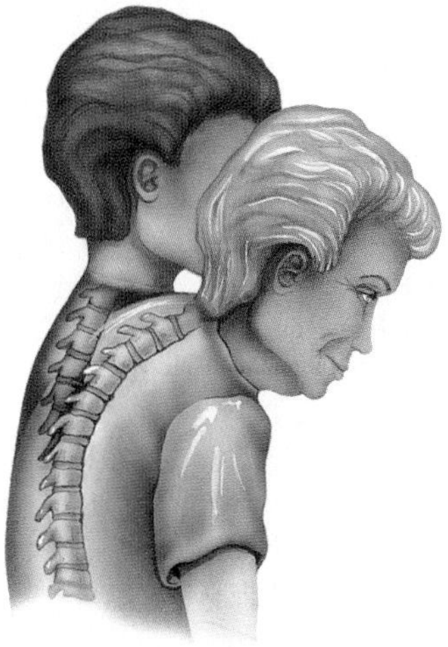

Figure 11-4 Photo showing deterioration of vertebral support. (Image provided by Anatomical Chart Co.)

low bone density at the hip. Women can lose up to 20% of their bone mass in the 5–7 years following menopause. The World Health Organization (2005) defines osteoporosis as a BMD value that is 2.5 standard deviations or more below the mean of a young adult of the same sex; therefore, the lower the BMD, the greater the fracture risk (Cummings et al, 2002).

Falls are associated with a higher risk of frailty fractures (Schwartz et al, 2005). Spinal or vertebral fractures may lead to loss of height, severe back pain, and spinal deformities such as kyphosis or stooped posture. Hip fractures require hospitalization and major surgery; they impair the ability to walk and may cause disability or death. By 2050, the number of hip fractures is expected to increase about three- or fourfold from the estimated 1.7 million in 1990 (World Health Organization, 2005).

Awareness and management of risk factors can be important for preventing osteoporosis and related disability. Both genetic and lifestyle factors play a role in BMD and risk for osteoporosis. Elevated plasma homocysteine levels are associated with both cardiovascular disease (CVD) and osteoporosis; statins stimulate bone formation (McFarlane et al, 2004). Postmenopausal women who have a history of diabetes are also at higher risk of osteoporosis (Nicodemus et al, 2001). Women may lose bone during lactation if their diets are low in calcium and other nutrients. Depression has been associated with decreases in BMD (Robbins et al, 2001). See Table 11-7, which lists risk factors for osteoporosis.

BMD is just one of many contributors to bone strength and fracture risk reduction (Cefalu, 2004). Interleukin-1 protein has been known for many years to be a stimulator of the immune system. In the skeleton, the protein causes an increase in the number and activity of osteoclastic cells—the cells that break down bone tissue and that develop from the same cells as those of the immune system.

Physical activity has different effects depending on its intensity, frequency, and duration, and the age at which it is started, with greater effects in adolescence and as a result of weight-bearing exercise (Branca and Vatuena, 2001). In addition, diet contributes significantly. See Table 11-8 for a list of nutrients and their respective roles in managing bone health.

Building strong bones during childhood and adolescence can be the best defense against developing osteoporosis later. By about age 20 years, most women have acquired 98% of total bone mass. Acquisition of a high peak bone mass (reaching genetic potential) by 30 years of age helps reduce bone losses later in life. To optimize bone health and to help prevent osteoporosis, include a balanced diet rich in calcium and vitamin D; weight-bearing and resistance-training exercises; a healthy lifestyle with no smoking or excessive alcohol intake; talking to one's health care professional about bone health; bone density testing; and medication when appropriate.

INTERVENTION: OBJECTIVES

- Preserve height, support independence, and improve functional status.
- Prevent osteoporosis and fractures (Tussing and Chapman-Novakofski, 2005).
- Lessen the risk of fractures by supporting dietary adequacy and adequate activity levels that are not excessive. Promote weight-bearing and muscle-strengthening exercises.
- Decrease precipitating factors, such as anticonvulsants, corticosteroids, lactase deficiency, low milk intake, general low intake of calcium or calcium malabsorption, sedentary lifestyle, and low weight for height.
- Provide adequate time for evaluating improvement (6–9 months at least).
- Assure adequate intake of protein.
- Intake of fruit and vegetables appears to be positively associated with bone health; magnesium and potassium are significantly related to total bone mass (New et al, 2000).
- Avoid excesses of caffeine (>300 mg) and alcohol (limit to 1 drink for women and 2 drinks for men per day).
- Soft drinks should not replace daily use of milk products.

INTERVENTION: FOOD AND NUTRITION

- Advise all patients to consume adequate amounts of calcium (≥1200 mg/d, including supplements if necessary) and vitamin D (400–800 IU/d for individuals at risk of deficiency). Women after menopause or over age 65 years will need 1500 mg calcium daily. For vitamin D, choose fortified milk, cod liver oil, egg yolks, and fatty fish; do not exceed 2000 IU/d.
- To fulfill the requirement, 1 quart of milk daily can be consumed. If fluid milk is not consumed, dry skim milk powder can be added to many foods. Aged cheeses and yogurt are sources as well.
- Calcium supplements can be used if dairy products are not tolerated; calcium absorption averages approximately 30–40% from most sources. Space the supplements throughout the day; take no more than 500–600 mg two or more times daily with meals. Use with vitamin D and magnesium.
- Higher doses than the current recommendation of vitamin D in persons over age 65 years may be required for

TABLE 11-7 Risk Factors for Osteoporosis

Factors That Cannot Be Changed:

- Female gender
- Family history of osteoporosis
- Being thin or having a slender frame; low body mass index (BMI) and low muscle mass
- Current low bone mass
- Caucasians, especially women of Northern European extraction, and Asian women
- Personal history of fracture after age 50 years
- History of fracture in a first-degree relative
- Advanced age

Factors That Might Be Altered:

- Estrogen deficiency from premature menopause, amenorrhea
- Excessive use of alcohol
- Current smoking
- Lifetime diet low in calcium (poor diet, excess fiber)
- Sedentary lifestyle or extended bed rest (immobilization)
- Low vitamin D intake or sunlight exposure
- Hypogonadism, as from low estrogen levels or anorexia nervosa
- Low testosterone levels in men
- Use of medications such as chemotherapy, tamoxifen, glucocorticoids, lithium, and some anticonvulsants
- Long-term total parenteral nutrition
- Depression, past or current
- Anorexia nervosa
- Hypertension or diabetes
- Elevated plasma homocysteine levels

Conditions or Diseases That May Lead to Osteoporosis:

- AIDS/HIV
- Amyloidosis
- Ankylosing spondylitis
- Celiac disease
- Chronic obstructive pulmonary disease
- Congenital porphyria
- Cushing's syndrome
- Diabetes, type 1
- Female athlete triad
- Gastrectomy
- Gaucher's disease
- Hemochromatosis
- Hemophilia
- Hyperparathyroidism
- Hypophosphatasia
- Idiopathic scoliosis
- Inflammatory bowel disease
- Liver disease, severe
- Lymphoma and leukemia
- Malabsorption syndromes
- Mastocytosis
- Multiple myeloma
- Multiple sclerosis
- Osteomalacia
- Pernicious anemia
- Primary biliary cirrhosis
- Rheumatoid arthritis
- Spinal cord transection
- Stroke (cerebrovascular accident)
- Thalassemia
- Thyrotoxicosis
- Tropical sprue

TABLE 11-8 Nutrients and Bone Health

Nutrient	Comments
Alcohol	Moderate drinking (1–2 glasses of wine daily) is associated with increased trochanteric bone mineral density (BMD), but higher intakes may be associated with lower BMD (Ganry et al, 2000; New et al, 2000). Use guidelines of 1 drink daily for women and no more than 2 for men.
B-complex vitamins	Folic acid and vitamins B_6 and B_{12} help to lower homocysteine when elevated.
Boron	Uncertain role.
Caffeine	Over 300 mg/d of caffeine can negatively impact the vitamin D receptor gene (*VDR*), and the Site Testing Osteoporosis Prevention and Intervention Trial (STOP-IT) found that greater amounts of caffeine affect BMD negatively (Rapuri et al, 2001). Limit intake to 3 cups of coffee daily and 5 servings of caffeinated soft drinks or tea; be sure to include adequate amounts of calcium.
Calcium and vitamin D	Dietary supplementation with calcium (1200 mg or more) and vitamin D (800–1000 IU) supports strong bone matrix, moderately reduces bone loss, and reduces the incidence of fractures. Vitamin D may actually be more important than calcium.
Magnesium and potassium	Low intakes of magnesium and potassium contribute to bone loss (New et al, 2000).
Protein and soy	70–100 g/d provides more bone building. Soy yields isoflavones for increasing bone density; use dietary sources. More soy in the diet may lead to fewer fractures.
Silicon	There may be a role for silicon in stimulation of collagen synthesis and osteoblast differentiation (Reffitt et al, 2003). Uncertain importance.
Sodium	Excesses can increase calcium excretion. Avoid using salt at the table, and limit total intake to 2400 mg/d.
Vitamin A	High intake of retinol may be associated with increased risk of fractures and osteoporosis.
Vitamin C	Part of collagen, which supports healthy bone structure. Tissues saturate at 200 mg/d.
Vitamin K	Supports osteocalcin for bone strength. Supplement with 120 μg may be needed.

optimal bone health; use 800–1000 IU/d (Nieves, 2005). Encourage use of vitamin D–fortified milk.
- Extra protein may be needed (Devine et al, 2005).
- For sufficient intake of vitamin B_{12}, include dairy products, meat, poultry, fish, and fortified cereals.
- Isoflavones may also prove to be beneficial (2–3 servings of soy foods daily).
- If patient is obese, use a calorie-controlled diet that provides adequate protein, vitamins, calcium, and other minerals.
- Adequate manganese, vitamins C and K, potassium, and magnesium also should be consumed to meet at least the DRI levels. Include dietary components (fruits and vegetables) that contribute to bone health.
- Beware of excesses of wheat bran because phytates may increase calcium excretion.
- Sodium must be controlled; keep sodium within desired limits while increasing potassium and magnesium.
- Intake of caffeine in coffee does not seem to be a problem if calcium (as from milk) is consumed in adequate amounts.
- Assure that folic acid and vitamins B_6 and B_{12} are adequate, especially if serum homocysteine levels are elevated.

CLINICAL INDICATORS

Clinical/History	Lab Work	
Height	Ca++	Serum P (may be decreased with hyperparathyroidism)
Weight	Urinary Ca++	Serum homocysteine
BMI	Mg++	Serum folate
Back pain	Na+, K+	Serum B_{12}
BP	Serum 25-OHD	
Bone densitometry, DEXA	Alb	
	CRP	
	PTH (useful in some patients)	

SAMPLE NUTRITION DIAGNOSTIC STATEMENT

Osteoporosis

PES: Inadequate intake of vitamin D related to poor dietary intake of food sources and no use of supplements as evidenced by very low bone mineral density and high fracture risk.

Assessment Data (sources of info): Food records, dual-energy x-ray absorptiometry (DEXA) scan.

Intervention: Counseling about good sources of vitamin D from diet and supplements, meal planning and shopping tips, dining out guide, referral to Meals-on-Wheels or other social agencies as appropriate, appropriate role for sunshine exposure.

Monitoring and Evaluation: Improvements in dietary and supplemental intake of vitamin D as shown in food records, lab values, and DEXA scan report.

Common Drugs Used and Potential Side Effects (see Tables 11-9 and 11-10)

- Adequate calcium and vitamin D intake are crucial to develop optimal peak bone mass and to preserve bone mass throughout life. Supplementation of these two components in bioavailable forms may be necessary in individuals who do not achieve recommended intake from dietary sources (National Institutes of Health, 2000).
- Oral alendronic acid is the reference drug for menopausal women with osteopenia. It may be used with parathormone as well, but this has a 2-year limit (Black et al, 2005).

Herbs, Botanicals, and Supplements

- Herbs and botanical supplements should not be used without discussing with physician. Cabbage, pigweed, dandelion, avocado, and parsley have been recommended, but there is no proof of efficacy.

INTERVENTION: NUTRITION EDUCATION, COUNSELING, CARE MANAGEMENT

- Prevention is the best medicine. Encourage patient to stand upright, rather than sit or recline, as often as feasible. Measures to decrease fall frequency and to slow down the rapid life pace of healthy people with low bone mass should prevent some fractures (Kelsey et al, 2005).
- Change a sedentary lifestyle. Regular exercise, especially resistance and high-impact activities, contributes to development of high peak bone mass and may reduce the risk of falls in older individuals (National Institutes of Health, 2000). Aerobic and strengthening exercises are beneficial. Walking or running is beneficial. However, excessive weight-bearing exercise can cause amenorrhea in premenopausal women when a low-calorie diet is consumed.
- An educational osteoporosis prevention program, using hands-on activities, can increase self-efficacy (Tussing and Chapman-Novakofski, 2005). Explain that calcium absorption declines with age. Adequate calcium and vitamin D are important throughout life.
- The overall benefit of healthful eating must be strongly emphasized. It may also be cost effective to consider public health initiatives, such as calcium and vitamin D supplementation in the elderly.
- Describe importance of the use of milk, cheeses, yogurt, broccoli, kale and other greens, and soybeans. Provide recipes and shopping tips.
- Decrease the use of alcohol and tobacco.
- Caffeine poses a minimal risk unless it replaces calcium-containing beverages; BMD is not affected by caffeine if at least 1 glass of milk is consumed daily.
- Encourage adequate exposure to sunlight (10–30 min/d), but be wary of sunburn and overexposure with its risks of skin cancer.
- Remind all teenagers that osteoporosis is "kid stuff" in that maintenance of weight-bearing activity is important during the growing years. Consumption of carbonated beverages instead of milk is a big concern.

TABLE 11-9 Tips on Calcium Supplements

Elemental calcium varies in different supplements:

- Calcium carbonate (Tums, Roxane, Os-Cal, Calciday, Oyst-Cal, Oystercal, Caltrate) contains 40%.
- Calcium chloride contains 36%.
- Tricalcium phosphate provides 39%.
- Calcium acetate (Phos-Ex, PhosLo) contains 25%.
- Calcium citrate (Citracal) contains 21%.
- Calcium lactate contains 13%.
- Calcium gluconate contains 9%.

Rates of calcium absorption vary, and dietary sources are the best absorbed. Calcium maleate is also well absorbed. Calcium carbonate temporarily decreases gastric acidity, which is needed for calcium absorption. Bone meal or Dolomite may include contaminants and should be avoided (even with a 33% calcium content). Excesses of calcium supplements can cause hypercalcemia; monitor intakes carefully and take no more than 500–600 mg two or more times daily with meals. Beware of excess vitamin D, which can cause vitamin D calcinosis, and avoid taking with iron supplements. Use extra water with supplements.

Product	Source of Calcium (mg)	No. of Tablets/Day to Provide About 900–1000 mg Calcium Per Tablet
Caltrate 600	Carbonate (600 mg)	1.5
Os-Cal 500	Carbonate from oyster shell (500 mg)	2
Os-Cal 500 + Vitamin D	Carbonate from oyster shell (500 mg)	2
Posture (600 mg)	Phosphate (600 mg)	1.5
Posture–Vitamin D	Phosphate (600 mg)	1.5
Citracal	Citrate (200 mg)	5
Citracal + Vitamin D	Citrate (315 mg)	3
Citracal Liquitab	Citrate (500 mg)	2
Tums 500 mg	Carbonate from limestone (500 mg)	2
Tums E-X	Carbonate from limestone (300 mg)	3.5
Tums Ultra	Carbonate from shell (400 mg)	2.5
Calcet + Vitamin D	Carbonate, lactate, gluconate (300 mg)	3.5
Fosfree	Carbonate, gluconate, lactate (175 mg)	6

Updated from: Shils M, et al, eds. *Modern nutrition in health and disease.* Baltimore: Lippincott Williams & Wilkins, 1999.

- Some mineral waters are excellent sources of calcium; bioavailability is good.
- Avoid long-term use of high doses of retinol from fortified foods or supplements (Feskanich et al, 2002).
- Persons with previous fractures are at risk and should be monitored carefully for osteoporosis (NIH Consensus Development Panel, 2001).
- The National Osteoporosis Foundation's Awareness and Prevention Month campaign (in May of each year) raises awareness of risk factors and prevention methods.
- When steroids are used, check on bone density changes; there is a high incidence of osteoporosis.

For More Information

- Clinical Guidelines–Osteoporosis
  http://www.nof.org/professionals/clinical.htm
- Medications for Osteoporosis
  http://www.nof.org/patientinfo/medications.htm
- National Bone Health Campaign
  http://www.nof.org/powerfulbones/index.htm
- National Institutes of Health Osteoporosis and Related Bones Diseases
  http://www.osteo.org/about.html
- National Osteoporosis Foundation
  http://www.nof.org/
- Osteopenia
  http://www.nlm.nih.gov/medlineplus/ency/article/007231.htm
- Osteoporosis Society of Canada
  http://www.osteoporosis.ca/english/home/default.asp?s=1

OSTEOPENIA AND OSTEOPOROSIS—CITED REFERENCES

Black DM, et al. One year of alendronate after one year of parathyroid hormone (1-84) for osteoporosis. *N Engl J Med.* 353:555, 2005.

Branca F, Vatuena S. Calcium, physical activity and bone health—building bones for a stronger future. *Public Health Nutri.* 4:117, 2001.

Budak N, et al. Bone mineral density and serum 25-hydroxyvitamin D level: is there any difference according to the dressing style of the female university students. *Int J Food Sci Nutr.* 55:569, 2004.

Cauley JA, et al. Effects of estrogen plus progestin on risk of fracture and bone mineral density. The Women's Health Initiative Randomized Trial. *JAMA.* 290:1729, 2003.

Cefalu CA. Is bone mineral density predictive of fracture risk reduction? *Curr Med Res Opin.* 20:341, 2004.

Chesnut CH, et al. A randomized trial of nasal spray salmon calcitonin in postmenopausal women with established osteoporosis: the Prevent Recurrence of Osteoporotic Fractures Study. PROOF Study Group. *Am J Med.* 109:267, 2000.

TABLE 11-10 Medications Commonly Used for Management of Osteoporosis

The FDA approves calcitonin, alendronate, raloxifene, and risedronate for the treatment of postmenopausal osteoporosis; alendronate, risedronate, and raloxifene are approved for the prevention of the disease.

Current pharmacological options for osteoporosis prevention and/or treatment are bisphosphonates (alendronate and risedronate), calcitonin, estrogens and/or hormone therapy, parathyroid hormone (PTH 1-34), and raloxifene.

Medication	Effects	Comments
Bisphosphonates; risedronate (Actonel); alendronate (Fosamax)	Effective agents for reducing vertebral and nonvertebral fracture risk (Reginster et al, 2000; McClung et al, 2001). Use of these medications with parathormone may be indicated for increasing bone density. Studies are under way. Alendronate is approved for the treatment of osteoporosis in men. Alendronate and risedronate are approved for use by men and women with glucocorticoid-induced osteoporosis. Zoledronic acid is under study. Bisphosphonates inhibit atherogenesis (McFarlane et al, 2004).	Risedronate may cause dysphagia, esophageal ulcer, and stomach ulcer. Take on an empty stomach 30 minutes before meals. Take additional vitamin D and calcium. Headache, gastrointestinal (GI) distress, diarrhea, nausea, constipation, and rash may occur, although rarely. Alendronate may cause metallic taste, nausea, diarrhea, and decreased potassium and magnesium. Take with plain water only first thing in the morning. Avoid in severe renal disease, pregnancy, or breastfeeding. Nausea, heartburn, irritation or pain of the esophagus, vomiting, dysphagia, sensation of fullness, and constipation or diarrhea may occur.
Calcitonin-salmon (Miacalcin)	Bone loss is reduced, and bone mass increases, although not in the hip. A modest increase in bone mass occurs. The Prevent Recurrence of Osteoporotic Fractures (PROOF) trial is a 5-year dose-ranging trial evaluating calcitonin-salmon nasal spray (100, 200, and 400 IU/d) in postmenopausal women with osteoporosis.	200 IU/d, the recommended regimen, reduces vertebral fracture risk by 33% in women with low bone mass (Chesnut et al, 2000). Calcitonin makes calcium more available to bones. It is given as an injection or nasal spray; it may cause allergic reactions and flushing of the face and hands, urinary frequency, nausea, and skin rash.
Calcitriol (1,25-dihydroxyvitamin D)	Active form of vitamin D hormone that increases GI absorption of calcium from the gut, kidney reabsorption of calcium, stimulates bone resorption, decreases PTH production, and stimulates skeletal osteoblasts/osteoclasts.	
Growth hormone and anabolic therapies	Anabolic therapy is being studied. Bone formation is directly stimulated by growth hormone, insulin-like growth factor I, the statins, and PTH (Rosen and Bilezikian, 2001).	
Hormone or estrogen replacement therapy (ERT)	Both merit and controversy are noted.	Estrogen tends to increase the risk of cancer of the endometrium if not opposed with progesterone (Cauley et al, 2003).
Ibandronate (Boniva)	Ibandronate is used to treat or prevent osteoporosis in women after menopause; it may increase bone mass by slowing loss of bone.	Should not be taken if hypocalcemia is a problem.
PTH (teriparatide; Forteo)	PTH is the only anabolic osteoporosis agent available for clinical use to lower vertebral fracture incidence by triggering formation of new bone (Michelotti and Clark, 1999; Neer et al, 2001).	Use only in ambulatory patients.
Raloxifene (Evista)	Significantly reduces vertebral fracture risk but not nonvertebral fracture risk (Maricic et al, 2002; Sarkar et al, 2002).	Protects against thin, weak bones and fractures; also lowers serum cholesterol by 7% and low-density lipoprotein (LDL) by 11%. It may trigger menopausal symptoms, including hot flashes, but is less likely to have an estrogen-like increase in cancer risk.
Sodium fluoride	The slow-release form may increase bone formation and decrease the risk of fractures.	In patients with mild to moderate osteoporosis, long-term supplements with fluoride plus calcium result in lower rates of vertebral fracture than supplementation with calcium alone. Intake of fluoride in drinking water at 1 ppm does not appear to be associated with increased risk of hip fracture (Hillier et al, 2000).
Statins	Statins, agents that reduce atherogenesis, stimulate bone formation (MacFarlane et al, 2004).	Cardiovascular disease and low bone mineral density have some common etiologies.

For more information, see the following National Osteoporosis Foundation website: http://www.nof.org/patientinfo/medications.htm.

Cummings SR, et al. Improvement in spine bone density and reduction in risk of vertebral fractures during treatment with antiresorptive drugs. *Am J Med.* 112:281, 2002.
Dawson-Hughes B, Harris SS. Calcium intake influences the association of protein intake with rates of bone loss in elderly men and women. *Am J Clin Nutr.* 75:773, 2002.
Devine A, et al. Protein consumption is an important predictor of lower limb bone mass in elderly women. *Am J Clin Nutr.* 81:1423, 2005.
Feskanich D, et al. Vitamin A intake and hip fractures among postmenopausal women. *JAMA.* 287:47, 2002.
Ganry O, et al. Effect of alcohol intake on bone mineral density in elderly women: the EPIDOS study. *Am J Epidemiol.* 151:773, 2000.
Hillier S, et al. Fluoride in drinking water and risk of hip fracture in the U.K. *Lancet.* 355:265, 2000.
Kelsey JL, et al. Reducing the risk for distal forearm fracture: preserve bone mass, slow down, and don't fall! *Osteoporos Int.* 16:681, 2005.
Maricic M, et al. Early effects of raloxifene on clinical vertebral fractures at 12 months in postmenopausal women with osteoporosis. *Arch Intern Med.* 162:1140, 2002.
McClung MR, et al. Effect of risedronate on the risk of hip fracture in elderly women. *N Engl J Med.* 344:333, 2001.
McFarlane SI, et al. Osteoporosis and cardiovascular disease: brittle bones and boned arteries, is there a link? *Endocrine* 23:1, 2004.
Michelotti J, Clark J. Femoral neck length and hip fracture risk. *J Bone Miner Res.* 14:1714, 1999.
National Institutes of Health. Osteoporosis prevention, diagnosis, and therapy. NIH Consensus Statement, 2000. Available at http://www.zosteo.org/osteo.html.
Neer RM, et al. Effect of parathyroid hormone (1-34) on fractures and bone mineral density in postmenopausal women with osteoporosis. *N Engl J Med.* 344:1434, 2001.
New S, et al. Dietary influences on bone mass and bone metabolism: further evidence of a positive link between fruit and vegetable consumption and bone health? *Am J Clin Nutr.* 71:142, 2000.
Nicodemus K, et al. Type 1 and type 2 diabetes and incident hip fractures in postmenopausal women. *Diabetes Care* 24:1192, 2001.
Nieves JW. Osteoporosis: the role of micronutrients. *Am J Clin Nutr.* 81:1232, 2005.
National Institutes of Health Consensus Development Panel on Osteoporosis Prevention, Diagnosis, and Therapy. Osteoporosis prevention, diagnosis, and therapy. *JAMA.* 285:785, 2001.
National Osteoporosis Foundation (NOF). National Osteoporosis Foundation. Accessed October 1, 2005 at http://www.nof.org/.
Rapuri P, et al. Caffeine intake increases the rate of bone loss in elderly women and interacts with vitamin D receptor genotypes. *Am J Clin Nutr.* 74:694, 2001.
Reffitt DM, et al. Orthosilicic acid stimulates collagen type 1 synthesis and osteoblastic differentiation in human osteoblast-like cells in vitro. *Bone* 32:127, 2003.
Reginster J, et al. Randomized trial of the effects of risedronate on vertebral fractures in women with established postmenopausal osteoporosis. Vertebral Efficacy with Risedronate Therapy (VERT) Study Group. *Osteoporos Int.* 11:83, 2000.
Robbins J, et al. The association of bone mineral density and depression in an older population. *J Am Geriatr Soc.* 49:732, 2001.
Rosen C, Bilezikian J. Clinical review 123: anabolic therapy for osteoporosis. *J Clin Endocrinol Metab.* 86:957, 2001.
Sarkar S, et al. Relationships between bone mineral density and incident vertebral fracture risk with raloxifene therapy. *J Bone Miner Res.* 17:1, 2002.
Schwartz AF, et al. Increased falling as a risk factor for fracture among older women: the study of osteoporotic fractures. *Am J Epidemiol.* 161:180, 2005.
Tussing L, Chapman-Novakofski K. Osteoporosis prevention education: behavior theories and calcium intake. *J Am Diet Assoc.* 105:92, 2005.
World Health Organization. Prevention and management of osteoporosis. Accessed August 31, 2005 at http://whqlibdoc.who.int/trs/WHO_TRS_921.pdf.

PAGET'S DISEASE (OSTEITIS DEFORMANS)

NUTRITIONAL ACUITY RANKING: LEVEL 1–2

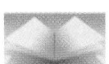

DEFINITIONS AND BACKGROUND

Paget's disease is a chronic disorder of the skeleton, where areas on bone grow abnormally, enlarging and becoming soft. It is of unknown etiology, with excessive bone destruction and repairing. Of all persons older than 50 years of age, 3% have an isolated lesion; actual clinical disease is much less common. Paget's disease of bone is the second most common bone disease in the world.

The disease tends to run in families. Genetic analysis indicates that 40% of patients with Paget's disease have an affected first-degree relative, and 1% of patients develop osteosarcoma (Reddy, 2004).

Approximately 3 million Americans have the disease, and it rarely occurs before age 40. The disease is higher in frequency in people who are aged 65 or older; there is a slight male predominance in the 45- to 74-year age group (Altman et al, 2000). Sarcoma can occur in this population (Mankin and Hornicek, 2005).

Juvenile Paget's disease, although very rare, is very debilitating. Osteoclasts are larger than normal and increased in size (Deftos, 2005). Juvenile Paget's disease usually presents in infancy or childhood and results in progressive deformity, growth retardation, and deafness.

Symptoms and signs include deep "bone pain," joint pain, neck pain, skull enlargement, hearing loss or headaches, thickening of long bones, bowing of limbs, reduced height, and spontaneous fractures. Prognosis is good in mild cases.

INTERVENTION: OBJECTIVES

- Prevent complications, especially related to the nervous system (e.g., fractures, spinal stenosis, paraplegia, cardiac failure, and deafness).
- Prevent side effects of drug therapy.
- Promote full recovery when possible.
- Differentiate from other conditions with bone lesions.

INTERVENTION: FOOD AND NUTRITION

- Adequate protein is important, with adequate calories to spare protein.
- Adequate levels of calcium and vitamins C and D may be needed.
- To correct anemia, monitor serum levels of iron and vitamin B_{12} to determine need for an altered diet.

CLINICAL INDICATORS

Clinical/History	Lab Work	
Height	Ca++, Mg++	Uric acid (UA) (often elevated)
Weight	Na+, K+	Transferrin
BMI	Urinary Ca++ (altered)	Serum P
X-rays (denser, expanded bones)	Alb, transthyretin	Alk phos (increased)
Bone scans	CRP	H & H
	PTH (abnormal)	Serum B_{12}
		Radiolabeled bisphosphonate

Common Drugs Used and Potential Side Effects

- Drugs that inhibit bone resorption—bisphosphonates (etidronate, pamidronate, clodronate, or alendronate)—may be used to slow the progression. Bisphosphonates are pyrophosphate analogs that bind to bone at active sites of remodeling (Theriault and Hortobagyi, 2001). Pamidronate (Aredia) may cause osteonecrosis of the jaw.
- Recent research suggests that a bisphosphonate drug, zoledronic acid (Zometa), given in a single injection yields a rapid and long-lasting improvement in bone health (Reid et al, 2005). Studies are ongoing.
- Risedronate (Actonel) can cause dysphagia, esophageal ulcer, and stomach ulcer. Take on an empty stomach 30 minutes before meals. Take additional vitamin D and calcium. Headache, diarrhea, nausea, constipation, and rash may occur, although they are rare.
- Osteoprotegerin may be useful in managing the juvenile form of Paget's disease (Cundy et al, 2005).
- Thyrocalcitonin or synthetic calcitonin may be used to decrease passage of calcium from bones to bloodstream. Monitor for nausea or vomiting. Newer methods of administration include a nasal spray.

Herbs, Botanicals, and Supplements

- Herbs and botanical supplements should not be used without discussing with physician.
- Unusual bone diseases may be associated with use of Chinese herbs (Hoshino et al, 2003).

INTERVENTION: NUTRITION EDUCATION, COUNSELING, CARE MANAGEMENT

- Discuss appropriate dietary alterations for patient's condition, individualized for the current condition and status. Include good food sources of calcium, B-complex vitamins, iron, protein, and vitamin D. Monitor carefully, if supplements are used, in addition to dietary guidance.
- Discuss side effects for the specific drugs ordered.

For More Information

- National Association for the Relief of Paget's Disease
  http://www.paget.org.uk/
- National Institute of Arthritis and Musculoskeletal and Skin Diseases
  http://www.niams.nih.gov/bone/hi/paget/diagnosed.htm
- National Institutes of Health Osteoporosis and Related Bones Diseases
  http://www.niams.nih.gov/bone/
- Paget's Disease
  http://www.nlm.nih.gov/medlineplus/ency/article/000414.htm
- Paget Foundation
  http://www.paget.org/

PAGET'S DISEASE—CITED REFERENCES

Altman R, et al. Prevalence of pelvic Paget's disease of bone in the United States. *J Bone Miner Res.* 15:461, 2000.

Cundy T, et al. Recombinant osteoprotegerin for juvenile Paget's disease. *N Engl J Med.* 353:918, 2005.

Deftos LJ. Treatment of Paget's disease—taming the wild osteoclast. *N Engl J Med.* 353:872, 2005.

Hoshino J, et al. Chinese herbs and bone disease. *Intern Med.* 42:345, 2003.

Mankin HJ, Hornicek FJ. Paget's sarcoma: a historical and outcome review. *Clin Orthop Relat Res.* 438:97, 2005.

Reddy SV. Etiology of Paget's disease and osteoclast abnormalities. *J Cell Biol.* 93:688, 2004.

Reid IR, et al. Comparison of a single infusion of zoledronic acid with risedronate for Paget's disease. *N Engl J Med.* 353:898, 2005.

Theriault R, Hortobagyi G. The evolving role of bisphosphonates. *Semin Oncol.* 28:284, 2001.

POLYARTERITIS NODOSA

NUTRITIONAL ACUITY RANKING: LEVEL 1–2

DEFINITIONS AND BACKGROUND

Polyarteritis nodosa (PAN) is a rare condition characterized by necrotizing inflammation of medium-sized or small arteries without glomerulonephritis or vasculitis in arterioles, capillaries, or venules (Colmegna and Maldonado-Cocco, 2005). In PAN, arteries become inflamed in several organs, causing damage (often in brain, heart, liver, gastrointestinal [GI] tract, and renal tissues).

PAN is rare and fatal if not treated. It is 2–3 times more common in men and usually develops in men aged 40–50 years. Viral or bacterial infections such as hepatitis B seem to trigger it, but the specific cause is not known.

Symptoms and signs include chest pains (heart), shortness of breath (lungs), abdominal pain (liver and intestines), weakness and numbness (nerves), edema, and hematuria (kidneys). Fatigue, aches and pains, persistent fever, anorexia, kidney damage, weight loss, and tachycardia may result. Some skin changes may occur, including rash, nodules, or Raynaud's syndrome.

Renal involvement develops and is accompanied by hypertension in half of patients. PAN also commonly involves the gut (abdominal angina, hemorrhage, perforation), heart (myocarditis, myocardial infarction), or eye (scleritis); rupture of renal or mesenteric microaneurysms can also occur.

INTERVENTION: OBJECTIVES

- Treat as soon as possible to decrease heart and renal damage.
- Improve appetite and intake.
- Prevent weight loss.
- Increase calorie intake when there is fever.
- Reduce edema, anorexia, hypertension, and other effects of the disorder.

INTERVENTION: FOOD AND NUTRITION

- A high-energy intake may be beneficial in case of weight loss.
- A normal to high protein intake generally is required.
- Fluid or sodium intake may be limited with hypertension, kidney disease, or edema or with use of steroids.
- Include phytochemicals derived from spices such as turmeric (curcumin); red pepper (capsaicin); cloves (eugenol); ginger (gingerol); cumin, anise, and fennel (anethol); basil and rosemary (ursolic acid); garlic (diallyl sulfide, *S*-allylmercaptocysteine, and ajoene); and pomegranate (ellagic acid) (Aggarwal and Shishodia, 2004).

CLINICAL INDICATORS

Clinical/History	Abdominal pain	Hepatitis B antigen
Height	BP (elevated)	Ca++, Mg++
Weight	Myalgias, weakness	Na+, K+
BMI	Neuropathy	Alb, transthyretin
Weight loss		BUN, Creat (may be elevated)
Hematuria	**Lab Work**	Transferrin
I & O	ESR (elevated)	H & H
Edema	CRP	
Temperature (fever)	Glucose	

Common Drugs Used and Potential Side Effects

- Steroids such as prednisone may be used. Side effects of long-term use include negative nitrogen and potassium balances; decreased calcium and zinc levels; CHO intolerance; and excessive sodium retention. Weight gain is also common; a calorie-controlled diet may be useful.
- Pain relievers may be needed; monitor individually for side effects such as GI distress.
- Immunosuppressive cyclophosphamide may be used; long-term effects can reduce the ability to fight infections. Corticosteroids plus cyclophosphamide is the standard of care, in particular for patients with more severe disease, in whom this combination prolongs survival (Colmegna and Maldonado-Cocco, 2005).
- Infliximab may be used as an alternative agent for the treatment of patients with PAN refractory to conventional therapy (Al-Bishri et al, 2005).

Herbs, Botanicals, and Supplements

- Herbs and botanical supplements should not be used without discussing with physician.

INTERVENTION: NUTRITION EDUCATION, COUNSELING, CARE MANAGEMENT

- Discuss alternate dietary guidelines as appropriate for medications and side effects of the disease.
- Discuss sources of nutrients as appropriate for the ordered diet.

For More Information

- Johns Hopkins Vasculitis Center
  http://vasculitis.med.jhu.edu/typesof/polyarteritis.html
- Polyarteritis Nodosa Foundation
  http://www.angelfire.com/pa3/autoimmunedisease/aifeindex.html
- Polyarteritis Nodosa
  http://www.emedicine.com/ped/topic1844.htm

POLYARTERITIS NODOSA—CITED REFERENCES

Aggarwal BB, Shishodia S. Suppression of the nuclear factor-kappa B activation pathway by spice-derived phytochemicals: reasoning for seasoning. *Ann N Y Acad Sci.* 1030:434, 2004.

Al-Bishri J, et al. Refractory polyarteritis nodosa successfully treated with infliximab. *J Rheumatol.* 32:1371, 2005.

Colmegna I, Maldonado-Cocco JA. Polyarteritis nodosa revisited. Polyarteritis nodosa revisited. *Curr Rheumatol Rep.* 7:288, 2005.

RHABDOMYOLYSIS

NUTRITIONAL ACUITY RANKING: LEVEL 3

DEFINITIONS AND BACKGROUND

Rhabdomyolysis (RML) is a clinical and biochemical syndrome resulting from skeletal muscle injury with release of myoglobin into the plasma and breakdown of muscle fibers with release into the circulation. Some of these changes are toxic to the kidney, often resulting in kidney damage or acute renal failure. A disturbance in myocyte calcium homeostasis takes place.

RML may occur in infants, toddlers, and adolescents who have inherited enzyme deficiencies of carbohydrate or lipid metabolism, Duchenne muscular dystrophy, or malignant hyperthermia. RML may also occur from extensive muscle damage as from a crushing injury, major burn, electrical shock, toxins, bacterial infections, excessive exercise (Olpin, 2005), seizures, alcoholism, overdose of cocaine, or use of drugs such as statins. Cholesterol-reducing statins lower the levels of cholesterol and triglycerides.

The most common causes of RML in adults include crush injury, overexertion, alcohol abuse, use of certain medicines, and toxic substances. Postoperative RML in bariatric surgery occurs with prolonged muscle compression; potential consequences may lead to death (de Menezes Ettinger et al, 2005).

Muscle pain caused by RML may involve specific symptoms of groups of muscles or may be generalized throughout the body; muscles in the calves and the lower back are commonly affected. Each patient is different. See Table 11-11 for symptoms.

Early complications of RML include severe hyperkalemia that causes cardiac arrhythmia and arrest; the most serious late complication is acute renal failure, which occurs in approximately 15% of patients with the syndrome (Sauret et al, 2002).

INTERVENTION: OBJECTIVES

- Preserve renal function.
- Eliminate myoglobin out of the kidneys with early and aggressive hydration. Medicines may also be needed to make the urine more alkaline.
- Treat kidney failure or hyperkalemia if needed.

INTERVENTION: FOOD AND NUTRITION

- Hydration needs with muscle necrosis may approximate the massive fluid volume needs of a severely burned patient.
- Special dietary advice is required if there is renal disease or the need for dialysis.
- It is important to offer advice according to the medical condition that preceded RML.

CLINICAL INDICATORS

Clinical/History

- Height
- Weight
- BMI
- I & O
- Tea-colored urine
- Temperature
- BP (elevated)
- Exposure to toxic substances or chronic alcohol use
- Use of medications such as statins

Lab Work

- Serum myoglobin test (positive)
- Urinary casts or hemoglobin
- Ca++, Mg++
- Na+
- K+ (may be high from muscle breakdown)
- Creatine phosphokinase (CPK) (very high)
- Alb, transthyretin
- CRP
- BUN
- Creat
- Transferrin
- H & H
- UA (elevated)

Common Drugs Used and Potential Side Effects

- Statins block the enzyme in the liver that is responsible for making cholesterol, hydroxy-methylglutaryl-coenzyme A reductase (HMG-CoA reductase). Serial muscle testing after initiation of statins may be suggested to manage a reversible muscle weakness (Dobkin, 2005).
- Despite the withdrawal of cerivastatin because of fatal RML, the risk of this complication with other statins is extremely low (Waters, 2005). Patients who are given statins may want to take coenzyme Q10 at the same time.
- Diuretic therapy may be needed if there is hypertension.
- If there is hyperkalemia, calcium chloride or calcium gluconate may be used.

TABLE 11-11 Symptoms of Rhabdomyolysis

- Muscle tenderness
- Weakness of the affected muscle(s)
- Generalized weakness
- Muscle stiffness or aching (myalgia)
- Weight gain (unintentional)
- Seizures
- Joint pain
- Fatigue
- Abnormally dark colored urine from excretion of myoglobin

Herbs, Botanicals, and Supplements

- Herbs and botanical supplements should not be used without discussing with physician.
- Even brief exposure to atorvastatin causes a marked decrease in blood coenzyme Q10 concentration, with commonly reported adverse effects of exercise intolerance, myalgia, and myoglobinuria (Rundek et al, 2004).

INTERVENTION: NUTRITION EDUCATION, COUNSELING, CARE MANAGEMENT

- Discuss alternate dietary guidelines as appropriate for medications and side effects of the disease.
- Discuss how to use diet and exercise to manage high serum cholesterol if this information has not been given before. Reinforce what the patient has been doing well.
- After damage to any muscles, extra fluid is needed to dilute urine and to eliminate myoglobin. Among soldiers, RML occurs in 25% of those who are injured (Carter et al, 2005).

For More Information

- E-medicine
  http://www.emedicine.com/emerg/topic508.htm
- Rhabdomyolysis
  http://www.nlm.nih.gov/medlineplus/ency/article/000473.htm

RHABDOMYOLYSIS—CITED REFERENCES

Carter R 3rd, et al. Epidemiology of hospitalizations and deaths from heat illness in soldiers. *Med Sci Sports Exerc.* 37:1338, 2005.

de Menezes Ettinger JE, et al. Prevention of rhabdomyolysis in bariatric surgery. *Obes Surg.* 15:874, 2005.

Dobkin BH. Underappreciated statin-induced myopathic weakness causes disability. *Neurorehabil Neural Repair.* 19:259, 2005.

Olpin SE. Fatty acid oxidation defects as a cause of neuromyopathic disease in infants and adults. *Clin Lab.* 51:289, 2005.

Sauret JM, et al. Rhabdomyolysis. *Am Fam Physician.* 65:907, 2002.

Rundek T, et al. Atorvastatin decreases the coenzyme Q10 level in the blood of patients at risk for cardiovascular disease and stroke. *Arch Neurol.* 61:889, 2004.

Waters DD. Safety of high-dose atorvastatin therapy. *Am J Cardiol.* 96:69, 2005.

RHEUMATOID ARTHRITIS

NUTRITIONAL ACUITY RANKING: LEVEL 1

DEFINITIONS AND BACKGROUND

Rheumatoid arthritis (RA) is a chronic polyarthritis mainly affecting the smaller peripheral joints and is accompanied by general ill health. Crippling deformities can occur. Arthritis and other rheumatic conditions are common conditions associated with ambulatory medical care (Hootman et al, 2000). Of all cases, 75% are women. Most patients are between ages 20–40 years, and RA affects 2.1 million Americans (www.arthritis.org).

To diagnose RA, symptoms must have been present for at least 6 weeks and four of eight criteria of the American Rheumatism Association (ARA) must be met. Table 11-12 lists these criteria. Table 11-13 provides a list of the variant forms of RA.

The cause of RA is increased inflammatory cytokine production, such as from mast cells, interleukin-6, tumor necrosis factor alpha (TNFα), and acute-phase proteins. Inflammation of synovial tissues is the dominant manifestation; hand involvement occurs in 85% of cases, and knees or ankles/feet are involved in 80% of cases (Kast, 2001). Supplements of gamma linolenic acid (GLA), as from borage oil, may reduce generation of mediators of inflammation and attenuate symptoms but may cause potentially harmful increases in serum arachidonic acid unless eicosapentaenoic acid (EPA) is also used (Barham et al, 2000). GLA increases prostaglandin E levels, which increase cyclic adenosine monophosphate (cAMP) levels which, in turn, suppress TNFα synthesis.

Omega-3 fatty acids reduce tenderness in joints, decrease morning stiffness, and reduce the amount of medication needed; they also downregulate T-cell proliferation (Arrington et al, 2001). People with RA who eat 4 oz of fish every day have less morning stiffness, swollen joints, and all-around

TABLE 11-12 Symptoms of Rheumatic Arthritis

- Morning stiffness in and around joints, lasting more than 1 hour
- Arthritis of 3 or more joint areas involved simultaneously
- Arthritis of at least 1 area in a wrist, metacarpophalangeal, or proximal interphalangeal joint
- Symmetric arthritis involving the same joint areas
- Rheumatoid nodules
- Positive serum rheumatoid factor
- Radiographic changes typical of rheumatoid arthritis on hand and wrist radiographs, including erosions, or unequivocal bony decalcification in or adjacent to the involved joints
- No evidence of other disease such as lupus

Source: National Institute of Arthritis and Musculoskeletal and Skin Diseases. Available at http://www.nih.gov/niams/healthinfo/info.htm.

TABLE 11-13 Variant Forms of Rheumatic Arthritis (RA)

Condition	Background	Nutritional Implications
Juvenile RA (JRA)	JRA causes joint inflammation and stiffness for more than 6 weeks in a child 16 years of age or less. It is classified into 3 types, depending on symptoms, number of joints involved, and presence or absence of antibodies in the blood. Pauciarticular JRA affects mainly the knees and is most common. The polyarticular form affects 30% of children with JRA. The systemic form tests negative for the usual antibodies, may affect internal organs, may become chronic in adulthood, affects 20% of children with JRA, and is known as Still's disease. Both genetic factors and environmental factors, such as a virus, can trigger JRA. Because JRA often affects knees, limping can occur. Salicylates, gold salts, or glucocorticoids may be used.	Children suffering from JCA may have reduced serum levels of beta-carotene, retinol, and zinc compared with healthy children (Helgeland, 2000).
Sjögren's syndrome	Dry eyes and dry mouth occur as a result of insufficient production of lacrimal and salivary secretions. Artificial tears and glucocorticoids may be needed. Sjögren's syndrome is a relatively common autoimmune disorder, striking 4 million Americans, mostly women. It is most often related to RA, lupus, scleroderma, or polymyositis. Debilitating pain and fatigue can occur. Sensitivity to sunlight is common; sunscreen is helpful.	Plan meals and use artificial saliva for easier swallowing. Chewing sugar-free gum can stimulate saliva production if any is available. Gel-based saliva substitutes are useful. Sip water often, and avoid caffeinated drinks, which can be dehydrating. Drink water during meals to help with swallowing. Mouth infections are common; good oral hygiene is essential. Aspiration pneumonia can be a problem if dry mouth causes dysphagia. With digestive problems, anorexia, diarrhea, and weight loss are prominent.
Felty's syndrome	A triad of RA, granulocytopenia, and splenomegaly. Painful, stiff, and swollen joints occur. Infections, leg ulcers, burning eyes, and anemia also can complicate the condition. Sometimes, splenectomy is indicated; drug therapy may be helpful to others. Felty's syndrome affects about 1% of patients with RA and is rare.	Fever, weight loss, and brown pigmentation may occur. Immunosuppressive drugs may be helpful; monitor for side effects.
Rheumatoid vasculitis	Rheumatoid vasculitis can be life threatening and usually occurs in patients with severe deforming arthritis and a high titer of rheumatoid factor. A majority have a strong human leukocyte antigen relationship. Vasculitic lesions include rheumatoid nodules, small nail fold infarcts, and purpura. Fatigue, weight loss, fever, organ ischemia, CNS infarctions, myocardial infarction, and peripheral neuropathy can occur.	Corticosteroids are the usual treatment. D-penicillamine and prednisone generally are used.

pain. Fish oil and aspirin are blood thinners, and they should not be taken together for a long time. Omega-3 fatty acid supplementation and reduction of omega-6 fatty acids can improve symptoms.

Epidemiological studies suggest that the antioxidant potential of dietary carotenoids may protect against the oxidative damage that can result in inflammation (Pattison et al, 2005). Proper antioxidant nutrients provide defense against increased oxidant stress. Supplementation of folate and vitamin B_{12} is needed in patients treated with methotrexate to reduce side effects and to offset elevated plasma homocysteine.

Complications of RA may include osteoporosis and chronic anemia. Calcium and vitamin D reduce the bone loss in patients who take steroids. An iron supplement may prevent anemia, and serum ferritin levels may be low. Patients benefit from a basic dietary supplement.

A study suggested that higher intakes of meat and total protein and lower intakes of fruit, vegetables, and vitamin C are associated with an increased risk of RA (Choi, 2005). However, dietary factors such as fruit, coffee, long-chain fatty acids, olive oil, vitamins A, E, C, and D, zinc, selenium, and iron need to be studied over a longer time period (Pedersen et al, 2005).

INTERVENTION: OBJECTIVES

- Preserve a high level of physical and social functioning to promote good quality of life; reduce the effects of pain and swelling.
- Maintain satisfactory nutritional status; malnutrition and loss of lean body mass are common in this condition. Monitor weight changes.

- Suggest ways of simplifying meal preparation.
- Consume foods rich in antioxidants, such as carotenoids (Pattison et al, 2005), vitamin E, selenium, and vitamin D (Cantorna and Mahon, 2004). A vegetarian diet may have significant benefits (Agren et al, 2001).
- Promote adequate growth in children who have RA; stunting can occur from glucocorticoids.
- Promote return of fat-free body mass and improvement in muscle strength.
- Restrict sodium intake, if needed.
- Modify patient's diet if hyperlipidemia is present or if there is elevated homocysteine.
- Avoid or correct constipation.

INTERVENTION: FOOD AND NUTRITION

- Use a high-protein and high-calorie diet if patient is malnourished. Cachexia is common (Marcora et al, 2005).
- A diet that lessens inflammation is useful; olive oil should be used often because it contains oleocanthal, a natural anti-inflammatory agent. Omega-3 fatty acids in foods such as salmon, tuna, mackerel, fish oils, and sardines should be consumed often. Try to acquire 3–6 g of omega-3 fatty acids per day for 4 months for an effective trial period.
- An uncooked vegan diet may be useful (Hanninen et al, 2000). This "living food" diet includes berries, fruits, vegetables, roots, nuts, and seeds. There is improvement in RA when eating a lactovegetarian, vegan, or Mediterranean diet (Skoldstam et al, 2005).
- Include phytochemicals derived from spices such as turmeric (curcumin); red pepper (capsaicin); cloves (eugenol); ginger (gingerol); cumin, anise, and fennel (anethol); basil and rosemary (ursolic acid); garlic (diallyl sulfide, *S*-allylmercaptocysteine, and ajoene); and pomegranate (ellagic acid) (Aggarwal and Shishodia, 2004).
- Adequate fluid, fiber, vitamins, and minerals are important. Use of foods high in beta-carotene, selenium, and vitamins C and E may be beneficial; choose nutrient-dense foods wisely. Antioxidants such as beta-cryptoxanthin (as from one glass of freshly squeezed orange juice daily) can reduce the risk of developing RA (Pattison et al, 2005).
- Increase vitamin D intakes to decrease the incidence and severity of RA and the rate of bone fracture (Cantorna and Mahon, 2004).
- Ensure diet provides adequate intake of calcium, magnesium, B-complex vitamins, potassium, and zinc.
- Increase folic acid if methotrexate is used; either use diet or folic acid supplements.
- Provide meals that are easy to tolerate when the drugs being used cause gastric irritation. Avoid acidic or highly spiced foods if needed.
- With dysphagia, tube feed or use soft/thick, pureed foods as needed.
- Identify and eliminate any food allergens. Individualize the diet accordingly.

CLINICAL INDICATORS

Clinical/History

Height
Weight
BMI
Temperature
Food allergies

Lab Work

RBC
CRP
LE prep
Creat (may be decreased)
ESR (increases with inflammation)
ANA
Rheumatoid factor (RF)
Antistreptococcal antibody titer
Immunoglobulins (may be elevated in Sjögren's)
Ceruloplasmin (may be increased)
H & H
Serum ferritin
Serum B_{12}
Transferrin
Serum folate, RBC folate
Serum copper
Alb, transthyretin
Gluc
BUN
Ca^{++}, Mg^{++}
Na^{+}, K^{+}

Common Drugs Used and Potential Side Effects (see Table 11-14)

- New research indicates that a new medication, abatacept, will sell under the trade name Orencia if it wins approval by the Food and Drug Administration.

Herbs, Botanicals, and Supplements

- Herbs and botanical supplements should not be used without discussing with physician. Some people have tried acupuncture and other alternatives to traditional medicine, but it is important not to neglect regular health care or treatment of serious symptoms.
- Younger female patients tend to use alternative treatments for RA more than males; perception of negative

SAMPLE NUTRITION DIAGNOSTIC STATEMENT

Rheumatoid Arthritis (RA)

PES: Inadequate calcium/vitamin D intake related to food records showing low daily intake and use of corticosteroid treatment for RA as evidenced by dual-energy x-ray absorptiometry (DEXA) scan of 80% desirable range for age and perimenopausal status.

Assessment Data (sources of info): Food records, lab reports, DEXA scan report.

Intervention: Counseling about good sources of calcium and vitamin D from diet and supplements, meal planning and shopping tips, dining out guide, referral to Meals-on-Wheels or other social agencies as appropriate.

Monitoring and Evaluation: Improvements in dietary and supplemental intake of vitamin D and calcium as shown in food records, lab values, and DEXA scan report.

TABLE 11-14 Medications Used in Rheumatoid Arthritis

Medications	Uses/Effects	Side Effects	Monitoring
Analgesics and nonsteroidal anti-inflammatory drugs (NSAIDs)	Analgesics relieve pain; NSAIDs relieve pain and reduce inflammation.	Upset stomach, peptic ulcer, bleeding, renal failure. Use of NSAIDs may increase rate of miscarriage for pregnant women.	For all traditional NSAIDs: avoid drinking alcohol or using blood thinners; avoid if there is sensitivity or allergy to aspirin or similar drugs, kidney or liver disease, heart disease, high blood pressure, asthma, or peptic ulcers.
Acetaminophen		Usually no side effects when taken as directed.	Not to be taken with alcohol or with other products containing acetaminophen. Not to be used for more than 10 days unless directed by a physician.
Aspirin: buffered, plain	Aspirin is used to reduce pain, swelling, and inflammation, allowing patients to move more easily and carry out normal activities. It is generally part of early and ongoing therapy.	Upset stomach; tendency to bruise easily; ulcers, pain, or discomfort; diarrhea; headache; heartburn or indigestion; nausea or vomiting.	Doctor monitoring is needed. Not used for children in whom Reye's syndrome is a risk, but otherwise useful in lessening inflammation.
Traditional NSAIDs: ibuprofen, ketoprofen, naproxen	NSAIDs help relieve pain within hours of administration in dosages available over the counter (available for all three medications). They relieve pain and inflammation in dosages available in prescription form (ibuprofen and ketoprofen). It may take several days to reduce inflammation.	For all traditional NSAIDs: abdominal or stomach cramps, pain, or discomfort; diarrhea; dizziness; drowsiness or light-headedness; headache; heartburn or indigestion; peptic ulcers; nausea or vomiting; possible kidney and liver damage (rare).	For all traditional NSAIDs: avoid drinking alcohol or using blood thinners; avoid if there is sensitivity or allergy to aspirin or similar drugs, kidney or liver disease, heart disease, high blood pressure, asthma, or peptic ulcers.
Cyclo-oxygenase (COX)-2 inhibitor NSAIDs: celecoxib, valdecoxib	COX-2 inhibitors, like traditional NSAIDs, block COX-2, an enzyme in the body that stimulates an inflammatory response. Unlike traditional NSAIDs, however, they do not block the action of COX-1, an enzyme that protects the stomach lining. Some, like Vioxx, have been withdrawn by FDA.	Stomach irritation, ulceration, and bleeding may occur. Caution is advisable for patients with a history of bleeding or ulcers, decreased renal function, hepatic disease, hypertension, or asthma.	Doctor monitoring for possible allergic responses to valdecoxib and celecoxib is important.
Corticosteroids	These are steroids given by mouth or injection. They are used to relieve inflammation and reduce swelling, redness, itching, and allergic reactions.	Increased appetite, indigestion, nervousness, or restlessness.	For all corticosteroids, advise the doctor if there is presence of the following: fungal infection, history of tuberculosis, underactive thyroid, herpes simplex of the eye, high blood pressure, osteoporosis, or stomach ulcer.
Methylprednisolone, prednisone	These steroids are available in pill form or as an injection into a joint. Improvements are seen in several hours up to 24 hours after administration. There is potential for serious side effects, especially at high doses. They are used for severe flares and when the disease does not respond to NSAIDs and disease-modifying antirheumatic drugs.	Osteoporosis, mood changes, fragile skin, easy bruising, fluid retention, weight gain, muscle weakness, onset or worsening of diabetes, cataracts, increased risk of infection, and hypertension (high blood pressure).	Doctor monitoring for continued effectiveness of medication and for side effects is needed.

(continued)

TABLE 11-14 **Medications Used in Rheumatoid Arthritis *(continued)***

Medications	Uses/Effects	Side Effects	Monitoring
Disease-modifying antirheumatic drugs (DMARDs)	These are common arthritis medications. They relieve painful, swollen joints and slow joint damage, and several DMARDs may be used over the disease course. They take a few weeks or months to have an effect and may produce significant improvements for many patients. Exactly how they work is still unknown.	Side effects vary with each medicine. DMARDs may increase risk of infection, hair loss, and kidney or liver damage.	Doctor monitoring allows the risk of toxicities to be weighed against the potential benefits of individual medications.
Azathioprine	This drug was first used in higher doses in cancer chemotherapy and organ transplantation. It is used in patients who have not responded to other drugs and in combination therapy.	Cough or hoarseness, fever or chills, loss of appetite, lower back or side pain, nausea or vomiting, painful or difficult urination, unusual tiredness or weakness.	Avoid with allopurinol or kidney or liver disease. May decrease immunity; contact doctor immediately with chills, fever, or a cough. Regular blood and liver function tests are needed.
Cyclosporine	This medication was first used in organ transplantation to prevent rejection. It is used in patients who have not responded to other drugs.	Bleeding, tender, or enlarged gums; high blood pressure; increase in hair growth; kidney problems; trembling and shaking of hands.	Avoid with sensitivity to castor oil (if receiving the drug by injection), liver or kidney disease, active infection, or high blood pressure. Using this drug may make you more susceptible to infection and certain cancers. Do not take live vaccines while on this drug. St. John's wort and echinacea should not be used.
Hydroxychloroquine	It may take several months to notice the benefits of this drug, which include reducing the signs and symptoms of rheumatoid arthritis.	Diarrhea, eye problems (rare), headache, loss of appetite, nausea or vomiting, and stomach cramps or pain.	Doctor monitoring is important, particularly with an allergy to any antimalarial drug or a retinal abnormality.
Gold sodium thiomalate (Ridaura)	This was one of the first DMARDs used to treat rheumatoid arthritis.	Redness or soreness of tongue; swelling or bleeding gums; skin rash or itching; ulcers or sores on lips, mouth, or throat; irritation on tongue. Joint pain may occur for 1 or 2 days after injection.	Avoid with lupus, skin rash, kidney disease, or colitis. Periodic urine and blood tests are needed to check for side effects.
Leflunomide	This drug reduces signs and symptoms and slows structural damage to joints caused by arthritis.	Bloody or cloudy urine; congestion in chest; cough; diarrhea; difficult, burning, or painful urination or breathing; fever; hair loss; headache; heartburn; loss of appetite; nausea and/or vomiting; skin rash; stomach pain; sneezing; and sore throat.	Doctor must monitor for the following: active infection, liver disease, known immune deficiency, renal insufficiency, or underlying malignancy. Regular blood tests, including liver function tests, are needed. Leflunomide must not be taken during pregnancy because it may cause birth defects in humans.
Methotrexate (Rheumatrex)	This drug can be taken by mouth or by injection and results in rapid improvement (it usually takes 3–6 weeks to begin working). It appears to be very effective, especially in combination with infliximab or etanercept. In general, it produces more favorable long-term responses compared with other DMARDs such as sulfasalazine, gold sodium thiomalate, and hydroxychloroquine. May be used in pediatrics.	Abdominal discomfort, chest pain, chills, nausea, mouth sores, painful urination, sore throat, and unusual tiredness or weakness.	Doctor monitoring is important, particularly with an abnormal blood count, liver or lung disease, alcoholism, immune system deficiency, or active infection. Methotrexate must not be taken during pregnancy because it may cause birth defects in humans. Avoid Echinacea. Extra folic acid is needed.

(continued)

TABLE 11-14 Medications Used in Rheumatoid Arthritis *(continued)*

Medications	Uses/Effects	Side Effects	Monitoring
Sulfasalazine	This drug works to reduce the signs and symptoms of rheumatoid arthritis by suppressing the immune system.	Abdominal pain, aching joints, diarrhea, headache, sensitivity to sunlight, loss of appetite, nausea or vomiting, and skin rash.	Doctor monitoring is important, particularly with allergy to sulfa drugs or aspirin or with a kidney, liver, or blood disease.
Biological response modifiers	These drugs selectively block parts of the immune system called cytokines. Cytokines play a role in inflammation. Long-term efficacy and safety are uncertain.	Increased risk of infection, especially tuberculosis. Increased risk of pneumonia, and listeriosis (a foodborne illness caused by the bacterium *Listeria monocytogenes*).	It is important to avoid eating undercooked foods (including unpasteurized cheeses, cold cuts, and hot dogs) because undercooked food can cause listeriosis for patients taking biological response modifiers.
Tumor necrosis factor inhibitors: etanercept, infliximab, adalimumab	These medications are highly effective for treating patients with an inadequate response to DMARDs. They may be prescribed in combination with some DMARDs, particularly methotrexate. Etanercept requires subcutaneous (beneath the skin) injections 2 times per week. Infliximab is taken intravenously (IV) during a 2-hour procedure. It is administered with methotrexate. Adalimumab requires injections every 2 weeks. Long-term efficacy and safety are uncertain.	Etanercept: Pain or burning in throat; redness, itching, pain, and/or swelling at injection site; runny or stuffy nose. Infliximab: Abdominal pain, cough, dizziness, fainting, headache, muscle pain, runny nose, shortness of breath, sore throat, vomiting, wheezing. Adalimumab: Redness, rash, swelling, itching, bruising, sinus infection, headache, nausea.	Long-term efficacy and safety are uncertain. Doctor monitoring is important, particularly with active infection, exposure to tuberculosis, or a central nervous system disorder. Evaluation for tuberculosis is necessary before treatment begins.
Interleukin-1 inhibitor: anakinra	This medication requires daily injections. Long-term efficacy and safety are uncertain.	Redness, swelling, bruising, or pain at the site of injection; headache; upset stomach; diarrhea; runny nose; and stomach pain.	Doctor monitoring is required.
Other medications	Pilocarpine hydrochloride (Salagen) and cevimeline (Evoxac).	Available to treat dry mouth associated with Sjögren's syndrome. They simulate the salivary glands.	

Source: National Institutes of Health. Health topics. Accessed September 7, 2005 at http://www.niams.nih.gov/hi/topics/arthritis/rahandout.htm.

impact of the disease on several aspects of life seems to play a large part (Jacobs et al, 2001). Psychosocial intervention may be beneficial.

- With borage oil, concomitant non-steroidal anti-inflammatory drug (NSAID) use may undermine the effects; borage oil would be contraindicated in pregnancy given the teratogenic and labor-inducing effects of prostaglandin E agonists (Kast, 2001).
- St. John's wort and echinacea should not be used with cyclosporine or methotrexate.

INTERVENTION: NUTRITION EDUCATION, COUNSELING, CARE MANAGEMENT

- Adoption of a Mediterranean diet confers health benefits in this population because of greater consumption of fruits and vegetables, lower consumption of animal products, and use of olive oil, which modulates immune function (Wahle et al, 2005). Inclusion of omega-3 fatty acids is also important (Berbert et al, 2005); herring, salmon, sardines, tuna, and mackerel are good dietary sources.
- Encourage nutrient-dense foods. If intake is poor, a vitamin-mineral supplement may be needed. Dietary quinones, phenolics, vitamins, amino acids, isoprenoids, and other compounds in functional foods may become very popular (Losso and Bawadi, 2005).
- Instruct patient about simplified planning and preparation tips.
- Discourage quackery and substitute sound health practices.
- Carbohydrate intolerance occurs because of chronic inflammation and use of steroids; planning must reflect individual needs.
- A support group may be helpful for coping.
- Physical therapy and exercise are beneficial for most patients. Strengthening exercises may help improve patient's ability to walk and may decrease joint pain and fatigue.
- Check on bone density; there is a high incidence of osteoporosis when steroids are used.

For More Information

- American Autoimmune Related Diseases Association
  http://www.aarda.org
- American College of Rheumatology
  http://www.rheumatology.org/
- Arthritis Foundation
  http://www.arthritis.org
- Felty Syndrome
  http://rarediseases.about.com/od/rarediseasesf/a/121104.htm
- Information on Rheumatoid Arthritis
  http://www.niams.nih.gov/hi/topics/arthritis/rahandout.htm
- Juvenile Rheumatoid Arthritis
  http://www.niams.nih.gov/hi/topics/juvenile_arthritis/juvarthr.htm
- National Institute of Dental and Craniofacial Research–Sjögren's Syndrome
  http://www.nidr.nih.gov/
- National Sjögren's Syndrome Association
  http://www.sjogrenssyndrome.org/index.html
- Rheumatoid Vasculitis
  http://vasculitis.med.jhu.edu/typesof/rheumatoid.html
- Sjögren's Syndrome Foundation
  http://www.sjogrens.org/

RHEUMATOID ARTHRITIS—CITED REFERENCES

Aggarwal BB, Shishodia S. Suppression of the nuclear factor-kappa B activation pathway by spice-derived phytochemicals: reasoning for seasoning. *Ann N Y Acad Sci.* 1030:434, 2004.

Agren J, et al. Divergent changes in serum sterols during a strict uncooked vegan diet in patients with rheumatoid arthritis. *Br J Nutr.* 85:137, 2001.

Arrington J, et al. Docosahexaenoic acid suppresses function of the CD28 costimulatory membrane receptor in primary murine and Jurkat T cells. *J Nutr.* 131:1147, 2001.

Barham J, et al. Addition of eicosapentaenoic acid to gamma-linolenic acid-supplemented diets prevents serum arachidonic acid accumulation in humans. *J Nutr.* 130:1925, 2000.

Berbert AA, et al. Supplementation of fish oil and olive oil in patients with rheumatoid arthritis. *Nutrition* 21:131, 2005.

Cantorna MT, Mahon BD. Mounting evidence for vitamin D as an environmental factor affecting autoimmune disease prevalence. *Exp Biol Med.* 229:1136, 2004.

Choi HK. Dietary risk factors for rheumatic diseases. *Curr Opin Rheumatol.* 17:141, 2005.

Hanninen O, et al. Antioxidants in vegan diet and rheumatic disorders. *Toxicology* 155:45, 2000.

Helgeland M, et al. Dietary intake and serum concentrations of antioxidants in children with juvenile arthritis. *Clin Exp Rheumatol.* 18:637, 2000.

Hootman J, et al. Characteristics of chronic arthritis and other rheumatic condition-related ambulatory care visits, United States, 1997. *Ann Epidemiol.* 10:454, 2000.

Jacobs J, et al. Why do patients with rheumatoid arthritis use alternative treatments? *Clin Rheumatol.* 20:192, 2001.

Kast R. Borage oil reduction of rheumatoid arthritis activity may be mediated by increased cAMP that suppresses tumor necrosis factor-alpha. *Int Immunopharmacol.* 1:2197, 2001.

Losso JN, Bawadi HA. Hypoxia inducible factor pathways as targets for functional foods. *J Agric Food Chem.* 53:3751, 2005.

Marcora S, et al. Dietary treatment of rheumatoid cachexia with beta-hydroxy-beta-methylbutyrate, glutamine and arginine: a randomised controlled trial. *Clin Nutr.* 24:442, 2005.

Pattison DJ, et al. Dietary beta-cryptoxanthin and inflammatory polyarthritis: results from a population-based prospective study. *Am J Clin Nutr.* 82:451, 2005.

Pedersen M, et al. Diet and risk of rheumatoid arthritis in a prospective cohort. *J Rheumatol.* 32:1249, 2005.

Skoldstam L, et al. Weight reduction is not a major reason for improvement in rheumatoid arthritis from lacto-vegetarian, vegan or Mediterranean diets. *Nutr J.* 4:15, 2005.

Wahle KW, et al. Olive oil and modulation of cell signaling in disease prevention. *Lipids* 39:1223, 2005.

RUPTURED INTERVERTEBRAL DISC

NUTRITIONAL ACUITY RANKING: LEVEL 1

DEFINITIONS AND BACKGROUND

Other names for a slipped or ruptured disc include cervical radiculopathy, herniated intervertebral disc, lumbar radiculopathy, or prolapsed intervertebral disc. In this condition, slipping or prolapse of a cervical or lumbar disc occurs, with neck, shoulder, or low back pain accordingly. Degenerating changes in the disks begin around 30 years of age.

With **lumbar radiculopathy,** ambulation may be painful, and limping can occur. Muscular weakness, severe back pain that radiates to buttocks or legs and feet, pain that worsens with coughing or laughing, tingling or numbness in legs or feet, and muscle contractions or spasms may also result.

With **cervical radiculopathy,** neck pain in back and sides is deep; pain may radiate to shoulders, upper arms, or forearms and worsens with coughing or laughing. Spasm of neck muscles and pain that worsens at night may occur.

A laminectomy surgically removes the lamina of a vertebra. Percutaneous automated discectomy (PAD) surgery can be performed in some cases; this surgery breaks up the disc and removes fragments. There is no convincing medical evidence to support routine use of lumbar fusion, but it may be useful in patients with associated spinal deformity, instability, or associated chronic low-back pain (Resnick et al, 2005). See Figure 11-5.

INTERVENTION: OBJECTIVES

- Maintain adequate rest and activity levels, as assigned by physician.
- Prevent weight gain from decreased activity.
- Encourage adequate hydration.
- Prevent constipation and straining.
- Assist with feeding, if patient is in traction.
- Relieve pain and promote healing.

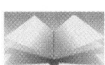

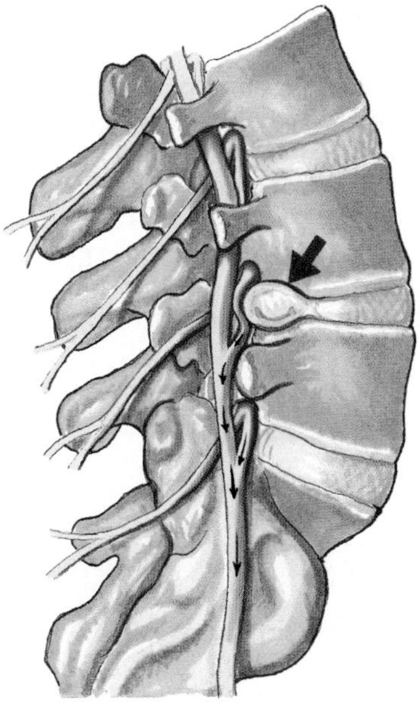

Figure 11-5 Herniated disc. (Image provided by Anatomical Chart Co.)

INTERVENTION: FOOD AND NUTRITION

- A regular diet generally is sufficient. For some, a more strict calorie-controlled diet may be beneficial to promote weight loss.
- Increased fluid and fiber intake can be helpful to reduce constipation. Fresh fruits and vegetables, bran, and other foods may be needed.

CLINICAL INDICATORS

Clinical/History	Constipation	Myelography
Height	Edema	Discography
Weight	MRI or computed tomography (CT) scan	Spinal or neck x-rays
BMI		Nerve conduction velocity test
I & O		
BP		

Lab Work	Na+, K+	Alk phos
H & H	Alb, transthyretin	Gluc
Ca++, Mg++	BUN, Creat	

Common Drugs Used and Potential Side Effects

- Anti-inflammatory drugs may be used. Nausea, gastrointestinal (GI) distress, and anorexia may result. Follow directions regarding when to take (e.g., before or after meals).
- Analgesics may be helpful to relieve pain. Chronic use of aspirin may cause GI bleeding.
- Muscle relaxants may be ordered. GI distress or nausea can occur.

Herbs, Botanicals, and Supplements

- Herbs and botanical supplements should not be used without discussing with physician.

INTERVENTION: NUTRITION EDUCATION, COUNSELING, CARE MANAGEMENT

- Instruct patient regarding effective methods of relieving constipation.
- Discuss role of nutrition and exercise in health maintenance. Weight loss may be needed.
- After surgery, the role of nutrition in wound healing should be discussed.

For More Information

- Lumbar Radiculopathy
  http://neuroland.com/spine/l_radiculo.htm

RUPTURED INTERVERTEBRAL DISC—CITED REFERENCES

Resnick DK, et al. Guidelines for the performance of fusion procedures for degenerative disease of the lumbar spine. Part 8: lumbar fusion for disc herniation and radiculopathy. *J Neurosurg Spine.* 2:673, 2005.

SCLERODERMA

NUTRITIONAL ACUITY RANKING: LEVEL 1–2

DEFINITIONS AND BACKGROUND

Approximately 2% of the population in Europe and North America suffers from systemic rheumatic diseases, such as scleroderma, rheumatoid arthritis, and lupus (Chen and von Mikecz, 2005). In systemic sclerosis (SSc), pathological deposition of fibrous connective tissue in the skin and visceral organs occurs. The gastrointestinal (GI) tract is affected, and Raynaud's syndrome (ischemia of fingers) is common.

Research suggests that the fibrosis involves an increase of hydroxylysine aldehyde collagen cross-linkages as well as an increase in inflammatory cytokines (Brinckmann et al, 2005). Genetic, immunological, hormonal, and environmental factors are considered to be important triggers of autoimmune disorders, including SSc (Molina and Shoenfeld, 2005).

Symptoms and signs include thickening and swelling of the ends of the fingers, dysphagia, heartburn, fibrosis of salivary and lacrimal glands, abdominal pains, flatulence, weight loss, nausea and vomiting, diarrhea, and constipation. The CREST syndrome (limited cutaneous sclerosis) is less severe than SSc and causes less internal organ damage. Calcium deposits, Raynaud's phenomenon, esophageal dysfunction, skin damage on fingers, and telangiectasia form the acronym for CREST.

As the disease progresses, large areas of the skin or just the fingers (sclerodactyly) may be affected. Skin on the face tightens and causes a mask-like appearance. Spider veins (telangiectasia) occur on the fingers, chest, face, lips, or tongue. Calcium deposits can occur on the fingers or other bony areas; sores or contractures may result from the scarring. Scarring of the esophagus may be especially detrimental, causing blockage or even cancer. Lungs can be affected, leading to shortness of breath with exercise.

Neurological involvement consists of epilepsy, central nervous system vasculitis, peripheral neuropathy, vascular malformations, headache, and neuroimaging abnormalities; ocular manifestations include uveitis, xerophthalmia, glaucoma, and papilledema (Zulian et al, 2005). Multiple organ system dysfunction may occur in the cardiac and renal systems; pulmonary hypertension, heart failure, and respiratory failure are major causes of morbidity and mortality (Bar et al, 2001). There is no known cure, and SSc can be fatal.

INTERVENTION: OBJECTIVES

- Prevent or correct protein–energy malnutrition and nutrient deficiencies.
- Correct xerostomia where present; decreased saliva, dysphagia, and difficulty in chewing will result.
- Monitor dysphagia with esophageal involvement; alter method of feeding as needed.
- Counteract vitamin B_{12} and fat maldigestion and absorption, which may be common.
- Monitor hypomotility and gastroparesis; alter fiber intake as appropriate. For many patients, nutritional support and relief of symptoms remain the primary management goals (Quigley, 1999).
- Improve quality of life and reduce fatigue; allow return to work or maintenance of energy levels.

INTERVENTION: FOOD AND NUTRITION

- Diets high in energy (30–40 kcal/kg) and adequate to high in protein are often necessary. A soft diet with moistened foods and extra fluids is useful. Add fiber if constipation is a problem (such as adding crushed bran to hot cereal).
- Small, frequent feedings may be needed.
- Tube feed if patient is dysphagic or has obstruction.
- Use total parenteral nutrition (TPN) if GI tract is highly affected, with intractable diarrhea and severe malabsorption.
- Reduce lactose if intolerance occurs. Extra calcium may be needed if lactose is not tolerated orally.
- Give supplements of fat- and water-soluble vitamins.
- With hypertension and multiple organ system dysfunction, reduced sodium or fluid restriction may be needed.

CLINICAL INDICATORS

Clinical/History

Height
Weight
BMI
Temperature
Skinfold measurements
BP
I & O

Lab Work

ANA (high)
RF (high)
Trig (may be low)
Serum folate
H & H
Serum B_{12}
Gluc
Prothrombin time (PT)
Alb, transthyretin
CRP
GFR
BUN, Creat
Homocysteine
Ca++, Mg++
Na+, K+
Alk phos
Fecal fat test, hydrogen breath test for malabsorption

Common Drugs Used and Potential Side Effects

- Current treatments include topical or systemic corticosteroids, vitamin D analogs (calcitriol and calcipotriol), photochemotherapy, laser therapy, antimalarials, phenytoin, D-penicillamine, and colchicine, all with varying degrees of success (Man and Dytoc, 2004). Topical tacrolimus cream may be useful as an immunosuppressive antibiotic.
- Anti-inflammatory agents, such as steroids, are often used. Monitor for nitrogen and calcium losses, altered electrolyte levels, and elevated glucose levels. Correct diet accordingly.
- Antihypertensives usually are needed; monitor blood pressure results. Potassium supplements may or may not be required; determine need according to medication selected. Angiotensin-converting enzyme (ACE) inhibitors are commonly used.
- Trental (pentoxifylline) is used for Raynaud's syndrome to improve circulation. Anorexia or GI distress may result.
- Treprostinil is a prostacyclin analog that is approved in the United States only for treatment of primary pulmonary hypertension. It has been found to be useful in healing digital ulcerations in scleroderma (Engel and Rockson, 2005).

Herbs, Botanicals, and Supplements

- Herbs and botanical supplements should not be used without discussing with physician.
- For Raynaud's disease, evening primrose, gingko, mustard, garlic, borage, and red pepper have been suggested, but there are no clinical trials that prove effectiveness.

INTERVENTION: NUTRITION EDUCATION, COUNSELING, CARE MANAGEMENT

- Artificial saliva (Xero-Lube) or lemon glycerine may be useful.
- Chew sugarless gum.
- If eating orally, adequate chewing time will be required.
- Consume adequate fluids. Choose moist foods or foods with sauces/gravies.
- For heartburn, keep head elevated after meals; decrease or limit intake of chocolate, caffeine, fatty foods, alcohol, citrus, and tomatoes.
- Physical therapy and exercise may help maintain muscle strength but cannot totally prevent joints from locking into stiffened positions.

For More Information

- Scleroderma Foundation
  http://www.scleroderma.org/
- Scleroderma Research Foundation
  http://www.srfcure.org

SCLERODERMA—CITED REFERENCES

Bar J, et al. Pulmonary-renal syndrome in systemic sclerosis. *Semin Arthritis Rheum.* 30:403, 2001.
Brinckmann J, et al. Interleukin 4 and prolonged hypoxia induce a higher gene expression of lysyl hydroxylase 2 and an altered cross-link pattern: important pathogenetic steps in early and late stage of systemic scleroderma? *Matrix Biol.* 24:459, 2005.
Chen M, von Mikecz A. Xenobiotic-induced recruitment of autoantigens to nuclear proteasomes suggests a role for altered antigen processing in scleroderma. *Ann N Y Acad Sci.* 1051:382, 2005.
Engel G, Rockson SG. Treprostinil for the treatment of severe digital necrosis in systemic sclerosis. *Vasc Med.* 10:29, 2005.
Man J, Dytoc MT. Use of imiquimod cream 5% in the treatment of localized morphea. *J Cutan Med Surg.* 8:166, 2004.
Molina V, Shoenfeld Y. Infection, vaccines and other environmental triggers of autoimmunity. *Autoimmunity* 38:235, 2005.
Quigley E. Chronic intestinal pseudo-obstruction. *Treat Options Gastroenterol.* 2:239, 1999.
Zulian F, et al. Localized scleroderma in childhood is not just a skin disease. Localized scleroderma in childhood is not just a skin disease. *Arthritis Rheum.* 52:2873, 2005.

SYSTEMIC LUPUS ERYTHEMATOSUS

NUTRITIONAL ACUITY RANKING: LEVEL 2

DEFINITIONS AND BACKGROUND

Systemic lupus erythematosus (SLE), or lupus, is an autoimmune disorder that involves areas of inflammation of the joints, tendons, other connective tissues, and skin. There are three types of lupus: discoid, systemic, and drug induced. Women in their late teens to thirties are most affected. See Table 11-15 for a list of symptoms used for diagnostic purposes.

Environmental factors that may trigger the disease include infections, antibiotics (especially sulfa and penicillin), other drugs, and exposure to phthalate in toys, plastics, and beauty products. There may also be a genetic tendency; persons with close family members who have lupus have a 10 times greater frequency than the general population. More people have lupus than AIDS; 1–2 million people have lupus, especially Latino, African American, and Native American women.

For most people, lupus is a mild disease affecting only a few organs. For others, it may cause serious and even life-threatening problems. Thousands of Americans die each year from related complications; a cure is not yet possible.

Because lupus has symptoms that mimic other disorders, careful diagnosis is important. For example, lupus may show symptoms similar to those of celiac disease. The immunological profile of immunoglobulin (Ig) A defi-

TABLE 11-15 Symptoms of Lupus Used for Diagnosis

Joints:	Achy joints (arthralgia) Swollen and painful joints (nonerosive arthritis)
Skin:	Butterfly rash across cheeks and nose Skin rashes, red raised patches Photosensitivity Painless mouth or nose ulcers Pale or purple fingers from cold or stress (Raynaud's syndrome) Unusual hair loss
Neurological system:	Seizures and cognitive dysfunction
Blood disorders:	Anemia, low platelet count, low white blood cell count Abnormal blood clotting
Immunological changes:	Positive antinuclear antibody test (ANA) Antibodies to double-stranded DNA
Cardiopulmonary disorders:	Pleuritis or pericarditis
Renal disorder:	Protein or cellular casts in urine Swollen ankles
Fever over 100°F	
Prolonged fatigue	

ciency or raised double-stranded DNA in the absence of antinuclear factor, elevated inflammatory markers, and symptoms suggestive of an immune disorder should alert the physician to the possibility of gluten sensitivity (Hadjivassiliou et al, 2004).

Patients with lupus experience excess morbidity and mortality due to coronary artery disease, and related oxidative stress is present (Tam et al, 2005). Antioxidant interventions are being studied extensively. Supplementation with fish oil may be beneficial in modifying symptomatic disease activity in patients with lupus; patients can reduce their intake of steroids (Duffy et al, 2004).

INTERVENTION: OBJECTIVES

- Counteract steroid therapy.
- Replenish potassium reserves.
- Reduce fever and replace nutrient losses and weight loss.
- Control disease manifestations.
- Manage cardiac effects. Pericarditis is the most common problem. Shortness of breath and chest pain can occur.
- Lupus nephritis is the term for the kidney disease (glomerulonephritis) that occurs in SLE; about a third of patients with lupus will develop it, requiring medical evaluation and nutritional management.
- Rule out gluten intolerance.

INTERVENTION: FOOD AND NUTRITION

- Diet should be adequate in protein and energy during fever.
- When renal disease is present, diet should be adjusted. Check lab values regularly.
- Alter diet, if needed, to lower blood pressure levels or excess weight. If needed, mildly restrict sodium intake and monitor for potassium and phosphorus changes.
- Dietary nutrients may modify clinical course of disease in female patients with SLE; vitamin C intake may prevent the occurrence of active disease (Minami et al, 2003). A multivitamin-mineral supplement may be needed.
- Anemia is often present and does not correlate with iron intake; vitamin B_{12}, dietary fiber, iron, calcium, and folate may be low in the diets of lupus patients (Shah et al, 2004). However, avoid excessive doses of supplements; use DRI levels.
- Use a nutrient-rich diet that includes nuts, fish and fish oils (Simopoulos, 2002), olive oil, fruits, vegetables, and whole grains that are rich in phytochemicals, omega-3 fatty acids, and antioxidants. Alter diet, if needed, when there is kidney disease.
- Include phytochemicals derived from spices such as turmeric (curcumin); red pepper (capsaicin); cloves (eugenol); ginger (gingerol); cumin, anise, and fennel (anethol); basil and rosemary (ursolic acid); garlic (diallyl sulfide, *S*-allylmercaptocysteine, and ajoene); and pomegranate (ellagic acid) (Aggarwal and Shishodia, 2004).
- If gluten intolerance is present, provide a gluten-free dietary plan.

CLINICAL INDICATORS

Clinical/History

Height
Weight
BMI
BP
I & O
Temperature

Lab Work

LE prep
ESR
Complement protein test (C3, C4, CH50, CH100)
CRP
ANA (increased)
Serum copper (increased)
Total protein (decreased)
WBC (decreased)
Gluc (increased)
Specific gravity, urine (decreased)
Chol (increased)
BUN, Creat
Alb, transthyretin
Transferrin
Ca++, Mg++
Na+, K+
H & H (decreased)
Transferrin
Serum ferritin

Common Drugs Used and Potential Side Effects

- Currently, nonsteroidal anti-inflammatory drugs (NSAIDs) and acetaminophen are useful. If sodium retention occurs, alter diet as necessary.
- Steroid therapy may cause sodium retention, hyperglycemia, potassium and calcium depletion, and negative nitrogen balance. Side effects include weight gain, a round face, acne, easy bruising, fractures or osteoporosis, hypertension, cataracts, hyperglycemia or onset of diabetes, increased risk of infection, and stomach ulcers. Take fish oil supplements for possible gradual reduction in use of steroids (Duffy et al, 2004).
- Sunscreens are needed to protect against the sun's harmful rays; there are no systemic side effects.
- Antimalarials, such as chloroquine (Aralen) or hydroxychloroquine (Plaquenil), may be used for skin and joint symptoms of lupus. Side effects are rare and consist of occasional diarrhea or rashes. Chloroquine can affect the eyes. Hydroxychloroquine may cause anorexia, nausea, abdominal cramps, and diarrhea.
- Immunosuppressive agents such as azathioprine (Imuran) and cyclophosphamide (Cytoxan) or methotrexate are used to control the overactive immune system. There are often gastrointestinal (GI) side effects.

Herbs, Botanicals, and Supplements

- Herbs and botanical supplements should not be used without discussing with physician.
- Coumestrol, a natural phytoestrogen, may relieve some symptoms (Schoenroth et al, 2004). Other dietary changes being studied include energy restriction and use of indoles, conjugated linolenic acid (CLA), and vitamins C, E, and D.

INTERVENTION: NUTRITION EDUCATION, COUNSELING, CARE MANAGEMENT

- Ensure patient has an adequate intake of fluids during febrile periods.
- Explain which foods are sources of sodium and potassium in the diet.
- Adequate rest is needed during flare-ups.
- Sunblock should be used outdoors.
- Cortisone creams may be needed for persistent skin rashes.
- Discuss how to manage diet if elevated blood glucose is present. Insulin may be needed, and carbohydrate counting should be used.
- Weight loss plans may be needed if there is obesity.
- Regular doctor visits and lab tests are important, especially blood and urine testing.
- Dietary strategies for the prevention of obesity, osteoporosis, and hyperlipidemia deserve attention.

For More Information

- Lupus Alliance of America
  http://www.lupusalliance.org/
- Lupus Canada
  http://www.lupuscanada.org/
- Lupus Foundation of America
  http://www.lupus.org/
- Lupus Library
  http://www.lupusny.org/library.php
- Office on Women's Health–Lupus Awareness Project
  http://www.womenshealth.gov/owh/minority.htm#Lupus%20Awareness%20Project
- Other Lupus Organizations
  http://www.lupusny.org/links.php#lupusorg
- SLE Foundation, Inc.
  http://www.lupusny.org/

SYSTEMIC LUPUS ERYTHEMATOSUS—CITED REFERENCES

Aggarwal BB, Shishodia S. Suppression of the nuclear factor-kappa B activation pathway by spice-derived phytochemicals: reasoning for seasoning. *Ann N Y Acad Sci.* 1030:434, 2004.

Duffy EM, et al. The clinical effect of dietary supplementation with omega-3 fish oils and/or copper in systemic lupus erythematosus. *J Rheumatol.* 31:1551, 2004.

Hadjivassiliou M, et al. Gluten sensitivity masquerading as systemic lupus erythematosus. *Ann Rheum Dis.* 63:1501, 2004.

Minami Y, et al. Diet and systemic lupus erythematosus: a 4 year prospective study of Japanese patients. *J Rheumatol.* 30:747, 2003.

Schoenroth LJ, et al. The effect of the phytoestrogen coumestrol on the NZB/W F1 murine model of systemic lupus. *J Autoimmun.* 23:323, 2004.

Shah M, et al. Nutrient intake and diet quality in patients with systemic lupus erythematosus on a culturally sensitive cholesterol lowering dietary program. *J Rheumatol.* 31:71, 2004.

Simopoulos A. Omega-3 fatty acids in inflammation and autoimmune diseases. *J Am Coll Nutr.* 21:495, 2002.

Tam LS, et al. Effects of vitamins C and E on oxidative stress markers and endothelial function in patients with systemic lupus erythematosus: a double blind, placebo controlled pilot study. *J Rheumatol.* 32:275, 2005.

SECTION 12

Hematology: Anemias and Blood Disorders

CHIEF ASSESSMENT FACTORS

- Concurrent Illness—Cerebrovascular Disease, Myocardial Infarction, Asthma, Hemorrhage, Cancers, Renal Disease
- Previous Blood Disorder, Bleeding Tendencies, Blood Transfusion, or Exposure to Radiation
- Blood Type
- Bruising
- Lymphadenopathy
- Surgery, Especially Gastric, Hepatic, or Renal
- Infections, Sepsis
- Family History of Leukemias, Cancer, Anemias, Immune Disorders, Allergies
- History of Alcohol and Nicotine Use
- Dietary Habits: Use of Heme and Nonheme Iron, Vitamin and Mineral Deficiencies, Protein Intake, Vegan Lifestyle, Other Factors (see Table 12-1)
- Medication Use (Prescriptions, Over-the-Counter) and Use of Herbal or Botanical Medications
- Anorexia, Fatigue
- Beefy, Red Tongue; Other Signs of Nutrient Deficiencies
- Occupational or Environmental Exposure to Toxic Substances
- Exposure to Lead Paint, Other Toxins

GENERAL INFORMATION ABOUT ANEMIAS

Anemias are a set of hematological disorders with a reduced number of red blood cells, reduced amount of hemoglobin, or reduced number of volume-packed red blood cells (hematocrit). The main consequences of these disorders include hypoxia and decreased oxygen-carrying capacity. Anemia is an effect of hypoxia and not a disease itself. Inflammations, infections, and cancers may all contribute to anemias. Causes of anemias include peptic ulcers, gastritis, liver disease, renal disease, hypothyroidism, history of blood transfusions, blood coagulation disorders, and poor diet. Overall, anemias affect over 3.4 million people in the United States alone.

Erythropoietin is a hormone that stimulates red blood cell production. The erythrocyte life span is 120 days, after which the cells are destroyed by the spleen. Anemia should not be accepted as inevitable; chronic disease and iron deficiency are the most common causes (Smith, 2000). Other causes of anemia include excessive bleeding, decreased red blood cell production, and increased red blood cell destruction. Anemias can be encountered with generalized or specific nutritional deficiencies (see Table 12-1). The nutritional anemias caused by deficits must be corrected by provision, but not all anemias require nutritional intervention; use caution when evaluating single laboratory analyses.

Inadequate intakes of many nutrients are now known to contribute to several chronic diseases that affect the populations of the industrialized nations, the long latency deficiency diseases (Heaney, 2003). Folic acid and vitamin B_{12} are among the key nutrients involved. Inadequate intakes of specific nutrients may produce more than one disease, may produce diseases by more than one mechanism, and may require several years for the consequent morbidity to be sufficiently evident to be clinically identified (Heaney, 2003).

Iron and copper participate in one-electron exchange reactions; the same property that makes them essential also generates free radicals that can be seriously deleterious to cells, and so a careful balance (homeostasis) is needed (Arredondo and Nunez, 2005). Iron is one of the most frequently lacking nutrients in populations in the developing world and in developed countries. Iron deficiency with anemia affects about 25% of infants worldwide. Adults, especially menstruating women, are also susceptible. Up to 10% of young women in developed countries are iron deficient. The problem is not easily resolved by adopting an iron-rich diet because absorption varies greatly.

Vitamin B_{12} deficiency, iron or folate deficiency, chronic gastrointestinal bleeding, and myelodysplastic syndrome are causes of anemia in the elderly. Anemias are more common in the hospitalized elderly than among those who live independently.

Dietary heme iron is important and is more readily absorbed than nonheme iron derived from vegetables and grain. Most heme is absorbed in the proximal intestine, and the newly identified HCP1 protein is the long-sought intestinal heme transporter (Shayeghi et al, 2005). Another interesting fact that has been identified recently is that probiotic products may help with digestion of phytates, allowing more iron to be absorbed (Sazawal et al, 2004). Table 12-2 indicates the relationship of iron to various types of anemias. Table 12-3 provides some key definitions used to describe and identify specific anemias. Table 12-4 lists signs and symptoms of common anemias.

TABLE 12-1 Nutritional Factors in Blood Formation

Protein	Folic acid
Iron	Vitamin B_6
Vitamin C	Vitamin B_{12}
Vitamin E	Vitamin K
Riboflavin (minute amounts)	Copper

CITED REFERENCES

Arredondo M, Nunez MT. Iron and copper metabolism. *Mol Aspects Med.* 26:313, 2005.

Heaney RP. Long-latency deficiency disease: insights from calcium and vitamin D. *Am J Clin Nutr.* 78:912, 2003.

TABLE 12-2 Significance of Iron Stores in Various Anemias

Type of Anemia	Ferritin	Total Iron-Binding Capacity (TIBC)	Marrow Iron	Treatment
Anemia of chronic disease	Normal or high	Normal or low	Normal or increased	Treat underlying disease.
Iron deficiency	Low	High	Absent	Iron supplements; treat sources of blood loss.
Megaloblastic anemia	Normal to high	Usually normal	Normal or low	Treat cause.
Renal disease	Normal	Normal or low	Normal	Give erythropoietin. Iron supplementation may also be needed.
Thalassemia minor	Normal	Normal	Normal	None specifically.

Adapted from: Abramson S, Abramson N. 'Common' uncommon anemias. *Am Fam Physician.* 59:851, 1999. See also: Iron Overload Disease Association. Iron tests. Available at http://www.irondisorders.org/Forms/irontests.pdf.

TABLE 12-3 Definitions and Iron Tests

Acute anemia—Precipitous drop in the red blood cell (RBC) population due to hemolysis or acute hemorrhage.

Anemia—Reduction in the number of circulating RBCs, the amount of hemoglobin, or the volume of packed RBCs (hematocrit).

Chronic anemia—Anemia that lasts 2 months or longer.

Hypochromia—Blood condition in which there is a low level of hemoglobin.

Hyperchromia—Blood that is excessively pigmented.

Microcytic anemias—Usually caused by or resulting in iron deficiency; RBCs are small in size.

Macrocytic anemias—Folic acid or vitamin B_{12} insufficiency; RBCs are larger than usual.

Megaloblastic anemias—Anemias in which there are large, nucleated abnormal RBCs that are irregular in shape, as in pernicious anemia. It may also result from use of certain immunosuppressive or antitumor drugs.

Normocytic anemias—From inhibition of marrow by infection or chronic disease; RBCs are of usual size.

Normochromia—Blood with a normal color and level of hemoglobin.

Iron Tests

Fasting serum iron, total iron-binding capacity (TIBC), serum ferritin, and hemoglobin.

Hemoglobin: reflects the level of functional iron. Low levels can indicate iron deficiency anemia or anemia of chronic disease. Hemoglobin values help determine if anemia is present and if a blood donation can be done.

Serum ferritin: measures the amount of iron in containment. One ferritin molecule can hold as many as 4500 iron atoms. Ferritin can be elevated when a person has an infection or inflammatory condition.

Serum iron (Fe): is free or unbound iron in serum. Ideal range is 40–180 μg/dL. Measurement is best done fasting because serum iron is sensitive to foods or supplements recently consumed, time of day, and menstruation.

Transferrin: is an iron-binding and transport protein that can bind to and transport 2 molecules of iron. Transferrin carries iron through the bloodstream to the bone marrow, the liver, and ferritin. Transferrin is no longer measured directly by most physicians, instead TIBC is used.

TIBC: demonstrates the iron-binding ability of transferrin. Serum iron divided by TIBC × 100% provides the transferrin-iron saturation percentage (Tsat%), which is also called iron saturation. Normally, Tsat% is 25–35%. Higher numbers are suggestive of iron loading. Lower numbers are suggestive of iron deficiency anemia. Serum ferritin measures iron in containment (or stored iron).

From: Iron Overload Disease Association. Iron tests. Accessed September 25, 2005 at http://www.irondisorders.org/Forms/irontests.pdf.

TABLE 12-4 General Signs and Symptoms of Anemia

- Anorexia
- Ascites
- Chest pain, palpitations
- Coldness of extremities
- Dizziness, especially postural
- Dyspnea, especially with increased physical activity (exercise intolerance)
- Decreased libido or impotence
- Decreased urine output/bowel irregularity
- Difficulty sleeping or concentrating
- Fatigue, weakness, irritability
- Headache
- Mental status changes
- Pale conjunctiva
- Tachycardia
- Thirst
- Tinnitus
- Vertigo, syncope

Sazawal S, et al. Efficacy of milk fortified with a probiotic *Bifidobacterium lactis* (DR-10TM) and prebiotic galacto-oligosaccharides in prevention of morbidity and on nutritional status. *Asia Pac J Clin Nutr.* 13:28S, 2004.

Shayeghi M, et al. Identification of an intestinal heme transporter. *Cell* 122:789, 2005.

Smith D. Anemia in the elderly. *Am Fam Physician.* 62:1565, 2000.

For More Information

- Anemia Information for Patients
  http://www.anemia.org/patients/educationsheets/
- Anemia Monograph
  http://www.anemia.org/pdf/mon_Anemia_Overview.pdf
- Anemia Resource Center
  http://www.emedicine.com/rc/rc/pfeatured/i30/anemia.htm
- Burden of Anemia Model
  http://chi.cerner.com/naac/homepage.asp
- National Anemia Action Center–Slide Series
  http://www.anemia.org/professionals/resources/slides/
- National Institutes of Health/National Heart, Lung, and Blood Institute Information Center
  http://www.nhlbi.nih.gov/
- National Organization for Rare Disorders
  www.rarediseases.org
- Public Advocacy Issues
  http://www.nhlbi.nih.gov/public/nhlbi-listens-a.pdf

ANEMIAS

ANEMIA OF CHRONIC DISEASE

NUTRITIONAL ACUITY RANKING: LEVEL 2

DEFINITIONS AND BACKGROUND

Anemia of chronic disease (ACD) is the condition of impaired iron utilization where functional iron (hemoglobin) is low, but tissue iron (such as in storage) is normal or high. ACD is known as hypoferremia of inflammatory disease or anemia of inflammation and is often diagnosed as mild iron deficiency anemia. The difference is that low hemoglobin, low total iron-binding capacity (TIBC), and low transferrin with elevated ferritin are identified.

ACD is seen in a wide range of chronic autoimmune, cancerous or leukemic, inflammatory, and infectious disease conditions. In rheumatoid arthritis, there is frequently coexistence of ACD and iron deficiency anemia resulting from gastrointestinal (GI) bleeding due to use of many drugs. ACD is very common in systemic lupus erythematosus; it is found in approximately 50% of patients (Giannouli et al, 2006). In the aging population, chronic severe anemia is actually tolerated (Aessopos et al, 2004).

Hemoglobin improvement is an independent predictor of quality of life improvement in anemic patients, yet supplementation with iron for those with ACD can be harmful and even result in death. Levels of erythropoietin are reduced in ACD; the genetically engineered form can correct anemia caused by cancer in about 50–60% of patients and may improve survival in human immunodeficiency virus (HIV) patients with anemia.

Genetically engineered erythropoietin (epoetin) may be helpful and can eliminate the need for transfusions; however, it is very expensive. Epoetin provides clinically significant improvement in hepatitis C–infected patients (Pockros et al, 2004). Anemia in chronic kidney disease is treated with erythropoiesis-stimulating agents (ESAs); they are safe and may forestall some of the target-organ damage of chronic kidney disease (Nurko, 2006).

INTERVENTION: OBJECTIVES

- Prevent infections or sepsis. Reduce fever and excessive inflammation.
- Reduce bleeding tendencies and hemorrhages.
- Ensure adequate periods of rest.
- Prepare for bone marrow transplantation.
- Prevent further complications and decline in organ functioning.

INTERVENTION: FOOD AND NUTRITION

- Provide a balanced diet that is easily prepared, with six small feedings.
- Provide extra fluid unless contraindicated.
- If steroids are used, limiting sodium intake may be needed.
- Correct iron overload where present.

CLINICAL INDICATORS

Clinical/History	Lab Work	
Height	Complete blood count (CBC)	Serum Fe
Weight	Red blood cell count (RBC)	Glucose (Gluc)
Body mass index (BMI)	Total iron-binding capacity (TIBC) (low)	Transferrin (low)
Diet history	Hemoglobin and hematocrit (H & H) (high)	Albumin (Alb)
Intake and output (I & O)	Serum ferritin (high)	C-reactive protein (CRP)
Blood pressure (BP)		
Fatigue and weakness		
Headache, irritability		

Common Drugs Used and Potential Side Effects

- Genetically engineered erythropoietin (epoetin) is often used; given weekly, it can improve quality of life and levels of energy.
- Avoid iron supplements in this condition; they can be harmful and even result in death.
- Corticosteroids may be used. Watch side effects of chronic use such as elevated serum sodium levels, decreased potassium and calcium levels, and negative nitrogen balance. Hyperglycemia may occur; alter diet accordingly.
- Antibiotics may be required when infections are present. Monitor for GI distress and other effects.

Herbs, Botanicals, and Supplements

- Herbs and botanical supplements should not be used without discussing with physician.

INTERVENTION: NUTRITION EDUCATION, COUNSELING, CARE MANAGEMENT

- Discuss needs of the patient that are specific for signs and symptoms and for side effects of any medications.
- Discuss nutritious meal planning. If patient has diabetes, heart failure, or cirrhosis, counsel specifically to those issues.

- Correcting anemia in heart failure patients improves quality of life and exercise capacity in both men and women (Fox and Jorde, 2005). Once improvement is noted, activity levels can be increased.
- Counsel about method for reduction of iron overload where present. For example, iron-fortified cereals and oral supplements containing iron should be avoided. Increasing grains, cheese, and dairy foods and using fewer heme iron sources will help.
- Being female is often independently associated with lower hemoglobin, so when deciding upon initiation of treatment in this population, sex-specific lab values should be assessed (Fox and Jorde, 2005).

For More Information

- Anemia of Chronic Disease
http://www.emedicine.com/emerg/topic734.htm

ANEMIA OF CHRONIC DISEASE—CITED REFERENCES

Aessopos A, et al. Cardiovascular adaptation to chronic anemia in the elderly: an echocardiographic study. *Clin Invest Med.* 27:265, 2004.

Giannouli S, et al. Anemia in systemic lupus erythematosus: from pathophysiology to clinical assessment. *Ann Rheum Dis.* 65:144, 2006.

Fox MT, Jorde UP. Anemia, chronic heart failure, and the impact of male vs. female gender. *Congest Heart Fail.* 11:129, 2005.

Nurko S. Anemia in chronic kidney disease: causes, diagnosis, treatment. *Cleve Clin J Med.* 73:289, 2006.

Pockros PJ, et al. Epoetin alfa improves quality of life in anemic HCV-infected patients receiving combination therapy. *Hepatology.* 40:1458, 2004.

ANEMIAS IN NEONATES

NUTRITIONAL ACUITY RANKING: LEVEL 2

DEFINITIONS AND BACKGROUND

Anemia of prematurity (AOP) is a normocytic, normochromic anemia that presents with very low hemoglobin and low erythropoietin level. Inadequate red blood cell production occurs, and the average lifespan of these cells is about 35–50 days (compared with 120 days for adults). AOP is very common in very low birth weight (VLBW) infants and among those born prematurely; it is especially common in those born with weight below 1500 g (Haiden et al, 2006). Critically ill, extremely premature infants develop anemia because of intensive laboratory blood testing and undergo multiple red blood cell (RBC) transfusions in the early weeks of life (Widness et al, 2005). Poor weight gain, apnea and tachypnea, lethargy, tachycardia, and pallor are symptoms.

Reducing anemia in infants may be a preventive measure to lower disease burden from infectious disease in this vulnerable population (Levy et al, 2005). Nutritional deficiencies of vitamin E, vitamin B_{12}, and folate exaggerate the degree of anemia. Vitamin E supplementation, however, when given to preterm infants, does not reduce the severity of this anemia (Fishman et al, 2000). Administration of vitamin B_{12} and folate with erythropoietin and iron may enhance erythropoietin-induced erythropoiesis more than erythropoietin alone (Haiden et al, 2006).

When detected early in pregnancy, iron deficiency anemia is associated with a greater risk of preterm delivery (Scholl, 2005). It is important not to overdo iron intake also. High levels of hemoglobin, hematocrit, and ferritin are associated with an increased risk of fetal growth restriction, preterm delivery, and preeclampsia (Scholl, 2005).

Diamond-Blackfan anemia (DBA) (erythrogenesis imperfecta, or congenital hypoplastic anemia) is a rare blood disorder characterized by deficiency of red blood cells at birth. Other symptoms including slow growth, abnormal weakness, fatigue, pallor, characteristic facial abnormalities, protruding shoulder blades, abnormal shortening of the neck due to fusion of cervical vertebrae, hand deformities, and congenital heart defects. DBA may be inherited as either an autosomal dominant or recessive genetic trait, where the body's bone marrow produces little or no red blood cells. A genetic error on chromosome 19 is associated with about 25% of cases, and there is a family history of the disorder in 10–20% of cases.

DBA affects approximately 600 to 700 million people worldwide, but DBA can be difficult to identify. The symptoms may also vary greatly, from very mild to severe and life threatening. DBA is usually diagnosed within the first 2 years of life, sometimes even at birth, based on symptoms. The diagnosis of this anemia might not be recognized right away, however, because it is rare.

The first line of treatment for DBA is prednisone. About 70% of children with DBA will respond to this lifelong treatment, where the medication stimulates the production of more red blood cells. If steroids do not work, the next treatment is blood transfusions. Regular blood transfusions will provide red blood cells but can lead to iron overloading. Normally, the body uses the iron when making new red blood cells, but since the person with DBA is not making many cells, the iron builds up. The person then needs to take medication that takes the excess iron out of the body.

Finally, the only cure available for DBA is bone marrow transplantation, which is used when steroid medications and blood transfusions do not help. Fortunately, there has been progress in the application of stem-cell transplantation with human leukocyte antigen (HLA)-matched stem cells for DBA (Kuliev et al, 2005).

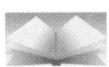

INTERVENTION: OBJECTIVES

- Prevent infections or sepsis. Reduce fever and excessive inflammation.
- Prevent further complications.
- Support growth.

INTERVENTION: FOOD AND NUTRITION

- Provide a balanced diet that is easily prepared, with small feedings given frequently.
- Provide extra fluid unless contraindicated.

CLINICAL INDICATORS

Clinical/History		
Height	BP	H & H
Weight	Weakness	Serum ferritin
BMI	Fatigue and pallor	Serum Fe
Diet history	I & O	Gluc
Slow growth in child (low height–weight percentiles)		Alb
	Lab Work	CRP
	CBC	Serum folic acid
	RBC count	Serum B_{12}
		K+, Na+
		Calcium

Common Drugs Used and Potential Side Effects

- If corticosteroids are used, watch side effects of chronic use such as elevated serum sodium levels, decreased potassium and calcium levels, and negative nitrogen balance. Hyperglycemia may occur; alter diet accordingly. Besides diabetes, glaucoma, bone weakening, and high blood pressure can occur, and the medication may suddenly stop working for that person at any point in time.
- Antibiotics may be required when infections are present. Monitor for gastrointestinal distress and other side effects.

Herbs, Botanicals, and Supplements

- Herbs and botanical supplements should not be used without discussing with physician.

INTERVENTION: NUTRITION EDUCATION, COUNSELING, CARE MANAGEMENT

- Discuss needs of the patient that are specific for signs and symptoms and for side effects of any medications.
- Discuss nutritious meal planning.
- If patient has diabetes, counsel specifically for nutritional management.
- Activity levels must be restricted to avoid accidents or falls that could promote bleeding.
- Referral to the Women, Infants, and Children (WIC) Program can be beneficial. WIC programs are helpful in improving hemoglobin concentration among young children (Altucher et al, 2005).

For More Information

- Anemia in Neonates
  http://www.anemia.org/professionals/research/articles/mild.jsp
- Anemia of Prematurity
  http://www.emedicine.com/ped/topic2629.htm
- Diamond Blackfan Anemia
  http://www.diamondblackfan.org.uk/
- Diamond Blackfan Anemia Registry
  http://www.dbar.org/

ANEMIAS IN NEONATES—CITED REFERENCES

Altucher K, et al. Predictors of improvement in hemoglobin concentration among toddlers enrolled in the Massachusetts WIC Program. *J Am Diet Assoc* 105:716, 2005.

Fishman S, et al. The role of vitamins in the prevention and control of anemia. *Public Health Nutr.* 3:125, 2000.

Haiden N, et al. A randomized, controlled trial of the effects of adding vitamin B12 and folate to erythropoietin for the treatment of anemia of prematurity. *Pediatrics* 118:180, 2006.

Kuliev A, et al. Preimplantation genetics: improving access to stem cell therapy. *Ann N Y Acad Sci.* 1054:223, 2005.

Levy A, et al. Anemia as a risk factor for infectious diseases in infants and toddlers: results from a prospective study. *Eur J Epidemiol.* 20:277, 2005.

Scholl TO. Iron status during pregnancy: setting the stage for mother and infant. *Am J Clin Nutr.* 81:1218S, 2005.

Widness JA, et al. Reduction in red blood cell transfusions among preterm infants: results of a randomized trial with an in-line blood gas and chemistry monitor. *Pediatrics* 115:1299, 2005.

ANEMIA OF RENAL DISEASES

NUTRITIONAL ACUITY RANKING: LEVEL 2

DEFINITIONS AND BACKGROUND

Anemia of renal disease occurs in both acute and chronic renal disease. This anemia is often normochromic and normocytic and sometimes microcytic. The buildup of uremic toxins and decreased erythropoietin production adversely affect erythropoiesis. The accumulation of toxic metabolites, which are normally excreted by the kidneys, shortens the life span of circulating red blood cells.

There is an inverse relationship between blood urea nitrogen (BUN) levels and red blood cell life span, but there is also diminished renal production of erythropoietin that results in decreased red blood cell production. If no cause for anemia other than chronic kidney disease is detected based on the workup and the serum creatinine is ≥2 mg/dL, anemia is most likely due to erythropoietin deficiency (National Kidney Foundation, 2001). Measurement of serum erythropoietin levels usually is not needed.

Short daily hemodialysis and daily home nocturnal hemodialysis are promising to improve quality of life, control blood pressure, and manage anemia in this population (Pierratos, 2005).

INTERVENTION: OBJECTIVES

- Prevent infections or sepsis. Reduce fever and excessive inflammation.
- Prevent further complications, such as heart disease.
- Support growth in children.
- Improve energy level and decrease fatigue, irritability, and infections.

INTERVENTION: FOOD AND NUTRITION

- Provide a balanced diet that is easily prepared, with small feedings given frequently.
- Provide extra fluid unless contraindicated.
- Provide iron-rich foods if appropriate for the individual (depending on lab values, current status, predialysis, or dialysis).

CLINICAL INDICATORS

Clinical/History

- Height
- Weight
- BMI
- Diet history
- BP
- I & O
- Weakness
- Fatigue and pallor

Lab Work

- CBC
- RBC count
- Blood urea nitrogen (BUN)
- Creatinine (Creat)
- Hemoglobin (Hgb) (desired level, 11–12 g/dL in chronic kidney disease [CKD])
- Hematocrit (desired level, 33–36% in CKD)
- Percent transferrin saturation (serum iron × 100 ÷ TIBC)
- Serum ferritin
- TIBC
- Test for occult blood
- Reticulocyte count
- Gluc
- Alb
- CRP
- Serum folic acid
- Serum B_{12}

Common Drugs Used and Potential Side Effects

- When oral iron is used, it may be given as 200 mg of elemental iron per day, in 2 to 3 divided doses in the adult patient, and 2–3 mg/kg/d in the pediatric patient (National Kidney Foundation, 2001). Take oral iron without food and separately from other medications.
- Epoetin is used when oral iron therapy fails in anemia of chronic renal disease (Nurko, 2006). In anemia of persistent nephrotic syndrome, anemia is common before the deterioration of kidney function. Nephrotic patients have erythropoietin (EPO) deficiency with a blunted response to anemia; EPO therapy is recommended for this group of patients (Feinstein et al, 2001).
- The most common cause of an incomplete response to epoetin is iron deficiency. In the iron-replete patient with an inadequate response to epoetin, the following conditions should be evaluated and treated, if reversible: infection or inflammation (access infections, surgical inflammation, acquired immunodeficiency syndrome [AIDS], lupus); chronic blood loss; aluminum toxicity; hemoglobinopathies (thalassemias, sickle cell anemia); folate or vitamin B_{12} deficiency; multiple myeloma; malnutrition; and hemolysis (National Kidney Foundation, 2001).

Herbs, Botanicals, and Supplements

- Herbs and botanical supplements should not be used without discussing with physician.

INTERVENTION: NUTRITION EDUCATION, COUNSELING, CARE MANAGEMENT

- Discuss needs of the patient that are specific for signs and symptoms and for side effects of any medications.
- Discuss simplified, but nutritious, meal planning.
- If patient has diabetes, heart failure, or cirrhosis, counsel specifically to those issues for nutritional management.
- Activity levels must be restricted to avoid accidents or falls that could promote bleeding.

For More Information

- American Association of Kidney Patients
  http://kidney.niddk.nih.gov/kudiseases/pubs/anemia/index.htm
- National Institute of Diabetes and Digestive and Kidney Diseases–Anemia
  http://kidney.niddk.nih.gov/kudiseases/pubs/anemia/index.htm
- Side Effects of Kidney Disease–Anemia
  http://www.aakp.org/AAKP/Forms/ckdbook.pdf

ANEMIA OF RENAL DISEASES—CITED REFERENCES

Feinstein S, et al. Erythropoietin deficiency causes anemia in nephrotic children with normal kidney function. *Am J Kidney Dis.* 37:736, 2001.

National Kidney Foundation. NKF-K/DOQI clinical practice guidelines for anemia of chronic kidney disease: update 2000. *Am J Kidney Dis.* 37:182S, 2001.

Nurko S. Anemia in chronic kidney disease: causes, diagnosis, treatment. *Cleve Clin J Med.* 73:289, 2006.

Pierratos A. New approaches to hemodialysis. *Annu Rev Med.* 55:179, 2005.

APLASTIC ANEMIA AND FANCONI'S ANEMIA

NUTRITIONAL ACUITY RANKING: LEVEL 1

DEFINITIONS AND BACKGROUND

Aplastic anemia is a rare bone marrow disorder with normocytic, normochromic anemia in which normal marrow is replaced with fat. Aplastic anemia, myelodysplastic syndromes, and paroxysmal nocturnal hemoglobinuria (PNH) are bone marrow failure diseases that occur when the bone marrow stops making healthy blood-forming stem cells. Stem cells produce red blood cells, white blood cells, and platelets.

In about 50% of cases, the cause may be inherited or autoimmunity. In other cases, exposure to toxic agents (e.g., radiation, heavy metals, inorganic arsenic) or use of drugs (e.g., phenylbutazone, chloramphenicol, anticonvulsants) may be the cause. Hematopoietic effects of interferon-gamma (IFN-γ) may be responsible for certain aspects of the pathology seen in bone marrow failure syndromes, including aplastic anemia (Zeng et al, 2006). Signs and symptoms are listed in Table 12-5.

Treatment includes blood transfusion, preventive antibiotics, careful hand washing, hormone therapy, immunosuppressive therapy, and medications to enhance bone marrow cell production.

Fanconi's anemia (FA) is a rare, genetic disorder characterized by multiple congenital anomalies, progressive bone marrow failure, and an increased prevalence of cancer (Fagerlie and Bagby, 2006). FA is characterized by delayed bone marrow failure with progression to aplastic anemia that requires bone marrow transplantation. It may be apparent at birth or during childhood and is characterized by deficiency of all bone marrow elements including red blood cells, white blood cells, and platelets (pancytopenia).

FA may also be associated with cardiac, kidney, or skeletal abnormalities as well as patchy, brown discolorations (pigmentation changes) of the skin. There are several different subtypes, each of which is thought to result from abnormal mutations of different genes. Prognosis is poor among those individuals with low blood counts.

Treatment of FA involves transfusions, bone marrow transplantation, or gene therapy. Individuals with FA are prone to cancers, even after transplantation. Currently, lifespan is not long, and many children do not survive to adulthood. However, National Institute on Aging (NIA) researchers have discovered the gene *FANCM*, the mutation of which is responsible for one form of FA; its protein provides a potential target for the development of drug therapy (Meetei et al, 2005).

TABLE 12-5 Signs and Symptoms of Aplastic Anemia

Blood in stool
Bronzing of skin
Dizziness
Hemorrhagic diathesis (gums, nose, gastrointestinal tract, urinary tract, vagina)
Hemosiderosis with resulting cirrhosis, diabetes, heart failure
Increasing fatigue and weakness
Increasing or persistent infections
Irritability
Nausea
Oral thrush
Petechiae, ecchymosis
Slow thought processes, headache
Tachycardia, tachypnea, dyspnea
Wax-like pallor

INTERVENTION: OBJECTIVES

- Prevent infections or sepsis. Reduce fevers.
- Reduce bleeding tendencies and hemorrhages.
- Ensure adequate periods of rest.
- Prepare for splenectomy or bone marrow transplantation.
- Prevent further complications, where possible, and decline in cardiovascular and hepatic functions.

INTERVENTION: FOOD AND NUTRITION

- Replenish nutrient stores.
- Provide a balanced diet that is easily prepared, with six small feedings.
- Provide extra fluid unless contraindicated (35 cc/kg or more).
- If patient has mouth lesions, avoid excesses of hot or cold foods, spicy or acidic foods, or foods with rough textures.
- If steroids are used, limiting sodium intake may be beneficial.

CLINICAL INDICATORS

Clinical/History

Height
Weight
BMI
Diet history
BP
Fatigue and weakness
Headache, irritability
Wax-like pallor
Petechiae, ecchymosis
Hemorrhagic diathesis (gums, nose, GI tract, urinary tract, vagina)
Tachycardia, tachypnea, dyspnea
Persistent infections
Oral lesions (aplastic)
Bronzing of skin
Small head, low birth weight (FA)
Skeletal anomalies of spine, hips, ribs (FA)

Lab Work

RBC count (decreased)

Prothombin time (PT)	Platelets (decreased)	Alanine aminotransferase (ALT)
Serum Fe	White blood cell (WBC) count (<1500)	Aspartate aminotransferase (AST)
Gluc	Alb, transthyretin	Bilirubin
Granulocytes (decreased)	CRP	
Transferrin		
H & H		

Common Drugs Used and Potential Side Effects

- Corticosteroids may be used. Watch for side effects of chronic use such as elevated serum sodium levels, decreased potassium and calcium levels, and negative nitrogen balance. Hyperglycemia may occur; alter diet accordingly.
- Aspirin should be avoided because it may aggravate blood losses.
- Antibiotics may be required when infections are present. Monitor for GI distress and other side effects.
- Other drugs that may aggravate the condition include chloramphenicol, phenylbutazone, sulfa drugs, and ibuprofen. Each of these has specific GI side effects that should be monitored (see index for more information).

Herbs, Botanicals, and Supplements

- Herbs and botanical supplements should not be used without discussing with physician.

INTERVENTION: NUTRITION EDUCATION, COUNSELING, CARE MANAGEMENT

- Discuss needs of the patient that are specific for signs and symptoms and for side effects of any medications.
- Discuss simplified, but nutritious, meal planning.
- If patient has diabetes, heart failure, or cirrhosis, counsel specifically to those issues for nutritional management.
- Activity levels must be restricted to avoid accidents or falls that could promote bleeding.
- Genetic counseling may be advisable for parents who have children with these deadly anemias.

For More Information

- America's Blood Centers
  http://www.americasblood.org/
- Aplastic Anemia Answer Book
  http://medic.med.uth.tmc.edu/ptnt/00001038.htm
- Aplastic Anemia and MDS International Foundation, Inc.
  http://www.aplastic.org/
- Bloodline
  http://www.bloodline.net/
- Fanconi's Anemia
  http://www.fanconi.org/aboutfa/diagnosis.htm
- Fanconi Anemia Handbook for Families
  http://www.fanconi.org/pubs/books/FAHandbook3.pdf
- Fanconi Anemia Research Fund
  http://www.fanconi.org
- Fanconi's Syndrome
  http://www.nlm.nih.gov/medlineplus/ency/article/000334.htm
- Fanconi Canada
  http://www.fanconicanada.org
- University of Maryland
  http://www.umm.edu/blood/aneaplas.htm

APLASTIC ANEMIA AND FANCONI'S ANEMIA—CITED REFERENCES

Fagerlie SR, Bagby GC. Immune defects in Fanconi anemia. *Crit Rev Immunol.* 26:81, 2006.

Meetei AR, et al. A human ortholog of archaeal DNA repair protein Hef is defective in Fanconi anemia complementation group M. *Nat Genet.* 37:958, 2005.

Zeng W, et al. Interferon-gamma–induced gene expression in CD34 cells. Identification of pathologic cytokine-specific signature profiles. *Blood* 107:167, 2006.

COPPER DEFICIENCY ANEMIA

NUTRITIONAL ACUITY RANKING: LEVEL 2

DEFINITIONS AND BACKGROUND

Copper is required for the function of over 30 proteins, including superoxide dismutase, ceruloplasmin, lysyl oxidase, cytochrome c oxidase, tyrosinase, and dopamine beta-hydroxylase (Arredondo and Nunez, 2005). Copper is found in trace amounts in all tissues in the body; it has a role in the production of hemoglobin (the main component of red blood cells), myelin (the substance that surrounds nerve fibers), collagen (a key component of bones and connective tissue), and melanin (a dark pigment that colors the hair and skin). Copper also works with vitamin C to make elastin.

Copper is also needed in minute amounts for the formation of hemoglobin. The metabolism of copper and iron are closely related; systemic copper deficiency generates cellular iron deficiency, which results in diminished work capacity, reduced intellectual capacity, diminished growth, alterations in bone mineralization, and diminished immune response (Arredondo and Nunez, 2005). Copper deficiency also results in reduced activity of white blood cells and reduced thymus hormone production, thus resulting in increased infection rates.

Marginal deficits of this element can contribute to the development and progression of a number of disease states including cardiovascular disease and diabetes (Urui-Adams and Keen, 2005; Li et al, 2005). Homocysteine thiolactone accumulates when homocysteine is high; it inhibits lysyl oxidase, which depends on copper to catalyze cross-linking of collagen and elastin in arteries and bone (Klevay, 2004). A copper deficiency should, therefore, be avoided. Betaine, copper, folate, pyridoxine, and vitamin B_{12} have proven to be beneficial in lowering serum homocysteine levels (Klevay, 2004). Overall, supplementation with 3–6 mg of copper per day can improve copper status in otherwise healthy individuals; increased intake could reduce the risk of atherosclerosis by promoting improved fibrinolytic capacity (Bugel et al, 2005).

Copper, along with zinc and iron, are essential metals for normal central nervous system development and function; imbalances can result in neuronal death (apoptosis), which may contribute to Alzheimer's disease, Parkinson's disease, amyotrophic lateral sclerosis (ALS), and Huntington's disease; imbalances can also result in neuron deaths in traumatic brain and spinal cord injury, stroke, and seizures (Levenson, 2005).

People with poor intake of protein or whose diets are very high in milk may become deficient in copper or iron. Infants fed an all cow's milk diet without copper supplements may develop copper deficiency. Acquired copper deficiency may be a delayed complication of gastric surgery and may result in a myelopathy similar to that seen with vitamin B_{12} deficiency (Kumar et al, 2004).

Zinc supplementation causes reduced copper absorption and potential for copper deficiency anemia. Other conditions that can lead to copper deficiency include burns, pancreatic or liver disease, kidney disease, diarrhea, and prematurity.

Hospitalized patients should be evaluated carefully. Although enteral feedings contain adequate concentrations of trace elements, problems with bioavailability may occur, and patients receiving long-term enteral feeding should be monitored to avoid anemia and leukopenia (Ito et al, 2005; Oliver et al, 2005).

Bicytopenia (anemia and neutropenia) with normal platelet count is a feature of hematological disorders caused by copper deficiency; abnormalities improve within a few months after copper supplementation therapy (Nagano et al, 2005). Ceruloplasmin (Cp) is a copper-containing plasma protein with an important role in iron homeostasis; levels are low when copper intake is deficient. Table 12-6 describes symptoms of copper deficiency and related anemia.

INTERVENTION: OBJECTIVES

- Correct copper deficiency and documented anemias.
- Instruct patient regarding good sources of protein, iron, and copper to prevent recurrences.
- Monitor use of zinc in supplements, diet, and enteral or parenteral sources to avoid overdosing and related copper depletion.

TABLE 12-6 Symptoms of Copper Insufficiency and Anemia

Fatigue
Edema
Slowed growth
Hair loss
Anorexia
Diarrhea
Dermatitis or loss of pigmentation of skin, pallor
Poor collagen formation and decreased wound healing
Skin sores
Reduced red blood cell function
Shortened red cell life span
Weakness
Labored respiration from decreased oxygen delivery
Reduced thyroid function
Cardiovascular disease, increased serum cholesterol levels
Irregular heart rhythms
Skeletal defects related to bone demineralization
Bone fractures
Poor nerve conductivity
Myeloneuropathy (Rowin and Lewis, 2005) and myelopathy (Kumar et al, 2004)
Persistent neurological and immunological abnormalities in newborns if mothers are deficient (Urui-Adams and Keen, 2005).

INTERVENTION: FOOD AND NUTRITION

- Good sources of copper include oysters, liver, nuts, dried legumes, and raisins. A typical diet provides about 2–3 mg copper/d, about half of which is absorbed. A supplement of 3–6 mg copper may be useful in adults.
- Protein should be at least 1 g/kg for adults; iron intake should be adequate for age and sex.
- Monitor use of multivitamin-mineral supplements to avoid large doses of zinc. Ascorbic acid can act as a prooxidant in the presence of metals such as iron or copper; large doses are not recommended (Gerster, 1999).
- Monitor tube-fed patients to ensure that they are receiving sufficient amounts of copper (Ito et al, 2005; Oliver et al, 2005).

CLINICAL INDICATORS

Clinical/History		Lab Work
Height	BP	CBC
Weight	Pallor	Serum copper (low)
BMI	Other symptoms (see Table 12-6)	
Diet history		

Ceruloplasmin (low)	Platelets (normal)	Homocysteine
H & H	Erythropoietin (EPO) levels (elevated)	Alb, transthyretin
Serum Fe	Serum zinc (Zn) (often elevated)	CRP
Serum ferritin (increased)		Retinol-binding protein (RBP)
Macrocytic, hypochromic anemia		

Common Drugs Used and Potential Side Effects

- Cupric sulfate is one brand of injectible copper supplement. Copper gluconate is given orally. Beware of excesses, which can be indicated by black or bloody vomit; bloody urine; diarrhea; heartburn; loss of appetite; lower back pain; metallic taste; nausea (severe or continuing); pain or burning while urinating; vomiting; yellow eyes or skin; dizziness or fainting; severe headache or even coma.
- Do not refrigerate this supplement. Discard when outdated.
- Avoid taking copper supplements with nonsteroidal anti-inflammatory drugs (NSAIDs), birth control pills, allopurinol, estrogen hormones, or cimetidine.

Herbs, Botanicals, and Supplements

- Herbs and botanical supplements should not be used without discussing with physician.

INTERVENTION: NUTRITION EDUCATION, COUNSELING, CARE MANAGEMENT

- Have patient avoid fad diets. Monitor vegetarian (nonheme iron) diets carefully.
- Zinc in large doses may deplete copper levels; discuss use of mineral supplements.
- Patients at risk for copper deficiency should be counseled on how to avoid this condition. For example, patients with muscular dystrophy may not consume adequate amounts, and muscle strength can diminish as a result (Motlagh et al, 2005).
- Indicate which foods are good sources of copper, iron, and protein. See Table 12-7.

TABLE 12-7 Food Sources of Copper

Blackstrap molasses
Black pepper
Chocolate (unsweetened or semisweet baker's chocolate and cocoa)
Enriched cereals (bran flakes, raisin bran, shredded wheat)
Fruits (such as dried fruits, bananas, grapes)
Legumes (such as soybeans, lentils, navy beans, and peanuts)
Nuts and nut butters (cashews, filberts, macadamia nuts, pecans, almonds, and pistachios)
Organ meats (beef liver, kidneys, and heart)
Seafood (oysters, squid, lobster, mussels, crab, and clams)
Vegetables (avocado, mushrooms, potatoes, sweet potatoes, tomatoes)

For More Information

- Merck Manual
  http://www.merck.com/mrkshared/mmanual/section1/chapter4/4j.jsp

COPPER DEFICIENCY ANEMIA—CITED REFERENCES

Arredondo M, Nunez MT. Iron and copper metabolism. *Mol Aspects Med.* 26:313, 2005.

Bugel S, et al. Effect of copper supplementation on indices of copper status and certain CVD risk markers in young healthy women. *Br J Nutr.* 94:231, 2005.

Gerster H. High-dose vitamin C: a risk for persons with high iron stores? *Int J Vitam Nutr Res.* 69:67, 1999.

Ito Y, et al. Latent copper deficiency in patients receiving low-copper enteral nutrition for a prolonged period. *J Parenter Enteral Nutr.* 29:360, 2005.

Klevay LM. Ischemic heart disease as deficiency disease. *Cell Mol Biol.* 50:877, 2004.

Kumar N, et al Acquired hypocupremia after gastric surgery. *Clin Gastroenterol Hepatol.* 2:1074, 2004.

Levenson CW. Trace metal regulation of neuronal apoptosis: from genes to behavior. *Physiol Behav.* 86:399, 2005.

Li Y, et al. Marginal dietary copper restriction induces cardiomyopathy in rats. *J Nutr.* 135:2130, 2005.

Motlagh B, et al. Nutritional inadequacy in adults with muscular dystrophy. *Muscle Nerve.* 31:713, 2005.

Nagano T, et al. Clinical features of hematological disorders caused by copper deficiency during long-term enteral nutrition. *Intern Med.* 44:554, 2005.

Oliver A, et al. Trace element concentrations in patients on home enteral feeding: two cases of severe copper deficiency. *Ann Clin Biochem.* 42:136, 2005.

Rowin J, Lewis SL. Copper deficiency myeloneuropathy and pancytopenia secondary to overuse of zinc supplementation. *J Neurol Neurosurg Psychiatry.* 76:750, 2005.

Urui-Adams JY, Keen CL. Copper, oxidative stress, and human health. *Mol Aspects Med.* 26:268, 2005

FOLIC ACID DEFICIENCY ANEMIA

NUTRITIONAL ACUITY RANKING: LEVEL 2

DEFINITIONS AND BACKGROUND

Folic acid is composed of a pterin ring connected to *p*-aminobenzoic acid (PABA). Humans do not generate folate because they cannot synthesize PABA. The amino acid histidine is metabolized to glutamic acid; formiminoglutamic acid (FIGLU) is an intermediary in this reaction, and tetrahydrofolic acid is the coenzyme that converts it to glutamic acid (Cooperman and Lopez, 2002).

Under normal conditions, sufficient intake of dietary histidine can prevent anemia. When dietary intake of histidine is diminished or urinary excretion is greatly increased, anemia results (Cooperman and Lopez, 2002). Folate deficiency depletes histidine with increased urinary excretion of this amino acid.

Folic acid is needed for the synthesis of DNA and maturation of red blood cells. Deficiency of folate can lead to many clinical abnormalities, including macrocytic anemia, cardiovascular diseases, birth defects, and carcinogenesis. For example, colorectal cancer has a relationship to folic aid deficiency (Duthie et al, 2004). The immune system is affected by deficiency because there is a reduced capacity of CD8+ cells to proliferate in response to activation (Courtemanche et al, 2004). Folic acid deficiency anemia generally is caused by inadequate diet, intestinal malabsorption, alcoholism, or pregnancy. See Table 12-8.

Folic acid deficiency yields a hyperchromic, macrocytic, megaloblastic anemia with signs and symptoms of weight loss, anorexia, malnutrition, smooth and sore red tongue, diarrhea, easy fatigue, lethargy, poor wound healing, and coldness of extremities. Because similar hematological changes occur with vitamin B_{12} deficiency, it is important to check the Schilling test and serum levels of vitamin B_{12} along with folate tests. Folate is best measured by red blood cell folate because serum levels are misleading.

Homocysteine elevation is a risk factor for vascular and thrombotic disease, and genetic or acquired influences are being sorted out (Carmel et al, 2003). Alzheimer's disease and cognitive decline have not been shown to improve with folic acid supplementation (Malouf et al, 2003).

While neural tube defects result from maternal folate insufficiency in the periconceptual period, there are also inborn errors of folate metabolism that aggravate the problem. Congenital folate malabsorption, methylenetetrahydrofolate reductase (MTHFR) deficiency, and formiminotransferase deficiency are several types. MTHFR deficiency causes neurological problems without megaloblastic anemia; it is the most common inborn error of folate metabolism (Carmel et al, 2003).

TABLE 12-8 Conditions and Medications That Deplete Folic Acid

Aging
Alcoholism
Burns
Cancers
Dialysis
Elevated homocysteine levels
Hemolytic anemias
Hepatitis
Infection
Inflammatory diseases
Malabsorptive states: celiac disease, blind-loop syndrome, megacolon, Crohn's disease
Pregnancy and lactation
Smoking
Stress
Surgery
Medications: anticonvulsants, metformin, methotrexate, pentamidine isethionate (antiprotozoal), pyrimethamine (antimalarial), triamterene (diuretic), trimethoprim (antibiotic), oral contraceptives, cimetidine (Tagamet), sulfasalazine (Azulfidine) for Crohn's disease, and isoniazid (INH) for tuberculosis

INTERVENTION: OBJECTIVES

- Increase folic acid in diet to alleviate anemia.
- Improve diet to provide nutrients needed to make red blood cells: folate and other B-complex vitamins, iron, and protein. Instruct patient to correct faulty diet habits if relevant.
- Check for malabsorption syndromes (celiac disease, blind-loop syndrome, congenital or acquired megacolon, Crohn's disease) and correct these as far as possible through use of medications and other treatments. Monitor folate status regularly.

INTERVENTION: FOOD AND NUTRITION

- Provide a diet that is high in folic acid, protein, copper, iron, and vitamins C and B_{12}. A combination of folic acid and histidine is beneficial for folate-deficient individuals (Cooperman and Lopez, 2002).
- Folic acid is distributed widely in green leafy vegetables, citrus fruits, and animal products. Ingestion of one fresh fruit or vegetable provides sufficient folic acid for most people, but other sources include fish, legumes (dried beans and peas), whole grains, leafy dark green vegetables, broccoli, citrus juices, berries, and meats.
- Food manufacturers in the United States have fortified grains with folic acid since 1998. These fortified foods include most enriched breads, flours, corn meal, rice, noodles, macaroni, and other grain products.
- Diets that provide bland, liquid, or soft foods may be needed for patients with a sore mouth; 6–8 small meals may be helpful.

CLINICAL INDICATORS

Clinical/History
- Height
- Weight
- BMI
- Diet history
- BP
- I & O
- Weight loss
- Anorexia, malnutrition
- Smooth and sore red tongue
- Diarrhea
- Fatigue, lethargy
- Poor wound healing
- Coldness of extremities
- History of alcohol abuse

Lab Work
- Serum folate (<3 ng/mL)
- RBC folate (more reliable than serum)
- Serum homocysteine (often elevated)
- Low RBC
- H & H
- CBC (macrocytic cells)
- Transferrin
- Serum B_{12}
- Serum Fe (increased)
- Mean cell volume (MCV)
- Leukopenia, WBC
- Urinary formiminoglutamic acid (FIGLU) after histidine load
- Schilling test

TABLE 12-9 Folic Acid Sources

Source	Folic Acid (mg)
Lentils or black-eyed peas, cooked ½ cup	179
Pinto beans, cooked, ½ cup	147
Chickpeas, cooked, ½ cup	141
Okra, frozen, cooked, ½ cup	135
Spinach, cooked and drained, ½ cup	13
Black or navy beans, cooked, ½ cup	128
Asparagus, frozen, cooked, ½ cup	122
Broccoli, cooked, ½ cup	84
Creamed corn, canned, ½ cup	58
Baked potato/skin, 1 medium	57
Orange, 1 medium	54
Strawberries, 1 cup	40
Orange juice, 6 fluid oz	34

Common Drugs Used and Potential Side Effects

- Supplements of folic acid (Folvite) are better than diet alone to alleviate the anemia. Folate deficiency is generally treated with 800–1000 μg of folic acid daily. Leucovorin is an active reduced form. **Beware of the interaction between vitamin B_{12} and folic acid.** Vitamin B_{12} helps folate travel into cells via transport form (5-methyltetrahydrofolate). High levels of folate may mask a vitamin B_{12} deficiency; this is especially important to evaluate in older individuals. Maintain dose below 1000 μg/d.
- The natural folate derivative, 5-methyltetrahydrofolate, is an option for supplementation and fortification without the potential disadvantage of masking the anemia of vitamin B_{12} deficiency (Pentieva et al, 2004).
- Folic acid antagonists (cancer treatments) affect the body's use of folic acid. Methotrexate is especially depleting; it is common to administer leucovorin at the same time as a "folinic acid rescue."
- Anticonvulsants (e.g., primidone, phenytoin, phenobarbital) also interfere with the body's use of folic acid. It is common to hold meals or a tube feeding for 1 hour before and after administration of phenytoin (Dilantin).

Herbs, Botanicals, and Supplements

- Herbs and botanical supplements should not be used without discussing with physician.

INTERVENTION: NUTRITION EDUCATION, COUNSELING, CARE MANAGEMENT

- Pregnant women should receive appropriate counseling; 30% may have a folate deficiency. Daily needs increase by approximately 200 mg over the adult requirements of 400 mg. Folate protects against neural tube defects in the first trimester.
- Large intakes of folate (>1 mg/d) can cure the anemia but may mask a correlated vitamin B_{12} anemia; monitor carefully.
- Attractive meals may help appetite.
- Fad and restrictive diets should be avoided.
- Alcoholic beverages interfere with folate metabolism and absorption.
- Food folates are oxidized easily and destroyed by lengthy cooking; advise patients accordingly.
- Vitamin C promotes absorption of folic acid from foods. See Table 12-9 for a list of folic acid sources.

For More Information

- E-medicine
  http://www.emedicine.com/med/topic802.htm
- Folic Acid Exams and Tests
  http://my.webmd.com/hw/diet_and_nutrition/hw152371.asp
- Folic Acid Supplements
  http://ods.od.nih.gov/factsheets/folate.asp
- March of Dimes–Folic Acid Deficiency
  http://www.marchofdimes.com/professionals/681_1151.asp

FOLIC ACID DEFICIENCY ANEMIA—CITED REFERENCES

Carmel R, et al. Update on cobalamin, folate, and homocysteine. *Hematology (Am Soc Hematol Educ Program)*. 62-81, 2003.
Cooperman JM, Lopez R. The role of histidine in the anemia of folate deficiency. *Exp Biol Med (Maywood)*. 227:998, 2002.
Courtemanche C, et al. Folate deficiency inhibits the proliferation of primary human CD8+ T lymphocytes in vitro. *J Immunol.* 173:3186, 2004.
Duthie SJ, et al. Folate, DNA stability and colorectal neoplasia. *Proc Nutr Soc.* 63:571, 2004.
Malouf M, et al. Folic acid with or without vitamin B12 for cognition and dementia. *Cochrane Database Syst Rev.* 4:CD004514, 2003.
Pentieva K, et al. The short-term bioavailabilities of [6S]-5-methyltetrahydrofolate and folic acid are equivalent in men. *J Nutr.* 134:580, 2004.

HEMOLYTIC ANEMIAS

NUTRITIONAL ACUITY RANKING: LEVEL 2–3

DEFINITIONS AND BACKGROUND

In **hemolytic anemia,** red blood cells have an abnormal membrane, which results in hemolysis. Red blood cells are destroyed faster than they can be produced in bone marrow. The incidence of all types of hemolytic anemias is 4 in 100,000 persons in the United States. Most are not affected specifically by vitamin E.

Types of hemolytic anemias include hemoglobin-SC disease, hemolytic anemia due to glucose-6-phosphate dehydrogenase (G6PD) deficiency, hereditary elliptocytosis, hereditary spherocytosis, idiopathic autoimmune hemolytic anemia, nonimmune hemolytic anemia caused by chemical agents, and secondary immune hemolytic anemia. This text covers aplastic anemia, sickle cell anemia, and thalassemia. Table 12-10 describes some of these types of anemias.

Symptoms and signs of hemolytic anemia include shortness of breath, rapid heart rate, jaundice, dark urine, splenomegaly, nosebleeds, chills, fatigue, bleeding gums, heart murmur, weakness, confusion, or dizziness, edema, pallor, intolerance for physical activity, and puffy eyelids. In severe cases in infancy, encephalomalacia can result. Treatment may involve splenectomy or steroid use.

INTERVENTION: OBJECTIVES

- Prevent further complications.
- Correct anemia or deficits of nutrients, such as vitamin E.

INTERVENTION: FOOD AND NUTRITION

- Provide diet as usual for age and sex.
- Avoid excesses of iron.
- Ensure adequate intake of vitamin E and zinc, which may become deficient.

CLINICAL INDICATORS

Clinical/History		
Height	BMI	BP
Weight	Diet history	Tachycardia
	Growth percentile	Shortness of breath

TABLE 12-10 Types of Hemolytic Anemia

Type	Description
Acquired autoimmune hemolytic anemia	A rare autoimmune disorder characterized by the premature destruction of red blood cells. Normally, red blood cells have a life span of 120 days before the spleen removes them, but in this condition, red blood cells are destroyed prematurely. Bone marrow production of new cells can no longer compensate. This anemia occurs in individuals who previously had a normal red blood cell system. Patients with autoimmune hemolytic anemia usually belong to a distinct category, which is associated with anticardiolipin antibodies, thrombosis, thrombocytopenia, and renal involvement, often in the context of secondary antiphospholipid syndrome (Giannouli et al, 2006).
Familial hemolytic jaundice (spherolytic anemia)	A hereditary anemia in which red blood cells are shaped like spheres rather than their normal, donut-like shape. Jaundice and anemia occur from destruction of the abnormal cells by the spleen. Surgical removal of the spleen usually is indicated. There is no permanent cure.
Glucose-6-phosphate dehydrogenase (G6PD) deficiency anemia	This anemia is seen in about 10% of African American males in the United States and is also common in persons from the Mediterranean area or Asia. The severity differs among different populations. In the most common form in the African American population, the deficiency is mild, and the hemolysis affects primarily older red blood cells. In Caucasians, G6PD deficiency tends to be more serious because even young red blood cells are affected. It affects about 400 million people worldwide, especially in malaria-prone areas (Matsuo et al, 2003).
Hereditary nonspherocytic hemolytic anemia	A group of rare genetic blood disorders characterized by defective red blood cells (erythrocytes) that are not abnormally "sphere shaped" (spherocytes). Membranes of red blood cells, abnormal metabolism of a chemical contained in hemoglobin (porphyrin), and deficiencies in certain enzymes such as G6PD or pyruvate kinase are thought to be the cause of these disorders.
Vitamin E–sensitive hemolytic anemia	This condition may occur in infants who receive polyunsaturated fatty acids (PUFAs) without adequate vitamin E. Children with cystic fibrosis should be screened for vitamin E–deficient hemolytic anemia.

Dizziness
Edema
Pallor
Nosebleeds
Dark urine
Puffy eyelids

Lab Work

RBC (low)
Hgb (low)
Reticulocyte count (increased)
Serum alpha-tocopherol levels
Hgb in urine
Hemosiderin in urine
TIBC
Bilirubin (elevated)
Transferrin
Gluc
AST (increased)
Blood test for G6PD
CRP

Common Drugs Used and Potential Side Effects

- For hemolytic anemia that is sensitive to vitamin E deficiency, water-soluble vitamin E (alpha-tocopherol) is likely to be given daily. Avoid taking with an iron supplement, which could interfere with utilization.
- Persons with G6PD deficiency need to avoid exposing themselves to certain medicines such as aspirin (acetylsalicylic acid), certain antibiotics used to treat infections, fava beans, and mothballs.

Herbs, Botanicals, and Supplements

- Herbs and botanical supplements should not be used without discussing with physician.
- Flavonoid preparations, marketed for a variety of effects and generally safe, should be evaluated carefully because there have been reports of toxic flavonoid–drug interactions, hemolytic anemia, and other problems (Galati and O'Brien, 2004).

INTERVENTION: NUTRITION EDUCATION, COUNSELING, CARE MANAGEMENT

- For hemolytic anemia that is sensitive to vitamin E deficiency, discuss, in layman's terms, the role of vitamin E in lipid oxidation and utilization. Discuss sources of polyunsaturated fatty acids (PUFAs) and why excesses should be controlled. Discuss sources of vitamin E in the diet; natural sources are more bioavailable than synthetic sources.
- Discuss exercise tolerance and ability to eat sufficient amounts of food as related to fatigue.

For More Information

- American Autoimmune Related Diseases Association, Inc. http://www.aarda.org

HEMOLYTIC ANEMIAS—CITED REFERENCES

Galati G, O'Brien PJ. Potential toxicity of flavonoids and other dietary phenolics: significance for their chemopreventive and anticancer properties. *Free Radic Biol Med.* 37:287, 2004.

Giannouli S, et al. Anemia in systemic lupus erythematosus: from pathophysiology to clinical assessment. *Ann Rheum Dis.* 65:144, 2006.

Matsuo M, et al. Glucose-6-phosphate dehydrogenase deficiency: molecular heterogeneity in Southeast Asian countries. *Southeast Asian J Trop Med Public Health.* 34:127, 2003.

IRON DEFICIENCY ANEMIA

NUTRITIONAL ACUITY RANKING: LEVEL 2

DEFINITIONS AND BACKGROUND

The nutrient most commonly deficient in the world is iron. Iron deficiency affects two billion people, most of whom live in developing countries (Lynch, 2005). Iron deficiency anemia (IDA) results from inadequate intake, impaired erythropoiesis or absorption of iron, blood loss, or demands from closely repeated pregnancies. Anemia limits productivity and causes economic losses where it prevails (Boccio and Iyengar, 2003). When caused by an inadequate diet, it may take years to produce symptoms when there are adequate iron stores. In the elderly, chronic blood loss is the most common cause of IDA.

Iron is the basic nutritional component of heme, a protein. Hemoglobin is the iron-containing protein in red blood cells that carries oxygen to all body cells. Hematocrit is the measure of red blood cells in a given volume of blood, packed by centrifuge. Transferrin is the carrier protein that picks up iron from the intestines (ferric state). Serum ferritin is the most useful test to differentiate IDA from anemia of chronic disease. Absorption of iron occurs in the ferrous form; storage is in the liver, spleen, and bone marrow. See Table 12-11 for content of iron in various body sources.

Symptoms and signs of IDA include weakness, fatigue, vertigo, headache, irritability, heartburn, dysphagia, flatulence, vague abdominal pains, anorexia, glossitis, stomatitis, pale skin, ankle edema, tingling extremities, and palpitations. Serious systemic consequences include impaired cognitive function, koilonychia, and impaired exercise tolerance.

Approximately 90% of the body's store of iron is reused. Diet replaces iron lost through sweat, feces, and urine. The duodenum (upper small intestine) is where iron is best absorbed. Damage or surgery of the duodenum can greatly inhibit total iron absorption, thus leading to greater risk of deficiency. Table 12-12 describes factors that can modify iron absorption.

Iron deficiency is relatively common in toddlers, adolescent girls, and women of childbearing age. Ingestion of cow's milk causes occult intestinal blood loss in young infants. The hemoglobin content of reticulocytes (young red blood cells)

TABLE 12-11 Iron Distribution in the Body

Forms	Men (mg iron/kg BW)	Women (mg iron/kg BW)
Storage—ferritin	9	4
Storage—hemosiderin	4	1
Transport protein: transferrin	<1	<1
Functional hemoglobin	31	31
Functional myoglobin	4	4
Enzymes	2	2
TOTAL	50	42

Based on data from: Insel P, Turner R, Ross D. *Nutrition*. Sudbury, MA: Jones & Bartlett Publishers, 2001.

is a good indicator of iron deficiency and IDA in children. Risk of iron deficiency may be underestimated in high-risk populations, even those served by the Women, Infants, and Children's (WIC) Supplemental Feeding Program. Efforts to prevent mild and moderate mental retardation should include adequate nutrition during early childhood. Celiac disease may be present in up to 1% of the general population and is associated frequently with IDA (Goel et al, 2005).

Menstruation increases iron losses each month; thus, women tend to become iron deficient more easily than men. When there is not enough hemoglobin, free erythrocyte protoporphyrin (FEP) accumulates. Another factor in iron deficiency involves athletics. Recreational athletes should be screened for iron deficiency using serum ferritin, serum transferrin receptor, and hemoglobin (Sinclair and Hinton, 2005).

Pica is seen in approximately 50% of patients with iron deficiency. Pica generally is a consequence, rather than a cause, of iron deficiency; it is relieved by iron supplementation. Exposure to lead also has a significant effect on hemoglobin and hematocrit levels. Lead poisoning reduces hemoglobin production, causes iron deficiency, and elevates FEP as the precursor.

TABLE 12-12 Factors That Modify Iron Absorption

Factor	Description
Physical state (bioavailability)	Heme > Fe^{2+} > Fe^{3+}
High gastric pH	Hemigastrectomy, vagotomy, pernicious anemia, histamine H_2-receptor blockers, calcium-based antacids
Disruption of intestinal structure	Crohn's disease, celiac disease (nontropical sprue)
Inhibitors	Phylates, tannins, soil clay, laundry starch, iron overload
Competitors	Cobalt, lead, strontium
Facilitators	Ascorbate, citrate, amino acids, iron deficiency

From: Information Center for Sickle Cell and Thalassemic Disorders. Iron deficiency. Available at http://sickle.bwh.harvard.edu/fe-def.html.

Postpartum anemia is associated with breathlessness, tiredness, palpitations, and maternal infections, and blood transfusions and iron supplementation have been used in the treatment of IDA. Erythropoietin may be found to be useful (Dodd et al, 2004).

One of the major causes of anemia in childhood worldwide is iron deficiency; prevalence is higher during infancy and adolescence, and a diet low in iron is the most common cause (Panagiotou and Douros, 2004). Iron fortification of food is a cost-effective method for reducing the prevalence of nutritional iron deficiency (Lynch, 2005). While iron deficiency is primary, altered intake of vitamins A, B_{12}, C, and E, folic acid, and riboflavin have also been linked to the development and control of IDA. Vitamin A can improve hematological indicators and enhance the efficacy of iron supplementation.

INTERVENTION: OBJECTIVES

- Alleviate cause of the anemia and associated anorexia.
- Provide adequate oral iron to replace losses or deficits, especially heme sources of protein (e.g., liver, beef, oysters, lamb, pork, ham, tuna, shrimp, other fish, chicken).
- Provide an acid medium to favor better absorption. Enhancers include gastric juice and ascorbic acid. Food sources of vitamin C should be included daily.
- Monitor and correct pica, including geophagia (clay eating), amylophagia (starch eating), ice eating, etc.
- Avoid or correct constipation.
- Screen for IDA or sports anemia in athletes (Sinclair and Hinton, 2005).
- Reduce iron inhibitors, such as excessive fiber (as in whole grains), phytic acid (as in spinach, bran, legumes, and soy products), tannins in tea, and polyphenols in coffee or red wine. In many developing countries, cereal and legume-based diets contain low amounts of bioavailable iron, which may increase the risk of iron deficiency (Zimmermann et al, 2005).

INTERVENTION: FOOD AND NUTRITION

- If IDA is related to inadequate iron in diet, usually adding three portions of lean red meat (heme iron sources) per week, along with all other essential vitamins and minerals, will correct the anemia. The average mixed diet contains approximately 6 mg of iron per 1000 kcal. Iron absorption increases as stores become depleted. Sources of iron include liver, eggs, kidney, beef, dried fruits, enriched wholegrain cereals, molasses, and oysters.
- Heme iron is found readily in beef, pork, and lamb; consume with fruit or fruit juice. Heme iron is absorbed well, regardless of other foods in the diet, whereas nonheme iron absorption is greatly affected by other foods. Absorption of nonheme iron is best in the presence of foods rich in vitamin C or with heme-containing sources.
- Increase intake of vitamin C (oranges, grapefruit, tomatoes, broccoli, cabbage, baked potatoes, strawberries, cantaloupe, and green peppers), especially when patient is taking an iron supplement.

- Detect pica and discuss with patient. Pica substance may displace other important foods, leading to nutrient malnutrition. The ingested substance may also be toxic.
- Tea, coffee, wheat brans, and soy products tend to inhibit absorption of nonheme iron. Monitor use carefully; avoid excesses. Serum ferritin is lowered by consumption of tea (Milman et al, 2004).

CLINICAL INDICATORS

Clinical/History

- Height
- Weight
- BMI
- Diet history
- BP
- I & O
- Pallor
- Brittle, spoon-shaped fingernails (koilonychia)
- Stool exam for occult blood
- Impaired cognitive function
- Blue sclerae
- Impaired exercise tolerance
- Weakness, fatigue
- Vertigo
- Headache, irritability
- Heartburn
- Dysphagia
- Flatulence, vague abdominal pains
- Anorexia
- Diarrhea
- Glossitis, stomatitis
- Ankle edema
- Tingling in extremities
- Palpitations
- Alopecia

Lab Work

- Ferritin (decreased stores in liver, spleen, bone marrow; levels are <20 g/L)
- Serum iron (low)
- H & H (hemoglobin more sensitive)
- Mean cell hemoglobin (MCH) (decreased)
- Mean cell hematocrit (MCHC) (decreased)
- CBC
- Transferrin (increased)
- MCV (<80)
- RBC (small, microcytic, hypochromic)
- WBC/differential (increased)
- TIBC (increased >350 μg/dL)
- Reticulocyte count
- Serum copper
- Cholesterol (Chol)

Common Drugs Used and Potential Side Effects (see Table 12-13)

- If anemia is caused by an increased demand for iron such as a growth spurt (toddlers, adolescents) or pregnancy, oral supplementation may be necessary. Short-term supplementation with moderate doses (30–60 mg daily) of oral iron combined with increased consumption of heme-rich sources of iron may be sufficient to address iron demands. It takes 4–30 days to note improvements after iron therapy, especially in hemoglobin levels.
- Regardless of source, large doses of supplemental oral iron have not proven to be beneficial. Iron stores are replaced after 1–3 months of treatment. Treat only when indicated; many individuals receive oral iron without justification. Increased supplementation in normal individuals can cause additional, unnecessary iron to go into storage as reflected by ferritin elevation.
- When hemoglobin levels are seriously low, the heart is particularly vulnerable. Whole-blood transfusion or intravenous iron may be needed to stabilize hemoglobin levels.
- Aspirin or corticosteroids can increase GI bleeding or cause peptic ulceration. Vitamin C and nutrient levels may be decreased.
- Some medications, including antacids, can reduce iron absorption. Iron tablets may also reduce the effectiveness of other drugs, including the antibiotics tetracycline, penicillamine, and ciprofloxacin and the anti-Parkinson's drugs methyldopa, levodopa, and carbidopa. Wait 2 hours between doses of these drugs and iron supplements.

Herbs, Botanicals, and Supplements

- Herbs and botanical supplements should not be used without discussing with physician.

INTERVENTION: NUTRITION EDUCATION, COUNSELING, CARE MANAGEMENT

- Hemoglobin is made from protein, iron, and copper. Red blood cells are made from vitamin B_{12}, folacin, and amino acids. Explain which foods are good sources of iron, protein, vitamin C, and these related nutrients.
- Temporary changes in stool color (green or tarry and black) are common with supplements; this is not cause for alarm. To avoid side effects of supplements, take them

TABLE 12-13 Medications to Correct Iron Deficiency Anemia

Medication	Description
Ferrous salts (Feosol, Fer-In-Sol, Mol-Iron)	Better used for iron therapy than other forms; a few studies have shown that prolonged-release ferrous sulfate (Slow Fe) improved iron absorption with fewer side effects than standard ferrous sulfate pills. Other forms include ferrous fumarate (Femiron, Feostat, Fumerin, Hemocyte, Ircon) and ferrous gluconate (Fergon, Ferralet, Simron).
Enteric-coated or sustained-release iron	More expensive and often carry the iron past maximal absorption site in the upper intestine.
Iron tablets (Feostat, Fergon, Feosol)	May cause gastric irritation and constipation.
Parenteral or intravenous iron	Can be administered by injection or infusion. This therapy is reserved for cases of trauma where blood loss is life threatening and is not used for insufficiency due to inadequate dietary iron intake. Imferon can be given intramuscularly, if oral iron is not tolerated; pain and skin discoloration may result.

with meals or milk; food iron has fewer side effects. Avoid excesses of phytates, phosphates, oxalates, fiber, alkalis, antacids, tannins, and calcium phosphates; discuss food sources.

- The average American diet contains 10–20 mg of iron daily, roughly 10% of which is absorbed. However, overdosing with iron supplements is to be avoided. The body can only synthesize 5–10 mg of hemoglobin per day, and excesses may work against the immune system.
- Local or systemic infections interfere with iron absorption and transport. The World Health Organization–initiated Integrated Management of Childhood Illness integrates nutrition into the care of both sick and well children, as does the Early Child Development Program of the World Bank and UNICEF (Neumann et al, 2004).
- In children under 2 years, it is useful to limit milk intake to no more than 500 mL/d for better iron status (Gunnarsson et al, 2004).
- Young people who follow a vegan diet should have their iron status monitored closely (Waldmann et al, 2004).
- Explain nonfood pica—clay, starch, plaster, paint chips—and the relationship to nutrition. In food pica in which singular foods are eaten instead of balanced meals, the foods chosen are often crunchy or brittle. Excessive consumption of lettuce, ice, celery, snack chips, and chocolate has been noted; after iron supplementation, cravings often become a revulsion.
- Iron deficiency is partly induced by plant-based diets containing low levels of poorly bioavailable iron; careful assessment will be important to offer dietary guidelines for the specific patient (Kesa and Oldewage-Theron, 2005). Use culturally appropriate nutrition counseling. In some cultures, boys may be fed iron-rich foods preferentially over girls, and counseling should be designed to encourage improved intake by girls (Shell-Duncan and McDade, 2005).

For More Information

- Iron Deficiency Anemia for Kids
  http://www.kidshealth.org/parent/medical/heart/ida.html
- National Institutes of Health–Iron Deficiency Anemia
  http://www.nlm.nih.gov/medlineplus/ency/article/000584.htm
- University of Maryland
  http://www.umm.edu/blood/aneiron.htm

IRON DEFICIENCY ANEMIA—CITED REFERENCES

Boccio JR, Iyengar V. Iron deficiency: causes, consequences, and strategies to overcome this nutritional problem. *Biol Trace Elem Res.* 94:1, 2003.

Dodd J, et al. Treatment for women with postpartum iron deficiency anaemia. *Cochrane Database Syst Rev.* 4:CD004222, 2003.

Goel NK, et al. Cardiomyopathy associated with celiac disease. *Mayo Clin Proc.* 80:674, 2005.

Gunnarsson BS, et al. Iron status in 2-year-old Icelandic children and associations with dietary intake and growth. *Eur J Clin Nutr.* 58:901, 2004.

Kesa H, Oldewage-Theron W. Anthropometric indications and nutritional intake of women in the Vaal Triangle, South Africa. *Public Health.* 119:294, 2005.

Lynch SR. The impact of iron fortification on nutritional anaemia. *Best Pract Res Clin Haematol.* 18:333, 2005.

Milman N, et al. Iron status in 358 apparently healthy 80-year-old Danish men and women: relation to food composition and dietary and supplemental iron intake. *Ann Hematol.* 83:423, 2004.

Neumann CG, et al. Child nutrition in developing countries. *Pediatr Ann.* 33:658, 2004.

Panagiotou JP, Douros K. Clinicolaboratory findings and treatment of iron-deficiency anemia in childhood. *Pediatr Hematol Oncol.* 21:521, 2004.

Shell-Duncan B, McDade T. Cultural and environmental barriers to adequate iron intake among northern Kenyan schoolchildren. *Food Nutr Bull.* 26:39, 2005.

Sinclair LM, Hinton PS. Prevalence of iron deficiency with and without anemia in recreationally active men and women. *J Am Diet Assoc.* 105:975, 2005.

Waldmann A, et al. Dietary iron intake and iron status of German female vegans: results of the German vegan study. *Ann Nutr Metab.* 48:103, 2004.

Zimmermann MB, et al. Iron deficiency due to consumption of a habitual diet low in bioavailable iron: a longitudinal cohort study in Moroccan children. *Am J Clin Nutr.* 81:115, 2005.

MEGALOBLASTIC ANEMIAS: PERNICIOUS ANEMIA AND VITAMIN B_{12} DEFICIENCY ANEMIA

NUTRITIONAL ACUITY RANKING: LEVEL 2

DEFINITIONS AND BACKGROUND

Megaloblastic anemias affect the nervous system if left untreated. Symptoms of megaloblastic anemias include fatigue, flatulence, nausea, vomiting, diarrhea, upset stomach, constipation, anorexia, weight loss, pale waxy skin, abnormal lemon-yellow jaundice, tachycardia, cardiomegaly, achlorhydria, impaired smell, and glossitis.

Pernicious anemia is a rare blood disorder characterized by inability of the body to properly utilize vitamin B_{12} (cobalamin), which is essential for development of red blood cells (RBCs). Pernicious anemia is thought to be an autoimmune disorder, and certain people may have a genetic predisposition. The three forms of pernicious anemia are congenital pernicious anemia, juvenile pernicious anemia, and adult-onset pernicious anemia. The forms are based on the age at onset and the precise nature of the defect causing impaired vitamin B_{12} utilization (e.g., absence of intrinsic factor). Defective RBC production occurs, caused by a lack of intrinsic factor of the stomach. If there is no intrinsic factor, extrinsic factor (vitamin B_{12}) is not absorbed.

Areas for research include intermittent vitamin B_{12} supplement dosing and better measurements of the bioavailability of vitamin B_{12} in fermented vegetarian foods and algae.

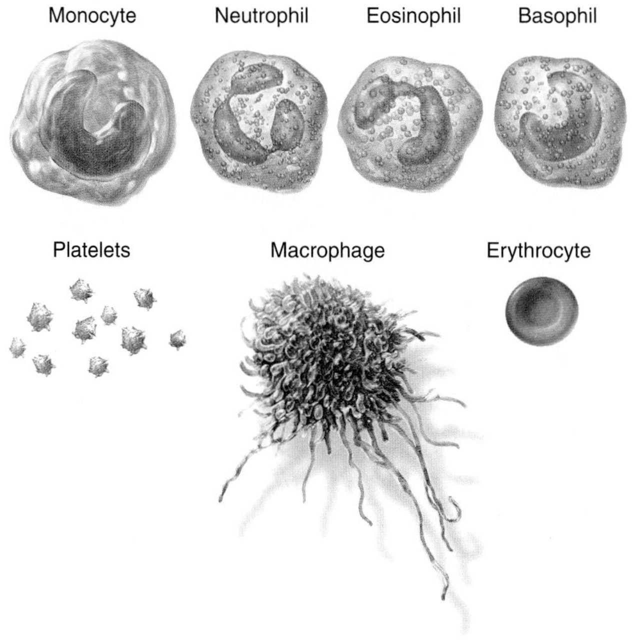

Figure 12-1 Types of blood cells. (Images provided by Anatomical Chart Co.)

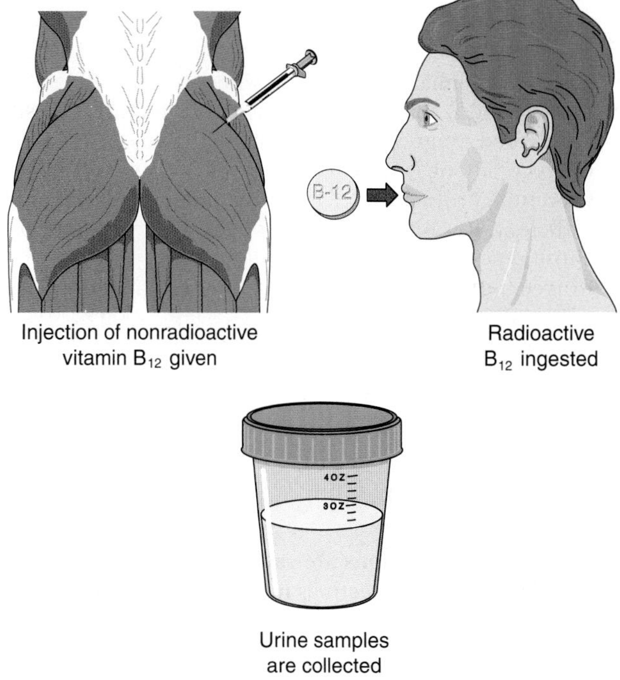

Figure 12-2 Schilling test.

Vitamin B_{12} deficiency anemia may take 5–6 years to appear. With poor intake of vitamin B_{12}, a megaloblastic anemia occurs. Megaloblastic anemia due to vitamin B_{12} deficiency is a reversible form of ineffective hematopoiesis (Drabick et al, 2001), corrected by use of oral cyanocobalamin once weekly for a month. Dietary vitamin B_{12} deficiency is a severe problem in the Indian subcontinent, Mexico, Central and South America, and selected areas of Africa; but it is not common in Asia, except in vegetarians (Stabler and Allen, 2004). See Figures 12-1 and 12-2.

There may be almost 800,000 older adults in the United States who have undiagnosed and untreated vitamin B_{12} deficiency, which is often masked by high folate intakes. Hidden blood loss, gastric atrophy, and poor dietary intake should be addressed. In addition, dietary deficiency of vitamin B_{12} from vegetarianism can lead to hyperhomocysteinemia, and this can contribute to heart disease (Stabler and Allen, 2004). See Table 12-14.

The Schilling test is used to detect vitamin B_{12} absorption; vitamin B_{12} levels are measured in the urine after the ingestion of radioactive vitamin B_{12}. With normal absorption, the ileum absorbs more vitamin B_{12} than the body needs and excretes excess into the urine. With impaired absorption, however, little or no vitamin B_{12} is excreted into the urine.

Low serum levels cannot identify all cases of vitamin B_{12} deficiency; serum methylmalonic acid level may also be needed. Holotranscobalamin (holoTC), when compared with the other markers of vitamin B_{12} deficiency and age, renal function, and thyroid status, shows promise for diagnosing early vitamin B_{12} deficiency (Hvas and Nexo, 2005).

Glutathione inhibits the reduction of hydroxocobalamin by formation of a complex called glutathionylcobalamin, which could protect against diseases related to vitamin B_{12} depletion (Watson et al, 2004). Therefore, selenium may play an important role in maintaining vitamin B_{12} adequacy.

TABLE 12-14 Risks and Causes of Pernicious Anemia or Vitamin B_{12} Deficiency Anemia

Pernicious Anemia	Vitamin B_{12} Deficiency Anemia
High risk: Family history of pernicious anemia; African, Scandinavian, or Northern European descent; autoimmune endocrine disorders.	High risk: Vegans; elderly; persons with intestinal malabsorption or gastric atrophy or hypochlorhydria; stomach removal surgery; drug use (colchicine, neomycin); metabolic disorders (homocystinuria, methylmalonic aciduria); breastfed infants of vitamin B_1-deficient mothers; poor diet in infancy or pregnancy.
Causes: Autoimmune endocrine diseases such as type 1 diabetes, hypoparathyroidism, Addison's disease, hypopituitarism, testicular dysfunction, Graves' disease, chronic thyroiditis, myasthenia gravis, secondary amenorrhea, vitiligo, gastric surgery, anorexia nervosa, or bulimia nervosa.	Causes: Poor intake of extrinsic factor (vitamin B_{12}). Chronic alcoholism. *Helicobacter pylori* infection with diminished production of intrinsic factor (Kaptan et al, 2000). *H. pylori* induces autoantibodies directed against the gastric proton pump $H+/K+$-ATPase; this causes gastritis, increased atrophy, and apoptosis in the mucosa (Bergman et al, 2005). Hidden blood loss. Fish tapeworm. Reduced intestinal absorption, as with celiac disease (Dahele and Ghosh, 2001) or Crohn's disease.

INTERVENTION: OBJECTIVES

- Alleviate anemia and causation where possible.
- Provide foods that will not hurt a sore mouth. Glossitis (beefy, red tongue) decreases the desire to eat.
- Correct patient's anorexia.
- Prevent neurological defects if treatment is delayed or insufficient. Psychiatric symptoms such as depression, psychosis, and mania can appear.
- Correct pernicious anemia to prevent progression to gastric cancer.
- Correct hyperhomocysteinemia.

INTERVENTION: FOOD AND NUTRITION

The following suggestions are supportive measures for the required vitamin B_{12} injections in pernicious anemia:

- Diet should make liberal use of high biological value (HBV) proteins. Supplement diet with iron, vitamin C, other B vitamins (folic acid), and copper.
- If patient has a sore mouth, use a soft or liquid diet, especially with bland foods.
- Good sources of vitamin B_{12} include liver, other meats, fish, poultry, eggs, and fortified products such as soy milk. The daily average intake is 2–30 mg.
- Adequate intake of selenium to provide glutathione may be useful (Watson et al, 2004).

CLINICAL INDICATORS

Clinical/History

- Height
- Weight
- BMI
- Diet history
- Weight loss?
- Fatigue
- Flatulence, nausea, and vomiting
- Diarrhea
- Constipation
- Anorexia
- Tachycardia, cardiomegaly
- Achlorhydria
- Glossitis
- Beefy, red tongue
- Yellow or waxy skin
- BP, postural hypotension

Lab Work

- RBC
- Serum B_{12}
- MCV, MCHC, MCH (increased)
- Macrocytic/nucleated cells
- Reticulocyte count (low)
- Hematocrit (low)
- Lactate dehydrogenase (LDH) (increased)
- CBC (altered platelets and WBC count)
- Gastrin (increased)
- TIBC
- Urinary methylmalonic acid for B_{12} status
- Serum folate
- Serum homocysteine (elevated?)
- Holotranscobalamin (holoTC)
- Bilirubin
- Transferrin
- Schilling test (decreased)

Common Drugs Used and Potential Side Effects

- Vitamin B_{12} deficiency is effectively treated with oral vitamin B_{12} supplementation (Smith, 2000). Crystamine or Rubramin PC is cyanocobalamin in drug form for vitamin B_{12} deficiency.
- For pernicious anemia, vitamin B_{12} injections are given daily until remission, after which 6–8 injections yearly will suffice. Vitamin B_{12} supplements may be as effective as injections for correcting deficiency; high doses, such as 1000 μg, are needed daily for about 18 months (Nyholm et al, 2003).
- Trinsicon contains vitamin B_{12}, ferrous fumarate, vitamin C, folacin, and intrinsic factor. It is less effective when taken with dairy products.

Herbs, Botanicals, and Supplements

- Herbs and botanical supplements should not be used without discussing with physician.

INTERVENTION: NUTRITION EDUCATION, COUNSELING, CARE MANAGEMENT

- Be aware that vegan diets do not contain vitamin B_{12}; it is found only in animal foods. Include eggs, meat, fish, shellfish, cheese, milk, and milk products. Some fad diets may be low in vitamins and proteins; monitor carefully.
- Pernicious anemia develops after total gastrectomy unless vitamin B_{12} is administered. The problem can occur in patients with only partial gastrectomy or in patients who have had gastrojejunostomies.
- Avoidance of fatigue is essential. Plan simple meals and snacks.
- Megaloblastic B_{12} anemia may be common in elderly individuals; careful food choices are essential.
- For pernicious anemia, lifelong vitamin B_{12} replacement or injections are necessary.
- Breastfed infants of vitamin B_{12}–deficient mothers are at risk for severe developmental abnormalities, growth failure, and anemia (Stabler and Allen, 2004). Counseling for lactating women is important.

For More Information

- Medline–Pernicious Anemia
  http://www.nlm.nih.gov/medlineplus/ency/article/000569.htm
- Schilling Test
  http://www.nlm.nih.gov/medlineplus/ency/article/003572.htm
- Vitamin B_{12} Deficiency Anemia
  http://www.nlm.nih.gov/medlineplus/ency/article/000574.htm

MEGALOBLASTIC ANEMIAS: PERNICIOUS ANEMIA AND VITAMIN B_{12} DEFICIENCY ANEMIA—CITED REFERENCES

Bergman MP, et al. The story so far: *Helicobacter pylori* and gastric autoimmunity. *Int Rev Immunol.* 24:63, 2005.

Dahele A, Ghosh S. Vitamin B12 deficiency in untreated celiac disease. *Am J Gastroenterol.* 96:745, 2001.

Drabick J, et al. Concurrent pernicious anemia and myelodysplastic syndrome. *Ann Hematol.* 80:243, 2001.

Hvas AM, Nexo E. Holotranscobalamin—a first choice assay for diagnosing early vitamin B deficiency? *J Intern Med.* 257:289, 2005.
Kaptan K, et al. *Helicobacter pylori*—is it a novel causative agent in vitamin B12 deficiency? *Arch Intern Med.* 160:1349, 2000.
Nyholm E, et al. Oral vitamin B12 can change our practice. *Postgrad Med J.* 79:218, 2003.
Smith D. Anemia in the elderly. *Am Fam Physician.* 62:1565, 2000.
Stabler SP, Allen RH. Vitamin B12 deficiency as a worldwide problem. *Annu Rev Nutr.* 24:299, 2004.
Watson WP, et al. A new role for glutathione: protection of vitamin B12 from depletion by xenobiotics. *Chem Res Toxicol.* 17:1562, 2004.

PARASITIC ANEMIA AND MALARIA

NUTRITIONAL ACUITY RANKING: LEVEL 1

DEFINITIONS AND BACKGROUND

Gastrointestinal infestation by parasitic worms that feed on blood (hookworm) or on nutrients (tapeworm) can occur, especially in tropical or subtropical areas. Intestinal parasites that affect nutrition in particular include soil-transmitted helminths, *Giardia duodenalis, Entamoeba histolytica,* other parasites such as the coccidia, *Schistosoma* sp., and malarial parasites (Hesham et al, 2004).

Prevalence of iron deficiency is found to be associated with diverse factors in tropical countries (Shell-Duncan and McDade, 2005). In addition, more than 1000 cases of malaria are reported to the Centers for Disease Control and Prevention each year in the United States from travelers or immigrants, who present with fever, chills, nausea, vomiting, headache, abdominal pain, severe anemia, and acute renal failure (Vicas et al, 2005).

Malaria affects 300–500 infections per year in over 90 countries of the world. Anemia in coastal East Africa may be related to impaired erythropoietin production caused by malarial parasites (Cusick et al, 2005). *Plasmodium falciparum* malaria in pregnancy poses substantial risk to a pregnant woman and her neonate through anemia and low birth weight (Newman et al, 2003).

Symptoms of parasitic anemia include fatigue, abdominal discomfort, nausea, vomiting, fever, and irritability. Eosinophilia and iron or folate deficiencies secondary to parasitic infections are largely preventable (Erber et al, 2005). Chemoprophylaxis or intermittent preventive treatment (IPT) with an effective antimalarial can ameliorate the effects of malaria (Newman et al, 2003).

INTERVENTION: OBJECTIVES

- Correct anemia from blood losses; eliminate parasitic infestation.
- Prevent gastrointestinal (GI) tract perforation or obstruction, when likely to exist.
- Improve nutritional status and appetite. Parasitic infections affect the intake of food, subsequent digestion and absorption, metabolism, and nutrient storage and cause subtle micronutrient deficiency, such as vitamin A deficiency (Hesham et al, 2004).
- Prevent low birth weight and other adverse effects in pregnant or postpartum women and their infants.

INTERVENTION: FOOD AND NUTRITION

- A diet high in protein, B-complex vitamins, and iron may be appropriate. Provide adequate energy to meet individual's needs for anabolism where needed.
- Foods rich in heme iron and vitamins C and A should be included in meals served or planned. Iron inhibitors should be excluded from diet as far as possible until recovery is complete.
- Include plenty of other nutrient-dense foods, such as good sources of zinc and other micronutrients. See Table 12-15.

CLINICAL INDICATORS

Clinical/History
- Height
- Weight
- BMI
- Diet history
- BP
- I & O
- Fatigue
- Abdominal discomfort
- Nausea, vomiting
- Fever
- Irritability

Lab Work
- Serum B_{12}
- TIBC
- Alb
- Serum Fe
- Ferritin
- Serum folic acid
- Hgb (often <5 g/dL)
- Hematocrit
- CRP
- Transferrin
- Gluc
- Serum Cu
- Serum Zn

Common Drugs Used and Potential Side Effects

- Sulphadoxine-pyrimethamine has the best overall effectiveness in preventing adverse outcomes from malaria, especially in pregnancy (Newman et al, 2003).
- If needed, oral or parenteral iron may be given to correct anemia more rapidly. Beware of excessive use of oral supplements because of their potential side effects with iron overloading; monitor all sources (including iron-enriched foods).

Herbs, Botanicals, and Supplements

- Herbs and botanical supplements should not be used without discussing with physician.

TABLE 12-15 Micronutrient Deficiencies in Parasitic Anemias Such as Malaria

Micronutrient	Deficiency Effects
Vitamin A	Increased susceptibility to malarial anemia, altered iron metabolism, deficit of retinol for synthesis of acute phase reactants
Vitamin C	Impaired T-lymphocyte response, delayed cutaneous hypersensitivity, impaired complement function, reduced phagocytic function
Vitamin E	Impaired T-lymphocyte response, altered B-cell function and impaired humoral response, delayed cutaneous hypersensitivity, impaired cytokine function or production, reduced phagocytic function; deficiency can contribute to oxidant damage to erythrocytes, leading to hemolysis, but deficiency can make the parasite more vulnerable to oxidation generated with some antimalarial drugs
Riboflavin	Decreased iron absorption, increased erythrocyte fragility, depressed erythropoiesis; deficiency may protect against malaria by diminished parasite multiplication and growth
Folate	Impaired erythropoiesis; deficiency may protect against malaria through impaired parasite metabolism
Copper	Involvement in acute phase response to infection
Iron	Impaired erythropoiesis, decreased T-lymphocyte response, altered B-cell function and impaired humoral response, delayed cutaneous hypersensitivity, impaired cytokine function or production, reduced phagocytic function; deficiency and associated microcytosis may reduce malaria parasite multiplication. Avoid excesses.
Selenium	Unknown role
Zinc	Impaired immune function including decreased T-lymphocyte response, altered B-cell function and impaired humoral response, delayed cutaneous hypersensitivity, impaired cytokine function or production, reduced phagocytic function; can contribute to increased parasitemia

From: Nussenblatt V, Semba, RD. Micronutrient malnutrition and the pathogenesis of malarial anemia. *Acta Trop.* 82:321, 2002; and Scrimshaw NS, Sangiovanni JP. Synergism of nutrition, infection, and immunity: an overview. *Am J Clin Nutr.* 66:464S, 1997.

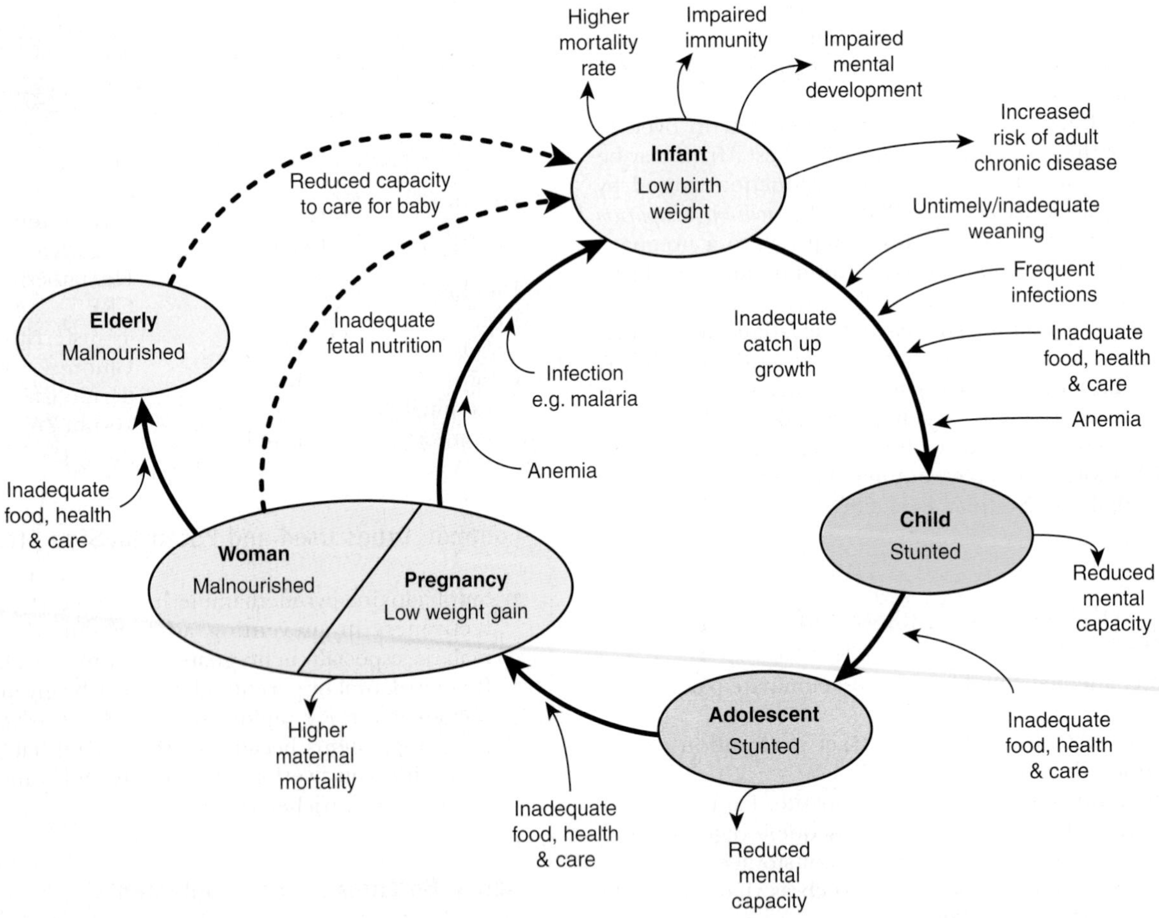

Figure 12-3 Cycle of parasitic infection and relationship to malnutrition. (Figure reprinted with permission from Steketee RW. Pregnancy, nutrition and parasitic diseases. *J Nutr.* 133:1662S, 2003.)

INTERVENTION: NUTRITION EDUCATION, COUNSELING, CARE MANAGEMENT

- Discuss ways to prevent further parasitic infestations, as with small children playing in soil. Pregnant women must be particularly careful, especially in developing countries where malaria, hookworm, and other parasites are common.
- Discuss ways to prepare foods high in necessary nutrients and methods to increase bioavailability (e.g., combining orange juice at breakfast with an iron-fortified cereal, etc.). In vulnerable populations, use of fortified beverages can help to correct micronutrient deficiency (Ash et al, 2003).
- In areas of malaria transmission, anemia is apparent from the first few months of life, and there is great need to target interventions at pregnant women and infants, which are the groups at highest risk (Crawley, 2004). Food-fortification programs can be very beneficial.

For More Information

- Anemia Control
  http://www.mostproject.org/IVACG/A%20Strategic%20Approach%20to%20Anemia%20Control.pdf#search='parasitic%20anemia'
- Multilateral Initiative on Malaria (MIM)
  http://www.mim.su.se/
- Parasitic Disorders
  http://www.oas.org/osde/publications/Unit/oea37e/ch10.htm
- World Health Organization–Malaria
  http://www.who.int/tdr/diseases/malaria/mim.htm

PARASITIC ANEMIA AND MALARIA—CITED REFERENCES

Ash DM, et al. Randomized efficacy trial of a micronutrient-fortified beverage in primary school children in Tanzania. *Am J Clin Nutr.* 77:891, 2003.
Crawley J. Reducing the burden of anemia in infants and young children in malaria-endemic countries of Africa: from evidence to action. *Am J Trop Med.* 71:25, 2004.
Cusick SE, et al. Short-term effects of vitamin A and antimalarial treatment on erythropoiesis in severely anemic Zanzibari preschool children. *Am J Clin Nutr.* 82:406, 2005.
Erber WN, et al. The haematology of indigenous Australians. *Hematology* 9:339, 2005.
Hesham MS, et al. Intestinal parasitic infections and micronutrient deficiency: a review. *Med J Malaysia.* 59:284, 2004.
Newman RD, et al. Safety, efficacy and determinants of effectiveness of antimalarial drugs during pregnancy: implications for prevention programmes in *Plasmodium falciparum*-endemic sub-Saharan Africa. *Trop Med Int Health.* 8:488, 2003.
Shell-Duncan B, McDade T. Cultural and environmental barriers to adequate iron intake among northern Kenyan schoolchildren. *Food Nutr Bulletin.* 26:39, 2005.
Vicas AE, et al. Imported malaria at an inner-city hospital in the United States. *Am J Med Sci.* 329:6, 2005.

SICKLE CELL ANEMIA

NUTRITIONAL ACUITY RANKING: LEVEL 1

DEFINITIONS AND BACKGROUND

Sickle cell disease (SCD) is the most common genetic disorder of the blood (Edwards et al, 2005). SCD involves anemia that is hereditary and hemolytic. Cells in SCD are crescent shaped and become rigid; they lodge themselves in the capillaries of the peripheral-blood system outside the heart. The sickling of red blood cells (RBCs) occurs when partially or totally deoxygenated hemoglobin molecules distort their normal disk shape, producing stiff, sticky, sickle-shaped cells that obstruct small blood vessels; this causes vaso-occlusion as well as deprivation of oxygen to body tissues (Edwards et al, 2005).

SCD has several forms including sickle cell anemia, sickle cell hemoglobin C disease, and sickle cell thalassemia disease. It is usually detected within the first year of life. Routine use of daily antibiotics until 5 years of age, immunization of children with pneumococcal vaccine, annual influenza vaccination after 6 months of age, and meningococcal vaccination after 2 years of age are important preventive measures (Mehta et al, 2006).

The largest population in the world with sickle cell anemia is in Africa. While this condition most commonly affects blacks of African descent, it is also found in people of Middle Eastern, East Indian, and Mediterranean origin. About 100,000 Americans have SCD (approximately 1 in every 400–500 African Americans). The origins of sickle cell anemia probably occurred thousands of years ago, and the trait helps people resist malaria.

Patients with SCD are at risk for delayed growth and sexual maturation; acute and chronic pulmonary dysfunction; stroke; aseptic necrosis of the hip, shoulders, or both; sickle cell retinopathy; dermal ulcers; and severe chronic pain (Edwards et al, 2005; Kirkham and DeBaum, 2004). The homozygous state (SS) is associated with complications and a reduced life expectancy (Cordeiro and Oniyangi, 2004).

Chronic anemia, pallor, and jaundice result because sickled cells do not last as long as normal blood cells. Bone marrow functions at six times the normal rate. Because there are fewer cells, the blood is thinner or anemic. When RBCs are destroyed, bilirubin is released into the blood and turns the whites of the eyes to a shade of yellow.

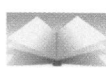

Inadequate dietary intakes of folate are common, while vitamin B_{12} intakes are usually adequate (Kennedy et al, 2001). Low RBC folate levels may occur. Serum total homocysteine (tHcy) levels may be elevated in this population; greater intakes than normal of folate may be needed to normalize serum tHcy levels, even if transfusions are used (Lowenthal et al, 2000). Elevated tHcy levels contribute to thrombosis, a frequent event in this population (Segal et al, 2004). Children with sickle cell anemia have lower vitamin B_6 concentrations, and further studies are needed to evaluate the implications (Nelson et al, 2002).

Infants and children who have sickle cell anemia are at risk for nutritional deficiencies and loss of body mass during acute illnesses, when inadequate intake of energy and macronutrients may occur (Malinauskas et al, 2000). Suboptimal vitamin A intake is common, with more frequent hospitalizations and poor growth (Schall et al, 2004). Low serum vitamin D status is highly prevalent in children with SCD; vitamin D status is associated with season and dietary intake (Buison et al, 2004). Prepubertal children with SCD may have zinc deficiency and may benefit from zinc supplementation to improve linear growth and weight gain (Zemel et al, 2002).

Dietary omega-3 fatty acids reduce the frequency of pain episodes in SCD by reducing prothrombotic activity (Tomer et al, 2001). It is prudent to include omega-3 fatty acids in diet and supplemental form.

Aggressive antibiotic therapy and transfusions can save lives. Although life saving, transfusion therapy has resulted in the majority of sickle cell anemia patients being at risk for hemosiderosis-induced organ damage (Vichinsky et al, 2005). Iron overloading may occur after transfusions. After 1–2 years of conventional transfusions, iron concentrations and tissue damage may be observed in patients with SCD. Iron deficiency, through reduction of mean cell hematocrit (MCHC), actually may be beneficial for longer RBC survival and oxygen affinity.

Patients with SCD have problems with surgery, including prolonged bleeding (Raffini et al, 2006). Vitamin K should be given preoperatively.

Acute chest syndrome, triggered by infections and fat clots in the lungs, is the leading cause of death in sickle cell anemia. Newer treatments include hydroxyurea therapy to decrease the frequency of painful episodes and associated comorbidities and hematopoietic cell transplantation for some patients (Mehta et al, 2006). Bone marrow transplantation is one consideration in which a perfect match must be available from a sibling.

A significant advance in stroke prevention is the use of transcranial Doppler ultrasonography to identify asymptomatic, at-risk children who should be considered for chronic blood transfusions (Mehta et al, 2006). Finally, studies of gene expression may bring new solutions to this complex condition.

INTERVENTION: OBJECTIVES

- Supplement diet with missing nutrients. Correct any malnutrition.
- Reduce oxygen debt. Improve patient's ability to participate in the activities of daily life.
- Reduce painful cramps, liver dysfunction, cholelithiasis, jaundice, and hepatitis.
- Lessen likelihood of pressure ulcers, infections, and renal failure.
- Promote normal growth and development, which tend to be stunted in children.
- Prevent chronic hypoxia, which can lead to lower intellectual performance.
- Improve quality of life, where possible.

TABLE 12-16 Equation to Predict Energy Needs in Adolescents with Sickle Cell Disease

Basal energy requirements are higher in adolescents with sickle cell anemia than in healthy control subjects (Buchowski et al, 2002).

Males: REE (kcal/d) = 1305 + 18.6.weight (kg) − 55.7.hemoglobin (g/dL)
REE (kJ/d) = 5461 + 77.7.weight (kg) − 233.2.hemoglobin (g/dL)

Females: REE (kcal/d) = 1100 + 13.3.weight (kg) − 30.2.hemoglobin (g/dL)
REE (kJ/d) = 4603 + 55.6.weight (kg) − 126.2.hemoglobin (g/dL)

INTERVENTION: FOOD AND NUTRITION

- Include food sources of omega-3 fatty acids; vitamins D, C, A, B_{12}, and B_6; folic acid; and high biological value (HBV) proteins; ensure adequate zinc and riboflavin.
- Estimate energy needs and increase diet accordingly (see Table 12-16).
- A multivitamin-mineral supplement should be recommended; one without excess iron is important when transfusions are used. Avoid excesses of iron, including from tube feedings or total parenteral nutrition (TPN).
- Energy deficits are common in this population (Singhal et al, 2002). Nightly tube feeding can help to improve nutritional status. While supplementation with arginine has been suggested, more studies in humans are needed (Fasipe et al, 2004).

CLINICAL INDICATORS

Clinical/History

Height
Weight
BMI
Diet history
BP
I & O
Chronic anemia, pallor
Jaundice

Lab Work

Hemoglobin (often low)
Hematocrit
Serum Fe (increased from hemolysis)
RBP (decreased)
tHcy (often elevated)
Transferrin saturation
Serum B_{12}
Serum folacin
Serum and urinary zinc
N balance
Alb
CRP
Cholesterol
Triglycerides (Trig) (decreased)
MCV
Serum ferritin
Partial pressure of oxygen (pO_2), partial pressure of carbon dioxide (pCO_2)
Uric acid (increased)
PT and INR

SAMPLE NUTRITION DIAGNOSTIC STATEMENT

Anemia: Sickle Cell Disease

PES: Involuntary weight loss related to sick cell anemia with inadequate caloric intake as evidenced by 10% loss of usual body weight in the last 2 months.

Assessment Data (sources of info): Weight pattern, percent desirable body weight, diet history, problems with meal planning or shopping, financial challenges.

Intervention: Nutrition counseling, encouraging energy-dense foods and favorites, referrals to social service agencies for help with meal preparation and delivery if needed.

Monitoring and Evaluation: Weight records, improvements in appetite and intake.

Common Drugs Used and Potential Side Effects

- Pain medicines (such as ibuprofen) may be used. Monitor for all side effects and gastrointestinal (GI) distress.
- Hydroxyurea therapy is used to increase hemoglobin production. It may curtail the hypermetabolic state observed in children with SCD, offering a secondary benefit (Fung et al, 2001).
- Rofecoxib is a cyclo-oxygenase-2 (COX-2) inhibitor approved for pain and has been tested in children with no adverse effects (Prescilla et al, 2004).

Herbs, Botanicals, and Supplements

- Herbs and botanical supplements should not be used without discussing with physician.
- A phytomedicine, Niprisan, reduces episodes of SCD crisis associated with severe pain over a 6-month period (Cordeiro and Oniyangi, 2004). More studies are needed.

INTERVENTION: NUTRITION EDUCATION, COUNSELING, CARE MANAGEMENT

- Indicate which foods are good sources of folic acid, high biological value (HBV) proteins, zinc, riboflavin, and vitamins A, C, D, E, B_6, and B_{12}.
- Discuss ways for easy meal preparation because fatigue tends to be a problem.
- Malaria may aggravate sickle cell crises; health professionals often recommend lifelong malaria chemoprophylaxis for people with SCD, but there is very little direct evidence to support or refute this practice (Oniyangi and Omari, 2003).
- Quality of life is often decreased among adults with SCD, and health professionals should try to offer assistance that will help improve this quality (McClish et al, 2005).

For More Information

- American Sickle Cell Association
  http://www.ascaa.org/
- March of Dimes
  http://www.marchofdimes.com/professionals/681_1221.asp
- National Institutes of Health (NIH)–Genes and Disease
  http://www.ncbi.nlm.nih.gov/disease/sickle.html
- NIH–Sickle Cell Anemia
  http://www.nlm.nih.gov/medlineplus/sicklecellanemia.html
- Sickle Cell Links
  http://www.sicklecellct.org/links/index.html
- Sickle Cell Disease Association of America
  http://www.sicklecellct.org/
- Sickle Cell Facts
  http://www.sicklecelldisease.org/about_scd/faqs.phtml

SICKLE CELL ANEMIA—CITED REFERENCES

Buchowski MS, et al. Equation to estimate resting energy expenditure in adolescents with sickle cell anemia. *Am J Clin Nutr.* 76:1335, 2002.

Buison AM, et al. Low vitamin D status in children with sickle cell disease. *J Pediatr.* 145:622, 2004.

Cordeiro NJ, Oniyangi O. Phytomedicines (medicines derived from plants) for sickle cell disease. *Cochrane Database Syst Rev.* 3:CD004448, 2004.

Edwards CL, et al. A brief review of the pathophysiology, associated pain, and psychosocial issues in sickle cell disease. *Int J Behav Med.* 12:171, 2005.

Fasipe FR, et al. Arginine supplementation improves rotorod performance in sickle transgenic mice. *Hematology* 9:301, 2004.

Fung EB, et al. Effect of hydroxyurea therapy on resting energy expenditure in children with sickle cell disease. *J Pediatr Hematol Oncol.* 23:604, 2001.

Kennedy T, et al. Red blood cell folate and serum vitamin B12 status in children with sickle cell disease. *J Pediatr Hematol Oncol.* 23:165, 2001.

Kirkham FJ, DeBaum MR. Stroke in children with sickle cell disease. *Curr Treat Options Neurol.* 6:357, 2004.

Lowenthal E, et al. Homocysteine elevation in sickle cell disease. *J Am Col Nutr.* 19:608, 2000.

Malinauskas B, et al. Impact of acute illness on nutritional status of infants and young children with sickle cell disease. *J Am Diet Assoc.* 100:330, 2000.

McClish DK, et al. Health related quality of life in sickle cell patients: the PiSCES project. *Health Qual Life Outcomes.* 3:50, 2005.

Mehta SR, et al. Opportunities to improve outcomes in sickle cell disease. *Am Fam Physician.* 74:303, 2006.

Nelson MC, et al. Vitamin B6 status of children with sickle cell disease. *J Pediatr Hematol Oncol.* 24:463, 2002.

Oniyangi O, Omari AA. Malaria chemoprophylaxis in sickle cell disease. Malaria chemoprophylaxis in sickle cell disease. *Cochrane Database Syst Rev.* 3:CD003489, 2003.

Prescilla RP, et al. Pharmacokinetics of rofecoxib in children with sickle cell hemoglobinopathy. *J Pediatr Hematol Oncol.* 26:661, 2004.

Raffini LJ, et al. Prolongation of the prothrombin time and activated partial thromboplastin time in children with sickle cell disease. *Pediatr Blood Cancer.* 47:589, 2006.

Schall JI, et al. Vitamin A status, hospitalizations, and other outcomes in young children with sickle cell disease. *J Pediatr.* 145:99, 2004.

Segal JB, et al. Concentrations of B vitamins and homocysteine in children with sickle cell anemia. *South Med J.* 97:149, 2004.

Singhal A, et al. Energy intake and resting metabolic rate in preschool Jamaican children with homozygous sickle cell disease. *Am J Clin Nutr.* 75:1093, 2002.

Tomer A, et al. Reduction of pain episodes and prothrombotic activity in sickle cell disease by dietary n-3 fatty acids. *Thromb Haemost.* 85:966, 2001.

Vichinsky E, et al. Comparison of organ dysfunction in transfused patients with SCD or beta thalassemia. *Am J Hematol.* 80:70, 2005.

Zemel BS, et al. Effect of zinc supplementation on growth and body composition in children with sickle cell disease. *Am J Clin Nutr.* 75:300, 2002.

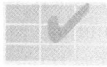

SIDEROBLASTIC ANEMIA

NUTRITIONAL ACUITY RANKING: LEVEL 1

DEFINITIONS AND BACKGROUND

Sideroblastic anemias are a group of blood disorders characterized by an impaired ability of the bone marrow to produce normal red blood cells. The iron inside red blood cells is inadequately used to make hemoglobin, despite adequate or increased amounts of iron. Abnormal red blood cells called sideroblasts are found in the blood of people with these anemias. This anemia is a microcytic, hypochromic anemia similar to that caused by iron deficiency, except that serum iron is normal or elevated. Copper deficiency is another, rare cause of sideroblastic anemia and neutropenia that often is not suspected clinically (Willis et al, 2005).

The disease X-linked sideroblastic anemia with ataxia is due to a mutation in the protein transporter that is thought to transfer iron clusters from the mitochondrion to the cytoplasm (Napier et al, 2005). Another name for the congenital type of anemia is hereditary iron-loading anemia. Another type is a vitamin B_6–responsive form. Vitamin B_6–responsive sideroblastic anemia responds to high pyridoxine doses. Vitamin B_6 is the main vitamin for processing amino acids. Vitamin B_6 is also needed to make melatonin, serotonin, and dopamine.

INTERVENTION: OBJECTIVES

- Correct problems and symptoms.
- Identify causes and solutions.
- Correct any suppression of bone marrow, iron loading, or related problems.

INTERVENTION: FOOD AND NUTRITION

- A diet high in vitamin B_6 may be beneficial (drugs are often used). Potatoes, bananas, raisin bran cereal, lentils, liver, turkey, and tuna are good sources of vitamin B_6.
- Protein and carbohydrate (CHO) intake should be adequate, and energy should also be adequate to spare protein.
- Folic acid and copper may also be needed.
- Alcohol intake should be severely limited.
- Balanced meals and snacks, as necessary, may be helpful.

CLINICAL INDICATORS

Clinical/History		Lab Work		
Height	BMI	B_6 levels	Transferrin saturation (often elevated)	Serum folic acid
Weight	Diet history	RBC		Serum homocysteine
	BP			WBC
	I & O			Serum Fe
				Serum Cu

Common Drugs Used and Potential Side Effects

- Vitamin B_6 may be ordered; age-dependent doses are specified. The National Academy of Sciences performed an analysis of vitamin B_6 studies. It is usually safe at intakes of up to 100 mg/d in adults, but neurological side effects can sometimes occur at or above that level. Vitamin B_6 toxicity damages sensory nerves, leading to numbness in the hands and feet as well as difficulty walking.
- Chloramphenicol may cause drug-induced bone marrow suppression, resulting in sideroblastic anemia.
- Isoniazid and cycloserine can cause abnormal vitamin B_6 metabolism. Monitor for gastrointestinal side effects.

Herbs, Botanicals, and Supplements

- Herbs and botanical supplements should not be used without discussing with physician.

INTERVENTION: NUTRITION EDUCATION, COUNSELING, CARE MANAGEMENT

- Discuss adequate sources of all needed nutrients such as vitamin B_6, especially if deficiency caused the anemia.
- Discuss attractive menu planning and balancing of meals because appetite and intake may be poor chronically. Discuss snacks and frequency.

For More Information

- Genetics Home Reference
  http://ghr.nlm.nih.gov/ghr/resource/health
- Medline Plus: Anemia
  http://www.nlm.nih.gov/medlineplus/anemia.html
- National Institutes Health: X-linked Sideroblastic Anemia
  http://ghr.nlm.nih.gov/condition=xlinkedsideroblasticanemia

SIDEROBLASTIC ANEMIA—CITED REFERENCES

Napier I, et al. Iron trafficking in the mitochondrion: novel pathways revealed by disease. *Blood* 105:1844, 2005.

Willis MS, et al. Zinc-induced copper deficiency: a report of three cases initially recognized on bone marrow examination. *Am J Clin Pathol.* 123:125, 2005.

THALASSEMIA

NUTRITIONAL ACUITY RANKING: LEVEL 1

DEFINITIONS AND BACKGROUND

Thalassemia (the most severe is Cooley's anemia or Mediterranean anemia) is a hereditary disease with an increased rate of destruction of red blood cells. Frequency of thalassemia is dependent on ethnic origins of the patient population; it is most common in persons with Mediterranean ancestry. Beta-thalassemia is well recognized in persons of Greek and Italian descent, whereas alpha-thalassemic syndromes have an increased frequency in African, American Indian, and Asian populations.

Collectively, the thalassemias are among the most common inherited disorders. The beta-thalassemias are more common and are a worldwide clinical problem due to an increasing immigrant population (Hahalis et al, 2005). Figure 12-4 shows how the trait is passed.

Signs and symptoms of thalassemia include anemia, bone abnormalities, jaundice, enlarged spleen, and leg ulcers. The red blood cells are fragile and contain abnormal hemoglobin. In thalassemia major, symptoms can begin as early as 3 months of age. In the first year or two of life and in the absence of transfusion, a child can demonstrate severe anemia and expansion of the facial and other bones. These children may be pale or jaundiced, have a poor appetite, fail to grow normally, and have an enlarged spleen, liver, or heart. The incidence of gallstones is unusually common in this population (Premawardhena et al, 2001).

Regular blood transfusions are necessary early in life (Hahalis et al, 2005). Blood transfusions and increased gastrointestinal (GI) iron absorption result in iron overload and tissue damage. Excess iron accumulates, leading to liver, heart, and pituitary damage and failure of these organs.

Cardiac complications caused by iron deposition are major causes of death in patients with beta-thalassemia (Anderson et al, 2004; Wu et al, 2004). Among these patients, cardiomyopathy remains the leading cause of mortality (Hahalis et al, 2005). If splenomegaly occurs, a splenectomy may be needed. Recent advances in gene therapy are expected to result in the long-awaited cure of this disease.

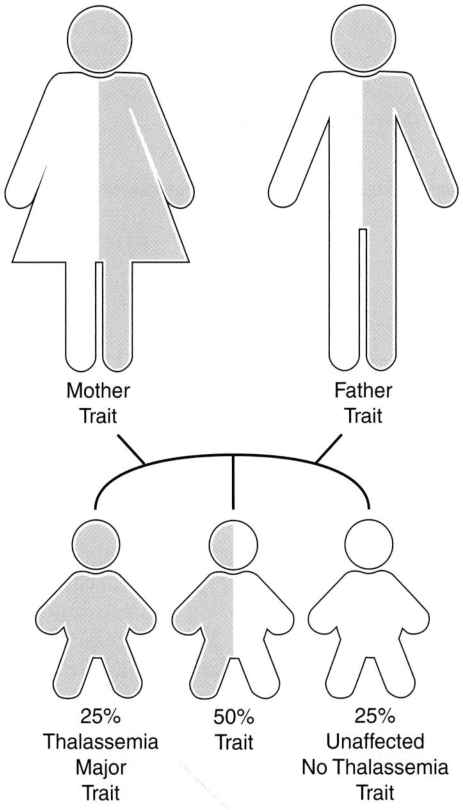

Figure 12-4 Thalassemia trait.

INTERVENTION: OBJECTIVES

- Offer temporary relief with blood transfusions; this will improve hematological status with oxygen availability.
- Correct failure to thrive and GI problems. Impaired growth is a problem; increased caloric dietary intake increases insulin-like growth factor I (IGF-I) levels, BMI, midarm circumference, and skinfold thickness in these children (Soliman et al, 2004).
- Reduce or correct infections.
- Promote healing of any ulcerations.
- Prevent or correct side effects of iron overloading from the necessary transfusions.
- Prevent slow or stunted growth.

INTERVENTION: FOOD AND NUTRITION

- A diet high in quality protein, energy, B-complex vitamins (especially folic acid and vitamin B_{12}), and zinc will be beneficial. To prevent iron overloading, avoid use of multivitamin-mineral supplements that contain iron and vitamin C in large amounts.
- Provide adequate fluid intake.
- If hyperglycemia and diabetes are present, use carbohydrate counting and other accepted techniques for managing glucose levels.

CLINICAL INDICATORS

Clinical/History		
Height	Diet history	Leg ulcers
Weight	BP	Bone abnormalities
BMI	Growth failure	Enlarged spleen
	Jaundice	Hypogonadism
	I & O	

Lab Work

- RBC
- CBC
- H & H
- Transferrin (decreased)
- Transferrin iron saturation percentage (increased)
- Serum Fe (increased)
- Superconducting Quantum Interference Device (SQUID) determines liver iron content by measuring magnetic fields
- Serum ferritin (increased)
- TIBC (decreased)
- Thyroid-stimulating hormone (TSH), thyroxine (T4) (hypothyroidism is common)
- Alkaline phosphatase (Alk phos)
- Gluc
- Vitamin B_{12}
- Serum zinc
- Alb
- CRP
- Hypoparathyroidism

Common Drugs Used and Potential Side Effects

- Iron-chelating therapy with deferoxamine in patients with thalassemia major has dramatically improved the prognosis of this disease (Taher et al, 2005). Side effects include allergic reactions, tinnitus, and erythematous rash. Overchelation may cause growth retardation and mineral deficiency.
- Future therapies for iron overload may include oral iron-binding agents capable of preventing dietary iron absorption from the diet (Murray et al, 2003). The oral chelator deferiprone (Ferriprox) is under FDA evaluation.

Herbs, Botanicals, and Supplements

- Herbs and botanical supplements should not be used without discussing with physician.

INTERVENTION: NUTRITION EDUCATION, COUNSELING, CARE MANAGEMENT

- Discuss ways to improve nutritional intake, when deficient.
- Discuss importance of diet in the maintenance of hematological health.

For More Information

- Cooley's Anemia Foundation
  www.thalassemia.org
- Cord Blood Information
  http://www.thalassemia.com/cord_blood.html
- International Support Groups
  http://www.thalassemia.com/inter_support.html
- Thalassemia International Federation
  http://www.thalassaemia.org.cy/
- Too Much Iron
  http://www.askaboutiron.com/index.jsp?usertrack.filter_applied=true&NovaId=2229644950362982731

THALASSEMIA—CITED REFERENCES

Anderson LJ, et al. Myocardial iron clearance during reversal of siderotic cardiomyopathy with intravenous desferrioxamine: a prospective study using T2* cardiovascular magnetic resonance. *Br J Haematol.* 27:348, 2004.

Hahalis G, et al. Heart failure in beta-thalassemia syndromes: a decade of progress. *Am J Med.* 118:957, 2005.

Murray KF, et al. Current and future therapy in haemochromatosis and Wilson's disease. *Expert Opin Pharmacother.* 4:2239, 2003.

Premawardhena A, et al. Genetic determinants of jaundice and gallstones in hemoglobin E beta-thalassaemia. *Lancet.* 357:1945, 2001.

Soliman AT, et al. The effect of high-calorie diet on nutritional parameters of children with beta-thalassaemia major. *Clin Nutr.* 23:1158, 2004.

Taher A, et al. Comparison between deferoxamine and deferiprone (L1) in iron-loaded thalassemia patients. *Eur J Haemetol.* 67:30, 2005.

Wu KH, et al. Combined therapy with deferiprone and desferrioxamine successfully regresses severe heart failure in patients with beta-thalassemia major. *Ann Hematol.* 83:471, 2004.

OTHER BLOOD DISORDERS

HEMOCHROMATOSIS (IRON OVERLOADING)

NUTRITIONAL ACUITY RANKING: LEVEL 2

DEFINITIONS AND BACKGROUND

Hereditary hemochromatosis is one of the most common autosomal recessive disorders among Caucasians; one in 200–400 individuals of Northern European ancestry is at risk for hemochromatosis (Camaschella and Merlini, 2005). The disorder is recessive, requiring the gene from two carrier parents. It is also common in Hispanics or people of Mediterranean descent and is 10 times more common in males than in females. Irish Americans and African Americans have double the usual frequency. Tragically, hemochromatosis remains underdiagnosed.

In hemochromatosis, iron stores are deposited in excess, often from excess intake or liver/pancreatic diseases, renal dialysis, or frequent and long-term transfusions. Healthy people may accumulate up to 1 g of iron, but people with this condition accumulate 15–30 g. Increased iron absorption leads to excessive accumulation of iron deposits within cells of the liver, heart, pituitary gland, pancreas, and other organs, gradually causing tissue damage.

Symptoms and signs of iron overloading include bronzing of the skin, profound fatigue, joint pain or arthritis, loss of body hair, loss of libido, lack of menstruation or early menopause, abdominal pain, chronic intermittent diarrhea,

TABLE 12-17 Facts About Hemochromatosis

1. Undetected or untreated excess iron kills after inflicting injury to a variety of body organs. The physician's concern must be to detect any excess iron instead of establishing the diagnosis.
2. Some literature suggests treatment when ferritin alone is elevated. Giving blood does no harm and, instead, is beneficial to health. About one fourth of patients have low hemoglobin; treatment is the same unless the anemia is so severe that blood transfusions are required. Severely anemic patients require iron removal by an iron chelator, Desferal.
3. Iron overloading is preventable. When diagnosis is in doubt, the patient should begin a trial of weekly phlebotomies at the blood bank. Four to 6 weeks will usually provide the answer, and getting rid of a little excess iron will improve health.
4. The patient should be taken to the blood bank upon physician's order for weekly phlebotomies.
5. A liver biopsy is not always necessary, and waiting can delay important treatment. DNA testing is not useful because it cannot detect all of the known mutations.
6. When iron levels test low, the cause must be found. It is dangerous to medicate with iron without testing first and then finding the reason for any deficiency.
7. Symptoms vary. Chronic fatigue, arthritis, anemia (iron-loading anemia is one symptom), and elevated liver enzymes must not be ignored. Hemoglobin level does not indicate iron status. A disorder of thyroid or any part of the body can be a symptom of iron overload.
8. Excess iron lowers immunity. Many diseases (such as cancer, hepatitis, and AIDS) will show a poor outcome unless any excess iron is removed. Excess iron stored in the brain exacerbates severity in Alzheimer's, multiple sclerosis, Lou Gehrig's disease, Parkinson's disease, psychological problems, autism, and other diseases.

Adapted from: Iron Overload Diseases Association. Accessed September 27, 2005 at http://www.ironoverload.org/.

irregular heartbeat, cardiomegaly with congestive failure, hepatomegaly, enlarged spleen, hypothyroidism, and depression.

Because hemochromatosis has so many possible symptoms, it often goes undiagnosed. However, early detection is important and may prevent organ failure that can occur if it is left untreated. Long-term complications include liver cirrhosis, diabetes, cardiomyopathy, hypogonadism, arthropathy, skin pigmentation, and susceptibility to liver cancer (Camaschella and Merlini, 2005). See Table 12-17.

INTERVENTION: OBJECTIVES

- Remove excess iron from body (usually with phlebotomies of 500 mL weekly, performed by the physician). This may take a few months or years, and then therapy is repeated several times annually for rest of life.
- Prevent liver cancer, heart attack, or stroke by unloading storage iron as fast as possible; keep serum ferritin below 10 ng/mL. If excess iron intake is a chronic problem, discontinue use in supplements and fortified foods (such as iron-fortified cereals). Read labels carefully.
- Teach principles of nutrition and menu planning to incorporate adequate intake of other nutrients that may be depleted with excessive phlebotomies (e.g., folate and other B-complex vitamins, protein).

INTERVENTION: FOOD AND NUTRITION

- Provide a normal diet unless renal or hepatic function is altered. Do not consume foods rich in vitamin C in large amounts; read cereal labels and avoid those with 100% or more of the daily allowance for these two nutrients.
- A low-iron diet is not recommended.
- Ensure adequate protein intake and provide sufficient energy to meet estimated needs and activity levels.
- Avoid alcohol because of potential damage to a vulnerable liver.
- *Vibrio vulnificus* in some raw seafood kills people every year, many are those with undetected iron overload. Avoid eating raw seafood.

CLINICAL INDICATORS

Clinical/History

Height
Weight
BMI
Diet history
BP
I & O

Lab Work

Serum iron saturation or transferrin saturation (best tests)
Transferrin (increased)
Serum Cu (increased)
Alb
Serum Fe
Ferritin (may be increased; normal, 5–150 ng/mL)
Hgb (desirable level, 10 g/dL)
Hematocrit (desirable level, 30–35%)
Gluc
Serum B_6
Serum B_{12}
Serum folic acid
Thyroid tests
Liver function tests
CRP
TIBC* (normal range, 12–45%)

*Divide total serum iron by TIBC for percentage of tissue saturation (TS). Divide the serum iron level by TIBC for percentage of transferrin saturation.

Common Drugs Used and Potential Side Effects

- Avoid use of multivitamin supplements that contain iron and vitamin C because these can increase iron absorption.

Herbs, Botanicals, and Supplements

- Herbs and botanical supplements should not be used without discussing with physician.

INTERVENTION: NUTRITION EDUCATION, COUNSELING, CARE MANAGEMENT

- All blood relatives of the patient must be evaluated and monitored yearly for iron overloading.
- Genetic testing of other family members is also recommended for those with inherited type.
- Discuss avoidance of alcohol and raw seafood.
- Discuss nutrient sources as appropriate for the individual.

For More Information

- Blood Banks
  http://www.ironoverload.org/bloodbanks.htm
- Centers for Disease Control and Prevention: Hemochromatosis for Health Professionals
  http://origin.cdc.gov/hemochromatosis/training/course_summary/
- Hemochromatosis
  http://origin.cdc.gov/hemochromatosis/training/pdf/hemochromatosis_diet.pdf
- Iron Disorders Institute
  http://www.irondisorders.org
- Iron Overload Diseases Association, Inc.
  http://www.ironoverload.org/
- Iron Tests
  http://www.irondisorders.org/Forms/irontests.pdf
- Phlebotomy for Patients
  http://origin.cdc.gov/hemochromatosis/training/pdf/phlebotomy_info.pdf

HEMOCHROMATOSIS—CITED REFERENCES

Camaschella C, Merlini R. Inherited hemochromatosis: from genetics to clinics. *Minerva Med.* 96:207, 2005.

HEMORRHAGE AND BLEEDING DISORDERS

NUTRITIONAL ACUITY RANKING: LEVEL 2

DEFINITIONS AND BACKGROUND

The circulatory system is a closed system, with low volume and high pressure. It provides efficient delivery of nutrients to all tissues. When there is volume loss, a large decrease in nutrient delivery occurs. **Hemorrhage** is the excessive discharge of blood from a ruptured vessel.

Bleeding (bright red and in spurts from an artery; dark red and in a steady flow from a vein) can be external, internal, or into skin or other tissue. When massive, a hemorrhage can cause such symptoms as rapid, shallow breathing; cold, clammy skin; thirst; visual disturbances; and extreme weakness. Loss of more than 20% of blood volume causes hypotension and tachycardia; loss of more than 1 quart of blood may lead to shock. Peptic ulcer, hemophilia, or stroke may be causes.

To stop a hemorrhage, blood must clot properly. Blood clots when its fibrinogen is converted to fibrin by action of thrombin. Vitamin K works as a coenzyme that converts glutamic acid to gamma-carboxyglutamic acid; this helps to bind calcium and is required for the activation of the seven vitamin K–dependent clotting factors in the coagulation cascade. Table 12-18 shows blood clotting and how nutritional factors play a role. See Figure 12-5.

INTERVENTION: OBJECTIVES

- Medical management is designed to control bleeding, take care of the underlying cause of the bleeding, and replace lost blood. Transfusions may be needed. Less severe hemorrhages may require iron, vitamin B_{12}, and folic acid to help replace red blood cells.
- Support erythropoiesis.
- Control intestinal impact of gastrointestinal (GI) bleeding, which can cause a protein overload.
- Prevent hypovolemic shock (low cardiac output, decreased blood pressure, and decreased urinary output) from uncontrolled bleeding.

INTERVENTION: FOOD AND NUTRITION

- Ensure that diet is rich in proteins, iron, folic acid, vitamin B_{12}, and copper.
- Check need for vitamin K. Patients with intestinal or liver disease may become deficient. If medications to replace vitamin K are used, diet should provide a balance without excess. Monitor content of meals or enteral feedings and multivitamin supplements carefully to ensure that all RDAs are met without excesses. See Table 12-19.

CLINICAL INDICATORS

Clinical/History	Diet history	I & O
Height	BP	Petechiae
Weight	Pulse	Hemophiliac arthropathy
BMI	Temperature	

Excessive bleeding
Excessive bruising
Easy bleeding
Nose bleeds
Abnormal menstrual bleeding

Lab Work

Coagulation testing
PT
Activated partial thromboplastin time (aPTT)
Thrombin time (thrombin added to plasma, and time to clot measured)
Fibrinogen
Platelet count
Bleeding time (international normalized ratio [INR])
Transferrin
RBC
Alb
BUN
CBC
H & H
Serum Fe
Serum B_{12}
Serum folate
TIBC (increased)
Creatinine
Occult blood
CRP

TABLE 12-18 Blood Clotting Factors That Involve Nutrition

The coagulation cascade involves a series of steps that stop bleeding through clot formation. Vitamin K–dependent coagulation factors are synthesized in the liver. Consequently, severe liver disease results in lower blood levels of vitamin K–dependent clotting factors and an increased risk of uncontrolled bleeding (hemorrhage).

In hemostatic (bleeding) disorders, it is important to evaluate for bleeding problems in the family history, history of heavy menses or easy bruising, and prior blood transfusions. Bleeding disorders include a number of conditions in which people tend to bleed longer. Clotting involves about 20 different plasma proteins (clotting factors). Normally, clotting factors form fibrin that stops bleeding. In bleeding disorders, the process does not occur normally.

Some bleeding disorders are present at birth (hemophilia and von Willebrand's disease), or they can be acquired (such as vitamin K deficiency, severe liver disease, use of anticoagulant drugs or prolonged use of antibiotics, bone marrow problems, leukemia, pregnancy-associated eclampsia, or snake bite). In these disorders, vision loss can occur from bleeding into the eye, or anemia may result, or there may be neurological problems or even death.

The following factors involve nutrition:

I. Fibrinogen
II. Prothrombin
III. Thromboplastin
IV. Calcium.

Gene therapy may one day be available to treat the bleeding disorders.

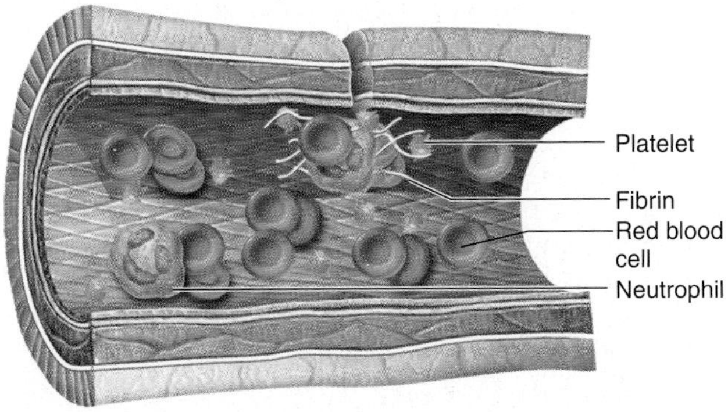

Figure 12-5 Blood clot formation. (Images provided by Anatomical Chart Co.)

TABLE 12-19 Food Sources of Vitamin K

Food	Serving	Vitamin K (μg)
Kale, raw	1 cup (chopped)	547
Broccoli, cooked	1 cup (chopped)	420
Parsley, raw	1 cup (chopped)	324
Swiss chard, raw	1 cup (chopped)	299
Spinach, raw	1 cup (chopped)	120
Leaf lettuce, raw	1 cup (shredded)	118
Watercress, raw	1 cup (chopped)	85
Soybean oil	1 tbsp	26
Canola oil	1 tbsp	20
Mayonnaise	1 tbsp	12
Olive oil	1 tbsp	7

Source: U.S. Department of Agriculture. USDA national nutrient database for standard reference, release 16. Available at http://www.nal.usda.gov/fnic/foodcomp/Data/SR16/wtrank/wt_rank.html.

Common Drugs Used and Potential Side Effects

- Vitamin K may be needed. In the United States, vitamin K is available in multivitamins and other supplements in doses that generally range from 10–120 μg/dose.
- Oral anticoagulants, such as warfarin, inhibit coagulation through antagonism of the action of vitamin K. Inadequate gamma-carboxylation of vitamin K–dependent proteins will inhibit clot formation. Patients taking these drugs are cautioned against consuming very large or highly variable quantities of vitamin K in their diets. A reasonably constant dietary intake of vitamin K is suggested.
- Avoid aspirin and other blood thinners.

Herbs, Botanicals, and Supplements

- Herbs and botanical supplements should not be used without discussing with physician.
- Evidence of bleeding effects and other potential adverse effects of high vitamin E intakes in humans is not convincing (Hathcock et al, 2005). In chronic myelogenous leukemia (CML), a slowly progressive disease, platelets are increased in number, and easy bleeding occurs; vitamins A, D_3, E, and B_{12} and *Curcuma longa* have been studied to determine whether they are helpful (Steriti, 2002).

INTERVENTION: NUTRITION EDUCATION, COUNSELING, CARE MANAGEMENT

- Blood donors should be alerted to the need to replace daily iron intake by 0.7 mg for a year. Every pint is equivalent to 250 mg of iron lost.
- Discuss adequate dietary replacement for lost nutrients. A multivitamin-mineral supplement may be indicated.

For More Information

- All About Bleeding
  http://www.allaboutbleeding.com/
- Anemia from Excessive Bleeding
  http://www.merck.com/mmhe/sec14/ch172/ch172b.html
- Bleeding Disorder Websites
  http://www.hemophilia.org/resources/wwwresources.htm#hemovon
- Blood Line
  http://www.bloodline.net/
- Hemophilia
  http://www.hemophilia.org/bdi/bdi_history.htm
- International Society on Thrombosis and Haemostasis
  http://www.med.unc.edu/isth/
- National Hemophilia Foundation
  http://www.hemophilia.org/about/programs.htm
  http://www.hemophilia.org/about/quickguide_2005.pdf

HEMORRHAGE AND BLEEDING DISORDERS—CITED REFERENCES

Hathcock JN, et al. Vitamins E and C are safe across a broad range of intakes. *Am J Clin Nutr.* 81:736, 2005.

Steriti R. Nutritional support for chronic myelogenous and other leukemias: a review of the scientific literature. *Altern Med Rev.* 7:404, 2002.

POLYCYTHEMIA VERA

NUTRITIONAL ACUITY RANKING: LEVEL 1

DEFINITIONS AND BACKGROUND

Polycythemia vera (PV) is a chronic, progressive disease in which increased blood volume and increased erythrocyte production occurs. Other names include erythemia, Osler-Vasquez disease, and polycythemia rubra vera. Signs and symptoms may include belching, fullness, thirst, flatulence, constipation, headache, vertigo, lassitude, tinnitus, blurred vision, diplopia, dyspnea on exertion, chest pain, paresthesias, pruritus, dusky reddish skin on face and hands, thrombosis, gout, hemorrhagic tendency, hypertension, enlarged spleen, seizures, confusion, slurred speech, peptic ulcer, and heart failure.

Hematological disorders like PV can result in elevated levels of cobalamin, which is released during hepatic cytolysis; elevated levels of cobalamin can also be caused by decreased cobalamin clearance by the affected liver (Ermens et al, 2003). The cause of PV is unknown, and the disease is considered a hematological malignancy. The disease develops slowly and may progress to acute myelogenous leukemia. The average age at diagnosis is 50–60 years. Incidence is highest among those of Jewish ancestry, occurring in 2.3 of 100,000 of the population.

Increased viscosity of the blood and the increased number of platelets can result in a high potential for clot formation, which can cause stroke, hemorrhage, or myocardial infarction. Patients with PV frequently develop hyperhomocysteinemia due to discrete depletion of cobalamin or folate; vitamin therapy should be considered, even though hyperhomocysteinemia does not seem to be of crucial importance for the thrombotic tendency (Faurschou et al, 2000). With treatment, individuals with this condition may live 15–20 years. Phlebotomy or medications may be useful.

INTERVENTION: OBJECTIVES

- Prepare patient for phlebotomy by ensuring adequate nutrient stores.
- Prepare, as needed, for chemotherapy or radiation therapy, which may be provided.
- Correct or control condition.
- Manage any side effects such as heart failure, peptic ulcer disease, gastric bleeding, gout, leukemia, and seizures.

INTERVENTION: FOOD AND NUTRITION

- A diet of preferred foods and balanced meals should be offered. Monitor for the need for vitamin or mineral supplementation.
- Extra fluids will be helpful (e.g., 3–4 L/d, unless contraindicated, as with heart failure).
- Changes in dietary texture or content may be needed if radiation or chemotherapy alters nutrient or dietary needs.

CLINICAL INDICATORS

Clinical/History

- Height
- Weight
- BMI
- Diet history
- BP
- I & O
- Belching, fullness
- Constipation
- Headache
- Vertigo
- Lassitude
- Tinnitus
- Pruritus after bathing
- Transient blurred vision, diplopia
- Dyspnea
- Chest pain
- Dusky reddish skin on face and hands
- Hemorrhagic tendency
- BP (hypertension)
- Seizures, confusion
- Splenomegaly

Lab Work

- Hgb (elevated, >18 g/dL)
- Hct (elevated, >52% for men and >47% for women)
- Platelets (elevated)

Leukocytes (elevated)	Leukocyte Alk phos	Alb, transthyretin
Serum B_{12} (elevated)	Serum ferritin	CRP
Erythropoietin (low)	Gluc	Chol, Trig
TIBC	RBC (7–12 million)	BUN, Creat
Erythrocyte sedimentation rate (ESR)	Oxygen saturation >92%	Uric acid (elevated)
	CRP	Bone marrow biopsy

Common Drugs Used and Potential Side Effects

- Myelosuppressive agents may be prescribed. Anagrelide hydrochloride (Agrylin) is an oral imidazoquinazoline agent that has been shown to reduce elevated platelet counts and the risk of thrombosis (Pescatore and Lindley, 2000). Interferon-alpha may be used in younger patients.
- The antimetabolite hydroxyurea may be used. Side effects include anemia and skin ulcers.
- Chemotherapeutic agents (busulfan, chlorambucil, and cyclophosphamide) may be used. Nausea and vomiting are common side effects. Weight loss can occur.
- Antihistamines can help reduce itching sensation.
- Low-dose aspirin is sometimes used in patients with thrombotic or ischemic conditions. It can relieve some of the burning sensations in the feet and hands.
- Other medications may be necessary based on complications.

Herbs, Botanicals, and Supplements

- Herbs and botanical supplements should not be used without discussing with physician.

INTERVENTION: NUTRITION EDUCATION, COUNSELING, CARE MANAGEMENT

- Discuss need to maintain a healthy lifestyle and to eat adequate protein and calories because of the frequent phlebotomies (where completed).
- Discuss ways to make meals that are nutritious yet simple to prepare.
- Oatmeal baths may help reduce pruritus (Stuart and Viera, 2004).

For More Information

- Merck Manual–Blood Disorders
  http://www.merck.com/mmhe/sec14.html
- Myeloproliferative Disorders
  http://www.acor.org/diseases/hematology/MPD/

POLYCYTHEMIA VERA—CITED REFERENCES

Ermens AA, et al. Significance of elevated cobalamin (vitamin B12) levels in blood. *Clin Biochem.* 36:585, 2003.

Faurschou M, et al. High prevalence of hyperhomocysteinemia due to marginal deficiency of cobalamin or folate in chronic myeloproliferative disorders. *Am J Hematol.* 65:136, 2000.

Pescatore SL, Lindley C. Anagrelide: a novel agent for the treatment of myeloproliferative disorders. *Expert Opin Pharmacother.* 1:537, 2000.

Stuart BJ, Viera AJ. Polycythemia vera. *Am Fam Physician.* 69:2146, 2004.

THROMBOCYTOPENIA

NUTRITIONAL ACUITY RANKING: LEVEL 1

DEFINITIONS AND BACKGROUND

Thrombocytopenia is the most common cause of bleeding. Bleeding is usually from small capillaries. Thrombocytopenia purpura, a myeloproliferative disorder, is a blood disease affecting the clotting factor (platelets) of the blood, with an abnormally low platelet count and shorter than normal (10 days) platelet survival time.

There are many reasons for the development of decreased marrow production or platelet destruction that causes thrombocytopenia, including some hereditary causes. These can sometimes be determined by examination of bone marrow. Idiopathic thrombocytopenic purpura (ITP) is caused by platelet destruction by antibodies. Thrombotic thrombocytopenic purpura (TTP) is a manifested by vascular lesions.

Headache, slurred speech, numbness and weakness of extremities, and increased temperature occur. Tendency to bleed excessively into the skin or mucous membranes (as from the nose), especially during menstruation, also occurs. In this illness, only after splenectomy is a complete remission obtained, which is defined as a normal platelet count and lifespan and sufficient platelet production (Louwes et al, 2001). Laparoscopic splenectomy (LS) patients have less postoperative pain, earlier general diet tolerance, and shorter hospital stay at no significant additional cost as compared with open splenectomy patients (Cordera et al, 2003).

INTERVENTION: OBJECTIVES

- Avoid infections, especially upper respiratory infections and flu to prevent coughing, which increases intracranial pressure.
- Rest frequently.

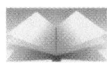

- Prepare patient for splenectomy, if indicated. Ensure adequate nutrient stores.
- Reduce bleeding tendency and complications, such as intracranial hemorrhage.

INTERVENTION: FOOD AND NUTRITION

- Maintain diet of preference or as ordered. Use small, frequent feedings if patient has nausea or vomiting.
- Adequate folic acid will be needed.
- Increase fluids (e.g., 3 L/d) unless contraindicated.
- After splenectomy, patient will need adequate protein, energy, zinc, and vitamins A and C for wound healing. Vitamin K from the diet and supplements may need to be monitored.

CLINICAL INDICATORS

Clinical/History		
Height	Bruising	RBP
Weight	Pinpoint red spots on skin	N balance
BMI	I & O	PT (normal)
Diet history	**Lab Work**	Casts in urine
BP	CBC (low platelets)	Proteinuria
Nosebleeds	Alb, transthyretin	CRP
Bleeding from other sites		H & H (decreased)
		Ca++
		Na+, K+

Common Drugs Used and Potential Side Effects

- Corticosteroids such as prednisone may be used to control bleeding. Side effects are numerous and may affect nutritional status (e.g., decreased serum calcium, potassium, and nitrogen; increased serum sodium; and glucose intolerance may occur).
- Myelosuppressive agents are often prescribed. Anagrelide hydrochloride (Agrylin) is an oral imidazoquinazoline agent that has been shown to reduce elevated platelet counts and the risk of thrombosis (Pescatore and Lindley, 2000). Interferon-alpha may be used.
- Recombinant human thrombopoietin (rhTPO) increases platelets, and the peak response of rhTPO is not uniformly effective when administered after chemotherapy; two doses of rhTPO (one before and one after chemotherapy) are required to significantly reduce the severity of chemotherapy-related thrombocytopenia (Vadhan-Raj et al, 2003).
- Most drugs are stopped because nearly any drug may aggravate the condition.
- Rituximab seems to be a promising drug in the treatment of refractory autoimmune thrombocytopenia even in patients with underlying lymphoproliferative disorders (Hensel and Ho, 2003).

Herbs, Botanicals, and Supplements

- Herbs and botanical supplements should not be used without discussing with physician.

INTERVENTION: NUTRITION EDUCATION, COUNSELING, CARE MANAGEMENT

- Discuss altering nutrients as needed, depending on medications ordered and their use over time; surgery, if required; and ability to eat adequately.

For More Information

- The ITP Society of the Children's Blood Foundation
http://www.childrensbloodfoundation.org/
- Platelet Disorder Support Foundation
http://www.itppeople.com/

THROMBOCYTOPENIA—CITED REFERENCES

Cordera F, et al. Open versus laparoscopic splenectomy for idiopathic thrombocytopenic purpura: clinical and economic analysis. *Surgery* 134:45, 2003.

Hensel M, Ho AD. Successful treatment of a patient with hairy cell leukemia and pentostatin-induced autoimmune thrombocytopenia with rituximab. *Am J Hematol.* 73:37, 2003.

Louwes H, et al. Effects of prednisone and splenectomy in patients with idiopathic thrombocytopenic purpura: only splenectomy induces a complete remission. *Ann Hematol.* 80:728, 2001.

Vadhan-Raj S, et al. Importance of predosing of recombinant human thrombopoietin to reduce chemotherapy-induced early thrombocytopenia. *J Clin Oncol.* 21:1358, 2003.

S E C T I O N 13

Cancer

CHIEF ASSESSMENT FACTORS

American Cancer Society's Seven Warning Signs of Cancer

- Change in Bowel/Bladder Habits
- Sore That Does Not Heal
- Unusual Bleeding or Discharge
- Thickening or Lump in Breast or Elsewhere
- Indigestion or Dysphagia
- Obvious Change in Wart or Mole
- Nagging Cough or Hoarseness

Other Factors:

- History of Tobacco Use, Excessive Alcohol Use, Carcinogen Exposure
- Weight Changes—Unintended Weight Loss or BMI Less Than 22
- Changes in Food Intake
- Fever of Unknown Origin (May Relate to Hematological, Liver, Pancreatic, Brain, or Kidney Cancers)
- Anorexia or Nausea
- Vomiting
- Dysphagia, Mucositis, or Esophagitis, Mouth Sores
- Dry Mouth
- Problems with Nauseating Odors
- Pain
- Changes in Usual Functional Capacity or Energy Levels
- Muscle Wasting
- Depression
- Edema or Ascites
- Diarrhea
- Side Effects of Medications
- Participation in Complementary and Alternative Medicine Treatments

Table 13-1 provides a list of cancer definitions, and Figure 13-1 shows types of cancers.

TABLE 13-1 Cancer Definitions

Term	Definition	Term	Definition
Adenocarcinoma	Cancer that starts in the glands.	Hormonal therapy	Treatment or prevention of cancer by removing, blocking, or adding hormones that affect the growth of a tumor.
Adenoma	Benign growth that may or may not transform to cancer.	Leukemia	Leukemia is cancer in the blood where bone marrow–produced abnormal white blood cells crowd out normal white blood cells, red blood cells, and platelets.
Basal cell carcinoma	Most common form of skin cancer, affecting 800,000 Americans each year. Chronic exposure to sunlight is the cause of almost all basal cell carcinomas, which occur most frequently on exposed parts (e.g., face, ears, neck, scalp, shoulders, and back).	Lymphoma	Lymphoma can include: AIDS-related lymphoma; cutaneous T-cell lymphoma; Hodgkin's lymphoma in adults, children, and during pregnancy; mycosis fungoides; non-Hodgkin's lymphoma (adult, childhood, and during pregnancy); primary central nervous system lymphoma; Sézary's syndrome; cutaneous T-cell lymphoma; and Waldenstrom's macroglobulinemia.
Biotherapy	Treatment to stimulate or restore the ability of the immune system to fight infection and disease and to lessen side effects that may be caused by some cancer treatments. It is also known as immunotherapy, biological therapy, or biological response modifier (BRM) therapy.	Male reproductive cancers	Penile and testicular cancers are diseases in which cancer (malignant) cells are found in the penis or testes. Prostate cancer is diagnosed when cancer (malignant) cells are found in the tissues of the prostate gland.
Cancer	Abnormal, uncontrolled growth of cells in a lump or mass that also destroys normal tissue. Oncogenes in a tumor cell may be identifying markers.	Meningiomas	Tumors affecting the meninges.
Carcinoma	A form of cancer involving epithelial tissue and coverings of internal and external surfaces. Lungs, colon, breast, stomach, uterus, skin, and tongue cancers are included in this group, which compose 80–90% of all cancers.	Mesothelioma	Mesothelioma is a rare type of cancer affecting the lining of the chest, heart, and abdominal cavity; exposure to asbestos is the usual cause.
Endocrine system cancers	Several types of cancers of the endocrine system exist: adrenocortical carcinoma; gastrointestinal carcinoid tumor; islet cell carcinoma (arising in the islet cells of the pancreas, a so-called "endocrine pancreatic cancer"); parathyroid cancer; pheochromocytoma; pituitary tumor; and thyroid cancer.	Metastasis	A transfer of disease from one organ to another that is not directly connected to it; especially the spread of carcinoma.
		Neuroma	A neuroma, a tumor composed of nerve cells, may occur along any nerve.
Epithelioma	Carcinoma consisting of many epithelial cells.	Oat cell carcinoma	A rapidly spreading, highly fatal cancer of the bronchus.
		Oncology	Scientific study of tumors.
Gastrointestinal (GI) cancers	GI cancers include: anal cancer; bile duct cancer; GI carcinoid tumor; colon cancer; esophageal cancer; gallbladder cancer; liver cancers; pancreatic cancer; rectal cancer; small intestine cancer; and stomach (gastric) cancer.	Osteosarcoma	The most common type of bone cancer, which develops in new tissue in growing bones, affecting young people and more often males than females.
		Sarcoma	Cancer arising from bone or connective tissue, which sometimes spreads into blood or lymphatic tissues.
Gynecological cancer	This is a group of diseases in which malignant cells form in the tissues of the specific organ in the female reproductive system and includes: cervical cancer; endometrial cancer; gestational trophoblastic tumor; ovarian epithelial cancer; ovarian germ cell tumor; ovarian low malignant potential tumor; sarcoma; vaginal cancer; and vulvar cancer.	Small cell carcinoma	A carcinoma that most commonly arises in the lung but can occur as a cancer in other body sites including the prostate, cervix, and head and neck; almost always responsive to chemotherapy and radiation therapy.

See also the following websites for more information: http://www.cancer.gov/dictionary/ and http://www.lillyoncology.com/; for types of cancers, see http://www.cancer.gov/cancertopics/alphalist/a-d.

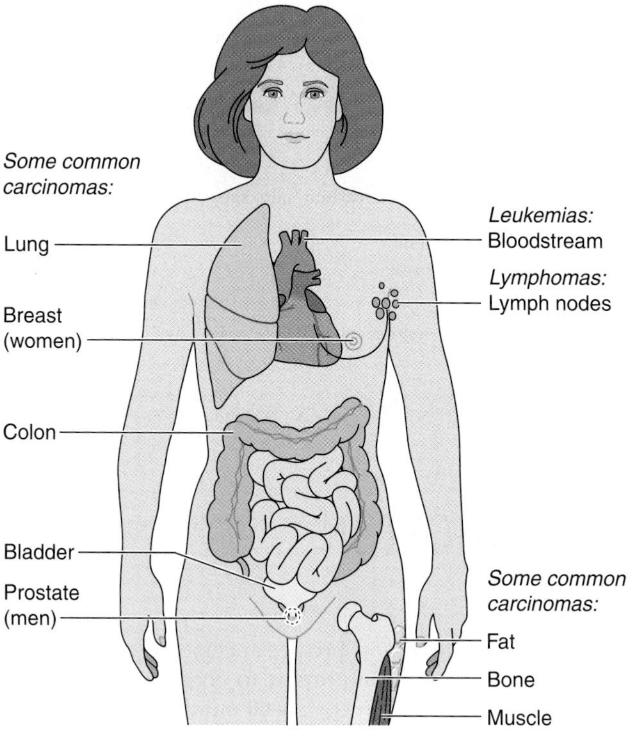

Figure 13-1 Types of cancer.

For More General Information on Cancer

- AMC Cancer Research Center and Foundation
  http://www.amc.org/
- American Cancer Society
  http://www.cancer.org/
- American Dietetic Association
  http://eatright.org/
- American Dietetic Association Oncology Nutrition Dietetic Practice Group
  http://www.oncologynutrition.org/
- American Institute for Cancer Research (AICR)
  http://www.aicr.org/
  Hotline: http://www.aicr.org/site/PageServer?pagename=dc_nh_home
- Cancer Care
  http://www.cancercare.org/
- Cancer Health Centers online
  http://cancer.healthcentersonline.com/conditionsdiseasescenter.cfm
- Cancer Screening Guidelines
  http://www.aafp.org/afp/20010315/1101.html
- Chemical Carcinogens
  http://www.state.nj.us/health/eoh/odisweb/ca_hsfs.htm
- Clinical Practice Guidelines in Oncology
  http://www.nccn.org/professionals/physician_gls/recently_updated.asp
- Genetics 101
  http://www.ornl.gov/sci/techresources/Human_Genome/project/info.shtml
- Harvard–Dana-Farber Cancer Institute
  http://www.dfci.harvard.edu/
- Harvard Center for Risk Analysis
  http://www.hcra.harvard.edu/#
- Herbs in Cancer
  http://www.cancer.med.umich.edu/learn/pwherbs.htm
- Herbs, Vitamins, and Minerals
  http://www.cancer.org/docroot/ETO/ETO_5_2_5.asp?sitearea=ETO
- Hospice Net
  http://www.hospicenet.org/
- Human Carcinogens
  http://www.cancer.org/docroot/PED/ped_1_1.asp
- International Center for Research on Cancer
  http://ntp-server.niehs.nih.gov/index.cfm
- Journal of the National Cancer Institute
  http://jncicancerspectrum.oxfordjournals.org/
- Lance Armstrong Foundation
  http://www.laf.org
- National Cancer Institute
  http://www.nci.nih.gov/
- National Coalition for Cancer Survivorship
  http://www.canceradvocacy.org/
- National Institutes of Health Gene Testing
  http://www.genetests.org/
- National Toxicology Program
  http://ntp-server.niehs.nih.gov/index.cfm
- North American Cancer Registry
  http://www.naaccr.org/
- Oncology Association of Naturopathic Medicine
  http://www.oncanp.org
- Oncology Nursing Society
  http://www.ons.org/
- Online Human Genome Resources
  http://www.genome.gov/10000464
- Recipes
  http://www.cancer.med.umich.edu/learn/nutrrec.htm
- Vital Options
  http://www.vitaloptions.org/

For More Information on Cancer Prevention

- Cancer Prevention and Control
  http://www.cdc.gov/cancer/
- Cancer Research and Prevention
  http://www.preventcancer.org/
- Complementary Treatments
  http://nccam.nih.gov/health/bytreatment.htm
- National Cancer Institute
  http://www3.cancer.gov/prevention/lifestyle.html
- Patient Advocate Foundation
  http://www.patientadvocate.org
- Wellness Community
  http://www.thewellnesscommunity.org/

For More Information on Cancer Treatments

- Anemia and Fatigue Guidelines
  http://www.nccn.org/patients/patient_gls/_english/_fatigue/contents.asp
- Antioxidants and Chemoradiotherapy
  http://nccam.nih.gov

- Cancer Information Page
  http://www.cancerguide.org/stats_home.html
- Cancer Pain
  http://www.nccn.org/patients/patient_gls/_english/_pain/contents.asp
- Cancer Treatments
  http://www.cancer.org/docroot/MBC/MBC_6.asp
- Clinical Trials
  http://www.cancer.gov/clinical_trials/
- Medicine Online
  http://www.meds.com/
- Nausea and Vomiting Guidelines
  http://www.nccn.org/patients/patient_gls/_english/_nausea_and_vomiting/contents.asp
- OncoLink: University of Pennsylvania Cancer Center
  http://oncolink.upenn.edu/
- Supportive Treatments
  http://www.cancer.gov/cancerinfo/pdq/supportivecare/
- Texas Cancer Data Center
  http://www.txcancer.org/
- Treatment Decisions
  http://www.cancer.org/docroot/ETO/eto_1_1a.asp

Cancer Prevention

CANCER: PREVENTION AND RISK REDUCTION

Cancer results from dysregulated cell growth control and is caused by an interaction of dietary, genetic, and environmental risk factors (Williams and Hord, 2005). There are over 100 variations of cancer. Cancer was the second most common cause of death in the United States in 2002 (http://www.cdc.gov/nchs/fastats/deaths.htm) and will surpass coronary heart disease by the year 2010 (Samoha and Arber, 2005).

Cancer has a strong genetic component, resulting in multiple events associated with initiation, promotion, and metastatic growth, equivalent to the loss of cellular homeostasis (Seth and Watson, 2005). Natural carcinogens include ultraviolet (UV) radiation, dyes, environmental chemicals from smoke or mines, viruses, nitrosamines, aflatoxins, and safrole. The most consistent carcinogen is tobacco use.

The Human Genome Project has identified 30,000 human protein-coding genes. Individualized DNA methylation helps to control gene expression. Knowledge about human genetic variation is unprecedented; genotyping resources allow cancer prevention investigators to identify in a more precise way which genetic subsets of patients are likely to benefit most from chemoprevention and screening interventions (Velasquez and Lipkin, 2005). Remarkable advances in carbohydrate and glycopeptide assembly techniques have allowed for the development of synthetic clinically effective, carbohydrate-based antitumor vaccines (Ouerfelli et al, 2005). This emerging science is very promising.

Many cancers have a nutrition or dietary component; functional food components impact greatly on incidence and treatment of cancer (Riezzo et al, 2005). Activation of nuclear transcription factor-κB has been linked with inflammatory diseases and cancer; spices are protective (Aggarwal and Shishodia, 2004).

Dietary factors and physical inactivity may contribute to approximately one third of all cancers (Williams and Hord, 2005). Prospective epidemiological studies have provided strong evidence supporting regular physical activity and minimal adult weight gain to lower risk of colorectal and breast cancer (Williams and Hord, 2005). Excess body weight increases the risk of cancers such as acute myelogenous leukemia (AML) and kidney, endometrium, colon, prostate, gallbladder, and breast cancers (Bergstrom et al., 2001). It is, therefore, important to control weight, avoid obesity, and exercise daily for 30–60 minutes.

Nutritive and nonnutritive dietary constituents can either promote or hinder development of cancer, individualized by genetic predisposition. Very low–fat diets have been tested for breast and colorectal cancer prevention with no benefit, except in estrogen receptor–positive, progesterone receptor–negative women who consumed high-fat diets, according to the Women's Health Initiative Randomized Controlled Dietary Modification Trial (Buzdar, 2006; Prentice et al, 2006). Omega-3 fatty acids are not indicated for cancer prevention (MacLean et al, 2006).

The strongest evidence linking specific foods to decreased risk of certain cancers is related to the consumption of fruits and vegetables and whole grains (Williams and Hord, 2005). Antioxidants protect against free radical damage, improving resistance of cells to oxidative stress. Diets rich in phytochemicals can reduce the risk of cancer; carotenoids, antioxidative vitamins, phenolic compounds, terpenoids, steroids, indoles, and fibers are responsible for risk reduction (Nishino et al, 2005). People who eat the most fruits and vegetables have approximately one half the rate of cancer of other members of the same population (Van Duyn and Pivonka, 2000). A diet rich in fruits and vegetables may be useful in secondary rather than primary prevention of breast cancer (Buzdar, 2006).

The nutritional message should be widely communicated. Key nutrients, chemoprotective phytochemicals, and functional food ingredients are listed in Table 13-2. Table 13-3 provides a list of important dietary factors in specific types of cancer. A complete "anticancer" grocery list includes dark green, yellow, and orange fruits or vegetables, red grapes, cruciferous vegetables, orange juice, tomatoes, olive and canola oils, garlic, legumes, strong coffee, whole grains, soy, and other plant estrogens.

Overall, nine factors increase the likelihood of having cancer: smoking, alcohol use, low fruit and vegetable intake, overweight and obesity, unsafe sex, urban air pollution, physical inactivity, contaminated injections in health care settings, and indoor smoke from household use of solid fuels.

TABLE 13-2 Nutritional Synergy: Phytochemicals and Functional Food Ingredients

Phytochemicals are functional food ingredients that occur naturally in fruits and vegetables and whole grains, often to protect against micro-organisms and to serve as antioxidants. They are not "essential" nutrients. Some phytochemicals function as antioxidants to squelch free radicals. Diets rich in phytochemicals (carotenoids, antioxidative vitamins, phenolic compounds, terpenoids, steroids, indoles, and fibers) may reduce the risk of cancer and related chronic diseases (Nishino et al, 2005). Protection against DNA damage by plant food products can now be demonstrated (Collins, 2005). Functional foods contain ingredients that provide additional physiological benefits beyond basic nutrition (Riezzo et al, 2005). The current emphasis remains on food sources, not supplements or pills.

The concept of delaying or preventing epithelial transformation is a viable goal for the future; use of specific foods, diet manipulation strategies, and nutraceuticals may be appropriate to delay or prevent carcinogenesis progression in healthy populations with genetic or epidemiological risks (Brenner and Gescher, 2005). Caution in interpreting studies is needed because there is limited information on the bioavailability and biotransformation of flavonoids; more controlled clinical trials are needed (Graf et al, 2005). Insulin-like growth factor (IGF) system is related to proliferation and tumor growth and is a risk factor for several types of cancer; more research aimed at the effects of specific food components or dietary strategies on the IGF system is warranted (Voskuil et al, 2005).

When doctors do not have the time to give advice about diet and cancer prevention (Ganry and Boche, 2005), referral to a registered dietitian is recommended. Dietary modification has shown its greatest beneficial effect when started prior to or immediately after the onset of disease (Jolly, 2005). The Bridge to Better Health (BRIDGE) project focuses on providing rural high school youth with use of motivation, knowledge, and skills; significant improvements have been noted in self-efficacy, intention to practice self-examinations (breast, testicular, and skin), and consumption of a high-fiber diet (Harmon et al, 2005).

Phytochemical	Roles	Food Sources
Antioxidants and Specific Nutrients	Health benefits associated with diets rich in vegetables and fruit (VF) are often attributed to the antioxidant activity of their constituent phytochemical (Thompson HJ et al, 2005). Cabbage and sauerkraut consumption provides glucosinolate and yields a lower risk of breast cancer after consuming high amounts beginning in adolescence and throughout adulthood (Fowke et al, 2003).	Black or green tea induces a significant rise in plasma antioxidant activity (Leenan et al, 2000). Currants and raisins contain high levels of isoflavones, genistein, and daidzein and can be included easily in the diet (Liggins et al, 2000).
Calcium and vitamin D_3	Higher intakes of vitamin D and calcium from food and supplements are related to lower levels of breast density among premenopausal women; increasing intakes of these nutrients provides a safe and inexpensive strategy for breast cancer prevention (Berube et al, 2005; Chen et al, 2005). Vitamin D intake is often too low to sustain healthy circulating levels of 25-hydroxyvitamin D (Whiting and Calvo, 2005). Individuals may need 1500 IU to be more protective.	Dairy foods and vitamin D–fortified milk
Coenzyme Q10 (ubiquinone)	Some small studies have suggested that coenzyme Q10 may help treat cancer or reduce chemotherapy-related heart damage, but these results need to be confirmed by larger randomized clinical trials.	Coenzyme Q10 occurs naturally in the body and can also be found in mackerel, salmon, sardines, beef, soybeans, peanuts, and spinach.
Folate	Folic acid holds a key position in DNA synthesis and mitosis as well as DNA methylation and regulation of gene expression (Strohle, 2005). It decreases cancer cell multiplication; contributes to efficient DNA synthesis and repair; and regulates cellular *S*-adenosylmethionine levels and gene expression. Folate may protect against breast cancer, especially when women consume alcohol (Baglietto et al, 2005).	Leafy greens, orange juice
Glutathione and selenium	Selenium increases immune cell functioning, DNA methylation, and regulation of cytokine production. Intake of 50–200 μg is recommended, mostly for people who are deficient. Avoid levels over 400 μg because of hair loss and gastrointestinal (GI) distress. Selenium status has been inversely associated with colorectal cancers and a significantly reduced risk of prevalent adenomas but only among individuals with low baseline selenium levels and smokers (Reid et al, 2006). Onion and garlic extracts, with sulfur constituents, can induce phase II detoxification enzymes like glutathione-*S*-transferases and quinone reductase, as well as influence cell cycle arrest and apoptosis in numerous cancer cells (Reed et al, 2005). Multiple components of broccoli, such as selenium, may inhibit cancer (Finley et al, 2005). The SELECT trial is evaluating the effectiveness of selenium and vitamin E in reducing onset of prostate cancer (Thompson IM et al, 2005).	Brazil nuts, lean meats, seafood, and potatoes (glutathione) Onions, garlic Methionine and cysteine are precursors for glutathione (Shoveller et al, 2005).
Potassium	Role in cancer not clear.	Leafy greens, broccoli, bananas, oranges, grapefruit, lemons, pineapple, apricots

(continued)

TABLE 13-2 Nutritional Synergy: Phytochemicals and Functional Food Ingredients *(continued)*

Phytochemical	Roles	Food Sources
Vitamin A and retinoids	Clinical studies are now being done to explore the role of vitamin A and other retinoids in cancer prevention and treatment. High doses of vitamin A are toxic, and long-term use of high-dose supplements may increase the risk of lung cancer among people at high risk, such as smokers. Vitamin A supplements have been ineffective in preventing cancer. High doses of vitamin A supplements can cause nausea, vomiting, diarrhea, loss of appetite, tiredness, headaches, dizziness, blurred vision, muscular incoordination, itchiness and scaling of the skin, bone pain, hair loss, irregular menstruation in women, birth defects if taken during pregnancy, and temporary or permanent liver damage. Retinoids are signaling molecules that play important roles in cell growth, differentiation, and death; they have been used successfully to cure acute promyelocytic leukemia (APL) and can suppress carcinogenesis in skin, lung, breast, and oral cancers (Clarke et al, 2004). There may be a role in preventing promyelocytic leukemia.	Liver, fish oils, dairy products
Vitamin B_6 and B-complex	Vitamin B_6 supports healthy immunity and increases lymphocyte numbers (Kwak et al, 2002). A few population-based studies have also shown a possible link between intake of vitamin B_6 and lower risks of colorectal and breast cancers in women. Otherwise, there is no evidence that B vitamins are an effective treatment for people who already have cancer.	Legumes, whole grains, chicken, pork, fish, liver, potatoes, wheat germ, bananas
Vitamin C	Minimizes damage to neutrophils. DRI is 75 mg for women and 90 mg for men. Body becomes saturated at ~200 mg, and levels above that may be not be useful Evidence indicates that vitamin C supplements do not reduce cancer risk. Preventing cancer is due to a combination of many vitamins and other phytochemicals and not to vitamin C alone. High doses of vitamin C can cause a number of side effects. Factors that increase potential for oxidative stress, such as higher intake of heme iron or higher intake of vitamin C in the presence of high intake of iron, might actually increase the risk of lung cancer (Lee and Jacobs, 2005). Antioxidant: As a pro-oxidant, vitamin C induces apoptosis; inhibits histamine; supports immune system; and might decrease stomach, mouth, and esophageal cancer; there is conflicting evidence with breast cancer; mostly administered intravenously in cancer trials (Kogut and Luthringer, 2005).	**Bioflavonoids:** Oranges, grapefruit, lemons, tangerines, clementines, peaches, papaya, apricots, nectarines, pears, pineapple, yellow raisins, yellow pepper, broccoli **Other:** Cranberries, pink grapefruit, raspberries, strawberries, watermelon, red cabbage, red pepper, radishes, tomatoes **Anthocyanins:** Blueberries, blackberries, purple grapes, black currants, elderberries
Vitamin E	Increases antibody production and B- and T-cell functioning. Supplements of 600 IU of natural-source vitamin E taken every other day provide no overall benefit, and data do not support recommending vitamin E supplementation for cancer prevention among healthy women (Lee et al, 2005). For natural sources, such as d-alpha-tocopherol, 22 IU/d for basic needs is needed. Synthetic sources, such as dl-alpha-tocopherol, are less available, and 33 IU for basic needs is required. Avoid supplementation beyond a basic multivitamin supplement if taking statin drugs. Antioxidant: Most trials used a combination of other antioxidants; vitamin E is used topically on chemotherapy-induced skin ulcers and prevents recurrence of colorectal, prostate, breast, and gastric cancer (Kogut and Luthringer, 2005).	Wheat germ, whole grains, mayonnaise, creamy salad dressings, pistachios, almonds, peanuts, walnuts, cereals, meats, egg yolks
Vitamin K	No specific role known for cancer prevention.	Swiss chard, kale, Brussels sprouts, spinach, turnip greens, watercress, endive, lettuce, mustard greens, cabbage
Zinc	Zinc in normal amounts increases neutrophil function and killer cell numbers; decreases cytokines; and increases T- and B-cell numbers. It is being studied for its role in prevention of esophageal cancers. Zinc may play a role in protecting against lung cancer (Zhou et al, 2005). High dietary zinc may decrease the risk of lung cancer among postmenopausal women who consume high-dose vitamin C supplements (Lee and Jacobs, 2005). Unfortunately, high doses of zinc may promote prostate cancer (Chan et al, 2005).	Wheat germ, lean beef, seafood, black-eyed peas

(continued)

TABLE 13-2 Nutritional Synergy: Phytochemicals and Functional Food Ingredients *(continued)*

Phytochemical	Roles	Food Sources
Fatty Acids	The Mediterranean-type dietary pattern helps to decrease risk of cancer (Williams and Hord, 2005).	Legumes, nuts, and seeds are protective (Williams and Hord, 2005).
Polyunsaturated fats	The essential polyunsaturated fatty acids (PUFAs), linoleic acid omega-6 (LA) and alpha linolenic acid (ALA) omega-3, obtained from the diet are precursors of the long-chain PUFAs (LC-PUFAs) arachidonic acid (AA) and docosahexaenoic acid (DHA), respectively. Promote consumption of PUFAs; include higher intake of omega-3 fatty acids and fewer saturated fats or fried foods. The World Health Organization supports intake of omega-6 to omega-3 at a ratio of 5–10:1.	**Omega-6 fatty acids** (corn, soy, and safflower oils)
Omega-3 fatty acids (alpha linolenic acid [ALA], docosahexaenoic acid [DHA], and eicosapentaenoic acid [EPA]); conjugated linoleic acid (CLA)	Reduce inflammation; support mental and visual functioning. May help reduce cancer cachexia. ALA supports mental and visual functioning. DHA and EPA reduce the risk of coronary heart disease and support mental and visual functioning. CLA may help maintain immune function and normal body composition; some antitumor properties are suggested.	**Omega-3 fatty acids:** seafood, canola oil, walnuts, flaxseed **ALA:** English walnuts, flaxseed oil, kidney beans, great northern beans, soybeans **DHA and EPA:** Salmon, tuna, sardines, mackerel, marine and other fish oils **CLA:** Beef, lamb, some cheeses and yogurt
Monounsaturated fats	Monounsaturated fats decrease tumorigenesis. Anticancer effects of virgin olive oil phenols reduce colorectal carcinogenesis (Gill et al, 2005).	Canola and olive oils; tree nuts
Grains, Herbs, and Miscellany		
Capsaicin	Capsaicin (8-methyl-*N*-vanillyl-6-nonenamide) is a major ingredient in red peppers of the genus *Capsicum;* it contains carotenoids that may be protective against cancer (Perez-Galvez et al, 2003).	Red peppers, paprika
Coumarins	Coumarins belong to a diverse group known as benzo-alpha-pyrones (Leung et al, 2005). Anticoagulant; inhibit proteolysis and lipoxygenase; anti-inflammatory agent and antitumor effects.	Coumarins
Fiber and whole grains	Whole grains are protective against some cancers (Williams and Hord, 2005). Insoluble fiber maintains a healthy digestive tract, but there is not a clear protection against rectal cancers (Bingham et al, 2005).	Fiber and whole grains
Herbs and spices	Astragalus increases macrophages. Echinacea increases immunity (interferon, killer cells, interleukin-2) PC-SPES is an herbal mixture that has often been used by prostate cancer patients; *Rabdosia rubescens* is the most potent component, and it may potentially be used to treat or prevent breast cancer (Sartippour et al, 2005). Silymarin may protect the liver. Spices such as anise, fennel, coriander, curcumin, and garlic may be beneficial.	Ethnic cuisines vary with available content (Indian—cumin, cardamom, chili; Italian—basil, oregano, etc.). Herbal supplements are primary sources.
Inositol hexaphosphate (IP6)	IP6 is found as phytic acid in plants or as phospholipid in animals. It is converted into compounds in the body that are used by all cells to relay outside messages to the cell nucleus; it aids in the metabolism of calcium and other minerals.	Inositol is found in cereals, legumes, nuts, sesame seeds, and soybeans (Singh and Agarwal, 2005). It is also found in brown rice, corn, and wheat bran.
Oligosaccharides and protease inhibitors	These increase short-chain fatty acid formation; decrease cholesterol and lower insulin levels; and inhibit action of protein-splitting enzymes. They may prevent cancer cell formation or decrease tumor size (Slavin, 2003).	Whole grains
Phytates	Phytates can decrease oxidative damage to cells.	Whole grains, beans, seeds (soybeans, oats, barley, brown rice, whole wheat, flaxseed)
Prebiotics and probiotics	**Prebiotics:** Support GI health and improve calcium absorption. Inulin may help protect against colon cancer (Pool-Zobel, 2005). **Probiotics:** Normalize the intestinal microflora, block the invasion of potential pathogens in the gut, prevent colon cancer, modulate immune function, inhibit *Helicobacter pylori*, and enhance calcium absorption (Lin, 2003). They also synthesize niacin, folic acid, vitamin B_6, and biotin.	**Prebiotics:** Inulin, onions, garlic, leeks, fructooligosaccharides (FOS), polydextrose in whole grains, some fruits, honey, fortified foods, and beverages. **Probiotics:** *Lactobacilli*, *Bifidobacteria* in yogurt and other dairy products; fermented milk such as Kefir.

(continued)

TABLE 13-2 Nutritional Synergy: Phytochemicals and Functional Food Ingredients *(continued)*

Phytochemical	Roles	Food Sources
Polyphenols: Flavonoids	Polyphenols are the most abundant antioxidants in the diet and are widespread constituents of fruits, vegetables, cereals, dry legumes, chocolate, tea, coffee, and wine (Scalbert et al, 2005). Polyphenols provide neuroprotection in adult animal models of ischemia and Alzheimer's disease (Loren et al, 2005). More human studies are needed to evaluate the possible risks from too high a polyphenol intake (Scalbert et al, 2005).	
Anthocyanins and proanthocyanidins	Anthocyanins bolster cellular antioxidant defenses especially against ultraviolet radiation and may contribute to maintenance of brain function and motor function. They neutralize free radicals and have antimicrobial action and help to keep heart and urinary tract healthy. Anthocyanins are protective because of their polyphenols (Kim, 2005).	**Anthocyanins:** Berries (especially blueberry skins), cherries, red grapes, red cabbage, eggplant, red onion, kidney beans, red beans, beets, black currants, elderberries **Proanthocyanidins:** Cinnamon, cocoa, apples, strawberries, purple grapes and wines, peanuts, cranberries
Catechins: epigallocatechin gallate (EGCG); glycyrrhizin catechins	Catechins decrease growth of hydroquinone oxidase; decrease *COX-2* gene expression and cancer cell growth; and neutralize free radicals. Antioxidant properties may help with hepatitis C. Flavonoid content decreases ascorbate-dependent free radical oxidation and decreases inflammation, tumorigenesis, and malarial impact.	Green, oolong, and black teas, dark chocolate, red wines, licorice root. Tea and coffee contain catechins and flavonoids, whereas caffeine may elevate cancer risk (Baker et al, 2005).
Flavonols: quercetin, kaempferol, myricetin, rutin, apigenin	Flavonols neutralize free radicals and support antioxidant defense system; they preserve alpha-tocopherol and decrease liver inflammation; they decrease ATPase and protect plasma DNA from radiation damage. Flavonols reduce inflammation, which leads to many chronic diseases (Pattison et al, 2005). When consumed daily, a woman's risk of breast cancer decreases. Apigenin, a flavone subclass of flavonoid widely distributed in many herbs, fruits, and vegetables, possesses a variety of biological activities including tumor growth inhibition and chemoprevention (Jeyabal et al, 2005). It may protect against skin cancer and ultraviolet damage. Myricetin may protect against prostate cancer (Ganry, 2005).	Apples, black tea, grapefruit, onions Citrus fruits, cantaloupe, pomegranate, watermelon, whole grains, potato skins, wild leafy greens, celery stalks, lettuce, sweet peppers, spinach, green chili peppers, lemon, parsley Herbs, spices (ginger, mint, rosemary, garlic, ginger, thyme, oregano, sage, basil, coriander, cumin and turmeric, caraway, fennel, chili powder, black pepper) Tea, cocoa, chocolate, apples, grapes, onions, broccoli
Phenolic acids	Superoxide anion radical (SOR) has scavenging activity; protects against oxidation of low-density lipoprotein and protects vision; and protects against *Salmonella* and *Staphylococcus aureus* infections (especially ellagitannins in raspberries). 1. Ellagic acid, ferulic acid 2. Gallic acid: anticancer properties (Dedoussis et al, 2005) 3. Chlorogenic acid (Ito et al, 2005) 4. Tannic acid: inhibits proliferation of cancer cells (Adhami et al, 2005; Fujiki, 2005). 5. Punicalagin: potent antioxidant (Seeram et al, 2005). Pomegranate juice may be protective against prostate cancer (Malik et al, 2005).	Grapes, berries, cherries, apples, cantaloupe, green tea extract, watermelon, prunes, raisins, plums, eggplant 1. Tomatoes, citrus fruits, carrots, whole grains, nuts; grapes and wine; raspberries 2. Green and black grape juices 3. Cherry juice 4. Green and black teas; strong coffee 5. Pomegranate fruit and juice
Resveratrol and other stilbenes	Resveratrol is a phytoalexin produced in plants in response to exposure to ultraviolet light or fungi (Husken et al, 2005). It decreases platelet activity, lowers cholesterol, and has anticancer properties by suppressing proliferation of a variety of tumor cells. Lymphoid and myeloid cancers; multiple myeloma; cancers of the breast, prostate, stomach, colon, pancreas, and thyroid; melanoma; head and neck squamous cell carcinoma; ovarian carcinoma; and cervical carcinoma are reduced (Aggarwal et al, 2004).	Red grapes, wine, grape juice, peanuts
Polyphenols: Phytoestrogens	Phytoestrogens are natural plant substances with anticarcinogenic potential; they include isoflavones, coumestans, and lignans (Ganry, 2005). Phytoestrogens occur in plants as part of their own defense system. The daily dietary intake of phytoestrogens in healthy postmenopausal Caucasian women in the United States is <1 mg (de Kleijn et al, 2001).	
Coumestans	Coumestrol is a coumestan with a high level of estrogenic activity. Phytoestrogens may reduce risk for lung cancer (Schabath et al, 2005). The estimated daily intake of coumestans is 0.6 μg, with broccoli as the main source (de Kleijn et al, 2001).	Clover, alfalfa, soybeans, broccoli, peas, beans, and other vegetables

(continued)

TABLE 13-2 Nutritional Synergy: Phytochemicals and Functional Food Ingredients *(continued)*

Phytochemical	Roles	Food Sources
Isoflavones: genistein, daidzein, biochanin A	Phytoestrogens attach to estrogen receptors and block real estrogen. Use soy in moderation with breast cancer (Maskarinec, 2005; Fang et al, 2005). Red clover and soy extracts contain isoflavones, with high affinity to estrogen receptor-alpha (ERα), estrogen receptor-beta (ERβ), progesterone receptor (PR), and androgen receptor (AR); 40–50 mg of isoflavones (biochanin A, daidzein, formononetin, and genistein) is recommended as a daily dose (Beck et al, 2005). Soy isoflavones do not seem to protect against colorectal (Adams et al, 2005), prostate (Ganry, 2005), or breast cancer (Keinan-Boker et al, 2004).	Soybeans (tofu, vegetable soy milk, soy nuts); legumes such as chick peas, beans, peas; nuts; grain products, coffee, tea; raisins and currants
Lignans: matairesinol and secoisolariciresinol	Phytoestrogens attach to estrogen receptors and block real estrogen, lower cholesterol levels, and decrease cancer activity. Lignans may play a role in the prevention and treatment of prostate cancer over the lifetime of an individual (McCann et al, 2005). High intake of the lignans enterolactone and enterodiol and use of hormone therapy have been associated with a 50% reduction in risk of lung cancer (Schabath et al, 2005). The median total intake of lignans is 578 μg; a main source is fruits (de Kleijn et al, 2001).	Flaxseed, rye, whole grains, berries, carrots, spinach, broccoli, tea, asparagus, linseeds; alcoholic beverages (red and white wines).
Plant Sterols	Phytoestrogens and vegetables may protect against lung cancer (van Breda et al, 2005; Schabath et al, 2005).	
Sterols: beta-sitosterol, campesterol, stigmasterol, squalene	Can reduce risk of lung cancer and may reduce tumor growth of other cancers. Sterols are found in vegetable oils; sitosterol is the most studied.	Soy, peanuts, rice bran; vegetable oils
Stanols	Stanols reduce risk of coronary heart disease by lowering low-density lipoprotein cholesterol but have no consistent role in reduction of cancer (de Jong et al, 2003).	Corn, soy, wheat, wood oils, fortified foods and beverages; fortified table spreads, stanol ester supplements
Terpenes		
Carotenoids: alpha-carotene, beta-carotene, lutein, lycopene, zeaxanthin, chlorophyll	Natural carotenoids have been studied extensively and proven to show beneficial effects on human cancer prevention (Fahey et al, 2005; Nishino et al, 2005). Beware of excesses of supplements; they may act as pro-oxidants. Dietary fat is needed for proper absorption of carotenoids. Carotenoids increase activity of killer cells slightly; they serve as a photoprotective agent and neutralize free radicals, which damage cells; they function as antioxidants and contribute to healthy vision (protect against macular degeneration). Increased tomato (lycopene) consumption reduces risk for prostate cancer (Canene-Adams et al, 2005; Fraser et al, 2005).	Beta carotene: Carrots, sweet potatoes, pumpkin, butternut squash, cantaloupe, mangoes, apricots, peaches, papaya, watermelon Lutein and zeaxanthin: Turnip, collard, and mustard greens, kale, spinach, lettuce, broccoli, green peas, kiwi, honeydew melon, cilantro, parsley Solanaceous vegetables: Tomatoes, peppers
Ginseng	Ginseng is a triterpene glycoside with radioprotective capability. This is attributed to the ginsenosides, which are saponins with antioxidant properties (Lee et al, 2005). Ginseng may increase lymphocyte production. Ginseng stimulates natural killer cells and other immune activity; inhibits cancer cell growth in stomach, lung, liver, ovarian, and skin cancers; and is an antioxidant (Kogut and Luthringer, 2005).	Not generally available from foods but often added to supplements
Ginkgo biloba (ginkgolide A and B)	Ginkgo biloba, taken for 6 months or longer, may lower the risk of ovarian cancer; ginkgo and ginkgolides are involved in anti-inflammation processes.	Supplements are the usual way in which ginkgo is acquired.
Limonoids (limonene)	Citrus glycosides decrease bacterial and fungal growth and decrease cancer cell growth by detoxifying enzymes in liver. They also cause cell apoptosis with certain types of cancers (Poulouse et al, 2005). Cancer-preventive effects of citrus fruits demonstrated in epidemiological studies may be due in part to stimulation of DNA repair by naringenin (Gao et al, 2006).	Citrus fruit oils (orange, grapefruit, lemon); cherries; citrus fruit peel
Saponins (oleanic acid, hedagenin)	Saponins are triterpene glycosides that decrease heart disease and cancer risks; neutralize enzymes in the intestine that may cause cancer; and boost immunity. With breast cancer risk or in survivors, the current recommendation is to consume only moderate amounts of soy as part of a healthy plant-based diet (Maskarinec, 2005).	Beans and legumes, soybeans, whole grains, alfalfa, lentils, bean sprouts

(continued)

TABLE 13-2 Nutritional Synergy: Phytochemicals and Functional Food Ingredients *(continued)*

Phytochemical	Roles	Food Sources
Thiols		
Allium and allicin (allyl sulfides, *S*-allylcysteine [SAC])	Organosulfurs decrease tumor cell growth; inhibit kinase activity; support healthy hearts as a vasodilator; and may protect the immune system, assist the liver in rendering carcinogens harmless, and reduce cholesterol production in the liver. Diallyl sulfide (DAS) inhibits the effects of PhIP that, when biologically active, can cause DNA damage or transform substances in the body into carcinogens, as when meat or eggs are cooked at high temperatures (Thomas et al, 2004). This seems to be protective against stomach cancer.	Onions, garlic (especially oil), leeks, chives, scallions, shallots
Indoles/glucosinolates and isothiocyanate/ thiocyanates (sulforaphane)	Indoles are antimutagenics that may enhance detoxification of undesirable compounds and may contribute to a healthy immune system and downregulate estrogen and tumor formation. Bioactive isothiocyanates (ITCs) protect the body from cancer by inducing detoxification enzymes such as quinone reductase (Hwang and Jeffery, 2005). They increase periods of cancer latency and are effective agents against fungi such as *Aspergillus*. Bioactive glucosinolates and phenolic acids are two of the most abundant and important in broccoli (Robbins et al, 2005). The bioactive ITC sulforaphane (SF) is the hydrolysis product of glucoraphanin, the predominant aliphatic glucosinolate in broccoli (Hwang and Jeffery, 2005; Finley et al, 2005). Sulphorophane may be protective against stomach and skin cancers (Fahey et al, 2005). Cabbage and sauerkraut consumption provides glucosinolate and yields a lower risk of breast cancer after consuming high amounts, beginning in adolescence and throughout adulthood (Fowke et al, 2003).	Cruciferous vegetables: Broccoli, cabbage, Brussels sprouts, bok choy, arugula, Swiss chard, turnips, rutabaga, watercress, cauliflower, kale, kohlrabi
Jasmonates	Jasmonates are plant signaling compounds; they activate the coordinated gene expression of factors involved in ascorbate and glutathione metabolic pathways and are important in defense responses to oxidative stress and biosynthesis of indole glucosinolate, a defense compound in the *Brassica* family (Sasaki-Sekimoto et al, 2005).	Cruciferous vegetables: Broccoli, cauliflower, cabbage, watercress, Brussels sprouts, kale, turnips, bok choy, kohlrabi, Chinese cabbages, sauerkraut

TABLE 13-3 Dietary Factors and Cancer Risk by Organ Site

Dietary changes may prevent up to 30–40% of cancers worldwide (American Institute of Cancer Research, 2005). Chemopreventive agents include selective estrogen receptor modulators (SERMS) such as tamoxifen, nonsteroidal anti-inflammatory drugs (NSAIDs), calcium compounds, glucocorticoids, and retinoids. Note that fruits and vegetables consistently show a protective effect against cancer when they include the entire "biological action package" (Meyskens and Szabo, 2005). One nutrient, or dietary ingredient, may enhance or cancel out the beneficial effects of another dietary ingredient (Jolly, 2005). For example, vitamin E derivatives that possess no antioxidant activity may be potent inhibitors of some but not all types of cancer (Jolly, 2005). In addition, the combination of foods that include garlic and tomatoes will yield an even better chemopreventive effect because of the *S*-allylcysteine (SAC) and lycopene.

Organ Site	Protective Factors (Protectors)	Risk Factors (Promoters)
Gastrointestinal Tract Cancers		
Salivary gland cancer	Fiber intake (beans) Vitamin C	Smoking, excessive alcohol intake Exposure to ionizing radiation
Oral cancer (mouth and pharynx)	Beta-carotene and lycopene (Levi et al, 2000) Fish intake (Guneri et al, 2005) Fruits, salad, raw vegetables, and red wine (Guneri et al, 2005; American Institute for Cancer Research [AICR], 2005) Zinc (Fong et al, 2005)	Alcohol (AICR, 2005) Tobacco use: smoking cigarettes, cigars, or pipes; chewing smokeless tobacco or betel Periodontitis or poor oral hygiene (Tezal et al, 2005; Guneri et al, 2005)

(continued)

TABLE 13-3 Dietary Factors and Cancer Risk by Organ Site *(continued)*

Organ Site	Protective Factors (Protectors)	Risk Factors (Promoters)
Esophageal cancer	Green leafy vegetables and citrus fruits (vitamin C and beta-carotene) and lycopene Physical activity and weight maintenance Whole grains Zinc (Abnet et al, 2005)	Smoking cigarettes; use of smokeless tobacco; alcohol Use of untreated well water
Laryngeal cancer	Dark green and orange vegetables and beta-carotene Whole grains (Levi et al, 2000)	High use of alcohol; smoking
Stomach cancer	Allium and garlic (raw or lightly cooked) Carotenoids and lycopene (Ito et al, 2005; Yuan et al, 2004) Fish Fruits Nonherbal tea Polyunsaturated fat, vitamin A, and ascorbic acid are protective (Qiu et al, 2005) Refrigeration of food decreases possible risks (AICR, 2005) Vegetables: indoles (cruciferous vegetables) and sulforaphane (Fahey et al, 2002); onions are protective; leeks and garlic supplements are not. Vitamin C: protective, especially against *Helicobacter pylori* Yellow onions and shallots for quercetin	Smoking High intakes of protein, saturated fat, cholesterol, and sodium (Qiu et al, 2005) High alcohol intake Low use of whole grains Salted foods and high intake of salt (AICR, 2005)
Liver cancer	Chronic, long-term use of oral contraceptives Vegetables (carotenoids)	Aflatoxins (AICR, 2005) High consumption of alcohol (AICR, 2005) Infection with hepatitis B or C viruses, especially with obesity
Gallbladder or biliary tract cancer	Vegetables	Obesity Untreated chronic gallstones
Pancreatic cancer	Lycopene, vegetables, and fruits (Chan et al, 2005); onions, garlic, orange and yellow vegetables, spinach, broccoli, kale, and raw vegetables are especially protective. Beans or legumes (phytoestrogens) Citrus fruit Fiber	Smoking Obesity, inactivity, and insulin resistance
Colorectal cancer	Aspirin and other nonsteroidal anti-inflammatory drugs Calcium: traps bile acids and limits harm to colon; over 800 mg of calcium may reduce risk by as much as 26–46%; take a supplement if needed. Carotenoids, lutein, and lycopene: reduces cellular damage; eat more tomato products, watermelon, spinach, kale, greens, broccoli, romaine lettuce, pink grapefruit. Curcumin may be an effective deterrent. Fiber and starch (AICR, 2005): increases stool bulk (use cereals, beans, vegetables, and fruits); recommend 20–35 g/d. Not found to prevent polyp recurrence. Flavonoids: diet containing fruits and vegetables, especially apples, onions, proanthocyanidins (green tea), and flavones in chamomile tea (Hoensch and Kirch, 2005). Folate (folic acid): aids DNA repair (use more spinach, broccoli, asparagus, avocado, orange juice, dried beans, and fortified cereals). Fruit and vegetable intake, including indoles and cruciferous vegetables (broccoli, cabbage, cauliflower, and kale) (Emmons et al, 2005; AICR, 2005). Low-meat diet; plant-based diet (AICR, 2005) Methylpyridinium in coffee may prevent colon cancer. Multivitamin supplements: long-term use (Emmons et al, 2005)	Alcohol, smoking, and physical inactivity (Emmons et al, 2005; AICR, 2005) B vitamin deficiency, insulin resistance, and colonic inflammation (Bruce et al, 2005) Excess calories and saturated fats; obesity; and frequent eating (elevated insulin and exposure to carcinogenic bile acids) Family history of colon cancer Nonsteroidal anti-inflammatory drugs Red meat consumption (Emmons et al, 2005; AICR, 2005) Refined carbohydrates: may trigger overproduction of insulin Soy: supplements of soy protein may cause proliferation of colon cancer cells (Adams et al, 2005). Heterocyclic aromatic amines (HAAs) formed in meat during high-temperature cooking: pan-fried fish, pork, and chicken; deep-fried chicken and fish, roasted/barbecued pork, and grilled minced beef (Wong et al, 2005)

(continued)

TABLE 13-3 Dietary Factors and Cancer Risk by Organ Site *(continued)*

Organ Site	Protective Factors (Protectors)	Risk Factors (Promoters)
	Omega-3 fatty acids: low-dose celecoxib with an omega-3 polyunsaturated fatty acid–rich diet is protective (Reddy et al, 2005). Physical activity: speeds intestinal time and reduces obesity (AICR, 2005) Plant-based diets: use more poultry, fish, tofu, and beans as primary protein sources. Removal of polyps (early) Selenium in high levels can reduce colorectal polyps. Statins were thought to be protective (Poynter et al, 2005), but a recent study questions this fact (Dale et al, 2006). Unsaturated fats: to slow growth of colon cancer cells. Eat more flaxseed, salmon and fatty fish, and olive or canola oil. Vitamin B_6 has a crucial role in DNA synthesis and DNA methylation; deficiency is implicated in colorectal carcinogenesis, particularly among women who drink alcohol (Larsson et al, 2005). Vitamin D: promotes calcium absorption; use at least 400 IU/d. Vitamin D deficiency can promote colon cancer growth (Spina et al, 2005; Kallay et al, 2005).	A high-fat diet containing mixed lipids promotes colorectal cancer (Reddy et al, 2005).
Reproductive System Cancers		
Breast cancer	Alcohol avoidance (AICR, 2005) Breastfeeding >2 years reduces risk by half (Zheng, 2001). Bromelain, curcumin Calcium and vitamin D (Berube et al, 2005) Carotenoids: alpha- and beta-carotene, zeaxanthin, lycopene, and vegetables Exercise can lower estrogen levels. Fiber: eating beans or lentils at least 2 times weekly may reduce the risk; fiber slows insulin response Folate aids DNA repair; multivitamin with 400–600 μg folic acid is effective, especially in women who consume alcohol (Baglietto et al, 2005). Fruits and vegetables and a plant-based diet (AICR, 2005). Garlic may be protective. Lower fat: Women's Intervention Nutrition Study found that a diet with 20% of energy from fat helps reduce risk in women whose diets are high in fat (>75 g/d). Monounsaturated fatty acids are good because they increase cancer cell apoptosis. Combinations of calorie restriction and omega-3 fatty acids may be a more potent anti-inflammatory diet for breast cancer reduction (Jolly, 2005). Red wine and resveratrol Soy and soy products in moderation (Fang et al, 2005; Maskarinec, 2005) Tamoxifen prophylaxis (Fisher et al, 2005) Vitamins A and C Vitamin E as alpha-tocopherol	Age (older is higher risk) Alcohol (AICR, 2005) Estrogen exposure: early onset of menses, late menopause Family genetics: *BRCA1* or *BRCA2* gene HAAs formed in meat during high-temperature cooking: pan-fried fish, pork, and chicken; deep-fried chicken and fish, roasted/barbecued pork, and grilled minced beef (Wong et al, 2005) Late age for delivery of first full-term infant Low exercise Obesity and excessive energy intake, which stimulates estrogen production, especially after menopause (AICR, 2005) Rapid early growth and early menarche (AICR, 2005) Refined carbohydrates (heightened insulin response)
Cervical cancer	Carotenoids and lycopene Chronic, long-term use of oral contraceptives Folate Fruit and vegetable intake Vitamin C Vitamin E	Smoking Low folate intake (implicated with human papilloma virus)

(continued)

TABLE 13-3 Dietary Factors and Cancer Risk by Organ Site *(continued)*

Organ Site	Protective Factors (Protectors)	Risk Factors (Promoters)
Endometrial cancer	Fiber	Obesity
	Fruits, vegetables: lycopene and carotenoids	Estrogen exposure
	Physical activity and walking	
Ovarian cancer	Early pregnancy	Chronic, long-term use of oral contraceptives
	High intake of green leafy vegetables	Nulliparity
	Lutein, beta-carotene	Frequent reporting of increased bloating, abdominal size, urgency to urinate, and pelvic pain may be indicative of onset.
	Oral contraceptive use	
	Menopause	
	Vitamin E	
Prostate cancer	Cruciferous vegetables (Joseph et al, 2004)	Obesity, lack of exercise
	Curcumin may be an effective deterrent.	High total and saturated fat intake
	Exercise: Men 65 and older who exercise vigorously 3 or more hours a week reduce the rate of advanced prostate cancer. Exercise 30–60 minutes most days of the week.	Red meats
	Grape seed extract	
	Green tea (beverage or tablets)	
	Herbs (Shenouda et al, 2004)	
	Lutein	
	Lycopene (tomato-based products such as salsa)	
	Lignans (McCann et al, 2005)	
	Omega-3 fatty acids (fish such as tuna and salmon, flaxseed, walnuts)	
	Red wine and resveratrol	
	Selenium and vitamin E: under study	
	Soy genistein (soy nuts, soy burgers, soy milk) (McCann et al, 2005)	
	Toremifene prophylaxis	
	Vegan, low-fat diet with vitamin D supplementation (Dunn-Emke et al, 2005)	
	Vitamin-mineral supplements (up to 400 IU vitamin E, 200 μg selenium, extra vitamin D)	
Other Cancers		
Bone cancer	Use of bisphosphonates (Clines and Guise, 2005)	Hypercalcemia
Brain cancer	Fish and poultry	Exposure to formaldehyde
	Fruit	
	Vegetables (Chinese cabbage and onion especially)	
Leukemia	Flavonoids in red wine and resveratrol; coffee and tea; fruits and vegetables	Exposure to formaldehyde or asbestos
	Isoflavones such as genistein in soy foods	
Lung cancer	Curcumin	Smoking
	Fruits, vegetables	Exposure to asbestos or radon
	Gamma-tocopherol may be protective whereas alpha-tocopherol is not. Eat more sesame seeds and pecans.	Exposure to frying oils at high temperatures
	Quercetin and other flavonoids, selenium, lycopene, and carotenoids (Michaud et al, 2002).	Higher body mass index (BMI) (Rauscher et al, 2000); low physical activity
	Natural estrogens: isoflavones, lignans, coumestans, and phytosterols	
	Vitamins E and C	
Lymphomas	Healthy immune system	Exposure to viruses and bacteria?
	Herbs such as *Coriolus versicolor* (yunzhi) may contain protective ingredients (Lau et al, 2004).	

(continued)

TABLE 13-3 Dietary Factors and Cancer Risk by Organ Site *(continued)*

Organ Site	Protective Factors (Protectors)	Risk Factors (Promoters)
Melanoma, skin cancers: basal cell cancer (BCC) and squamous cell cancer (SCC)	Retinol (McNaughton et al, 2005) Green and black tea and other flavonols (McNaughton et al, 2005) Omega-3 fatty acids Red wine and resveratrol Soy proteins (isoflavones) Vitamin B_6	Excessive sun exposure High fat intake (McNaughton et al, 2005)
Non-Hodgkin's lymphoma (NHL)	Drinking alcohol may lower risk Dietary fiber Polyunsaturated fatty acids Some fruits and vegetables	High protein/meat intake and a high intake of saturated fat from animal sources Untreated celiac disease with gluten exposure
Renal cancer	Plant-based diets; high vegetable intake Selenium	Exposure to asbestos and tobacco smoke High-protein, high–animal fat diet? Obesity (Chow et al, 2000)
Urinary tract or bladder cancer	Fruits, vegetables Nonherbal tea drinking Retinol, vitamin C, and multivitamin use (Kamat and Lamm, 2002)	Smoking
Thyroid cancer	Fruit and vegetable intake	High iodine exposure

CANCER: PREVENTION AND RISK REDUCTION—CITED REFERENCES

Abnet CC, et al. Zinc concentration in esophageal biopsy specimens measured by x-ray fluorescence and esophageal cancer risk. *J Natl Cancer Inst.* 97:301, 2005.

Adams KF, et al. Soy protein containing isoflavones does not decrease colorectal epithelial cell proliferation in a randomized controlled trial. *Am J Clin Nutr.* 82:620, 2005.

Adhami VM, et al. Molecular targets for green tea in prostate cancer prevention. *J Nutr.* 133:2417S, 2003.

Aggarwal BB, Shishodia S. Suppression of the nuclear factor-kappaB activation pathway by spice-derived phytochemicals: reasoning for seasoning. *Ann N Y Acad Sci.* 1030:434, 2004.

Aggarwal BB, et al. Role of resveratrol in prevention and therapy of cancer: preclinical and clinical studies. *Anticancer Res.* 24:2783, 2004.

American Institute of Cancer Research. Accessed November 10, 2005 at http://www.aicr.org/

Baglietto L, et al. Does dietary folate intake modify effect of alcohol consumption on breast cancer risk? Prospective cohort study. *Br Med J.* 331:807, 2005.

Baker JA, et al. Associations between black tea and coffee consumption and risk of lung cancer among current and former smokers. *Nutr Cancer.* 52:15, 2005.

Beck V, et al. Phytoestrogens derived from red clover: an alternative to estrogen replacement therapy? *J Steroid Biochem Mol Biol.* 94:499, 2005.

Bergstrom A, et al. Overweight as an avoidable cause of cancer in Europe. *Int J Cancer.* 91:421, 2001.

Berube S, et al. Vitamin D and calcium intakes from food or supplements and mammographic breast density. Vitamin D and calcium intakes from food or supplements and mammographic breast density. *Cancer Epidemiol Biomarkers Prev.* 14:1653, 2005.

Bingham SA, et al. Is the association with fiber from foods in colorectal cancer confounded by folate intake? *Cancer Epidemiol Biomarkers Prev.* 14:1552, 2005.

Brenner DE, Gescher AJ. Cancer chemoprevention: lessons learned and future directions. *Br J Cancer.* 93:735, 2005.

Bruce WR, et al. A pilot randomised controlled trial to reduce colorectal cancer risk markers associated with B-vitamin deficiency, insulin resistance and colonic inflammation. *Br J Cancer.* 93:639, 2005.

Buzdar AU. Dietary modification and risk of breast cancer. *JAMA.* 295:691, 2006.

Canene-Adams K, et al. The tomato as a functional food. *J Nutr.* 135:1226, 2005.

Chan JM, et al. Role of diet in prostate cancer development and progression. *J Clin Oncol.* 23:8152, 2005.

Chan JM, et al. Vegetable and fruit intake and pancreatic cancer in a population-based case-control study in the San Francisco bay area. *Cancer Epidemiol Biomarkers Prev.* 14:2093, 2005.

Chen WY, et al. Associations between polymorphisms in the vitamin D receptor and breast cancer risk. *Cancer Epidemiol Biomarkers Prev.* 14:2335, 2005.

Chow W, et al. Obesity, hypertension, and the risk of kidney cancer in men. *N Engl J Med.* 343:1305, 2000.

Clarke N, et al. Retinoids: potential in cancer prevention and therapy. *Expert Rev Mol Med.* 6:1, 2004.

Clines GA, Guise TA. Hypercalcaemia of malignancy and basic research on mechanisms responsible for osteolytic and osteoblastic metastasis to bone. *Endocr Relat Cancer.* 12:549, 2005.

Collins AR. Antioxidant intervention as a route to cancer prevention. *Eur J Cancer.* 41:1923, 2005.

Dale KM, et al. Statins and cancer risk: a meta-analysis. *JAMA.* 295:74, 2006.

Dedoussis GV, et al. Effect of phenols on natural killer (NK) cell-mediated death in the K562 human leukemic cell line. *Cell Biol Int.* 29:884, 2005.

de Jong A, et al. Why whole grains are protective: biological mechanisms. *Proc Nutr Soc.* 62:129, 2003.

de Kleijn MJ, et al. Intake of dietary phytoestrogens is low in postmenopausal women in the United States: the Framingham study. *J Nutr.* 131:1826, 2001.

Dunn-Emke SR, et al. Nutrient adequacy of a very low-fat vegan diet. *J Am Diet Assoc.* 105:1442, 2005.

Emmons KM, et al. Project PREVENT: a randomized trial to reduce multiple behavioral risk factors for colon cancer. *Cancer Epidemiol Biomarkers Prev.* 14:1453, 2005.

Fahey JW, et al. Chlorophyll, chlorophyllin and related tetrapyrroles are significant inducers of mammalian phase 2 cytoprotective genes. *Carcinogenesis* 26:1247, 2005.

Fahey JW, et al. Sulforaphane inhibits extracellular, intracellular, and antibiotic-resistant strains of *Helicobacter pylori* and prevents benzo[a]pyrene-induced stomach tumors. *Proc Natl Acad Sci U S A.* 99:7610, 2002.

Fang CY, et al. Correlates of soy food consumption in women at increased risk for breast cancer. *J Am Diet Assoc.* 105:1552, 2005.

Finley JW, et al. Selenium enrichment of broccoli: interactions between selenium and secondary plant compounds. *J Nutr.* 135:1236, 2005.

Fisher B, et al. Tamoxifen for the prevention of breast cancer: current status of the National Surgical Adjuvant Breast and Bowel Project P-1 Study. *J Natl Cancer Inst.* 97:1652, 2005.

Fong LY, et al. Dietary zinc modulation of COX-2 expression and lingual and esophageal carcinogenesis in rats. *J Natl Cancer Inst.* 97:40, 2005.

Fowke JH, et al. Urinary isothiocyanate levels, brassica, and human breast cancer. *Cancer Res.* 63:3980, 2003.

Fraser ML, et al. Lycopene and prostate cancer: emerging evidence. *Expert Rev Anticancer Ther.* 5:847, 2005.

Fujiki H. Green tea: Health benefits as cancer preventive for humans. *Chem Rec.* 5:119, 2005.

Ganry O. Phytoestrogens and prostate cancer risk. *Prev Med.* 41:1, 2005.

Ganry O, Boche T. Prevention practices and cancer screening among general practitioners in Picardy, France. *Public Health* 119:1023, 2005.

Gao K, et al. The citrus flavonoid naringenin stimulates DNA repair in prostate cancer cells. *J Nutr Biochem.* 17:89, 2006.

Gill CI, et al. Potential anti-cancer effects of virgin olive oil phenols on colorectal carcinogenesis models in vitro. *Int J Cancer.* 117:1, 2005.

Graf BA, et al. Flavonols, flavones, flavanones, and human health: epidemiological evidence. *J Med Food.* 8:281, 2005.

Guneri P, et al. Primary oral cancer in a Turkish population sample: association with sociodemographic features, smoking, alcohol, diet and dentition. *Oral Oncol.* 41:1005, 2005.

Harmon AL, et al. Cancer prevention among rural youth: building a "bridge" to better health with genealogy. *J Cancer Educ.* 20:103, 2005.

Hoensch HP, Kirch W. Potential role of flavonoids in the prevention of intestinal neoplasia: a review of their mode of action and their clinical perspectives. *Int J Gastrointest Cancer.* 35:187, 2005.

Husken A, et al. Resveratrol glucoside (Piceid) synthesis in seeds of transgenic oilseed rape (*Brassica napus* L). *Theor Appl Genet.* 111:1553, 2005.

Hwang ES, Jeffery EH. Induction of quinone reductase by sulforaphane and sulforaphane N-acetylcysteine conjugate in murine hepatoma cells. *J Med Food.* 8:198, 2005.

Ito H, et al. Polyphenol levels in human urine after intake of six different polyphenol-rich beverages. *Br J Nutr.* 94:500, 2005.

Ito Y, et al. Cancer mortality and serum levels of carotenoids, retinol, and tocopherol: a population-based follow-up study of inhabitants of a rural area of Japan. *Asian Pac J Cancer Prev.* 6:10, 2005.

Jeyabal PV, et al. Apigenin inhibits oxidative stress-induced macromolecular damage in N-nitrosodiethylamine (NDEA)-induced hepatocellular carcinogenesis in Wistar albino rats. *Mol Carcinog.* 44:11, 2005.

Jolly CA. Diet manipulation and prevention of aging, cancer and autoimmune disease. *Curr Opin Clin Nutr Metab Care.* 8:382, 2005.

Joseph MA, et al. Cruciferous vegetables, genetic polymorphisms in glutathione s-transferases m1 and t1, and prostate cancer risk. *Nutr Cancer.* 50:206, 2004.

Kallay E, et al. Colon-specific regulation of vitamin D hydroxylases: a possible approach for tumor prevention. *Carcinogenesis* 26:1581, 2005.

Kamat AM, Lamm DL. Chemoprevention of bladder cancer. *Urol Clin North Am.* 29:157, 2002.

Keinan-Boker L, et al. Dietary phytoestrogens and breast cancer risk. *Am J Clin Nutr.* 79:282, 2004.

Kim H. New nutrition, proteomics, and how both can enhance studies in cancer prevention and therapy. *J Nutr.* 135:2715, 2005.

Kogut VJ, Luthringer SL, eds. *Nutritional issues in cancer care.* Pittsburgh: Oncology Nursing Society, 2005

Kwak HK, et al. Improved vitamin B-6 status is positively related to lymphocyte proliferation in young women consuming a controlled diet. *J Nutr.* 132:3308, 2002.

Larsson SC, et al. Vitamin B6 intake, alcohol consumption, and colorectal cancer: a longitudinal population-based cohort of women. *Gastroenterology* 128:1830, 2005.

Lau CB et al. Cytotoxic activities of *Coriolus versicolor* (Yunzhi) extract on human leukemia and lymphoma cells by induction of apoptosis. *Life Sci.* 75:797, 2004.

Lee DH, Jacobs DR Jr. Interaction among heme iron, zinc, and supplemental vitamin C intake on the risk of lung cancer: Iowa Women's Health Study. *Nutr Cancer.* 12:130, 2005.

Lee IM, et al. Vitamin E in the primary prevention of cardiovascular disease and cancer: the Women's Health Study—a randomized controlled trial. *JAMA.* 294:56, 2005.

Leenan R, et al. A single dose of tea with or without milk increases plasma antioxidant activity in humans. *Euro J Clin Nutr.* 54:87, 2000.

Leung KN, et al. Immunomodulatory effects of esculetin (6,7-dihydroxycoumarin) on murine lymphocytes and peritoneal macrophages. *Cell Mol Immunol.* 2:181, 2005.

Levi F, et al. Refined and whole grain cereals and the risk of oral, esophageal, and laryngeal cancer. *Euro J Clin Nutr.* 54:487, 2000.

Liggins J, et al. Daidzein and genistein content of fruits and nuts. *J Nutr Biochem.* 11:326, 2000.

Lin DC. Probiotics as functional foods. *Nutr Clin Pract.* 18:497, 2003.

Loren DJ, et al. Maternal dietary supplementation with pomegranate juice is neuroprotective in an animal model of neonatal hypoxic-ischemic brain injury. *Pediatr Res.* 57:858, 2005.

MacLean CH, et al. Effects of omega-3 fatty acids on cancer risk: a systematic review. *JAMA.* 295:403, 2006.

Malik A, et al. Pomegranate fruit juice for chemoprevention and chemotherapy of prostate cancer. *Proc Natl Acad Sci U S A.* 102:14813, 2005.

Maskarinec G. Soy foods for breast cancer survivors and women at high risk for breast cancer. *J Am Diet Assoc.* 105:1524, 2005.

McCann MJ, et al. Role of mammalian lignans in the prevention and treatment of prostate cancer. *Nutr Cancer.* 52:1, 2005.

McNaughton SA, et al. Role of dietary factors in the development of basal cell cancer and squamous cell cancer of the skin. *Cancer Epidemiol Biomarkers Prev.* 14:1596, 2005.

Meyskens FL Jr, Szabo E. Diet and cancer: the disconnect between epidemiology and randomized clinical trials. *Cancer Epidemiol Biomarkers Prev.* 14:1366, 2005.

Michaud D, et al. Intake of specific carotenoids and risk of lung cancer in two prospective U.S. cohorts. *Am J Clin Nutr.* 72:990, 2000.

Nishino H, et al. Cancer prevention by phytochemicals. *Oncology* 69:38S, 2005.

Ouerfelli O, et al. Synthetic carbohydrate-based antitumor vaccines: challenges and opportunities. *Expert Rev Vaccines.* 4:677, 2005.

Pattison DJ, et al. Dietary beta-cryptoxanthin and inflammatory polyarthritis: results from a population-based prospective study. *Am J Clin Nutr.* 82:451, 2005.

Perez-Galvez A, et al. Incorporation of carotenoids from paprika oleoresin into human chylomicrons. *Br J Nutr.* 89:787, 2003.

Pool-Zobel BL. Inulin-type fructans and reduction in colon cancer risk: review of experimental and human data. *Br J Nutr.* 93:73S, 2005.

Poulouse SM, et al. Citrus limonoids induce apoptosis in human neuroblastoma cells and have radical scavenging activity. *J Nutr.* 135:870, 2005.

Poynter JN, et al. Statins and the risk of colorectal cancer. *N Engl J Med.* 352:2184, 2005.

Prentice RL, et al. Low-fat dietary pattern and risk of invasive breast cancer: the Women's Health Initiative Randomized Controlled Dietary Modification Trial. *JAMA.* 295:629, 2006.

Qiu JL, et al. Nutritional factors and gastric cancer in Zhoushan Islands, China. *World J Gastroenterol.* 11:4311, 2005.

Rauscher G, et al. Relation between body mass index and lung cancer risk in men and women never and former smokers. *Am J Epidemiol.* 152:506, 2000.

Reddy BS, et al. Prevention of colon cancer by low doses of celecoxib, a cyclooxygenase inhibitor, administered in diet rich in omega-3 polyunsaturated fatty acids. *Cancer Res.* 65:8022, 2005.

Reed GA, et al. A phase I study of indole-3-carbinol in women: tolerability and effects. *Cancer Epidemiol Biomarkers Prev.* 14:1953, 2005.

Reid ME, et al. Selenium supplementation and colorectal adenomas: an analysis of the nutritional prevention of cancer trial. *Int J Cancer.* 118:1777, 2006.

Riezzo G, et al. Functional foods: salient features and clinical applications. *Curr Drug Targets Immune Endocr Metabol Disord.* 5:331, 2005.

Robbins RJ, et al. Cultivation conditions and selenium fertilization alter the phenolic profile, glucosinolate, and sulforaphane content of broccoli. *J Med Food.* 8:204, 2005.

Samoha S, Arber N. Cyclooxygenase-2 inhibition prevents colorectal cancer: from the bench to the bed side. *Oncology* 69:33S, 2005.

Sartippour MR, et al. *Rabdosia rubescens* inhibits breast cancer growth and angiogenesis. *Int J Oncol.* 26:121, 2005.

Sasaki-Sekimoto Y, et al. Coordinated activation of metabolic pathways for antioxidants and defense compounds by jasmonates and their roles in stress tolerance in Arabidopsis. *Plant J.* 44:653, 2005.

Scalbert A, et al. Dietary polyphenols and the prevention of diseases. *Crit Rev Food Sci Nutr.* 45:287, 2005.

Schabath MB, et al. Dietary phytoestrogens and cancer risk. *JAMA.* 294:1550, 2005.

Seeram NP, et al. In vitro antiproliferative, apoptotic and antioxidant activities of punicalagin, ellagic acid and a total pomegranate tannin extract are enhanced in combination with other polyphenols as found in pomegranate juice. *J Nutr Biochem.* 16:360, 2005.

Seth A, Watson DK. ETS transcription factors and their emerging roles in human cancer. *Eur J Cancer.* 41:2462, 2005.

Shenouda NS, et al. Phytoestrogens in common herbs regulate prostate cancer cell growth in vitro. *Nutr Cancer.* 49:200, 2004.

Shoveller AK, et al. Nutritional and functional importance of intestinal sulfur amino acid metabolism. *J Nutr.* 135:1609, 2005.

Singh RP, Agarwal R. Prostate cancer and inositol hexaphosphate: efficacy and mechanisms. *Anticancer Res.* 25:2891, 2005.

Slavin J. Why whole grains are protective: biological mechanisms. *Proc Nutr Soc.* 62:129, 2003.
Spina C, et al. Colon cancer and solar ultraviolet B radiation and prevention and treatment of colon cancer in mice with vitamin D and its Gemini analogs. *J Steroid Biochem Mol Biol.* 97:111, 2005.
Strohle A, et al. Folic acid and colorectal cancer prevention: molecular mechanisms and epidemiological evidence. *Int J Oncol.* 26:1449, 2005.
Tezal M, et al. Is periodontitis associated with oral neoplasms? *J Periodontol.* 76:406, 2005.
Thomas RD, et al. Diallyl sulfide inhibits the oxidation and reduction reactions of stilbene estrogens catalyzed by microsomes, mitochondria and nuclei isolated from breast tissue of female ACI rats. *Carcinogenesis* 25:787, 2004.
Thompson HJ, et al. 8-Isoprostane F2alpha excretion is reduced in women by increased vegetable and fruit intake. *Am J Clin Nutr.* 82:768, 2005.
Thompson IM, et al. Phase III prostate cancer prevention trials: are the costs justified? *J Clin Oncol.* 23:8161, 2005.
Van Breda SG, et al. Vegetables affect the expression of genes involved in carcinogenic and anticarcinogenic processes in the lungs of female C57BL/6 mice. *J Nutr.* 135:2546, 2005.
Van Duyn M, Pivonka E. Overview of the health benefits of fruit and vegetable consumption for the dietetics professional: selected literature. *J Am Diet Assoc.* 100:1511, 2000.
Velasquez JL, Lipkin SM. What are SNPs and haplotypes and how will they help us manage the prevention of adult cancer? *Curr Oncol Rep.* 7:475, 2005.
Voskuil DW, et al. The insulin-like growth factor system in cancer prevention: potential of dietary intervention strategies. *Cancer Epidemiol Biomarkers Prev.* 14:195, 2005.
Whiting SJ, Calvo MS. Dietary recommendations to meet both endocrine and autocrine needs of Vitamin D. *J Steroid Biochem Mol Biol.* 97:7, 2005.
Williams MT, Hord NG. The role of dietary factors in cancer prevention: beyond fruits and vegetables. *Nutr Clin Pract.* 20:451, 2005.
Wong KY, et al. Dietary exposure to heterocyclic amines in a Chinese population. *Nutr Cancer.* 52:147, 2005.
Yuan JM, et al. Prediagnostic levels of serum micronutrients in relation to risk of gastric cancer in Shanghai, China. *Cancer Epidemiol Biomarkers Prev.* 13:1772, 2004.
Zheng T, et al. Lactation and breast cancer risk: a case-control study in Connecticut. *Br J Cancer.* 84:1472, 2001.
Zhou W, et al. Dietary iron, zinc, and calcium and the risk of lung cancer. *Epidemiology.* 16:772, 2005.

CANCER, TREATMENT AND TIPS FOR LONG-TERM SURVIVAL

CANCER: TREATMENT GUIDELINES

DEFINITIONS AND BACKGROUND

Cancer patients can be divided into three groups: those receiving standard or experimental therapy, those who have become unresponsive to these therapies, and those in remission who are at risk for recurrence or a second new cancer. Cancer cachexia, a wasting syndrome characterized by weight loss, anorexia, early satiety, progressive debilitation, and malnutrition, may lead to organ dysfunction and death in cancer patients (Mattox, 2005). Fatigue is the most common experience among patients with cancer. Otherwise, each type of cancer has its own set of treatments and side effects.

Weight loss and cachexia are common in most cancer patients. Malnourished cancer patients commonly have high protein turnover and loss of nitrogen. Cancer cachexia may lead to significant loss of muscle mass and impaired physical capacity. Tumor factors such as proteolysis-inducing factor (PIF), tumor necrosis factor (TNF), and lipid mobilizing factor (LMF) all tend to promote catabolism. Nutritional inadequacy mobilizes protein stores and thus causes loss of lean body mass, and altered nutrient utilization causes glucose intolerance, insulin resistance, increased glucose turnover, lipolysis, hyperlipidemia, and increased protein turnover. Properly nourishing patients, especially when malnourished, is essential therapy. Figure 13-2 provides the Subjective Global Assessment tool and scoring sheet used for cancer patients. Indications for use of tube feeding (enteral nutrition [EN]) are listed in Table 13-4.

Total parenteral nutrition (TPN) should not be used to prolong life for patients at the end stages of disease but may be appropriate for patients with responsive cancers when enteral and oral feedings are poorly tolerated. Table 13-5 defines the types of side effects and treatments in cancer therapy. Tables 13-6 and 13-7 list drugs and common side effects.

Patients unresponsive to standard or experimental therapies have few treatment options and usually experience poor quality of life for the remainder of their lives. An active nutritional protocol including high doses of multiple dietary antioxidants (vitamin C, alpha-tocopherol, and natural beta-carotene), when administered as an adjunct to other therapies, may increase tumor response and decrease toxicity. A maintenance nutritional protocol with lower doses of antioxidants, in addition to a modified diet and lifestyle, may reduce the risk of recurrence of the original tumor and development of a second cancer among survivors.

Use of complementary and alternative medicine (CAM) therapy is common in the cancer population. Some products are harmless, but some may lead to serious problems. Table 13-8 describes herbs commonly used by cancer patients, with some general comments.

OVERALL OBJECTIVES IN CANCER TREATMENT

- Diminish toxicity of treatments. Improve quality of life through resolution of treatment-related side effects.
- Coordinate total care plan with doctor, nurse, patient, family, caregivers, and other team members.
- Review each case individually and honor patient's wishes regarding more aggressive intervention.
- Correct cachexia from weakness, anorexia, redistribution of host nutrients, and nutritional depletion.
- Prevent depletion of humoral and cellular immunity from malnutrition. Improved nutritional status may allow neoplastic cells to become more susceptible to medical treatment.

Patient's Name: ______________________ Patient ID: __________ Date: __________

SGA Score

Part 1: Medical History

1. Weight Change

A. Overall change in past 6 months: __________ kgs.

B. Percent change: _____ gain - < 5% loss
_____ 5-10% loss
_____ > 10% loss

C. Change in past 2 weeks: _____ increase
_____ no change
_____ decrease

2. Dietary Intake

A. Overall change: _____ no change
_____ change

B. Duration: _____ weeks

C. Type of change:
_____ suboptimal solid diet or full liquid diet
_____ hypocaloric liquid
_____ starvation

3. Gastrointestinal Symptoms (persisting for > 2 weeks)

_____ none
_____ nausea _____ vomiting _____ diarrhea _____anorexia

4. Functional Impairment (nutritionally related)

A. Overall impairment: __________ none
__________ moderate
__________ severe

B. Change in past 2 weeks: __________ improved
__________ no change
__________ regressed

A	B	C

Score _____ _____ _____

Part 2: Physical Examination

5. Evidence of:

	Normal	Mild	Moderate	Severe
Loss of subcutaneous fat				
Muscle wasting				
Edema				
Ascites (hemo only)				

Part 3: Choose SGA Rating ☐ Well-Nourished ☐ Mildly-Moderately Malnourished ☐ Severely malnourished

Figure 13-2 Subjective Global Assessment scoring sheet for cancer.

TABLE 13-4 Use of Enteral Feeding in Cancer Patients

Indications	Contraindications
Inability to consume 50% of estimated needs orally for 1 week or longer—estimated or actual	Severe malabsorption that cannot be corrected with enteral nutrition
Functioning gastrointestinal (GI) tract with adequate capacity for nutrient absorption	Intestinal obstruction below feeding placement site
Patient willingness to use tube feeding method	Condition such as high-output fistula or high aspiration risk

Adapted from: Dixon SW. Nutrition care issues in the ambulatory (outpatient) head and neck cancer. *Support Line* 27:3, 2005.

TABLE 13-5 Side Effects of Treatment and Common Problems of Cancer

Side Effect	Comments
Anemias	About 40–60% of patients coming to cancer treatment are anemic (Varlotto and Stevenson, 2005). For anemias, use a balanced diet with high-quality proteins, B-complex vitamins, and vitamin C. Heme sources of iron will increase iron bioavailability. Avoid long-term excesses of iron. Use beef, chicken, fortified grains, dried fruits such as prunes, nuts, and seeds, and blackstrap molasses.
Anorexia	Anorexia may be caused by coping with the diagnosis and treatment-related side effects, medications, gastrointestinal (GI) distress, altered sensory experiences, or tumors. The condition often leads to cachexia. Determine specific factors contributing to symptom, such as pain, constipation, and GI symptoms, and treat appropriately. Encourage small, frequent feedings. Consider pharmacological therapy with appetite-enhancing medications.
Aversion to foods or flavors	For some patients, a lower threshold for urea causes aversion to meat; these patients may say that the meat "smells rotten." Substitute milk, cottage cheese, eggs, peanut butter, legumes, poultry, fish, and cheese. In addition, patient may have a decreased ability to taste salt and sugar. Add other seasonings, sauces, and more salt or sugar as desired by the patient; however, do not allow sweet foods to replace nourishing foods. Some people are "super tasters" and have a lot of taste buds, with extra sensitivity to sweet and sour foods; some are normal; and some are nontasters, with dull sensitivity to foods. Ensure adequate zinc intake. Foods served at cool or cold temperatures often have a less offensive taste and aroma. Clear palate prior to meals by brushing teeth, gums, and oral cavity and rinsing with baking soda and salt water
Cachexia	Cachexia is the clinical consequence of a chronic, systemic inflammatory response; depletion of skeletal muscle and redistribution of the body's protein are major changes that occur (Kotler, 2000). Nutritional deprivation at diagnosis can lead to further depletion with treatments. **Anorexia cachexia syndrome (ACS)** is caused by numerous factors; altered glucose metabolism may be one of them. Use small, frequent feedings and supplements. Teach ways to increase calories and protein. Fortify foods when possible. Relieve symptoms before meals whenever possible. Anabolic and anticatabolic agents, such as Megace and Oxandrin, may be able to mitigate cachexia (Kotler, 2000). The most recent studies suggest that use of omega-3 fatty acids (EPA and DHA) can disrupt the disordered metabolism of cachexia (Mattox, 2005; Tisdale, 2005).
Chemotherapy	With all types (given daily, weekly, monthly for 1–2 months or even years), prompt attention to side effect management and appropriate use of supportive care (medications, nutrition, etc., will be needed). Increase fluid intake for adequate hydration. After chemotherapy, cardiac, kidney, or
Chemotherapy (cont.)	pulmonary toxicity may occur. Some chemotherapy agents may cause infertility in both men and women. Nausea and vomiting can now be well controlled; drugs include Zofran (ondansetron), Kytril (granisetron), and Anzemet (dolasetron). Hemopoietic agents (e.g., Neupogen, Procrit, granulocyte colony-stimulation factor, granulocyte-macrophage colony-stimulating factor) may be needed if red blood cell production is too low; transfusions are used as a last resort. Avoid risk of infection and cuts during chemotherapy. Monitor for nosebleeds, bruising, black or bloody stools, or reddish urine. Use of glutamine supplementation has been used with some success.
Cold food preference	Cold foods may be better accepted than hot foods. Use cold, clear fluids, carbonated beverages, ices, gelatin, watermelons, grapes and peeled cucumbers, cold meat platters, ice cream, and salted nuts. Serve supplements over ice between meals. Shakes, puddings, and custards are other alternatives.
Constipation	Establish an appropriate bowel program, including regular use of pharmacological agents. Constipation requires fiber and fluids (8 cups) to be added to the diet. Milk also may be beneficial, if tolerated. Fresh or dried fruits, all vegetables, and bran may help. A hot drink may help. Get adequate exercise. Use of over-the-counter bulking agents may be useful in some cases. Avoid gas-forming foods or beverages in excess.
Diarrhea	Assess severity, including hydration status and associated symptoms. Alter fiber in diet. Beware of lactose intolerance secondary to disease process, drug therapy, or abdominal or pelvic radiation therapy. Decrease fatty foods. Increase fluids that contain sodium and potassium; a clear liquid diet for 24 hours may be helpful. Use cool or room temperature foods instead of very hot or very cold foods. Evaluate all medications carefully. Avoid dairy products if they increase indigestion or diarrhea. Consume small amounts of fluid and food throughout the day. Use of oral glutamine has been used with some success.
Difficulty swallowing (dysphagia)	Modify diet consistency and follow swallowing techniques provided by speech pathologist. Consider feeding tube if unable to obtain adequate nourishment orally. For difficulty in swallowing (dysphagia), use moist foods. Add gravies and sauces to foods. Some patients tolerate semisolid foods better than liquids. Patient should sip fluids throughout meal. To prevent aspiration, patient should try placing liquid under tongue. Some patients may also find that tilting their heads will be useful. Thickeners are available for liquids, if thin beverages are not tolerated well (as with choking, coughing with each swallow). Use of a straw may be beneficial. Spoons are easier to control than forks in the mouth. Avoid very hot or very cold foods. Pureed foods may be better tolerated than regular foods.

(continued)

TABLE 13-5 Side Effects of Treatment and Common Problems of Cancer (*continued*)

Side Effect	Comments
Dental caries or poor dentition	Avoid sweets and use sodium fluoride three times daily. Mouth care should be provided several times daily. Persons receiving irradiation to the head and neck area may benefit from use of fluoride trays and stannous fluoride.
Dry mouth (xerostomia)	Dry mouth from surgical removal of salivary glands, atrophy of mucous membranes, or from permanent damage from radiation to salivary glands may cause difficulty in eating and swallowing. Use salivary substitutes, lip balm, sugarless gum and candies, gravies, and sauces. Increase fluids and use softened, moist foods (custard, stews, and soups). Sip beverages with each bite of food. Cut food into small pieces. Ice chips and popsicles also can help. Pureed or baby foods often are useful. Avoid salty foods. Tart foods and beverages such as lemonade may help to stimulate saliva production. Sucking on popsicles, lemon drops, and hard candy can also help. Sip on water or other fluids frequently throughout the day. Synthetic saliva products such as Optimoist or MouthKote may help. Use caution with tart foods if oral lesions are present. Radiation therapy patients benefit from a thorough dental examination before treatment. Use of fluoride trays, rinses, and other measures may be helpful. Avoid caffeine, alcohol, and tobacco products.
Early satiety	Early satiety can be a problem. Rather than serving plain water, encourage a calorie-containing beverage. Take liquids between meals. Avoid fatty, greasy foods because they are more slowly digested and absorbed. Use small meals and frequent snacks between meals. Add protein and calories to favorite foods using extra butter, margarine, cheese, and nonfat dry milk powder.
Fatigue	Fatigue is probably the most common experience of patients with cancer. Assess the treatable causes of fatigue such as anemia, infection, pain, neutropenia, depression, and medication side effects, and manage appropriately. For fatigue, meals may be prepared in quantity when the patient is less tired. To prevent further fatigue, foods that require less chewing may be used. Provide frequent rest periods, especially before meals.
Fluid retention (edema)	Fluid retention may require elevating the legs at rest, staying physically active (walking, etc.), and reducing salt intake overall. The doctor will prescribe diuretics, if indicated.
Graft-versus-host disease (GVHD)	Total lymphoid irradiation plus antithymocyte globulin decreases the incidence of acute GVHD in patients with lymphoid malignant diseases or acute leukemia treated with hematopoietic-cell transplantation (Lowsky et al, 2005).
Insulin resistance	Insulin resistance is common from the tumor itself. Control of CHO intake may be indicated when this occurs. Various medications also may be used to treat insulin resistence, such as oral agents. Common after pancreatic surgery.
Loneliness	Loneliness may affect eating habits. Social eating may improve food intake. Visitors should be encouraged to bring gifts of food, as appropriate.
Loss of lean body mass	Protein wasting and unintentional weight loss are common with cancer treatments. Exercise is extremely helpful. Endurance activities can counteract loss of physical performance and improve lower and upper body strength. Patients who exercise also have less fatigue and depression. Taking hormones such as growth hormone, insulin-like growth factor (IGF-I), thyroid hormone, androgens, and cortisol makes a difference as well. Muscle protein synthesis can be increased accordingly.
Malabsorption	In the case of malabsorption, elemental diets can only be used if patient has an intact duodenum and jejunum. Total parenteral nutrition (TPN) can be used only in some cases, considering risks of infection. Elemental diets are often prescribed by mouth with poor patient compliance; work with patient on ways to improve compliance. Use of tart beverages with mixed product can be useful (e.g., lemonade).
Meal interruptions	If meals are interrupted by treatment, encourage a good breakfast and snacks to make up for interrupted meals. Keep kitchen well stocked. Meals-on-Wheels may be a useful way to serve meals to this population.
Mouth blindness (dysgeusia)	Mouth blindness (dysgeusia) is defined as disinterest and aversion to foods. Emphasize the aroma and colors of foods. Provide a variety of foods and use garnishes. Acidic foods (e.g., lemonade) may help stimulate patient's ability to taste foods. Use highly flavored foods and sauces. Try milk shakes that are coffee or mint flavored. Fresh vegetables, special breads, highly flavored snacks, olives, and pickles may be well received by the patient. Add sauces to meats. Foods that are served warm or hot have more flavor and aroma.
Mouth or throat soreness (stomatitis, mucositis, or esophagitis)	Sore mouth and throat results from local bleeding, mucosal irritation, and lesions. Pain and inflammation are common. Modify the texture and consistency of foods as needed. Use a diet with fewer spices and seasonings including chili powder and red and black pepper. Have patient rinse mouth with water and sodium bicarbonate. Avoid acidic juices, salty foods or soups, dry toast, and coarse or grainy breads or cereals. Grind meats. Use the "mechanical soft diet" as needed. Offer fluids frequently and by straw—cold or tepid. Popsicles and cold liquid foods may help. Smaller meals are useful. Cut foods into smaller pieces; grind or puree if needed. Mix food with sauces or gravies to make it easier to swallow. Swish mouth with lidocaine before meals; some changes in taste or enjoyment of foods may result. Avoid smoking and use of alcohol. Use of oral glutamine has been used with some success. Rinse mouth and gargle frequently with mild saline solution. Avoid alcohol-based mouthwashes.

(*continued*)

TABLE 13-5 Side Effects of Treatment and Common Problems of Cancer (*continued*)

Side Effect	Comments
Muscle wasting	Muscle weakness is frequently associated with tumor growth. Depression, altered moods, immobility, and bed rest may all contribute to loss of muscle mass. Structured exercise, including resistance training and aerobic exercises, can improve muscle mass and strength. Increased physical activity will allow the cancer patient to gain in emotional stability, self-confidence, and independence. Active patients often also have less fatigue, nausea, and insomnia. Quality of life seems to improve as well. If possible, include adequate amounts of protein and amino acids in the diet or in enteral feeding. Arginine, glutamine, leucine, and other specific amino acids can stimulate muscle protein synthesis. Encourage ambulation whenever possible, even taking a few steps each day.
Nausea	Nausea can be treated by slow, deep breathing, ice chips, or sips of carbonated beverages. Try a dry diet (liquids between meals). Eat small meals; rest afterward. Keep crackers or salty potato chips handy. Eat toast, yogurt, sherbet, popsicles, pretzels, angel food cake, canned fruit, baked chicken, and hot cereal such as oatmeal, clear liquids, or broth. Cut down on greasy, spicy, and fried or fatty foods. Some people prefer tart lemonade to sweetened beverages. Foods with strong odors and excessive sweetness may not be tolerated. Sit upright for meals and snacks. Avoid tight clothing. If breakfast is the best meal, it can also be the largest of the day. Encourage patients to use antiemetics as directed by physician; underusage may contribute to nausea. Sip on ginger ale, tea, or candied dried ginger.
Pain	Give pain medications with the first few bites of a meal or have patient eat when pain is lowest. Encourage trying foods again after time lapse. Try biofeedback or muscle relaxation.
Radiation enteritis or colitis	Serious injury to the intestinal epithelium and arterioles of the small or large intestines results in cell death, fibrosis, and obstruction after radiation therapy. Radiation to the ileum is especially devastating. If radiation must be given chronically, resection may be needed. The ability of the intestines to become hyperplastic and to increase absorptive capacity is thus prevented. Of patients who are given abdominal or pelvic radiotherapy, 5–40% will develop radiation enteritis or colitis. Of these persons, many will require home TPN or chronic parenteral nutrition (PN) because of the effects on the intestinal tract. About 50–80% of patients who have radiation to the pelvis end up with radiation enteritis; onset can occur up to years later. Symptoms and signs of radiation enteritis or colitis include nausea, vomiting, mucoid diarrhea, abdominal pain, and bleeding (later effects include colic, decrease in stool caliber, and progressive obstipation with stricture and fibrosis).
Radiation therapy	**Radiotherapy** may involve high-energy radiation from x-rays, cobalt-60, or radium. **Brachytherapy** provides internal, continuous local delivery of radiation to site of malignancy (concealed). **Teletherapy** provides external radiation to a localized area; 7000 rads usually causes damage, especially to small intestine (radiation enteritis). Radiation therapy (usually given daily for 2–8 weeks) can cause nausea or vomiting if administered to the brain or abdominal/pelvic fields. A light meal is encouraged before treatment. Diarrhea may occur in radiation enteritis; glutamine may be useful in supplements or in tube feeding (TF)/TPN. Formulas containing multiple antioxidants for biological protection against radiation damage in humans are needed, and this can reduce potential risks of ionizing radiation (Prasad, 2004). Use of oral glutamine has been used with some success. Radiation treatment to the GI tract may cause the following side effects: **Head and neck cancer:** Anorexia, dysgeusia, weight loss, odynophagia, dysphagia, difficulty chewing, xerostomia **Thorax:** Nausea, esophagitis, vomiting **Abdominal, intestinal:** Early: lactose intolerance, diarrhea, distention, abdominal pain, nausea and vomiting. Later: intestinal stenosis, edema, fluid and electrolyte loss, weight loss
Surgery, curative	Direct efforts at restoring nutritional health to pre-illness status. Common problems after GI surgery include: **Oropharynx:** Difficulty with chewing and swallowing, dysgeusia, xerostomia **Esophagus:** Heartburn, loss of normal swallowing, decreased motility, obstruction **Stomach:** Dumping syndrome, delayed emptying, anemia, malabsorption **Small intestines:** Lactose intolerance, bile acid depletion, steatorrhea, fat malabsorption, vitamin B_{12} deficiency and anemia, short-gut syndrome **Colon:** Loss of electrolytes and water, diarrhea, constipation, gas, bloating
Thick saliva	Thick, ropy saliva can produce more caries. Use less bread, milk, gelatin, and oily foods. Blenderize foods such as fruits and vegetables. Encourage intake of plenty of fluids to decrease viscosity of oral secretions. Encourage good oral intake and regular oral rinses.
Tooth loss	Loss of teeth makes the patient's mouth more sensitive to cold, heat, and sweets. Try serving foods at room temperature. Use ground, chopped, or pureed foods as needed until dental repair is possible.
Vomiting	During periods of vomiting, use sips of clear liquids every 10–15 minutes after vomiting episodes cease; keep head elevated. "Flat" carbonated beverages are useful. Call doctor if abdominal pains persist. Give antiemetic medications prior to meals, use small feedings, avoid foods with strong odor, use liquids between meals, and try lower fat diet.

(continued)

TABLE 13-5 **Side Effects of Treatment and Common Problems of Cancer *(continued)***

Side Effect	Comments	Side Effect	Comments
Weight loss	Weight loss can be treated by adding fats to foods, dry milk to mashed potatoes and shakes, and extra sugar to coffee and cereals. Use small, frequent feedings and the patient's favorite foods.		Use 40–45 kcal/kg for repletion. Add cream sauces, extra meat or cheeses in casseroles, and gravies. Encourage patients to be as physically active as possible, especially using long muscles to promote lean body mass.

See also Cancer Nutrition Info at http://web.cancernutritioninfo.com/main.cfm?ID=1349.

TABLE 13-6 **Cancer Drugs and Chemotherapy Agents**

When chemotherapy is required, patients may suffer severe side effects such as nausea and vomiting, hair loss, infection, and injury to the gastrointestinal (GI) tract. Medications that may increase appetite include progestational agents, glucocorticoids, cannabinoids, cyproheptadine, olanzapine, mirtazapine, and anabolic agents such as testosterone derivatives (Mattox, 2005). Other agents have been investigated for their anti-inflammatory properties, including thalidomide, pentoxyphylline, melatonin, and omega-3 fatty acids (Mattox, 2005). Serotonin antagonists such as Anzemet (dolasetron), if administered at the same time as chemotherapy, can prevent nausea and vomiting, but abdominal pain, headache, and constipation may occur. When antineoplastic agents are used, side effects include nausea, anorexia, stomatitis, diarrhea, taste alterations, some vomiting, and possibly sloughing of colonic mucosa (see Table 13-7 also).

Drug	Description
Alkylating agents: cyclophosphamide, fluorouracil	These drugs kill cancer cells by stopping their growth or by making it hard for cancer cells to repair damage. Nausea, vomiting, hyperuricemia.
Antiangiogenic agent: humanized monoclonal antibody bevacizumab (Avastin)	Tumors require nutrients and oxygen in order to grow; angiogenesis provides access to these nutrients. The key mediator of angiogenesis is vascular endothelial growth factor (VEGF), which is induced by many characteristics of tumors, most importantly hypoxia (Ferrara, 2005).
Antimetabolites: flucytosine	This small molecule is a DNA substrate analog that leads to incorrect DNA synthesis to affect the cancer cells. Nausea, vomiting, diarrhea, and stomatitis can occur.
Antiemetics: granisetron or ondansetron, medical cannabis, Marinol, domperidone, promethazine (Phenergan), metoclopramide (Reglan)	May be useful for anorexia/cachexia syndrome. Also used to relieve nausea and vomiting after chemotherapy. Headache may result. Other side effects include nausea, diarrhea, increased gastric emptying, or drowsiness.
Aspirin and anti-inflammatory agents	May prevent some types of cancer, including colon cancer. Use of herbal nonsteroidal anti-inflammatory drugs (NSAIDs) may eventually be recommended along with these medications to enhance effectiveness.
Irinotecan (Camptosar)	For the treatment of stage I–IV breast, lung, prostate, colon, skin, and most other metastatic or nonmetastatic forms of cancer.
Corticosteroids: prednisone	Hyperglycemia, sodium and fluid retention, weight gain, and calcium losses can occur.
Folate antagonist: methotrexate	Use of folate preparations can alter drug response. Folate, lactose, vitamin B_{12}, and fat are less well absorbed. Mouth sores are common.
Immunotherapy: interleukin-2 and interferon	Lymphokine is administered to decrease tumor growth. Nausea, vomiting, abdominal pain, fatigue, and anorexia can result. In addition, low levels of folate and vitamins A and B_6 may result.
Monoclonal antibodies (MAbs): cetuximab, Campath-1H, rituximab (Rituxan), and Bexxar	These attack only abnormal elements of cells ("kinder and gentler" cancer therapies). These drugs correct the abnormal enzyme that causes cancerous cells to grow out of control. Cetuximab specifically binds to the epidermal growth factor receptor with high affinity, blocking growth factor binding, receptor activation, and subsequent signal transduction events leading to cell proliferation (Baselga, 2001).
Vinca alkaloids: vincristine, vinblastine	Nausea and vomiting can occur.

See also the Food and Drug Administration Drug List at http://www.fda.gov/cder/cancer/druglistframe.htm.

TABLE 13-7 Antineoplastic Agents: Generic and Brand Names

Generic	Brand	Generic	Brand
Altretamine	Hexalen	Interferon-α2a	Roferon-A
Asparaginase	Elspar	Interferon-α2b	Intron-A
Bevacizumab	Avastin	Interferon-αn3	Alferon-N
BCG	TheraCys, TICE BCG	Irinotecan	Camptosar
Bleomycin sulfate	Blenoxane	Leucovorin calcium	Wellcovorin
Busulfan	Myleran	Leuprolide	Lupron, Lupron-Depot
Carboplatin	Paraplatin	Levamisole	Ergamisol
Carmustine	BiCNU	Lomustine	CeeNU
Chlorambucil	Leukeran	Megestrol	Megace
Cisplatin (*cis*-platinum, *cis*-diammine-dichloroplatinum)	Platinol, Platinol-AQ	Melphalan, L-phenylalanine mustard, L-sarcolysin	Alkeran (R)
Cladribine, 2-chlorodeoxyadenosine	Leustatin	Melphalan hydrochloride	IV Alkeran
Cyclophosphamide	Cytoxan, Neosar	Mercaptopurine	Purinethol Tablets
Cytarabine, cytosine arabinoside	Cytosar-U	Mesna	Mesnex
Dacarbazine, imidazole carboxamide	DTIC-DME	Mechlorethamine, nitrogen mustard	Mustargen
Dactinomycin	Cosmegen	Methylprednisolone	Solumedrol, Medrol
Daunorubicin, daunomycin	Cerubidine	Methotrexate, amethopterin	Trexall
Dexamethasone	Decadron, Tobradex	Mitomycin	Mutamycin
Doxorubicin	Adriamycin	Mitoxantrone	Novantrone
Erlotinib	Tarceva	Paclitaxel	Taxol
Etoposide (epipodophyllotoxin)	VePesid	Plicamycin, mithramycin	Mithracin
Floxuridine	FUDR	Prednisone	Deltasone
Fludarabine	Fludara	Procarbazine	Matulane
Fluorouracil	Fluorouracil Injection	Streptozocin, streptozotocin	Zanosar
Fluoxymesterone	Halotestin	Tamoxifen	Nolvadex
Flutamide	Eulexin	6-Thioguanine	Tabloid
Goserelin	Zoladex	Thiotepa, triethylene thiophosphoramide	Thiotepa
Hydroxyurea	Hydrea	Vinblastine	Velban
Idarubicin HCL	Idamycin	Vincristine	Oncovin
Ifosfamide	IFEX	Vinorelbine tartrate	Navelbine Injection
Interferon-alfa	Roferon-A, Intron-A		

Source: Medicine Online. Antineoplastic agents generic abbreviations. Accessed at http://www.meds.com/dosecalc/reg_agents.html.

TABLE 13-8 Herbs, Dietary Supplements, and Cancer

Over 50% of all patients diagnosed with cancer explore complementary and alternative medicine (CAM), especially herbal medicine (Boon and Wong, 2004). Popular CAM methods related to dietary intervention should be carefully addressed (Kronenberg et al, 2005). The Natural Product Cancer Chemopreventive Agents study through the National Cancer Institute has found about 200 active chemical ingredients in over 15,000 products. Naturopathic physicians often use dietary counseling (94%), botanical medicines (88%), antioxidants (84%), and supplemental nutrition (84%) with vitamin C, coenzyme Q10, and Hoxsey formula (Standish et al, 2002). The dietetics professional must evaluate the risks and benefits of the use of herbs and botanical products in various cancers; indicate whether **"guidance" or "promotion"** is being offered. Alternative therapies should be reviewed in light of potential harm.

The activation of nuclear transcription factor-κB has been linked with a variety of inflammatory diseases, including cancer (Aggarwal and Shishodia, 2004). Spices can suppress this pathway. Research has demonstrated that the commonly used herbs and spices such as allspice, bay leaves, cumin, cloves, cinnamon, garlic, mustard, rosemary, and thyme possess antimicrobial properties; saffron, turmeric, tea (green or black), and flaxseed contain potent phytochemicals, including carotenoids, curcumins, catechins, and lignans, respectively, which provide significant protection against cancer (Lai and Roy, 2004). Phenolic compounds and flavonoids contain antimutagenic and antioxidant properties. Studies have been done with turmeric (curcumin), red pepper (capsaicin), cloves (eugenol), ginger (gingerol), fennel (anethol), basil and rosemary (ursolic acid), pomegranate (ellagic acid), garlic (diallyl sulfide, *S*-allylmercaptocysteine, and ajoene), and anise (Aggarwal and Shishodia, 2004). Herbs should be appropriately labeled to alert consumers to potential interactions when used with drugs, and consultation with a general practitioner is recommended (Hu et al, 2005). While vitamin and mineral preparations represent 90% of all pharmacologic CAM used by the public, green tea, echinacea, and Essiac are the most popular herbs (Dy et al, 2004).

Herb or Supplement	Uses/Actions	General Comments
Ashwagandha (*Withania somnifera*)	Used for cancer treatment, diabetes, epilepsy, fatigue, gastrointestinal (GI) disorders, pain, rheumatoid arthritis (RA), skin infections, and stress.	Should not be used in pregnant women because it is an abortifacient.
Astragalus	Stimulates interferon and positively impacts the immune system. Possibly reduces the effectiveness of chemotherapy. Strong immune booster.	A type of legume used for years in Chinese medicine. No convincing evidence in cancer.
Black cohosh (Remifemin)	May relieve symptoms of menopause. No known side effects with chemotherapy. Source of vitamin A and pantothenic acid. Drug interactions: may increase the toxicity of doxorubicin and docetaxel.	Used to lower hot flashes, which can be a challenge for breast cancer patients (Osmers et al, 2005).
Bromelain	Bromelain (from pineapple extract) positively impacts the immune system. Improved tumor boundaries.	Studies have not demonstrated evidence in cancer therapy.
Cat's claw	May have some effect on immune system, but more comprehensive studies are needed. Antioxidant.	Contains alkaloids.
Chamomile	No proven efficacy in cancer. May promote sedation or allergic reactions.	
Chili powder	Capsaicin may actually have tumor-promoting effects; chili powder has been implicated in several GI cancers, but the results are conflicting.	In Mexico, higher use of chili powder is related to more stomach cancer.
Chinese herbal medicine	Chinese herbal medicine uses a variety of herbs, in different combinations, to restore balance to the body.	See Astragalus, Ginkgo, Ginseng, Green tea, and Siberian ginseng.
Chinese PC-SPES	Contains chrysanthemum, isatis, licorice, Panax ginseng, saw palmetto, skullcap, and two other herbal products of which *Rabdosia rubescens* is the most potent (Sartippour et al, 2005). PC-SPES contains flavonoids, alkaloids, polysaccharides, amino acids, and trace minerals such as selenium, calcium, magnesium, zinc, and copper.	Antiestrogenic effects; being studied in clinical trials for prostate and breast cancers as adjuvant therapy (Sartippour et al, 2005).
Cloves	Contains eugenol, which reduces lipid peroxidation and reduces cancer cell proliferation (Aggarwal and Shisohda, 2004).	
Dehydroepiandrosterone (DHEA)	DHEA is a steroid hormone produced by the adrenal gland and converted into estrogen and testosterone.	It is normally found in humans, plants, and animals. DHEA extracted from a wild yam plant is available as a dietary supplement.
Echinacea	No evidence of usefulness in reducing incidence or symptoms of cancer.	May reduce colds or flu for some people.
Eleuthero (Siberian ginseng)	May boost energy. More studies are needed.	
Essiac	Mixture of four herbs: burdock root (*Arctium lappa*), sheep sorrel (*Rumex acetosella*), slippery elm bark (*Ulmus rubra*), and Indian rhubarb root (*Rheum officinale*) to make a tea. Watercress (*Nasturtium officinale R.Br.*), blessed thistle (*Cnicus benedictus L.*), red clover (*Trifolium pratense L.*), and kelp (*Laminaria digitata [Hudson] Lamx.*) have been added to later recipes for a product sold as Flor Essence. Possibly estrogenic, antioxidant, anti-inflammatory, antimicrobial, and anticarcinogenic.	Essiac tea possesses potent antioxidant and DNA-protective activity, making it a natural anticancer agent (Leonard et al, 2006). More studies are needed (Boon and Wong, 2004)).

(continued)

TABLE 13-8 Herbs, Dietary Supplements, and Cancer *(continued)*

Herb or Supplement	Uses/Actions	General Comments
Evening primrose oil or gamma linolenic acid (GLA)	Proposed to reduce effects of cancer treatments. GLA is an omega-6 unsaturated fatty acid made in the human body from other essential fatty acids. The main supplemental sources of GLA are oils of the seeds of evening primrose, borage, and black currant plants. GLA is claimed to slow cancer cell growth. Increases effectiveness of chemotherapy; boost efficiency of tamoxifen; antioxidant; boost immune system.	Additional research is needed about the efficacy of evening primrose oil (Boon and Wong, 2004). GLA is found in human breast milk.
Falcarinol	A cancer-fighting substance found only in carrots; it seems to reduce the development of cancer in rats (Yoshikawa et al, 2006).	Human studies are needed.
Flaxseed	There is some evidence that flaxseed supplements along with low-fat diets may be useful in men with early-stage prostate cancer.	Controlled clinical studies are needed.
Garlic	Seems to have reduced gastric cancer in China and Italy. May also reduce prostate cancer (Xiao and Singh, 2006). Sulfur compounds tend to be the most chemoprotective. Useful in treatment as well as prevention. Garlic appears to induce cytochrome P-450 3A4 and may enhance metabolism of many medications such as cyclosporine and saquinavir. Antimicrobial properties are helpful.	Supplements are not as effective as real garlic for allicin and *S*-allylcysteine activity. Garlic poultices may cause burns in infants. Used as spice and to treat hyperlipidemia, hypertension, atherosclerosis, cancer, and infections, but sustained response has not been found. Mixed effects regarding reduction of blood glucose levels, blood pressure, or cardiovascular diseases. Garlic should not be used in patients on anticoagulants and patients with platelet dysfunction.
Ginger (6-gingerol)	May help to reduce the side effects of cancer treatments as an antiemetic, anti-inflammatory agent. Effective in preventing nausea and vomiting in some patients. It is a relatively safe herb, but patients taking blood thinners or about to undergo surgery should avoid ginger supplements. Interaction with many drugs including antacids, anticoagulants and antiplatelets, antidiabetics, antihypertensives, H_2 blockers, proton pump inhibitors (PPI), and barbiturates.	Ginger may be effective in treating chemotherapy-induced nausea and vomiting (Boon and Wong, 2004).
Ginkgo biloba (maidenhair tree)	Antioxidant and anti-inflammatory effects; role in cancer is being studied (see Table 13-2). Stimulates blood circulation and helps improve memory.	Ginkgo biloba (ginkgo) causes bleeding when combined with warfarin or aspirin (acetylsalicylic acid), raises blood pressure when combined with a thiazide diuretic, and causes coma when combined with trazodone in patients (Hu et al, 2005). Known to lower the threshold for seizures in seizure-prone individuals.
Ginseng, Asian (Panax ginseng)	The dried roots of the plants are used in some traditional medicines to treat a variety of conditions, including cancer. Rh2 is a ginsenoside extracted from ginseng that has effects on cell proliferation, induction of apoptosis, and positive support of conventional chemotherapy agents (Jia et al, 2004). Stimulates natural killer cells and other immune activity.	Asian ginseng may prevent various cancers (Boon and Wong, 2004). Proposed to give strength and stamina. Interactions with monoamine oxidase (MAO) inhibitors. American ginseng (*Panax quinquefolius*), a plant with similar (but not exactly the same) properties, is grown mainly in the United States. Siberian ginseng (*Acanthopanax senticosus*) has chemotherapy side effects; used for health maintenance, strength, stamina, and immunostimulation. Contraindicated in patients with hypertension and in premenopausal women.
Glucarate (calcium glucarate)	Proponents claim that glucarate may reduce the risk of colon, lung, liver, skin, prostate, and other cancers by increasing the body's ability to eliminate cancer-causing toxins that come from diet and the environment. Supporters also suggest that glucarate may hinder the formation of breast and uterine cancers by helping the body remove excess estrogen and other hormones that promote these diseases. These claims are now being studied.	Glucarate is found in many fruits and vegetables, including apples, grapefruit, broccoli, Brussels sprouts, and bean sprouts. It also occurs naturally in the body in very small amounts.

(continued)

TABLE 13-8 Herbs, Dietary Supplements, and Cancer *(continued)*

Herb or Supplement	Uses/Actions	General Comments
Green tea (*Camellia sinesis*)	Green tea contains polyphenols and may slow the delivery of nutrients to cancer cells by inhibiting the formation of new blood vessels (angiogenesis). Recent research has focused on green tea for the prevention of breast, prostate, skin, esophagus, stomach, colon, pancreas, lung, and bladder cancers. Current evidence suggests that green tea as part of the diet is useful in preventing various cancers (Boon and Wong, 2004). Antioxidant.	Use of skin products that contain green tea may be somewhat protective against skin cancers. Green tea contains epigallocatechin gallate (EGCG). EGCG may cause cancer cells to die and may stop new blood vessels from forming, thereby cutting off the supply of blood to cancer cells. Do not use with pregnant or lactating mothers. Use with caution with many drugs especially anticoagulants.
Herbal NSAIDs	Herbs are being studied for their anti-inflammatory effects that are less detrimental than COX-2 inhibitors (Block, 2005).	See Table 13-2.
Hoxsey herbal treatment	Contains arsenic and cascara, which can be toxic (Standish et al, 2002).	Not recommended.
Isatis root (Ban lan gen, *Radix isatidis baphicacanthi, Isatis tinctoria, Isatis indigotica*)	Used for common cold, sore throat, mumps, respiratory ailments, and malignant tumors. Leaves are used in one of the herbal formulas to treat prostate cancer. No adverse reactions known.	This herb is also used to treat chronic myelogenous leukemia. Studies also indicate that this plant has antiviral and immunostimulatory effects.
Kava (*Piper methysticum*)	Said to promote a reduction in anxiety. Avoid if liver disease exists. Banned by the Canadian and United Kingdom governments due to its hepatotoxic side effects. NOT RECOMMENDED.	Kava increases the "off" periods in patients taking levodopa and induces a semicomatose state when given with alprazolam (Hu et al, 2005).
Kombucha tea	Proposed role in stress reduction and in hepatic protection. There may be serious side effects. NOT RECOMMENDED.	No clear evidence to support a role in cancer treatment.
Licorice	Licorice root is an ingredient in many traditional Chinese herbal remedies. More research is needed to find out whether licorice extract has any role in cancer prevention or treatment.	May cause serious side effects, including hypertension or muscle weakness or paralysis.
Lipoic acid (alpha lipoic acid)	Lipoic acid plays an important role in metabolism. Recent research has shown that it is beneficial in treating nerve damage in diabetics. It may be helpful for other conditions as well. There is currently no evidence that lipoic acid prevents the development or spread of cancer.	Lipoic acid is an antioxidant found in certain foods, including red meat, spinach, broccoli, potatoes, yams, carrots, beets, and yeast. It is also made in small amounts in the human body. Its possible role as a form of complementary therapy to reduce the side effects of radiation therapy or chemotherapy is still unclear.
Lyprinol (green-lipped mussel)	This is a fatty acid complex extracted from *Perna canaliculus,* a green-lipped mussel (shellfish) native to New Zealand. It contains omega-3 fatty acids. Lyprinol is promoted as a dietary supplement with anti-inflammatory properties to work against leukotrienes.	It is available in capsule form as a dietary supplement.
Macrobiotic diet	The standard macrobiotic diet today consists of 50–60% organically grown whole grains, 20–25% locally and organically grown fruits and vegetables, and 5–10% soups made with vegetables, seaweed, grains, beans, and miso (a fermented soy product). Early versions of the diet included no animal products at all.	Some vegetables such as potatoes, tomatoes, eggplant, peppers, asparagus, spinach, beets, zucchini, and avocados are excluded. The diet also advises against eating fruits that do not grow locally, such as bananas, pineapples, and other tropical fruits. The use of dairy products, eggs, coffee, sugar, stimulant and aromatic herbs, red meat, poultry, and processed foods is discouraged.
Melatonin	May aid in the effectiveness of chemotherapy and in improving survival in numerous types of cancer. Melatonin inhibits tumorigenesis with suppression of tumor linoleic acid (LA) uptake and its metabolism; nocturnal dietary supplementation has the potential to be a new strategy to optimize survival and quality of life (Blask et al, 2005). Melatonin may also stimulate natural killer cells, which attack tumors. Inhibits cachexia.	Circadian rhythm may be enhanced with use of melatonin; this may help to alleviate fatigue associated with cancer (Levin et al, 2005).

(continued)

TABLE 13-8 **Herbs, Dietary Supplements, and Cancer *(continued)***

Herb or Supplement	Uses/Actions	General Comments
Milk thistle	Silymarin, an antioxidant, may be useful for treating liver diseases such as cirrhosis or chronic hepatitis. Early studies in test tubes have suggested that silymarin may help with cancer prevention. Human studies are needed. Milk thistle has been used as a cytoprotectant for the treatment and prevention of cancer; it appears to be safe for up to 41 months of use (Rainone, 2005).	It contains flavorlignans and 80% silymarin and perhaps has a role in decreasing skin or prostate cancer.
Mistletoe (Iscador)	Lectin-rich mistletoe extract should be further evaluated in patients with inoperable locally advanced pancreatic cancer (Rostock et al, 2005).	Additional research is needed (Boon and Wong, 2004). There may be toxic side effects.
Mulberry	Anthocyanins in mulberry have an anticancer effect (Chen et al, 2006).	More research is needed.
Mustard seed (*Brassica compestris*)	Mustard seeds enhance the antioxidant defense system and provide protection against the toxic effects of carcinogens (Gagandeep et al, 2005).	May protect against stomach and uterine cancers.
Nerium odorum (oleandrin, odoroside)	Raw leaves are toxic. In vitro studies have shown that Anvirzel (proprietary product) causes apoptosis in various cancer cell lines. It increases the sensitivity of human prostate cells to radiotherapy.	Anvirzel is used in cancer treatment, congenital heart diseases, hepatitis, HIV and AIDS, psoriasis, and rheumatoid arthritis. Side effects include nausea, vomiting and diarrhea, tachycardia, and arrhythmia.
Noni juice (*Morinda citrifolia*)	An immunomodulatory polysaccharide-rich substance (Noni-ppt) from the fruit juice of *Morinda citrifolia* has both prophylactic and therapeutic potentials (Furusawa et al, 2005). It is rich in potassium. Juice contains a high amount of sugar.	Noni juice is common in Polynesian diets.
Pokeweed (Poke salad)	Pokeweed antiviral protein has anti-tumor effects in mice and laboratory studies. Clinical trials have not yet been done.	All parts of the mature plant contain chemically active substances such as phytolaccine, formic acid, tannin, and resin acid, and all are mildly poisonous when eaten.
Probiotics	Evidence suggests the following beneficial effects: normalization of the intestinal microflora, ability to block the invasion of potential pathogens in the gut, prevention of colon cancer, modulation of immune function, inhibition of *Helicobacter pylori*, and possible enhancement of calcium absorption (Lin, 2003).	Regular use of yogurt and other naturally functional foods may be useful for cancer patients. Daily intake of *Bifidobacterium lactis* enhances natural immune function (Arunachalam et al, 2000). Acidophilus has been promoted for cancer prevention, but there have been no studies with humans.
Pycnogenol (pine bark extract)	Pycnogenol is the name of a group of compounds that contain proanthocyanidins taken from a number of natural sources, such as grape seeds. They contain bioflavonoids and function as an antioxidant (Huang et al, 2005).	The maritime pine tree (*Pinus pinaster*) contains naturally occurring proanthocyanidins.
Quercetin	Quercetin is promoted to help prevent or treat different types of cancer. It has also been promoted to help with the symptoms of chronic prostatitis and to relieve some of the neurological complications of diabetes.	See Table 13-2.
Reishi mushroom (*Ganoderma lucidum*)	The medicinal mushroom Reishi (*Ganoderma lucidum*) has been widely used to treat cancer, diabetes, and neurasthenia in many Asian countries (Tang et al, 2005). Used for fatigue, high cholesterol, HIV and AIDS, hypertension, immunostimulation, inflammation, strength and stamina, and viral infections.	Additional research is needed about the efficacy of Reishi (Boon and Wong, 2004). Can interfere with immunosuppressants and chemotherapeutic drugs. Adverse reactions may include dry throat and nose, GI upset, itchiness, nausea, and vomiting.
Rosemary and marjoram	Terpinoids in these spices provide anticancer effects	Ursolic acid (UA) is a triterpenoid compound that occurs naturally in a large variety of vegetarian foods, medicinal herbs, and plants.
Saffron (*Crocus sativus*)	This spice contains glutathione and crocetin, which will decrease tumor growth and also protects platelets from aggregation.	Being studied for effects on depression and Parkinson's disease also.
Saw palmetto (*Serenoa repens*)	Permixon, a phytotherapeutic agent derived from the saw palmetto plant, is a lipid/sterol extract; mixed research results suggest that further work is needed to be sure that there are anticancer effects (Hill and Kyprianou, 2004). No side effects are seen with chemotherapy in patients using saw palmetto.	Often used to prevent prostate cancer.

(continued)

TABLE 13-8 Herbs, Dietary Supplements, and Cancer *(continued)*

Herb or Supplement	Uses/Actions	General Comments
Shark cartilage	It seems to have a role in inhibiting angiogenesis. Frequently recommended to cancer patients by family members (Hyodo et al, 2005).	No evidence that it plays a role in cancer (Finkelstein, 2005; Loprinzi et al, 2005). Part of the pseudoscience related to cancer and CAM therapy (Ostrander et al, 2004). Prolonged use can have adverse side effects.
Shark oil	Alkylglycerols, found in shark liver oil, may fight cancer by killing tumor cells indirectly and activating the immune system by stimulating macrophages.	Depending on the supplement, it may be rich in omega-3 fatty acids and vitamin A.
Shiitake mushrooms	Contains lentin, which stimulates T-cell and natural killer cell production; this may have a role in leukemia (Ngai and Ng, 2003). Animal studies have found antitumor, cholesterol-lowering, and virus-inhibiting effects of the active compounds in shiitake mushrooms.	Additional research is needed about the efficacy of shiitake (Boon and Wong, 2004).
Skullcap (*Scutellaria*)	Do not take skullcap orally. Being studied for various treatments, including liver cancer (de Boer et al, 2005; Goh et al, 2005). It seems to play a role in reduction of aflatoxin toxicity (de Boer et al, 2005).	*Scutellaria barbata* (SB) is a medicinal plant that contains flavonone compounds such as scutellarein, scutellarin, carthamidin, isocarthamidin, and wogonin (Goh et al, 2005).
Soy isoflavones	Role in cancer prevention is not clear. Exact dosage and effects on specific genes are not currently known; the best advice is to encourage usual dietary use and not to change drastically. Reduces menopausal symptoms.	Soy should not be used in estrogen-dependent breast cancer or with endometrial cancer. Avoid with use of tamoxifen.
Spirulina (*Spirulina* spp; blue-green algae)	Adverse effects are uncommon unless contaminated; if contaminated, it is hepato-, nephro-, and neurotoxic.	Used to treat cancers, viral infections, weight loss, oral leukoplakia, increased cholesterol, and attention-deficit hyperactivity disorder.
St. John's wort (*Hypericum perforatum*)	Not been proven effective against acute depression. Avoid with all types of chemotherapy. St John's wort decreases the blood concentrations of cyclosporine, midazolam, tacrolimus, amitriptyline, digoxin, indinavir, warfarin, and theophylline (Hu et al, 2005).	It accelerates the effects of tamoxifen and must be used cautiously. *Hypericum* may cause breakthrough bleeding and unplanned pregnancy when used with oral contraceptives (Hu et al, 2005). Avoid use in combination with selective serotonin reuptake inhibitors and in pregnancy or lactation.
Turkey tail mushroom (*Coriolus versicolor;* Yunzhi)	*Coriolus versicolor* is a mushroom used in traditional Asian herbal remedies. Two substances (extracted from the mushroom using hot water), polysaccharide K (PSK) and polysaccharide peptide (PSP), are being studied as possible complementary cancer treatments.	
Turmeric (*Curcuma longa*)	Turmeric and other phenols have an anticancer effect (Cole et al, 2005; Yang et al, 2006). Warn breast cancer patients on cyclophosphamide to restrict the intake because it inhibits the antitumor action of these chemotherapeutic agents.	Additional research is needed about the efficacy of turmeric as a cancer treatment (Boon and Wong, 2004).
Valerian	Used to promote natural sleep; 2–4 weeks of use is needed. People who are going to have surgery should not use valerian or should taper down slowly, starting several weeks before surgery.	Avoid taking with alcohol, certain antihistamines, muscle relaxants, mental health drugs, sedatives, antiseizure drugs, or narcotics. People on cancer treatment medicines should talk with their doctors or pharmacists about possible drug interactions before taking valerian.
Wheatgrass	There have been almost no scientific studies in humans to support claims made for wheatgrass; one very small study suggested that it may help people with colitis.	Proponents suggest that wheatgrass strengthens the immune system.
White Birch (betulinic acid)	Betulinic acid may hold promise as an anticancer agent. Studies are under way to determine its potential role in treating melanoma and certain brain cancers. Randomized clinical trials are needed.	Birch bark, buds, and leaves are used as folk medicines but have not been studied to find out if they are safe or effective.

(continued)

TABLE 13-8 Herbs, Dietary Supplements, and Cancer *(continued)*

	Herbs and Treatments Associated with Toxic Side Effects
	aconite (bushi, monkshood)
	aloe vera, oral use
	arnica (wolfbane, mountain tobacco)
	aveloz (pencil cactus)
	belladonna (deadly nightshade)
	blue cohosh (squaw root)
	borage
	broom (broom tops, Irish broom)
	calamus (sweet root/flag)
	cesium chloride
	chaparral (creosote bush; *Larrea tridentate*)
	coltsfoot
	comfrey (bruisewort; *Symphytuen officinale*)
	Convallaria (lily of the valley)
	DiBella (DMB)
	ephedra (ma huang)
	germander
	germanium
	horse chestnut
	Hoxsey herbal treatment
	jimson weed
	jin bu huan
	krebiozin (creatine)
	laetrile (amygdalin)-cyanide toxicity
	licorice (*Glycyrrhiza glabra*)
	liferoot (golden senecio, ragwort)
	lobelia (Indian or wild tobacco)
	mandrake
	oleander
	Pau d'Arco (Taebuia)
	pennyroyal
	periwinkle
	poke root
	sassafras
	sea cucumber
	tea tree oil
	wormwood (madder, mug or Ming wort, *Artemisia*)
	yohimbe

Table was developed with assistance of Dr. Vijay Erankl and Valerie Kogut, MS, RD. See also: American Cancer Society. Herbs, vitamins, and minerals. http://www.cancer.org/docroot/ETO/ETO_5_2_5.asp?sitearea=ETO

- An improved nutritional status reduces side effects, promotes better rehabilitation, and improves quality of life while perhaps increasing survival rates. Malnutrition can potentiate toxicity of antineoplastic agents.
- Prevent infection or sepsis, further morbidity, or death.
- Control complications such as anemia or multiple organ dysfunction.
- In general, intake of protein should be high (1–1.5 g/kg body weight to maintain; 1.5–2 g/kg body weight to replete lean body mass) to protect from muscle wasting, malnutrition, cachexia, and treatments
- Intake of energy should be 25–35 kcal/kg body weight to maintain and 35–45 kcal/kg body weight to replete lost stores. Add calories if the patient is febrile or septic.
- Prevent or minimize weight changes. Some patients are hypometabolic; others are hypermetabolic by 10–30% above normal rates. Greatest losses occur from protein stores and body fat. Good nutritional status early is a good prognostic indicator.
- Provide structured exercise programs and specialized nutritional supplementation to preserve body mass.
- Provide appropriate and adequate, but not excessive, micronutrient supplementation. Use more foods high in phytochemicals and antioxidants. Avoid excesses of iron, but correct anemias when diagnosed.
- Schedule larger meals earlier in the day. If needed, schedule five to six small meals daily, tube feeding, or intravenous feeding. If the gut works, use it.
- Control gastrointestinal symptoms, which are more common with weight loss greater than 10%.
- After surgery or abdominal radiation, glutamine may be useful to protect from enteropathy, lower morbidity,

TABLE 13-9 General Patient Education Tips

For **cancer therapy**, start "where the patient is." Instruct patient to use unscientific treatments with caution. Discuss these issues with compassion and understanding of patient's perspective. Patients want *faith* in their doctor's expertise, *hope* for coping and for strength, and *respect* for their wishes.

For **cancer survivors**, optimal attention to nutrition should continue. Because there are different phases of cancer survivorship, from active treatment to advanced disease, existing evidence must be reviewed from which informed decisions can be made regarding dietary choices.

For **terminal, palliative care**, emotional support and comfort may be the best treatment. The patient must be included in all decisions. Hydration is the priority rather than meeting protein and energy requirements. The counselor should be aware of the stages of death and dying to identify where patient is: (a) denial, (b) anger, (c) bargaining, (d) depression and loss, or (e) acceptance.

For **family member counseling**, a "systems biology" or "functional genomics" approach teaches that nutrition is fundamental in the molecular basis of cancer (Kauwell, 2005). This "metabolomics approach" is further delineated with these principles of **nutrigenomics** (German et al, 2005):

Gene expression or DNA structure is modified by the action of nutrients and other bioactive food substances on the human genome.

Diet is a risk factor for certain diseases in individuals under specific circumstances. Cancer, heart disease, and metabolic disorders are examples.

Chronic disease onset, incidence, progression, and severity are affected by diet-regulated genes and their variants.

Diet influences health and disease through a relationship to genetic make-up.

Nutrition interventions should be tailored to the individual according to nutritional status, genotype, current health status, and nutritional requirements to prevent or to alleviate the consequences of chronic disease.

Metabolomics will allow practitioners to recognize metabolic shifts in individuals and to allow them to adapt according to shifts in environment, lifestyle, and normal progression of maturation and aging.

Food safety tips for immunosuppressed individuals (Cahruhas, 1998):

- Use safe food handling practices, including frequent hand washing, prompt and appropriate food storage, use of leftovers within 1–2 days or freezing after preparation, avoidance of public salad bars or buffets, use of safe drinking water supplies, and avoidance of ice cubes in areas where water safety is unknown (such as underdeveloped countries and well sources).
- Avoid high risk foods, such as:
  - All raw and undercooked meats, poultry, fish, and game meats
  - Sushi, raw seafood, and shellfish
  - Raw or undercooked eggs and foods made with raw eggs (such as Caesar dressing, homemade eggnog)
  - Unpasteurized milk, dairy products, juices, and cider
  - All fresh sprouts such as bean or alfalfa
  - Raw, moldy, and spoiled food items
  - Foods contaminated with *Salmonella* or other foodborne illness

augment tumor cell kill, and boost natural killer (NK) cell activity.

- Use adequate fluid for hydration.
- Use TPN if enteral nutrition is contraindicated. Parenteral nutrition (PN) is not likely to benefit advanced cancer patients who are unresponsive to treatment and should be used with caution in current or potentially septic patients because of the risks.
- Educate family about special patient needs (Dixon, 2005). Answer questions about the use of herbs and botanicals in cancer treatment plans. See Table 13-9 for more guidance and patient education tips.

SAMPLE NUTRITION DIAGNOSTIC STATEMENT

Oncology: Food–Drug Interaction

PES: Food–medication interaction related to methotrexate use with low intake of folate as evidenced by decreased serum folate level and medically diagnosed macrocytic anemia.

Assessment Data: Food records, lab reports, physician diagnosis of anemia, medication records.

Intervention: Discuss importance of increasing folic acid from diet and supplements during and after chemotherapy treatment to improve serum levels and correct the anemia; counsel about excellent food sources and recommended changes in recipes or meal planning.

Monitoring and Evaluation: Improvements in dietary and supplemental intake of folate (from food records, supplement use), lab values, and physician follow-up report about anemia status.

SAMPLE NUTRITION DIAGNOSTIC STATEMENT

Cancer: Use of Herbs and Botanicals

PES: Knowledge deficit as evidenced by patient requesting information regarding the proper use of herbs and botanicals in conjunction with cancer treatment.

Assessment: Medications, lab values, current use of herbs and botanical products.

Intervention: Education and counseling about herbs and botanical products in cancer, resources and websites, label reading.

Monitoring and Evaluation: Reports of adverse side effects with herbs and botanicals, medications, or foods (such as allergic reactions).

SAMPLE NUTRITION DIAGNOSTIC STATEMENT

Hospice Patient

PES: Inadequate oral food and beverage intake related to poor appetite as evidenced by patient and family refusing solid food and only requesting liquids for hydration.

Assessment: Palliative care order; discuss desires with patient or family.

Intervention: Liquids and requested foods on demand.

Monitoring and Evaluation: Needed only if patient improves and leaves hospice.

CANCER: TREATMENT GUIDELINES—CITED REFERENCES

Aggarwal BB, Shishodia S. Suppression of the nuclear factor-kappaB activation pathway by spice-derived phytochemicals: reasoning for seasoning. *Ann N Y Acad Sci.* 1030:434, 2004.

Arunachalam K, et al. Enhancement of natural immune function by dietary consumption of *Bifidobacterium lactis* (HN109). *Euro J Clin Nutr.* 54:263, 2000.

Baselga J. The EGFR as a target for anticancer therapy-focus on cetuximab. *Eur J Cancer.* 37:16S, 2001.

Blask DE, et al. Putting cancer to sleep at night: the neuroendocrine/circadian melatonin signal. *Endocrine* 27:178, 2005.

Block KI. The demise of the super-aspirins: an opportunity for integrative medicine? *Integr Cancer Ther.* 4:5, 2005.

Boon H, Wong J. Botanical medicine and cancer: a review of the safety and efficacy. *Expert Opin Pharmacother.* 5:2485, 2004.

Cahruhas P. Bone marrow trabnsplantation. In: Skipper A, ed. *Dietitian's handbook of enteral and parenteral nutrition.* 2nd ed. Gaithersburg, MD: Aspen Publishers, 1998, pp. 280–281.

Chen PN, et al. Mulberry anthocyanins, cyanidin 3-rutinoside and cyanidin 3-glucoside, exhibited an inhibitory effect on the migration and invasion of a human lung cancer cell line. *Cancer Lett.* 235:248, 2006.

Cole GM, et al. Prevention of Alzheimer's disease: omega-3 fatty acid and phenolic anti-oxidant interventions. *Neurobiol Aging.* 26:133, 2005.

De Boer JG, et al. Protection against aflatoxin-B1-induced liver mutagenesis by *Scutellaria baicalensis. Mutat Res.* 578:15, 2005.

Dixon SW. Nutrition care issues in the ambulatory (outpatient) head and neck cancer. *Support Line* 27:3, 2005.

Dy GK, et al. Complementary and alternative medicine use by patients enrolled onto phase I clinical trials. *J Clin Oncol.* 22:4810, 2004.

Ferrara N. VEGF as a therapeutic target in cancer. *Oncology* 69:11S, 2005.

Finkelstein JB. Sharks do get cancer: few surprises in cartilage research. *J Natl Cancer Inst.* 97:1562, 2005.

Furusawa E, et al. Antitumour potential of a polysaccharide-rich substance from the fruit juice of *Morinda citrifolia* (Noni) on sarcoma 180 ascites tumour in mice. *Phytother Res.* 17:1158, 2003.

Gagandeep DM, et al. Chemopreventive effects of mustard (*Brassica compestris*) on chemically induced tumorigenesis in murine forestomach and uterine cervix. *Hum Exp Toxicol.* 24:303, 2005.

German JB, et al. Metabolomics in practice: emerging knowledge to guide future dietetic advice toward individualized health. *J Am Diet Assoc.* 105:1425, 2005.

Goh D, et al. Inhibitory effects of a chemically standardized extract from *Scutellaria barbata* in human colon cancer cell lines, LoVo. *J Agric Food Chem.* 53:8197, 2005.

Hill B, Kyprianou N. Effect of permixon on human prostate cell growth: lack of apoptotic action. *Prostate* 61:73, 2004.

Hu Z, et al Herb-drug interactions: a literature review. *Drugs* 65:1239, 2005

Huang WW, et al. Pycnogenol induces differentiation and apoptosis in human promyeloid leukemia HL-60 cells. *Leuk Res.* 29:685, 2005.

Hyodo I, et al. Nationwide survey on complementary and alternative medicine in cancer patients in Japan. *J Clin Oncol.* 23:2645, 2005.

Jia WW, et al. Rh2, a compound extracted from ginseng, hypersensitizes multidrug-resistant tumor cells to chemotherapy. *Can J Physiol Pharmacol.* 82:431, 2004.

Kauwell GP. Emerging concepts in nutrigenomics: a preview of what is to come. *Nutr Clin Pract.* 20:75, 2005.

Kotler D. Cachexia. *Ann Intern Med.* 133:622, 2000.

Kronenberg F, et al. The future of complementary and alternative medicine for cancer. *Cancer Invest.* 23:420, 2005.

Lai PK, Roy J. Antimicrobial and chemopreventive properties of herbs and spices. *Curr Med Chem.* 11:1451, 2004.

Leonard SS, et al. Essiac tea: scavenging of reactive oxygen species and effects on DNA damage. *J Ethnopharmacol.* 103:288, 2006.

Levin RD, et al. Circadian function in patients with advanced non-small-cell lung cancer. *Br J Cancer.* 93:1202, 2005.

Lin DC. Probiotics as functional foods. *Nutr Clin Pract.* 18:497, 2003.

Loprinzi CL, et al. Evaluation of shark cartilage in patients with advanced cancer: a North Central Cancer Treatment Group trial. *Cancer* 104:176, 2005.

Lowsky R, et al. Protective conditioning for acute graft-versus-host disease. *N Engl J Med.* 353:1321, 2005.

Mattox TW. Treatment of unintentional weight loss in patients with cancer. *Nutr Clin Pract.* 20:400, 2005.

Ngai PH, Ng TB. Lentin, a novel and potent antifungal protein from shitake mushroom with inhibitory effects on activity of human immunodeficiency virus-1 reverse transcriptase and proliferation of leukemia cells. *Life Sci.* 73:3363, 2003.

Osmers R et al. Efficacy and safety of isopropanolic black cohosh extract for climacteric symptoms. *Obstet Gynecol.* 105:1074, 2005.

Ostrander GK, et al. Shark cartilage, cancer and the growing threat of pseudoscience. *Cancer Res.* 64:8485, 2004.

Prasad KN. Multiple dietary antioxidants enhance the efficacy of standard and experimental cancer therapies and decrease their toxicity. *Integr Cancer Ther.* 3:310, 2004

Rainone F. Milk thistle. *Am Fam Physician.* 72:1285, 2005.

Rostock M, et al. Anticancer activity of a lectin-rich mistletoe extract injected intratumorally into human pancreatic cancer xenografts. *Anticancer Res.* 25:1969, 2005.

Sartippour MR, et al. *Rabdosia rubescens* inhibits breast cancer growth and angiogenesis. *Int J Oncol.* 26:121, 2005.

Standish LJ, et al. Complementary and alternative medical treatment of breast cancer: a survey of licensed North American naturopathic physicians. *Altern Ther Health Med.* 8:68, 2002.

Tang W, et al. A randomized, double-blind and placebo-controlled study of a *Ganoderma lucidum* polysaccharide extract in neurasthenia. *J Med Food.* 8:53, 2005.

Tisdale MJ. Molecular pathways leading to cancer cachexia. *Physiology* 20:340, 2005.

Varlotto J, Stevenson MA. Anemia, tumor hypoxemia, and the cancer patient. *Int J Radiat Oncol Biol Phys.* 63:25, 2005.

Xiao D, Singh SV. Diallyl trisulfide, a constituent of processed garlic, inactivates Akt to trigger mitochondrial translocation of BAD and caspase-mediated apoptosis in human prostate cancer cells. *Carcinogenesis.* 27:533, 2006.

Yang X, et al. Curcumin inhibits platelet-derived growth factor-stimulated vascular smooth muscle cell function and injury-induced neointima formation. *Arterioscler Thromb Vasc Biol.* 26:85, 2006.

Yoshikawa M, et al. Inhibitory effects of coumarin and acetylene constituents from the roots of *Angelica furcijuga* on d-galactosamine/lipopolysaccharide-induced liver injury in mice and on nitric oxide production in lipopolysaccharide-activated mouse peritoneal macrophages. *Bioorg Med Chem.* 14:456, 2006.

BONE CANCER AND OSTEOSARCOMA

NUTRITIONAL ACUITY RANKING: LEVEL 3

DEFINITIONS AND BACKGROUND

Bone represents a fertile ground for cancer cells to flourish (Clines and Guise, 2005). Bone cancers include osteosarcomas, chondrosarcomas, and the Ewing family of tumors. Osteosarcoma involves a rapidly growing malignant bone tumor of unknown origin, occurring most often in the long bones of young people. Osteosarcoma is most common in males between 10 and 25 years of age. People who have had previous high doses of radiotherapy to a bone or Paget's disease have an increased risk of developing bone cancer. This type of cancer often spreads to the lung.

Metastases from other organs, such as from breast or prostate, may occur (a secondary bone cancer). Use of soy foods with genistein may slow down or prevent progression (Li et al, 2004).

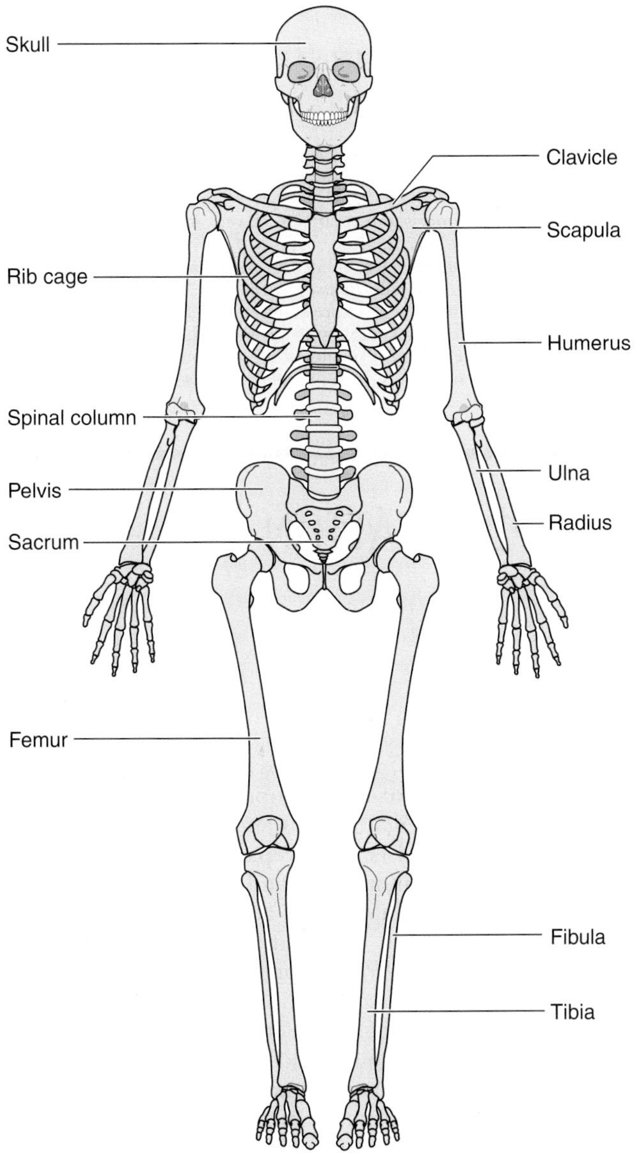

Figure 13-3 Major bones.

Symptoms and signs of bone cancer include pain over one affected extremity, weight loss, limited use of the extremity, fatigue, warmth in a local area, fever, and cough. Patients with metastasis to the spine may present with pain, neurological deficit, or both; optimal treatment should include consideration of the patient's neurological status, anatomical extent of disease, general health, age, and quality of life (Ecker et al, 2005).

The most common treatment for bone cancer pain is radiation. Radiation decreases bone cancer pain by direct effects on tumor cells (Goblirsch et al, 2005). Surgery is reserved for neurological compromise, radiation failure, or spinal instability (Ecker et al, 2005). Quality of life in this population is affected by factors such as depression, socialization problems, and physical limitations, with depression being most common (Rustoen et al, 2005).

INTERVENTION: OBJECTIVES

- Prevent dehydration; correct fever.
- Relieve pain; prolong and improve quality of life.
- Counteract effects of surgery (perhaps limb amputation), radiation therapy, or chemotherapy.
- Meet needs related to growth or elevated metabolic rate in children.

INTERVENTION: FOOD AND NUTRITION

- A balanced diet (high in energy and protein) will be needed.
- Extra fluids are used, unless contraindicated.
- Supplement with nutrients that are low in patient's dietary intake. A diet rich in zinc, vitamins A and C, and other key nutrients will help with wound healing after surgery.
- Small, frequent feedings may be better tolerated than large meals.

CLINICAL INDICATORS

Clinical/History		
Height	Pain and limited use of affected area	Cough
Weight	Fatigue	Input and output (I & O)
Weight changes	Warmth in a local area	Bone x-ray or dual-energy x-ray absorptiometry (DEXA) scan
Body mass index (BMI)	Fever, temperature	
Diet history		

Computed tomography (CT) scan or magnetic resonance imaging (MRI)	Alkaline phosphatase (Alk phos) (increased)	C-reactive protein (CRP)
Lab Work	Glucose (Gluc)	Total lymphocyte count (TLC) (varies)
Hemoglobin and hematocrit (H&H)	Ca++ (increased)	Alanine aminotransferase (ALT) (increased)
	Mg++	
	Na+, K+	
	Albumin (Alb)	

Common Drugs Used and Potential Side Effects

- Hormone therapy may be given, usually with temporary results.
- Doxorubicin may be used with side effects affecting intake. Dry mouth, anemia, stomatitis, nausea, esophagitis, or vomiting may occur.
- Bisphosphonates may be used to restrict the action of the osteoclasts, help reduce the breakdown of the bone, reduce the risk of fracture and hypercalcemia, and reduce bone pain.

Herbs, Botanicals, and Supplements (see Table 13-8)

- Herbs and botanical supplements should not be used without discussing with physician.

INTERVENTION: NUTRITION EDUCATION, COUNSELING, CARE MANAGEMENT

- Discuss ways to make meals more attractive and appetizing.
- Discuss with patient and family how to adjust diet for therapies given.
- Encourage patient to address depression or other issues that affect quality of life.

For More Information

- American Cancer Society's Bone Cancer
  http://www.cancer.org/docroot/LRN/LRN_0.asp?dt=2
- Bone Cancer Information
  http://www.cancerbacup.org.uk/Cancertype/Bone
- Bone Tumor
  http://www.bonetumor.org/
- Clinical Guidelines for Bone Cancer
  http://www.nccn.org/professionals/physician_gls/PDF/bone.pdf
- National Cancer Institute
  http://www.cancer.gov/cancer_information/cancer_type/bone/

BONE CANCER AND OSTEOSARCOMA—CITED REFERENCES

Clines GA, Guise TA. Hypercalcaemia of malignancy and basic research on mechanisms responsible for osteolytic and osteoblastic metastasis to bone. *Endocr Relat Cancer.* 12:549, 2005.

Ecker RD, et al. Diagnosis and treatment of vertebral column metastases. *Mayo Clin Proc.* 80:1177, 2005.

Goblirsch M, et al. Radiation treatment decreases bone cancer pain through direct effect on tumor cells. *Radiat Res.* 164:400, 2005.

Li Y, et al. Regulation of gene expression and inhibition of experimental prostate cancer bone metastasis by dietary genistein. *Neoplasia* 6:354, 2004.

Rustoen T, et al. Predictors of quality of life in oncology outpatients with pain from bone metastasis. *J Pain Symptom Manage.* 30:234, 2005.

HEMATOPOIETIC STEM-CELL TRANSPLANTATION

NUTRITIONAL ACUITY RANKING: LEVEL 4

DEFINITIONS AND BACKGROUND

Hematopoietic stem cells are cells from which all blood cells evolve. Since bone marrow contains the greatest concentration of blood stem cells, most transplantations historically have been bone marrow transplantations. However, with the administration of an artificial growth factor called granulocyte colony-stimulating factor (G-CSF), stem cells are stimulated to grow and leave marrow and can be collected from the bloodstream by a process called apheresis. The terms "hematopoietic stem-cell transplantation" and "peripheral-blood stem-cell transplantation" often are now used when referring to bone marrow transplantation. Currently, peripheral-blood stem-cell transplantations are being used with increased frequency. This process is much less invasive. Traditional bone marrow harvest requires the use of general anesthesia.

The objectives of bone marrow or stem-cell transplantation are to replace the malignant or defective hematopoietic system (the production and development of blood cells) and to restore normal hematopoiesis and immunological function. Treatment consists of a preparative regimen that includes high-dose chemotherapy and may also include total-body irradiation. An infusion of autologous (the patient's own), syngeneic (from an identical twin), or allogeneic (from a histocompatible related or unrelated donor) marrow follows.

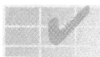

Hematological malignancies, including leukemias, lymphomas, multiple myeloma, and aplastic anemia, are the main indications for stem-cell transplantation. Nonhematological malignancies, such as testicular cancer and some autoimmune conditions, are also indications for stem-cell transplantation. Stem-cell transplantations are performed in both adult and pediatric populations. Stem-cell transplantations in patients with matched siblings versus unrelated donors have been associated with significantly better long-term survival (Talano et al, 2006). After transplantation, the patient is often neutropenic, and nutritional status may decline rapidly.

Children undergoing bone marrow transplantation may have suboptimal nutritional status; body mass index (BMI) is not an accurate indication of nutritional status in these cases (White et al, 2005). Hospitalized transplantation patients resume oral intake sooner than ambulatory patients, but no differences exist in time spent on total parenteral nutrition (TPN) or days it takes to resume good protein intake (Stern, 2000).

Treatment is aggressive and has many side effects. Early side effects are basically the same as those of any other type of high-dose chemotherapy and are caused by damage to bone marrow and other rapidly reproducing tissues of the body. Long-term side effects could include radiation damage to the lungs with shortness of breath, graft-versus-host disease (GVHD), damage to the ovaries causing infertility and loss of menstrual periods, damage to the thyroid gland causing problems with metabolism, cataracts, bone damage, and growth changes in children. Hemolytic uremic syndrome (HUS) is an uncommon but potentially life-threatening complication of stem-cell transplantation.

INTERVENTION: OBJECTIVES

Pretransplantation

- Provide adequate nutrient stores (glucose, calories, vitamins, minerals, and protein).
- Assure adequate hydration.

Posttransplantation

- Individualize needs; promote engraftment of marrow. Rejection occurs less often in well-nourished patients.
- Prevent infections, mucositis, gastroenteritis, and pneumocystosis.
- Reduce nausea, vomiting, and diarrhea, when present.
- Improve weight status; promote anabolism.
- Correct anorexia, stomatitis, xerostomia, and depression, all of which reduce total intake. Early satiety is also common.
- GVHD causes erythroderma, jaundice, abdominal pain, emaciation, pneumonitis, infections, and gastrointestinal tract problems. Hepatic veno-occlusive disease (VOD) occurs after high doses of chemotherapy in preparation for bone marrow transplantation. Rapid weight gain, elevated bilirubin, right upper quadrant (RUQ) pain, ascites, jaundice, and hepatomegaly can occur. Patients may require nutrition support during these times due to hypermetabolism and side effects of these conditions, which makes it difficult for them to achieve adequate oral intake.
- Promote positive nitrogen balance when possible.
- Correct hyperglycemia from metabolic stress, insulin resistance, and medication side effects.
- Monitor closely for renal insufficiency and necessary changes for diet.
- Prevent or prepare for long-term complications such as hyperphagia and obesity, insulin resistance and diabetes, hyperlipidemia, hypertension, and osteoporosis.
- Maximize quality of life.

INTERVENTION: FOOD AND NUTRITION

- In some cases, use of a low-bacteria (neutropenic) diet may be useful for several months before and after transplantation. A neutropenic diet guide is found in Table 13-10. Protective isolation may be needed.
- TPN may be needed to initiate recovery after transplantation. Parenteral nutrition (PN) supports long-term survival but not short-term survival; tube feeding (TF) has fewer complications. Glutamine may be an additive for both TPN and TF products. TPN may be needed with severe intestinal GVHD.
- A naso-jejunal (NJ) feeding is associated with less risk of loss due to vomiting and less risk of aspiration (Sefcick et al, 2001).
- Provide 30–35 kcal/kg to maintain weight or 35–45 kcal/kg for infection, GVHD, or neutropenia.
- Protein intake should be 1.5–2 g/kg of weight; increase during corticosteroid therapy.
- Fat intake should be 10–30% of total kcal. Monitor for hyperlipidemia over time, and modify dietary intake of fat and cholesterol as needed.

TABLE 13-10 Neutropenic Diet Guidelines

To reduce the introduction of pathogenic organisms into the gastrointestinal (GI) tract of immunocompromised patients, food safety practices and dietary changes are in order. The following are practices that may be helpful to patients after bone marrow transplantation (for 3 months or until immunosuppressive therapies are complete):

- Products may require special preparation (as with a laminar flow hood).
- Keep foods at a temperature that is safe to prevent food infection.
- Microwave hot foods immediately before service.
- Ensure careful hand washing.
- Avoid foods such as:
  - Raw or undercooked meats, fish, shellfish, poultry, eggs, game meats
  - Hot dogs, bacon, sausage, luncheon meats
  - Tofu
  - Pickled fish, cold smoked salmon, and lox
  - Raw or unpasteurized milk and dairy products
  - Deli cheeses and foods
  - Soft cheeses such as brie or blue
  - Salad dressings made with raw eggs
  - Unrefrigerated cheese-based salad dressings
  - Raw vegetable sprouts
  - Unwashed fruits or vegetables
  - Raw honey
  - Miso and tempeh products
  - Raw brewer's yeast
  - Unboiled well water
  - Powdered infant formula
  - All moldy or outdated food products
  - Unpasteurized beer

Adapted from: Oncology Nutrition Practice Group. *The clinical guide to oncology nutrition*. 2nd ed. Chicago, IL: American Dietetic Association, 2006.

SAMPLE NUTRITION DIAGNOSTIC STATEMENT

Hematopoietic Stem-Cell Transplantation

PES: Decreased oral intake related to pain and mucositis as evidenced by the refusal of food.

Assessment Data: Analysis of oral intake compared to requirements from nursing flow sheet, patient statements of pain with eating, and results of physical examination of the oral cavity.

Intervention: Diet modification for consistency.

Monitoring and Evaluation: Follow-up in 24 hours to evaluate changes in oral intake.

- If there is hyperglycemia, keep carbohydrate intake at a steady amount each day.
- Sterile water may be used to keep hydration at an adequate level to prevent renal problems. Maintain 1 mL/kcal of intake.
- A multivitamin-mineral supplement will be useful. Assure adequate intake of vitamin D and calcium with long-term steroid use. Potassium and magnesium can be depleted by some medications; monitor needs carefully. Avoid iron in supplements if transfusions have been frequent; iron overload may occur.
- Patient may need a low-lactose, low-fiber, low-fat diet. Progress, as tolerated, to a normal diet over time.
- As patient recovers and no longer requires a protective setting, use of live-culture pasteurized yogurt may be beneficial to increase bowel flora. *Lactobacillus acidophilus* therapy also can be helpful.

TABLE 13-11 Drugs Commonly Used in Bone Marrow or Stem-Cell Transplantation

Drug	Comments
Analgesics, antihistamines, and antidepressants	Monitor for specific side effects.
Antibiotics	Amphotericin may be used to fight infections. Nausea, stomach pain, or vomiting may occur.
Antivirals	Acyclovir may be given prophylactically to resolve oral ulcers. Headaches, gastrointestinal (GI) distress, or diarrhea may occur.
Bisphosphonates	These may be needed if there is osteopenia or osteoporosis.
Chemotherapy	Busulfan (to destroy marrow stem cells) or cyclophosphamide (Cytoxan) can cause nausea, vomiting, diarrhea, and anorexia.
	Methotrexate, fludarabine, carmustine, and cyclophosphamide may cause anorexia, mucositis, and esophagitis; some also cause diarrhea.
	Gleevec interferes with an abnormal enzyme that sends signals to the nucleus of a cancer cell. Nausea, extensive diarrhea, and vomiting are potential side effects. Useful for leukemia or advanced stomach cancer.
Immunosuppressive therapy (graft-versus-host disease [GVHD] prophylaxis)	GVHD prophylaxis consists of T-cell depletion (antibody T10B9 or OKT3 and complement) with posttransplantation cyclosporine (Talano et al, 2006).
	Antithymocyte globulin may cause vomiting, nausea, diarrhea, and stomatitis.
	Azathioprine may cause vomiting, nausea, diarrhea, mucosal ulceration, esophagitis, and steatorrhea.
	Beclomethasone can lead to thrush, nausea, and xerostomia.
	Corticosteroids cause sodium and fluid retention, weight gain, hyperglycemia, skeletal muscle wasting, growth retardation in children, peptic ulceration, and elevated triglycerides.
	Cyclosporine (as Sandimmune) may cause nausea and vomiting, skin rashes, hemorrhagic cystitis, and altered potassium metabolism.
	Methotrexate causes nausea and vomiting, mucositis, esophagitis, diarrhea, renal and liver changes, decreased absorption of vitamin B_{12}, fat, and D-xylose, and taste changes.
	Monoclonal antibodies cause nausea and vomiting.
	Sirolimus elevates triglycerides.
	Tacrolimus can be nephrotoxic or cause hyperglycemia, hyperkalemia, or hypomagnesemia.
	Ursodeoxycholic acid can cause nausea and vomiting, diarrhea, and GI distress.
Insulin	May be needed if there is hyperglycemia.
Filgrastim (Neupogen)	Neutropenia secondary to immune suppression may be managed with Neupogen and a low-bacteria diet.
Oral hygiene	Clotrimazole (Mycelex) may cause nausea or vomiting; it is used for oral hygiene and prevention of oral candidiasis.
Total-body irradiation (TBI)	Side effects vary for each individual, but anorexia, diarrhea, and mucositis or esophagitis are common.

CLINICAL INDICATORS

Clinical/History
- Height
- Weight
- BMI
- Weight changes
- Diet history
- Temperature
- Ascites, jaundice
- I & O

Lab Work
- H & H
- Bilirubin
- Gluc
- Mg++, Ca++
- Complete blood count (CBC)
- Absolute neutrophil count (ANC) to evaluate engrafting
- Na+, K+
- Alb, transthyretin
- CRP
- Retinol-binding protein (RBP)
- Serum phosphorus (low from cyclosporine A)
- Uric acid
- Cholesterol (Chol), triglycerides (Trig)
- TLC (varied reliability)
- Ferritin
- Transferrin
- Blood urea nitrogen (BUN), creatinine (Creat)

Common Drugs Used and Potential Side Effects

- See Table 13-11.

Herbs, Botanicals, and Supplements (see Table 13-8)

- Herbs and botanical supplements should not be used without discussing with physician.
- St. John's wort and echinacea should not be taken with cyclosporine because they alter drug functioning.

INTERVENTION: NUTRITION EDUCATION, COUNSELING, CARE MANAGEMENT

- Discuss needed protection against environmental infections (e.g., safe food handling and preparation, keeping foods at proper temperatures, use of sterile water, reheating foods properly).
- The neutropenic, low-bacteria diet includes careful use of raw fruits and vegetables, milk, and shellfish—all of which may be contaminated easily with bacteria. These diets are often used in bone marrow transplantation units.
- Small, frequent meals of bland, cold consistency may be well tolerated.
- Discuss any necessary nutritional support methods and procedures to be used at home or in discharge planning. Transition from TPN and PN to enteral nutrition or oral diet will be helpful.
- Physical therapy may be helpful to maintain strength and to regain mobility.

Patient Education—Food Safety

- Educate about food safety issues.

For More Information

- Bone Marrow Support Group
http://www.bmtsupport.ie/

HEMATOPOIETIC STEM-CELL TRANSPLANTATION—CITED REFERENCES

Sefcick A, et al. Naso-jejunal feeding in allogeneic bone marrow transplant recipients: results of a pilot study. *Bone Marrow Transplant.* 28:1135, 2001.

Stern J. Impact of a randomized, controlled trial of liberal vs conservative hospital discharge criteria on energy, protein, and fluid intake in patients who received marrow transplants. *J Am Diet Assoc.* 2100:1015, 2000.

Talano JM, et al. Alternative donor bone marrow transplant for children with Philadelphia chromosome ALL. *Bone Marrow Transplant.* 37:135, 2006.

White M, et al. Nutritional status and energy expenditure in children pre-bone-marrow-transplant. *Bone Marrow Transplant.* 35:775, 2005.

BRAIN TUMOR

NUTRITIONAL ACUITY RANKING: LEVEL 3

DEFINITIONS AND BACKGROUND

Tumors are either primary or secondary when they are found in the brain. Primary brain tumors start their growth in the brain and can be benign or malignant. They can occur in children, especially girls between the ages of 5 and 9. About 17,000 Americans each year are diagnosed with a primary brain tumor.

Secondary brain tumors are more common, with about 90,000 cases diagnosed each year. These tumors result from cancer that has metastasized to the brain from the lung, breast, or other part of the body. Constituting 50% of brain tumors, a glioma is a tumor of neurological origin.

Glioblastoma multiforme (GBM) is a central nervous system (CNS) neoplasm, especially related to the cerebrum. Tarceva and Iressa are epidermal growth factor receptor (EGFR) kinase inhibitors that were developed with treatment possibilities in a range of cancers in which EGFR plays a role. Some glioblastomas respond to these medications.

TABLE 13-12 Types of Brain Tumors

Type of Tumor	Cell Origin and Function
Oligodendroglioma	Produces a substance called myelin, which covers the nerves and helps information to travel quickly between the brain and other parts of the body.
Ependymoma	Lines the ventricles and aids in the circulation of cerebrospinal fluid.
Meningioma	Covers and protects the brain and spinal cord.
Lymphoma	Part of the immune system, the body's primary defense against infection and foreign substances.
Schwannoma	Produces the myelin that protects the acoustic nerve for hearing.
Medulloblastoma	These cells normally do not remain in the body after birth.

Source: OncoLink. Accessed November 16, 2005 at http://www.oncolink.org.

Headache is the most common symptom in brain tumor illness (Stewart-Amidei, 2005). Other symptoms and signs include vertigo, altered consciousness, convulsions, inability to follow commands, mental or personality changes, unequal pupil response, hemianopsia, blurred or decreased vision, ptosis, tinnitus, altered gait, dysphagia, vomiting with or without nausea, aphasia, elevated blood pressure, and loss of sense of smell. Depression, fatigue, and memory and personality changes may complicate care (Stewart-Amidei, 2005).

Because malignant brain tumors are largely dependent on glycolysis for energy, normal neurons and glia readily transition to ketone bodies (beta-hydroxybutyrate) for energy when glucose levels are reduced; dietary energy restriction and the ketogenic diet may have a role in managing malignant brain tumors (Seyfried and Mukherjee, 2005). Several types of brain tumors can be treated successfully with multiple treatment methods, including surgery, radiation therapy, and chemotherapy. Emerging and new technologies allow physicians to target and treat brain tumors more precisely. Genomic deletion of chromosomes 6, 21, and 22 represents new targets for further research (Lassman et al, 2005). Table 13-12 describes types of brain tumors and cells of origin.

INTERVENTION: OBJECTIVES

- Provide adequate energy (30 kcal/kg or more if needed).
- Provide adequate protein: surgery: 1.2–1.5 g/kg body weight; radiation: 1.0–1.2 g/kg body weight. Consider: adjust for renal/hepatic dysfunction; obesity (>25% ideal body weight [IBW]) using IBW; and skin breakdown and/or wound healing.
- Avoid constipation and straining.
- Prevent lower respiratory infections with coughing, which can increase intracranial pressure.
- Counteract side effects of therapy (e.g., radiation, surgery).
- Monitor carefully for elevated blood glucose levels, which may occur secondary to corticosteroids that are used to control brain edema.

INTERVENTION: FOOD AND NUTRITION

- Maintain diet, as ordered, with extra fluid, unless contraindicated.
- If oral diet is possible, use a protective diet by including fish, fruits, vegetables, and adequate fiber.
- Alter texture and liquids, if necessary, for dysphagia. If necessary, tube feed or offer TPN.
- Limit sodium to 4–6 g/d to correct cerebral edema.
- Offer meal setup and assistance with eating, altered liquid/food textures, and/or enteral tube feedings for patients with cognitive deficits, swallowing difficulties, or limited function of upper extremity.

CLINICAL INDICATORS

Clinical/History

Height
Weight
BMI
Weight changes
Diet history
Aphasia
Blood pressure (BP)
Cerebral edema, headaches
Vertigo
Altered consciousness or convulsions
Inability to follow commands
Mental or personality changes
Unequal pupil response
Hemianopsia, blurred or decreased vision
Tinnitus
Altered gait
Dysphagia
Vomiting (with or without nausea)
Loss of sense of smell
Temperature
CT scan
Diffusion MRI
Skull x-ray
Electroencephalogram (EEG)
Immobility

Lab Work

Gluc (elevated)
Cerebrospinal fluid (CSF)—elevated protein levels
Alb, transthyretin
CRP
TLC, white blood cell count (WBC) (altered)
WBC in CSF (normal or increased)
Transferrin
ALT (elevated)
NA+, K+
Serum folate

Common Drugs Used and Potential Side Effects

- Seizures are best managed with antiepileptic drug therapy (Stewart-Amidei, 2005). Levetiracetam (Keppra), an anticonvulsant, reduces seizures in malignant brain tumors and may help improve chemotherapy outcomes. Side effects may include a decrease in serum folacin levels and other nutrients; monitor carefully.
- Use of procarbazine (an antineoplastic) may warrant restriction of tyramine-containing foods secondary to its monoamine oxidase (MAO) inhibitor–like action.
- Nonsteroidal anti-inflammatory agents may help to reduce inflammation (Byrne, 2005).
- Steroid therapy may be used. Decrease sodium and increase potassium if appropriate. Negative nitrogen balance or hyperglycemia may result over time. Maintain near-normal blood glucose levels if possible.
- Temozolomide (Temodar) was recently approved for brain cancer and GBM in particular.

Herbs, Botanicals, and Supplements (see Table 13-8)

- Herbs and botanical supplements should not be used without discussing with physician.

INTERVENTION: NUTRITION EDUCATION, COUNSELING, CARE MANAGEMENT

- The importance of regular and attractive meals should be stressed to help appetite if fair or poor. Keep in mind that sense of smell may have declined recently.
- Discuss importance of a balanced diet with good sources of protein at meals.
- Early discussion about end-of-life issues is necessary because the disease can impair decision-making ability (Stewart-Amidei, 2005).
- A multidisciplinary approach using physical, occupational, and speech therapies is essential to maximize neurological function and activities of daily living.

For More Information

- Brain Tumor Clinical Trials: Musella Foundation
http://www.virtualtrials.com/musella.cfm
- National Brain Tumor Foundation
http://www.braintumor.org/
- OncoLink—Brain Cancer
http://cancer.med.upenn.edu/disease/brain/

BRAIN TUMOR—CITED REFERENCES

Byrne TN. Cognitive sequelae of brain tumor treatment. *Curr Opin Neurol.* 18:662, 2005.

Lassman AB, et al. Molecular study of malignant gliomas treated with epidermal growth factor receptor inhibitors: tissue analysis from North American Brain Tumor Consortium Trials. *Clin Cancer Res.* 11:7841, 2005.

Seyfried TN, Mukherjee P. Targeting energy metabolism in brain cancer: review and hypothesis. *Nutr Metab (London).* 2:30, 2005.

Stewart-Amidei C. Managing symptoms and side effects during brain tumor illness. *Expert Rev Neurother.* 5:71S, 2005.

BREAST CANCER

NUTRITIONAL ACUITY RANKING: LEVEL 2–3

DEFINITIONS AND BACKGROUND

Breast cancer (mammary carcinoma) is the second most common site of cancer in women, with over 200,000 cases diagnosed annually in the United States. It affects one in nine women at some point in their lives. Breast cancer in men is less common and generally is preceded by gynecomastia.

Mutations in the *BRCA1* gene result in an elevated risk of breast cancer and ovarian cancer (Kroiss et al, 2005). *BRCA1* is located on chromosome 17. Primary care physicians should not routinely refer all women for genetic counseling and DNA testing to detect the presence of specific gene mutations, according to the U.S. Preventive Services Task Force. When a woman has specific family history patterns that put her at risk for these gene mutations, her primary care physician should suggest DNA testing; only about 2% of women have this level of risk. Having routine breast screenings for cancer is more important.

Onset of breast cancer is more common after age 30. Age and health history can affect the risk of developing breast cancer. Fertility, ovarian function, and estrogen exposure play a role in the onset of breast cancer. Exposure to diets that produce high levels of estrogen seems to be most important in utero and after menopause; high estrogen levels during reproductive years seem to be protective. American Institute for Cancer Research (AICR) has found that a higher intake of sugary and refined carbohydrates is connected with breast cancer; fiber curbs insulin secretion and should be encouraged.

Breast cancer may be related to oxidative stress. Obesity and Western dietary patterns may independently provoke hyperinsulinemic insulin resistance at puberty. In teen girls, anovulation may decrease breast cancer. Weight gain in the years preceding onset of menses is a promoter: increased fat cell adiposity increases estrogen availability at this time.

An increased risk of breast cancer may be observed among woman who frequently consumed French fries at preschool age; whole milk intake slightly decreases risk, and these data suggest a possible association between diet before puberty and the subsequent risk of breast cancer (Michels et al, 2006). Monounsaturated fats (e.g., olive oil, canola oil) may cause cancer cells to commit "cell suicide."

Soy is found to be most protective in younger women. Eating soy foods yields greater benefits than taking isoflavone supplements (Li et al, 2005). Being physically active is also protective against breast cancer.

Alcohol intake is a problem, especially if folic acid intake is low (need about 600 μg to be protective). Limit alcohol to no more than one drink per day.

Total duration of breastfeeding is associated with a reduced risk of breast cancer (Lipworth et al, 2000). Women with deleterious *BRCA1* mutations who breastfed for a cumulative total of more than 1 year had a statistically significantly reduced risk of breast cancer; no such association was seen for *BRCA2* (Jernstrom et al, 2004).

Breast cancer can be treated very effectively, especially when it is diagnosed in early stages. Staging of breast cancer is described in Table 13-13. Tumors are frequently found in the upper/outer quadrant of the breast (45%) and nipple area (25%), with 30% identified in other breast areas. In early stages, a single nontender, firm, or hard mass with poorly defined margins may exist. Later, skin or nipple re-

TABLE 13-13 Staging of Breast Cancer

- Stage 0: In situ—Cancer cells are present in either the lining of a breast lobule or a duct, but they have not spread to the surrounding fatty tissue.
- Stage I: Rarely metastasizing/noninvasive (<2 cm or 1 inch in diameter)—Cancer has spread from the lobules or ducts to nearby tissue in the breast; cancer has not spread to the lymph nodes.
- Stage II: Rarely metastasizing/invasive—The tumor can range from 2 cm to <5 cm in diameter (approximately 1–2 inches); sometimes, cancer may have spread to the lymph nodes.
- Stage III: Moderately metastasizing/invasive (≥2 inches)—Cancer cells have grown extensively into axillary (underarm) lymph nodes.
- Stage IV: Highly metastasizing/invasive into other parts of the body, such as bone, liver, lung, or brain.

traction, axillary lymphadenopathy, breast enlargement, redness, mild edema, and pain may occur. In late stages, ulceration, moderate edema, and metastases to bone, liver, or brain are common.

Four standard types of therapy are used to treat breast cancer: surgery for removal of cancerous tissue and, sometimes, other tissue; radiation therapy; chemotherapy; and hormonal therapy. New types of therapy are being researched through clinical trials.

INTERVENTION: OBJECTIVES

- Control side effects of therapy and treatments (e.g., local or extensive mastectomy, chemotherapy, external-beam radiation therapy, brachytherapy).
- Promote good nutritional status to reduce future incidents and recurrence.
- Encourage regular breast self-examinations.
- Maintain or attain appropriate weight for height. Patient should lose weight before treatment, if obese, but be careful not to lose lean body mass (LBM).
- Increase likelihood of survival, wellness, and improved quality of life. Promote protective foods.
- For mastectomy patients, promote wound healing and prevent infection.
- Monitor genetic responsiveness to 6-n-propylthiouracil (PROP) and preferences for fruits and vegetables. Generally, lower acceptance of cruciferous and selected green and raw vegetables occurs in women who report disliking such foods; they tend to be medium or super tasters of PROP (Drewnowski, 2000). PROP-sensitive tasters may seek to reduce bitterness by adding fat, sugar, or salt to their vegetables.
- Women undergoing hormonal therapies are prone to unwanted weight gain, and weight management or counseling may be needed.

INTERVENTION: FOOD AND NUTRITION

- A diet with controlled total energy and fat may be helpful. Obesity may promote original tumor growth, and extra calories seem to play a key role. A 10–20% fat intake, with a decrease in saturated fatty acids to 7%, has been suggested. Overall, the Western style of diet should be discouraged (Adebamowo et al, 2005).
- A protective diet should be encouraged, such as a Mediterranean diet (Masala et al, 2006).
- At least 5–9 fruits and vegetables (Ahn et al, 2005; Rock et al, 2005) and 6 grain foods daily should be encouraged for access to important nutrients, fiber, and phytochemicals. Use of olive or canola oils, grape juice or red wine, and cheese seems to be beneficial. The fruits and vegetables should include sources of alpha- and beta-carotene, zeaxanthin, and lycopene. Garlic, bromelain, and curcumin should be used often for seasoning foods. Calorie restriction and use of omega-3 fatty acids may be potent as an anti-inflammatory diet (Jolly, 2005). Include fiber from beans and lentils frequently.
- Alcoholic beverages in amounts greater than one drink per day should be discouraged because alcohol has a role in promoting estrogen receptor–positive tumors (Suzuki et al, 2005). Red wine and resveratrol may be acceptable.
- The use of phytoestrogens (e.g., soy foods, flaxseed) has been encouraged to decrease the risk of developing breast cancer or to lengthen the disease-free period. Because there is conflicting research regarding the role that phytoestrogens play in promoting breast cancer cell growth, patients with breast cancer should limit concentrated sources of phytoestrogens in their diet.
- Intake of soy seems to be protective for most women unless they are estrogen sensitive (Fang et al, 2005; Li et al, 2005). An isoflavone-rich diet might include wild leafy greens (as in the Greek diet), celery stalks, shredded lettuce, sweet peppers, raw spinach, fresh lemon, and sprigs of fresh parsley.
- Dietary sources of vitamins and minerals that meet Dietary Reference Intake (DRI) and recommended dietary allowance (RDA) levels are usually adequate, but a general supplement also may be safely recommended. This is especially important for folic acid (Zhang et al, 2005), calcium, vitamin D, vitamin A, vitamin C, and vitamin E as alpha-tocopherol.

CLINICAL INDICATORS

Clinical/History

Height
Weight
BMI
Weight changes
Diet history
Anorexia, nausea
Breast self-examination—masses
Calcifications
Biopsy
Skin or nipple retraction
Axillary lymphadenopathy
Breast enlargement
Redness, mild edema, pain
Ulceration, moderate edema
I & O
Temperature

Lab Work

Serum estrogen
Estrogen receptors (positive or negative)
Carcinoembryonic antigen (CEA)
Prolactin
Serum carotenoid levels
Mg++, Ca++
H & H
Gluc
Alk phos

Erythrocyte sedimentation rate (ESR) to evaluate	metastasis Complete blood cell count (CBC)	Chol, Trig Alb, transthyretin CRP Mammography

Common Drugs Used and Potential Side Effects

- For patients who are **estrogen receptor positive**, hormonal therapy may be a breast cancer promoter; oral contraceptive use should be monitored or discontinued. Estrogen replacement (to prevent osteoporosis) increases risk levels by 2.5% annually but reduces risks for stroke, hip fracture, and coronary heart disease (CHD).
- Antiestrogen therapy with tamoxifen (Noraldex) may be prescribed to treat estrogen-dependent breast cancer or be used in women at high risk. Nausea, vomiting, and hot flashes are common side effects.
- For patients who are **estrogen receptor negative**, hormonal therapy actually may be recommended (e.g., progesterone and androgen therapy). Megestrol acetate (a hormonal antineoplastic drug and a synthetic derivative of progesterone) can reverse anorexia and weight loss in some women. Appetite improvement often is noted.
- Chemotherapy also may be used. Taste alterations are common for beef, chicken, and coffee. Cyclophosphamide (Cytoxan) requires extra fluid intake. Doxorubicin, fluorouracil, and methotrexate are also commonly used; many gastrointestinal (GI) side effects are noted.
- Anastrozole (Arimidex) can cause anorexia, weight changes, nausea, vomiting, dry mouth, constipation, and diarrhea.
- Gemcitabine (Gemzar) in combination with paclitaxel is indicated for the first-line treatment of patients with metastatic breast cancer after failure of other chemotherapy.
- Trastuzumab (Herceptin) helps with early-stage HER2 breast cancer as an adjunct to chemotherapy to decrease recurrence.

Herbs, Botanicals, and Supplements (see Table 13-8)

- Herbs and botanical supplements should not be used without discussing with physician.
- Grape seed extract may be protective, but more studies are needed (Kim, 2005).
- Omega-3 fatty acids in combination with other nutrients (namely, vitamin C, vitamin E, beta-carotene, selenium, and coenzyme Q10) may prove to be of particular value for preventing and treating breast cancer. Dietary intake is recommended over supplements at this time.
- Dehydroepiandrosterone (DHEA; taken to delay aging) may stimulate late promotion of breast cancer in postmenopausal women and should be avoided.
- With use of methotrexate (Rheumatrex), avoid echinacea because of potential damage to liver.
- The following herbal/botanical supplements should be avoided by patients with breast cancer because of their phytoestrogen content:

  Ginseng
  Gingko biloba
  Licorice root
  Black cohosh
  Wild yam root
  DHEA

INTERVENTION: NUTRITION EDUCATION, COUNSELING, CARE MANAGEMENT

- For prevention and to reduce risk of recurrence, breast cancer detection projects are available throughout the United States. Check with local chapter of the National Cancer Institute (NCI) and the American Cancer Society (ACS). Early detection of new tumors is crucial because lower stage tumors are much easier to control.
- Attain or maintain healthy body weight.
- Discuss ways to make meals more appetizing, especially if appetite is poor.
- Counsel patient regarding a prudent diet to prevent weight gain or to lose weight if needed. Eat a diet high in whole grains, fruits, and vegetables. Diets rich in fruit intake, rather than supplement use, help to reduce breast cancer risk (Ahn et al, 2005). Low total energy or lower fat dietary patterns may also be helpful (Elias et al, 2005).
- Reduced intake of sweet and high-glycemic index foods is recommended (Tavani et al, 2006).
- Use of moderate amounts of soy should be encouraged. Consumers of soy foods are more likely to have higher levels of education and report eating five or more daily servings of fruits and vegetables (Fang et al, 2005).
- Exercise is an important preventive factor.
- Daughters of women with breast cancer should have a first mammogram before 40 years of age as a baseline and annually every 1–2 years thereafter. Lumps and changes should be reported immediately to a physician.
- Reduce intake of alcoholic beverages; limit to no more than one alcoholic drink per day (Suzuki et al, 2005).
- Calcium supplementation at 500–1000 mg/d may be indicated for patients who are menopausal or postmenopausal. These patients may be unable to take hormone replacement therapy, putting them at increased risk for developing osteoporosis.

For More Information

- Clinical Practice Guidelines for Breast Cancer
  http://www.nccn.org/professionals/physician_gls/PDF/breast.pdf
- Cornell University
  http://envirocancer.cornell.edu/factsheet/diet/fs49.BCRisk.cfm
- National Alliance of Breast Cancer Organizations
  http://www.nabco.org/
- National Breast Cancer Coalition
  http://www.stopbreastcancer.org/
- National Breast Cancer Risk Assessment
  http://www.cancer.gov/clinicaltrials/NCI-00-C-0039
- Program on Breast Cancer and Environmental Risk Factors
  http://envirocancer.cornell.edu/learning

- Onco-Link
  http://oncolink.upenn.edu/
- Sisters Network
  http://www.sistersnetworkinc.org/
- Treatment Decisions
  http://www.nccn.org/patients/patient_gls/_english/_breast/contents.asp
- Y-Me National Breast Cancer Organization
  http://www.y-me.org/

BREAST CANCER—CITED REFERENCES

Adebamowo CA, et al. Dietary patterns and the risk of breast cancer. *Ann Epidemiol.* 15:789, 2005.

Ahn J, et al. Associations between breast cancer risk and the catalase genotype, fruit and vegetable consumption, and supplement use. *Am J Epidemiol.* 162:943, 2005.

Drewnowski A, et al. Genetic taste markers and preferences for vegetables and fruit of female breast cancer patients. *J Am Diet Assoc.* 100:191, 2000.

Elias SG, et al. The 1944–1945 Dutch famine and subsequent overall cancer incidence. *Cancer Epidemiol Biomarkers Prev.* 14:1981, 2005.

Fang CY, et al. Correlates of soy food consumption in women at increased risk for breast cancer. *J Am Diet Assoc.* 105:1552, 2005.

Jernstrom H, et al. Breast-feeding and the risk of breast cancer in BRCA1 and BRCA2 mutation carriers. *J Natl Cancer Inst.* 96:1094, 2004.

Jolly CA. Diet manipulation and prevention of aging, cancer and autoimmune disease. *Curr Opin Clin Nutr Metab Care.* 8:382, 2005.

Kim H. New nutrition, proteomics, and how both can enhance studies in cancer prevention and therapy. *J Nutr.* 135:2715, 2005.

Kroiss R, et al. Younger birth cohort correlates with higher breast and ovarian cancer risk in European BRCA1 mutation carriers. *Hum Mutat.* 26:583, 2005.

Li Y, et al. Inactivation of nuclear factor kappaB by soy isoflavone genistein contributes to increased apoptosis induced by chemotherapeutic agents in human cancer cells. *Cancer Res.* 65:6934, 2005.

Lipworth L, et al. History of breastfeeding in relation to breast cancer risk: a review of the epidemiological literature. *J Natl Cancer Inst.* 92:302, 2000.

Masala G, et al. Dietary and lifestyle determinants of mammographic breast density. A longitudinal study in a Mediterranean population. *Int J Cancer.* 118:1782, 2006.

Michels KB, et al. Preschool diet and adult risk of breast cancer. *Int J Cancer.* 118:749, 2006.

Rock CL, et al. Plasma carotenoids and recurrence-free survival in women with a history of breast cancer. *J Clin Oncol.* 23:6631, 2005.

Suzuki R, et al. Alcohol and postmenopausal breast cancer risk defined by estrogen and progesterone receptor status: a prospective cohort study. *J Natl Cancer Inst.* 97:1601, 2005.

Tavani A, et al. Consumption of sweet foods and breast cancer risk in Italy. *Ann Oncol.* 17:341, 2006.

Zhang SM, et al. Folate intake and risk of breast cancer characterized by hormone receptor status. *Cancer Epidemiol Biomarkers Prev.* 14:2004, 2005.

CHORIOCARCINOMA

NUTRITIONAL ACUITY RANKING: LEVEL 3

DEFINITIONS AND BACKGROUND

Choriocarcinoma involves a highly malignant neoplasm of the placenta with secretion of human chorionic gonadotropin (hCG). It may develop in women after a molar pregnancy (where the fetus does not develop but a tumor develops instead), a miscarriage, or a full-term delivery. Rarely, it may occur in males. Gestational choriocarcinoma occurs in approximately 1 in 20,000–40,000 pregnancies (Alvarez et al, 2005).

Diet may affect the development of this type of cancer because the placenta has such a large role in nutrient availability (Briese et al, 2005). Placental trophoblasts and newly identified proteins known as B7 immunomodulatory molecules are under investigation (Petroff et al, 2005).

Symptoms and signs in women include profuse or intermittent vaginal bleeding, discharge between menses, cough, hemoptysis, headache, nausea and vomiting, hypertension, tachypnea, vaginal or vulvar lesion, anemia, sepsis, weight loss, and cachexia. Alternative names include chorioblastoma, trophoblastic tumor, chorioepithelioma, invasive/malignant mole, gestational trophoblastic disease, and gestational trophoblastic neoplasia

After an initial diagnosis, a careful history and examination are done to rule out metastasis. Gestational choriocarcinoma is responsive to chemotherapy; surgical excision is reserved for acute emergencies (Alvarez et al, 2005). A hysterectomy is rarely indicated but may be used for some women under age 40.

INTERVENTION: OBJECTIVES

- Maintain appropriate weight for height. Correct weight loss and cachexia.
- Correct side effects of chemotherapy if used.
- Treat and correct all other side effects of therapy and disease state.
- Prepare patient for surgery, if necessary.

INTERVENTION: FOOD AND NUTRITION

- Modify diet to patient preferences.
- Increase liquids as needed.
- Provide adequate protein, B-complex vitamins, iron, calories, and other nutrients for wound healing, as appropriate. Use RDA and DRI levels as a guide.
- Alter texture of diet if patient is fatigued at mealtimes or if stomatitis occurs after chemotherapy.

CLINICAL INDICATORS

Clinical/History

- Height
- Weight
- BMI
- Weight loss?
- Diet history
- Nausea, vomiting
- Temperature
- I & O
- BP; hypertension?
- Vaginal bleeding
- Discharge between menses
- Cough, hemoptysis
- Headache
- Nausea and vomiting
- Tachypnea
- Vaginal or vulvar lesion
- Sepsis?
- Cachexia?

Lab Work

- Human chorionic gonadotropin (hCG) titer
- Alb, transthyretin
- CRP
- Transferrin
- Gluc
- H & H
- Serum Fe
- Mg++, Ca++
- TLC (varies)
- Na+, K+
- ALT (increased)

Common Drugs Used and Potential Side Effects

- Methotrexate may be used; nausea and vomiting are common side effects. Administer with glucose to reduce toxicity.
- Vincristine or dactinomycin may also be used. Constipation or dysphagia can occur with vincristine. Dry mouth or stomatitis/esophagitis may occur with dactinomycin.

Herbs, Botanicals, and Supplements (see Table 13-8)

- Herbs and botanical supplements should not be used without discussing with physician.

INTERVENTION: NUTRITION EDUCATION, COUNSELING, CARE MANAGEMENT

- Nausea or vomiting may require small, frequent feedings and control of fluid intake at mealtimes.
- See general cancer entry for more suggestions specific to individual patient's side effects from therapy.

For More Information

- Family Practice Notebook–Choriocarcinoma http://www.fpnotebook.com/OB65.htm

CHORIOCARCINOMA—CITED REFERENCES

Alvarez NR, et al. Metastatic choriocarcinoma to the pancreas. *Am Surg.* 71:330, 2005.

Briese J, et al. Osteopontin expression in gestational trophoblastic diseases: correlation with expression of the adhesion molecule, CEACAM1. *Int J Gynecol Pathol.* 24:271, 2005.

Petroff MG, et al. The immunomodulatory proteins B7-DC, B7-H2, and B7-H3 are differentially expressed across gestation in the human placenta. *Am J Pathol.* 167:465, 2005.

COLORECTAL CANCER

NUTRITIONAL ACUITY RANKING: LEVEL 3–4

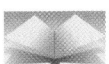

DEFINITIONS AND BACKGROUND

Colorectal cancer currently is the second most common type of cancer in the United States. Family history of colorectal cancer is a risk factor in 25% of cases. High risk also exists among patients with ulcerative colitis and Crohn's disease after 8 or more years of duration. Incidence of colorectal cancer rises significantly after age 50 and doubles with each successive decade. Cyclooxygenase-2 (COX-2) and its proinflammatory metabolite, prostaglandin E_2 (PGE2), enhance colon cancer progression, but this remains poorly understood (Castellone et al, 2005). The inflammatory stress response is a complex, integrated biological network in which several key molecules regulate gene expression (Staib et al, 2005).

Purine synthesis may be a relevant biological mechanism linking folate metabolism to colon cancer risk (Ulrich et al, 2005). The PREVENT intervention trial found the following to potentially reduce the risk for colorectal cancer: reducing alcohol and red meat consumption; increasing fruit and vegetable and multivitamin intake; reducing smoking; and increasing physical activity (Emmons et al, 2005). Table 13-14 lists factors that either promote or prevent the risks of colon cancer.

Fecal occult blood test and flexible sigmoidoscopy are methods of choice for diagnosis. Standard colonoscopy (optical) may be replaced by computed tomography (CT) colonoscopy (virtual) eventually because CT is less invasive and requires less sedation. A virtual colonoscopy is not available in all facilities.

In **cancer of the small intestine**, malignancy generally is found in the lower duodenum and lower ileum, with a high rate of mortality and few early symptoms; it presents in only 5% of cases. The adenomatous polyp is the precursor of most, if not all, colorectal cancers (see Fig. 13-4). In the **colon,** slow-growing malignancies are usually found in the cecum, lower ascending colon, and sigmoid colon; prognosis is optimistic, but few early symptoms are found.

TABLE 13-14 Risks and Preventive Factors for Colorectal Cancer

Preventive Factors	Risk Factors
Aspirin or nonsteroidal anti-inflammatory drugs (Gao et al, 2005; Samoha and Arber, 2005).	Alcohol excess is a risk.
Calcium intake seems to be important to reduce polyp proliferation by binding bile acids.	Abdominal obesity and its metabolic effects of increased blood glucose and insulin levels
Chicken may be protective.	Processed meats (bacon, sausage, hot dogs, ham, and lunch meats).
Folate is protective (Bingham et al, 2005; Choi and Mason, 2000). Dietary supplements of folic acid, omega-3 fatty acids, and calcium may reduce colon cancer risk (Bruce et al, 2005).	Overweight and obesity increase the risk of developing colon cancer (McTiernan, 2005).
Green tea seems to be protective (Ju et al, 2005).	Red meat and low intake of green vegetables are risks (deVogel et al, 2005).
Lutein (spinach, broccoli, lettuce, tomatoes, oranges, orange juice, carrots, celery, and greens) may help prevent colon cancer.	A Western-style diet that is high in fat and low in calcium and vitamin D can dramatically increase and accelerate tumor formation (Yang et al, 2005).
Omega-3 fatty acids appear to reduce the risk of colorectal cancer (Reddy et al, 2005).	
Selenium in high levels can reduce colorectal polyps.	
Sulforaphane (broccoli) may be protective (Myzak et al, 2006).	
Vitamin D and lactose may also play a role (Spina et al, 2005; Ma et al, 2001).	

Rectal cancer is more common in men than in women and often occurs after middle age, with bleeding, pain, and irregular bowel habits.

Symptoms and signs of colorectal cancers include: weakness, weight loss, anorexia, anemia, dehydration, electrolyte imbalance, intestinal obstruction, bowel abscess, fistula, altered bowel habits, rectal bleeding, abdominal cramping, pain, and distention. The right side of the colon (ascending) absorbs fluids and salts; cancer spreads upward here; obstruction is rare. The left side of the colon (the descending colon) stores feces; cancer here tends to encircle the bowel and cause obstructions. If surgery is required, maintaining the ileocecal valve is crucial.

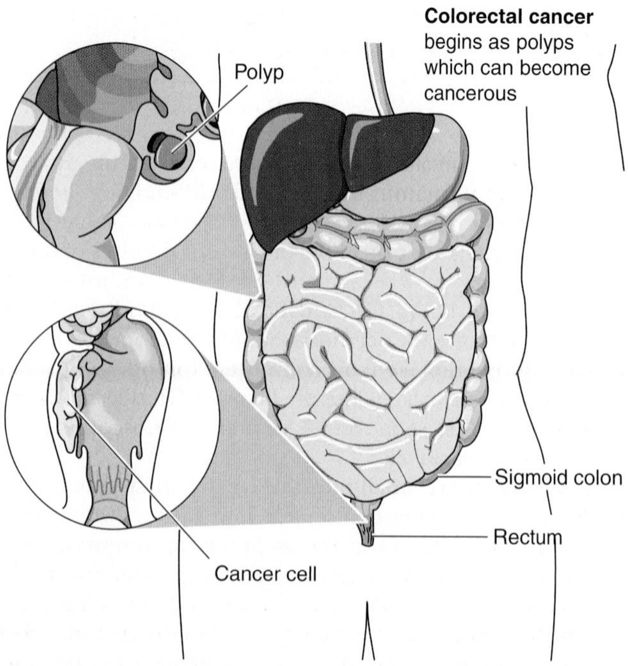

Figure 13-4 Colorectal cancer.

INTERVENTION: OBJECTIVES

- Decrease residue, especially with obstruction, until fiber is better tolerated.
- Prevent further weight loss; correct anemia and dehydration.
- Counteract side effects of therapies; resection is common. Chemotherapy or radiation is also used.
- Provide nutrients in a tolerable form—oral, parenteral, or enteral.
- Provide sufficient calcium, vitamin D, and dairy products. Calcium may block tumor-producing effects of dietary fats by binding free fatty acids in the lumen.
- Prevent or ameliorate starvation diarrhea.
- Protect against recurrence by dietary changes indicated in Table 13-14.
- Maintain adequate hydration.

INTERVENTION: FOOD AND NUTRITION

- TPN or TF may be needed for an extended period of time. Include glutamine in either type of solution.
- Administer parenteral fluids with adequate electrolytes, vitamins C and K, and selenium (if used over a long time). Vitamin D, calcium, iron, zinc, and fat intakes also should be monitored for adequacy.
- With ileal resection, vitamin B_{12} deficiency can occur, bile salts may be lost in diarrhea, and hyperoxaluria and renal oxalate stones can be a problem. With massive bowel resection, malabsorption, malnutrition, metabolic acidosis, and gastric hypersecretion may result.

- With ileostomy and colostomy, salt and sodium/water balance are problems. Ostomy diets may be needed (see ileostomy and colostomy entries in Section 7). Increase energy and ensure adequate protein.
- As needed, decrease fiber until tolerated. Eventually increase whole grains including rye bread, cereals, fruits, and vegetables. Eat less meat (use more poultry, fish, tofu, and beans as primary protein sources), more fiber such as cereal, and more vitamin D.
- If oral diet is possible, discuss protective foods, such as chicken and other poultry; calcium-rich foods; carotenoid-rich foods for lutein and lycopene (tomato products, watermelon, spinach, kale, greens, broccoli, romaine lettuce, and pink grapefruit); use of cumin; cereal, bean, vegetable, and fruit fiber; flavonoids (apples, onions, green tea, and chamomile tea); folic acid in spinach, broccoli, asparagus, avocado, orange juice, dried beans, and fortified cereals; cruciferous vegetables; coffee; less red meat; omega-3 fatty acid foods such as fish and walnuts; selenium foods such as Brazil nuts; and unsaturated fats such as flaxseed, salmon, and canola and olive oils. In addition, a multivitamin supplement is beneficial, especially for vitamins B_6 and D.
- Monitor carefully for possible lactose intolerance. Decrease intake of lactose or use lactase enzyme products when indicated.
- Physical activity should be encouraged as much as possible.

CLINICAL INDICATORS

Clinical/History

- Height
- Weight (loss?)
- BMI
- Diet history
- Rectal bleeding, pain
- Irregular bowel habits
- Weakness
- Anorexia
- Dehydration, electrolyte imbalances
- Intestinal obstruction, bowel abscess
- Fistula
- Proctoscopy
- Colonoscopy
- Digital rectal examination

Lab Work

- CEA level (CEA 125)
- Colon lavage cytology
- Melena (stool test)
- H & H (decreased)
- Serum Fe
- Transferrin
- Na+
- K+ (often decreased)
- Chol, Trig
- TLC (varies)
- WBC, ESR (increased)
- Alb, transthyretin
- CRP
- RBP
- Mg++, Ca++
- Serum zinc

Common Drugs Used and Potential Side Effects

- Bevacizumab (Avastin) use leads to a significant decrease in colon cancer deaths.
- Cetuximab (Erbitux), when added to chemotherapy, will shrink tumors and delay progression.
- COX-2 inhibitors are helpful because 50% of polyps and 85% of colonic tumors in humans overexpress COX-2 (Samoha and Arber, 2005). Regular low doses of aspirin may help prevent colon cancer by reducing prostaglandin production. Nitric oxide–donating aspirin (NO-ASA) is a promising chemopreventive agent against colon cancer and other cancers (Gao et al, 2005).
- Chemotherapy may be used; monitor side effects accordingly because these agents may further impact bowel function. Fluorouracil plus levamisole, methotrexate, mitomycin, lomustine, vincristine, and similar agents are used commonly. Diarrhea, nausea, vomiting, low WBC, and mouth sores can occur.
- The multidrug combination of oxaliplatin, fluorouracil, and leucovorin is currently considered as the gold standard treatment for metastatic colorectal carcinoma (Caraglia et al, 2005).

Herbs, Botanicals, and Supplements (see Table 13-8)

- Herbs and botanical supplements should not be used without discussing with physician.
- With use of methotrexate (Rheumatrex), avoid echinacea for potential damage to the liver.
- Low-dose fish oil supplementation may be useful to reduce inflammation.

INTERVENTION: NUTRITION EDUCATION, COUNSELING, CARE MANAGEMENT

- Discuss appropriate dietary regimen for specific problems generated by therapy.
- Encourage family participation in all levels of care.
- Discuss how to prevent further tumors or polyps. Increasing intake of berries, vitamin D and calcium in dairy products, chocolate, coffee, soy foods, folate from foods and supplements, lutein and carotenoids from fruits or vegetables, and rye and whole grains should be suggested. Medical advice may include frequent use of aspirin or nonsteroidal anti-inflammatory drugs (NSAIDs).
- Encourage consumption of milk for its useful calcium, vitamin D, and lactose content. If necessary, use lactase enzymes if intolerance exists; monitor also for verified milk allergy and avoid milk in those cases.
- Encourage physical activity when feasible.
- Surveillance following curative cancer treatment generally includes interval history and physical examinations every 6 months for 5 years, then every 3 months for 2 years, and then every 6 months for 3–5 years for colorectal cancer (Sunga et al, 2005).
- Limit foods that may cause gas, such as corn, broccoli, cauliflower, beans, cabbage, melon, and carbonated beverages.
- Provide instruction on the use of fiber to help with bowel management, especially for rectal cancer patients.
- Provide education on signs and symptoms of dehydration.
- Family members (offspring and other first-degree relatives) should have a digital examination annually at 40 years of age, stool tests for blood after 50 years of age, and sigmoidoscopy or colonoscopy after age 50 every 3–5 years. An annual fecal occult blood test (FOBT) can also be useful.

For More Information

- Clinical Practice Guidelines for Anal Cancer
  http://www.nccn.org/professionals/physician_gls/PDF/anal.pdf
- Clinical Practice Guidelines for Colon Cancer
  http://www.nccn.org/professionals/physician_gls/PDF/colon.pdf
- Clinical Practice Guidelines for Rectal Cancer
  http://www.nccn.org/professionals/physician_gls/PDF/rectal.pdf
- Colorectal Cancer Network
  http://www.colorectal-cancer.net/
- Colorectal Cancer Prevention and Control Initiatives
  http://www.cdc.gov/cancer/colorctl/colorect.htm
- Colorectal Cancer Screening
  http://www.gastro.org/public/cc_screening.html#Diagnosed
- Medline Information–Colorectal Cancer
  http://www.nlm.nih.gov/medlineplus/colorectalcancer.html
- National Colorectal Cancer Action Campaign
  http://www.cdc.gov/cancer/screenforlife/
- Treatment Options
  http://www.nccn.org/patients/patient_gls/_english/_colon/contents.asp

COLORECTAL CANCER—CITED REFERENCES

Bingham SA, et al. Is the association with fiber from foods in colorectal cancer confounded by folate intake? *Cancer Epidemiol Biomarkers Prev.* 14:1552, 2005.

Bruce WR, et al. A pilot randomised controlled trial to reduce colorectal cancer risk markers associated with B-vitamin deficiency, insulin resistance and colonic inflammation. *Br J Cancer.* 93:639, 2005.

Caraglia MD, et al. Chemotherapy regimen GOLF induces apoptosis in colon cancer cells through multi-chaperone complex inactivation and increased Raf-1 ubiquitin-dependent degradation. *Cancer Biol Ther.* 4:1159, 2005.

Castellone MD, et al. Prostaglandin E2 promotes colon cancer cell growth through a novel Gs-axin-beta-catenin signaling axis. *Science* 310:1504, 2005.

Choi S, Mason J. Folate and carcinogenesis: an integrated scheme. *J Nutr.* 130:129, 2000.

de Vogel J, et al. Natural chlorophyll but not chlorophyllin prevents heme-induced cytotoxic and hyperproliferative effects in rat colon. *J Nutr.* 135:1995, 2005.

Emmons KM, et al. Project PREVENT: a randomized trial to reduce multiple behavioral risk factors for colon cancer. *Cancer Epidemiol Biomarkers Prev.* 14:1453, 2005.

Gao J, et al. Nitric oxide-donating aspirin induces apoptosis in human colon cancer cells through induction of oxidative stress. *Proc Natl Acad Sci U S A.* 102:17207, 2005.

Ju J, et al. Inhibition of intestinal tumorigenesis in apcmin/+ mice by (-)-epigallocatechin-3-gallate, the major catechin in green tea. *Cancer Res.* 65:10623, 2005.

Ma J, et al. Milk intake, circulating levels of insulin-like growth factor-I, and risk of colorectal cancer in men. *J Natl Cancer Inst.* 93:1330, 2001.

McTiernan A. Obesity and cancer: the risks, science, and potential management strategies. *Oncology* 19:871, 2005.

Myzak MC, et al. Sulforaphane inhibits histone deacetylase activity in BPH-1, LnCaP, and PC-3 prostate epithelial cells. *Carcinogenesis* 27:811, 2006.

Reddy BS, et al. Prevention of colon cancer by low doses of celecoxib, a cyclooxygenase inhibitor, administered in diet rich in omega-3 polyunsaturated fatty acids. *Cancer Res.* 65:8022, 2005.

Samoha S, Arber N. Cyclooxygenase-2 inhibition prevents colorectal cancer: from the bench to the bed side. *Oncology* 69:33S, 2005.

Spina C, et al. Colon cancer and solar ultraviolet B radiation and prevention and treatment of colon cancer in mice with vitamin D and its Gemini analogs. *J Steroid Biochem Mol Biol.* 97:111, 2005.

Staib F, et al. The p53 tumor suppressor network is a key responder to microenvironmental components of chronic inflammatory stress. *Cancer Res.* 65:10255, 2005.

Sunga AY, et al. Care of cancer survivors. *Am Fam Physician.* 71:699, 2005.

Ulrich CM, et al. Polymorphisms in the reduced folate carrier, thymidylate synthase, or methionine synthase and risk of colon cancer. *Cancer Epidemiol Biomarkers Prev.* 14:2509, 2005.

Yang K, et al. Dietary components modify gene expression: implications for carcinogenesis. *J Nutr.* 135:2710, 2005.

ESOPHAGEAL, HEAD AND NECK, AND THYROID CANCERS

NUTRITIONAL ACUITY RANKING: LEVEL 3–4

DEFINITIONS AND BACKGROUND

Head and neck cancers include the following cancers: hypopharyngeal cancer; laryngeal cancer; lip and oral cavity cancer; metastatic squamous neck cancer with occult primary; nasopharyngeal cancer; oropharyngeal cancer; paranasal sinus and nasal cavity cancer; parathyroid cancer; salivary gland cancer; and esophageal cancer. Annually, about 38,000 people in the United States are diagnosed with a head or neck cancer, and the highest overall incidence rate is in black males.

Thyroid cancer affects about 26,000 people in the United States. Thyroid-stimulating hormone (TSH) from the pituitary causes the thyroid gland to produce thyroid hormones and to release thyroglobulin. TSH is likely to cause most thyroid tumors. Thyroxine medicine (Synthroid, Levoxyl, and Unithroid) is needed to keep TSH levels low (Spencer, 2005).

Etiology is linked to tobacco use and alcohol for all tumor sites (see Table 13-15). Viruses such as human papillomavirus (HPV) and the herpes viruses are now considered possible contributors to some cases of oral cancer. A diet lacking fruits and vegetables may play a role; low vitamin C intake, low use of whole grains, and high use of refined grains are implicated (Levi et al, 2000). High doses of vitamin E do not protect against head and neck cancers; in fact, supplementation with 400 IU/d may promote cancer progression. Zinc deficiency has been associated with esophageal cancer. Folate insufficiency may be important in the pathogenesis of squamous cell carcinomas of the head and neck (SCCHN); folate repletion may be effective for chemoprevention, especially in susceptible individuals who use alcohol and tobacco (Kane, 2005).

Prognosis for cure worsens as the depth of tumor invasion increases. Surgery is possible for some cases. Cervicofacial and cervicothoracic rotation flaps provide a reliable means to reconstruct complex defects of the face, lateral skull base, and neck, with the potential for excellent results (Moore et al, 2005). Radiation therapy side effects may include odynophagia, dysphagia, mucositis, esophagitis, xerostomia (with occasional osteoradionecrosis), dental caries, weight loss, taste changes, and decreased appetite. Many head and neck cancer

TABLE 13-15 Key Factors in Types of Head and Neck Cancer

Site	Comments
Oral cavity	May present with gingival swelling, pain, bleeding, and loosening teeth. Oral cancer is more prevalent in persons with chronically unclean mouths or in persons with poorly fitting dentures. A goal includes elimination of irritation and infections. The disorder is rare in persons younger than age 40. Risk of metastasis is great; only about half of these individuals will live longer than 5 years.
Nasopharynx	Signs include unilateral obstruction, epistaxis, pain, otological changes, and nasal obstruction.
Oropharynx	There may be a dull ache, dysphagia, referred otalgia, and trismus.
Larynx	Symptoms include voice changes, dysphagia, odynophagia, and dyspnea.
Parotid and salivary glands	Unilateral symptoms and impaired jaw mobility can occur. The parotid gland is the largest salivary gland. Cancer here is rare. Surgery is often curative.
Esophageal cancer	Develops in the middle or lower third of the esophagus. It is one of the more common types of head and neck cancer; primarily presents as adenocarcinoma or squamous cell cases that require surgical resection. This condition is more common in persons older than 50 years of age, especially males. Barrett's esophagus (BE) is a premalignant condition associated with esophageal cancer; cyclooxygenase-2 (COX-2) is an inducible enzyme that is overexpressed. Aspirin and other nonsteroidal anti-inflammatory drugs may help prevent esophageal cancer from developing in patients with BE because of the reduction in inflammation. Signs and symptoms include dysphagia, painful swallowing, substernal pain, feeling of fullness, weight loss, malaise, malnutrition, dehydration, anemia, regurgitation after eating, electrolyte imbalance, hiccups, foul breath, aspiration, increased salivation, hoarseness, coughing, and hepatomegaly.
	Stage 0: Very early cancer, found only in the first layer of cells in the lining of the esophagus.
	Stage I: Cancer is found in only a small part of the esophagus and has not spread to nearby tissues, lymph nodes, or other organs.
	Stage II: Cancer is found in a large portion of the esophagus and has spread to all sides of the esophagus and may have spread to local lymph nodes, but has not spread to other tissues.
	Stage III: Cancer has spread to tissues or lymph nodes near the esophagus but has not spread to other parts of the body.
	Stage IV: Cancer has metastasized.
Thyroid cancer	A lump on the side of the neck, hoarseness, and dysphagia can be signs. Thyroidectomy may be used, or radioactive iodine (RDI) can be used to destroy cancerous cells that remain after surgery. A low-iodine diet may be needed about 2 weeks before the RDI treatment.

patients are malnourished before treatment begins, and those who are treated with radiotherapy are at an increased risk of malnutrition due to the severe side effects (Moore et al, 2005; Wood, 2005). Prophylactic placement of a gastrostomy feeding tube is recommended (Anwander et al, 2004).

INTERVENTION: OBJECTIVES

- Prevent malnutrition, further weight loss, cachexia, and aspiration. Weight loss, caused by acute mucositis and dysphagia, is common during concurrent chemotherapy and irradiation (chemoradiotherapy) of head and neck cancer (Lin et al, 2005).
- Hydrate adequately; encourage fluids between meals and limit fluid intake at meals to improve intake of other foods.
- Promote positive nitrogen balance and prevent loss of lean body mass (LBM).
- Prepare for treatments, such as surgery, radiation, or chemotherapy.
- Correct anemia.
- Prevent sepsis, abscesses, and infection; provide good mouth care.
- Monitor for dysphagia, difficulty chewing, mucositis, xerostomia, fibrosis, and dental caries after treatments.
- Omit alcoholic beverages and abstain from tobacco, including chewing snuff.
- In patients with advanced cancer, goals are to reduce the symptoms of large tumors, preserve organ function, and improve quality of life.
- Maintain adequate hydration.
- Minimize weight loss.
- Promote adequate bowel function.
- Promote adequate wound healing.
- Provide 100% of the RDA with tube feeding and oral intake. Progress to tube feeding goal with minimal signs and symptoms of intolerance (i.e., nausea, fullness). Transition to full or partial oral intake when feasible.
- If resection is needed, fat malabsorption, reflux, dumping syndrome, increased mediastinal pressure, and increased food transit time may be side effects. Nutrition support for patients with head and neck cancer is associated with a significant increase in total energy ingestion (Moore et al, 2005). Placing gastrostomy tubes prophylactically prevents disruption to treatment plans (Wood, 2005).

INTERVENTION: FOOD AND NUTRITION

- After radiation: xerostomia, ulceration, bleeding, and pain may result; after chemotherapy, nausea, vomiting, weakness, and fatigue may occur (Dixon, 2005).
- A dysphagia diet (thick pureed foods, decrease in thin liquids) may be needed if swallowing is difficult. Provide a

diet high in energy and protein with bland or pureed foods as required. Adjust diet individually to meet patient's needs: 30–35 kcal/kg; 1.0–1.5 g protein/kg may be needed.

- Tolerance will vary for hot and cold foods and drinks. Monitor and alter intake accordingly.
- Patients are often fed with gastrostomy or jejunostomy feedings. Cellular and morphological changes follow a period of malnutrition; enteral feeding is an important strategy for maintaining gut integrity and function (Sica et al, 2005). Use of immediate enteral feeding with formulas that are high in omega-3 fatty acids can be helpful (Aiko et al, 2005).
- Increase fluid intake as tolerated; dehydration is common.
- Increase intake of vitamins A and C, zinc, and other nutrients that may be low. A diet rich in fruits and vegetables is associated with a reduced risk of head and neck cancer (Falciglia et al, 2005). Otherwise, a multivitamin-mineral supplement is indicated if oral intake is not possible.
- Initiation of oral feeding 48 hours after total laryngectomy is a safe clinical practice (Medina and Khafif, 2001).
- If esophagectomy has been performed, gastric stasis can occur. The use of needle catheter jejunostomy (NCJ) is safe, with an extremely low rate of complications over a prolonged period of time at low costs; routine use in patients undergoing esophagectomy is recommended (Sica et al, 2005).
- Decrease use of irritants when oral diet is possible (e.g., black pepper, chili powder) and dilute acidic fruits or juices, such as orange, grapefruit, and tomato.
- Use protective foods to prevent recurrence (if oral diet is possible). These include fiber-rich foods such as beans, vegetables, fish, foods rich in zinc and lycopene, whole grains, citrus fruits, and vitamin C–rich foods.
- If the patient has thyroid cancer, a low-iodine diet may be needed prior to treatment.
- In advanced cases, palliative care may be needed.

CLINICAL INDICATORS

Clinical/History

Height
Weight
BMI
Usual weight
Weight changes
Diet history
BP
I & O
Dehydration?
Temperature
Dysphagia, painful swallowing
Substernal pain or feeling of fullness
Malaise
Malnutrition
Anemia
Regurgitation after eating
Hiccups, foul breath
Aspiration
Increased salivation
Hoarseness and coughing
Gingival swelling, pain, bleeding, or hyperplasia
Nonhealing ulcerative oral lesions
Mucositis, esophagitis
Xerostomia
Dental caries
Taste changes, decreased appetite
Loosening teeth
Oral biopsy
Esophageal webs with achalasia?
Palpable mass
Barium swallow
Endoscopy
Nasopharyngoscopy
Direct laryngoscopy, esophagoscopy
Biopsy

Lab Work

Alb, transthyretin
CRP
Transferrin
H & H
ALT (increased)
Gluc
Triiodothyronine (T3), thyroxine (T4), thyroid-stimulating hormone (TSH)
Ca++, Mg++
Na+, K+
Alb, transthyretin
Chol
Bicarbonate

Common Drugs Used and Potential Side Effects

- Aspirin can lower esophageal cancer risk by 90% by reducing prostaglandin production. Some doctors will prescribe a low daily dose to prevent recurrence.
- Chemotherapy with cisplatin may be used, along with radiation therapy. Cisplatin can cause nausea, vomiting, altered taste, changes in renal function, and diarrhea. Weight loss during cisplatin-containing chemoradiotherapy is associated with reduced kidney function; findings highlight the importance of intensive supportive measures of nutrition and hydration beyond standard measures, and these steps should be started before 10% weight loss occurs (Lin et al, 2005).
- Bleomycin and methotrexate can lead to nausea, vomiting, anorexia, or stomatitis.
- Tarceva is being investigated for use in head and neck cancers.
- Steroids may be used to reduce inflammation; hyperglycemia, sodium retention, potassium depletion, and negative nitrogen balance can result.

Herbs, Botanicals, and Supplements (see Table 13-8)

- Herbs and botanical supplements should not be used without discussing with physician.
- With methotrexate (Rheumatrex), avoid echinacea because of potential damage to the liver.
- With cyclosporine, avoid use with echinacea and St. John's wort because of counterproductive effects on the drug.

INTERVENTION: NUTRITION EDUCATION, COUNSELING, CARE MANAGEMENT

- Discuss a diet rationale that is appropriate for patient's condition. If patient can eat orally, encourage him or her to chew slowly.
- If jejunostomy feeding is required after esophagastric surgery, teach patient/family/caretaker how to prepare feedings and how to produce the item in a clean environment.
- Encourage help from speech therapy services.
- Hypothyroid status can cause dysphagia; counsel accordingly.

- If oral diet is possible, discuss use of protective foods, including fiber-rich foods (such as beans), vegetables, fish, foods rich in zinc and lycopene, whole grains, citrus fruits, and vitamin C–rich foods.
- Relaxation therapy or biofeedback can be beneficial.
- During radiation therapy/surgical recovery, patients with gastrostomy tubes should be encouraged to practice swallowing exercises, as prescribed by the speech pathologist, to maintain swallowing function and reduce the risk of fibrosis.
- Radiation-induced fibrosis (RIF) is caused by reduced blood supply months or years later; rinse with vitamin E solutions and use 1000 IU tocopherol with pentoxifylline to decrease mucositis (Chiao and Lee, 2005; Haddad et al, 2005). Use small frequent feedings and oral supplements.

For More Information

- American Oral Cancer Clinic
  http://www.tonguecancer.com/oral_cancer.htm
- CancerLinks USA–Esophageal Cancer
  http://www.cancerlinksusa.com/esophagus/wynk/
- Medline–Esophageal Cancer
  http://www.nlm.nih.gov/medlineplus/esophagealcancer.html
- National Cancer Institute–Esophageal Cancer
  http://www.cancer.gov/cancerinfo/wyntk/esophagus
- National Institutes of Health Cancer Information
  http://www.nidr.nih.gov/Spectrum/NIDCR3/3menu.htm
- Oncology Channel
  http://www.oncologychannel.com/esophagealcancer/
- OnTumor.com
  http://www.ontumor.com/esophageal.htm
- Oral Cancer Consortium
  http://www.oral-cancer.org/
- Thyroid Cancer Survivors' Association
  http://www.thyca.org/

ESOPHAGEAL, HEAD AND NECK, AND THYROID CANCERS—CITED REFERENCES

Aiko S, et al. The effects of immediate enteral feeding with a formula containing high levels of omega-3 fatty acids in patients after surgery for esophageal cancer. *J Parent Enter Nutr.* 29:141, 2005.

Anwander T, et al. Percutaneous endoscopic gastrostomy for long-term feeding of patients with oropharyngeal tumors. *Nutr Cancer.* 50:40, 2004.

Chiao TB, Lee AJ. Role of pentoxifylline and vitamin E in attenuation of radiation-induced fibrosis. *Ann Pharmacother.* 39:516, 2005.

Dixon SW. Nutrition care issues in the ambulatory (outpatient) head and neck cancer. *Support Line* 27:3, 2005.

Falciglia GA, et al. A clinical-based intervention improves diet in patients with head and neck cancer at risk for second primary cancer. *J Am Diet Assoc.* 105:1609, 2005.

Haddad P, et al. Pentoxifylline and vitamin E combination for superficial radiation-induced fibrosis: a phase II clinical trial. *Radiother Oncol.* 77:324, 2005.

Kane MA. The role of folates in squamous cell carcinoma of the head and neck. *Cancer Detect Prev.* 29:46, 2005.

Levi F, et al. Refined and whole grain cereals and the risk of oral, esophageal, and laryngeal cancer. *Euro J Clin Nutr.* 54:487, 2000.

Lin A, et al. Metabolic abnormalities associated with weight loss during chemoirradiation of head-and-neck cancer. *Int J Radiat Oncol Biol Phys.* 63:1413, 2005.

Medina J, Khafif A. Early oral feeding following total laryngectomy. *Laryngoscope* 111:368, 2001.

Moore BA, et al. Cervicofacial and cervicothoracic rotation flaps in head and neck reconstruction. *Head Neck.* 27:1092, 2005.

Sica GS, et al. Needle catheter jejunostomy at esophagectomy for cancer. *J Surg Oncol.* 91:276, 2005.

Spencer C. Thyroglobulin (Tg) and Tg antibody (TgAb) testing for patients treated for thyroid cancers. Accessed November 25, 2005 at http://www.thyca.org/thyroglobulin.htm.

Wood K. Audit of nutritional guidelines for head and neck cancer patients undergoing radiotherapy. *J Hum Nutr Diet.* 18:343, 2005.

GASTRIC CANCER

NUTRITIONAL ACUITY RANKING: LEVEL 3–4

DEFINITIONS AND BACKGROUND

Gastric cancer is a carcinoma that most commonly occurs in the pyloric segment and along the lesser curvature. Often, no early definitive signs are evident. Symptoms and signs include a feeling of fullness, indigestion, dysphagia, anorexia, weight loss, anemia, occasional vomiting, belching, and melena. Gastric cancer often follows long-term pernicious anemia, Ménétrier's disease, or chronic gastritis. It is generally found in males aged 50–70 years, often among smokers. Vitamin C seems to be protective, but green tea does not appear to be protective. Physical activity may protect against gastric adenocarcinoma; more studies are needed (Vigen et al, 2006). Risks of gastric cancer are listed in Table 13-16. It is believed that *Helicobacter pylori* infection plays a role. The mechanism underlying *H. pylori*–induced carcinogenesis is not clear; chemokine production and antiapoptosis seem to be mediated by *H. pylori*–induced processing of nuclear factor-kappa B, which drives lymphocytes to acquire malignant potential (Ohmae et al, 2005). Genetic predisposition may be another risk factor in gastric cancer. *P65* gene expression is connected with poor prognosis for patients suffering from gastric cancer; this expression does not depend on *H. pylori* infection (Balcerczak et al, 2005).

A diet rich in sulforaphane from broccoli sprouts significantly reduces *H. pylori* infection (Fahey et al, 2002; Galan et al, 2004). High intake of antioxidant vitamins contributes to the reduction of gastric cancer risk (Kim et al, 2005).

In a rare form of previously incurable stomach cancer known as gastrointestinal stromal tumor (GIST), imatinib (Gleevec) may shrink tumors by more than half with minimal side effects, leading to an extended remission (Heinrich and Corless, 2005).

TABLE 13-16 Risks for Gastric Cancer

Advanced age
Chronic atrophic gastritis, pernicious anemia, gastric polyps, family history of gastric cancer, Ménétrier's disease, intestinal metaplasia
Diet high in salt, salted foods, smoked and preserved foods
Ethnicity—young white and Hispanic males more commonly; and African Americans from poor socioeconomic backgrounds
Helicobacter pylori gastric infection
High intakes of protein, saturated fat, cholesterol, and sodium (Qiu et al, 2005)
High alcohol intake
Low use of fruits and vegetables
Male gender
Smoking
Occupational exposures

INTERVENTION: OBJECTIVES

- Prevent or reverse weight loss and further malnutrition.
- Encourage fluids.
- Counteract side effects of chemotherapy, radiation, or gastrectomy. If gastrectomy is performed, dumping syndrome or hypochlorhydria may result.
- Correct protein-losing enteropathy.
- Improve quality of life.
- Prevent cancer recurrence by including protective foods.
- Promote wound healing. Replete visceral proteins as stress level decreases.

INTERVENTION: FOOD AND NUTRITION

- Parenteral therapy or total parenteral nutrition (TPN) may be used, especially before surgery. After removal of parts of the stomach, patients are often volume sensitive and need small meals and snacks with fluids between meals.
- If oral intake is allowed, try light meals that are nutrient dense and well balanced. A high-protein/high-energy diet will be needed.
- Generally, 2–3 L of fluid is required throughout the day, unless contraindicated for other reasons.
- If stomach has not been resected, include protective foods such as *Allium* in garlic (raw or lightly cooked); carotenoids and lycopene (Ito et al, 2005; Yuan et al, 2004); fish; fruits; nonherbal tea; polyunsaturated fat, vitamin A, and ascorbic acid (Qiu et al, 2005); indoles (cruciferous vegetables) and sulforaphane (Fahey et al, 2002); and yellow onions and shallots for quercetin.
- After gastrectomy, prepare for dumping syndrome (see gastrectomy entry in Section 7). Small, frequent feedings may be better tolerated; concentrated carbohydrates, alcohol, and use of carbonated beverages should be limited or omitted.
- Jejunostomy at time of resection may be indicated.
- Be sure that dietary intake (or supplementation) includes selenium and other key nutrients for wound healing and correction of anemia. Take supplements with food because they are often not tolerated on an empty stomach. If the stomach was resected, vitamin B_{12} anemia is likely to occur within several years; monitor carefully.
- Drink fluids between meals.

CLINICAL INDICATORS

Clinical/History		Lab Work
Height	Dysphagia, anorexia	Alb, transthyretin
Weight	Anemia, pallor	CRP
BMI	Vertigo	Ca++, Mg++
Weight losses	Nausea or vomiting	Na+, K+
Diet history	Temperature	Gluc
I & O, dehydration?	Anorexia	H & H
BP	MRI or CT scan	Transferrin
Feelings of fullness, indigestion	Barium swallow	ALT (increased)
	Endoscopy	Melena, occult blood
		Serum B_{12}

Common Drugs Used and Potential Side Effects

- Cytotoxic drugs such as mitomycin C may cause fever, nausea, vomiting, anorexia, and stomatitis.
- Imatinib (Gleevec) interferes with an abnormal enzyme that sends signals to the nucleus of a cancer cell. Nausea and vomiting are potential side effects. Imatinib is useful in advanced stomach cancer.
- Sunitinib (Sutent) is another new drug useful in stomach cancer when imatinib is not effective.
- With fluorouracil (FU), anorexia and nausea are common. Sore mouth, taste changes, and vomiting also may result. Added thiamine is recommended with FU treatment. Leucovorin is often used with FU.
- Antibiotic therapy to eradicate *H. pylori* bacteria may be needed, if present.

Herbs, Botanicals, and Supplements (see Table 13-8)

- Herbs and botanical supplements should not be used without discussing with physician.

INTERVENTION: NUTRITION EDUCATION, COUNSELING, CARE MANAGEMENT

- Instruct patient on postgastrectomy diet.
- Encourage patient to chew slowly and well, when and if oral intake is possible.
- Feeding tubes may be useful in home setting (e.g., jejunostomy).

- Discuss protective foods if oral diet is possible, including *Allium* and garlic (raw or lightly cooked), carotenoids, lycopene, fish, fruits, nonherbal tea, polyunsaturated fat, vitamin A, ascorbic acid, indoles (cruciferous vegetables), sulforaphane, and yellow onions and shallots for quercetin.

For More Information

- Health Center Online
http://cancer.healthcentersonline.com/gastrointestinalsystemcancers/stomachcancer.cfm
- Memorial Sloan-Kettering Cancer Center
http://www.mskcc.org/mskcc/html/1467.cfm
- National Cancer Institute–Gastric Cancer
http://www.cancer.gov/cancerinfo/pdq/treatment/gastric/healthprofessional
- OncoLink–Gastric Cancer
http://cancer.med.upenn.edu/types/

GASTRIC CANCER—CITED REFERENCES

Balcerczak E, et al. Expression of the P65 gene in gastric cancer and in tissues with or without *Helicobacter pylori* infection. *Neoplasma* 52:464, 2005.
Fahey JW, et al. Sulforaphane inhibits extracellular, intracellular, and antibiotic-resistant strains of *Helicobacter pylori* and prevents benzo[a]pyrene-induced stomach tumors. *Proc Natl Acad Sci USA.* 99: 7610, 2002.
Galan MV, et al. Oral broccoli sprouts for the treatment of *Helicobacter pylori* infection: a preliminary report. *Dig Dis Sci.* 49:1088, 2004.
Heinrich MC, Corless CL. Gastric GI stromal tumors (GISTs): the role of surgery in the era of targeted therapy. *J Surg Oncol.* 90:195, 2005.
Ito H, et al. Polyphenol levels in human urine after intake of six different polyphenol-rich beverages. *Br J Nutr.* 94:500, 2005.
Kim HJ, et al. Effect of nutrient intake and *Helicobacter pylori* infection on gastric cancer in Korea: a case-control study. *Nutr Cancer.* 52:138, 2005.
Ohmae T, et al. *Helicobacter pylori* activates NF-kappaB via the alternative pathway in B lymphocytes. *J Immunol.* 175:7162, 2005.
Qiu JL, et al. Nutritional factors and gastric cancer in Zhoushan Islands, China. *World J Gastroenterol.* 11:4311, 2005.
Vigen C, et al. Occupational physical activity and risk of adenocarcinomas of the esophagus and stomach. *Int J Cancer.* 118:1004, 2006.
Yuan JM, et al. Prediagnostic levels of serum micronutrients in relation to risk of gastric cancer in Shanghai, China. *Cancer Epidemiol Biomarkers Prev.* 13:1772, 2004.

HEPATIC (LIVER) CANCER

NUTRITIONAL ACUITY RANKING: LEVEL 3–4

DEFINITIONS AND BACKGROUND

Hepatocellular carcinoma is the fifth most common cancer and causes 1 million deaths per year (Cahill, 2005). Primary hepatic tumors are common with alcohol abuse, aflatoxin ingestion, and chronic hepatitis (see Table 13-17). Hepatic cancer may develop after years of chronic inflammation and persistent mucosal or epithelial cell colonization by hepatitis B or C viruses (Moss and Blaser, 2005). Advise patients who are at risk for hepatocellular carcinoma from hepatitis C infection that maintaining a lean weight may help to prolong life. This is new research, and more studies are warranted.

TABLE 13-17 Risk Factors for Liver Cancer

Aflatoxins (Voight, 2005)
Anabolic steroids
Arsenic in drinking water
Cirrhosis from alcohol abuse or hemochromatosis (Kuper et al, 2001)
Male gender
Liver disease: hepatitis B virus (HBV) and hepatitis C virus (HCV)
Obesity
Oral contraceptive use (higher dose estrogen)
Tobacco use
Vinyl chloride and thorium dioxide (Voight, 2005)

Malignant hepatic tumors are common due to metastatic lesions from other organs. Hepatocellular cancer accounts for almost half a million cancer deaths a year, and the incidence is escalating in the Western world (Voight, 2005). Liver cancer is also a major cause of cancer deaths in Asia and Africa, especially in developing countries (McGlynn et al, 2001).

Symptoms and signs of hepatic cancer include gradual and silent onset with anorexia, weakness, progressive weight loss, nausea or vomiting, increased flatulence, steatorrhea, diarrhea, abdominal fullness, low-grade fever, dehydration, anemia, malnutrition, abnormal liver function tests (LFTs), decreased albumin levels, portal hypertension, dyspnea, jaundice, ascites, and hepatic coma.

Hepatic cancer progresses in a stepwise manner, mostly regulated by gene expression (Nam et al, 2005). Untreated liver cancer may rapidly lead to death within a year.

Surgical resection is sometimes possible in some cases; laparoscopic procedures are being evaluated. Laser-induced thermotherapy for treatment of liver metastases may be an option. Chemotherapy may be administered as well. Systemic chemotherapy may lead to immunosuppression and possible reactivation of hepatitis B virus, suggesting that prophylactic antiviral therapy may also be needed (Park et al, 2005).

Where radiation is used, new treatments involve sending radioactive substances into the artery that leads directly to the liver. Computed tomography–guided focal liver irradiation combined with chemotherapy delivered via the hepatic artery may extend the lives of patients with unresectable cancer.

INTERVENTION: OBJECTIVES

- Reduce fluid retention and ascites.
- Correct serum protein levels and improve hepatic production capacity.
- Prevent further nausea and vomiting, weight loss, anorexia, and malnutrition.
- Counteract side effects of therapy (e.g., surgery, chemotherapy, radiation).
- Improve overall nutritional and hematologic status.
- Maintain adequate hydration.
- Improve prognosis and prolong life as long as possible.
- Improve quality of life.

INTERVENTION: FOOD AND NUTRITION

- Avoid total parenteral nutrition (TPN) when possible, and tube feed if possible; patients with hepatic cancer usually have significant fluid balance/overload/retention problems.
- Progress, if and when tolerated, to high-protein diet with sufficient carbohydrate intake. Managing weight will be important to prolong life; a carefully planned weight loss diet is needed in those patients who are obese.
- If hepatic coma occurs, decrease protein and supplement with amino acids (see hepatic encephalopathy in Section 8). Branched-chain amino acids may be beneficial; studies are ongoing (Togo et al, 2005).
- Reduce sodium if ascites and edema are significant. Monitor need for extra protein if albumin is also low. Monitor serum levels of other electrolytes to determine if other restrictions are needed.
- Supplemental vitamins may be beneficial. Be careful of toxic levels of vitamins A, D, or K because of poor hepatic clearance.
- With surgery, monitor nutritional intake for adequate wound healing and recovery.
- Encourage regular meals and snacks. Manage anorexia by offering small meals or snacks every few hours or as tolerated.
- Decreased calcium absorption secondary to duodenal bypass can occur; calcium supplementation is needed, especially in postmenopausal women.

CLINICAL INDICATORS

Clinical/History

Height
Weight
BMI
Diet history
Progressive weight loss
Gastrointestinal (GI) bleeding
I & O, dehydration
Anorexia, weakness
Nausea and/or vomiting
Increased flatulence
Steatorrhea, diarrhea
Abdominal fullness
Low-grade fever
Anemia, malnutrition
Portal hypertension
Dyspnea
Jaundice, ascites, or hepatic coma
Melena
Hepatomegaly
Temperature (fever?)

Lab Work

Alpha-fetoprotein (AFP)
Prothrombin time (PT) (prolonged)
H & H
Transferrin
Aspartate aminotransferase (AST), ALT (abnormal)
Sedimentation rate (increased)
Ca++, Mg++
Na+, K+
Ammonia
Alb (decreased), transthyretin
CRP
RBP
Gluc (decreased)
Alk phos
TLC (varies)

Common Drugs Used and Potential Side Effects

- Antiemetics may be used for vomiting.
- Diuretics are used commonly; monitor side effects carefully.
- Chemotherapy may include cisplatin, interferon, doxorubicin, and fluorouracil (Yeo et al, 2005).

Herbs, Botanicals, and Supplements (see Table 13-8)

- Herbs and botanical supplements should not be used without discussing with physician.
- Use of prebiotics (inulin and oligosaccharides) and silymarin may be protective. Studies are needed.

INTERVENTION: NUTRITION EDUCATION, COUNSELING, CARE MANAGEMENT

- Hepatic cancer from hepatitis C virus infection warrants maintaining a lean weight to prolong life.
- Teach patient about signs of deficiency of vitamins K and C such as bleeding gums.
- Discuss signs of hepatic coma that require dietary alterations.
- Encourage hepatitis B virus vaccination. Where needed, offer information and educational sessions (Wai et al, 2005).
- Provide education related to diet (regular, six small feedings) and jejunostomy tube feeding.

Patient Education—Food Safety

- Educate about food safety issues.

For More Information

- American Liver Foundation
  http://www.liverfoundation.org/
- Medline–Liver Cancer
  http://www.nlm.nih.gov/medlineplus/livercancer.html
- OncoLink–Liver Cancer
  http://cancer.med.upenn.edu/disease/liver/

HEPATIC CANCER—CITED REFERENCES

Cahill BA. Management of patients who have undergone hepatic artery chemoembolization. *Clin J Oncol Nurs.* 9:69, 2005.

Kuper H, et al. The risk of liver and bile duct cancer in patients with chronic viral hepatitis, alcoholism, or cirrhosis. *Hepatology* 34:714, 2001.
McGlynn K, et al. International trends and patterns of primary liver cancer. *Int J Cancer.* 94:290, 2001.
Moss SF, Blaser MJ. Mechanisms of disease: inflammation and the origins of cancer. *Nat Clin Pract Oncol.* 2:90, 2005.
Nam SW, et al. Molecular changes from dysplastic nodule to hepatocellular carcinoma through gene expression profiling. *Hepatology* 42:809, 2005.
Park JW, et al. Risk of hepatitis B exacerbation is low after transcatheter arterial chemoembolization therapy for patients with HBV-related hepatocellular carcinoma: report of a prospective study. *Am J Gastroenterol.* 100:2194, 2005.
Togo S, et al. Usefulness of granular BCAA after hepatectomy for liver cancer complicated with liver cirrhosis. *Nutrition* 21:480, 2005.
Voight MD. Alcohol in hepatocellular cancer. *Clin Liver Dis.* 9:151, 2005.
Wai CT, et al. Misperceptions among patients with chronic hepatitis B in Singapore. *World J Gastroenterol.* 11:5002, 2005.
Yeo W, et al. A randomized phase III study of doxorubicin versus cisplatin/interferon alpha-2b/doxorubicin/fluorouracil (PIAF) combination chemotherapy for unresectable hepatocellular carcinoma. *J Natl Cancer Inst.* 97:1532, 2005.

KIDNEY, BLADDER, AND URINARY TRACT CANCERS

NUTRITIONAL ACUITY RANKING: LEVEL 3

DEFINITIONS AND BACKGROUND

Renal cell cancer (renal adenocarcinoma, or hypernephroma) accounts for about 2% of cancers worldwide. It is most common in persons over age 45 years. Incidence has increased in North America and northern Europe but not in other areas of the world (McLaughlin and Lipworth, 2000). In the United States, the highest rates are now seen among blacks. Blood in the urine and increased frequency of urination are the most common symptoms. Smoking; exposure to dyes, rubber, and leather products at work; long-term dialysis; and obesity are risk factors (Chow et al, 2000). Renal cancer can often be cured if it is diagnosed and treated when still localized to the kidney, and a majority of patients are diagnosed at that time. Surgical resection is possible when early diagnosis is made; nephrectomy may be needed. The management of metastatic renal cell carcinoma remains a therapeutic challenge; less than 10% of patients survive for longer than 5 years (Arya et al, 2004). See Figure 13-5.

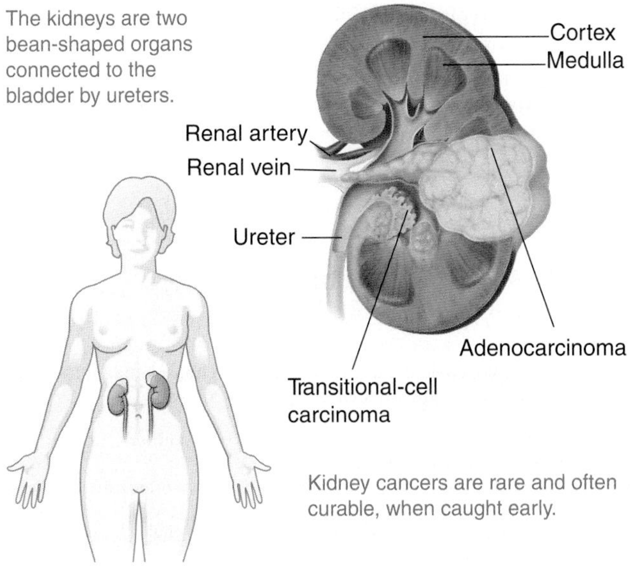
The kidneys are two bean-shaped organs connected to the bladder by ureters.
Cortex
Medulla
Renal artery
Renal vein
Ureter
Adenocarcinoma
Transitional-cell carcinoma
Kidney cancers are rare and often curable, when caught early.

Figure 13-5 Kidney cancers.

Wilms' tumor (nephroblastoma or embryoma of the kidney) is a highly malignant tumor occurring almost exclusively in children younger than 6 years of age. Metastasis to lungs, liver, and brain can occur. Symptoms and signs include weight loss, anorexia, enlarged kidney, hypertension, fever, anemia, and abdominal pain. A cure may be possible if metastasis has not occurred before nephrectomy. There is now an overall survival rate of 85%, and treatment-related morbidity has been reduced by chemotherapy (Gommersall et al, 2005).

Bladder cancer can be caused by factors such as smoking, exposure to chemicals at work (such as hair dyes, textiles, and paint), old age, and infectious parasites. It can often be cured in early stages. Surgery, radiation, chemotherapy, or immunotherapy may be used. Photodynamic therapy is being tested in individuals with renal tumors.

Urinary tract cancers affect more than 50,000 Americans each year. Men are more prone to this type of cancer than women. Surgery is usually required for removal of urinary tract tumors; prognosis with early intervention is good. Survival has improved. Fruit, extra fluids, vitamin C, retinol, daily multivitamin supplements, and green and nonherbal tea tend to be protective.

INTERVENTION: OBJECTIVES

- If needed, prepare patient for surgery and for postsurgical wound healing.
- Control side effects of radiotherapy and chemotherapy.
- Promote normal growth and development, as far as possible, in children and teens.
- Control hypertension; correct anemia, which is common.
- Maintain adequate hydration.
- Minimize weight loss.
- Promote adequate bowel function.

INTERVENTION: FOOD AND NUTRITION

- Provide adequate energy and protein according to age and to compensate for weight loss that has occurred. In

obese adults, weight loss regimens are not recommended until several months after surgery.
- Restrict excessive sodium with hypertension. Monitor calcium and magnesium levels as well; supplement if necessary.
- Monitor protein tolerance and adjust according to lab values, blood pressure, edema, and other signs of renal failure.
- Ensure adequate fluid intake, especially water, unless restriction is needed for some other medical reason.

CLINICAL INDICATORS

Clinical/History		Lab Work
Height	Abdominal or lower back pain	Urinalysis
Weight	I & O	Ca++, Mg++
Weight changes	Smoking history	Na+, K+
BMI (obesity?)	Painful urination	Alb, transthyretin
Diet history	Frequent urinary tract infections	CRP
Growth percentile in child	Incontinence	Creat
Hematuria	Abdominal CT scan	Gluc
BP (increased)	Cystoscopy	TLC (varies)
Anorexia	X-ray (intravenous pyelogram)	BUN
Enlarged kidney?	Bone scan for metastasis	H & H
Fever, temperature		Serum Fe
Anemia		Serum ferritin
		Transferrin
		Liver function tests
		ALT

Common Drugs Used and Potential Side Effects

- Dactinomycin or vincristine may be used for **renal cancer**. These drugs may cause dry mouth, dysphagia, stomatitis, esophagitis, diarrhea, nausea, and other side effects. Monitor accordingly.
- Doxorubicin also may be used for renal tumors. Dry mouth, nausea, vomiting, esophagitis, or stomatitis may occur.
- Interferon and interleukin-2 may be used in advanced kidney cancer. Interferon often causes patients to have flu-like symptoms, and nausea and vomiting are common; interleukin-2 can cause nausea and vomiting or fluid retention.
- Sunitinib (Sutent) is a new drug useful in advanced kidney cancer where chemotherapy has not been effective.
- Sorafenib can reduce progression of kidney cancer; this drug awaits Food and Drug Administration (FDA) approval.
- Tarceva and Avastin are being investigated for kidney cancers.
- Zoledronic acid is a bisphosphonate that is approved for preventing fractures after bone metastasis from renal cancer.
- For **bladder cancer,** chemotherapy often involves fluorouracil, cisplatin, cyclophosphamide, methotrexate, or vinblastine. Many gastrointestinal (GI) side effects are common, including nausea, anorexia, diarrhea, or vomiting.
- Treatments for **Wilms' tumor** include perioperative vincristine and dactinomycin, with or without doxorubicin or radiotherapy (Gommersall et al, 2005).

Herbs, Botanicals, and Supplements (see Table 13-8)

- Herbs and botanical supplements should not be used without discussing with physician.
- Herbal preparations are subject to contamination with metals such as mercury or may contain potassium, all of which can be harmful to the kidney.

INTERVENTION: NUTRITION EDUCATION, COUNSELING, CARE MANAGEMENT

- Discuss side effects patient is experiencing in light of therapies used (e.g., radiation therapy, chemotherapy, or surgery).
- Discuss normal growth and/or desirable weight for patient.
- Highlight meals that are attractive so patient eats as well as possible.
- Discuss how to manage anemia through appropriate medications or dietary measures.

For More Information

- Cancer Information Network
  http://www.ontumor.com/kidney.htm
- Clinical Practice Guidelines for Kidney Cancer
  http://www.nccn.org/professionals/physician_gls/PDF/kidney.pdf
- Kidney Cancer Association
  http://www.kidneycancerassociation.org/
- Medline–Kidney Cancer
  http://www.nlm.nih.gov/medlineplus/kidneycancer.html
- National Cancer Institute Kidney Cancer Web
  http://web.ncifcrf.gov/research/kidney/
- National Kidney Foundation
  http://www.kidney.org/
- Treatment Decisions for Bladder Cancer
  http://www.nccn.org/patients/patient_gls/_english/_bladder/contents.asp

KIDNEY, BLADDER, AND URINARY TRACT CANCERS—CITED REFERENCES

Arya M, et al. Allogeneic hematopoietic stem-cell transplantation: the next generation of therapy for metastatic renal cell cancer. *Nat Clin Pract Oncol.* 1:32, 2004.

Chow W, et al. Obesity, hypertension, and the risk of kidney cancer in men. *N Engl J Med.* 343:1305, 2000.

Gommersall LM, et al. Current challenges in Wilms' tumor management. *Nat Clin Pract Oncol.* 2:298, 2005.

McLaughlin J, Lipworth L. Epidemiologic aspects of renal cell cancer. *Semin Oncol.* 27:115, 2000.

LEUKEMIAS

NUTRITIONAL ACUITY RANKING: LEVEL 3–4

DEFINITIONS AND BACKGROUND

Leukemia involves uncontrolled proliferation of leukocytes and their precursors in blood-forming organs, with infiltration into other organs. The blood has a grayish-white appearance. Leukemia incidence is highest among Hispanic whites and lowest among American Indians and Alaskan natives.

Since various specific chromosome rearrangements are found in acute myeloid leukemia (AML) and in childhood acute lymphocytic leukemia (ALL), most childhood leukemias begin before birth (Smith et al, 2005). Persons with Down syndrome, Fanconi's anemia, and other genetic disorders tend to have a risk of leukemia. Because chromosomal abnormalities are present at birth in children who later develop leukemia, factors such as nutrition during pregnancy might affect the risk of acute lymphoblastic leukemia among young children. There is no evidence that breastfeeding affects onset (Kwan et al, 2005).

Leukemia risk in children is lowered by increased maternal intake of fruits, vegetables, fish, and seafood, and risk is increased with higher maternal intake of sugars, syrups, meat, and meat products (Petridou et al, 2005). Polymorphisms in the 5,10-methylenetetrahydrofolate reductase (*MTHFR*) gene have been associated with adult and childhood ALL; low folate intake may be important in elevating leukemia risk in children (Smith et al, 2005). Proteasome activity is required for cancer cell survival; consumption of fruits, vegetables, and phytochemicals, such as grape extract, apigenin, quercetin, kaempferol, and myricetin, may target the proteasome and be protective (Chen et al, 2005).

Primary treatment of leukemias currently involves chemotherapy to kill attacking abnormal blood cells. Bone marrow transplantation may be feasible in some cases. Table 13-18 lists various types of leukemias, relevant signs and symptoms, and treatments.

INTERVENTION: OBJECTIVES

- Prevent hemorrhage and infections.
- Promote recovery and stabilization before bone marrow transplantation, if performed.
- Correct anorexia and nausea or vomiting.
- Prevent complications and further morbidity, such as veno-occlusive disease (VOD).

TABLE 13-18 Various Forms of Leukemia

Form	Description
Acute Leukemias	Symptoms and signs include easy fatigue, malaise, irritability, fever, pallor, petechiae, bruising, purpura, hemorrhage, palpitations, shortness of breath, slight weight loss, bone or joint pain, painless lumps in underarm or stomach, cough, sternal tenderness, splenomegaly, hepatomegaly, anemia, hemorrhages such as nosebleeds, headache, nausea and vomiting, and mouth ulcers.
Acute lymphocytic leukemia (ALL)	Primarily affects bone marrow and lymph nodes. This condition is rapidly progressing and mainly affects children, accounting for 50% of all childhood leukemias. Central nervous system treatment: ALL often spreads to the coverings of the brain and spinal cord, and patients often receive chemotherapy in the spinal fluid or radiation therapy of the head as a method of prevention. The toxicity of bone marrow transplantation (BMT) treatment or peripheral-blood stem-cell transplant (PBSCT) may lead to bloody diarrhea, fever, and other symptoms of graft-versus-host disease (GVHD).
Acute myelogenous leukemia (AML)	AML starts in the bone marrow but moves into the blood and to the lymph nodes, liver, spleen, central nervous system, and testes. AML consists of proliferation of myeloblasts, which are immature polynuclear leukocytes. AML is more common in adult males but also accounts for just under half of cases of childhood leukemia. Average onset of AML is the sixth decade. Smoking, obesity, and chronic exposure to benzene, usually in the workplace, have been established as causes. Extraordinary doses of irradiation can also increase the incidence of AML.
Chronic Leukemias	Symptoms and signs include anemia, increased infections, bleeding, enlarged lymph nodes (in lymphatic form), night sweats, fever, weight loss, and anorexia.
Chronic lymphocytic leukemia (CLL)	Affects adults and is almost twice as common as chronic myelogenous leukemia (CML). CLL involves a crowding out of normal leukocytes in lymph glands, interfering with the body's ability to produce other blood cells. CLL is more common in people older than 50 years of age and in males.
Chronic myelogenous leukemia (CML)	Affects mostly adults and is very rare in children. It is half as common as CLL.
Chronic granulocytic leukemia	Has similar overproduction of white blood cells in the bone marrow and is often believed to be developed through an abnormal acquired chromosome (Philadelphia chromosome, Ph1), perhaps as a result of ionizing radiation; less common than the other types.

- Alter diet according to medications and therapies such as chemotherapy.
- Maintain weight that is appropriate for height. Correct weight loss in cachexia.
- Maintain adequate hydration.

INTERVENTION: FOOD AND NUTRITION

- Serve attractive meals at temperatures that are tolerated.
- Small meals may be better tolerated to avoid overwhelming patient.
- In some cases, cold or iced foods may be preferred.
- A high-protein, high-energy, high-vitamin/mineral intake should be offered. The use of tube feeding (TF) in these patients is often useful. Intolerance due to treatment side effects may be an obstacle.
- Extra fluids will be important during febrile states or with use of interferon, but avoid overload.
- Vitamins A and D may be beneficial (Oren et al, 2003; Trump et al, 2005). Avoid excesses.
- Include protective foods such as isoflavones in soy and flavonoids in grapes, coffee, tea, nuts, seeds, fruits, and vegetables.

CLINICAL INDICATORS

Clinical/History

Height
Weight
BMI
Weight changes (slight weight loss?)
Diet history
Fever (over 101°F?)
Frequent infections
Malaise, irritability
Pallor
Hemorrhage
Petechiae, ecchymosis, purpura
Palpitations
Shortness of breath
Bone or joint pain
Cough, sternal tenderness
Splenomegaly, hepatomegaly
Hemorrhages, such as nosebleeds
Headache
Anorexia
Nausea and vomiting
Mouth ulcers
Blood pressure
Bleeding
Enlarged lymph nodes (in lymphatic form)
Night sweats

Lab Work

WBC (increased)
Alb, transthyretin
CRP
N balance
Serum copper (increased)
Gluc
H & H
Serum Fe
Platelets
Lactate dehydrogenase (LDH) (elevated)
Zinc (decreased)
Uric acid (increased)
Transferrin
Ferritin (increased)
Lumbar puncture
Cytochemistry
Immunocytochemistry
Cytogenetics
Molecular genetic studies
PT or international normalized ratio (INR)
Na+, K+
Ca++, Mg++

TABLE 13-19 Medications for Acute Leukemias

Acute Leukemia Treatments
Induction: The purpose of the first phase is to destroy as many cancer cells as quickly as possible and bring about a remission.
Consolidation: The goal of this phase is to get rid of leukemia cells from where they reside.
Maintenance: After the number of leukemia cells has been reduced by the first two phases of treatment, lower doses of chemotherapy drugs are given over a period of about 2 years.
CEP-701 (lestaurtinib) inhibits the receptor tyrosine kinase FLT3 in acute myelogenous leukemia patients
Chemotherapy often includes methotrexate, 5-azacitidine, cytarabine, thioguanine, and daunorubicin, which may cause stomatitis, nausea, or vomiting. Coadministration of these agents with glucose may help. Adequate fluid is needed. When methotrexate is used, neurotoxicity is a concern; current protocols that use low-dose folinic acid rescue can be recommended (Cohen, 2004).
Gemtuzumab ozogamicin (Mylotarg) may be added. Granulocyte colony-stimulating factors (Neupogen, Leukine) may improve response to chemotherapy. This intensive therapy, which usually takes place in the hospital, typically lasts 1 week.
L-asparaginase (Elspar) may be used; hepatitis or pancreatitis may result; watch carefully.
Pegaspargase (Oncaspar) can cause nausea, vomiting, anorexia, and glucose changes.
Interferon may be used.
Prednisone may be used, with side effects related to steroids with chronic use. Alter diet and intake accordingly to manage hyperglycemia, hypokalemia, and nitrogen losses. Children on steroid therapy for acute lymphoblastic leukemia (ALL) may be at greater risk for a more severe *Varicella* infection, possibly resulting in death, if they were exposed to the virus within 3 weeks of receiving steroids.

Common Drugs Used and Potential Side Effects

- See Tables 13-19 and 13-20.

Herbs, Botanicals, and Supplements (see Table 13-8)

- Herbs and botanical supplements should not be used without discussing with physician.
- Several nutrients and botanicals have been studied for use in chronic myelogenous leukemia, including bioflavonoids, vitamin A, all-*trans*-retinoic acid (Retin-A), vitamin D_3, vitamin E, vitamin B_{12}, indirubin (found in herbs including *Indigofera tinctoria* and *Isatis tinctoria*), and *Curcuma longa* (Matsui, 2005; Steriti, 2002).

INTERVENTION: NUTRITION EDUCATION, COUNSELING, CARE MANAGEMENT

- A well-balanced diet is essential; discuss ways to improve or increase intake.

TABLE 13-20 **Medications for Chronic Leukemias**

Chronic Leukemia Treatments
Chemotherapeutic agents may be used with varying side effects. Chlorambucil (Leukeran) and busulfan are common; nausea, severe fatigue, flu-like symptoms, low-grade temperature, vomiting, glossitis, and cheilosis may occur. Avoid hot, spicy, or acidic foods, if not tolerated.
Pegaspargase (Oncaspar) can cause nausea, vomiting, anorexia, and glucose changes.
Imatinib (Gleevec), which is useful for chronic myelogenous leukemia, interferes with an abnormal enzyme that sends signals to the nucleus of a cancer cell. Nausea and vomiting are potential side effects.
For chronic lymphocytic leukemia, palliation has changed to potential cure, especially in younger patients. Multiple treatment options have emerged, including purine analogs, monoclonal antibodies, and potentially stem-cell transplantation (Yee and O'Brien, 2006).
Antifungals, antivirals, or antibiotic drugs may be also be used. Side effects vary with specific medication used.

- Tumor lysis syndrome is a side effect caused by rapid breakdown of leukemia cells. When these cells die, they release substances into the bloodstream that can affect the kidneys, heart, and nervous system. Giving patient extra fluids or certain drugs that help rid the body of these toxins can prevent this problem.
- Offer guidelines to transition from TPN or PN to enteral nutrition and oral intake.
- Discuss guidance for graft-versus-host disease (acute vs. chronic symptoms). The nutrition team must recognize that short- and long-term outcomes are affected by transplantation type, preparative regimens, diagnosis, disease stage, age, and nutritional status (Lenssen et al, 2001).
- Discuss alternative ways to make meals more attractive and appealing.
- Instruct patient on nutrition repletion if appropriate.

Patient Education—Food Safety

- Educate about food safety issues.

For More Information

- Clinical Practice Guidelines–Acute Myeloid Leukemia
  http://www.nccn.org/professionals/physician_gls/PDF/aml.pdf
- Clinical Practice Guidelines–Chronic Myelogenous Leukemia
  http://www.nccn.org/professionals/physician_gls/PDF/cml.pdf
- Leukemia and Lymphoma Society
  http://www.leukemia-lymphoma.org

LEUKEMIAS—CITED REFERENCES

Chen D, et al. Dietary flavonoids as proteasome inhibitors and apoptosis inducers in human leukemia cells. *Biochem Pharmacol.* 69:1421, 2005.

Cohen IJ. Defining the appropriate dosage of folinic acid after high-dose methotrexate for childhood acute lymphatic leukemia that will prevent neurotoxicity without rescuing malignant cells in the central nervous system. *J Pediatr Hematol Oncol.* 26:156, 2004.

Kwan ML, et al. Breastfeeding patterns and risk of childhood acute lymphoblastic leukaemia. *Br J Cancer.* 93:379, 2005.

Lenssen P, et al. Nutrient support in hematopoietic cell transplantation. *J Parenter Enteral Nutr.* 25:219, 2001.

Matsui J, et al. Dietary bioflavonoids induce apoptosis in human leukemia cells. *Leuk Res.* 29:573, 2005.

Oren T, et al. Hematopoiesis and retinoids: development and disease. *Leuk Lymphoma.* 44:1881, 2003.

Petridou E, et al. Maternal diet and acute lymphoblastic leukemia in young children. *Cancer Epidemiol Biomarkers Prev.* 14:1935, 2005.

Smith MT, et al. Molecular biomarkers for the study of childhood leukemia. *Toxicol Appl Pharmacol.* 206:237, 2005.

Steriti R. Nutritional support for chronic myelogenous and other leukemias: a review of the scientific literature. *Altern Med Rev.* 7:404, 2002.

Trump DL, et al. Anti-tumor activity of calcitriol: pre-clinical and clinical studies. *J Steroid Biochem Mol Biol.* 89–90:519, 2005.

LUNG CANCER

NUTRITIONAL ACUITY RANKING: LEVEL 3 (MAY OFTEN BE 4)

DEFINITIONS AND BACKGROUND

Lung (bronchial) cancer begins in the lungs and is the most common type of cancer in the Western world. Cancer cells of the lung often spread to the brain, bone, liver, and skin. For most cases, radiation and chemotherapy are needed because the cancer is discovered too late for surgical intervention or surgery is not clinically indicated. Lung cancer's 5-year survival rate is only 15%, which is worse than many other types of cancer. Signs and symptoms are listed in Table 13-21.

There are two main types of lung cancer: non–small-cell lung cancer and small-cell lung cancer. **Non–small-cell lung cancer (NSCLC)** has three major subtypes: adenocarcinoma (40% of cases), squamous carcinoma (30–35% of cases, slow growing, and formerly called epidermoid carcinoma), and large-cell carcinoma (affecting 5–15% of cases). NSCLC is the leading cause of cancer-related death in the United States (Budde and Hanna, 2005).

Small-cell lung cancer (SCLC) is a more aggressive type of lung cancer that composes 15% of all lung cancer diagnoses. It is highly correlated to smoking. SCLCs grow quickly but tend to respond to specific chemotherapy protocols. Oat cell cancer is a highly fatal lung cancer; aggressive chemotherapy is needed.

In 85% of cases, smoking causes lung cancer. Heavy tobacco or marijuana smokers are 25 times more susceptible

TABLE 13-21 Signs and Symptoms of Lung Disease

Depression	Recurring pneumonia or bronchitis
Dyspnea	Hoarseness
Fatigue	Shortness of breath
Fever of unknown cause	Persistent cough
Bloody sputum	Swelling of neck or face
Chest pain	Weight loss

to lung cancer. High lung cancer rates in Taiwanese women, despite a low prevalence of smoking, are positively related to Chinese quick-frying cooking without using fans to ventilate the oils (Ko et al, 2000). Other causes include exposure to industrial chemicals, radon, and passive smoke. Nickel depletes intracellular ascorbate, which inhibits cellular hydroxylases that are important for lung surfactant; depletion of ascorbate by chronic exposure to nickel could be deleterious for lung cells and may lead to lung cancer (Salnikow and Kasprzak, 2005). Cyclooxygenase-2 (COX-2) and prostanoid production play a role in the pathogenesis of lung carcinoma (Saha et al, 2003).

Key dietary factors play a protective role. Foods rich in flavonoids may protect against certain types of lung cancer, possibly by inhibiting P450 enzymes, which decrease bioactivation of carcinogens (Le Marchand et al, 2000). Onions and apples have quercetin; white grapefruit provides naringin.

Smoking is associated with lower levels of vitamin C (Lykkesfeldt et al, 2000). Two large randomized trials with a lung cancer endpoint, the Alpha-Tocopherol, Beta-Carotene (ATBC) Prevention Study and the Beta-Carotene and Retinol Efficacy Trial (CARET), suggested that antioxidants might be harmful in smokers; however, the results of the Linxian study were significantly different in this respect, and the relationship between antioxidants and carcinogenesis remains open to debate (Lee and Park, 2003).

Vitamin E food sources are important; gamma-tocopherol seems protective, whereas alpha-tocopherol from supplements is not. Studies with omega-3 fatty acids are needed as well.

INTERVENTION: OBJECTIVES

- Patient must be encouraged to stop smoking.
- Prepare patient for therapy (e.g., surgery, radiation, or chemotherapy).
- Meet energy needs, which are often elevated as much as 30% above normal.
- Counteract side effects such as cachexia, infections, atelectasis, syndrome of inappropriate antidiuretic hormone (SIADH), weight loss, and anorexia.
- Maximize pulmonary health and improve quality of life.
- Increase disease-free time.
- Minimum weight loss.
- Maximize intake through side-effects management.

INTERVENTION: FOOD AND NUTRITION

- Increase intake of protein, CHO, energy, and fluids.
- Alter diet as appropriate for side effects (see general cancer entry).
- Small, frequent meals may be beneficial.
- If oral diet is possible, promote a protective diet by including fruits, vegetables, sesame seeds and pecans (for gamma-tocopherol), foods rich in quercetin (apples and onions) and other flavonoids, selenium, lycopene, carotenoids, and natural estrogens (such as soy foods). Use curcumin as seasoning if tolerated. Adequate vitamin-mineral provision will be needed, especially from diet.
- Include good sources of phytosterols such as sunflower seeds, pistachio nuts, sesame seeds, and wheat germ (Phillips et al, 2005).
- Include more omega-3 fatty acids from fish, shellfish, flaxseed, and walnuts.
- Tube feedings are highly recommended if weight loss, decreased appetite, dehydration, or electrolyte imbalance occurs.

CLINICAL INDICATORS

Clinical/History

Height
Weight
Weight changes
BMI
Diet history
I & O
Persistent cough
Bloody sputum
Chest pain
Recurring pneumonia or bronchitis
Bronchoscopy
Biopsy
MRI, CT scan
Chest x-ray

Lab Work

CEA
Alb, transthyretin
Gluc
CRP
Partial pressure of carbon dioxide (pCO_2), partial pressure of oxygen (pO_2)
Ca^{++}, Mg^{++}
Na^+, K^+
ALT (increased)
Sputum cytology
Thoracentesis

Common Drugs Used and Potential Side Effects

- Cytotoxic drugs are often used. Vincristine can cause severe constipation; with methotrexate, nausea and vomiting are common; doxorubicin (Adriamycin) causes stomatitis, anorexia, hair loss, and diarrhea. Coadministration of methotrexate with intravenous glucose may alleviate some of the toxic gastrointestinal (GI) effects.
- Cyclophosphamide (Cytoxan) and other combinations of therapy may be used. Anorexia, stomatitis, nausea, or vomiting may occur.
- Pemetrexed, a multitargeted antifolate, has activity as a single agent and as part of combination chemother-

apy against NSCLC; toxicity with the use of vitamin B_{12} and folate supplementation is far less than with docetaxel (Budde and Hanna, 2005).
- Tarceva modestly improves survival in NSCLC patients.
- Inhibitors of COX-2 in combination with chemoradiation therapy may be an alternative strategy (Laskin and Sandler, 2003; Saha et al, 2003).
- With immunotherapy, bacillus Calmette-Guérin (BCG) vaccine often is used.

Herbs, Botanicals, and Supplements (see Table 13-8)

- Herbs and botanical supplements should not be used without discussing with physician.
- Avoid beta-carotene supplementation, which tends to promote lung cancer. Diet is more protective.

INTERVENTION: NUTRITION EDUCATION, COUNSELING, CARE MANAGEMENT

- Discuss alternate methods of eating if meals are not consumed as usual.
- A diet high in antioxidant-rich foods such as fruits, vegetables, and spices would be both protective and a prudent preventive strategy for smokers (Kelly, 2002).
- Discuss side effects of drugs being used.
- Smokers who quit will allow their lung tissues to repair much of the damage. Those who cannot quit should use a brand of cigarettes with lower nicotine and low tar. Chewing tobacco and snuff is also carcinogenic. Avoid smoking prior to or with meals; smoking may decrease appetite.
- Offer tube feeding education.
- Offer nutritional build-up education as appropriate.

For More Information

- Alliance for Lung Cancer
  http://www.alcase.org/
- Cancer Net–Lung Cancer
  http://cancernet.nci.nih.gov/cancertopics/wyntk/lung/page1
- Clinical Practice Guidelines–Small-Cell Lung Cancer
  http://www.nccn.org/professionals/physician_gls/PDF/sclc.pdf
- Clinical Practice Guidelines—Non–Small-Cell Lung Cancer
  http://www.nccn.org/professionals/physician_gls/PDF/nscl.pdf
- Focus on Lung Cancer
  http://www.lungcancer.org/
- Lung Cancer Information Library
  http://www.meds.com/lung/lunginfo.html
- Lung Cancer Online
  http://www.lungcanceronline.org/
- OncoLink–Lung Cancer
  http://cancer.med.upenn.edu/disease/lung1/
- Treatment Decisions
  http://www.nccn.org/patients/patient_gls/_english/_lung/contents.asp

LUNG CANCER—CITED REFERENCES

Budde LS, Hanna NH. Antimetabolites in the management of non-small cell lung cancer. *Curr Treat Options Oncol.* 6:83, 2005.
Kelly GS. The interaction of cigarette smoking and antioxidants. Part I: diet and carotenoids. *Altern Med Rev.* 7:370, 2002.
Ko Y, et al. Chinese food cooking and lung cancer in women nonsmokers. *Am J Epidemiol.* 151:140, 2000.
Laskin JJ, Sandler AB. The importance of the eicosanoid pathway in lung cancer. *Lung Cancer* 41:73S, 2003.
Lee BM, Park KK. Beneficial and adverse effects of chemopreventive agents. *Mutat Res.* 523–524:265, 2003.
Le Marchand L, et al. Intake of flavonoids and lung cancer. *J Natl Cancer Inst.* 92:154, 2000.
Lykkesfeldt J, et al. Ascorbate is depleted by smoking and replanted by moderate supplementation: a study in male smokers and nonsmokers with matched dietary antioxidant intakes. *Am J Clin Nutr.* 71:530, 2000.
Phillips KM, et al. Phytosterol composition of nuts and seeds commonly consumed in the United States. *J Agric Food Chem.* 53:9436, 2005.
Saha D, et al. COX-2 inhibitor as a radiation enhancer: new strategies for the treatment of lung cancer. *Am J Clin Oncol.* 26:70S, 2003.
Salnikow K, Kasprzak KS. Ascorbate depletion: a critical step in nickel carcinogenesis? *Environ Health Perspect.* 113:577, 2005.

LYMPHOMAS

NUTRITIONAL ACUITY RANKING: LEVEL 3

DEFINITIONS AND BACKGROUND

Hodgkin's disease is a malignant tumor of the lymphatic system. Patients present with enlarged lymph nodes that are firm and rubbery, severe pruritus, jaundice, night sweats, fatigue and malaise, weight loss, slight fever, alcohol-induced pain, cough, dyspnea, and chest pain. Patients who have human immunodeficiency virus (HIV) infection are more prone to Hodgkin's disease. Hodgkin's disease presents most commonly between ages 15 and 34 and after age 60. Treatment involves radiation and chemotherapy. Stage I is limited to one body part; stage II involves two or more areas on the same side of the diaphragm; stage III involves lymph nodes above and below the diaphragm; and stage IV involves lymph nodes and other areas such as the lungs, marrow, and liver.

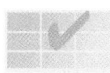

Patients who present with weight loss initially have a worse prognosis than those without weight loss. The 5-year survival rate for Hodgkin's disease is 83%; it is one of the more curable forms of cancer. Unfortunately, surviving Hodgkin's lymphoma in childhood quadruples the risk of a stroke later in life. Young women who receive high-dose radiation for Hodgkin's disease are more at risk for breast cancer later in life.

Non-Hodgkin's lymphomas (NHL) are malignant tumors of lymphoid tissue, resulting from invasion of the lymph nodes and other tissues by lymphocytes. The bacterium *Helicobacter pylori* is associated with the development of lymphoma in the stomach wall. Burkitt's lymphoma is associated with prior infection with the Epstein-Barr virus. Burkitt's lymphoma is most common in children, young adult males, and patients with acquired immunodeficiency syndrome (AIDS); it originates from a B lymphocyte and requires chemotherapy. NHL is relatively common among individuals whose immune system is suppressed. Exposure to certain chemicals (such as nitrates) in herbicides and pesticides promotes risk. In one large study, intake of alcohol and one-carbon nutrients, particularly vitamin B_6 and methionine, was found to be protective (Lim et al, 2005).

Enteropathy-associated T-cell lymphoma (EATL) is a rare form of high-grade, T-cell NHL of the upper small intestine that is specifically associated with celiac disease (Catassi et al, 2005). Capsule endoscopy is now used to evaluate celiac disease–associated enteropathy in intestinal T-cell lymphoma (Joyce et al, 2005). Studies suggest that strict adherence to the gluten-free diet (GFD) protects from cancer development, especially if started during the first years of life (Hervonen et al, 2005). Unraveling the relationships between NHL and celiac disease may help increase understanding of oncogenesis (Holmes, 2002).

Symptoms and signs of NHL are similar to those of Hodgkin's disease and those of enlarged tonsils and adenoids. Difficulty breathing, swelling of face, thickened or dark, itchy skin areas, increased incidence of bacterial infections, night sweats, weight loss, fever, anemia, and pleural effusion can occur. It is possible, as well, to develop chylous ascites or chyloperitoneum. By the time of NHL diagnosis, it is often widely spread. It may spread to the cervix, uterus, and vagina in women. Radiation is a common treatment for early stages. A cure is less likely for those over age 60. The 5-year survival rate for NHL is 52%. Figure 13-6 shows an image of lymphoma.

INTERVENTION: OBJECTIVES

- Prevent or correct weight loss, fever, malaise, and infections such as candidiasis.
- Correct dysphagia, nausea and vomiting, and anorexia.
- Control protein-losing enteropathy, chylous ascites, and other side effects.
- Control enteropathy in patients who also have celiac disease; doing so can reduce malignancy in this population (Leffler et al, 2003).
- Modify diet according to side effects of therapy (e.g., radiation or chemotherapy).

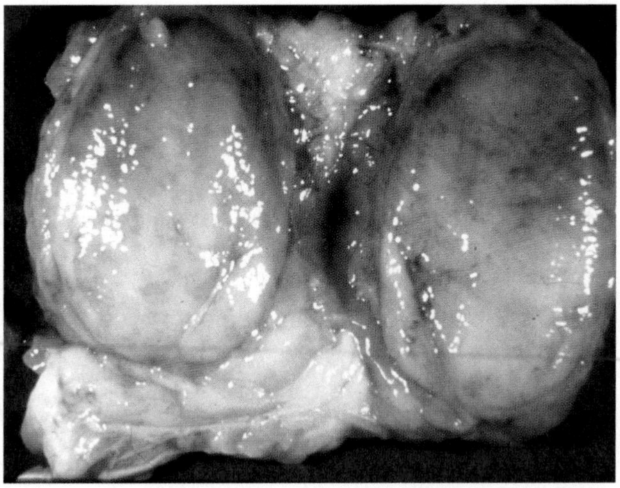

Figure 13-6 Lymphoma. (Image from Rubin E, Farber JL. *Pathology*. 3rd ed. Philadelphia: Lippincott Williams & Wilkins, 1999.)

INTERVENTION: FOOD AND NUTRITION

- A diet as tolerated is acceptable. Bland foods may be better accepted for awhile. With celiac disease, the GFD is required.
- Increase protein, energy intake, and fluids.
- Six small feedings are generally better tolerated than three large meals.
- Alter diet according to symptoms.
- With hyperglycemia, control carbohydrates and overall energy intake.
- To prevent relapse, eating a diet with lots of vegetables and legumes is recommended. Folate may play a protective role (Skibola et al, 2004).

CLINICAL INDICATORS

Clinical/History

Height
Weight
BMI
Weight loss?
Diet history
Enlarged, rubbery lymph nodes
Painless adenopathy
Pruritus, severe
Jaundice
Night sweats
Fatigue and malaise
Slight fever, temperature
Alcohol-induced pain
Cough, dyspnea, and chest pain
Diarrhea
I & O
Lymphangiogram
X-ray or CT scan
Bone marrow biopsy

Lab Work

Ceruloplasmin (increased)
Reed-Sternberg cells (more than one nucleus)
ESR
Uric acid (increased)

PT (increased)	Bilirubin (increased)	ALT (increased)
Gluc	Alk phos (often increased)	Serum lipids—Chol, Trig
CRP	Ferritin (increased)	Ca++, Mg++
Serum Cu (increased)		Na+, K+
H & H		

Common Drugs Used and Potential Side Effects

Hodgkin's Disease

- Chemotherapy is often given in combination. The regimen MOPP, which includes mechlorethamine (nitrogen mustard), vincristine (Oncovin), procarbazine, and prednisone, may cause nausea, vomiting, diarrhea, weakness, constipation, and mouth sores. The regimen ChlVPP, which includes chlorambucil, vinblastine, procarbazine, and prednisone, may cause similar side effects. After chemotherapy, young women may have amenorrhea.
- Corticosteroids can aggravate electrolyte status and will decrease calcium, potassium, and nitrogen balance over time. Hyperglycemia also may occur; monitor blood glucose levels.

NHL

- Chemotherapy is often given as regimen known as CHOP, which includes cyclophosphamide, doxorubicin, vincristine (Oncovin), and prednisone. CHOP may cause nausea, vomiting, anorexia, diarrhea, and other gastrointestinal (GI) side effects. Single agents may also be used. Methotrexate causes GI pain, mouth ulcers, nausea, and folic acid depletion.

Herbs, Botanicals, and Supplements (see Table 13-8)

- Herbs and botanical supplements should not be used without discussing with physician.
- Studies suggest that acupuncture, coenzyme Q10, and polysaccharide K may have positive results (Leukemia and Lymphoma Society, 2005).

INTERVENTION: NUTRITION EDUCATION, COUNSELING, CARE MANAGEMENT

- Discuss methods of improving appetite by use of attractive meals.
- Encourage rest periods before and after meals to reduce fatigue.
- Encourage diet that is protective with plenty of vegetables and legumes.
- Vitamin D may protect against NHL (Hughes et al, 2004).

Patient Education—Food Safety

- Educate about food safety issues.

For More Information

- Cancer Information Network
  http://www.ontumor.com/
- Cancer Links
  http://www.ontumor.com/lymphoma/index.asp
- Lymphoma Information Network
  http://www.lymphomainfo.net/lymphoma.html
- National Cancer Institute–Hodgkin's Lymphoma
  http://www.cancer.gov/cancerinfo/types/hodgkinslymphoma
- National Library of Medicine
  http://www.nlm.nih.gov/medlineplus/hodgkinsdisease.html
- Non-Hodgkin's Lymphoma
  http://www.nlm.nih.gov/medlineplus/ency/article/000581.htm
- Treatment Decisions
  http://www.nccn.org/patients/patient_gls/_english/_non_hodgkins/contents.asp
- Wellness After Treatment
  http://www.cancer.gov/cancertopics/life-after-treatment/page4

LYMPHOMAS—CITED REFERENCES

Catassi C, et al. Association of celiac disease and intestinal lymphomas and other cancers. *Gastroenterology* 128:S79, 2005.

Hervonen K, et al. Lymphoma in patients with dermatitis herpetiformis and their first-degree relatives. *Br J Dermatol.* 152:82, 2005.

Holmes GK. Coeliac disease following high-dose chemotherapy. *Clin Oncol (R Coll Radiol).* 14:494, 2002.

Hughes AM, et al. Sun exposure may protect against non-Hodgkin lymphoma: a case-control study. *Int J Cancer.* 112:865, 2004.

Joyce AM, et al. Capsule endoscopy findings in celiac disease associated enteropathy-type intestinal T-cell lymphoma. *Endoscopy* 37:594, 2005.

Leffler D, et al. Celiac disease. *Am J Manag Care.* 9:825, 2003.

Leukemia and Lymphoma Society. Integrative medicine and complementary and alternative therapies as part of blood cancer care. Accessed December 2, 2005 at http://www.leukemia-lymphoma.org/all_mat_toc.adp?item_id=9882.

Lim U, et al. Dietary determinants of one-carbon metabolism and the risk of non-Hodgkin's lymphoma: NCI-SEER case-control study, 1998–2000. *Am J Epidemiol.* 162:953, 2005.

Skibola CF, et al. Polymorphisms and haplotypes in folate-metabolizing genes and risk of non-Hodgkin lymphoma. *Blood* 104:2155, 2004.

Yee KW, O'Brien SM. Chronic lymphocytic leukemia: diagnosis and treatment. *Mayo Clin Proc.* 81:1105, 2006.

MELANOMA AND SKIN CANCERS

NUTRITIONAL ACUITY RANKING: NOT RANKED

DEFINITIONS AND BACKGROUND

Skin cancer is the most common cancer in the United States, and the incidence is increasing. Skin cancer and photoaging are thought to be the result of excessive ultraviolet radiation exposure (Uliasz and Spencer 2004). Vitamin D is made in the skin on exposure to solar radiation; regular use of a tanning bed that emits vitamin D–producing ultraviolet radiation is associated with higher 25-hydroxyvitamin D concentrations, which may benefit the skeleton but not the skin (Tangpricha et al, 2004). Ultraviolet B–induced skin damage places individuals more at risk for basal cell and squamous cell carcinomas than for malignant melanoma.

Since carcinogenesis and photoaging are multistep processes, tumor development may be halted at several points of intervention (Uliasz and Spencer 2004). Intake of flavonols may be protective (McNaughton et al, 2005).

Excessive ultraviolet B light exposure in childhood seems to promote development of skin cancer in adulthood (Wolpowitz and Gilchrest, 2006; Greer, 2004). Approximately 65–90% of melanomas may be caused by ultraviolet radiation, especially exposure during childhood. Interesting research now suggests that occupational sun exposure rate is positively correlated with a lower risk of overall organ mortality; adequate vitamin D is protective, and the health benefits of sunlight may outweigh some risks (Krause et al, 2006). Table 13-22 describes risk factors for skin cancers.

Basal cell tumors start as small, shiny, firm nodules that enlarge slowly; they may bleed and scab then heal and then repeat the cycle. Basal cell tumors should be removed to avoid destruction to other tissues. Low intake of total fat and high intake of vitamins may reduce risk of basal cell carcinoma (van Dam et al, 2000).

Squamous cell carcinoma originates in the middle layer of epidermis and may develop on sun-damaged skin or even in the mouth lining or tongue. This type begins as a reddened area with a scaly, crusted surface that does not heal. It may have the appearance of a wart and eventually becomes an open sore. Removal is important before it can spread.

Melanoma, the deadliest type of skin cancer, originates in the melanocytes and tends to spread rapidly. Biopsy is essential. It is the most common cancer for women aged 25–29 years and the second most common cancer for women aged 30–34 years. One study suggests that abnormal intake or metabolism of copper and iron might be implicated in the etiology of melanoma (Bergomi et al, 2005). Disfiguring surgery is no longer necessary to remove a melanoma. Treatments include chemotherapy, and adding glutamine to the diet may be beneficial (Benlloch et al, 2006).

TABLE 13-22 Risk Factors for Skin Cancer

History of sunburns early in life
Chronic exposure to the sun and ultraviolet light with susceptible vitamin D receptor genes
Light skin color, hair color, or eye color
Family or personal history of skin cancer
Certain types of moles or a large number of moles
Freckles, which indicate sun sensitivity and sun damage

INTERVENTION: OBJECTIVES

- Maintain appropriate weight for height.
- General healthy dietary guidelines should be followed.
- Prevent or correct nutritional deficiencies and improve patient tolerance of treatment.
- Minimize potential treatment side effects.
- Optimize immune function to increase effectiveness of therapy.
- Enhance quality of life.
- Ensure appropriate healing of surgical sites (if applicable).

INTERVENTION: FOOD AND NUTRITION

- Eat a variety of foods.
- Choose a diet moderate in fat while controlled in saturated fat and cholesterol. Include good sources of omega-3 fatty acids regularly (i.e., salmon, tuna, mackerel, herring, and sardines).
- Choose a diet with plenty of vegetables, fruits, grain products, and flavonols such as tea and coffee. Micronutrients can act as ultraviolet absorbers or as antioxidants, or they can modulate signaling pathways elicited upon ultraviolet exposure (Sies and Stahl, 2004).
- Use sugars, salt, and alcoholic beverages in moderation.
- If anemic, a diet that meets at least DRI requirements for blood-forming nutrients will be needed.
- Weight gain caused by fluid retention is commonly seen in patients receiving biological therapy (immunotherapy). Fluid retention can be improved with 2–4 g of sodium in the diet and/or fluid restriction.

CLINICAL INDICATORS

Clinical/History

Height
Weight
Weight changes
BMI
Diet history
Changes in skin or mole
Itching, bleeding of mole
Nausea and vomiting
Anorexia

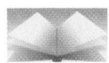

Lab Work	H & H	Ca++, Mg++
Alb	Serum ferritin	Na+, K+
CRP	Transferrin	

Common Drugs Used and Potential Side Effects

- Aldara skin cream reduces basal cell lesions without surgery
- Interferon-α2b (Intron-A) is used in adult patients who have surgically treated melanoma considered at high risk of recurrence.
- Immunomodulating agent histamine dihydrochloride (Maxamine), when used in combination with interleukin-2 (IL-2), improves survival for stage IV malignant melanoma patients compared with those treated with the same doses of IL-2 alone.

Herbs, Botanicals, and Supplements (see Table 13-8)

- Herbs and botanical supplements should not be used without discussing with physician.

INTERVENTION: NUTRITION EDUCATION, COUNSELING, CARE MANAGEMENT

- Discuss rationale for spacing meals throughout day to avoid fatigue.
- Offer recipes and meal plans that provide nutrients required to improve status and immunological competence.
- Patients undergoing treatment should be allowed flexibility in their food selections, while focusing on high-energy, high-quality protein and phytochemical-rich choices whenever possible.
- Offer recipes and menu options for individual planning.
- Patient should apply sunscreen after about 15 minutes in the sun.
- Biofeedback and stress management techniques may be useful.
- Dietary protection is provided by carotenoids, tocopherols, ascorbate, flavonoids, or omega-3 fatty acids, contributing to lifelong protection (Sies and Stahl, 2004). A variety of potential chemopreventive agents may be considered, including vitamins, diet, aspirin, nonsteroidal anti-inflammatory drugs, and topical agents (Uliasz and Spencer, 2004).

Patient Education—Food Safety

- Education on food safety may be needed.

For More Information

- Clinical Guidelines for Melanoma
  http://www.nccn.org/professionals/physician_gls/PDF/melanoma.pdf
- Melanoma Research Foundation
  http://www.melanoma.org/
- Treatment Decisions
  http://www.nccn.org/patients/patient_gls/_english/_melanoma/contents.asp

MELANOMA AND SKIN CANCERS—CITED REFERENCES

Benlloch M, et al. Bcl-2 and MnSOD antisense oligodeoxynucleotides and a glutamine-enriched diet facilitate elimination of highly resistant B16 melanoma cells by TNF-alpha and chemotherapy. *J Biol Chem.* 281:69, 2006.

Bergomi M, et al. Trace elements and melanoma. *J Trace Elem Med Biol.* 19:69, 2005.

Greer FR. Issues in establishing vitamin D recommendations for infants and children. *Am J Clin Nutr.* 80:1759S, 2004.

Krause R, et al. UV radiation and cancer prevention: What is the evidence? *Anticancer Res.* 26:2723, 2006.

McNaughton SA, et al. Role of dietary factors in the development of basal cell cancer and squamous cell cancer of the skin. *Cancer Epidemiol Biomarkers Prev.* 14:1596, 2005.

Sies H, Stahl W. Nutritional protection against skin damage from sunlight. *Annu Rev Nutr.* 24:173-200, 2004.

Tangpricha V, et al. Tanning is associated with optimal vitamin D status (serum 25-hydroxyvitamin D concentration) and higher bone mineral density. *Am J Clin Nutr.* 80:1645, 2004.

Uliasz A, Spencer JM. Chemoprevention of skin cancer and photoaging. *Clin Dermatol.* 22:178, 2004.

van Dam R, et al. Diet and basal cell carcinoma of the skin in a prospective cohort of men. *Am J Clin Nutr.* 71:135, 2000.

Wolpowitz D, Gilchrest BA. The vitamin D questions: how much do you need and how should you get it? *J Am Acad Dermatol.* 54:301, 2006.

MYELOMA, MULTIPLE

NUTRITIONAL ACUITY RANKING: LEVEL 3

DEFINITIONS AND BACKGROUND

Multiple myeloma is a malignant plasma cell cancer of the hematopoietic system in which plasma cells proliferate, invade bone marrow, and produce abnormal immunoglobulin. The condition is rare, affecting four in 100,000 persons. Males are affected more often than females, and the disorder usually strikes after 50 years of age. It represents only 1% of all cancers. Obesity promotes this type of cancer (Pan et al, 2004). Greater use of vitamin C supplements by whites and the higher frequency of obesity among blacks may explain why the incidence of multiple myeloma among blacks is higher compared to whites in the United States (Brown et al, 2001).

Multiple myeloma affects several areas of bone marrow. Symptoms and signs include bone pain, anemia, weight loss, hypercalcemia with pathological fractures, shortened stature, fatigue, weakness, renal disorders, bleeding tendency (especially gums), nausea and vomiting, pneumonia, and urinary tract infections. If significant bone lesions, renal failure, or hypercalcemia occur, chemotherapy or transplantation is recommended (Pan, 2004). Stem-cell transplantation or radiation therapy may be administered to the right candidate.

INTERVENTION: OBJECTIVES

- Avoid fasting. Space meals and snacks adequately.
- Counteract episodes of fatigue and weakness.
- Manage pain effectively.
- Counteract side effects of antineoplastic therapy, steroid therapy, and radiotherapy.
- Avoid infections and febrile states.
- Prevent spontaneous fractures, as far as possible.
- Correct anorexia, nausea and vomiting, and weight loss.

INTERVENTION: FOOD AND NUTRITION

- Provide diet as usual, with six small feedings rather than large meals.
- A higher protein intake may be useful to counteract losses.
- Provide adequate energy to meet requirements of weight control, preventing unnecessary losses.
- Avoid dehydration by including adequate fluid intake (e.g., 3 L daily). This is important.
- Ensure sufficient intake of omega-3 fatty acids, vitamins, minerals, and phytochemicals, especially from fruits and vegetables.

CLINICAL INDICATORS

Clinical/History		Lab Work
Height	Renal disorders	Ca++ (increased)
Weight, weight loss	Bleeding tendency (especially gums)	Mg++
BMI	Frequent infections, urinary or respiratory	Na+, K+
Diet history	Skeletal survey	Total protein
Bone pain	I & O	Parathormone (PTH) (increased)
Infections	BP	TLC (varies)
Fractures, shortened stature	Nausea and vomiting	Hypercalciuria
Paraplegia	Anorexia	Alb (often increased)
Fatigue, weakness, apathy	History of bleeding	CRP
Sudden confusion		Transferrin

H & H	Sedimentation rate (increased)	Uric acid (increased)
Proteinuria (Bence Jones proteins)		RBP
		ALT (increased)

Common Drugs Used and Potential Side Effects

- Arsenic trioxide (Trisenox), carmustine (BiCU, BCNU), cyclophosphamide (Cytoxan), doxorubicin (Adriamycin, Rubex), idarubicin (Idamycin), interferon-alpha (Roferon-A, Intron-A), lenalidomide (Revlimid), pamidronate (Aredia), vincristine (Oncovin), or zoledronic acid (Zometa) may be given as chemotherapy, often with several in a mixture. Melphalan (Alkeran) or nitrosoureas may also be used; monitor for anorexia, anemia, nausea, vomiting, and stomatitis.
- Bisphosphonates may be used to prevent bone fractures.
- Pamidronate may be used. Ensure adequate fluid intake but not excess. Avoid use with calcium and vitamin D supplements. Extra phosphorus may be needed. Nausea, vomiting, gastrointestinal bleeding or distress, and constipation can occur.
- Prednisone, if used chronically, can increase nitrogen losses and potassium and magnesium depletion and can cause hyperglycemia and sodium retention.
- Lenalidomide delays disease progression in late-stage multiple myeloma. It also helps reduce the need for blood transfusions.
- Thalidomide has shown some benefit.
- Bortezomib (Velcade), a proteasome inhibitor, delays disease progression and extends survival.

Herbs, Botanicals, and Supplements (see Table 13-8)

- Herbs and botanical supplements should not be used without discussing with physician.

INTERVENTION: NUTRITION EDUCATION, COUNSELING, CARE MANAGEMENT

- Discuss rationale for spacing meals throughout day to avoid fatigue.
- Offer recipes and meal plans that provide nutrients required to improve status and immunological competence.

Patient Education—Food Safety

- Education on food safety may be needed.

For More Information

- Cleveland Clinic–Multiple Myeloma Programs
  http://www.clevelandclinic.org/myeloma/
- Clinical Guidelines for Multiple Myeloma
  http://www.nccn.org/professionals/physician_gls/PDF/myeloma.pdf

- International Myeloma Foundation
  http://www.myeloma.org/
- Mayo Clinic Myeloma
  http://www.mayoclinic.com/health/multiple-myeloma/DS00415
- Multiple Myeloma Education Network
  http://www.healthtalk.com/mmen/
- Multiple Myeloma Foundation
  http://www.multiplemyeloma.org/
- National Library of Medicine
  http://www.nlm.nih.gov/medlineplus/multiplemyeloma.html

MYELOMA, MULTIPLE—CITED REFERENCES

Brown LM, et al. Diet and nutrition as risk factors for multiple myeloma among blacks and whites in the United States. *Cancer Causes Control.* 12:117, 2001.

Pan SL, et al. Association of obesity and cancer risk in Canada. *Am J Epidemiol.* 159:259, 2004.

PANCREATIC CANCER

NUTRITIONAL ACUITY RANKING: LEVEL 3–4

DEFINITIONS AND BACKGROUND

Pancreatic cancer is the fourth most common cause of death from cancer in men and the fifth for women, primarily occurring between 65 and 79 years of age. Development of pancreas cancer progresses over many years before symptoms appear, and most people with pancreatic cancer die within 6 months of diagnosis (Hine et al, 2003). Nearly all pancreatic cancers are primary pancreatic adenocarcinomas. Incidence is increasing. Table 13-23 lists known risk factors for this type of cancer; symptoms and interventions are listed in Table 13-24.

Exercise, such as walking 4 hours or more weekly, may protect against this cancer. Good folate and pyridoxine status helps reduce risk of pancreatic cancer. Intake of omega-3 fatty acids may reduce tumor growth (Gregor et al, 2006).

TABLE 13-23 Risk Factors for Pancreatic Cancer

Smoking is the major known risk factor, found in 20–30% of all cases (Lowenfels and Maisonneuve, 2005)
History of diabetes mellitus (Qiu et al, 2005; Schernhammer et al, 2005)
Age (over 60 years) and being male
Rare hereditary disorders (such as familial pancreatic cancer, Peutz-Jeghers disease, familial melanoma, hereditary nonpolyposis colorectal cancer, hereditary pancreatitis)
African Americans in the United States have rates that are about 50% higher than Caucasians (Lowenfels and Maisonneuve, 2005)
Inheriting the *BRCA2* gene, common among the Jewish population
Chronic pancreatitis
Partial gastrectomy for peptic ulcer surgery
Underlying insulin resistance (Chari et al, 2005; Schernhammer et al, 2005; Silvera et al, 2005; Stolzenberg-Solomon et al, 2005)
Diet high in meat, cholesterol, and fried foods (Lin et al, 2005)
Diet low in vitamin C, fruits, and vegetables (Lin et al, 2005)
Consumption of dietary nitrite from animal products, but not from drinking water, may increase risk (Coss et al, 2004)
Occupational exposures

Nutrition intervention together with chemotherapy improved outcomes in patients with pancreatic cancer over 8 weeks; supplement intake does not inhibit meal intake (Bauer and Capra, 2005).

About 50–70% of patients have cancer in the head of the pancreas, and 50% have cancer in the body and tail. Patients who have cancer in the head of the pancreas often present with cholangitis, nausea, anorexia, weight loss, new-onset diabetes, light-colored stools, dark urine, steatorrhea, jaundice, and pruritus. Those who have cancer in the body or tail of the pancreas present with vague abdominal pain, dyspepsia, nausea, intermittent diarrhea, unexpected diabetes, and constant back pain.

Medical treatment consists of radiation, chemotherapy, immunotherapy, or vaccine therapy. Unfortunately, only about 10% of patients with pancreatic cancer have a form that can be resected with pancreaticoduodenectomy; it has many nutritional implications (Petzel, 2005; Tang et al, 2005). **Whipple's procedure** (pancreaticoduodenectomy) involves many operations; the entire duodenum is usually removed, and the pancreas, gallbladder, and spleen may also be removed. After surgery, the diet can be liberalized after 10–14 days, adding one new food at a time and using supplements when appetite is poor.

In the United States, the cumulative mortality or lifetime risk of dying from pancreatic cancer is about 1–2% (Lowenfels and Maisonneuve, 2005). Malignancy in the pancreas has a high mortality rate from lack of early symptoms, symptoms that mimic other conditions, and rapid metastasis to other organs. Survival rate of 1 year or longer is only 25%.

INTERVENTION: OBJECTIVES

- Reduce nausea and vomiting; control future episodes.
- Prevent or correct weight loss, which is associated with poor outcomes (Davidson et al, 2004), and restore lean body mass.
- Control side effects of therapies and the disease such as diabetes, anemia, pancreatic fistula, wound infection, bile leak, cholangitis, dumping syndrome, weight loss, and lactose intolerance (Petzel, 2005).
- Provide foods or supplements that include all necessary nutrients to prolong health.

TABLE 13-24 Symptoms, Side Effects, Causes, and Interventions for Pancreatic Cancer

Condition	Frequency	Cause	Intervention
Abdominal distention (ascites)	Not uncommon during advanced disease	Spread of the cancer to the abdominal cavity Liver disease Portal vein thrombosis	Treatment varies depending on the cause.
Abdominal pain	Very common Occurs in approximately three fourths of patients with advanced disease	Often caused by the tumor growing large enough to push against surrounding organs and nerves. May worsen after eating or when lying down. Also common during recovery from surgery.	Pain medication (analgesics) Opiates are very effective if taken regularly and at correct dosage. Opiates frequently cause constipation and may be taken with laxatives. If pain persists, a celiac nerve block may be considered. This involves the injection of alcohol into the nerves near the pancreas to block the sensation of pain. The injection can be given through the skin, during surgery, or during an endoscopic ultrasound.
Anemia	Occasional	Often related to chemotherapy.	Medication: erythropoietin
Anorexia	Common during advanced disease	Loss of appetite and signs of physical weight loss Weight loss is common to almost all types of cancer. The cancer cells compete with normal cells for nutrients. Also, tumors of the pancreas often interfere with digestion, which further contributes to weight loss.	It is difficult to treat this weight loss, especially loss of muscle mass. Nutritional supplements may be of benefit. Appetite stimulants such as Megace (medroxyacetate) may be of modest benefit. Occasionally a percutaneous endoscopic gastrostomy (PEG) feeding tube is placed in the stomach during endoscopy.
Back pain	Very common especially during advanced disease	Often caused by the tumor growing large enough to push against surrounding organs and nerves. May worsen after eating or when lying down.	Pain medication (analgesics) Opiates are very effective if taken regularly and at correct dosage. Opiates frequently cause constipation and may be taken with laxatives. If pain persists, a celiac nerve block may be considered.
Bone pain	Uncommon	Spread of the cancer to bone Osteomalacia can occur.	Medication (bisphosphonates) may be helpful. Adequate vitamin D and calcium are needed.
Bruising	Uncommon	The anticancer drugs given during chemotherapy affect normal cells as well as cancer cells. When normal blood cells are affected, they may not clot well, which can lead to easy bruising.	If severe, platelet and blood transfusions may be administered.
Bleeding	Uncommon	The anticancer drugs given during chemotherapy affect normal cells as well as cancer cells. When normal blood cells are affected, the blood cells may not clot well, which may cause the patient to bleed easily.	If severe, platelet and blood transfusions may be administered.
Cachexia	Common	Usually caused by metastatic disease	It is difficult to treat this weight loss, especially loss of muscle mass. Nutritional supplements may be of benefit. Appetite stimulants such as Megace (medroxyacetate) may be of modest benefit.
Chills	Common	Infection caused by obstruction of the bile ducts and/or biological therapy (vaccines)	Antibiotics May require a stent to relieve obstruction. The stent can be placed endoscopically or percutaneously through the liver. Hospitalization may be required.

(continued)

TABLE 13-24 Symptoms, Side Effects, Causes, and Interventions for Pancreatic Cancer *(continued)*

Condition	Frequency	Cause	Intervention
Cramping	Fairly common	May be present after surgery due to electrolyte imbalances and/or resumption of bowel function	Only intervention is to correct electrolyte balance.
Diabetes	New onset is not uncommon.	Due to impaired insulin secretion by the pancreas May also occur after surgical removal of entire pancreas or a portion of it	Removal of part of the pancreas with the cancer may cure the diabetes. Insulin replacement
Diarrhea	Very common after surgery	Many patients have diarrhea after surgery. This is caused by a lack of pancreatic enzymes, which affects digestion. Adjuvant chemotherapy may aggravate preexisting diarrhea.	Medication to replace pancreatic enzymes taken with meals and possibly dietary changes If diarrhea is not due to fat malabsorption or *Escherichia coli*, use antidiarrheal agent. Oral calcium may be used to slow gastrointestinal transit time.
Depression	Common	Related both to the emotional reaction to the diagnosis and to direct effects of the cancer	Supportive therapy and/or antidepressant medication
Fatigue and weakness	Very common after surgery	Surgery, radiation therapy, chemotherapy, and malnutrition are all a strain on the body and often cause fatigue. Anemia also contributes.	There is not much to do other than resting as necessary. Exercise improves stamina. A healthy diet and psychological support can also help.
Fever	Common during advanced disease Rare during vaccine therapy	Obstruction of bile ducts can lead to infection in the bile ducts and possibly the liver. The body's immune response to the infection results in a fever.	Surgical relief of obstruction, stent placement, and antibiotics Antipyretics may be needed.
Hair thinning and hair loss	Uncommon with drugs used for pancreatic cancer	Anticancer drugs used in chemotherapy are chosen because they affect cells that divide rapidly, such as cancer cells and hair root cells. However, this is uncommon (<5%) during pancreatic cancer treatment. Radiation therapy can cause hair loss in affected area.	There is no way to prevent hair from falling out as a result of chemotherapy. Hair usually begins growing back within 1 month after the treatment ends.
Itchiness (pruritus)	Common May be a symptom of a bile duct obstruction caused by pancreatic cancer	Occurs due to obstruction of bile ducts (see Jaundice below)	Surgical relief, stent placement
Jaundice	Very common	The last portion of the bile duct joins with the pancreatic duct in the back of the head of the pancreas and empties into the duodenum. As a tumor grows in the head of the pancreas, the bile duct becomes blocked. When the duct becomes blocked (obstructed), bile backs up into the liver and enters the bloodstream. This leads to a visible yellowing of the eyes and the skin. As bile is not getting to the digestive tract, stool becomes light or clay colored.	Stent placement either endoscopically or percutaneously
Mouth sores	Uncommon Occur in patients during chemotherapy treatment	The anticancer drugs used in chemotherapy are chosen because they affect cells that divide rapidly, such as cancer cells. The cells of the digestive tract also divide rapidly and are therefore strongly affected by these drugs. More often occur during fluorouracil chemotherapy. Also occurs with gemcitabine but not quite as often.	Antiseptic and analgesic mouthwashes may be prescribed to numb the discomfort. The sores will heal on their own without medication.

(continued)

TABLE 13-24 Symptoms, Side Effects, Causes, and Interventions for Pancreatic Cancer *(continued)*

Condition	Frequency	Cause	Intervention
Muscle aches	Rare	Biological therapy (vaccines)	Probably reflects a flu-like reaction and therefore may respond to acetaminophen (e.g., Tylenol)
Nausea	Common in 30–50% depending on stage	Obstruction of digestive tract by tumor	Surgical relief or duodenal stent
		Radiation or chemotherapy	Reglan (metoclopramide) or other antivomiting drugs may be prescribed.
Rash	Uncommon	Due to obstruction Biological therapy (vaccines)	There is currently no treatment for rashes due to obstruction. Topical steroids may be prescribed for rashes developing during vaccine therapy.
Skin irritation		Radiation therapy may cause red, dry, tender, itchy skin in affected area. Darkening of skin may also occur.	Patients should consult their doctor before using lotion or cream on the affected area.
Stool discoloration	Very common	See Jaundice.	
Swelling during vaccine therapy	Very common	Occurs near injection site	None; typically goes away in about a week
Thrombophlebitis	Uncommon	This condition is marked by inflammation and clotting of veins in the skin. This is the body's response to the cancer or direct spread of the cancer to blood vessels	Prescription of anticoagulants to prevent clots from forming and potentially causing a stroke
Urine discoloration	Very common	Jaundice The accumulation of bile in the urine makes it appear darker than usual.	Stent placement either endoscopically or percutaneously
Vomiting	Uncommon More common during advanced disease	Also may be caused by chemotherapy	Medication such as metoclopramide (Reglan), lorazepam (Ativan), steroids, ondansetron, granisetron, and tetrahydrocannabinol

Adapted from: Johns Hopkins Pathology. Pancreas cancer. Accessed December 4, 2005 at http://pathology2.jhu.edu/pancreas/symptom.cfm.

- Augment nutritional intake; correct anemia. Include protective vegetables.
- Monitor for depression and encourage use of antidepressants if needed to help with appetite.
- Manage problems such as lactose intolerance, pancreatic cancer–related diabetes, and malabsorption. Eventually, vitamin B_{12} malabsorption occurs.
- Total parenteral nutrition (TPN) is indicated mainly for perioperative use in patients with known malnutrition preoperatively. Postoperatively, tube feeding is the nutrition support method of choice.
- Wean off tube feeding with increasing oral intake and resolving gastroparesis, usually 4–6 weeks postoperatively.

INTERVENTION: FOOD AND NUTRITION

- **For pancreatic insufficiency:** Medium-chain triglycerides (MCT) and fat-soluble vitamins (water-miscible form) may be added to the diet. Essential fatty acids (EFAs) should also be included. Calcium, zinc, and iron may become deficient unless supplemented. Selenium may also be needed.
- Use of omega-3 fatty acids can reduce inflammation and pain, thus improving quality of life (Bauer and Capra, 2005). It may be helpful to take 2 g/d, especially of eicosapentaenoic acid (EPA).
- TPN may be beneficial for short-term use, altering nutrients according to serum values. There are few studies that support the long-term use of parenteral nutrition (PN) after surgery (Gupta and Ihmaidat, 2003).
- After Whipple's procedure, TPN or tube feeding may be required. If pain is severe, tube feeding should be tried before TPN.
- Small, frequent meals may be better tolerated when and if the patient can eat orally. Include protective foods, especially tomato products for lycopene and other vegetables and fruits (Nkondjock et al, 2005). Onions, garlic, beans, orange and yellow vegetables, spinach, broccoli, kale, and raw vegetables are especially protective.
- Increased energy intake and protein should be provided to restore lost weight, unless patient is currently hyperglycemic or has extensive liver impairment. Eventually, a carbohydrate-controlled diet may be needed to manage diabetes if patient is able to eat.
- After Whipple's procedure, feed after bowel sounds return, and use a low-fat diet (40–60 g) that is low in lactose.

Avoid fatty and fried foods, nuts, and seeds. Small meals are best tolerated; 6–8 feedings may be better tolerated than three large meals. Pancreatic enzyme replacement will be needed. Delayed gastric emptying is common, so avoidance of simple sugars and hot liquids may also be needed.

CLINICAL INDICATORS

Clinical/History

Height
Weight
BMI
Rapid weight loss
Diet history
Midepigastric pain
Signs of biliary obstruction
Anorexia
Pancreatic insufficiency (indigestion, cramping, bloating)
Belching
Steatorrhea or loose stools
Nausea and vomiting
Fatigue
Ascites
Thrombophlebitis
Hepatomegaly
Temperature
BP
Angiography
CT scan
Endoscopic ultrasound
Fine-needle biopsy
Endoscopic retrograde cholangiopancreatography (ERCP)

Lab Work

Ca 19-9
Alk phos (increased)
PT (increased)
Gluc (increased)
Serum lipase (increased)
Secretin
PSCA levels
Transferrin
Serum insulin
TLC (varies)
Bilirubin (increased)
Cholecystokinin
Alb
CRP
Chol, Trig
Serum amylase (increased)
H & H
ALT, AST (increased)
Ca++, Mg++
Na+, K+
Serum B_{12}
Serum folate

Common Drugs Used and Potential Side Effects

- Chemotherapy may include gemcitabine.
- Pancreatic enzymes (pancrelipase and pancreatin) are given. Enteric coating aids in maintaining integrity of enzymes until they reach small intestine. If pork allergy is present, there may be a reaction to these enzymes; a pork-free product is PAN-2400. As much as 20,000–30,000 units of lipase may be needed per meal; 10,000 units may be needed with snacks. They must be swallowed whole and not chewed.
- Insulin may be needed if patient is hyperglycemic. In islet cell tumors, hypoglycemia may occur instead. Monitor with meal timing.
- Acid-reducing medications (such as proton-pump inhibitors or H_2 blockers) are usually needed.
- Vitamin B_{12} supplements may be required with total pancreatectomy, especially with steatorrhea.
- Water-miscible fat-soluble vitamins A, D, E, and K will be needed until intake of pancreatic enzymes is sufficient. Brands may include Vitamax, Source CF, and ADEKs.
- Antiemetics, diuretics, and analgesics may be needed. Monitor side effects according to medications prescribed.
- Calcium carbonate twice daily may be useful to help bulk stools that are loose. Antidiarrheal medications (e.g., Lomotil, opiates, or Imodium) may be needed if loose stools are persistent. Guar gum and psyllium can be used to add soluble fiber.
- Streptozocin and other antibiotics can cause or aggravate nausea.

Herbs, Botanicals, and Supplements (see Table 13-8)

- Herbs and botanical supplements should not be used without discussing with physician.

INTERVENTION: NUTRITION EDUCATION, COUNSELING, CARE MANAGEMENT

- Discuss specific dietary recommendations appropriate for patient's condition and therapies.
- With pancreatectomy, a diabetic diet may be absolutely essential. Discuss rationale with patient.
- Explain how diet affects malabsorption in regard to fat, protein, vitamins, and minerals.
- Lactase enzymes may be helpful if lactose intolerance persists.
- Use supplements that contain omega-3 fatty acids (Moses et al, 2004).
- Family members may need genetic counseling (Vimalachandran et al, 2004).
- Discuss use of pancreatic enzymes.
- Provide education for diet and jejunostomy feeding.

Patient Education—Food Safety

- Educate about food safety issues.

For More Information

- Cancer Net–Pancreatic Cancer
  http://cancernet.nci.nih.gov/templates/doc.aspx?viewid=e70b3e33-2d56-4084-8ded-8336fe72d157
- Diet and Nutrition
  http://www.pancan.org/Patient/Pancreatic/Diet/more.html
- Hospice
  http://www.hospicenet.org/index.html
- Johns Hopkins–Pancreatic Cancer Home Page
  http://www.path.jhu.edu/pancreas
- Lustgarten Foundation for Pancreatic Cancer Research
  http://www.lustgartenfoundation.org/
- Medline–Pancreatic Cancer
  http://www.nlm.nih.gov/medlineplus/pancreaticcancer.html
- National Pancreas Foundation
  http://www.pancreasfoundation.org/
- Pancreatic Cancer Action Network
  http://www.pancan.org/

PANCREATIC CANCER—CITED REFERENCES

Bauer JD, Capra S. Nutrition intervention improves outcomes in patients with cancer cachexia receiving chemotherapy—a pilot study. *Support Care Cancer.* 13:270, 2005.

Chari ST, et al. Beta-cell function and insulin resistance evaluated by HOMA in pancreatic cancer subjects with varying degrees of glucose intolerance. *Pancreatology* 5:229, 2005.

Coss A, et al. Pancreatic cancer and drinking water and dietary sources of nitrate and nitrite. *Am J Epidemiol.* 159:693, 2004.

Davidson W, et al. Weight stabilisation is associated with improved survival duration and quality of life in unresectable pancreatic cancer. *Clin Nutr.* 23:239, 2004.

Gregor JI, et al. Does enteral nutrition of dietary polyunsaturated fatty acids promote oxidative stress and tumour growth in ductal pancreatic cancer? Experimental trial in Syrian Hamster. *Prostaglandins Leukot Essent Fatty Acids.* 74:67, 2006.

Gupta R, Ihmaidat H. Nutritional effects of oesophageal, gastric and pancreatic carcinoma. *Eur J Surg Oncol.* 29:634, 2003.

Hine RJ, et al. Nutritional links to plausible mechanisms underlying pancreatic cancer: a conference report. *Pancreas* 27:356, 2003.

Lin Y, et al. Nutritional factors and risk of pancreatic cancer: a population-based case-control study based on direct interview in Japan. *J Gastroenterol.* 40:297, 2005.

Lowenfels AB, Maisonneuve P. Risk factors for pancreatic cancer. *J Cell Biochem.* 95:649, 2005.

Moses AW, et al. Reduced total energy expenditure and physical activity in cachectic patients with pancreatic cancer can be modulated by an energy and protein dense oral supplement enriched with n-3 fatty acids. *Br J Cancer.* 90:996, 2004.

Nkondjock A, et al. Dietary intake of lycopene is associated with reduced pancreatic cancer risk. *J Nutr.* 135:592, 2005.

Petzel M. Nutrition support of the patient with pancreatic cancer. *Nutr Support.* 27:11, 2005.

Qiu D, et al. Overview of the epidemiology of pancreatic cancer focusing on the JACC Study. *J Epidemiol.* 15:157S, 2005.

Schernhammer ES, et al. Sugar-sweetened soft drink consumption and risk of pancreatic cancer in two prospective cohorts. *Cancer Epidemiol Biomarkers Prev.* 14:2098, 2005.

Silvera SA, et al. Glycemic index, glycemic load, and pancreatic cancer risk (Canada). *Cancer Causes Control.* 16:431, 2005.

Stolzenberg-Solomon RZ, et al. Insulin, glucose, insulin resistance, and pancreatic cancer in male smokers. *JAMA.* 294:2872, 2005.

Tang CN, et al. Endo-laparoscopic approach in the management of obstructive jaundice and malignant gastric outflow obstruction. *Hepatogastroenterology* 52:128, 2005.

Vimalachandran D, et al. Genetics and prevention of pancreatic cancer. *Cancer Control.* 11:6, 2004.

PROSTATE CANCER

NUTRITIONAL ACUITY RANKING: LEVEL 2

DEFINITIONS AND BACKGROUND

Prostate cancer has the third highest incidence of all cancers in men worldwide and is the most common neoplasm diagnosed among men beyond middle age in many developed countries (Fraser et al, 2005). Prostate cancer is the second leading cause of cancer-related death in the United States (Lamb and Zhang, 2005). Prevalence is higher in northwestern Europe and the United States. Incidence among African Americans is the highest in the world. Adult height may be a predictor of risk among black males, representative of hormonal activity and dietary intakes (Freedland et al, 2005).

Men at greatest risk are those with abdominal obesity; those with family history of the disease; those with African American heritage; and those whose diets are low in fiber, high in saturated fats, and high in red meats. Overexpression of the *AMACR* gene is associated with prostate cancer risk, as are increased levels of phytanic acid, which comes from overconsumption of dairy products and red meat (Xu et al, 2005). Obesity in prostate cancer progression suggests a link to the biological basis (Strom et al, 2005).

An effective chemoprevention strategy for prostate cancer will likely serve as a model for chemoprevention of other adult malignancies (Canby-Hagino and Thompson, 2005). Diets rich in specific vitamins, grains, fruits, and vegetables may be associated with lower cancer rates than high-fat diets (Lamb and Zhang, 2005). Preventive factors are listed in Table 13-25. A diet consisting of a wide variety of plant-based foods and fish is prudent (Chan et al, 2005).

Protective dietary elements include tomatoes/lycopene, other carotenoids, cruciferous vegetables, vitamin E, selenium, fish/marine omega-3 fatty acids, soy, isoflavones, and polyphenols (Chan et al, 2005). Vitamin E as gamma-tocopherol interrupts the synthesis of sphingolipids, important components of cell membranes. Vitamin D in its active form of cholecalciferol (1,25-hydroxyvitamin D_3) may inhibit the spread of prostate cancer cells (Tokar and Webber, 2005).

Signs and symptoms of prostate cancer include urinary dribbling, frequency, pain, or burning. Persistent pain in the pelvis, lower back, or upper thighs also may occur. The new normal prostate-specific antigen (PSA) level should be 2.6 ng/mL to catch prostate cancer at an earlier stage.

High-intensity focused ultrasound (HIFU) has been developed and shows promise as treatment. Surgical intervention, radiation, and hormonal therapy are also used. Radiation therapy may cause temporary changes in bowel habits (such as increased frequency, increased flatulence, and bowel cramping). Brachytherapy is internal radiation therapy in which small radioactive pellets are inserted or implanted into the prostate gland.

INTERVENTION: OBJECTIVES

- Prepare patient for therapies (surgery, radiation, medications, chemotherapy, or hormone therapy).
- Prevent or correct side effects such as nausea, vomiting, and diarrhea.
- Prevent or correct weight loss.
- Maintain weight that is appropriate for height. If patient is obese, a weight control plan may be needed.
- Promote intake of protective foods and phytochemicals.

TABLE 13-25 Preventive Dietary Factors for Prostate Cancer

Apigenin
Cruciferous vegetables (Joseph et al, 2004)
Curcumin
Epigallocatechin gallate (EGCG)
Gamma-tocopherol (walnuts, pecans, sesame seed, corn and sesame oils)
Grains, nuts, cereals, soy products
Grape seed extract
Green tea
Herbs and herbal supplements (saw palmetto)
Lignans
Lower fat diet with the addition of omega-3 fatty acids from fish or fish oil (specifically DHA and EPA)
Lutein
Lycopene—antioxidant abundant in red tomatoes and processed tomato products (such as salsa)
Multivitamins including selenium and vitamin E as gamma-tocopherol only (Klein et al, 2001)
Omega-3 fatty acids (fish such as tuna and salmon, flaxseed, walnuts)
Physical activity and exercise (Jian et al, 2005; Zeegers et al, 2005)
Quercetin
Resveratrol
Soy genistein
Vegan diet
Vitamin D (Schwartz, 2005; Tokar and Webber, 2005)

INTERVENTION: FOOD AND NUTRITION

- Provide adequate calories and protein; avoid excesses.
- If surgery has been performed, a multiple vitamin–mineral supplement may be indicated to promote wound healing.
- Monitor need for lowering sodium if corticosteroids are prescribed.
- Increase use of fruits and vegetables, especially green and yellow-orange, and sources of folic acid. Tomatoes, pizza sauce, strawberries, salsa, and tomato products are important for their lycopene content. Drink pomegranate juice often to reduce likelihood of recurrence (Malik et al, 2005).
- Increase use of isoflavonoids (Haddad et al, 2006). Choose often from beans, soybeans, lentils, tofu, tempeh, soy nuts, soymilk, and dried fruit.
- Low-fat, vegan, and high-fiber diets may be indicated (Dunn-Emke et al, 2005; Ornish et al, 2005). Increased use of omega-3 fatty acids has been shown in some preliminary studies to be useful; include salmon, sardines, tuna, mackerel, and herring in diet.
- Take supplements of natural vitamin E (800 IU) and vitamin C (500 mg) daily.
- Vitamin D should be consumed; drink fortified milk, get modest exposure to the sun, and take a vitamin pill.

CLINICAL INDICATORS

Clinical/History

Height
Weight
BMI
Weight changes
Diet history
I & O
Urine testing (infections, enlarged prostate)
Urinary dribbling, frequency, pain, burning
Persistent pain (pelvis, lower back, or upper thighs)
BP
Transrectal ultrasound
Doppler scan
Digital rectal examination
Bone scan, chest x-ray
CT scan, MRI

Lab Work

PSA levels (>2.5 ng/mL is a concern)
Alb, transthyretin
CRP
BUN, Creat
Serum vitamin D
Transferrin
H & H
Ca++, Mg++
Na+, K+

Common Drugs Used and Potential Side Effects

- Aspirin improves survival after prostate cancer.
- Chemotherapy drugs have varying side effects; monitor closely. Fatigue, nausea and vomiting, mouth sores, hair loss, and a low white blood cell count are common.
- Hormonal therapy may be used as the treatment of choice (Bracarda et al, 2005). Luteinizing hormone–releasing hormone (LH-RH) agonists can decrease the amount of testosterone produced by a man's testicles as effectively as surgical removal of the testicles. Lupron Depot (leuprolide acetate for depot suspension), one of the LH-RH agonists, is used in the palliative treatment of advanced prostate cancer.
- Vitamin D: Patients should not take large amounts of vitamin D without medical supervision because it increases blood calcium levels and may cause kidney problems.

Herbs, Botanicals, and Supplements (see Table 13-8)

- Complementary and alternative medicine (CAM) use is common. In the Cancer of the Prostate Strategic Urologic Research Endeavor (CaPSURE), a large, community-based national registry of men with prostate cancer, common practices included vitamin and mineral supplements (26%), herbs (16%), antioxidants (13%), and CAM for prostate health (12%) with use of saw palmetto, selenium, vitamin E, and lycopene (Chan, Elkin et al, 2005). Herbs and botanical supplements should not be used without discussing with the physician.
- Antiandrogen activities of decursin and decursin-containing herbal extracts have significant implications for the chemoprevention and treatment of prostate cancer and other androgen-dependent diseases (Jiang et al, 2006).

- Saw palmetto has some proven efficacy. Avoid taking with estrogens, testosterone, anabolic steroids, oral contraceptives, or finasteride because the herb and drugs function in similar ways and additive effects are possible.
- Pygeum, nettle, and isoflavones in soy and red clover are being studied at this time.
- Phytoestrogens found in common herbal products are effective inhibitors of prostate tumor cell growth through different mechanisms; these include quercetin, baicalein, genistein, epigallocatechin gallate (EGCG), curcumin, apigenin, and resveratrol (Shenouda et al, 2004).

INTERVENTION: NUTRITION EDUCATION, COUNSELING, CARE MANAGEMENT

- Discuss side effects of any specific therapy offered and long-term plans for recovery.
- Discuss lifestyle and dietary changes that are recommended (i.e., lowering intake of red meats and saturated fats, increasing fruits and vegetables and tomato products, increasing fiber and whole grains, and consuming vitamin D–fortified milk).
- Discuss menu plans for sufficient intakes of all protective nutrients. Lycopene can be found in foods such as tomatoes, watermelon, guava, and red grapefruit. Include pomegranates, soy, fish, and plant-based choices. A vegan diet may be especially beneficial (Dunn-Emke et al, 2005).
- Maintain adequate hydration.
- Strategies for prevention include hormonal manipulation and limiting accumulation of genetic damage with anti-inflammatory agents and/or dietary antioxidants (Canby-Hagino and Thompson, 2005).
- Lifestyle changes tend to correlate with quality of life after prostate cancer treatments (Sheriff et al, 2005). Diet and exercise changes are important (Jian et al, 2005).
- Maintaining a positive, optimistic outlook yields more favorable results than giving in to negative emotions (Kronenwetter et al, 2005).

For More Information

- Association for the Cure of Prostate Cancer
  http://www.capcure.org/
- Cancer Nutrition Tips
  http://www.cancer.med.umich.edu/learn/nutrprev.htm
- Medline
  http://www.nlm.nih.gov/medlineplus/prostatecancer.html
- Memorial-Sloan Kettering
  http://www.mskcc.org/mskcc/html/2904.cfm
- Minorities and Underserved Populations
  http://www.ustoo.org/Minority_Program.asp
- Prostate Cancer Research Institute
  http://www.prostate-cancer.org/
- Prostate Cancer Support Group
  http://www.ustoo.com/
- Prostate Information
  http://www.prostate.com/
- Treatment Decisions
  http://www.nccn.org/patients/patient_gls/_english/_prostate/contents.asp
- Urologic Oncology Program
  http://www.cancer.med.umich.edu/prostcan/prostcan.html
- Virtual Prostate
  http://www.virtualprostate.com/

PROSTATE CANCER—CITED REFERENCES

Bracarda S, et al. Cancer of the prostate. *Crit Rev Oncol Hematol.* 56:379, 2005.

Canby-Hagino ED, Thompson IM. Mechanisms of disease: prostate cancer—a model for cancer chemoprevention in clinical practice. *Nat Clin Pract Oncol.* 2:255, 2005.

Chan JM, et al. Role of diet in prostate cancer development and progression. *J Clin Oncol.* 23:8152, 2005.

Chan JM, Elkin EP, et al. Total and specific complementary and alternative medicine use in a large cohort of men with prostate cancer. *Urology* 66:1223, 2005.

Dunn-Emke SR, et al. Nutrient adequacy of a very low-fat vegan diet. *J Am Diet Assoc.* 105:1442, 2005.

Fraser ML, et al. Lycopene and prostate cancer: emerging evidence. *Expert Rev Anticancer Ther.* 5:847, 2005.

Freedland SJ, et al. Racial differences in prognostic value of adult height for biochemical progression following radical prostatectomy. *Clin Cancer Res.* 11:7735, 2005.

Haddad AQ, et al. Novel antiproliferative flavonoids induce cell cycle arrest in human prostate cancer cell lines. *Prostate Cancer Prostatic Dis.* 9:68, 2006.

Jian L, et al. Moderate physical activity and prostate cancer risk: a case-control study in China. *Eur J Epidemiol.* 20:155, 2005.

Jiang C, et al. Potent antiandrogen and androgen receptor activities of an *Angelica gigas*-containing herbal formulation: identification of decursin as a novel and active compound with implications for prevention and treatment of prostate cancer. *Cancer Res.* 66:453, 2006.

Joseph MA, et al. Cruciferous vegetables, genetic polymorphisms in glutathione s-transferases m1 and t1, and prostate cancer risk. *Nutr Cancer.* 50:206, 2004.

Klein E, et al. SELECT: the next prostate cancer prevention trial. Selenium and Vitamin E Cancer Prevention Trial. *J Urol.* 166:1311, 2001.

Kronenwetter C, et al. A qualitative analysis of interviews of men with early stage prostate cancer: the Prostate Cancer Lifestyle Trial. *Cancer Nurs.* 28:99, 2005.

Lamb DJ, Zhang L. Challenges in prostate cancer research: animal models for nutritional studies of chemoprevention and disease progression. *J Nutr.* 135:3009S, 2005.

Malik A, et al. Pomegranate fruit juice for chemoprevention and chemotherapy of prostate cancer. *Proc Natl Acad Sci USA.* 102:14813, 2005.

Ornish D, et al. Intensive lifestyle changes may affect the progression of prostate cancer. *J Urol.* 174:1065, 2005.

Schwartz GG. Vitamin D and the epidemiology of prostate cancer. *Semin Dial.* 18:276, 2005.

Shenouda NS, et al. Phytoestrogens in common herbs regulate prostate cancer cell growth in vitro. *Nutr Cancer.* 49:200, 2004.

Sheriff SK, et al. Lifestyle correlates of health perception and treatment satisfaction in a clinical cohort of men with prostate cancer. *Clin Prostate Cancer.* 3:239, 2005.

Strom SS, et al. Obesity, weight gain, and risk of biochemical failure among prostate cancer patients following prostatectomy. *Clin Cancer Res.* 11:6889, 2005.

Tokar EJ, Webber MM. Cholecalciferol (vitamin D3) inhibits growth and invasion by up-regulating nuclear receptors and 25-hydroxylase (CYP27A1) in human prostate cancer cells. *Clin Exp Metastasis.* 22:275, 2005.

Xu J, et al. Serum levels of phytanic acid are associated with prostate cancer risk. *Prostate* 63:209, 2005.

Zeegers MP, et al. Physical activity and the risk of prostate cancer in the Netherlands cohort study, results after 9.3 years of follow-up. *Cancer Epidemiol Biomarkers Prev.* 14:1490, 2005.

SECTION 14

Surgical Disorders

CHIEF ASSESSMENT FACTORS

Presurgical Status:

- History of Illness—Acute or Chronic (Such as Diabetes, Cerebrovascular Disease, Coronary Heart Disease)
- Recent Weight Changes, Especially Unintentional Loss
- Serum Albumin, Transferrin, Retinol-Binding Protein, and C-Reactive Protein (Inflammation)
- Hydration Status
- Electrolyte Status
- Blood Pressure, Abnormal
- Anemia, Blood Loss
- Nausea, Vomiting
- Surgical Procedure with Gastrointestinal Impact
- Obesity and Anesthesia Risk
- Infections
- Respiratory Function, Oxygen Saturation
- Recent Starvation Status

Postsurgical Status:

- Breathing Rate, Pneumonia
- Labs Such as Glucose, CRP, and Electrolyte Balance
- Pain, Sleep Disturbance
- Nausea, Vomiting, Constipation
- Impaired Skin Integrity, Wound Dehiscence
- Urinary Tract Infection, Sepsis
- Atelectasis
- Paralytic Ileus, Abdominal Distention
- Respiratory Function, Oxygen Saturation
- Fever

General Surgical Guidelines

SURGERY

NUTRITIONAL ACUITY RANKING: LEVEL 2

DEFINITIONS AND BACKGROUND

Nutritional risk from surgery is related to the extent of surgery, prior nutritional state of the patient, and the effect of surgery on the patient's ability to digest and absorb nutrients. Weight loss is one of the most important assessment tools to predict surgical risk as related to nutritional status (Parekh and Steiger, 2004). Techniques to assess body composition help to quantify weight loss and clarify the impact of malnutrition on postsurgical status.

After surgery or injury, plasma cortisol generally increases rapidly, with an acceleration in the breakdown of fat to fatty acids and glycerol. The metabolic response to surgical or accidental injury is characterized by the breakdown of skeletal muscle protein and the transfer of amino acids to visceral organs and the wound, where the substrate serves to enhance host defenses and support vital organ function and wound repair (Wilmore, 2001). Increased excretion of nitrogen and sodium retention occur, but these are reversed in approximately 5–7 days or as late as 12–14 days in elderly individuals and after severe burns. Increased excretion of potassium occurs but begins to reverse itself 1–2 days after surgery.

Malnutrition is prevalent among surgical patients and is associated with higher surgical complication rates and mortality. Some causes of poor nutritional status are related to the underlying disease, socioeconomic factors, age, and length of hospitalization. Because medical teams often overlook malnutrition and screening of these patients is not routine, patients are at risk for malnutrition and complications (Patel, 2005). In a population of patients preparing for gastrointestinal (GI) or hernia surgery, use of Subjective Global Assessment identifies malnutrition in half of the patients, with almost 20% being severely malnourished (Correia et al, 2001).

Elective surgery involves minimal increases in nitrogen loss and a 10–15% increase in energy requirements. Major surgery involves greater intensity and duration that will increase catabolic effects. Prevention of hypoxia in surgical wounds is especially important and preventable; fluid and temperature management are key factors (Ueno et al, 2006). Table 14-1 defines the average length of time and stages of catabolic response after surgery, followed by anabolism. See Figure 14-1 for a surgeon at work.

TABLE 14-1 Postsurgical Phases in Nutrition

3–7 days	Marked catabolic response
2–5 weeks	Turning point and anabolic phase at which spontaneous improvement begins
>6 weeks	Fat gain phase; vigorous nutritional support could promote excessive fat stores

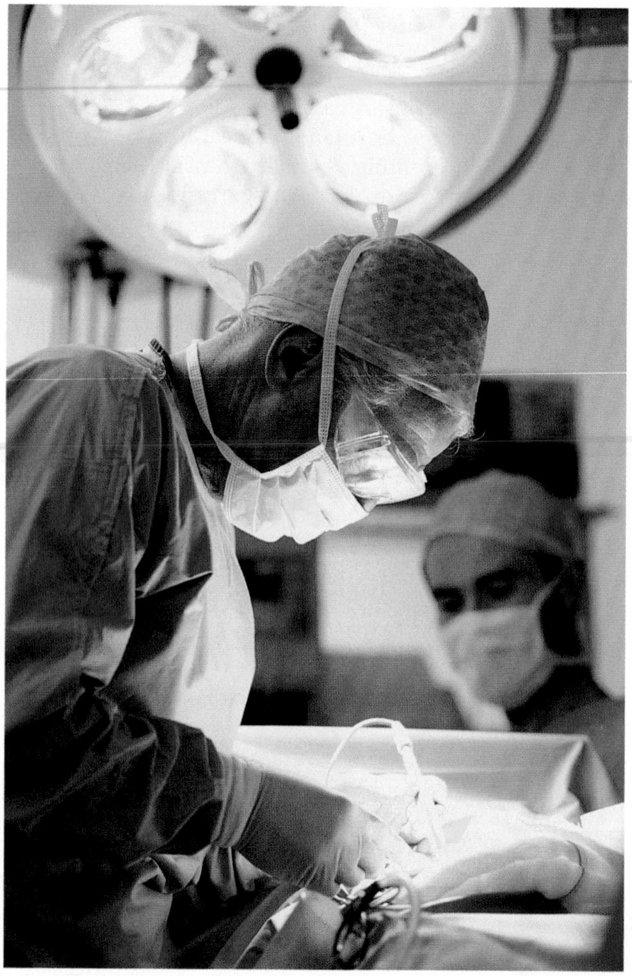

Figure 14-1 Surgeon at work. (Image from Flying Colours Ltd/Digital Vision/Getty Images.)

The presence of cancer, infection, age over 60 years, upper GI disease, and longer length of hospital stay all negatively influence nutritional status. Nutritional status plays an important role in determining outcome after many types of operations. Early postoperative enteral nutrition with a formula supplemented with arginine, omega-3 fatty acids, and RNA increases hydroxyproline synthesis and improves surgical wound healing in patients undergoing gastrectomy for gastric cancer (Farreras et al, 2005; Daly et al, 1992). Enteral immunonutrition is an important consideration preoperatively as well, if time permits.

Fever causes increased nutritional needs; for every 1°F increase, there is an increased energy requirement of 7–8%. Fluids should be increased as well. Optimum healing of a wound requires integration of responses to inflammatory mediators, growth factors, cytokines, and mechanical forces

(Falanga, 2005). Extra protein is needed for wounds, burns, and hemorrhage; major wounds and burns can cause a loss of greater than 50 g protein/d. With hemorrhage or major blood loss, or even when much blood is drawn for laboratory tests, loss of iron and plasma protein may be significant; loss of 1 L of blood equals a loss of 500 mg of iron and 50 g of plasma protein.

C-reactive protein (CRP) is a risk factor for cardiovascular outcomes and mortality in the general population; it predicts all-cause mortality (Winklemayer et al, 2005). Preoperative serum albumin concentration predicted surgical outcomes such as sepsis, renal failure, and major infections in the National Veterans Affairs Surgical Risk Study (Gibbs et al, 1999). Early identification of high-risk patients undergoing major surgery can result in aggressive management; after the surgery, the presence of systemic inflammatory response syndrome is a predictor of later sepsis (Mokart et al, 2005). Other patient risk factors predictive of postoperative morbidity include anesthesia classification, complexity of operation, and other preoperative variables (Daly et al, 1997).

A complete, balanced therapeutic diet is recommended after surgery. After surgery, patients fed a regular diet have less morbidity than those fed a clear liquid diet (Martindale, 1998). D5W solution has only 170 kcal/L, and clear liquid diets may have as few as 600 kcal/d.

Early postoperative oral feeding has been demonstrated to be safe and does not increase postoperative morbidity (Lucha et al, 2005). Enhanced rate of recovery can be achieved by an approach focused on enhancing the metabolic status of the patient before (e.g., carbohydrate and fluid loading), during (e.g., epidural anesthesia), and after (e.g., early oral feeding) surgery, and this may reduce length of stay (Fearon and Luff, 2003).

Healing of wounds involves blood cells, tissues, cytokines, growth factors, and metabolic demand for nutrients. Vitamin A is required for epithelial and bone formation, cellular differentiation, and immune function; vitamin C is necessary for collagen formation, for proper immune function, and as a tissue antioxidant (MacKay and Miller, 2003).

Adequate dietary protein is absolutely essential for proper wound healing. Tissue levels of the amino acids arginine and glutamine may influence wound repair and immune function (Stechmiller et al, 2005; MacKay and Miller, 2003). Arginine is especially helpful in wound healing after trauma (Wittman et al, 2005), but its use as a single nutrient needs further study (Stechmiller et al, 2005; Wilmore, 2004).

Patients who receive enteral immunonutrition with multiple nutrients before and after major GI surgery have lower treatment costs (Sax, 2005). Glutamine plays a role in fibrinogen utilization and wound strength (Weisel, 2005). Glutamine (GLN) supplementation has important effects in catabolic surgical patients (Wilmore, 2001). Its use in various enteral or parenteral products is accepted in many facilities.

Increased excretion of calcium is seen after skeletal trauma and during immobilization. Major surgery or stress to soft tissue is followed by increased calcium excretion in children and adults and decreased calcium excretion in the elderly. Vitamin C may be destroyed by extensive inflammation in postoperative conditions. Table 14-2 indicates the extent of body reserves of nutrients. Higher nutrient reserves serve as an advantage in most surgeries (Heyland et al, 2001).

TABLE 14-2 Extent of Body Reserves of Nutrients: Nutrient Time Required to Deplete Reserves in Well-Nourished Individuals

Nutrient	Time
Amino acids	Several hours
Carbohydrate	13 hours
Sodium	2–3 days
Water	4 days
Zinc	5 days
Fat	20–40 days
Thiamin	30–60 days
Vitamin C	60–120 days
Niacin	60–180 days
Riboflavin	60–180 days
Vitamin A	90–365 days
Iron	125 days (women); 750 days (men)
Iodine	1000 days
Calcium	2500 days

From: Guthrie H. *Introductory nutrition.* 7th ed. St Louis: Times Mirror/Mosby College Publishers, 1989.

INTERVENTION: OBJECTIVES

Preoperative

- Maintain or enhance reserves. Half of patients admitted to hospitals are malnourished; therefore, proper presurgical assessment and nourishment should be emphasized to prepare for surgical stress, wound healing, hemorrhage, and potential dehydration (Patel, 2005). Some authors suggest glucose/potassium intravenous loading in nondiabetic, nonrespiratory patients for preoperative preparation.
- Identify risks for cardiac events after surgery, which are common and costly (Maddox, 2005).
- Monitor patients who are morbidly obese. Fatty tissues are not resistant to infections; they are hard to suture, and dehiscence may occur. A large amount of anesthesia is needed in the morbidly obese, and it is difficult to awaken them. Controlled weight loss should be instituted before surgery whenever possible.
- Elevated serum glucose on admission is an accurate predictor of postoperative infection, length of stay, and mortality (Bochicchio et al, 2005). Reducing hyperglycemia is important.

Postoperative

- Replete nutrient stores, such as protein and iron from hemorrhage or other blood losses. Replace important vitamins and minerals (vitamin C, 100–200% recommended amounts; vitamin K, zinc, and vitamin A).

- Correct imbalances in fluid, sodium, potassium, and other electrolytes.
- Promote wound healing. The surgical wound has priority for the first 5–10 days; tensile strength peaks at 40–50 days.
- Use enhanced immunonutrition where needed to provide sufficient amount of protein and energy to preserve muscle function; stimulate and protect enterocytes while limiting bacterial translocation; keep liver function as normal as possible; prevent or compensate for disturbances in the immune response. Arginine triggers anabolic hormones (e.g., insulin, growth hormone) and speeds wound healing (Zaloga et al, 2004; Basu and Liepa, 2002). Arginine is important for growth, wound healing, cardiovascular function, immune function, inflammatory responses, energy metabolism, urea cycle function, and other metabolic processes (Zaloga et al, 2004). While somewhat controversial, it may be helpful to select an immune-enhanced tube feeding product for GI surgeries.
- Attend to special needs such as fever, trauma, pregnancy, and growth in infants and children.
- Prevent infection and sepsis, which can occur in more than 10% of surgical cases.
- Prevent aspiration, a leading cause of pneumonia and the most serious complication of enteral tube feeding. Traditional clinical monitors of glucose oxidase strips and blue food coloring (BFC) should no longer be used; evaluation of gastric residual volumes is recommended (McClave et al, 2002).
- Minimize weight loss, which is not obligatory. Prevent or correct protein–energy malnutrition (PEM). Table 14-3 describes the use of estimated energy requirement calculations when indirect calorimetry is not available.

INTERVENTION: FOOD AND NUTRITION

Preoperative

- Use a high-protein/high-energy diet. Perioperative enteral nutrition is more effective than postoperative nutrition (Grimble, 2005). Use tube feeding (TF) or total parenteral nutrition (TPN) if needed. Enteral nutrition is effective, poses lower risks than parenteral nutrition, reduces infection rates, and shortens intensive care unit and hospital length of stay of critically ill patients (Grimble, 2005).
- If patient is obese, use a low-energy diet that includes carbohydrates adequate for glycogen stores and protein to protect lean body mass. Elevated serum glucose on admission is an accurate predictor of postoperative infection, length of stay, and mortality (Bochicchio et al, 2005).
- Ensure that intakes of zinc and vitamins C and K are adequate.
- Bowel cleansing regimens commonly require adherence to liquid diets for 24–48 hours before examination, which often leads to poor compliance; offering patients a regular breakfast and a low-residue lunch before bowel cleansing with sodium phosphate oral solution may be better accepted and tolerated (Scott et al, 2005).
- Gradually restrict diet to clear liquids and then NPO, nothing by mouth.

Postoperative

- Immediately after surgery, use intravenous glucose, insulin, or electrolytes as needed (Bossingham et al, 2005). As treatment progresses, diet should progress as tolerated to a combination of liquid and solid items (Travis and Barr, 1997).
- If oral feeding is not possible, use enteral nutrition. Initiate TF within 12–18 hours for less sepsis and fewer complications. The gut can generally tolerate early feedings (Lucha et al, 2005; Martin et al, 2005; Gabor et al, 2005). Total enteral nutrition is well tolerated, even in pancreatitis, and gastric feeding is acceptable for most patients (Marek and Zaloga, 2004; Marek and Zaloga, 2003).
- When necessary, because of prolonged GI compromise or short bowel syndrome, use TPN. Parenteral immunonutrition carries a higher risk but can be efficacious in selected patient groups for whom enteral nutrition is problematic (Grimble, 2005).
- A complete, balanced diet with a mix of nutrients is best. Excessive vitamin and mineral supplements do not increase rate of healing; in fact, zinc and iron are bacterial nutrients, and excesses may be detrimental.
- Intravenous lipids may be deleterious due to the proinflammatory effects of omega-6 fatty acids.
- Omega-3 fatty acids are anti-inflammatory; olive oil is being studied for beneficial effects as well (Grimble, 2005).
- After elective GI surgery, early postoperative feeding is generally safe and effective, resulting in a shorter hospital stay than traditional feeding. Costs and morbidity are also reduced (Braga and Gianotti, 2005). Glutamine-enhanced products are useful, especially in malnourished patients (Grimble, 2005). Supplemental glutamine granules with oral feeding or TF will support glutamine repletion, promote protein synthesis, inhibit protein decomposition, improve wound healing, and reduce hospital stay (Peng et al, 2005). The adaptive role of the small intestine is described in Table 14-4.
- With increased appetite and capacity for oral diet, offer increased fluid and include sources of protein, zinc, and vitamins C and A for wound healing. Use of 25–45 kcal/kg and 1–1.5 g protein/kg may be needed (Reid, 2004); this varies depending on extent of surgical intervention and degree of catabolism since losses of 5–15 g of nitrogen daily may occur.

TABLE 14-3 Measuring Energy Expenditure in Critical Illness

Measuring energy expenditure via indirect calorimetry (IC) is the most accurate method of determining needs. For short-term use, predictive equations such as the Harris-Benedict equation multiplied by a stress factor of 1.6 may be accurate enough for short-term nutrition support of critically ill patients when IC is unavailable (MacDonald and Hildebrandt, 2003).

Ireton-Jones Equations for Estimated Energy Expenditure (EEE) (Ireton-Jones and Jones, 1998)

(1) Spontaneously Breathing Patient: $EEE = 629 - 11(A) + 25(W) - 609(O)$

(2) Ventilator-Dependent Patient: $EEE = 1784 - 11(A) + 5(W) + 244(G) + 239(T) + 804(B)$

Key: A = age in years; W = weight in kg; O = obesity (>130% ideal body weight); G = gender (female = 0, male = 1); T = diagnosis of trauma (absent = 0, present = 1); B = diagnosis of burn (absent = 0, present = 1).

TABLE 14-4 Absorptive Role of Small Intestine

- The small intestine has a large adaptive capacity, with resection of small segments generally not causing nutritional problems.
- If the terminal ileum is removed, vitamin B_{12} and bile salts will not be reabsorbed. Diarrhea can be massive if the ileocecal valve is removed with the terminal ileum, with great electrolyte losses and hypovolemia.
- Cholestyramine may be needed to bind bile salts. Fat malabsorption with steatorrhea and inadequate vitamin A, D, E, and K absorption may also occur. Medium-chain triglycerides (MCT) and water-miscible supplements may be necessary. Hyperoxaluria and renal stones may occur. Calcium supplements, altered polyunsaturated fatty acid (PUFA) intake, and aluminum hydroxide binders may be needed.

- An analysis of clinical studies using enteral formulas with supplemental arginine suggests benefits without detrimental effects (Zaloga et al, 2004). Arginine food sources include shrimp, lean ground beef, pumpkin seeds, garbanzo beans, cottage cheese, peanuts, and soymilk; use where oral diet is possible.
- Hyperglycemia is associated with risks for poorer wound healing, increased susceptibility to infection, and loss of administered nutrients through glycosuria (Hoogwerf, 2001). Manage patients who have hyperglycemia carefully because they often have complications. Adverse outcomes are related to preexisting complications of diabetes, especially atherosclerotic disease, nephropathy, and peripheral and autonomic neuropathy (Hoogwerf, 2001).
- Electrolyte imbalances, which are common after surgery, are described in Table 14-5.

CLINICAL INDICATORS

Clinical/History

Height
Weight
Body mass index (BMI)
Weight changes
Diet history
Blood pressure (BP)
Intake and output (I & O)
Nausea, vomiting
Constipation
Anorexia
Urinary tract infection
Skin integrity; pressure ulcers
History of dehydration or slow wound healing
Transfusions

Lab Work

Glucose (Gluc)
C-reactive protein (CRP)
Platelet count
Albumin (Alb), transthyretin
Blood urea nitrogen (BUN)
Creatinine (Creat)
Na+
K+
Ca++
Mg++
Phosphorus (P)
Urinary electrolytes
Serum osmolality (Osm)
N balance
Transferrin
Prothrombin time (PT) or international normalized ratio (INR)
Hemoglobin and hematocrit (H & H)
Serum Fe
Vitamin B_{12}

Common Drugs and Anesthesia Used with Surgery and Potential Side Effects

- Anesthesia delays peristalsis; nausea is common. Patient may eat ice chips or sip carbonated beverages until nausea subsides.
- Analgesics should provide effective pain relief. Epidural analgesia in GI surgery yields shorter duration of postoperative ileus, attenuation of the stress response, fewer pulmonary complications, and improved postoperative pain control and recovery (Fotiadis et al, 2004). Pain medications should be taken sufficiently in advance of meals to allow a pleasant, pain-free mealtime.
- Antibiotics may be needed; monitor specific side effects for selected medication.
- Insulin may be needed if hyperglycemia occurs or persists. Insulin use has the flexibility of timing and dose in the postoperative management of most diabetic patients (Hoogwerf, 2001).
- Laxatives may deplete electrolytes. When able to progress, use a higher fiber intake and plenty of liquids.
- Metoclopramide (Reglan) may help with postoperative ileus (Chan et al, 2005). Dry mouth or nausea can result after prolonged use.
- Nitrous oxide anesthesia may cause neurological damage in patients with a vitamin B_{12} deficiency (Flippo and Holder, 1993).
- Vitamin K can help with clotting. There are generally no side effects with this injection.
- Warfarin (Coumadin), a blood thinner used to prevent emboli, requires that patient maintain steady intake of vitamin K foods (cabbage, kale, and spinach) to control levels. Heparin has no dietary consequences.

Herbs, Botanicals, and Supplements

- Interactions between herbs, anesthesia, and surgery must be noted. Bromelain may reduce edema, bruising, pain, and healing time following trauma and surgical procedures (MacKay and Miller, 2003). For surgical patients, herbs can affect sedation, pain control, bleeding, heart function, metabolism, immunity, and recovery. As many as one third of presurgical patients take herbal medications, and many of those patients fail to disclose herbal use during preoperative assessment, even when prompted (Ang-Lee et al, 2001). Table 14-6 describes these potential interactions.

INTERVENTION: NUTRITION EDUCATION, COUNSELING, CARE MANAGEMENT

- Immobilization of patient can produce unwanted side effects. Have patient drink plenty of fluids and ambulate as soon as possible.
- Patients tend to lose 0.5 lb daily early in postoperative period. Weight gain during this time suggests fluid excess.
- Eat and drink slowly to prevent gas formation from swallowed air.
- Discuss the role of surgery as "planned trauma," allowing adequate time for return to homeostasis. Discuss wound healing priority, tensile strength, role of nutrients (zinc,

TABLE 14-5 Managing Electrolyte Imbalances

Three independent variables regulate pH in blood plasma: carbon dioxide, relative electrolyte concentrations, and total weak acid concentrations; all changes in blood pH occur through changes in these variables (Kellum, 2005). As many as 50% of older adults may have hypertonic plasma, an indication of cell dehydration that leads to consequences such as glucose dysregulation (Dunmeyer Stookey et al, 2005).

Condition and Clinical Indicators	Causes	Signs and Symptoms	Nutritional Concerns
Hyponatremia Serum Na+ (<135 mEq/L) Urinary Na+ Osm (<285 mOsm/kg)	Low serum sodium concentration can occur as a result of loss of sodium in excess of osmotically obligated water (primary salt depletion), dehydration in which sodium loss is greater than water loss. Heavy exercise may also induce a rare form of hyponatremia (Montain et al, 2001). Retention of water in excess of sodium may cause water intoxication, dilutional hyponatremia, or syndrome of inappropriate antidiuretic hormone (SIADH). Furosemide (Lasix) and vigorous diuretic therapy may cause hyponatremia.	Lethargy, anorexia, nausea, vomiting, cramping, muscular twitching, confusion, fingerprinting over the breastbone, seizures, and coma.	Distinguish between the different types of hyponatremia and their treatments. Contracted extracellular fluid volume may occur; a hypertonic or isotonic saline solution is given (perhaps along with salty broths). Avoid giving large water flushes with isotonic tube feeding. Fluid restriction and low-sodium diet with diuretics may cause hyponatremia. D5W used in excess can cause hyponatremia with cases of water intoxication. Hyponatremia is associated with increased morbidity and mortality; treatment in heart failure includes hypertonic saline solution, loop diuretics, fluid restriction, and other pharmacological agents, such as demeclocycline, lithium carbonate, and urea (Goldsmith, 2005).
Hypernatremia Serum Na+ (>135 mEq/L) Urinary Na+ Osm (>295 mOsm/kg) Urinary-specific gravity (>1.015)	Hypernatremia usually occurs in water deprivation or in persons who cannot obtain sufficient water to replace losses (after head trauma, carbon monoxide poisoning, or diabetes insipidus). Sodium intoxication may result from excess intake of NaCl or sodium bicarbonate. Steroids also can cause hypernatremia. In infants, severe prolonged hypernatremia can impair intellectual and physical development (Birnbaumer, 2001).	Thirst, dry and sticky mucous membranes, fever, dry and swollen tongue, disorientation, and seizures. Flushing, fever, loss of sweating, dry tongue and mucous membranes, tachycardia, hallucinations, or coma.	High-protein tube feedings without adequate water flushes, excessive diaphoresis, diabetes insipidus, or watery diarrhea may cause problems. Correct dehydration. Monitor thirst, the first sign of water loss. High doses of steroids can cause hypernatremia; monitor carefully. Monitor solutions that contain NaCl and other sodium additives closely. Over-the-counter (OTC) analgesics that contain sodium should not be used without physician's awareness. Determine patient's fluid needs (generally 30 mL/kg or 1 mL/kcal given in tube feeding [TF] or total parenteral nutrition [TPN]). Elderly individuals may need more or less according to their renal or cardiovascular status. Monitor use of all tube feedings carefully; high-protein formulas can cause simple dehydration. Patients with dysphagia may have difficulty obtaining enough fluid if they cannot tolerate thin liquids; monitor closely.
Hypokalemia K+ (<3.5 mEq/L) Osmolality (Osm) Na+	Results from inadequate intake, excessive gastrointestinal (GI) losses from diarrhea, gastric suction, vomiting, or fistulas, and urinary losses of adrenal or renal origin. Diuretic therapy is a common cause. Chronic use of aspirin and penicillin, refeeding syndrome after starvation (Crook et al, 2001), alcoholism, and anorexia nervosa are also potential causes. Diuretics such as furosemide and steroids, penicillin, and aspirin can cause or aggravate potassium depletion.	Severe muscle weakness, electrocardiogram (EKG) changes and arrhythmias, lethargy, hypotension, shallow breathing, fatigue, anorexia, constipation, confusion, and impaired CHO tolerance. Chloride depletion usually accompanies hypokalemia; alkalosis also is common.	Replace potassium (generally done with intravenous or oral KCl, except in renal tubular acidosis). Kaochlor, Kay-Ciel, K-Lor, K-Lyte, K Tab, Klotrix, Micro-K, K-Dur, Klor-Con, Ten-K, and Slow-K are all sources of potassium. Some products are slow release. Be aware that an overdose of potassium may cause blood in the stools or even cardiac arrest. There have been reports of GI bleeding unless taken with meals. Diarrhea, nausea, or vomiting also may occur; take with meals. A potassium-rich diet includes bananas, oranges, grapefruit, lima beans, baked potatoes, and most other fruits and vegetables. In addition, most salt substitutes contain potassium (read labels); avoid overuse. Monitor potassium intake to prevent under- and overdoses. Discuss fiber sources if constipation is a problem. Fluid intake should be adequate.

(continued)

TABLE 14-5 Managing Electrolyte Imbalances *(continued)*

Condition and Clinical Indicators	Causes	Signs and Symptoms	Nutritional Concerns
Hyperkalemia Serum K+ (>5.5 mEq/L) Na+ Cl−	Because the distal nephron has such a large capacity for secreting potassium, even in advanced renal failure, hyperkalemia occurs only when an additional problem exists (e.g., oliguria, tissue catabolism, potassium supplementation, use of penicillin G, severe acidosis, excessive spironolactone or triamterene therapy, deficiency of endogenous steroids, chronic kidney disease, crush injury, or adrenal insufficiency).	Weakness, anxiety, altered EKGs (with >7 mEq/L, a fatal arrhythmia can occur), flaccid muscle paralysis, or even respiratory arrest, if severe.	Immediate treatment is needed to prevent arrhythmias, bradycardia, heart block, and respiratory arrest. If all else fails, dialysis may be needed. Intravenous feedings are likely to be used (glucose, insulin, bicarbonate) to shift potassium intracellularly. Sodium or calcium may also be needed as physical antagonists; infusions will be given until serum potassium is corrected. Monitor closely. When patient can eat orally, a controlled potassium intake will be needed to avoid further exacerbation. Avoid dried fruits, bananas, orange juice, baked potatoes, dried beans, milk, milk-based products, cocoa, coffee, and whole-grain breads in excess of planned amounts. Sodium polystyrene sulfonate (Kayexalate) may also be needed and should be given with sorbitol to prevent constipation and taken separately from calcium or antacids. Discuss how potassium-sparing diuretics can cause problems if not carefully monitored. Discuss potassium sources from diet, how medications affect serum levels, and use of salt substitutes sparingly, if at all. Read labels of all supplements to avoid overdoses of potassium.
Hypocalcemia Ca++ Osm Urinary Ca++ Mg++ Phosphorous T3, T4 Alkaline phosphatase (Alk phos)	Vitamin D deficiency caused by nutritional deficiency or malabsorption, renal insufficiency, hepatic dysfunction, hypoparathyroidism, hyperphosphatemia, acute pancreatitis, or calcitonin-producing tumors of the thyroid will cause hypocalcemia. In addition, malnutrition or hypoalbuminemia may aggravate hypocalcemia because calcium is transported bound to serum albumin. This is pseudohypocalcemia due to the low albumin levels; once albumin is corrected, Ca++ levels will rise. Corticosteroids, furosemide, isoniazid (INH), and tetracycline can reduce calcium availability. Aluminum in antacids can reduce calcium bioavailability. Citrated blood transfusions may cause hypocalcemia.	Tetany, seizures, and cardiac arrest. In the long term, bone demineralization with bone pain and compression fractures may result.	Correct symptomatic condition (usually calcium gluconate intravenously). Be careful when correcting coexisting acidosis with sodium bicarbonate. Provide adequate vitamin D_3 supplementation, as needed. Once able to eat, offer calcium-rich foods. Calcium is found in milk, cheese, leafy greens, and yogurt. Dry milk can be added to foods. Beware of excesses of caffeine, oxalates, fiber, and aluminum-containing antacids. Increase consumption of vitamin D and lactose-containing foods, if tolerated. Calcium carbonate (as in Tums) provides 40% elemental calcium. Drink extra water and avoid use of iron supplements at the same time. Beware of bone meal and dolomite because of their toxic metal content.

(continued)

TABLE 14-5 Managing Electrolyte Imbalances *(continued)*

Condition and Clinical Indicators	Causes	Signs and Symptoms	Nutritional Concerns
Hypercalcemia Ca++ Osm Urinary Ca++ Mg++ Phosphorous T3, T4 Alk phos	Hypercalcemia can be caused by increased parathormone activity, increased vitamin D activity (as in tuberculosis or sarcoidosis), enhanced bone resorption from bone tumors, multiple myeloma, immobilization, milk-alkali syndrome, adrenal insufficiency, breast cancer, or head/neck cancer. Malignant disease produces hypercalcemia via bone destruction or metastasis with resulting release of calcium into the bloodstream. Lithium and thiazides may increase serum calcium levels; monitor carefully. Be aware of high calcium levels in Tums, which is available over the counter.	Drowsiness, lethargy, stupor, muscle weakness, decreased reflexes, nausea and vomiting, anorexia, constipation, ileus, polyuria, renal stones, azotemia, nocturia, hypertension, bradycardia, pruritus, and eye abnormalities.	Correct nausea, vomiting, constipation, other side effects. Correct underlying condition with rehydration (usually with normal saline) and hemodilution. Intravenous organic phosphate can help remove excess calcium. Neutra-Phos or Phospho-Soda may be used. Be careful not to provide excesses of milk, vitamins D or A, calcium supplements or antacids, and lactose until condition has been normalized. Caffeine, oxalates, fiber, and phytates will decrease calcium absorption and help promote greater excretion. Monitor potassium and magnesium losses with treatment since these are common; correct diet accordingly. Furosemide and ethacrynic acid can help increase calcium excretion; avoid in renal failure, and monitor potassium carefully. Prednisone can be used to decrease vitamin D–mediated calcium absorption; monitor serum glucose, sodium, and side effects such as nausea, metallic taste, diarrhea, and vomiting. Didronel (intravenous) can decrease calcium levels; nausea and vomiting may result. Antacids with aluminum can also be used to increase excretion.
Hypomagnesemia Mg++ Ca++ Parathormone (PTH) Osm	Hypomagnesemia is usually seen with diarrhea, protein–calorie malnutrition (PCM), malabsorption, or alcoholism. Of patients in tertiary care units, 10% may have this condition. Hypomagnesemia may contribute to development of foot ulcers in patients with diabetes (Rodriguez-Moran and Guerrero-Romero, 2001). Many medications can cause hypomagnesemia, including furosemide, ethacrynic acid, thiazides, some antibiotics, cisplatin, and cyclosporine.	Anxiety, hyperirritability, confusion, hallucinations, seizures, tremor, hyperreflexia, tetany, tachycardia, hypertension, arrhythmias, vasomotor changes, profuse sweating, muscle weakness, grimaces of facial muscles, and refractory hypocalcemia.	Correct low serum magnesium levels to prevent sudden death. Chocolate, nuts, fruits and green vegetables, beans, potatoes, wheat, and corn are considered good sources. Discuss long-term measures to prevent further episodes. Long-term use of magnesium-free TPN can be one aggravating source of the problem. Monitor intake from all sources—oral, TF, and TPN. Normal renal function is needed for use of $MgSO_4$; diarrhea can occur. Milk of magnesia (MOM) can be used for liquid form of magnesium hydroxide; nausea, cramps, or diarrhea may result.
Hypermagnesemia	Hypermagnesemia is usually found in patients with renal failure who are treated with antacids such as Maalox or Gelusil or with cathartics such as MOM.	Lethargy, hyporeflexia, and respiratory depression. Fatal effects include bradycardia, myocardial infarction, and respiratory failure (Schelling, 2000).	Reduce or eliminate sources of exogenous magnesium. No specific dietary alterations are required, except omission of magnesium-rich sources until condition is corrected. Discuss effects of magnesium on the body, sources from diet, and as OTC medications and supplements. Treat respiratory depression with calcium, gluceptate, or other medications. Calcium-containing medications may be given to help with excretion of excessive magnesium. Use caution with multivitamin-mineral supplement in megadoses (McGuire et al, 2000). TPN solutions should be monitored carefully for all electrolytes.

(continued)

TABLE 14-5 Managing Electrolyte Imbalances *(continued)*

Condition and Clinical Indicators	Causes	Signs and Symptoms	Nutritional Concerns
Hypophos-phatemia Serum phosphate Alk phos Creatine phospho-kinase (CPK) Serum Ca++ Mg++	Ingestion of CHO acutely depresses serum phosphorus levels, probably resulting from cellular uptake and phosphate formation. Lowered plasma phosphorus can occur from alkalosis, hyperparathyroidism, hypovitaminosis D, malabsorption syndrome, starvation or cachexia, chronic alcoholism, renal tubular defects, acid–base disturbances, diabetic ketoacidosis, and genetic hypophosphatemia. Hypophosphatemia also can occur as a result of unmonitored TPN. Rapid delivery of intravenous glucose, such as with TPN, may accentuate phosphorus depletion syndrome and can lead to convulsions, muscle weakness, and hemolytic anemia (known as refeeding syndrome).	Hypophosphatemia may result in sudden death, rhabdomyolysis, red cell dysfunction, and respiratory insufficiency (Marinella, 2005). Anorexia, weakness, bone pain, dizziness, and waddling gait may be observed. In severe cases, elevated CPK levels are seen, with rhabdomyolysis superimposed on myopathy. Heart failure can result if phosphorus is not administered. Low serum phosphorus levels will result in lowered 2,3-diphosphoglyceric acid (2,3-DPG), which facilitates oxyhemoglobin dissociation (leading to tissue hypoxia and low partial pressure of oxygen).	Phosphorus is a major component of bone and is one of the most abundant constituents of all metabolic processes and tissues; 85% is found in the skeleton. Only about 12% is bound to proteins, so a typical laboratory assessment is of elemental phosphorus, with some additional values for HPO_4 and $NaHPO_4$ as well. Prevent further abnormalities and complications. Control phosphorus delivery to all tissues. Appropriate measures should be provided to patient according to his or her condition. For example, a low-phosphorus diet with high calcium and adequate vitamin D will be needed for patients with renal osteodystrophy. Patient may be advised that approximately 50–60% of dietary phosphorus is absorbed from dietary intakes (more in depleted persons). Potassium acid phosphate (K-Phos Original), an acidifier, can be used; it may cause nausea, vomiting, or diarrhea. For conditions causing hypophosphatemia (such as Reye's syndrome and other infectious illnesses), adequate dietary phosphorus would be warranted. Balance is required.
Hyperphos-phatemia Serum phosphate Alk phos CPK Serum Ca++ Mg++	Hyperphosphatemia can result from renal insufficiency, hypoparathyroidism, or hypervitaminosis D. In hyperphosphatemia, calcium phosphate may be deposited in abnormal sites. In addition, abnormal renal phosphorus clearance occurs.	Phosphorus levels tend to be higher in children and to rise in women after menopause.	Provide appropriate levels of phosphorus according to age and serum status. Monitor glucose intake, especially from parenteral nutrition (PN) or TPN. Check all tube feedings for phosphorus content as well. Monitor dietary intake of milk, meat, and other foods high in phosphorus. Observe serum levels regularly, especially in renal patients. Antacids containing aluminum will prevent phosphorus absorption in intestinal lumen. Calcium acetate is useful in dialysis patients (Friedman, 2005).

TABLE 14-6 Herbal Medications and Recommendations for Discontinued Use before Surgery

Herb	Relevant Effects	Perioperative Concerns	Recommendations
Echinacea	Boosts immunity	Allergic reactions, impairs immune system, especially for transplantation patients	Discontinue as far in advance as possible.
Ephedra (ma huang)	Increases heart rate and increases blood pressure	Risk of heart attack, arrhythmias, stroke, kidney stones, interaction with other drugs	Discontinue 24 hours before surgery.
Garlic	Prevents clotting	Risk of bleeding, especially when combined with other drugs that inhibit clotting	Discontinue at least 7 days before surgery.
Ginkgo	Prevents clotting	Risk of bleeding, especially when combined with other drugs that inhibit clotting	Discontinue at least 36 hours before surgery.
Ginseng	Lowers blood glucose, inhibits clotting	Increases risk of bleeding; interferes with warfarin (an anticlotting drug)	Discontinue at least 7 days before surgery.
Kava	Sedates, decreases anxiety	May increase sedative effects of anesthesia	Discontinue 24 hours before surgery.
St. John's wort	Inhibits reuptake of neurotransmitters	Alters metabolisms of other drugs	Discontinue at least 5 days before surgery.
Valerian	Sedates	Could increase effects of sedatives. Long-term use could increase amount of anesthesia needed.	If possible, taper dose weeks before surgery. Withdrawal symptoms resemble Valium addiction.

Source: Ang-Lee M, et al. Herbal medicines and perioperative care. *JAMA.* 286:208, 2001. Reprinted with permission.

TABLE 14-7 Percentage of Body Weight and Amputations

Body weight is a good indicator of a person's size and is widely used in assessments. Body mass index (BMI) values in subjects with limb amputation are less than those in healthy control subjects without limb amputation because the lost weight of the limbs is not considered in calculating BMI (Modan et al, 1998). To reduce the underestimation of nutritional status in persons with limb amputation, estimation of body weight is necessary so that BMI can be reliably estimated for persons with limb amputation. Estimated body weight is more reliable than observed weight in patients with limb amputation (Mozumdar and Roy, 2004). Estimates of body weight after amputation is often calculated by the use of the following formula (Osterkamp, 1995):

Estimated Ideal Body Weight (IBW) = (100 − % amputation)/100 × IBW for original height

Body Part Lost	Percentage
Trunk without limbs	50%
Entire leg	16%
Thigh	10%
Lower leg with foot	5.9%
Entire arm	5.0%
Forearm with hand	2.3%
Foot	1.5%
Hand	0.7%

vitamin C, vitamin A, and amino acids). Note that poor nutrient intake can decrease anabolism, delaying scar formation. B-complex vitamins are also beneficial (Neiva et al, 2005). While zinc deficiency impairs wound healing, supplementation in people who are not deficient does not accelerate wound-healing rates. Zinc supplementation excess can interfere with immune system function and copper absorption and may cause GI distress.

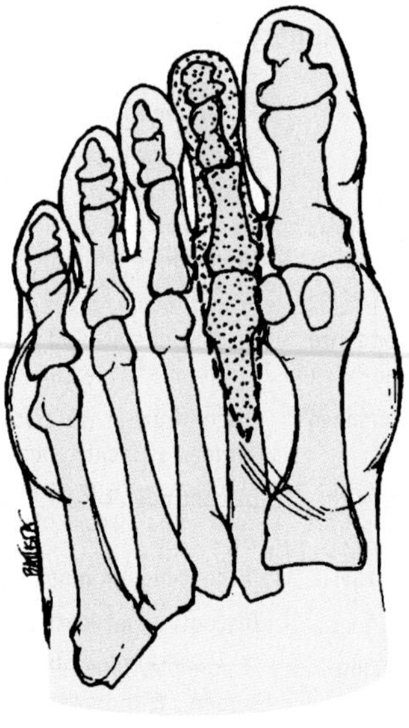

Figure 14-2 Amputated toe. (From Blackbourne LH. *Advanced surgical recall.* 2nd ed. Baltimore: Lippincott Williams & Wilkins, 2004.)

SAMPLE NUTRITION DIAGNOSTIC STATEMENT

Amputation

PES: Involuntary weight loss related to above the knee amputation as evidenced by weight loss of >6% in past 2 weeks and poor oral intake related to depression and diabetes.

Assessment Data (sources of info): Food records, input and output reports, medication history, assessment of depression.

Intervention: Review status of depression with medications or counseling, counseling about desired food and beverage intake for wound healing and management of diabetes.

Monitoring and Evaluation: Food records, weight status, rate of wound healing, medications used, symptoms of depression.

- Enteral nutrition is preferred over parenteral nutrition when the GI tract is functional (Zaloga, 2006).
- During the rehabilitative anabolic stage (3 months to 1 year postoperatively), energy intake should be adequate but not excessive.
- Provide medical nutrition therapy and general diabetes education for newly diagnosed diabetic patients to ensure long-term, excellent surgical and medical outcomes (Hoogwerf, 2001).
- With amputation, determine the percentage of body mass lost and decrease estimated energy needs accordingly. See Table 14-7. Figure 14-2 shows an amputated toe.
- Table 14-8 lists types of surgeries and their specific nutritional impact.

For More Information

- American Academy of Physical Medicine and Rehabilitation
  http://www.aapmr.org/
- Amputees
  http://www.nlm.nih.gov/medlineplus/amputees.html
- Amputee Coalition of America
  http://www.amputee-coalition.org/
- Amputee Resource Foundation of America
  http://www.amputeeresource.org/
- Family Practices
  http://www.fpnotebook.com/SUR131.htm

SAMPLE NUTRITION DIAGNOSTIC STATEMENT

Coronary Artery Bypass Graft (CABG)

PES: Inadequate oral intake following CABG related to poor intake for past 48 hours as evidenced by complaints of nausea at mealtime.

Assessment Data (sources of info): Diet history, mealtime observations, premeal medications.

Intervention: Timing of antinausea medicines to precede meals.

Monitoring and Evaluation: Improvement in meal intake, length of stay in cardiac care unit.

TABLE 14-8 Surgeries and Specific Nutritional Impact

Surgery and Nutritional Acuity Ranking	Background	Specific Objectives	Food and Nutrition Recommendations
Amputation, Level 2	Amputations may result from poorly controlled diabetes, trauma, peripheral artery disease, congenital deformity, chronic infections, gangrene, or tumors such as osteosarcoma. In rare cases, tropical diabetic hand syndrome may occur in patients with diabetes who have an insect bite with resulting cellulitis, which must be treated quickly to avoid the need for amputation (Abbas and Archibald, 2005). "AK" denotes above the knee and "BK" denotes below the knee amputation. In amputation, the percentage of total body weight lost depends on body part lost. See Table 14-7 regarding calculations of body weight percentages for amputated limbs.	Immediately Postoperative: Determine percentage of body weight of amputated area and calculate changes from preoperative to postoperative status in height, weight, and body mass index (BMI). Provide adequate protein and calories for healing. Provide adequate intake of vitamins and minerals (zinc, and vitamins C, K, and A). Low albumin levels, serum carotene, zinc, and vitamin C are commonly found. Long Term: Patients with an AK amputation who walk (with/without prosthesis) use 25% more energy than a normal person who walks at the same speed. These patients may have difficulty maintaining weight. Otherwise, immobilized patients may tend to gain weight and will need control measures.	Immediately Postoperative: Use a high-protein/high-energy diet for healing. Supplement diet with vitamins and minerals, especially zinc, vitamins A, C, and K, and arginine. Use tube feeding (TF) if necessary; consider use of an immune-enhanced product. Long Term: Provide a low-calorie diet, if needed. For patients who lose too much weight, a higher energy diet should be used. Discuss how to control or increase calories in diet for energy use. For hand or arm amputations, consider use of adaptive feeding equipment. Occupational therapy (OT) specialists can help.
Appendectomy, Level 1	Appendectomy generally is an uncomplicated procedure with minimal recovery time. It is believed that a low-fiber diet contributes to appendicitis. White blood cell count and erythrocyte sedimentation rate may be increased.	Reduce fever. Lower risks of infection or sepsis, peritonitis, or abscess formation.	Use a balanced diet with adequate amounts of zinc and vitamins C, K, and A. When patient is able to eat fiber, include more fruits, vegetables, and whole grains.
Cesarean delivery (C-section), Level 1	Cesarean delivery (C-section) is performed for numerous reasons, including HIV infection, maternal diabetes, or edema-proteinuria-hypertensive (EPH) gestosis. Delivery of a fetus through a uterine incision could have such complications as hemorrhage, infection, fever, drainage, cystitis, or pneumonia after the operation. Monitor for signs of anemia.	Replenish stores of nutrients from blood and fluid losses. Reduce fever or correct infections.	NPO with intravenous or clear liquids will be given until nausea subsides. Progress to usual diet, with increased fiber to soften stools. Increase fluids unless contraindicated. Promote wound healing with protein and energy; include vitamins C and A and zinc in diet or supplemental form. Anesthesia delays peristalsis; nausea is common. If permitted, patient may eat ice chips or sip carbonated beverages until nausea subsides. A prenatal supplement can be used for several months postpartum, or an iron supplement may be given; ferrous salts are more beneficial and bioavailable than ferric salts.
Coronary Artery Bypass Graft (CABG) or Valve Replacement, Level 3	Open heart procedures require use of a cardiopulmonary machine for extracorporeal circulation. In CABG surgery, narrowed or blocked arteries are bypassed. The vein usually comes from the leg. Blood can then flow directly into the heart muscle. CABG usually takes 4–5 hours. Valve replacement is not as extensive; it involves replacing the damaged valve with a mechanical prosthesis (St. Jude valve) or biological tissue valve.	Preoperative: Monitor serum levels of electrolytes, albumin, and glucose. Provide the diet as prescribed by physician (diet may be sodium, energy, or fluid restricted). Provide ample amounts of glycogen for stores. Use parenteral nutrition (PN) support, as needed, for malnourished cardiac patients. Postoperative: Promote wound healing and restore normal fluid and electrolyte balance. Promote weight control. Wean from ventilator support when possible. Prevent hyperglycemia or coma, sepsis, renal failure, cardiac tamponade, atelectasis, or wound dehiscence. Maintain comfort and educate regarding follow-up.	Control fluid intake by measuring previous day's output plus 500 mL for insensible losses. Control sodium and potassium intake by monitoring serum levels, controlling edema, and measuring blood pressure; modify diet as needed. As treatment progresses, control intake of cholesterol in diet (check serum levels and discuss history with patient). Modify sodium intake as needed. At home, 2–4 g of sodium is reasonable. The National Cholesterol Education Program guidelines may be used.

(continued)

TABLE 14-8 Surgeries and Specific Nutritional Impact *(continued)*

Surgery and Nutritional Acuity Ranking	Background	Specific Objectives	Food and Nutrition Recommendations
Coronary Artery Bypass Graft (CABG) or Valve Replacement, Level 3		Long Term: Avoid excessive weight gain, which can further aggravate heart condition. Teach appropriate measures for changes in daily diet to prevent further problems while wound is healing. Discuss need to alter lifestyle (diet, exercise, and stress) to prevent additional problems; many patients continue to have atherogenic effects even after heart surgery. Control carbohydrates in patients with diabetes or hypertriglyceridemia.	Provide adequate protein and energy for wound healing; provide adequate zinc and vitamins A, C, and K as well. TF or use total parenteral nutrition (TPN) if severely malnourished. Replete slowly and keep head of bed elevated 30° to prevent worsening of heart failure. Low-sodium, high-calorie, low-volume TF products may be useful. Diuretics and digoxin may deplete potassium; anorexia, nausea, and diarrhea may occur. Beta-blockers, ace inhibitors, and other cardiac drugs may be used; some require use of low-sodium, low-calorie diets for effectiveness. Hypoalbuminemia may cause digoxin toxicity.
Craniotomy, Level 2	Craniotomy involves removing and replacing the bone of the skull to provide access to intracranial structures, usually for a brain tumor. Monitor altered states of consciousness, nausea and vomiting, seizures, paralysis of face or extremities, drainage from the site, shock, aspiration, hyperthermia, dysphagia, thrombophlebitis, diabetes insipidus, or syndrome of inappropriate antidiuretic hormone (SIADH). Monitor indicators such as computed tomography (CT) scan, consciousness, input and output (I & O), nausea, vomiting, gag reflex, electroencephalogram, and cerebrospinal fluid (CSF) levels.	Prevent aspiration. Prevent or correct dysphagia, constipation, urinary tract infection (UTI), nausea and vomiting, and diabetes insipidus. Normalize electrolyte levels. Anticoagulants may be used to prevent venous thromboembolic disease (Knovich and Lesser, 2004). Anticonvulsants may be used; with phenytoin, folic acid depletion is common.	NPO is needed until nausea and vomiting subside. Progress from liquids to soft diet as ordered; patient should be fed while lying on his/her side or with his/her head elevated 30° to prevent aspiration. Check swallowing reflex. Assist with feeding if needed, and TF may be required. Adequate fiber may be beneficial. If steroids are used, reduce sodium intake to 4–6 g/d (or less). Discuss importance of diet in correcting any malnutrition or anemia. As needed, teach family about a diet for dysphagia (e.g., thick, pureed foods with reduced thin liquids). When and if patient can eat, teach him or her to chew slowly and thoroughly. Promote eventual self-feeding. Discuss anxiety related to pain, poor vision, headaches, and seizures. Some patients may be aphasic.
Hip Arthroplasty, Total, Level 2	A total hip replacement (arthroplasty) is the formation of an artificial hip joint. Prostheses are either cemented in place or uncemented. The procedure is performed in cases of severe degenerative joint disease, rheumatoid arthritis, or congenital deformities. Those persons with a prior wrist fracture may be twice as likely to break a hip later in life. Nutritional status before arthroplasty is a good predictor of surgical outcomes after surgery; albumin levels over 3.4 predict a better outcome (Lavernia et al, 1999).	Replenish stores pre- and postoperatively. Prevent side effects of immobilization (renal calculi, pressure ulcers, and UTIs). Promote adequate wound healing. Regain maximum mobility. Ambulation, when possible, will promote healing and increase strength. Have patient eat small, frequent meals if nausea is a problem.	Use a high-protein/high-energy diet. Supplement diet with zinc and vitamins A, C, and K. Check patient's iron stores to determine whether replenishing is needed after blood loss. If weight loss is needed, provide a balanced, low-energy diet after wound healing is completed. Diet should provide adequate amounts of calcium and phosphorus—prevent calculi. Promote bone tissue adaptation to the new joint.

(continued)

TABLE 14-8 Surgeries and Specific Nutritional Impact *(continued)*

Surgery and Nutritional Acuity Ranking	Background	Specific Objectives	Food and Nutrition Recommendations
Hysterectomy, Abdominal, Level 1	An abdominal hysterectomy is the surgical removal of the uterus through an abdominal incision. An abdominal approach is used if the uterus is enlarged or if an oophorectomy (ovary removal) and salpingectomy (removal of the fallopian tubes) are performed at the same time. In extensive surgery, 5–10 pints of blood may be lost. Laser surgery for some women may prevent need for a more extensive surgery. Diverticular colovaginal fistulas arise in patients who have previously undergone a hysterectomy; a careful multidisciplinary approach can improve outcomes (Bahadursingh and Longo, 2003).	Promote wound healing and rapid recovery. Replete nutrient reserves and glycogen stores. Replace protein, iron, and vitamin K from heavy blood losses (when they occur). Prevent complications such as UTIs, incisional infections, fever, nausea, and vomiting. Explain that resumption of normal activity may be slow but exercise improves nutrient repletion and tissue repair. Emphasize importance of nutrition for wound healing.	Use a high-protein/high-calorie diet. Increase fluid intake. Ensure adequate fiber is provided for alleviation of constipation. Supplement diet with iron, zinc, and vitamins K, C, and A.
Pancreatic Surgery, Level 3	Indications for major pancreatic surgery are complications of chronic and acute pancreatitis and pancreatic malignancies (Kahl and Malfertheiner, 2004). Surgery of the pancreas may include total pancreatectomy with or without islet cell autotransplantation for chronic pancreatitis and cancer and subtotal or pancreatoduodenectomy (Whipple's procedure) for islet cell tumors. Postoperative pancreatic function is determined by type of resection, resection of adjacent organs, the underlying disease, and preoperative pancreatic function (Kahl and Malfertheiner, 2004). The standard Whipple's procedure results in dumping syndrome, diarrhea, dyspepsia, ulceration at gastroenterostomy site, and postoperative weight loss of 10–40 kg (Kozuschek et al, 1994). A new pylorus-preserving method is more protective of the upper intestine. Distal pancreatectomy and pancreaticojejunostomy are effective treatments for this difficult group of patients, with long-term pain relief and reduced need for rehospitalization (Weber and Keller, 2001).	Monitor any history of ethanol (ETOH) abuse with resulting malnutrition and malabsorption. Prevent or correct sepsis, which is a common complication. Encourage nourishing, well-balanced meals, if ordered and tolerated. Monitor medications and replacement enzymes or hormones, if ordered. Postoperatively, most patients also develop diabetes mellitus, which requires insulin; hypoglycemia is the most difficult clinical problem to handle following total pancreatectomy (Kahl and Malfertheiner, 2004). Offer resources to help with diabetes. If patient has a history of ETOH abuse, discuss how alcohol affects the pancreas.	<u>Preoperatively:</u> Total enteral nutrition or TPN to prepare patient for a major operation. <u>Postoperatively:</u> Enteral nutrition, TPN, or oral intake may progress as tolerated. Enteral nutrition has no adverse effect compared with parenteral nutrition during the course of acute pancreatitis and is probably beneficial in regard to outcome (Mayerle et al, 2004). Clear liquid to soft diet is a common order. A carbohydrate-controlled diet may be needed if there is diabetes. Small, frequent feedings may be helpful. Force fluids unless contraindicated. Alter fat source with malabsorption or if steatorrhea occurs. Standard treatment following major pancreatic surgery includes the administration of pancreatic enzyme preparations and inhibition of acid secretion by proton pump inhibitors (Kahl and Malfertheiner, 2004).
Parathyroidectomy, Level 1	Surgical removal of the parathyroid glands may cause hypoparathyroidism (with tingling, tetany, hoarseness, and seizures).	Prepare patient preoperatively for surgery. Force fluids unless contraindicated. Alter calcium, vitamin D, and phosphorus intake if needed. Vitamin D, calcium, chemotherapy, and a low-phosphorus diet with aluminum hydroxide (Amphojel) may be ordered for hypoparathyroidism; constipation is one side effect. Counsel patient regarding follow-up measures according to prescribed dietary regimen or medication side effects.	Immediately after surgery, intravenous feeding or TF may be needed. TPN may not be used because of potential for sepsis in the neck area. Extra fluids are necessary. A high-calcium/low-phosphorus diet may be necessary. Monitor carefully.

(continued)

TABLE 14-8 Surgeries and Specific Nutritional Impact *(continued)*

Surgery and Nutritional Acuity Ranking	Background	Specific Objectives	Food and Nutrition Recommendations
Pelvic Exenteration Surgery, Level 1	Pelvic exenteration surgery involves removal of all reproductive organs and adjacent tissues in the female patient (i.e., radical hysterectomy, pelvic node dissection, cystectomy and formation of an ileal conduit, vaginectomy, and rectal resection with colostomy). Cancer is usually the reason for this surgery. Postoperative colonic stasis occurs after major abdominal surgery and persists for approximately 3 days; early feeding after major gynecological surgery results in emesis but does not increase incidence of aspiration pneumonia, dehiscence, or intestinal leaks; after radical hysterectomy, postoperative bowel stimulation decreases length of hospital stay (Fanning and Andrews, 2001).	Preoperatively, a low-residue or elemental diet may be needed, regressing to clear liquids, NPO. Vitamin K may be needed 24–48 hours before the procedure. Postoperatively, promote wound healing and recovery. Prevent hemorrhage, infection, urinary or GI problems, shock, fever, and sepsis. Correct anemia or other problems. Provide colostomy teaching if needed.	Parenteral fluids with electrolytes may be needed (3–4 L/d unless contraindicated). TPN or TF may also be appropriate. Progress, as tolerated, to a high-protein/high-calorie intake with snacks (eggnog, custard, oral supplements). If nausea is an extensive problem, using fluids between, instead of with, meals may help. Adequate iron, zinc, and vitamins A and C will help with wound-healing process.
Spinal Surgery, Level 2	Spinal surgery generally is performed to relieve pressure on spinal nerves or cord due to herniated discs, trauma, displaced fractures, osteoporosis, or incomplete vertebral dislocation from rheumatoid arthritis. A laminectomy, discectomy, or spinal fusion may be performed.	Preoperatively, nutrients may be needed for adequate stores (e.g., glucose, protein, vitamins A, C, and K, and zinc). Correct nausea and vomiting if a problem. Avoid weight gain. Prevent calculi, UTIs, and pressure ulcers. Discuss importance of hydration in prevention of UTIs and other problems such as renal stones. Discuss how fiber can prevent or correct constipation.	Parenteral fluids may be given as ordered. A balanced diet, when patient is ready, with control of total energy intake to prevent excessive weight gain, may be used. If patient has been malnourished, a gradual increase in calories may be beneficial. Adequate hydration will be necessary unless contraindicated; monitor to prevent overhydration. Increasing fiber intake may be helpful if constipation is a problem. Prune juice, crushed bran, and other items may be used if chewing is a problem for patient; otherwise, extra fruits and raw vegetables may be used.
Tonsillectomy and Adenoidectomy, Level 1	Removal of tonsils and adenoids is less common than a few decades ago. This tissue is considered to be part of the protective immune system, and removal is less common than in the past. It may be used for children with chronic ear, throat, and sinus infections.	Supply adequate nourishment for glycogen stores preoperatively. Postoperatively provide cold liquids that will not produce discomfort and progress to nonirritating foods. Prevent or correct vomiting and nausea. Help patient select nonirritating foods for use at home. Avoidance of hot, spicy foods, raw vegetables, toast and crackers, citrus juices, and other related foods until full recovery is recommended. Taking large swallows of water causes less pain than small swallows. Patient should remain on cool liquids until pain subsides. Some doctors recommend avoidance of red gelatin to distinguish from blood.	Postoperatively, give cold liquids (sherbet, ginger ale, nectars, and gelatin). Avoid milk products only if patient cannot tolerate them. On second or third day, use soft, smooth foods (pudding, strained cereals, soft-cooked eggs). Progress to regular diet as tolerated. A soft diet may be preferred for a few more days. Use supplements of vitamin C if patient cannot tolerate juices. Evaluate zinc intake and encourage dietary sources when possible. Use extra fluid intake.

- Merck–Surgery
http://www.merck.com/mmhe/sec25/ch301/ch301a.html
- National Library of Medicine–Surgery
http://www.nlm.nih.gov/medlineplus/surgery.html
- OSHA Amputation Facts
http://www.osha.gov/OshDoc/data_General_Facts/amputation-factsheet.pdf
- Refeeding Syndrome
http://www.ccmtutorials.com/misc/phosphate/page_07.htm

SURGERY—CITED REFERENCES

Abbas ZG, Archibald LK. Tropical diabetic hand syndrome. Epidemiology, pathogenesis, and management. *Am J Clin Dermatol.* 6:21, 2005.

Ang-Lee M, Moss J, Yuan C. Herbal medicines and perioperative care. *JAMA.* 286:208, 2001.

Bahadursingh AM, Longo E. Colovaginal fistulas. Etiology and management. *J Reprod Med.* 48:489, 2003.

Basu HN, Liepa SU. Arginine: a clinical perspective. *Nutr Clin Pract.* 17:218, 2002.

Birnbaumer M. The V2 vasopressin receptor mutations and fluid homeostasis. *Cardiovasc Res.* 51:409, 2001.

BOCHICCHIO GV, et al. Admission preoperative glucose is predictive of morbidity and mortality in trauma patients who require immediate operative intervention. *Am Surg.* 71:171, 2005.

Bossingham MJ, et al. Water balance, hydration status, and fat-free mass hydration in younger and older adults. *Am J Clin Nutr.* 81:1342, 2005.

Braga M, Gianotti L. Preoperative immunonutrition: cost-benefit analysis. *JPEN J Parenter Enteral Nutr.* 29:S57, 2005.

Chan DC, et al. Preventing prolonged post-operative ileus in gastric cancer patients undergoing gastrectomy and intra-peritoneal chemotherapy. *World J Gastroenterol.* 11:4776, 2005.

Correia M, et al. Risk factors for malnutrition in patients undergoing gastroenterological and hernia surgery: an analysis of 374 patients. *Nutr Hosp.* 16:59, 2001.

Crook M, et al. The importance of the refeeding syndrome. *Nutrition* 17:632, 2001.

Daly J, et al. Enteral nutrition with supplemental arginine, RNA and omega-3 fatty acids in patients after operation: immunologic, metabolic and clinical outcome. *Surgery* 112:56, 1992.

Daly J, et al. Risk adjustment of the postoperative morbidity rate for the comparative assessment of the quality of surgical care: results of the National Veterans Affairs Surgical Risk Study. *J Am Col Surg.* 185:328, 1997.

Dunmeyer Stookey J, et al. Is the prevalence of dehydration among community-dwelling older adults really low? Informing current debate over the fluid recommendation for adults aged 70+ years. *Public Health Nutr.* 8:1275, 2005.

Falanga V. Wound healing and its impairment in the diabetic foot. *Lancet* 366:1736, 2005.

Fanning J, Andrews S. Early postoperative feeding after major gynecologic surgery: evidence-based scientific medicine. *Am J Obstet Gynecol.* 185:1, 2001.

Farreras N, et al. Effect of early postoperative enteral immunonutrition on wound healing in patients undergoing surgery for gastric cancer. *Clin Nutr.* 24:55, 2005.

Fearon KC, Luff R. The nutritional management of surgical patients: enhanced recovery after surgery. *Proc Nutr Soc.* 62:807, 2003.

Flippo T, Holder W. Neurologic degeneration associated with nitrous oxide anesthesia in patients with vitamin B12 deficiency. *Arch Surg.* 128:1391, 1993.

Fotiadis RJ, et al. Epidural analgesia in gastrointestinal surgery. *Br J Surg.* 91:828, 2004.

Friedman EA. An introduction to phosphate binders for the treatment of hyperphosphatemia in patients with chronic kidney disease. *Kidney Int Suppl.* 96:S2, 2005.

Gabor S, et al. Early enteral feeding compared with parenteral nutrition after oesophageal or oesophagogastric resection and reconstruction. *Br J Nutr.* 93:509, 2005.

Gibbs J, et al. Preoperative serum albumin level as a predictor of operative mortality and morbidity: results from the National VA Surgical Risk Study. *Arch Surg.* 134:36, 1999.

Goldsmith SR. Current treatments and novel pharmacologic treatments for hyponatremia in congestive heart failure. *Am J Cardiol.* 95:14B, 2005.

Grimble RF. Immunonutrition. *Curr Opin Gastroenterol.* 21:216, 2005.

Heyland D, et al. Should immunonutrition become routine in critically ill patients? A systematic review of the evidence. *JAMA.* 286:944, 2001.

Hoogwerf BJ. Postoperative management of the diabetic patient. *Med Clin North Am.* 85:1213, 2001.

Ireton-Jones CS, Jones JD. Should predictive equations or indirect calorimetry be used to design nutrition support regimens? Predictive equations should be used. *Nutr Clin Pract.* 13:141, 1998.

Kahl S, Malfertheiner P. Exocrine and endocrine pancreatic insufficiency after pancreatic surgery. *Best Pract Res Clin Gastroenterol.* 18:947, 2004.

Kellum JA. Determinants of plasma acid-base balance. *Crit Care Clin.* 21:329, 2005.

Knovich MA, Lesser GJ. The management of thromboembolic disease in patients with central nervous system malignancies. *Curr Treat Option Oncol.* 5:511, 2004.

Kozuschek W, et al. A comparison of long term results of the standard Whipple procedure and the pylorus preserving pancreatoduodenectomy. *J Am Col Surg.* 178:443, 1994.

Lavernia C, et al. Nutritional parameters and short-term outcome in arthroplasty. *J Am Coll Nutr.* 18:274, 1999.

Lucha PA Jr, et al. The economic impact of early enteral feeding in gastrointestinal surgery: a prospective survey of 51 consecutive patients. *Am Surg.* 71:187, 2005.

MacDonald A, Hildebrandt L. Comparison of formulaic equations to determine energy expenditure in the critically ill patient. *Nutrition* 19:233, 2003.

MacKay D, Miller AL. Nutritional support for wound healing. *Altern Med Rev.* 8:359, 2003.

Maddox TM. Preoperative cardiovascular evaluation for noncardiac surgery. *Mt Sinai J Med.* 72:185, 2005.

Marek PE, Zaloga GP. Meta-analysis of parenteral nutrition versus enteral nutrition in patients with acute pancreatitis. *BMJ.* 328:1407, 2004.

Marek PE, Zaloga GP. Gastric versus post-pyloric feeding: a systematic review. *Crit Care.* 7:46-51, 2003.

Marinella MA. Refeeding syndrome and hypophosphatemia. *J Intensive Care Med.* 20:155, 2005.

Martin TJ, et al. Abdominal surgery decreases food-reinforced operant responding in rats: relevance of incisional pain. *Anesthesiology* 103:629, 2005.

Martindale R. Clear liquid diets: tradition or intuition? *Nutr Clin Pract.* 13:186, 1998.

Mayerle J, et al. Medical treatment of acute pancreatitis. *Gastroenterol Clin North Am.* 33:855, 2004.

McClave SA, et al. North American Summit on Aspiration in the Critically Ill Patient: consensus statement. *J Parenter Enteral Nutr.* 26:S80, 2002.

McGuire J, et al. Fatal hypermagnesemia in a child treated with megavitamin/megamineral therapy. *Pediatrics* 105:18, 2000.

Modan M, Peles E, Halkin H, et al. Increased cardiovascular disease mortality rates in traumatic lower limb amputees. *Am J Cardiol.* 82:1242, 1998.

Modzumar A, Roy SK. Method for estimating body weight in persons with lower-limb amputation and its implication for their nutritional assessment. *Am J Clin Nutr.* 80:868, 2004.

Mokart D, et al. Predictive perioperative factors for developing severe sepsis after major surgery. Predictive perioperative factors for developing severe sepsis after major surgery. *Br J Anaesth.* 95:776, 2005.

Montain S, et al. Hyponatremia associated with exercise: risk factors and pathogenesis. *Exerc Sport Sci Rev.* 29:113, 2001.

Neiva RF, et al. Effects of vitamin-B complex supplementation on periodontal wound healing. *J Periodontol.* 76:1084, 2005.

Osterkamp LK. Current perspective on assessment of human body proportions of relevance to amputees. *J Am Diet Assoc.* 95:215, 1995.

Parekh NR, Steiger E. Percentage of weight loss as a predictor of surgical risk: from the time of Hiram Studley to today. *Nutr Clin Pract.* 19:471, 2004.

Patel GK. The role of nutrition in the management of lower extremity wounds. *Int J Low Extrem Wounds.* 4:12, 2005.

Peng X, et al. Clinical and protein metabolic efficacy of glutamine granules-supplemented enteral nutrition in severely burned patients. *Burns* 31:342, 2005.

Reid CL. Nutritional requirements of surgical and critically-ill patients: do we really know what they need? *Proc Nutr Soc.* 63:467, 2004.

Rodriguez-Moran M, Guerrero-Romero F. Low serum magnesium levels and foot ulcers in subjects with type 2 diabetes. *Arch Med Res.* 32:300, 2001.

Sax HC. Immunonutrition and upper gastrointestinal surgery: what really matters. *Nutr Clin Pract.* 20:540, 2005.

Schelling J. Fatal hypermagnesemia. *Clin Nephrol.* 53:61, 2000.

Scott SR, et al. Efficacy and tolerance of sodium phosphates oral solution after diet liberalization. Efficacy and tolerance of sodium phosphates oral solution after diet liberalization. *Gastroenterol Nurs.* 28:133, 2005.

Stechmiller JK, et al. Arginine supplementation and wound healing. *Nutr Clin Pract.* 20:52, 2005.

Travis K, Barr S. Rethinking postoperative diets for short-stay orthopedic patients. *J Am Diet Assoc.* 97:971, 1997.

Ueno C, et al. Using physiology to improve surgical wound outcomes. *Plast Reconstr Surg.* 117:59S, 2006 (suppl 7).
Weber T, Keller M. Operative management of chronic pancreatitis in children. *Arch Surg.* 136:550, 2001.
Weisel JW. Fibrinogen and fibrin. *Adv Protein Chem.* 70:247, 2005.
Wilmore D. The effect of glutamine supplementation in patients following elective surgery and accidental injury. *J Nutr.* 131:2543S, 2001.
Wilmore D. Enteral and parenteral arginine supplementation to improve medical outcomes in hospitalized patients. *J Nutr.* 134:2863S, 2004.
Winkelmayer WC, et al. C-reactive protein and body mass index independently predict mortality in kidney transplant recipients. *Am J Transplant.* 4:1178, 2005.
Wittman F, et al. L-arginine improves wound healing after trauma-hemorrhage by increasing collagen synthesis. *J Trauma.* 59:162, 2005.
Zaloga GP, et al. Arginine: mediator or modulator of sepsis? *Nutr Clin Pract.* 19:201, 2004.
Zaloga GP. Parenteral nutrition in adult inpatients with functioning gastrointestinal tracts: assessment of outcomes. *Lancet* 367:1101, 2006.

GASTROINTESTINAL SURGERIES

BOWEL SURGERY

NUTRITIONAL ACUITY RANKING: LEVEL 3

DEFINITIONS AND BACKGROUND

Small bowel surgery may be needed for inflammatory bowel disease, intestinal blockage, precancerous polyps, cancer, necrotizing enterocolitis, and other problems. Emergency surgical procedures in patients with inflammatory bowel disease are rare but can have a high morbidity unless carefully managed (Berg et al, 2002).

Contrast-enhanced computed tomography (CT) has decreased the use of barium studies and often replaces ultrasound and magnetic resonance imaging in the diagnostic management of small bowel obstruction patients (Hayanga et al, 2005).

Small bowel transplantation has become the treatment of choice for patients with chronic intestinal failure, whose illness cannot be managed with medications or who cannot be maintained on home parenteral nutrition (PN). Rejection, bacterial translocation, and sepsis rates are higher for these patients than for those who have received other organs (Ghanekar and Grant, 2001). After small bowel surgery, short bowel syndrome (SBS) occurs.

Residual small bowel length remains an important predictor of duration of the need for PN. Most people with SBS experience spontaneous small bowel adaptation over time, when they can be weaned from PN. There are some individuals who cannot be weaned and are potential candidates for techniques to promote intestinal adaptation and intestinal lengthening (Vernon and Georgeson, 2001). Prompt restoration of intestinal continuity is associated with lowered risk of cholestatic liver disease (Andorsky et al, 2001).

Patients who have had a **colectomy** have part or all of the colon removed. A colostomy or ileostomy creates an opening on the abdomen (stoma) for the drainage of feces. It may be permanent or temporary. Patients who have had an **ileostomy** lose a considerable amount of fluid that contains sodium and potassium. Fat and vitamin B_{12} absorption is reduced.

Patients who have had a **hemorrhoidectomy** usually tolerate a low-residue diet to delay defecation and allow healing at operative site. After patient is healed, it is important to have patient return to a high-fiber diet to prevent constipation. See Figure 14-3 for bleeding hemorrhoids.

INTERVENTION: OBJECTIVES

Preoperative

- Replenish depleted reserves by using special immune-enhanced formulas. Uninterrupted enteral nutrition (before, during, and after surgery) is popular in practice to achieve energy intake goals.
- Mechanical bowel preparation before surgery offers no major benefits.

Postoperative

- Restore enteral autonomy with complex surgical history, posttransplantation immunosuppressive regimen, and newly created surgical anatomy (Weseman and Gilroy, 2005). Early enteral feeding is generally recommended,

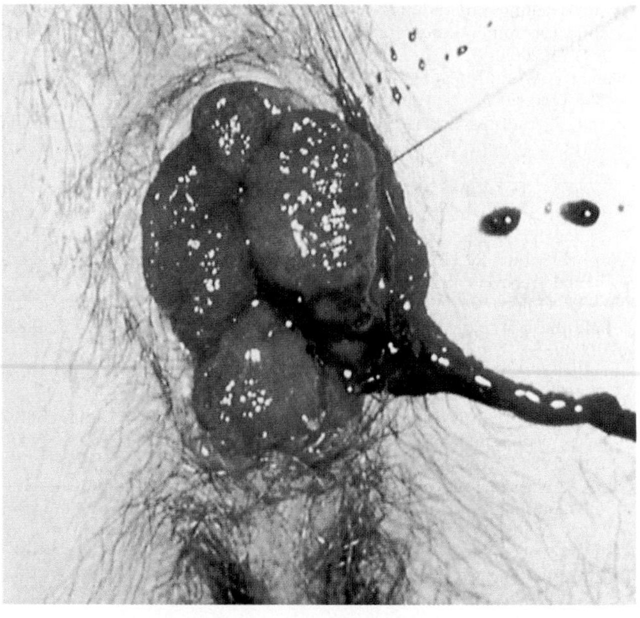

Figure 14-3 Bleeding hemorrhoids. (From Yamada T, et al. *Atlas of gastroenterology.* 3rd ed. Philadelphia: Lippincott Williams & Wilkins, 2003.)

although both enteral nutrition and PN have good results after bowel surgery (Pacelli et al, 2001). Enteral nutrition is cheaper than PN, and it reduces the impact of cytokines on surgical patients with related infectious complications.

- Slowly progress back to a normal diet. Progress from clear liquids to soft–solid diet and avoid dairy products as needed (Stike et al, 2001). Modify diet, as needed, for part of bowel that was affected.
- Correct inadequate digestion or absorption of fluid, electrolytes, and nutrients (Matarese et al, 2005).
- Prevent complications, such as peritonitis or ileus. Chewing gum can prevent ileus in some patients.
- Coordinate efforts with a transplantation team to restore nutritional autonomy to transplantation recipients and free them from PN (Weseman and Gilroy, 2005). Routine use of nasogastric tubes after abdominal operations do not necessarily speed the return of bowel function. They may be useful temporarily. Successful small bowel transplantation recipients can resume unrestricted oral diets (Ghanekar and Grant, 2001).
- Fight surgical infections by adding probiotics to enteral nutrition in order to improve the immune status of the colon.

INTERVENTION: FOOD AND NUTRITION

Preoperative

- Regress from soft diet to full liquids and then clear liquids.
- If needed, use a hydrolyzed formula or jejunostomy.

Postoperative

- Enteral nutrition may be primary therapy. Growth hormone, glutamine, short-chain fatty acids, and fermentable fiber sources are often useful.
- Intestinal rehabilitation regimens provide specialized oral diets, soluble fiber, oral rehydration solutions (ORS), and tropic factors to enhance absorption (Matarese et al, 2005).
- Probiotics may be beneficial (Floch et al, 2006).
- Slowly progress from a low-residue diet to a normal diet. Suggest that patient eat slowly and chew foods well. Excesses of fiber should be avoided. Probiotics may be included (Jenkins et al, 2005).
- Include fluids in adequate amounts; needs are usually above normal levels.
- Long-term nutritional support may be needed. This may include total PN for a short time.

For More Information

- American College of Gastroenterology
  http://www.acg.gi.org/
- Atlas of Gastrointestinal Endoscopy
  http://www.endoatlas.com/atlas_1.html
- Bowel Obstruction
  http://www.cancer.gov/cancertopics/pdq/supportivecare/gastrointestinalcomplications/HealthProfessional/page4
- Bowel Sounds
  http://www.nlm.nih.gov/medlineplus/ency/article/003137.htm
- Crohn's and Colitis Foundation
  http://www.ccfa.org/
- Ileostomy, Colostomy, and Other Surgery
  http://digestive.niddk.nih.gov/ddiseases/pubs/ileostomy/index.htm
- Inflammatory Bowel Diseases Journal
  http://www.ccfa.org/myccfa/IBD_journal
- Mechanical Bowel Prep before Surgery
  http://www.medscape.com/viewarticle/501745
- National Digestive Diseases Information Clearinghouse
  http://digestive.niddk.nih.gov/index.htm
- Ostomy
  http://www.cpmc.org/learning/documents/crm-ostomysurg-ws.html
- Preparation for Endoscopy
  http://www.asge.org/nspages/practice/patientcare/preparation.cfm
- Preparation for Lower Gastrointestinal Endoscopy
  http://www.asge.org/nspages/practice/patientcare/lgeindex.cfm
- Small Bowel Resection
  http://www.nlm.nih.gov/medlineplus/ency/article/002943.htm
- Society for American Gastroenterological and Endoscopic Surgeons
  http://www.sages.org/
- Society for Surgery of the Gastrointestinal Tract
  http://www.ssat.com/

BOWEL SURGERY—CITED REFERENCES

Andorsky D, et al. Nutritional and other postoperative management of neonates with short bowel syndrome correlates with clinical outcomes. *J Pediatr.* 139:27, 2001.

Berg DF, et al. Acute surgical emergencies in inflammatory bowel disease. *Am J Surg.* 184:45, 2002.

Floch MH, et al. Recommendations for probiotic use. *J Clin Gastroenterol.* 40:275, 2006.

Ghanekar A, Grant D. Small bowel transplantation. *Curr Opin Crit Care.* 7:133, 2001.

Hayanga AJ, et al. Current management of small-bowel obstruction. *Adv Surg.* 39:1, 2005.

Jenkins B, et al. Probiotics: a practical review of their role in specific clinical scenarios. *Nutr Clin Pract.* 20:262, 2005.

Matarese LE, et al. Short bowel syndrome: clinical guidelines for nutrition management. *Nutr Clin Pract.* 20:493, 2005.

Pacelli F, et al. Enteral vs parenteral nutrition after major abdominal surgery: an even match. *Arch Surg.* 136:933, 2001.

Stike R, et al. Dairy product-induced diarrhea after bowel surgery: a performance improvement opportunity. *Nutr Clin Pract.* 16:147, 2001.

Vernon A, Georgeson K. Surgical options for short bowel syndrome. *Semin Pediatr Surg.* 10:91, 2001.

Weseman RA, Gilroy R. Nutrition management of small bowel transplant patients. *Nutr Clin Pract.* 20:509, 2005.

GASTRIC BYPASS

NUTRITIONAL ACUITY RANKING: LEVEL 3

DEFINITIONS AND BACKGROUND

Over 10 million Americans are severely obese. Bariatric surgery is a viable option for the treatment of severe obesity, resulting in long-term weight loss and improved health risk factors (Buchwald et al, 2004; Sjostrom et al, 2004). **Gastric bypass surgery** produces greater weight loss and improvement in endothelial function (Gokce et al, 2005). Results show lower incidence rates of diabetes, hypertriglyceridemia, and hyperuricemia.

The production of inflammatory mediators by abdominal adipose tissue may link obesity and insulin resistance (Gletsu et al, 2005). In addition, the hormone ghrelin has a role in the long-term regulation of body weight, and gastric bypass is associated with markedly suppressed ghrelin levels, possibly contributing to the weight-reducing effect of the procedure (Cummings et al, 2002).

The most widely performed procedure, Roux-en-Y gastric bypass, achieves permanent and significant weight loss in over 90% of patients (Blackburn, 2005; Mun et al, 2001). Gastric bypass procedures induce physiological and neuroendocrine changes that appear to affect the weight regulatory centers in the brain; researchers have begun to explore the molecular pathways responsible for these outcomes (Blackburn, 2005).

Laparoscopic Roux-en-Y gastric bypass (LRYGB) has fewer side effects than more invasive procedures; one side effect may be anastomotic leak. Procedures reduce capacity to 40–60 mL. Roux-en-Y gastric bypass that is performed with at least a 150-cm Roux limb results in significantly greater weight loss but not more nutritional sequelae than shorter (<100 cm) procedures in superobese patients with a body mass index (BMI) >50 (Brolin, 2005).

According to Pories and Albrecht (2001), the Roux-en-Y gastric bypass induces long-term remission of type 2 diabetes mellitus in morbidly obese patients, returning those with impaired glucose tolerance to euglycemia in a matter of days. Exclusion of food and alteration in signals from the antrum, duodenum, and proximal jejunum to the islet cells of the pancreas seem to be the cause of improved glucose tolerance. Metabolic syndrome is also resolved after gastric bypass (Madan et al, 2006).

Use of a multidisciplinary clinical pathway, preprinted orders, discharge home instruction sheet, and daily guidelines for patients has been shown to decrease length of stay, average total charges, and percentage of wound infections (Rouse et al, 1998).

Rhabdomyolysis is a risk in this population from extended immobilization and is accompanied by pain in the region of the referred muscle group, increase in creatine phosphokinase levels, myoglobinuria, severe renal failure, multiorgan system failure, and death, if not treated in time (Filis et al, 2005). Another rare complication is nesidioblastosis, which is hyperfunction of the pancreatic beta cells; this can lead to a life-threatening hypoglycemia (Service et al, 2005).

Most patients lose more than 60% of their excess weight after surgery. Expected long-term outcomes after this surgery include improvement or resolution of diabetes (Torquati et al, 2005), coronary artery disease, dyslipidemia, gastroesophageal reflux disease (GERD), sleep apnea, hypertension, and osteoarthritis. The evidence for management of child and adolescent overweight and obesity is limited (Steinbeck, 2005). In the severely obese adolescent with obesity-related comorbidity, the use of very low–energy diets and antiobesity agents could be considered; bariatric surgery may be indicated in carefully selected, older, severely obese adolescents (Steinbeck, 2005).

Deficiencies in protein, iron, vitamin B_{12}, folate, calcium, fat-soluble vitamins (A, D, E, and K), and other micronutrients are common and may become clinically significant if not recognized and treated with supplementation (Carlin et al, 2006; Bloomberg et al, 2005). Copper deficiency, for example, has been noted in this population with cardiovascular and neurological changes (Tan et al, 2006). Monitoring and follow-up with a dietitian should be standard procedure. See Table 14-9.

Bariatric surgery is expensive, costing between $20,000 and $35,000. However, it is an effective weapon against the consequences of morbid obesity (Karmali and Shaffer, 2005). The consensus that obesity surgery is superior to medical intervention is growing and is supported by abundant evidence (Puzziferri, 2005). Candidates should be 100 lb or more over ideal weight range, have a BMI >40, or a BMI >35 in addition to serious medical comorbidities (Albrecht and Pories, 1999). See Figure 14-4.

INTERVENTION: OBJECTIVES

Preoperative

- Provide adequate glycogen stores and vitamins C and K for surgical procedure. Consider enteral immunonutrition.
- Patients with diabetes should be under fairly good glucose control or at least stable.

Postoperative

- Promote wound healing and restoration of depleted glycogen in the liver.
- Prevent side effects during weight loss. The weight loss results of gastric bypass surgery average 10 lb per month and stabilize somewhere between 18 and 24 months after surgery.
- Prevent complications such as alkaline reflux gastritis, esophagitis, perforation, gastric dilation, stomal obstruction, peptic ulcer, staple line disruption, and excessive vomiting.
- Monitor for rare conditions such as rhabdomyolysis and nesidioblastosis and manage as needed. Bowel obstruction (Capella et al, 2006) and acute renal failure (Sharma et al, 2006) are other rare complications.
- At 4–6 weeks postoperatively, patients often report that foods taste sweet and will modify intakes accordingly.

TABLE 14-9 Tips for Diet after Gastric Bypass

- Allow 30–45 minutes for each meal.
- Take small bites, and chew food until fairly liquefied before swallowing.
- Choose low-fat foods (<5g fat per serving)
- Stay away from concentrated sweets and sugar (>10 g sugar per serving).
- Sip at least 48–64 oz of liquid (preferably water) each day.
- Take a prescribed multivitamin every day.

Progression of Steps: diet will progress from:

Clear Liquids (*no more than ½ cup total*)	1–2 days after surgery
Full Liquids (*gradually increase from ½ cup to no more than ¾ cup total*)	days 3–21
Pureed (*meals should be from ¾ cup to no more than 1 cup total*)	3–6 weeks after surgery
Regular (small meals and snacks) (*no more than 1 cup total; meat should be no more than 2 oz*)	6 weeks on

Sometimes progression takes longer than usual; each person is different.

Food Suggestions for Each Step

Clear Liquid Step

Choose from the following:

- Water
- Diluted (pulp-free) juices (1 part juice to 10 parts water)
- Diet gelatin
- Unsweetened drinks
- Sugar-free popsicles
- Clear broth
- Decaffeinated tea
- **No carbonated drinks**

Full Liquid Step

Choose from the following:

The foods listed above plus:

- Nonfat acidophilus milk**
- Plain soy milk**
- Sugar-free yogurt
- Sugar-free pudding
- No sugar added Carnation Instant Breakfast drink**
- Low-fat cream soups
- Cream of wheat
- Cream of rice
- Unsweetened applesauce
- Infant strained fruits
- Sugar-free powdered drinks
- Sugar-free iced tea

** Good sources of protein during this step.

Pureed Diet Step

Choose from the following:

The foods listed above plus:

- Regular unflavored oatmeal
- Baby food or toddler fruits and vegetables
- Baby food chicken or turkey**
- Chicken or vegetable broth
- Low-fat cottage cheese
- Eggs**
- Humus
- Tofu**
- Blended fruit smoothies

** Good sources of protein during this step.

Regular Diet Step

Choose from the following:

The foods listed above plus:

- Well-cooked pasta
- Rice
- Most foods except for tough meats like beef as long as they are reduced in sugar and fat
- Protein is an important part of the diet; be sure to eat a balanced diet.

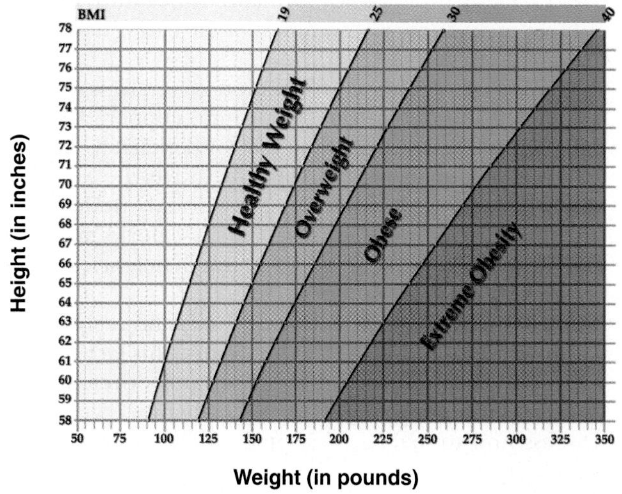

Figure 14-4 Body mass index (BMI) table showing obesity range. (Asset provided by Anatomical Chart Co.)

Aversions to meat may occur. Recent studies have found pica in some patients who also have iron deficiency anemia (Kushner and Shanta Retelny, 2005).

- Have patient eat and sip liquids slowly to prevent vomiting. Meat and bread/toast should be taken in small bites.
- Prevent neurological, hematological, and cardiovascular side effects of thiamine and vitamin B_{12} deficiency and other nutrients that may be inadequate (Bloomberg et al, 2005).
- In teens, use dietary change with lower fat intake and smaller portions; increased physical activity; decreased sedentary behavior; behavioral change; and parental involvement (Steinbeck, 2005).

INTERVENTION: FOOD AND NUTRITION

Preoperative

- Use a balanced diet with adequate energy, protein, vitamins, and minerals. Enteral immunonutrition may be useful.

- Diet should regress from liquids to NPO, nothing by mouth.

Postoperative

- Over a period of several days, progress from clear to full liquids. Enteral feeding with a high-protein intake may be useful to promote healing. Provide at least 1000 kcal/d with 1.5–2.0 g protein/kg.
- Until weight loss is achieved, add semisolid or pureed foods in small amounts. Initial gastric capacity is 30–60 mL; progression is up to 250 mL. Three meals and two snacks are well tolerated.
- Include 60–80 g of protein per day when possible. High-protein, low-fat foods such as milk, eggs, yogurt, boneless fish, and skinless poultry are important for maintaining adequate lean body mass while losing weight.
- Carbohydrate should be consumed at less than 30 g total per meal. A minimum of 130 g of carbohydrate per day should be included to meet DRIs.
- Some patients have problems with vomiting if they eat too rapidly, drink fluids right after eating, lie down after eating, or overeat. Recommend chewing slowly and consuming liquids separately from meals (30 minutes before or after).
- Dumping syndrome also can occur. Avoid alcoholic beverages and soft drinks; high-fat food such as fried foods and pastries; and high-carbohydrate foods such as cookies, cake, and candies.
- Assure adequate fluid intake to prevent dehydration. Use at least 6–8 cups (48–64 oz) of noncaffeinated/noncaloric fluid a day (water).
- Meet micronutrient requirements, such as a daily multivitamin-mineral supplement; calcium with vitamin D supplement (Johnson et al, 2005); and vitamin B_{12} injection monthly. Monitor for iron and calcium deficiencies; correct through supplemental sources. A liquid multivitamin-mineral supplement that provides 100% of the DRI levels is a recommendation early; progress to a chewable supplement.
- Avoid obstructive foods, such as popcorn, celery, nuts, seeds, and membranes of citrus fruits.

CLINICAL INDICATORS

Clinical/History

Height
Weight
Postoperative weight
BMI
Diet history
Waist circumference
Vomiting
I & O
BP
Sleep apnea
Endoscopy

Lab Work

Gluc
Hemoglobin A1c
CRP
Interleukin-6
Na+, K+
Ca++, Mg++
Alb, transthyretin
H & H
Serum Fe
Serum B_{12}
Serum folic acid
Serum vitamin D
Serum copper
Alkaline phosphatase
Cholesterol
Triglycerides

SAMPLE NUTRITION DIAGNOSTIC STATEMENT

Bariatric Surgery

PES: Inadequate vitamin B_{12} intake related to limited adherence to nutrition-related recommendations as evidenced by history of not taking vitamin supplement.

Assessment Data: Medication history.

Intervention: Nutrition-related medication management and discussion of importance of vitamin B_{12} from supplemental intake.

Monitoring and Evaluation: Pill count and changes in vitamin B_{12} lab values.

INTERVENTION: NUTRITION EDUCATION, COUNSELING, CARE MANAGEMENT

- **Preoperative evaluations** include: all weight loss attempts and outcomes; usual eating patterns and nutritional intake evaluations; frequency of eating away from home; cooking and shopping habits; reasons and motives for surgery; knowledge about protein, vitamins, and minerals; awareness of signs of dehydration; and food allergies and intolerances. Keeping a food diary and sharing it with the dietitian is important. Continuous nutrition monitoring can prevent poor outcomes if the patient and dietitian work together.
- **Postoperative education** includes: use of high-protein supplemental beverages, especially for wound healing. Thinned baby food, low-fat and sugar-free milkshakes, thinned hot cereals, blenderized soups, vegetable juices, and sugar-free instant breakfast drinks are useful.
- Patients require close monitoring, with special regard to the rapidity of weight loss and vigilant screening for signs and symptoms of subclinical and clinical nutritional deficiencies (Bloomberg et al, 2005; Shuster and Vasquez, 2005).
- Indicate appropriate quantities and qualities of foods that will be consumed; overeating may stretch the stoma or cause dumping syndrome. Have patient eat and sip liquids slowly to prevent vomiting. Meat and bread/toast should be taken in small bites, chewed thoroughly.
- Help patient progress to normalized diet with 120–200 mL per meal. Increase awareness of the eating and satiety process.
- A multivitamin-mineral preparation generally is needed. Vitamin B_{12}, folacin, iron, potassium, copper, and vitamins A and D are especially at risk for deficiency. The nutritional adequacy of the postoperative diet has frequently been overlooked. Nutritional deficiencies become apparent, including protein–calorie malnutrition and various vitamin and mineral deficiencies (Shuster and Vasquez, 2005).
- Discuss methods for blenderizing foods and recipes.
- Fasting can cause hypoglycemia; discuss this fact.
- Promote adequate sleep, exercise, and other lifestyle measures that support a sense of well-being.
- Discuss how to manage dumping syndrome by avoiding simple sugars.
- Most patients lose a significant amount of weight and maintain their weight loss long term and thus have

improved quality of life with decreased comorbidities and enhanced psychosocial functioning (Puzziferri, 2005). Unfortunately, between 5% and 30% of patients lose little weight or are unable to maintain their weight loss postoperatively (Puzziferri, 2005). Encourage exercise to help with weight loss and self-esteem.

- The American Society for Bariatric Surgery and the bariatric community promote use of quality assurance to produce the best outcomes (Rendon and Pories, 2005).

For More Information

- American Society for Bariatric Surgery
  http://www.asbs.org/
- BMI Charts
  http://win.niddk.nih.gov/publications/gastric.htm#bmichart
- Cleveland Clinic
  http://cms.clevelandclinic.org/bariatricsurgery/
- Fitness
  http://www.fitness.gov/
- Gastric Bypass
  http://www.nlm.nih.gov/medlineplus/ency/article/007199.htm
- Longitudinal Assessment of Bariatric Surgery (LABS)
  http://www.niddklabs.org
- Mayo Clinic
  http://www.mayoclinic.com/health/gastric-bypass/HQ01465
- Presurgical Psychological Assessment
  http://www.asbs.org/html/pdf/PsychPreSurgicalAssessment.pdf
- Weight Control Information Network
  http://win.niddk.nih.gov/

GASTRIC BYPASS—CITED REFERENCES

Albrecht R, Pories W. Surgical intervention for the severely obese. *Baillieres Best Pract Res Clin Endocrinol Metab.* 13:149, 1999.

Blackburn GL. Solutions in weight control: lessons from gastric surgery. *Am J Clin Nutr.* 82:248S, 2005.

Bloomberg RD, et al. Nutritional deficiencies following bariatric surgery: what have we learned? *Obes Surg.* 15:145, 2005.

Brolin RE. Long limb Roux en Y gastric bypass revisited. *Surg Clin North Am.* 85:807, 2005.

Buchwald H, et al. Bariatric surgery: a systematic review and meta-analysis. *JAMA.* 292:1724, 2004.

Capella RF, et al. Bowel obstruction after open and laparoscopic gastric bypass surgery for morbid obesity. *J Am Coll Surg.* 203:328, 2006.

Carlin AM, et al. Prevalence of vitamin D depletion among morbidly obese patients seeking gastric bypass surgery. *Surg Obes Relat Dis.* 2:98, 2006.

Cummings DE, et al. Plasma ghrelin levels after diet-induced weight loss or gastric bypass surgery. *N Engl J Med.* 346:1623, 2002.

Filis D, et al. Rhabdomyolysis following laparoscopic gastric bypass. *Obes Surg.* 15:1496, 2005.

Gletsu N, et al. Changes in C-reactive protein predict insulin sensitivity in severely obese individuals after weight loss surgery. *J Gastrointest Surg.* 9:1119, 2005

Gokce N, et al. Effect of medical and surgical weight loss on endothelial vasomotor function in obese patients. *Am J Cardiol.* 95:266, 2005.

Johnson JM, et al. Effects of gastric bypass procedures on bone mineral density, calcium, parathyroid hormone, and vitamin D. *J Gastrointest Surg.* 9:1106, 2005.

Karmali S, Shaffer E. The battle against the obesity epidemic: is bariatric surgery the perfect weapon? *Clin Invest Med.* 28:147, 2005.

Kushner RF, Shanta Retelny V. Emergence of pica (ingestion of non-food substances) accompanying iron deficiency anemia after gastric bypass surgery. *Obes Surg.* 15:1491, 2005.

Madan AK, et al. Metabolic syndrome: yet another co-morbidity gastric bypass helps cure. *Surg Obes Relat Dis.* 2:48, 2006.

Mun E, et al. Current status of medical and surgical therapy for obesity. *Gastroenterology* 120:669, 2001.

Pories W, Albrecht R. Etiology of type II diabetes mellitus: role of the foregut. *World J Surg.* 25:527, 2001.

Puzziferri N. Psychologic issues in bariatric surgery—the surgeon's perspective. *Surg Clin North Am.* 85:741, 2005.

Rendon SE, Pories WJ. Quality assurance in bariatric surgery. *Surg Clin North Am.* 85:757, 2005.

Rouse A, et al. Meeting the challenge of managed care through clinical pathways for bariatric surgery. *Obes Surg.* 8:530, 1998.

Service GJ, et al. Hyperinsulinemic hypoglycemia with nesidioblastosis after gastric-bypass surgery. *N Engl J Med.* 353:249, 2005.

Sharma SK, et al. Acute changes in renal function after laparoscopic gastric surgery for morbid obesity. *Surg Obes Relat Dis.* 2:389, 2006.

Shuster MH, Vasquez JA. Nutritional concerns related to Roux-en-Y gastric bypass: what every clinician needs to know. *Crit Care Nurs Q.* 28:227, 2005.

Sjostrom L, et al. Lifestyle, diabetes, and cardiovascular risk factors 10 years after bariatric surgery. *N Engl J Med.* 351:2683, 2004.

Steinbeck K. Childhood obesity. Treatment options. *Best Pract Res Clin Endocrinol Metab.* 19:455, 2005.

Tan JC, et al. Severe ataxia, myelopathy, and peripheral neuropathy due to acquired copper deficiency in a patient with history of gastrectomy. *J Parenter Enteral Nutr.* 30:446, 2006.

Torquati A, et al. Is Roux-en-Y gastric bypass surgery the most effective treatment for type 2 diabetes mellitus in morbidly obese patients? *J Gastrointest Surg.* 9:1112, 2005.

SECTION 15

AIDS and Immunology, Infections, Burns, and Trauma

CHIEF ASSESSMENT FACTORS

- Recent Illnesses, Surgery
- Presence of Chronic Diseases
- Medications (Prescription and Over-the-Counter)
- Anemia, Anorexia, Malnutrition
- Fever, Chills
- Accidents or Trauma
- Metabolic Rate (Estimated or Indirect Calorimetry)
- Infection or Sepsis (Heat, Pain, Redness, Swelling, or Drainage in Any Area)
- Rapid Pulse Rate
- Altered Breathing
- Urinary Changes (Frequency, Urgency, Burning)
- Altered White Blood Cell Count (WBC) and Differential
- Indicators of Immunity Such as T Cells, Other Lymphocytes
- Culture Results, Specimens
- Fluid Status, Edema
- Multiple Organ System Function
- Nutritional Status for Zinc, Iron, Selenium; Vitamins A, C, E; Albumin
- Environmental Sanitation and Level of Personal Hygiene

OVERVIEW OF NUTRITION AND IMMUNOCOMPETENCE

The interdependency between the disciplines of nutrition and immunology was recognized in the 1970s when immunological measures were introduced as a component of assessing nutritional status (Field, 2000). The fetal and early infant origins of adult cardiovascular and metabolic diseases have also been studied. Fetal and early infant programming of thymic function suggests that early environments may have long-term implications for immunocompetence and adult disease risk (McDade et al, 2001).

Chandra (2000) verified that nutrition and physical growth affect immunocompetence and morbidity from infections. Reduced numbers of lymphocytes in the peripheral immune system appear to be a significant cause of the loss in host defense capacity in humans that are zinc deficient; both marrow and thymus are affected, with large losses noted among the pre-B and pre-T cells (Fraker and King, 2001).

Common diseases such as atopy and allergy, autoimmunity, chronic infections, and sepsis are characterized by a dysregulation of the pro- versus anti-inflammatory and T helper (Th) 1 versus Th2 cytokine balance; proinflammatory cytokines promote atherosclerosis, major depression, visceral-type obesity, metabolic syndrome, and sleep disturbances (Elenkov et al, 2005).

Studies regarding the role of nutrients on gene expression and related cytokine production have established the importance of maintaining a balanced immune system throughout life (Field, 2000). Lack of adequate macronutrients or selected micronutrients, especially zinc, selenium, iron, and the antioxidant vitamins, can lead to clinically significant immune deficiency and infections, especially in childhood (Cunningham-Rundles et al, 2005).

There are large variations in many immune functions between individuals, related to genetics, age, gender, smoking habits, habitual levels of exercise, alcohol consumption, diet, stage in the female menstrual cycle, stress, history of infections and vaccinations, and early life experiences (Calder and Kew, 2002). Adopting sound nutritional practices, reducing life stressors, maintaining good hygiene and sanitation, obtaining adequate rest, and maintaining a healthy exercise routine can enhance immunocompetence and reduce risks of infection in any population.

Older adults are at special risk for malnutrition, which contributes to their increased risk of infection. Nutritional supplementation strategies have been proposed to reduce this risk and reverse some of the immune dysfunction associated with advanced age.

Hospital admission screening information that best identifies patients who are at risk for malnutrition-related complications (MRCs) are occurrence of a wound, poor oral intake, malnutrition-related admission diagnosis, serum albumin value, hemoglobin value, and total lymphocyte count (Brugler et al, 2005). The ability of admission information to accurately reflect MRC risk is crucial to early initiation of restorative medical nutritional therapy (Brugler et al, 2005).

Table 15-1 defines how the immune system works. Table 15-2 describes more specifics about nutrition and its role in maintaining immunocompetence. Table 15-3 provides a list of key nutrients for immunocompetence. Table 15-4 provides important nutritional factors to consider in patients who are critically ill. Figure 15-1 provides a summary of how injury impacts metabolic rate. Table 15-5 lists nutritional implications in infections and febrile conditions. Table 15-6 lists virulence increased by iron supplementation.

TABLE 15-1 How the Immune System Works

The immune system is designed to provide protection from invading organisms, including bacteria and viruses, tumor cells, dirt, pollen, and other foreign material. Normally, barriers—including the skin and the lining of the lungs and gastrointestinal and reproductive tracts—protect the underlying delicate tissues from the outside environment. However, when there is a breakdown in that protective lining, germs and other irritants can enter the body. The immune system's function is to conquer these foreign molecules by engulfing them or by destroying them with enzymes or other detoxifying means. In addition to fighting off these foreign invaders, the immune system has evolved to destroy abnormal cells (such as tumor cells) but occasionally reacts against the body's own normal tissues (autoimmunity).
Innate and Acquired Immunity
There are two principal types of immune response, innate and adaptive (or acquired) immunity, which are distinguished from one another by both their speed and specificity. The innate immune system, present from birth, involves nonspecific responses that are the first line of defense against common infectious agents, including bacteria and viruses. This system is generally able to recognize foreign organisms but is unable to distinguish between particular invaders. Thus, an innate response does not require stimulation by sophisticated cell to cell interactions to remove bacteria or other foreign material and degrade it.
In contrast to the innate immune system, the more specific adaptive (acquired) immune system must be triggered by a specific virus, bacterium, or other foreign material, which stimulates lymphocytes to produce antibodies that can combat the foreign substance. At the next exposure, the preformed antibodies will allow the person to respond with an even stronger, more specific response. This is called immunological memory.
Cells of the Immune System
The immune system consists of white blood cells (leukocytes), which are produced in the bone marrow and mature there or in the thymus and other lymphoid organs. Leukocytes circulate in the blood along with oxygen-carrying red blood cells. Under normal conditions, leukocytes leave the circulation and migrate into organs, including the skin, lungs, intestine, and reproductive tract, where germs can appear. There, they can wait for infectious agents, or they can migrate back through the circulation to other organs. There are three major types of leukocytes. (See next page.)

(continued)

TABLE 15-1 How the Immune System Works *(continued)*

Neutrophils are the most plentiful of the white blood cells in humans. They are the immune system's first line of defense, as they contain an arsenal of preformed chemicals known as enzymes, which are capable of destroying bacteria. In addition, they are phagocytic, meaning that they can engulf viruses, bacteria, or other foreign material, protecting the host from further damage. Neutrophils are very short lived and are often destroyed during the process of fighting infection.

Monocytes are leukocytes that, after migrating to tissues, mature into macrophages. Macrophages are phagocytic and can remove foreign material and parts of dead cells from the tissues. They contain enzymes that can destroy infectious material but live longer than neutrophils and do not tend to self-destruct as easily. The tissue macrophage in the liver is called the Kupffer cell.

Lymphocytes, the most selective cells of the immune system, are specialized white blood cells that can combat specific infectious agents. There are two types of lymphocyte: B cells and T cells. B cells, which are responsible for humoral immunity (so called because it takes place in the body fluids, classically known as the humors), release specialized, soluble proteins known as antibodies into the blood and other body fluids. The antibodies recognize and bind to the surface of foreign substances (i.e., pathogens), immobilizing them and further labeling them as foreign so that they can be more readily taken up by phagocytic cells.

T cells, in contrast, act directly on other cells rather than manufacturing antibodies to combat infectious agents. Because of this direct interaction with other cells, T cells are responsible for cellular immunity. They can be further divided into helper T cells, which recognize foreign invaders and stimulate immune responses from other cells, and cytotoxic T cells, which destroy infected cells. Whereas some of these cells survive only briefly, others are extremely long lived, including "memory cells," which are capable of remembering certain features on the foreign molecules so that, if the organism encounters that foreign molecule in the future, it can quickly stimulate its response team.

Communication between Immune Cells: Cytokines

One form of communication between immune cells is direct cell-to-cell contact, which can occur either as a loose, transient association or as a tighter, long-lasting encounter. Either way, cells must make physical contact with one another.

In the second form of contact, cells release small proteins called cytokines, which bind to specific receptors on the surface of target cells. Cytokines interact only with the appropriate target cell with no effect on surrounding cells. Although many of the effects of cytokines are local, they have been called the hormones of the immune system because they are transported by the circulating blood. Cytokines can affect the same cell that produced them, a neighboring cell, or a cell far away. They stimulate or dampen cell proliferation (replication), production of other cytokines, killing of damaged cells or tumor cells (cytotoxicity), and cell migration (chemotaxis). The latter response is controlled by a subset of cytokines called chemokines. Just as there are cells that can stimulate or inhibit immune response, cytokines produced by those cells can regulate a variety of cell functions either positively or negatively.

Interleukin-6 is an important cytokine in immunity. Excessive production of proinflammatory cytokines or their production in the wrong biological context may lead to situations of chronic inflammation and negative health consequences (Philpott and Ferguson, 2004).

Gut Immunity

An extremely important function of the gastrointestinal tract is its ability to regulate the flow of macromolecules between the environment and the host through a barrier mechanism (Fasano and Shea-Donohue, 2005). The gastrointestinal immune response maintains critical pathways (Cunningham-Rundles et al, 2005). Together with the gut-associated lymphoid tissue and the neuroendocrine network, the intestinal epithelial barrier, with its intercellular tight junctions, controls the equilibrium between tolerance and immunity to nonself-antigens (Fasano and Shea-Donohue, 2005).

TABLE 15-2 Immunocompetence and Immunity Concerns

Almost all nutrients in the diet play a crucial role in maintaining an "optimal" immune response, such that deficient and excessive intakes can have negative consequences on immune status and susceptibility to a variety of pathogens. In addition, use of botanical and herbal products can be a concern, as indicated (Bielory, 2004):

- Echinacea is a common herb used to treat symptoms of the "common cold" or upper respiratory tract allergies; there is a risk of hepatotoxicity, exacerbation of allergies and asthma, and anaphylactic reactions.
- Garlic is often used to relieve cough, colds, and rhinitis; gastrointestinal (GI) disturbances, change in body odor through the sweat and breath, and rarely allergic reactions or hypoglycemia can occur.
- Other complementary and alternative medicine (CAM) agents, including angelica, German chamomile flower, ephedra, ginkgo, grape seed extract, licorice root, St. John's wort, kava kava rhizome, peppermint, stinging nettle, and ginseng, may have undesirable side effects (see Section 2).

Groups at greatest risk for infectious illness	Nutrition and dietary patterns have been shown to have direct impact on health of the population and of selected patient groups, related to a reduction of oxidative damage from free radical production (Berger, 2005). Infants; the elderly; and malnourished, immunocompromised, and hospitalized persons are at high risk. Alcoholics are also prone to frequent infections (Happel and Nelson, 2005). Antioxidant vitamin and trace element intakes are particularly important in the prevention of cancer, cardiovascular diseases, age-related ocular diseases, and aging (Berger, 2005).
Infants and children	Undernutrition in critical periods of gestation and neonatal maturation and during weaning impairs the development and differentiation of a normal immune system (Cunningham-Rundles et al, 2005). There is a high prevalence of micronutrient deficiencies and infectious diseases in infants in developing countries; weekly use of a micronutrient mix containing 20 mg iron, 20 mg zinc, 1 mg riboflavin along with other minerals and vitamins reduces risk of diarrhea in all infants (Baqui et al, 2003). Breastfed infants have lower morbidity and mortality due to diarrhea than those fed artificially (Newburg et al, 2005). Human milk oligosaccharides protect against pathogens, primarily due to their inhibition of pathogen binding to host cell ligands (Newburg et al, 2005).

(continued)

TABLE 15-2 Immunocompetence and Immunity Concerns *(continued)*

	There are beneficial effects of moderate amounts of zinc given in the first 6 months of life, especially for small-for-gestational age and low birth weight infants; this helps cell-mediated immunity, antibody responses, and phagocyte function (Chandra, 2000). Vitamin C and zinc reduce the incidence and improve the outcome of pneumonia, malaria, and diarrhea infections, especially in children in developing countries (Wintergerst et al, 2005).
Older adults	Interleukin-6 (IL-6), a cytokine, is tightly controlled by hormonal feedback (estrogen, testosterone) that is lost in the aging process. Elevated IL-6 levels progressively increase and promote tumorigenesis (e.g., breast, prostate, lung, colon, ovarian) and conditions such as osteoporosis, rheumatoid arthritis, multiple myeloma, neurodegenerative diseases, and frailty (Dijsselbloem et al, 2004). Adults aged 65 years and older comprise the fastest-growing segment of the United States population, and older adults experience greater morbidity and mortality due to infection than do young adults (High et al, 2005). Data support use of a daily multivitamin or trace mineral supplement that includes elemental zinc (>20 mg/d) and selenium (100 mg/d), with additional vitamin E to achieve a daily dose of 200 mg/d (High, 2001).
Common cold	The role of large doses of vitamin C to reduce duration or severity of cold symptoms has been inconclusive. Several clinical trials support the evidence against taking large amounts of vitamin C to treat the common cold (Audera et al, 2001). Vitamin E supplementation has been shown to be helpful in reducing the incidence of respiratory infections among the elderly (Meydani et al, 2004). Echinacea and ginseng may be modestly protective (Predy et al, 2005; Block and Mead, 2003). Chilling of the feet does seem to contribute to the onset of colds; research is ongoing (Johnson and Eccles, 2005).
Gut-associated lymphoid tissue (GALT)	GALT is the dominant location for initiation of mucosal immune response, which is dependent on nutritional elements, including fats, amino acids, and micronutrients (Cunningham-Rundles, 2001). A healthy gastrointestinal mucosal immune system provides barriers against systemic access for food antigens and microbes. Changes in the GALT immune response may contribute to intestinal dysfunction and increase susceptibility to postinjury gut-derived sepsis (Bastian and Weimann, 2002).
Immunocompromised persons (cancer, human immunodeficiency virus [HIV], tuberculosis)	Supplementation of vitamin C improves antimicrobial and natural killer cell activities, lymphocyte proliferation, chemotaxis, and delayed-type hypersensitivity (Wintergerst et al, 2005). Glutamine, arginine, fatty acids, and vitamin E provide additional benefits for immunocompromised persons or patients who suffer from various infections (Bastian and Weimann, 2002; Field et al, 2002). Avoid excesses of arginine in sepsis (Bistrian, 2004). Zinc, epigallocatechin galate (EGCG), omega-3 polyunsaturated fatty acids, and probiotics appear to have the potential to protect against cancer development and progression (Philpott and Ferguson, 2004). Chronic undernutrition and infection further weakens the immune response, leading to altered immune cell populations and a generalized increase in inflammatory mediators (Cunningham-Rundles et al, 2005).
Nutrition support	Assessment of immunocompetence by available methods can identify individuals who are most in need of appropriate nutritional support to enhance host defense to infectious pathogens (Field et al, 2002).
Public health	Iron and vitamin A deficiencies and protein–energy malnutrition are highly prevalent worldwide and are important to public health in terms of immunocompetence (Field et al, 2002). Vitamin A and zinc play important roles in protecting individuals from severity in illnesses such as diarrhea and HIV infection. Zinc undernutrition or deficiency impairs cellular phagocytosis, natural killer cell activity, and the generation of oxidative burst (Wintergerst et al, 2005). CAM is very common in the public arena; allergic reactions may occur; and these should be carefully monitored (Bielory, 2005). Risks and adverse functional and health outcomes may be associated with deficient and excessive intakes and nutrition status of iron, iodine, zinc, vitamins A and D, folate, vitamin B_{12}, and riboflavin in children (Viteri and Gonzalez, 2002). Outcomes may be altered in growth and development, mental and neuromotor performance, immunocompetence, physical working capacity, and morbidity (Viteri and Gonzalez, 2002).
Obesity	Obesity caused by excess nutrition or excess storage of fats relative to energy expenditure is a form of malnutrition that is increasingly seen; leptin is a cytokine-like immune regulator that has complex effects in both overnutrition and in the inflammatory response in malnutrition (Cunningham-Rundles et al, 2005).
Surgical patients	Preoperative oral intake of immunonutrition containing omega 3-fatty acids, arginine, and nucleotides at home may prevent the risks of hospitalization and may lead to immunomodulating effects, which can improve nutritional status (see Section 14). Postsurgical or septic patients given branched-chain amino acids (BCAA) intravenously show improved immunity and improved outcomes (Calder, 2006).
Trauma	Sepsis and multiple organ failure have mortality rates of up to 80%; limitation of the inflammatory response of immunocompetent cells must be achieved as quickly as possible (<72 hours), and immunonutrition should be strongly considered (Bastian and Weimann, 2002). Vitamin C concentrations in the plasma and leukocytes rapidly decline during infections and stress (Wintergerst et al, 2005).

TABLE 15-3 Nutritional and Host Factors in Immunity

Nutrient status is an important factor contributing to immune competence; undernutrition impairs the immune system, suppressing immune functions that are fundamental to host protection (Calder and Kew, 2002). In recent studies, vitamin D_3 (1,25-dihydroxyvitamin D) has been found to regulate the differentiation, growth, and function of a broad range of immune system cells, including monocytes, dendritic cells, and T and B lymphocytes (Equils et al, 2006). In addition, branched-chain amino acids (BCAA) are absolutely essential for lymphocytes to synthesize protein, RNA, and DNA and to respond to pathogens (Calder, 2006).

Infectious Disease Determinants

- Environmental sanitation
- Host immunity, including nutritional status
- Micro-organismic virulence
- Personal hygiene

Host-Resistance Factors

- Cell-mediated immunity (T cells) from thymus gland
- Complement system
- Immunoglobulins and antibodies (B cells) from bone marrow
- Monocytes and dendritic cells
- Mucus and cilia on epithelial surfaces
- Oligosaccharides and other prebiotics (Newburg et al, 2005)
- Phagocytes (leukocytes, macrophages)
- Physical barriers (skin, mucous membranes)
- Probiotic bacteria (Calder and Kew, 2002)

Immune System

- Bone marrow
- Lymphoid tissue (Peyer's patches in gut and gut-associated lymphoid tissue; Luster patches in bronchioles)
- Lymph nodes
- Spleen
- Thymus
- Tonsils

Nutrients of Immunocompetence

- Macronutrients
  - Amino acids such as arginine and glutamine (Field et al, 2002)
  - Essential amino acids (Calder and Kew, 2002); dietary nucleotides (RNA)
  - Linoleic acid, as essential fatty acid (Field et al, 2002)
  - Omega-3 fatty acids (Watson et al, 2005; Calder, 2004)
- Vitamins
  - Vitamin A (Field et al., 2002); beta-carotene
  - Folic acid, vitamin B_6, vitamin B_{12} (Calder and Kew, 2002)
  - Vitamin C
  - Vitamin D (Equils et al, 2006).
  - Vitamin E (Meydani et al, 2004; Calder and Kew, 2002; Field et al, 2002)
- Minerals
  - Copper (Calder and Kew, 2002)
  - Iron (Calder and Kew, 2002; Fraker and King, 2001)
  - Magnesium
  - Selenium (Calder and Kew, 2002)
  - Zinc (Calder and Kew, 2002)

Immunonutrition

To be immunonutrition, enteral feeding is supplemented with specific nutrients such as arginine, glutamine, omega-3 polyunsaturated fatty acids (PUFAs), and nucleotides (Bastian and Weimann, 2002). Immunonutrition may provide a less invasive alternative to immunotherapy in protection against cancers associated with chronic inflammation (Philpott and Ferguson, 2004).

Intravenous lipids may be deleterious due to the proinflammatory effects of omega-6 fatty acids; omega-3 fatty acids are anti-inflammatory, and combined with medium-chain triglycerides (MCT) and olive oil, they may provide a more efficacious form of intravenous lipid (Grimble, 2005).

Antioxidants, plant fibers, and live lactic acid bacteria are especially important for boosting the immune system (Bengmark, 2005). The systemic inflammatory response syndrome and multiorgan dysfunction syndrome can be reduced if much higher doses of bioactive lactic acid bacteria (synbiotics) are used (Bengmark, 2005).

Nutrient–Nutrient Interactions, Excesses, and Immunocompetence

- A prenatal multiple micronutrient supplement may provide no added advantage over iron and folate in reducing outcomes such as low birth weight; data also suggest that adding zinc may negate the beneficial effect of iron and folic acid on birth weight (Christian, 2003).
- Although under most circumstances the systemic inflammatory response is beneficial to the host, improving the eventual outcome of injury, infection, or inflammation, excessive proinflammation may lead to cardiac, hepatic, and mitochondrial dysfunction, and excessive counterinflammation leads to immune depression (Bistrian, 2004).
- Excesses of iron, zinc, vitamin E, and PUFA may interfere with immunity, especially when given intravenously or intramuscularly.
- Whereas enteral nutrition improves immune function, parenteral nutrition reduces immune functions (Bengmark, 2005). Parenteral iron and zinc are to be used with great caution in sepsis. Total parenteral nutrition (TPN) is contraindicated in septic patients.
- Excess calcium interferes with leukocyte function by displacing magnesium (Kubena and McMurray, 1996).
- Figure 15-1 shows the impact of injury on metabolic rate.

TABLE 15-4 Factors of Importance in Critical Care

1. Estimated energy needs in critical illness uses 25–30 kcal/kg current body weight (CBW). In intensive care, 20–25 kcal/kg CBW with 30% kcal as fat is recommended. In a retrospective analysis conducted to compare four energy prediction equations versus measured resting energy expenditure (MREE) determined via indirect calorimetry, the following results were identified (Campbell et al, 2005):
   - The Harris-Benedict (HB) equation was calculated for patients <90% of ideal body weight (IBW) using both CBW and IBW; using the CBW or IBW in the HB underestimated the patient's energy needs.
   - Energy needs were estimated with an Ireton-Jones formula for all mechanically ventilated patients; this calculation tended to overestimate their energy needs.
   - For patients <85% IBW, an adjusted body weight was determined ([CBW + IBW]/2) and used in the HB formula; values were significantly different than MREE. The average caloric need was 31.2 ± 6.0 kcal/kg CBW.
   - **Indirect calorimetry remains the best method of determining a patient's energy needs.** Until a large prospective trial is conducted, a combination of prediction equations tempered with clinical judgment and monitoring of the appropriateness of the nutrition prescription remains the best approach to quality patient care.
2. Metabolic complications can occur from overfeeding critically ill patients. In general, current practice is to underfeed slightly rather than to overfeed. Indirect calorimetry decreases complications from overfeeding and saves costs by reducing length of stay (Headley, 2003).
3. Maintain protein at approximately 1.5 g/kg. In critical illness, glutamine levels are much higher in the duodenal mucosa than in starvation; glutamine supplementation may be beneficial (De-Souza and Greene, 2005). Arginine is a conditionally essential amino acid; it is a substrate for protein synthesis but can also be metabolized to various compounds, including nitric oxide, ornithine, and creatine phosphate, that are important for growth, wound healing, cardiovascular function, immune function, inflammatory responses, energy metabolism, urea cycle function, and other metabolic processes (Zaloga et al, 2004). Arginine supplementation improves outcomes with sepsis, wounds, ischemia-reperfusion injury, and burns (Zaloga et al, 2004). Although there is controversy surrounding this issue, use of arginine may be better for surgical patients than for septic patients (Grimble, 2005; Ochoa et al, 2004; Wilmore, 2004).
4. The use of specific nutrients to modify immune, inflammatory, and metabolic processes also offers new possibilities for reducing morbidity following major surgery (Heys et al, 2005). Trace elements and antioxidant nutrients, especially selenium, are important for use in critical care and may reduce mortality (Grimble et al, 2005; Heyland et al, 2005). Vitamin E levels also tend to be low and may be supplemented accordingly (Bulger and Maier, 2003). Use of omega-3 fatty acids is important in this population (Grimble, 2005).
5. Enteral nutrition (EN) is more efficacious and poses lower risks than parenteral nutrition; EN reduces infection rates and shortens intensive care unit and hospital length of stay in critically ill patients (Grimble, 2005).
6. Control of hyperglycemia is very important, especially to lessen infection and sepsis (Butler et al, 2005).

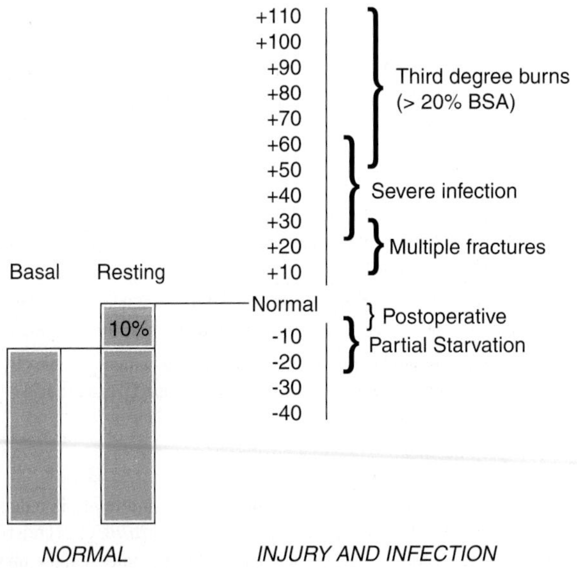

Figure 15-1 The impact of injury on metabolic rate.

TABLE 15-5 Infections and Febrile Conditions and Nutritional Implications

Emergence of new infectious diseases and old diseases with new properties affects the world; severe acute respiratory syndrome (SARS) and avian flu are just two examples in which the nutritional status of the host can also influence the genetic makeup of the viral genome (Beck et al, 2004).

Condition and Nutritional Acuity Ranking	Background	Nutritional Implications
Bacterial endocarditis, Level 3	Bacterial endocarditis is an infection (often *Streptococcus*) of the membrane lining the heart chambers. Bacterial endocarditis accounts for 2% of all cases of organic heart disease. Symptoms and signs include fever, chills, joint pain, lassitude, and malaise. Acute forms have rapid onset; the subacute form begins slowly. Anorexia and weight loss are common. Most afflicted persons have had a previous heart condition such as rheumatic fever.	Restore patient's nutritional status to normal. Replenish electrolytes and fluids. Reduce edema, if present. Prevent heart failure, infections, anemia, embolism, and nephritis. Use a high-energy and high-protein diet. If patient's appetite is poor, encourage intake of favorite foods. Ensure adequate intake of vitamins and minerals, especially vitamins A and C. Ensure intake of an adequate amount of fluids, especially fruit juices. Penicillin, erythromycin, and other combinations may be used; monitor for appropriate timing of meals and drugs.
Candidiasis, Level 2	*Candida albicans* is found in the mouth, feces, and vagina normally. A greater colonization occurs in debilitated persons, in whom thrush or vaginitis or cutaneous lesions are common. Persons who are susceptible include patients with hematological malignancy, those who are on long-term total parenteral nutrition (TPN), immunosuppressed patients, postoperative patients, people receiving antibiotic therapy, and people who are obese or have diabetes.	Prevent or treat systemic infections. Prevent endocarditis, emboli, splenomegaly, and other complications. Correct underlying conditions when possible. Ensure balanced intake for all nutrients; diet should be high in quality proteins and adequate in calories. Adequate fluid intake is beneficial. Increase vitamin and mineral intake from tolerated fruits and vegetables, especially for vitamins A and C. Nystatin or amphotericin B may be used; diarrhea, nausea, and stomach pain may occur. Extended use of antibiotics may have caused or aggravated condition. For patients with malignant disease, a discussion about the importance of nutrition in maintaining good health status is essential. Meals should be consumed regularly with smaller, frequent meals or snacks. Avoid fasting and skipping meals.
Clostridium difficile–associated disease, Level 3	The incidence of this condition is rising, with more colectomy and mortality. This condition is also hard to treat. The common name is recurrent *Clostridium difficile*–associated disease (RCDAD). Suppression of gastric acid with proton pump inhibitor drugs like Prilosec (omeprazole) or Nexium (esomeprazole) is associated with a two- to three-fold increase in the risk of community-acquired *Clostridium difficile* (Dial et al, 2004). *Clostridium difficile* causes approximately 25% of nosocomial antibiotic-associated diarrheas and most cases of pseudomembranous colitis (Zheng et al, 2004).	Repeat antibiotics are usually indicated, either metronidazole or vancomycin; tapering the antibiotic dose after a 10-day standard course decreases the incidence of recurrences compared with abruptly stopping antibiotics (Surawicz, 2004). Long-term use of metronidazole may cause neurotoxicity. Probiotics may be important in the treatment of RCDAD; *Saccharomyces boulardii* has been shown to decrease recurrences by about 50%, especially when combined with high-dose vancomycin (Surawicz, 2004).
Chronic fatigue and immune dysfunction syndrome (CFIDS), Level 1	Chronic fatigue syndrome is a serious health concern affecting over 800,000 Americans of all ages, races, socioeconomic groups, and genders (Gerrity et al, 2004). CFIDS, formerly called the chronic Epstein-Barr virus (EBV) syndrome, involves severe exhaustion and weakness, headaches, sore throat, tender lymph nodes, unrefreshing sleep, fever, muscle aches, inability to concentrate, and depression. Symptoms tend to mimic depression, lupus, or even cancer. A thorough physical examination is suggested. The etiology and pathophysiology are unknown; studies have suggested an involvement of the immune system (Gerrity et al, 2004). Etiology suggests a chronic mononucleosis caused by a herpes virus (perhaps human B-lymphotrophic virus). Research suggests a link to Hodgkin's disease or multiple sclerosis a few years after diagnosis. The patient often has "neurally mediated hypotension." Testing for viral load is helpful. For more information on CFIDS, see http://www.cfids.org/.	Improve immunological status and prevent malnutrition. Lessen severity of symptoms. Avoid infections and stress to prevent recurrent attacks, where possible. Adequate protein should be consumed (0.8–1 g/kg); 35 kcal/kg may be needed. Adequate vitamin and mineral intake should be ensured; antioxidant foods should be included regularly in diet. Extra salt or fluids may be needed for hypotension. Fludrocortisone promotes sodium retention. Analgesics may be used for relief of muscle aches and other types of pain. If zinc is taken as an immunostimulant; avoid use with immunosuppressants, tetracycline, ciprofloxacin, levofloxacin, or ofloxacin; antagonistic effects or binding can occur. Purslane, spinach, ginseng, and wheat grass have been suggested but are not proven; avoid dandelion, fennel, or khat with ciprofloxacin or ampicillin. Discuss importance of maintaining adequate nutritional intake to optimize immunological status. Discourage use of fad diets and special supplements.

(continued)

TABLE 15-5 Infections and Febrile Conditions and Nutritional Implications *(continued)*

Condition and Nutritional Acuity Ranking	Background	Nutritional Implications
Encephalitis and Reye's syndrome, Level 2	**Encephalitis** involves an inflammation of brain cells, usually by a virus such as measles, mumps, mononucleosis, or herpes simplex. It may also be caused by the tsetse fly (African sleeping sickness). **Reye's syndrome** is a disease of the brain and some abdominal organs (e.g., liver), affecting mostly children and teenagers after viral illness. Etiology is unknown, but some linkage to aspirin has been suggested. Symptoms are similar to those of encephalitis, including headache, loss of energy, anorexia, irritability, restlessness, drowsiness, double vision, impaired speech and hearing, and possibly even seizures or coma. Lactate dehydrogenase (LDH), creatine phosphokinase (CPK), aspartate aminotransferase (AST) and alanine aminotransferase (ALT), blood urea nitrogen (BUN), uric acid, and ammonia may be increased; glucose can be low.	Ease symptoms. Allow natural defense system to work. Assist breathing with respirator if necessary. Control any pernicious vomiting. Tube feed if patient is comatose. With seizures, a ketogenic diet may be helpful (Bautista, 2003). When patient can eat again, a high-protein/high-calorie diet should be provided, including vitamins and minerals in adequate amounts. Vitamins A and C should be provided from dietary sources. Adequate fluid intake will be important. Steroids are provided commonly; long-term use may affect nitrogen balance, cause hyperglycemia, deplete potassium, or retain sodium. Alter diet as necessary. Stress importance of consuming a balanced diet with adequate fluids. Help patient accept speech therapy or physical therapy, if needed.
Fever, Level 2	Fever represents disturbed thermoregulation, controlled by the hypothalamus. Fever higher than 102°F is pyrexia, and the cause may be acute (pneumonia, measles, flu, or chicken pox) or chronic (tuberculosis, hepatitis, or malaria). Fever of unknown origin (FUO) involves illness of 3 weeks in duration with a fever higher than 100.4°F; testing is needed. Results show that 40% of FUO is from infections; 20% from neoplasms, 15% from connective tissue disease, and 25% from undetermined causes. Parenteral zinc supplementation significantly increases fever in patients with recent injury or infection, showing an exaggerated acute-phase response (Braunschweig et al, 1997).	Meet increased nutrient needs caused by patient's hypermetabolic state, especially energy requirements. Each 1°F elevation causes a 7% increase in basal metabolic rate (BMR). Replace nitrogen losses and replenish tissue. Replenish carbohydrate since liver stores only last 24 hours. "Feed a cold, feed a fever." Discuss how fever affects metabolic rate. Normalize electrolyte status; replace losses from perspiration, and facilitate toxin elimination through increased urine output. Prevent water retention from syndrome of inappropriate antidiuretic hormone (SIADH) and hypertonic dehydration. Treat anorexia, nausea, and vomiting when present. Adults need 30–40 kcal/kg/d; infants and children need additional calories as well. Monitor weight changes closely. Adults need 1.5–2 g protein/kg if fever is high and chronic. If fever is acute, patient may prefer liquids. As treatment progresses, a diet with small, frequent feedings can be used. Offer preferred foods according to appetite, such as puddings, shakes, and soups. With longer duration, thiamin and vitamins A and C may be depleted, and a supplement may be used. Antipyretics/aspirin can cause gastrointestinal (GI) distress; take with food or milk and avoid alcoholic beverages. Erythromycin should be taken with a full glass of water on an empty stomach; it may cause sore mouth, diarrhea, and nausea. Penicillins should not be taken with acidic food or fluids such as fruit juice. Penicillin binds with serum albumin; adequate protein repletion is needed. Tetracycline should be taken on an empty stomach with a full glass of water. Do not give with milk or 2 hours before or after use of calcium-containing foods. Avoid use in pregnancy and in children because tetracycline can mottle teeth. Medicinal plants are proving to be useful sources of new treatments for fever, but they need to be tested in larger trials. Willow, elder, peppermint, meadow sweet, ginger, and red pepper have been suggested for clinical trials.
Herpes simplex, Level 1	Herpes simplex involves a viral infection of skin or mucous membranes (herpes simplex I usually involves oral infections, whereas herpes simplex II usually involves genital/anal infections) with vesicular eruptions of repeated frequency. It is related to the chicken pox virus.	High-quality protein and adequate calories will be essential. Increase intakes of vitamins A and C. Discuss relationship of nutrition to immune status.

(continued)

TABLE 15-5 Infections and Febrile Conditions and Nutritional Implications *(continued)*

Condition and Nutritional Acuity Ranking	Background	Nutritional Implications
	Testing may include polymerase chain reaction (PCR), herpes simplex virus (HSV) test, and swollen lymph nodes. Herpetic outbreaks are common in HIV-positive and other immunocompromised patients. Oral lesions ("cold sores" or "fever blisters") are latent in the nerve cell ganglia of the trigeminal nerve and are triggered by stress. A herpes vaccine is being tested; the target will be young adolescent girls.	Acyclovir (Zovirax) and antiviral agents (Valtrex) are currently available; nausea, vomiting, or headaches may occur. Interferon studies are being conducted; GI distress, stomatitis, nausea and vomiting, abdominal pain, and diarrhea may occur. Immediate use of medication at signs of a breakout may be helpful to reduce severity. Reduce inflammation and duration. Lessen recurrences and virulence. Reduce stress, febrile states, or further complications such as encephalitis or aseptic meningitis. Relaxation and stress reduction techniques should be highlighted. Herbs and botanical supplements are not proven for effectiveness. St. John's wort, lysine, lemon balm, echinacea, garlic, red pepper, tea, and mint have been suggested but are not proven through clinical trials.
Herpes zoster (shingles; see Fig. 15-2), Level 1	Herpes zoster is an acute viral infection with vesicles, usually confined to a specific nerve tract, and neuralgic pain in the area of the affected nerve. It is a reactivation of the *Varicella* virus (chicken pox); severity correlates with age. Symptoms and signs include pain along the affected nerve tract, fever, malaise, anorexia, and enlarged lymph nodes. Bacterial infection of the lesions, poor nutritional status, and risk of dehydration may occur if rehabilitation requires a long period of time. There is a sensitive assay that detects simultaneous HSV-1, HSV-2, varicella-zoster virus (VZV), human cytomegalovirus (CMV), and EBV (Markoulatos et al, 2001). This more comprehensive approach to testing is useful. A herpes zoster vaccine is effective (Oxman et al, 2005).	A balanced diet with frequent, small feedings may be needed. Increased fiber may be useful to correct constipation. Facial nerves may be affected; alter diet as needed. Adequate vitamin E has been suggested for postherpetic neuralgia. Vitamin B_{12} has also been prescribed for recovery of the damaged nerve and for pain relief. Be sure vitamins A and C meet at least the DRI levels from dietary sources. Prevent further systemic infection; reduce fever. Correct or prevent malnutrition, constipation, and encephalitis. Hydrate adequately. Prevent or correct unplanned weight loss. Prevent or reduce severity of postherpetic neuralgia, a very painful complication. Discuss need to increase fluid intake. A balanced diet will be essential in recovery. Include foods that contain vitamins E and B_{12}. Infectious precautions should be discussed with patient and family. There is a link to chickenpox, and this condition may spread to others during the early stage. Narcotics and analgesics are needed to reduce pain. Capsaicin cream from hot peppers has proven to be useful for pain relief. Injecting lidocaine and prednisone directly into spinal column for pain relief of postshingles neuralgia has been tested in Japan. Oral prednisone may be used in some cases; alter sodium intake and monitor for glucose intolerance. Acyclovir is helpful if administered immediately. Newer medications such as famciclovir may shorten duration and decrease pain. Monitor for GI distress, nausea and vomiting, or diarrhea. Valacyclovir is more effective than acyclovir at facilitating cutaneous healing and healing of zoster-associated pain and postherpetic neuralgia (Baker, 2002). Herbs and botanical supplements should not be used without discussing with physician. Lemon balm, Chinese angelica, red pepper, passionflower, and licorice have been suggested but are not yet proven through clinical trials.
Infection, Levels 1–2	Infection results from successful invasion, establishment, and growth of micro-organisms in a host. Responses involve general and antigen-specific immunological defense systems. In infectious processes, vitamin A is excreted in large amounts from the urine. Correct iron-deficiency anemia, but do not use excesses. Microbes depend on iron for growth and proliferation; iron is mostly protein bound as transferrin.	Provide adequate nourishment to counteract hypermetabolic state. Support body's host defense system. Prevent or correct dehydration, hypoglycemia, complications, and anorexia. Replace nutrient losses (potassium, nitrogen, magnesium, phosphorus, and sulfur).

(continued)

TABLE 15-5 Infections and Febrile Conditions and Nutritional Implications *(continued)*

Condition and Nutritional Acuity Ranking	Background	Nutritional Implications
	Iron and zinc supplements serve as bacterial nutrients. Wait until fever is down before providing these supplements, especially by intravenous administration, intramuscular administration, or total parenteral nutrition (TPN). Parenteral zinc supplementation significantly increases fever in patients with recent injury or infection, showing an exaggerated acute-phase response (Braunschweig et al, 1997). Avoid zinc supplementation until the infection is under control.	Discuss role of nutrients in maintaining skin and mucous membrane integrity and preventing bacterial invasion and subsequent infections. Use a high-protein, high-calorie diet. Needs increase 0–20% in mild infections, 20–40% in moderate conditions, and 40–60% in sepsis. Increase patient's fluid intake. Enhance diet with foods rich in vitamin A, folate, vitamin C, and B-complex vitamins. Emphasize importance of eating to counteract infection and prevent new infections. Administration of antibiotics with or without food is specific to the type of drug used: Avoid caffeine, sodas, and fruit juices when taking penicillins. For tetracycline, avoid milk and dairy products 2 hours before and after taking drug. With amoxicillin (Augmentin), diarrhea, nausea, and vomiting may occur. Cephalosporins (e.g., Ceclor, Cephalexin, Duricef) may cause diarrhea, nausea and vomiting, sore mouth, hypokalemia, and vitamin K deficiency. Griseofulvin for fungal infections should be taken with a high-fat meal. Dry mouth, nausea, and diarrhea are common effects. Ketoconazole (Nizoral) is used in fungal infections and should be taken with an acidic liquid such as orange juice; avoid taking ketoconazole within 2 hours of use of calcium or magnesium supplement. Metronidazole (Flagyl) may cause nausea and vomiting, diarrhea, and anorexia; avoid alcoholic beverages.
Influenza (flu) and the common cold, Level 1	The common cold and influenza are the most common syndromes of infection in human beings (Eccles, 2005). Influenza virus is transmitted by respiratory route, generally in the fall and winter months. Incubation is 1–4 days, with abrupt onset. Signs and symptoms include chills, fever for 3–5 days, malaise lasting 2–3 weeks, muscular aching, substernal soreness, nasal stuffiness, sore throat, some nausea, nonproductive cough, and headache. New knowledge of the effects of cytokines helps to explain some of the symptoms of colds and flu such as fever, anorexia, malaise, chilliness, headache, and muscle aches and pains (Eccles, 2005). Annual vaccinations are suggested for high-risk populations, including elderly individuals and those individuals with pulmonary diseases. Low humidity, cold weather, and psychological stress may increase susceptibility. Low-dose supplementation of zinc and selenium provides significant improvement in elderly patients by increasing humoral response after flu vaccination; this could be important by reducing morbidity from respiratory tract infections (Girodon et al, 1999). Discuss need for rest and adequate hydration to promote rapid recovery. Discuss infection control, hand washing, and personal hygiene, if necessary.	Reduce fever and relieve symptoms. Chicken soup is actually useful by providing potassium and sodium, as well as fluid; it increases mucus flow. Prevent complications such as Reye's syndrome, secondary bacterial infections (especially pneumonia), otitis media, and bronchitis. Promote bed rest, adequate hydration, and calorie intake. Replace fluid and electrolyte losses. Increase fluids from salty broths, juices, and other fluids. A high-energy and protein intake should be encouraged. Small meals and snacks may be better tolerated than three large meals. Adequate sodium and potassium should be considered. Ensure adequate intakes of vitamins A and C, especially from fruits and vegetables. Citrus fruits and juices are recommended, if tolerated. Antibiotics may be needed if secondary bacterial infections occur; monitor for proper timing of administration with food and beverages. Amantadine or rimantadine may be helpful, especially in type A flu. Nausea, dry mouth, and constipation may occur. Aspirin should not be used because of potential for Reye's syndrome in children; other analgesics and pain relievers can be used. Zinc nasal gel can reduce the duration and severity of symptoms of the common cold (Hulisz, 2004).

(continued)

TABLE 15-5 Infections and Febrile Conditions and Nutritional Implications *(continued)*

Condition and Nutritional Acuity Ranking	Background	Nutritional Implications
Meningitis, Level 1	Infection of the meninges (meningitis) causes inflammatory reactions, usually in the pia mater or arachnoid membranes. The condition may be viral or bacterial. Bacterial forms are more likely to be fatal if left untreated. Bacterial forms include *Listeria monocytogenes, Neisseria meningitidis, Haemophilus influenzae,* or *Streptococcus pneumoniae.* Meningitis can be caused by lung or ear infections or by a skull fracture. Symptoms and signs include headache, neck rigidity, fever, tachycardia, tachypnea, nausea and/or vomiting, disorientation, diplopia, altered consciousness, photophobia, petechial rash, irritability, malaise, seizure activity, and dehydration. Spinal tap or lumbar puncture is needed to assess cerebrospinal fluid. Meningitis could lead to septic shock, respiratory failure, or death. It most commonly affects children aged 1 month to 2 years old.	Prevent or correct weight loss. Force fluids but do not overhydrate, especially if there is cerebral edema. Prevent or correct constipation, fever, and other symptoms. In the long term, control obesity, which may occur. Maintain intravenous feedings as appropriate; prevent overhydration. Progress diet, as possible, to high-calorie/high-protein intake. Unless contraindicated, provide 2–3 L of fluid. Adequate fiber will be beneficial to correct or prevent constipation. Gradually return to normal caloric intake for age. Ensure adequate intake of vitamins A and C from fruits, juices, and vegetables. Discuss methods to promote recovery and emphasize adequate rest. Discuss role of nutrition in immunological status. Chronic meningitis can affect people with cancer, HIV/ AIDS, and other severe disorders. Antibiotics (penicillin, ampicillin, and cephalosporin) may be used in bacterial forms or to prevent complications in viral forms; nausea, vomiting, and diarrhea can result. Corticosteroids may be used; side effects may include nitrogen and calcium losses and sodium retention.
Mononucleosis, Level 1	Infectious mononucleosis is an acute disease that is believed to be caused by EBV herpes virus and causes gland swellings in the neck and elsewhere (giving it its other name, "glandular fever"). It causes fatigue, malaise, headache, chills, and other symptoms such as sore throat, fever, abdominal pain, jaundice, stiff neck, chest pain, breathing difficulty, cough, and hepatitis. Incubation is 5–15 days. It is most common in those between ages 10 and 35 years. Lab work may include evaluation of increased cerebrospinal fluid (CSF) pressure, EBV titer, uric acid and liver enzymes. It is also useful to evaluate a serum agglutination test. Restore fluid balance. Replenish glucose stores. Spare protein. Restore lost weight. Reduce fever. Prevent complications such as myocarditis, hepatitis, and encephalitis.	Use a high-protein, high-calorie diet. Use liquids when swallowing solid foods is difficult. Use small, frequent feedings to improve overall nutritional quality and quantity. Ensure adequate intakes of vitamins A and C, especially from fruits and vegetables. Modify food textures when swallowing is difficult. Emphasize importance of exercise in restoring lean body mass. Acyclovir (Zovirax) may be useful in initial infection, preventing typical persistence; nausea, anorexia, and vomiting may occur. Other antibiotics may be needed for related infections.
Pelvic inflammatory disease (PID), Level 1	PID involves inflammation of the pelvic cavity, which may affect the fallopian tubes (salpingitis) and ovaries (oophoritis). Symptoms and signs include acute pelvic and abdominal pain, low back pain, fever, purulent vaginal discharge, nausea and vomiting, urinary tract infection (UTI), diarrhea, maceration of the vulva, and leukocytosis. Long-term sequelae may include tubal infertility or chronic pelvic pain.	Promote good nutritional status to maintain weight and immunity. Increase hydration as tolerated. Lessen diarrhea, nausea, and vomiting. Discuss role of nutrition in immunity. If nausea or vomiting is extensive, discuss need for small meals and consumption of fluids separately from meals. Provide diet as tolerated with small, frequent feedings until nausea and vomiting subside. Alter fiber and fluid, as needed. Increase energy and protein if needed to improve patient's nutritional status. Ensure adequate intake of all vitamins and minerals, especially vitamins A and C. Use more fruits and vegetables when possible. Antibiotics may be used; monitor for side effects. Quinolones, cephalosporins, metronidazole, and doxycycline may be prescribed. Analgesics are generally used to reduce pain; chronic use may cause GI distress.

(continued)

TABLE 15-5 Infections and Febrile Conditions and Nutritional Implications *(continued)*

Condition and Nutritional Acuity Ranking	Background	Nutritional Implications
Poliomyelitis, Level 1	A highly contagious enterovirus, poliomyelitis attacks the motor neurons of the brain stem and spinal cord; it may or may not cause paralysis (infantile paralysis). Polio is transmitted by personal contact, by eating contaminated food, or by drinking contaminated fluids. Polio is rare in areas where the vaccine is available, but there are risks in areas where the vaccine is not administered to all members of the population. Extra immunization may be needed for persons traveling to tropical areas. Symptoms and signs include headache, sore throat, fever, and neck and back pain. For breathing problems, a ventilator may be needed. Postpolio syndrome produces neuromuscular symptoms 25–30 years after attack; serious swallowing difficulties can ensue. Beware of possible choking or aspiration in the bulbar type of paralysis; patient may be unable to swallow. Provide adequate nourishment. Correct electrolyte imbalances. Prevent complications of prolonged immobilization: renal stones, pressure ulcers, and negative N balance.	For patient with acute paralysis, use a high-protein, high-calorie diet in liquid form. Use intravenous feeding and tube feeding (TF) when needed. Use vitamin supplements with 1–2 times the DRI; extra calcium and potassium may be needed to replace losses. As treatment progresses, diet may be changed from a liquid to a solid diet as tolerated. A dysphagia diet may be useful, with varying levels of thickened liquids to enhance swallowing. Wean to oral diet as intake increases. Frequent high nutrient-density snacks are recommended. Instruct patient regarding how to puree or blenderize foods as needed, including how to add thickeners to liquids. Discuss appropriate recipes for high-energy and high-protein foods. Current antiviral drugs do not work; polio has no cure.
Rheumatic heart disease (rheumatic fever), Level 1	Rheumatic fever is an inflammatory condition affecting the connective tissues that causes joint pain, swelling, fever, rash, jerky movements (Sydenham's chorea), facial grimacing, and carditis. It usually ensues 3 weeks after streptococcal infection. Lab work includes testing for serum antibodies to streptococci; albumin, transthyretin, and cholesterol may be decreased; erythrocyte sedimentation rate (ESR) and white blood cells (WBCs) may be increased. Heart inflammation usually disappears but may cause permanent damage to the valves (especially the mitral valve), with a resulting heart murmur. Long-term effects are called rheumatic heart disease. Electrocardiogram (EKG) is needed to assess for heart rhythm problems and echocardiograms may identify heart valve problems. Children and adults younger than 30 years of age are more susceptible; it is rare before age 4 and after age 18. Cure the infection and prevent its recurrence. Reduce inflammation in joints and heart. Decrease physical activity and encourage rest while heart is inflamed. Recover lost weight. Reduce fluid retention, if present. Prevent complications such as bacterial endocarditis, atrial fibrillation, and heart failure.	Use a full liquid diet for acute rheumatic fever. As treatment progresses, gradually change diet, first to a soft diet, then to a regular diet. Restrict sodium intake if edema is present or if steroids are used. Increase intake of vitamin C, protein, and calories. Include adequate vitamin A as well. Explain increased need for calories and protein. Adequate rest, exercise, and nutrition are essential to prevent recurrence. Restrict sodium if prednisone or adrenocorticotropic hormone (ACTH) is given for severe heart inflammation. Side effects include depletion of nitrogen, calcium, potassium, and hyperglycemia. Antibiotics are used. Monitor for specific side effects such as GI distress. Penicillin may be needed for 10 days. Aspirin and nonsteroidal anti-inflammatory drugs (NSAIDs) in high doses are often needed to reduce joint pain and inflammation. Lifelong use of antibiotics before surgery and dental work is needed to protect against bacterial invasion of heart valves.
Staphylococcus aureus and methicillin-resistant *Staphylococcus aureus* (MRSA) infection, Level 1	*Staphylococcus aureus* is a gram-positive bacterium that developed resistance to the penicillin derivative methicillin; MRSA emerged as a bacterium that became less susceptible to the actions of methicillin and thus developed the ability to colonize and cause life-threatening infections (Banning, 2005). *S. aureus* and MRSA population estimates are in the millions of persons.	MRSA colonization should be contained by infection control measures and not treated (Cunha, 2005). Hand washing technique is very important. The most potent anti-MRSA drug at the present time is daptomycin, especially to treat endocarditis (Cunha, 2005).
Toxic shock syndrome (TSS), Level 1	TSS is an acute bacterial infection caused by *Staphylococcus aureus* and most often is associated with prolonged use of tampons during menses. Symptoms and signs include sudden onset of high fever, severe headache, red eyes, myalgia, vomiting, watery diarrhea, red rash on palms and soles (with desquamation), decreased circulation to fingers and toes, disorientation, peripheral edema, pulmonary edema, respiratory distress syndrome, and sudden hypotension progressing to shock. Anemia, kidney, liver, and muscle damage can occur.	Progress, as tolerated, from clear liquids to diet as usual. Small, frequent feedings are best tolerated. Ensure adequate intakes of vitamins A and C from dietary sources, including fruits, juices, and vegetables. Increase fluids to 3 L daily, unless contraindicated. Discuss need for adequate fluid intake and small meals, especially with vomiting or nausea.

(continued)

TABLE 15-5 Infections and Febrile Conditions and Nutritional Implications *(continued)*

Condition and Nutritional Acuity Ranking	Background	Nutritional Implications
	Treat patient for septic shock or respiratory distress or for other complications. Control diarrhea and vomiting. Improve well-being. Stabilize hydration and electrolyte balance. Prevent renal, heart, and lung problems and other complications. Monitor labs for increased levels of WBC, BUN, creatinine, bilirubin, liver enzymes, and CPK. Platelets may be decreased.	Antibiotics are required. Monitor for GI side effects. Determine how to administer specific drugs (such as with food, water, or milk).
Typhoid fever (enteric fever), Level 2	Enteric fever is a more inclusive term for typhoid fever and paratyphoid fever; it is a systemic infection caused by *Salmonella enterica,* and it is most common among travelers (Connor and Schwartz, 2005). This infectious fever is spread by contamination of food, water, or milk with *Salmonella typhi or paratyphi,* which can come from sewage, flies, or faulty personal hygiene. Most infections are found in people who are in contact with carriers who have persistent gallbladder or urinary tract infections. Incubation is 5–14 days. Symptoms include malaise, headache, cough, sore throat, "pea soup" diarrhea, constipation, rose spots, and splenomegaly. The problem practically has been eradicated in areas of proper sanitary practices. Lab work includes stool and urine for Widal test. Reduce fever and prevent irritation. Replace nutrient losses from diarrhea. Replace tissue losses. Prevent complications such as intestinal hemorrhage or shock and pulmonary or cardiac side effects.	For patients with acute fever, use a diet of high-protein, high-calorie liquids. A low-residue diet may be needed temporarily. As treatment progresses, gradually add soft, bland foods. Try small, frequent feedings. Gradually add pectin and other fiber. Include good dietary sources of vitamins A and C especially. Explain which foods are high-protein, high-calorie sources. Discuss how to prevent future reinfection. First-line therapy is ceftriaxone, and fluoroquinolones can also be given (Connor and Schwartz, 2005). Monitor for GI distress. Preventive measures are educating travelers about hygiene precautions and vaccination (Connor and Schwartz, 2005).

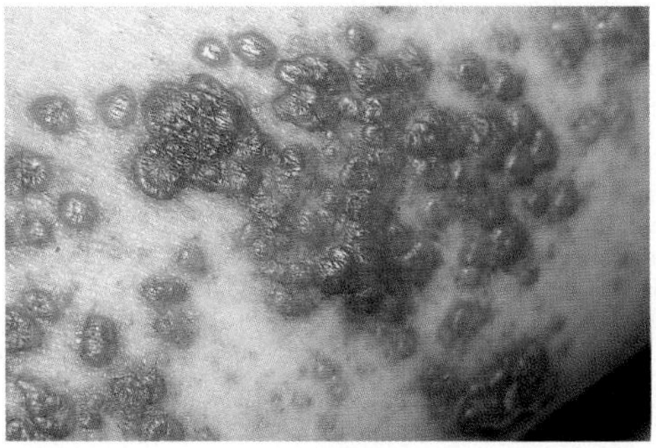

Figure 15-2 Shingles. (From Goodheart HP. *Goodheart's photoguide of common skin disorders.* 2nd ed. Philadelphia: Lippincott Williams & Wilkins, 2003.)

TABLE 15-6 Virulence Increased by Iron

Iron is an essential nutrient for most organisms because it serves as a cofactor in oxidative-reduction reactions.

Acid-fast and gram-positive bacteria	*Bacillus, Clostridium, Listeria, Mycobacterium, Staphylococcus, Streptococcus*
Fungi	*Candida, Cryptococcus, Histoplasma, Mucor, Pneumocystis, Rhizopus*
Gram-negative bacteria	*Campylobacter, Chlamydia, Escherichia, Klebsiella, Legionella, Proteus, Pseudomonas, Salmonella, Shigella, Vibrio, Yersinia*
Protozoa	*Entamoeba, Leishmania, Plasmodium, Toxoplasma, Trypanosoma*

Based on data from: Robien M. Iron and microbial infection. *Support Line* 22:23, 2000.

CITED REFERENCES

Audera C, et al. Mega-dose vitamin C in treatment of the common cold: a randomized controlled trial. *Oncology* 175:359, 2001.

Baker D. Valacyclovir in the treatment of genital herpes and herpes zoster. *Expert Opin Pharmacother.* 3:51, 2002.

Banning M. Transmission and epidemiology of MRSA: current perspectives. *Br J Nurs.* 14:548, 2005.

Baqui AH, et al. Simultaneous weekly supplementation of iron and zinc is associated with lower morbidity due to diarrhea and acute lower respiratory infection in Bangladeshi infants. *J Nutr.* 133:4150, 2003.

Bastian L, Weimann A. Immunonutrition in patients after multiple trauma. Immunonutrition in patients after multiple trauma. *Br J Nutr.* 87:133S, 2002.

Bautista RE. The use of the ketogenic diet in a patient with subacute sclerosing panencephalitis. *Seizure* 12:175, 2003.

Beck MA, et al. Host nutritional status: the neglected virulence factor. *Trends Microbiol.* 12:417, 2004.

Bengmark S. Bio-ecological control of acute pancreatitis: the role of enteral nutrition, pro and synbiotics. *Curr Opin Clin Nutr Metab Care.* 8:557, 2005.

Berger MM. Can oxidative damage be treated nutritionally? *Clin Nutr.* 24:172, 2005.

Bielory L. Complementary and alternative interventions in asthma, allergy, and immunology. *Ann Allergy Asthma Immunol.* 93:45S, 2004.

Bistrian BR. Immunonutrition. *J Nutr.* 134:2868S, 2004.

Block KI, Mead MN. Immune system effects of echinacea, ginseng, and astragalus: a review. *Integr Cancer Ther.* 2:247, 2003.

Braunschweig C, et al. Parenteral zinc supplementation in adult humans during the acute phase response increases the febrile response. *J Nutr.* 127:70, 1997.

Brugler L, et al. A simplified nutrition screen for hospitalized patients using readily available laboratory and patient information. *Nutrition* 21:650, 2005.

Bulger EM, Maier RV. An argument for Vitamin E supplementation in the management of systemic inflammatory response syndrome. *Shock* 19:99, 2003.

Butler SO, et al. Relationship between hyperglycemia and infection in critically ill patients. *Pharmacotherapy* 25:963, 2005.

Calder PC. Branched-chain amino acids and immunity. *J Nutr.* 136:288S, 2006.

Calder PC. Omega-3 fatty acids, inflammation, and immunity—relevance to postsurgical and critically ill patients. *Lipids* 39:1147, 2004

Calder PC, Kew S. The immune system: a target for functional foods? *Br J Nutr.* 88:165S, 2002.

Campbell CG, et al. Predicted vs measured energy expenditure in critically ill, underweight patients. *Nutr Clin Pract.* 20:276, 2005.

Chandra R. Food allergy and nutrition in early life: implications for later health. *Proc Nutr Soc.* 59:273, 2000.

Christian P. Micronutrients and reproductive health issues: an international perspective. *J Nutr.* 133:1969S, 2003.

Connor BA, Schwartz E. Typhoid and paratyphoid fever in travelers. *Lancet Infect Dis.* 5:623, 2005.

Cunha BA. Methicillin-resistant *Staphylococcus aureus:* clinical manifestations and antimicrobial therapy. *Clin Microbiol Infect.* 11:33S, 2005.

Cunningham-Rundles S. Nutrition and the mucosal immune system. *Curr Opin Gastroenterol.* 17:171, 2001.

Cunningham-Rundles S, et al. Mechanisms of nutrient modulation of the immune response. *J Allergy Clin Immunol.* 115:1119, 2005.

De-Souza DA, Greene LJ. Intestinal permeability and systemic infections in critically ill patients: effect of glutamine. *Crit Care Med.* 33:1125, 2005.

Dial S et al. Risk of *Clostridium difficile* diarrhea among hospital inpatients prescribed proton pump inhibitors: cohort and case-control studies. *CMAJ.* 171:33, 2004.

Dijsselbloem N, et al. Soy isoflavone phyto-pharmaceuticals in interleukin-6 affections. Multi-purpose nutraceuticals at the crossroad of hormone replacement, anti-cancer and anti-inflammatory therapy. *Biochem Pharmacol.* 68:1171, 2004.

Eccles R. Understanding the symptoms of the common cold and influenza. Lancet *Infect Dis.* 5:718 2005.

Elenkov IJ, et al. Cytokine dysregulation, inflammation and well-being. *Neuroimmunomodulation* 12:255, 2005.

Equils O, et al. 1,25-Dihydroxyvitamin D inhibits lipopolysaccharide-induced immune activation in human endothelial cells. *Clin Exp Immunol.* 143:58, 2006.

Fasano A, Shea-Donohue T. Mechanisms of disease: the role of intestinal barrier function in the pathogenesis of gastrointestinal autoimmune diseases. *Nat Clin Pract Gastroenterol Hepatol.* 2:416, 2005.

Field CJ. Use of T cell function to determine the effect of physiologically active food components. *Am J Clin Nutr.* 71:1720S, 2000.

Field CJ, et al. Nutrients and their role in host resistance to infection. *J Leukoc Biol.* 71:16, 2002.

Fraker P, King L. A distinct role for apoptosis in the changes in lymphopoiesis and myelopoiesis created by deficiencies in zinc. *FASEB J.* 15:2572, 2001.

Gerrity TR, et al. Immunologic aspects of chronic fatigue syndrome. Report on a Research Symposium convened by The CFIDS Association of America and co-sponsored by the US Centers for Disease Control and Prevention and the National Institutes of Health. *Neuroimmunomodulation* 11:351, 2004.

Girodon F, et al. Impact of trace elements and vitamin supplementation on immunity and infections in institutionalized elderly patients: a randomized controlled trial. *Arch Intern Med.* 159:748, 1999.

Grimble RF. Immunonutrition. *Curr Opin Gastroenterol.* 21:216, 2005.

Happel KI, Nelson S. Alcohol, immunosuppression, and the lung. *Proc Am Thorac Soc.* 2:428, 2005.

Headley JM. Indirect calorimetry: a trend toward continuous metabolic assessment. *AACN Clin Issues.* 14:155, 2003.

Heyland DK, et al. Antioxidant nutrients: a systematic review of trace elements and vitamins in the critically ill patient. *Intensive Care Med.* 31:327, 2005.

Heys SD, et al. Nutrition and the surgical patient: triumphs and challenges. *Surgeon* 3:139, 2005.

High K. Nutritional strategies to boost immunity and prevent infection in elderly individuals. *Clin Infect Dis.* 33:1892, 2001.

High KP, et al. A new paradigm for clinical investigation of infectious syndromes in older adults: assessment of functional status as a risk factor and outcome measure. *Clin Infect Dis.* 40:114, 2005.

Hulisz D. Efficacy of zinc against common cold viruses: an overview. *J Am Pharm Assoc.* 44:594, 2004.

Johnson C, Eccles R. Acute cooling of the feet and the onset of common cold symptoms. *Fam Pract.* 22:608, 2005.

Kubena K, McMurray D. Nutrition and the immune system: a review of nutrient–nutrient interactions. *J Am Diet Assoc.* 96:1156, 1996.

Markoulatos P, et al. Laboratory diagnosis of common herpesvirus infections of the central nervous system by a multiplex PCR assay. *J Clin Microbiol.* 39:4426, 2001.

McDade T, et al. Prenatal undernutrition and postnatal growth are associated with adolescent thymic function. *J Nutr.* 131:1225, 2001.

Meydani SN, et al. Vitamin E and respiratory infection in the elderly. *Ann N Y Acad Sci.* 1031:214, 2004.

Newburg DS, et al. Human milk glycans protect infants against enteric pathogens. *Annu Rev Nutr.* 25:37, 2005.

Ochoa JB, et al. A rational use of immune enhancing diets: when should we use dietary arginine supplementation? *Nutr Clin Pract.* 19:216, 2004.

Oxman MN, et al. A vaccine to prevent herpes zoster and postherpetic neuralgia in older adults. *N Engl J Med.* 352:2271, 2005.

Philpott M, Ferguson LR. Immunonutrition and cancer. *Mutat Res.* 551:29, 2004.

Predy GN, et al. Efficacy of an extract of North American ginseng containing poly-furanosyl-pyranosyl-saccharides for preventing upper respiratory tract infections: a randomized controlled trial. *CMAJ.* 173:1043, 2005.

Surawicz CM. Treatment of recurrent *Clostridium difficile*-associated disease. *Nat Clin Pract Gastroenterol Hepatol.* 1:32, 2004.

Viteri FE, Gonzalez H. Adverse outcomes of poor micronutrient status in childhood and adolescence. *Nutr Rev.* 60:77S, 2002.

Watson RR, et al. Nutritional regulation of immunosenescence for heart health. *J Nutr Biochem.* 16:85, 2005.

Wilmore D. Enteral and parenteral arginine supplementation to improve medical outcomes in hospitalized patients. *J Nutr.* 134:2863S, 2004.

Wintergerst ES, et al. Immune-enhancing role of vitamin C and zinc and effect on clinical conditions. *Ann Nutr Metab.* 50:85, 2005.

Zaloga GP, et al. Arginine: mediator or modulator of sepsis? *Nutr Clin Pract.* 19:201, 2004.

Zheng L, et al. Multicenter evaluation of a new screening test that detects *Clostridium difficile* in fecal specimens. *J Clin Microbiol.* 42:3837, 2004.

AIDS AND HIV INFECTION

NUTRITIONAL ACUITY RANKING: LEVEL 4

DEFINITIONS AND BACKGROUND

Acquired immunodeficiency syndrome (AIDS) is a viral infection caused by human immunodeficiency virus (HIV) that has progressed to AIDS after the infected person developed an opportunistic infection, a tumor that might not have developed if HIV had not been present, or a helper T-cell count in the blood of less than 200 cells/mm^3. Levels of CD41 (helper) and CD81 (nonhelper) subsets of T cells are used to evaluate immunological competency in HIV/AIDS. After levels have been identified, staging of the HIV infection is identified from which to plan therapeutic interventions.

HIV is not easily transmitted but can be transmitted through exchange of bodily fluids during sexual contact, by receipt of infected blood through a blood transfusion or blood products, by sharing contaminated needles for intra-

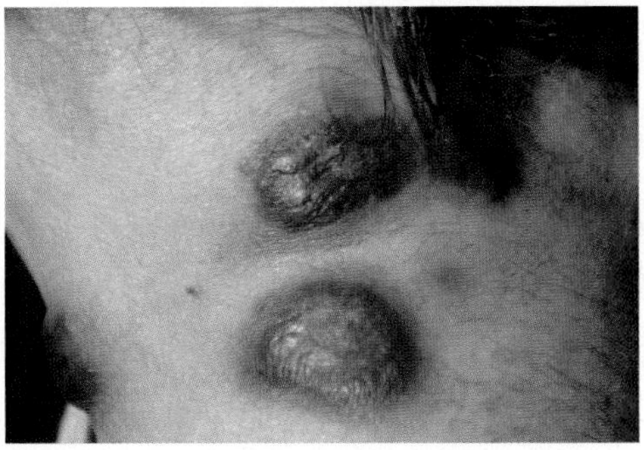

Figure 15-3 Kaposi's sarcoma. (From Goodheart HP. *Goodheart's photoguide of common skin disorders*. 2nd ed. Philadelphia: Lippincott Williams & Wilkins, 2003.)

venous drug abuse, or from an HIV-infected mother to neonate (children represent 15–20% of the affected population). Persons at higher risk include homosexual or bisexual males, hemophiliacs, intravenous drug addicts, heterosexuals with multiple partners, and infants of HIV-positive mothers (especially those who are breastfed). Breastfeeding by HIV-infected mothers results in HIV transmission to the infant, especially if there is mastitis (Dorosko, 2005). In some environments or developing countries, the relative seriousness for risk of HIV transmission may be of lower significance than malnutrition when the infant is not breastfed. The risks and benefits of breastfeeding must be weighed individually.

HIV infection involves multiple organs. Symptoms and signs include fever, chills, sore throat, headache, tachypnea, anxiety, fatigue, night sweats, hypoxemia, dyspnea on exertion, rales or rhonchi, cyanosis, pneumonia, diarrhea, cryptococcosis, frequent viral infections, ulcerating herpes simplex lesions, meningitis, anorexia, inflamed mouth or esophagus, malabsorption, weight loss, and poor nutritional status.

HIV targets the immune system and makes an infected person susceptible to infection and neoplasm because of an impaired ability to mount an adequate immune response. Malnutrition and its complications further impair the body. Immune reconstitution inflammatory syndrome (IRIS) develops in a substantial percentage of HIV-infected patients who have an underlying opportunistic infection and receive highly active antiretroviral therapy (HAART) (Shelburne et al, 2006). AIDS-related malignancies are another major complication. Kaposi's sarcoma (KS), Hodgkin's disease (HD), and non-Hodgkin's lymphoma (NHL) are most common (Wood and Harrington, 2005). See Figure 15-3.

HIV has infected more than 60 million people worldwide and has led to more than 23 million deaths; there are approximately 40 million people who are living with HIV infection, with 5 million new infections in 2004 (Fauci et al, 2005). Worldwide, hepatitis B virus (HBV) accounts for an estimated 370 million chronic infections, hepatitis C virus (HCV) accounts for an estimated 130 million, and HIV accounts for an estimated 40 million; in HIV-infected persons, an estimated 2–4 million have chronic HBV co-infection, and 4–5 million have HCV co-infection (Alter, 2006). Vertically acquired HIV infection has been virtually eliminated in developed countries through the use of HAART, reducing mother-to-child transmission rates to below 1–2% (Thorne and Newell, 2005).

Although effective antiretroviral treatments are available, HIV-infected people face a lifetime of vigilant polypharmacy. Nutrition has both direct effects (immune-cell triggering) and indirect effects (on DNA and protein synthesis) on progression of HIV disease. Decline in body cell mass and deficiencies in vitamins and minerals have been reported in asymptomatic patients with HIV disease. Some clinicians have recommended a series of antioxidant supplements to augment antioxidant activity in the cells. Because of the crucial role that nutrition plays throughout the course of HIV, medical nutrition therapy should be considered an integral part of disease management at all stages.

In starvation, there generally is loss of adipose tissue with maintenance of lean body mass (LBM); in HIV/AIDS, there is loss of LBM while maintaining body fat (wasting). Wasting syndrome is defined by the World Health Organization (WHO) as the involuntary loss of at least 10% of body weight and is a common AIDS-defining diagnosis. Weight loss is an independent prognostic indicator of outcome and mortality. Weight loss, fatigue, anorexia, diarrhea, and low-grade fevers may occur. Failure to monitor body weight may further contribute to malnutrition and wasting. As long as an infection remains untreated, nutritional support regimens will meet with only limited success.

Fat redistribution as part of a syndrome known as peripheral lipodystrophy has been seen in patients receiving HAART. Etiology is unknown; patients experience loss of facial and extremity fat with redeposition into visceral and truncal adiposity. Abnormal fatty deposits, which may be disfiguring, have been reported in the neck and dorsocervical area ("buffalo hump"). These changes may or may not be accompanied by development of hyperlipidemia and/or diabetes mellitus. Body composition measures should be accurate and should ideally be taken prior to initiation of antiretroviral therapy. Bioelectrical impedance analysis (BIA) has been found to be useful. Skinfold measurements tend to overestimate fat-free mass and underestimate fat mass.

Gastrointestinal (GI) complications are common in AIDS. Weight loss is often multifactorial in etiology, but reduced oral intake is common. Malnutrition has been associated with an increased risk of transmission of HIV from infected mothers to infants, and malnutrition may further compromise HIV-infected individuals who have tuberculosis or persistent diarrheal disease (Wanke, 2005). Nutritional supplements, dietary counseling, tube feeding (TF), and, if needed, parenteral nutrition may be used. Studies on specific nutrients, such as vitamin D, continue to be critically important (Villamor, 2006).

While total parenteral nutrition (TPN) is often indicated with HIV patients experiencing severe GI dysfunction, there is a concern over infection with use of central venous catheters in patients with advanced HIV/AIDS. Medication interactions, co-infection with other infections and diseases, wasting, lipodystrophy, and other issues make individualized nutrition care plans extremely important (American Dietetic Association, 2004). Although the incidence of most AIDS-defining opportunistic infections, including HIV wasting syndrome, has dramatically decreased since the introduction of HAART, weight loss and wasting are still common in HIV-infected persons who use injection drugs; live below the federal poverty level; have a BMI over 25; have a lower CD4 cell count or higher HIV viral load; or have presence of diarrhea, nausea, or fever (Tang et al, 2005).

Medical nutrition therapy for HIV/AIDS patients can reduce illness, hospital stays, and related medical costs. The American Dietetic Association has recommended 3 medical nutrition therapy visits per year for adults with stage 1 HIV/AIDS; 3–6 per year for adults with stage 2 or 3 HIV/AIDS; and a minimum of 5 per year for children or adolescents with HIV/AIDS.

Work on an HIV vaccine continues. The International AIDS Vaccine Initiative has established a consortium to elucidate mechanisms of protection conferred by live attenuated immunodeficiency virus vaccines in monkeys (Koff et al, 2006).

INTERVENTION: OBJECTIVES

- Improve nutrition-related immunity to prevent opportunistic infections, such as oral candidiasis; cirrhosis or hepatocellular carcinoma (HCC) from chronic infection with hepatitis B or C; and other conditions such as IRIS.
- Enhance response to therapy through continuous counseling to manipulate diet and enhance drug effectiveness.
- Maintain body weight at 95–100% of usual body weight levels. LBM is especially affected. Prevent additional weight loss from fever, poor intake with oral pain, infection, nausea, diarrhea, and vomiting by early nutritional intervention.
- Reduce mealtime fatigue to encourage better intake. Avoid unnecessary distractions and stresses.
- Lower temperature to normal when febrile.
- Diagnose and treat diarrhea, malabsorption, vomiting, and HIV-induced enteropathy.
- If necessary, use TPN to prevent further weight loss and potential malnutrition. TPN will stop weight loss, but it will not prevent further immunodeficiency.
- Keep body well hydrated. Fluids are critical to keeping body well hydrated as well as to prevent kidney stones and other complications.
- Support depleted levels of nutrients such as linoleic acid, selenium, and vitamin B_{12}.
- Counteract such problems as dysphagia, mouth pain, difficulty swallowing, taste alterations (dysgeusia), and difficulty chewing.
- Alleviate nutritional effect of fatigue, anemia, anorexia, depression, and dyspnea. Optimize nutritional status.
- Maintain fat intake at prudent levels (30–35% total kcal) to maintain normal lipid levels.
- Alter dietary regimen if there is renal or hepatic impairment.
- Maintain honest discussions regarding use of alternative therapies such as herbs, special diets, and megavitamin therapy.
- Comply with food and water safety guidelines.

INTERVENTION: FOOD AND NUTRITION

- Maintain diet as appropriate for patient's condition (high-energy/high-protein diet with adequate nutritional supplements). Weight gain or maintenance is possible in patients with HIV infection and early stages of AIDS by use of oral liquid supplements.
- From 2–2.5 g protein/kg and 35–45 kcal/kg are needed. Fever and infection may further elevate need for these nutrients. Increase energy intake in cases of infection, fever, and pneumonia. Use indirect calorimetry when available since estimates are often incorrect (Frankenfield et al, 2005).
- Keep the body well hydrated. Estimate 35–40 cc/kg unless there is a reason to restrict fluids.
- Use TF, especially gastrostomy, if warranted. Low-lactose/low-fat TF products may need to be fed continuously to reduce gastroenteritis or reflux. TPN may be necessary for weight loss exceeding 20% of usual body weight.
- Increase use of omega-3 fatty acids and decrease saturated fats. There may be advantages to using a medium-chain triglyceride formula in the presence of AIDS-associated malabsorption.
- Small, frequent feedings (6–9 times daily) are usually better tolerated but may be difficult to achieve given complex medication regimens, which must be adhered to as well.
- A general multivitamin-mineral supplement should be recommended, not to exceed 100% of the recommended dietary allowances. Low serum micronutrient levels are common in HIV-positive individuals and have been associated with immune impairment, HIV disease progression, and increased mortality (Lanzillotti and Tang, 2005). Vitamin K deficiency is common with antibiotic use.
- Nutrient-dense snacks may be beneficial (such as pudding, if tolerated, nonacidic juices for sore mouth, ices made with tolerated juices, and sandwiches made with cold meat salads, while following safe food handling recommendations). Add protein powders and glucose polymers, if desired. Oral supplements are useful when needed.
- With bouts of diarrhea, use small meals and avoid extremes in temperatures; room temperature is often best. Avoid excesses of caffeine, alcohol, and fried and high-fat foods. Use soft cooked chicken, turkey, fish, and lean beef. Replace electrolytes with foods such as broth soups or Gatorade for sodium, potassium, magnesium, and chloride.
- If lactose intolerant, avoid milk and use a low-lactose or lactose-free diet.

SAMPLE NUTRITION DIAGNOSTIC STATEMENT

HIV/AIDS

PES: Inadequate food and beverage intake related to use of multiple medications for HIV infection as evidenced by poor appetite and 10% weight loss over past 2 months.

Assessment Data (sources of info): Food records and input and output, weight status, and medication records.

Intervention: Counseling about potential food–medication interactions and timing of meals/medications, tracking of gastrointestinal (GI) symptoms related to meal or snack intake, counseling about simplified food preparation and useful snacks for improving intake.

Monitoring and Evaluation: Weight records, reports of GI distress and symptoms, food and intake records.

- Sucrose may not be tolerated by some individuals, and gluten intolerance may also be present.
- Children present unique nutritional needs, which are further compounded by HIV infection. See Section 3.

CLINICAL INDICATORS

Clinical/History

- Height
- Pre-illness weight
- Current weight
- Waist to hip ratio
- Body mass index (BMI)
- Diet history
- Weight changes
- Head circumference (up to age 3 years)
- Subjective Global Assessment (useful tool)
- Nausea, vomiting
- Temperature (fever, chills)
- Night sweats
- Dysphagia
- Chewing problems
- Stomatitis
- Blood pressure (BP)
- Intake and output (I & O)
- Diarrhea
- Herpes outbreaks
- Fecal fat test
- Biopsies (lymph nodes, skin lesions)
- Dual-energy x-ray absorptiometry (DEXA) scan

Lab Work

- Complete blood count (CBC) with differential
- Platelets
- Cholesterol (Chol)
- Triglycerides (Trig) (increased)
- Glucose (Gluc)
- CD4 lymphocytes (active AIDS, <200)
- CD8 lymphocytes
- Total lymphocyte count (TLC)
- Viral load
- Polymerase chain reaction (PCR) for herpes virus
- P24 antigen
- Albumin (Alb) or transthyretin (decreased)
- C-reactive protein (CRP)
- Liver function tests: aspartate aminotransferase (AST), alanine aminotransferase (ALT), bilirubin, prothrombin time (PT)
- Hemoglobin and hematocrit (H & H) (decreased)
- Ferritin (increased)
- Creatine (Creat), blood urea nitrogen (BUN)
- Transferrin
- Lactose test
- Schilling test
- Serum B_{12} (decreased)
- Serum folate (decreased)
- Serum vitamin A
- Serum testosterone

Common Drugs Used and Potential Side Effects (see Table 15-7)

- Antiretroviral regimens are complicated and difficult for patients to follow, and they can have serious side effects, such as osteonecrosis and bone demineralization (Lesho and Gey, 2003). Because nonalcoholic fatty liver disease is a prominent feature in HIV-positive patients, induced by HAART, hepatitis A and B virus vaccinations and close monitoring of liver parameters are suggested (Kahraman et al, 2005). Malabsorption can occur if antiretroviral agents are taken improperly with regard to meals or if they are taken with certain other drugs or herbal remedies. Suboptimal exposure to antiretrovirals because of noncompliance or malabsorption can result in viral resistance and loss of future treatment options (Lesho and Gey, 2003).

Herbs, Botanicals, and Supplements

- Ethical dilemmas surround the use of complementary and alternative medicine (Maillet et al, 2004). HIV-infected people and AIDS patients often seek complementary therapies including herbal medicines due to reasons such as unsatisfactory effects, high cost, nonavailability, or adverse effects of conventional medicines (Liu et al, 2005).
- There may be risk for herb–drug and herb–nutrient interactions. Many herbals may also interact with prophylactic medicines to prevent bacterial infections such as antibiotics. Therefore, herbs and botanical supplements should not be used without discussing with physician. Licorice, oregano, curcumin, capsaicin, astragalus, and burdock have been tested but are not yet proven. Potential beneficial effects need to be confirmed in large, rigorous trials (Liu et al, 2005).
- Ursolic acid and oleanolic acid in rosemary or marjoram are pentacyclic triterpenoic acids with a similar chemical structure to medical herbs wildly distributed all over the world; they have anti-inflammatory, hepatoprotective, gastroprotective, antiulcer, anti-HIV, cardiovascular, hypolipidemic, antiatherosclerotic, and immunoregulatory effects (Ovesna et al, 2004). There would be no harm in seasoning foods with these herbs.
- Echinacea is often consumed as an antiviral agent. Do not use with warfarin or immunosuppressants.
- Garlic and St. John's wort may make saquinavir or indinavir less effective.

INTERVENTION: NUTRITION EDUCATION, COUNSELING, CARE MANAGEMENT

- The role of nutrition in infection and immunity should be discussed. In addition, patients should be encouraged to decrease use of drugs and alcohol and cigarette smoking because of their effects on overall health status and immunocompetence.
- Patients and caregivers should report all weight loss, anorexia, and fever to doctor. Continue to pay attention to weight loss; even a 5% weight loss in 6 months markedly increases the risk of death (Tang et al, 2005).
- Diet must be altered whenever necessary. Evaluation of nutrition assessment parameters on a regular basis requires a comprehensive process (Earthman, 2005). Continuing contact with a dietitian is essential regarding alternative feeding methods, changes in medications, need for home-delivered meals, simplified menu planning, and treatment of GI side effects.
- Aversion to meat may be countered by use of cold protein foods such as cottage cheese, yogurt, skim milk, and cheeses.

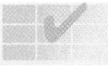

TABLE 15-7 Medications Used for HIV Infections and AIDS

Class	Generic Name	Brand and Other Names	Nutritional Implications and Comments
Nonnucleoside reverse transcriptase inhibitors (NNRTIs) *NNRTIs bind to and disable reverse transcriptase, a protein that HIV needs to make more copies of itself.* *NNRTIs can cause rashes and hepatotoxicity.*			Nausea, vomiting, and diarrhea are common side effects. Liver inflammation may occur; avoid alcohol and St. John's wort.
	Delavirdine	Rescriptor, DLV	Monitor for abnormal liver enzymes. Headaches are common.
	Efavirenz	Sustiva, EFV	Acceptable for use in children. Hyperlipidemia can occur.
	Nevirapine	Viramune, NVP	Take with food or on an empty stomach; fever, headache, hepatitis, general fatigue, mouth sores, and rash can occur.
Nucleoside reverse transcriptase inhibitors (NRTIs) (hepatitis B virus [HBV] polymerase inhibitors) *NRTIs are faulty versions of building blocks that HIV needs to make more copies of itself. When HIV uses an NRTI instead of a normal building block, reproduction of the virus is stalled. NRTIs can cause lactic acidosis, hypersensitivity reactions, neuropathies, pancreatitis, anemia, and neutropenia.*			Can cause severe bone marrow depletion and anemia, altered taste, constipation, nausea, indigestion, or vomiting. Adequate folate and vitamin B_{12} may prevent toxicity.
	Abacavir	Ziagen, ABC	Diarrhea may be a side effect. Malaise, fever, rash, and liver inflammation can occur.
	Abacavir, Lamivudine	Epzicom	Diarrhea may be a side effect. Malaise, fever, rash, and liver inflammation can occur.
	Abacavir, Lamivudine, Zidovudine	Trizivir	Diarrhea may be a side effect. Malaise, fever, rash, and liver inflammation can occur.
	Adefovir	Hepsera, ADV, Preveon	Often used in chronic HBV treatments. Has nephrotoxic potential. Nausea, diarrhea, and vomiting can occur.
	Aptivus	Tipranivir	For the adjunctive treatment of HIV-1 infections.
	Didanosine	Videx, ddI Videx EC	May cause liver toxicity in low-weight patients. Neuropathy and pancreatitis may result.
	Emtricitabine	Emtriva, FTC, Coviracil	Well tolerated. Anorexia and fatigue are side effects.
	Emtricitabine, Tenofovir DF	Truvada	May cause diarrhea, nausea, and vomiting. Take with food.
	Lamivudine	Epivir, 3TC	May cause nausea and vomiting, pancreatitis, and depression. Lamivudine is well tolerated and safe (Mauss, 2006). Avoid alcohol. Take without regard for meals.
	Lamivudine, Zidovudine	Combivir	Headache, liver inflammation, and fatigue can occur. Take with meals.
	Stavudine	Zerit, d4T	Severe anemia may occur. Avoid alcohol.
	Tenofovir DF	Viread, TDF	Gastrointestinal side effects and hypophosphatemia may occur; may have a nephrotoxic potential (Mauss, 2006). Acute renal failure is possible (Zimmerman et al, 2006).
	Zalcitabine	Hivid, ddC	Can cause oral ulcers, nausea and vomiting, and dry mouth. Neuropathy may result. Take on empty stomach. Avoid taking with antacids.
	Zidovudine	Retrovir, AZT, ZDV	Can cause severe bone marrow depletion and anemia, altered taste, constipation, nausea, indigestion, or vomiting. It works better in sequence with acyclovir. Adequate folate and vitamin B_{12} may prevent toxicity. Take with food.
Protease inhibitors (PI) *PIs disable protease, a protein that HIV needs to make more copies of itself. PI therapy has been associated with hyperlipidemia, hyperglycemia, gastrointestinal symptoms, and body fat distribution abnormalities.*			Disguising their taste is important; add a small amount to cold foods such as ice cream, shakes, and fruit ices; thick sweet foods such as honey, jellies, and frozen juice; or small amounts of peanut butter, pudding, applesauce, or yogurt.
	Amprenavir	Agenerase, APV	May cause a tendency to bleed. Hyperglycemia may result.
	Atazanavir	Reyataz, ATV	May cause a tendency to bleed. Take with food.
	Fosamprenavir	Lexiva, FPV	May cause a tendency to bleed. Take without regard for meals.
	Indinavir	Crixivan, IDV	Best absorbed on an empty stomach or with a light, nonfat snack and increased fluids (but not skim milk, coffee, or tea), even juice if calories are needed. Nausea and vomiting, change in taste, and diarrhea can occur.
	Lopinavir, Ritonavir	Kaletra, LPV/r	Elevated lipids and gastrointestinal distress may occur. Take with food. Abnormal mouth sensations are noted. Hyperglycemia can occur.
	Nelfinavir	Viracept, NFV	Take with food; flatulence, loose stools, or diarrhea can occur. Hyperglycemia may result.

(continued)

TABLE 15-7 Medications Used for HIV Infections and AIDS *(continued)*

Class	Generic Name	Brand and Other Names	Nutritional Implications and Comments
	Ritonavir	Norvir, RTV	Take with a high-energy, high-fat meal; side effects include weakness, diarrhea, nausea and vomiting, loss of appetite, abdominal pain, abnormal mouth sensations of burning or prickling, and high cholesterol or triglyceride levels. Ritonavir-boosted PI regimens have provided substantial benefits in the treatment of HIV/AIDS, resulting in improved clinical outcomes; unfortunately, dyslipidemia is highly prevalent, and coronary events are possible (Cohen, 2005).
	Saquinavir	Fortovase, SQV Invirase	Best absorbed after a high-energy, high-fat meal; contains some lactose; may cause gastrointestinal distress, diarrhea, or nausea.
Fusion inhibitors			
Fusion inhibitors prevent HIV entry into cells.			
	Enfuvirtide	Fuzeon, T-20	Pneumonia has been one side effect. Take without regard for meals. Nausea, diarrhea, fatigue, and pancreatitis are possible side effects.
Antineoplastic agents			
For Kaposi's sarcoma.			
	Adriamycin, Bleomycin, Vincristine		Numerous side effects occur, including nausea and vomiting, diarrhea, anorexia, stomatitis, and weight loss.
	Doxorubicin		Administer with riboflavin to decrease toxicity. Dry mouth, esophagitis, stomatitis, nausea, and vomiting are common.
Other medications			
To manage other side effects of HIV.			
	Acyclovir	Zovirax	May cause headache, nausea, anorexia, sore throat, fatigue, altered taste, and diarrhea.
	Antidepressants	Zoloft, Wellbutrin, others	May be useful before interferon therapy if there is a history of depression.
	Antifungals	Amphotericin-B, clotrimazole, flucytosine, ketoconazole	May cause nausea and vomiting, diarrhea, weight loss, metallic taste, and gastrointestinal distress.
	Antioxidants	Multivitamin-mineral supplement that meets 100% DRI levels	Antioxidant supplementation may decrease markers of oxidative stress, and selenium may enhance immune function by modulating cytokine production; current knowledge supports the use of a multivitamin supplement (without extra vitamin A) as a low-cost adjunct to antiretroviral treatment (Lanzillotti and Tang, 2005).
	Cidofovir	Vistide	A cytosine nucleotide analog, used for treatment of cytomegalovirus (CMV), herpes type II, papilloma, and pox viruses.
	Corticosteroids	Prednisone, others	Sodium retention and potassium, calcium, and vitamin C depletion can occur; protein malnutrition can occur with extended use. Glucose intolerance also may result.
	Foscarnet	Foscavir	Used for CMV retinitis (used by IV only) and may cause anorexia, nausea and vomiting, abdominal pain, and diarrhea.
	Ganciclovir	Cytovene	Approved for use with CMV. May cause diarrhea, fever, neuropathy, elevated blood urea nitrogen and creatinine, and hypoglycemia.
	Pancreatic enzymes	Various	May be used with malabsorption.
	Peginterferon alpha plus ribavirin		For hepatitis C virus/HIV co-infection, this is standard of care; flu-like symptoms, fatigue, and depressive mood changes are frequent (Mauss, 2006). Weight loss is common.
	Topical microbicides	Currently, 62 microbicides are in development. Alkyl sulfate microbicides, such as sodium dodecyl sulfate (SDS) agents	Proposed to break the chain of transmission by providing chemical, biological, and physical barriers to infection by blocking or inactivating pathogens at the mucosal surface where infection can occur (Howett and Kuhl, 2005).
	Trimethoprim-sulfamethoxazole	Bactrim, Septra	Used for *Pneumocystis carnii* pneumonia (PCP) for approximately 1 month. Drug may cause hepatitis, azotemia, anorexia, stomatitis, and thrombocytopenia. Monitor carefully. Folate may be needed.
	Valganciclovir	Valcyte	Approved for CMV.

(continued)

TABLE 15-7 **Medications Used for HIV Infections and AIDS** ***(continued)***

Class	Generic Name	Brand and Other Names	Nutritional Implications and Comments
Appetite stimulants and anabolic steroids *To improve appetite and intake.*			Combined treatment with appetite stimulants (such as megestrol acetate) and anabolic steroids leads to significant increase in body weight and fat-free mass (Cuerda et al, 2005).
	Dronabinol	Marijuana derivative	Takes 4–6 weeks to show effects; somnolence and impaired memory can occur.
	Megestrol acetate (MA)	Megace	Useful for stimulating appetite.
	Anabolic steroids: oxandrolone, nandrolone decaonoate (ND)	Oxandrin	Synthetic testosterone (anabolic steroid) that promotes weight gain, linear growth in children, and increased muscle mass. Hepatic changes or tumors have been reported. Elevation of low-density lipoprotein (LDL) can occur with prolonged use; this may have cardiovascular effects. Nutritional status and quality of life can improve in HIV-infected individuals receiving a therapeutic approach that includes oxandrolone (Earthman et al, 2002).

- Adequate education should address any decline in self-care abilities, as well as alternative therapies and consequences.
- Resistance and strengthening exercises should be maintained to keep LBM intact (Evans, 2004).
- New mothers who are HIV positive will want to use formula or milk from a surrogate mother instead of breastfeeding.
- In home care, TPN may be used. Adequate and continuing education should be offered to caregivers to prevent transmission of the disease and to reduce other infections.
- In the short term, nutrition counseling and oral supplements can achieve a substantial increase in energy intake. Importance of maintaining a balanced, nutritious diet should be addressed. Rest periods before and after meals are suggested.
- Patients are living longer because of HAART therapy, and they may be susceptible to other age-related diseases such as diabetes, cardiovascular disease, and obesity (Gerrior and Neff, 2005). They should receive appropriate nutrition counseling to meet their individual needs.
- Use of stress management and coping mechanisms will be important to maintain nutritional health (Tromble-Hoke et al, 2005).

Patient Education—Food Safety

- Educate about food safety issues. Reducing infections is very important.
- Exceptional hand washing techniques should be used by all caregivers and by patient. Safe food-handling techniques are imperative to reduce exposure to *Cryptosporidia, Giardia,* and *Salmonella.*

For More Information

- AEGIS (AIDS Education Global Information System)
  http://www.aegis.com/
- AIDS Info
  http://www.aidsinfo.nih.gov
- AIDS Research Information Center
  http://www.critpath.org/aric/
- American Foundation for AIDS Research
  http://www.amfar.org/
- Body: An AIDS and HIV Information Resource
  http://www.thebody.com/
- HIV and Hemophilia
  http://www.hivpositive.com/f-HIVyou/f-Hemophilia/3-HemoSubMenu.html
- HIV and Hepatitis
  http://www.hivandhepatitis.com/index.html
- HIV InSite
  http://hivinsite.ucsf.edu/InSite
- HIV and Solid Organ Transplant Multi-Site Study
  http://www.hivtransplant.com
- International AIDS Vaccine Initiative
  http://www.iavi.org
- National AIDS Information Clearinghouse (NAIC)
  http://www.cdcnpin.org/

AIDS AND HIV INFECTION—CITED REFERENCES

Alter MJ. Epidemiology of viral hepatitis and HIV co-infection. Epidemiology of viral hepatitis and HIV co-infection. *J Hepatol.* 44:S6, 2006.

American Dietetic Association. Position of the American Dietetic Association and Dietitians of Canada: nutrition intervention in the care of persons with human immunodeficiency virus infection. *J Am Diet Assoc.* 104:1425, 2004.

Cohen CJ. Ritonavir-boosted protease inhibitors. Part 2: cardiac implications of lipid alterations. *AIDS Read.* 15:528, 2005.

Cuerda C, et al. Treatment with nandrolone decanoate and megestrol acetate in HIV-infected men. *Nutr Clin Pract.* 20:93, 2005.

Dorosko SM. Vitamin A, mastitis, and mother-to-child transmission of HIV-1 through breast-feeding: current information and gaps in knowledge. *Nutr Rev.* 63:332, 2005.

Earthman CP. Evaluation of nutrition assessment parameters in the presence of human immunodeficiency virus infection. *Nutr Clin Pract.* 19:330, 2004.

Earthman CP, et al. Body cell mass repletion and improved quality of life in HIV-infected individuals receiving oxandrolone. *J Parenter Enteral Nutr.* 26:357, 2002.

Evans WJ. Protein nutrition, exercise and aging. *J Am Coll Nutr.* 23:601S, 2004.

Fauci AS, et al. NK cells in HIV infection: paradigm for protection or targets for ambush. *Nat Rev Immunol.* 5:835, 2005.

Frankenfield D, et al. Comparison of predictive equations for resting metabolic rate in healthy nonobese and obese adults: a systematic review. *J Am Diet Assoc.* 105:775, 2005.

Gerrior JL, Neff LM. Nutrition assessment in HIV infection. *Nutr Clin Care.* 8:6, 2005.

Howett MK, Kuhl JP. Microbicides for prevention of transmission of sexually transmitted diseases. *Curr Pharm Des.* 11:3731, 2005.

Kahraman A, et al. Non-alcoholic fatty liver disease in HIV-positive patients predisposes for acute-on-chronic liver failure: two cases. *Eur J Gastroenterol Hepatol.* 18:101, 2006.
Koff WC, et al. HIV vaccine design: insights from live attenuated SIV vaccines. *Nat Immunol.* 7:19, 2006.
Lanzillotti JS, Tang AM. Micronutrients and HIV disease: a review pre- and post-HAART. *Nutr Clin Care.* 8:16, 2005.
Lesho EP, Gey DC. Managing issues related to antiretroviral therapy. *Am Fam Physician.* 68:675, 2003.
Liu JP, et al. Herbal medicines for treating HIV infection and AIDS. *Cochrane Database Syst Rev.* 3:CD003937, 2005.
Maillet JO, et al. Ethical issues in nutrition and human immunodeficiency virus. *Nutr Clin Pract.* 19:365, 2004.
Mauss S. Treatment of viral hepatitis in HIV-coinfected patients—adverse events and their management. *J Hepatol.* 44:S144, 2006.
Ovesna Z, et al. Pentacyclic triterpenoic acids: new chemoprotective compounds. Minireview. *Neoplasma* 51:327, 2004.
Shelburne SA, et al. Immune reconstitution inflammatory syndrome: more answers, more questions. *J Antimicrob Chemother.* 2006. In press.
Tang AM, et al. Increasing risk of 5% or greater unintentional weight loss in a cohort of HIV-infected patients, 1995 to 2003. *J Acquir Immune Defic Syndr.* 40:70, 2005.
Thorne C, Newell ML. Treatment options for the prevention of mother-to-child transmission of HIV. *Curr Opin Investig Drugs.* 6:804, 2005.
Tromble-Hoke SM, et al. Severe stress events and use of stress-management behaviors are associated with nutrition-related parameters in men with HIV/AIDS. *J Am Diet Assoc.* 105:1541, 2005.
Villamor E. A potential role for vitamin D on HIV infection? *Nutr Rev.* 64:226, 2006.
Wanke C. Nutrition and HIV in the international setting. *Nutr Clin Care.* 8:44, 2005.
Wood C, Harrington W Jr. AIDS and associated malignancies. *Cell Res.* 15:947, 2005.
Zimmerman AE, et al. Tenofovir-associated acute and chronic kidney disease: a case of multiple drug interactions. *Clin Infect Dis.* 42:283, 2006

BURNS (THERMAL INJURY)

NUTRITIONAL ACUITY RANKING: LEVEL 3 (MINOR), LEVEL 4 (MAJOR BURNS)

DEFINITIONS AND BACKGROUND

Electrical, thermal, chemical, or radioactive agents can cause burns. Burns are the third leading cause of accidental death in the United States; 35% of burn victims are children. With a first-degree burn, simple redness of epidermis occurs. In a second-degree burn, redness and blistering occur. In a third-degree burn, skin and tissue destruction occurs. See Figures 15-4, 15-5, and 15-6.

The hypermetabolic response to burn injury (mediated by hugely increased levels of circulating catecholamines, prostaglandins, glucagon, and cortisol) causes profound skeletal muscle catabolism, immune deficiency, peripheral lipolysis, reduced bone mineralization, reduced linear growth, and increased energy expenditure (Murphy et al, 2003). The metabolic rate is markedly increased in burns (Jeejeeboy, 2004). Estimating the percentage of total body burned is important. Figure 15-7 shows how the estimates are made.

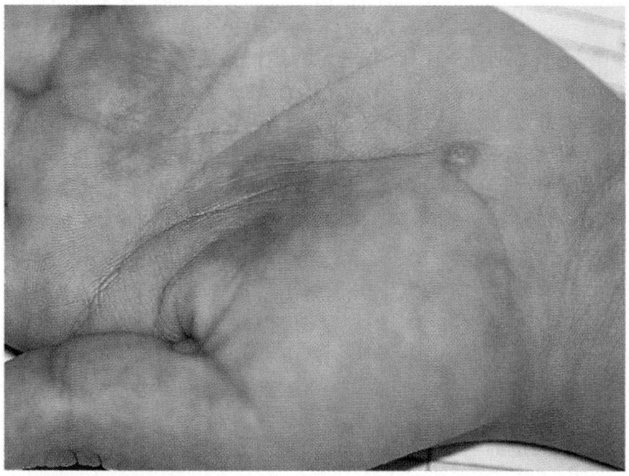

Figure 15-4 First-degree burn. (From Reece RM, Ludwig S. *Child abuse: medical diagnosis and management.* 2nd ed. Philadelphia: Lippincott Williams & Wilkins, 2001.)

Total burn thickness affects metabolic rate more than body surface area (BSA). Increased catecholamine production, body temperature, evaporative losses, and infections may occur. Local mediators (cytokines) are released from inflammatory cells, attracting more to the affected area. Interleukin-1 and interleukin-6 as well as tumor necrosis factor (TNF) are involved. A 25–30% total BSA (TBSA) burn leads to systemic edema and catabolic responses. A 90% TBSA burn is usually fatal; 60% or more in an older person is also usually fatal.

Much of the morbidity and mortality of severely burned patients is connected with catabolism and hypermetabolism (Andel et al, 2003). The development of systemic inflammation, acute lung injury, and multiple organ failure are common (Magnotti and Deitch, 2005). Before the modern era of early enteral nutrition support, significant weight loss led to impaired wound healing, infectious morbidity, and increased mortality (Lee et al, 2005). Loss of 1 g of nitrogen equals a 30-g loss of lean body mass; nitrogen balance becomes a matter of life and death in a major burn victim. Survival depends on medical treatment and early, effective nutritional support. Weight loss of up to 10% is acceptable; 40–50% can lead to mortality.

Early institution of enteral feeding can attenuate the stress response, abate hypermetabolism, and improve patient outcome (Lee et al, 2005). Despite adequate nutritional support, severe thermal injury leads to decreased anabolic hormones over a prolonged period of time and longer intensive care unit (ICU) stays (Jeschke et al, 2005). If the gastrointestinal (GI) tract becomes nonfunctional, use of parenteral support may be needed.

Addition of high doses of ascorbic acid (rate of 25 mg/mL) to resuscitation fluid administered during the first

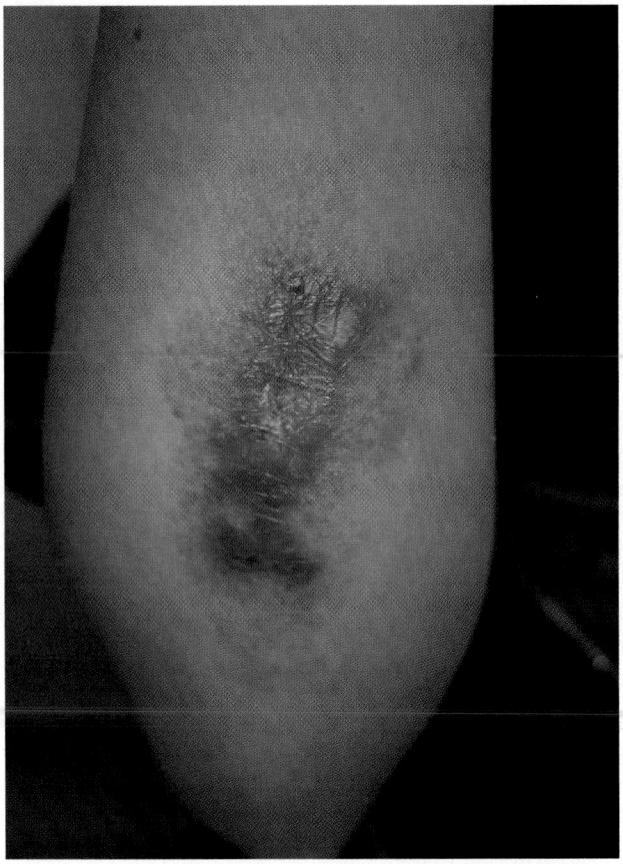

Figure 15-5 Second-degree burn. (Image provided by Stedman's.)

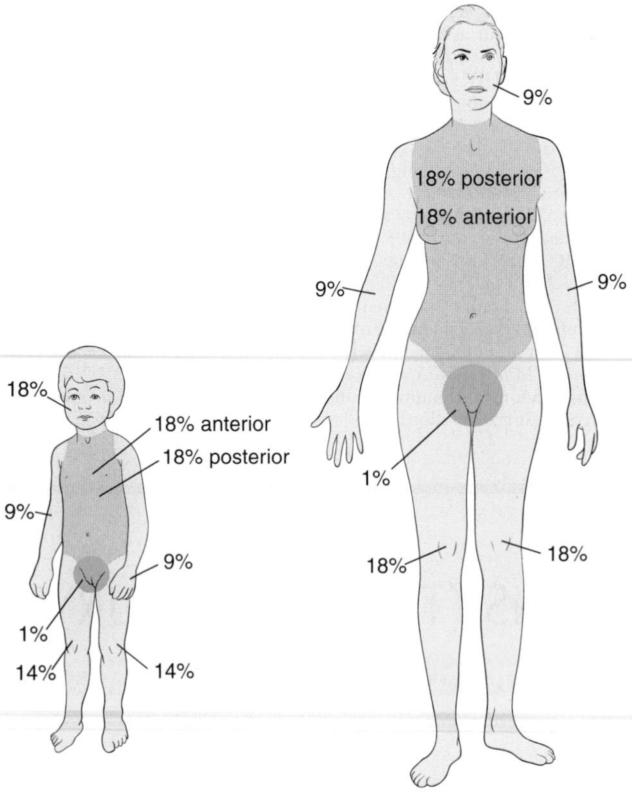

Figure 15-7 Percentage of body burned. (From LifeART image, copyright © 2006 Lippincott Williams & Wilkins. All rights reserved.)

24 hours after severe burns significantly reduces resuscitation fluid volume, body weight gain, wound edema, and severity of respiratory dysfunction (Tanaka et al, 2000). Growth hormone (GH) may be used to decrease the catabolic effect of burns.

Eschars cut off blood supply to an extremity or may impair breathing; they are often cut open in a surgical escharotomy. Bleeding occurs, but because the burn causing the eschar has destroyed the nerve endings in the skin, there is little pain. Healing takes place in three stages: establishment of the epithelial barrier, scar tissue formation (dermal replacement), and contraction (shrinkage). Severity of thermal injury and presence of systemic infection increase risk for developing ischemic bowel disease.

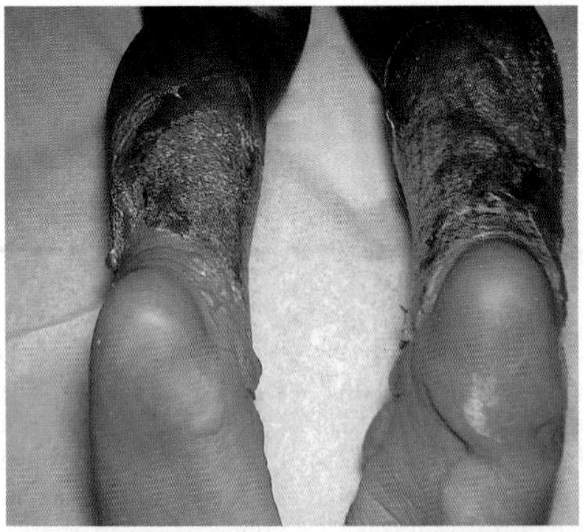

Figure 15-6 Third-degree burn. (From Fleisher GR, Ludwig S, Baskin MN. *Atlas of pediatric emergency medicine.* Philadelphia: Lippincott Williams & Wilkins, 2004.)

INTERVENTION: OBJECTIVES

- Restore fluid and electrolyte balance to prevent hypovolemic shock and to stabilize body temperature. Beware of exudate losses, which may be 20–25% of total daily nitrogen losses. Prevent renal insufficiency or failure from decreased plasma volume, cardiac output, and excessive pigment overload (from necrosis, toxins, and hemolysis). Correct syndrome of inappropriate antidiuretic hormone (SIADH), hypertonic dehydration, or overhydration.
- Promote wound healing while minimizing loss of lean body mass (Lee et al, 2005). Close wound surface with grafts to reduce likelihood of organ failure. Grafts may be autograft (own body) or from cultured keratinocytes; promote graft retention.
- Minimize catabolism of protein tissues to avoid consequences of protein–energy malnutrition including impaired immunity, decreased wound healing, decreased vigor and muscle strength, retarded synthesis of blood proteins and hemoglobin, and increased likelihood of infection. Patients with burns have an elevated measured metabolic rate 1.2–1.3 times normal rate, which is increased further by percentage of burn surface. Use indirect calorimetry where possible.

- Avoid weight losses greater than 10% of preburn weight. In children, growth must continue.
- Achieve positive nitrogen balance and minimize losses. One indication for which albumin therapy is considered is in burn therapy; reviews have documented the advantages of albumin therapy in the management of ascites and volume resuscitation (Mendez et al, 2005).
- Reduce evaporative water losses, especially with occlusive wound dressings.
- Relieve pain.
- Alleviate problems such as postburn pruritus, deep venous thrombosis, peptic ulceration, and psychosocial problems such as acute stress syndrome, depression, and posttraumatic stress syndrome (Murphy et al, 2003). Prevent pressure ulcers (Gordon et al, 2004).
- Prevent ischemic gut, which may contribute to the development of sepsis and organ failure (Magnotti and Deitch, 2005). Use enteral nutrition, starting as early as possible without any supplemental parenteral nutrition, as the preferred feeding method (Andel et al, 2003).
- The possibility of overfeeding is a consideration when using high-energy nutrition in burned patients (Andel et al, 2003). Minimize the negative consequences of hyperglycemia and unnecessary energy expenditures by the patient (Flynn, 2004).
- Restore skin's protection to reduce infection. Sepsis is a major cause of mortality, often occurring 2–3 weeks after injury.

INTERVENTION: FOOD AND NUTRITION

- Immediately use intravenous fluids to replace deficits; prevent gastric distention and paralytic ileus. Prevent overhydration. Add vitamin C (25 mg/mL) to promote healing.
- Tube feeding (TF) may be possible; start within a few hours for best results to decrease hypermetabolic response to injury (Magnotti and Dietch, 2005). A duodenal placement, especially in the early postburn phase, seems to be superior to gastric feeding (Andel et al, 2003). Use specialty immunoenhanced products with peptides rather than amino acids. Glutamine may help to preserve gut function (De-Souza and Greene, 2005).
- Protein intake should be from 2–3 times the RDA or 1.5–3 g/kg body weight; adjust for children (De-Souza and Greene, 1998). Add modular protein supplements as needed, especially glutamine. Leucine-supplemented nutrition is also very promising, even more than use of all three branched-chain amino acids (De Bandt and Cynober, 2005).
- Use 20% protein, 60% carbohydrates (CHO), and 20% fat (2–4% essential fatty acids and slight increase in omega-3 fatty acids). CHO may be given at rate of 5 mg/kg/min; intravenous lipids can be given at 4 g/kg maximum in pediatrics. Add Polycose or other CHO supplements as needed.
- Gradually progress to oral diet when possible; use a high-calorie, high-protein diet with 5–6 small meals and snacks. Suitable snacks may include peanut butter cookies, brownies, cake, shakes, pasteurized eggs in milkshakes or eggnog, protein in broths, and dextrins added to coffee. (See tips for adding protein and calories to the diet in Section 5.)
- Supplemental glutamine granules with oral feeding or TF can abate the degree of glutamine depletion, promote protein synthesis, inhibit protein decomposition, improve wound healing, and reduce hospital stay (Peng et al, 2005).
- Provide adequate fluid intake: encourage intake of fruit juices (cranberry, grapefruit, prune, or orange juice) for adequate supplies of potassium. Water losses may be 10–12 times normal during first few weeks.
- Supplement diet with 5–10 times the RDA of vitamin C; 2 times the RDA of zinc sulfate; and 2–3 times the RDA of B-complex vitamins. Two times the RDA for vitamins A and D may be useful at first. Vitamins K and B_{12} may need to be given weekly; check serum levels as needed.
- For children, vitamins should be given at twice the RDA until recovery.
- Provide adequate copper (for collagen cross-linkage). Arginine (up to 2% of kilocalories) and carnitine also may be beneficial. Phosphorus should be added intravenously as potassium phosphate, enterally, or orally as Neutra-Phos.
- Include omega-3 fatty acids. Essential fatty acids have been used to reduce inflammation and promote wound healing. Omega-3 fatty acids help promote a healthy balance of proteins in the body, and protein balance is important for recovery after sustaining a burn. Further research is necessary (Jeschke et al, 2001).
- Administration of high-calorie total enteral nutrition in any later septic phase should be avoided (Andel et al, 2003). Avoid excesses of linoleic acid, which can depress immunocompetence. Be careful about iron and zinc excesses in patients with sepsis.
- Do not alter nutritional support because of watery diarrhea; this type of diarrhea is likely to occur for reasons other than carbohydrate intolerance (Thakkar et al, 2005).

SAMPLE NUTRITION DIAGNOSTIC STATEMENT

Burn

PES: Inadequate nutrient intake related to burns of 45% of total body surface (mostly upper extremities) as evidenced by weight loss of 10 lb in past 14 days.

Assessment Data: Analysis of preferences, dislikes, and allergies; intake compared to measured or estimated requirements; confirmation of severity and extent of burn from medical record; recorded weights.

Intervention: If needs cannot be met by oral route due to extent and severity of burn, patient will need nutrition support or feeding assistance. Eliminate distractions at mealtime and avoid lab work and painful procedures before meals. Discourage use of empty-calorie foods or beverages, and use nutrient-dense beverages with medication passes.

Monitoring and Evaluation: Monitor and evaluate weights, and meet nutritional needs. Anticipate 2–3 months total for optimal recovery time.

CLINICAL INDICATORS

Clinical/History

Height
Preburn weight
Weight changes
Daily weight (beware of heavy exudate, edema)
BMI
Diet history
Measured energy expenditure (MEE)
% Body burned
Burn classification (1st, 2nd, 3rd, 4th)
Edema
I & O
BP
Temperature
Urine acetone, sugars
Ability to chew
Ability to swallow
Hypovolemic shock: tachycardia, low BP, decreased urinary output

Lab Work

Alb
Transthyretin (decreased)
CRP
BUN, Creat
H & H
Gluc (increased)
AST (increased)
Na+ (decreased)
Chloride
K+
Total urinary N (TUN)
Ca++, Mg++
Partial pressure of carbon dioxide (pCO_2)
Partial pressure of oxygen (pO_2)
Transferrin
Chol, Trig
White blood cell count (WBC), TLC
Serum catecholamines (increased)
Ceruloplasmin
Alkaline phosphatase (Alk phos)
N balance

Common Drugs Used and Potential Side Effects

- See Table 15-8.

Herbs, Botanicals, and Supplements

- Herbs and botanical supplements should not be used without discussing with physician.
- St John's wort, echinacea, garlic, gotu kola, and plantain have been suggested but are not yet proven through clinical trials.

INTERVENTION: NUTRITION EDUCATION, COUNSELING, CARE MANAGEMENT

- Considering possible consequences of long-term immobilization (renal calculi, pneumonia, contractures, and pressure ulcers), increase activity as pain tolerance allows. Discuss importance of the balance between appetite, nutritional intake, and physical activity.
- Review the fact that fat is high in energy while low in volume. Fat is helpful in normalizing elimination; however, excesses may negatively affect immunocompetence.
- Explain that adequate intake of fiber is important.
- The family's attitude toward patient's dietary intake should be firm but also patient and understanding. A daily nutrient intake record may be a good way to track goals and to assess total intake.
- Discuss problems to monitor and report, such as fever or wound drainage.
- Offer a written care plan for home use.

TABLE 15-8 Pharmacotherapy for Burns

Antimicrobial control, analgesia, sedation, and anxiety management are required (Murphy et al, 2003).

Medication	Description
Analgesics	Pain medications may have some effect on gastrointestinal (GI) function and appetite.
Antacids	Used to prevent Curling's ulcer. Cimetidine also is useful.
Antibiotics	Topical antibiotics are used. Early burn wound excision and complete coverage with autograft, cadaver skin, synthetic dressings, and amnion markedly reduce septic complications (Murphy et al, 2003). Beware of nutrient leaching of sodium, copper, potassium, magnesium, calcium, and B-complex vitamins with Silvazine; added salt or supplements of potassium and calcium may be needed. Acticoat results in a reduced incidence of burn wound cellulitis, antibiotic use, and cost when compared with Silvazine in the treatment of early burn wounds (Fong et al, 2005). When using Acticoat, average length of stay (LOS) in hospital dropped by 4.75 days, saving $30,450 (Fong et al, 2005).
Insulin	Used for stress-induced hyperglycemia.
Interferon-gamma or -alpha-2b	Used to decrease keloid formation. Dry mouth, stomatitis, nausea and vomiting, diarrhea, and abdominal pain may result.
Supportive therapy	Given acutely and during rehabilitation using growth hormone, insulin and related proteins, oxandrolone, and propranolol. This can ameliorate the hypermetabolic response, improving survival and long-term outcome (Murphy et al, 2003).

Patient Education—Food Safety

- Educate about food safety issues. Reducing infections is very important.
- Meticulous hand washing will be essential.

For More Information

- American Burn Association
  http://www.ameriburn.org/
- Burn Care Foundation
  http://www.burnsurvivor.com/index.html
- Burn Incidence Fact Sheet
  http://www.ameriburn.org/pub/BurnIncidenceFactSheet.htm
- Burn Prevention
  http://kidshealth.org/parent/firstaid_safe/sheets/burns_sheet.html
- Burn Survivors
  http://www.burnsurvivor.com/index.html
- Centers for Disease Control and Prevention Emergency Treatment of Burns
  http://www.bt.cdc.gov/masscasualties/burns.asp

- Fire Safety
  http://www.nlm.nih.gov/medlineplus/firesafety.html
- Mayo Clinic
  http://www.mayoclinic.com/health/first-aid-burns/FA00022
- National Library of Medicine–Burns
  http://www.nlm.nih.gov/medlineplus/burns.html

BURNS—CITED REFERENCES

Andel H, et al. Nutrition and anabolic agents in burned patients. *Burns* 29:592, 2003.

De Bandt JP, Cynober L. Therapeutic use of branched-chain amino acids in burn, trauma, and sepsis. *J Nutr.* 136:308S, 2006.

De-Souza DA, Greene LJ. Intestinal permeability and systemic infections in critically ill patients: effect of glutamine. *Crit Care Med.* 33:1125, 2005.

De-Souza DA, Greene LJ. Pharmacological nutrition after burn injury. *J Nutr.* 128:797, 1998.

Flynn MB. Nutritional support for the burn-injured patient. *Crit Care Nurs Clin North Am.* 16:139, 2004.

Fong J, et al. A silver coated dressing reduces the incidence of early burn wound cellulitis and associated costs of inpatient treatment: comparative patient care audits. *Burns* 31:562, 2005

Gordon MD, et al. Review of evidenced-based practice for the prevention of pressure sores in burn patients. *J Burn Care Rehabil.* 25:388, 2004.

Jeejeeboy KN. Permissive underfeeding of the critically ill patient. *Nutr Clin Pract.* 19:477, 2004.

Jeschke MG, et al. Endogenous anabolic hormones and hypermetabolism: effect of trauma and gender differences. *Ann Surg.* 241:759, 2005.

Jeschke MG, et al. Nutritional intervention high in vitamins, protein, amino acids, and omega-3 fatty acids improves protein metabolism during the hypermetabolic state after thermal injury. *Arch Surg.* 136:1301, 2001.

Lee JO, et al. Nutrition support strategies for severely burned patients. *Nutr Clin Pract.* 20:325, 2005.

Magnotti LJ, Deitch EA. Burns, bacterial translocation, gut barrier function, and failure. *J Burn Care Rehabil.* 26:383, 2005.

Mendez CM, et al. Albumin therapy in clinical practice. *Nutr Clin Pract.* 20:314, 2005.

Murphy KD, et al. Effects of long-term oxandrolone administration in severely burned children. *Surgery* 136:219, 2004.

Peng X, et al. Clinical and protein metabolic efficacy of glutamine granules-supplemented enteral nutrition in severely burned patients. *Burns* 31:342, 2005.

Tanaka H, et al. Reduction of resuscitation fluid volumes in severely burned patients using ascorbic acid administration: a randomized, prospective study. *Arch Surg.* 135:326, 2000.

Thakkar K, et al. Diarrhea in severely burned children. *J Parenter Enteral Nutr.* 29:8, 2005.

FRACTURES

NUTRITIONAL ACUITY RANKING: LEVEL 2

DEFINITIONS AND BACKGROUND

Broken bones result from a physical force greater than stress that cannot be withstood. **Fatigue fractures** occur from prolonged stress on normal bones. *Simple* fractures involve bones that do not protrude. A *compound* fracture allows bone to protrude. With multiple fractures, metabolic rate may increase by 20% or more for several weeks. A *long-bone fracture* generally is an emergency and may be complicated by shock, wound infection, bleeding, or inadequate hydration. Traction is usually needed for internal immobilization. See Table 15-9 for a list of the most commonly broken bones and Figure 15-8 for a fractured bone.

Pathological fractures involve weakened bones breaking from old age, osteoporosis, and bone cancer. Incidence increases after 60 years of age, especially in women. Aggressive refeeding of malnourished patients is useful in decreasing morbidity and mortality in fracture patients (Bonjour, 2005). One in two women and one in four men over age 50 will have an osteoporosis-related fracture in their remaining lifetime. A previous vertebral or hip fracture is the primary predictor of fracture risk; bone density is the best predictor of fracture risk for those without prior adult fractures; age, weight, certain medications, and family history also help establish a person's risk for osteoporotic fractures (Cosman, 2005). Low birth weight and poor childhood growth are directly linked to later risk of hip fracture (Cooper et al, 2006). Optimizing nutrition throughout life is protective.

Osteoporosis is responsible for more than 1.5 million fractures annually, including:

- over 300,000 hip fractures; and approximately
- 700,000 vertebral fractures;
- 250,000 wrist fractures; and
- 300,000 fractures at other sites.

Experimental and clinical published data concur to indicate that poor nutrition negatively affects bone health. Deficiency in dietary proteins causes marked deterioration in bone mass, microarchitecture, and strength, the hallmark of osteoporosis (Bonjour, 2005). Dietary proteins enhance insulin-like growth factor I (IGF-I), a factor that exerts positive activity on skeletal development and bone formation (Bonjour, 2005). Vitamin D is another nutritional factor; recent evidence suggests that an increase in current recommendations should be considered to prevent fractures (Bischoff-Ferrari et al, 2006).

Broken hip includes fractures of the femur head (intracapsular), femur neck (extracapsular), and greater Hesser trochanter. Relative risk for hip fracture is related to many

TABLE 15-9 Most Commonly Broken Bones

1. Forearm (ulna, radius)
2. Hands and feet (carpals, metacarpals, tarsals, and metatarsals)
3. Ribs
4. Fingers and thumbs (phalanges)
5. Shin bones (tibia, fibula)
6. Thigh bones (femur)
7. Skull
8. Upper arm (humerus)
9. Collar bone (clavicle)
10. Back bone (spinal bones or vertebrae)

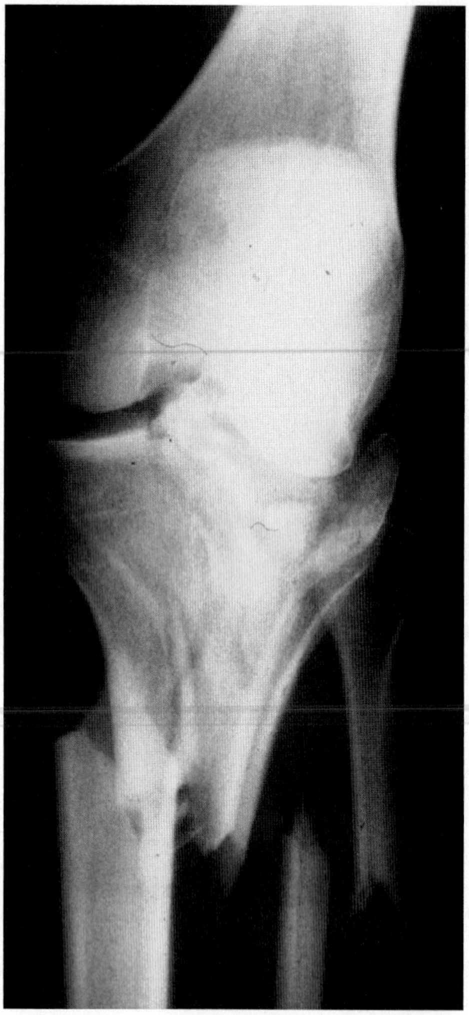

Figure 15-8 Fractured bone. (From Bucholz RW, Heckman JD. *Rockwood & Green's fractures in adults.* 5th ed. Philadelphia: Lippincott Williams & Wilkins, 2001.)

factors, such as low body mass index (BMI), low calcium intake, high alcohol intake, prevalent vertebral fracture, early age at menarche, and high number of children. For some reason, those who sustain a wrist fracture are twice as likely to have hip fracture later in life. Hip fracture risk is increasing most rapidly among Hispanic women. Women with a hip fracture are at a four-fold greater risk of having a second one, and the risk factors are similar to those for the first hip fracture. Osteoporotic fractures lower a patient's quality of life.

Vitamin A in amounts greater than 5000 IU/d may cause increased risk of hip fractures. In surgical cases after hip fracture, open reduction with internal fixation (ORIF) may be necessary; adequate nutrition must be provided for wound healing and to reduce infectious processes.

INTERVENTION: OBJECTIVES

- Support formation of bone matrix. Complete union may take 4–8 months.
- Supply adequate nutrition for collagen formation and calcium deposition.
- Prevent side effects of long-term immobilization, such as renal calculi, pressure ulcers, urinary tract infections, embolus, contractures, and neurovascular dysfunction.
- Maintain optimal systemic functioning.
- Use fluoridated water. Hip fracture is not increased in areas where water is fluoridated (Phipps et al, 2000). Monitor bottled waters and well water, which are often not fluoridated.
- For long-bone fracture, meet energy needs, which are increased by 20–25%. Keep nearby joints as active as possible and prevent complications such as pressure ulcers, renal calculi, and effects from spinal anesthesia.

INTERVENTION: FOOD AND NUTRITION

- Use a high-protein, high-energy diet; needs increase by 20–25%. There is no consistent evidence for superiority of vegetable protein over animal protein on calcium metabolism, bone loss prevention, and risk reduction of fragility fractures (Bonjour, 2005).
- Use adequate levels of calcium, phosphorus, vitamin D, and vitamin C. Encourage these nutrients to be taken in diet and a supplement that gives no more than 100% of vitamins A and D.
- Although the main source of dietary calcium is dairy products, calcium contained in mineral water, which is highly bioavailable, can provide another valuable source of calcium.
- Supply zinc for wound healing after surgical procedures. Watch for fever, pneumonia, and possible embolism.
- Ensure adequate fluid intake to excrete calcium excesses.

CLINICAL INDICATORS

Clinical/History	Lab Work	
Height	Serum Ca++	Gluc
Weight (may need chair scales)	Urinary Ca++	WBC, TLC
Weight changes	Mg++	CRP
BMI	BUN, Creat	Total iron-binding capacity (TIBC)
Diet history	H & H	Alk phos (increased)
I & O	Serum Fe	Na+, K+
BP	N balance	
Temperature	Alb, transthyretin	
	CRP	

Common Drugs Used and Potential Side Effects

- Analgesics may be needed for pain. Monitor for gastrointestinal distress or bleeding.
- Anticonvulsants and opioids (but not benzodiazepines or antidepressants) are associated with significantly reduced bone mineral density; these findings have implications for fracture-prevention strategies (Kinjo et al, 2005).

- Antiresorptive medications, such as estrogens, selective estrogen receptor modulators (raloxifene), bisphosphonates (alendronate, risedronate, and ibandronate), and calcitonins, work by reducing rates of bone remodeling (Cosman, 2005).
- Pain medications such as meperidine (Demerol) may cause vomiting, nausea, and constipation.
- Teriparatide (parathyroid hormone) is an anabolic agent that stimulates new bone formation, repairing architectural defects and improving bone density (Cosman, 2005).

Herbs, Botanicals, and Supplements

- Herbs and botanical supplements should not be used without discussing with physician.

INTERVENTION: NUTRITION EDUCATION, COUNSELING, CARE MANAGEMENT

- Emphasize importance of nutrition for healing. Indicate which foods are good sources of protein in diet.
- Encourage activity and use of physical therapy after healing has progressed. Use of oral supplements with resistance training can be very beneficial (Milkler et al, 2006).
- Refer to appropriate agencies, such as home health, Visiting Nurses Association, or Meals-on-Wheels, as needed.
- All women should have a bone density test by the age of 65 or younger (at the time of menopause) if risk factors are present (Cosman, 2005).
- Discourage smoking. Smoking cigarettes hinders healing of bones by decreasing collagen production and oxygen availability.
- Osteoporosis and fracture prevention requires adequate calcium and vitamin D intake, regular physical activity, and avoidance of smoking and excessive alcohol ingestion (Cosman, 2005). Encourage frequent fish consumption, especially in winter, for vitamin D (Nakamura, 2006).

FRACTURES—CITED REFERENCES

Bischoff-Ferrari HA, et al. Estimation of optimal serum concentrations of 25-hydroxyvitamin D for multiple health outcomes. *Am J Clin Nutr.* 84:18, 2006.

Bonjour JP. Dietary protein: an essential nutrient for bone health. *J Am Coll Nutr.* 24:526S, 2005.

Cooper C, et al. Review: developmental origins of osteoporotic fracture. *Osteoporos Int.* 17:337, 2006.

Cosman S. The prevention and treatment of osteoporosis: a review. *Med Gen Med.* 7:73, 2005.

Kinjo M, et al. Bone mineral density in subjects using central nervous system-active medications. *Am J Med.* 118:1414, 2005.

Miller MD, et al. Nutritional supplementation and resistance training in nutritionally at risk older adults following lower limb fracture: a randomized controlled trial. *Clin Rehabil.* 20:311, 2006.

Nakamura K. Vitamin D insufficiency in Japanese populations: from the viewpoint of the prevention of osteoporosis. *J Bone Miner Metab.* 24:1, 2006.

Phipps K, et al. Community water fluoridation, bone mineral density, and fractures: prospective study of effects in older women. *Br Med J.* 321:860, 2000.

INTESTINAL PARASITES

NUTRITIONAL ACUITY RANKING: LEVEL 1

DEFINITIONS AND BACKGROUND

Intestinal parasite infections (IPI) cause significant morbidity and mortality (Kucik et al, 2004). Protein–energy malnutrition is by far the most important cause of immune deficiency in developing countries (Gendrel et al, 2005). Newborns are especially vulnerable; in the developing world, morbidity is often secondary to infectious diseases such as intestinal parasites (Steer, 2005). Diseases caused by *Enterobius vermicularis, Giardia lamblia, Ancylostoma duodenale, Necator americanus,* and *Entamoeba histolytica* occur in the United States. See Table 15-10.

INTERVENTION: OBJECTIVES

- Differentiate symptoms and correctly identify condition as rapidly as possible; treat as needed.
- Diarrhea is only one of the many manifestations of intestinal parasites; when host defenses are weakened, parasitic diarrhea is frequent and severe (Gendrel et al, 2003). Treat infections and diarrhea.
- Prevent complications such as anemia, pneumonia, and cardiac failure.
- Prevent or correct malnutrition; prevent stunting and allow growth in children.
- Prevent blockage, inflammation, volvulus, and bowel perforation.
- Teach ways to prevent further infections.

INTERVENTION: FOOD AND NUTRITION

- Provide balanced intake of all macronutrients. Protein intake, especially lysine, is important (Kurpad et al, 2003). Adequate, but not excessive, iron and zinc are also useful.
- Diet as usual can be provided. Encourage adequate intake of food sources of vitamins A and C, especially from

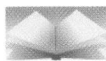

TABLE 15-10 Intestinal Parasites and Treatments

Parasite	Description and Treatment
Ancylostoma duodenale, Necator americanus (hookworms)	Cause blood loss, anemia, pica, and wasting. Finding eggs in the feces is diagnostic. Treatments include albendazole, mebendazole, pyrantel pamoate, iron supplementation, and blood transfusion. Preventive measures include wearing shoes and treating sewage.
Ascariasis (intestinal roundworms)	Common in warm or humid climates or when personal hygiene is inadequate. Adult worms live in the small intestine, with eggs that pass out in human feces. These eggs become infective within 2–3 weeks. When ingested by humans through fecally contaminated food or water, the eggs hatch and penetrate the intestines. Eventually, they reach the heart. Larvae mature within 2–3 months, and adult worms may live for 1 year or longer. Hemorrhage can occur in lung tissue and cause pneumonitis. Vague abdominal discomfort can occur with small intestine involvement. Malnutrition can cause an imbalance in T-cell subpopulations that may lead to a defective T-cell maturation and decreased specific anti-*Ascaris* immunoglobulin E response, thus increasing the susceptibility to parasitic infections (Hagel et al, 2003).
Enterobius vermicularis (pinworm)	Causes irritation and sleep disturbances. Diagnosis can be made using the "cellophane tape test." Treatment includes mebendazole and household sanitation.
Giardia	*Giardia intestinalis* is one of the most common intestinal parasites in the world, and it contributes to diarrhea, nutritional deficiencies, stunting, and cognitive impairment in children in developing regions (Ali and Hill, 2003). It causes nausea, vomiting, malabsorption, diarrhea, and weight loss. Stool ova and parasite studies are diagnostic. Treatment includes metronidazole. Sewage treatment, proper hand washing, and consumption of bottled water can be preventive.
Entamoeba histolytica	Can cause intestinal ulcerations, bloody diarrhea, weight loss, fever, gastrointestinal obstruction, and peritonitis. Amebas can cause abscesses in the liver that may rupture into the pleural space, peritoneum, or pericardium. Stool and serological assays, biopsy, barium studies, and liver imaging have diagnostic merit. Therapy includes luminal and tissue amebicides to attack both life-cycle stages. Metronidazole, chloroquine, and aspiration are treatments for liver abscess. Careful sanitation and use of peeled foods and bottled water are preventive.
Trichinella spirali (see Fig. 15-9)	*Trichinella spirali* is a roundworm that causes an acute infection (trichinosis) and is usually acquired by eating encysted larvae in raw or undercooked pork. Larvae mature and mate in the small intestine; larvae reaching striated muscle will encyst and live for years. Usual incubation is 5–15 days. The disorder has a 4% prevalence in the United States. Symptoms and signs include swelling of the upper eyelids, bleeding under the nails, skin rash, diarrhea, abdominal cramps, and malaise; later, low-grade fever, edema, sweating, dyspnea, cough, and muscle pain occur. In nonstriated muscle tissues such as the heart, brain, kidney, or lung, death can follow in 4–6 weeks, if untreated. Most symptoms disappear by the third month.

fruits, juices, and vegetables. Vitamin E and selenium may be especially protective (Smith et al, 2005).
- Ensure an adequate fluid intake, especially with diarrheal losses. Replace electrolytes with broths and juices.
- With poor appetite, offer small, frequent meals and snacks to correct malnutrition or weight loss that is undesirable.
- Ensure safe food handling at all meals.

CLINICAL INDICATORS

Clinical/History

Height
Weight
BMI
Diet history
Temperature
I & O
BP

Lab Work

Stool examination
Positive skin and serological tests for eosinophilia and leukocytosis
Trichinosis—biopsy of skeletal muscle after 4th week (for larvae or cysts)
Alb, transthyretin
CRP
H & H
Serum Fe
Transferrin
Na+, K+, Cl−
Ca++, Mg++
TLC, WBC
Gluc
TIBC
Transferrin

Common Drugs Used and Potential Side Effects

- Parasites require specific treatment in the malnourished; and the well-nourished should have preventive treatment when they are to receive corticosteroids or immunosuppressive agents (Gendrel et al, 2003).
- The albendazole-praziquantel combined regimen is a useful single-dose therapy for **giardiasis** in children.
- Pyrantel pamoate (Povan) may be used for **ascariasis.** Rarely, vomiting or diarrhea may occur.

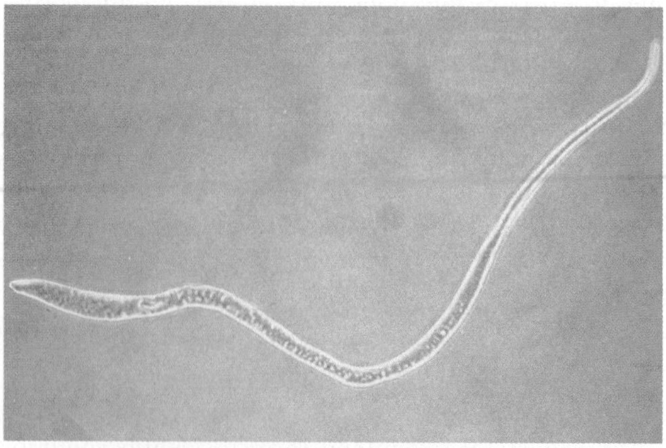

Figure 15-9 Roundworm. (From Sun T. *Parasitic disorders: pathology, diagnosis, and management.* 2nd ed. Baltimore: Lippincott Williams & Wilkins, 1999.)

- For **trichinosis,** mebendazole or thiabendazole may be used. Gastrointestinal (GI) distress is a common side effect. Aspirin or analgesics may be needed for muscular pain.
- Corticosteroids such as prednisone are often used temporarily to reduce inflammation of the heart or brain.

Herbs, Botanicals, and Supplements

- Herbs and botanical supplements should not be used without discussing with physician. Chincona, elecampane, golden seal, ipecac, and papaya have been suggested but are not proven through clinical trials.

INTERVENTION: NUTRITION EDUCATION, COUNSELING, CARE MANAGEMENT

- Discuss importance of personal hygiene in maintaining a sanitary environment and in preventing reinfestation. Children who play outside should always wash their hands before eating meals or snacks.
- Diarrhea caused by parasites such as *Cryptosporidium* may be severe in malnourished or immunodeficient children, and recovery is achieved only after renutrition or treatment of the immunodeficiency (Gendrel et al, 2003).

Patient Education—Food Safety

- Discuss safe handling and cooking methods for pork and other meats.
- Discuss proper use of thermometers, hand washing, food holding, and storage.

INTESTINAL PARASITES—CITED REFERENCES

Ali SA, Hill DR. Intestinal parasites increase the dietary lysine requirement in chronically undernourished Indian men. *Am J Clin Nutr.* 78:1145, 2003.

Gendrel D, et al. Parasitic diarrhea in normal and malnourished children. *Fundam Clin Pharmacol.* 17:189, 2003.

Hagel I, et al. Defective regulation of the protective IgE response against intestinal helminth *Ascaris lumbricoides* in malnourished children. *J Trop Pediatr.* 49:136, 2003.

Kucik CJ, et al Common intestinal parasites. *Am Fam Physician.* 69:1161, 2004.

Kurpad AV, et al. Intestinal parasites increase the dietary lysine requirement in chronically undernourished Indian men. *Am J Clin Nutr.* 78:1145, 2003.

Smith A, et al. Deficiencies in selenium and/or vitamin E lower the resistance of mice to *Heligmosomoides polygyrus* infections. *J Nutr.* 135:830, 2005.

Steer P. The epidemiology of preterm labor—a global perspective. *J Perinat Med.* 33:273, 2005.

MULTIPLE ORGAN DYSFUNCTION SYNDROME

NUTRITIONAL ACUITY RANKING: LEVEL 4

DEFINITIONS AND BACKGROUND

Multiple organ dysfunction syndrome (MODS) involves two or more systems in failure at the same time (e.g., renal, hepatic, cardiac, or respiratory). The condition is also called multiple organ failure (MOF). Sepsis is the leading cause of admission to intensive care units in the United States; MOF warrants hospitalization and intensive care unit support (Marik, 2004).

Although the treatment of sepsis is complex and multimodal, nutrition support plays an important role in the management of these patients. The diagnosis of sepsis, disease category, severity of illness, and change in sepsis severity and organ function over time affect the delivery of nutrition support.

Gut injury and impaired gut barrier function have a high impact on the development of MODS. Enteral nutrition using the physiological pathway (the gastrointestinal [GI] tract) provides the intestinal mucosa with nutrients, which is thought to reduce bacterial translocation and septic complications. Studies have suggested beneficial effects of immune-enhancing diets for systemic inflammatory response syndrome (SIRS) and MOF, especially after trauma or surgery.

In critical illness, glutamine levels are much higher in the duodenal mucosa than during starvation; glutamine supplementation may be beneficial (De-Souza and Greene, 2005). While arginine supplementation may improve outcomes, controversy continues surrounding its long-term use in septic patients (Grimble, 2005; Ochoa et al, 2004; Wilmore, 2004; Zaloga et al, 2004).

The use of specific nutrients to modify immune, inflammatory, and metabolic processes has been favorable (Heys et al, 2005). Trace elements and antioxidant nutrients, especially selenium, are important in critical care and may reduce mortality (Grimble et al, 2005; Heyland et al, 2005). Vitamin E levels tend to be low and may be supplemented accordingly (Bulger and Maier, 2003). Use of omega-3 fatty acids is also important in this population (Grimble, 2005).

Cytokines are direct mediators for MOF (Halbertsma et al, 2005). Mucosal lesions and increased intestinal permeability may cause translocation of bacteria and endotoxins, initiating local or systemic inflammatory response syndrome (SIRS). MOF is often triggered by tumor necrosis factor alpha and by a cytokine cascade (interleukin-6 and perhaps other interleukins). Stress hyperglycemia potentiates the proinflammatory response, while insulin has the opposite effect; tight glycemic control is important (Marik and Raghavan, 2004).

Lactate level is often used as a prognostic indicator of problems with tissue perfusion and may be predictive of a favorable outcome if it normalizes within 48 hours (Fall and

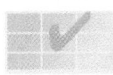

Szerlip, 2005). High baseline serum cortisol level is also a marker of severity and poor prognosis; random cortisol level <20 g/dL in a highly stressed patient (with respiratory failure, hypotension) may diagnose adrenal insufficiency, which should be treated (Marik et al, 2005). Early aggressive resuscitation of critically ill patients limits or reverses tissue dysoxia and may prevent progression to organ dysfunction and improve outcome (Marik, 2005).

INTERVENTION: OBJECTIVES

- Stabilize electrolyte and hemodynamic balances. Remove or control sources of organ dysfunction, such as bacterial translocation. Early identification and aggressive management of MOF is essential (Rivers et al, 2005).
- Provide continuous administration of at least minimal enteral nutrition in order to prevent gut mucosa atrophy. Provide nutritional support in appropriate mode(s); progress to enteral or oral nutrition as rapidly as possible to preserve gut and promote immune system integrity.
- Support organs with appropriate substrate. "Immunonutrition" uses special formulas supplemented with arginine, omega-3-fatty acids, ribonucleic acids, and glutamine.
- Control of hyperglycemia is very important to lessen infection and sepsis (Butler et al, 2005; Marik and Raghavan, 2004).
- Promote prompt and immediate responses to all changing parameters. Until organ dysfunction resolves, monitoring of weight, relevant laboratory parameters, and adequacy of nutrient intake will be important
- Consider short-term as well as long-term consequences of all actions (e.g., treatments must incorporate a consensus of opinions about which therapy precedes another).
- Manage complications, such as anemia, gastric reflux, and delayed bowel motility.
- Promote wound healing if surgery is required.
- Prevent additional sepsis. Promote recovery and improved well-being.

INTERVENTION: FOOD AND NUTRITION

- If there is gastric reflux or delayed bowel motility, a nasoduodenal or jejunal feeding tube or feeding jejunostomy is required. With enteral nutrition (EN), ensure that feeding is appropriate. Evaluate organ function and provide a correctly calculated feeding for patient's diagnosis and condition (e.g., a patient with hepatic and renal failure will require a carefully chosen feeding product). Consider using an immunoenhanced or glutamine-enriched product to preserve gut integrity and to restore normal organ functioning.
- Review current vitamin and mineral intakes; adjust according to changing needs. Antioxidants may play a role in supporting recovery.
- Do not use excesses of iron, zinc, polyunsaturated fatty acids (PUFAs), and linoleic acid—especially parenterally—because of their effects on the immune system.
- When possible, return to oral feeding to acquire the benefits of phytochemicals from whole foods.
- Patients requiring ventilator support may need a higher lipid content in their feeding, even with cardiac failure.

CLINICAL INDICATORS

Clinical/History

- Height
- Weight
- BMI
- Dry weight
- Weight changes
- Edema, ascites
- Diet history
- Temperature
- I & O
- BP
- Ultrasonography
- Echocardiography
- Electroencephalogram (EEG)

Lab Work

- Serum procalcitonin (PCT)
- BUN (often elevated)
- Creat (often elevated)
- ALT, AST (elevated)
- CRP
- Na+, K+
- Ca++, Mg++
- Cl−
- Creatine kinase (CK)
- Phosphorus
- Gluc—serum, urine
- Serum insulin
- Lactic acid (elevated)—imbalance between production and clearance of lactate
- Serum pH <7.35 (acidosis)
- Alanine, pyruvate (accumulation or retention)
- Alb, transthyretin
- CRP
- pCO_2, pO_2
- Chol—high-density lipoprotein, low-density lipoprotein profile
- Trig
- Glomerular filtration rate (GFR)
- TLC, WBC
- H & H
- Serum Fe
- TIBC
- Serum phosphorous (PO_4)
- Serum folate
- Serum zinc

Common Drugs Used and Potential Side Effects

- Hypertonic saline solution is commonly used to attenuate MOF (Cielsa et al, 2000).
- Anti-inflammatory treatment is vital for intervention in severe infectious disease.
- All medications should be reviewed for potential drug–nutrient incompatibility and stability with formulas. Try to avoid inclusion of medications with EN products because of drug–nutrient interactions and because drugs may then be less available to patient.
- Drug metabolism with the liver cytochrome P-450 (CYP) system is important in interactions that can result in drug toxicities, reduced pharmacological effect, and adverse drug reactions (Fujita, 2004). Foods consisting of complex chemical mixtures, such as fruits, alcoholic beverages, teas, and herbs, possess the ability to inhibit or induce the activity of CYP3A4 (Fujita, 2004). Avoid use of grapefruit or other citrus juices because they inhibit intestinal CYP3A4, which may promote drug toxicity (Flanagan, 2005).
- Review all vitamin-mineral supplements and enteral products to determine whether potential of hypervitaminosis and mineral toxicities exists.

- Insulin may be required because of the hyperglycemia that occurs with stress.
- With continuous seizures, lorazepam or anticonvulsants may be needed. Weight and appetite changes are common if used long term.

Herbs, Botanicals, and Supplements

- Herbs and botanical supplements should not be used without discussing with physician. Herbs often possess the ability to inhibit or induce the activity of CYP3A4 (Fujita, 2004).
- Use of Chinese herbs for reducing inflammatory reaction is being studied for enhancement of Western medicines.

INTERVENTION: NUTRITION EDUCATION, COUNSELING, CARE MANAGEMENT

- When possible, discuss implications of organ system dysfunction in relation to nutritional support. Include a realistic assessment of potential for recovery and use of EN in the home setting, as discussed with physician.
- Family should be included in discussions about nutritional support measures that are taken. As appropriate, prepare patient and family for home nutritional needs and total parenteral nutrition/EN/oral diet requirements.
- Alleviate fears associated with eating or nutritional support therapies.
- Discuss any signs or problems that should require professional intervention.

MULTIPLE ORGAN DYSFUNCTION SYNDROME—CITED REFERENCES

Bulger EM, Maier RV. An argument for vitamin E supplementation in the management of systemic inflammatory response syndrome. *Shock* 19:99, 2003.
Butler SO, et al. Relationship between hyperglycemia and infection in critically ill patients. *Pharmacotherapy* 25:963, 2005.
Cielsa DJ, et al. Hypertonic saline inhibits neutrophil (PMN) priming via attenuation of p38 MAPK signaling. *Shock* 14:265, 2000.
De-Souza DA, Greene LJ. Intestinal permeability and systemic infections in critically ill patients: effect of glutamine. *Crit Care Med.* 33:1125, 2005.
Fall PJ, Szerlip HM. Lactic acidosis: from sour milk to septic shock. *J Intensive Care Med.* 20:255, 2005.
Flanagan D. Understanding the grapefruit-drug interaction. *Gen Dent.* 53:282, 2005.
Fujita K. Food-drug interactions via human cytochrome P450 3A (CYP3A). *Drug Metabol Drug Interact.* 20:195, 2004.
Grimble RF. Immunonutrition. *Curr Opin Gastroenterol.* 21:216, 2005.
Halbertsma FJ, et al. Cytokines and biotrauma in ventilator-induced lung injury: a critical review of the literature. *Neth J Med.* 63:382, 2005.
Heyland DK, et al. Antioxidant nutrients: a systematic review of trace elements and vitamins in the critically ill patient. *Intensive Care Med.* 31:327, 2005.
Heys SD, et al. Nutrition and the surgical patient: triumphs and challenges. *Surgeon* 3:139, 2005.
Marik PE. Monitoring therapeutic interventions in critically ill septic patients. *Nutr Clin Pract.* 19:423, 2004.
Marik PE. Regional carbon dioxide monitoring to assess the adequacy of tissue perfusion. *Curr Opin Crit Care.* 11:245, 2005.
Marik PE, et al. The hepatoadrenal syndrome: a common yet unrecognized clinical condition. *Crit Care Med.* 33:1254, 2005.
Marik PE, Raghavan M. Stress-hyperglycemia, insulin and immunomodulation in sepsis. *Intensive Care Med.* 30:748, 2004.
Ochoa JB, et al. A rational use of immune enhancing diets: when should we use dietary arginine supplementation? *Nutr Clin Pract.* 19:216, 2004.
Rivers EP, et al. Early and innovative interventions for severe sepsis and septic shock: taking advantage of a window of opportunity. *CMAJ.* 173:1054, 2005.
Wilmore D. Enteral and parenteral arginine supplementation to improve medical outcomes in hospitalized patients. *J Nutr.* 134:2863S, 2004.
Zaloga GP, et al. Arginine: mediator or modulator of sepsis? *Nutr Clin Pract.* 19:201, 2004.

SEPSIS AND SYSTEMIC INFLAMMATORY RESPONSE

NUTRITIONAL ACUITY RANKING: LEVEL 4

DEFINITIONS AND BACKGROUND

Sepsis involves a systemic inflammatory response with infection that has spread to other areas. Sepsis may be a complication of vascular access devices or intravenous catheters and may be bacterial or fungal in origin. Like the stress response, the inflammatory reaction is crucial for survival and is meant to be tailored to the stimulus and time (Elenkov et al, 2005). Severe sepsis leading to shock is a common cause of death in critically ill patients.

A systemic inflammatory reaction results in stimulation of four major programs: the acute-phase reaction, the sickness syndrome, the pain program, and the stress response, mediated by the hypothalamic-pituitary-adrenal axis and the sympathetic nervous system (Elenkov et al, 2005). In sepsis, activated phagocytes release leukocytic endogenous mediators; hepatic uptake of amino acids and increased prostaglandin synthesis occur. Symptoms and signs of sepsis include fever, elevated white blood cells (WBC), pus, catabolism of lean body mass (LBM), and decreased glucose tolerance.

Called septicemia when involving the bloodstream, sepsis usually occurs from gram-negative or gram-positive bacteria (bacteremia). Diseases caused by group A *Streptococcus* (GAS) include acute rheumatic fever, rheumatic heart disease, poststreptococcal glomerulonephritis, and invasive infections; GAS is an important cause of morbidity and mortality, and new prevention strategies are needed (Carapetis et al, 2005). Pathogenic *Escherichia coli* cause infections such as urinary tract infection and meningitis, which are prevalent and associated with considerable morbidity (Kim et al, 2005).

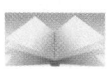

Predictors of bacteremia in elderly individuals include poor immune response and poor functional status (Gavazzi et al, 2005). *Yersinia enterocolitis* can cause bacteremia or abdominal abscess, especially in states of iron overload. Neonatal sepsis is a major cause of death among infants, especially those who are low in birth weight. In addition, while sepsis during pregnancy is uncommon, it is potentially fatal (Fernandez-Perez et al, 2005).

Natural killer cells are a crucial component of the innate immune response to various viruses, fungi, parasites, and bacteria (Fauci et al, 2005). Cytokines (tumor necrosis factor [TNF] and interleukin [IL]-1 and IL-6) regulate hepatic protein responses, with nitrogen turnover and loss from skeletal muscle, connective tissue, and gut (Elenkov et al, 2005). Immune status is altered in patients with sepsis or systemic inflammatory response syndrome (SIRS); reduced TNF production occurs (Cavaillon et al, 2005). This is a major shift in our understanding about sepsis (i.e., the immunosuppression rather than an excessive inflammatory response).

Host defense peptides have a role in feedback modulation of inflammation (Bowdish and Hancock, 2005). While albumin, transthyretin, and transferrin have a transport role in the body, acute-phase proteins (C-reactive protein, alpha-acid glycoprotein, and alpha-trypsin) help with host defense. These parameters go down in sepsis independent of nutritional status; monitor all protein levels as markers of inflammation in this population.

Metabolic responses in sepsis include increases in adrenocorticotropic hormone (ACTH), aldosterone, and catecholamines (with increased gluconeogenesis, glycolysis, proteolysis, and lipolysis). Decreased triiodothyronine (T3) may reflect increased tissue levels that occur with tissue degradation and increased mobilized triglycerides. Improvements in the management of respiratory failure, sepsis, and multiple organ system failure have frequently resulted from improvement in oncology and critical care practices (Sullivan et al, 2005).

Vitamin D as 1,25-dihydroxyvitamin D may play a role in immune activation of endothelial cells during gram-negative bacterial infections and may play a role in adjuvant treatment of gram-negative sepsis (Equils et al, 2006).

Acute renal failure is often a complication of underlying conditions such as sepsis, trauma, and multiple-organ failure in critically ill patients (Wooley et al, 2005). Dietary manipulation will be needed.

Enteral feeding is preferred over parenteral feeding in septic patients. Catheter infection is a risk with total parenteral nutrition (TPN) in septic patients. Overfeeding, which is easy with TPN, may explain why TPN sometimes increases sepsis (Jeejeeboy, 2001).

INTERVENTION: OBJECTIVES

- Treat the infection or drain a local site when possible.
- Support the body's antimicrobial defense system and keep the environment as germ free as possible. Use strict guidelines and protocols for insertion, care, and maintenance of any catheters and feeding tubes.
- Prevent septic shock with increased cardiac output, tachycardia, low blood pressure, decreased renal output, and warm flushed skin. Prevent multiple organ system dysfunction.
- Meet increased energy needs (mild infection elevates resting energy expenditure between 15–40%; sepsis increases it by 40–70% and doubles nitrogen losses). Do not overfeed.
- Promote tissue repair and wound healing. Protein turnover is often 30–50% higher than normal.
- Treat nausea, vomiting, and anorexia.
- Prevent or treat metabolic derangements during feeding process, such as hyperglycemia, glycosuria, hyperosmolar/nonketotic coma, electrolyte abnormalities (e.g., decreased potassium, decreased phosphate, elevated chloride), osmotic diarrhea, and fluid overload.
- Correct anemia, which prevents tissue oxygenation.

INTERVENTION: FOOD AND NUTRITION

- Protein should be provided in levels of 1.5–2.0 g/kg daily. Branched-chain amino acids (BCAAs) are useful for energy because they do not need to be metabolized to glucose. Use BCAAs and a higher percentage of arginine compared with a lower percentage of taurine/methionine/cysteine and a lower percentage of aromatic amino acids (phenylalanine, tyrosine, and threonine).
- Provide calories at 30–35 kcal/kg (approximately 350–450 g of carbohydrates as a daily average, and 20% kcal as fat).
- When patient can eat, soft diet and liquids of high nutrient and energy value are beneficial.
- Vitamins A, C, D, and K, thiamin, and folic acid may become depleted with infection. Supplement or include in oral intake.
- Urinary excretion of phosphorus, potassium, magnesium, zinc, and chromium also occur; monitor for signs of malnutrition. Replace in feedings or diet as appropriate.
- Include omega-3 fatty acids (Babcock et al, 2005; Calder, 2004). With oral diet, increase use of salmon, tuna, sardines, herring, and mackerel; include walnuts and flaxseed when possible.
- Monitor fluid requirements and intake carefully. There must be adequate levels to excrete wastes properly.

CLINICAL INDICATORS

Clinical/History

Height
Weight
BMI
Diet history
I & O
BP
Tachycardia
Temperature

Lab Work

CRP
Chol (decreased)
pO_2, pCO_2
Gluc (altered)
Glucagon (increased)
Serum insulin
Plasma lactate
WBC, TLC
Transferrin
Trig (increased)
AST (increased)
BUN, Creat
Urinary urea nitrogen (UUN)
Alb, transthyretin
Retinol-binding protein (RBP)
Na+, K+
Ca++, Mg++
Cl−
H & H
Serum Fe
N balance
T3 (decreased)
5-Hydroxyindole acetic acid (5-HIAA) (increased)
Phosphate (decreased)
Ketones
Osmolality

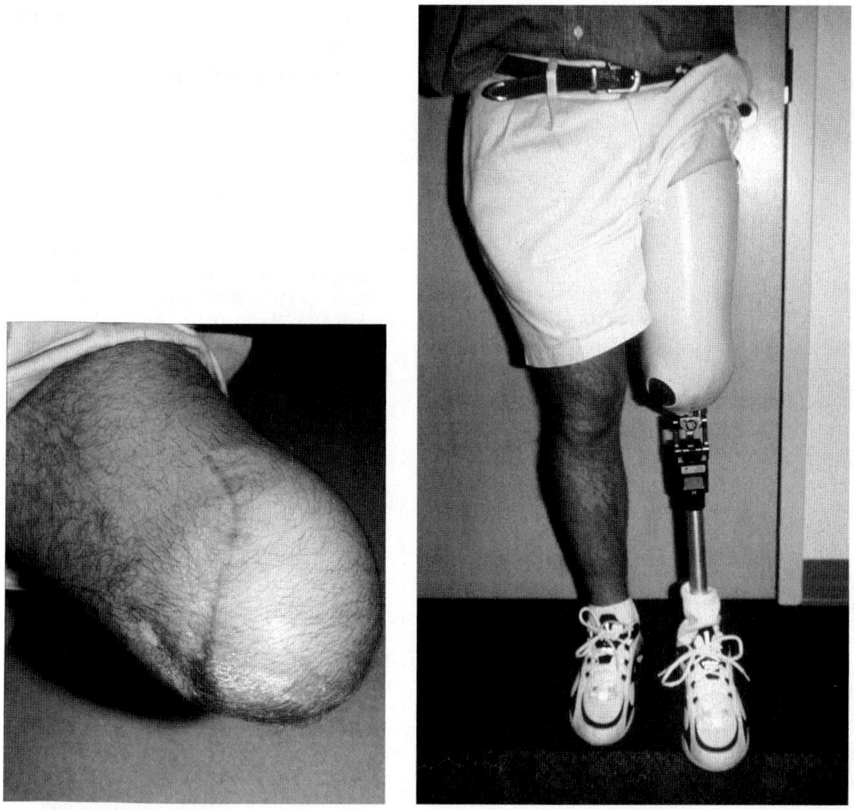

A B

) **(A)** Trauma resulting in below knee amputation. **(B)** Leg prosthesis after traumatic injury. (From Bucholz RW, Heckman JD. *Rock-'s fractures in adults.* 5th ed. Philadelphia: Lippincott, Williams & Wilkins, 2001.)

INTERVENTION: OBJECTIVES

nd monitor extent of injury and resulting prob-
store hemodynamic and metabolic functions and
se and fluid balance.
infection, respiratory failure, shock, sepsis, and
ion injury.
ing, use gut if possible. Enteral nutrition is more
us and poses lower risks than parenteral nutri-
educes infection rates and shortens intensive care
U) and hospital length of stay of critically ill pa-
rimble, 2005). Determine gastrointestinal (GI)
; provide nutrients in most effective mode.
healing and rapid recovery.
eus, fistula, glucose abnormalities, and other
ations.
nosocomial infections that are commonly associ-
increased use of ICU resources and length of
ber et al, 2005).
nitrogen losses; promote nitrogen balance. In-
f glutamine and arginine may be indicated (Pan
4).
evated energy requirements (up by 20–45%).
oteins and lean body mass.
overfeeding with respiratory distress from in-
arbon dioxide production.
ne and monitor fluid requirements and balance.
adequately but do not overhydrate because per-
ositive fluid balance in older surgical patients
prolongs mechanical ventilation (Epstein and Peerless, 2006).

- Promote rehabilitation.
- Correct anorexia and depression; improve quality of life.

INTERVENTION: FOOD AND NUTRITION

- **Day 1: Immediately**—Intravenous feedings are given for fluid resuscitation for approximately 24 hours until stable. Life support measures and careful monitoring will be offered.
- **Days 2–5: Transition Phase**—Assess changing status. Implement nutrition by the most effective means (oral, enteral, or parenteral). Injury location and extent will dictate most desirable mode. Controversy exists regarding the optimal nutrition regimen; therefore, individualize for each patient (Thompson and Fuhrman, 2005). Data support the use of enteral over parenteral nutrition to reduce infectious complications and cost; initiation of enteral feedings within 24–48 hours of injury or admission to ICU generally reduces infectious complications (Kattelmann et al, 2006). Feeding patients in the semirecumbent rather than supine position is associated with reduced aspiration pneumonia and pharyngoesophageal formula reflux (Kattelmann et al, 2006). Provide adequate energy and nutrients: 35–45 kcal/kg and 1.5–2 g protein/kg. Advance feeding rate over several days; gastrostomy may be useful in head/neck trauma. Actual

Common Drugs Used and Potential Side Effects

- Antibiotics are used for bacterial sepsis; monitor for side effects and GI distress.
- Antiseptic-impregnated catheters, such as those with minocycline-rifampicin or chlorhexidine/silver sulfadiazine, may be needed to reduce catheter-related blood stream infections.
- Biological agents, such as IL-2, IL-12, IL-11, and/or IL-18, should be studied to identify new approaches to enhance host defense and thereby decrease the incidence of sepsis and high risk of morbidity and mortality in neonates (Satwani et al, 2005).
- Insulin may be needed. Monitor for signs of hyper- and hypoglycemia.
- Iron and zinc are bacterial nutrients and should not be used automatically in TPN or parenteral nutrition solutions if patient is septic or at risk for sepsis.
- Steroids may be used and can cause greater nitrogen depletion and hyperglycemia, sodium retention, and potassium losses. Monitor carefully.

Herbs, Botanicals, and Supplements

- Herbs and botanical supplements should not be used without discussing with physician.

INTERVENTION: NUTRITION EDUCATION, COUNSELING, CARE MANAGEMENT

- Use of aseptic techniques for feedings and meals will be essential.
- Need for a well-managed convalescence and gradual refeeding process will be needed to support patient's resistance and immunity. Terminat malnutrition, and reinfection energy malnutrition.

SEPSIS AND SYSTEMIC INFLAMM CITED REFERENCES

Babcock TA, et al. Experimental studies defi flammatory mechanisms and abrogation *Nutr Clin Pract.* 20:62, 2005.
Bowdish DM, Hancock RE. Anti-endotoxin fence peptides and proteins. *J Endotoxin I*
Calder PC. Omega-3 fatty acids, inflammatio postsurgical and critically ill patients. *Lip*
Carapetis JR et al. The global burden of g *Lancet Infect Dis.* 5:685, 2005.
Cavaillon JM, et al. Reprogramming of circ *J Endotoxin Res.* 11:311, 2005.
Elenkov IJ, et al. Cytokine dysregulation, inf *roimmunomodulation* 12:255, 2005.
Equils O, et al. 1,25-Dihydroxyvitamin D inhi immune activation in human endothelia 2006.
Fauci AS, et al. NK cells in HIV infection: pa for ambush. *Nat Rev Immunol.* 5:835, 20
Fernandez-Perez ER, et al. Sepsis during pr 2005.
Gavazzi G, et al. Nosocomial bacteremia ir mortality. *Aging Clin Exp Res.* 17:337, 20
Jeejeeboy KN. Enteral and parenteral nut *Proc Nutr Soc.* 60:399, 2001.
Kim BY, et al. Invasion processes of patho *crobiol.* 295:463, 2005.
Satwani P, et al. Dysregulation of express tokine genes and its association with t cytic and cellular immunity. *Biol Neon*
Sullivan KJ, et al. Critical care of the p recipient in 2005. *Pediatr Transplant.* 9
Wooley JA, et al. Metabolic and nutrition critically ill patients requiring contir *Nutr Clin Pract.* 20:176, 2005.

TRAUMA

NUTRITIONAL ACUITY RANKING: LEVEL 3

DEFINITIONS AND BACKGROUND

Trauma is caused by major injury or accidents (50% are related to traffic accidents). Trauma is now the third leading cause of death and the number one killer of people younger than 45 years of age (Compton and Rhee, 2005).

Multiple traumas involve at least two injuries. Long-bone fractures, pelvis or vertebral fractures, and damage to body cavities (head, thorax, or abdomen) generally are involved. Vascular injuries comprise 3% of all traumas (Compton and Rhee, 2005). See Figure 15-10.

Elevated plasma catecholamines, glucocorticoids, glucagon, and glucose occur in response to injury. Reperfusion injury (RI), a potential life-threatening disorder, represents an acute inflammator ischemia resulting from my surgery, and trauma (Zhang et are the organs most affected b

Nutritional support must b agement of trauma victims (I caused by hypercatabolism a the severity of illness (Wooley a major protein source for amino acids (BCAAs) are m 2005). Nitrogen excretion in 7 days, and eventually stabili increase synthesis and decre cle protein when amino acid

delivery of 14–18 kcal/kg/d or 60–70% of goal is associated with improved outcomes, whereas greater intake may not be beneficial in some populations (Kattelmann et al, 2006). Blue food coloring should not be used with enteral feedings due to its limited sensitivity for aspiration and some risk of mortality (Kattelmann et al, 2006).

- **Days 5–10: Adaptive Phase**—Use products with glutamine, arginine, and high percentage of branched-chain amino acids; include lipids. Osmolarity should be monitored to be close to 300 mOsm. In general, 25 kcal/kg/d is an acceptable and achievable target intake, but patients with trauma may require almost twice as much energy during the acute phase of their illness (Reid, 2004). Provide 1.5–2 g protein/kg. Carbohydrate (CHO) should be given as 5 mg/kg/min. A diet providing 50% CHO, 15% protein, and 35% fat should be adequate. A slight increase in vitamin-mineral intake should be addressed, with B-complex vitamins, zinc, and vitamins A and C in particular.
- **Day 11 Onward: Rehabilitative Phase**—Patient can be weaned to oral diet, if possible, and off ventilator support. Liquid to regular diets are usually tolerated at this time.

CLINICAL INDICATORS

Clinical/History	BP	Serum Fe
Height	Arteriography	TLC
Weight before trauma	X-rays, computed tomography	WBC
Weight after trauma		Chol, Trig
% weight change	**Lab Work**	Phosphorus
Resting energy expenditure from indirect calorimetry	CRP	BUN, Creat
BMI	Alb, transthyretin (fluid shifts can affect serum levels)	Gluc (increased)
Diet history	Na+, K+	Creatine phosphokinase (CPK) (increased)
Temperature	Ca++, Mg++	pCO_2, pO_2
I & O	Cl−	Bilirubin, AST (increased)
	H & H	Serum amino acids
		N balance

Common Drugs Used and Potential Side Effects

- Albumin therapy is considered in trauma, hypovolemia, shock, burns, hypoalbuminemia, cardiopulmonary bypass, acute respiratory distress syndrome, hemodialysis, and volume resuscitation (Mendez et al, 2005).
- Analgesics may have an effect on nutritional status. Evaluate individually. Lidocaine can be used to alleviate neuropathic pain.
- Antibiotics generally are used to reduce bacterial infection. Monitor for GI distress and side effects.
- Insulin may be used for hyperglycemia. Monitor for meal and snack timing.
- Barbiturates are often used for closed head injury; they will decrease metabolic rate.
- Promotility agents are associated with reduced gastric residual volume in tube-fed patients (Kattelmann et al, 2006).

Herbs, Botanicals, and Supplements

- Herbs and botanical supplements should not be used without discussing with physician.
- Capsaicin and resveratrol have been used for some patients to decrease inflammation after trauma, but more studies are needed.

INTERVENTION: NUTRITION EDUCATION, COUNSELING, CARE MANAGEMENT

- Need for specific nutrients should be discussed, according to the mode tolerated.
- Rehabilitation should progress according to individual requirements and injury sites, side effects, and complications.

TRAUMA—CITED REFERENCES

Compton C, Rhee R. Peripheral vascular trauma. *Perspect Vasc Surg Endovasc Ther.* 17:297, 2005.

Epstein CD, Peerless JR. Weaning readiness and fluid balance in older critically ill surgical patients. *Am J Crit Care.* 15:54, 2006.

Farber MS, et al. Reducing costs and patient morbidity in the enterally fed intensive care unit patient. *J Parenter Enteral Nutr.* 29:62S, 2005.

Fox VJ, et al. Nutritional support in the critically injured. *Crit Care Nurs Clin North Am.* 16:559, 2004.

Grimble RF. Immunonutrition. *Curr Opin Gastroenterol.* 21:216, 2005.

Kattelmann KK, et al. Preliminary evidence for a medical nutrition therapy protocol: enteral feedings for critically ill patients. *J Am Diet Assoc.* 106:1226, 2006.

Laviano A, et al. Branched-chain amino acids: the best compromise to achieve anabolism? *Curr Opin Clin Nutr Metab Care.* 8:408, 2005.

Mendez CM, et al. Albumin therapy in clinical practice. *Nutr Clin Pract.* 20:314, 2005.

Pan M, et al. Arginine transport in catabolic disease states. *J Nutr.* 134:2826S, 2004.

Reid CL. Nutritional requirements of surgical and critically-ill patients: do we really know what they need? *Proc Nutr Soc.* 63:467, 2004.

Thompson C, Fuhrman MP. Nutrients and wound healing: still searching for the magic bullet. *Nutr Clin Pract.* 20:331, 2005.

Wooley JA, et al. Metabolic and nutritional aspects of acute renal failure in critically ill patients requiring continuous renal replacement therapy. *Nutr Clin Pract.* 20:176, 2005.

Zhang M, et al. Identification of the target self-antigens in reperfusion injury. *J Exp Med.* 203:141, 2006.

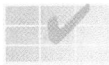

SECTION 16

Renal Disorders

CHIEF ASSESSMENT FACTORS

Seven Warning Signs of Kidney and Urinary Tract Disease

- Burning or Difficulty During Urination
- High Blood Pressure
- More Frequent Urination, Especially at Night
- Pain in Small of Back Just Below Ribs, Not Aggravated by Movement
- Passage of Bloody-Appearing Urine
- Puffiness Around Eyes
- Swelling of Hands and Feet, Especially in Children

Other Factors

- Proteinuria (Microalbuminuria)
- Uremia
- Bone Pain, Altered Height or Lean Body Mass
- Unbalanced Calcium:Phosphorus Ratios
- Altered Lipid and Amino Acid Levels
- Abnormal Blood Urea Nitrogen (BUN):Creatinine Ratio
- Presence or History of Urinary Tract Infections
- Frequent Weight Shifts
- Leg Cramps
- Weakness, Pallor, Anemia
- Itching and Dry Skin
- Loss of Appetite
- Difficulty Sleeping
- Serum Creatinine >1.7 mg/dL (Chronic Kidney Disease)
- Changes in Glomerular Filtration Rate (GFR)
- Protein–Energy Malnutrition or Wasting

OVERVIEW OF RENAL NUTRITION

According to the National Institute of Diabetes and Digestive and Kidney Diseases (NIDDK), an estimated 4.5% of adults 20 years of age and older have physiological evidence of chronic kidney disease (7.4 million adults), determined as a moderately or severely reduced glomerular filtration rate. Increased serum levels of inflammation contribute to development of protein–energy malnutrition in renal patients (Mehrotra and Kopple, 2001). Inflammation causes increased levels of specific cytokines (interleukin-6 and tumor necrosis factor alpha) and acute-phase proteins (C-reactive protein and serum amyloid A); loss of muscle mass; changes in plasma composition; and decreases in serum albumin, transthyretin, and transferrin (Kaysen, 2001). Inflammation alters lipoprotein structure and function as well as endothelial structure and function to favor atherogenesis; it also increases atherogenic proteins in serum such as fibrinogen and lipoprotein. Because most renal patients have cardiovascular disease and many have diabetes, a multifactorial approach is important.

The Kidney Disease Outcomes Quality Initiative (KDOQI) guidelines introduced a classification of chronic kidney disease (CKD) based on the level of kidney function (Mariat et al, 2005). They also suggest the use of standardized practices in renal nutrition and that a dietitian with special expertise provide those services. A registered dietitian with renal experience should be a central and integral part of the dietary management of both pediatric and adult patients (National Kidney Foundation, 2000). Registered dietitians are proficient in assessment and ongoing evaluation of patient's nutrition status and development of the nutrition plan of care and diet prescription. All anthropometric indices (weight, height, and body mass index), laboratory values, and dietary intakes deteriorate with worsening renal function (Norman et al, 2000).

In pediatrics, a registered dietitian skilled in the evaluation of growth as well as in physical, developmental, educational, and social needs will be needed. Assessing the child's nutritional status, developing the nutrition plan of care, providing education and counseling at the appropriate age level for patients, family, or caretakers, monitoring patient's nutritional status, evaluating adherence to nutrition prescription, assessing and monitoring adequacy of dialysis, and documentation of these services is all part of the job of the registered dietitian. Registered dietitians should manage the nutrition care and provide nutrition counseling for patients prior to starting dialysis and for those who have lost a kidney transplant and are returning to dialysis.

Tables 16-1 to 16-3 give a brief background of the functions of the kidneys and effects of renal activity. Figure 16-1 shows the anatomy of the kidney.

TABLE 16-1 Human Kidney Functions

1. Excretion of waste products of metabolism (urea, uric acid, creatinine)
2. Homeostasis:

Acid–Base Balance

The kidneys regulate the pH by eliminating excess H ion concentration, called augmentation mineral ion concentration, and water composition of the blood. By exchanging hydronium ions and hydroxyl ions, the blood plasma is maintained by the kidney at a neutral pH of 7.4. Urine is either acidic (pH 5) or alkaline (pH 8).

The pH is maintained through four main protein transporters: NHE3 (a sodium-hydrogen exchanger), V-type H-ATPase (an isoform of the hydrogen ATPase), NBC1 (a sodium-bicarbonate cotransporter), and AE1 (an anion exchanger that exchanges chloride for bicarbonate).

Potassium and phosphate require renal control as well.

Blood Pressure

Sodium ions are controlled in a homeostatic process involving aldosterone, which increases sodium ion absorption in the distal convoluted tubules. When blood pressure becomes low, renin is secreted by cells of the distal convoluted tubule, which are sensitive to pressure. Renin acts on a blood protein, angiotensinogen, converting it to angiotensin I. Angiotensin I is then converted by the angiotensin-converting enzyme (ACE) in the lung capillaries to angiotensin II, which stimulates the secretion of aldosterone by the adrenal cortex, which then affects the kidney tubules.

Aldosterone stimulates an increase in the reabsorption of sodium ions from the kidney tubules, which causes an increase in the volume of water that is reabsorbed from the tubule. This increase in water reabsorption increases the volume of blood, which ultimately raises the blood pressure.

Plasma Volume

Any rise or drop in blood osmotic pressure due to a lack or excess of water is detected by the hypothalamus, which notifies the pituitary gland via negative feedback. A lack of water causes the posterior pituitary gland to secrete antidiuretic hormone, which results in water reabsorption and an increase in urine concentration. Tissue fluid concentration thus returns to a mean of 98%. The kidneys therefore regulate osmolality of body fluid; body fluid is two-thirds extracellular and one-third intracellular.

3. Hormone secretion:

Erythropoietin secretion for red blood cell (RBC) production. Erythropoietin deficiency is common in chronic renal anemia.

Urodilatin is a natriuretic peptide that mediates natriuresis.

Vitamin D_3 conversion, for calcium:phosphorus homeostasis: the kidney accomplishes the final stage of conversion of vitamin D to its active form, 1,25-dihydroxyvitamin D, in the proximal tubule.

4. Carnitine synthesis to carry fatty acids from cytoplasm to mitochondria, for heart and skeletal muscle fuel. Note: lysine, methionine, vitamin C, iron, vitamin B_6, and niacin are needed to produce carnitine.
5. Glucose homeostasis: Gluconeogenesis and glucose counterregulation (Gerich et al, 2001)
6. Prostaglandin E_2 is a major renal cyclooxygenase metabolite of arachidonate that impacts renal hemodynamics and salt and water excretion.

Information from: Gerich J, et al. Renal gluconeogenesis: its importance in human glucose homeostasis. *Diabetes Care.* 24:382, 2001; and Wikipedia. Kidney. Accessed September 9, 2006 at http://en.wikipedia.org/wiki/Kidney.

TABLE 16-2 Stages of Chronic Kidney Disease

Stage	Description	GFR (mL/min/1.73 m^2 body surface area)
1	Kidney damage with normal or increased GFR	≥90
2	Kidney damage with mildly decreased GFR	60–89
3	Moderately decreased GFR	30–59
4	Severely decreased GFR	15–29
5	Kidney failure	<15 or dialysis

Reference: National Kidney Foundation. K/DOQI clinical practice guidelines for chronic kidney disease: evaluation, classification, and stratification. *Am J Kidney Dis.* 39:S266, 2002 (suppl 1).
GFR, glomerular filtration rate.

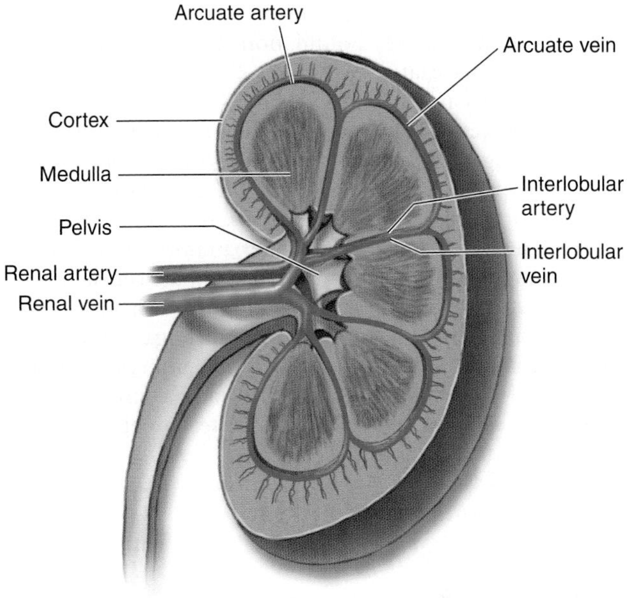

Figure 16-1 Anatomy of the normal kidney. (From Premkumar K. *The massage connection anatomy and physiology.* Baltimore: Lippincott Williams & Wilkins, 2004.)

TABLE 16-3 Management of Protein–Energy Malnutrition (PEM) in Renal Patients

Factors	Comments
Anorexia	Chronic inflammation, cardiovascular disease, diabetes mellitus, and other superimposed illnesses may produce anorexia and malnutrition; diminished appetite was associated with higher concentrations of proinflammatory cytokines.
Inflammation	Dyslipidemia and inflammation may promote renal disease via mechanisms of vascular endothelial cell dysfunction in type 2 diabetes mellitus (Lin et al, 2006).
	Serum albumin is altered by systemic inflammation, and a low serum albumin concentration is strongly associated with cardiac disease and mortality in chronic kidney disease (CKD) patients. Inflammatory cytokines, such as tumor necrosis factor (TNF)-α and interleukin-6, are associated with protein synthesis and catabolism in the body, and they downregulate albumin synthesis. Nonnutritional factors actually may be more important in determining serum albumin levels than dietary intake in CKD patients.
Lab Values	Serum creatinine concentration reflects muscle mass, somatic protein stores, and dietary protein intake. Because it predicts outcome in CKD, it may be another useful marker of nutritional status in CKD. However, creatinine levels are also affected by inflammation and other factors such as age, sex, race, residual kidney function, variation in creatinine metabolism, and dialysis dose. Clearly, other nutritional indices are needed to assess nutritional status in CKD. The assessment of dietary intake has been commonly used to assess nutritional status.
	Glomerular filtration rate (GFR) is the best measure of kidney function. GFR is the number used to figure out a person's stage of kidney disease. A math formula using the person's age, race, gender, and serum creatinine is used to calculate a GFR. A doctor will order a blood test to measure the serum creatinine level. Creatinine is a waste product that comes from muscle activity. When kidneys are working well, they remove creatinine from the blood. As kidney function slows, blood levels of creatinine rise.
	Transthyretin (transthyretin) is a good index of liver protein synthesis, but it is reabsorbed and metabolized by the proximal tubule, and serum levels rise as kidney function declines. Transthyretin levels correlate strongly with serum albumin; they provide prognostic value independent of albumin in most hemodialysis patients.
Management of Other Symptoms	Sleep disturbances, pain, erectile dysfunction, patient dissatisfaction with care, depression, symptom burden, and perception of intrusiveness of illness may all lead to poor quality of life (Kimmel and Patel, 2006), with resulting poor appetite and intake. Use of psychotherapy or antidepressants and other treatments may be indicated.
Oxidative Stress	PEM and low body mass index have been associated with increased oxidative stress and impaired endothelium-dependent vasodilation with reduced bioavailability of nitric oxide. Elevated C-reactive protein is a risk factor for mortality in CKD (Menon et al, 2005).
Wasting	Wasting may be due to anorexia, nausea, emesis, uremia, inflammation, infections, diabetes, underdialysis, or dental problems. Supplementation with branched-chain amino acids spares lean body mass during weight loss, promotes wound healing, may decrease muscle wasting with aging, and may have beneficial effects in renal disease (Tom and Nair, 2006).

Subjective Global Assessment may be used for renal patients (National Kidney Foundation, 2000). Items used to assess nutritional status are weight change over the past 6 months, dietary intake and gastrointestinal (GI) symptoms, visual assessment of subcutaneous tissue, and muscle mass. Weight change is assessed by evaluating the patient's weight during the past 6 months: loss of ≥10% of body weight over the past 6 months is severe, 5–10% is moderate, and <5% is mild; edema might obscure a greater amount of weight loss. Dietary intake is evaluated using a comparison of the patient's usual or recommended intakes to current intake. Duration and frequency of GI symptoms (e.g., nausea, vomiting, and diarrhea) are also assessed. The interviewer rates a 7-point scale with higher scores if the patient has little or no weight loss, a better dietary intake, better appetite, and the absence of GI symptoms.

REFERENCES

Kaysen G. The microinflammatory state in uremia: causes and potential consequences. *J Am Soc Nephrol.* 12:1549, 2001.

Kimmel PL, Patel SS. Quality of life in patients with chronic kidney disease: focus on end-stage renal disease treated with hemodialysis. *Semin Nephrol.* 26:68, 2006.

Lin J, et al. The association of serum lipids and inflammatory biomarkers with renal function in men with type II diabetes mellitus. *Kidney Int.* 69:336, 2006.

Mariat C, et al. Predicting glomerular filtration rate in kidney transplantation: are the K/DOQI guidelines applicable? *Am J Transplant.* 5:2698, 2005.

Mehrotra R, Kopple J. Nutritional management of maintenance dialysis patients: why aren't we doing better? *Annu Rev Nutr.* 21:343, 2001.

Menon V, et al. C-reactive protein and albumin as predictors of all-cause and cardiovascular mortality in chronic kidney disease. *Kidney Int.* 68:766, 2005.

National Kidney Foundation. Clinical practice guidelines for nutrition in chronic renal failure. K/DOQI, National Kidney Foundation. *Am J Kidney Dis.* 35:1S, 2000.

Norman L, et al. Nutrition and growth in relation to severity of renal disease in children. *Pediatr Nephrol.* 15:259, 2000.

Tom A, Nair KS. Assessment of branched-chain amino acid status and potential for biomarkers. *J Nutr.* 136:324S, 2006.

For More Information

- American Association of Kidney Patients
  http://www.aakp.org/
- American Kidney Fund
  http://www.kidneyfund.org/
- American Society of Pediatric Nephrology
  http://www.aspneph.com/
- American Urological Foundation
  http://www.afud.org
- Cyber Nephrology
  http://www.cybernephrology.org/
- Dialysis and Transplantation
  http://www.eneph.com/
- European Dialysis and Transplant Association
  http://www.era-edta.org/
- Forum of End-Stage Renal Networks
  http://www.esrdnetworks.org/index.htm
- Home Dialysis
  http://www.homedialysis.org/
- International Society of Nephrology
  http://www.isn-online.org/
- International Society for Peritoneal Dialysis
  http://www.ispd.org/
- Kidney Disease Outcomes Quality Initiative
  http://www.kidney.org/professionals/doqi/index.cfm
- Kidney Options Diet and Nutrition
  http://www.kidneyoptions.com/dietnutrition.html
- Kidney School
  http://www.kidneyschool.org/
- Medicare Dialysis Sites
  http://www.medicare.gov/Health/Dialysis.asp
- National Kidney Foundation (NKF)
  http://www.kidney.org/
- National Institutes of Health—National Kidney and Urologic Diseases Information Clearinghouse
  http://www.niddk.nih.gov
- Nephrology Calculator
  http://www.tinkershop.net/nephro.htm
- Nephrology News and Issues
  http://www.nephnews.com/
- Nephrology Links
  http://nephrologylinx.com/
- Nephron Information Center
  http://www.nephron.com/
- Nephro World
  http://www.nephroworld.com/
- Northwest Kidney Centers
  http://www.nwkidney.org/
- Renal Links
  http://www.aakp.org/AAKP/linksmall.htm
- Renal Net—Kidney Information Clearinghouse
  http://www.renalnet.org/
- Renal Physicians Association
  http://www.renalmd.org/
- Renal World
  http://www.renalworld.com/
- U.S. Renal Data System
  http://www.usrds.org/
- World Kidney Fund
  http://www.worldkidneyfund.org/

ALPORT SYNDROME, BRIGHT'S DISEASE, AND NEPHRITIS

NUTRITIONAL ACUITY RANKING: LEVEL 2–3

DEFINITIONS AND BACKGROUND

Alport syndrome (ATS) is a progressive inherited (usually X-linked) nephropathy, also called hereditary nephritis. The cause is a mutation in a gene for collagen, and this affects mostly males, in whom symptoms progress more rapidly.

ATS is characterized by irregular thinning, thickening, and splitting of the renal glomerular basement membrane and is often associated with hearing loss and ocular symptoms (Longo et al, 2006). Chronic glomerulonephritis causes progressive destruction of the glomeruli, blood in the urine, and decreased effectiveness of the kidney. Kidney function is lost, and fluids and wastes accumulate, with eventual progression to end-stage renal disease (between adolescence and age 40 years).

Hypertension, proteinuria, and edema and their relationship to kidney disease were first described by Richard Bright in the early 1800s. Subsequent studies established the central role of the kidney in hypertension through the renin-angiotensin system and extracellular volume control (Eknoyan, 2004). **Nephritis** (**Bright's disease**) involves kidney inflammation that results from a diffuse, progressive lesion affecting the renal parenchyma, interstitial tissue, and renal vascular system. The inflammation can become acute or chronic; it may result from scarlet fever, flu, or tonsillitis. Fish oils may decrease loss of renal function by affecting eicosanoid and cytokine production, altering renal dynamics, and decreasing inflammation.

INTERVENTION: OBJECTIVES

- Reduce renal workload to allow healing.
- Improve or control excretion of waste products such as urea and sodium.
- Prevent edema resulting from sodium and fluid retention.
- Prevent uremia from nitrogen retention.
- Adjust electrolyte levels as needed (e.g., sodium, potassium, and chloride).
- Prevent systemic complications, where possible, and protein catabolism, as from poor intake.
- Manage hypertension.

INTERVENTION: FOOD AND NUTRITION

- Determine fluid intake (measured output plus 500 mL insensible losses).
- Restrict sodium intake to 2–3 g if patient has hypertension or edema.
- In the case of renal failure, protein intake should be low (0.6 g/kg of adjusted edema-free body weight [BW]). Use 50% high biological value proteins to ensure positive nitrogen balance.
- Check need for vitamin A, which may be low.
- Decrease phosphorus with a low-phosphate diet (5–10 mg/kg/d).
- Provide adequate energy intake (35 kcal/kg BW).
- Use of fish oils may be beneficial to reduce inflammation.

CLINICAL INDICATORS

Clinical/History

Height
Weight
Edema-free adjusted body weight (aBWef)
Edema
Body mass index (BMI)
Diet history
Input and output (I & O)
Blood pressure (BP)
Temperature

Lab Work

Blood urea nitrogen (BUN), creatinine (Creat)
Chloride (Cl_2)
Glomerular filtration rate (GFR), creatine clearance (CrCl)
Cholesterol (Chol) (may be increased)
Albumin (Alb), transthyretin
C-reactive protein (CRP)
Na+, K+
Retinol-binding protein (RBP)
Phosphorus
Aspartate aminotransferase (AST)
Ca++
Proteinuria
Hemoglobin and hematocrit (H & H)
Serum Fe
Total iron-binding capacity (TIBC), percent saturation, serum ferritin
Parathormone (PTH)
Serum Cu (may be decreased)

Common Drugs Used and Potential Side Effects

- Antihypertensive and immunosuppressive medications are commonly used. Monitor for specific side effects, especially with long-term use.

Herbs, Botanicals, and Supplements

- Herbs and botanical supplements should not be used without discussing with physician.

INTERVENTION: NUTRITION EDUCATION, COUNSELING, CARE MANAGEMENT

- Ensure dietary measures are appropriate for patient's current status.
- Discuss ways to include more fish oils in diet.

For More Information

- Hearing Loss
  http://www.entnet.org/
- Hereditary Nephritis Foundation (Alport Syndrome)
  http://www.cc.utah.edu/~cla6202/HNF.htm

ALPORT SYNDROME, BRIGHT'S DISEASE, AND NEPHRITIS—CITED REFERENCES

Eknoyan G. On the central role of studies on the kidney in the recognition, conceptual evolution, and understanding of hypertension. *Adv Chronic Kidney Dis.* 11:192, 2004.
Longo I, et al. Autosomal recessive Alport syndrome: an in-depth clinical and molecular analysis of five families. *Nephrol Dial Transplant.* 21:665, 2006.

CHRONIC KIDNEY DISEASE AND RENAL FAILURE

NUTRITIONAL ACUITY RANKING: LEVEL 4

DEFINITIONS AND BACKGROUND

Chronic kidney disease (CKD) is characterized by the inability of kidney function to return to normal after acute kidney failure or progressive renal decline from disease. CKD causes permanent reduction in function, eventually leading to end-stage renal disease (ESRD). Excess urea and nitrogenous wastes accumulate in the bloodstream (azotemia).

Nearly 20 million Americans have some degree of CKD, which is defined as an estimated glomerular filtration rate (GFR) of less than 60 mL/min or as evidence of kidney damage by imaging study, biopsy, biochemical testing, or urine tests with an estimated GFR of more than 60 mL/min (Toto, 2005). CKD also includes kidney damage for 3 or more months involving structural or functional abnormalities.

Almost 80% of all persons with CKD have hypertension (Toto, 2005). The National Kidney Foundation clinical practice guidelines recommend a blood pressure goal of <130 mm Hg systolic and <80 mm Hg diastolic for all CKD patients (Toto, 2005). Other risk factors include diabetes, autoimmune diseases, systemic infections, urinary tract infections, kidney stones, cancer, family history of CKD, exposure to certain drugs, and low birth weight. In addition, CKD is characterized by many features of the metabolic syndrome (Shen et al, 2006).

Undiagnosed CKD is common in diabetes; incorporating estimated GFR into screening for CKD would identify individuals earlier in the natural history of the disease and enable early effective treatment (Middleton et al, 2006). The Pima Indians of Arizona have the world's highest incidence of type 2 diabetes; incidence of ESRD is 20 times higher in this group than the general U.S. population.

Current literature suggests that a low-protein, low-phosphorus diet may retard the progression of kidney disease (Kent, 2005). Potentially modifiable risk factors in CKD include: proteinuria, hypertension, dyslipidemia, anemia, oxidative stress, infections, and depression. Other modifiable risk factors affecting CKD include hyperglycemia, bone disease, and obesity (Kent, 2005).

Depending on the form of disease, renal function may be lost in a matter of days or weeks or may deteriorate slowly and gradually over the course of decades. Stages of CKD, including renal failure, are shown in Figure 16-2.

Acute renal failure (ARF) involves abrupt decline in renal function with waste retention. ARF occurs when the kidneys fail to function because of circulatory, glomerular, or tubular deficiency resulting from an abrupt cause. ARF is caused by diabetes in 43% of cases; hypertension in 23%; glomerulonephritis in 12%; polycystic kidney disease in 3%; and other causes in 18% (e.g., burns, severe crushing injuries, transfusions, antibiotics, nephrotoxicity, surgery or anesthesia, cardiac transplantation, shock, or sepsis). ARF occurs in about 5% of surgical or trauma cases; frequently, this is reversible. The patient gradually improves, although some loss of function may be permanent. ARF in acute care may be reversible, but mortality is still 50–75%. When toxic accumulation occurs, it may be fatal. In children, a cause recently has been hemolytic uremic syndrome (HUS) caused by a specific strain of *Escherichia coli* bacteria. The phases of ARF include:

- Anuric (14 days)
- Oliguric (8–14 days)
- Diuretic (10 days)
- Recovery (from 10 days to 3 months or up to 1 year)

Chronic renal failure (CRF) is the slow, gradual loss of kidney function. Some forms of CRF can be controlled or slowed down but never cured. Diabetic nephropathy may be delayed by tightly controlling blood glucose levels and using angiotensin-converting enzyme (ACE) inhibitors. Partial loss of renal function means that some portion of the patient's nephrons has been scarred, and scarred nephrons cannot be repaired. In patients with progressive CRF who consume uncontrolled diets, progressive declines in spontaneous protein and energy intake, serum proteins, cholesterol, total creatinine excretion, and anthropometric values are evident below a creatinine clearance level (CrCl) of about 25 mL/min (National Kidney Foundation, 2000).

Mortality increases greatly with serum albumin levels below 3.5 g/dL in renal patients. A low cholesterol level is a key indicator of malnutrition in this population. Individuals undergoing dialysis who have a low-normal (<150–180 mg/dL) nonfasting serum cholesterol have higher mortality than do those with higher cholesterol levels (National Kidney Foundation, 2000).

Glutathione peroxidase helps prevent generation of free radicals and decreases risk of oxidative damage to tissues, including the kidney and its vascular supply. Poor selenium status is common in patients with CKD who adhere to low-protein diets because selenium is found in protein foods. Poor selenium status exacerbates comorbid conditions such

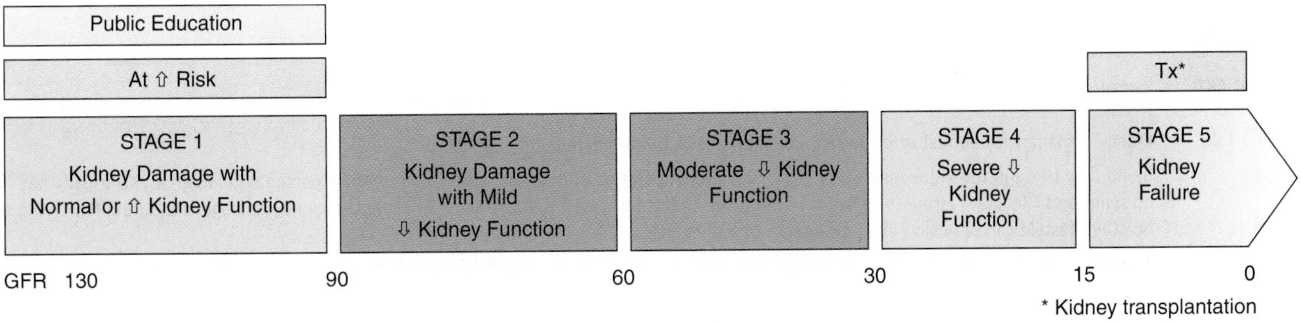

Figure 16-2 Stages of kidney disease through renal failure.

as congestive cardiomyopathy, skeletal myopathy, anemia, risk of cancer, and cardiac disease; therefore, it is important to correct poor selenium intake.

End-Stage Renal Disease (ESRD) care involves early detection of progressive renal disease, interventions to retard its progression, prevention of uremic complications, control of related conditions, adequate preparation for renal replacement therapy, and timely initiation of dialysis. Adherence to practices known to be of clinical benefit for patients with CKD not only improves patient outcomes but also reduces costs of care (Nissenson et al, 2001). A multidisciplinary effort is needed.

Higher blood pressure and lower income are associated with a higher incidence of ESRD in both white and African American men. The African American Study of Kidney Disease and Hypertension (AASK) supports lower blood pressure goals in terms of reduction of proteinuria; tight blood pressure control (<130/80 mm Hg) in patients with CKD appears reasonable (Rahman et al, 2005). Mortality is remarkably high in the ESRD population; cardiovascular disease is the leading problem (Shen et al, 2006). Decreasing risks such as smoking, chronic anemia, and hypertension in renal patients may reduce death rates.

Postmenopausal women may show signs of cognitive impairment when they have CKD (Kurella et al, 2005). Almost all patients with ESRD have elevated serum total homocysteine (tHcy) levels as well, and a multivitamin supplement that contains 800 μg folic acid should be taken (Dierkes et al, 2001). Renal failure patients, including predialysis, ESRD, and transplantation patients, need specialized supplementation to meet the requirements of disease management. Figure 16-2 shows the progressive stages of CKD that lead to ESRD, and Figure 16-3 shows how CKD can lead to kidney failure and death.

Protein–energy malnutrition (PEM) is common in CKD. Biochemical and anthropometric indicators of PEM present at the initiation of dialysis are predictive of future morbidity and mortality risk (National Kidney Foundation, 2000). Mechanisms of cachexia in CKD are poorly understood; anorexia, acidosis, and inflammation are frequently related (Mak et al, 2005). The decline in nutritional status during the course of progressive kidney failure may be caused by disturbances in protein and energy metabolism, hormonal derangement, and spontaneous reductions in dietary energy and protein intake. Worsening of PEM over time is associated with a greater risk for cardiovascular death in renal patients.

Early nutritional intervention may delay or prevent rapid progression of disease in some patients. Subjective Global Assessment (SGA) and other nutritional indicators, such as body mass index (BMI), handgrip strength (for measures of muscle mass), waist circumference, serum albumin, and serum creatinine, may be a good approach to provide useful information about the nutritional status of CKD patients. See Table 16-3 for management of PEM in renal patients, and see Table 16-4, which describes the stages of CKD and preventive measures.

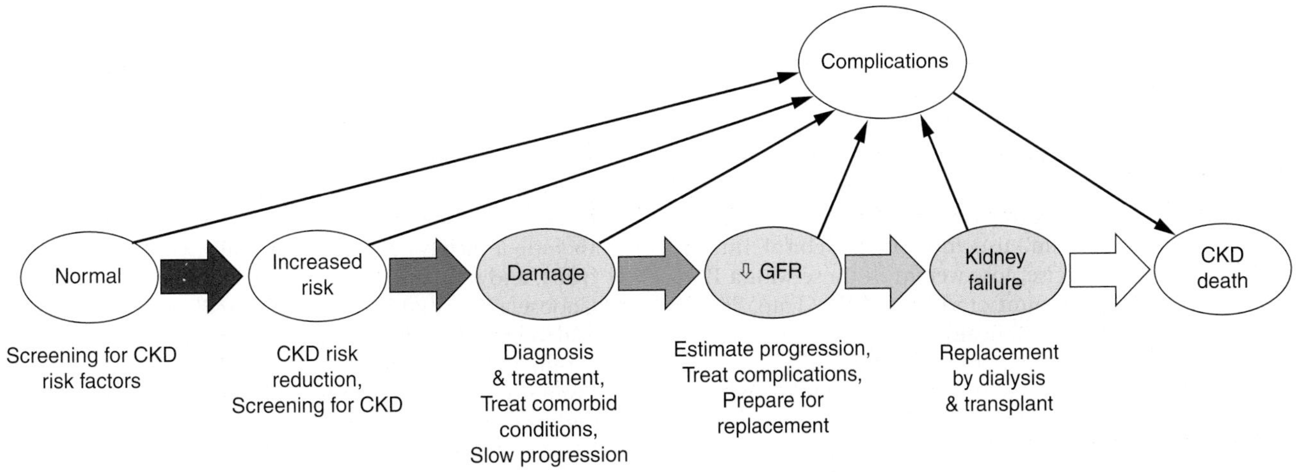

Figure 16-3 The pathway of untreated CKD.

TABLE 16-4 Symptoms and Preventive Measures for Stages of Chronic Kidney Disease (CKD)

Stage of CKD	Symptoms and Preventive Measures
Stage 1 CKD	Kidney damage with normal or increased GFR occurs. **GFR is 90 mL/min.** Blood flow through the kidney increases (hyperfiltration), and the kidneys are larger than usual. A person with stage 1 CKD usually has no symptoms. Regular testing for protein in the urine and serum creatinine can show whether the kidney damage is progressing. Living a healthy lifestyle can help slow the progression of kidney disease.
Stage 2 CKD	A person with stage 2 CKD has kidney damage with a mild decrease in their **GFR of 60–89 mL/min.** Filtration rate remains elevated or nearly normal. Glomeruli are showing signs of damage. Blood pressure is usually normal. Albuminuria is <30 mg/d. If someone finds out they have stage 2 CKD, it is usually because they were being tested for another condition such as diabetes or high blood pressure (the two leading causes of kidney disease).
Stage 3 CKD	A person with stage 3 CKD has kidney damage with a moderate decrease in the **GFR of 30–59 mL/min.** Microalbuminuria becomes constant. Losses increase to 30–300 mg/d. This can occur after about 7 years of having diabetes. As kidney function declines, uremia occurs. Complications of kidney disease such as high blood pressure, anemia, and early bone disease may occur. Consult a nephrologist to perform specific lab tests. Limit protein from diet to 0.8 g/kg.
Stage 4 CKD	A person with stage 4 CKD has advanced kidney damage with a severe decrease in the **GFR to 15–29 mL/min.** Nephropathy occurs at this stage. There is passage of large amounts of protein in the urine (>300 mg/d), and blood pressure continues to rise. Creatinine also rises above normal (which is 1.1–1.3 mg/dL or less). Someone with stage 4 CKD will need dialysis or a kidney transplantation. As kidney function declines, waste products build up in uremia. New symptoms include nausea, taste changes, uremic breath, anorexia, difficulty concentrating, and numbness in fingers and toes. Visits to the nephrologist every 3 months will be needed to test for creatinine, hemoglobin, calcium, and phosphorus levels as well as for management of hypertension and diabetes. An arteriovenous (AV) fistula and AV graft are created surgically and need a few months or so to mature before dialysis is needed. By doing everything possible to help prolong kidney function and overall health, the goal is to put off dialysis or transplantation for as long as possible. Limit protein from diet to 0.8 g/kg.
Stage 5 CKD	A person with stage 5 CKD has end-stage renal disease (ESRD) with a **GFR of 15 mL/min or less.** Kidney failure occurs. Renal replacement therapy (RRT) is initiated with hemodialysis, peritoneal dialysis, or renal transplantation. The National Kidney Foundation Dialysis Outcomes Quality Initiative recommends that dialysis be started when renal Kt/V (urea) falls below 2.0/wk (Jansen et al, 2001). At this advanced stage of kidney disease, the kidneys have lost nearly all their ability to do their job effectively, and eventually dialysis or a kidney transplantation is needed to live. When the kidneys are no longer able to remove waste and fluids from the body, toxins build up in the blood, causing an overall ill feeling. The National Kidney Foundation guidelines recommend starting dialysis when kidney function drops to 15% or less. The nephrologist will help the patient decide which treatment is best. New symptoms that can occur in stage 5 CKD include anorexia, nausea or vomiting, headaches, fatigue, anuria, swelling around eyes and ankles, muscle cramps, tingling in hands or feet, and changing skin color and pigmentation.

Derived from: National Kidney Foundation. Clinical practice guidelines for nutrition in chronic renal failure. Accessed January 17, 2006 at http://www.kidney.org/professionals/kdoqi/guidelines_updates/doqi_nut.html.

INTERVENTION: OBJECTIVES

- Work with high-risk conditions (such as diabetes) when urine albumin to creatinine ratio is abnormal (>30). Start working with other patients when serum creatinine is >1.5 mg/dL (women) or >2.0 mg/dL (men) to limit further renal impairment and reduce kidney workload. Patients should see a team, including a renal dietitian.
- Treat hypertension aggressively (DeNicola et al, 2006). Limit dietary sodium, use moderate alcohol intake, obtain regular exercise, lose weight in those with a BMI >25, and reduce amount of saturated fat (Toto, 2005). Keep blood pressure at a healthy level:
  - 125/75 mm Hg for patients with diabetes
  - 130/85 mm Hg for patients without diabetes and proteinuria
  - 125/75 mm Hg for patients without diabetes but with proteinuria
- Keep blood sugar or diabetes under control; goal is hemoglobin A1c of 7. Control carbohydrate intake if needed.
- Have regular checkups with the doctor and include a serum creatinine test to measure GFR; take medicines as prescribed.
- Exercise regularly, stop smoking, and eat a healthy diet.
- Maintain or improve nutritional status; protect lean body mass, minimize tissue catabolism, and spare protein.
- Include a variety of grains, especially whole grains, fresh fruits, and vegetables.
- Choose a diet that is low in saturated fat and cholesterol and moderate in total fats to achieve a normal lipid profile.
- Limit intake of refined and processed foods high in sugar and sodium.
- Choose and prepare foods with less salt or fewer high-sodium ingredients.

- Aim for a healthy weight and include physical activity each day; obesity is a known factor in decline in kidney function (Gelber et al, 2005).
- Keep protein intake at 0.6–0.75 g/kg/d if not on dialysis or at 1.2 g/kg/d if on dialysis.
- Consume adequate calories to spare protein.
- Consume the DRI for vitamins and minerals; goal includes a normal serum calcium while preventing osteodystrophy.
- Potassium and phosphorus are usually not restricted unless blood levels are above normal.
- Normalize amino acid repletion. Control uremic symptoms and reduce complications from accumulation of nitrogenous waste. Evaluate the blood urea nitrogen (BUN) to creatinine ratio; typically, a 10:1 ratio is desirable (creatinine doubles when renal function decreases by 50%). Provide amino acids in proportion to minimal DRI levels and protein status. Goal is to have a serum albumin level of 4.0 g/dL.
- Postpone dialysis as long as possible.
- Maintain growth in children with adequate calories, vitamins, and minerals.
- Restore and maintain electrolyte balance; correct acidosis.
- Treat anemia. Anemia is defined as a hematocrit <36% in women and <39% in men (Weiner et al, 2005).
- Correct other physiological changes (e.g., constipation, diarrhea, blurred vision, pruritus, ecchymosis, pallor, crackles in the lungs, loss of muscle tone, and tingling of lips or fingertips).

INTERVENTION: FOOD AND NUTRITION

- Aim for a healthy weight by consuming adequate calories and including physical activity each day. Nondialyzed patients with advanced CKD (GFR <25 mL/min) should be prescribed a dietary energy intake of 35 kcal/kg/d for patients who are <60 years of age and 30–35 kcal/kg for patients over age 60 years (Kopple, 2001). Carbohydrate (CHO) supplements may be needed; use fat additives if lipid levels are under control.
- In stage 1, 2, or 3 of CKD, protein intake may be limited to 12–15% of calorie intake each day. In stage 4 of CKD, reduce protein to 10% of calorie intake each day.
- For early CKD patients, use protein at the DRI level of 0.8 g protein/kg body weight and use high-quality protein. For nondialyzed patients with GFR <25 mL/min, 0.6 g protein/kg/d should be prescribed; at least 50% should come from high–biological value sources (Kopple, 2001). Amino acid analogs (CHO skeleton of amino acids minus the amino group) may also be used.
- CHO intolerance is common. Fructose, galactose, and sorbitol may be better tolerated than sucrose.
- Use a diet that is low in saturated fat and cholesterol and moderate in total fats, especially if cholesterol is high or if there is diabetes or heart disease.
- Fluid intake should be equivalent to patient's output plus 500–1000 mL for insensible losses. Monitor regularly.
- Calcium may be limited if blood levels are too high; limit elemental calcium to <2000 mg (including phosphorus binders).
- Phosphorus may be limited to help keep blood phosphorus or parathormone (PTH) normal and prevent renal bone disease. Controlling phosphorus may also help preserve existing kidney function. Limit phosphorus to <1000 mg.
- Initiate vitamin D therapy if PTH is greater than target, calcium is <9.5 mg/dL, or phosphorous is <4.6 mg/dL.
- Use a diet low in sodium for those with high blood pressure or fluid retention. Limit intake of refined and processed foods high in sodium, and use prepared foods with less salt or fewer high-sodium ingredients. A limit of 2 g sodium may be needed.
- Avoid over-the-counter dietary supplements unless approved by the nephrologist. The typical renal failure diet is low in B vitamins (especially folate and vitamin B_6); uremic factors affect folate and pyridoxine activities. Supplementation with water-soluble vitamins may be recommended; consume the DRI for the water-soluble vitamin B complex, and limit vitamin C to 100 mg/d from supplements.
- Fat-soluble nutrients like vitamin A and some minerals may not be recommended because levels can build up in the blood as kidney function declines.
- Iron must be tailored to individual requirements
- Include a variety of grains, fruits, and vegetables, but some may be limited if blood tests show phosphorus or potassium levels are above normal. When elevated, limit potassium to 2000–3000 mg, and limit use of salt substitutes, but liberalize diet when there is diarrhea or vomiting.
- Enteral nutrition may help infants and children overcome malnutrition and promote catch-up growth. Enteral multinutrient support significantly increases serum albumin concentrations and improves total dietary intake (Stratton et al, 2005).
- Renal-specific enteral products may be needed; monitor content according to serum protein levels and other lab data. If total parenteral nutrition (TPN) is needed, be careful not to use excesses of micronutrients.

CLINICAL INDICATORS

Clinical/History

Height
Weight
aBWef
Pitting edema, hands and legs
BMI (goal >24)
Waist circumference
Waist–hip ratio
Diet history
BP (increased)
I & O
Severe headache
Dyspnea
Failing vision
Poor appetite
Nausea and vomiting
Abdominal pain
Mouth ulcers, hiccups
Bone and joint pain
Fatigue
Uremic convulsions
Pericarditis
Skin changes and pigmentation
Electrocardiogram (EKG)
Renal biopsy
Dual-energy x-ray absorptiometry (DEXA) scan

Lab Work

Urine flow (normal, 1–1.5 L/d; nonoliguria, >500 mL/d; oliguria, <500 mL/d; anuria, <100 mL/d; polyuria, 3 L/d)

- Azotemia (excess urea and nitrogenous wastes in blood)
- Alb (goal, >4.0 g/dL)
- Transferrin saturation (goal, >20%)
- CRP
- BUN
- Creatinine
- BUN:creatinine ratio (altered by catabolic stress, low urine volume, and muscle mass changes)
- GFR (<10–15 mL/min consider dialysis)
- Glucose (Gluc) (goal, <140–160 mg/dL random)
- Hemoglobin A1c (HbA1c) <7%
- Na+
- K+ (goal, 3.5–5.5 mEq/L)
- Ca++ (goal, 8.5–10.2 mg/dL)
- Phosphorus (increased)
- Uric acid (increased)
- Mg++ (increased)
- PTH
- Hemoglobin (goal, 12 g/L for males; 11 g/L for females)
- Serum Fe
- Serum ferritin, mean cell volume (MCV), percent saturation
- RBC folate (≥ 200 ng/mL)
- Serum 23-hydroxyvitamin D (may be <30ng/mL)
- pH
- CO_2 (goal, 24–32 mEq/L)
- Serum chloride
- Chol (goal, >160 to <200 mg/dL)
- Triglycerides (Trig) (goal, <150 mg/dL)
- Body composition (SGA score)

Common Drugs Used and Potential Side Effects

- See Table 16-5.

Herbs, Botanicals, and Supplements

- Herbs and botanical supplements should not be used without discussing with physician.

INTERVENTION: NUTRITION EDUCATION, COUNSELING, CARE MANAGEMENT

- Counseling interventions should include aggressive blood pressure control, reduction of dietary protein to recommended levels for the American diet, weight loss, and control of hyperlipidemia (McClellan, 2005). Referral to a renal dietitian is suggested.
- Managing heart disease requires a healthy diet. Most CKD patients have a 10-year risk of coronary heart disease events, placing them in the highest risk category according to the National Cholesterol Education Program Adult Treatment Panel III guidelines (Farbakhsh and Kasiske, 2005).
- If the patient has diabetes, provide tips on limiting carbohydrates in the diet.
- Reading food labels, measuring portions, reading restaurant menus, planning for box lunches, and dining away from home should be discussed.
- Discuss that low-protein diets are nutritionally safe, they reduce the accumulation of metabolic products, and they can suppress progressive loss of kidney function (Mitch, 2005). Have patient consume the designated amount of proteins throughout the day. Low-protein wheat starch, hard candy, and jelly can be used.
- Taste changes may occur in patients with CKD. Foods with sharp, distinct flavors may be needed, and lack of interest in red meats is common.
- Manage high levels of phosphorus by dietary changes and prescribed medicines.
- Have patient weigh him or herself daily. Offer the following tips for maintaining fluid balance and managing thirst (from http://www.Davita.com):
  - Reduce intake of salty and spicy foods.
  - Limit foods that contain hidden or large amounts of fluid (e.g., popsicles, soup, gravy, watermelon, ice cream).
  - Stay cool in warm weather; drink cool instead of warm beverages.
  - Sipping beverages will make them last longer.
  - Using ice instead of beverages may seem more satisfying; freeze the allotted amount of beverages (such as fruit juice) and track intake accordingly.
  - Take medicines with applesauce instead of beverages; time intake according to doctor's orders.
  - Rinse often with mouthwash or suck on a lemon to decrease dry mouth.
  - Control high blood glucose with diabetes, since thirst is a side effect of hyperglycemia.

SAMPLE NUTRITION DIAGNOSTIC STATEMENT

Chronic Kidney Disease

PES: Excessive mineral intake related to recent increased intake of fresh fruit as evidenced by an increase in serum potassium by 10% since last report.

Assessment Data: Dietary recall and laboratory potassium measurements.

Intervention: Education on dietary sources of potassium.

Monitoring and Evaluation: Labs and dietary intake.

SAMPLE NUTRITION DIAGNOSTIC STATEMENT

Acute Renal Failure

PES: Inadequate intake from enteral nutrition infusion related to fluid restriction as evidenced by recorded infusion of 900 mL of enteral formula over the past 24 hours, providing only 70% of estimated energy and protein needs (1950 kcal and 78 g protein in 1.3 L of formula).

Assessment Data: Input and output (I/O) records, nursing flow sheets.

Intervention: Increase tube feeding by concentrating formula, increasing protein, and concentrating medications.

Monitoring and Evaluation: Monitor by I/O intake to monitor change in enteral formula administration, output, and serum creatinine levels.

TABLE 16-5 Drugs Used in Chronic Kidney Disease (CKD)

Medication	Comments
Angiotensin-converting enzyme inhibitor or angiotensin receptor blocker	First-line pharmacological intervention should be an angiotensin-converting enzyme inhibitor or angiotensin receptor blocker in those with diabetes or nondiabetics with more than 200 mg protein/g creatinine on a random urine sample (Toto, 2005).
Iron supplements	If recombinant human erythropoietin (r-HuEPO) is used to treat anemia, an iron supplement will be necessary. Be careful not to overload with excesses, and do not take supplements at the same time as calcium.
Lipid-lowering medications and statins	Lipid-lowering medications may be used if cholesterol or triglyceride levels are high. Lipoprotein metabolism is often impaired in CKD. The National Kidney Foundation Kidney Disease Outcomes Quality Initiative guidelines for managing dyslipidemia suggest that CKD patients with low-density lipoprotein ≥100 mg/dL should be treated with diet and a statin (Farbakhsh and Kasiske, 2005).
Phosphate binders	Phosphate binders, such as calcium acetate or calcium carbonate, are used to control serum phosphate levels. Nausea or vomiting may occur. Calcium medications (gluconate, carbonate, or lactate) may increase calcium intake, which may be otherwise inadequate if milk is limited.
	Fosrenol (lanthanum carbonate) was approved by the FDA in 2004.
Ruboxistaurin	Ruboxistaurin may add benefit to established therapies for diabetic nephropathy by reducing albuminuria and maintaining estimated glomerular filtration rate for a year (Tuttle et al, 2005).
Vitamin supplement	Renal multivitamins (such as Diatx) may be useful in providing B-complex vitamins (especially folic acid, B_6, and B_{12}) for hyperhomocysteinemia and CKD.
Vitamin D	In CKD, the patient's kidney is unable to convert vitamin D to its active form; osteodystrophy can result from the inability to use calcium. Ergocalciferol is a useful vitamin D analog. Extra water is needed to prevent constipation; monitor fluids carefully if urine output is decreased.
	The active form of vitamin D (calcitriol) should not be taken if calcium or phosphorus levels are too high because it will increase the risk of phosphorus deposits in soft tissues such as arteries, lungs, eyes, and skin.

- In addition to eating right and taking prescribed medicines, exercising regularly and not smoking are helpful to prolonging kidney health. Patients should talk to their doctors about an exercise plan.
- Discuss dietary sources of vitamin D:
  1 tablespoon cod liver oil = 1360 IU
  3.5 oz salmon = 360 IU
  3.5 oz mackerel = 345 IU
  3 oz tuna, canned in oil = 200 IU
  1.75 oz sardines, canned in oil = 250 IU
  8 oz fortified milk = 98 IU
  1 tablespoon fortified margarine = 60 IU
  1 whole egg = 20 IU
  3.5 oz beef liver = 15 IU
- Teach the patient how to monitor for signs of hyperkalemia, including nausea, weakness, numbness, tingling, slow pulse, or irregular heartbeat. See Table 16-6 for tips on managing potassium levels.

TABLE 16-6 Tips for Managing Potassium (K+) Levels

Category	Tip	High Sources of K+	Low Sources of K+
Fruit	Choose apples, berries, or grapes, instead of bananas, oranges, or kiwi.	Avocados	Apples
	Select a small piece of watermelon, instead of cantaloupe or honeydew.	Bananas	Berries
	Eat a peach, plum, or pineapple, instead of nectarines, mangos, or papaya.	Cantaloupe	Fruit cocktail
	Choose dried cranberries, instead of raisins or other dried fruit.	Dried fruits	Grapes
	Drink apple, cranberry, or grape juice, instead of orange juice or prune juice.	Honeydew	Lemon
	Use lower potassium canned pears, peaches, or fruit cocktail, instead of fresh fruit.	Kiwi	Peaches
		Mangos	Pears, canned
		Oranges and orange juice	Pineapple
		Papaya	Plums
		Prune juice	Watermelon

(continued)

TABLE 16-6 **Tips for Managing Potassium (K+) Levels *(continued)***

Category	Tip	High Sources of K+	Low Sources of K+
Vegetables	Choose green beans, wax beans, or snow peas, instead of dried beans or peas. Leach potatoes by cooking in water first to lower potassium content. Prepare mashed potatoes or hash browns from leached potatoes, instead of eating baked potatoes or French fries. Use summer squashes like crookneck or zucchini, instead of winter squashes like acorn, banana, or hubbard squash. Cook with onion, bell peppers, mushrooms, or garlic, instead of tomatoes, tomato sauce, or chili sauce. Drink ice water with sliced lemon and cucumber, instead of drinking vegetable juices.	Artichoke Dried beans and peas Pumpkin Potatoes, French fries Spinach (cooked) Sweet potatoes, yams Tomatoes, tomato juice and sauce Vegetable juice Winter squash	Carrots Cabbage Cauliflower Cucumber Eggplant Green beans Lettuce Onion Summer squash Sweet peppers
Dairy	Use nondairy creamer or unenriched rice milk, instead of milk. Prepare pudding with nondairy creamer, instead of eating yogurt or pudding made with milk. Enjoy sherbet, sorbet, or a popsicle, instead of ice cream or frozen yogurt.	Eggnog Ice cream Milk Pudding Yogurt	Nondairy creamer Rice milk, unenriched Popsicles Sorbet
Miscellaneous	Choose vanilla- or lemon-flavored desserts, instead of chocolate desserts. Eat unsalted popcorn or pretzels, rice cakes, jelly beans, or hard candies, instead of nuts or seeds. Season with pepper, lemon, or low-sodium herb and spice blends, instead of salt substitutes.	Chocolate Molasses Nuts Salt substitute Seeds	Donut, plain Hard candies Jelly beans Red licorice Unsalted pretzels Unsalted popcorn

Developed from: Davita Dialysis Centers. All about dialysis. Accessed January 20, 2006 at http://www.davita.com/articles/dialysis/.

For More Information

- American Dietetic Association
  Pre–End-Stage Renal Disease Protocol
  www.eatright.org
- End-Stage Renal Disease Clinical Performance Measures (CPMs) Project
  http://www.cms.hhs.gov/CPMProject/
- National Institute of Diabetes and Digestive and Kidney Diseases
  Patient Nutrition Guide
  http://www.niddk.nih.gov/health/kidney/pubs/kidney-failure/eat-right/eat-right.htm

CHRONIC KIDNEY DISEASE AND RENAL FAILURE—CITED REFERENCES

DeNicola L, et al. Global approach to cardiovascular risk in chronic kidney disease: reality and opportunities for intervention. *Kidney Int.* 69:538, 2006.

Dierkes J, et al. Homocysteine lowering effect of different multivitamin preparations in patients with end-stage renal disease. *J Renal Nutr.* 11:67, 2001.

Farbakhsh K, Kasiske BL. Dyslipidemias in patients who have chronic kidney disease. *Med Clin North Am.* 89:689, 2005.

Gelber RP, et al. Association between body mass index and CKD in apparently healthy men. *Am J Kidney Dis.* 46:871, 2005.

Jansen M, et al. Renal function and nutritional status at the start of chronic dialysis treatment. *J Am Soc Nephrol.* 12:157, 2001.

Kent PS. Integrating clinical nutrition practice guidelines in chronic kidney disease. *Nutr Clin Pract.* 20:213, 2005.

Kopple J. National kidney foundation K/DOQI clinical practice guidelines for nutrition in chronic renal failure. *Am J Kidney Dis.* 37:66S, 2001.

Kurella M, et al. Chronic kidney disease and cognitive impairment in menopausal women. *Am J Kidney Dis.* 45:66, 2005.

Mak RH, et al. Orexigenic and anorexigenic mechanisms in the control of nutrition in chronic kidney disease. *Pediatr Nephrol.* 20:427, 2005.

McClellan WM. Epidemiology and risk factors for chronic kidney disease. *Med Clin North Am.* 89:419, 2005.

Middleton RJ, et al. The unrecognized prevalence of chronic kidney disease in diabetes. *Nephrol Dial Transplant.* 21:88, 2006.

Mitch WE. Beneficial responses to modified diets in treating patients with chronic kidney disease. *Kidney Int Suppl.* 94:S133, 2005.

National Kidney Foundation. Clinical practice guidelines for nutrition in chronic renal failure. K/DOQI, National Kidney Foundation. *Am J Kidney Dis.* 35:1S, 2000.

Nissenson A, et al. Opportunities for improving the care of patients with chronic renal insufficiency: current practice patterns. *J Am Soc Nephrol.* 12:1713, 2001.

Rahman M, et al. The African American Study of Kidney Disease: do these results indicate that 140/90 mm hg is good enough? *Curr Hypertens Rep.* 7:363, 2005.

Shen Y, et al. Should we quantify insulin resistance in patients with renal disease? *Nephrology* 10:599, 2006.

Stratton RJ, et al. Multinutrient oral supplements and tube feeding in maintenance dialysis: a systematic review and meta-analysis. *Am J Kidney Dis.* 46:387, 2005.

Toto RD. Treatment of hypertension in chronic kidney disease. *Semin Nephrol.* 25:435, 2005.

Tuttle KR, et al. The effect of ruboxistaurin on nephropathy in type 2 diabetes. *Diabetes Care.* 28:2686, 2005.

Weiner DE, et al. Effects of anemia and left ventricular hypertrophy on cardiovascular disease in patients with chronic kidney disease. *J Am Soc Nephrol.* 16:1803, 2005.

GLOMERULAR DISORDERS

NUTRITIONAL ACUITY RANKING: LEVEL 2 ACUTE; LEVEL 3 CHRONIC

DEFINITIONS AND BACKGROUND

Glomerulonephritis (GN) is a form of autoimmunity; resolution of GN can be promoted by apoptosis of infiltrating leukocytes and excess resident glomerular cells, leading to efficient anti-inflammatory clearance by macrophages and mesangial cells (Watson et al, 2006). Unscheduled apoptosis in glomerular cells, especially epithelial cells, may drive progression of GN to nonfunctional scarring (Watson et al, 2006). **Glomerulosclerosis** involves scarring (sclerosis) of the glomeruli, often from lupus or diabetes. This may be stimulated by molecules called growth factors, which may be made by glomerular cells themselves or may be brought to the glomerulus by the circulating blood that enters the glomerular filter. Albumin is lost in the urine, nitrogen waste products are retained, and retinal changes occur.

Acute glomerulonephritis occurs when there is damage to the glomeruli, causing proteinuria. Causes include diabetes, hypertension, and other forms of kidney disease. Research shows that the level and type of proteinuria (whether the urinary proteins are only albumin or include other proteins) strongly determine the extent of damage and whether a patient is at risk for developing chronic kidney disease. Proteinuria is common in cardiovascular disease, where damaged blood vessels may lead to heart failure, stroke, or kidney failure. Untreated streptococcal infection can also cause acute GN, where antigen–antibody complex reactions become trapped in the glomeruli with resulting edema, scarring, and inflamed glomeruli.

Signs and symptoms of acute GN include a decrease in urine volume (oliguria), urine smell on breath and in perspiration, itching, vomiting, convulsions, rust-colored urine, proteinuria, yellowish-brown skin discoloration, and uremia (accumulation in the blood of waste substances ordinarily eliminated in the urine). This happens when the kidneys have lost their filtering ability, either as a result of temporary poisoning or from severe kidney disease. Anuria is a term that implies <400 cc/24 hours of urinary output, and this may require temporary dialysis. Most acute conditions resolve after 3–12 months.

The Acute Dialysis Quality Initiative Workgroup has outlined criteria for defining renal failure: the RIFLE classification identifies severity of renal impairment as Risk, Injury, Failure, Loss, and End-stage kidney disease (Kuitunen et al, 2006). There is very high mortality and morbidity and low quality of life among renal patients because hemodialysis (HD) currently provides less than 10% of the clearance power of the natural kidneys (Francisco and Pinera, 2006). Screening high-risk populations is effective in detecting renal disease, despite potential inaccuracy of serum creatinine concentrations and the preference for glomerular filtration rate estimates that take age and gender into account (Baumelou et al, 2005).

In **chronic glomerulonephritis,** repeated episodes of nephritis lead to loss of renal tissue and kidney function; glomeruli disappear, and normal filtering is lost. The kidneys can no longer concentrate urine; more urine is voided in an effort to rid the body of wastes. Protein and blood are lost in the urine. Blood pressure rises, causing vascular changes and chronic kidney disease (CKD). Conservative treatment promotes protein restriction (0.6 g protein/kg body weight) to correct metabolic and hormonal derangements. Decreased proteinuria indicates an improved prognosis, whereas hypertension can delay improvement. Protein restriction is contraindicated in protein malnutrition, neoplasm, growth, and infections. Sufficient energy intake is essential to prevent malnutrition.

INTERVENTION: OBJECTIVES

- Improve renal functioning; prevent systemic complications where possible.
- Monitor abnormal protein status and serum nitrogen retention.
- Spare protein for tissue repair. Prevent further catabolism of protein to lessen production of urea and other protein waste products.
- Control hypertension and edema.
- Prevent systemic complications.
- Control hyperglycemia and dyslipidemia.
- Correct metabolic abnormalities. Improve nutritional status and appetite.
- Prevent complications and growth failure in children.
- Reduce inflammation and workload of circulatory system by decreasing excess weight, where needed.

INTERVENTION: FOOD AND NUTRITION

- Modify patient's diet according to disease progression; maintain sufficient levels of protein as long as kidneys can eliminate waste products of protein metabolism.
- Use sufficient energy to spare protein (60% carbohydrates [CHO], 30% fat). Support patient's energy requirements with CHO and fat. For adults, 30–40 kcal/kg adjusted edema-free body weight (BW) may be needed to spare protein for tissue synthesis, wound healing, and other purposes.
- Vegetarian diets, soy products, and use of omega-3 fatty acids may be beneficial for dyslipidemia. Restrict fat and cholesterol if needed; monitor diet carefully.
- Control CHO intake with diabetes or hyperglycemia.
- If patient is obese, use an energy-controlled diet but avoid fasting and very low–calorie diets.
- In **oliguria,** restrict fluid intake to 500–700 mL. Restrict protein intake (0.6–0.8 g/kg) when urinary output is <400 cc/24 hours or as physician deems necessary.
- In **uremia,** diet should include 50% high–biologic value proteins (such as from cheese, eggs, and dairy foods), or

essential amino acids (EAAs) 2–3 times normal should be included. Protein may be restricted to 0.6–0.8 g/kg.
- With **edema or high blood pressure,** restrict sodium intake to 2–3 g/d. In a child, a restriction of 500–1000 mg may be needed. Carefully monitor sodium levels because sodium depletion can occur during the diuretic phase of chronic glomerulonephritis.
- When urinary output is reduced greatly, restrict phosphorus intakes if needed. Potassium is often controlled by medications but monitor serum values closely and adjust as needed. Some patients will require dialysis to remove waste products.
- Determine vitamins and nutrients provided by therapeutic diet and supplement to meet daily requirements, especially for calcium and B vitamins, which are easily lost in urine.
- Children with uremia require vitamin D_3 replacement to promote growth and improve appetite; adults will need it to maintain bone health.
- See CKD entry for more details.

CLINICAL INDICATORS

Clinical/History

Height
Weight
aBWef
Edema
BMI
Diet history
Waist–hip circumference
BP
Temperature
I & O
Oliguria or decrease in urine volume
Urine smell on breath and sweat
Itching
Vomiting
Convulsions
Rust-colored urine
Yellowish-brown skin discoloration
Renal x-rays

Lab Work

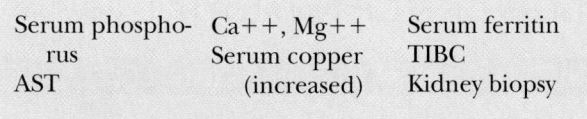

CRP
GFR
CrCl level
Uremia
Alb, transthyretin
Transferrin
BUN
Creat
Proteinuria
Gluc
Urinary ketones
Chol (often increased from proteinuria)
Trig
White blood cell count (WBC)
H & H
MCV
Serum Fe
Specific gravity (often decreased)
PTH
Na+, K+
Serum phosphorus
AST
Ca++, Mg++
Serum copper (increased)
Serum ferritin
TIBC
Kidney biopsy

Common Drugs Used and Potential Side Effects

- When diuretics such as furosemide are used to reduce edema, watch for potassium wasting. Dehydration can elevate BUN; assess carefully.
- Antihypertensives have various effects; evaluate individually.
- Immunosuppressants may be used to block the body's immune system.
- See Table 16-5 for more specific medications.

Herbs, Botanicals, and Supplements

- Herbs and botanical supplements should not be used without discussing with physician.

INTERVENTION: NUTRITION EDUCATION, COUNSELING, CARE MANAGEMENT

- A renal dietitian should provide nutrition therapy and counseling. A diet controlled in protein, fluid, phosphorus, sodium, and potassium may be needed; it must be individualized and is likely to change frequently. Table 16-7 describes the findings of the Modified Diet in Renal Disease (MDRD) Study and its various forms of dietary guidance.
- Commitment from the patient and family is needed; extra expense may be incurred for low-protein foods and amino acid analogs.
- Fluid intake should be distributed carefully throughout the patient's waking hours. Check for changes according to diarrhea and related problems. The patient should not avoid drinking fluid to prevent nocturia.
- Encourage frequent doctor or clinic visits to monitor renal functioning.
- Edema is better controlled by sodium restriction than by fluid restriction; monitor patient carefully. See Table 16-8. Patients with edema are often thirsty; edema water is trapped and unavailable for body's use.

TABLE 16-7 Tips from the Modified Diet in Renal Disease (MDRD) Study

Eight hundred forty adult patients with renal disease followed a low-protein (usually 0.6 g/kg for advanced disease) and low-phosphate diet (5–10 mg/kg/d). Results show that:

Keto and amino acid analogs are very useful.

Evaluations of quality of life find that among the usual-protein, low-protein, and very low-protein groups, the very low–protein diet is clearly the least palatable.

The imprecision of using exchange lists is difficult; counting grams of protein is easier.

Although many types of counseling strategies can be used, the most beneficial are psychosocial and behavioral approaches.

Time spent by registered dietitians averages from 183–116 minutes over a few to 25–36 months; more time is required for very low–protein diets.

Resources: National Institute of Diabetes and Digestive and Kidney Disease. Modified Diet in Renal Disease Study. Accessed September 9, 2006 at http://www.niddk.nih.gov/fund/divisions/kuh/kdcsi/MDRDS.pdf; and Songer T, et al. Cost-effectiveness of nutrition therapy in the MDRD study. Accessed September 9, 2006 at http://www.pitt.edu/~tjs/mdrd/mdrd.pdf#search=%22MDRD%20study%22.

TABLE 16-8 **Substitutes for Salt: Spices and Condiments**

Allspice	Dry mustard	Paprika
Bay leaf	Garlic, fresh or powder	Rosemary
Black pepper	Ginger	Scallions
Caraway seeds	Green bell pepper	Shallots
Celery seed	Lemons and limes	Sugar substitute
Chili powder	Mint	Sweet basil
Chives	Mrs. Dash	Tabasco sauce
Cinnamon	Nutmeg	Thyme
Cloves	Onions	Turmeric or cumin
Curry powder	Oregano	Vanilla extract
Dill	Pan spray, nonstick	Vinegar

- Patients with ascites may become anorexic in the upright position. Position patient carefully for food intake.

For More Information

- Acute Glomerulonephritis
  http://www.nephrologychannel.com/agn/

GLOMERULAR DISORDERS—CITED REFERENCES

Baumelou A, et al. Renal disease in cardiovascular disorders: an underrecognized problem. *Am J Nephrol.* 25:95, 2005.

Francisco AL, Pinera C. Challenges and future of renal replacement therapy. *Hemodial Int.* 10:19S, 2006.

Kuitunen A, et al. Acute renal failure after cardiac surgery: evaluation of the RIFLE classification. *Ann Thorac Surg.* 81:542, 2006.

Watson S, et al. Apoptosis and glomerulonephritis. *Curr Dir Autoimmun.* 9:188, 2006.

INBORN ERRORS OF RENAL METABOLISM: VITAMIN D–RESISTANT RICKETS AND HARTNUP DISORDER

NUTRITIONAL ACUITY RANKING: LEVEL 3–4

DEFINITIONS AND BACKGROUND

Vitamin D–resistant rickets is X-linked familial hypophosphatemia (XLH) associated with decreased renal tubular reabsorption of phosphorous. Mutations of the metalloproteinase PHEX are responsible (Schmitt and Mehls, 2004). Incidence is 1 in 20,000 births.

XLH is characterized by low to normal serum levels of 1,25-dihydroxyvitamin D_3 [1,25(OH)(2)D(3)], normocalcemia, and hypophosphatemia (Schmitt and Mehls, 2004). There is also abnormal regulation of production and/or degradation of parathyroid hormone (PTH).

Because vitamin D is metabolized abnormally, skeletal and dental structures are affected. Hypophosphatemia is responsible for most of the clinical manifestations, which vary with the age of the patient and the severity of wasting in vitamin D–resistant rickets (Laroche and Boyer, 2005). In poorly growing patients, growth hormone therapy combined with conventional treatment improves final height, phosphate retention, and radial bone mineral density (Baroncelli et al, 2001).

Hartnup disorder is an autosomal recessive abnormality of renal and gastrointestinal neutral amino acid transport, especially tryptophan and histidine (Broer et al, 2005). It is a rare familial condition characterized by hyperaminoaciduria. A red, scaly, photosensitive pellagra-like skin rash is seen on the face, neck, hands, and legs, and cerebellar changes occur, including delirium. The failure to resorb amino acids in this disorder is thought to be compensated by a protein-rich diet (Broer et al, 2005). The tryptophan-loading test is used to diagnose the disorder.

INTERVENTION: OBJECTIVES

- **Vitamin D–resistant rickets.** Correct malabsorption of vitamin D, calcium, and phosphorus in persons with vitamin D–resistant rickets. Regulate phosphorus to establish homeostasis with adequate bone and skeletal mineralization (Bielesz et al, 2004).
- **Hartnup disorder.** Correct skin changes and behavioral side effects. Ensure adequacy of protein. Support measures such as psychiatric treatment as needed.

INTERVENTION: FOOD AND NUTRITION

- **Vitamin D–resistant rickets.** Diet should include 4800 IU of 1,25-dihydroxyvitamin D_3 plus oral phosphate in a quantity of 1.5–2 g phosphorus/d. Ensure that diet provides adequate amounts of calcium. Monitor to avoid mineral toxicities.
- **Hartnup disorder.** Patient should be given oral nicotinamide therapy (40–200 mg/d) plus a high-protein diet or supplements. Oral neomycin should also be given.

CLINICAL INDICATORS

Clinical/History		
Birth weight	Length	Diet history
Present weight	Growth percentile	BP
	BMI	Red, scaly rash
		Signs of rickets

Skeletal x-rays	**Lab Work**	H & H
Tryptophan-loading test	Serum vitamin D	Serum ferritin
Delayed growth or short stature	Ca++	Chol
Ultrasound	Phosphorus	Trig
Psychiatric evaluation	PTH	K+
	Hyperphosphaturia (rickets)	Na+
	BUN	Gluc
		Alb, transthyretin
		CRP

Common Drugs Used and Potential Side Effects

- In **vitamin D–resistant rickets,** ergocalciferol is a vitamin D analog that is used with phosphate supplements. After growth is completed, the drug is often reduced. Hyperparathyroidism is regularly seen in patients treated with phosphate supplements, although circulating serum phosphate levels do not reach the normal range (Schmitt and Mehls, 2004). Phosphate supplements may include dibasic sodium phosphate.
- Growth hormone therapy may be used; monitor for untoward side effects.

Herbs, Botanicals, and Supplements

- Herbs and botanical supplements should not be used without discussing with physician.

INTERVENTION: NUTRITION EDUCATION, COUNSELING, CARE MANAGEMENT

- Explain measures that are appropriate to specific condition. Encourage regular medical visits and nutritionist follow-up.
- Patients with **rickets** will need counseling about desired intake of phosphorus, vitamin D, and calcium to ensure adequate growth and development.
- Patients with **Hartnup disorder** should use sunscreen and avoid sun exposure as much as necessary. They will need counseling about high-protein diets.

For More Information

- American Academy of Bone and Mineral Research
  http://www.asbmr.org/
- Hartnup Disorder
  http://www.nlm.nih.gov/medlineplus/ency/article/001201.htm
- National Resource Center–Osteoporosis and Related Disorders
  http://www.niams.nih.gov/bone/
- Office of Rare Diseases
  http://rarediseases.info.nih.gov/
- XLH (Vitamin D–Resistant Rickets)
  http://www.xlhnetwork.org/site/Diagnosis.html

INBORN ERRORS OF RENAL METABOLISM—CITED REFERENCES

Baroncelli G, et al. Effect of growth hormone treatment on final height, phosphate metabolism, and bone mineral density in children with X-linked hypophosphatemic rickets. *Pediatrics* 138:236, 2001.

Bielesz B, et al. Renal phosphate loss in hereditary and acquired disorders of bone mineralization. *Bone* 35:1229, 2004.

Broer S, et al. Neutral amino acid transport in epithelial cells and its malfunction in Hartnup disorder. *Biochem Soc Trans.* 33:233, 2005.

Laroche M, Boyer JF. Phosphate diabetes, tubular phosphate reabsorption and phosphatonins. *Joint Bone Spine.* 72:376, 2005.

Schmitt CP, Mehls O. The enigma of hyperparathyroidism in hypophosphatemic rickets. *Pediatr Nephrol.* 19:473, 2004.

KIDNEY STONES

NUTRITIONAL ACUITY RANKING: LEVEL 1–2

DEFINITIONS AND BACKGROUND

The modern lifestyle, dietary habits, and obesity promote idiopathic stone disease (Straub and Hautmann, 2005). Kidney stones are, therefore, common. The official process is called urolithiasis or nephrolithiasis. Signs and symptoms include excruciating groin or flank pain, nausea, vomiting, burning, urinary frequency, fever, hematuria, mild pyuria, abnormal urine color, and excessive urination at night.

While all humans form calcium oxalate crystals, most do not form stones (Lemann, 2002). Prevalence has been rising in both sexes (Moe, 2006). The lifetime risk for a white man is 12–15%, and for white women, it is 5–6%, with lifetime recurrence rates of up to 50% (Reynolds, 2005).

A person who has had kidney stones often gets them again in the future. Untreated calcium oxalate stones can lead to a greater chance of forming additional stones within later decades. A person with a family history of kidney stones is more likely to develop stones. Annually, nearly 400,000 people are treated for this problem. In the South where there is a slightly higher prevalence, a history of hypertension and low intake of calcium and magnesium have been found among older women (Hall et al, 2001). Finally, kidney stones may occur in premature infants.

Kidney stones develop when salt and minerals in urine form crystals that coalesce and grow in size. Stones are formed by progressive deposition of crystalline material around an organic nidus. Decreased fluid intake and consequent urine

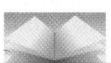

TABLE 16-9 Causes of and Predisposition to Kidney Stones

Climate—Hot climate and dehydration during summer months
Diet—Low intakes of dietary calcium and fluid, high intakes of sodium in susceptible individuals
Diminished water intake—During sleep, travel, or illness, or from poor habits
Family history of kidney stones
Genetic disorders—Gout, primary hyperoxaluria, hyperparathyroidism, renal tubular acidosis, cystinuria, hypercalciuria
Gender—Three times more common in males
Inflammatory bowel disease, intestinal bypass surgery, ostomy surgery
Medications such as certain diuretics; use of the protease inhibitor indinavir
Medication misuse, such as excessive intake of supplemental vitamin D
Urinary tract infection or stagnation from blockage

Reference: National Institute of Diabetes and Digestive and Kidney Diseases. Kidney stones in adults. Accessed September 9, 2006 at http://kidney.niddk.nih.gov/kudiseases/pubs/stonesadults/.

concentration are among the most important factors influencing stone formation. Stones ultimately arise because of an unwanted phase change of these substances from a liquid to solid state (Coe et al, 2005).

The major causes of renal stones are urinary tract infections, cystic kidney diseases, certain metabolic disorders such as hyperparathyroidism, and renal tubular acidosis (see Table 16-9).

Many stones can be prevented through changes in diet (Grases et al, 2006). About 75% of stones formed are from calcium oxalate (Reynolds, 2005). While dietary oxalate is another possible cause, the role of dietary calcium is less clear. Certain medications, such as triamterene (Dyrenium), indinavir (Crixivan), and acetazolamide (Diamox), are also associated with urolithiasis.

Approximately 80% of stones are composed of calcium oxalate and calcium phosphate; 10% are composed of struvite (magnesium ammonium phosphate produced during infection with bacteria that possess the enzyme urease); 9% are composed of uric acid; and the remaining 1% are composed of cystine or ammonium acid urate or are diagnosed as drug-related stones (Coe et al, 2005).

Fluid is a key factor (Parks et al, 2003). It is not the quantity of fluid consumed that should be measured, but rather the fluid voided that is important. Extra fluid intake will be needed by those who live in hot, dry conditions and by those who exercise and perspire significantly. Because there may be a modest positive relationship between caffeine intake and urinary calcium levels in stone formers, they should drink more water and avoid excess caffeine (Massey and Sutton, 2004). While it is thought that wine and beer consumption may decrease risk, apple or grapefruit juices actually may aggravate risk.

Adequate calcium intake is associated with decreased stone formation in young women (Curhan et al, 2004). Additionally, a 5-year randomized clinical trial of men with a history of calcium oxalate stones found that a normal calcium, decreased sodium, and decreased animal protein diet was more effective for reducing stone events than was a restricted calcium diet (Borghi et al, 2002). High intake of dietary calcium generally decreases the risk of oxalate kidney stones, while supplements of calcium may increase risk (Williams et al, 2001).

Because calcium and sodium compete for reabsorption in the renal tubules, excess sodium intake and consequent excretion result in loss of calcium in the urine. High-sodium diets are associated with greater calcium excretion in the urine (Lemann, 2002). Modern diets containing a lot of animal protein, refined carbohydrates, and salt act on the metabolism like an acid load; a sufficient supply of potassium and alkali is required (Straub and Hautmann, 2005).

Balanced diets containing moderate amounts of either beef or plant protein (legumes, seeds, nuts, and grains) may keep urinary composition within guidelines (Massey and Kynast-Gales, 2001). However, high dietary protein is associated with increased urinary calcium; vegetarians form stones at one third of the rate of those eating a mixed diet (Lemann, 2002). Overall, adequate calcium plus decreased sodium and protein intake has a significantly more protective effect against stones than decreased calcium intake alone (Curham et al, 2004; Borghi et al, 2002).

Resulting from purine metabolism, uric acid stones may require a reduction in foods that are high in purines (such as sardines). Uric acid stones may also result from gout, leukemia, or cancer. Urate stones are common after colectomy (Reynolds, 2005). Creating an alkaline urine is the goal (Reynolds, 2005).

Figures 16-4 and 16-5 show types and shapes of actual kidney stones.

INTERVENTION: OBJECTIVES

- Determine predominant components and prevent recurrence. Preventive concepts include normalization of body mass index, adequate physical activity, balanced nutrition, and sufficient daily fluid intake (Straub and Hautmann, 2005).
- Modify diet according to predominant components; there is seldom a single cause.
- To increase excretion of salts, dilute urine by increasing fluid volume to at least 2 L/24 h.
- Prevent scarring, recurrence of stones, obstruction, or kidney damage.
- Repeat urinary studies approximately 6–8 weeks after initial metabolic testing recommendations are implemented to evaluate effectiveness of dietary changes.
- Once stable, where the patient's urine demonstrates decreased risk of stone formation, metabolic testing and x-rays should be performed at least annually.

INTERVENTION: FOOD AND NUTRITION

- General guidelines: Fluid intake should be high, as tolerated (2 L/d). Colorless urine is sought. Individuals with cystinuria will need 3.5 L/d (Reynolds, 2005). Limit use of apple or grapefruit juices.
- A weight loss and exercise plan may be needed if the patient is overweight.
- Calcium should not be restricted, except in absorptive hypercalciuria where calcium restriction remains beneficial

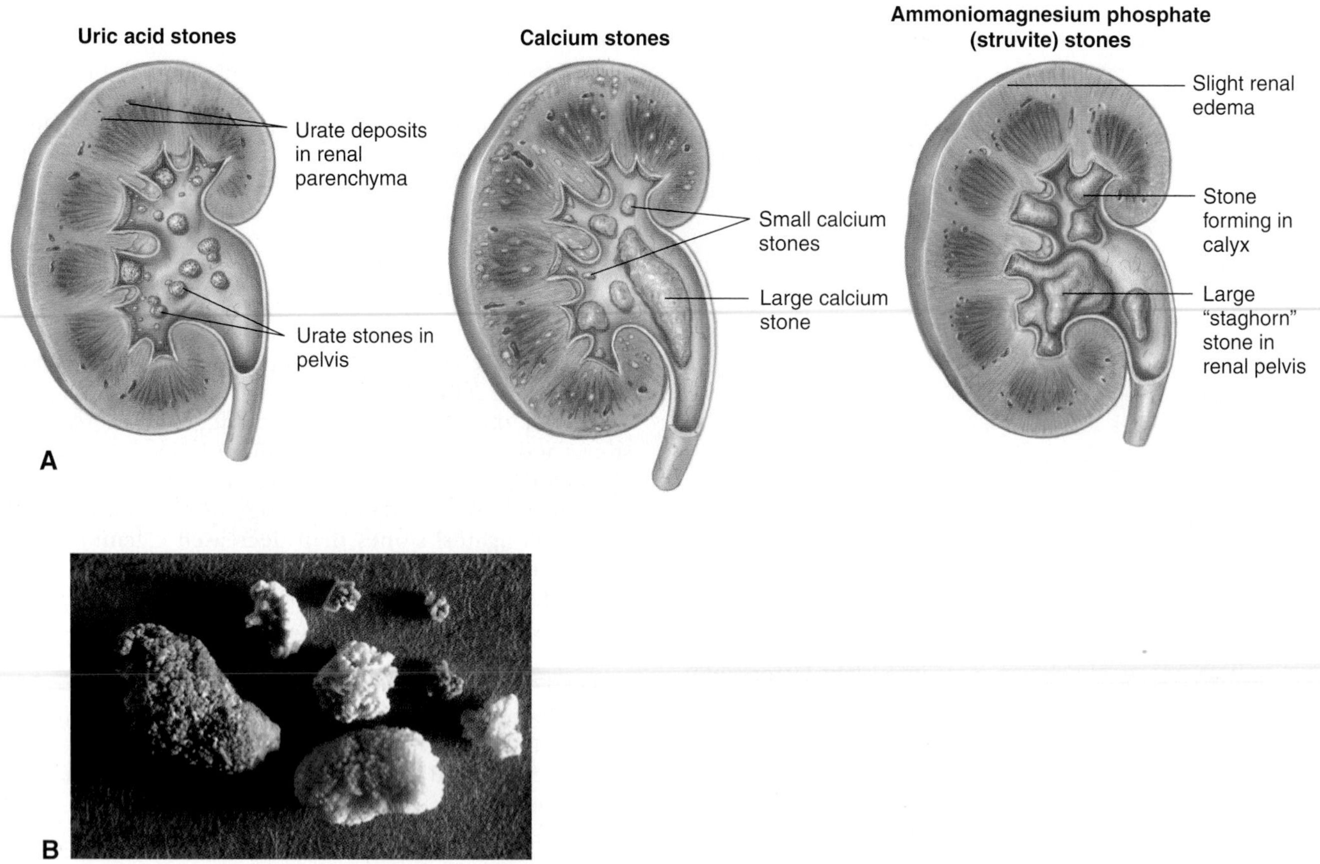

Figure 16-4 Types and shapes of kidney stones. A. Asset provided by Anatomical Chart Co.

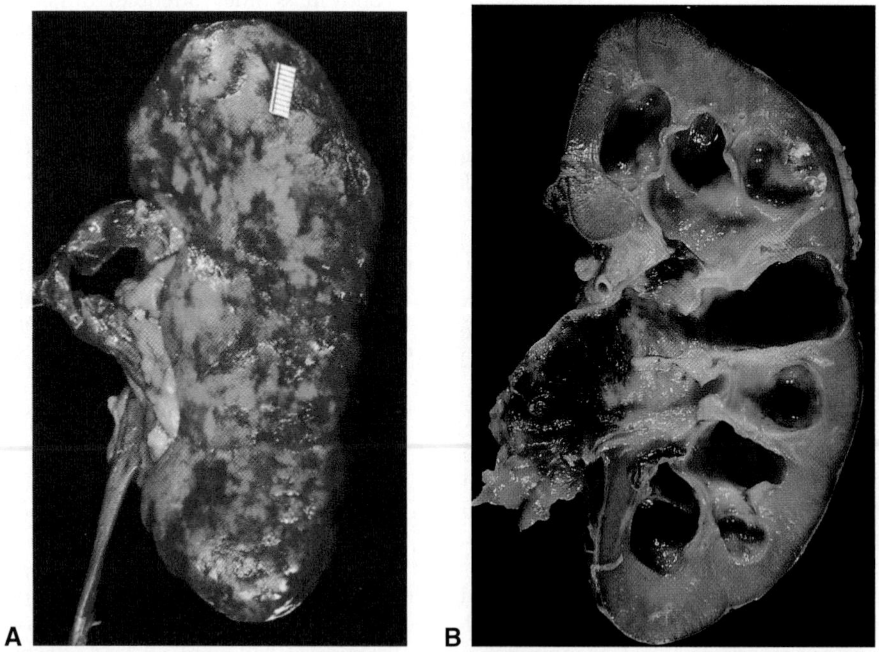

Figure 16-5 Kidney stones. (From Rubin E. *Rubin's pathology: clinicopathologic foundations of medicine*. 4th ed. Philadelphia: Lippincott Williams & Wilkins, 2005.)

TABLE 16-10 Dietary Treatment of Specific Renal Stones

Type	Treatment
Calcium oxalate stones	Calcium intake should be increased to >1000 mg/d; good sources include skim milk, yogurt, low-fat dairy products, broccoli, fortified orange juice, and ricotta or cheese. Green leafy vegetables, broccoli, fortified foods, and almonds are sources for those who do not like dairy products. Moderate protein intake decreases calcium excretion, mainly through a reduction in bone resorption and renal calcium loss, probably due to a decrease in exogenous acid load. Reducing urinary oxalates may have a more powerful effect on stone formation than reduction of urinary calcium (Morton et al, 2002). A diet reduced in oxalates is often needed, especially if patient hyperabsorbs oxalates. Although only 10–20% of urinary oxalates come from dietary sources (Morton et al, 2002), dietary limits are commonly advised. High amounts of oxalates are found in spinach, strawberries, rhubarb, beets, nuts, chocolate, coffee, black tea, cola, beans and soybeans, and beets. Vitamin B_6 intake may help lower urinary oxalates, but no controlled trials have been done yet (Reynolds, 2005). An inverse relation between nephrolithiasis and vitamin B_6 intake (>40 mg/d) in women has been shown; more studies are needed (Reynolds, 2005). Vitamin C is a precursor to endogenous production of oxalates, so some clinicians recommend avoiding mega-doses of vitamin C. A normal diet or daily supplement that contains the DRI level may be suggested. A specific epidemiological study of vitamin intake and renal stones in women found no positive link (Reynolds, 2005).
Citrate stones	Hypocitraturia is found in up to 20% of stone formers and may be idiopathic or secondary to intestinal, renal, dietary, or pharmacological causes (Reynolds, 2005).
Cystine stones	Individuals with cystinuria will need 3.5 L of fluid daily (Reynolds, 2005). Use a diet low in cystine, methionine, and cysteine. Protein intake should be lessened but not severely restricted. Cystine stones usually are the result of a hereditary defect. Alkalize urine with agents like D-penicillamine. These stones are rare.
Struvite stones	Struvite stones (magnesium ammonium phosphate) (15%) may form after an infection in the urinary system. Treatment of this type of infection must be done at the same time as removal of the stone. They can grow very large and may obstruct the kidney, ureter, or bladder if not removed.
Uric acid stones	Urate stones can be dissolved by urine alkalinization, with a reported success rate of 80% (Reynolds, 2005). Alkalinize urine with citrate or bicarbonate. There is no inhibitor of uric acid crystal formation; dietary measures focus on reducing uric acid and increasing urine volume. Reduction of animal and fish protein to 12 oz/d for adults is recommended (Menon and Resnick, 2002). Nonfat milk, low-fat yogurt, and other dairy products may have clinically meaningful antihyperuricemic effects; fruits such as cherries and high intakes of vegetable protein may reduce serum urate levels (Schlesinger et al, 2005).

in combination with thiazide and citrate therapy (Straub and Hautmann, 2005). Prevent bone demineralization.

- Consume a diet that is balanced, with fruits and vegetables for potassium to alleviate the association between low potassium intake and increased sodium chloride intake in stone formers (Reynolds, 2005). The DASH diet is a good recommendation (He and MacGregor, 2003).
- Include legumes and dried beans often for their health-promoting components, saponins, which are useful in the treatment of hypercalciuria (Shi et al, 2004).
- Essential fatty acid intake is proposed, but this is an area that requires further research (Reynolds, 2005).
- Specific guidelines are provided in Table 16-10.

CLINICAL INDICATORS

Clinical/History

Height
Weight
BMI
Diet history
BP
I & O
Excruciating pain
Nausea, vomiting
Burning and urinary frequency
Kidney ultrasound
Computed tomography (CT), urography
Abdominal x-rays

Lab Work

Urinalysis (crystals, red blood cells)
24-hour urine studies, including total urine volume, urinary calcium (normal, 300–400 mg), urinary sodium, urinary citrate, uric acid, urinary pH, and supersaturation of critical compounds
Serum oxalate levels
Gluc
Ca++, Mg++
Alb
CRP
Lactose intolerance
Serum Na+, K+
BUN
Creat
H & H
Serum Fe

Common Drugs Used and Potential Side Effects

- About 15% of patients forming stones require additional specific pharmacological prevention (Straub and Hautmann, 2005).
- For **calcium oxalate or uric acid stones,** allopurinol (Zyloprim) and probenecid usually are used in conjunction with a purine-restricted diet. Drink 10–12 glasses of fluid daily; avoid concomitant intake of vitamin C supplements. Maintain alkaline urine (may need to use sodium bicarbonate). Side effects include nausea, vom-

iting, diarrhea, and abdominal pain. Monitor renal and hepatic side effects. Oxalate absorption can be blocked by magnesium carbonate or cholestyramine; therefore, it may be logical to use them to prevent stone recurrence (Reynolds, 2005).

- For **citrate stones,** only potassium citrate and potassium-magnesium citrate have been tested in randomized trials for alkalinizing the urine (Reynolds, 2005).
- For **cystine stones:** D-penicillamine requires vitamin B_6 and zinc supplementation. Increase fluid intake. Take 1–2 hours before or after meals. Stomatitis, diarrhea, nausea, vomiting, and abdominal pain may occur.
- **Struvite** stones will require use of antibiotics.
- In **hypercalciuria:** Thiazide diuretic drugs can affect urine calcium excretion; treatment with thiazides is probably effective and worthwhile in the prevention of recurrence in patients with hypercalciuria (Reynolds, 2005).

Herbs, Botanicals, and Supplements

- Herbs and botanical supplements should not be used without discussing with physician.
- The use of probiotics has been suggested. Use of *Oxalobacter formigenes* in the prevention of calcium oxalate stone disease needs further investigation.

INTERVENTION: NUTRITION EDUCATION, COUNSELING, CARE MANAGEMENT

- The most important lifestyle change to prevent stones is to drink more liquids, especially water; try to produce at least 2 quarts of urine in every 24-hour period.
- A patient's 24-hour urine chemistry profile should guide the dietary adjustments (Taylor and Curhan, 2004).
- Use dietary measures that are appropriate for condition and content of the stone. Cranberry juice is a favorite beverage used to produce a more acidic urine; 2–3 glasses daily are recommended. Cranberry concentrate tablets are not beneficial for patients with a history of oxalate stones (Terris et al, 2001).
- Vitamin B_6 reduces production of oxalates and may help treatment. Include good dietary sources daily.
- Discuss occupational risks for stone formation, including working in hot, dry environments or working with metals such as cadmium.
- Discuss the principles of a healthy DASH diet.

For More Information

- American Foundation for Urologic Disease
http://www.auafoundation.org/
- Kidney Stone Diet
http://www.gicare.com/pated/edtgs29.htm.
- Low-Oxalate Diet
http://www.ohf.org/diet.html
- Kidney Stones in Adults
http://www.niddk.nih.gov/health/kidney/pubs/stonadul/stonadul.htm
- National Library of Medicine
http://www.nlm.nih.gov/medlineplus/ency/article/000458.htm
- Oxalosis and Hyperoxaluria Foundation
http://www.ohf.org/

KIDNEY STONES—CITED REFERENCES

Borghi L, et al. Comparison of two diets for the prevention of recurrent stones in idiopathic hypercalciuria. *N Engl J Med.* 346:77, 2002.

Curhan GC, et al. Dietary factors and the risk of incident kidney stones in young women: Nurses' Health Study II. *Arch Intern Med.* 164:885, 2004.

Grases F, et al. Renal lithiasis and nutrition. *Nutr J.* 5:23, 2006.

Hall W, et al. Risk factors for kidney stones in older women in the southern United States. *Am J Med Sci.* 322:12, 2001.

He FJ, MacGregor GA. Potassium: more beneficial effects. *Climacteric* 6:36S, 2003.

Lemann J. Idiopathic hypercalciuria. In: Coe FL, Favus MJ, eds. *Disorders of bone and mineral metabolism.* Philadelphia: Lippincott Williams & Wilkins, 2002; pp. 673–697.

Massey L, Kynast-Gales S. Diets with either beef or plant proteins reduce risk of calcium oxalate precipitation in patients with a history of calcium kidney stones. *J Am Diet Assoc.* 101:326, 2001.

Massey LK, Sutton RA. Acute caffeine effects on urine composition and calcium kidney stone risk in calcium stone formers. *J Urol.* 172:555, 2004.

Menon M, Resnick MI. Urinary lithiasis: etiology, diagnosis and medical management. In Walsh PC, et al, eds. *Campbell's urology.* Philadelphia: Saunders, 2002; pp. 3229–3305.

Moe OW. Kidney stones: pathophysiology and medical management. *Lancet* 367:333, 2006.

Morton AR, et al. Nephrology: 1. Investigation and treatment of recurrent kidney stones. *Can Med Assoc J.* 166:213, 2002.

Parks JH, et al. Changes in urine volume accomplished by physicians treating nephrolithiasis. *J Urol.* 169:863, 2003.

Reynolds TM. ACP Best Practice No 181: chemical pathology clinical investigation and management of nephrolithiasis. *J Clin Pathol.* 58:134, 2005.

Schlesinger N, et al. Dietary factors and hyperuricaemia. *Curr Pharm Des.* 11:4133, 2005.

Shi J, et al. Saponins from edible legumes: chemistry, processing, and health benefits. *J Med Food.* 7:67, 2004.

Straub M, Hautmann RE. Developments in stone prevention. *Curr Opin Urol.* 15:119, 2005.

Taylor EN, Curhan GC. Role of nutrition in the formation of calcium-containing kidney stones. *Nephron Physiol.* 98:55, 2004.

Terris M, et al. Dietary supplementation with cranberry concentrate tablets may increase the risk of nephrolithiasis. *Urology* 57:26, 2001.

Williams C, et al. Why oral calcium supplements may reduce renal stone disease: report of a clinical pilot study. *J Clin Pathol.* 54:54, 2001.

NEPHROTIC SYNDROME

NUTRITIONAL ACUITY RANKING: LEVEL 2–3

DEFINITIONS AND BACKGROUND

Nephrotic syndrome is not a disease; it causes massive proteinuria, with 3.5 g or more of protein lost within 24 hours. As much as 30 g can be lost as a result. Albumin is especially affected.

Idiopathic membranous nephropathy is a common cause of nephrotic syndrome (du Boef-Vereijken et al, 2005). The common form of nephrotic syndrome in children is called "minimal change disease," and its cause is unknown.

In about 20% of children with nephrotic syndrome, kidney biopsy reveals scarring or deposits in the glomeruli. The two most common diseases that damage these filtering units are focal segmental glomerulosclerosis (FSGS) and membranoproliferative glomerulonephritis (MPGN). Rarely, a child may be born with a condition that causes nephrotic syndrome (congenital nephropathy). Patients with renal insufficiency (serum creatinine level >1.5 mg/dL [>135 µmol/L]) are at risk for the development of end-stage renal disease and should receive immunosuppressive therapy (du Boef-Vereijken et al, 2005).

Signs and symptoms of nephrotic syndrome include weight gain, hyperlipidemia, edema, chest pains, hypovitaminosis D, hypokalemia, and weakness. Adults who have nephrotic syndrome usually have some form of glomerulonephritis, with renal failure not far behind. Elevated low-density lipoprotein (LDL) cholesterol is also common from altered lipoprotein production.

Nutrition therapy centers on the problem of salt and water retention, protein depletion, hyperlipidemia, and loss of carrier proteins for vitamins and minerals. A very high–protein diet will alter glomerular filtration rate (GFR); limit protein to decrease hyperfiltration. A moderate-protein diet that provides adequate energy can maintain nitrogen balance in nephrotic syndrome. These patients have normal anabolic responses to dietary protein restriction (decreased amino acid oxidation) and feeding (increased protein synthesis and decreased degradation).

INTERVENTION: OBJECTIVES

- Ensure efficient utilization of fed proteins, spared by use of adequate calories. Prevent muscle catabolism. If protein losses are severe, albumin infusion may be needed; this is rare.
- Reduce edema.
- Control sodium intake with otherwise uncontrolled hypertension (HPN).
- Monitor hypercholesterolemia and elevated triglycerides.
- Monitor patient for potassium deficits with certain diuretics.
- Replace any other nutrients, especially those at risk (e.g., calcium, vitamin D, etc.).
- Prevent or control renal failure.
- Correct anorexia.

INTERVENTION: FOOD AND NUTRITION

- Use a diet of modest protein restriction (0.8 g/kg in adults, with 50% of high biological value). Children should be given the RDA for their age because high protein levels may worsen proteinuria and will not improve serum albumin levels (Hogg et al, 2000).
- Diet should provide 35 kcal/kg/d unless patient is obese.
- With dyslipidemia, limit saturated fats and cholesterol; decrease intake of concentrated sugars and alcohol. Encourage use of linoleic acid and omega-3 fatty acids. A vegetarian, soy-based diet with amino acid replacements may be beneficial.
- Carbohydrate intake should be high to spare protein for lean body mass; use high–complex carbohydrate and high-fiber foods.
- If patient has edema, sodium intake should be restricted to 2–3 g.
- Provide adequate sources of potassium, vitamin D, and calcium as tolerated. Replace zinc, vitamin C, folacin, and other nutrients. Monitor iron according to laboratory values.
- Fluid restrictions may be necessary if edema is refractory to diuretic therapy.
- Offer appetizing meals to increase intake.
- If required, use tube feedings (specialty renal products if needed). Total parenteral nutrition may also be beneficial.

CLINICAL INDICATORS

Clinical/History	Lab Work	
Height	Alb, transthyretin	Ceruloplasmin (decreased)
Weight (gains?)	Proteinuria, uremia	AST (increased)
aBWef	CRP	Na+, K+ (hypokalemia?)
Edema	Trig (increased)	Serum phosphorus
BMI	Chol	Serum vitamin D
Diet history	H & H	Hypovitaminosis D
BP	Serum Fe	Ca++, Mg++
I & O	TIBC, percent saturation, serum ferritin	BUN, Creat
Chest pains	Transferrin (increased)	GFR
Weakness		CrCl

SAMPLE NUTRITION DIAGNOSTIC STATEMENT

Nephrotic Syndrome

PES: Excessive protein intake related to protein intake of 110 g/d as evidenced by worsening proteinuria over the past month by a factor of 10%.

Assessment Data: Dietary recall and laboratory analysis.

Intervention: Education on protein needs and sources.

Monitoring and Evaluation: Lab values and dietary intake.

Common Drugs Used and Potential Side Effects

- Thiazide diuretics such as furosemide deplete potassium. Other diuretics may spare or retain potassium (e.g., spironolactone, angiotensin-converting enzyme [ACE] inhibitors). Check need for dietary alterations.
- With corticosteroids such as prednisone, sodium restrictions may be needed. Potassium, nitrogen, or calcium losses may result. Muscle wasting or weight gain and other side effects are common.
- High-risk patients likely benefit from immunosuppressive therapy. Cyclophosphamide has fewer side effects (du Boef-Vereijken et al, 2005). Side effects include gastrointestinal distress, nausea, and vomiting.
- ACE inhibitors (blood pressure–lowering drugs) may help prevent protein from leaking into urine and keep kidneys from being damaged.

Herbs, Botanicals, and Supplements

- Herbs and botanical supplements should not be used without discussing with physician.
- With cyclosporine, avoid use with echinacea and St. John's wort because of counterproductive effects on drug.

INTERVENTION: NUTRITION EDUCATION, COUNSELING, CARE MANAGEMENT

- Help patient plan appetizing meals. Sodium restriction is common.
- If patient has abdominal edema, careful positioning may increase comfort at mealtimes.
- Weight management plans will be needed if steroid use will be long term.

NEPHROTIC SYNDROME—CITED REFERENCES

du Boef-Vereijken PW, et al. Idiopathic membranous nephropathy: outline and rationale of a treatment strategy. *Am J Kidney Dis.* 46(6):1012, 2005.

Hogg R, et al. Evaluation and management of proteinuria and nephrotic syndrome in children: recommendations from a pediatric nephrology panel established at the National Kidney Foundation Conference on Proteinuria, Albuminemia, Risk, Assessment, Detection, and Elimination (PARADE). *Pediatrics* 105:1242, 2000.

PYELONEPHRITIS AND URINARY TRACT INFECTIONS

NUTRITIONAL ACUITY RANKING: LEVEL 1 (3 IF CHRONIC)

DEFINITIONS AND BACKGROUND

Pyelonephritis, which is bacterial invasion of the kidneys and the most common cause of urinary tract infections (UTIs), may lead to fibrosis, scarring, and dilatation of the tubules, which impair renal function. *Escherichia coli* most often cause upper UTIs; other organisms are found in complicated infections associated with diabetes mellitus, instrumentation, urinary stones, and immunosuppression. With effective antibacterial therapy, the immune response by both T and B lymphocytes leads to antibodies that assist in bacterial eradication.

There are approximately 250,000 cases of acute pyelonephritis each year, resulting in more than 100,000 hospitalizations; the most common etiological cause is infection with *E. coli* (Ramakrishnan and Scheid, 2005). Pyelonephritis does not require extensive medical nutrition therapy. Indications for inpatient treatment include complicated infections, sepsis, persistent vomiting, failed outpatient treatment, or extremes of age (Ramakrishnan and Scheid, 2005). When the patient is septic, hospitalization and treatment with parenteral antibiotics may be needed.

If patient does not improve rapidly, studies, including ultrasound and computed tomography (CT), are used to diagnose obstruction, abscess, or emphysematous pyelonephritis. Most of these complications are now rapidly treated percutaneously, followed by surgical therapy as needed. Treatment failure may be caused by resistant organisms, underlying anatomic/functional abnormalities, or immunosuppressed states (Ramakrishnan and Scheid, 2005).

Scarring of chronic pyelonephritis leads to loss of renal tissue and function; it sometimes progresses to end-stage renal disease. Hypertension is often present in chronic pyelonephritis.

Although not always a cause of UTIs, **urinary incontinence** requires attention. Check for vitamin B_{12} deficiency;

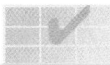

decrease caffeine intake; and try bladder training (use of toilet every 2 hours). It also may be useful to maintain an adequate level of fluid intake to prevent onset of any UTIs.

Interstitial cystitis (painful bladder syndrome) causes an inflamed bladder wall and has no specific link to diet. But omission of alcohol, caffeine, citrus beverages, and tomatoes may give relief to some individuals.

INTERVENTION: OBJECTIVES

- Preserve kidney function.
- Control blood pressure.
- Acidify urine to decrease additional bacterial growth.
- Force fluids unless contraindicated.

INTERVENTION: FOOD AND NUTRITION

- Restrict excess sodium to control elevated blood pressure. However, some patients lose excessive amounts of sodium in their urine and must be monitored for depletion.
- Restrict protein intake if renal function is decreased. Otherwise, use sufficient amounts of high biological value proteins, including foods such as meat, fish, poultry, eggs, and cheese.
- Restrict potassium when serum levels are elevated; check drugs first.
- Cranberries, plums, and prunes produce hippuric acid, which helps to acidify urine. Corn, lentils, breads/starches, peanuts, and walnuts also tend to acidify urine. Cranberry juice contains hippuric acid and another substance that seems to prevent adherence of bacteria to urinary tract epithelial cells (Kontiokari et al, 2001). It is often suggested to consume 3 glasses daily of cranberry juice cocktail for this purpose.
- Although vitamin C is not necessarily effective in lowering urinary pH, sufficient levels of intake are needed to stimulate the anti-infective process.
- Avoid an excess of caffeine because of its diuretic effect. Stimulants such as caffeine rapidly leave the bladder, a vulnerable site in which additional infections may begin.
- Vitamin A may be low; encourage improved intake, especially from carotenoid foods.

CLINICAL INDICATORS

Clinical/History	I & O	H & H
	BP (increased)	Serum Fe
Height		Serum ferritin
Weight	**Lab Work**	Ca++, Mg++
BMI		
Edema	Alb, transthyretin	Serum phosphorus
Diet history	CRP	
Temperature	Transferrin	
Na+, K+	RBP	Intravenous pyelogram
Urinary Na+	BUN, Creat	
Gluc		

Common Drugs Used and Potential Side Effects

- Outpatient oral antibiotic therapy with a fluoroquinolone is successful in most patients with mild uncomplicated pyelonephritis (Ramakrishnan and Scheid, 2005).
- Ceftriaxone and gentamicin are cost effective because only once-daily dosing is needed. With urinary anti-infectives, sufficient water and fluids should be ingested. Be careful with forced water diuresis, which impairs antibiotic effectiveness. Monitor responses to glucose changes in people with diabetes. Avoid use with alcohol.
- Nitrofurantoin (Furadantin, Macrodantin) should be consumed with food or milk. A diet adequate in protein is needed. Nausea, vomiting, and anorexia are common. Diarrhea is less common.
- Penicillin products such as amoxicillin (Amoxil, Trimox, Wymox) and ampicillin may be used. If penicillin allergy exists, vancomycin may be used.
- Quinolones include ofloxacin (Floxin), norfloxacin (Noroxin), ciprofloxacin (Cipro), and trovafloxin (Trovan). If Cipro (ciprofloxacin) is used, avoid taking with calcium supplements, milk, and yogurt; limit use of caffeine; monitor for nausea. If a fluoroquinolone (Floxin, Maxaquin) is used, nausea is one side effect. Take separately from vitamin supplements.
- Sulfisoxazole (Gantrisin) can deplete folacin and vitamin K. Nausea and vomiting may also occur.
- Trimethoprim (Trimpex) and trimethoprim/sulfamethoxazole (Bactrim, Septra, Cotrim) may cause diarrhea, gastrointestinal distress, and stomatitis. Use adequate fluid.

Herbs, Botanicals, and Supplements

- Herbs and botanical supplements should not be used without discussing with physician.
- Blueberry, parsley, bearberry, yogurt, birch, and couch grass have been suggested for kidney and bladder infections, but no clinical trials have shown efficacy.

INTERVENTION: NUTRITION EDUCATION, COUNSELING, CARE MANAGEMENT

- Indicate which foods are palatable as sources of nutrients for dietary restrictions and for nutrients that tend to be low.
- Encourage appropriate fluid intake.
- Discuss acid ash diets as adjunct therapy only; medical therapy must be first.

- Limit caffeine and oral fluid intake at night, if needed.
- Showers, instead of baths, may be preventive.

For More Information

- Interstitial Cystitis Association (ICA) http://www.ichelp.org/
- National Bladder Foundation http://www.bladder.org/

PYELONEPHRITIS AND URINARY TRACT INFECTIONS—CITED REFERENCES

Kontiokari T, et al. Randomized trial of cranberry-lingonberry juice and *Lactobacillus* GG drink for the prevention of urinary tract infections in women. *BMJ.* 322:1571, 2001.

Ramakrishnan K, Scheid DC. Diagnosis and management of acute pyelonephritis in adults. *Am Fam Physician.* 71:933, 2005.

RENAL DIALYSIS

NUTRITIONAL ACUITY RANKING: LEVEL 4

DEFINITIONS AND BACKGROUND

Renal replacement therapy (RRT) includes hemodialysis, peritoneal dialysis, and renal transplantation; the goal is to normalize the volume and composition of the body fluids and to remove uremic toxins. **Dialysis** specifically involves artificial filtering of blood by a machine; this is a catabolic process. Morbidity is largely related to physical fitness at the start of therapy. Among patients on dialysis, 33% have diabetes, and 50% of deaths are related to cardiovascular disease.

Chronic long-term dialysis can aggravate bone disease, anemia, and endocrine disorders and can lead to malnutrition if not monitored carefully. About 40% of patients undergoing maintenance dialysis suffer from varying degrees of protein–energy malnutrition (PEM) (Mehrotra and Kopple, 2001). Causes of PEM include the catabolic effects of hemodialysis treatments, acidemia associated with end-stage renal disease (ESRD), common comorbid conditions, and uremia-induced anorexia (Ohlrich et al, 2005). Toxins accumulate with renal failure that suppress appetite and contribute to nutritional decline (Mehrota and Kopple, 2001). Pica (mostly ice but also starch, dirt, flour, and aspirin intake) has also been found in many dialysis patients. A better nutritional status is associated with higher dialysis doses (Cano et al, 2006).

The National Kidney Foundation (NKF) recommends that strict criteria be used to diagnose malnutrition in patients maintained on dialysis, including serum albumin <3.4 g/dL, average body weight (ABW) <90% of desired goal, or documented protein intake <0.8 g/kg. The NKF Kidney Disease Guidelines for Nutrition provide many clinical practice guidelines for adults and separate guidelines for children. Protein–energy nutritional status in these patients should be assessed by a panel of measures rather than by any single measure (Kopple, 2001).

Nutritional intervention can decrease malnutrition and mortality. The first step is careful evaluation of protein—energy status, followed by intensive nutrition counseling and then by oral nutrition supplementation, appetite stimulation, or enteral tube feedings (Ohlrich et al, 2005). Parenteral nutrition should be initiated for the small number of dialysis patients who do not respond to other medical, psychiatric, and nutritional interventions.

Chronic, long-term dialysis can aggravate bone problems, anemia, and endocrine disorders and can lead to malnutrition. Chronic kidney disease (CKD) patients who do not respond to erythropoietin replacement may suffer from malnutrition and inflammation (Locatelli et al, 2006). Anemia can lead to chronic fatigue and debility if not corrected. Dialysis patients may be hospitalized frequently. Higher hemoglobin, higher albumin, and fistula or graft use are independently associated with fewer hospitalizations, fewer hospital days, and decreased Medicare inpatient reimbursement (O'Connor et al, 2005). Enteral multinutrient support significantly increases serum albumin concentrations and improves total dietary intake in dialysis patients (Stratton et al, 2005). Intensive diet counseling and use of enteral supplements may not be effective alone; aggressive nutrition options such as enteral and parenteral support may be needed (Moore and Celano, 2005).

Treatment of secondary hyperparathyroidism (HPT) in patients with chronic renal disease has improved in recent years; skeletal pain, disabling fractures, tendon ruptures, and myriad other symptoms associated with HPT can now be avoided, thus improving quality of life (Yudd and Llach, 2000). In another scenario, the side effects of elevated calcium levels are becoming more apparent. In contrast to recent Kidney Disease Outcomes Quality Initiative (KDOQI) recommendations, an upper dialysate concentration of 1.25 mmol/L may not be ideal for every patient; dialysate concentrations should be prescribed with reference to plasma calcium levels (Sigrist and McIntyre, 2006).

Dyslipidemia is common in ESRD, and dialysis patients have increased cardiovascular morbidity and mortality. The high frequency of cardiovascular disease in dialysis patients may originate from disturbed carbohydrate and lipid metabolism, oxidants and antioxidants, and the immunoinflammatory system (Schwedler et al, 2001). Elevated CRP levels can predict cardiovascular and overall mortality in these patients (Schwedler et al, 2001). Nutrition indicators are associated with subsequent mortality, with greatest effects at <6 months of follow-up (Dwyer et al, 2005).

An intensive program of dialysis and nutrition intervention can promote normal growth in children on maintenance RRT. Children need adequate protein to encourage growth. Monitor potassium and phosphorus restrictions because protein food choices may be high in these nutrients.

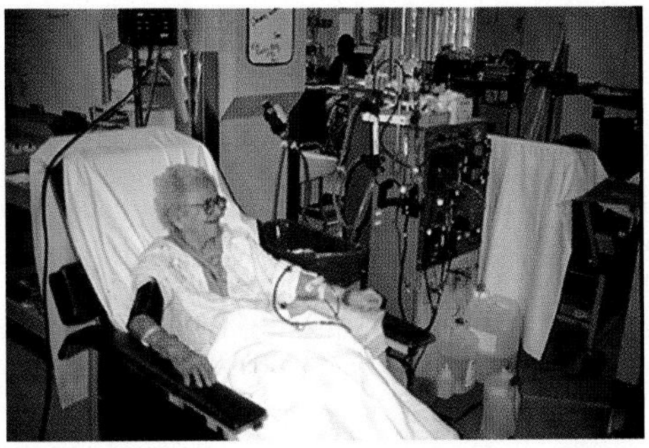

Figure 16-6 Hemodialysis.

With **hemodialysis,** less protein is lost than with peritoneal dialysis; nevertheless, amino acid losses still occur. See Figure 16-6. The Health Care Financing Administration's ESRD Core Indicators Project collects clinical information on prevalent adult patients receiving in-center hemodialysis care in the United States; quality of patient care could be improved, especially in anemia management (Frankenfield et al, 2000). Hemodialysis patients often have poor appetites; to correct poor nutritional status, use of favorite foods may be an important intervention. Decreased taste sensitivity has been shown to contribute to poor nutritional status in patients with chronic uremia or on maintenance hemodialysis. Developing palatable meals with appropriate seasoning enhancements is one step. Selection of dietary supplements for this population may require use of sugar-free, lactose-free renal supplements.

Peritoneal dialysis (PD) involves artificial filtering of the blood by a hyperosmolar solution (with osmosis to remove water and diffusion for glucose exchange/waste removal). Peritoneal dialysis removes metabolic wastes and excess fluid from the body but not so thoroughly that diet therapy is unnecessary. Types of peritoneal dialysis include intermittent, continuous cycling (used in nearly 100% of children), and continuous ambulatory. In continuous ambulatory peritoneal dialysis, there is fluid in the abdomen nearly 100% of the time; dialysis is performed four times daily, and no partner is necessary. Between dialysis treatments, the patient must return to a strict renal diet. Electrolytes (i.e., potassium, phosphorus, sodium) need not be restricted as much; intake of proteins is somewhat liberalized. Considerable losses of protein and amino acids occur, but peritoneal dialysis may yield fewer growth problems in children than hemodialysis. See Figure 16-7 for a peritoneal dialysis set.

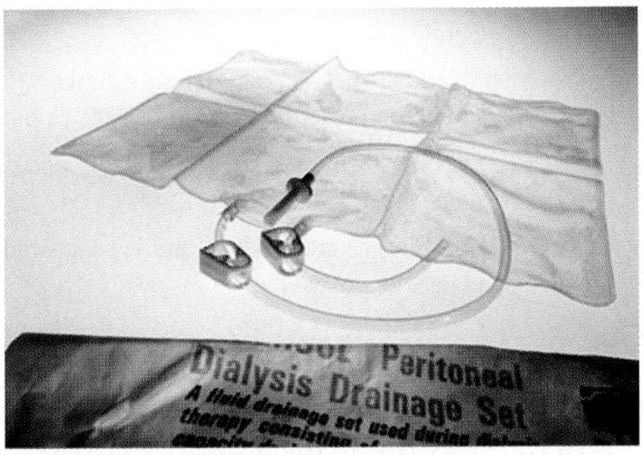

Figure 16-7 Peritoneal dialysis set.

INTERVENTION: OBJECTIVES

- Preserve residual renal function as long as possible.
- Compensate for protein losses. Replace lost amino acids without causing uremic symptoms.
- Spare protein adequately to allow for tissue repair and synthesis; assure sufficient total energy intake. Inflammation may elevate resting energy expenditure levels (Utaka et al, 2005); monitor accordingly.
- Promote growth in children.
- Maintain fluid balance; modify electrolytes and fluid intake according to patient's tolerance and lab values.
- Prevent or correct anorexia, constipation, growth delay, muscle weakness, cardiac arrhythmias, and hypertriglyceridemia. Excessive cardiovascular mortality of dialysis patients is at least in part related to chronic inflammation that is mediated by proinflammatory cytokines and leads to a reduction in appetite, increased muscle catabolism, and malnutrition (Kuhlmann and Levin, 2005).
- Manage hyperphosphatemia in patients with renal insufficiency, which causes hypocalcemia and secondary hyperparathyroidism. Bone demineralization in secondary hyperparathyroidism may induce fractures, while joint and subcutaneous precipitations of calcium pyrophosphate limit mobility and may cause crippling (Friedman, 2005).
- Prevent major shifts in serum calcium levels. Dialysate concentrations should be prescribed with reference to plasma calcium levels (Sigrist and McIntyre, 2006).
- Improve patient survival, reduce patient morbidity, increase efficiency of care, and improve quality of life. Provide follow-up for consistency of care in other settings or at home.
- **Peritoneal dialysis only:** Alter calorie intake according to glucose absorption from the solution (e.g., 20 kcal/L of 1.5% solution; 60 kcal/L of 2.5% solution; and 126 kcal/L of 4.5% solution).

INTERVENTION: FOOD AND NUTRITION

- See Table 16-11.

CLINICAL INDICATORS

Clinical/History

Height
Weight
aBWef
Edema
BMI
Diet history
Waist circumference
Waist–hip ratio
BP
I & O
Temperature
DEXA scan

Lab Work

BUN
Creat
GFR and CrCl (on hemodialysis, it will be <10)
Urine urea nitrogen (UUN) or Kt/V
Serum phosphorus (goal, <5.5 mg/dL)
CRP (usually elevated)

TABLE 16-11 Nutrition Therapy for Dialysis Patients

Nutrient	Hemodialysis (HD)	Peritoneal Dialysis (PD)
Protein	1.2 g protein/kg/d; at least 50% should come from high-biological value (HBV) sources. Urea kinetic modeling may also be used to devise a protein prescription. For children, base initial protein intake on RDA for age plus an increment of 0.4 g/kg/d.	1.2–1.3 g protein/kg/d, at least 50% from HBV sources (Kopple, 2001). If there is peritonitis, 1.5 g/kg may be needed until infection subsides. Children undergoing PD should be given RDA levels of protein, plus increments based on anticipated losses.
Energy	35 kcal/kg/d for patients who are <60 years of age and 30–35 kcal/kg for patients ≥ 60 years of age (Kopple, 2001). For children, follow RDA levels by age for energy.	35 kcal/kg/d for patients who are <60 years of age and 30–35 kcal/kg for patients ≥ 60 years of age (Kopple, 2001). Include dialysate kcals. In peritonitis, extra energy may be needed until infection subsides. For children, follow RDA levels by age for energy.
Carbohydrate (CHO) and Fat	After protein is calculated, assess patient needs (e.g., less CHO in diabetes, fewer lipids with dyslipidemia), and calculate percentages accordingly. Try oral supplements before using other modes of feeding such as enteral or parenteral nutrition.	Total energy intake increases from glucose in the dialysate in continuous ambulatory PD (CAPD). This extra 300–450 kcal of glucose can increase weight and triglyceride levels. CHO absorption calculations must be individualized and altered as the diet prescription changes. Limit simple sugars and saturated fats.
Fluid	≥ 1 L fluid output = 2 L fluid needed <1 L fluid output = 1–1.5 L fluid needed Anuria = 1 L fluid needed	Fluid restriction is less common in PD; 1–3 L/d is suggested. Fluid intake should be determined by patient's state of hydration; encourage or restrict according to intake and output; no more than 1 kg should be gained in 1 day.
Potassium and Phosphorus	Check levels of potassium and phosphorus; modify diet accordingly. Dialysis removes very little phosphorus; use 800–1000 mg or ≤ 17 mg/kg ideal body weight (BW). Potassium = 40 mg/kg BW	Check levels of potassium and phosphorus; modify diet accordingly. Adjust phosphorus intake according to serum levels; 800–1000 mg phosphorus or 10–15 mg phosphorus/g protein.
Sodium	Limit sodium intake unless there are large losses in dialysate or through vomiting or diarrhea. Restriction to 2–4 g of sodium is common and realistic.	Intake of sodium should be liberal, pending assessment of hydration, blood pressure, losses in dialysate,vomiting, and diarrhea. 2–4 g sodium is common; some patients need no restriction.
Vitamins	Use water-soluble vitamin supplementation to replace dialysate losses. Daily replacement may not be needed. Folic acid (often need 1 μg), vitamin B_6 (1.3–1.7 mg), vitamin C (75–90 mg), and vitamin B_{12} (2.4 μg) Active vitamin D should be monitored and replaced at recommended levels. Avoid vitamin A excesses. For children use DRI levels for age.	Supplement diet with water-soluble vitamins, especially vitamin B_6 and folic acid. Active vitamin D should be monitored and replaced at recommended levels. Avoid vitamin A excesses.
Minerals	Monitor serum labs as available. Individualize calcium; dialysate concentrations should be prescribed with reference to plasma calcium levels. Magnesium = 0.2–0.3 g Monitor zinc status; 8–11 mg is suggested.	Monitor serum labs as available. Individualize calcium; dialysate concentrations should be prescribed with reference to plasma calcium levels. Magnesium = 0.2–0.3 g Monitor zinc status; 8–11 mg is suggested.

(continued)

TABLE 16-11 Nutrition Therapy for Dialysis Patients *(continued)*

Enteral Nutrition	Try oral supplements first. If tube feeding (TF) is necessary, use an appropriate product to meet protein, energy, electrolyte, and volume needs. If low volume is needed, use a product with 1.5–2.0 kcal/mL with small free-water flushes. Monitor electrolytes.	If TF is needed, the formula should be carefully chosen considering the protein, energy, volume, and mineral needs of the patient.
Parenteral Nutrition	Before considering parenteral nutrition as a nutrition intervention in a dialysis patient, all other efforts to promote optimal nutrition need to be exhausted (Ohlrich et al, 2005). Use caution with parenteral solutions, especially for excesses of zinc and vitamins D and A.	Before considering parenteral nutrition as a nutrition intervention in a dialysis patient, all other efforts to promote optimal nutrition need to be exhausted (Ohlrich et al, 2005). Use caution with parenteral solutions, especially for excesses of zinc and vitamins D and A.
Omega-3 Fatty Acids and the Mediterranean Diet	Fish oil supplementation may help reduce prostaglandin synthesis and may help improve hematocrit levels. A Mediterranean dietary pattern and regular soy intake may be considered (Kuhlmann and Levin, 2005).	Fish oil supplementation may help reduce prostaglandin synthesis and may help improve hematocrit levels. A Mediterranean dietary pattern and regular soy intake may be considered (Kuhlmann and Levin, 2005).

Serum PTH (goal, 100–200 pg/mL)
Serum Ca++ (goal, 9.2–9.6 mg/dL)
Mg++
Gluc
Transferrin
Na+
K+ (levels >6 mg/dL can trigger heart failure)
Metabolic acidosis, hyperchloremia
Uric acid
Alb, transthyretin
RBP
Triceps skinfold, midarm circumference, and midarm muscle circumference (in nonaccess arm for hemodialysis)
Urea
Serum folacin
Serum B_{12}
Chol, Trig
AST (decreased)
Serum bicarbonate (may be low)
Hemoglobin
Hematocrit—target of 33–36% is acceptable (Collins et al, 2000)
Serum Fe
Serum ferritin, percent saturation
N balance
Serum zinc

Common Drugs Used and Potential Side Effects

- See Table 16-12.

Herbs, Botanicals, and Supplements

- Herbs and botanical supplements should not be used without discussing with physician. These products contain pharmacologically active compounds that may be hazardous to kidney patients (Burrowes and Van Houten, 2005).
- Noni juice should be avoided because of its high potassium content (Burrowes and Van Houten, 2005).
- Bulk-forming laxatives such as flaxseed should be used with caution because of the need for increased fluid intake (Burrowes and Van Houten, 2005).

INTERVENTION: NUTRITION EDUCATION, COUNSELING, CARE MANAGEMENT

Dialysis: General

- Public Law 92–603 provides financial assistance via Medicaid to all persons covered by Social Security who have ESRD with dialysis.
- Discuss signs of uremia (nausea, vomiting, hiccups, fatigue, and weakness).
- Discuss high-energy, low-protein, electrolyte-controlled food choices and supplements. Adequate care must be taken to ingest the designated protein and energy levels, according to current lab reports. See Table 16-13 concerning the role of a renal dietitian in these patient cases.
- When patients participate in an exercise program, appetites often improve, and protein and total energy intake are often improved.
- Counsel patient regarding managing a healthy diet to prevent or control heart disease or diabetes. A Mediterranean dietary pattern and regular soy intake both have been shown to attenuate chronic inflammation, and this may be useful in CKD patients (Kuhlmann and Levin, 2005).
- If avoiding potassium-rich foods is needed, salt substitutes should be monitored closely. Use of longer cooking times and extra water may help leach out excess potassium.
- Taste alterations are common. Distaste for red meats, fish, poultry, eggs, sweets, and vegetables is common. Work individually with patient to plan meals to ensure adequacy of protein intake.
- Provide information about dining away from home, home-delivered meals, and meals while traveling.

TABLE 16-12 Drugs Commonly Used in Dialysis Patients

Medication	Comments
Angiotensin-converting enzyme (ACE) inhibitor or angiotensin receptor blocker	First-line pharmacological intervention should be an ACE inhibitor or angiotensin receptor blocker in those with diabetes or nondiabetics with more than 200 mg protein/g creatinine on a random urine sample (Toto, 2005).
Antidepressants	Depression is common in this population. Chronic kidney disease (CKD) and end-stage renal disease (ESRD) patients with anemia, hypoalbuminemia, and higher serum C-reactive protein (CRP) and ferritin concentrations should be evaluated for depression after potential somatic causes have been eliminated; antidepressant treatment may be needed to improve appetite and intake (Kalender et al, 2005).
Carnitine	Carnitine is formed from lysine and methionine, requiring adequate vitamin C, niacin, iron, and vitamin B_6. Red meat and dairy products are typical dietary sources. Supplements of carnitine may be needed.
Growth hormone	Pharmacological doses of recombinant human growth hormone constitute a new anabolic therapy; its use improves whole-body protein homeostasis in chronic hemodialysis patients (Pupim et al, 2005).
Insulin	Insulin may be needed to control blood glucose levels. It serves as an anabolic hormone in that it can protect lean body mass for some patients.
Iron supplements	If recombinant human erythropoietin (r-HuEPO) is used to treat anemia, an iron supplement will be necessary. Be careful not to overload with excesses and do not take supplements at the same time as calcium.
Lipid-lowering medications and statins	Lipid-lowering medications may be used in dyslipidemia. Cerivastatin, a statin with powerful low-density lipoprotein (LDL) cholesterol–lowering capabilities, may contribute to a reduction of coronary events in dialysis patients (Keane et al, 2001). The National Kidney Foundation Kidney Disease Outcomes Quality Initiative guidelines for managing dyslipidemia suggest that CKD patients with LDL $\geq$100 mg/dL should be treated with diet and a statin (Farbakhsh and Kasiske, 2005).
Phosphate binders	Control of hyperphosphatemia, maintenance of normocalcemia, and appropriate dosing of vitamin D analogs can prevent hyperparathyroidism (HPT) in many cases. If severe HPT develops, many patients can still be controlled medically with correction of hyperphosphatemia and high doses of intravenous calcitriol.
	Fosrenol (lanthanum carbonate) was approved by the FDA in 2004. Aluminum products should be used for a short time period only.
	Phosphate binders containing calcium (calcium acetate, lactate, carbonate, or gluconate) may be prescribed and can cause nausea or vomiting. Monitor calcium levels carefully to prevent high levels of calcium over time.
Potassium excretion	Kayexalate may be needed to deplete excess serum potassium until serum levels return to normal. Anorexia, constipation, or diarrhea can occur. Take separately from calcium supplements or antacids.
Ruboxistaurin	Ruboxistaurin may add benefit to established therapies for diabetic nephropathy by reducing albuminuria and maintaining estimated glomerular filtration rate for a year (Tuttle et al, 2005).
Vitamin D_3	Vitamin D_3 supplements may be prescribed; avoid long-term high doses.
Water-soluble vitamins	Supplements should be used to replace water-soluble vitamins. Use of a low-potassium diet creates the potential risk for low vitamin C intake. Use caution with generic multivitamin-mineral supplements, which may supply higher doses of vitamin A, phosphorus, and potassium than are possible to remove with dialysis.

TABLE 16-13 Role of the Dietitian in Care of Dialysis Patients

Patients with end-stage renal disease often experience malnutrition as a result of decreased dietary intake; inadequate dialysis; loss of nutrients into the dialysate; abnormal protein, carbohydrate, and lipid metabolism; and concomitant diseases, which may contribute to an increase in morbidity and mortality (How and Lau, 2004).

Close monitoring of nutritional status is completed by evaluating serum albumin and relevant biochemical data, appetite assessments, dietary energy and protein intakes, consumption of vitamins and minerals, and intake of oral supplemental foods, tube feeding, and parenteral nutrition. Anthropometry is performed at baseline and on a yearly basis (Leung et al, 2001).

Specified changes in serum albumin level or body weight trigger action by the dietitian to prevent protein–energy malnutrition.

Multiple diet parameters are necessary to provide optimal nutritional health, including monitoring of calories, protein, sodium, fluid, potassium, calcium, and phosphorus, as well as other individualized nutrients. Consider all modes of nutritional intervention; use that which is best accepted by the patient and the least invasive.

Consider the role of intradialytic parenteral nutrition (IDPN), with its benefits and shortcomings (How and Lau, 2004). The biggest advantage of IDPN is probably its convenience since it is administered during dialysis treatment. The disadvantage is that it is not currently covered by Medicare.

The rising incidence of chronic kidney disease will increase the probability of the nonrenal specialist dietetics professional delivering care to this patient population (Beto and Bansal, 2004).

TABLE 16-14 Fluid Equivalents

Equivalent Measures

30 mL = 1 fluid oz = 2 tablespoons
240 mL = 8 fluid oz = 1 cup
2 cups = 1 lb fluid weight
2.2 lb = 1 kg fluid weight or 4 cups liquid

Sample Fluid Content

1 whole popsicle = 90 mL
4 oz soup = 120 mL
6 oz juice = 180 mL
8 oz beverage = 240 mL
12 oz soda = 360 mL
16 oz milkshake = 480 mL

TABLE 16-15 Phosphorus Foods and Suggested Alternatives

High-Phosphorus Foods	Phosphorus Content (mg)	Suggested Alternatives	Phosphorus Content (mg)
1 cup yogurt	353	1 cup sorbet	19
½ cup nuts	315	1 cup unsalted popcorn or 1 oz pretzels	24
1 cup milk	236	1 cup nondairy creamer	132
½ cup macaroni and cheese	220	½ cup pasta noodles with margarine and garlic	150
1 oz chocolate	200	1 oz hard candy, jelly beans, or marshmallows	1
1 oz cheese	150	1 oz cream cheese or Neufchatel cheese	34
½ cup bran cereal	143	½ cup cornflakes, rice or corn cereals	19
½ cup dried beans or peas	143	½ cup green or wax beans	19
½ cup custard	142	½ cup custard made with nondairy creamer	110
2 slices pizza	246	1 slice pizza plus 1 cup lettuce with Italian dressing	149
12 oz cola soda	44	12 oz lemon-lime or ginger ale or grape or root beer soda	0

Moe SM. *Calcium and phosphorus balance in ESRD: implications and management.* Cambridge, MA: Genzyme Corporation, 2001.

- Establishing trust, mutual respect, and emotional support are essential to promote a successful set of nutritional outcomes.
- For fluid management, see Table 16-14.

Hemodialysis

- Discuss maximum fluid gain (usually 3–5% of body weight) between dialysis sessions. Noncompliance with fluid intake restrictions is common in patients with renal disease using hemodialysis and can lead to systemic and cardiac overload.
- Teach fluid management to motivate patients to comply with their regimens; patients report that they feel better when their weight gains are within acceptable limits.

Peritoneal Dialysis

- Fluid restrictions are not always needed with peritoneal dialysis. Patient should learn how to recognize significant changes in dry weight (adjusted edema-free body weight) or food intake. Discuss actions to be taken. Usually, 3–4 lb between intermittent peritoneal dialysis is allowed.
- Teach the patient and family about managing diet to control phosphorus levels (goal is <5.5 mg/dL). See Table 16-15. Increasing patient knowledge of hyperphosphatemia and its treatment may enhance dietary adherence to phosphorus restriction and use of phosphate binders. Instruct patient to avoid use of carbonated beverages that contain phosphates, such as colas.

For More Information

- Hemodialysis
  http://www.kidney.org/professionals/KDOQI/guidelines_updates/doqi_uptoc.html#hd
- National Kidney Foundation–Nutrition Guidelines
  http://www.kidney.org/professionals/doqi/guidelines/doqi_nut.html
- Peritoneal Dialysis
  http://www.kidney.org/professionals/KDOQI/guidelines_updates/doqi_uptoc.html#pd

RENAL DIALYSIS—CITED REFERENCES

Burrowes JD, Van Houten G. Use of alternative medicine by patients with stage 5 chronic kidney disease. *Adv Chronic Kidney Dis.* 12:312, 2005.

Cano F, et al. Kt/V and nPNA in pediatric peritoneal dialysis: a clinical or a mathematical association? *Pediatr Nephrol.* 21:114, 2006.

Dwyer JT, et al. Are nutritional status indicators associated with mortality in the Hemodialysis (HEMO) Study? *Kidney Int.* 68:1766, 2005.

Farbakhsh K, Kasiske BL. Dyslipidemias in patients who have chronic kidney disease. *Med Clin North Am.* 89:689, 2005.

Frankenfield D, et al. Anemia management of adult hemodialysis patients in the U.S. results: from the 1997 ESRD Core Indicators Project. *Kidney Int.* 57:578, 2000.

Friedman EA. Consequences and management of hyperphosphatemia in patients with renal insufficiency. *Kidney Int Suppl.* 95:1S, 2005.

How PP, Lau LH. Malnutrition in patients undergoing hemodialysis: is intradialytic parenteral nutrition the answer? *Pharmacotherapy* 24:1748, 2004.

Kalendar B, et al. Association of depression with markers of nutrition and inflammation in chronic kidney disease and end-stage renal disease. *Nephron Clin Pract.* 102:115, 2005.

Keane W, et al. The CHORUS (Cerivastatin in Heart Outcomes in Renal Disease: Understanding Survival) protocol: a double-blind, placebo-controlled trial in patients with ESRD. *Am J Kidney Dis.* 37:48S, 2001.

Kopple J. National kidney foundation K/DOQI clinical practice guidelines for nutrition in chronic renal failure. *Am J Kidney Dis.* 37:66S, 2001.
Kuhlmann MK, Levin NW. Interaction between nutrition and inflammation in hemodialysis patients. *Contrib Nephrol.* 149:200, 2005.
Leung J, et al. The role of the dietitian in a multicenter clinical trial of dialysis therapy: The Hemodialysis (HEMO) Study. *J Ren Nutr.* 11:101, 2001.
Locatelli F, et al. Nutritional-inflammation status and resistance to erythropoietin therapy in haemodialysis patients. Nephrol Dial Transplant. 21:991, 2006.
Mehrotra R, Kopple J. Nutritional management of maintenance dialysis patients: why aren't we doing better? *Annu Rev Nutr.* 21:343, 2001.
Moe SM. *Calcium and phosphorus balance in ESRD: implications and management.* Cambridge, MA: Genzyme Corporation, 2001.
Moore E, Celano J. Challenges of providing nutrition support in the outpatient dialysis setting. *Nutr Clin Pract.* 20:202, 2005.
O'Connor AS, et al. The morbidity and cost implications of hemodialysis clinical performance measures. *Hemodial Int.* 9:349, 2005.
Ohlrich H, et al. The use of parenteral nutrition in a severely malnourished hemodialysis patient with hypercalcemia. *Nutr Clin Pract.* 20:559, 2005.
Pupim LB, et al. Recombinant human growth hormone improves muscle amino acid uptake and whole-body protein metabolism in chronic hemodialysis patients. *Am J Clin Nutr.* 82:1235, 2005.
Schwedler S, et al. Inflammation and advanced glycation end products in uremia: simple coexistence, potentiation, or causal relationship? *Kidney Int.* 59:32S, 2001.
Sigrist M, McIntyre CW. Calcium exposure and removal in chronic hemodialysis patients. *J Ren Nutr.* 16:41, 2006.
Stratton RJ, et al. Multinutrient oral supplements and tube feeding in maintenance dialysis: a systematic review and meta-analysis. *Am J Kidney Dis.* 46:387, 2005.
Toto RD. Treatment of hypertension in chronic kidney disease. *Semin Nephrol.* 25:435, 2005.
Tuttle KR, et al. The effect of ruboxistaurin on nephropathy in type 2 diabetes. *Diabetes Care.* 28:2686, 2005.
Utaka S, et al. Inflammation is associated with increased energy expenditure in patients with chronic kidney disease. *Am J Clin Nutr.* 82:801, 2005.
Yudd M, Llach F. Current medical management of secondary hyperparathyroidism. *Am J Med Sci.* 320:100, 2000.

POLYCYSTIC KIDNEY DISEASE

NUTRITIONAL ACUITY RANKING: LEVEL 2

DEFINITIONS AND BACKGROUND

Polycystic kidney diseases (PKD) are disorders that cause multiple, fluid-filled, bilateral cysts in the kidneys and may also affect the liver, pancreas, colon, blood, and heart valves. Fluid-filled sacs or cysts of varying sizes that become larger as the disease progresses replace normal kidney tissue.

PKD in its autosomal dominant form (ADPKD) affects 600,000 people in the United States at a rate of 1 in 400–1000 persons and is caused by mutations in the *PKD1* gene in 85% of cases and the *PKD2* gene in the rest of the cases (Wilson, 2004). The rare autosomal recessive form occurs in 1 per 44,000 births. Infants who are not treated may die before 1 month of age. An acquired form occurs in patients on dialysis and often affects adults in midlife.

ADPKD is one of the most common human genetic disorders (Kleymenova et al, 2001). Children with autosomal recessive PKD experience high blood pressure, urinary tract infections, and frequent urination; their disease affects the liver, spleen, and pancreas, resulting in low blood cell counts, varicose veins, and hemorrhoids. Because kidney function is crucial for early physical development, children with autosomal recessive PKD are usually smaller than average size.

PKD results from loss of function of either of two novel proteins, polycystin-1 or polycystin-2. Recent studies show that intracellular calcium signaling is important in kidney development, and defects in this signaling pathway are the basis of cyst formation in PKD (Somlo and Ehrlich, 2001).

Increased understanding of genetic and pathophysiologic mechanisms responsible for development of ADPKD, made possible by the advances of the last three decades, has laid the foundation for development of effective therapies (Qian et al, 2001). The concept that a polycystic kidney is a neoplasm in disguise is becoming increasingly accepted; therapies will benefit from information on cancer chemoprevention and chemosuppression.

Signs and symptoms include back or side pain, abnormally high blood pressure, progressive loss of kidney function, hematuria, vomiting, and chronic headaches. Most infants with autosomal recessive PKD also have unusual facial features (Potter's face) and failure to thrive. People with ADPKD can also experience urinary tract infections, liver and pancreatic cysts, abnormal heart valves, kidney stones, aneurysms in the brain, and diverticulosis. Proteinuria and microalbuminuria occur with a highly variable severity and are associated with progression of the autosomal form (Nakamura et al, 2001).

Treatment of PKD involves efforts to identify patients at greatest risk for disease progression, thus allowing targeted therapy and combination therapy to retard disease progression and renal functional deterioration (Cowley, 2004). Half of patients with PKD will require dialysis. Laparoscopic surgery to remove the cysts may be beneficial for some patients. For others, transplantation is needed. Figure 16-8 shows a polycystic kidney.

INTERVENTION: OBJECTIVES

- Prevent renal failure; manage chronic kidney disease.
- Minimize or alleviate nausea, vomiting, and anorexia.
- Bring hypertension under control where present.
- Correct or alleviate proteinuria or microalbuminuria.
- Manage dialysis when and if needed.
- Prepare for transplantation, if planned.

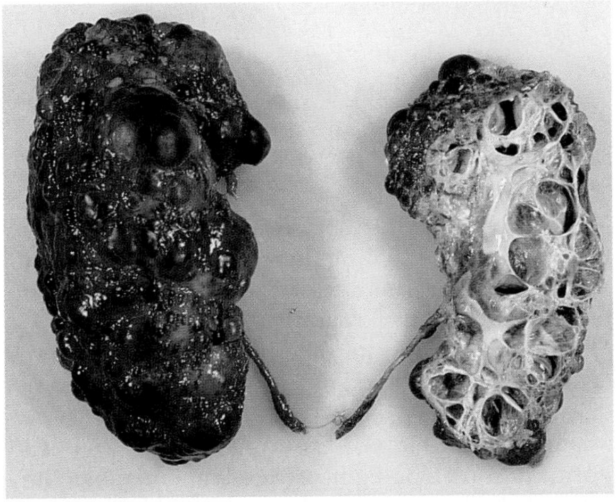

Figure 16-8 Polycystic kidney. (From Rubin E. *Rubin's pathology: clinicopathologic foundations of medicine*. 4th ed. Philadelphia: Lippincott Williams & Wilkins, 2005.)

INTERVENTION: FOOD AND NUTRITION

- Modify diet according to symptoms; sodium restriction may be beneficial for lowering blood pressure. Controlled protein intake (meeting dietary allowance for age) is recommended unless proteinuria is excessive, in which case lower levels are needed.
- Reduce or eliminate caffeine.

CLINICAL INDICATORS

Clinical/History	Vomiting	Na+, K+
Length or height	Chronic headaches	Chol, Trig
Birth weight	**Lab Work**	Gluc
Present weight	BUN, Creat	Serum vitamin D
Growth percentile	H & H	Alb, transthyretin
BMI	Serum Fe, percent saturation	CRP
Diet history	Serum ferritin	Proteinuria, microalbuminuria
Back or side pain	MCV	Ca++, Mg++
BP (very high)	Ultrasound	Serum phosphorus
Hematuria		

Common Drugs Used and Potential Side Effects

- New experimental drug therapies for PKD are being tested.
- Angiotensin-converting enzyme (ACE) inhibitors are most frequently prescribed for hypertension; calcium channel blockers, diuretics, and beta-blockers may also be used.
- A common combined therapy is a diuretic plus an ACE inhibitor. Antihypertensive regimens with ACE inhibitors are more effective in lowering urine protein excretion in patients with advanced PKD compared with regimens without ACE inhibitors; benefits are greater in patients with higher levels of baseline urine protein excretion (Jafar et al, 2005).
- Dilazep dihydrochloride, an antiplatelet drug, is effective in patients with immunoglobulin A nephropathy or diabetic nephropathy; it may be effective in reducing urinary albumin excretion in normotensive ADPKD patients with microalbuminuria (Nakamura et al, 2001).
- Antibiotics may be used to treat infections; monitor specific medicines for nutritional side effects.
- Analgesics may be useful for pain management.

Herbs, Botanicals, and Supplements

- Herbs and botanical supplements should not be used without discussing with physician.

INTERVENTION: NUTRITION EDUCATION, COUNSELING, CARE MANAGEMENT

- Explain measures that are appropriate to specific condition.
- Encourage regular medical visits and nutritionist follow-up.

For More Information

- National Kidney and Urologic Diseases Information Clearinghouse
  http://kidney.niddk.nih.gov/
- Polycystic Kidney Disease Foundation
  http://www.pkdcure.org

POLYCYSTIC KIDNEY DISEASE—CITED REFERENCES

Cowley BD Jr. Recent advances in understanding the pathogenesis of polycystic kidney disease: therapeutic implications. *Drugs* 64:1285, 2004.

Jafar TH, et al. The effect of angiotensin-converting-enzyme inhibitors on progression of advanced polycystic kidney disease. *Kidney Int.* 67:265, 2005.

Kleymenova E, et al. Tuberin-dependent membrane localization of polycystin-1: a functional link between polycystic kidney disease and the TSC2 tumor suppressor gene. *Mol Cell.* 7:823, 2001.

Nakamura T, et al. Effect of dilazep dihydrochloride on urinary albumin excretion in patients with autosomal dominant polycystic kidney disease. *Nephron* 88:80, 2001.

Qian Q, et al. Treatment prospects for autosomal-dominant polycystic kidney disease. *Kidney Int.* 59:2005, 2001.

Somlo S, Ehrlich B. Human disease: calcium signaling in polycystic kidney disease. *Curr Biol.* 11:356, 2001.

Wilson PD. Polycystic kidney disease: new understanding in the pathogenesis. *Int J Biochem Cell Biol.* 36:1868, 2004.

RENAL TRANSPLANTATION

NUTRITIONAL ACUITY RANKING: LEVEL 4

DEFINITIONS AND BACKGROUND

Renal transplantation is completed in ESRD when GFR drops to 10 mL/min. Persons with poor health or history of cancer often cannot receive a transplantation. Pediatric kidney transplantation has become an option for children with ESRD. A child must reach a certain body surface area or weight (such as 20 kg) to receive a parent's kidney; siblings younger than 18 years of age generally are not allowed to donate a kidney.

Patient and graft survival rates, as well as long-term quality of life, have improved dramatically, a result of advances in surgical techniques, immunosuppression, and pre- and postoperative care (Papalois and Najarian, 2001). Laparoscopic living-donor nephrectomy has improved the possibility of live renal donations.

Malnutrition that exists prior to transplantation may be associated with an increased risk of infection, delayed wound healing, and muscle weakness (Martins et al, 2004). Because uremic men before transplantation display undernutrition indices and slow anthropometric recovery during the first 3 months posttransplantation (whereas women start close to normal and have significantly increased body weight and fat content posttransplantation), nutritional requirements after kidney grafting may be significantly different between male and female patients (Coroas et al, 2005). An adequate nutritional status may improve outcomes after transplantation (Martins et al, 2004).

After a renal transplantation, the patient has a functioning donor kidney. High doses of glucocorticoid drugs are given to prevent rejection. The acute posttransplantation phase lasts up to 2 months; the chronic phase starts after 2 months. After transplantation, the usual equations to predict GFR decline may be impaired and may potentially compromise the validity of the Kidney Disease Outcomes Quality Initiative (KDOQI) guidelines if implemented in their current form (Mariat et al, 2005). Additional forms of evaluation should be used.

Complications of corticosteroid use include new-onset diabetes, osteoporosis, and hyperlipidemia. In the long term, cardiovascular morbidity remains the greatest risk (Roberts et al, 2006), followed by infections and malignancy. It is expected that cancer will become the leading cause of death in transplantation patients within the next two decades (Buell et al, 2005).

Complications are listed in Table 16-16. Prognosis is good for transplantation patients who take care of themselves and attend to medical follow-up. Early intensive dietary advice and follow-up helps control complications after renal transplantation.

INTERVENTION: OBJECTIVES

- Promote healing and prevent infections, especially during acute phase. Alleviate rejection episodes. Support immunity to prevent additional infections.
- Normalize diet to meet specific needs of patient and modify diet according to drug therapy to enhance outcome.
- Watch for abnormalities in calcium or phosphorus metabolism with hyperparathyroidism.
- Monitor for abnormal electrolyte levels (sodium, potassium). Control blood pressure carefully to prevent cardiac problems.
- Maintain good blood pressure control as well as near-normal fasting blood glucose levels and hemoglobin A1c levels (Schiel et al, 2005). Manage carbohydrate (CHO) intake, but make sure diet provides enough energy to spare protein for healing.
- Manage fluid intake according to intake and output. Most patients can return to a normal or increased fluid intake after transplantation.
- Help patient adjust to a lifelong medical regimen during chronic phase. Improve survival rate by supporting immune response.
- Correct or manage complications that occur, such as posttransplantation anemia (Molnar et al, 2005).
- Minimize weight gain.

INTERVENTION: FOOD AND NUTRITION

- Progress to solids as quickly as possibly postoperatively. Monitor fluid status and adjust as needed.
- Energy should be calculated as 30–35 kcal/kg. Needs may increase with postoperative complications.
- Daily intake of protein should be 1.3–2.0 g/kg in the acute phase and 0.8–1.0 g/kg in the chronic phase. Soy proteins can be used in most cases and may help lower low-density lipoprotein (LDL) cholesterol (Cupisti et al, 2004).
- Control CHO intake; 50% of total kcal is usual. Limit concentrated sweets and encourage use of complex CHO.
- Limit fat to 30% of total kcal; encourage monounsaturated fats and omega-3 fatty acids. Use of the Mediterranean diet principles has been recommended with some success (Stachowska et al, 2005). Use more fish and fish oils and olive oil.
- Fluid is not restricted unless there are problems with graft functioning.
- Daily intake of sodium should be 2–4 g until drug regimen is reduced. Careful management of sodium efficiently controls blood pressure in patients who are hypertensive (Keven et al, 2006).
- Adjust potassium levels as needed (2–4 g if hyperkalemic).
- Daily intake of calcium should be 1200–1500 mg. Children especially will need adequate calcium for growth.
- Supplement diet with vitamin D, magnesium, phosphorus, and thiamine if needed. If homocysteine-lowering multivitamin therapy is needed; folic acid and vitamins B_6 and B_{12} are essential (Winkelmayer et al, 2005).
- Reduce gastric irritants as necessary, if gastrointestinal distress or reflux occurs.

TABLE 16-16 Complications after Renal Transplantation

Many possible complications may be prevented or treated through early nutritional intervention and follow-up (Martins et al, 2005).

Complication	Description
Anemia	Posttransplantation anemia is a prevalent and undertreated condition; protein–energy malnutrition and/or chronic inflammation may be independently associated with anemia (Molnar et al, 2005).
Cancer	Lymphomas may occur. Malignancies are rapidly becoming a major cause of mortality in transplantation patients (Buell et al, 2005).
Cardiovascular complications	Hyperlipidemia is one of the consequences of long-term use of corticosteroids. Elevated triglycerides and metabolic syndrome can also persist. Diet alone may be sufficient in this population (Zaffari et al, 2004). Renal transplantation recipients (RTRs) are at high risk for ischemic heart disease and heart failure and will benefit from lifestyle modifications (e.g., smoking cessation, maintenance of ideal body mass index, healthy diet), aggressive blood pressure control (<130/80 mm Hg), use of angiotensin-converting enzyme inhibitors or angiotensin receptor blockers, lipid lowering with statins, antiplatelet therapy for diabetics and those with established coronary disease, and use of beta-blockers for congestive heart failure or after myocardial infarction (Rigatto, 2005).
Diabetes	A high number of patients are at risk for posttransplantation diabetes because of the use of corticosteroids. The most important parameter associated with new-onset diabetes is higher BMI, and the most important parameter associated with transplantation rejection is an elevated fasting blood glucose level (Schiel et al, 2005). Protocols with minimal steroid use and/or steroid withdrawal may be beneficial for the kidney recipient population. It is also important to manage high blood pressure (Schiel et al, 2005).
Infection	Acute meningitis caused by *Listeria monocytogenes* or Guillain-Barré syndrome triggered by cytomegalovirus (CMV) or *Campylobacter jejuni* infection can occur (Ponticelli and Campise, 2005).
Neurological complications	Neurotoxic immunosuppressive medications such as the calcineurin inhibitors may cause mild symptoms, such as tremors and paresthesia, or severe symptoms, such as disabling pain syndrome and leukoencephalopathy (Ponticelli and Campise, 2005). Monoclonal antibody OKT3 may also cause neuronal changes.
	Peripheral neuropathies: An acute femoral neuropathy may occur in about 2% of patients as a result of nerve compression after operation (Ponticelli and Campise, 2005).
Osteoporosis	Bone density declines after long-term use of corticosteroids. Tertiary hyperparathyroidism (THPT) may occur in patients after kidney transplantation.
Pulmonary complications	Infectious pulmonary complications may occur. Noninfectious pulmonary complications arise because of numerous factors, including the underlying conditions that preceded transplantation, the transplantation surgery itself, and toxicity of posttransplantation medications (Kotloff, 2005).
Stroke	Stroke may occur in about 8% of renal transplantation patients, caused by hypertension, diabetes, and accelerated atherosclerosis, which may be acquired during dialysis or after transplantation (Ponticelli and Campise, 2005).
Weight gain	Obesity decreases effectiveness of insulin receptors, increasing the tendency for glucose intolerance. It may also delay wound healing.

- Encourage exercise and a weight control plan for the long-term recovery phase.

CLINICAL INDICATORS

Clinical/History

Height
Present weight
aBWef
Edema
BMI
Weight changes
Diet history
I & O
BP
Temperature
DEXA

Lab Work

CRP
Alb
Ca++, Mg++
Phosphorus
Na+, K+
H & H
Serum Fe
BUN
Creat
GFR
WBC, total lymphocyte count (TLC)
Gluc
Total homocysteine (tHcy) levels
Chol and lipid profile (LDL goal <100 mg/dL)
Trig
N balance
GFR, CrCl
Serum phosphorus
AST, alanine aminotransferase (ALT)
Bilirubin
PTH

Common Drugs Used and Potential Side Effects

- See Table 16-17.
- Kidney transplantation is a routine phenomenon with excellent 1-year graft survival in most centers, but chronic allograft nephropathy (CAN) remains a common cause of graft attrition over time (Afzali et al, 2005). Mycophenolate mofetil and sirolimus may have useful antitumor properties (Buell et al, 2005).
- Switching to tacrolimus due to cyclosporine-related side effects improves disease-specific quality of life indicators within a short time (Franke et al, 2006).

TABLE 16-17 Drugs Commonly Used in Renal Transplantation

Medication	Comments
Calcium and vitamin D supplements	Even if serum calcium and phosphorous levels are in the normal range after kidney transplantation, calcium or vitamin D supplements may be needed to correct osteopenia.
Corticosteroids (prednisone, Solu-Cortef)	Used for immunosuppression. Side effects include increased catabolism of proteins, negative nitrogen balance, hyperphagia, ulcers, decreased glucose tolerance, sodium retention, fluid retention, and impaired calcium absorption and osteoporosis. Cushing's syndrome, obesity, muscle wasting, and increased gastric secretion may result. A higher protein intake and controlled carbohydrates may be needed.
Immunosuppressants: cyclosporine	Cyclosporine does not retain sodium as much as corticosteroids. Nausea, vomiting, and diarrhea are common side effects. Hyperlipidemia, hypertension, and hyperkalemia also may occur; decrease sodium and potassium as necessary. Elevated glucose and lipids may occur. The drug is also nephrotoxic; a controlled renal diet may be beneficial.
	Implicated in fibrotic processes that are the hallmarks of chronic allograft nephropathy (CAN) (Afzali et al, 2005).
Immunosuppressants: monoclonal antibodies (mAbs) (basiliximab, daclizumab)	Less nephrotoxic than cyclosporine but can cause nausea, anorexia, diarrhea, and vomiting. Monitor carefully. Fever and stomatitis also may occur; alter diet as needed. Anti-CD25 mAbs (basiliximab and daclizumab) are well tolerated; other recently developed mAbs, like anti-CD52 (Campath-1H), anti-CD20 (rituximab), anti-LFA-1, anti-ICAM-1, and anti-tumor necrosis factor (TNF)-alpha (infliximab), are currently being tested and show encouraging potential (Buhaescu et al, 2005).
Immunosuppressants: azathioprine (Imuran)	May cause leukopenia, thrombocytopenia, oral and esophageal sores, macrocytic anemia, pancreatitis, vomiting, diarrhea, and other complex side effects. Folate supplementation and other dietary modifications (liquid or soft diet, use of oral supplements) may be needed. The drug works by lowering the number of T cells; it often is prescribed along with prednisone for conventional immunosuppression.
Immunosuppressants: tacrolimus (Prograf, FK506)	Suppresses T-cell immunity; it is 100 times more potent than cyclosporine, thus requiring smaller doses. Side effects include gastrointestinal distress, nausea, vomiting, hyperkalemia, and hyperglycemia.
	May cause fibrotic processes that are the hallmarks of chronic allograft nephropathy (Afzali et al, 2005).
Statins	At least 60% of adult renal transplantation recipients develop dyslipidemia, which occurs within 1 month of the initiation of immunosuppressive therapy (mostly cyclosporine, sirolimus, and prednisone) and continues indefinitely unless treated with statins and diet therapy (Mathis et al, 2004).

NOTE. Patients are generally on three to four of the five drugs listed.

Herbs, Botanicals, and Supplements

- Herbs and botanical supplements should not be used without discussing with physician.
- With cyclosporine, avoid use with echinacea and St. John's wort because of counterproductive effects on the drug.

INTERVENTION: NUTRITION EDUCATION, COUNSELING, CARE MANAGEMENT

- Share, as appropriate, details of the DASH diet and Mediterranean diet; indicate which foods are sources of protein, calcium, magnesium, potassium, and sodium.
- If patient does not drink milk, describe other sources of calcium. Calcium supplementation may be needed.
- Alcohol and smoking should be avoided.
- Patients should learn how to apply self-management and when to seek medical attention.
- Encourage moderation in diet; promote adequate exercise.
- Rigorous efforts should be made to optimize weight before and after solid-organ transplantation by a judicious combination of diet, exercise, minimization of steroid therapy, surgery, and psychological therapies (Jindal and Zawada, 2004).
- Discuss the importance of bone health and how diet affects prevention of osteoporosis.

For More Information

- Nephrology Channel
  http://www.nephrologychannel.com/rrt/transplant.shtml
- University of Maryland Transplant Center
  http://www.umm.edu/transplant/kidney/index.html

RENAL TRANSPLANTATION—CITED REFERENCES

Afzali B, et al. What we CAN do about chronic allograft nephropathy: role of immunosuppressive modulations. *Kidney Int.* 68:2429, 2005.

Buell JF, et al. Malignancy after transplantation. *Transplantation* 80:254S, 2005.

Buhaescu I, et al. New immunosuppressive therapies in renal transplantation: monoclonal antibodies. *J Nephrol.* 18:529, 2005.

Coroas A, et al. Nutritional status and body composition evolution in early post-renal transplantation: is there a female advantage? *Transplant Proc.* 37:2765, 2005.

Cupisti A, et al. Effect of a soy protein diet on serum lipids of renal transplant patients. *J Ren Nutr.* 14:31, 2004.

Franke GH, et al. Switching from cyclosporine to tacrolimus leads to improved disease-specific quality of life in patients after kidney transplantation. *Transplant Proc.* 38:1293, 2006.
Jindal RM, Zawada ET Jr. Obesity and kidney transplantation. *Am J Kidney Dis.* 43:943, 2004.
Keven K, et al. The impact of daily sodium intake on posttransplant hypertension in kidney allograft recipients. *Transplant Proc.* 38:1323, 2006.
Kotloff RM. Noninfectious pulmonary complications of liver, heart, and kidney transplantation. *Clin Chest Med.* 26:623, 2005.
Mariat C, et al. Predicting glomerular filtration rate in kidney transplantation: are the K/DOQI guidelines applicable? *Am J Transplant.* 5:2698, 2005.
Martins C, et al. Nutrition for the post-renal transplant recipients. *Transplant Proc.* 36:1650, 2004.
Mathis AS, et al. Drug-related dyslipidemia after renal transplantation. *Am J Health Syst Pharm.* 61:565, 2004.
Molnar MZ, et al. Anemia in kidney transplanted patients. *Clin Transplant.* 19:825, 2005.
Papalois V, Najarian J. Pediatric kidney transplantation: historic hallmarks and a personal perspective. *Pediatr Transplant.* 5:239, 2001.
Ponticelli C, Campise MR. Neurological complications in kidney transplant recipients. *J Nephrol.* 18:521, 2005.
Rigatto C. Management of cardiovascular disease in the renal transplant recipient. *Cardiol Clin.* 23:331, 2005.
Roberts MA, et al. Cardiovascular biomarkers in CKD: pathophysiology and implications for clinical management of cardiac disease. *Am J Kidney Dis.* 48:341, 2006.
Schiel R, et al. Post-transplant diabetes mellitus: risk factors, frequency of transplant rejections, and long-term prognosis. *Clin Exp Nephrol.* 9:164, 2005.
Stachowska E, et al. Elements of Mediterranean diet improve oxidative status in blood of kidney graft recipients. *Br J Nutr.* 93:345, 2005.
Winkelmayer WC, et al. Fasting plasma total homocysteine levels and mortality and allograft loss in kidney transplant recipients: a prospective study. *J Am Soc Nephrol.* 16:255, 2005.
Zaffari D, et al. Effectiveness of diet in hyperlipidemia in renal transplant patients. *Transplant Proc.* 36:889, 2004.

SECTION 17

Enteral and Parenteral Nutrition Interventions

CHIEF ASSESSMENT FACTORS

- Inability to Eat Orally (Mechanical, Gastrointestinal, Surgical Procedures)
- Therapies Such as Radiation or Chemotherapy, Past or Concurrent
- Benefits of Nutritional Intervention Outweigh Risks?
- Availability of Appropriate Lab Work
- Serial Anthropometric Measures
- Other Planned Procedures and Impact of Delayed Nutrition Support
- Unwillingness to Eat (Anorexia Nervosa, Fear, Anxiety, Psychosis)
- Disorder or Disease State:
  - GI Obstruction, Chronic Diarrhea, Crohn's Disease, Short Bowel Syndrome
  - GI Disease from HIV Infection or AIDS
  - Pancreatic Disease
  - Pulmonary Aspiration or Complications; Ventilator Use
  - Cystic Fibrosis
  - Failure to Thrive, Chronic Malnutrition
  - Cancer
  - Surgery (Preoperative or Postoperative Status)
  - Organ Transplantation
  - Sepsis, Trauma, Burns, or Other Causes of High Rates of Catabolism

OVERVIEW OF ENTERAL AND PARENTERAL NUTRITION AS AN INTERVENTION

The role of nutrition support has grown over the past few decades. Initially, total parenteral nutrition (TPN) was the ultimate standard of care and then enteral nutrition (EN) was found to protect against translocation of intestinal bacteria, protecting gut function. TPN was then considered to be a detrimental form of therapy when, in truth, data show neither mucosal atrophy from use of TPN nor increased bacterial translocation (Jeejeebhoy, 2001).

Nutrition support is not always applied effectively or consistently, despite available scientific evidence and treatment protocols; obstacles include lack of time, inadequate research skills, and information overload (Hise et al, 2005). Parenteral nutrition (PN) should be especially carefully managed (Fessler, 2001). While overfeeding may aggravate sepsis in TPN patients, TPN is an effective alternative to EN in patients who cannot be fed using the gastrointestinal (GI) tract (Jeejeebhoy, 2001). Advances in technology have contributed to improved quality of life for many patients under long-term home PN.

Nutrition support is often used in the care of infants and children, both for acute and chronic conditions; monitoring tolerance is an ongoing challenge (Weckwerth, 2004). Special standards should be used in pediatrics (Wessel et al, 2005) and in home care.

Many healthy elderly persons do not desire to be tube fed, especially in advanced disease or dementia. In fact, tube feeding (TF) has not necessarily improved outcomes in end-stage cancer, dementia, or other terminal illnesses. Selection of patients receiving TF must include consideration of long-term goals and ethical issues (American Dietetic Association, 2002). Due to the potential complications of permanent enteral access, percutaneous gastrostomy (PEG) or jejunostomy (PEJ) should be considered only when anticipated length of use is 1 month or longer (McMahon et al, 2005). When considering initiation of feedings, the treatment goal should be taken into account, whether palliative, curative, or rehabilitative. Additionally, the patient's wishes should be foremost in the decision-making process (McMahon et al, 2005).

Full authorization to write diet and TF orders expedites patient-centered care and expands the dietitian's responsibilities beyond traditional dietetic practice (Braga et al, 2006). When dietitians are granted full authority to implement nutritional recommendations, they write diet and TF orders on the physician's order sheets, change existing physician orders, and implement orders immediately (Wildish, 2001).

Critically ill patients are at high risk for infections, organ dysfunction, and death; their long, expensive stays in intensive care units may be shortened by use of carefully selected specialty products (Farber et al, 2005). Payments for PN and EN and services furnished under the prosthetic device are under federal guidelines (Federal Register, 2001). Therefore, reasonable and prudent use of expensive products and supplies is expected in dietetic practice.

Dietitians sometimes need to help decide whether or not to initiate, withhold, or withdraw medically assisted nutrition and hydration. A **persistent vegetative state** is defined as a condition of complete unawareness of self and the environment accompanied by sleep–wake cycles with complete or partial preservation of hypothalamic and brainstem autonomic functions (Quality Standards Subcommittee, 1995). While medically assisted nutrition can maintain life, it may be considered futile if it cannot improve the prognosis, comfort, or general status of health of an individual (Andrews and Marian, 2006). Autonomy and the patient's self-determination must always be the overriding principle.

Evidence-based practice merges the best and most relevant clinical research data with clinician experience, pathophysiology of disease state, and the specifics of individual patient care (Hise et al, 2005). See Table 17-1.

TABLE 17-1 Clinical Practice Guidelines for Nutrition Support

Evidence-based clinical practice guidelines for nutrition support (enteral nutrition [EN] and parenteral nutrition [PN]) should consider:

Issue	Considerations or Evidence
EN versus PN	When considering nutrition support in critically ill patients, strongly recommend that EN be used in preference to PN (Hise et al, 2006; Heyland et al, 2003).
Early versus late EN	Recommend that standard, polymeric enteral formula be initiated within 24–48 hours after admission to intensive care unit (ICU) (Heyland et al, 2003; Hise et al, 2006).
Positioning of patient for EN	When clinically feasible, patients should be placed in a 45° head of bed elevation during gastric feedings to decrease reflux of gastric contents into pharynx and esophagus and possibly to decrease pneumonia (Hise et al, 2006).
Dose and actual delivery of EN	Actual delivery of threshold intake of approximately 14–18 kcal/kg/d or 60–70% of enteral feeding goal in the first week of ICU admission is associated with improved outcomes (e.g., length of hospital stay, time on ventilator, infectious complications), particularly when initiated within 48 hours of injury or admission (Hise et al, 2006).
Composition of EN (protein, carbohydrates, lipids, immune-enhancing additives)	Standard formula is acceptable for most patients.
	Use of products with fish oils, borage oils, and antioxidants should be considered for patients with acute respiratory distress syndrome (Heyland et al, 2003).
	A glutamine-enriched formula should be considered for patients with severe burns and trauma (Heyland et al, 2003).

(continued)

TABLE 17-1 Clinical Practice Guidelines for Nutrition Support *(continued)*

Issue	Considerations or Evidence
Strategies to optimize delivery of EN	Start at the target rate, use a feeding protocol with a higher threshold of gastric residual volumes, use motility agents, and use small bowel feeding (Heyland et al, 2003). Promotility agents (metoclopramide) or postpyloric feeding should be considered to reduce the gastric residual volume (Hise et al, 2006).
Strategies to minimize risks in EN	Manage rate of advancement, check residuals, use bedside algorithms, consider motility agents, use small bowel versus gastric feedings when needed, elevate head of the bed, use closed delivery systems, consider use of probiotics, and evaluate bolus administration (Heyland et al, 2003).
EN in combination with supplemental PN	When initiating EN, strongly recommend that PN not be used in combination with EN (Heyland et al, 2003; Hise et al, 2006).
Use of PN and gastrointestinal tract immunity	When PN is used, supplement with glutamine, where available (Heyland et al, 2003).
Dose of PN and composition of PN	Calculate needs for protein, carbohydrates, intravenous lipids, additives, vitamins, trace elements, and immune-enhancing substances.
Strategies that maximize the benefits and minimize the risks of PN	Hypocaloric dose, withholding lipids, and the use of intensive insulin therapy to achieve tight glycemic control should be considered (Heyland et al, 2003).
Use of intensive insulin therapy	With elevated glucose levels (as in diabetes, infection, and sepsis), insulin therapy will help to achieve better control.
Clinical outcomes	Length of stay (ICU and hospital), quality of life, and specific complications should be considered: Enteral feeding is associated with decreased infectious complications compared with PN (Hise et al, 2006). Enteral feeding should be started within 24–48 hours following injury or admission to the ICU in fluid resuscitated patients to decrease infectious complications and to decrease the length of hospital stay (Hise et al, 2006). Placement of the tip of the feeding tube in the postpyloric position is associated with decreased gastric residual volume, a factor that has been associated with reduced reflux of formula; postpyloric feeding tube placement may not be necessary or feasible for all patients but may be useful in patients with large gastric residual volumes (Hise et al, 2006). Markers such as serum levels of albumin, transthyretin, transferrin, insulin-like growth factor I, delayed hypersensitivity, and total lymphocyte count may be valid to help stratify levels of nutritional risk, but they are not effective markers of adequacy of nourishment in the sick patient (Seres, 2005).
Costs	Charge for PN may be $200–$1000 per day, whereas EN costs $25 per day (Kirby, 2001).
Nutrition support protocol	An enteral feeding protocol for use by dietitians in the ICU should include the following topics (Hise et al, 2006). • When to use enteral vs. parenteral feeding • When initiation of enteral feeding should be initiated • Positioning of patient • Caloric goal per kilogram per day • Use of blue dye (omit or use very minimally) • Indications for holding feedings • Tube placement • Prokinetic/promotility agents
Insufficient data	There are insufficient data to generate recommendations in the following areas (Heyland et al, 2003): • Use of indirect calorimetry • Optimal pH of EN • Supplementation with trace elements, antioxidants, or fiber • Optimal mix of fats and carbohydrates • Use of closed feeding systems • Continuous vs. bolus feedings • Use of probiotics • Type of lipids • Mode of lipid delivery
Percutaneous gastrostomy (PEG) tube placement recommendation (Rabeneck et al, 1997) See Figure 17-1	Rationale: Start feeding upon being medically stable and continue until treatment is futile (American Dietetic Association, 2002). Anorexia-cachexia syndrome: Do not recommend, patient unable to benefit. Dysphagia with complications: Discuss, patient equivocally benefits. Dysphagia without complications: Recommend, patient usually benefits. Persistent vegetative state: Do not recommend; patients unable to experience satisfying quality of life

(continued)

TABLE 17-1 Clinical Practice Guidelines for Nutrition Support ***(continued)***

Issue	Considerations or Evidence
Artificial nutrition and hydration at the end of life	Treat each case individually. Base feeding choice on patient's wishes.
	Consider: What is the potential benefit for the patient and do risks outweigh the benefits?
	When oral feeding is medically appropriate as per swallowing exam, do not artificially feed.
	Consider a family conference with the physician, nurse, case manager, social worker, dietitian, and patient representative to present the necessary information for making the best decision for the patient when there is no legal document describing patient wishes.
	Minimize suffering and discomfort; provide comfort foods without dietary restrictions (American Academy of Hospice and Palliative Medicine, 2006).
	Contrary to expectations, most patients with complex medical conditions at the end of life do not experience hunger even with low energy intake, but they do experience dry mouth (American Academy of Hospice and Palliative Medicine, 2006). It is not common to hydrate in the presence of symptoms of edema or vomiting (American Nurses Association, 2006).
Dying process and hospice considerations (Dickinson Law School, 2006)	Starvation is a long, drawn out (and typically painful) process that can take anywhere from 30–60 days; dying patients who stop taking in food and fluids *do not* starve to death. While the body can sustain itself for up to 2 months without food, it can sustain itself no more than about 2 weeks (at most) without fluid intake. Unlike starvation, dehydration is typically not a painful or even an uncomfortable process, especially when good comfort care measures are undertaken. Many patients report less discomfort, and there is less request for pain medication as dehydration runs its course.
	Patients who stop taking in food and fluids drift into a state of unconsciousness. This phase of the process may take 5–8 days if the patient is fully hydrated when food and fluid intake is stopped. Patients will typically die peacefully several days after that. If the patient is already partly dehydrated when fluid intake is stopped, the dying process will be compressed and may only last a couple of days or less.
Pediatric end of life issues	There is a need for more ethics education and more interdisciplinary discussion of inherently complex and stressful pediatric end of life cases; appropriate goals of care and use of medically supplied nutrition and hydration are part of this educational process (Solomon et al, 2005).

CITED REFERENCES

American Academy of Hospice and Palliative Medicine. Statement on the use of nutrition and hydration. Accessed February 13, 2006 at http://www.aahpm.org/positions/nutrition.html.

American Dietetic Association. Position of the American Dietetic Association. Ethical and legal issues in nutrition, hydration, and feeding. *J Am Diet Assoc.* 102:716, 2002.

American Nurses Association. Position statement on foregoing nutrition and fluid. Accessed February 13, 2006 at http://www.nursingworld.org/readroom/position/ethics/etnutr.htm.

Andrews M, Marian M. Ethical framework for the registered dietitian in decisions regarding withholding/withdrawing medically assisted nutrition and hydration. *J Am Diet Assoc.* 106:206, 2006.

Braga JM, et al. Implementation of dietitian recommendations for enteral nutrition results in improved outcomes. *J Am Diet Assoc.* 106:281, 2006.

Dickinson Law School. Tube feeding options at the end of life. Accessed February 13, 2006 at http://www.dickinson.edu/endoflife/.

Farber MS, et al. Reducing costs and patient morbidity in the enterally fed intensive care unit patient. *J Parenter Enteral Nutr.* 29:62S, 2005.

Federal Register. Medicare program; replacement of reasonable charge methodology by fee schedules for parenteral and enteral nutrients, equipment, and supplies. Final rule. *Federal Register* 66:45173, 2001.

Fessler T. Appropriateness of adult parenteral nutrition use in a large hospital. *Nutr Clin Pract.* 16:153, 2001.

Jeejeebhoy K. Total parenteral nutrition: potion or poison? *Am J Clin Nutr.* 74:160, 2001.

Heyland DK, et al. Canadian clinical practice guidelines for nutrition support in mechanically ventilated, critically ill adult patients. *J Parenter Enteral Nutr.* 27:355, 2003.

Hise M, et al. Enteral feedings in the intensive care unit: a systematic review. Preliminary report for the ADA Medical Nutrition Therapy Evidence-Based Guide for Practice. Accessed October 20, 2006 at http://www.dnsdpg.org/documents/1079117807_Evidence_Analysis_Summary.pdf.

Hise ME, et al. Evidence-based clinical practice: dispelling the myths. *Nutr Clin Pract.* 20:294, 2005.

Kirby DF. Decisions for enteral access in the intensive care unit. *Nutrition* 17:776, 2001.

McMahon M, et al. Medical and ethical aspects of long-term enteral tube feeding. *Mayo Clin Proc.* 80:1461, 2005.

Quality Standards Subcommittee. American Academy of Neurology. Practice parameters: Assessment and management of patients in the persistent vegetative state. *Neurology* 45:1015, 1995.

Rabeneck L, et al. Ethically justified, clinically comprehensive guidelines for percutaneous endoscopic gastrostomy tube replacement. *Lancet* 349:496, 1997.

Seres DS. Surrogate nutrition markers, malnutrition, and adequacy of nutrition support. *Nutr Clin Pract.* 20:308, 2005.

Solomon MZ, et al. New and lingering controversies in pediatric end-of-life care. *Pediatrics* 116:872, 2005.

Weckwerth JA. Monitoring enteral nutrition support tolerance in infants and children. *Nutr Clin Pract.* 19:496, 2004.

Wessel J, et al. Standards for specialized nutrition support: hospitalized pediatric patients. *Nutr Clin Pract.* 20:103, 2005.

Wildish D. Medical directive: authorizing dietitians to write diet and tube-feeding orders. *Can J Diet Pract Res.* 62:204, 2001.

For More Information

- American Society for Parenteral and Enteral Nutrition (ASPEN)
  http://clinnutr.org/
- Artificial Nutrition–Family Doctor
  http://familydoctor.org/629.xml
- Determining Prognosis in Hospice Patients
  http://aspe.hhs.gov/daltcp/reports/impquesa.htm
- Pikes Peak Forum on Artificial Nutrition
  http://www.epcms.org/forumanhques.htm

ENTERAL NUTRITION

NUTRITIONAL ACUITY RANKING: LEVEL 4 (HOME)

DEFINITIONS AND BACKGROUND

There are approximately 1000 kcal available in the muscles, liver, and bloodstream as glucose or glycogen; daily replacement is crucial for brain and red blood cell survival. When oral feeding is not possible or is not safe, nutrients should be replaced by other means. Specialized nutrition support includes both enteral and parenteral feeding methods. Enteral nutrition (EN) involves nutrition support via nasogastric tube, orogastric tube, gastrostomy, nasoduodenal or nasoenteric feeding, or jejunostomy for patients who are unable to consume adequate nutrients and fluid orally (see Fig. 17-1). Candidates must have a functioning gastrointestinal (GI) tract for enteral feedings. Parenteral nutrition (PN) is reserved for conditions in which EN is contraindicated, unsuccessful, or inadequate.

EN is more economical than most parenteral feedings. EN yields better nutrient utilization by helping to maintain gut mucosal integrity. Trophic stimulation of the gut occurs with EN rather than PN. Use of EN has also been associated with a reduction in hospital-associated infectious complications, a decrease in overall infection rate, and a decrease in ventilator and intensive care unit (ICU) days (Bernard et al, 2004). EN has other advantages: immunoglobulin A (IgA) prevents absorption of enteric antigens; IgA increases with EN but not PN. Immunoenhancement from tube feeding (TF) occurs when increased intakes of arginine, glutamine, long-chain polyunsaturated fatty acids (PUFAs), omega-3 fatty acids, and other related nutrients (vitamins A, C, and E and ribonucleic acids) have pharmacological effects.

Pneumonia, sepsis, and bacteremia are less common in patients who receive enteral feedings supplemented with glutamine (Wischmeyer et al, 2001). Glutamine supplementation in surgical patients may be associated with a decrease in infectious complications and shorter hospital stays. In critically ill patients, parenterally administered glutamine may result in decreased complication and mortality rates (Novak et al, 2002).

It is often thought that enteral feeding should be initiated slowly in those who are severely malnourished, but malnourished patients at risk for refeeding syndrome can be fed early without observed negative clinical consequences (Flesher et al, 2005). Early enteral feeding is beneficial if the patient is hemodynamically stable, depending on where the tube must be placed. Improved clinical outcomes, including lower rates of infection and decreased hospital stay, have been observed when EN was initiated within 24–72 hours of admission to an ICU. Furthermore, implementation of an ICU nutrition protocol has been observed to increase the likelihood of patients receiving EN and decrease the duration of mechanical ventilation (Barr et al, 2004).

Judicious use of EN should be considered in the low birth weight premature infant because feeding intolerance is common among these infants. Caution should be taken when starting EN in infants with conditions that would inhibit adequate intestinal blood flow because this could increase the risk of necrotizing enterocolitis (Mayhew and Gonzalez, 2003). Gastrostomy buttons have minimal complications and acceptable longevity; they are preferred devices of long-term enteral feeding in children (Ruangtrakool and Ong, 2000).

Although TF is often started to prevent aspiration pneumonia from oral diet in stroke or demented patients, it may also increase risks. Because tube-fed patients in long-term acute-care facilities are routinely over- or underfed, monitoring how much feeding is actually given to a patient should be done to determine if needs are being met. Both underfeeding and overfeeding affect ventilatory status. Therefore, it is ideal to measure a patient's energy requirements using indirect calorimetry (IC) at least once. Uses of IC include assessing energy expenditure in patients who are critically ill, obese, or in whom estimation of requirements are difficult.

Feeding the obese, critically ill patient has become a widespread challenge due to the unique metabolic demands. It has been suggested that critically ill obese patients are at higher risk for infectious complications including postoperative wounds, nosocomial infections, as well as increased posttraumatic mortality and ICU mortality (Dickerson, 2005). Protein stores will be mobilized and less protein is synthesized during critical illness. The goals for feeding the critically ill obese patient should be to attenuate hypermetabolism and minimize catabolic losses. Because the increase in body fat poses a unique challenge when estimating nutritional needs, indirect calorimetry is particularly useful. A hypocaloric, high-nitrogen regimen may be beneficial to promote protein anabolism and glycemic control (Elamin, 2005).

The definition of what constitutes gastric residual volumes as indicators of TF tolerance will vary. Volume of gastric residuals, which prompts holding or cessation of TF, varies from one facility to the next; one high volume should probably not prompt the clinician to stop TF but to monitor carefully and recheck frequently (McClave et al, 2002). Optimal patient positioning, use of prokinetic agents to improve gastric emptying, and careful abdominal examinations to evaluate for distention are important steps to consider.

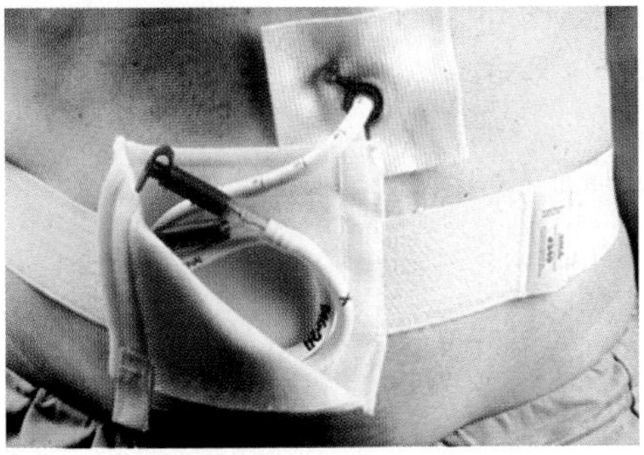

Figure 17-1 Percutaneous gastrostomy tube feeding.

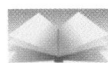

For terminally ill individuals, consideration of a patient's advance directives or medical care guidelines must be part of the plan. When a patient's wishes are not known, TF is viewed as humane by many internists. When life-sustaining care includes nutrition and hydration, families and other surrogate decision makers sometimes reach different conclusions; a multidisciplinary group can help with this important decision.

Home nutrition support is the fastest growing segment of health care, usually for the management of short bowel syndrome, bowel obstruction, chronic pancreatitis, enterocutaneous fistula, cancer, and severe dysphagia. Long-term enteral feeding optimizes body weight among ambulatory patients who are dependent on EN (Schattner et al, 2005).

Use of clinical practice guidelines or pathways may help practitioners to standardize nutrition support for patients. The American Dietetic Association recommends four or more medical nutrition therapy (MNT) visits for adults who are receiving EN. A multidisciplinary approach works well for consideration of medical, nutritional, and ethical principles for care of these patients (McMahon et al, 2005).

Cost Savings and Issues: MNT for patients who are tube fed saves thousands of dollars per case each year. Nutrition support teams are associated with improved quality and cost-effective care. Teams are often able to decrease complications, decrease lengths of stay, and decrease readmission rates (Saalwachter et al, 2004). Registered dietitians with special training and demonstrated competency in nutrition support are able to evaluate, write, or recommend TF or TPN orders (American Society for Parenteral and Enteral Nutrition, 2006).

INTERVENTION: OBJECTIVES

- Prevent or reverse malnutrition, cachexia, impaired immunity, and loss of lean body mass.
- Write or edit TF prescription to provide adequacy of protein, carbohydrate, fat, vitamins, minerals, and water. Nitrogen needs will increase for burn or trauma patients, and the percentage of total kilocalories from protein should be increased in these cases.
- Calculate order to meet 100% of DRIs for vitamins and minerals, or provide explanation for increased provision. Additional liquid vitamins and minerals may be needed if volume of formula prescribed is not sufficient.
- Conduct nutritionally focused physical exams on the patient, including state of hydration, abdominal exam for possible GI intolerance, state of consciousness, general overall appearance, body composition, presence of respiratory distress, nausea, vomiting, abdominal distention, diarrhea, abdominal cramping, constipation, weight changes, hydration status, and abnormal laboratory values. Alter TF prescriptions accordingly.

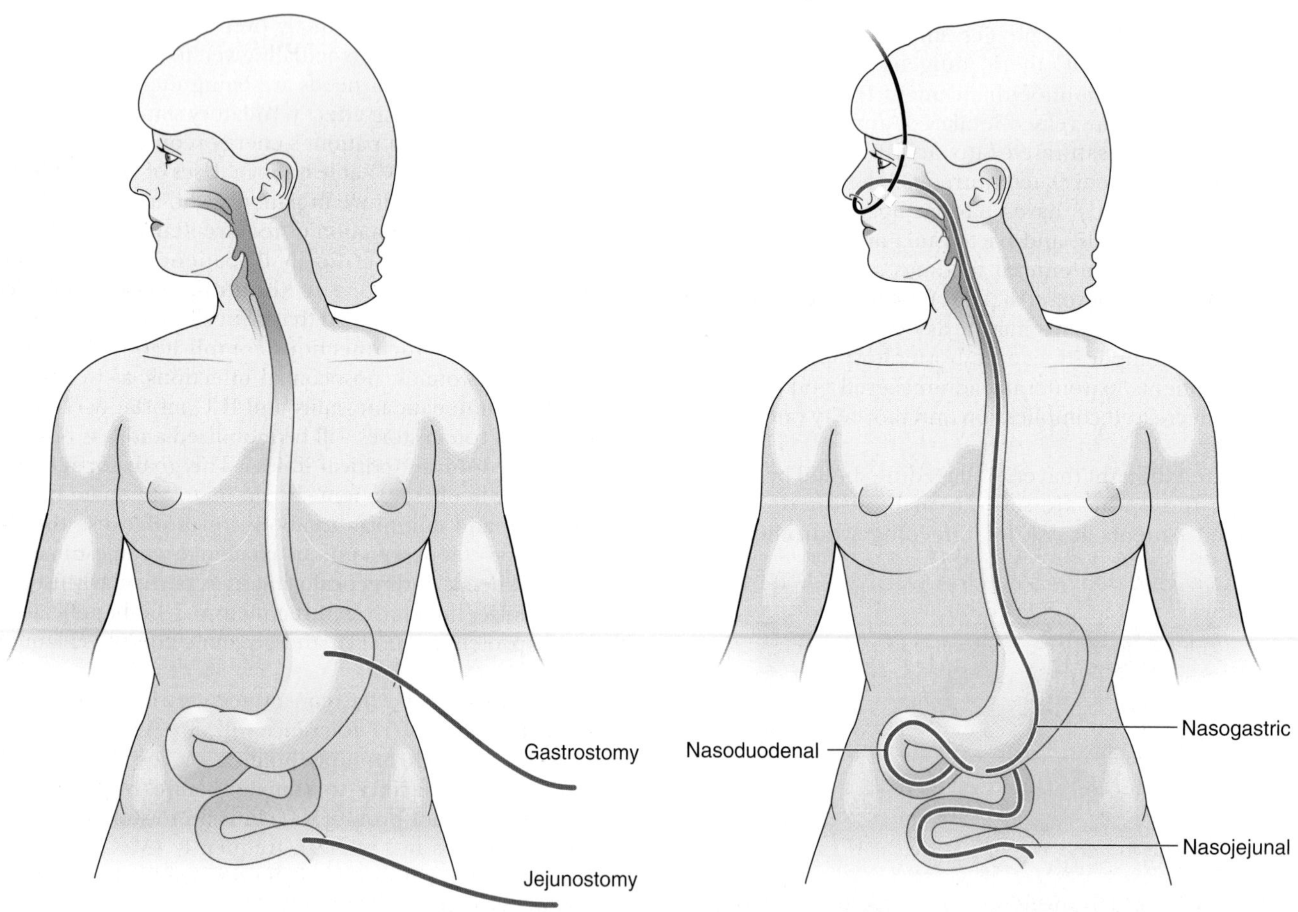

Figure 17-2 Enteral tube placement sites. (Modified from Cohen BJ. *Medical terminology*. 4th ed. Philadelphia: Lippincott Williams & Wilkins, 2003.)

TABLE 17-2 Sample Formulas

Blenderized	Compleat
Polymeric 1 kcal/mL	Ensure, Osmolite, Isocal, Nutren
Added Fiber	Ensure with fiber, Boost/Fiber, Jevity, Impact with fiber, Nutren, Replete with fiber, Fibersource
Energy Dense	Ensure Plus, Boost Plus, Magnacal, Two Cal HN, Novasource 2.0, Nutren 2.0
High Nitrogen	Osmolite 1.5, Two Cal HN, Impact, Isocal HN, Nutren Replete
Critical Care	Impact, Traumacal, Pivot
Predigested or Elemental	Vivonex TEN, Optimental, Tolerex
Disease Specific	Nutrihep, Nepro, Pulmocare, Oxepa, Suplena, TraumaCal, Nutren Glycol, Glucerna, Nutrivent, Novasource
Peptide Based	Peptamen, Vital HN, Perative, Subdue
Modular Protein Products	Prosource, ProMod, Beneprotein
Immune Enhancing	Oxepa, Pivot, Impact, Crucial

- Recommend or select feeding tube and site/location based on clinical condition, GI anatomy, and anticipated length of treatment.
- Formula selection includes type of feeding needed by individual and disorder, viscosity, and kcal/mL. Elemental formulas should be limited to specific conditions in which digestion or absorption is impaired or in which polymeric diets have failed. See Table 17-2 for content selection.
- Monitor patient positioning. Head of bed should be elevated 30–45° during feeding. With impaired gastric emptying, feeding tube may be placed in a reverse Trendelenburg, right lateral decubitus position, and 250 mg of erythromycin may be administered intravenously (Komenaka et al, 2000). For the unconscious patient, turn to side to help with gastric emptying.
- Once feeding has started, check residuals; if greater than 200 mL, hold feeding for 2 hours, conduct bedside evaluation, and reassess tolerance. Replace aspirate to reduce loss of electrolytes and gastric juices (McClave et al, 2002).
- For intermittent or bolus feedings, keep patient on his/her right side, or keep head of bed elevated for 30 minutes after feeding to prevent aspiration.
- For patients at high risk for aspiration, who will be fed longer than 1 month, try a percutaneous gastrostomy (PEG) tube with continuous feeding. If aspiration persists, try a transjejunal tube with lower placement in the GI tract.
- Optimal oral health, tight glycemic control, minimal use of narcotics, and continuous feedings are recommended for patients at high risk for aspiration (McClave et al, 2002).
- Patient should be weighed on same scale at regular intervals, wearing similar clothing. Check twice if weights differ significantly from previous weights.
- Adjust formula, as needed, for constipation, diarrhea, abdominal distention, and other signs of intolerance. Type, volume, and concentration may be altered.
- With diabetic gastroparesis, tube feeding may not be well tolerated. Insulin may be required.
- Fiber-added formulas may be appropriate with diarrhea or constipation, especially if formula will be used over time.
- Ensure adequate free water is provided (usually 30 mL/kg in young adults with normal renal function). Determine percentage of free water in formula (usually 70–85%), and subtract this amount from estimated needs; flushes can provide the difference. Monitor fluid carefully in heart, renal, or liver failure where fluid restriction may be needed; a more concentrated product may be needed to achieve energy and protein goals.
- Evaluate medications or infection as cause for diarrhea or feeding intolerance.
- Use feeding at safe temperatures: commercially prepared formulas do not require refrigerated storage. Hang time for open-system containers (feeding bags) is 4 hours; hang time for closed-system containers is 24–48 hours.
- Although it is possible to use homemade, blenderized feedings, they are no longer recommended. Table 17-3 describes critical control points in a Hazard Analysis Critical Control Points (HACCP) procedure for maintaining a clean TF product in a hospital setting.

INTERVENTION: FOOD AND NUTRITION

- See Table 17-4 for major considerations with enteral feeding.
- Calculate energy requirements and protein, fluid, and nutrient needs according to age, sex, and medical status.
- For weight loss, 20 kcal/kg is recommended. Use 25 kcal/kg to maintain weight, 30 kcal/kg with mild stress factors, and 35–40 kcal/kg in moderately stressed patients.
- Protein is generally 0.8–1.0 g/kg to maintain status, 1.25 g/kg for mild stress, 1.5 g/kg for moderate stress, and 1.75–2.0 g/kg for severe stress, trauma, or burns. The critically ill may need more calories and protein than other patients.
- Estimate fluid needs at 30–35 mL free H_2O/kg body weight (BW) or 1 mL/kcal.
- Check patient's tolerance and side effects; alter formula content as appropriate.
- Flush tubing with water (25–100 mL) every 3–6 hours for tube patency and before/after medications are given.
- With a gastrostomy tube, bolus or intermittent feeding is possible. For postpyloric or transpyloric placement, cyclic feedings may be better tolerated than continuous feedings.
- When patient is in transition back to oral diet or works during the day, night feeding may be used. It may be more energy efficient than continuous feeding over 24 hours.
- Sample new products to determine costs and convenience for home or institutional use.
- See Table 17-5 for the role of the dietitian in nutrition support.

TABLE 17-3 Critical Control Point Checklist for a Hazard Analysis and Critical Control Point Procedure for Tube Feedings

Purchasing, Receiving, and Storage

- Enteral feeding product(s) received according to specification.
- Temperature standards for refrigeration and dry storage of enteral feeding product(s) met.
- Product usage according to FIFO (first in, first out); those exceeding expiration date returned/discarded.
- Liquid protein module and frozen shakes thawed under refrigeration; products labeled with date placed in refrigerator for thawing.
- Open cartons discarded after 48 hours.
- Unopened and unused thawed liquid protein module discarded after 5 days.
- Unopened and unused thawed shakes discarded after 12 days.
- Medium-chain triglyceride oil, dry carbohydrate powder, and protein powder stored at room temperature; labeled with date opened. Opened cases and unused bottles/cans discarded after 1 month.
- Inventory of reconstituted, mixed enteral formulas and portioned protein, fat, and carbohydrate modules reveals none are past expiration date.
- Prepared enteral feedings kept separate from raw or processed food items and cleaning compounds.

Preparation and Delivery

- Employees wash hands prior to preparing enteral feedings or modular components.
- Cleaned and sanitized surface and equipment used to prepare enteral feedings or modular components.
- Enteral formula prepared according to recipe.
- Tap water used to reconstitute pediatric powdered formulas and Ceralyte; distilled or sterile water used in the preparation of enteral formulas upon specific order.
- Reconstituted mixed enteral formulas and portioned protein, fat, and carbohydrate modules sealed and labeled (formula, rate of administration, patient name and room number, date prepared).
- Temperature standards for refrigerated storage of reconstituted, mixed enteral formulas and portioned protein, fat, and carbohydrate modules met.
- Nursing staff washes hands prior to handling feedings and administration systems.
- Nursing staff avoids touching any part of the container or administration system that will come in contact with the feeding.
- Nursing staff assembles feeding system on a disinfected surface and inspects seals/reservoirs for damage.
- Medications are not added to feeding unless necessary. If added, tube is flushed with tap water (or as specified) after administration.
- Date/time each component of feeding system; also feeding bag is labeled with patient name and formula.
- Hang time of feeding limited to 4 hours.
- Feeding bags completely emptied of product prior to pouring newly opened product into the bag.
- Disconnected sets are capped.
- Container is positioned to prevent reflux of feeding up set.
- Feeding tube is irrigated with tap water (or as specified).
- Administration sets changed every 24 hours.

Adapted with permission from New York-Presbyterian Hospital/New York Weill Cornell Medical Center.

CLINICAL INDICATORS

Clinical/History

Height
Weight
Body mass index (BMI)
Intake and output (I & O)
Blood pressure (BP)
Diarrhea
Temperature
Nausea, vomiting
Chest x-ray
Residuals

Lab Work

Albumin (Alb), transthyretin
Transferrin
C-reactive protein (CRP)
Cholesterol (Chol)
Triglycerides (Trig)
Ca++
Mg++
Glucose (Gluc)
Hemoglobin and hematocrit (H & H)
Na+
K+
Chloride
Phosphorus
Respiratory quotient (RQ) (>1.0 may indicate that energy delivery is excessive)
Blood urea nitrogen (BUN)
Creatinine (Creat)
Prothrombin time (PT) and international normalized ratio (INR)
Serum insulin
Partial pressure of carbon dioxide (pCO_2)
Partial pressure of oxygen (pO_2)
Total lymphocyte count (TLC)
Urine acetone

TABLE 17-4 Key Enteral Issues

Issue	Comments
Feeding Site Selection	Consider any gastrointestinal (GI) impairments or inability to absorb nutrients, vomiting, severe and persistent diarrhea, respiratory disease or skull surgery/fracture, or tendency to remove tubes by choice or inadvertently.
Nasogastric	Often used for temporary needs; tube placed into stomach from the nose.
Nasoenteric	For patients with impaired gastric emptying or in whom a gastric feeding is contraindicated.
Nasojejunal	For patients at risk of pulmonary aspiration or with GI problems that preclude stomach placement such as mechanical problems or problems with gastric emptying or tolerance.
Gastrostomy	Surgical incision or endoscopically placed percutaneous gastrostomy (PEG). Allows long-term feeding. A low-profile device (button) can be used for long-term feedings or for improved body image.
Jejunostomy	Surgical incision into the jejunum to bypass inaccessible areas of the duodenum such as with short bowel syndrome or obstructions from cancer, adhesions, stricture, or inflammatory disease. Percutaneous jejunostomy (PEJ) is a PEG with a transjejunal limb. A jejunostomy tube may cause some bowel necrosis; monitor carefully.
Gastrojejunostomy	Good for small bowel feeding when stomach must be decompressed.
Contraindications for Tube Feeding	
Malabsorption	Impaired ability to digest or absorb nutrients (e.g., severe malabsorption disorders, short bowel syndrome).
Diarrhea	Severe and intractable diarrhea.
Formula Selection	
Generic versus brand-name orders	It is generally more cost effective to have an enteral formulary established, including multiple products, but one main brand of each category (e.g., standard/isotonic, isotonic with fiber, high nitrogen isotonic, elemental, high protein/high calorie for stress, critical care products, concentrated for patients with volume intolerance, malabsorption, specialty products for pulmonary or diabetes or immunocompromised, renal, or hepatic patients).
Substrates	Carbohydrate, protein, and fat (consider patient's ability to digest and absorb nutrients).
Elemental versus intact formulas	No superiority has been documented for elemental; if not sure of ability to digest fats, use medium-chain triglycerides (e.g., Osmolite or Isocal). Peptides and amino acids may be used for most patients.
Tolerance factors	Osmolality, calorie, and nutrient densities. In general, more free water is needed with a more concentrated formula.
Fluid Needs	Generally, 1 mL/kcal is recommended, unless patient needs fluid restriction; 30 mL/kg is most common for adults. Elderly individuals may require slight alterations, depending on organ function.
Organ failure	Heart failure, renal failure, or liver failure with ascites; 20 mL/kg can also be used initially, progressing to 25 mL/kg as tolerated.
Risk for dehydration or losses	Risk of abnormal losses due to GI drainage, diarrhea, and dehydration, and for those with other needs for extra water, 35–40 mL/kg may be used.
Pediatrics	Children must receive adequate fluid, calculated by their body weight.
Delivery Methods	Patient tolerance is key. Goal: meet needs without complications such as nausea, vomiting, diarrhea, or glucosuria.
Bolus	Set amount given every 3–4 hours as a rapid syringe feeding; this closely resembles an oral diet for patients who are ambulatory or with long-term and well-established feedings.
Intermittent	Prescribed amount given every 3–4 hours by drip over 20–30 minutes.
Continuous	Controlled delivery of feeding over 24 hours. Less nausea and diarrhea are likely. Once stable, most patients may transfer to intermittent.
Cycled	Controlled delivery over 8–16 hours, allowing some rest periods for patient during 24 hours. Cyclic is well tolerated by ambulatory patients.
Complications	Evaluate for metabolic complications. Electrolyte shifts and elevated glucose may occur. Patient may require addition of an insulin regimen until hyperglycemia is resolved.
Pulmonary aspiration	Proper positioning greatly reduces risks of pulmonary aspiration.
Mechanical ventilation	Use enteral nutrition with H_2 antagonists to facilitate gastric emptying.
Clogging of tubes	Small-bore tubes are associated with clogging. To prevent or correct mechanical clogging in small-bore tubes, flush regularly with water before and after all medications.
GI side effects	For GI concerns, check for residuals and hold feedings for amounts greater than 150 mL; stop for 4 hours and recheck. For diarrhea, check osmolality of feeding, rate, albumin level, and medications (e.g., sorbitol, magnesium).
PEG tube problems	Possible complications include pain at the PEG site, leakage of stomach contents around the tube site, dislodgment or malfunction of the tube, aspiration, bleeding, and perforation.

TABLE 17-5 Roles of the Nutrition Support Dietitian

The role of the nutrition support dietitian (NSD) is a specialty practice. The goal of this position, working in conjunction with other health care professionals including a pharmacist, nurse, and physician, is to support, restore, and maintain optimal nutritional health for individuals with potential or known alterations in nutritional status.

The NSD is a registered dietitian with clinical expertise or credentialing in nutrition support obtained through education, training, or experience in this field. The NSD assures optimal nutrition support through implementation of the Nutrition Care Process related to delivery of enteral (EN) and parenteral nutritional (PN) support (Fuhrman et al, 2001). The Nutrition Care Process has established a standardized series of steps by which dietitians can (Lacey and Pritchett, 2003):

- review individualized nutrition screening and complete thorough **nutrition assessments;**
- select all essential **nutrition diagnoses,** which can be resolved by the dietitian and nutrition team members
- implement appropriate **interventions,** especially early enough to support recovery and repletion
- **monitor** and reassess an individual's response to the nutrition care delivered;
- **evaluate** outcomes, including the need for a transitional feeding care plan or for termination of a nutrition support intervention.

The NSD may interpret laboratory reports, change medication orders, use herbs or botanicals, and decide to alter a nutrition prescription, in collaboration with the medical team.

- There are no labs mandated solely because of a patient's age; in assessing a patient's overall physiological state, an organ systems–based approach focusing on the cardiac, respiratory, renal, hepatic, endocrine, nutritional, and neurological systems may be beneficial (John and Sieber, 2004).
- While serum hepatic protein (albumin, transferrin, and transthyretin) levels have been linked in clinical practice to nutritional status, evidence about the effects of inflammation on hepatic protein metabolism is now recognized, and low serum levels are correlated with morbidity and mortality rather than nutritional repletion (Fuhrman et al, 2004). Low serum levels indicate that a patient is very ill and most likely requires aggressive, closely monitored medical nutrition therapy (Fuhrman et al, 2004).
- Patient use of herbs or botanical products must be assessed because this affects the outcomes of treatments, including use of nutrition support measures.
- Medications affect nutrient absorption and delivery. The NSD must stay current about medications and their impact on EN and PN products, intolerances, and nutrient absorption.

Other roles may include but are not limited to:

- Identification and application of the most valid primary research and evidence summaries (clinical guides to practice and meta-analyses) as an integral part of appropriate nutrition care (Hise et al, 2005).
- Management of nutrition support services, including developing policies and procedures, supervising personnel, and maintaining budgets.
- Recommending and maintaining current enteral and parenteral formularies.
- Evaluating equipment for enteral feeding delivery.
- Leading nutrition support committees.
- Assuring optimal reimbursement for nutrition support measures.
- Education and training of patients, caregivers, and health care professionals concerning theories, principles, and practices of specialized nutrition support.
- Research activities with participation in or generation of research and outcomes studies, with evaluation, interpretation, and application of research results. The limitations of the research that forms the scientific basis of many nutrition recommendations must be realized; there are few rigorously performed clinical studies (Thompson and Fuhrman, 2005).
- Participation in ethics decisions of whether or not to feed a patient or remove a tube feeding (see Table 17-6).

The NSD may practice in a variety of settings (acute facilities, subacute facilities, ambulatory/outpatient clinics, long-term care facilities, home care, and hospice) and care for patients of all age groups and across all developmental stages.

The NSD works with a coordinated multidisciplinary team approach. This approach is critical to the success of the concurrent use of medical nutrition therapy and pharmacotherapy because of the long-term duration of the treatments, the necessity of monitoring compliance and effectiveness, and the likelihood of multiple medication–nutrient interactions (McCaffree, 2003).

Common Drugs Used and Potential Side Effects

Drug–nutrient interactions are complex and can cause malabsorption of either the drug or the nutrient in tube feedings. Depending on the physical properties of a drug, it may be absorbed in a limited area of the GI tract or along much of the entire length. Monitor carefully for toxicity. Flush with 5–10 mL water after each medication is administered to prevent clogging.

- Antibiotics, H_2-receptor antagonists, and sorbitol elixirs alter gut flora and can cause diarrhea because of their high osmolality.
- Antidiarrheal drugs (kaolin, Lomotil) can be used to slow GI motility. Their use should not preclude a carefully planned fiber intake. Dry mouth is one common side effect.
- Metoclopramide (Reglan) has been used to prevent gastroesophageal (GE) reflux and aspiration in patients who are tube fed. Administration 10 minutes before tube insertion seems to increase success rate of tube passage. Gastric motility and relaxation of the pyloric sphincter are improved with this drug. However, chronic use may dislodge gastrostomy tubes; monitor closely. Combining prokinetic effects of

TABLE 17-6 Consequences Statement: Not Feeding a Resident/Patient by Tube When Oral Intake Is Insufficient

"The clinical manifestations of protein-energy undernutrition are related to length of time and extent of nutritional deprivation and the prior health status of the person. Based on both animal and human studies, there are serious detrimental effects on the function of every organ system, including the **heart, respiratory muscles, and the brain.** When maintained on a prolonged semi-starvation diet, otherwise healthy individuals experience a **loss of heart tissue** that parallels their loss of body mass. Respiratory rate, vital capacity and minute volume of ventilation also decrease. These **changes in pulmonary function** are thought to result from reduced basal metabolic rate that accompanies starvation. In addition, **liver function declines, kidney filtration rates decline, and nearly every aspect of the immune system is compromised.** Defective ability to fight bacterial and viral infections occurs. Starvation therefore leads to **increased susceptibility to infection, delayed wound healing, reduced rate of drug metabolism, and impairment of both physical and cognitive function.** If starvation is prolonged, complications develop, **leading eventually to death."**

—Sullivan, D. The role of nutrition in increased morbidity and mortality. Clin Geriatr Med. 11:663, 1995.

Other documented consequences of not tube feeding a resident/patient who *will not* or *cannot* eat sufficiently orally include:

- possibility of **dehydration** with increased risk of urinary tract infections, fever, swollen tongue, sunken eyeballs, decreased urine output, constipation, nausea and vomiting, decreased blood pressure, mental confusion, electrolyte disturbances
- **decreased awareness** of environment from decreased glucose availability for the brain
- possibility of **development of pressure ulcers** over bony prominences from lack of sufficient protein, calorie, vitamin, and mineral intakes and decreased body fat
- **decreased ability to participate in activities of daily living** (self-feeding, dressing, bathing, toileting)
- **low body weight and rapid, involuntary weight loss** which are highly predictive of illness and imminent death in the elderly (note: the elderly are especially unable to regain weight after a stress situation).

****

I, the undersigned, understand and acknowledge that these consequences have been reviewed with me. I am deciding not to tube feed ________________ (resident/patient) and accept the outcome of this decision.

Signed:________________ Witness:________________

Power of Attorney, Guardian or Other Representative

Date:________________ Witness:________________

erythromycin with proper patient positioning allows a rapid bedside transpyloric placement of feeding tubes (Komenaka et al, 2000).
- Phenytoin (Dilantin) administration should be separated from TF by 1–2 hours to prevent decreased medication absorption. TF rate may need to be recalculated, accounting for time TF is held before and after phenytoin administration, and adjusted accordingly.

Herbs, Botanicals, and Supplements

- Herbs and botanical supplements should not be used with enteral feedings without discussing with physician and pharmacist.

INTERVENTION: NUTRITION EDUCATION, COUNSELING, CARE MANAGEMENT

- Patient/caretaker should be taught to review signs and symptoms of intolerance, how to manage simple problems, when to call for guidance, and when to call the physician.
- At least one follow-up phone call or home visit should be made to patients on home EN.
- Patient should be allowed and encouraged to maintain social contacts at mealtime.
- When transitionally weaning young children to an oral diet, oral–motor, sensory, and developmental feeding problems may occur. Check for feeding readiness via oral stimulation, and develop a feeding plan.

Patient Education—Food Safety

- Safe preparation of TF is essential.
- Some ready-to-hang products may remain at room temperature for up to 48 hours after opening; read product labels carefully.
- Homemade TFs are not recommended in most cases.
- Temperature standards for refrigeration and storage of enteral feeding product must be met. See Table 17-3 for other tips that may be adapted for a home-monitoring safety checklist for EN patients and their caregivers.

For More Information

- American Dietetic Association–Ethical and Legal Issues in Nutrition, Hydration, and Feeding
http://www.eatright.org/cps/rde/xchg/ada/hs.xsl/advocacy_adar0502_ENU_HTML.htm
- American Society for Gastrointestinal Endoscopy
http://www.askasge.org/pages/brochures/peg.cfm
- American Society for Parenteral and Enteral Nutrition–Standards
http://www.nutritioncare.org/profdev/stnds.html
- Cleveland Clinic–Feeding Tubes
http://www.clevelandclinic.org/health/health-info/docs/2800/2825.asp?index=10348
- End of Life Decisions–Brown University
http://www.chcr.brown.edu/dying/CONSUMERFEEDINGTUBE.HTM
- Home Enteral Nutrition
http://www.mayoclinic.org/gi-jax/enteral.html

ENTERAL NUTRITION—CITED REFERENCES

American Society for Parenteral and Enteral Nutrition. Standards and guidelines. Accessed October 4, 2006 at http://www.nutritioncare.org/profdev/stnds.html.

Barr J, et al. Outcomes in critically ill patients before and after the implementation of an evidence-based nutritional management protocol. *Chest* 125:1446, 2004.

Bernard A, et al. Defining and assessing tolerance in enteral nutrition. *Nutr Clin Pract.* 19:481, 2004.

Dickerson RN. Hypocaloric feeding of obese patients in the intensive care unit. *Curr Opin Clin Nutr Metab Care.* 8:189, 2005.

Elamin M. Nutritional care of the obese intensive care unit patient. *Curr Opin Crit Care.* 11:300, 2005.

Flesher ME, et al. Assessing the metabolic and clinical consequences of early enteral feeding in the malnourished patient. *J Parenter Enteral Nutr.* 29:108, 2005.

Fuhrman MP, et al. Hepatic proteins and nutrition assessment. *J Am Diet Assoc.* 104:1258, 2004.

Fuhrman MP, et al. The American Society for Parenteral and Enteral Nutrition (A.S.P.E.N). Standards of Practice for nutrition support dietitians. *J Am Diet Assoc.* 101:825, 2001.

Hise M, et al. Evidence-based clinical practice: dispelling the myths. *Nutr Clin Pract.* 20:294, 2005.

John AD, Sieber FE. Age associated issues: geriatrics. *Anesthesiol Clin North Am.* 22:45, 2004.

Komenaka I, et al. Erythromycin and position facilitated placement of postpyloric feeding tubes in burned patients. *Dig Surg.* 17:578, 2000.

Lacey K, Pritchett E. Nutrition Care Process and Model: ADA adopts road map to quality care and outcomes management. *J Am Diet Assoc.* 103:1061, 2003.

Mayhew S, Gonzalez E. Neonatal nutrition: a focus on parenteral nutrition and early enteral nutrition. *Nutr Clin Pract.* 18:406, 2003.

McCaffree J. Position of the American Dietetic Association: Integration of medical nutrition therapy and pharmacotherapy. *J Am Diet Assoc.* 103: 1363, 2003.

McClave S, et al. North American summit on aspiration in the critically ill patient: consensus statement. *J Parenter Enteral Nutr.* 26:S80, 2002.

McMahon M, et al. Medical and ethical aspects of long-term enteral tube feeding. *Mayo Clin Proc.* 80:1461, 2005.

Novak F, et al. Glutamine supplementation in serious illness: a systematic review of the evidence. *Crit Care Med.* 30:2022, 2002.

Ruangtrakool R, Ong T. Primary gastrostomy button: a means of long-term enteral feeding in children. *J Med Assoc Thai.* 83:151, 2000.

Saalwachter AR, et al. A nutrition support team led by general surgeons decreases inappropriate use of total parenteral nutrition on a surgical service. *Am Surg.* 70:1107, 2004.

Schattner MA, et al. Long-term enteral nutrition facilitates optimization of body weight. *J Parenter Enteral Nutr.* 29:198, 2005.

Thompson C, Fuhrman MP. Nutrients and wound healing: still searching for the magic bullet. *Nutr Clin Pract.* 20:331, 2005.

Wischmeyer P, et al. Glutamine administration reduces Gram-negative bacteremia in severely burned patients: a prospective, randomized, double-blind trial versus isonitrogenous control. *Crit Care Med.* 29:2075, 2001.

PARENTERAL NUTRITION

NUTRITIONAL ACUITY RANKING: LEVEL 4 (HOME)

DEFINITIONS AND BACKGROUND

Parenteral nutrition (PN) refers to intravenous feeding. It is an intravenous nutrient admixture administered into the blood with a catheter placed in a vein; it contains protein, carbohydrate, fat, vitamins, minerals, and other nutrients needed and is referred to as total parenteral nutrition (TPN) if it meets the needs of the patient. It is difficult to determine whether PN makes a significant difference in patient outcomes and should not be automatically used in all surgical patients (Heyland et al, 2001).

Critical review of the data (Jeejeebhoy, 2001) suggests that TPN does not cause mucosal atrophy or increase translocation of bacteria through the small intestine. Overfeeding, which is easy with TPN, can explain why TPN increases sepsis for some patients. Overall risks of TPN-induced complications have been exaggerated. When there is risk of malnutrition and enteral nutrition (EN) is not tolerated or there is gut failure, TPN is an equally effective and safe alternative (Jeejeebhoy, 2001).

In general, PN is more expensive than EN and oral diets. Inappropriate initiation of PN, short-term use of PN, and metabolic complications associated with PN are best managed by an expert in nutrition support. Specially trained registered dietitians may write TPN orders if granted clinical privileges by their institution or facility. The skills of specialists distinguish them from other practitioners. These skills include competency in fluid and electrolyte monitoring, acid–base monitoring, metabolic monitoring, and related areas.

To determine energy and nutrient requirements accurately, use of a programmed calculation may help to prevent administration of excessive glucose and energy in solutions.

PN may be most useful in patients undergoing surgery for esophageal or stomach cancers, in preoperative patients who are severely malnourished, and in patients with prolonged gastrointestinal (GI) tract failure. Other indications are listed in Table 17-7.

Adequate nutrition support criteria include reaching a nutritional goal within 72 hours after initiation. PN may be given by continuous or cyclic infusion, altered according to patient tolerance. In most cases, gradual transition from PN to EN or oral nutrition is required. This prevents periods of inadequate nutrition where TPN might be discontinued before oral nutrition or EN is adequate. Central PN, partial PN, peripheral PN (PPN), and TPN are options for intravenous feeding. Placement sites are shown in Figure 17-3. Indications for PPN include temporary losses of GI function (e.g., acute ileus) and occasions when short-term use is indicated such as after minor GI surgery.

PN may be performed safely at home with proper patient and family training and follow-up. TPN will drip through a needle or catheter placed into the central vein for 10–12 hours, once a day or five times a week.

Dependence on PN significantly impacts quality of life (Fish et al, 2000). Travel, sleep, exercise, and leisure activities are most often cited as being altered by home PN. Quality of life has to be addressed for each individual (Winkler, 2005).

TABLE 17-7 Indications for Total Parenteral Nutrition (TPN) in Adults (developed from ASPEN, 2006)

General: Standard TPN is indicated for:

1. A nonfunctional or inaccessible gastrointestinal tract
2. Someone who cannot be adequately nourished with an oral diet or enteral nutrition (EN)
3. Inadequate oral or enteral intake anticipated to persist for at least 7–14 days

Specific: Standard TPN is routine for:

1. Dysfunction because of short bowel syndrome, radiation enteritis, ischemic bowel, or chronic malabsorption
2. Severely catabolic patients whose gut cannot be used within 3–5 days (such as closed head trauma, fractures, burns)
3. Disorders of the small bowel (inflammatory bowel disease, gastrointestinal obstruction, inflammatory adhesions, severe diarrhea)
4. After bone marrow transplantation, specifically in cases of graft versus host disease accompanied by inadequate oral intake
5. Cases with a high risk of aspiration
6. Severe acute necrotizing pancreatitis when EN fails after a trial of 5–7 days
7. High-output enterocutaneous fistula
8. Acquired immunodeficiency syndrome (AIDS) or AIDS-related complex (ARC) with intractable diarrhea when enteral feeding is not successful
9. Short intervals during pregnancy when oral intake is compromised and when EN is not tolerated, as with short bowel syndrome
10. After major surgery when enteral access cannot be established

Recommendations for home parenteral nutrition (HPN) in adult cancer patients (Schneider et al., 2001):

1. HPN may be offered to cancer patients with malnutrition or with inadequate/impossible oral intake
2. Patients need a multidisciplinary follow-up (oncologists, nutritionists, and pain specialists), and this follow-up will make treatment adaptations according to nutritional status possible; active participation of patients and/or their family is important
3. The benefit of HPN on the quality of life of terminally ill patients (vs. hydration) has not been clearly demonstrated. When life expectancy is below 3 months and the Karnofsky index is below 50, the drawbacks of home artificial nutrition are more significant than the advantages; in this case, HPN is not recommended.
4. Prospective clinical trials are recommended to evaluate the impact of PN on quality of life in cancer patients.
5. Use of educational booklets that mention the telephone number of referring health care and what to do when a problem happens (e.g., fever on HPN) are recommended.

From: American Society for Parenteral and Enteral Nutrition. Standards and guidelines. Accessed October 4, 2006 at http://www.nutritioncare.org/profdev/stnds.html.

INTERVENTION: OBJECTIVES

- Maintain or replete lean body mass, avoiding or correcting malnutrition and its consequences.
- Assess calculations using height, weight, and age; or use indirect calorimetry. Determine appropriate patient requirements for calories, protein, vitamins, minerals, and fluid. Some studies suggest use of hypocaloric feedings in obese patients to meet basic needs. Fat and carbohydrate (CHO) make the balance of nonprotein calories after protein needs are estimated.
- Avoid substrate excesses and prevent refeeding syndrome (dextrose infusion followed by increased insulin release, causing shifts in phosphorus, potassium, and magnesium).
- Maintain aseptic technique in all procedures for safe parenteral support. Lipid emulsions support rapid growth of most micro-organisms and the Centers for Disease Control and Prevention (CDC) suggests that lipid-containing PN solutions should be changed every 12 hours. For this reason, total nutrient admixtures (TNA) with all key nutrients in one bag have been discontinued in some institutions. All PN solutions regardless of lipid content should be used within 24 hours.
- Prevent or correct complications associated with PN (e.g., weight gain over 2 lb or 1 kg daily, indicating syndrome of inappropriate antidiuretic hormone; mouth sores; skin changes; poor night vision; fluid overload; elevated glucose levels; cardiac arrhythmias; metabolic bone disease).
- PN-associated liver disease (PNALD) is the most devastating complication of long-term PN therapy; progression is typically insidious, and its long-term consequences are generally underappreciated (Buchman et al, 2006).
- Manage fluid requirements and monitor urinary and enteric outputs or extraneous losses. Avoid fluid overload, which actually may be more common than dehydration in these patients.
- Prevent essential fatty acid deficiency, which may occur when lipids are not administered. Prevent excessive use of linoleic acid, which can cause inflammation and immunosuppression in patients with infection or sepsis.
- Formulate PN solutions according to patient conditions: for renal, review fluid and electrolytes, and monitor essential amino acids (EAAs) in the solution; for hepatic, evaluate needs for fluid, electrolytes, and specialty amino acid solutions. For pulmonary conditions and diabetes, increased lipids and decreased dextrose may be needed.

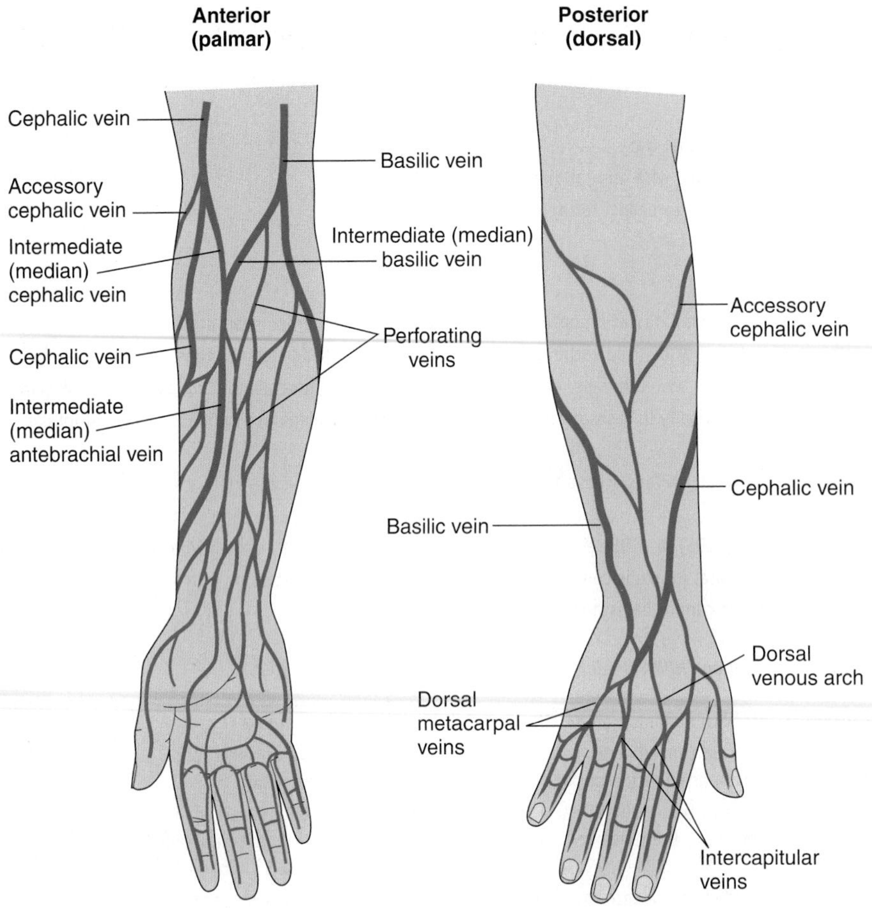

Figure 17-3 Parenteral access sites. (From Smeltzer SC, Bare BG. *Textbook of medical-surgical nursing.* 9th ed. Philadelphia: Lippincott Williams & Wilkins, 2000.)

- For home PN, allow patient to continue usual activity, employment, and a usual daily life.
- Monitor for long-term complications such as liver failure and metabolic bone disease. Parathyroid gland function may be abnormal in patients who receive long-term TPN; this may contribute to disturbed bone metabolism (Goodman et al, 2000).
- Transition back to EN or oral intake, when and if feasible.

INTERVENTION: FOOD AND NUTRITION

- Calculate needs for PN related to present requirements (energy, protein, fluid, vitamins, and minerals). Usually, 30–35 kcal/kg body weight is used, starting with estimates such as 20–25 kcal/kg to determine basal requirements.
- Fat should be given daily as an energy source. If tolerated, 4% total kilocalories should be given as fat to prevent essential fatty acid deficiency (EFAD). A 10% lipid emulsion generally yields 1.1 kcal/mL. Use of omega-3 fatty acids is controversial, but some studies suggest a role in maintaining a healthy immune function (Sweeney et al, 2005).
- Be careful not to overfeed because of risk of hyperglycemia, fatty liver, and excessive CO_2 production. Maximum rate of glucose infusion should not exceed 5–6 mg/kg/min, the rate of glucose oxidation or utilization.
- Provide weaning when patient is ready; use TF for interim nourishment if necessary. Early enteral feeding reduces postoperative septic complications for many patients (Moore et al, 1992). Progress to liquids and solids when patient is ready (return of bowel sounds, appropriate gag reflex). Infusion of PN nutrients may suppress appetite, excessively prolonging PN use.
- Monitor phosphate carefully in relation to anabolism, refeeding syndrome, and malnutrition.
- Glutamine infusion may be helpful (DeSouza and Greene, 2005). It is often used in inflammatory bowel disease or for stressed patients but not in hepatic encephalopathy.
- Short-chain fatty acids, soy, and fermentable fiber may be needed to reduce TPN-induced bowel atrophy.
- Osmolality is important to monitor to prevent dehydration and other complications: for example, D5W 5 has an osmolality of 252 mOsm/L; D20W 5 has an osmolality of 1008 mOsm/L.
- Dextrose monohydrate in TPN yields 3.4 kcal/g, not 4 kcal/g. For unstable blood glucose, use fat at 10–20% of energy intake; avoid overfeeding and consider use of insulin.
- Major mineral and micronutrient requirements in adult parenteral use are listed in Table 17-8. Intravenous vita-

TABLE 17-8 Major Mineral and Micronutrient Requirements in Normal Adults

Nutrient	Recommended Daily Parenteral Intake in Normal Adults
Major minerals	
Sodium	60–150 mEq
Potassium	40–100 mEq
Magnesium	8–24 mEq
Calcium	5–15 mEq
Phosphorus	10–30 mmol
Trace minerals	
Chromium	10–20 mg
Copper	0.3–1.2 mg
Iodine	70–140 mg
Iron	1–1.5 mg
Manganese	0.2–0.8 mg[a]
Molybdenum	19 mg
Selenium	20–80 mg
Zinc	2.5–4 mg
Fat-soluble vitamins	
A	3300 IU
D	200 IU
E	10 IU
K	150 mg
Water-soluble vitamins	
Thiamine (B_1)	6 mg
Riboflavin (B_2)	3.6 mg
Pantothenic acid (B_5)	15 mg
Niacin (B_3)	40 mg
Pyridoxine (B_6)	6 mg
Biotin (B_7)	60 mg
Folic acid (B_9)	600 mg
Cobalamin (B_{12})	5 mg
Ascorbic acid (C)	200 mg

[a] Recent evidence suggests that manganese toxicity, manifesting as extrapyramidal manganese deposition and parkinsonian-like symptoms and/or chronic liver disease may develop with long-term PN. Many clinicians now limit manganese addition to PN solutions to 0.1 mg or eliminate it entirely.

Based on data from: American Gastroenterological Association medical position statement: parenteral nutrition. *Gastroenterology* 121:966, 2001.

min A is only one fourth to one third available because it attaches to the plastic bags; vitamin E may also be less available. Vitamin D is given as ergocalciferol in PN form; beware of excesses because they may contribute to bone disease that may occur in long-term TPN. Vitamin K is part of the multivitamin infusate. Water-soluble vitamins are needed daily; see Table 17-9.

- For mineral and electrolyte administration, see Table 17-10. Choline is important in metabolic pathways but is not generally used in daily solutions.
- Follow practice guidelines, especially for home care (Kovacevich et al, 2005) and pediatrics (Wessel et al, 2005).
- Dialysis patients may benefit from intradialytic PN (IDPN), but currently, reimbursement is not available (Bossola et al, 2005).
- TPN is sometimes used in cancer patients. It must be used judiciously in metastatic cancer patients because of its effects on quality of life, complications, and cost (Joque and Jatoi, 2005). TPN may also not show improvements when used in chronic obstructive pulmonary disease patients (Ferreira et al, 2005).
- For management of complications of PN, see Table 17-11.

CLINICAL INDICATORS

Clinical/History

Height
Weight (measure daily)
BMI
Resting energy expenditure (REE)
BP
I & O
Edema
Skin turgor
Physical signs of malnutrition

Lab Work

Gluc (check daily or several times weekly once stable)
Urinary Gluc (check daily or several times weekly once stable)
Alb
Transthyretin (check weekly once stable)
CRP
Retinol-binding protein (RBP)
K+, Na+ (daily, then at least 3 times weekly when stable)
Serum Osmolality
BUN
Creat (check weekly once stable)
Alkaline phosphatase
Acetone
Chol, Trig
Transferrin
PT or INR (check weekly once stable)
Chest x-ray
Ca++
Mg++
N balance
Serum triglycerides (check weekly if receiving lipids)
Serum phosphorus (check weekly once stable)
Serum selenium
Amylase, lipase
Bilirubin
Serum ammonia
H & H
Serum Fe
Serum folacin
Serum B_{12}
Aspartate aminotransferase, alanine aminotransferase
White blood cell count, TLC
pCO_2, pO_2

Common Drugs Used and Potential Side Effects

- Contact pharmacy for drugs that are stable and compatible with PN solutions or nutrient additives. Often, H_2-blockers, steroids, and insulin may be added to PN solutions.
- TPN does not reduce toxicity associated with chemotherapy.
- Use of intestinal tropic factors, such as recombinant human growth hormone (r-hGH), is being tested in some patients. In the past, short bowel syndrome

TABLE 17-9 Daily Parenteral Multivitamin Requirements

Vitamin	Adult Intake	Pediatric Intake (ages 1–11)
Vitamin A	3300 IU	2300 IU
Vitamin D	200 IU	400 IU
Vitamin E	10 IU	7 IU
Vitamin K	150 μg	200 μg
Ascorbic acid	200 mg	80 mg
Thiamine	6 mg	1.2 mg
Riboflavin	3.6 mg	1.4 mg
Niacin	40 mg	17 mg
Folic acid	400 mg	140 mg
Pantothenic acid	15 mg	5 mg
Vitamin B_6	6 mg	1 mg
Vitamin B_{12}	5 mg	1 mg
Biotin	60 mg	20 mg

Derived from: American Society for Parenteral and Enteral Nutrition. Safe practices for parenteral nutrition. *J Parenter Enteral Nutr.* 28:S38, 2004.

(<200 cm of functional small intestine) required long-term home PN; but now patients may be given intestinal rehabilitation regimens with specialized oral diets, soluble fiber, oral rehydration solution, and tropic factors to enhance absorption (Matarese et al, 2005).

Herbs, Botanicals, and Supplements

- Herbs and botanical supplements should not be added to any intravenous feedings.

INTERVENTION: NUTRITION EDUCATION, COUNSELING, CARE MANAGEMENT

- Discuss with patient/caretakers the goals of the PN, especially if home TPN will be used. Discuss aseptic technique, input and output records, TPN pump use, medications, additives, and complications.
- Long-term consequences should be discussed (such as trace element deficiencies and metabolic problems).
- Teach transition processes when and if patient is ready. Assistance from a registered dietitian is recommended. Nausea and vomiting may occur; eating some type of concentrated CHO during transition is helpful.
- Transition may be possible from TPN to TF if patient tolerates one third to one half of kilocalorie needs by that route. To wean from TPN to oral diet, start with sips of clear liquids and advance, if tolerated, to full liquids by the second day; use lactose-free liquids at first. When intake is greater than 500 kcal orally, reduce TPN by 50%. When patient is consuming two thirds to three fourths of estimated needs orally, discontinue TPN by tapering (first hour by 50%, second hour by 75%, and third hour 100%).
- Discuss problems such as when to call the doctor, when to call the dietitian, and when to call the pharmacist or nurse.
- Discuss psychosocial issues related to adaptation to PN, oral deprivation, and lifestyle changes. Quality of life tends to decline with long-term TPN use (Baxter et al, 2005). Encourage patient to participate in favorite activities as much as possible.
- Promote positive communications and collaboration among members of the health care team. Nutrition therapy is challenging; the objective is to restore enteral autonomy to a patient with a complex medical and surgical history, and a coordinated team effort is needed to wean from PN eventually (Weseman and Gilroy, 2005).

TABLE 17-10 Daily Parenteral Electrolyte and Trace Element Requirements

Electrolytes	Adult Intake	Preterm Neonates	Infants/Children	Teens
Acetate	AN[a]	AN	AN	AN
Calcium	10–15 mEq	2–4 mEq/kg	0.5–4 mEq/kg	10–20 mEq
Chloride	AN	AN	AN	AN
Magnesium	8–20 mEq	0.3–0.5 mEq/kg	0.3–0.5 mEq/kg	10–30 mEq
Phosphorus/phosphate	20–40 mmol	1–2 mmol/kg	0.5–2 mmol/kg	10–40 mmol
Potassium	1–2 mEq/kg as needed	2–4 mEq/kg	2–4 mEq/kg	1–2 mEq/kg
Sodium	1–2 mEq/kg as needed	2–5 mEq/kg	2–5 mEq/kg	1–2 mEq/kg
Trace Element	**Adult Intake**	**Term Neonates**	**Under Age 5**	**Ages 5–18**
Chromium	10–15 mg	0.05–0.2 mcg/kg	0.14–0.2 mcg/kg	5–15 mg
Copper	0.3–0.5 mg	20 mcg/kg	5–20 mcg/kg	200–500 mg
Manganese	60–100 mg	1 mcg/kg	1 mcg/kg	50–150 mg
Selenium	20–60 mcg	2–3 mcg/kg	1–2 mcg/kg	40–60 mg
Zinc	2.5–5 mg	400 mcg/kg	50–125 mcg/kg	2–5 mg

[a] As needed to maintain acid-base balance.

Derived from: Amerian Society for Parenteral and Enteral Nutrition. Safe practices for parenteral nutrition. *J Parenter Enteral Nutr.* 28:S38, 2004.

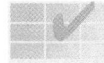

TABLE 17-11 **Complications in Parenteral Nutrition (PN)**

Complication	Comments
Pulmonary complications	Calculate needs and avoid overfeeding (minimal kilocalories may be best, e.g., 20–25 kcal/kg); carbohydrate (CHO) provision should not exceed 4–5 mg/kg/min; avoid fluid excesses. Respiratory failure may occur in patients with limited pulmonary reserve. Prolonged mechanical ventilation can occur with carbon dioxide retention associated with overfeeding.
Lipid abnormalities	Decrease lipids if triglycerides are higher than 300 mg/dL; infuse over a longer time period; calculate that total kilocalories are not greater than 60% from lipids. Lipids over 2 g/kg/d can increase congestion of reticuloendothelial system and impair clearance of triglycerides.
Dehydration	Calculate needs as 30 mL/kg body weight or as 1 mL/kcal given; alter as needed for diarrhea, medications used, ostomy, and losses from exudates such as burns or pressure ulcers. Include intravenous fluids from other non-PN sources.
Fluid overload	Calculate needs and decrease volume to meet needs; diuretics or dialysis may be needed; a higher concentration of dextrose or lipids may be needed if fluid restriction is required.
Hyperglycemia or blood glucose abnormalities	Hyperglycemia is no longer considered a normal response to stress, and it should be managed carefully (Digman et al, 2005). Reduce total grams of dextrose in the solution; add or increase insulin; consider use of lipids as partial substrate; advance feedings more slowly. Intensive insulin therapy to achieve euglycemia reduces mortality and morbidity in critically ill patients (Digman et al, 2005). Blood glucose >220 mg/dL can cause hyperinsulinemia, increased intracellular transport of potassium and phosphate with hypokalemia, and hypophosphatemia. Impaired phagocytosis and neutrophil clearance may also occur.
Hypoglycemia	Administer more dextrose; reduce or discontinue insulin use; gradually taper infusion rate during weaning.
Electrolyte abnormalities	Monitor fluid status, organ system function, and serum sodium, potassium, phosphorus, calcium and magnesium regularly. Determine relevant cause or mechanism. Hypernatremia: Replace fluids with a more dilute total PN (TPN) solution; decrease sodium. Hyponatremia: Diuretic therapy with or without fluid restriction. Sometimes this occurs with fluid overload and total body water excess. Only occasionally is added sodium required. Hyperkalemia: Evaluate renal function; decrease potassium in solution, and evaluate medications used; reduce exogenous supplements. Hypokalemia: Increase potassium in solution and monitor potassium-depleting diuretic use such as furosemide. Add additional potassium if needed. Hyperphosphatemia: Evaluate renal function; decrease phosphate in solution, and use phosphate binders if necessary. Hypophosphatemia: Increase phosphate in solution and monitor for refeeding syndrome. Hypermagnesemia: Decrease magnesium in solution. Hypomagnesemia: Increase magnesium in solution and monitor refeeding. Consider if magnesium-wasting medications are being used. Additional magnesium may be needed. Hypercalcemia: Consider endocrine causes. Evaluate vitamin D, use isotonic saline, and add inorganic phosphate to solution until normal. Hypocalcemia: Consider endocrine causes. Evaluate for hypoalbuminemia. Add additional calcium if needed.
Altered liver function	Altered liver function from excess energy may cause fatty infiltration and increased alkaline phosphatase. Occasionally, aspartate aminotransferase (AST) and alanine aminotransferase (ALT) will be elevated as well. Hepatomegaly and cholestasis may also result at levels of 150% or more beyond total energy needs.
Renal function changes	Protein excesses >2 g/kg daily can increase ureagenesis and decrease renal function or cause dehydration.
Catheter occlusion, venous thrombosis, phlebitis, sepsis	Contact physician or designated member of health care team for evaluation, diagnosis, and treatment of lines. For air embolism, place patient on his or her left side and lower head of the bed until resolved. Monitor for pneumothorax and ensure that trained staff handles catheters.

Adapted from: American Society for Enteral and Parenteral Nutrition. Guidelines for the use of parenteral and enteral nutrition in adult and pediatric patients. *J Parenter Enteral Nutr.* 26:18, 2002 (suppl 1).

TABLE 17-12 **Enteral and Parenteral Feeding Order Audit**

DATE	FEEDING ORDER	ROUTE	VOLUME AND FREQUENCY	FLUSH

NUTRITION SUPPORT SUMMARY

	ESTIMATED NEEDS	ORDER PROVIDES		
		Date:	Date:	Date:
TOTAL CALORIES	kcals/d			
	kcals/kg			
PROTEIN	g/d			
	g/kg			
FLUID	mL/d			
(including flush)	mL/kg			

ORAL INTAKE: ____________

OTHER FACTORS:

Dehydration _____	Edema _____	Ascites _____
Pressure Ulcer_____	Surgical wounds _____	Skeletal trauma _____
Infection/fever _____	Nausea _____	Vomiting _____
Diarrhea _____	Constipation _____	Bowel sounds _____
Accuchecks _____	Ventilator_____	Residuals _____

CURRENT FEEDING MEETS CALCULATED NEEDS. ____________

RECOMMENDATIONS: ____________

Patient Education—Food Safety

- Solutions must always be prepared and handled under sterile conditions.
- Home TPN requires aseptic technique and meticulous catheter care. Infection control measures should be discussed because catheter-related bloodstream infections are the most critical complication.
- Change bag, tubing, and cassette every 24 hours or as recommended by home care agency.
- Audits of the TF or PN are important. See Table 17-12.

For More Information

- American Society of Health-System Pharmacists http://www.safemedication.com/about/index.cfm

PARENTERAL NUTRITION—CITED REFERENCES

Baxter JP, et al. A review of the instruments used to assess the quality of life of adult patients with chronic intestinal failure receiving parenteral nutrition at home. *Br J Nutr.* 94:633, 2005.

Bossola M, et al. Malnutrition in hemodialysis patients: what therapy? *Am J Kidney Dis.* 46:371, 2005.

Buchman AL, et al. Parenteral nutrition-associated liver disease and the role for isolated intestine and intestine/liver transplantation. *Hepatology* 43:9, 2006.

De Souza DA, Greene LJ. Intestinal permeability and systemic infections in critically ill patients: effect of glutamine. *Crit Care Med.* 33:1125, 2005.

Digman C, et al. Hyperglycemia in the critically ill. *Nutr Clin Care.* 8:93, 2005.

Ferreira IM, et al. Nutritional supplementation for stable chronic obstructive pulmonary disease. *Cochrane Database Syst Rev.* 2:CD000998, 2005.

Fish J, et al. Recent developments in home total parenteral nutrition. *Gastroenterology* 2:327, 2000.

Goodman W, et al. Altered diurnal regulation of blood ionized calcium and serum parathyroid hormone concentrations during parenteral nutrition. *Am J Clin Nutr.* 71:560, 2000.

Heyland D, et al. Total parenteral nutrition in the surgical patient: a meta-analysis. *Can J Surg.* 44:102, 2001.

Jeejeebhoy K. Enteral and parenteral nutrition: evidence-based approach. *Proc Nutr Soc.* 60:399, 2001.

Kovacevich DS, et al. Standards for specialized nutrition support: home care patients. *Nutr Clin Pract.* 20:579, 2005.

Joque L, Jatoi A. Total parenteral nutrition in cancer patients: why and when? *Nutr Clin Care.* 8:89, 2005.

Matarese LR, et al. Short bowel syndrome: clinical guidelines for nutrition management. *Nutr Clin Pract.* 20:493, 2005.

Moore FA, et al. Early enteral feeding, compared with parenteral, reduces postoperative septic complications. The results of a meta-analysis. *Ann Surg.* 216:172, 1992.

Schneider S, et al. Standards, options, and recommendations for home parenteral or enteral nutrition in adult cancer patients. *Bull Cancer.* 288:605, 2001.

Sweeney B, et al. Modulation of immune cell function by polyunsaturated fatty acids. *Pediatr Surg Int.* 21:335, 2005.

Weseman RA, Gilroy R. Nutrition management of small bowel transplant patients. *Nutr Clin Pract.* 20:509, 2005.

Wessel J, et al. Standards for specialized nutrition support: hospitalized pediatric patients. *Nutr Clin Pract.* 20:103, 2005.

Winkler MF. Quality of life in adult home parenteral nutrition patients. *J Parenter Enteral Nutr.* 29:162, 2005.

APPENDIX A

Nutritional Review

MACRONUTRIENTS

Carbohydrates and Fiber

Carbohydrates are essential for life. The brain and central nervous system require a continuously available glucose supply. When it is necessary, lean body mass is metabolized to provide glucose for these tissues. Generally, 90% of carbohydrates are absorbed from a mixed diet.

Sugar replacers are sugar-free sweeteners; they are carbohydrates (usually sugar alcohols) but not sugars (McNutt, 2000). Unlike calorie-free intense sweeteners such as saccharin and aspartame, they are used in the same amount as sugars. Sugar replacers have the same bulk and volume. Sugar replacers are usually labeled as "sugar free" or "no sugar added." These products include mannitol, erythritol, isomalt, lactitol, maltitol, xylitol, sorbitol, and hydrogenated starch hydrolysate.

Both soluble and insoluble fiber play an important role in maintenance of health. Except in a few therapeutic situations, fiber should be obtained from food sources. Between 20 and 35 g/d is recommended (American Dietetic Association, 2002). All dietary fibers, regardless of type, are readily fermented by microflora of the small intestines, producing short-chain fatty acids (acetate, propionate, and butyrate). Insoluble fibers (e.g., bran, cereal, vegetables) increase fecal volume (bulk) and decrease colonic transit time by virtue of their ability to increase water-holding capacity. They are useful in reducing appendicitis, constipation, diverticulosis, and perhaps colon cancer; mineral depletion may occur with excesses. Soluble fibers (e.g., fruit, barley, oat bran, legumes) decrease serum cholesterol by decreasing the enterohepatic recycling of bile acids resulting in increased use of cholesterol for bile synthesis, which in turn alters enzyme activities related to cholesterol synthesis, stabilizes blood glucose levels, and helps maintain mineral nutriture. They have little effect on fecal bulk or transit time. An overview of carbohydrate and fiber classifications is provided in Table A-1.

Fats, Lipids, and Fatty Acid Review

The usual American diet contains 35–40% fat kilocalories. Fats are carriers for fat-soluble vitamins and essential fatty acids (EFAs). Fat is essential for cell membranes (including the brain), serves as an insulating agent for organ padding, and is a rich energy source. Generally, 95% of fat from the diet is absorbed. One to 2% of calories should be available as linoleic acid, which prevents EFA deficiency. At risk for EFA deficiency are people with low body fat stores, very malnourished persons, psychiatric patients, and premature low birth weight (LBW) infants.

Lipase is needed for long-chain triglycerides (LCT) to metabolize into free fatty acids (FFAs). Many parenteral fat emulsions contain LCT and can compromise immune function, elevate serum lipids, impair alveolar diffusion capacity, or decrease reticular endothelial system function. Medium-chain fatty acids (MCFAs) are produced from medium-chain triglycerides (MCTs) and are transported to the liver via the portal vein and, therefore, do not require micelle or chylomicron formation.

Omega-3 fatty acids reduce inflammation and help prevent certain chronic diseases such as arthritis. These essential fatty acids are highly concentrated in the brain. Uses for omega-3 fatty acids may include management of heart disease, neurological and psychiatric conditions, rheumatic conditions, and asthma. People with diabetes or schizophrenia may lack the ability to convert alpha linoleic acid (ALA) to eicosapentaenoic acid (EPA) and docosahexaenoic acid (DHA) and should obtain their omega-3 fatty acids from dietary sources rich in EPA and DHA. Two to three servings of fatty fish per week (about 1250 mg EPA and DHA per day) are beneficial for most people.

Fish oil supplements should provide 3000–4000 mg standardized fish oils per day. The safe and effective doses of all types of omega-3 fatty acid supplements in children have not been established. Fish oil can cause flatulence and diarrhea unless coated preparations are used.

EPA and arachidonic acids are transformed into eicosanoids for prostaglandin, leukotriene, thromboxane, and prostacyclin synthesis. Prostaglandins are used in many diverse hormone-like compounds. Thromboxanes are vasoconstrictors (in platelets); leukotrienes are for chemotaxis (in leukocytes); and prostacyclins are vasodilators (in blood vessels). Drugs like antihypertensives, diuretics, anti-inflammatories, and antithrombotics interfere with this transformation process.

Omega-3 fatty acids should be used cautiously by people who bruise easily, have a bleeding disorder, or take blood thinners such as warfarin because excessive amounts of omega-3 fatty acids may lead to bleeding. People who eat

TABLE A-1 Carbohydrate and Fiber Classifications

Category	Type	Food Sources
Monosaccharides	Glucose	Corn syrup, honey, fruits, vegetables
	Fructose	High-fructose corn syrup, honey, fruits, vegetables
	Galactose	Milk sugar (as a part of lactose)
	Mannose	Of little nutritional value; found in poorly digested fruit structures
Disaccharides	Sucrose	Table sugar, cane or beet sugars, maple sugar, some natural fruits and vegetables
	Lactose	Milk, cream, whey
	Maltose	Malt sugar, sprouting grains, partially digested starch
Oligosaccharides	Raffinose and stachyose	Beans and other legumes
Polysaccharides —digestible	Starch (amylose and amylopectin)	Modified food starch, potatoes, beans, breads, rice, pasta, starchy products such as tapioca
	Glycogen	Muscle and liver storage form of glucose
Polysaccharides —indigestible (fiber)	Insoluble fibers —cellulose	Soybean hulls, fruit membranes, legumes, carrots, other vegetables
	Lignin (noncarbohydrate)	Wheat straw, alfalfa stems, tannins, cottonseed hulls
	Cutin (noncarbohydrate)	Apple or tomato peels, seeds in berries, peanut or almond skins, onion skins
	Insoluble hemicelluloses	Corn hulls, wheat and corn brans, brown rice
	Soluble fibers —pectin	Citrus pulp, apple pulp, sugar beet pulp, banana, cabbage and *Brassica* foods, legumes (such as kidney beans), alfalfa leaves, sunflower heads
	Soluble hemicelluloses	Soy fiber concentrate, barley hulls
	Gums and mucilages	Oats, gum arabic, guar gum from legumes, psyllium from plantains, xanthan from prickly ash trees

Adapted from Wardlaw GM, Hampl J, Disilvestro RA. *Perspectives in nutrition*. 7th ed. New York: McGraw-Hill, 2004.

more than 3 g of omega-3 fatty acids per day may be at an increased risk for hemorrhagic stroke.

It is very important to maintain a balance between omega-3 and omega-6 fatty acids in the diet. Most omega-6 fatty acids are proinflammatory. The Mediterranean diet consists of a healthier balance between omega-3 and omega-6 fatty acids than the typical American diet.

Sphingolipids all have a sphingoid base backbone such as D-erythro-sphingosine. These lipids include ceramides, sphingomyelins, cerebrosides, gangliosides, and sulfatides. Sphingolipids in plants, fungi, and yeasts include mainly cerebrosides and phosphoinositides. Dairy products, eggs, and soybeans contain the most in our diet; fruit has a tiny bit. They are hydrolyzed throughout the gastrointestinal tract to regulate growth, differentiation, apoptosis, and other cellular functions.

Sphingolipids inhibit colon carcinogenesis, reduce low-density lipoprotein (LDL) levels, and increase high-density lipoprotein (HDL) levels. Dietary constituents such as cholesterol, fatty acids, and mycotoxins alter their metabolism.

Table A-2 describes more details about lipids.

Other Fatty Acid Issues and Substances

Carnitine When carnitine is in short supply, production of ATP slows down or halts altogether. Deficiency in heart or skeletal muscle reduces muscle efficiency. In renal failure, carnitine may actually be a useful additive to the diet to improve fatty acid metabolism. Carnitine does not enhance athletic performance and is not a "fat burner."

Function: Carnitine transports fatty acids into mitochondria, where they undergo beta-oxidation.

Sources: Carnitine is normally produced in the liver from essential amino acids lysine and methionine.

Myo-Inositol Myo-inositol has been distributed as a "vitamin," but there is no current evidence that dietary intake is necessary for good health.

Functions: Inositol phosphates liberated from glycerophosphatides acts as a secondary messenger in the release of intracellular of calcium, which in turn causes activation of certain cellular enzymes and produces hormonal responses; they have a possible role in diabetes mellitus or in renal failure.

Sources: Found as phytic acid in plants and as phospholipid in animals.

Proteins and Amino Acids

Amino acids and proteins are the building blocks of life. All growth and repair functions of the body require utilization and availability of amino acids in the proper proportion and amounts. The main protein source in the American diet is animal protein; beef contributes the most, followed by poultry. Average total protein needs are as follows: infants, 1700 mg/kg body weight (40% essential); children, 700 mg/kg body weight (36% essential); and adults, 425 mg/kg body weight (19% essential).

TABLE A-2 Lipid Categories and Sources

Class	Fatty Acid Component	Key Food Sources	Comments
Fatty acids:[a] Omega-3 family	Alpha linolenic acid (ALA) (polyunsaturated)	Vegetable oils (soybean, canola, or rapeseed), flaxseeds, flaxseed oil, soybeans, pumpkin seeds, pumpkin seed oil, purslane, perilla seed oil, walnuts, walnut oil Flaxseed and flaxseed oil should be kept refrigerated. Whole flaxseeds must be ground within 24 hours of use, otherwise the ingredients lose their activity. Flaxseeds are also available in ground form in a special mylar package so that the components in the flaxseeds stay active.	**An essential fatty acid.** Once eaten,the body converts ALA to eicosapentaenoic acid and docosahexanoic acid, the two types of omega-3 fatty acids more readily used by the body. The adequate daily intake of ALA should be 1.6 and 1.1 grams for men and women, respectively. Diets rich in ALA may increase the risk of macular degeneration and prostate cancer.
	Eicosapentaenoic acid (EPA) (polyunsaturated)	Cold-water fish such as salmon, mackerel, eel, tuna, halibut, sardines, and herring. Fish oil capsules should be refrigerated.	EPA and DHA (1 g/d) from fatty fish can reduce CHD
	Docosahexanoic acid (DHA) (polyunsaturated)	Cold-water fish such as salmon, mackerel, eel, tuna, halibut, sardines, and herring. Fish oil capsules should be refrigerated.	Infants who do not get enough DHA from their mothers during pregnancy are at risk for developing vision and nerve problems.
Omega-6 family	Linoleic acid (polyunsaturated)	Vegetable oils (safflower, sunflower, corn, soybean, peanut)	**An essential fatty acid**
	Conjugated linoleic acid (CLA)	Naturally rich in milk fat	Group of isomers produced by rumen bacteria. CLA may inhibit atherosclerosis, increase bone formation, reduce inflammatory joint disease, and reduce body fat accumulation (Scimeca and Miller, 2000)
	Arachidonic acid (polyunsaturated)	Animal tissues (very low). There is no good dietary source.	**An essential fatty acid**
Omega-9 family	Oleic acid (monounsaturated)	Vegetable oils and lipids	
Acyl -glycerols	Triglycerides (triacylglycerols)	Fats and oils	Glycerol with 3 esterified fatty acids
	Mono- and diglycerides	Additive in low-fat foods	Glycerol with 1 or 2 esterified fatty acids
Phospholipids	Glycerophosphatides	Egg yolks, liver, wheat germ, peanuts (lecithin)	Glycerol with 2 fatty acids and a nitrogen
	Sphingophosphatides	Found in myelin of nerve tissue (low in food supply)	Sphingosine with one esterified fatty acid (a ceramide)
Glycolipids	Cerebrosides, gangliosides	A ceramide linked to a monosaccharide or an oligosaccharide	Found in nerve and brain tissue (low in food supply)
Sterols	Cholesterol	Liver, heart, and other organ meats	Steroid nucleus (synthesized from acetyl-coenzyme A)
Fat-soluble vitamins	A,D, E, and K	Various food sources	Lipid soluble; some are esterified with 1 fatty acid
Trans fatty acids		Margarines, some cookies and crackers. The new food label includes the amount of trans fat in a serving of a food (Stahl, 2000).	These are made by hydrogenation of vegetable oils to form more solid products (i.e., margarine). The process increases the amount of saturation and converts natural *cis*-double bonds to *trans*-double bonds

[a]Recommended intakes of total fat per day equal 20–35% of kcals. Of this, consume 1–2% from omega-3 fatty acids and 5–8% from omega-6 fatty acids

TABLE A-3 Amino Acid Classification

Essential Amino Acids (must be consumed from diet)	Conditional Amino Acids (generally nonessential except in illness, stress)	Nonessential Amino Acids (generally made by the body if adequate nitrogen is available)
Histidine (aromatic)	Arginine (basic)	Alanine (neutral)
Isoleucine (neutral)	Cysteine (sulfur)	Asparagine (acidic)
Leucine (neutral)	Glutamine (acidic)	Aspartic acid (acidic)
Lysine (basic)	Tyrosine (aromatic)	Glutamic acid (acidic)
Methionine (sulfur)	Glycine (neutral)	
Phenylalanine (aromatic)	Ornithine (basic)	
Threonine (neutral)	Proline (cyclic)	
Tryptophan (aromatic)	Serine (neutral)	
Valine (neutral)		

Source: Shils M, et al. *Modern nutrition in health and disease*. 9th ed. Baltimore: Lippincott Williams & Wilkins, 1999.

To produce the nonessential amino acids from dietary intake of the essentials, it is recommended that the limited amino acids be consumed within a 24-hour period of each other. Protein synthesis requires all amino acids; an insufficient amount of any one may impede or slow formation of the polypeptide chain. For valine, leucine, and isoleucine, the requirement of each is increased by excess of the other branched-chain amino acids (BCAAs).

Protein requirement is inversely related to calories when the latter are deficient. Generally, more than 90% of protein is absorbed from the diet. Foods of high biological value (HBV) contain approximately 40% EAAs. Table A-3 indicates which amino acids are essential and which can be made by the body (nonessential). See Table A-4 for biological value of proteins; see Table A-5 for the top sources of protein.

MICRONUTRIENTS

Minerals

Minerals are inorganic compounds containing no carbon structures. There are 22 essential minerals known to be needed from the diet. Macrominerals (needed in large amounts) include calcium, phosphorus, magnesium, potassium, sodium, chloride, and sulfur. Trace minerals include iron, copper, selenium, fluoride, iodine, chromium, zinc, manganese, molybdenum, cobalt, and others.

Major Minerals

Minerals that are needed at levels of 100 mg daily or more are known as macrominerals. Estimated intakes of 12 differ-

TABLE A-4 Biological Value of Proteins

Protein	Biological Value
Whey protein	104
Egg	100
Cow's milk	95
Cottonseed	81
Beef	80
Fish	79
Casein	77
Soybean	74
Rice, white	67
Wheat, whole	53
Sesame	50
Corn	49

Derived from the Joint FAO/WHO Ad Hoc Expert Committee. Energy and protein requirements. WHO technical report no. 522. Geneva: World Health Organization, 1973, p. 67.

TABLE A-5 Top Sources of Protein

Source	Protein (g)
Fish, poultry, lean meat (3 oz)	20–30
Cottage cheese, 1/2 cup	14
Tofu, 3 oz	13
Yogurt, 6–8 oz	11
Kashi cereal	10
Lentils, cooked 1/2 cup	9
Milk, 8 oz	8
Peanut butter, 2 tablespoons	8
Pudding 1 cup	8
Cheese, 1 oz	7
Nuts, 1 oz	7
Egg, 1	6

From: U.S. Department of Agriculture. Nutrient database. Accessed July 1, 2005 at http://www.nal.usda.gov/fnic/foodcomp/search/.

ent minerals have been studied and reported by Hunt and Meacham (2001); where available, these data are included in the following mineral descriptions.

Calcium Calcium absorption is dependent upon the calcium needs of the body, foods eaten, and the amount of calcium in foods eaten. Vitamin D, whether from diet or exposure to the ultraviolet light of the sun, increases calcium absorption. Calcium absorption tends to decrease with increased age for both men and women. *New RDA for calcium is 1000 mg for most adults, 1300 mg for teenagers, and 1200 mg for those over age 50 years.*

Roles: For strong bones and teeth, nerve irritability, muscle contraction, heart rhythm, blood coagulation, enzymes, osmotic pressure, intercellular cement, maintenance of cell membranes, and helps protect against high blood pressure. About 60% is bound to protein, mostly albumin. About 30–60% absorption occurs with intakes of 400–1000 mg.

Sources: Milk and cheese products remain the primary source of calcium for Americans (Hunt and Meacham, 2001). Foods that contain small amounts of calcium but are not considered good sources can contribute significant amounts of calcium to an individual's diet if these foods are eaten often or in large amounts—oysters, dried fruit, green leafy vegetables, salmon and sardines with bones, molasses, and tofu. Some foods, such as orange juice, bread, and ready-to-eat cereals, are not normally good sources of calcium but may have had calcium added. Most instant-prepared cereals are fortified with calcium; check labels on the carton or package for the percentage of the U.S. RDA. Phytates and excessive protein or zinc decrease absorption. Calcium-fortified soy milk does not provide as much calcium as cow's milk, and the calcium from soy milk is absorbed only 75% as efficiently as from cow's milk (Heaney et al, 2000). Calcium is lost in cooking some foods, even under the best conditions. To retain calcium, cook foods in a minimal amount of water and for the shortest possible time. Table A-6 lists nonmilk calcium sources.

Signs of Deficiency: Hypocalcemia, tetany, paresthesia, hyperirritability, muscle cramps, convulsions, and stunting in growth. Premenstrual syndrome (PMS) is associated with a calcium deficiency, and calcium supplements often alleviate the symptoms of PMS (Schrezenmeir and Miller, 2000).

Signs of Excess: Hypercalcemia, loss of intestinal tone, kidney failure, and psychosis. Recommending excessive calcium use in the general, unsupervised public is not advisable.

Chloride Chloride constitutes about 3% of total mineral content in the body. It is the main extracellular ion, along with sodium. *No RDA levels have been established for chloride. The upper limit (UL) for adults is 3.6 g/d.*

Roles: Digestion (HCl in stomach), acid–base balance, O_2/CO_2 exchange in red blood cells (RBCs), and fluid balance.

Sources: Table salt, salt substitutes containing potassium chloride, processed foods made with table salt, sauerkraut, snack chips, and green olives.

TABLE A-6 Nonmilk Calcium Sources

Source	Calcium (mg)
1 cup plain nonfat yogurt	452
3 oz sardines, canned, with bones	372
1 cup fruited low-fat yogurt	345
1 cup almonds	332
1 cup Brazil nuts	260
1 cup frozen yogurt	240
1 cup oysters	226
1 cup rhubarb	174
3 oz salmon, canned, with bones	167
1 cup pork and beans	138
1 cup spinach, cooked	138
1 tbsp blackstrap molasses	137
1 cup tofu	130
1 cup dates	130
1 cup peanuts	107
1 cup cranberry sauce	104
1 cup dried apricots	100
1/2 cup turnip greens	99
1/2 cup kale, cooked	90
1 cup broccoli, cooked	72

Signs of Deficiency: Hypochlorhydria and disturbed acid–base balance.

Signs of Excess: Disturbed acid–base balance.

Magnesium Magnesium is a mineral needed by every cell of the body; half of the stores are found inside cells of body tissues and organs, and half are combined with calcium and phosphorus in bone. Only 1% of magnesium in the body is found in blood. The body works hard to keep blood levels of magnesium constant. Results of two national surveys indicated that the diets of most adult men and women do not provide the recommended amounts of magnesium. Adults aged 70 years and over eat less magnesium than younger adults, and non-Hispanic black subjects consume less magnesium than either non-Hispanic white or Hispanic subjects. Despite poor intakes, magnesium deficiency is rarely seen in the United States in adults. *RDA varies by age but is typically 420 mg for men and 320 mg for women. UL for supplemental magnesium for adolescents and adults is 350 mg/d.*

Roles: Magnesium is needed for more than 300 biochemical reactions in the body. It helps maintain normal muscle contraction, nerve transmission and function, heart rhythm, energy metabolism and protein synthesis, enzyme activation (ADP, ATP), glucose utilization, prevention of atherosclerosis, bone matrix and growth, and normal Na^+/K^+ pump. Maintaining an adequate magnesium intake is a positive lifestyle modification for preventing and managing high blood pressure. Magnesium deficiency can cause metabolic changes that may contribute to heart attacks and strokes;

population surveys have associated higher blood levels of magnesium with lower risk of coronary heart disease. Magnesium deficiency may also be a risk factor for postmenopausal osteoporosis. Elevated blood glucose levels increase the loss of magnesium in the urine, which in turn lowers blood levels of magnesium; this explains why low blood levels of magnesium (hypomagnesemia) are seen in poorly controlled type 1 and type 2 diabetes.

Sources: Green vegetables such as spinach and beet greens provide magnesium because the center of the chlorophyll molecule contains magnesium. Nuts (e.g., almonds, cashews), peanut butter, lentils, avocado, pumpkin seeds, and whole grains (e.g., oatmeal, wheat germ, bran) are also good sources of magnesium. Although magnesium is present in many foods, it usually occurs in small amounts. As with most nutrients, daily needs for magnesium cannot be met from a single food. Eating a wide variety of foods, including five servings of fruits and vegetables daily and plenty of whole grains, helps to ensure an adequate intake. Other sources include cocoa, chocolate, soybeans, meats, seafood, milk, tofu, and chili. Intake from a meal may be 45–55% absorbed. Beware of excess phytates. In the United States, milk and cheese contribute to the diets of infants and toddlers, as well as adolescents; beverages such as instant coffee are often contributors of magnesium to the diets of adults and seniors (Hunt and Meacham, 2001).

Water can provide magnesium, but the amount varies according to the water supply. "Hard" water contains more magnesium than "soft" water. Dietary surveys do not estimate magnesium intake from water, which may lead to underestimating total magnesium intake and its variability.

Signs of Deficiency: Hypomagnesemia. Poor growth, confusion, disorientation, loss of appetite, depression, tetany with muscle contractions and cramps, tingling, numbness, abnormal heart rhythms, coronary spasm, abnormal nerve function with seizures or convulsions, hyperirritability, and even death. When magnesium deficiency does occur, it is usually due to excessive loss of magnesium in urine from diabetes, antibiotics, diuretics, or excessive alcohol use; gastrointestinal (GI) system disorders that cause a loss of magnesium or limit magnesium absorption; or chronically low intake of magnesium. Chronic or excessive vomiting, diarrhea, and fat malabsorption may also result in magnesium depletion.

Signs of Excess: Hypermagnesemia. Mental status changes, nausea, diarrhea, appetite loss, muscle weakness, difficulty breathing or respiratory failure, extremely low blood pressure, and irregular heartbeat. High doses of magnesium supplements, which may be added to laxatives, can promote diarrhea. Magnesium toxicity is more often associated with kidney failure, when the kidney loses the ability to remove excess magnesium. Very large doses of laxatives also have been associated with magnesium toxicity, even with normal kidney function. The elderly are at risk of magnesium toxicity because kidney function declines with age and they are more likely to take magnesium-containing laxatives and antacids.

Phosphorus Phosphorus is second only to calcium in quantity in the human body. About 80% is in the skeleton and teeth as calcium phosphate; 20% is in extracellular fluid and cells. About 10% is bound to protein. *RDA for adult men and women is 700 mg/d. UL for adults varies from 3–4 g/d.*

Roles: Energy metabolism (ADP, ATP); fat, amino acid, and carbohydrate metabolism; calcium regulation; vitamin utilization; bones and teeth; osmotic pressure; DNA coding; buffer salts; fatty acid transport; oxygen transport and release; leukocyte phagocytosis; and microbial resistance.

Sources: Protein-rich foods such as meat, poultry, fish, egg yolks, dried beans and nuts, whole grains, enriched breads and cereals, milk, cheese, and dairy products. Also found in peas, corn, chocolate, and seeds. Excessive intake of soft drinks increases phosphorus intake, often causing an unbalanced intake of calcium. About 70% of oral intake is absorbed. In the United States, milk and cheese products contribute the main sources of phosphorus for infants, toddlers, and adolescents; meat, poultry, and fish products contribute more to the diets of adults and seniors (Hunt and Meacham, 2001).

Signs of Deficiency: Hypophosphatemia, neuromuscular and hematological changes, rickets, osteomalacia, and renal changes. Deficiency is rare but may occur in those persons who take phosphate binders, persons receiving total parenteral nutrition without phosphate, and prematurity.

Signs of Excess: Hyperphosphatemia, especially problematic in renal failure. Nutritional secondary hyperparathyroidism may occur, with fragile bones and fractures.

Potassium Potassium constitutes about 5% of total mineral content in the body. It is the main intracellular ion. *No specific RDA exists.*

Roles: Nerve conduction, muscle contraction, glycolysis, glycogen formation, protein synthesis and utilization, acid–base balance, cellular enzyme functioning, and water balance.

Sources: Fruits and vegetables, dried beans and peas, whole grains, and whole and skim milk. In the United States, milk and cheese products contribute the main sources of potassium for infants, toddlers, and adolescents; meat, poultry, and fish products contribute more to the diets of adults and seniors, with vegetables being a secondary source (Hunt and Meacham, 2001). Table A-7 provides a list of foods that contain over 500 mg potassium per serving.

Signs of Deficiency: Hypokalemia. Muscle weakness, cardiac arrhythmia, paralysis, bone fragility, decreased growth, weight loss, and even death.

Signs of Excess: Hyperkalemia. Paralysis, muscular weakness, arrhythmias and heart disturbances, and even death.

Sodium Sodium constitutes about 2% of total mineral content in the body. It is the main extracellular ion, along with chloride. *No specific RDA exists; 2300 mg/d is the UL for adults.*

Roles: Nerve stimulation, muscle contraction, acid–base balance, regulation of blood pressure, and glucose transport into cells. Sodium is the major extracellular fluid cation.

TABLE A-7 Foods That Contain >500 mg Potassium Per Serving

1 tsp cream of tartar (on cereal, etc.)
1 cup prune or tomato juice
1-1/4 cup orange or citrus juice
1 medium banana (1 small banana, 400 mg)
7-8 dates or 4 figs
7 large prunes or 1/2 cup dark raisins
6 fresh apricots
1-1/2 cups milk (any kind)
1/2 cantaloupe
1 cup broccoli
3/4 cup winter squash
1 large white or sweet potato
1/2 avocado (600 mg)
2 tbsp molasses
1/2 cup nuts
1/2 cup dry beans, cooked
1/2 tsp salt substitute (most brands)

Sources: Milk, cheese, eggs, meat, fish, poultry, beets, carrots, celery, spinach, chard, seasoned salts, baking powder and soda, table salt (NaCl), many drugs and preservatives, some drinking water, and processed foods with salt added. More than 95% of sodium from a mixed diet is absorbed. In the United States, infants receive the greatest amount of sodium from milk and cheese products; grain products are the primary source for all other age groups, and meat, poultry, and fish are secondary sources for adults and seniors (Hunt and Meacham, 2001).

Signs of Deficiency: Hyponatremia, water intoxication, anorexia, nausea, muscle atrophy, poor growth, weight loss, confusion, coma, and even death.

Signs of Excess: Hypernatremia. Confusion, coma. High blood pressure and calcium excretion from bones may result. Heart failure and edema may also result from excesses.

Sulfur Sulfur exists as part of the amino acids methionine, cystine, and cysteine and as part of the antioxidant glutathione peroxidase and other organic molecules. *No specific RDA exists.*

Roles: Amino acids (methionine, cystine, cysteine), thiamin molecule, coenzyme A, biotin and pantothenic acid, connective tissue metabolism, penicillin, sulfa drugs, insulin molecule, heparin, and keratin of skin, hair, and nails.

Sources: Meat, poultry, fish, eggs, dried beans and legumes, *Brassica* family vegetables (broccoli, cabbage, cauliflower, Brussels sprouts), and wheat germ.

Signs of Deficiency: Not specific but likely to occur with hypoalbuminemia.

Signs of Excess: Uncommon because excess is excreted in the urine as sulfate, usually in combination with calcium. This may result in hypercalciuria (often after a high-protein meal).

Trace Minerals

Trace minerals are elements that are found in minute amounts in body tissues and are specific to the function of certain enzymes. They are typically not found in free ionic state but are bound to other proteins.

Copper Copper is an antioxidant. Concentrations of copper are highest in the liver, brain, heart, and kidney; skeletal muscle also contains a large percentage because of total mass (Anderson, 2000). About 90% of copper is bound as ceruloplasmin and is transported to other tissues, mainly by albumin. *New RDA is 900 μg daily for men and women. UL was set at 10 mg/d.*

Roles: Skeletal development, immunity, formation of red blood cells and leukopoiesis, phospholipid synthesis, electron transport, pigmentation, aortic elasticity, connective tissue formation, and central nervous system and myelin sheath structure.

Sources: Barley and whole grains, oysters and shellfish, nuts, dried beans and legumes, cocoa, eggs, prunes, and potatoes. Note: Milk is low in copper. Daily intake of copper in the United States is 2–5 mg; however, many persons have a lower intake than this because fresh foods are low in copper. Meat, poultry, and fish are primary sources in the United States for all age groups except infants, for whom infants' foods are the primary source of copper (Hunt and Meacham, 2001). Approximately 30–60% of oral intake is absorbed. Absorption is enhanced by acid and decreased by calcium. Approximately 94% of copper is tightly bound to ceruloplasmin.

Signs of Deficiency: Hypochromic anemia, cardiomyopathy, aortic aneurysms, elevated cholesterol levels, neutropenia, skeletal abnormalities and osteoporosis, decreased skin and hair pigmentation, Menke's disease or kinky-hair syndrome, dermatitis, anorexia, diarrhea, and reduced immune responses. Deficiency is rare in adults, except with celiac sprue, protein-losing enteropathies, and nephrotic syndrome. Requirement is increased by excessive zinc intake.

Signs of Excess: Excess is rare, but liver cirrhosis, biliary cirrhosis, and other liver disorders (including Wilson's disease) may contribute to the retention of copper. Abnormalities in red blood cell formation, copper deposits in the brain, and liver damage occur. Excesses may decrease vitamin A absorption.

Fluoride Fluoride is found in nearly all drinking waters and soils. The American Dietetic Association affirms that fluoride is an important element for all mineralized tissues and that appropriate consumption aids bone and tooth health (American Dietetic Association, 2005). Eighty percent to 90% of oral intake is absorbed. *RDA is 3–4 mg/d for men and women. UL is set at 10 mg/d.*

Roles: Calcium uptake; some role in prevention of calcified aortas; resistance to dental caries, collapsed vertebrae, and osteoporosis; formation of hydroxyapatite; and enamel growth.

Sources: Fluoridated water, tea, mackerel, salmon with bones, infant foods to which bone meal has been added.

Signs of Deficiency: Dental caries, calcification of aorta, and anemia. Possibly bone thinning and osteoporosis.

Signs of Excess: Bony outgrowths at the spine. Tooth mottling, pitting, and discoloration (fluorosis) occur at doses of greater than 2–3 ppm in the drinking water. Excess can result in neurological problems; this feature is valuable in rat poison, for example.

Iron Iron deficiency anemia is the most common nutrient deficiency in the world, especially among toddlers, teenage girls, and women of childbearing age. Functional iron is found in hemoglobin, myoglobin, and enzymes. Storage iron is found in ferritin, hemosiderin, and transferrin. Iron is conserved and reused at a rate of 90% daily; the rest is excreted, mainly in bile. Dietary iron must be consumed to meet the 10% gap to prevent deficiency. Sulfur amino acids and vitamin C increase iron absorption. Excessive calcium intake and oxalic, tannic, and phytic acids can reduce absorption. Serum iron is largely bound to transferrin. About 5–15% is absorbed as ferrous iron; 15–25% of oral intake of heme iron is absorbed (meat, fish, and poultry); 2–20% of oral intake of nonheme iron is absorbed (legumes, grains, and fruit). *The RDA is 8 mg for men and postmenopausal women and 18 mg for premenopausal women. Pregnant women need 27 mg/d. UL for iron is 45 mg/d.*

Roles: Responsible for carrying oxygen to cells through hemoglobin and myoglobin, skeletal muscle functioning, cognitive functioning, leukocyte functions and T-cell immunity, cellular enzymes, and cytochrome content for normal cellular respiration.

Sources: Beans, beef, dried fruit, enriched grains, fortified cereals, pork. In the United States, grain products provide the highest amount of dietary iron for all age groups except infants, for whom infant foods are the best source (Hunt and Meacham, 2001). See Table A-8.

Signs of Deficiency: Hypochromic anemia, fatigue and weakness, pallor, dyspnea, decreased resistance to infection, koilonychia, spoon-shaped nails, impaired learning ability, headache, tachycardia, glossitis, cheilosis, and dysphagia. Deficiency is defined as having an abnormal value for two of three laboratory tests of iron status (erythrocyte protoporphyrin, transferrin saturation, or serum ferritin). Iron deficiency anemia is defined as iron deficiency plus low hemoglobin.

Signs of Excess: Iron deposits, liver damage (cirrhosis), diabetes mellitus, and skin pigmentation; GI distress (Trumbo, 2001); hereditary or secondary hemochromatosis. Transfusion overload is rare but may be found in persons with sickle cell anemia or thalassemia major. Excess may occur from taking iron supplements daily or from multiple sources.

Zinc Zinc is so prevalent in cellular metabolism that even minor impairment in supply is likely to have multiple biological and clinical effects. Zinc deficiency causes a reduction in antibody responses and cell-mediated responses of the immune system. Zinc absorption is affected by level of zinc in the diet and any interfering substances, such as phytates, calcium, cadmium, folic acid, excessive fiber, and copper. Albumin is the major plasma carrier. *New RDA is 11 mg for men and 8 mg for women. UL is 40 mg.*

Roles: ACTH-stimulated steroidogenesis in adrenals and sexual maturation; fatty acid, carbohydrate, protein, and nucleic acid metabolism; CO_2 transport; amino acid breakdown from peptides; oxidation of vitamin A; reproduction; growth; enzymes (such as alcohol dehydrogenase, alkaline phosphatase, and lactic acid dehydrogenase); wound healing; catalyst for hydrogenation; immunity; night vision; alcohol detoxification in the liver; heme synthesis; taste and smell acuity; synthesis of glutathione; and collagen precursors.

Zinc supplementation has been shown to be effective in reducing morbidity and mortality from diarrhea, malaria, HIV infection, sickle cell anemia, renal disease, and GI disorders by preventing the immune system response from being diminished (Fraker et al, 2000). Zinc gluconate lozenges do not always alleviate cold symptoms in children and adolescents but may be somewhat helpful.

Sources: Beans, seafood (e.g., lobster, shrimp, oysters), poultry, meat (red meat such as beef and liver especially), eggs, milk, peanuts, oatmeal, whole grains (e.g., whole wheat, rye bread, wheat germ), and yeast. The average American diet contains 10–15 mg/d. Meat, poultry, and fish are the primary sources of zinc for all age groups of Americans except infants, for whom infant foods provide the richest source (Hunt and Meacham, 2001). Zinc is distributed in the body with proteins such as albumin, transferrin, ceruloplasmin, and gamma-globulin. Animal sources are better utilized; vegetarian diets must be monitored for zinc deficiency. Phytates, excess copper, and fiber can decrease absorption by forming complexes. Calcium and phosphate salts also decrease absorption; 10–40% from meals is absorbed in the duodenum and the jejunum. Vitamin D can increase bioavailability.

Signs of Deficiency: Dermatitis and skin lesions, hypoglycemia, growth failure and hypogonadism, mild anemia, decreased taste acuity, alopecia, diarrhea, apathy, depression, and impaired wound healing. Zinc deficiency has a significant impact on development and on immune function; premature infants and children are at greatest risk (Costello and Grumstrup-Scott, 2000). In children with zinc deficiency, severe growth depression is seen. Strict vegetarians, preschoolers who do not eat meat, adolescent females, and those on a chronically high-phytate diet may also be at risk, especially if other disease states are present.

Signs of Excess: Low levels of serum copper and lowered HDL cholesterol may result. Excessive zinc intake is probably self-limiting because of GI distress that occurs. Zinc toxicity can occur in renal dialysis if not carefully monitored.

TABLE A-8 Food Sources of Heme and Nonheme Iron

Food Sources	Milligrams per Serving	% Daily Value	Food Sources	Milligrams per Serving	% Daily Value
Heme Iron			**Nonheme Iron**		
Chicken liver, cooked, 3-1/2 oz	12.8	70	Ready-to-eat cereal, 100% iron fortified, 3/4 cup	18.0	100
Oysters, breaded and fried, 6 pieces	4.5	25	Oatmeal, instant, fortified, prepared with water, 1 cup	10.0	60
Beef, chuck, lean only, braised, 3 oz	3.2	20	Soybeans, mature, boiled, 1 cup	8.8	50
Clams, breaded, fried, 3/4 cup	3.0	15	Lentils, boiled, 1 cup	6.6	35
Beef, tenderloin, roasted, 3 oz	3.0	15	Beans, kidney, mature, boiled, 1 cup	5.2	25
Turkey, dark meat, roasted, 3-1/2 oz	2.3	10	Beans, lima, large, mature, boiled, 1 cup	4.5	25
Beef, eye of round, roasted, 3 oz	2.2	10	Beans, navy, mature, boiled, 1 cup	4.5	25
Turkey, light meat, roasted, 3-1/2 oz	1.6	8	Ready-to-eat cereal, 25% iron fortified, 3/4 cup	4.5	25
Chicken, leg, meat only, roasted, 3-1/2 oz	1.3	6	Beans, black, mature, boiled, 1 cup	3.6	20
Tuna, fresh bluefin, cooked, dry heat, 3 oz	1.1	6	Beans, pinto, mature, boiled, 1 cup	3.6	20
Chicken, breast, roasted, 3 oz	1.1	6	Molasses, blackstrap, 1 tablespoon	3.5	20
Halibut, cooked, dry heat, 3 oz	0.9	6	Tofu, raw, firm, 1/2 cup	3.4	20
Crab, blue crab, cooked, moist heat, 3 oz	0.8	4	Spinach, boiled, drained, 1/2 cup	3.2	20
Pork, loin, broiled, 3 oz	0.8	4	Spinach, canned, drained solids, 1/2 cup	2.5	10
Tuna, white, canned in water, 3 oz	0.8	4	Black-eyed peas (cowpeas), boiled, 1 cup	1.8	10
Shrimp, mixed species, cooked, moist heat, 4 large	0.7	4	Spinach, frozen, chopped, boiled, 1/2 cup	1.9	10
			Grits, white, enriched, quick, prepared with water, 1 cup	1.5	8
			Raisins, seedless, packed, 1/2 cup	1.5	8
			Whole wheat bread, 1 slice	0.9	6
			White bread, enriched, 1 slice	0.9	6

Source: U.S. Department of Agriculture nutrient database. Accessed February 1, 2006 at http://www.nal.usda.gov/fnic/foodcomp/search/.

Ultra-Trace Minerals

Boron Boron can be found in the brain and the bone; it is also found in the spleen and thyroid. It is found in foods such as sodium borate; it is absorbed at a rate of 90%. *No RDA has been set, but a UL of 20 mg was established.*

Roles: Mineral metabolism in animals and humans, cell membrane functioning. It may function in a role similar to estrogen in bone metabolism and strengthening (Anderson, 2000).

Sources: Drinking water, wine, cider and beer, noncitrus fruits, leafy vegetables, nuts, and legumes. Note: Protein foods and grains are low in boron. In the United States, infant foods provide the most for infants; fruits and fruit juices provide the most for toddlers; milk and cheese foods provide the most in adolescent diets; and beverages provide the most for adults and seniors (Hunt and Meacham, 2001).

Signs of Deficiency: None known at this time.

Signs of Excess: Reproductive and developmental effects (Trumbo, 2001).

Chromium Chromium is closely related to insulin action. Absorption ranges from 0.5–2%. Chromium needs transferrin for distribution. *No specific RDA exists.*

Roles: Insulin molecule (part of glucose tolerance factor [GTF]); some inhibition of vascular disorders from aortic plaque, fatty acid, triglyceride, and cholesterol metabolism; normal glucose metabolism; nucleic acid stability; regulation of gene expression; and peripheral nerve functioning.

Sources: Oysters, liver, potatoes, eggs, vegetable oil, brewer's yeast, whole grains and bran, shortening, nuts, and peanuts. Dairy products, fruits, and vegetables are low in chromium. Phytates and oxalates can decrease absorption.

Signs of Deficiency: Glucose intolerance, increased FFA levels, low respiratory quotient, peripheral neuropathy, impaired fertility and growth, and perhaps elevated cholesterol and triglycerides. Deficiency may be found in severe malnutrition, in diabetes, or in elderly patients with cardiovascular disease.

Signs of Excess: None known.

Cobalt Most cobalt appears in the body with vitamin B_{12} stores in the liver (Anderson, 2000). Cobalt may share intestinal transport with iron and is increased in patients with low iron intake and iron stores. *No specific RDA exists.*

Roles: Treatment of some anemias, part of structure of cobalamin in vitamin B_{12}, role in immunity, and healthy nerves and red blood cells.

Sources: Seafood (such as oysters and clams), meats (such as liver), poultry, some grains, and cereals. Note: Cow's milk is very low. More than 50% of dietary cobalt is absorbed.

Signs of Deficiency: Weakness, anemia, and emaciation. Deficiency is usually in conjunction with vitamin B_{12} deficiency and low intake of protein foods. Lack of intrinsic factor, gastrectomy, or malabsorption syndromes may also cause deficiency.

Signs of Excess: Polycythemia, bone marrow hyperplasia, reticulocytosis, and increased blood volume may result.

Iodine With the iodization of salt, iodine deficiency has been almost eliminated in the United States and Western nations. Fortification results in fewer goiters and less cretinism, stillbirths, spontaneous abortions, and mental or growth retardation. Millions of people are at risk in other nations. The thyroid gland maintains 75% of the body's iodine; the rest is throughout the body, as in the gastric mucosa and blood. Iodide content of vegetables varies by the content of the local soil. Absorption is 50–100% from the gut. *New RDA is 150 μg/d for both men and women. UL is 1.1 mg/d.*

Roles: Energy metabolism, proper thyroid functioning, normal growth and reproduction, prevention of goiter, and regulation of cellular metabolism and temperature. Iodine is found with T3 and T4 distribution.

Sources: Iodized salt, seaweed, and seafood (clams, oysters, sardines, lobster, and saltwater fish). Other lesser sources may include cream (in milk), eggs, drinking water in various areas, plant leaves (broccoli, spinach, and turnip greens), cranberries, and legumes. Iodized salt should be encouraged for pregnant women. Goitrogens in cabbage, turnips, rapeseeds, peanuts, cassava, and soybeans may block uptake of iodine by body cells; heating and cooking inactivate them.

Signs of Deficiency: Enlarged thyroid gland and related goiter and hypothyroidism, cretinism, deaf-mutism, abnormal fetal growth, and brain development.

Signs of Excess: Excess may depress thyroid activity or can lead to elevated thyroid-stimulating hormone (TSH) levels (Trumbo, 2001), hyperthyroidism, high levels of thyroid hormone, and possibly a hyperthyroidism goiter.

Manganese Manganese affects reproductive capacity, pancreatic function, and carbohydrate metabolism. Less than 5% is absorbed from diet. It is transported bound to a macroglobulin, transferrin, or transmanganin. Human milk tends to be low in manganese levels. *An adequate intake (AI) level has been set at 2.3 mg for men and 1.8 mg for women. The UL has been established at 11 mg.*

Roles: Polysaccharide and fatty acid metabolism, enzyme activation, tendon and skeletal development, possible role in hypertension, fertility and reproduction (role with squalene as a precursor of cholesterol and sex hormones), melanin and dopamine production, energy and glucose production, and possible roles in blood and ear labyrinth formation.

Sources: Tea, coffee, whole grains, wheat germ and bran, blueberries, peas, beans and dried legumes, nuts, spinach, and cocoa powder. Sources of manganese are plant foods, not animal foods. In the United States, infant foods provide the highest amount of manganese for infants; grain products are primary sources for all other age groups, and beverages, fruits, vegetables, desserts, and mixed dishes are secondary sources (Hunt and Meacham, 2001).

Signs of Deficiency: Nausea, vomiting, transient dermatitis, color changes in hair, hypocholesterolemia, growth retardation, weight loss, and slow growth of hair and beard. In animals, sterility and striking skeletal abnormalities occur. Beware of excess calcium, phosphorus, iron, or magnesium supplementation. Manganese, cobalt, and iron compete for pathways.

Signs of Excess: Excess can rarely occur in those who mine manganese for a living. Excesses accumulate in the liver and CNS; neurological side effects like Parkinson's tremors may occur.

Molybdenum Molybdenum is important mostly for its role in xanthine oxidase. About 40–100% of intake is absorbed from the duodenum in protein-bound form. It is readily absorbed from the stomach and small intestine and excreted in the urine. *New RDA is 45 μg for both men and women. The UL was set at 2 mg.*

Roles: Flavoproteins; copper antagonist; component of sulfite oxidase, aldehyde oxidase, and xanthine oxidase; iron storage; energy metabolism; and degradation of cysteine and methionine through sulfite oxidase.

Sources: Legumes, whole-grain breads and cereals, dark green leafy vegetables, milk and dairy products, and organ meats. Milk and cheese products provide the most molybdenum for infants, toddlers, and adolescents; grain products provide the most for adults and seniors (Hunt and Meacham, 2001).

Signs of Deficiency: Tachycardia, tachypnea, visual and mental changes, headache, nausea, and vomiting. This has been seen in patients with long-term total parenteral nutrition (TPN) that is deficient in molybdenum.

Signs of Excess: Impaired reproduction and growth and gout-like syndrome can occur. Excess is rare because it is usually just excreted in the urine.

Selenium Cellular and plasma glutathione are the functional parameters for measuring selenium status. Selenium intake in the United States is generally very good; deficiency is not seen here. More than 50% dietary intake is absorbed (average range, 35–85%). It is transported protein-bound to albumin from the duodenum. *A new RDA level for selenium was set at 55 μg/d for both men and women to achieve the best antioxidant levels; UL was set at 400 μg.*

Roles: Protein biosynthesis, spares vitamin E, cell wall protection as an antioxidant (glutathione peroxidase), protein matrix of teeth, protection against mercury toxicity, some role in fertility, liver function, heart muscle function, and growth. Selenium functions within mammals primarily as selenoproteins, which contain selenium as selenocysteine. Glutathione catalyzes the reduction of peroxides that can cause cellular damage.

Sources: Seafood and fish, chicken, egg yolks, meats (especially kidney and liver), whole-grain breads and cereals, wheat germ, foods grown in selenium-rich soil including garlic, dairy products, Brazil nuts, and onions. Dietary selenium is found with protein in animal tissue. Muscle meats, organ meats, and seafood are dependable sources of selenium. Grains and seeds have variable amounts dependent on the soil.

Signs of Deficiency: Muscle weakness and pain, carcinogenesis, and cardiomyopathy. Keshan's disease is a selenium deficiency that occurs in China where soil levels are quite low; cardiomyopathy is the main symptom. Kashin-Beck's disease is common in preadolescents and adolescents; it is caused by a virus and has effects similar to osteoarthritis with stiffness and swelling of the elbows, knees, and ankles.

Signs of Excess: Symptoms of toxicity have been reported in China with selenosis (skin and nail changes, decaying of teeth, and neurological abnormalities).

Less Studied Ultra-trace Minerals

Aluminum, Arsenic, Cadmium, Lead, Lithium, and Tin Not much is known about the roles, functions, or purpose in the human body of these minerals. For all age groups, grain products (mainly cornbread, pancakes, biscuits, muffins, and yellow cake) provide the highest amount of aluminum in the diet; beverages contribute secondarily (Hunt and Meacham, 2001).

Nickel *No RDA has been set, but UL was established at 1 mg/d because decreased body weight can occur with excess as noted in animal studies (Trumbo, 2001).*

Suspected Roles: Growth, reproduction, iron and zinc metabolism, hematopoiesis, DNA and RNA, and enzyme activation.

Sources: Grains and vegetables. Note: Less than 10% is absorbed. It is transported by serum albumin.

Silicon *No RDA or UL have been established.*

Suspected Roles: Normal bone growth and calcification, normal collagen and connective tissue formation (especially in the presence of calcium), and development of atherosclerosis with decreased silicon in aorta is experimental.

Sources: Most foods; only minute amounts are needed. Grains and beer are good sources.

Vanadium *No RDA has been set, but UL was established at 1.8 mg/d because renal lesions have been noted in animal studies (Trumbo, 2001).*

Suspected Roles: Possible roles in growth, lipid metabolism, and reproduction. Early trials with vanadium indicate that there may be a role in treatment of diabetes mellitus; it has the ability to mimic insulin and lower blood pressure and glucose levels.

Sources: Leafy green vegetables and cereal grains.

Vitamins

Vitamins were first named "vital amines" in 1912 because they seemed to be important to life. Once it was known that they contain few amine groups, the "e" was dropped. There are 13 known vitamins (four fat soluble and nine water soluble). They are organic compounds, containing carbon structures.

Inadequate intake of several vitamins has been linked to chronic diseases including coronary heart disease, cancers, and osteoporosis (Fairfield and Fletcher, 2002). The best nutritional strategy for promoting optimal health and reducing the risk of chronic disease is to obtain adequate nutrients from a wide variety of foods. Eating more fruits and vegetables rather than taking supplements is currently the recommendation. Supplements are needed in special cases, such as during pregnancy and in some medical conditions. Supplements are most useful when taken as a whole, such as a multivitamin supplement that meets 100% of the DRI values. Because many physicians are unaware of the food sources of specific vitamins and because fat-soluble vitamins should not be consumed in large doses, this recommendation of meeting 100% DRI levels is safest (Fairfield and Fletcher, 2002).

Fat-Soluble Vitamins

Vitamin A (Retinol, Retinal, Retinoic Acid) Vitamin A is best known for its role in vision and skin integrity. Its provitamins include beta-carotene and cryptoxanthin. From 7–65% of vitamin A from the diet is absorbed. Dietary retinyl esters are hydrolyzed in the intestine by the pancreatic enzyme, pancreatic triglyceride lipase (PTL), and the intestinal brush border enzyme, phospholipase B (Harrison and Hussain, 2001). Once in the cell, retinol is complexed with cellular retinol-binding protein type 2 (CRBP2), a substrate for reesterification of the retinol by the enzyme lecithin:retinol acyltransferase (LRAT); retinol not bound is esterified by acyl-coenzyme A (CoA) acyltransferase (Harrison and Hussain, 2001). Retinol-binding protein (RBP) is used to evaluate transport. Retinyl esters are incorporated into chylomicrons.

Stress can increase excretion; zinc or protein deficiency can decrease transport. Dietary vitamin A is transported via chylomicrons; 90% of vitamin A is stored in the liver. *New RDA is 900 mg for men and 700 mg for women. UL is 3000 mg/d.*

Functions: Vision (especially night), gene regulation, growth, prevention of early miscarriage, immunity against infection (measles and many others), corticosterones, weight gain, proper bone, tooth, and nerve development, membrane functions, and epithelial tissue integrity in lungs and trachea especially. Vitamin A supplementation is used to treat some forms of cancer and degenerative retinitis pigmentosa.

Sources: Beef liver, fish liver oil, fortified cereal, egg yolk, animal livers, dairy products, butter and fortified margarine, cheddar cheese, and cream.

Signs of Deficiency: Xerophthalmia, night blindness, follicular hyperkeratosis or thickening of skin around hair follicles, drying of the whites of the eyes, eventual blindness, spots on the whites of the eyes, risk of infections, and death.

Vulnerable Populations: Anorexia nervosa, burns, biliary obstruction, cancer, cirrhosis, celiac disease, cystic fibrosis, drug use (cholestyramine, mineral oil, and neomycin), hookworm, hepatitis of infectious origin, giardiasis, kwashiorkor, malaria, measles, pancreatic disease, pneumonia, pregnancy, prematurity, rheumatic fever, tropical sprue, and zinc deficiency.

Signs of Excess: Headache, peeling of skin, enlarged spleen and kidneys, bone thickening and joint pain, drying of the mucous membranes, and liver damage. Vitamin A is known for its teratogenic affects; if pregnant women are using a supplement, they should consider taking it in the form of beta-carotene (Voyles et al, 2000). Caution should be given to supplement use in women of childbearing age because many women don't know they are pregnant in the earliest stages; supplements with retinol should be avoided during the first trimester if vitamin A deficiency is not present. Long-term supplementation with retinol (such as 25,000 IU/d) may have adverse effects on blood lipid levels and bone health.

Carotenoids There are more than 500 natural carotenoids. Two beta-carotene molecules are equivalent to one molecule of vitamin A. The bioavailability of carotenoids from vegetables is low, and the fat required for adequate absorption is low (van het Hof et al, 2000). Between 9% and 17% of dietary carotenes are absorbed. Dietary carotenoids may prevent some types of cancer through enhancement of immune response, inhibition of mutagenesis, and protection against oxidative damage to cells; alpha-carotenes, beta-cryptoxanthin, lutein, zeaxanthin, and lycopenes may contribute to these important functions. Persons at risk for developing lung cancer (i.e., current smokers and workers exposed to asbestos) should be discouraged from taking beta-carotene supplements. With new RDA levels, no recommendations were made for beta-carotene because there is not enough evidence to support a specific RDA.

Sources: Beta-carotene is found in deep yellow, orange, or dark green fruits and vegetables such as pumpkin, sweet potato, carrots, spinach, kale, turnip greens, cantaloupe, apricots, romaine lettuce, broccoli, papaya, mango, and tangerine.

Signs of Excess: Hypercarotenodermia (yellowing of skin with clear whites of eyes).

Vitamin D (Ergocalciferol or D_2, Cholecalciferol or D_3) The main function of vitamin D is bone metabolism and calcium homeostasis. Vitamin D is actually a prohormone. Total-body sun exposure provides the equivalent of 250 mg (10,000 IU) vitamin D daily, suggesting that this is a physiological limit. Bile salts are required for absorption; 90% of dietary intake is absorbed. There is decreased production with aging. Active metabolite is 1,25-dihydroxyvitamin D_3. Transport occurs via chylomicrons to the liver. *New RDA is 200 IU for most people and 400 IU for people age 51–70 years. UL is 50 μg/d for adults.*

Functions: Utilization of calcium and phosphorus, volume and acidity of gastric secretions, growth of soft tissues, bone calcification, growth and repair, tooth formation, effects on parathormone (PTH), and renal/intestinal phosphate absorption. Supplemental vitamin D may also help prevent some cancers, osteoarthritis progression, multiple sclerosis, and hypertension.

Sources: Canned pink salmon (3 oz = 530 IU), canned tuna (3 oz = 200 IU), cod liver oil, sunshine, eggs (one yolk = 27 IU), herring (3 1/2 oz = 330 IU), vitamin D–fortified milk (8 oz = 100 IU), fortified orange juice (8 oz = 100 IU), fortified cereal (1 cup = 40–60 IU), fortified margarine (1 tablespoon = 60 IU), sardines, and fish roe. Brief and casual exposure to sunlight can be safely encouraged. Sunlight and vitamin D exposure tend to be low in northern climates during winter months.

Signs of Deficiency: Bowed legs, rickets in children, and osteomalacia in adults. Hypovitaminosis D is related to lowered vitamin D intake, less exposure to ultraviolet light, anticonvulsant use, renal dialysis, nephrotic syndrome, hypertension, diabetes, winter season, and high PTH and alkaline phosphatase levels. Hypovitaminosis D is common in general medical in-patients.

Vulnerable Populations: Biliary obstruction, celiac disease, cystic fibrosis, diabetes, drug use (bile salt binders, glucocorticoids, phenobarbital, primidone, and mineral oil), end-organ failure, Fanconi's disease, hepatic disease, hypertension, primary hypophosphatemia, hypoparathyroidism, inflammatory bowel disease, intestinal malabsorption, lack of exposure to sunlight, lymphatic obstruction, multiple sclerosis, nephrotic syndrome, neurological and psychiatric conditions such as depression and bipolar disorders, pancreatitis, parathyroid surgery, postmenopausal status, prematurity, renal disease and dialysis, small bowel resection, and tropical sprue. Pregnant women should enjoy a few minutes in the sun each day, if possible.

Signs of Excess: Poor appetite, nausea, vomiting, increased urination, weakness, thirst, itchy skin, kidney failure, calcium deposits throughout the body, and nervousness.

Vitamin E (Alpha-Tocopherol, Gamma-Tocopherol) The main function of vitamin E is as a membrane antioxidant. Tocotrienols plus other forms affect cholesterol metabolism, carotid arteries, and immunity against cancer. The natural form is *d*-alpha-tocopherol (need 22 IU). The *dl*-alpha-tocopherol form is synthetic and less effective. *The new RDA is 15 mg for adults. UL is 1000 mg.*

Functions: Antioxidant along with vitamin C and selenium; anticoagulant and vitamin K antagonist; intracellular respiration; hemopoietic agent; roles in muscular, vascular, reproductive, and central nervous system (CNS) systems; some role in reproduction; neutralizes free radicals; protects against cataracts; may relieve discomforts of rheumatoid arthritis; protects against effects of the sun, smog, and lung disease; protects brain cell membranes.

Sources: Salad oils (safflower, corn, and sunflower oils), wheat germ oil, margarine, grain products, seeds and nuts, mayonnaise, green leafy vegetables (spinach, asparagus, broccoli, and turnip greens), avocado, dried prunes, and mango. Note: Normal requirements increase with use of PUFAs. Normal needs are 15 mg/d, but with PUFAs, normal requirements double daily. Overall, 20–40% is absorbed with meals. Bile and pancreatic secretions are needed. Very low–density lipoproteins (VLDL) and LDL carry it to tissues. Gamma-tocopherol is more common in the U.S. food supply (as from soybean oil); it is less useful to the body.

Signs of Deficiency: Rupture of red blood cells, nerve damage, impaired bone mineralization, impaired vitamin A storage, and prolonged blood coagulation. Vitamin E is one of the least toxic vitamins, but at high doses, it can antagonize the utilization of other fat-soluble vitamins.

Vulnerable Populations: Alzheimer's disease, arthritis, biliary cirrhosis, bronchopulmonary dysplasia, cardiovascular diseases, cystic fibrosis, drug use (cholestyramine, clofibrate, oral contraceptives, and triiodothyronine), high intake of PUFA in diet, malabsorption syndromes, malnutrition, musculoskeletal disorders, pancreatic diseases, pregnancy, prematurity, pulmonary diseases, and steatorrhea.

Signs of Excess: Excessive intake does not seem to cause hypervitaminosis but has caused isolated cases of dermatitis, fatigue, pruritus ani, acne, vasodilation, hypoglycemia, GI symptoms, increased requirement for vitamin K and impaired coagulation, and muscle damage.

Vitamin K (Phylloquinone K_1, Menaquinone K_2, Menadione K_3) First isolated from alfalfa, vitamin K is also known as phylloquinone in green plants and as menaquinone in bacterial synthesis. It is important for normal blood clotting and calcium metabolism. *The new RDA is 120 μg for men and 90 μg for women. No UL was established.*

Functions: Antihemorrhagic factor, normal blood coagulation, calcium metabolism, and bone mineralization. Low vitamin K intakes are associated with an increased incidence of hip fractures (Booth et al, 2000).

Sources: Plant foods are better sources of vitamin K. Broccoli, kale, Brussels sprouts, spinach, cauliflower, cabbage, large amounts of lettuce. Fish, liver, meat, eggs, cereal, and some fruits contain smaller amounts. Because intestinal bacteria make about 50% of the bodily requirement, a sterile gut or malabsorption can create deficiency. Vitamin K absorption is optimal with bile and pancreatic juice; 10–70% of dietary intake is usually absorbed. Vitamin E excesses can reduce absorption of vitamin K. Warfarin (Coumadin) blocks regeneration of active, reduced vitamin K, thus prolonging clotting time, which is best monitored through international normalized ratio (INR) where 2–3 is desired.

Signs of Deficiency: Bleeding and hypoprothrombinemia. Vitamin K deficiency is rare but can be found in lipid malabsorption, chronic antibiotic therapy, and liver disease. Giving an injection of vitamin K upon birth prevents hemorrhagic disease of the newborn.

Vulnerable Populations: Calcium disorders, medication use (anticoagulants, cholestyramine, mineral oil, neomycin, and other antibiotics), hepatic biliary obstruction, hepatocellular disease, malabsorption syndromes, postmenopausal women at risk for hip fractures, prematurity, and small bowel disorders.

Signs of Excess: Prolonged bleeding time. Menadione can be toxic if given in excessive dose; severe jaundice in infants or hemolytic anemia may result.

Water-Soluble Vitamins

Thiamin (Vitamin B_1) Known as the "morale" vitamin, thiamin is beneficial for nerve and heart function and for carbohydrate (CHO) metabolism. Thiamin is mainly a coenzyme for decarboxylations of 2-keto acids and transketolations. High-CHO intakes, pregnancy, lactation, increased basal metabolic rate, and antibiotic use will increase needs. As energy intake from protein and fat increases, thiamin requirement decreases. The extent of absorption varies widely. Thiamin hydrochloride is the common supplemental form. *RDA is 1.2 mg/d for men and 1.1 mg/d for women. No UL was established.*

Functions: Prevents beriberi; role in cell respiration, RNA and DNA formation, protein catabolism, growth, appetite, normal muscle tone in cardiac and digestive tissues, neurological functioning, CHO metabolism as coenzyme in energy-producing Krebs' cycle, and thiamin pyrophosphate (TPP) at the pyruvic acid step. Magnesium, manganese, riboflavin, and vitamin B_6 are synergists. Acetylcholine synthesis requires thiamin.

Sources: Pork, fortified cereals, dried legumes such a split peas, brown rice, organ and lean meats, whole grains such as oats and whole wheat, nuts, cornmeal, enriched flour or bread, dried milk, wheat germ, dried egg yolk or whole egg, green peas, and seeds. Note: Two slices of bread or one slice of bread and one serving of cereal will provide 15% of the daily RDA. Some nutrients are thiamin sparing; others destroy the nutrient. Thiamin is spared by fat, protein, sorbitol, and vitamin C; antagonists include raw fish, tea, coffee, blueberries, and red cabbage. Avoid cooking with excessive water and alkaline products such as baking soda; thiamin is lost readily.

Signs of Deficiency: Anorexia, calf muscle weakness, weight loss, and cardiac and neurological signs (mental confusion, muscular wasting, edema in wet beriberi, peripheral neuropathy, and tachycardia). In dry beriberi, energy deprivation and inactivity are causes. Wernicke's encephalopathy is due to thiamin deficiency and often associated with malnutrition and alcoholism. TPN without multivitamin use can lead to symptoms of Wernicke's encephalopathy.

Vulnerable Populations: Alcoholism, cancers, cardiomyopathies, CHO (high intakes), celiac disease, children with congenital heart disease before and after surgery (Shamir, 2000), congestive heart failure, fever, high parenteral glucose loading, lactation and pregnancy, tropical sprue, and thyrotoxicosis.

Signs of Excess: Respiratory failure and death with large doses (1000 times nutritional needs). With 100 times the normal dose, headache, convulsions, muscular weakness, cardiac arrhythmia, and allergic reactions have been noted.

Riboflavin (Vitamin B_2) Riboflavin is important in CHO metabolism and maintenance of healthy mucous membranes. It is the main coenzyme in redox reactions of fatty acids and the tricarboxylic acid (TCA) cycle. *RDA is 1.3 mg/d for men and 1.1 mg/d for women. No UL was established.*

Functions: Cell respiration, oxidation reduction, conversion of tryptophan to niacin, component of retinal pigment, involvement in all metabolisms (especially fat), purine degradation, adrenocortical function, coenzyme in electron transport as flavin adenine dinucleotide (FAD) and flavin mononucleotide (FMN), healthy mucous membranes, skin and eyes, growth, and proper functioning of niacin and pyridoxine.

Sources: Milk, yogurt, cheese, egg whites, liver, beef, chicken, fish, legumes, peanuts, enriched grains and fortified cereals. Body size, growth, activity excesses, and fat metabolism affect daily requirements. Avoid excesses of niacin and methylxanthines. Light destroys riboflavin; buy milk in opaque cartons. As protein intake increases, the need for riboflavin decreases. Riboflavin is spared by dextrins and starch and is found in greater amounts in protein foods. Cheilosis causes a magenta-colored tongue.

Signs of Deficiency: Photophobia; lacrimation; itchy and burning eyes or lips, mouth, and tongue; fissures and scaling of lips; angular stomatitis; dermatitis; greasy nasolabial folds; purple, swollen tongue; and peripheral neuropathy. Riboflavin deficiency is most commonly found in developing countries like India and can lead to deficiency of vitamins B_6 and B_2 and impairment of psychomotor function. Riboflavin metabolism is affected by infections, drugs, and hormones.

Vulnerable Populations: Alcoholism, cancers, chronic infections, drug use (broad-spectrum antibiotics and chloramphenicol), gastrectomy, and low oral intake during childhood, pregnancy, or lactation.

Signs of Excess: There is no known toxicity.

Niacin (Nicotinic Acid, Nicotinamide) Niacin serves as coenzyme for several dehydrogenases. Niacin requirements are related to protein and calorie intake. *RDA is 16 mg/d for men and 14 mg/d for women. UL was established at 35 mg for men and women.*

Functions: Prevention of pellagra (along with other B-complex vitamins); needed to treat tuberculosis with isoniazid; part of nicotinamide adenine dinucleotide (NAD) in metabolism; use of CHO, protein, and fat in energy metabolism; growth; conversion of vitamin A to retinol; and metabolism of fatty acids, serum cholesterol, and triglycerides. Nicotinic acid is used as a vasodilator; nicotinamide is less vasodilating.

Sources: Beef and meats, organ meats, poultry, tuna and salt water fish, peanut butter, nuts and legumes, enriched breads and fortified cereals. Sixty milligrams of tryptophan is equivalent to 1 mg of niacin. Diet supplies 31% of niacin intake as tryptophan. Milk and eggs are good sources of tryptophan but not niacin.

Signs of Deficiency: Muscular weakness, inflammation of the tongue, anorexia, abnormal intestinal function and indigestion, skin eruptions, abnormal brain functioning. Severe deficiency leads to pellagra; one sign of pellagra is Casal's collar, a rough, red dermatitis; others include diarrhea, dementia, or even death (the three D's of pellagra). Pellagra is commonly seen in undernourished people in Africa.

Vulnerable Populations: Alcoholism, cancers, chronic diarrhea, cirrhosis, diabetes, and tuberculosis.

Signs of Excess: Histamine release, causing flushing of skin (when using 1–2 g of nicotinic acid daily in an effort to lower cholesterol levels). Megadoses should be avoided.

Vitamin B_6 (Pyridoxol, Pyridoxal, Pyridoxamine) Vitamin B_6 is primarily known for its role in amino acid metabolism. *RDA is 1.3–1.7 mg/d for men and 1.3–1.5 mg/d for women. UL was established at 100 mg/d for adult men and women.*

Functions: Protein metabolism, coenzymes (-ases), conversion of tryptophan to niacin, fat metabolism (changing linoleic to arachidonic acid), CHO metabolism, synthesis of folic acid with possible role in homocysteine metabolism and atherosclerosis, glandular and endocrine functions, nerve and brain energy, antibodies, dopamine and serotonin metabolism, glycogen phosphorylase, healthy red blood cells, and immunity.

Sources: Bananas, red meat, organ meats, poultry, fish, whole-grain cereals (such as oatmeal), legumes (garbanzo beans, soybeans, and peanuts). Note: Enteric bacteria can make vitamin B_6 in healthy persons. About 96% of dietary vitamin B_6 is absorbed. Infants need three times as much vitamin B_6 as adults. Needs increase with increased protein intake, decrease with fatty acids, or decrease with other B-complex vitamins. High-protein intakes may deplete vitamin B_6 levels.

Signs of Deficiency: Convulsions in infants, anemias, skin disorders, weakness, sleeplessness, peripheral neuropathies, cheilosis, stomatitis, and impaired immunity. The vitamin is widely distributed throughout the diet; deficiency is rare, except in alcoholics, individuals taking isoniazid without B_6 supplementation, women taking oral contraceptives, and persons who have schizophrenia.

Vulnerable Populations: Alcoholism, use of certain medications (cycloserine, dilantin, hydralazine, isoniazid, oral contraceptives, and penicillamine), elderly status, pregnancy, schizophrenia, and tuberculosis with isoniazid treatment and no vitamin replacement.

Signs of Excess: Sensory neuropathy with gait changes and peripheral sensation and muscle incoordination.

Vitamin B_{12} (Cobalamin, Cyanocobalamin) Vitamin B_{12} is known for its role as a coenzyme in metabolism of propionate, amino acids, and single-carbon fragments. It is known as a growth stimulator and is informally called "extrinsic factor." Many people over age 50 lose the ability to absorb vitamin B_{12} from foods and should consider using more fortified foods. *New RDA is 2.4 mg for adults. No UL was established.*

Functions: Coenzymes, blood cell formation, nucleoproteins and genetic material, nutrient metabolism, growth, nerve tissue, thyroid functions, metabolism, transmethylation, myelin formation, and possible role in homocysteine metabolism and control of atherosclerosis.

Sources: Milk, eggs, liver, kidney, muscle meats, cheese, shellfish, fish, and fortified foods such as soy milk. Vitamin B_{12} is not found in plant foods; monitor vegetarian diets. For best absorption, riboflavin, niacin, magnesium, and vitamin B_6 are needed.

Signs of Deficiency: Pernicious anemia, poor vision, and some psychiatric disturbances. Monitor persons after total gastrectomy for megaloblastic anemia when intrinsic factor is not available.

Vulnerable Populations: Adolescents with poor diets, disorders of gastric mucosa, gastric bypass or gastrectomy, genetic defects (apoenzymes, absence of transcobalamin II, and absence of ileal receptors), intestinal infections, malabsorption due to ileal resection or disease, prolonged daily intake of megadoses of folic acid, and strict vegetarians or vegans.

Signs of Excess: No toxicity is known.

Folate (Folic Acid, Polyglutamyl Folacin) Folic acid works primarily as a coenzyme in single-carbon metabolism. Folic acid can be made in the intestines with help from biotin, protein, and vitamin C. Synthetic folic acid increases blood folate levels more effectively than food sources of folate. Pteroylglutamic acid is the pharmacological form. Only 25–50% of dietary sources are bioavailable. Fortification of more commonly eaten foods has been implemented to provide adequate folic acid for vulnerable populations. *New RDA is 400 mg for adults. UL is 1000 mg/d.*

The Dietary Reference Intakes (DRIs) express folate in "folate equivalents," which account for the difference between natural sources and more bioavailable supplemental sources. Dietary folate equivalents from fortified foods provide 1.7 times the micrograms of added folic acid; use of this term is recommended for planning and evaluating people's intake (West Suitor and Bailey, 2000).

About 90% of circulating folacin is bound to albumin. Some drugs interfere with utilization such as sulfasalazine (Azulfidine), phenytoin (Dilantin), and methotrexate.

Functions: Prevents megaloblastic and macrocytic anemias; needed for growth; hemoglobin; amino acid metabolism; prevents excessive buildup of homocysteine in the body, which may be a precursor of atherosclerosis; and reduces the incidence of neural tube defects. Protective roles against cervical and colon cancer are under study.

Folate is required for many one-carbon reactions involved in synthesis of phospholipids, DNA, proteins, and neurotransmitters. Metabolism of folate and choline is interdependent; choline is used as a methyl donor (to convert homocysteine to methionine) when folate intake is low.

Sources: Foods with highest folate content include fortified cereals, pinto and navy beans (cooked), lentils, beets, asparagus, spinach, romaine lettuce, broccoli, and oranges. Major contributors also include brewer's yeast, orange juice, nuts, whole grains, kidney beans, lima beans, and wheat germ.

Signs of Deficiency: Decrease in total number of cells (pancytopenia) and large red blood cells with a macrocytic or megaloblastic anemia. Neural tube defects in newborns may result. Deficiency is common, especially during pregnancy, with oral contraceptive use, in malabsorption syndromes, in alcoholics, in teens, and in elderly individuals.

Vulnerable Populations: Alcoholism, cancers, medication use (aspirin, cycloserine, dilantin, methotrexate, oral contraceptives, primidone, and pyrimethamine), hematological diseases (pernicious anemia, sickle cell anemia, and thalassemia), vitamin B_{12} deficiency, malabsorption syndromes, and pregnancy.

Signs of Excess: May cause zinc deficiency by forming nonabsorbable complexes in gut.

Pantothenic Acid Pantothenic acid is a coenzyme in fatty acid metabolism. Pantothenic acid is digested "from everywhere." *RDA for adult men and women is 5 mg/d. UL is not established.*

Functions: Coenzyme A, metabolism, synthesis of cholesterol and fatty acids, adrenal gland activity, acetyl transfer, antibodies, normal serum glucose, electrolyte control and hydration, prevents premature graying in some animals, heme synthesis, choline to acetylcholine, and healthy red blood cells.

Sources: Liver, organ meats, egg yolks, legumes, peanuts, yeast, salmon, mushrooms, broccoli, kale, avocado, whole grains, lean muscle meats, poultry, milk, yeast, and molasses. Needs increase by one third in pregnancy and lactation; 50% is bioavailable from diet.

Signs of Deficiency: Deficiency is rare, but patient complaints may include burning feet syndrome, vomiting, paresthesias, and leg cramps. People at risk for deficiency include persons with chronic ulcerative colitis.

Vulnerable Populations: Alcoholism, elderly women, liver disease, and pregnancy.

Signs of Excess: Mild GI distress and diarrhea.

Biotin Biotin is a coenzyme for carboxylations. *RDA is 30 mg/d for adult men and women. UL is not established.*

Functions: Coenzyme in CO_2 fixation, deamination, decarboxylation, synthesis of fatty acids, CHO metabolism, oxidative phosphorylation, leucine catabolism, and carboxylation of pyruvic acid to oxaloacetate.

Sources: Liver, kidney, pork, milk, egg yolk, yeast, cereal, nuts, legumes, and chocolate. Note: Synthesized by intestinal bacteria. Biotin is called the "anti–raw egg white" factor because raw egg white decreases biotin availability with avidin. Be wary of extended antibiotic use or prolonged unsupplemented TPN use. Probably, 50% of dietary biotin is absorbed from the small intestine.

Signs of Deficiency: Inflammation of the skin and lips. The biotin-binding protein avidin can cause problems if raw egg whites are consumed. Other symptoms include dermatitis, alopecia, paralysis, depression, nausea, hepatic steatosis, hypercholesterolemia, and glossitis.

Vulnerable Populations: Individuals who have excessive intake of avidin from raw egg whites, genetic conditions (beta-methylcrotonylglycinuria and propionic acidemia), and inadequate provision with long-term parenteral nutrition.

Signs of Excess: There are no known toxic effects.

Choline Choline is a methyl-rich nutrient that is required for phospholipid synthesis and neurotransmitter function. Internal synthesis of phosphatidylcholine is insufficient to maintain choline status when intakes of folate and choline are low. *AI is set at 550 mg/d for adult men and 425 mg/d for adult women. UL level has been set at 3.5 g/d.*

Functions: Lipotropic agent, some role in muscle control and in short-term memory with the neurotransmitter acetylcholine, component of sphingomyelin, emulsifier in bile, and component of pulmonary surfactant (CO_2/O_2 exchange). It helps the body absorb and use fats, especially for cell membranes. Choline is used as a methyl donor to convert homocysteine to methionine when folate intake is low.

Sources: Eggs, high-protein animal products such as liver, dairy foods, soybeans, peanuts, cauliflower, lettuce, and chocolate. Lecithin is a choline precursor, as is phosphatidylcholine. Liver can synthesize or resynthesize. Average daily intake is 400–900 mg. High-fat intake accelerates deficiency.

Signs of Deficiency: Insufficient phospholipid synthesis occurs; neurotransmitter function and liver damage might occur.

Signs of Excess: None known at this time.

Vitamin C (Ascorbic Acid, Dehydroascorbic Acid) Vitamin C is a reductant in hydroxylations in biosynthesis of collagen and carnitine and in metabolism of drugs and steroids. Vitamin C is needed via an exogenous source by all humans and is found in fruits and vegetables. About 90% of dietary intake is absorbed. *RDA for vitamin C is 75 mg for women and 90 mg for men to reach saturation levels. UL for vitamin C is 2000 mg/d.*

Concentration of vitamin C in plasma and other body fluids does not increase in proportion to increasing daily doses of vitamin C. There is no pharmacokinetic justification for use of megadoses of vitamin C over 200 mg/d since bioavailability is complete at 200 mg.

Functions: Hydroxylation (lysine and proline) in collagen formation and wound healing, norepinephrine metabolism, tryptophan to serotonin transformation, folic acid metabolism, antioxidant as a scavenger of superoxide radicals and to protect vitamins A and E, changing ferric iron to ferrous iron, prevention of infection, intracellular respiration, tyrosine metabolism, intercellular structures of bone, teeth, and cartilage, prevention of scurvy, may defer aging through the collagen turnover process, serves as a reducing agent, elevates HDL cholesterol in the elderly, and lowers serum cholesterol. Dietary antioxidants, including vitamins C and E, may protect against atherosclerotic disease and cognitive impairment. High serum levels of ascorbic acid are independently inversely associated with blood lead levels.

Sources: Sweet red and green peppers, apricot nectar, oranges, orange juice, strawberries, kiwifruit, grapefruit juice, cantaloupe, vegetable juice cocktail, broccoli, Brussels sprouts, raspberries, grapefruit, pineapple, cauliflower, tangerine, tomatoes, and baked potato. Note: No more than 1 g/d is stored in liver tissue. Body reserves may be up to 1500 mg, or a 30- to 40-day supply. An excretion of 50% is normal. Men are found to have lower serum levels than women. Smoking decreases serum levels; increasing the intake of vitamin C is recommended for smokers. Increased intake removes greater amounts of nicotine. Avoid high levels of pectin, iron, copper, and zinc from the diet.

Signs of Deficiency: The first symptom of deficiency is fatigue; treatment with vitamin C results in quick recovery and alleviation of symptoms. Scurvy reveals swollen, bleeding gums, eventual tooth loss, lethargy, fatigue, poor wound healing, edema, hemorrhages, weak bones or cartilage and connective tissues, rheumatic pains in the legs, muscular atrophy, skin lesions, and psychological changes including depression and hypochondria.

Vulnerable Populations: Achlorhydria, alcoholism, Alzheimer's disease, burns, cancers, chronic diarrhea, diabetes, elevated serum cholesterol, nephrosis, pregnancy, severe trauma, surgical wounds, and tuberculosis.

Signs of Excess: GI distress and diarrhea. Excesses do not produce a hypervitaminosis but have been linked to oxalate kidney stones or gout in susceptible persons.

Dietary Reference Intakes (DRIs): Recommended Intakes for Individuals, Vitamins

Food and Nutrition Board, Institute of Medicine, National Academies

Life Stage Group	Vit A (μg/d)[a]	Vit C (mg/d)	Vit D (μg/d)[b,c]	Vit E (mg/d)[d]	Vit K (μg/d)	Thiamin (mg/d)	Riboflavin (mg/d)	Niacin (mg/d)[e]	Vit B_6 (mg/d)	Folate (μg/d)[f]	Vit B_{12} (μg/d)	Pantothenic Acid (mg/d)	Biotin (μg/d)	Choline[g] (mg/d)
Infants														
0–6 mo	400*	40*	5*	4*	2.0*	0.2*	0.3*	2*	0.1*	65*	0.4*	1.7*	5*	125*
7–12 mo	500*	50*	5*	5*	2.5*	0.3*	0.4*	4*	0.3*	80*	0.5*	1.8*	6*	150*
Children														
1–3 y	**300**	**15**	5*	**6**	30*	**0.5**	**0.5**	**6**	**0.5**	**150**	**0.9**	2*	8*	200*
4–8 y	**400**	**25**	5*	**7**	55*	**0.6**	**0.6**	**8**	**0.6**	**200**	**1.2**	3*	12*	250*
Males														
9–13 y	**600**	**45**	5*	**11**	60*	**0.9**	**0.9**	**12**	**1.0**	**300**	**1.8**	4*	20*	375*
14–18 y	**900**	**75**	5*	**15**	75*	**1.2**	**1.3**	**16**	**1.3**	**400**	**2.4**	5*	25*	550*
19–30 y	**900**	**90**	5*	**15**	120*	**1.2**	**1.3**	**16**	**1.3**	**400**	**2.4**	5*	30*	550*
31–50 y	**900**	**90**	5*	**15**	120*	**1.2**	**1.3**	**16**	**1.3**	**400**	**2.4**	5*	30*	550*
51–70 y	**900**	**90**	10*	**15**	120*	**1.2**	**1.3**	**16**	**1.7**	**400**	**2.4**[i]	5*	30*	550*
> 70 y	**900**	**90**	15*	**15**	120*	**1.2**	**1.3**	**16**	**1.7**	**400**	**2.4**[i]	5*	30*	550*
Females														
9–13 y	**600**	**45**	5*	**11**	60*	**0.9**	**0.9**	**12**	**1.0**	**300**	**1.8**	4*	20*	375*
14–18 y	**700**	**65**	5*	**15**	75*	**1.0**	**1.0**	**14**	**1.2**	**400**[i]	**2.4**	5*	25*	400*
19–30 y	**700**	**75**	5*	**15**	90*	**1.1**	**1.1**	**14**	**1.3**	**400**[i]	**2.4**	5*	30*	425*
31–50 y	**700**	**75**		**15**	90*	**1.1**	**1.1**	**14**	**1.3**	**400**[i]	**2.4**	5*	30*	425*
51–70 y	**700**	**75**	10*	**15**	90*	**1.1**	**1.1**	**14**	**1.5**	**400**	**2.4**[h]	5*	30*	425*
> 70 y	**700**	**75**	15*	**15**	90*	**1.1**	**1.1**	**14**	**1.5**	**400**	**2.4**[h]	5*	30*	425*
Pregnancy														
14–18 y	**750**	**80**	5*	**15**	75*	**1.4**	**1.4**	**18**	**1.9**	**600**[j]	**2.6**	6*	30*	450*
19–30 y	**770**	**85**	5*	**15**	90*	**1.4**	**1.4**	**18**	**1.9**	**600**[j]	**2.6**	6*	30*	450*
31–50 y	**770**	**85**	5*	**15**	90*	**1.4**	**1.4**	**18**	**1.9**	**600**[j]	**2.6**	6*	30*	450*
Lactation														
14–18 y	**1,200**	**115**	5*	**19**	75*	**1.4**	**1.6**	**17**	**2.0**	**500**	**2.8**	7*	35*	550*
19–30 y	**1,300**	**120**	5*	**19**	90*	**1.4**	**1.6**	**17**	**2.0**	**500**	**2.8**	7*	35*	550*
31–50 y	**1,300**	**120**	5*	**19**	90*	**1.4**	**1.6**	**17**	**2.0**	**500**	**2.8**	7*	35*	550*

NOTE: This table (taken from the DRI reports, see www.nap.edu) presents Recommended Dietary Allowances (RDAs) in **bold type** and Adequate Intakes (AIs) in ordinary type followed by an asterisk (*). RDAs and AIs may both be used as goals for individual intake. RDAs are set to meet the needs of almost all (97 to 98 percent) individuals in a group. For healthy breastfed infants, the AI is the mean intake. The AI for other life stage and gender groups is believed to cover needs of all individuals in the group, but lack of data or uncertainty in the data prevent being able to specify with confidence the percentage of individuals covered by this intake.

[a] As retinol activity equivalents (RAEs). 1 RAE = 1 μg retinol, 12 μg β-carotene, 24 μg α-carotene, or 24 μg β-cryptoxanthin. The RAE for dietary provitamin A carotenoids is twofold greater than retinol equivalents (RE), whereas the RAE for preformed vitamin A is the same as RE.

[b] As cholecalciferol. 1 μg cholecalciferol = 40 IU vitamin D.

[c] In the absence of adequate exposure to sunlight.

[d] As α-tocopherol. α-Tocopherol includes *RRR*-α-tocopherol, the only form of α-tocopherol that occurs naturally in foods, and the *2R*-stereoisomeric forms of α-tocopherol (*RRR*-, *RSR*-, *RRS*-, and *RSS*-α-tocopherol) that occur in fortified foods and supplements. It does not include the *2S*-stereoisomeric forms of α-tocopherol (*SRR*-, *SSR*-, *SRS*-, and *SSS*-α-tocopherol), also found in fortified foods and supplements.

[e] As niacin equivalents (NE). 1 mg of niacin = 60 mg of tryptophan; 0–6 months = preformed niacin (not NE).

[f] As dietary folate equivalents (DFE). 1 DFE = 1 μg food folate = 0.6 μg of folic acid from fortified food or as a supplement consumed with food = 0.5 μg of a supplement taken on an empty stomach.

[g] Although AIs have been set for choline, there are few data to assess whether a dietary supply of choline is needed at all stages of the life cycle, and it may be that the choline requirement can be met by endogenous synthesis at some of these stages.

[h] Because 10 to 30 percent of older people may malabsorb food-bound B_{12}, it is advisable for those older than 50 years to meet their RDA mainly by consuming foods fortified with B_{12} or a supplement containing B_{12}.

[i] In view of evidence linking folate intake with neural tube defects in the fetus, it is recommended that all women capable of becoming pregnant consume 400 μg from supplements or fortified foods in addition to intake of food folate from a varied diet.

[j] It is assumed that women will continue consuming 400 μg from supplements or fortified food until their pregnancy is confirmed and they enter prenatal care, which ordinarily occurs after the end of the periconceptional period—the critical time for formation of the neural tube.

Dietary Reference Intakes (DRIs): Recommended Intakes for Individuals, Elements

Food and Nutrition Board, Institute of Medicine, National Academies

Life Stage Group	Calcium (mg/d)	Chromium (μg/d)	Copper (μg/d)	Fluoride (mg/d)	Iodine (μg/d)	Iron (mg/d)	Magnesium (mg/d)	Manganese (mg/d)	Molybdenum (μg/d)	Phosphorus (mg/d)	Selenium (μg/d)	Zinc (mg/d)	Potassium (g/d)	Sodium (g/d)	Chloride (g/d)
Infants															
0–6 mo	210*	0.2*	200*	0.01*	110*	0.27*	30*	0.003*	2*	100*	15*	2*	0.4*	0.12*	0.18*
7–12 mo	270*	5.5*	220*	0.5*	130*	**11**	75*	0.6*	3*	275*	20*	**3**	0.7*	0.37*	0.57*
Children															
1–3 y	500*	11*	**340**	0.7*	**90**	**7**	**80**	1.2*	**17**	**460**	**20**	**3**	3.0*	1.0*	1.5*
4–8 y	800*	15*	**440**	1*	**90**	**10**	**130**	1.5*	**22**	**500**	**30**	**5**	3.8*	1.2*	1.9*
Males															
9–13 y	1,300*	25*	**700**	2*	**120**	**8**	**240**	1.9*	**34**	**1,250**	**40**	**8**	4.5*	1.5*	2.3*
14–18 y	1,300*	35*	**890**	3*	**150**	**11**	**410**	2.2*	**43**	**1,250**	**55**	**11**	4.7*	1.5*	2.3*
19–30 y	1,000*	35*	**900**	4*	**150**	**8**	**400**	2.3*	**45**	**700**	**55**	**11**	4.7*	1.5*	2.3*
31–50 y	1,000*	35*	**900**	4*	**150**	**8**	**420**	2.3*	**45**	**700**	**55**	**11**	4.7*	1.5*	2.3*
51–70 y	1,200*	30*	**900**	4*	**150**	**8**	**420**	2.3*	**45**	**700**	**55**	**11**	4.7*	1.3*	2.0*
> 70 y	1,200*	30*	**900**	4*	**150**	**8**	**420**	2.3*	**45**	**700**	**55**	**11**	4.7*	1.2*	1.8*
Females															
9–13 y	1,300*	21*	**700**	2*	**120**	**8**	**240**	1.6*	**34**	**1,250**	**40**	**8**	4.5*	1.5*	2.3*
14–18 y	1,300*	24*	**890**	3*	**150**	**15**	**360**	1.6*	**43**	**1,250**	**55**	**9**	4.7*	1.5*	2.3*
19–30 y	1,000*	25*	**900**	3*	**150**	**18**	**310**	1.8*	**45**	**700**	**55**	**8**	4.7*	1.5*	2.3*
31–50 y	1,000*	25*	**900**	3*	**150**	**18**	**320**	1.8*	**45**	**700**	**55**	**8**	4.7*	1.5*	2.3*
51–70 y	1,200*	20*	**900**	3*	**150**	**8**	**320**	1.8*	**45**	**700**	**55**	**8**	4.7*	1.3*	2.0*
> 70 y	1,200*	20*	**900**	3*	**150**	**8**	**320**	1.8*	**45**	**700**	**55**	**8**	4.7*	1.2*	1.8*
Pregnancy															
14–18 y	1,300*	29*	**1,000**	3*	**220**	**27**	**400**	2.0*	**50**	**1,250**	**60**	**13**	4.7*	1.5*	2.3*
19–30 y	1,000*	30*	**1,000**	3*	**220**	**27**	**350**	2.0*	**50**	**700**	**60**	**11**	4.7*	1.5*	2.3*
31–50 y	1,000*	30*	**1,000**	3*	**220**	**27**	**360**	2.0*	**50**	**700**	**60**	**11**	4.7*	1.5*	2.3*
Lactation															
14–18 y	1,300*	44*	**1,300**	3*	**290**	**10**	**360**	2.6*	**50**	**1,250**	**70**	**14**	5.1*	1.5*	2.3*
19–30 y	1,000*	45*	**1,300**	3*	**290**	**9**	**310**	2.6*	**50**	**700**	**70**	**12**	5.1*	1.5*	2.3*
31–50 y	1,000*	45*	**1,300**	3*	**290**	**9**	**320**	2.6*	**50**	**700**	**70**	**12**	5.1*	1.5*	2.3*

NOTE: This table presents Recommended Dietary Allowances (RDAs) in **bold type** and Adequate Intakes (AIs) in ordinary type followed by an asterisk (*). RDAs and AIs may both be used as goals for individual intake. RDAs are set to meet the needs of almost all (97 to 98 percent) individuals in a group. For healthy breastfed infants, the AI is the mean intake. The AI for other life stage and gender groups is believed to cover needs of all individuals in the group, but lack of data or uncertainty in the data prevent being able to specify with confidence the percentage of individuals covered by this intake.

SOURCES: *Dietary Reference Intakes for Calcium, Phosphorous, Magnesium, Vitamin D, and Fluoride* (1997); *Dietary Reference Intakes for Thiamin, Riboflavin, Niacin, Vitamin B_6, Folate, Vitamin B_{12}, Pantothenic Acid, Biotin, and Choline* (1998); *Dietary Reference Intakes for Vitamin C, Vitamin E, Selenium, and Carotenoids* (2000); *Dietary Reference Intakes for Vitamin A, Vitamin K, Arsenic, Boron, Chromium, Copper, Iodine, Iron, Manganese, Molybdenum, Nickel, Silicon, Vanadium, and Zinc* (2001); and *Dietary Reference Intakes for Water, Potassium, Sodium, Chloride, and Sulfate* (2004). These reports may be accessed via http://www.nap.edu.

Dietary Reference Intakes (DRIs): Tolerable Upper Intake Levels (UL[a]), Vitamins

Food and Nutrition Board, Institute of Medicine, National Academies

Life Stage Group	Vitamin A (μg/d)[b]	Vitamin C (mg/d)	Vitamin D (μg/d)	Vitamin E (mg/d)[c,d]	Vitamin K	Thiamin	Ribo-flavin	Niacin (mg/d)[d]	Vitamin B_6 (mg/d)	Folate (μg/d)[d]	Vitamin B_{12}	Pantothenic Acid	Biotin	Choline (g/d)	Carote-noids[e]
Infants															
0–6 mo	600	ND[f]	25	ND	ND	ND	ND	ND	ND	ND	ND	ND	ND	ND	ND
7–12 mo	600	ND	25	ND	ND	ND	ND	ND	ND	ND	ND	ND	ND	ND	ND
Children															
1–3 y	600	400	50	200	ND	ND	ND	10	30	300	ND	ND	ND	1.0	ND
4–8 y	900	650	50	300	ND	ND	ND	15	40	400	ND	ND	ND	1.0	ND
Males, Females															
9–13 y	1,700	1,200	50	600	ND	ND	ND	20	60	600	ND	ND	ND	2.0	ND
14–18 y	2,800	1,800	50	800	ND	ND	ND	30	80	800	ND	ND	ND	3.0	ND
19–70 y	3,000	2,000	50	1,000	ND	ND	ND	35	100	1,000	ND	ND	ND	3.5	ND
> 70 y	3,000	2,000	50	1,000	ND	ND	ND	35	100	1,000	ND	ND	ND	3.5	ND
Pregnancy															
14–18 y	2,800	1,800	50	800	ND	ND	ND	30	80	800	ND	ND	ND	3.0	ND
19–50 y	3,000	2,000	50	1,000	ND	ND	ND	35	100	1,000	ND	ND	ND	3.5	ND
Lactation															
14–18 y	2,800	1,800	50	800	ND	ND	ND	30	80	800	ND	ND	ND	3.0	ND
19–50 y	3,000	2,000	50	1,000	ND	ND	ND	35	100	1,000	ND	ND	ND	3.5	ND

[a] UL = The maximum level of daily nutrient intake that is likely to pose no risk of adverse effects. Unless otherwise specified, the UL represents total intake from food, water, and supplements. Due to lack of suitable data, ULs could not be established for vitamin K, thiamin, riboflavin, vitamin B_{12}, pantothenic acid, biotin, carotenoids. In the absence of ULs, extra caution may be warranted in consuming levels above recommended intakes.

[b] As preformed vitamin A only.

[c] As α-tocopherol; applies to any form of supplemental α-tocopherol.

[d] The ULs for vitamin E, niacin, and folate apply to synthetic forms obtained from supplements, fortified foods, or a combination of the two.

[e] β-Carotene supplements are advised only to serve as a provitamin A source for individuals at risk of vitamin A deficiency.

[f] ND = Not determinable due to lack of data of adverse effects in this age group and concern with regard to lack of ability to handle excess amounts. Source of intake should be from food only to prevent high levels of intake.

SOURCES: *Dietary Reference Intakes for Calcium, Phosphorous, Magnesium, Vitamin D, and Fluoride* (1997); *Dietary Reference Intakes for Thiamin, Riboflavin, Niacin, Vitamin B_6, Folate, Vitamin B_{12}, Pantothenic Acid, Biotin, and Choline* (1998); *Dietary Reference Intakes for Vitamin C, Vitamin E, Selenium, and Carotenoids* (2000); and *Dietary Reference Intakes for Vitamin A, Vitamin K, Arsenic, Boron, Chromium, Copper, Iodine, Iron, Manganese, Molybdenum, Nickel, Silicon, Vanadium, and Zinc* (2001). These reports may be accessed via http://www.nap.edu.

Dietary Reference Intakes (DRIs): Tolerable Upper Intake Levels (UL[a]), Elements

Food and Nutrition Board, Institute of Medicine, National Academies

Life Stage Group	Arsenic[b]	Boron (mg/d)	Calcium (g/d)	Chromium	Copper (μg/d)	Fluoride (mg/d)	Iodine (μg/d)	Iron (mg/d)	Magnesium (mg/d)[c]	Manganese (mg/d)	Molybdenum (μg/d)	Nickel (mg/d)	Phosphorus (g/d)	Potassium	Selenium (μg/d)	Silicon[d]	Sulfate	Vanadium (mg/d)[e]	Zinc (mg/d)	Sodium (g/d)	Chloride (g/d)
Infants																					
0–6 mo	ND[f]	ND	ND	ND	ND	0.7	ND	40	ND	ND	ND	ND	ND	ND	45	ND	ND	ND	4	ND	ND
7–12 mo	ND	ND	ND	ND	ND	0.9	ND	40	ND	ND	ND	ND	ND	ND	60	ND	ND	ND	5	ND	ND
Children																					
1–3 y	ND	3	2.5	ND	1,000	1.3	200	40	65	2	300	0.2	3	ND	90	ND	ND	ND	7	1.5	2.3
4–8 y	ND	6	2.5	ND	3,000	2.2	300	40	110	3	600	0.3	3	ND	150	ND	ND	ND	12	1.9	2.9
Males, Females																					
9–13 y	ND	11	2.5	ND	5,000	10	600	40	350	6	1,100	0.6	4	ND	280	ND	ND	ND	23	2.2	3.4
14–18 y	ND	17	2.5	ND	8,000	10	900	45	350	9	1,700	1.0	4	ND	400	ND	ND	ND	34	2.3	3.6
19–70 y	ND	20	2.5	ND	10,000	10	1,100	45	350	11	2,000	1.0	4	ND	400	ND	ND	1.8	40	2.3	3.6
>70 y	ND	20	2.5	ND	10,000	10	1,100	45	350	11	2,000	1.0	3	ND	400	ND	ND	1.8	40	2.3	3.6
Pregnancy																					
14–18 y	ND	17	2.5	ND	8,000	10	900	45	350	9	1,700	1.0	3.5	ND	400	ND	ND	ND	34	2.3	3.6
19–50 y	ND	20	2.5	ND	10,000	10	1,100	45	350	11	2,000	1.0	3.5	ND	400	ND	ND	ND	40	2.3	3.6
Lactation																					
14–18 y	ND	17	2.5	ND	8,000	10	900	45	350	9	1,700	1.0	4	ND	400	ND	ND	ND	34	2.3	3.6
19–50 y	ND	20	2.5	ND	10,000	10	1,100	45	350	11	2,000	1.0	4	ND	400	ND	ND	ND	40	2.3	3.6

[a] UL = The maximum level of daily nutrient intake that is likely to pose no risk of adverse effects. Unless otherwise specified, the UL represents total intake from food, water, and supplements. Due to lack of suitable data, ULs could not be established for arsenic, chromium, silicon, potassium, and sulfate. In the absence of ULs, extra caution may be warranted in consuming levels above recommended intakes.

[b] Although the UL was not determined for arsenic, there is no justification for adding arsenic to food or supplements.

[c] The ULs for magnesium represent intake from a pharmacological agent only and do not include intake from food and water.

[d] Although silicon has not been shown to cause adverse effects in humans, there is no justification for adding silicon to supplements.

[e] Although vanadium in food has not been shown to cause adverse effects in humans, there is no justification for adding vanadium to food and vanadium supplements should be used with caution. The UL is based on adverse effects in laboratory animals and this data could be used to set a UL for adults but not children and adolescents.

[f] ND = Not determinable due to lack of data of adverse effects in this age group and concern with regard to lack of ability to handle excess amounts. Source of intake should be from food only to prevent high levels of intake.

SOURCES: *Dietary Reference Intakes for Calcium, Phosphorous, Magnesium, Vitamin D, and Fluoride* (1997); *Dietary Reference Intakes for Thiamin, Riboflavin, Niacin, Vitamin B_6, Folate, Vitamin B_{12}, Pantothenic Acid, Biotin, and Choline* (1998); *Dietary Reference Intakes for Vitamin C, Vitamin E, Selenium, and Carotenoids* (2000); *Dietary Reference Intakes for Vitamin A, Vitamin K, Arsenic, Boron, Chromium, Copper, Iodine, Iron, Manganese, Molybdenum, Nickel, Silicon, Vanadium, and Zinc* (2001); and *Dietary Reference Intakes for Water, Potassium, Sodium, Chloride, and Sulfate* (2004). These reports may be accessed via http://www.nap.edu.

Dietary Reference Intakes (DRIs): Estimated Energy Requirements (EER) for Men and Women 30 Years of Age[a]

Food and Nutrition Board, Institute of Medicine, National Academies

Height (m [in])	PAL[b]	Weight for BMI[c] of 18.5 kg/m² (kg [lb])	Weight for BMI of 24.99 kg/m² (kg [lb])	EER, Men[d] (kcal/day)		EER, Women[d] (kcal/day)	
				BMI of 18.5 kg/m²	BMI of 24.99 kg/m²	BMI of 18.5 kg/m²	BMI of 24.99 kg/m²
1.50 (59)	Sedentary	41.6 (92)	56.2 (124)	1,848	2,080	1,625	1,762
	Low active			2,009	2,267	1,803	1,956
	Active			2,215	2,506	2,025	2,198
	Very active			2,554	2,898	2,291	2,489
1.65 (65)	Sedentary	50.4 (111)	68.0 (150)	2,068	2,349	1,816	1,982
	Low active			2,254	2,566	2,016	2,202
	Active			2,490	2,842	2,267	2,477
	Very active			2,880	3,296	2,567	2,807
1.80 (71)	Sedentary	59.9 (132)	81.0 (178)	2,301	2,635	2,015	2,211
	Low active			2,513	2,884	2,239	2,459
	Active			2,782	3,200	2,519	2,769
	Very active			3,225	3,720	2,855	3,141

[a] For each year below 30, add 7 kcal/day for women and 10 kcal/day for men. For each year above 30, subtract 7 kcal/day for women and 10 kcal/day for men.

[b] PAL = physical activity level.

[c] BMI = body mass index.

[d] Derived from the following regression equations based on doubly labeled water data:

Adult man: $EER = 662 - 9.53 \times \text{age (y)} + PA \times (15.91 \times \text{wt [kg]} + 539.6 \times \text{ht [m]})$

Adult woman: $EER = 354 - 6.91 \times \text{age (y)} + PA \times (9.36 \times \text{wt [kg]} + 726 \times \text{ht [m]})$

Where PA refers to coefficient for PAL

PAL = total energy expenditure ÷ basal energy expenditure

PA = 1.0 if PAL ≥ 1.0 < 1.4 (sedentary)

PA = 1.12 if PAL ≥ 1.4 < 1.6 (low active)

PA = 1.27 if PAL ≥ 1.6 < 1.9 (active)

PA = 1.45 if PAL ≥ 1.9 < 2.5 (very active)

Dietary Reference Intakes (DRIs): Acceptable Macronutrient Distribution Ranges

Food and Nutrition Board, Institute of Medicine, National Academies

Macronutrient	Range (percent of energy) Children, 1–3 y	Children, 4–18 y	Adults
Fat	30–40	25–35	20–35
n-6 polyunsaturated fatty acids[a] (linoleic acid)	5–10	5–10	5–10
n-3 polyunsaturated fatty acids[a] (α-linolenic acid)	0.6–1.2	0.6–1.2	0.6–1.2
Carbohydrate	45–65	45–65	45–65
Protein	5–20	10–30	10–35

[a] Approximately 10% of the total can come from longer-chain *n*-3 or *n*-6 fatty acids.

SOURCE: *Dietary Reference Intakes for Energy, Carbohydrate, Fiber, Fat, Fatty Acids, Cholesterol, Protein, and Amino Acids* (2002).

Dietary Reference Intakes (DRIs): Recommended Intakes for Individuals, Macronutrients
Food and Nutrition Board, Institute of Medicine, National Academies

Life Stage Group	Total Water[a] (L/d)	Carbohydrate (g/d)	Total Fiber (g/d)	Fat (g/d)	Linoleic Acid (g/d)	α-Linolenic Acid (g/d)	Protein[b] (g/d)
Infants							
0–6 mo	0.7*	60*	ND	31*	4.4*	0.5*	9.1*
7–12 mo	0.8*	95*	ND	30*	4.6*	0.5*	**13.5**
Children							
1–3 y	1.3*	**130**	19*	ND	7*	0.7*	**13**
4–8 y	1.7*	**130**	25*	ND	10*	0.9*	**19**
Males							
9–13 y	2.4*	**130**	31*	ND	12*	1.2*	**34**
14–18 y	3.3*	**130**	38*	ND	16*	1.6*	**52**
19–30 y	3.7*	**130**	38*	ND	17*	1.6*	**56**
31–50 y	3.7*	**130**	38*	ND	17*	1.6*	**56**
51–70 y	3.7*	**130**	30*	ND	14*	1.6*	**56**
> 70 y	3.7*	**130**	30*	ND	14*	1.6*	**56**
Females							
9–13 y	2.1*	**130**	26*	ND	10*	1.0*	**34**
14–18 y	2.3*	**130**	26*	ND	11*	1.1*	**46**
19–30 y	2.7*	**130**	25*	ND	12*	1.1*	**46**
31–50 y	2.7*	**130**	25*	ND	12*	1.1*	**46**
51–70 y	2.7*	**130**	21*	ND	11*	1.1*	**46**
> 70 y	2.7*	**130**	21*	ND	11*	1.1*	**46**
Pregnancy							
14–18 y	3.0*	**175**	28*	ND	13*	1.4*	**71**
19–30 y	3.0*	**175**	28*	ND	13*	1.4*	**71**
31–50 y	3.0*	**175**	28*	ND	13*	1.4*	**71**
Lactation							
14–18 y	3.8*	**210**	29*	ND	13*	1.3*	**71**
19–30 y	3.8*	**210**	29*	ND	13*	1.3*	**71**
31–50 y	3.8*	**210**	29*	ND	13*	1.3*	**71**

NOTE: This table presents Recommended Dietary Allowances (RDAs) in **bold** type and Adequate Intakes (AIs) in ordinary type followed by an asterisk (*). RDAs and AIs may both be used as goals for individual intake. RDAs are set to meet the needs of almost all (97 to 98 percent) individuals in a group. For healthy infants fed human milk, the AI is the mean intake. The AI for other life stage and gender groups is believed to cover the needs of all individuals in the group, but lack of data or uncertainty in the data prevent being able to specify with confidence the percentage of individuals covered by this intake.

[a] *Total* water includes all water contained in food, beverages, and drinking water.

[b] Based on 0.8 g/kg body weight for the reference body weight.

Dietary Reference Intakes (DRIs): Additional Macronutrient Recommendations
Food and Nutrition Board, Institute of Medicine, National Academies

Macronutrient	Recommendation
Dietary cholesterol	As low as possible while consuming a nutritionally adequate diet
Trans fatty acids	As low as possible while consuming a nutritionally adequate diet
Saturated fatty acids	As low as possible while consuming a nutritionally adequate diet
Added sugars	Limit to no more than 25% of total energy

SOURCE: *Dietary Reference Intakes for Energy, Carbohydrate, Fiber, Fat, Fatty Acids, Cholesterol, Protein, and Amino Acids* (2002).

Dietary Reference Intakes (DRIs): Estimated Average Requirements for Groups
Food and Nutrition Board, Institute of Medicine, National Academies

Life Stage Group	CHO (g/d)	Protein (g/d)	Vit A (μg/d)[a]	Vit C (mg/d)	Vit E (mg/d)[b]	Thiamin (mg/d)	Riboflavin (mg/d)	Niacin (mg/d)[c]	Vit B_6 (mg/d)	Folate (μg/d)[d]	Vit B_{12} (μg/d)	Copper (μg/d)	Iodine (μg/d)	Iron (mg/d)	Magnesium (mg/d)	Molybdenum (μg/d)	Phosphorus (mg/d)	Selenium (μg/d)	Zinc (mg/d)
Infants																			
7–12 mo		10												6.9					2.5
Children																			
1–3 y	100	11	210	13	5	0.4	0.4	5	0.4	120	0.7	260	65	3.0	65	13	380	17	2.5
4–8 y	100	15	275	22	6	0.5	0.5	6	0.5	160	1.0	340	65	4.1	110	17	405	23	4.0
Males																			
9–13 y	100	27	445	39	9	0.7	0.8	9	0.8	250	1.5	540	73	5.9	200	26	1,055	35	7.0
14–18 y	100	44	630	63	12	1.0	1.1	12	1.1	330	2.0	685	95	7.7	340	33	1,055	45	8.5
19–30 y	100	46	625	75	12	1.0	1.1	12	1.1	320	2.0	700	95	6	330	34	580	45	9.4
31–50 y	100	46	625	75	12	1.0	1.1	12	1.1	320	2.0	700	95	6	350	34	580	45	9.4
51–70 y	100	46	625	75	12	1.0	1.1	12	1.4	320	2.0	700	95	6	350	34	580	45	9.4
> 70 y	100	46	625	75	12	1.0	1.1	12	1.4	320	2.0	700	95	6	350	34	580	45	9.4
Females																			
9–13 y	100	28	420	39	9	0.7	0.8	9	0.8	250	1.5	540	73	5.7	200	26	1,055	35	7.0
14–18 y	100	38	485	56	12	0.9	0.9	11	1.0	330	2.0	685	95	7.9	300	33	1,055	45	7.3
19–30 y	100	38	500	60	12	0.9	0.9	11	1.1	320	2.0	700	95	8.1	255	34	580	45	6.8
31–50 y	100	38	500	60	12	0.9	0.9	11	1.1	320	2.0	700	95	8.1	265	34	580	45	6.8
51–70 y	100	38	500	60	12	0.9	0.9	11	1.3	320	2.0	700	95	5	265	34	580	45	6.8
> 70 y	100	38	500	60	12	0.9	0.9	11	1.3	320	2.0	700	95	5	265	34	580	45	6.8
Pregnancy																			
14–18 y	135	50	530	66	12	1.2	1.2	14	1.6	520	2.2	785	160	23	335	40	1,055	49	10.5
19–30 y	135	50	550	70	12	1.2	1.2	14	1.6	520	2.2	800	160	22	290	40	580	49	9.5
31–50 y	135	50	550	70	12	1.2	1.2	14	1.6	520	2.2	800	160	22	300	40	580	49	9.5
Lactation																			
14–18 y	160	60	880	96	16	1.2	1.3	13	1.7	450	2.4	985	209	7	300	35	1,055	59	10.9
19–30 y	160	60	900	100	16	1.2	1.3	13	1.7	450	2.4	1,000	209	6.5	255	36	580	59	10.4
31–50 y	160	60	900	100	16	1.2	1.3	13	1.7	450	2.4	1,000	209	6.5	265	36	580	59	10.4

NOTE: This table presents Estimated Average Requirements (EARs), which serve two purposes: for assessing adequacy of population intakes, and as the basis for calculating Recommended Dietary Allowances (RDAs) for individuals for those nutrients. EARs have not been established for vitamin D, vitamin K, pantothenic acid, biotin, choline, calcium, chromium, fluoride, manganese, or other nutrients not yet evaluated via the DRI process.

[a] As retinol activity equivalents (RAEs). 1 RAE = 1 μg retinol, 12 μg β-carotene, 24 μg α-carotene, or 24 μg β-cryptoxanthin. The RAE for dietary provitamin A carotenoids is two-fold greater than retinol equivalents (RE), whereas the RAE for preformed vitamin A is the same as RE.

[b] As α-tocopherol. α-Tocopherol includes *RRR*-α-tocopherol, the only form of α-tocopherol that occurs naturally in foods, and the 2*R*-stereoisomeric forms of α-tocopherol (*RRR*-, *RSR*-, *RRS*-, and *RSS*-α-tocopherol) that occur in fortified foods and supplements. It does not include the 2*S*-stereoisomeric forms of α-tocopherol (*SRR*-, *SSR*-, *SRS*-, and *SSS*-α-tocopherol), also found in fortified foods and supplements.

[c] As niacin equivalents (NE). 1 mg of niacin = 60 mg of tryptophan.

[d] As dietary folate equivalents (DFE). 1 DFE = 1 μg food folate = 0.6 μg of folic acid from fortified food or as a supplement consumed with food = 0.5 μg of a supplement taken on an empty stomach.

SOURCES: *Dietary Reference Intakes for Calcium, Phosphorous, Magnesium, Vitamin D, and Fluoride* (1997); *Dietary Reference Intakes for Thiamin, Riboflavin, Niacin, Vitamin B_6, Folate, Vitamin B_{12}, Pantothenic Acid, Biotin, and Choline* (1998); *Dietary Reference Intakes for Vitamin C, Vitamin E, Selenium, and Carotenoids* (2000); *Dietary Reference Intakes for Vitamin A, Vitamin K, Arsenic, Boron, Chromium, Copper, Iodine, Iron, Manganese, Molybdenum, Nickel, Silicon, Vanadium, and Zinc* (2001), and *Dietary Reference Intakes for Energy, Carbohydrate, Fiber, Fat, Fatty Acids, Cholesterol, Protein, and Amino Acids* (2002). These reports may be accessed via www.nap.edu.

Recommended Dietary Allowances and Dietary Reference Intakes

The Dietary Reference Intakes (DRIs) are nutrient-based reference values for use in planning and assessing diets and for other purposes. They replace the RDAs that were first published by the National Academy of Sciences in 1941. The DRI values comprise seven reports and give more detailed guidance than the old system. The DRIs are composed of:

- **Estimated average requirements** (EAR), expected to satisfy the needs of 50% of the people in that age group.
- **Recommended dietary allowances** (RDA). After computing the EARs for each age/gender category, the Food and Nutrition Board (FNB) then established RDAs to meet the nutrient requirements of each category.
- **Adequate intake** (AI), where no RDA has been established
- **Tolerable upper intake levels** (UL), to caution against excessive intake of nutrients (like vitamin D) that can be harmful in large amounts.

See also the U.S. Government Food and Nutrition Information Center list of DRIs and RDAs at http://fnic.nal.usda.gov/nal_display/index.php?info_center=4&tax_level=3&tax_subject=256&topic_id=1342&level3_id=5141.

CITED REFERENCES

American Dietetic Association. Position of The American Dietetic Association: health implications of dietary fiber. *J Am Diet Assoc.* 102:993, 2002.

American Dietetic Association. Position of The American Dietetic Association: the impact of fluoride on health. *J Am Diet Assoc.* 105:1620, 2005.

Anderson J. Minerals. In: Mahan L, Escott-Stump S. *Krause's food, nutrition, and diet therapy.* 10th ed. Philadelphia: WB Saunders, 2000.

Booth S, et al. Dietary vitamin K intakes are associated with hip fracture but not with bone mineral density in elderly men and women. *Am J Clin Nutr.* 71:1201, 2000.

Costello R, Grumstrup-Scott J. Zinc: what role might supplements play? *J Am Diet Assoc.* 100:371, 2000.

Fairfield KM, Fletcher RH. Vitamins for chronic disease prevention in adults. *JAMA.* 287:3116, 2002.

Fraker P, et al. The dynamic link between the integrity of the immune system and zinc status. *J Nutr.* 130:1399S, 2000.

Harrison E, Hussain M. Mechanisms involved in the intestinal digestion and absorption of dietary vitamin A. *J Nutr.* 131:1405, 2001.

Heaney R, et al. Bioavailability of the calcium in fortified soy imitation milk, with some observations on method. *Am J Clin Nutr.* 71:1166, 2000.

Hunt C, Meacham S. Aluminum, boron, calcium, copper, iron, magnesium, manganese, molybdenum, phosphorus, potassium, sodium and zinc: concentrations in common Western foods and estimated daily intakes by infants, toddlers, and male and female adolescents, adults, and seniors in the United States. *J Am Diet Assoc.* 101:1058, 2001.

McNutt K. What clients should know about sugar replacers. *J Am Diet Assoc.* 100:466, 2000.

Schrezenmeir J, Miller G. Calcium. *J Am Col Nutr.* 19:83S, 2000.

Scimeca J, Miller G. Health benefits of conjugated linoleic acid. Proceedings of a symposium held October 2, 1999, at the 40th Annual Meeting of the American College of Nutrition in Washington, DC. *J Am Col Nutr.* 19:469S, 2000.

Shamir R. Thiamine deficiency in children with congenital heart disease before and after corrective surgery. *J Parenter Enteral Nutr.* 24:154, 2000.

Stahl P. What's new at the FDA: informing consumers about trans fat labeling. *JAMA.* 100:1133, 2000.

Trumbo P, et al. Dietary Reference Intakes: vitamin A, vitamin K, arsenic, boron, chromium, copper, iodine, iron, manganese, molybdenum, nickel, silicon, vanadium, and zinc. *J Am Diet Assoc.* 101:294, 2001.

van het Hof K, et al. Dietary factors that affect the bioavailability of carotenoids. *J Nutr.* 130:503, 2000.

Voyles L, et al. High levels of retinol intake during the first trimester of pregnancy result from use of over-the-counter vitamin/mineral supplements. *J Am Diet Assoc.* 100:1068, 2000.

West Suitor C, Bailey L. Dietary folate equivalents: interpretation and results. *J Am Diet Assoc.* 100:88, 2000.

APPENDIX B

Dietetic Process, Forms, and Counseling Tips

INTRODUCTION TO THE PRACTICE OF DIETETICS

The American Dietetic Association maintains responsibility for establishing required education, practice guidelines, and standards of professional performance for dietetic professionals. The Commission on Dietetic Registration maintains credentialing authority. A formal scope of practice framework has been established to assist dietetic professionals in the performance of their responsibilities (Kieselhorst et al, 2005).

Practice and job analyses are conducted every few years to determine current trends as well as future goals. A majority of dietitians and dietetic technicians continue to practice in clinical dietetics (Rogers, 2005.) Key factors in health care dietetics practice include the following points:

1. **Standards** from the Joint Commission on Accreditation of Healthcare Organizations (JCAHO) and other organizations set the expectation that quality care will lead to positive outcomes. Leadership and continuous performance improvement are two areas that are critical for maintaining quality of services (Escott-Stump et al, 2000).
2. Dietitians and dietetic technicians work in a variety of settings but tend to be **concentrated in health care settings:** acute care, long-term care, dialysis units, psychiatric facilities, community sites, and home health. They perform a variety of tasks including clinical services, food systems management, nutrition education, and public health functions. Levels of responsibility tend to increase with years of experience. Because they possess strong knowledge and skills in both nutrition and management, dietetics professionals are in an ideal position to advance to all kinds of **management positions**, including foodservice director roles and patient case management.
3. Most dietitians work in settings that are supportive of **interdisciplinary teamwork**. Dietitians must be proactive, take on new skills, acquire more knowledge, readily market their services, take risks, and overcome traditional stereotypes (Dahlke et al, 2000). **Business skills**, such as marketing and negotiation skills, help to maintain a competitive edge.
4. **Order-writing privileges** by dietitians allow orders for tube feeding (TF) and total parenteral nutrition (TPN) to be implemented quickly and effectively (Ceres et al, 2006; Braga et al, 2006; Moreland et al, 2002; Myers et al, 2002). Many positions now include responsibilities such as nutritionally focused physical assessment, certification for cardiopulmonary resuscitation, needs assessment for adaptive feeding equipment, worksite wellness, exercise prescription and education, and home care services.
5. Changes in hospital foodservice operation include serving fewer meals to inpatients, employing fewer staff, having smaller expense budgets, and generation of more revenue (Silverman et al, 2000). **Customer satisfaction** must meet or exceed basic patient expectations.
6. Two tiers of nutrition services include **basic nutrition education**, where advice can be provided by most health care professionals, and **medical nutrition therapy (MNT)**, which is an intensive approach to the nutritional management of chronic disease. MNT requires significantly more training in food and nutrition science than is commonly provided by the curriculum of other health professionals to translate complex diet prescriptions into meaningful individualized dietary modifications for the public (Fox, 2000). Registered dietitians are the single identifiable group of health care professionals with the most standardized education, clinical training, continuing education, and national credentialing requirements necessary to be directly reimbursed as a provider of MNT.
7. Application of newly **standardized language** and the **Nutrition Care Process** enables dietitians to perform at a higher level of comprehensive care than previously. Demonstration of effectiveness is necessary in evidence-based care (Barr et al, 2001).
8. Evaluation of outcomes is significant; **health-related quality of life (HRQL)** is an outcome measure of patient evaluations of care. Quality of life and nutritional status of older residents in long-term care facilities may be enhanced by **liberalization of diet prescriptions** (Neidert, 2005.)
9. **Person-centered or resident-centered care** involves residents in decisions about schedules, menus, and dining locations; allowing residents to participate in diet-related decisions can provide nutrient needs, allow alterations contingent on medical conditions, and simultaneously increase the desire to eat and the enjoyment of food, thus decreasing the risks of weight loss, undernutrition, and other potential negative effects of poor nutrition and hydration (Neidert, 2005).
10. The best patient care emphasizes **coordinated, comprehensive care along the continuum of disease and across health care delivery systems**. Evidence-based care integrates pathophysiological rationale, diagnosis, etiology, and prognosis with valid and current clinical research evidence (Meakins, 2002).

TABLE B-1 Sample Nutrition Department Scope of Services

PURPOSE

In order to provide care consistent with the mission of the XYZ Hospital System, the Nutrition Department defines its scope of services and goals.

POLICY

It is the policy of Hospital System for each department to provide care and/or services based on defined scope of services and goals and set policies and procedures based on the scope of services and goals.

DEPARTMENT MISSION

The Nutrition Department commits itself to enhancing the quality of life throughout the life cycle, promoting and restoring health through the provision of quality nutritional care services in an environment that ensures dignity and respect for each person. The Nutrition Department has an obligation to continuous quality improvement in the care and services it provides.

PROCEDURE

Care/services provided

The department provides timely nutrition assessment, monitoring, counseling, education, discharge planning, and diet instruction, as defined in department policies, to meet the needs of patients' various backgrounds, which affect nutritional preferences and habits. The division evaluates the activities of the department as to the provision of quality dietary intervention, patient treatment and outcomes, and quality of meal service.

Types of patients/customers served

Nutrition Services are available for all ages of hospital population—newborn, infant, children, adolescent, adult, and geriatrics—including outpatient services, cardiopulmonary rehabilitation, emergency department, corporate wellness, and community events.

Timeliness

Clinical Dietitians are scheduled Monday through Saturday, with shift availability at all meal periods. One Dietitian is scheduled for weekend coverage; Sunday coverage is an on-call procedure. Nursing staff is responsible to notify the on-call dietitian for Level 1 patients. When appropriate, formula calculations, calorie counts or nutrient analyses, and basic nutrition assessments can be completed via the computer system and telephone from within the system to facilitate timely treatments.

STAFFING

The Clinical Nutrition Manager sets a staffing plan to meet the needs of the patient population. A staffing assessment is completed every 2 years and when deemed necessary. The department administration is involved in all staffing decisions. Dietitian schedules are prepared in advance and are distributed to food service personnel and the hospital operator. Dietitian hours and on-call schedules are scheduled in advance.

STAFF CREDENTIALS AND REQUIREMENTS

Dietitians are registered through the American Dietetic Association, and each must maintain their registration through continuing education. The education requirement is 75 hours during each 5-year period. Competency standards follow the national Commission on Dietetic Registration requirements and are reviewed by the Clinical Nutrition Manager to meet the specific needs of the Hospital and circulated to each nursing unit.

ASSIGNMENTS

Full-Time Equivalents of Clinical Dietitian are staffed to the patient care areas and to the Medical Nutrition Therapy ambulatory clinic. One Full-Time Equivalent of Clinical Nutrition Manager leads the clinical/outpatient staff. Staff are assigned to Community Education Programs upon request and scheduling. Based on the daily census and acuity, Clinical and Outpatient Dietitians may adjust daily staffing pattern to meet needs working from Level 1 to Level 3 priority.

The staffing plan meets average hospital census and nutrition outpatient census. With high census, increased acuity, emergency/disaster, or dietitian vacation, patient care prioritization is as follows: Level 1 Inpatient (all units) and supervision of food service patient meals. During periods of high patient census and acuity, basic patient education needs will be completed; patients may be offered additional outpatient nutrition services with an MD referral and patient consent for follow-up. Outpatient nutrition consultation appointments may be limited to highest risk patients with adjunct classroom education experiences offered for others.

During low census periods, the Clinical Dietitian will participate in wellness/community program development, patient education literature update, and clinical nutrition skill development. A minimum of two Clinical Dietitians will be necessary to staff the department during an emergency. The priority will be patient food production (using emergency menu) at both hospitals. When this priority is met, the clinical dietitians will focus on patient nutrition assessment beginning from Level 1 to Level 3 nutrition risk. Patients who are discharged will be given the opportunity for outpatient consult/classroom education if need is identified by dietitian, doctor, or nursing.

STANDARDS OF CARE

The Clinical Dietitians provide care in accordance with Standards of Nutritional Care approved for use by the Hospital System.

SCREENING

Patients receive nutrition intervention based on priority and acuity levels. All inpatients are screened by nursing within 24 hours of admission to determine need for further nutrition assessment. The clinical dietitians develop the screening triggers that are approved by the Medical Staff.

The clinical dietitian performs subsequent re-screening according to daily schedule. The dietitian assigns patients a level of care as Level 1, 2, or 3 based upon the re-screening information.

ASSESSMENT

The clinical dietitians assess patients using the timelines and guidelines illustrated in the standards of care. The Medical Staff approves the standards of care.

EDUCATION

The clinical dietitian performs a nutrition education needs assessment to determine patient/family/significant other educational needs. The patient's age, barriers to learning, assessed needs, abilities, readiness, and length of stay will determine the level of education to provide. Lifestyle factors, financial concerns, patient/family expectations, and food preferences will affect the individualized education plan.

(continued)

TABLE B-1 Sample Nutrition Department Scope of Services *(continued)*

INTERDISCIPLINARY TEAM MEETINGS

The Clinical Dietitian will participate in weekly and as-needed patient care meetings on assigned units. Discharge planning needs will be identified throughout the assessment, re-assessment, and education process. These needs will be referred to social worker/case manager for the unit/patient and communicated to the team during planning meetings. The Dietitian will communicate with referring agency/facility when specialized care plan is needed.

DEPARTMENT GOALS

In support of the hospital mission to provide high-quality health care through continuous improvement to exceed the expectations of patients and customers, the Clinical Nutrition staff of the Food and Nutrition Department have the following goals:

1. To staff qualified, progressive Registered Dietitians who exceed baseline knowledge proficiency standards set by the American Dietetic Association. To accomplish this, each Registered Dietitian will set annual professional development goals on their performance evaluations. These goals are supported by the Clinical Nutrition Manager, funded by Food and Nutrition Services, and tracked by the Professional Development Portfolio of the Commission on Dietetic Registration.
2. To provide timely nutrition therapy that results in measurable improvements to patient/customer health. Timeliness is measured from time of admission/registration to time of discharge/exit from therapy. Dietitians will follow outcomes of therapy via objective measures (such as weight, verbalization of learning, and blood glucose improvements) and chart them in their documentation.
3. Outpatient Medical nutrition therapy and diabetes education, combined, will meet break-even financial status. Billing and accounts receivable will be monitored by the program coordinator and areas for improvement identified.
4. Community education nutrition programs will be offered yearly to local county residents.
5. Patients will be 90% or more satisfied with their inpatient nutrition care and 90% or more satisfied with ambulatory services.

11. Multidisciplinary teams are suited to develop, lead, and implement **evidence-based disease management** programs. Dietitians are able to incorporate an evidence-based approach, determined by their education and training, work experience, and professional association involvement (Byham-Gray et al, 2005).
12. **Unique nutritional care guidelines** should be used in specialty areas, such as cancer (Robien et al, 2006) and diabetes (Reader et al, 2006; Swift and Boucher, 2006). Nutrition support providers should use specialized guidelines to optimize care (Kattelmann et al, 2006). In addition, current specialty guidance should be used in areas such as cardiology and pulmonary (Anker et al, 2006), gastroenterology (Lochs et al, 2006), geriatrics (Volkert et al, 2006), HIV-AIDS (Ockenga et al, 2006), liver disease (Plauth et al, 2006), pancreatic disease (Meier et al, 2006), renal failure (Cano et al, 2006), surgical or transplantation units (Weimann et al, 2006), and intensive care (Kreymann et al, 2006).
13. **Age-specific competencies** are needed in the various populations and settings. For example, children and adolescents require different meal plans and interventions from those given to adults (Stang et al, 2006). Residents in long-term care facilities who need assistance should be given sufficient time and attention (Simmons and Schnelle, 2006), and those on nutrition support require monitoring using available guidelines (Durfee et al, 2006).
14. **Ongoing intervention** is needed to support continued progress by patients (Lemon et al, 2004). Difficulty obtaining current laboratory values, lack of time, and inability to reach subjects for follow-up present the greatest obstacles for dietitians who provide nutritional services to patients in various settings.
15. **Combatting nutrition misinformation** is another important role of the dietetics professional (Wasink and the American Dietetic Association, 2006). Use of science and evidence-based education can help to overcome the potentially dangerous perceptions of consumers, or even misunderstanding by members of the medical community (Krebs and Primak, 2006).
16. **Clinical nutrition managers are in special positions** of opportunity in the health care arena. They have power and leadership roles and can influence other managers, increase the capacity to acquire resources, identify opportunities, and use available information productively (Mislevy et al, 2000). To begin, they must write a **scope of practice** for their operation and services. See Table B-1.

STANDARDIZED NUTRITION CARE PROCESS: IMPLEMENTING A-D-I-M-E

The use of the standardized Nutrition Care Process promotes the best, most predictable outcomes of care. This process has been established by task forces of the American Dietetic Association from 2001 to the present. Figure B-1 provides the accepted nutritional care process and flow chart.

Nutritional Risk Screening JCAHO requires screening for moderate to high nutritional risk for patients. The need to screen patients during the first hours after admission has resulted in frequent use of preadmission screenings. Critical pathways may be developed; patients are called at home prior to admission, leading to greater patient satisfaction and better screening outcomes (Baird Schwartz and Gudzin, 2000). Screening factors should be developed for the specific setting and type of population typically seen. Identify priority patients from nutritional screening in Table B-2; assign screenings as low risk (level 1), moderate risk (level 2), and high risk (level 3). A trained professional can then identify nutritional risk factors and the level of dietitian involvement (see Appendix D).

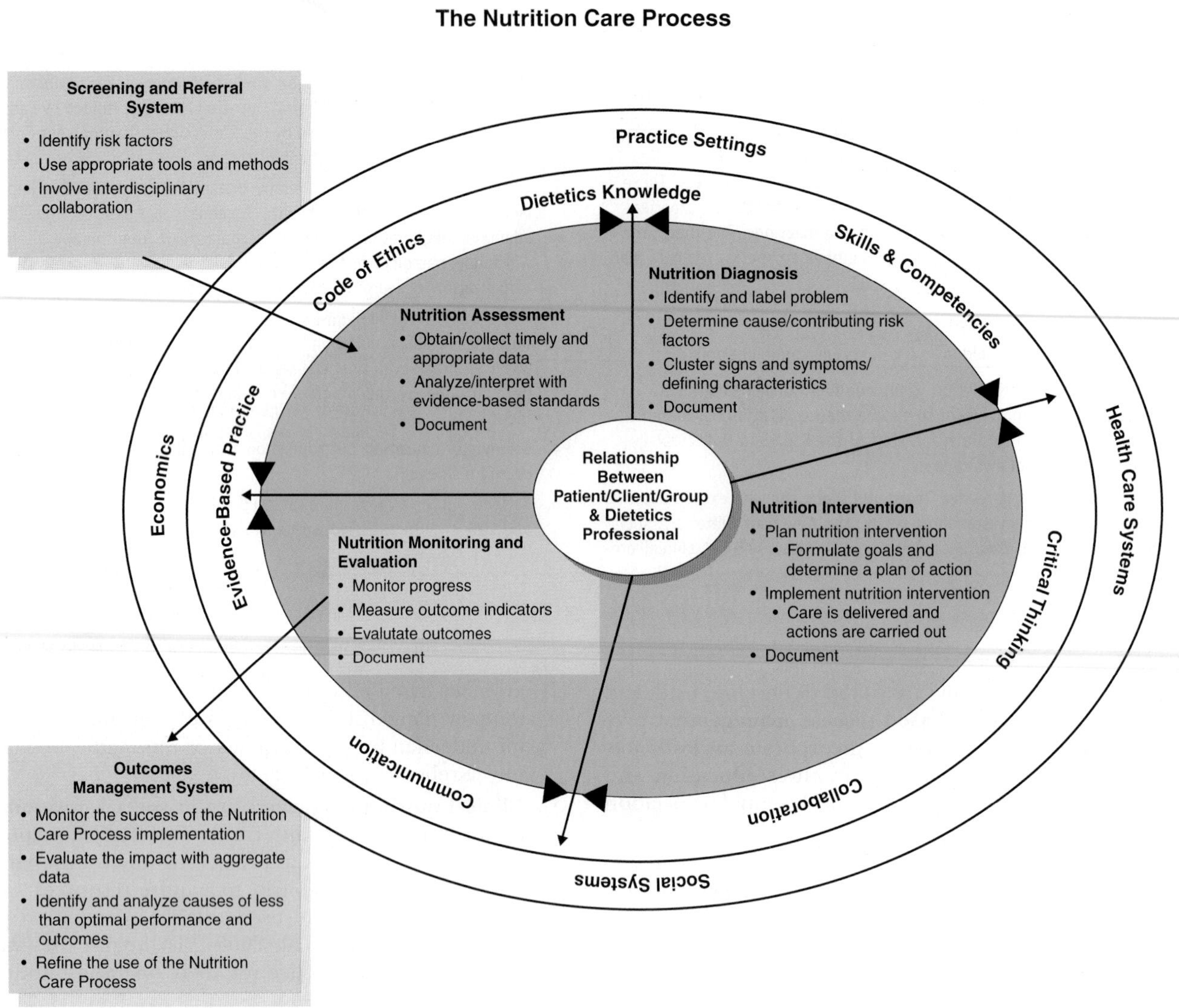

Figure B-1 Nutritional Care Process (From Lacey K, Pritchett E. Nutrition Care Process and Model: ADA adopts road map to quality care and outcomes management. *J Am Diet Assoc.* 103:1061, 2003.)

TABLE B-2 Identifying Priority Patients from Nutrition Screening

1. High-risk admitting diagnosis: 1 POINT EACH

   Pediatrics: failure to thrive, necrotizing enterocolitis, or phenylketonuria

   Neurological: brain trauma or coma

   Pulmonary: respiratory failure and ventilator dependency

   Celiac disease, inflammatory bowel disease: Crohn's disease or ulcerative colitis, short bowel syndrome, or intestinal fistula

   Transplantation: bone marrow, heart, heart-lung, liver, pancreatic, renal, or intestinal transplantation

   Diabetes: complex type 1 diabetes, or type 2, gestational

   Obesity: medical with comorbidities or surgical (gastric bypass surgery)

   Protein–energy malnutrition: moderate or severe energy malnutrition or unintentional weight loss >10% usual body weight

   Gastrointestinal challenge: refeeding syndrome, tube feeding, or parenteral nutrition initiation or complexity

   Cancer: head and neck, gastric, intestinal, pancreatic

   Major stress: burns, major thermal injury, major trauma, multiple organ dysfunction

   Renal: chronic kidney disease with or without dialysis

2. Other factors: 1 POINT EACH

   Albumin <3.0 g/dL

   Unintentional weight loss

   Dysphagia, or mouth sores

   Clear liquid diets or nothing by mouth >5 days

   Complex modified diets

3. Nutritional Priority Score:

   a. high risk (4+ points)____

   b. moderate risk (2–3 points)_____

   c. low risk (0–1 point)_____

NOTE: If problems are identified by the screening process, complete the Nutrition Assessment step. (See Appendix D also.)

TABLE B-3 Nutritional Assessment Factors

Step 1. Assessment Nutrition Assessment is the first step of the Nutrition Care Process. Nutrition assessment is a systematic process of obtaining, verifying, and interpreting data in order to make decisions about the nature and cause of nutrition-related problems.

Category	Tests and Procedures and Tools
Anthropometric Measurements	Weight Height Body mass index Circumferences (head, waist, hip, mid arm circumference) Skinfold measurements (multiple locations) Body composition: estimated/measured • Bioelectrical impedance analysis • Infrared interaction • Dual-energy x-ray absorptiometry • Underwater weighing • Air displacement (Bod Pod)
Diet or Nutrition History	Review dietary intake for factors that affect health conditions and nutrition risk. See Table B-4B for a Nutrition History Form. With a food diary, have patient list everything he/she eats or drinks during a 24-hour period, recording the amount of each food, time food was consumed, method of preparation and ingredients, related activities or symptoms, with whom patient dined, and emotional atmosphere at the time. Feeding modality Dietary Intake Measurement • Food Frequency Questionnaire (FFS) • 24-hour recall • Food record or diary • Calorie count • Plate waste Food preferences, aversion, allergy Special diet Supplement use (vitamin, mineral, herbals) Supplemental food and formulas Bioactive substance use Cultural, religious food practices Meal pattern, feeding schedule Food preparation practices Nutrient and energy adequacy
	Energy requirement: estimated or measured • Indirect calorimetry • Metabolic cart • Hand-held calorimetry • Room calorimetry
Examination	Evaluate physical exam and disease condition for nutrition-related consequences; see Table B-5 for signs of malnutrition. Nutrition-focused clinical exam Review of systems Blood pressure, temperature
Lab and Biochemical Data	Evaluate biochemical data, compare with normal ranges for age and sex; see Table B-8. Laboratory analysis of any body fluid or tissue
Nutrient–Drug Interactions	Evaluate medications and potential for food–drug interactions; see Table B-9.
Patient History	Evaluate psychosocial, functional, and behavioral factors related to food access, selection, preparation, physical activity, and understanding of health condition. Physical activity history Food and nutrition knowledge Willingness to change, stage of change Cognitive status—Mini Mental Functional status—Karnofsky Performance scale Vision, hearing, sensory limitations Living environment, where, who, safety Food safety and security Capability to implement Knowledge of community resources Medical condition and comorbidities
Readiness for Education and Change	Evaluate patient/client/group's knowledge, readiness to learn, and potential for change behaviors. See Table B-11 for tips on patient education and counseling.
Documentation	Quality and timely documentation should occur. See Figure B-5 for a sample nutrition documentation form using A-D-I-M-E format.

Adapted from: Lacey K, Pritchett E. Nutrition Care Process and Model: ADA adopts road map to quality care and outcomes management. *J Am Diet Assoc.* 103:1061, 2003.

TABLE B-4 Dietary Intake Assessment and Nutrition History

Methods for Assessing Dietary Intake	Advantages	Disadvantages
24-Hour Recall: An informal, qualitative method in which you ask the patient to recall all of the foods and beverages that were consumed in the last 24 hours, including the quantities and methods of preparation.	An *advantage* of this method is that dietary information is easily obtained. It is also good during a first encounter with a new patient in which there are no other nutritional data. Patients should be able to recall all that they have consumed in the last 24 hours.	A *disadvantage* of this method is that it is very limited and may not represent an adequate food intake for the patient. Data achieved using this method may not represent the long-term dietary habits of the patient. Estimating food quantities and food ingredients may be difficult especially if the patient ate in restaurants.
Usual Intake/Diet History: This method asks the patient to recall a typical daily intake pattern, including amount, frequencies, and methods of preparation. This intake history should include all meals, beverages, and snacks. Include discussion of usual intake and lifestyle recall. This consists of asking the patient to run through a typical day in chronological order, describing all food consumption as well as activities. This method is very helpful because it may reveal other factors that can affect the patient's nutritional and overall health.	*Advantages* of this method are that it evaluates long-term dietary habits and is quick and easy to do. Based on the information acquired, you may identify patients who would benefit from meeting with a registered dietitian.	A *disadvantage* of this method is that a limited amount of information on the actual quantities of food and beverages is obtained. Also, this method only works if a patient can actually describe a "typical" daily intake, which is difficult for those who vary their food intake greatly. In these patients, it is would be advisable to use the 24-hour recall method. Another disadvantage is that patients may not include foods that they know are unhealthy.
Food Frequency Questionnaire: This method makes use of a standardized written checklist where patients check off the particular foods or type of foods they consume. It is used to determine trends in patients' consumption of certain foods. The checklist puts together foods with similar nutrient content, and frequencies are listed to identify daily, weekly, or monthly consumption.	An *advantage* of this method is that it makes it possible to identify inadequate intake of any food group, so that dietary and nutrient deficiencies may be identified. The questionnaire can be geared to a patient's pre-existing medical conditions.	*Disadvantages* include patient error in filling out the questionnaire and no way to find out how foods are prepared. Patients may over- or underestimate food quantities.
Dietary Food Log: This method asks the patient to record all food, beverage, and snack consumption for a 1-week period. Specific foods and quantities should be recorded. The data from the food log may later be entered into a computer program, which will analyze the nutrient components of the foods eaten according to specific name brands or food types. Patients are asked to enter data into the food log immediately after food is consumed so they do not forget.	The most important *advantage* of this method is that a computer can objectively analyze data obtained. Data on calorie, fat, protein, and carbohydrate consumption can be obtained. Also, since patients are asked to enter data immediately after eating, the data are more accurate than other methods.	*Disadvantages* include patient error in entering accurate food quantities. In addition, it is possible that the week-long food log does not accurately represent a patient's normal eating habits since they know the foods they eat will be analyzed and thus may eat healthier.

TABLE B-4A Summary of Factors Leading to Potential Nutrition Diagnoses

EXCESS INTAKE OF:

alcohol; binge drinking

amino acid intake from food, supplements, parenteral or enteral sources

carbohydrate that is consistently above recommended amounts

convenience foods, preprepared meals, and foods prepared away from home resulting in an inability to adhere to nutritional prescription

energy-dense or high-fat foods/beverages or larger portions of foods/beverages

energy (foods/beverages, food groups, or specific food items)

energy from food, total parenteral nutrition (TPN) or enteral nutrition above estimated or measured expenditure

fast food or restaurant food

fat, phosphorus, sodium, protein, fiber

fat from high-risk lipids (saturated fat, trans fat, cholesterol)

fat from foods, foods prepared with added fat

fiber intake higher than tolerated or generally recommended for current medical condition

fluid intake in excess of recommended intake

(continued)

TABLE B-4A Summary of Factors Leading to Potential Nutrition Diagnoses *(continued)*

foods that do not contain available vitamins

foods and supplements containing vitamins consistently above requirements

food prepared with added fat of a nondesirable type

food in a defined time period; sense of lack of control of overeating during the episode

hunger (extreme) with or without palpitations, tremor, sweating

iron supplement

manganese

mercury from food

minerals (foods or supplements) compared to DRIs

plant foods containing soluble fiber, soy protein, beta-glucan, or plant sterol and stanol esters

protein

protein, type

sodium

substances that interfere with digestion or absorption of foodstuffs

zinc

Factors associated with excess intake

binge eating patterns

change in way clothes fit

ready access to available foods/products with bioactive substance

respiratory quotient >1.0

use of alcohol, narcotics

INSUFFICIENT INTAKE OF:

carbohydrate below recommended amounts

energy compared to estimated or measured resting metabolic rate

fiber

fluid

fat, essential fatty acids (<10% of calories)

fat, monounsaturated, polyunsaturated, or omega-3 fatty acids

food and nutrients

food or foods from specific foods/groups due to gastrointestinal symptoms

foods/supplements

micronutrients

parenteral or enteral nutrition based on estimated or measured resting metabolic rate

protein to meet requirements

vitamin D intake/sunlight exposure

Factors associated with insufficient intake

alterations in food intake from usual

anorexia, nausea, vomiting

avoidance of food or calorie-containing beverages

avoidance of foods of age-appropriate texture

changes in appetite or taste

changes in recent food intake level

chronic dieting behavior

cultural or religious practices that limit protein intake

decreased appetite

decreased intake or avoidance of food difficult to form into a bolus

failure to recognize foods

fasting

fewer than six wet diapers in 24 hours

forgetting to eat

hunger

infant coughing, crying, latching on and off, pounding on breasts

infant lethargy

infant with decreased feeding frequency/duration, early cessation of feeding, and/or feeding resistance

infant with hunger, lack of satiety after feeding

intake of foods that do not contain sufficient quantities of available nutrient

lack of interest in food

limited supply of food in the home

mother does not hear infant swallowing

mother is concerned about breastfeeding/lack of support

mother with lack of confidence in ability to breastfeed

mother with small amount of milk when pumping

normal intake in the face of illness

recent food avoidance and or/lack of interest in food

refusal to eat; chew

respiratory quotient <0.7

spitting food out or prolonged feeding time

swallowing, difficulty

thirst

INTAKE DIFFERENT FROM RECOMMENDED:

carbohydrate intake that is different from recommended types

carbohydrate, protein, and/or fat intake from enteral and/or parenteral nutrients consistently above or below recommendations

food, inappropriate use of

food choices, inappropriate

food group/nutrient imbalance

food intake includes raw eggs, unpasteurized milk products, soft cheeses, and undercooked meats

food variety, limited

medication (over the counter or prescribed), herbal, botanical, or dietary supplement intake that is problematic or inconsistent with recommended foods

nutrient intake consistently above or below recommendations

protein or other supplementation that is inappropriate

U.S. Dietary Guidelines, intake inconsistent with

FOOD AND NUTRIENT TOLERANCE:

allergic reactions to certain carbohydrate foods or food groups

coughing and choking with eating

diminished joint mobility or wrist, hand, or digits that impair ability to independently consume food

diarrhea in response to high refined carbohydrate intake

(continued)

TABLE B-4A Summary of Factors Leading to Potential Nutrition Diagnoses *(continued)*

dropping cups, utensils
dropping food from utensil on repeated attempts to feed
inability to eat due to foods provided not conducive to self-feeding
inability to tolerate solid foods necessitating a liquid diet
nausea, vomiting, diarrhea, high gastric residual volume
poor lip closure, drooling
prolonged chewing
shortness of breath or abdominal distention resulting in inability to consume full meals
Utensil biting

PHYSICAL ACTIVITY:

decreased or sedentary activity level (due to barriers or other reasons)
increased physical activity
excessive physical activity (ignoring family, job; exercising without rest/rehabilitation days or while injured or sick)

FOOD AND NUTRIENT BELIEFS, ATTITUDES, AND PRACTICES:

belief that aging can be slowed by dietary limitations and extreme circumstances
cultural or religious practices that do not support modification of dietary carbohydrate intake
defensiveness, hostility, or resistance to change
denial of hunger
denial of need for food- and nutrition-related changes
dieting, food faddism
eating alone because of feeling embarrassed by the amount of food eaten
eating much more rapidly than normal, eating until feeling uncomfortably full, consuming large amounts of food when not feeling hungry
embarrassment or anger at need for self-monitoring
emotional distress, anxiety, or frustration surrounding mealtimes
excessive reliance on nutrition terming and preoccupation with nutrient content of food
expected food/nutrition-related outcomes are not achieved
failure to complete any agreed homework
failure to keep appointments, schedule follow-up appointments, or engage in counseling
fear of foods or dysfunctional thoughts regarding food or food experiences
feeling disgusted with oneself, depressed, or guilty after overeating
food faddism
food fetish, pica
food preoccupation
frustration or dissatisfaction with medical nutrition therapy recommendations
incomplete self-monitoring records
inflexibility with food selection
irrational thoughts about food's affect on the body
knowledge about current fad diets
lack of appreciation of the importance of making recommended nutrition-related changes
mealtime resistance
previous failures to effectively change target behavior
unwillingness or disinterest in applying nutrition-related recommendations
verbalizes unwillingness/disinterest in learning
weight preoccupation

Developed from tools used by the American Dietetic Association in standardized language, 2006.

TABLE B-4B Nutrition History Questions

Patient Name ____ Date__________

1. How much weight have you gained or lost in the past month?____ 3 months?____ year?________
   Height ______ft. ______inches
   Present Weight ________ BMI_______ Usual weight________ Desirable weight for height_____
2. Have you ever had problems with your weight? Overweight Underweight Comment:_________________
3. How would you generally describe your eating habits? Good Fair Poor
4. How often do you skip meals? Daily Seldom Never
5. How would you rate your appetite recently? Hearty Moderate Poor
6. If you snack between meals, what is your typical kind of snack?_______________ How often?______________
7. When you chew your food, do you have problems or take a long time? No Yes
8. Do you wear dentures at meatime? Yes No If yes, do they fit comfortably? Yes No
9. What vitamin/mineral supplements/herbs and botanicals do you take?____________________________________
10. How much alcohol do you consume in a day? None 1–2 drinks More than 2 drinks

(continued)

TABLE B-4B Nutrition History Questions *(continued)*

11. What foods do you **NOT** tolerate: ______________________ Why?____________
12. What foods do you especially dislike?______________________________
13. What are your favorite foods?______________________________
14. What foods are you **ALLERGIC** to?______________________
15. What type of modified diet are you following now?__________ What types in the past?__________ Who prescribed or suggested this diet for you? Doctor Friend Self-selected
16. How many meals do you eat at home each week?_____ How many at schools____ restaurants____?
17. What is your current occupation?__________ How active are you? Sedentary___ Moderate___ Active___

Calculations: Estimated Energy Needs:_______ Estimated Protein Needs:______ Estimated Fluid Needs:__________

TABLE B-5 Physical Assessment for Clinical Signs of Malnutrition

Certain risk factors and signs of nutrient deficiency or excess can be identified during the physical examination. Any one sign is rarely diagnostic; the more signs present, the more likely they reflect a malnourished individual.

Body System	Normal	Abnormal	Severe
Weight for age	At ideal BMI, or normal	Thin Recent illness? Overweight/obese	Emaciated Starvation, severe PEM Morbid obesity
Hair	Firmly attached Normal distribution Lustrous, shiny	Thin Sparse Protein or biotin deficits? Dull, dry	Depigmented Chemotherapy? Easily pluckable, shedding Lanugo body hair Brittle, very dry Corkscrew hairs
Eyes	Bright, clear Pink conjunctiva	Sunken, dull Pale, dry conjunctiva Poor vision Bitot's spots Cloudiness Vitamin A or riboflavin deficiency	Xerophthalmia Keratomalacia Dull or red Night blindness Conjunctival inflammation
Lips	Good color, moist	Swollen, red Riboflavin, pyridoxine, niacin deficiencies? Dry, cracked at sides	Fissured, lesions Bleeding
Gums	Pink, firm	Sore, spongy Vitamin C deficiency? Red, swollen	Bleed easily Inflamed
Tongue	Pink Papillae present	Purple or magenta White or gray coating Smooth, slick Atrophic lingual papillae Deficiency of riboflavin, niacin, folate, vitamin B_{12} Deficiency of protein or iron	Beefy red, glossitis Burning, swollen Fissured, cheilosis
Teeth	Clean, intact	Dentures Poor dietary habits	Edentulous Rampant caries
	All present	Missing, loose, or chipped teeth Calcium deficiency?	Poorly fitted or loose dentures Enamel erosion in bulimia
Neck	No swelling	Small nodule	Goiter Iodine excess or deficiency?
Skin	Smooth, slightly moist Good color	Pale (iron deficiency?) Dry, flaky or scaly Vitamin A or C or zinc deficiency? Nasolabial seborrhea Bruises easily, petechiae Essential fatty acid or protein deficiency? Pressure ulcer stage 1–2 Acanthosis nigricans Facila pallor or darkening skin	Pellagrous dermatitis Pressure ulcers stage 3–4 Impaired wound healing, low protein Xanthomas from increased lipids Hyperpigmented (niacin excess?)

(continued)

TABLE B-5 Physical Assessment for Clinical Signs of Malnutrition *(continued)*

Certain risk factors and signs of nutrient deficiency or excess can be identified during the physical examination. Any one sign is rarely diagnostic; the more signs present, the more likely they reflect a malnourished individual.

Body System	Normal	Abnormal	Severe
Bloodstream	Normal lab values	Anemia, mild Vitamin E, iron, copper, folate, vitamin B_{12} deficiencies? Vitamin K deficiency?	Anemia, severe or chronic Prolonged bleeding time
General	Normal development Calorie or fluid deficits?	Loss or excessive subcutaneous fat Altered body temperature	Severe emaciation with sunken or hollow cheeks
Heart	Strong, regular heartbeat	Arrhythmias Potassium excess or deficits? Prehypertension Palpitations Thiamin or selenium deficiency? Bradycardia, tachycardia	High output failure Severe hypertension Cardiomegaly Hypotension
Lungs	Adequate breathing Protein, phosphorus deficiency	Respiratory muscle weakness Increased RQ	Respiratory failure Pneumonia
Legs	Well developed Firm muscles No joint/bone pain	Calf tenderness Protein deficiency? Flaccid muscles Vitamins A, C, or D, calcium deficiency? Aches	Edema Bowed legs or rickets Bone or joint pain
Genitourinary	Normal function	Kidney stones	Polycystic ovaries
GI and abdomen	No swelling or pain	Mildly edematous Protein or fat deficiencies? Nausea Diarrhea Niacin or zinc deficiencies?	Hepatomegaly Vomiting, excessive Ascites, distention Colon polyps
Hands and nails	Normal, smooth	Brittle, thin or ridged nails Iron deficiency, mild Atrophied fine muscles	Spoon-shaped nails Transverse depigmentation Smooth areas on backs of fingers from induced vomiting (bulimia)
Musculoskeletal	Normal muscles and bone	Calf muscle tenderness Thiamin, protein, vitamin C deficiency? Wasted, weak Muscle pain or soreness Decreased grip strength Bone alterations, osteopenia Cyanosis of hands and feet	Paralysis Edematous extremities Osteoporosis Bone fractures Rickets
Neurologic	Normal reflexes No developmental delay	CVA Limited reflexes B-complex or calcium deficiency? Irritability, depression, apathy Mild disorientation, confusion Fatigue, lethargy Peripheral neuropathy Motor or gait changes	Convulsions Comatose Paresthesia Seizures Psychotic episodes Dementia, memory loss

From: Halsted C, et al. Preoperative nutritional assessment. In Quigley E, Sorrell M, eds. *The gastrointestinal surgical patient: preoperative and postoperative care.* Baltimore: Williams & Wilkins, 1994; pp. 27–49; and Shils M, et al. *Modern nutrition in health and disease.* 9th ed. Baltimore: Williams & Wilkins, 1999; p. 886.

TABLE B-6 Calculations of Energy Requirements

Basal metabolic rate (BMR) is energy expenditure at rest. It involves energy required to maintain minimal physiological functioning (i.e., heart beating, breathing). Factors affecting BMR and energy include:

1. Age. Infants need more energy per square meter of body surface than any other age groups. BMR declines after maturity.
2. Body Size. Total BMR relates to body size; large persons require more energy for basal needs and for activity.
3. Body Composition. Lean tissue is more active than adipose tissue.
4. Climate. A damp or hot climate decreases BMR, and a cold climate increases BMR slightly.
5. Hormones. Thyroxine increases BMR; sex hormones and adrenalin alter BMR mildly; low zinc intake may lower BMR.
6. Fever. BMR increases by 7% for each degree above normal, Fahrenheit; 10% for each degree Centigrade.
7. Growth. BMR increases during anabolism (pregnancy, childhood, teen years, and the anabolic phase of wound healing).

TABLE B-6A Adult Assessments

Various methods are used to determine basal metabolic rate (BMR) and calorie needs for sick individuals. Several of the most common methods include indirect calorimetry: calculation of energy expenditure by measuring gas exchange (VO_2 and VCO_2 represent intracellular metabolism). Resting energy expenditure (REE) includes specific dynamic action for digestion and absorption (slightly above basal) and is considered relatively equivalent in clinical context. REE can be from normal to below normal in mild starvation such as that which occurs in the hospital setting. It may be useful to defer weight repletion until a patient's critical episode subsides; keep in mind that needs generally normalize again in 20–50 days. Overfeeding can cause fluid overload, increased CO_2 production, and hepatic aberrations. The energy needs of critically ill or injured adults are not as high as previously thought.

Harris Benedict Formulas For Determining Basal Energy Expenditure (BEE) (Harris, Benedict, 1919)

Males: BEE = 66.4 + 13.7 (W) + 5 (H) − 6.8 (A)

Females: BEE = 655 + 9.6 (W) + 1.8 (H) − 4.7 (A)

Note: W is actual weight in kilograms (weight in lb divided by 2.2 = weight in kg)

H is height in centimeters (height in inches × 2.54 = height in cm)

A is age in years

TOTAL ENERGY REQUIREMENTS = BEE × Activity Factor × Injury Factor

Activity Category	Activity Factor (AF)
Confined to bed	1.2
Out of bed	1.3
Sedentary: Seated work, little movement, little leisure activity	1.4–1.5
Seated work with requirement to move, little leisure activity	1.6–1.7
Standing work	1.8–1.9
Strenuous work or highly active leisure activity	2.0–2.4
30–60 minutes strenuous leisure activity 4–5 times/week	AF + 0.3

(continued)

TABLE B-6A Adult Assessments *(continued)*

Injury Factors	Factor
Postoperative (no complication), elective surgery	1.05–1.15
Simple starvation	0.85
Pressure ulcers:	
Stage I	1.0–1.1
Stage II	1.2
Stage III	1.3–1.4
Stage IV	1.5–1.6
Closed head injury	1.3
Multiple trauma	1.4
Systemic inflammatory response syndrome	1.5
Sepsis	1.2–1.4
Major burns	1.8–2.5
Refeeding syndrome	1.2–1.5

For Healthy Persons (Shils, 1999)	Sedentary	Moderate	Active
Overweight	20–25 kcal/kg	30 kcal/kg	35 kcal/kg
Normal weight	30 kcal/kg	35 kcal/kg	40 kcal/kg
Underweight	30 kcal/kg	40 kcal/kg	45–50 kcal/kg

For Hospitalized Patients (American Gastroenterological Association, 2001)

Use estimates based on body mass index (BMI). Feeding programs should support a patient being within 10–15 lb of desirable weight range, such as BMI.

BMI (kg/m^2)	Energy Required (kcal/kg/d)
<15	35–40
15–19	30–35
20–29	20–25
>30	15–20

Assessment of Unintentional Weight Loss

Unplanned weight loss can affect morbidity and mortality; problematic % weight change equals:

- more than 2% in 1 week
- more than 5% in 1 month
- more than 7.5% in 3 months
- more than 20% in unlimited period of time
- more than 40% usually incompatible with life

TABLE B-6B Pediatric Assessment

Date of Birth__________ Hx of LBW or other birth problems__________

Present Illness:__________ Medical History:__________

Social History:__________

Family Medical Hx:__________

Height (Length):______(cm) Height for Age:______(%ile)

Current weight:______(kg) Weight for Age:______(%ile)

% Weight for Height:__________ Interpretation:__________

% Height for Age:__________ Interpretation:__________

Ideal Weight for Height:______(kg) Ideal Height for Age:______(cm)

If weight change? (days, weeks, or months)__________

Head circumference (cm):
(%ile)______(For children < 3 years old, use growth chart)

Review of Systems for Nutritional Deficiencies:

General:__________

Skin:__________ Hair:__________ Nails:__________

Head:__________

Eyes:__________

Mouth:__________

GI/Abdomen:__________

Cardiac:__________

Extremities:__________

Neurological:__________

Musculoskeletal:__________

Laboratory Test Results:__________

(continued)

TABLE B-6B Pediatric Assessment *(continued)*

Child allergic to any food or drinks? Yes / No   Rash or eczema? Yes / No

If yes, allergic reaction to what?________________________________

Does the child avoid any specific foods such as milk or meats? Yes / No   If yes, which ones?________________

Child take any vitamins / minerals or food supplements? Yes / No

If yes, which ones?________ With fluoride Yes / No

If not taking a vitamin, does the water supply contain fluoride? Yes / No

Using formula?______ How much given and how much water is added?_______

Put to bed with a bottle? Yes / No

What type of milk?__________ # ounces/day?_____

Other beverages during the day? Ice tea   Soda   Diet soda   Kool-aid   Juice   Water   Other_____

If eating foods, when were solid foods introduced into their diet?_______________

How many meals eaten during the day?_____________

How many snacks eaten during the day?_____________ What types?_____________

Does the child usually eat the food that is prepared for the family? Yes / No

Does the child chew on any: Dirt   Clay   Paint chips   Woodwork   Ice   Plaster   Newspaper

How old is the house? Are there lead pipes? Yes / No   Has the water been tested for lead? Yes / No

Estimated Energy Needs:__________ Protein Needs:________ Fluid Needs:____________

Patient Age	Energy Requirements	Fluid
Infants, up to 6 months	108 kcal/kg	1–10 kg = 100 cc/kg body weight
Infants, 6 months to 1 year	98 kcal/kg	11–20 kg = 1,000 cc plus 50 cc/kg body weight >10 kg
Children	Requirements increase to 102 kcal/kg from 1–3 years of age. Requirements gradually decline with age to 70 kcal/kg at age 10 years	≥21 kg = 1,500 cc plus 20 cc/kg body weight >20 kg
Adolescents	45–55 kcal/kg male; 40–47 kcal/kg female	Can use 30 cc/kg body weight; increase with fever, illness, diseases

Adapted from: University of California, Los Angeles Nutrition Department. Pediatric Nutrition Assessment Checklist. Accessed February 26, 2006 at http://apps.medsch.ucla.edu/nutrition/chklst2.htm.

TABLE B-7 Calculations of Adult Protein Requirements

It requires 6.25 g of dietary protein to equal 1 g of nitrogen; therefore, estimated nitrogen requirements × 6.25 = estimated protein needs in grams. If energy is not provided in adequate amounts, protein tissues become a substrate. Extra protein intake may be needed to compensate for excess protein loss in specific patient populations such as those with burn injury, open wounds, and protein-losing enteropathy or nephropathy. Lower protein intake may be necessary in patients with chronic renal insufficiency not treated by dialysis and certain patients with hepatic encephalopathy.

Clinical Condition	Protein Requirement (g/kg body weight/d)
Normal	0.8
Metabolic stress (illness/injury)	1.0–1.5
Acute renal failure (undialyzed)	0.8–1.0
Hemodialysis	1.2–1.4
Peritoneal dialysis	1.3–1.5

Adapted from the American Gastroenterological Association. Medical Position Statement: parenteral nutrition. *Gastroenterology* 121:966, 2001.

TABLE B-8 Lab Values

Many lab tests can provide useful information on patients' nutritional status along with information on their medical status. The following ranges are typical tests that are done. The table provides estimated and sample normal values. Normal ranges will vary by the techniques used by the laboratory completing the tests. Age-specific criteria should also be used to evaluate data.

Allergy Antibody Assessment

Immunoglobulins: IgG, IgM, IgA, IgD, and IgE; specific IgE for molds, IgG for spices and herbs
Helicobacter pylori antibodies test
Allergy blood and skin testing
C-reactive protein
Rheumatoid factor (RF)
Celiac profile: IgA-antitissue transglutaminase (tTG); IgA-antiendomysial antibodies (IgA-EMA); IgA-antigliadin antibodies (IgA-AGA)

Cardiopulmonary System

Arterial blood gases
Cardiac enzymes
Creatine kinase
Lactate dehydrogenase
Aspartate transaminase (AST)
Homocysteine
Lipid profile: Cholesterol, lipoproteins, triglycerides

Blood Chemistry and Renal Tests

Albumin
Total protein
Serum creatinine
Creatinine clearance/glomerular filtration rate
Blood urea nitrogen (BUN)
Nitrogen balance
Serum proteins

Coagulation Tests

Bleeding or coagulation time
International normalized ratio (INR)
Prothrombin time (PT)

Endocrine System

Aldosterone
Antidiuretic hormone
Blood glucose
C-peptide
Calcium
Calcitonin
Glucose tolerance test (GTT)
Insulin
Triiodothyronine (T3)
Thyroxine (T4)
Thyroid-stimulating hormone (TSH)
Phosphorus
Parathormone (PTH)

Gastrointestinal System and Stool Tests

Comprehensive digestive stool analysis
Parasitology assessment
Lactose intolerance breath test
Bacterial overgrowth of small intestine breath test
Gastric analysis
Serum gastrin

Hepatic System

Ammonia
Aspartate aminotransferase (AST)
Alanine aminotransferase (ALT)
Alkaline phosphatase (ALP)
Gamma-glutamyl transpeptidase (GGT)
Albumin, gamma-globulin, A-G ratio
Hepatitis virus
Blood
Albumin
Bilirubin
Total protein
Urine
Bilirubin
Urobilinogen
Prothrombin time
Partial thromboplastin time

Musculoskeletal System

Enzymes
Alkaline phosphatase (ALP)
Acid phosphatase
Isoenzymes
Lactate dehydrogenase (LDH)
Creatine phosphokinase (CPK)

Pancreatic Tests

Serum amylase
Serum lipase

Red Cell Indices

Mean cell volume (MCV)
Mean cell hemoglobin (MCH)
MCH concentration

(continued)

TABLE B-8 **Lab Values *(continued)***

Reticulocyte cell count
Serum ferritin
Serum iron and total iron-binding capacity
Electrolytes
Sodium
Potassium
Chlorine
Carbon dioxide

Vitamin and Mineral Assessment

Calcium
Zinc
Vitamin A
Vitamin C
Vitamin B_6
Folate
Vitamin B_{12}

Urinary System

Physical observation
Color, clarity, odor
Chemical tests
Specific gravity
pH
Protein
Glucose
Ketones
Blood
Bilirubin
Urobilinogen
Nitrite
Leukocyte esterase
Urine volume
Microscopic examination: Cells, casts, crystals, bacteria, yeast

Value	Normal Range	Purpose or Comment	Increased In	Decreased In
Hematology: Coagulation Tests and Bleeding Time				
Prothrombin time (PT), international normalized ratio (INR)	11–16 seconds control; 70–110% of control value Patients on anticoagulant drugs should have an INR of 2.0–3.0 for basic "blood thinning" needs. For some patients who have a high risk of clot formation, the INR needs to be higher—about 2.5–3.5.	Since PT and INR evaluate the ability of blood to clot properly, they can be used to assess both bleeding and clotting tendencies. One common use is to monitor the effectiveness of blood thinning drugs such as warfarin (Coumadin). Anticoagulant drugs must be carefully monitored to maintain a balance between preventing clots and causing excessive bleeding.	A prolonged or increased prothrombin time means that blood is taking too long to form a clot. Antibiotics, aspirin, and cimetidine can increase the PT/INR.	Too much anticoagulation (warfarin, for example). Barbiturates, oral contraceptives, hormone-replacement therapy (HRT), and vitamin K (either in a multivitamin or liquid nutrition supplement) can decrease PT. Beef and pork liver, green tea, broccoli, chickpeas, kale, turnip greens, and soybean products contain large amounts of vitamin K and can alter PT results if consumed in large amounts.
Hematology: Blood Cell Values				
Erythrocyte count (red blood cells [RBC])	4.5–6.2 million/mm^3 in males; 4.2–5.4 million/mm^3 in females	Made in bone marrow; production controlled by erythropoietin.	Polycythemia, dehydration, severe diarrhea	Anemias such as vitamin B_{12}, iron, folic acid, and protein; chronic infections; hemorrhage
Erythrocyte sedimentation rate	0–15 mm/hour in males; 0–25 mm/hour in females	Sedimentation rate measures how quickly RBCs (erythrocytes) settle in a test tube in 1 hour. Often used with C-reactive protein (CRP) for testing of inflammation.	Inflammation, pneumonia, appendicitis, pelvic inflammatory disease, lymphoma, multiple myeloma, lupus, rheumatoid arthritis (RA), osteomyelitis, temporal arteritis	
Ferritin	20–300 mg/mL in males; 20–120 mg/mL in females	Chief iron storage protein in the body. Reflects reticuloendothelial iron storage. Usually 23% of total iron stores.	Hemochromatosis, leukemias, anemias other than iron deficiency, Hodgkin's disease, liver diseases	Iron deficiency anemia

(continued)

TABLE B-8 Lab Values *(continued)*

Value	Normal Range	Purpose or Comment	Increased In	Decreased In
Folate, serum	0.3 μg/dL (7 nmol/L)	Important for DNA functioning	Blind loop syndrome	Pregnancy, lactation, macrocytic anemia, intestinal malabsorption syndrome, alcoholism, use of goat's milk in childhood, use of anticonvulsants, cycloserine, methotrexate, and oral contraceptives
Iron, serum	75–175 mg/dL in males; 65–165 mg/dL in females; 40–100+ mg/dL in children up to age 2 years; 50–120 mg/dL in children >2 years.	Iron found in blood, largely in hemoglobin	Hemochromatosis, acute or chronic liver disease, hemolytic anemia, leukemia, lead poisoning, thalassemia, vitamin B_{12} or folate deficiency, dehydration, small bowel surgery	50 μg/dL (9 mmol/L) may indicate iron deficiency anemia or blood loss. Chronic diseases, pregnancy, cancer, end-stage renal disease (ESRD) or chronic renal disease, malnutrition or poor dietary intake, sickle cell disease, viral hepatitis, thalassemia
Iron-binding capacity, total (TIBC)	240–450 mg/dL	Measure of the capacity of serum transferrin. 18–59% transferrin saturation is normal. As serum iron decreases, TIBC goes up, at least initially.	Iron deficiency, blood loss, later in pregnancy, oral contraceptive use, hepatitis, low serum iron, gastrectomy	High serum iron, renal disease, hemochromatosis, pernicious anemia, cancer, thalassemia, hemolytic diseases, small bowel surgery, sepsis, liver disease; may be low in malnutrition
Hematocrit (% packed cell volume)	40–54% in males; 37–47% in females; 33–35% in children; 37–49% in 12- to 18-year-old males; 36–46% in 12- to 18-year-old females	Cell volume % of RBCs in whole blood. Elevated when iron level is low.	Polycythemia	Anemias, prolonged dietary deficiency of protein and iron, sepsis, small bowel surgery, gastrectomy, renal or liver disease, blood loss
Hemoglobin, whole blood	14–17 g/dL in males; 12–15 g/dL in females; ≥10 g/dL in babies 6–23 months old; ≥11 in children 2-5 years old; 11.5–15.5 g/dL in children 6–12 years old; 13.0–16.0 g/dL in 12- to 18-year-old males; 12.0–16.0 g/dL in 12- to 18-year-old females	Oxygen carrier from lung to tissues. Binds CO_2 on return to the lung.	Polycythemia, dehydration, hemolysis, sickle cell anemia, recent blood transfusions, chronic obstructive pulmonary disease (COPD) heart failure, high altitude, burns, dehydration	Anemias, prolonged dietary deficiency of iron, excessive bleeding, cancer, lupus, overhydration, Hodgkin's disease, protein–calorie malnutrition, renal or liver disease, pregnancy, lead poisoning, sepsis, small bowel surgery, gastrectomy
Mean corpuscular hemoglobin (MCH)	26–32 pg; concentration is 32–36%	High concentration of individual RBCs (Hgb/RBC)	Macrocytic anemia	Hemoglobin deficiency, hypochromic anemia
Mean corpuscular volume (MCV)	80–94 cu/μm	Individual RBC size	High MCV or macrocytosis: folate, vitamin B_{12} deficiency. Alcoholic or liver disease, blood loss, hypothyroidism, small bowel surgery	Low MCV or microcytosis: iron, copper, pyridoxine deficiency. Thalassemia, anemia of chronic disease, cancer, blood loss
Transferrin (siderophilin)	170–370 mg/dL (1.7–3.7 g/L)	Glycoprotein in blood plasma that transports iron to liver and spleen for storage and to bone marrow for hemoglobin synthesis	Iron deficiency, acute hepatitis, oral contraceptive use, pregnancy, chronic blood loss, dehydration, gastrectomy	Acute or chronic inflammation, chronic liver disease, lupus, zinc deficiency, sickle cell anemia, pernicious anemia with vitamin B_{12} or folate deficiency, chronic infection and inflammatory diseases, malnutrition, burns, iron overload, nephrotic syndrome, sepsis, small bowel surgery

(continued)

TABLE B-8 Lab Values *(continued)*

Value	Normal Range	Purpose or Comment	Increased In	Decreased In
White blood cells (WBC), leukocytes	4.8–11.8 thousand/mm^3	Highly variable lab value; protect against disease or infection	Metabolic acidosis, acute hemorrhage, acute bacterial infections, leukemias, burns, gangrene, exercise, stress, eclampsia	Chemotherapy, ABT. Neutropenia is often seen in deficiency states. Some viral conditions, cachexia, anaphylactic shock, bone marrow suppression, pernicious or aplastic anemia, diuretic use
Hematology and Lymphatic System: Differential				
Lymphocytes	Total lymphocyte count (TLC) = normal, 12,000/mm^3; deficient, <900/mm^3; 24–44% total WBC count	Made in thymus and lymph nodes; produce antibodies	Infectious mononucleosis, mumps, German measles, convalescence from acute infections	Infections, malnutrition
Leukocytes: basophils	0–1.5% total WBC count	They release substances that cause smooth muscle contraction, vasoconstriction, and an increased permeability of small blood vessels. Basophils are stimulated by allergens.	Postsplenectomy, chronic myelogenous leukemia, polycythemia, Hodgkin's disease, chicken pox	Hyperthyroidism, acute infections, pregnancy, anaphylaxis
Leukocytes: eosinophils	0.5–4% total WBC count	Eosinophils are stimulated by parasites and some bacteria. They release substances that cause vasoconstriction, smooth muscle contraction, and an increased permeability of small blood vessels. Related to allergies.	Allergies, parasitic infections, pernicious anemia, ulcerative colitis, Hodgkin's disease	Use of β-blockers, corticosteroids, stress, and bacterial and viral infections including trichinosis
Leukocytes: monocytes	4–8% total WBC count	Phagocytosis. Produced in bone marrow.	Monocytic leukemia, lipid storage disease, protozoan infection, chronic ulcerative colitis	
Leukocytes: neutrophils	60–65% total WBC count	Phagocytosis	Wound sepsis in burns, bacterial infections, inflammation, cancer, traumas, stress, diabetes, acute gout	Folate or vitamin B_{12} deficiency, sickle cell anemia, steroid therapy, postsurgical status
Platelets (thrombocytes)	125,000–300,000 mm^3	Largely polysaccharides and phospholipids. Role in coagulation.	Malignancy, polycythemia vera, splenectomy, iron deficiency anemia, cirrhosis, chronic pancreatitis	Thrombocytopenic purpura
General Serum Values and Enzymes				
Amylase	60–180 Somogyi units/dL	Pancreatic enzyme for hydrolysis of starch and glycogen	Increased in perforated peptic ulcer, acute pancreatitis, mumps, cholecystitis, renal insufficiency, alcohol poisoning, partial gastrectomy	Decreased in hepatitis, severe burns, pancreatic disease, advanced cystic fibrosis, toxemia of pregnancy, hepatitis
Bicarbonate	22–28 mEq/L	Acid–base balance	Metabolic alkalosis, large intake of sodium bicarbonate, excessive vomiting, potassium deficiency, respiratory acidosis, emphysema	Diabetic acidosis, starvation, chronic diarrhea, renal insufficiency, respiratory alkalosis (hyperventilation), fistula drainage
Bilirubin	Direct: ≤0.3 mg/dL; total: ≤1 mg/dL	Hemoglobin is converted to bilirubin when RBCs are destroyed.	Hepatitis, jaundice, biliary obstruction, drug toxicity, hemolytic disease, prolonged fasting	Seasonal affective disorder

(continued)

TABLE B-8 Lab Values *(continued)*

Value	Normal Range	Purpose or Comment	Increased In	Decreased In
Calcium	9–11 mg/dL (2.3–2.8 mmol/L); 3.9–5.4 mg/dL serum ionized	50% is protein bound, so protein intake affects serum calcium level more than dietary calcium itself. Regulated by parathormone (PTH) and thyrocalcitonin. Coma above 13 mg/dL; death below 7 mg/dL.	Hyperparathyroidism, renal calculi, vitamin D excess, osteolytic disease, milk-alkali syndrome, immobilization, tuberculosis, Addison's disease, antibiotic therapy, cancer	Steatorrhea, renal failure, malabsorption, vitamin D deficiency, hypoparathyroidism, sprue, celiac disease, overhydration, hypoalbumenia, hyperphosphatemia
Ceruloplasmin	27–37 mg/dL	Form of copper found in bloodstream	Leukemias, anemias, cirrhosis of the liver, hypo/hyperthyroidism, collagen diseases, pregnancy	Wilson's disease, severe copper deficiency, nephrosis, leukemia remission, prolonged total parenteral nutrition (TPN) without copper, cystic fibrosis
Copper	70–140 μg/dL in males; 80–155 μg/dL in females	Found bound to albumin or as ceruloplasmin	Leukemias, anemias, cirrhosis of the liver, hypo/hyperthyroidism, collagen diseases, pregnancy	Wilson's disease, severe copper deficiency, nephrosis, leukemia remission, prolonged TPN without copper, cystic fibrosis
Creatine phosphokinase (CPK)	0–145 IU/L	Catalyst for phosphorylation of creatine by adenosine triphosphate (ATP). Mostly found in skeletal and cardiac muscle. Increases 2–4 hours after myocardial infarction (MI), returning to normal after 3 days.	Hepatic or uremic coma, striated muscle disease, muscular dystrophy, MI, cerebrovascular accident (CVA), trauma, alcoholic liver disease, encephalitis	
D-xylose, 25 g dose	30–40 mg/dL	This test measures the intestines' ability to absorb D-xylose, a simple sugar, as an indicator of whether nutrients are being properly absorbed.		Xylose malabsorption
Gamma-glutamyl transpeptidase (GGT)	5–40 IU/L	GGT participates in the transfer of amino acids across the cellular membrane and in glutathione metabolism. Used to detect diseases of the liver, bile ducts, and kidney and to differentiate liver or bile duct (hepatobiliary) disorders from bone disease.	Coronary heart failure (CHF), MI, cholecystitis, liver disease, alcoholism, hepatic biliary disease, pancreatitis, nephritic syndrome	
Lactic acid dehydrogenase (LDH)	200–680 IU/mL	Catalyzes conversion between pyruvate and lactic acid in glycolytic cycle. Has 5 isoenzymes. Increases 8–10 hours after MI, returning to normal after 7–14 days.	Untreated pernicious anemia, acute MI, heart failure, malignancy, alcoholic liver damage, cardiovascular surgery, hepatitis, pulmonary embolus, leukemia, cancer, renal failure, hemolytic or megaloblastic anemia, muscular dystrophy, nephrotic syndrome	Radiation therapy
Lipase	0.2–1.5 IU/mL	Synthesized by the pancreas	Pancreatic disease, acute pancreatitis, perforated ulcer, pancreatic duct obstruction, biliary tract infection, renal insufficiency	

(continued)

TABLE B-8 **Lab Values *(continued)***

Value	Normal Range	Purpose or Comment	Increased In	Decreased In
Phenylalanine, serum	<3 mg/dL	An amino acid of importance in phenylketonuria (PKU) patients	Levels might be high in PKU	Severe protein deficiency and protein-calorie malnutrition (PCM)
Phosphatase, acid	0.5–2 Bodansky units	A blood test that measures prostatic acid phosphatase (an enzyme found primarily in men in the prostate gland and semen) to determine the health of the prostate gland	Prostate dysfunction results in the release of prostatic acid phosphatase into the blood.	
Phosphatase, alkaline (ALP)	2–4.5 Bodansky units (30–135 IU/L); children = 3× that of adults	ALP is an enzyme found in all tissues. Tissues with particularly high concentrations of ALP include the liver, bile ducts, placenta, and bone. Indirect test for calcium, phosphorus, vitamin D nutriture. Used to determine presence of liver or bone cell disorders.	Anemia, Paget's disease, biliary obstruction, leukemia, hyperparathyroidism, rickets, bone disease, healing fracture	Malnutrition, protein deficiency
Sulfate, inorganic	0.5–1.5 mg/dL	Usual sulfur intake is 0.6–1.6 g on a mixed diet containing 100 g protein.	Supplemental overdose; high sulfate intake from water supply	Protein deficiency; injury to bones, cartilage, tendons
Transaminase: aspartate aminotransferase (AST)	5–40 IU/mL	Found in liver, muscle, and brain. Functional measure of vitamin B_6 nutriture. Released in tissue injury. Formerly SGOT (serum glutamic oxaloacetic transaminase).	Hepatic cancer, shock/trauma, cirrhosis, neoplastic disease, MI	Uncontrolled diabetes mellitus (DM), beriberi
Transaminase: alanine aminotransferase (ALT)	4–36 IU/L	Found in the liver. Generally parallels AST levels. Functional measure of vitamin B_6 nutriture. Formerly SGPT (serum glutamic pyruvic transaminase).	Hepatitis, cirrhosis, trauma, hepatic cancer, shock, mononucleosis	Wilson's disease
Glucose Control				
Glucose, fasting serum	70–110 mg/dL (3.9–6.1 mmol/L)	Principal fuel for cellular function, especially brain and RBCs.	DM, hyperthyroidism pancreatitis, MI, hyperfunction of endocrine, stress, CHF infection, surgery, CVA, hepatic dysfunction, cancer Cushing's syndrome, burns, steroids, chromium deficiency	Postprandial hypoglycemia, sepsis, cancer, malnutrition, hypothyroid, gastrectomy, liver damage or disease, Addison's disease
Glucose tolerance test (GTT)	2-hour post load glucose <200 mg/dL	Test done when blood glucose levels are >120 mg/dL.	Diabetes, hyperthyroidism, pancreatic cancer, Cushing's syndrome, acromegaly, pheochromocytoma.	Hypoglycemia, hypothyroidism, malabsorption, malnutrition, insulinoma, hypopituitarism
Glycosylated hemoglobin–HbA1C	4–7% (nondiabetic); good, <9%; fair, 9–12%; poor >12%	May reflect poor glucose control over past 2–4 months	Poor blood sugar control, newly diagnosed diabetes, pregnancy	Low RBC (chronic blood loss, hemolytic anemia), chronic renal failure (CRF), sickle cell anemia

(continued)

TABLE B-8 Lab Values *(continued)*

Value	Normal Range	Purpose or Comment	Increased In	Decreased In
Protein Factors				
Albumin	3.5–5 g/dL (35–50 g/L); 3.2–5.1 g/dL in infants up to 1 year old; 3.2–5.7 in children aged 1–2 years; 3.5–5.8 for ages 2 years to adult.	Nonspecific protein nutriture measure. Mostly synthesized in the liver. Transports fatty acids, thyroxin, bilirubin, and many drugs.	Dehydration, multiple myeloma	Decreased with inflammation and severity of illness, acute stress, starvation, PCM, malabsorption of protein, cirrhosis, nephritis with edema, liver disease
	Albumin is usually 40% of proteins.	Albumin-globulin ratio (A:G) is 1.2–1.9; low in renal or liver diseases.		
C-reactive protein (CRP)	0	Elevated in inflammation	Systemic inflammation, obesity, diabetes, heart disease, arthritis, smoking	Vitamin C supplements may lower an elevated CRP. Marathon runners may have very low levels.
Creatinine	0.6–1.2 mg/dL	A basic creatine anhydride, nitrogenous end product of skeletal muscle metabolism. Indirect measure of renal filtration rate.	Hyperthyroidism, CHF, diabetic acidosis, dehydration, muscle disease, some cancers, nephritis, urinary obstruction	Overhydration, multiple sclerosis (MS), pregnancy, eclampsia, increased age, severe wasting
Creatinine–height index (CHI)	CHI = (measured 24-hour creatine excretion × 100) / predicted 24-hour creatine excretion	Estimates skeletal muscle mass. CHI values of 60–80% represent mild marasmus. CHIs of 40–59% represent moderate marasmus. CHIs of <40% represent severe marasmus.	High doses of creatine supplementation	Marasmus, malnutrition
Globulin	2.3–3.5 g/dL	5 fractions; transport antibodies	Infections, leukemia, dehydration, shock, tuberculosis (TB), chronic alcoholism, Hodgkin's disease	Malnutrition, immunological deficiency
Nitrogen balance	Goal of 1–4 g/24 hours urinary urea nitrogen (UUN)	Nitrogen balance is the result of nitrogen intake (from the diet) and nitrogen losses, which consists of nitrogen recovered in urine and feces and miscellaneous losses.	Severe liver disease	Nephrosis
Prealbumin (transthyretin)	16–35 mg/dL	Reflects past 3 days of protein intake but is affected by inflammation	Renal failure, Hodgkin's disease, pregnancy, dehydration	Acute catabolic states, hepatic disease, stress infection, surgery, low protein intake, malnutrition, hyperthyroidism, nephritic syndrome, overhydration, inflammation
Proteins, total serum	6–8 g/dL; 5.6–7.2 in infants to 1 year; 5.4–7.5 in children 1–2 years old; 5.3–8.0 in ages 2 years to adult	Amount of protein in the bloodstream. Reflects depletion of tissue proteins. Act as buffers in acid–base balance. Plasma proteins equal about 7% of total plasma volume.	Dehydration, shock	Hepatic disease, leukemia, malnutrition, infection, pregnancy, malabsorption, severe burns
Nutrient Values				
Ascorbic acid (vitamin C)	0.2–2.0 mg/dL	Serum levels of vitamin C	Oxalate stones, diarrhea, high uric acid	Large doses of aspirin, barbiturates, stress, anemia, tetracycline, oral contraceptives, cigarette smoking, alcoholism, dialysis

(continued)

TABLE B-8 Lab Values *(continued)*

Value	Normal Range	Purpose or Comment	Increased In	Decreased In
Essential fatty acids (EFA) (triene to tetraene [T/T] ratio)	0.2 is normal; a ratio >0.4 in serum phospholipids indicates EFA deficiency in healthy people	Ratio 20:39/20:46 (T/T ratio) are measured. T/T ratios are assessed in RBCs, RBC phospholipids, and serum phospholipids.		EFA deficiency occurs in starvation, marasmus, and strict low-fat diets.
Niacin: *N*-methylnicotinamide	5.8 μmol/d	For niacin assessment. Usual dietary intake is 16–33 mg/d.	Large doses of nicotinic acid	Pregnancy, lactation, Hartnup's disease, pellagra, schizophrenia
Riboflavin: glutathione reductase, erythrocyte	1.2 IU/g hemoglobin	Dietary intake is related to CHO and total energy intake.		Tetracycline or thiazide diuretic use, probenecid, oral contraceptives, sulfa drugs, pellagra, cheilosis, some forms of glossitis, vegetarians using no dairy products or supplements
Selenium: glutathione peroxidase	Serum enzyme levels	Works with vitamin E to protect RBCs as part of the enzyme.	Excessive lipid peroxidation	PCM, hypoproteinemia
Thiamin: transketolase activity, erythrocyte	1.20 μg/mL/hr	Dietary requirements increase when CHO intake is high.		Use of baking soda in cooking, high CHO intake, infantile beriberi, dry or edematous (cardiac) beriberi, excessive intake of caffeic or tannic acids, pellagra, chronic alcoholism, lactic acidosis in metabolic disorders such as maple syrup urine disease (MSUD)
Vitamin B_6: pyrodoxal 5′phosphate, plasma	5 ng/mL (20 nmol/L)	Usual dietary intake is 2 mg, assuming 100 g of protein is consumed.		Acute celiac disease, chronic alcoholism, pellagra, high protein intake, pregnancy, oral contraceptive use, isoniazid (INH) and other TB drug use, use of anticonvulsants, malarial drugs
Vitamin A: carotene; retinol, serum	48–200 mg/dL; 10–60 μg/dL	Serum levels of carotenoids	Excessive intake, such as from carrots, postprandial hyperlipidemia, diabetes, hypothyroidism	High fever, liver disease, malabsorption syndrome
Retinol-binding protein	2.6–7.6 mg/dL	Used less often to determine status of retinol	May be high in renal failure	Protein deficiency
Serum vitamin A	125–150 IU/dL or 20–80 mg/dL		Hypervitaminosis A	Cirrhosis, infectious hepatitis, myxedema, night blindness, PCM, malabsorption, starvation, infections such as measles
Vitamin B_{12}: serum B_{12}	24.4–100 ng/dL (180 pmol/L)	Vitamin B_{12} is less well absorbed in the elderly and in persons who have less intrinsic factor or the ability to reabsorb in the intestines.	Leukemia such as acute myelogenous leukemia (AML) or CML, leukocytosis, polycythemia vera, liver metastasis, hepatitis, cirrhosis	Macrocytic anemia, iron or vitamin B_6 deficiency, gastritis, dialysis, congenital intrinsic factor deficiency, pernicious anemia, tapeworm, ileal resection, strict vegetarian diets, pregnancy
Vitamin D: 1,25-HCC, blood	0.7–3.3 IU/dL	Indirect measures are available from serum alkaline phosphatase, calcium levels, and serum phosphorus.	Hypervitaminosis D	Rickets, osteomalacia, steroid therapy, fracture, poorly calcified teeth, drug therapy such as anticonvulsants, cholestyramine, and barbiturates

(continued)

TABLE B-8 Lab Values *(continued)*

Value	Normal Range	Purpose or Comment	Increased In	Decreased In
Vitamin E: alpha-tocopherol; plasma vitamin E	<18 μmol/g (41.8 μmol/L); 0.5–2.0 mg/dL	Usual dietary intake is 14 mg of d-alpha-tocopherol	High vitamin E intake (this affects coagulation because it works against vitamin K)	High polyunsaturated fatty acid (PUFA) intake, premature infants, cystic fibrosis, hemolytic anemia
Vitamin K: INR or PT	PT, 10–15 seconds	Combined low levels of prothrombin activity, serum calcium, and serum carotene may indicate abnormal fat and fat-soluble vitamin absorption.	Menadione use, intravenous (IV) administration of vitamin K, parenchymal liver disease	PT is prolonged in salicylates, sulfa, and tetracycline use. Liver disease, fat malabsorption, prematurity, small bowel disorders.
Zinc: serum zinc	0.75–1.4 mg/mL or up to 79 μg/dL in plasma; 100–140 μg/dL in serum	Large amounts are found in liver, skeletal muscle, and bone. Part of the insulin molecule. Usual intake is 10–15 mg/d.	Eating foods stored in galvanized containers. Excesses from supplements.	Wounds, geophagia, high-calcium or high-phytate diets, growth, stress, skin lesions, poor taste or olfactory acuity, upper respiratory infections, MI, oral contraceptive use, cancer, pregnancy, cirrhosis, sickle cell or pernicious anemias
Electrolytes				
Chloride	95–105 mEq/L	Acid–base balance. Major anion. Follows sodium passively in its transport.	Eclampsia, metabolic acidosis, dehydration, pancreatitis, anemia, renal insufficiency, Cushing's syndrome, head injury, hyperventilation, hyperlipidemia, hypoproteinemia	Diabetic acidosis, metabolic alkalosis, gastroenteritis, fever, potassium deficiency, excessive sweating, CHF, hyponatremia, infection, diuretics, overhydration
Magnesium	1.8–3 mg/dL	Influences muscular activity. Coenzyme in CHO and protein metabolism.	Renal insufficiency, uncontrolled diabetes, Addison's disease, hypothyroidism, ingestion of magnesium-containing antacids or salts	Malnutrition, potassium-depleting diuretics, Malabsorption, alcohol abuse, starvation, renal disease, acute pancreatitis, severe diarrhea, ulcerative colitis
Phosphorous phosphate (PO_4)	2.3–4.7 mg/dL	Influenced by diet and absorption; regulated by kidneys.	Liver disease, bone tumors, hypervitaminosis D, end-stage renal disease, renal insufficiency, hypoparathyroidism, diabetic ketoacidosis (DKA), Addison's disease, childhood	Malnutrition, gout, hyperparathyroidism, osteomalacia, hyperinsulinism, hypovitaminosis D, alcoholism, overuse of phosphate-binding antacids, rapid refeeding after prolonged starvation
Potassium, serum	3.5–5.5 mEq/L (16–20 mg/dL)	Intracellular. Cellular metabolism; muscle protein synthesis. Enzymes.	Renal insufficiency or failure, overuse of potassium supplements, Addison's disease, dehydration, acidosis, cell damage, poorly controlled diabetes	Decreased potassium intake, renal disease, burns, trauma, diuretics, steroids, vomiting, stress, diarrhea, crash diet, overhydration, malnutrition, estrogen, steroid therapy, cirrhosis, hemolysis, fistula drainage
Sodium, serum	136–145 mEq/L	Absorbed almost 100% from gastrointestinal (GI) tract. Major cation; extracellular ion. Controls osmotic pressure. Acid–base balance.	Vitamin K deficiency, vomiting, heart failure, hypervitaminosis, dehydration, diabetes insipidus, Cushing's disease, primary aldosteronism, diarrhea, steroids	Decreased sodium intake, diuretic use, burns, diarrhea, vomiting, nephritis, diabetic acidosis, hyperglycemia, overhydration

(continued)

TABLE B-8 Lab Values *(continued)*

Value	Normal Range	Purpose or Comment	Increased In	Decreased In
Lipids				
Total serum cholesterol (TC)	Adults: Desirable: 120–199 mg/dL; borderline high: 200–239 mg/dL; high: ≥240 mg/dL Child: Desirable: 70–175 mg/dL; borderline: 170–199 mg/dL; high: ≥200 mg/dL	Fat-related compound; component of plaque. Need fasting sample. Usually 30% high-density lipoprotein (HDL) and 70% low-density lipoprotein (LDL).	High: >200 mg/dL. Hyperlipidemia, diabetes, MI, hypertension (HTN), high-cholesterol diet, nephrotic syndrome, hypothyroidism, pregnancy, cardiovascular disease (CVD)	Low: < 160 mg/dL. Low fat ingestion, malnutrition, malabsorption or starvation, fever, acute infections, liver damage, steatorrhea, hyperthyroidism, cancer, pernicious anemia
High-density lipoprotein (HDL)	Males: >45mg/dL; females: >55 mg/dL	Usually higher in females. Low levels may indicate risk for heart disease.	Vigorous exercise, weight reduction, liver disease, alcoholism	Starvation, obesity, liver disease, DM, smoking, hyperthyroidism
Low-density lipoprotein (LDL)	Desirable: <130 mg/dL; borderline high: 130–159 mg/dL; high: ≥160 mg/dL	May indicate cardiac risk when elevated.	Familial hyperlipidemia, diet high in saturated fat and cholesterol, hypothyroidism, MI, DM, nephrotic syndrome, pregnancy, hepatic disease	Nephritic syndrome
Phospholipids	60–350 mg/dL	Measure of EFAs, indirect. Includes lecithin, sphingomyelins, cephalins, and plasmogens.		EFA deficiency
Triglycerides (TG)	Desirable: 10–190 mg/dL; borderline high: 200–400 mg/dL; high: 400–1000 mg/dL; very high: >1000 mg/dL	Neutral fats are the main transport form of fatty acids. Need fasting sample.	High-carbohydrate diet, alcohol abuse (secondary), hyperlipoproteinemias, nephrotic syndrome, CRF MI, HTN, DM, respiratory distress, pancreatitis, hypothyroidism	Malnutrition, COPD, malabsorption, hyperthyroidism, hyperparathyroidism, brain infarct
Osmolality and pH				
pH, arterial, plasma	7.36–7.44	Hydrogen ion concentration. Enzymes work within narrow pH ranges.	Alkalosis (uncompensated), hyperventilation, pyloric obstruction, HCl losses, diuretic use	Acidosis (uncompensated), emphysema, diabetic acidosis, renal failure, vomiting, diarrhea, intestinal fistula
Osmolality, serum	270–280 mOsm/L	Maintaining normal serum level is desirable.	Elevated in dehydration	Low in overhydration
Respiratory Factors				
Respiratory quotient (RQ)	0.85 from mixed diet	1.0 from CHO; 0.80 from protein; 0.70 from fat	High-CHO diet	High-fat diet
Oxygen: partial pressure of oxygen (pO_2)	80–100 mm Hg	Reflects hemoglobin concentration. Arterial blood is used.	Hyperoxia	Hypoxia (anemic, stagnant, chronic, anoxic)
Carbon dioxide: partial pressure of carbon dioxide (pCO_2)	35–45 mm Hg; 24–30 mEq/L		Pulmonary problems, metabolic alkalosis due to ingestion of excess sodium bicarbonate, protracted vomiting with potassium deficiency, Cushing's syndrome, heart failure with edema	Diabetic ketosis or ketoacidosis, starvation, renal insufficiency, persistent diarrhea, lactic acidosis, respiratory alkalosis, diarrhea
Renal Values				
Glomerular filtration rate (GFR)	110–150 mL/min in males; 105–132 mL/min in females	GFR reflects kidney function		Renal failure: < 90 mL/min/1.73 m^2 indicates renal decline
Urea clearance	40–65 mL/min standard; 60–100 mL/min maximum	Part of assessment of renal status		Uremia

(continued)

TABLE B-8 Lab Values *(continued)*

Value	Normal Range	Purpose or Comment	Increased In	Decreased In
Blood urea nitrogen (BUN) to creatinine ratio	>10:1	Measure of impaired renal function.	Renal disease, excess protein intake, bleeding in small intestine, burns, high fever, steroid therapy, decreased renal blood flow, urinary tract obstruction	Low-protein intake, repeated dialysis without repletion, severe vomiting and diarrhea, hepatic insufficiency
BUN	8–18 mg/dL (3–6.5 mmol/L); slightly higher in males	Urea is the end product of protein metabolism. Varies directly with dietary intake. Formed in the liver from amino acids and other ammonia-containing compounds.	Renal failure, azotemia, DM, burns, dehydration, shock, heart failure, infection, chronic gout, excessive protein intake, catabolism, GI bleed, MI, urinary obstruction, starvation, steroid therapy, trauma	Hepatic failure, malnutrition, malabsorption, overhydration, pregnancy, acromegaly, low-protein diet
Uric acid	4.0–9.0 mg/dL in men; 2.8–8.8 mg/dL in women	Metabolite from purine metabolism. Excreted by kidney. Serum level reflects balance between production and excretion.	Higher in winter, stress, gout, leukemia, hypoparathyroidism, total fasting, toxemia of pregnancy, elevated triglycerides, DKA, hypertension, hemolytic or sickle cell anemia, renal disease, alcoholism, multiple myeloma, polycythemia, use of vincristine or mercaptopurine	Acute hepatitis, Wilson's disease, celiac disease, Fanconi's syndrome, Hodgkin's disease, use of allopurinol or large doses of coumadin, folic acid anemia, burns, pregnancy, malabsorption, lead poisoning
Hormones				
Adrenocorticotropic hormone (ACTH)	5–95 pg/mL at 9 AM; 0–35 pg/mL at midnight		Cushing's syndrome, secondary hypoadrenalism	Pituitary Cushing's syndrome, primary adrenal insufficiency
Cortisol	5–25 μg/dL at 8 AM; 10 μg/dL at 8 PM	Lower in women	Extreme stress, elevated in patients with night-eating syndrome	
Gastrin	0–200 pg/mL		Zollinger-Ellison syndrome, pyloric obstruction, short bowel syndrome, pernicious anemia, atrophic gastritis	
Growth hormone (GH)	<6 ng/mL in men; <10 ng/mL in women	Being administered in some medical conditions		
Insulin	6–26 IU/mL, fasting	Serum levels are useful.	Untreated obese patients who have diabetes, metabolic syndrome, insulinoma	Severe diabetic acidosis with ketosis and weight loss
Iodine, total	8–15 mEq/L	Affects activity of the thyroid gland, usual intake with 10 g NaCl is 1000 μg iodine.	Hyperthyroidism	Cretinism, simple goiter, low-iodine diet or high-goitrogenic dietary intake
Protein-bound iodine (PBI)	3.6–8.8 mg/dL	Most iodine is protein bound in the thyroid hormones.	Hyperthyroidism, thyroiditis, pregnancy, oral contraceptive use, hepatitis	Cretinism, simple goiter, low-iodine diet or high-goitrogenic dietary intake
Serotonin (5-HIAA)	0.05–0.20 μg/mL	Neurotransmitter		Depression
Thyroxine (T4); triiodothyronine (T3)	T4: 4–12 μg/100 mL; T3: 75–95 μg/100 mL	Tests of thyroid function	Myasthenia gravis, nephrosis, pregnancy, preeclampsia, Graves' disease, hyperthyroidism	Increased thyroid-stimulating hormone (TSH), decreased T4, T3 (hypothyroidism); malnutrition; hypothyroidism; nephrosis; cirrhosis; Simmonds' disease
Thyroid-stimulating hormone (TSH)	≤0.2 μU/L	Thyroid function tests (TSH, T4, T3)	Primary untreated hypothyroidism, post subtotal thyroidectomy	Hyperthyroidism

(continued)

TABLE B-8 Lab Values *(continued)*

Value	Normal Range	Purpose or Comment	Increased In	Decreased In
Stool Values				
Fat, fecal	<7 g/24 hr		Fat malabsorption	
Nitrogen	<2.5 g/d			
Urinalysis	Normal is pale golden yellow	Abnormal color changes: orange = high level of bile; red = blood, porphyria, urates, or bile; or ingestion of beets, blackberries, or food dyes; brown = blood; melanin may turn black on standing.	Dehydration: dark golden color	Overhydration: clear color (diluted)
Acetone, ketones	0	Elevation indicates ketosis.	Diabetic ketoacidosis, starvation, fever, prolonged vomiting, high-protein/high-fat or low-CHO diet, diarrhea, anorexia	
Aldosterone	6–16 mg/24 hr			
Ammonia	20–70 mEq/L		Hepatic disease or coma, renal failure, severe heart failure, high-protein diet	Essential hypertension
Amylase	260–950 Somogyi units/24 hr		Perforated peptic ulcer, acute pancreatitis, mumps, cholecystitis, renal insufficiency, alcohol poisoning	Hepatitis, pancreatic insufficiency, severe burns
Calcium, normal diet	<250 mg/24 hr		Hyperparathyroidism, high calcium or vitamin D in diet, immobilization, metastatic bone disease, multiple myeloma, renal tubular acidosis	Decreased levels may reflect poor intake. Hypoparathyroidism, rickets, renal failure, steatorrhea, osteomalacia
Cortisol, urinary free	10–100 μg/dL		Elevated in stress	Adrenal insufficiency
Creatinine clearance	Males (20 years old): 90 mL/min/SA; females (20 years old): 84 mL/min/SA; decreases by 6 mL/min/SA per decade		Pregnancy, childhood, exercise.	Ascites, dehydration, renal failure, CHF, shock, cirrhosis
Epinephrine, norepinephrine	Epinephrine: <10 μg/24 hr; Norepinephrine <100 μg/24 hr		Stress	
Estrogens	4–25 mg/24 hr in males; 4–60 mg/24 hr in females, higher in pregnancy			
Hemoglobin, myoglobin	0	Any amount	Blood loss, urinary tract injury	
5-Hydroxyindoleacetic acid	0	Serotonin excretion		
(5-HIAA)	20–60 mg/24 hr		Calcium oxalate stones	
Oxalate pH	4.6–8; average of 6 (dependent on diet)	Depends on time of sampling and food ingested	Alkaline: metabolic alkalemia, proteus infection, aged specimen, large amount of fruits and vegetables eaten	Acidic: high-protein intake
Protein (albumin)	<30 mg/24 hr (0 qualitative)	Amino acids in urine should be 0.4–1 g/L.	Nephrotic syndrome	
Specific gravity	1.003–1.030	Ability to concentrate urine	High in antidiuretic hormone deficiency	Low in renal tubular dysfunction
Sugar	0		Hyperglycemia, ketosis, DKA	

(continued)

TABLE B-8 Lab Values *(continued)*

Value	Normal Range	Purpose or Comment	Increased In	Decreased In
3-Methyl histidine, urine		Indicator of lean body mass turnover	Increased levels may reflect loss of lean body mass.	
Urea	20–35 g/L			
Uric acid	0.2–2.0 g/L			
Vanillylmandelic acid (VMA)	<6.8 mg/24 hr	Metabolite of both epinephrine and norepinephrine		
Volume	1000–1500 mL	Varies slightly between individuals	Diabetes insipidus	Dehydration

From: Pagana KD, Pagana TJ. *Mosby's manual of diagnostic and laboratory tests*. 2nd ed. Philadelphia: Mosby, 2002; and American Dietetic Association. *Handbook of clinical dietetics*. 2nd ed. New Haven, CT: Yale University Press, 1992, p. 21.

TABLE B-9 Quick Reference: Food–Drug Interactions

Drugs	Effects and Precautions
Antibiotics	
Cephalosporins, penicillin	Take on an empty stomach to speed absorption of the drugs.
Erythromycin	Do not take with fruit juice or wine, which decrease the drug's effectiveness.
Sulfa drugs	Increase the risk of vitamin B_{12} deficiency.
Tetracycline	Dairy products reduce the drug's effectiveness. Lowers vitamin C absorption.
Anticonvulsants	
Dilantin, phenobarbital	Increase the risk of anemia and nerve problems due to deficiency of folate and other B vitamins.
Antidepressants	
Fluoxetine	Reduces appetite and can lead to excessive weight loss.
Lithium	A low-salt diet increases the risk of lithium toxicity; excessive salt reduces the drug's efficacy.
Monoamine oxidase (MAO) inhibitors	Foods high in tyramine (aged cheeses, processed meats, legumes, wine, beer, among others) can bring on a hypertensive crisis.
Tricyclics	Many foods, especially legumes, meat, fish, and foods high in vitamin C, reduce absorption of the drugs.
Antihypertensives, Heart Medications	
Angiotensin-converting enzyme (ACE) inhibitors	Take on an empty stomach to improve the absorption of the drugs.
Alpha-blockers	Take with liquid or food to avoid excessive drop in blood pressure.
Antiarrhythmic drugs	Avoid caffeine, which increases the risk of irregular heartbeat.
Beta-blockers	Take on an empty stomach; food, especially meat, increases the drug's effects and can cause dizziness and low blood pressure.
Digitalis	Avoid taking with milk and high-fiber foods, which reduce absorption; increases potassium loss.
Diuretics	Increase the risk of potassium deficiency.
Potassium-sparing diuretics	Unless a doctor advises otherwise, do not take diuretics with potassium supplements or salt substitutes, which can cause potassium overload.
Thiazide diuretics	Increase the reaction to MSG.
Asthma Drugs	
Pseudoephedrine	Avoid caffeine, which increases feelings of anxiety and nervousness.
Theophylline	Charbroiled foods and high-protein diet reduce absorption. Caffeine increases the risk of drug toxicity.
Cholesterol-Lowering Drugs	
Cholestyramine	Increases the excretion of folate and vitamins A, D, E, and K.
Gemfibrozil	Avoid fatty foods, which decrease the drug's efficacy in lowering cholesterol.
Heartburn and Ulcer Medications	
Antacids	Interfere with the absorption of many minerals; for maximum benefit, take medication 1 hour after eating.
Cimetidine, famotidine, sucralfate	Avoid high-protein foods, caffeine, and other items that increase stomach acidity.

(continued)

TABLE B-9 Quick Reference: Food–Drug Interactions *(continued)*

Drugs	Effects and Precautions
Hormone Preparations	
Oral contraceptives	Salty foods increase fluid retention. Drugs reduce the absorption of folate, vitamin B_6, and other nutrients; increase intake of foods high in these nutrients to avoid deficiencies.
Steroids	Salty foods increase fluid retention. Increase intake of foods high in calcium, vitamin K, potassium, and protein to avoid deficiencies.
Thyroid drugs	Iodine-rich foods may lower the drug's efficacy.
Laxatives	
Mineral oils	Overuse can cause a deficiency of vitamins A, D, E, and K.
Painkillers	
Aspirin and stronger nonsteroidal anti-inflammatory drugs	Always take with food to lower the risk of gastrointestinal irritation; avoid taking with alcohol, which increases the risk of bleeding. Frequent use of these drugs lowers the absorption of folate and vitamin C.
Codeine	Increase fiber and water intake to avoid constipation.
Sleeping Pills, Tranquilizers	
Benzodiazepines	Never take with alcohol. Caffeine increases anxiety and reduce drug's effectiveness.
Weight Loss–Inducing Drugs	Many drugs cause weight loss because of changes in appetite or other side effects.

Step 2. Nutrition Diagnosis

Following a thorough assessment of patient history and current status, identify a list of nutrition problems. Using the latest edition of the Nutrition Diagnostic language from the American Dietetic Association, available from the research section at http://www.eatright.org, select the key nutrition diagnosis that will be addressed immediately and those that will be handled another time (see examples in Table B-10.)

Write a PES statement (problem, etiology, and signs and symptoms). Then select the appropriate interventions according to the etiology of the problem. Finally, identify the ways in which monitoring and evaluation will occur.

TABLE B-10 Nutrition Diagnoses

DOMAIN: CLINICAL	Self-monitoring deficit
Class: Functional Balance	Disordered eating pattern
Swallowing difficulty	Low adherence to nutrition-related recommendations
Chewing (masticatory) difficulty	Undesirable food choices
Breastfeeding difficulty	**Class: Physical and Environmental Balance**
Altered gastrointestinal (GI) function	Physical inactivity
Class: Biochemical Balance	Excessive physical activity
Impaired nutrient utilization	Inability to manage physical self-care
Altered nutrition-related laboratory values	Impaired ability to prepare foods/meals
Food medication interaction	Poor nutrition quality of life
Altered metabolic status (hyper)	Self-feeding difficulty
Altered metabolic status (hypo)	**Class: Food Safety and Access**
Class: Weight Balance	Intake of unsafe food
Underweight	Limited access to food
Involuntary weight loss	**DOMAIN: INTAKE**
Overweight/obesity	**Class: Caloric Energy Balance**
Involuntary weight gain	Increased energy needs
DOMAIN: BEHAVIORAL-ENVIRONMENTAL	Decreased energy needs
Class: Knowledge and Beliefs	Inadequate energy intake
Food and nutrition-related knowledge deficit	Excessive energy intake
Harmful beliefs/attitudes about food or nutrition-related topics	**Class: Nutrient Intake Balance**
Not ready for diet/lifestyle change	Increased nutrient (specify) needs

(continued)

TABLE B-10 Nutrition Diagnoses *(continued)*

Evident protein–energy malnutrition	Inadequate fiber intake
Inadequate protein–energy intake	Excessive fiber intake
Decreased nutrient (specify) needs	**Class: Vitamin Intake Balance**
Imbalance of nutrients	Inadequate vitamin intake (specify)
Class: Oral Intake Balance	Excessive vitamin intake (specify)
Inadequate oral food/beverage intake	**Class: Mineral Intake Balance**
Excessive oral food/beverage intake	Inadequate mineral intake (specify)
Class: Fat and Cholesterol Balance	Excessive mineral intake
Inadequate fat intake	**Class: Fluid Intake Balance**
Excessive fat intake	Inadequate fluid intake
Inappropriate intake of food fats (specify)	Excessive fluid intake
Class: Protein Balance	**Class: Bioactive Substances Balance**
Inadequate protein intake	Inadequate bioactive substance intake
Excessive protein intake	Excessive bioactive substance intake
Inappropriate intake of amino acids (specify)	Excessive alcohol intake
Class: Carbohydrate and Fiber Intake Balance	**Class: Nutrition Support**
Inadequate carbohydrate intake	Inadequate intake from enteral/parenteral nutrition infusion
Excessive carbohydrate intake	Excessive intake from enteral/parenteral nutrition
Inappropriate intake of types of carbohydrate (specify)	Inappropriate infusion of enteral/parenteral nutrition
Inconsistent carbohydrate intake	

Step 3. Intervention

Plan Establish a nutritional **care plan** to give directional stimulus to treatment efforts. Work with other disciplines for the best plan. Include evaluation of previous nutritional practices, knowledge of diet and of normal nutrition, and need for further instructions. Formulate objectives with patient and physician. Contact family when appropriate. Determine **short-term and long-term goals** (such as weight maintenance, anabolism, and correction of sodium-sensitive hypertension). Consider quality of life factors that are relevant to the patient. Consider all nutritional problems, and determine course of action. Request more data as needed (e.g., food diary, laboratory or other available tests, nutrient or energy intake analyses, or even a home visit).

Treat Select foods and dietary adjustment to meet goals, including oral, enteral, or parenteral methods. Consider underlying malnutrition, medications, chronic or acute illnesses, and patient goals. Carry out plans; this may include use of established care maps or clinical pathways. Complete anthropometric measurements. Participate in medical rounds. Consult and advise physician about necessary referrals, adaptive feeding equipment, and special wishes or needs of patient. Maintain medical team communication by making rounds or actively participating in conferences. Write and edit nutritional orders. Coordinate transitional feedings.

Educate and Counsel Assess what the patient already knows. Identify areas in which nutrition education and counseling are needed:

Inability or unwillingness to select, or disinterest in selecting food consistent with the guidelines
Inability to maintain weight or desired losses
Inability to apply food- and nutrition-related information
Inability to apply guideline information
Inability to apply nutrition-related recommendations
Inability to change food- or activity-related behavior
Inability to interpret data or self-management tools
Lack of meal preparation skill
Inability to recall agreed upon changes
Inaccurate or incomplete understanding/information related to guidelines or needed changes
Inaccurate or incomplete written response to questionnaire/written tool, or is unable to read written tool
Insufficient knowledge of breastfeeding or infant hunger/satiety signals
Limited food and nutrition-related knowledge
Limited knowledge of carbohydrate composition of foods or of carbohydrate metabolism
Lack of compliance or inconsistent compliance with plan
Lack of efficacy to make changes or to overcome barriers to change
Relates concerns about previous attempts to learn information
Uncertainty as to how to consistently apply food/nutrition information

Uncertainty of how to complete monitoring records
Uncertainty regarding appropriate foods to prepare based upon nutrition prescription
Uncertainty regarding changes that could/should be made in response to data in self-monitoring records
Uncertainty regarding nutrition-related recommendations

Using a client-centered approach, explain the relationship of diet to disorder and disease and the patient's/client's role in management. Explain the diet, including dietary principles, ways to change and improve habits, written materials, sample menus, and meal patterns. Evaluate potential food–drug interactions; counsel accordingly.

Use nutrition counseling skills. The goal is to promote desirable outcomes by promoting healthful behavior and involving patient and family in care decisions (Escott-Stump et al, 2000). Conduct group classes and outpatient conferences when needed. Use appropriate audiovisual aids and teaching tools. Teach using principles of adult education, lifestyle change management, and stages of change. Table B-11 provides many tips for planning educational sessions. The Health Belief Model is shown in Table B-12 and Figure B-2. Active learning is shown in Figure B-3.

TABLE B-11 Patient Education and Counseling Tips

Concept of the Adult Learner (Knowles, 1980)	During the process of maturation, a person moves from dependency toward increasing self-directedness, but at different rates for different people and in different dimensions of life. Teachers have a responsibility to encourage and nurture this movement. Adults have a deep psychological need to be generally self-directing, but they may be dependent in certain temporary situations.
Role of the Learner's Experience (Knowles, 1980)	As people grow and develop, they accumulate an increasing reservoir of experience that becomes and increasingly rich resource for learning—for themselves and for others. Furthermore, people attach more meaning to learnings they gain from experience than those they acquire passively. Accordingly, the primary techniques in education are experiential ones—laboratory experiments, discussion, problem-solving cases, field experiences, etc.
Readiness to Learn (Knowles, 1980)	People become ready to learn something when they experience a need to learn it in order to cope more satisfyingly with real-life tasks and problems. The educator has a responsibility to create conditions and provide tools and procedures for helping learners discover their "needs to know." Learning programs should be organized around life-application categories and sequenced according to the learners' readiness to learn. Key: Attend to learners' developmental readiness.
Orientation to Learning (Knowles, 1980)	Learners see education as a process of developing increased competence to achieve their full potential in life. They want to be able to apply whatever knowledge and skill they gain today to living more effectively tomorrow. Accordingly, learning experiences should be organized around competency-development categories. People are performance-centered in their orientation to learning.
Assumptions (Knowles, 1980)	1. All learners can think; critical and creative thinking are goals. 2. There needs to be a safe, risk-taking environment and sufficient time to learn. 3. The environment for learning should be rich and responsive. 4. Offer challenging problem solving opportunities.
Chief Assessment Factors	1. Socioeconomic factors. 2. Cultural, religious beliefs and background. 3. Age and sex of patient and significant others (SOs). 4. Birth order of patient and family involvement. 5. Occupation. 6. Medical status and medical history. 7. Marital status; number and ages of children. 8. Cognitive status; educational level. 9. Readiness to learn and staging: precontemplation, contemplation, preparation, action, or maintenance. 10. Emotional status (stress, acceptance of illness, chronic disease, or condition).
Health Literacy and Teaching Tools	Low health literacy (the ability to read, understand, and act on health information) is a public health issue. One out of five American adults reads at the 5th grade level or below, and the average American reads at the 8th to 9th grade level. Most consumers need help understanding health care information. Patients prefer medical information that is easy to read and understand. Easy-to-read health care materials are *essential*. Provide important information first. Highlight the need to know versus nice to know.
Written Materials	1. Print very clearly and avoid handwritten messages. Use large print; font size should be a minimum of 12 points. 2. Double space text to avoid crowding. Avoid using all capital letters. Use headings to introduce the upcoming topic. 3. Avoid abbreviations, and use black ink on light-colored paper.

(continued)

TABLE B-11 Patient Education and Counseling Tips *(continued)*

	4. Information must be current and accurate. Provide important information first. 5. Highlight the need to know versus nice to know. 6. Present information in a "how to" manner. 7. Use conversational style. 8. Spell out numbers less than 10. 9. Keep syllables to 1–2 per word. Keep sentences short, and use bullets when possible.
Tools	1. Newsletters and bulletin boards. 2. Demonstrations or role playing. 3. Laboratory reports, flip charts. 4. Food recall or intake records with feedback. 5. Educational games and fun quizzes. 6. Group classes or supermarket tours. 7. Educational video and audio tapes.
Visual Aids	1. Visuals should be able to stand alone, without words. 2. Use photographs and realistic images. 3. Use culturally appropriate food models, empty packages of real foods, and measuring cups and spoons. 4. Work with restaurant menus where needed. 5. Share simple recipes.
Principles of Learning	1. The recipient must value information. 2. Pace should be adequate for learner; take small steps. 3. Environment should be conducive to learning (free of distractions and stress), and patient should be ready to learn (free from pain). 4. Information must be meaningful, relevant, and organized. Material should be logical in sequence. 5. Counselor must be truly interested in sharing the information. 6. Adequate follow-up should be available for reinforcement of facts and principles. 7. For adult learners, information that is useful in the present is more meaningful than facts learned for the "future." 8. Adults tend to prefer problem-solving information (e.g., survival skills) over learning facts alone.
Principles of Teaching	1. Counselor must first listen to patient. Involve patient in setting mutual objectives. 2. Small segments of information should be presented in understandable language in small, manageable "sound bites." 3. An organized plan should be used to teach. Clear objectives should be established, with timelines and short- and long-term outcomes. 4. Feedback should be used with each step. Be prepared to receive evaluation (peer review) from patient; improve as needed. 5. Good eye contact should be maintained with patient. Be aware, however, that direct or prolonged eye contact would be seen as rude or threatening by some cultures; know your client. 6. Appropriate teaching tools or audiovisual aids should be used as appropriate. Using a 6th–8th grade reading level is suggested with easy layout, visual appeal, and illustrations. 7. Questions must be allowed for clarification. 8. Praise and positive reinforcement should be offered to learner. Carl Rogers emphasizes use of "unconditional positive regard" for all persons.
Counseling Tips	1. Knowledge does not automatically ensure compliance. Behavioral change takes time and encouragement. 2. Trial and error will be common for patient in learning new behaviors. 3. Increase in self-esteem comes with improvement in behavior. 4. Counselor should appropriately foster independence. 5. Empathy is an important part of humanistic care. 6. Counselor serves as an intervention specialist. The "patient-centered" approach to counseling is effective. 7. Steps include assessing stage of change and motivation level of client, assessing past experiences with dietary changes, assessing anticipated challenges, identifying challenges and obstacles, identifying coping strategies and skills, setting goals, identifying steps needed for follow-up, and anticipating lapses and relapses (Rosal et al, 2001). 8. Goal setting as a strategy for behavioral change requires that the patient recognize the need for change, establish a goal, monitor goal-related activity, and use self-reward for goal attainment (Cullen et al, 2001).

(continued)

TABLE B-11 Patient Education and Counseling Tips *(continued)*

Health Belief Model	The Health Belief Model (HBM) is a psychological model that attempts to explain and predict health behaviors by focusing on the attitudes and beliefs of individuals; it was originally introduced in the 1950s by psychologists working in the U.S. Public Health Service. See Table B-12 and Figure B-2.
Patient Assessment of Chronic Illness Care (PACIC tool)	Patient-centered model of behavioral counseling using the **5As**: **Assess:** Beliefs, behavior, and knowledge. **Advise:** Provide specific information about health risks and benefits of change. **Agree:** Collaboratively set goals based on patient's interest and confidence in their ability to change the behavior. **Assist:** Identify personal barriers, strategies, problem-solving techniques and social/environmental support. **Arrange:** Specify plan for follow-up (e.g., visits, phone calls, mailed reminders). Figure B-3 shows an ideal flow for active learning.
Counseling for End-of-Life or Hospice Patients (Lattanzi-Licht and Gallagher-Allred, 2001)	1. Attempt to reduce fears related to eating. 2. Recognize stages of terminal illness: fear of abandonment, finding a natural and realistic approach, building bridges, and ownership of the experience. 3. Pain management is most important for quality of life. 4. Respect individual's cultural beliefs and needs. 5. Identify a patient advocate who will address concerns as care progresses. 6. Help maintain self-esteem and dignity. 7. Comfort foods can be important to patient satisfaction; identify and address these needs on a meal-to-meal basis. 8. Look for hidden messages from patient; communicate with other health care team members.

TABLE B-12 Health Belief Model

Concept	Definition	Application
Perceived Susceptibility	One's opinion of chances of getting a condition.	Define population(s) at risk, risk levels. Personalize risk based on a person's features or behavior. Heighten perceived susceptibility if too low.
Perceived Severity	One's opinion of how serious a condition and its sequelae are.	Specify consequences of the risk and the condition.
Perceived Benefits	One's opinion of the efficacy of the advised action to reduce risk or seriousness of impact.	Define action to take: how, where, when; clarify the positive effects to be expected.
Perceived Barriers	One's opinion of the tangible and psychological costs of the advised action.	Identify and reduce barriers through reassurance, incentives, and assistance.
Cues to Action	Strategies to activate readiness.	Provide how-to information, promote awareness, reminders.
Self-Efficacy	Confidence in one's ability to take action.	Provide training, guidance in performing action.

From: Family Health International. Behavior change: a summary of four major theories. Accessed February 23, 2006 at http://www.fhi.org/NR/rdonlyres/ei26vbslpsidmahhxc332vwo3g233xsqw22er3vofqvrfjvubwyzclvqjcbdgexyzl3msu4mn6xv5j/BCCSummaryFourMajorTheories.pdf; and National Institutes of Health, National Cancer Institute. Theory at a glance: a guide for health promotion practice. Accessed February 23, 2006 at http://www.cancer.gov/theory/pdf.

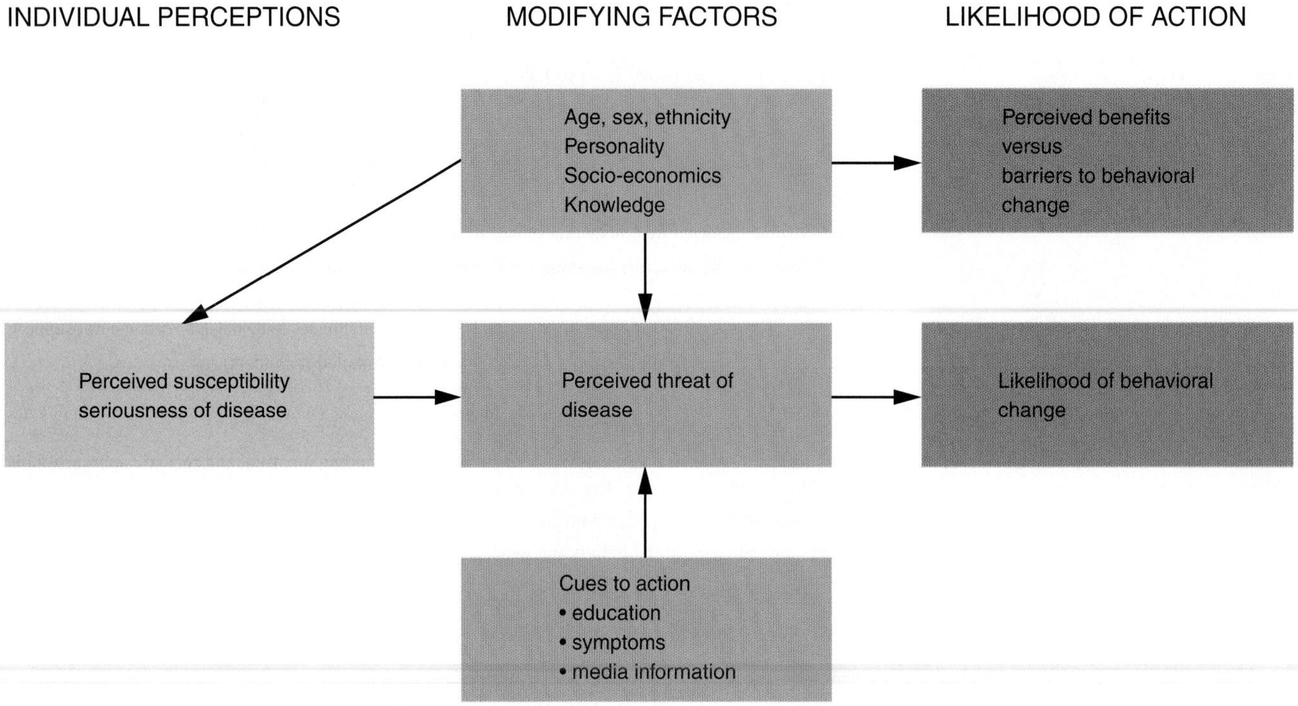

Figure B-2 Health Behavior Model. (Reprinted with permission from Glanz K, et al. *Health behavior and health education. Theory, research and practice*. San Francisco, CA: Wiley & Sons, 2002.)

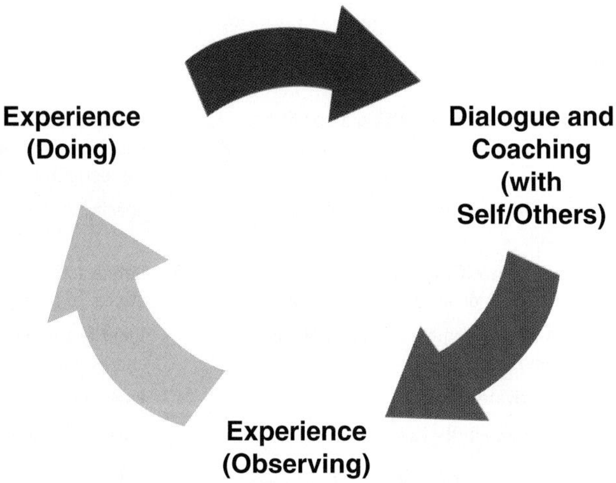

Figure B-3 Active Learning Process.

ASSESSMENT: Summary of subjective and objective data from chart review and patient/caregiver.

Ht____Wt____ IBW or IBW %____ Estimated needs for Energy______Protein______Fluid______Other Nutrients________

Intake approximately _________% at meals and/or _______% from TF and/or _______% from PN

Abnormal lab values______________________________ Liquids, Nausea, Vomiting, Diarrhea > 5 days Yes/No

Usual Meds____Side effects? Yes/No

Current Meds____Side effects? Yes/No

Food allergies____________________________Food intolerances:____________________________

Other Comments:____

NUTRITION DIAGNOSIS:	ETIOLOGY:	INTERVENTIONS:

MONITORING:

Previous Wt_______Current Wt_______%Change_______Comment on Progress_____________________

Previous labs compared with current labs:

Food-drug interaction potential and status:

EVALUATION:

Previous Problems -- Clinical Concerns: Comment on Progress_________________

Previous Problems -- Behavioral - Environmental Concerns: Comment on Progress_________________

Previous Intake compared with Current Intake:_______________ Comment on Progress_________________

Previous Educational Needs and Sessions Provided:______________Comment on Progress_________________

Other Evaluations and Plans or Recommendations:

Date:_____________ Dietitian (RD) ______________________________ Nutrition Provider #_______________

Figure B-4 Sample nutrition chart form using A-D-I-M-E format.

Document Use the Nutrition Care Process, preferably with A-D-I-M-E content: **A**ssessment, Nutrition **D**iagnosis, **I**ntervention, **M**onitoring, and **E**valuation. See Figure B-4. Use Figure B-5 to evaluate patient contact effectiveness.

Step 4. Monitoring

Monitor food intake, nitrogen balance, and laboratory values. Monitor patient's nutritional progress, including portion control, ingredient control, meal quality, and delivery system (oral, tube feeding, or parenteral nutrition). Monitor efficacy of therapy and nutritional interventions. See Table B-13 for Patient Care Audit.

Step 5. Evaluation

Evaluate care plan and outcomes; determine which goals, if any, have been met. Evaluate using comparisons with JCAHO, state, other federal and local regulations and accrediting agencies. Evaluate according to evidence-based practice guides (Myers et al, 2001). Evaluate number and depth of changes that have occurred—weight, dietary behavior, and laboratory data. Provide reassessment of nutritional problems and etiologies as needed. When feasible, give a follow-up call to patient after discharge or conduct a home visit. Evaluate or test knowledge of patient/client and family members; see Table B-14 for Sample Patient Education Outcomes. Figure B-6 shows how a registered dietitian practices at advanced levels.

Rubric for Evaluating Patient Contact Effectiveness

Key: Score the behaviors in categories related to rapport, screening and gathering data, transition, and documentation.

Establishing Rapport

A. Introduction: **Patient's Name**

4	Inquires about patient's name. Verifies correct name. Uses appropriate formality.
3	Makes an error about the name or formality, but corrects it and goes on.
2	Does not use name or uses inappropriate level of formality, but not continuously.
1	Continuously gets name wrong and/or uses inappropriate level of formality. Interviews wrong patient even after verification of name.

SCORE____

Provider's Name

4	States full name and that he or she is a dietetic professional.
3	States name clearly, but omits full name. Role not clear.
2	Gives name, but not understandably.
1	Does not give name or role.

SCORE____

Non-Verbal Communication

4	Establishes and maintains eye contact. Attentive posture. Appropriate personal space.
3	Generally appropriate, but has difficulty with one of the items.
2	Has difficulty with two of the items.
1	Wraps self up in arms to create a shell. Gestures wildly. Doesn't keep appropriate personal space. No eye contact. Poor posture.

SCORE____

B. Outline of Visit: **Nature and Focus of the Visit**

4	Reminds patient about the nature of the visit. If the patient has a problem that requires immediate attention from the preceptor, it is handled immediately.
3	Vaguely mentions the nature of the visit. Delays in helping situations that require immediate attention.
2	Does not give an accurate or clear account of the nature of the visit. Tries to deal with urgent situation.
1	Misrepresents the nature of the clinic. Ignores situations that are urgent.

SCORE____

Screening/Data Gathering **Questions**

4	Begins with open-ended question. Allows patient to fully express self. Uses additional open-ended questions to encourage conversation. Uses closed questions to complete the information needed.
3	Developing a comfort level with open and closed questions. Uses correct questions most of the time.
2	Interrupts the patient too often to get a complete story. Uses too many closed questions and not enough open ones.
1	Asks multiple closed questions together and does not give patient time to answer. For example, asking the patient "Do you have difficulty preparing meals, shopping and getting to the doctor?" all in one question.

SCORE____

Components

4	Gets all of the following information: chief complaint, prior medical history, dietary history, anthropometrics, physical exam results, lab data, drugs, activity level, social/family history, screening level.
3	Gets at least 8 out 10 of the components.
2	Gets at least 5 of 10 of the components.
1	Not yet getting 5 of 10 of the components.

SCORE____

Responses

4	Responds with head nodding and appropriate gestures. Responds to emotional situations with acknowledgement and empathy (the capacity for participation in another's feelings or ideas).
3	Encourages patient with nods and gestures but the response is not empathic.
2	Remarks, while not judgmental or offensive, do not acknowledge the patient. Avoids acknowledging patient emotion.
1	Makes judgmental remarks in response to patient situation. Completely skips acknowledgement of patient. Makes light of patient perspective.

SCORE____

Figure B-5 Rubric for evaluating patient contact effectiveness.

Closure

4	Seeks common ground. Asks patient's sense of what is going on. Asks if they can think of any reason for what is happening. Asks if there is anything else that the patient wants to share.	
3	Asks two of the questions, but doesn't really give credence to what the patient says.	
2	Ask one of these questions, but doesn't really allow the patient to have his or her say.	
1	Has hand on the door while still talking. Wraps up too quickly. Communicates lack of respect.	SCORE____

Handwashing before Exam

4	Done before any skinfold measurement or examination. Good contact with soap and warm water. Dry with towel.	
3	Uses soap and warm water, but not enough diligence to contact and not long enough.	
2	Sloppy or cursory manner. Sloppy about soap. Wet hands.	
1	Not done.	SCORE____

Response to Patient Inquiries

4	Limits responses to what they know. Gives information with evidence as appropriate.	
3	Limits responses to what they know and doesn't expand beyond their capabilities, but doesn't provide evidence with the information.	
2	Expands slightly beyond what they know.	
1	Clearly does not limit responses to what they know. May bluff or give incorrect information.	SCORE____

Progression to Treatment

4	Presents good information to patient. Does not recommend treatment beyond what has been planned.	
3	Listens, but does not actively partner with patient. Stays within comfort limits.	
2	May mention treatments before decisions have been made.	
1	Recommends treatments without evaluation of whole plan.	SCORE____

Transition

Leaving

4	Expresses gratitude to patient. Clear explanation of follow-up plans.	
3	Does both things, but neither are as clear as needed.	
2	Does only one of the two things.	
1	Leaves room abruptly with no explanation.	SCORE____

Ending Patient Encounter

4	Asks patient to summarize encounter. Check understanding with patient. Asks "Where are we now?" Uses common ground and ties up loose ends.	
3	Asks patient to summarize encounter, but doesn't check for understanding or tie up loose ends.	
2	Can summarize encounter, but doesn't include patient in the process.	
1	Leaves patient hanging with no clear understanding of encounter.	SCORE____

Documentation

Computer or Cardex Entry

4	Documents encounter on computer. Includes all assessment data.	
3	Documents most of record but content incomplete.	
2	Documentation delayed.	
1	Does not follow protocols for documentation.	SCORE____

Total Possible Score 56 Provider Score:

Figure B-5 *(continued)*

TABLE B-13 Patient Care Audit

Dietitian:_______________ Reviewed by_______________ Date:___________

Nutrition Care Evaluation	Poor	Fair	Good	Excellent
ASSESSMENT				
Pertinent medical and surgical histories reviewed and documented				
Medications with potential food/drug interactions are assessed and documented				
Relevant laboratory values are noted and assessed for age/sex				
Relevant findings that may effect nutritional status are assessed and documented				
Height and weight are documented				
Subjective nutritional data are obtained and documented				
Nutritional requirements for energy/protein/fluid are assessed and calculated based on established standards or DRI for age/sex				
Appropriate nutritional priority and risk identified				
NUTRITION DIAGNOSIS				
Appropriate nutrition diagnosis selected				
Correct PES statement written (problem-etiology-signs/symptoms)				
INTERVENTIONS				
Nutrition care plan established that includes patient/family goals and objectives				
Meal plan established and implemented when needed				
Nutrition recommendations are appropriate for patient condition				
Education assessment and plans are completed when appropriate.				
Identified preferred method of learning: visual__ auditory___ reading___ hands-on___.				
When education is provided, patient/family understanding is documented				
MONITORING AND EVALUATION				
Outpatient nutrition clinic referral completed				
Other referral(s) completed for MD/social worker/dental/other:				
Documented need and time frame for follow-up to occur				
Nutrition recommendations/interventions are appropriate, based on assessed data of disease state, medical goals of therapy, biochemical parameters				
Follow-up notes re-evaluate nutritional problems and plan with supporting documentation				
Documentation completed for all steps				
Please rate the chart for overall assessment, nutrition diagnosis, intervention, monitoring, evaluation, and documentation.				

TABLE B-14 Sample Outcome Audits—Patient Education

This patient education audit identifies the ability of the patient to demonstrate or verbalize how he or she will or has changed behaviors after nutritional instructions.

Any Patient

1. Patient is able to personalize the MyPyramid food guidance system.
2. Patient is able to explain importance of his or her diet to his or her health.
3. Patient is able to plan ____ day's menus and snacks from his/her dietary pattern.
4. Patient is able to incorporate desirable economic/ethnic food choices into his/her prescribed diet.
5. Patient has been following _____diet at home for period of time and is able to describe elements of this diet with accuracy.
6. Patient expresses recognition of need to lose/gain weight.
7. Patient is able to describe specific food allergies and food ingredients to avoid.
8. Patient is able to describe the reasons for following _______diet (e.g., improve appearance, increase energy, reduce chances for complications, improve quality of life).
9. Patient is able to describe the role of appropriate activity or exercise on health and nutritional well-being.

(continued)

TABLE B-14 Sample Outcome Audits—Patient Education *(continued)*

Cardiac Diet

1. Patient is able to name three beverages that are high in caffeine.
2. Patient is able to describe modifications in his or her diet that will be needed to prevent further coronary complications: saturated versus poly- and monounsaturated fats, sodium and potassium, fiber, and use of the DASH diet.
3. Patient is able to categorize correctly into the proper food pyramid lists.
4. Patient is able to plan menus for home use that include appropriate modifications.
5. Patient is able to name snack foods that can be included in dietary plan.

Diabetes Diet

1. Patient is able to explain relationship of diet to complications of diabetes.
2. Patient is able to name foods that contain CHO.
3. Patient is able to preplan meals for _____weeks.
4. Patient is able to verbalize a simple definition of diabetes.
5. Patient is able to describe role of medications related to food intake.
6. Patient is able to explain rationale for following a prudent diet to prevent complications such as heart disease.
7. Patient is able to explain how proper spacing of meals affects his/her disorder.
8. Patient is able to describe symptoms of ketoacidosis and insulin shock and can name foods to take or avoid for each condition.
9. After looking at several food labels, patient is able to point out ingredients that mean carbohydrate.
10. Patient is able to describe techniques for managing special events (travel, parties, restaurants, holiday meals, weekends).
11. Patient is able to describe his or her personal exercise prescription as ___ minutes of activity ___ times per week.
12. Patient is able to describe 1–2 items to carry in case of episodes of low blood glucose.
13. Patient is able to define when to call his or her health provider (e.g., when glucose is above/below normal ___ times).
14. Patient is able to discuss proper foot care, the need for eye exams, and the need for foot exams.

Dumping Syndrome Diet

1. Patient is able to verbalize effects of diet on dumping syndrome.
2. Patient is able to explain guidelines to be followed to prevent dumping syndrome (e.g., beverages are served 30 minutes before or after meals; concentrated sweets omitted or severely limited).

Gliadin-Free/Gluten-Restricted Diet

1. Patient is able to examine food labels and to name ingredients that must be avoided.
2. Patient is able to list products that must be avoided in diet.
3. Patient is able to plan menus that can be used at home.
4. Patient is able to adapt recipes for use at home.

High-Fiber Diet

1. Patient is able to verbalize foods that can be used to increase fiber in his or her diet, to desired level of ___ g daily.
2. Patient is able to explain role of fiber in his or her particular disorder.
3. Patient is able to describe purpose of adequate fluids in dietary regimen and is able to consume ___ mL daily.

Lactose Intolerance Diet

1. Patient is able to name foods or beverages that must be avoided.
2. Patient is able to plan menus that are nutritionally complete for calcium but are lactose restricted.
3. Patient demonstrates awareness that he or she can tolerate up to ___ mL of lactose per day at this time.
4. Patient is able to discuss difference between lactose intolerance and milk allergy.

Low-Cholesterol and Dyslipidemia Diets

1. Patient is able to describe simple definitions for cholesterol and saturated, polyunsaturated, and monounsaturated fats.
2. Patient is able to identify foods that have high cholesterol content.
3. Patient is able to name vegetable oils that may be used in diet.
4. Patient is able to describe three cooking methods that are acceptable for dietary regimen.
5. Patient is able to name foods that are good sources of monounsaturated fats.

(continued)

TABLE B-14 Sample Outcome Audits—Patient Education *(continued)*

Low-Fat Diet

1. Patient is able to name foods that he or she must omit for the low-fat diet.
2. Patient is able to explain role of fat in his or her condition.
3. Patient is able to note grams of fat from a given food label.

Mineral-Altered Diets (Iron, Potassium, Calcium, Sodium)

1. Patient is able to name foods that are high/low in mineral.
2. Patient is able to accurately select menu choices for days that include/exclude foods that are high in mineral.
3. Patient is able to plan menus for home that are high/low in mineral.

Pregnancy Diet

1. Patient is able to describe nutritional changes to her diet in order to have a healthy baby.
2. Patient is able to describe why breastfeeding is an important consideration.

Protein-Altered Diets

1. Patient can identify foods that contain protein of high biological value.
2. Patient can name foods to include/omit in diet to increase/decrease protein content of meals and snacks.

Renal Diets

1. Patient is able to describe restrictions that are needed in regard to protein, sodium, potassium, fluid, calories, and phosphorus.
2. Patient is able to plan menus that are balanced for the restricted nutrients.
3. Patient is able to name "free" foods that he or she can eat as desired.
4. Patient is able to discuss how foods, nutrients, and prescribed medications may interact.

Sodium Restrictions

1. Patient is able to name foods that are naturally high in sodium.
2. Patient is able to name foods that have been processed or prepared with excesses of sodium.
3. Patient is able to explain difference between "salt" and "sodium" in foods.
4. Patient is able to list seasonings that can be used at home in place of salt and salt-containing seasonings.
5. Patient is able to plan menus for home that will be low in sodium.
6. Patient is able to identify salt substitutes that he or she can use for his or her condition.
7. Patient is able to discuss how other minerals (potassium, calcium, magnesium) play a role in the specific condition.

Vegetarian Diet

1. Patient is able to identify correctly two or more complementary protein foods.
2. Patient is able to plan menus that provide adequate protein and vitamin B_{12}, zinc, etc., for age and sex.

Weight Management Diet

1. Patient is able to verbalize his or her primary motivation for losing weight and current readiness for change in behaviors.
2. Patient is able to describe his or her realistic goal for weight loss—either short term or long term, including a timetable.
3. Patient is able to list foods that are low in energy that may be eaten as snacks.
4. Patient is able to categorize foods into the proper pyramid food categories.
5. Patient is able to demonstrate proper technique for recording food intake at home.
6. Patient has demonstrated weight loss over a certain time frame.

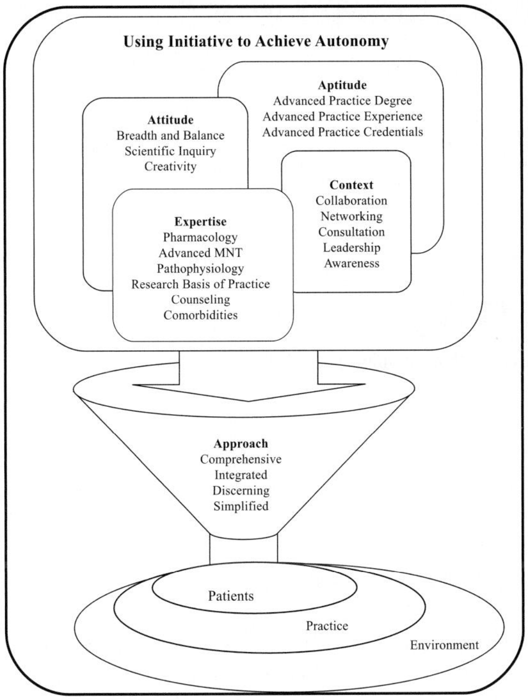

Figure B-6 Using initiative to achieve autonomy: A model of advanced medical nutrition therapy (MNT) practice. (From Skipper AL, Lewis NM. Using initiative to achieve autonomy: a model for advanced practice in medical nutrition therapy. *J Am Diet Assoc.* 106:1219, 2006.

REFERENCES

American Gastroenterological Association. Medical Position Statement: parenteral nutrition. *Gastroenterology* 121:966, 2001.

Anker SD, et al. ESPEN Guidelines on Enteral Nutrition: cardiology and pulmonology. *Clin Nutr.* 25:311, 2006.

Baird Schwartz D, Gudzin D. Preadmission nutrition screening: expanding hospital-based nutrition services by implementing earlier nutrition interventions. *J Am Diet Assoc.* 100:81, 2000.

Bandura A. Self-efficacy: toward a unifying theory of behavioral change. *Psychol Rev.* 84:191, 1977.

Bandura A. *Social foundations of thought and action: a social cognitive theory.* Englewood Cliffs, NJ: Prentice-Hall, 1986.

Bandura A. *Self-efficacy: the exercise of control.* New York: W. H. Freeman, 1997.

Barr J, et al. Case problem: quality of life outcomes assessment—how can you use it in medical nutrition therapy? *J Am Diet Assoc.* 101:1064, 2001.

Braga JM, et al. Implementation of dietitian recommendations for enteral nutrition results in improved outcomes. *J Am Diet Assoc.* 106:281, 2006.

Byham-Gray LD, et al. Evidence-based practice: what are dietitians' perceptions, attitudes, and knowledge? *J Am Diet Assoc.* 105:1574, 2005.

Cano N, et al. ESPEN Guidelines on Enteral Nutrition: adult renal failure. *Clin Nutr.* 25:295, 2006.

Ceres D, et al. Parenteral nutrition safe practices: results of the 2003 American Society for Parenteral and Enteral Nutrition survey. *J Parenter Enteral Nutr.* 30:259, 2006.

Cullen KW, et al. Using goal setting as a strategy for dietary behavior change. *J Am Diet Assoc.* 101:562, 2001.

Dahlke R, et al. Focus groups as predictors of dieticians' roles on interdisciplinary teams. *J Am Diet Assoc.* 100:455, 2000.

Durfee SM, et al. Standards for specialized nutrition support for adult residents of long-term care facilities. *Nutr Clin Pract.* 21:96, 2006.

Escott-Stump S, et al. Joint Commission on Accreditation of Healthcare Institutions: friend or foe? *J Am Diet Assoc.* 100:839, 2000.

Family Health International. Behavior change: a summary of four different theories. Accessed February 23, 2006 at http://www.fhi.org/NR/rdonlyres/ei26vbslpsidmahhxc332vwo3g233xsqw22er3vofqvrfjvubwyzclvqjcbdgexyzl3msu4mn6xv5j/BCCSummaryFourMajorTheories.pdf#search='Behavior%20Change%3A%20A%20Summary%20of%20Four%20Major%20Theories'.

Fox T. Institute of Medicine urges Medicare coverage of medical nutrition therapy. *J Am Diet Assoc.* 100:166, 2000.

Harris J, Benedict F. *A biometric study of basal metabolism in man.* Publication no. 279. Washington, DC: Carnegie Institute of Washington, 1919.

Kattelmann K, et al. Preliminary evidence for a medical nutrition therapy protocol: enteral feedings for critically ill patients. *J Am Diet Assoc.* 106:1226, 2006.

Kieselhorst K, et al. American Dietetic Association: standards of practice in nutrition care and updated standards of professional performance. *J Am Diet Assoc.* 105:641, 2005.

Knowles M. *The modern practice of adult education: from pedagogy to andragogy.* 2nd ed. New York: Association Press, 1980.

Krebs NF, Primak LE. Comprehensive integration of nutrition into medical training. *Am J Clin Nutr.* 83:945S, 2006.

Kreymann KG, et al. ESPEN Guidelines on Enteral Nutrition: intensive care. *Clin Nutr.* 25:210, 2006.

Lattanzi-Licht M, Gallagher-Allred C. End of life nutrition. Presentation at Food and Nutrition Conference and Exhibition, October 23, 2001.

Lemon CC, et al. Outcomes monitoring of health, behavior, and quality of life after nutrition intervention in adults with type 2 diabetes. *J Am Diet Assoc.* 104:1805, 2004.

Lochs H, et al. ESPEN Guidelines on Enteral Nutrition: gastroenterology. *Clin Nutr.* 25:260, 2006.

Meakins JL. Innovation in surgery: the rules of evidence. *Am J Surg.* 183:399, 2002.

Meier R, et al. ESPEN Guidelines on Enteral Nutrition: pancreas. *Clin Nutr.* 25:275, 2006.

Mislevy J, et al. Clinical nutrition managers have access to sources of empowerment. *J Am Diet Assoc.* 100:1038, 2000.

Moreland K, et al. Development of implementation of the Clinical Privileges for Dietitian Nutrition Order Writing program at a long-term acute care hospital. *J Am Diet Assoc.* 102:72, 2002.

Myers E, et al. Clinical privileges: missing piece of the puzzle for clinical standards that elevate responsibilities and salaries for registered dietitians? *J Am Diet Assoc.* 102:123, 2002.

Myers E, et al. Evidence-based practice guides vs. protocols: what's the difference? *J Am Diet Assoc.* 101:1085, 2001.

National Institutes of Health, National Cancer Institute. Theory at a glance: a guide for health promotion practice. Accessed February 23, 2006 at http://www.cancer.gov/theory/pdf.

Neidert K. Position of the American Dietetic Association: liberalization of the diet prescription improves quality of life for older adults in long-term care. *J Am Diet Assoc.* 105:1955, 2005.

Ockenga J, et al. ESPEN Guidelines on Enteral Nutrition: wasting in HIV and other chronic infectious diseases. *Clin Nutr.* 25:319, 2006.

PACIC. Patient Assessment of Chronic Illness Care Tool. Accessed February 23, 2006 at http://www.improvingchroniccare.org/tools/PACIC26itemscale.pdf.

Plauth M, et al. ESPEN Guidelines on Enteral Nutrition: liver disease. *Clin Nutr.* 25:285, 2006.

Reader D, et al. Impact of gestational diabetes mellitus nutrition practice guidelines implemented by registered dietitians on pregnancy outcomes. *J Am Diet Assoc.* 106:1426, 2006.

Robien K, et al. American Dietetic Association: standards of practice and standards of professional performance for registered dietitians (generalist, specialty, and advanced) in oncology nutrition care. *J Am Diet Assoc.* 106:946, 2006.

Rogers D. Report on the American Dietetic Association/ADA Foundation/Commission on Dietetic Registration 2004 Dietetics Professionals Needs Assessment. *J Am Diet Assoc.* 105:1348, 2005.

Rosal M, et al. Facilitating dietary change: the patient-centered counseling model. *J Am Diet Assoc.* 101:332, 2001.

Silverman M, et al. Current and future practices in hospital foodservice. *J Am Diet Assoc.* 100:76, 2000.

Simmons SF, Schnelle JF. Feeding assistance needs of long-stay nursing home residents and staff time to provide care. *J Am Geriatr Soc.* 54:919, 2006.

Stang J, et al. Position of the American Dietetic Association: child and adolescent food and nutrition programs. *J Am Diet Assoc.* 106:1467, 2006.

Swift CS, Bouchrr JL. Nutrition therapy for the hospitalized patient with diabetes. *Endocr Pract.* 12:61S, 2006.

Volkert D, et al. ESPEN Guidelines on Enteral Nutrition: geriatrics. *Clin Nutr.* 25:330, 2006.

Wasink B, The American Dietetic Association. Position of the American Dietetic Association: food and nutrition misinformation. *J Am Diet Assoc.* 106:601, 2006.

Weimann A, et al. ESPEN Guidelines on Enteral Nutrition: surgery including organ transplantation. *Clin Nutr.* 25:224, 2006.

A P P E N D I X C

Standardized Language, Nutrition Diagnosis, Problem-Based Learning, and Case Studies

NUTRITION CARE PROCESS AND STANDARDIZED LANGUAGE

This appendix provides practice in using the new Standardized Language for the profession. Tables C-1 and C-2 summarize the nutrition diagnoses and interventions used by the dietetics profession.

PROBLEM-BASED LEARNING

In problem-based learning (PBL), you can work in small groups to discuss the following cases and to add other interesting conditions or dietary recall information in order to make the cases more challenging and interesting.

TABLE C-1 Nutrition Diagnostic Labels and Definitions

Nutrition Diagnostic Label	Label Number	Definition of Diagnostic Label
DOMAIN: CLINICAL	NC	
Defined as "nutritional findings/problems identified that relate to medical or physical conditions"		
Class: Functional Balance (1)		
Defined as "change in physical or mechanical functioning that interferes with or prevents desired nutritional consequences"		
Swallowing difficulty	NC-1.1	Impaired movement of food and liquid from the mouth to the stomach
Chewing (masticatory) difficulty	NC-1.2	Impaired ability to manipulate or masticate food for swallowing
Breastfeeding difficulty	NC-1.3	Inability to sustain nutrition through breastfeeding
Altered GI function	NC-1.4	Changes in ability to digest or absorb nutrients
Class: Biochemical Balance (2)		
Defined as "change in capacity to metabolize nutrients as a result of medications, surgery, or as indicated by altered lab values"		
Impaired nutrient utilization	NC-2.1	Changes in ability to absorb or metabolize nutrients and bioactive substances
Altered nutrition-related laboratory values	NC-2.2	Changes in ability to eliminate byproducts of digestive and metabolic processes
Food medication interaction	NC-2.3	Undesirable/harmful interaction(s) between food and over-the-counter (OTC) medications, prescribed medications, herbals, botanicals, and/or dietary supplements that diminishes, enhances, or alters effect of nutrients and/or medications
Class: Weight Balance (3)		
Defined as "chronic weight or changed weight status when compared with usual or desired body weight"		
Underweight	NC-3.1	Low body weight compared to established reference standards or recommendations
Involuntary weight loss	NC-3.2	Decrease in body weight that is not planned or desired

(continued)

TABLE C-1 Nutrition Diagnostic Labels and Definitions *(continued)*

Nutrition Diagnostic Label	Label Number	Definition of Diagnostic Label
Overweight/obesity	NC-3.3	Increased adiposity compared to established reference standards or recommendations
Involuntary weight gain	NC-3.4	Weight gain above that which is desired or expected
DOMAIN: BEHAVIORAL-ENVIRONMENTAL		
Defined as "nutritional findings/problems identified that relate to knowledge, attitudes/beliefs, physical environment, or access to food and food safety"	NB	
Class: Knowledge and Beliefs (1)		
Defined as "actual knowledge and beliefs as reported, observed, or documented"		
Food and nutrition-related knowledge deficit	NB-1.1	Incomplete or inaccurate knowledge about food, nutrition, or nutrition-related information and guidelines (e.g., nutrient requirements, consequences of food behaviors, life stage requirements, nutrition recommendations, diseases and conditions, physiological function, or products)
Harmful beliefs/attitudes about food or nutrition-related topics	NB-1.2	Beliefs/attitudes and practices about food, nutrition, and nutrition-related topics that are incompatible with sound nutrition principles, nutrition care, or disease/condition
Not ready for diet/lifestyle change	NB-1.3	Lack of perceived value of nutrition-related care benefits compared to consequences or effort required to making the change; inconsistencies with other value structure/purpose; antecedent to behavior change
Self-monitoring deficit	NB-1.4	Lack of data recording to track personal progress
Disordered eating pattern	NB-1.5	Beliefs, attitudes, thoughts, and behaviors related to food, eating, and weight management, including classic eating disorders as well as less severe, similar conditions that negatively impact health
Limited adherence to nutrition-related recommendations	NB-1.6	Lack of nutrition-related changes as per intervention agreed upon by client or population
Undesirable food choices	NB-1.7	Food and/or beverage choices that are inconsistent with U.S. Recommended Dietary Intake, U.S. Dietary Guidelines, or the Food Guide Pyramid or with targets defined in the nutrition prescription or nutrition care process
Class: Physical Activity Balance and Function (2)		
Defined as "actual physical activity, self-care, and quality of life problems as reported, observed, or documented"		
Physical inactivity	NB-2.1	Low level of activity/sedentary behavior to the extent that it reduces energy expenditure and impacts health
Excessive exercise	NB-2.2	An amount of exercise that exceeds that which is necessary to improve health and/or athletic performance
Inability to manage self-care	NB-2.3	Lack of capacity or unwillingness to implement methods to support healthful food and nutrition-related behavior
Impaired ability to prepare foods/meals	NB-2.4	Cognitive or physical impairment that prevents preparation of foods/meals
Poor nutrition quality of life (NQOL)	NB-2.5	Diminished NQOL scores related to food impact, self-image, psychological factors, social/interpersonal, physical, or self-efficacy
Self-feeding difficulty	NB-2.6	Impaired actions to place food in mouth
Class: Food Safety and Access (3)		
Defined as "actual problems with food access or food safety"		
Intake of unsafe food	NB-3.1	Intake of food and/or fluids intentionally or unintentionally contaminated with toxins, poisonous products, infectious agents, microbial agents, additives, allergens, and/or agents of bioterrorism
Limited access to food	NB-3.2	Diminished ability to acquire food from sources (e.g., shopping, gardening, meal delivery) due to financial constraints, physical impairment, caregiver support, or unsafe living conditions (e.g., crime hinders travel to grocery store). Limitation to food because of concerns about weight or aging.

(continued)

TABLE C-1 Nutrition Diagnostic Labels and Definitions *(continued)*

Nutrition Diagnostic Label	Label Number	Definition of Diagnostic Label
DOMAIN: INTAKE		
Defined as "actual problems related to intake of energy, nutrients, fluids, bioactive substances through oral diet, or nutrition support (enteral or parenteral nutrition)"	NI	
Class: Caloric Energy Balance (1)		
Defined as "actual or estimated changes in energy (kcal)"		
Hypermetabolism (increased energy needs)	NI-1.1	Resting metabolic rate (RMR) above predicted requirements due to stress, trauma, injury, sepsis, or disease. Note: RMR is the sum of metabolic processes of active cell mass related to the maintenance of normal body functions and regulatory balance during rest.
Increased energy expenditure	NI-1.2	Resting metabolic rate (RMR) above predicted requirements due to body composition, medications, or endocrine, neurological, or genetic changes. Note: RMR is the sum of metabolic processes of active cell mass related to the maintenance of normal body functions and regulatory balance during rest.
Hypometabolism (decreased energy needs)	NI-1.3	Resting metabolic rate (RMR) below predicted requirements due to body composition, medications, or endocrine, neurological, or genetic changes
Inadequate energy intake	NI-1.4	Energy intake that is less than energy expenditure, established reference standards, or recommendations based upon physiological needs. Exception: when the goal is weight loss or during end of life care.
Excessive energy intake	NI-1.5	Caloric intake that exceeds energy expenditure, established reference standards, or recommendations based upon physiological needs. Exception: when weight gain is desired.
Class: Oral or Nutrition Support Intake (2)		
Defined as "actual or estimated food and beverage intake from oral diet or nutrition support compared with patient goal"		
Inadequate oral food/beverage intake	NI-2.1	Oral food/beverage intake that is less than established reference standards or recommendations based on physiological needs. Exception: when recommendation is weight loss or during end of life care.
Excessive oral food/beverage intake	NI-2.2	Oral food/beverage intake that exceeds energy expenditure, established reference standards, or recommendations based upon physiological needs. Exception: when weight gain is desired.
Inadequate intake from enteral/parenteral nutrition infusion	NI-2.3	Enteral or parenteral infusion that provides fewer calories or nutrients compared to established reference standards or recommendations based on physiological needs. Exception: when recommendation is for weight loss or during end of life care.
Excessive intake from enteral/parenteral nutrition	NI-2.4	Enteral or parenteral infusion that provides more calories or nutrients compared to established reference standards or recommendations based on physiological needs
Inappropriate infusion of enteral/parenteral nutrition	NI-2.5	Enteral or parenteral infusion that provides either fewer or more calories and/or nutrients or is of the wrong composition or type, is not warranted because the patient is able to tolerate an enteral intake, or is unsafe because of the potential for sepsis or other complications
Class: Fluid Intake Balance (3)		
Defined as "actual or estimated fluid intake compared with patient goal"		
Inadequate fluid intake	NI-3.1	Lower intake of fluid-containing foods or substances compared to established reference standards or recommendations based on physiological needs
Excessive fluid intake	NI-3.2	Higher intake of fluid compared to established reference standards or recommendations based on physiological needs

(continued)

TABLE C-1 Nutrition Diagnostic Labels and Definitions *(continued)*

Nutrition Diagnostic Label	Label Number	Definition of Diagnostic Label
Class: Bioactive Substances Balance (4)		
Defined as "actual or observed intake of bioactive substances, including single or multiple functional food components, ingredients, dietary supplements, and alcohol"		
Inadequate bioactive substance intake	NI-4.1	Lower intake of bioactive substance–containing foods or substances compared to established reference standards or recommendations based on physiological needs
Excessive bioactive substance intake	NI-4.2	Higher intake of bioactive substances other than traditional nutrients, such as functional foods, bioactive food components, dietary supplements, or food concentrates compared to established reference standards or recommendations based on physiological needs
Excessive alcohol intake	NI-4.3	Intake above the suggested limits for alcohol
Class: Nutrient Balance (5)		
Defined as "actual or estimated intake of specific nutrient groups or single nutrients as compared with desired levels"		
Increased nutrient (specify) needs	NI-5.1	Increased need for a specific nutrient compared to established reference standards or recommendations based on physiological needs
Evident protein–energy malnutrition	NI-5.2	Inadequate intake of protein and/or energy
Inadequate protein–energy intake	NI-5.3	Inadequate intake of protein and/or energy compared to established reference standards or recommendations based on physiological needs of short or recent duration
Decreased nutrient (specify) needs	NI-5.4	Decreased need for a specific nutrient compared to established reference standards or recommendations based on physiological needs
Imbalance of nutrients	NI-5.5	An undesirable combination of ingested nutrients, such that the amount of one nutrient ingested interferes with or alters absorption and/or utilization of another nutrient
Subclass: Fat and Cholesterol Balance (51)		
Inadequate fat intake	NI-51.1	Lower fat intake compared to established reference standards or recommendations based on physiological needs. Exception: when recommendation is for weight loss or during end of life care.
Excessive fat intake	NI-51.2	Higher fat intake compared to established reference standards or recommendations based on physiological needs
Inappropriate intake of food fats (specify)	NI-51.3	Intake of wrong type or quality of food fats compared to established reference standards or recommendations based on physiological needs
Subclass: Protein Balance (52)		
Inadequate protein intake	NI-52.1	Lower intake of protein-containing foods or substances compared to established reference standards or recommendations based on physiological needs
Excessive or unbalanced protein intake	NI-52.2	Intake above the recommended level and/or type of protein compared to established reference standards or recommendations based on physiological needs
Inappropriate intake of amino acids (specify)	NI-52.3	Intake that is more or less than recommended level and/or type of amino acids compared to established reference standards or recommendations based on physiological needs
Subclass: Carbohydrate and Fiber Balance (53)		
Inadequate carbohydrate intake	NI-53.1	Lower intake of carbohydrate-containing foods or substances compared to established reference standards or recommendations based on physiological needs
Excessive carbohydrate intake	NI-53.2	Intake above the recommended level and type of carbohydrate compared to established reference standards or recommendations based on physiological needs
Inappropriate intake of types of carbohydrate (specify)	NI-53.3	Intake or the type or amount of carbohydrate that is above or below the established reference standards or recommendations based on physiological needs
Inconsistent carbohydrate intake	NI-53.4	Inconsistent timing of carbohydrate intake throughout the day, day to day, or a pattern of carbohydrate intake that is not consistent with recommended pattern based on physiological needs

(continued)

TABLE C-1 Nutrition Diagnostic Labels and Definitions *(continued)*

Nutrition Diagnostic Label	Label Number	Definition of Diagnostic Label
Inadequate fiber intake	NI-53.5	Lower intake of fiber-containing foods or substances compared to established reference standards or recommendations based on physiological needs
Excessive fiber intake	NI-53.6	Higher intake of fiber-containing foods or substances compared to recommendations based on patient/client condition
Subclass: Vitamin Balance (54)		
Inadequate vitamin intake (specify)	NI-54.1	Lower intake of vitamin-containing foods or substances compared to established reference standards or recommendations based on physiological needs
Excessive vitamin intake (specify)	NI-54.2	Higher intake of vitamin-containing foods or substances compared to established reference standards or recommendations based on physiological needs
Subclass: Mineral Balance (55)		
Inadequate mineral intake (specify)	NI-55.1	Lower intake of mineral-containing foods or substances compared to established reference standards or recommendations based on physiological needs
Excessive mineral intake	NI-55.2	Higher intake of mineral from foods, supplements, medications, or water compared to established reference standards or recommendations based on physiological needs

Revised January 20, 2006. Used with permission from the American Dietetic Association, 2006.

TABLE C-2 Nutrition Interventions

NUTRITION EDUCATION **CATEGORY: E**

Meal and Snacks ND-1

Regular eating event (meal); food served between regular meals (snack).

- ❑ General/healthful diet
- ❑ Modify distribution, type, or amount of food and nutrients within meals or at specified time
- ❑ Specific foods/beverages or groups
- ❑ Other

*(specify)*________________

Enteral and Parenteral Nutrition ND-2

Nutrition provided through the GI tract via tube, catheter, or stoma (enteral) or intravenously, centrally, or peripherally (parenteral).

- ❑ Initiate enteral or parenteral nutrition
- ❑ Modify rate, concentration, composition or schedule
- ❑ Discontinue enteral or parenteral nutrition
- ❑ Insert enteral feeding tube
- ❑ Site care
- ❑ Other

*(specify)*________________

Medical Food Supplement ND-3.1

Commercial or prepared foods or beverages that supplement energy, protein, carbohydrate, fiber, fat intake.

Type

- ❑ Commercial beverage
- ❑ Commercial food
- ❑ Modified beverage
- ❑ Modified food

Purpose

*(specify)*________________

Vitamin and Mineral Supplement ND-3.2

Supplemental vitamins or minerals.

- ❑ Multivitamin/mineral
- ❑ Vitamin
  - ❑ A
  - ❑ Thiamin
  - ❑ Riboflavin
  - ❑ Niacin
  - ❑ Folate
  - ❑ Other ______
  - ❑ C
  - ❑ D
  - ❑ E
  - ❑ K
  - ❑ Multivitamin
- ❑ Mineral
  - ❑ Calcium
  - ❑ Potassium
  - ❑ Phosphorus
  - ❑ Multi-trace elements
  - ❑ Other ________
  - ❑ Iron
  - ❑ Zinc
  - ❑ Magnesium

Bioactive Substance Supplement ND-3.3

Supplemental bioactive substances.

- ❑ Initiate
- ❑ Dose change
- ❑ Form change
- ❑ Route change
- ❑ Administration schedule
- ❑ Discontinue

*(specify)*________________

(continued)

Table C-2 Nutrition Interventions *(continued)*

FOOD AND/OR NUTRIENT DELIVERY CATEGORY: ND

Feeding Assistance ND-4

Accommodation or assistance in eating.

- ❑ Adaptive equipment
- ❑ Feeding position
- ❑ Meal set-up
- ❑ Mouth care
- ❑ Other

*(specify)*____________________

Feeding Environment ND-5

Adjustment of the factors where food is served that impact food consumption.

- ❑ Lighting
- ❑ Odors
- ❑ Distractions
- ❑ Table height
- ❑ Table service/set-up
- ❑ Room temperature
- ❑ Other

*(specify)*____________________

Nutrition-Related Medication Management ND-6

Modification of a drug or herbal to optimize patient/client nutritional or health status.

- ❑ Initiate
- ❑ Dose change
- ❑ Form change
- ❑ Route change
- ❑ Administration schedule
- ❑ Discontinue

*(specify)*____________________

NUTRITION EDUCATION CATEGORY: E

Initial/Brief Nutrition Education E-1

Reinforcement of basic or essential nutrition-related knowledge.

- ❑ Purpose of the nutrition education
- ❑ Priority modifications
- ❑ Survival information
- ❑ Other

*(specify topic)*____________________

Comprehensive Nutrition Education E-2

Instruction or training leading to in-depth nutrition-related knowledge or skills.

- ❑ Purpose of the nutrition education
- ❑ Recommended modifications
- ❑ Advanced or related topics
- ❑ Result interpretation
- ❑ Other

*(specify topic)*____________________

NUTRITION COUNSELING CATEGORY: C

Nutrition-Related Behavior Modification Therapy C-1

An approach that attempts to identify and disconnect the triggers (antecedents) of undesirable behaviors and reinforce desirable behaviors.

- ❑ Self-monitoring
- ❑ Stimulus control/contingency management
- ❑ Plan rewards
- ❑ Other

*(specify)*____________________

Nutrition-Related Cognitive-Behavioral Therapy C-2

A method that assumes that thinking affects behavior and that relevant beliefs may be identified and altered.

- ❑ Motivational interviewing
- ❑ Problem solving
- ❑ Stimulus control/contingency management
- ❑ Cognitive restructuring
- ❑ Other

*(specify)*____________________

Other Nutrition-Related Counseling Approaches C-3

Alternate nutrition counseling methods employed to change nutrition-related behavior and attitudes.

*(specify)*____________________

COORDINATION OF NUTRITION CARE CATEGORY: RC

Coordination of Other Care During Nutrition Care RC-1

Facilitating services with other professionals, institutions, or agencies during nutrition care.

- ❑ Team meeting
- ❑ Referral to RD with different expertise
- ❑ Collaboration/referral to other providers
- ❑ Referral to community agencies/programs

*(specify)*____________________

Discharge and Transfer of Nutrition Care to New Setting or Provider RC-2

Discharge planning and transfer of nutrition care from one level or location of care to another.

- ❑ Collaboration/referral to other providers
- ❑ Referral to community agencies/programs

*(specify)*____________________

Nutritional assessment is important. In the following cases, note if the patient has nutritional "red flags," such as:

- No regular exercise regimen and/or sedentary lifestyle
- Recent loss of 10% or more of usual body weight
- Alcoholism
- Taking drugs such as steroids, immunosuppressants
- Infection, protracted fever, trauma
- Malabsorption syndromes, draining abscesses, renal dialysis
- Receiving simple intravenous solutions without oral intake for >10 days
- Older age

Family and Social History

- Family history of cancer, diabetes, heart disease, hypertension, obesity, and osteoporosis
- Parents, siblings, children, spouse: include ages, current health status, and cause of death if deceased
- Occupation, daily exercise pattern, marital and family status
- Economic status, educational level, residence, emotional response to illness, and coping skills
- Duration and frequency of use of substances, including tobacco, alcohol, illegal drugs, and caffeine

Past Medical History

- Immunizations, hospitalizations, operations, major injuries, chronic illnesses, and significant acute illnesses
- Current or recent prescription medications, vitamins and minerals, laxatives, topical medications, over-the-counter medications, and nutritional supplements
- Potential drug–nutrient interactions, such as those caused by potassium-wasting diuretics
- Food allergies or lactose intolerance

CASE STUDIES AND CONCEPT MAPS

You may use the Concept Map format from Figure C-1 as you work through each case. Insert as many details as needed to make the case complete. The concept map will help to identify key areas and to visualize the nutrition diagnoses, plans, and interventions more clearly. Figure C-2 is a sample charting form that uses the new standardized language; you may copy this document and practice writing chart notes accordingly.

SAMPLE CASE: Chronic Diarrhea and Weight Loss in Elderly Woman

First Visit

Marian J. has entered the acute-care facility where you work as a clinical dietitian. She is a 79-year-old white female who has been widowed and living alone for the past 7 years. Her only son lives near her and visits her in the hospital each evening. From a review of her medical records, it is noted that she has been admitted for chronic diarrhea and weight loss of 10 lb (she currently weighs 145 lb). She is 5′2″, and her weight has been 155 lbs all of her married life. Diarrhea seems to be related to recent use of antibiotics.

She has osteoarthritis in her wrists and ankles, hypertension with a current reading of 170/100, and history of a cerebrovascular accident (CVA) 5 years ago with minimal residual deficits. She is relatively sedentary because of her osteoarthritis and takes Trilisate when it flares up.

Marian did not take her prescribed diuretics on a regular basis before her stroke; since that time, she does take them faithfully. The current reading of 170/100 is "high normal" for her while on medication; it usually runs 145/95.

Marian previously was prescribed a low-sodium diet and was given a diet instruction sheet at the doctor's office. She has her own teeth, which are in good condition. Recently, she has complained to her son of being more "sad" than usual. The doctor has prescribed Kaopectate for the diarrhea, and it seems to be effective. He also ordered a general 2-g sodium diet. Marian is not eating well in the facility and seems depressed. She does not eat pork and dislikes fish intensely.

Prescribed Medications:

Trilisate for osteoarthritis
Bumex for hypertension
Kaopectate for diarrhea
Other: self-prescribed use of mineral oil for "regularity"

Diet History: Usual Intake at Home

Breakfast (7:30 AM)
Corn flakes/whole milk and 2 tsp sugar
Black coffee
Lunch (11:30 AM)
Peanut butter/jelly sandwich
1 cup canned tomato soup
½ cup canned pears
Snack (3:00 PM)
½ cup sherbet
Black coffee
Dinner (6:00 PM)
Chicken or beef/gravy
Buttered noodles
½ cup green beans
1 cup whole milk

Primary Concern:

Diarrhea with resulting weight loss of 10 lb

Secondary Concerns:

Osteoarthritis, which makes it difficult to eat and to walk quickly

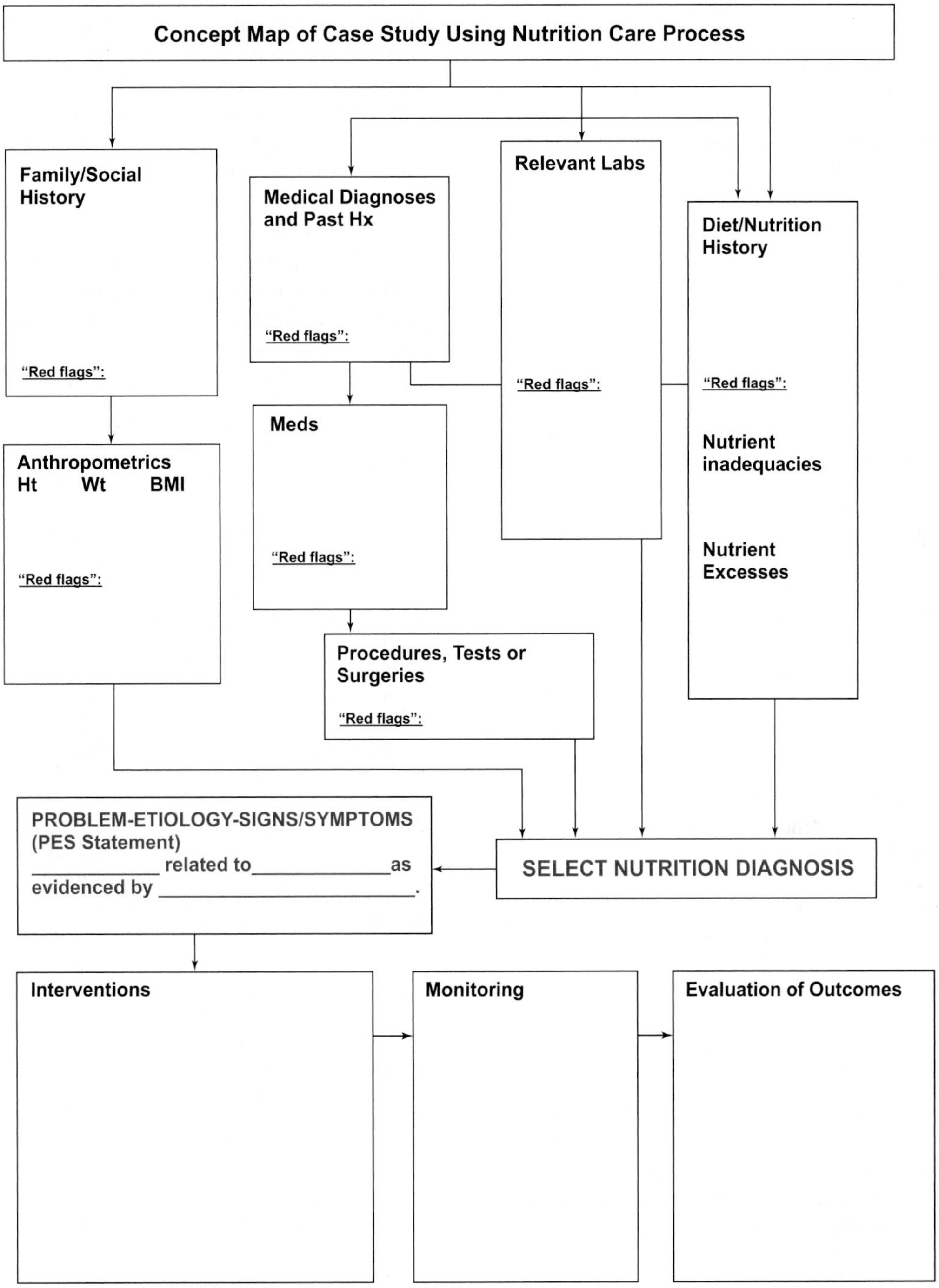

Concept Map of Case Study Using Nutrition Care Process
Family/Social History
"Red flags":
Medical Diagnoses and Past Hx
"Red flags":
Relevant Labs
"Red flags":
Diet/Nutrition History
"Red flags":
Nutrient inadequacies
Nutrient Excesses
Anthropometrics
Ht Wt BMI
"Red flags":
Meds
"Red flags":
Procedures, Tests or Surgeries
"Red flags":
PROBLEM-ETIOLOGY-SIGNS/SYMPTOMS
(PES Statement)
__________ related to ____________ as evidenced by ______________________.
SELECT NUTRITION DIAGNOSIS
Interventions
Monitoring
Evaluation of Outcomes

Figure C-1

Medical Nutrition Therapy Consultation

Nutrition Assessment

Subjective: Patient states the following—

____

____

Objective: Patient is a __ y/o ____ _____ referred by ________ for.
Ht. ____Wt. ____BMI ____

Pertinent Labs:

Pertinent Medications:

Nutrition Diagnosis/es P ____ E ____ S ____

Nutrition Interventions

Individualized Treatment Goals to Address Nutrition Diagnosis

1.

2.

3.

4.

Implementation of Intervention

1. Food/nutrient delivery:
2. Nutrition education:
3. Nutrition counseling:
4. Care management:

Education Materials Provided

1.

2.

3.

RD Follow Up Plan for Monitoring and Evaluation

1.

2.

3.

Signature:____________________________Date:____________

Figure C-2

Hypertension, which is regulated by medications
History of CVA
Mild depression of recent onset

After completing your assessment, what is the nutritional diagnosis, what interventions will you provide, and what outcomes are you seeking for Marian?

Nutrition Diagnosis and PES Statement:

Involuntary weight loss related to (RT) chronic diarrhea and altered appetite as evidenced by (AEB) actual intake less than assessed requirements.

Interventions:

Goal—resolve diarrhea and increase fiber intake from the diet.

Action—Request that the doctor change the diet order to high fiber/no added salt so that Marian's intake can improve with more flavorful foods. Diarrhea and weight loss may be attributed to the use of Trilisate. The doctor has changed her medication to Lodine, with less likelihood of causing any anorexia or diarrhea. Use yogurt or acidophilus milk to recolonize flora in the intestinal tract. Extra fluids are essential during this time.

Patient Education and Counseling:

- Discuss with Marian the effects of mineral oil on fat-soluble vitamin absorption and how it may also contribute to some diarrhea. Advise her that the high-fiber diet she has been given will help normalize bowel function.
- When her appetite returns, some suggested alterations in her dietary pattern may include: use of a high-fiber cereal at breakfast; use of more fresh fruits each day (especially oranges, bananas, and apples for potassium, pectin fiber, and low sodium content); use of skim milk instead of whole milk with at least 3 cups daily, if tolerated; addition of a salad or some raw vegetables with lunch or dinner to enhance vitamin and mineral content of her diet, as well as fiber.
- For her blood pressure, it may be recommended that she try some of the lower sodium/lower fat soups that are now available on the market. Easy-to-prepare foods are now available from the grocery store at reasonable prices so that she can readily plan her meals and maintain her independence.

Outcomes to Monitor and Evaluate:

Check electrolyte status until diarrhea resolves.

Monitor weights to see if rehydration helps Marian to recover a few of the lost pounds.

The doctor has ordered an antidepressant temporarily; depression is common after a CVA. Monitor to determine if the antidepressant helps Marian recover her appetite.

Follow-Up Session:

Approximately 2 weeks after returning home, Marian sees you in the Ambulatory Nutrition Clinic for a follow-up visit. She feels much better and has regained 3 lb that were lost from the diarrhea, which has resolved. Her son brings her dinner meals approximately three times weekly. He also has made contact with the local Meals-on-Wheels program to enroll his mother at your suggestion. They provide a hot meal that generally is lower in sodium and fat upon request.

Long-Term Objectives:

Discuss with Marian how to maintain weight after diarrhea has resolved. To help her mobility and reduce stress on the joints, additional weight gain should not be the plan. For her goal weight of 140 lb (minimal planned weight loss), a plan of 1500–1600 calories would be shared, using simplified exchange lists that also are low in added salt.

Although her activity level is not significantly improved, she does try to participate in daily exercises for strengthening and stretching. This has improved her range of motion and energy level. She sees the physical therapist each week for some resistance training exercises that she can follow at home. Her spirits also have improved, and her doctor has discontinued the antidepressant medication.

Marian no longer uses mineral oil as a laxative and has faithfully adopted high-fiber foods into her daily pattern. She indicates that your advice about fiber foods has not been as difficult as she expected. She is now including 3–4 fruits and vegetables daily, with the long-range goal of 5 or more per day. This is beneficial not only for her hypertension and for normal bowel function but also to protect against future CVAs as far as possible.

Marian agrees to call you if she has other questions or concerns about her diet. The high-fiber diet remains the emphasis, with consideration also to lower sodium foods but not so low that she loses her appetite. She and her son are pleased with your interventions; you plan to stay in contact once every 6 months by telephone.

PRACTICE CASE STUDIES

SECTION 1 CASE STUDY: Normal Life-Cycle Conditions

Josie is a 15-year-old white teen who is pregnant. She has a history of disordered eating and was hospitalized for this problem approximately 2 years ago. Her weight before the pregnancy was 95 lb and she was 5 feet 1 inch in height. She is now 24 weeks pregnant and weighs 102 lb. Her serum albumin level is 3.4 g/dL; blood glucose is 110 mg/100 mL; and HbA1c is 5. There is no other blood work available at this time. You are her outpatient dietitian and are now scheduled to see her twice a month until she delivers. You request a serum prealbumin for a more global marker due to the history of disordered eating.

Nutrition Diagnosis and PES Statement:

Disordered eating patterns RT patient's desire to regulate weight AEB failure to gain appropriate weight during pregnancy.

Interventions:

You will want intake and diet records; assess any fears and limitations or requirements she feels surround her, the "why" behind it all. Track appropriate weight gain and discuss the healthy and much needed aspects of weight gain as they pertain to her pregnancy. Prenatal vitamin will be needed.

What other assessment data do you ask for?
What are essential aspects to include in her care plan?
What counseling tips will you consider as you talk with her, considering both the pregnancy and the history of disordered eating?

Outcomes to Monitor and Evaluate:

How will you follow up her care and nutritional status?

SECTION 2 CASE STUDY: Dietary Practices and Miscellaneous Conditions

Nathan is a 24-year-old black male who presents at your nutrition office with gastrointestinal (GI) distress, recent acute gastroenteritis, and low albumin and serum electrolytes. His doctor has diagnosed food allergies, including wheat and egg allergies. He is also lactose intolerant. He has brought a 7-day food diary for you to review, which includes frequent consumption of fried foods, barbecued meats, and few vegetables. You need a calcium level and will need to monitor electrolytes and weight. He is 6′2″ and weighs 190 lb currently; his usual weight is 215 lb.

Nutrition Diagnosis and PES Statement:

Food and nutrition-related knowledge deficit RT lack of prior exposure to or knowledge about allergies AEB diet recall.

Interventions:

Review diary and make adjustments for intolerances and recommendations for other options and places to attain other options. Review issues related to cooking, eating out, and food preparation history. Suggest use of Lactaid milk and Lactaid pills.

What additional assessment data do you need?
What nutritional care plan will you develop?
What guidance will you offer in regard to label reading, dining in restaurants, packing a lunch for work, and holiday meals?

Outcomes to Monitor and Evaluate:

How will you follow up his care and nutritional status?

SECTION 3 CASE STUDY: Special Pediatric Conditions

Kyle is a 6-month-old white male with cerebral palsy and failure to thrive. He is below the 5th percentile on the growth charts for height and weight. His mother is 20 years old, and the father is absent. Kyle and his mother have been referred to your services by the pediatrician to conquer the failure to thrive. Kyle has a low hemoglobin and hematocrit (H & H), low blood glucose level, and low blood urea nitrogen and creatinine. You find that Kyle's mother started cow's milk at 6 weeks because it was "supposed to be good for him." She has not introduced any cereal, fruits, vegetables, or meats into his diet; she feeds him 4 oz of milk four times daily. Kyle requires use of a special nipple because he cannot close his lips completely around a bottle. After discussion, you determine that Mom has a knowledge deficit about feeding Kyle, especially related to the use of special feeding nipples.

Nutrition Diagnoses and PES Statements:

Knowledge deficit RT feeding techniques for cerebral palsy infant AEB failure to thrive and altered nutrition-related lab values. Inadequate protein-energy intake RT food and nutrition knowledge deficit AEB dietary recall and failure to thrive.

Interventions:

What additional assessment data do you need?

What nutritional care plan factors should be considered? Design a nutritional care plan, and establish goals for Kyle's recovery and growth.

Need to intervene and establish appropriate diet patterns and requirements. Why is Mom only using cow's milk, for example.

Outcomes to Monitor and Evaluate:

How will you follow up his care and nutritional status?

SECTION 4 CASE STUDY: Neurological and Psychiatric Conditions

Stanley is a 42-year-old male with a history of schizophrenia and tardive dyskinesia. He has taken many types of antipsychotics during the previous 20 years. He has lived in a nursing home since suffering a mild stroke. He is paralyzed on the right side and has mild dysphagia. You are assigned to his floor in the Veterans Administration Medical Center. Stanley's medical record indicates that he has a blood pressure that averages 150/95, blood glucose levels of 135 mg/100 mL, H & H slightly below normal, and other normal laboratory values. He is 5′6″ and currently weighs 152 lb. For Stanley's current status, the doctor has ordered a mechanical soft diet, but you note some coughing with meals and that he cannot feed himself well at all.

Nutrition Diagnosis and PES Statement:

Swallowing difficulty RT paralysis from stroke AEB coughing and self-feeding difficulty.

Interventions:

What additional nutritional information and food recall data do you need?

Should you ask for a speech therapy consult?

What other nutritional care plan factors will you need to know?

What are some common medications that cause tardive dyskinesia?

What are some risks noted for stroke patients who must also take antipsychotics?

Outcomes to Monitor and Evaluate:

How will you follow up his care and nutritional status?

SECTION 5 CASE STUDY: Pulmonary Disorders

Marlissa is a 28-year-old black female with cystic fibrosis, which was diagnosed when she was 12 years old. She now has extensive problems with chronic pneumonia and bouts of atelectasis. She takes three or four antibiotics to prevent additional pulmonary infections. Recently, elevated blood sugar levels have been noted on doctor's visits. Although a diagnosis of diabetes has not been made, Marlissa has been advised to see you in the outpatient clinic to discuss management of hyperglycemia along with the cystic fibrosis. Her recent blood glucose levels have averaged 210 mg/dL. She is 5′8″ in height and weighs 125 lb. She is on prednisone prophylactically for exacerbations of her condition. She lives alone.

Nutrition Diagnosis and PES Statement:

Hypermetabolism RT diagnosis of cystic fibrosis AEB low weight status for height.

Interventions:

Because shopping is a tedious prospect for Marlissa, what suggestions do you have to simplify the shopping and meal preparation process for her?

Develop recipe adaptations to her favorite meal of barbecued chicken with fried potatoes, greens, and sweet potato pie.

Consider meal delivery/order online. What else might you suggest?

Outcomes to Monitor and Evaluate:

How will you follow up her care and nutritional status?

SECTION 6 CASE STUDY: Cardiovascular Disorders

Sonny is a youthful 72-year-old man with arteriosclerosis and a recent valve replacement surgery. He has come to see you in your clinic office upon referral by his physician. He has experienced a 10-lb weight loss since his surgical procedure and has lost his appetite. He is experiencing postoperative pain issues as well. He wants to return to his usual practice of walking 5 miles per day but does not have the energy to do so. His lab work reveals a low H & H, normal glucose, albumin level of 3.2 g/dL, serum cholesterol of 275 g/dL, and high homocysteine level with low serum folate. Sonny has been taking a supplement from a local Chinese market, containing several herbs that you are not familiar with. He wants your help in designing a diet plan that includes his favorite foods of scrambled eggs and bacon.

Nutrition Diagnosis and PES Statement:

Involuntary weight loss RT pain associated status post surgery AEB percent weight loss (need usual weight) and reports of poor po.

Interventions:

What suggestions do you have for Sonny's dietary regimen?
What shopping tips do you have for him?
Who should you contact to find out more about the content of these supplements?
Should you talk with his doctor about this practice?
Sonny wants you to advise him about incremental increases in his activity program. Should you offer advice on this subject?

Outcomes to Monitor and Evaluate:

How will you follow up his care and nutritional status?

SECTION 7 CASE STUDY: Gastrointestinal Disorders

Naomi is a 52-year-old white female who is married and has two grown children. Recently, her daughter called you to make an appointment regarding Naomi's GI complaints. She has suffered for 10 years with Crohn's disease and has recently been diagnosed with acute pancreatitis. She is unable to consume solid foods with liquids at the same meal; she has nausea after meals and cannot sleep if she has eaten too close to bedtime. Naomi also has high blood pressure and a family history of cardiovascular disease. She is 5′3″ and weighs 102 lbs. Her lab work is not available because she is from another state. She takes Lasix for her blood pressure and prednisone for the inflammatory bowel disease.

Nutrition Diagnosis and PES Statement:

Inadequate oral food and beverage intake RT GI pain AEB nausea and difficulty eating.

Interventions:

What nutritional assessment data should you seek?
What types of nutritional guidance would you offer to Naomi regarding: nausea, liquid and solid food consumption, foods to limit for lowering blood pressure and reducing cardiovascular risks, and other nutritional issues related to inflammatory bowel disease and pancreatitis?
What side effects do her medications have? What suggestions can you offer?

Outcomes to Monitor and Evaluate:

How will you follow up her care and nutritional status?

SECTION 8 CASE STUDY: Pancreatic, Hepatic, and Biliary Disorders

William is a 65-year-old male with liver failure and recent encephalopathy. His current blood work reveals a low H & H, albumin of 2.5 mg/dL, glucose of 160 mg/100 mL, elevated serum ammonia levels, and blood urea nitrogen (BUN) and creatinine that are slightly elevated. William's doctor advises you that he probably has early renal failure. His height is 6′2″ and his weight is 220 lb. He takes ferrous sulfate, Glynase, and lactulose. William's appetite is poor, and he is uncomfortable at meals because of his ascites, so he has only been consuming 25% on most days.

Nutrition Diagnosis and PES Statement:

Inadequate protein and energy intake RT ascites and inability to eat oral diet recently AEB altered nutritional labs and diet recall indicating 25% intake at most meals.

Interventions:

What other information should you seek to develop a nutritional care plan?
What dietary advice may be useful to William?
If William is allowed to go home from the hospital, what type of diet should be prescribed for use at home? It is tricky with encephalopathy and beginning renal failure; how should you handle this?
What medication side effects are likely?

Outcomes to Monitor and Evaluate:

How will you follow up his care and nutritional status?

SECTION 9 CASE STUDY: Endocrine Disorders

Tyler is a 60-year-old white male with a recent diagnosis of hyperthyroidism; he has long-term diabetes. His doctor referred him to you and indicates that he has lost approximately 25 lb in a 6-month period. He is 5′10″ and weighs 142 lb. He is taking Tapazole and Humulin insulin. From a diet history, you find that Tyler consumes approximately 2500 kcal and 50 g of protein each day. He does not consume excessive amounts of carbohydrate, and his blood glucose levels tend to be easily controlled by the current insulin. He has a stage 1 pressure ulcer on his left hip. His laboratory work indicates a low H & H, slightly low BUN and creatinine, and normal glucose. You have estimated his protein needs to be 1 g/kg because of recent weight loss and skin changes.

Nutrition Diagnosis and PES Statement:

Inadequate protein RT hypermetabolic needs AEB intake of 50 g versus estimated needs of >64 g and stage 1 pressure ulcer.

Interventions:

What type of nutritional care plan would you design?

Because Tyler enjoys dining in restaurants, especially Italian and Mexican, what types of foods would you recommend for him?

What choices can he make if he stops at restaurants often?

Tyler travels a lot on business and skips breakfast regularly. What suggestions do you have for him while he is "on the road?"

Outcomes to Monitor and Evaluate:

How will you follow up his care and nutritional status?

SECTION 10 CASE STUDY: Weight Control

Sarai is a 32-year-old female who has been referred by her doctor to your weight control clinic. Her height is 5′1″, and her weight is 182 lb. She has a history of diabetes controlled by diet, current diagnosis of gallstones, and recent knee replacement surgery. Sarai is willing to work with you at this time on a nutritional plan that allows her to lose 1–1.5 lb weekly over the next 6 months. She needs support because her family does not think she needs any weight loss; she is "just fine as she is." Her laboratory work is normal at this time for all factors other than a slightly low H & H. Sarai works in a factory where she must stand all day on her feet. She gets hungry and takes frequent breaks.

Nutrition Diagnosis and PES Statement:

Obesity/excessive intake RT undesirable food choices/high-fat food intake AEB diet recall and body mass index (BMI) of 34.

Interventions:

What types of questions would you ask regarding her dietary habits?

What suggestions do you have for Sarai's snack breaks?

With her knee replacement, Sarai is not able to walk great distances without pain. What type of referral might be useful for her to inquire about reasonable exercises?

Outcomes to Monitor and Evaluate:

How will you follow up her care and nutritional status?

SECTION 11 CASE STUDY: Musculoskeletal Disorders

Suzanne is a 50-year-old white female with a diagnosis of lupus and multiple allergies, including milk allergy. She has come to see you in the outpatient clinic of the hospital where you work. She has no available lab work but tells you that she tends to fatigue easily and to have a lot of GI distress. Recently, she has had chronic mild diarrhea after meals. Her height is 5′6″, and she weighs 120 lb. She is curious about whether there is a special diet for lupus. Suzanne has copies of four diets that she uses in sequence to try to cure her disease. From her intake records and patterns, you identify that she is consuming hidden milk products (in cheese sauces, cream sauces, and salad dressings) and does not read labels or ask about food ingredients at restaurants.

Nutrition Diagnosis and PES Statement:

Knowledge deficit RT milk allergy and dietary management for lupus AEB mild diarrhea and GI distress and low BMI of 19.

Interventions:

Assess recent hydration and weight loss associated with diarrhea. Add fiber for diarrhea.

What additional information should you request from her physician?

What type of nutritional care plan might you begin to design for Suzanne?

What types of foods are tolerable for diarrhea? List several suggestions.

What advice would you offer to her about these diets?

Outcomes to Monitor and Evaluate:

How will you follow up her care and nutritional status?

SECTION 12 CASE STUDY: Anemias and Blood Disorders

Lenora is a 14-year-old black female who has sickle cell anemia. She eats well but has pain and no energy for her after-school sports activities. She takes a multivitamin supplement twice a week. She currently is using nighttime standard tube feedings from 8 PM to 8 AM that meets 25% of her daily requirements. Lenora weighs 120 lb and is 5′8″; she recently lost 12 lbs after a bout of influenza. She tends to lose weight easily. Her doctor has diagnosed Lenora with GI malabsorption problems this past month and referred her to your clinic.

Nutrition Diagnosis and PES Statement:

Involuntary weight loss and impaired nutrient utilization RT sickle cell anemia and malabsorption AEB low BMI of 18.

Interventions:

What nutritional parameters do you need to assess her nutritional status further?

What suggestions do you have for Lenora to include more fruits, vegetables, and nutrients needed for added vitamins B_6, A, and E and folic acid?

What suggestions do you have for Lenora to be able to participate in sports more regularly?

Outcomes to Monitor and Evaluate:

How will you follow up her care and nutritional status?

SECTION 13 CASE STUDY: Cancer

Ed is a 68-year-old retired farmer. He recently has been diagnosed with throat cancer and severe anemia. He is unable to swallow thin liquids and uses thickened beverages for most of his meals. His height is 5′10″, and his current weight is 140 lb; his usual weight is 182 lb. He has had radiation therapy to his throat and will have another few months of this treatment. His prognosis is poor, and he wants advice on how to make meals more appealing. He has significant anorexia and mouth sores.

Nutrition Diagnosis and PES Statement:

Swallowing difficulty RT throat cancer AEB involuntary weight loss, inability to drink thin liquids, and current BMI of 20.

Interventions:

What nutritional assessment factors should you seek?

What type of nutritional care plan would be useful for Ed? Plan a high-calorie, high-protein diet that uses thickened liquids and soft foods that he can tolerate.

What other suggestions would you offer besides sauces, gravies, and supplements?

He may need a tube feeding later; how would you approach this subject with him?

Outcomes to Monitor and Evaluate:

How will you follow up his care and nutritional status?

SECTION 14 CASE STUDY: Surgical Disorders

Matt is a white 12-year-old boy who has recently undergone surgery for a fractured femur. He has a history of asthma, takes theophylline, and uses inhalers. He eats poorly and skips all fruits and vegetables. His surgical wound is not healing well, and his doctor has not prescribed any vitamin-mineral supplements. His lab work indicates a low serum ferritin and low serum zinc level. The diet recall indicates that he consumes about 50% of his estimated protein requirements because he does not eat enough protein-rich foods and eats a diet high in concentrated sweets and fats. When Matt goes home, he will return to school, where he likes to play hockey.

Nutrition Diagnosis and PES Statement:

Inadequate mineral intake RT undesirable food choices/limited adherence to nutrition recommendations AEB diet recall and low serum ferritin and zinc levels.

Interventions:

What nutritional parameters do you need to assess Matt's nutritional status further?

What side effects are common from his asthma medications?

What suggestions do you have for Matt to include more fruits, vegetables, and nutrients needed for wound healing?

How can you use Matt's desire to play hockey as a reinforcer for improving his diet and ensuring a faster recovery?

Outcomes to Monitor and Evaluate:

How will you follow up his care and nutritional status?

SECTION 15 CASE STUDY: Hypermetabolic, Infectious, Traumatic, and Febrile Conditions

Marcus is a 35-year-old male who has been diagnosed as HIV positive. He has made an appointment to see you in the outpatient nutrition clinic because he wants advice on how to stay healthy. His height is 6′4″, and his weight is 240 lb. Currently, his total lymphocyte count (TLC) is low, as is his H & H. He has an albumin level of 3.5 mg/dL, elevated C-reactive protein, and normal laboratory values for other parameters. He has begun taking zidovudine (AZT) and two experimental medications, under doctor's supervision. Marcus has asked you for information about supplemental herbs and botanical products.

Nutrition Diagnosis and PES Statement:

Knowledge deficit RT use of herbs and botanical products AEB request for information.

Interventions:

What factors should you monitor for Marcus?
What side effects might he experience on AZT related to his appetite?
What are some common long-term problems associated with being HIV positive?
What tips can you offer to provide symptom relief for problems such as diarrhea?

Outcomes to Monitor and Evaluate:

How will you monitor his care for changes in nutritional diagnoses?

SECTION 16 CASE STUDY: Renal Disorders

Aaron is a 75-year-old male in your skilled nursing facility. He has chronic kidney disease and is blind. He uses adaptive feeding equipment and receives dialysis three times weekly. Recently, his renal dietitian has called you to note that his albumin level has dropped to 2.4 g/dL; his phosphorus level is normal, but the serum potassium is elevated slightly. He is 5′7″ and weighs 130 lb. Because of his osteoarthritis, Aaron takes a lot of pain medication. He wears dentures and follows a mechanical soft diet. From dietary recall, it is noted that Aaron eats 50–75% of his entrees, about 75–100% of the fruits and vegetables in his meals, and 50% of the beverages (including milk and juices). He likes ice cream for snacks and is able to handle finger foods.

Nutrition Diagnosis and PES Statement:

Inadequate protein intake RT chronic kidney disease and poor protein intake at meals AEB albumin of 2.4 g/dL.

Interventions:

What nutritional information should you address first?
What tips are useful for Aaron to maintain his self-feeding ability despite his blindness?
What guidance will you offer regarding his nutritional care plan?

Outcomes to Monitor and Evaluate:

How will you follow up his care and nutritional status?

SECTION 17 CASE STUDY: Enteral and Parenteral Nutrition

Sophie is an 80-year-old grandmother of six. She lives with her daughter, who provides her with a gastrostomy tube feeding without problems at home. Sophie has had problems with elevated lipid levels recently, and her doctor is concerned. You have been called as the home-care dietitian to make a visit and to discuss Sophie's needs. Her height is 4′11″, and her weight is 140 lb; her serum cholesterol is 250 mg/dL. Her tube feeding runs 90 mL/hr of standard product, yielding 1 kcal/mL. Her daughter wants the doctor to give lipid medications.

Nutrition Diagnosis and PES Statement:

Excessive energy intake RT overfeeding AEB tube feeding providing 2160 kcal/d compared with estimated needs of about 1590 kcal/d, using 25 kcal/kg calculation.

Interventions:

What is Sophie currently receiving in calories?
How would you suggest making adjustments for her elevated lipid levels?
At Sophie's age, would you support the daughter's request to aggressively treat the hypercholesterolemia with medications?
Because Sophie is nonambulatory, what other suggestions do you have for her nutritional care plan?

Outcomes to Monitor and Evaluate:

How will you follow up her care and nutritional status?

APPENDIX D

Acuity Ranking for Dietitian Services

Over 100 dietitians, clinical nutrition managers, and specialists were surveyed regarding this acuity ranking for dietitian services, and a summary is given below. Consensus levels about acuity are indicated for the medical diagnoses and conditions in this text. Where strong consensus of agreement was available, this table provides the acuity ranking for nutritional involvement needed from a registered dietitian. The survey asked the questions listed in Table D-1.

TABLE D-1 Nutrition Acuity and Medical Diagnosis–Related Survey Questions

Rate your opinion about the level of dietitian involvement (over time, not just per visit) for the following diagnoses on the 1 to 5 rating scale where:

1 = Little involvement; minimal, can be delegated to others

2 = Some roles in oversight of nutrition care

3 = Moderate involvement needed over time

4 = Extensive involvement needed over time

5 = Unable to determine; no opinion or experience

TABLE D-2 Acuity for Dietitian Roles in Medical Diagnoses

Minimal Role of Dietitian–1	Some Roles of Dietitian–2	Moderate Role of Dietitian–3	Extended Role of Dietitian–4
SECTION 1: NORMAL LIFE-CYCLE CONDITIONS			
Pregnancy, normal Lactation Infant, normal (birth up to 6 months) Infant, normal (6–12 months) (1–2)	Child, normal (1–2) Teenager, normal Adult male, normal Adult female, normal Elderly male, normal Elderly female, normal	Pregnancy, high risk	
SECTION 2: DIETARY PRACTICES AND MISCELLANEOUS CONDITIONS			
Periodontal disease (1–2) Temporomandibular joint (TMJ) dysfunction Skin disorders (acne, rosacea, eczema, psoriasis) Ménière's syndrome	Complementary medicine and herbal/botanical counseling Cultural food pattern, advisement and planning Vegetarian diet advisement or planning Religious dietary patterns, advisement/planning Dental difficulties (caries, wired jaw, mouth pain, xerostomia) (2–3) Vision and self-feeding problems (low vision, blindness, coordination or chewing problems) (1–2) Food allergy, simple (2–3) Foodborne illness, prevention or counseling	Pressure ulcer, stage 1 or 2 (2–3) Vitamin deficiency prevention or counseling Food allergy, multiple or complex (3–4)	Pressure ulcer, stage 3 or 4 or multiple

(continued)

TABLE D-2 Acuity for Dietitian Roles in Medical Diagnoses *(continued)*

Minimal Role of Dietitian–1	Some Roles of Dietitian–2	Moderate Role of Dietitian–3	Extended Role of Dietitian–4
SECTION 3: PEDIATRICS: BIRTH DEFECTS AND GENETIC AND ACQUIRED DISORDERS			
Attention deficit disorders Autism spectrum disorders (1–2) Adrenoleukodystrophy (variable) Leukodystrophies (variable) Otitis media	Abetalipoproteinemia (variable) Biliary atresia (2–3) Congenital heart disease Cystinosis and Fanconi's syndrome (variable) Down syndrome Fetal alcohol syndrome (1–2) Large for gestational age infant (variable)	Bronchopulmonary dysplasia (3–4) Cerebral palsy Cleft palate Homocystinuria (3–4) Maple syrup urine disease (MSUD) (3–4) Medium-chain acyl-CoA dehydrogenase deficiency (MCADD) Myelomeningocele (variable) Obesity, childhood (prevention, treatment) (3–4) Prader-Willi syndrome (3–4) Rickets, nutritional Spina bifida and neural tube defects Wilson's disease (hepatolenticular degeneration)	Failure to thrive, pediatric Inborn errors of carbohydrate metabolism Hirschsprung's disease (congenital megacolon) HIV infection and AIDS, pediatric Low birth weight or premature infant (3–4) Necrotizing enterocolitis Phenylketonuria (PKU) Tyrosinemia (variable) Urea cycle disorders (variable)
SECTION 4: NEUROLOGICAL AND MENTAL CONDITIONS			
Neurological Disorders			
Migraine headache, prevention or counseling Trigeminal neuralgia (1–2)	Epilepsy or seizure disorders Multiple sclerosis Myasthenia gravis and neuromuscular junction disorders Parkinson's disease Tardive dyskinesia	Amyotrophic lateral sclerosis Cerebral aneurysm Guillain-Barré syndrome Huntington's chorea (variable) Spinal cord injury Stroke (cerebrovascular accident)	Brain trauma Coma
Eating Disorders			
		Anorexia nervosa Binge eating disorder (3–4) Bulimia (3–4) Other disordered eating patterns (3–4)	
Psychiatric Disorders			
Bipolar disorder (1–2) Depression with numerous medications (1–2) Schizophrenia and psychoses (1–2) Substance use disorders		Alzheimer's disease or other dementias	

(continued)

TABLE D-2 Acuity for Dietitian Roles in Medical Diagnoses *(continued)*

Minimal Role of Dietitian–1	Some Roles of Dietitian–2	Moderate Role of Dietitian–3	Extended Role of Dietitian–4
SECTION 5: PULMONARY DISORDERS			
Asthma Bronchiectasis Bronchitis, acute Pneumonia (1–2) Pulmonary embolism (1–2)	Cor pulmonale (variable) Interstitial lung disease (1–2) Sarcoidosis Sleep apnea Thoracic empyema Tuberculosis	Chronic obstructive pulmonary diseases (emphysema or chronic bronchitis) Cystic fibrosis Respiratory distress syndrome (3–4) Transplantation, lung (3–4)	Chylothorax Respiratory failure and ventilator dependency
SECTION 6: CARDIOVASCULAR DISORDERS			
Angina pectoris Arteritis Pericarditis and cardiac tamponade Thrombophlebitis	Peripheral artery disease	Atherosclerosis, coronary heart disease, and dyslipidemias Cardiomyopathies Heart failure Hypertension Myocardial infarction	Cardiac cachexia Heart transplantation or heart-lung transplantation
SECTION 7: GASTROINTESTINAL DISORDERS			
Upper GI			
Dyspepsia or indigestion (1–2)	Esophageal varices (2–3) Hiatal hernia, esophagitis, and gastroesophageal reflux (GERD) (2–3) Gastric retention or gastroparesis (2–3) Peptic ulcer	Dysphagia (3–4) Esophageal stricture or spasm, achalasia, or Zenker's diverticulum Esophageal trauma (3–4) Gastritis and gastroenteritis Giant hypertrophic gastritis (Ménétrier's disease) Gastrectomy and/or vagotomy (3–4) Vomiting, pernicious	
Lower GI			
Lactose malabsorption (lactase deficiency) (variable) Constipation (1–2) Fecal incontinence Hemorrhoids, hemorrhoidectomy Proctitis	Diarrhea, dysentery, and traveler's diarrhea Diverticular diseases (2–3) Peritonitis Colostomy (2–3)	Fat malabsorption syndrome Megacolon, acquired Irritable bowel disease Carcinoid syndrome Ileostomy Intestinal lymphangiectasia (variable) Whipple's disease (intestinal lipodystrophy) (3–4)	Tropical sprue Celiac disease Crohn's disease (3–4) Ulcerative colitis Short bowel syndrome Intestinal fistula Intestinal transplantation
SECTION 8: HEPATIC, PANCREATIC, AND BILIARY DISORDERS			
Jaundice	Ascites and chylous ascites Hepatitis Pancreatic insufficiency (2–3)	Alcoholic liver disease Hepatic cirrhosis Hepatic encephalopathy, failure or coma (3–4)	Liver transplantation

(continued)

TABLE D-2 Acuity for Dietitian Roles in Medical Diagnoses *(continued)*

Minimal Role of Dietitian–1	Some Roles of Dietitian–2	Moderate Role of Dietitian–3	Extended Role of Dietitian–4
SECTION 8: HEPATIC, PANCREATIC, AND BILIARY DISORDERS			
	Gallbladder disease, surgical or nonsurgical Biliary cirrhosis Cholestatic liver disease (2–3)	Pancreatitis, acute (3–4) Pancreatitis, chronic Zollinger-Ellison syndrome (variable)	
SECTION 9: ENDOCRINE DISORDERS			
Adrenocortical insufficiency chronic Addison's disease (variable) Cushing's syndrome (variable) Acromegaly (variable) Hyperaldosteronism (variable) Hypopituitarism (variable) Pheochromocytoma (variable) Hyperthyroidism Hypothyroidism	Pregnancy-induced hypertension and preeclampsia Syndrome of inappropriate antidiuretic hormone (SIADH) Parathyroid disorders (altered calcium)	Metabolic syndrome (3–4) Prediabetes (3–4) Diabetic gastroparesis (3–4) Diabetic ketoacidosis (3–4) Hyperosmolar hyperglycemic state (3–4) Hypoglycemia, iatrogenic Hyperinsulinism and spontaneous hypoglycemia (3–4) Diabetes insipidus	Type 1 diabetes Pancreatic transplantation Type 2 diabetes mellitus, adults Type 2 diabetes mellitus, children and teens Gestational diabetes
SECTION 10: WEIGHT MANAGEMENT, UNDERNUTRITION, AND MALNUTRITION			
		Underweight or unintentional weight loss (3–4) Protein–calorie malnutrition, mild (3–4)	Overweight or uncomplicated obesity Obesity, medical (with comorbidities) Protein–calorie malnutrition, moderate or severe Energy malnutrition Refeeding syndrome
SECTION 11: MUSCULOSKELETAL AND COLLAGEN DISORDERS			
Ankylosing spondylitis (variable) Myofascial pain syndromes: fibromyalgia or polymyalgia rheumatica Osteomyelitis, acute (1–2) Paget's disease (osteitis deformans) (variable) Polyarteritis nodosa (variable) Rheumatoid arthritis Ruptured intervertebral disc Scleroderma (systemic sclerosis) (1–2)	Immobilization, extended Muscular dystrophy Osteoarthritis and degenerative joint disease Osteopenia and osteomalacia Osteoporosis Systemic lupus erythematosus	Rhabdomyolysis	

(continued)

TABLE D-2 Acuity for Dietitian Roles in Medical Diagnoses *(continued)*

Minimal Role of Dietitian–1	Some Roles of Dietitian–2	Moderate Role of Dietitian–3	Extended Role of Dietitian–4
SECTION 12: HEMATOLOGY: ANEMIAS AND BLOOD DISORDERS			
Aplastic anemia Anemia from parasitic infestation Anemia, sickle cell Anemia, sideroblastic Polycythemia vera (Osler's disease) Thalassemia (Cooley's anemia) Thrombocytic purpura	Anemia, hemolytic from vitamin E deficiency (2–3) Anemia, iron deficiency Anemia, nutritional (folic acid, copper, etc.) Anemia, pernicious or vitamin B_{12} deficiency Hemochromatosis (iron overloading) Hemorrhage, acute or chronic		
SECTION 13: CANCER			
	Breast cancer Choriocarcinoma Leukemia, chronic Lung cancer Myeloma (simple or multiple) (2–3) Prostate cancer	Brain tumor Esophageal cancer (3–4) Gastric carcinoma (3–4) Hepatic carcinoma Intestinal carcinoma (3–4) Leukemia, acute Lymphoma, Hodgkin's disease Lymphoma, non-Hodgkin's Oral cancer (3–4) Osteosarcoma (2–3) Pancreatic carcinoma Radiation colitis or enteritis (3–4) Wilms' tumor (embryoma of kidney)	Bone marrow transplantation
SECTION 14: SURGICAL DISORDERS			
Appendectomy Cesarean delivery Hysterectomy, abdominal Pelvic exenteration Spinal surgery (1–2) Total hip arthroplasty Tonsillectomy and adenoidectomy	Surgery, general Sodium imbalances: hyponatremia or hypernatremia Potassium imbalances: hypokalemia or hyperkalemia Calcium imbalances: hypocalcemia or hypercalcemia Magnesium imbalances: hypomagnesemia or hypermagnesemia Phosphate imbalances: hypophosphatemia or hyperphosphatemia Amputation, one or more limbs Parathyroidectomy	Bowel surgery Open heart surgery Pancreatic surgery (3–4)	Gastric bypass surgery

(continued)

TABLE D-2 Acuity for Dietitian Roles in Medical Diagnoses *(continued)*

Minimal Role of Dietitian–1	Some Roles of Dietitian–2	Moderate Role of Dietitian–3	Extended Role of Dietitian–4
SECTION 15: AIDS AND IMMUNOLOGY, INFECTIONS, BURNS, AND TRAUMA			
Candidiasis Chronic fatigue syndrome (1–2) Fever >102°F Herpes simplex 1 or 2 Herpes zoster (shingles) Infection, general Influenza (flu, respiratory) Intestinal parasites Meningitis Mononucleosis Pelvic inflammatory disease Poliomyelitis Rheumatic fever Toxic shock syndrome Trichinosis Typhoid fever	Bacterial endocarditis Burns, minor thermal injury Encephalitis or Reye's syndrome Fracture, hip or long bone Trauma, minor	AIDS and HIV infection, adult (3–4) Sepsis or septicemia Trauma, major	Burns, major thermal injury Multiple organ dysfunction
SECTION 16: RENAL DISORDERS			
Pyelonephritis Urolithiasis (renal stones) (1–2)	Inborn errors: polycystic kidney disease Glomerulonephritis, acute Glomerulonephritis, chronic Nephritis (Bright's disease) (2–3) Nephrotic syndrome (2–3)	Inborn errors: vitamin D–resistant rickets (3–4) Inborn errors: Hartnup's disease (variable) Nephrosclerosis (2–3) Renal failure, acute	Chronic kidney disease Hemodialysis Peritoneal renal dialysis Renal transplantation
SECTION 17: ENTERAL AND PARENTERAL NUTRITION			
			Tube feeding, initiation, monitoring, or home Parenteral nutrition, initiation, monitoring, or home

Thanks to Matthew Dallas, MS, RD, for summarizing this table.

TABLE D-3 Medical Nutrition Therapy/Activities Care Plan

Using the ranking system in Table D-2, a clinical nutrition director may develop a tool such as the one given below to establish staffing related to nutrition acuity for a facility. This form is to be used in identifying a patient's nutrition acuity level and corresponding interventions.

NUTRITION ACUITY 4

One of the Following Criteria Met

a. Weight for height below the 5th percentile
b. Weight for age below the 5th percentile
c. Diagnosis of:
    i. Chronic gastrointestinal disorder
    ii. Acute/chronic renal disease
    iii. Cystic fibrosis
    iv. Diabetes mellitus
    v. Eating disorder
    vi. Prematurity/low birth weight
    vii. Burns
    viii. Liver failure
    ix. Malnutrition
    x. Trauma
    xi. Metabolic disorder
    xii. AIDS
    xiii. Carcinoma/leukemia
    xiv. Respiratory failure
d. Present diet order:
    i. Tube feeding
    ii. Total parenteral nutrition
    iii. Multiple food allergies

Nutrition Care Plan

a. RD LD will assess 3 times a week and post a medical nutrition therapy note in the medical record
b. Reassess nutrition acuity status
c. Specialized formula recommendations and calculations as needed; coordinate with nutrition services
d. Assist with menu selections as needed
e. Provide education as appropriate

NUTRITION ACUITY 3

One of the Following Criteria Met

a. Percent height/length for age 5–10th percentile
b. Percent weight for age 5–10th percentile
c. Weight for height 5–10th percentile
d. Two or more of the following:
    i. Nausea/vomiting
    ii. Feeding intolerance
    iii. Weight change
    iv. Swallowing problem
e. Present diet order:
    i. Specialized formula
    ii. Two or more diet restrictions

Nutrition Care Plan

a. RD LD will assess 2 times a week and post a medical nutrition therapy note in the medical record
b. Reassess nutrition acuity status
c. Specialized formula recommendations/calculations as needed; coordinate with nutrition services
d. Assist with menu selections as needed
e. Provide education as appropriate

NUTRITION ACUITY 2

One of the Following Criteria Met

a. Weight for height >85th percentile
b. BMI >85th percentile
c. Percent weight for age >95th percentile
d. One of the following:
    i. Nausea/vomiting
    ii. Feeding intolerance
    iii. Weight change
    iv. Swallowing problem
e. Present diet order: one diet restriction (i.e., low fat, vegetarian, or low sodium)

Nutrition Care Plan

a. RD LD/DTR will assess once a week and post a medical nutrition therapy note in the medical record
b. Assist with menu selections as needed
c. Reassess nutrition acuity status
d. Provide education as appropriate

NUTRITION ACUITY 1

No medical condition identified affecting nutrition status on the *Interdisciplinary Admission Assessment* form.

Nutrition Care Plan

a. RD LD/DTR re-screen within 7 days
b. RD LD/DTR available by consult by the medical team

Used with permission from Children's Hospital of Dayton, Dayton, OH, February 1, 2006.

APPENDIX E

Herbs and Botanicals

TABLE E-1 Medicinal Herbs: Patient Information Sheet

- Plants have been used throughout history to improve health. Many modern medicines come from plants; an example is aspirin from willow bark.
- Herbs used for health purposes are drugs; they are chemicals that affect the human body.
- Plant products are not necessarily safe, even if they are "natural." Some commonly used herbal remedies are unsafe.
- Individual reports of safety for any herbal product are not reliable. This is because some people who use an herb will feel better even if there is no evidence of its efficacy.
- Unlike drugs, the Food and Drug Administration does not regulate the safety and efficacy of herbs.
- Select herbal products carefully. Check with www.consumerlab.com first to identify brand names that are reliable to purchase.
- Check also with NIH Herbal Listing: http://www.nlm.nih.gov/medlineplus/druginfo/herb_All.html

Adapted from: O'Hara M, et al. A review of 12 commonly used medicinal herbs. *Arch Fam Med.* 7:523, 1998.

TABLE E-2 Herbal, Botanical, and Dietary Supplement Intake Form

NAME ______________ AGE ________ DATE ________

1. What kind of supplements do you use? (Check all that apply)

___ None
___ Multivitamin/mineral supplement
___ Herbal or botanical supplement
___ Amino acid or protein supplement
___ Fiber supplement
___ Other (such as aloe, black cohosh, calcium, ginseng, gingko biloba, valerian) ______________

2. How long have you used this supplement(s)?

___ 1 month or less
___ 3–6 months
___ 6–12 months
___ More than 1 year (specify) ______________

3. How long do you plan to use this supplement(s)?

___ Indefinitely
___ 1–6 months
___ 6–12 months

4. What are your primary reason(s) for taking this supplement(s)?

___ For its preventive effect against disease/medical condition
___ To help treat a disease/medical condition
___ General wellness
___ Energy
___ Weight loss
___ Other (specify)

If used to *treat* specific medical condition: What are your medical symptoms? ______________

5. How long have you had these symptoms/medical conditions?

___ 1 week or less
___ 1–3 months
___ 3–6months
___ 6–12 months
___ More than 1 year (specify)

(continued)

TABLE E-2 Herbal, Botanical, and Dietary Supplement Intake Form *(continued)*

6. Have symptoms improved since you started taking this supplement?

___ Yes (explain how) ________________________

___ No

7. Are you currently taking or have you recently taken any over-the-counter or prescription medications, including oral contraceptives?

___ Yes (specify)

___ No

8. Do you have any additional illnesses or medical conditions?

___ Yes (specify) ________________________

___ No

9. Are you pregnant or breastfeeding?

___ Yes

___ No

10. Do you drink alcohol?

___ Yes (If yes, how often? Rarely___ Occasionally___ Often___ Never___)

___ No

If yes, how much at one sitting?

___ 1 glass ___ 2 glasses ___ 3 glasses or more

11. Do you smoke?

___ Yes (If yes, how often and how many per day? ________)

___ No

12. Are you allergic to any medications, foods, plants, or flowers?

___ Yes (specify) ____________________

___ No

13. Are you on a self- or medically prescribed eating plan/diet?

___ Yes (specify) ____________________

___ No

Sources: American Dietetic Association. *Sports nutrition: a guide for the professional working with active people.* Chicago: American Dietetic Association, 2000; and American Dietetic Association. Special report from the Joint Working Group on Dietary Supplements, 2000. Used with permission.

TABLE E-3 Adverse Effects of Herbal Supplements Commonly Used

Supplement	Adverse Effects
Barberry	Coagulant herb. May inhibit effects of anticoagulant medications such as warfarin.
Bilberry	Exhibits antiplatelet activity. May enhance effects of anticoagulant medications such as warfarin and potentiate bleeding.
Bromelain	From pineapple stem. Exhibits antiplatelet activity. May enhance effects of anticoagulant medications such as warfarin and (*Ananas comosus*) potentiate bleeding.
Buckthorn bark	Laxative herbs speed digestion, which reduces absorption time of drugs. Chronic use results in a loss of potassium, thereby strengthening effects of cardiac glycosides and antiarrhythmic agents. Simultaneous use of thiazide diuretics, corticosteroids, or licorice root may increase potassium loss.
Cayenne	Exhibits anticoagulant activity. May enhance effects of anticoagulant medications such as warfarin and potentiate bleeding.
Chamomile	Exhibits anticoagulant activity. May enhance effects of anticoagulant medications such as warfarin and potentiate bleeding.
Coleus, or forskolin	Exhibits antiplatelet activity. May enhance effects of anticoagulant medications such as warfarin and potentiate bleeding.
Dong quai	Exhibits anticoagulant activity. May enhance effects of anticoagulant medications such as warfarin and potentiate bleeding.
Feverfew	Exhibits antiplatelet activity. May enhance effects of anticoagulant medications such as warfarin and potentiate bleeding.
Flaxseed oil	Exhibits antiplatelet activity. May enhance effects of anticoagulant medications such as warfarin and potentiate bleeding.
Garlic	Exhibits antiplatelet activity. May enhance effects of anticoagulant medications such as warfarin and potentiate bleeding.
Ginger	Exhibits antiplatelet activity. May enhance effects of anticoagulant medications such as warfarin and potentiate bleeding.
Ginkgo	Exhibits antiplatelet activity. May enhance effects of anticoagulant medications such as warfarin and potentiate bleeding.
Ginseng, American	May increase side effects of stimulants. Exhibits antiplatelet activity. May enhance effects of anticoagulant medications such as warfarin and potentiate bleeding.
Green tea	Exhibits antiplatelet activity. May enhance effects of anticoagulant medications such as warfarin and potentiate bleeding.
Horse chestnut	Exhibits anticoagulant activity. May enhance effects of anticoagulant medications such as warfarin and potentiate bleeding.
Kava	May cause drowsiness, dizziness, and intoxication. May enhance effects of sedatives or hypnotics.
Licorice	May impair action of drugs that cause potassium loss. May enhance action of corticosteroids. May counteract effectiveness of drugs used to treat hypertension. Licorice contains a substance known as glycyrrhizic acid, which can affect the hormone aldosterone that helps regulate blood pressure. For people with high blood pressure, edema, or electrolyte imbalance, use of licorice root or its products can lead to sodium retention, excessive potassium excretion, and water retention. Some licorice products have the glycyrrhizic acid removed and are sold sometimes as DGL (deglycyrrhizinated licorice).

(continued)

TABLE E-3 Adverse Effects of Herbal Supplements Commonly Used *(continued)*

Supplement	Adverse Effects
Meadowsweet	Exhibits antiplatelet activity. May enhance effects of anticoagulant medications such as warfarin and potentiate bleeding.
Motherwort	Exhibits antiplatelet activity. May enhance effects of anticoagulant medications such as warfarin and potentiate bleeding.
Oregon grape root	Coagulant herb. May inhibit effects of anticoagulant medications such as warfarin and potentiate bleeding.
Poplar	Exhibits antiplatelet activity. May enhance effects of anticoagulant medications such as warfarin and potentiate bleeding.
Senna	Laxative herbs speed digestion, which reduces absorption time of drugs. Chronic use results in a loss of potassium, thereby strengthening effects of cardiac glycosides and antiarrhythmic agents. Simultaneous use of thiazide diuretics, corticosteroids, or licorice root increases potassium loss.
Shepherd's purse	Coagulant herb. May inhibit effects of anticoagulant medications such as warfarin and potentiate bleeding.
St. John's wort	May enhance effects of narcotics and selective serotonin reuptake inhibitors (SSRIs). Increases side effects of photosensitizing drugs, alcohol, and melatonin. Laboratory reports have suggested but not confirmed that the mechanism of action for St. John's wort may involve monoamine oxidase (MAO) inhibition, SSRI reuptake inhibition, increased melatonin production, and others. This herb has been shown to induce the drug-metabolizing enzyme cytochrome p4503A4 and has the potential to interact with many medications.
Turmeric	Exhibits antiplatelet activity. May enhance effects of anticoagulant medications such as warfarin and potentiate bleeding.
Valerian	Enhances the effects of sedatives and hypnotic drugs.

Source: Kumar NB, et al. Perioperative herbal supplement use in cancer patients: potential implications and recommendations for presurgical screening. *Cancer Control.* 12:149, 2005.

I N D E X

Note: Page numbers followed by f refer to illustrations; those followed by t refer to tables; and those followed by b refer to boxes.